TEXTBOOK OF

Radiographic Positioning and Related Anatomy

Sixth Edition

TEXTBOOK OF

Radiographic Positioning and Related Anatomy

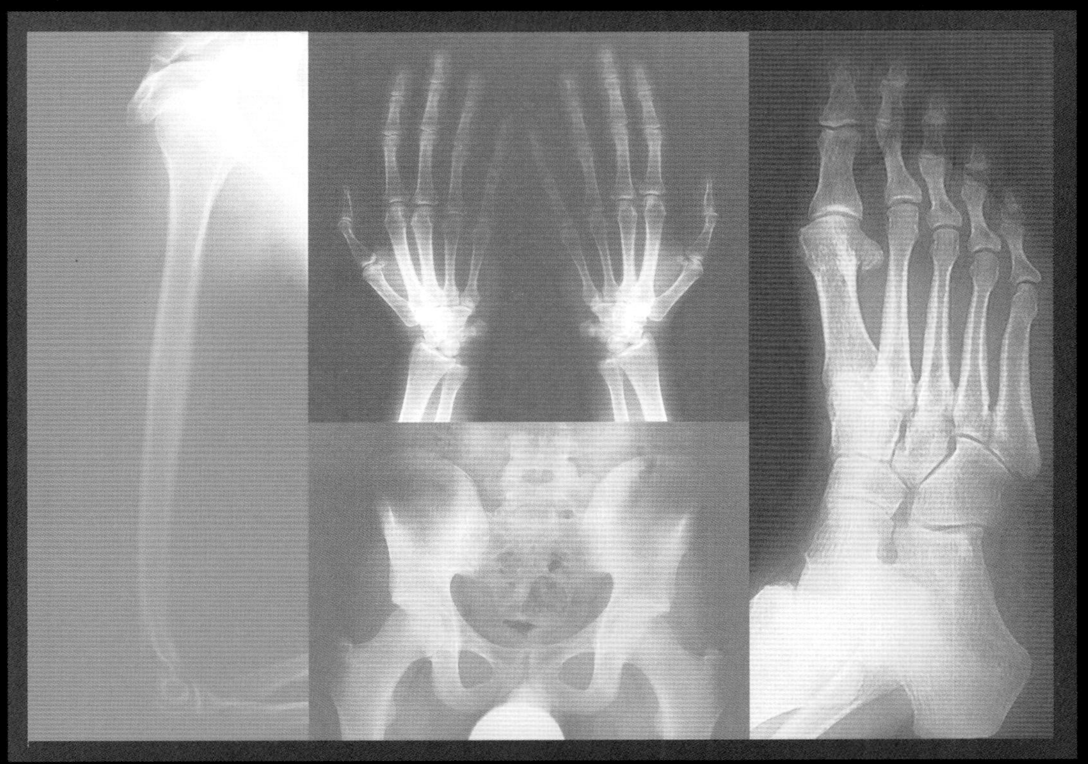

Kenneth L. Bontrager, MA, RT(R)
John P. Lampignano, MEd, RT(R)(CT)

With approximately 2,300 illustrations

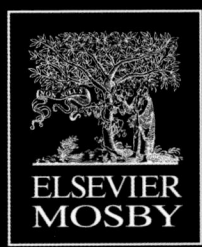

ELSEVIER
MOSBY

11830 Westline Industrial Drive
St. Louis, Missouri 63146

TEXTBOOK OF RADIOGRAPHIC POSITIONING
AND RELATED ANATOMY, 6th EDITION

ISBN 0-323-02507-2

NOTICE

Pharmacology is an ever-changing field. Standard safety precautions must be followed, but as new research and clinical experience broaden our knowledge, changes in treatment and drug therapy may become necessary or appropriate. Readers are advised to check the most current product information provided by the manufacturer of each drug to be administered to verify the recommended dose, the method and duration of administration, and contraindications. It is the responsibility of the licensed prescriber, relying on experience and knowledge of the patient, to determine dosages and the best treatment for each individual patient. Neither the publisher nor the author assumes any liability for any injury and/or damage to persons or property arising from this publication.

Previous editions copyrighted 2001, 1997, 1993, 1987, 1982

Executive Editor: Jeanne Wilke
Developmental Editor: Becky Swisher
Editorial Assistant: Christina Pryor
Publishing Services Manager: Pat Joiner
Senior Project Manager: Karen M. Rehwinkel
Senior Designer: Kathi Gosche
Photography: Kenneth L. Bontrager
Rocky McPherson
Facilities for Photography: Energized Laboratory, Gateway Community College, Phoenix, Arizona
Phoenix Baptist Hospital and Medical Center, Phoenix, Arizona
St. Joseph's Hospital and Medical Center, Phoenix, Arizona
University of Iowa Hospitals and Medical Clinics, Iowa City, Iowa

Printed in China

Last digit is the print number: 9 8 7 6 5 4 3 2 1

Acknowledgments and Dedication

By Kenneth L. Bontrager

This edition is again the culmination of a team effort by numerous contributors and reviewers. I appreciate more and more the advantage of new editions of the same works with the opportunity to correct, add to, and improve from each previous edition. For this reason, and with increased contributions by specialty contributors, I really believe this new sixth edition is the best and most complete text on radiographic positioning that I have seen or been involved with.

It is virtually impossible for me to acknowledge all those who made contributions to all the previous editions and thus by accumulation to this edition also. However, I must start with **Barry Anthony**, RT(R), for his early contribution in the areas of anatomy and special procedures for the first edition of this text and the associated audiovisual series that provided the foundation for this textbook. **Derrick McPhee,** MD, FRCPC, also contributed through his reviews and suggestions on the anatomy and pathology sections for past editions.

I also want to acknowledge and thank **Karen Brown, Nancy Johnson, Beth Vealé, Patti Ward, Rene Tossel, Gene Frank, Daniel Bandy,** and other unnamed contributors for their help with locating new radiographic images and/or photos for this sixth edition.

Two persons who have made major contributions to this edition are **David Hall** and **Cindy Murphy.** David has advised us and proofed various drafts of the last several editions. He is one of the best proofers and reviewers that I have worked with. He not only proofs and reviews critically but also makes positive suggestions that we can incorporate. Cindy has joined us as a major contributor to numerous chapters in the last two editions, such as those on angiography and computed tomography (CT). She, along with **Joe Popovitch,** also contributed much of the new information in Chapter 2, including providing new images on the various aspects of digital imaging.

John Lampignano, who has been a key contributor for the past several editions, is a gifted and popular RT educator with keen knowledge and an astute memory of anatomy, positioning, and imaging facts and principles. I have been blessed by working with him and experienced first hand his exceptional dedication and work ethics as applied to each task and assignment that he has undertaken. I'm pleased and honored that he is now joining me as coauthor of both the workbooks and this textbook.

I thank **Jeanne Wilke,** Executive Editor, **Rebecca Swisher,** Developmental Editor, and **Karen Rehwinkel,** Senior Project Manager from Elsevier (Mosby) for their support and assistance in the planning and completion of this complex project. Each of these persons, along with other graphics personnel at Elsevier, has been very helpful and encouraging and has functioned well as a team to meet author and editor requests for the complex color graphics and page layout requirements for this new edition.

I also want to recognize and thank all those contributors and reviewers of this edition and past editions as listed elsewhere in the front matter of this text. I thank each of you for the significant contributions you have made in your area of expertise. Your efforts will be greatly appreciated by the many students, technologists, and educators who will be using this text worldwide over the coming years in both English and numerous non-English translations.

Lastly, as always, I am most indebted to my family—not only for their love, support, and encouragement but also for their assistance in the various production aspects of these works. My wife, **Mary Lou,** as my life partner, continues to be my most valuable assistant and helpmate. Our two sons, **Neil** and **Troy,** not only literally grew up with "the book" but also spent time between their college years and between college and graduate school in the graphics and literal page-by-page layout of early editions of this textbook and accompanying ancillaries. I thank each of you for your continuing help, support, and advice, and I'm so glad that both of you can experience the satisfaction of knowing that you are making a difference in the careers you have chosen.

I'm sure our two daughters-in-law, **Kim** and **Robyn,** didn't fully realize that marrying into the Bontrager family also included being part of the family publishing efforts. I sincerely thank both of you for your continuing help and support and also for giving us those special grandchildren, which now include **Hallie, Alexis, Ashton,** and **Jonathan.** I love and appreciate each and every one of you very much.

Finally, as I look back over the past 35 plus years of my involvement in radiologic technology education, I realize that my most significant contributions to this field may be behind me. Therefore I dedicate this book to those future generations of students, and to those educators and graduate technologists who will be helping these students reach their goal of serving in a helping profession and thus make a difference in this world, each in their own way.

KLB

Acknowledgments

By John P. Lampignano

First, I must acknowledge the current and past Diagnostic Medical Imaging students from Gateway Community College. Their thirst for knowledge has driven me to ensure that we write the most complete and accurate text possible. They remain my inspiration. This text is a reflection of each student's dedication to the profession that we love dearly.

The Diagnostic Medical Imaging faculty at Gateway are incredible role models for the students and the profession. **Alex Backus, Nancy Johnson, Mary Carrillo, Kathleen Murphy,** and **Jeanne Dial** were instrumental in providing images and allowing us to use the imaging labs for many photo shoots and phantom work. Special thanks to **Jerry Olson** for teaching me radiography 30 years ago and his assistance during this project. Special thanks also to **Mark Richard** for being my inspiration and spiritual leader every day.

Ken Bontrager, with the help and support of his family, has been dedicated to this text and other instructional media in radiologic technology for approximately 35 years. They have given of themselves fully to this text and ancillaries; it has always been more than just another project to them. As a co-author, I will dedicate myself to maintaining the same standards as have been established by Ken and his wife Mary Lou. Ken has taken the time to develop me as an author. His mentoring has always been positive, gentle, and constant. To be tutored by one of the best humbles me and I'm grateful to have been given this opportunity to work with Ken.

Special thanks to **Susan K. Wallen** for her tireless efforts in assisting us with the Surgical Radiography section of the sixth edition. Susan made arrangements for the surgical equipment, drapes, prosthetic devices, and facilities for the photo shoot. Thanks to St. Joseph's Medical Center for allowing us to use their surgical suites and radiology facilities during the photo shoots as well. Thanks to **Karen Brown** for making the arrangements to use St. Joseph's radiography facilities and for acquiring images. **Daniel Bandy** of Banner Good Samaritan Medical Center was instrumental in the creation of the new section on positron emission tomography (PET) in Chapter 24. Dan wrote and edited countless drafts and acquired images to ensure that the PET section was the very best.

Ellie Arispe and **Timothy Jasper** served as models for many of the new photographs taken for this sixth edition. Thanks to both of them for hours of posing for countless photographs. They maintained a high degree of professionalism and humor throughout the process.

Finally, thanks to the Lampignano clan for their ongoing support. **Deborah, Daniel,** and **Molly** have provided me the encouragement and unconditional love to meet every task that I have faced in my life, including this text. Thanks to **Frankie** for providing the computer support and companionship throughout this project.

JPL

Contributors

Daniel J. Bandy, MS, CNMT
Chapter 24
Technical Director
Banner Good Samaritan PET Center
Phoenix, Arizona

Eugene D. Frank, MA, RT(R), FASRT, FAERS
Chapter 18
Program Director
Riverland Community College
Austin, Minnesota;
Retired, Assistant Professor of Radiology
Mayo Clinic
College of Medicine
Rochester, Minnesota

Richard Geise, PhD, FACR, FAAPM
Chapter 2
Director, Radiation Therapy Physics
Abbott Northwestern Hospital
Minneapolis, Minnesota

Brenda K. Hoopingarner, MS, RT(R)(CT)
Chapter 23
Chairman and Associate Professor
Department of Allied Health
Fort Hays State University
Hays, Kansas

Nancy Johnson, BA, RT(R)(CV)(CT)(QM)
Chapters 3, 5, and 6
Faculty, Medical Radiography
Gateway Community College
Phoenix, Arizona

Cindy Murphy, RT R, ACR, BHSc
Chapters 2, 21, and 22
Faculty
School of Health Sciences
Dalhousie University
Halifax, Nova Scotia, Canada

Sandra J. Nauman, RT(R)(M)
Chapter 18
Clinical Coordinator/Instructor
Riverland Community College
Radiography Program
Austin, Minnesota

Joseph Popovitch, RT R, ACR, DHSA
Chapter 2
Sessional Lecturer
School of Health Sciences
Dalhousie University
Halifax, Nova Scotia, Canada;
Product Specialist
Philips Medical Systems
Canada

Renee F. Tossell, PhD, RT(R)(M)(CV)
Chapters 12 and 13
Instructional Faculty/Clinical Coordinator
Pima Community College
Tucson, Arizona

Beth L. Vealé, MEd, RT(R)(QM)
Chapters 7 and 8
Associate Professor
Midwestern State University
Wichita Falls, Texas

Patti Ward, MEd, RT(R)
Chapters 9, 10, and 11
Associate Professor
Mesa State College
Grand Junction, Colorado

Charles R. Wilson, PhD, FAAPM, FACR
Chapter 23
Associate Professor of Radiology
Medical College of Wisconsin
Milwaukee, Wisconsin

Contributors to Past Editions

Barry T. Anthony, RT(R)
Swedish Medical Center
Englewood, Colorado

Patrick Apfel, MEd, RT(R)
University of Nevada
Las Vegas, Nevada

April Apple, RT(R)
Senior Staff Technologist
Duke University Health Systems
Durham, North Carolina

Alex Backus, MS, RT(R)
Gateway Community College
Phoenix, Arizona

Karen Brown, RT(R)
St. Josephs's Hospital and Medical Center
Phoenix, Arizona

Claudia Calandrino, MPA, RT(R)
Signa Health Plans of California
Los Angeles, California

Donna Davis, MEd, RT(R)(CV)
Assistant Professor
Department of Radiologic Technology
University of Arkansas for Medical Sciences
Little Rock, Arkansas

Nancy L. Dickerson, RT(R)(M)
Radiography Program
Mayo Clinic
Rochester, Minnesota

Eugene D. Frank, MA, RT(R), FASRT
Mayo Clinic
Rochester, Minnesota

Richard Geise, PhD
University of Minnesota Hospitals
Minneapolis, Minnesota

Cecilie Godderidge, BS, RT(R)
Consultant and Lecturer in Pediatric Imaging
Boston, Massachusetts

Jeannean Hall-Rollins, MRC, BS, RT(R) (CV)
Assistant Professor
Department of Radiologic Sciences
Arkansas State University
Jonesboro, Arkansas

Jessie R. Harris, RT(R)
Signa Health Plans of California
Los Angeles, California

Brenda K. Hoopingarner, MS, RT(R)
Assistant Professor
Allied Health Department,
Fort Hays State University
Hays, Kansas

Jenny A. Kellstrom, MEd, RT(R)
Assistant Professor/Advising Coordinator
Department of Medical Imaging
Oregon Institute of Technology
Klamath Falls, Oregon

John P. Lampignano, MEd, RT(R)(CT)
Diagnostic Medical Imaging
Gateway Community College
Phoenix, Arizona

Linda S. Lingar, MEd, RT(R)(M)
Assistant Professor
Department of Radiologic Technology
University of Arkansas for Medical Sciences
Little Rock, Arkansas

James D. Lipcamon, RT(R)
Harbor-UCLA Diagnostic Imaging Center
Torrance, California

Kathy M. Martensen, BS, RT(R)
University of Iowa Hospitals and Clinics
Iowa City, Iowa

J. Fred Price, MS, RT(R), FASRT
Garland Community College
Hot Springs, Arkansas

Joan Radke, BS, RT(R)
University of Iowa Hospitals and Clinics
Iowa City, Iowa

E. Russel Ritenour, PhD
University of Minnesota Hospitals
Minneapolis, Minnesota

James A. Sanderson, BS, RT(R)
St. Joseph's Hospital and Medical Center
Phoenix, Arizona

Marianne Tortorici, EdD, RT(R)
San Diego City College
San Diego, California

Donna L. Wright, EdD, RT(R)
Associate Professor
Department of Radiologic Science
College of Health and Human Services
Midwestern State University
Wichita Falls, Texas

Reviewers

Laura L. Alipoon, EdD, RT(R)
Associate Professor
Loma Linda University
Loma Linda, California

Deanna Butcher, MA, RT(R)
Program Director
Department of Radiology Education
St. Luke's College
Sioux City, Iowa

Charles Francis, MEd, RT(R)(QM)
Department Chairperson and Associate Professor
Radiographic Science
Idaho State University
Pocatello, Idaho

Cynthia F. Griffith, MEd, RT(R)(CV)
Assistant Director of Education
Advanced Health Education Center
Houston, Texas

Astor Halcomb Jr., AAS, BUS, ARRT(R)(CT)
Associate Professor of Radiography and Clinical Coordinator
Hazard Community College/Southeast Community College Regional Radiography Program
Whitesburg, Kentucky

David S. Hall, MS, RT(R)
Associate Professor, Radiography
Broward Community College
Davie, Florida

Nancy Johnson, BA, RT(R)(CV)(CT)(QM)
Faculty, Medical Radiography
Gateway Community College
Phoenix, Arizona

Donna S. Laird, BS, RT(R)(M)
Instructor
St. Philip's College
San Antonio, Texas

Linda S. Lingar, MEd, RT(R)(M)(ARRT)
Associate Professor
Radiologic Technology Department
University of Arkansas for Medical Sciences
Little Rock, Arkansas

Galen Miller, RT(R), BS
Radiography Clinical Coordinator
Mid Michigan Community College
Harrison, Michigan

Cindy Murphy, RT R, ACR, BHSc
Faculty
School of Health Sciences
Dalhousie University
Halifax, Nova Scotia, Canada

Barbara Smith, RT(R)(QM), FASRT
Instructor, Radiologic Technology
Portland Community College
Portland, Oregon

Patricia Ann Stoddard, MS, RT(R), MT, CMA
Academic Program Director II
Western Business College, Vancouver
Vancouver, Washington

Gloria Strickland, EdS, RT(R)(M)(QM)
Assistant Professor in Radiologic Sciences
Armstrong Atlantic State University
Savannah, Georgia

Homer Terry, RT(R)(M)(QM), BUS
Associate Professor and Program Director
Hazard Community College/Southeast Community College Regional Radiography Program
Hazard, Kentucky

Renee F. Tossell, PhD, RT(R)(M)(CV)
Instructional Faculty/Clinical Coordinator
Pima Community College
Tucson, Arizona

Beth L. Vealé, MEd, RT(R)(QM)
Associate Professor
Midwestern State University
Wichita Falls, Texas

Patti Ward, MEd, RT(R)
Associate Professor
Mesa State College
Grand Junction, Colorado

Gary Lee Zimmerman, ARRT(R)(CT)(MR), MS Curriculum and Supervision
Associate Professor
Oregon Institute of Technology
Klamath Falls, Oregon

Foreword

Simply stated, the new sixth edition of the respected and immensely popular *Textbook of Radiographic Positioning and Related Anatomy* establishes the standard for texts of this type. It is the best of the best! John Lampignano joins Ken Bontrager as co-author of this updated edition. Like Ken Bontrager, John is a well-known and respected educator in the field of radiography. He has been actively involved as a contributor and reviewer of the Bontrager Positioning and Related Anatomy series for years and, with Ken, co-authored the fifth edition workbook and laboratory manuals and accompanying slide series.

Together, Ken and John have produced a text that is exceptionally well organized and structured for teaching and learning radiographic positioning and related anatomy. The entire text has been updated and made even easier to read and understand. Numerous diagrams, images, and radiographs have been relabeled or replaced to improve clarity. A new chapter on image quality in digital imaging thoroughly describes the basic principles and applications associated with digital radiographic imaging. In addition, each chapter now includes a section relating specifically to digital imaging considerations. Together these two additions ensure that all the positioning considerations required for employment in a film-based or filmless radiography department are presented in this text.

The totally new section on surgical radiography is also a welcome addition to the text. The coverage of this area is exemplary and fills a void found in many texts and programs relating to the difficult task of teaching surgical radiography. An expanded section on bone densitometry, along with a new introduction to positron emission tomography (PET) and updated and revised chapters on angiography, interventional procedures, and computed tomography (CT) also ensures that educators and students will have the very latest information relating to these rapidly changing modalities.

After thoroughly reviewing this text I can only add that it will be the text that I use personally as my reference and will remain the required text I use in teaching radiographic positioning at the college level. I wholeheartedly recommend this text to anyone teaching or learning radiographic positioning. In as much as this text is now published in English, Portuguese, Spanish, Taiwanese/Chinese, and Russian, I know that an ever-increasing number of educators and students worldwide will benefit from the extensive knowledge and expertise of Ken Bontrager and John Lampignano.

David S. Hall, MS RT(R)
Associate Professor, Radiography
Broward Community College
Davie, Florida

Preface

Purpose and History

Early in my teaching career, first at a hospital-based program and then at a citywide college-affiliated program in radiologic technology, I discovered that other allied health programs were far ahead of us in the type and quality of instructional media available in their fields of study. We had no audiovisuals or teaching ancillaries at that time, and many of our textbooks were outdated, incomplete, and difficult to read and comprehend. In the late 1960s and early 1970s, as I was completing my graduate degree in education and instructional media, I began to develop audiovisuals and self-paced instructional programs for my students, which later turned out to be the first commercially available programmed audiovisual education media in radiologic technology. I chose as my subject radiographic anatomy and positioning because it is the one subject that all radiography students need to master.

This comprehensive audiovisual series was soon being widely used throughout the United States and Canada. It became apparent, however, that students also needed a thorough, clearly written, and easy-to-understand textbook on the important subject of radiographic anatomy and positioning. In the early 1980s the first edition of this textbook took shape, and it too was soon being widely used to supplement our audiovisual self-paced instructional series. Students and instructors now for the first time had access to a comprehensive audiovisual package, a three-volume student workbook, a five-volume instructor's manual, and a new, clearly written textbook.

Thus began my writing and publishing career nearly 35 years ago. My motivation for writing and developing instructional media remains the same today—to provide students and instructors with thorough, easy-to-use resources that are current and necessary for understanding the art and science of radiographic anatomy and positioning.

Unique Features

DISTINCTIVE PRESENTATION

I believe the most unique and distinctive feature of *Textbook of Radiographic Positioning and Related Anatomy* is its "show-and-tell" style of presentation. I have used the principle of presenting information from simple to complex, from known to unknown, and showing what is being talked about as it is being talked about. This maximizes the potential for comprehension and retention. Most of us remember best through mental images; we remember much more of what we see than what we hear. When we *see* with our eyes and *hear* as we read and *do* as we complete the positioning and workbook exercises, we gain the greatest opportunity for understanding and retaining what we have learned.

RADIOGRAPHIC CRITERIA AND CRITIQUE

A unique feature of this textbook is the inclusion of radiographs for critique at the end of each positioning chapter. This provides a great opportunity for students to use their knowledge of radiographic anatomy as related to positioning to **evaluate radiographs for errors.** They will begin to learn the difficult task of determining which errors are cause for repeats and which are acceptable but can still be improved.

This critiquing concept is made easier by the organization of the radiographic criteria section on each positioning page into subheads and grouping of information as related to specific aspects of positioning. This will help students develop a systematic routine for evaluating radiographic quality.

RADIATION PROTECTION, PATIENT DOSAGE, AND POSITIONING

As described in the ARRT code of ethics, radiologic technologists are responsible for controlling and "limiting the radiation exposure to the patient, self, and others of the health care team."* This requires a **good understanding and application of radiation protection practices** and an **awareness of radiation dose ranges** received by the patient for each body part being radiographed. The **relationship between patient doses and specific projections** (AP or PA) and **various combinations of exposure factors** needs to be understood. This awareness of specific dose ranges can be an additional motivating factor for careful positioning and technique selection to prevent unnecessary repeats. This is achieved by detailed shielding descriptions and by including patient dose icon boxes on positioning pages indicating specific **skin doses** as well as **midline** and **organ doses** when such radiosensitive organs are in or near the primary x-ray beam.

ALTERNATIVE MODALITIES, PATHOLOGY, AND POSITIONING

Today's health care workers are expected to expand their roles and be more "cross-functional" in their duties and responsibilities. Therefore all imaging technologists should understand at least the **basic principles** and the **possible procedures and exams** that can be performed in each of the imaging modalities as described in Chapter 24.

With these expanding roles for technologists also comes more responsibility for determining and understanding the **clinical** and **pathologic indications** for the exam or procedure being ordered. Technologists are expected to do more than just position a patient to demonstrate the anatomic part being examined per the order chart or exam requisition. They need to understand **why** the procedure is being ordered to ensure that the best projections or positions are obtained. They also need to know which pathologies affect the exposure factors required. Evaluating and critiquing obtained radiographic images requires knowledge and some understanding of how that disease or condition should appear on the radiographic image.

*Code of Ethics, Chapter 1, p. 32

SURVEY INFORMATION

Readers familiar with this textbook know that earlier editions included results of current practices by surveys of exams performed in the United States. The survey for the fifth edition was expanded to include both accredited radiologic technology programs and all clinical affiliates in the United States and Canada. Publishing the results of these surveys reinforces the importance of learning all of the most common positioning routines for each anatomic body part so that technologists will be well prepared to function in any geographic region that they may choose for employment. A description of these surveys is included in Appendix A.

New To This Edition

The entire text has been updated with numerous improved drawings and radiographic images. This edition now also includes both film-screen imaging considerations as well as principles and applications of digital imaging.

The new extensive section on **surgical radiography** now provides important and thorough coverage of those surgical radiographic procedures as performed by students and technologists. Information on **bone density** has been expanded to make it a more complete resource for performing these procedures and for studying for certification in this specialty.

New Content as Listed by Chapter

- Chapter 2. New chapter to include **Image Quality in Digital Imaging, Basic Principles and Applications**
- Chapters 3-18. New sections in all positioning chapters on **Digital Imaging Considerations**
- Chapter 5. New projection—**Skier's Thumb (Folio method)**
- Chapter 19. Totally new section on **Surgical Radiography**
- Chapters 21 and 22. Updated and revised chapters on **Angiography and Interventional Procedures,** and **Computed Tomography**
- Chapter 23. New expanded section on **Bone Densitometry**
- Chapter 24. New introductory section on **Positron Emission Tomography (PET)**

Ancillaries

WORKBOOK SET, COMPUTERIZED TEST BANK, ELECTRONIC IMAGE COLLECTION

The two-volume workbook set has been fully revised to coordinate with all the changes in the sixth edition of this textbook. This edition contains many new learning-exercise and self-test questions, including more situation-based questions and new questions on digital imaging.

A computerized test bank is available to instructors who use this textbook in their classrooms. The test bank features over 1200 questions. They have been expanded and fully revised into registry-type questions for the test bank. These questions can be used as final evaluation exams for each chapter or they can be put into custom exams that educators create.

Also available again is an electronic image collection featuring over 2000 images that are fully coordinated with the sixth edition textbook and workbooks. Instructors can make up their own customized classroom presentations using these electronic images, which closely follow the textbook and workbook, chapter by chapter.

KLB

How to Use the Positioning Pages

1 **PROJECTION TITLE BAR** The projection title bar describes the specific position/projection to be radiographed, including the proper name of the position, if such applies.

2 **PATHOLOGY DEMONSTRATED** The pathology demonstrated section gives a summary of conditions or pathologies that may be demonstrated by the exam and/or projection. This summary helps the technologist understand the purpose of the exam and which structures or tissues should be most clearly demonstrated.

3 **PROJECTION SUMMARY BOX** The projection summary box lists all the specific **basic** or **special projections** most commonly performed for that body part. The projection highlighted in blue is the projection described on that page.

4 **TECHNICAL FACTORS** The technical factors section lists the technical factors for the projection. Technical factors include the **image receptor (IR) size** recommended for the average adult; whether the IR should be placed **crosswise** or **lengthwise** in relation to the patient; a **grid,** if one is needed; and the **kV range** for the projection.

5 **TECHNIQUE AND DOSE BAR** The technique and dose bar summarizes a suggested starting technique for the projection for an average adult and the **approximate patient dose** for the exposure and the size of the exposure field. This is given in millirads of skin dose, midline dose, and specific radiosensitive organ dose. See Chapter 2, p. 73, for a more complete discussion of patient dosages.

6 **IMAGE RECEPTOR ICON** The image receptor icon gives a visual display of the **IR relative size (cm) and orientation (crosswise or lengthwise), patient ID blocker location, relative collimated field size, location of R and L markers,** and **the recommended AEC cell location** if AEC is used.

7 **SHIELDING** The shielding section describes shielding that should be used for the projection. See Chapter 2, p. 71, for more information on specific area shielding.

8 **PATIENT POSITION** The patient position section indicates the **general body position** required for the projection.

9 **PART POSITION** The part position section gives a clear, **step-by-step description** of how the body part should be positioned in relation to the IR and/or tabletop. The **CR icon,** ⌖, is included for all those projections in which the **CR is of primary importance** to remind the technologist to pay special attention to the CR during the positioning process for that projection.

10 **CENTRAL RAY** The central ray section provides a description of the **precise location of the CR** in relation to both the IR and the body part. The **minimum SID** (source-to-image receptor distance) is listed. See Chapter 2, p. 48, for the advantages of increasing the SID from 40 inches (100 cm) to 44 or 48 inches (110 to 120 cm) for general tabletop procedures.

11 **COLLIMATION** The collimation section describes the collimation of the x-ray field recommended for that projection.

12 **RESPIRATION** The respiration section lists the breathing requirements for that projection.

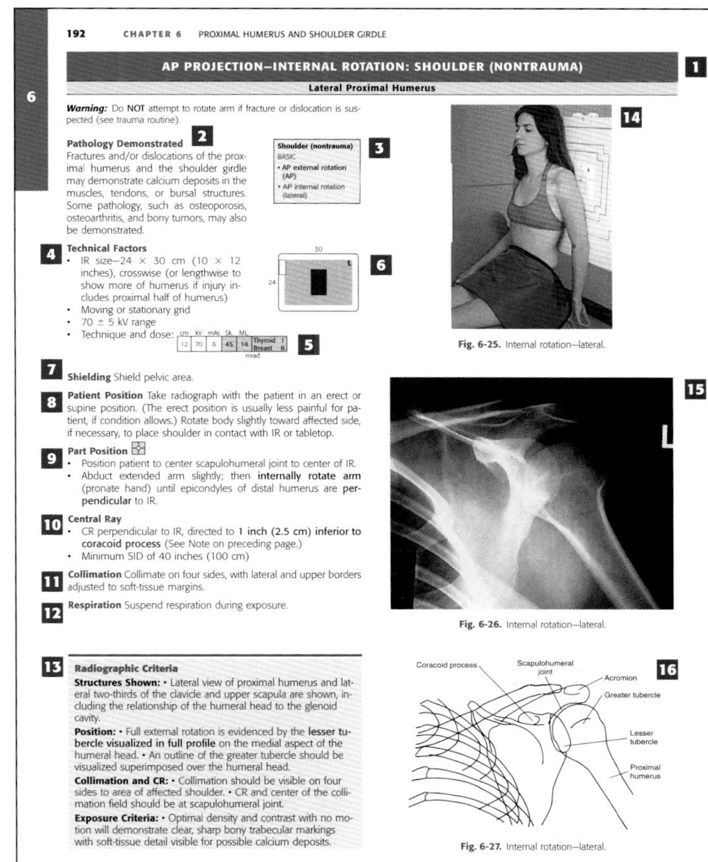

13 **RADIOGRAPHIC CRITERIA BOX** The radiographic criteria box describes the four-step evaluation/critique process that should be completed for each processed radiographic image. This process is divided into four categories of information as related to the following: (1) **structures that should be shown;** (2) **evidence of correct positioning;** (3) **correct collimation and CR location;** and (4) **acceptable exposure factors.**

14 **POSITIONING PHOTOGRAPH** The positioning photograph demonstrates the correct patient and part position in relation to the CR and IR.

15 **RADIOGRAPHIC IMAGE** The radiographic image demonstrates a correctly positioned and correctly exposed radiographic image of the featured projection.

16 **ANATOMY LINE DRAWING** The anatomy line drawing indicates and interprets the specific anatomic parts visible on the radiographic image shown on the page.

Contents

TEXTBOOK OF

Radiographic Positioning and Related Anatomy

How to Use the Positioning Pages

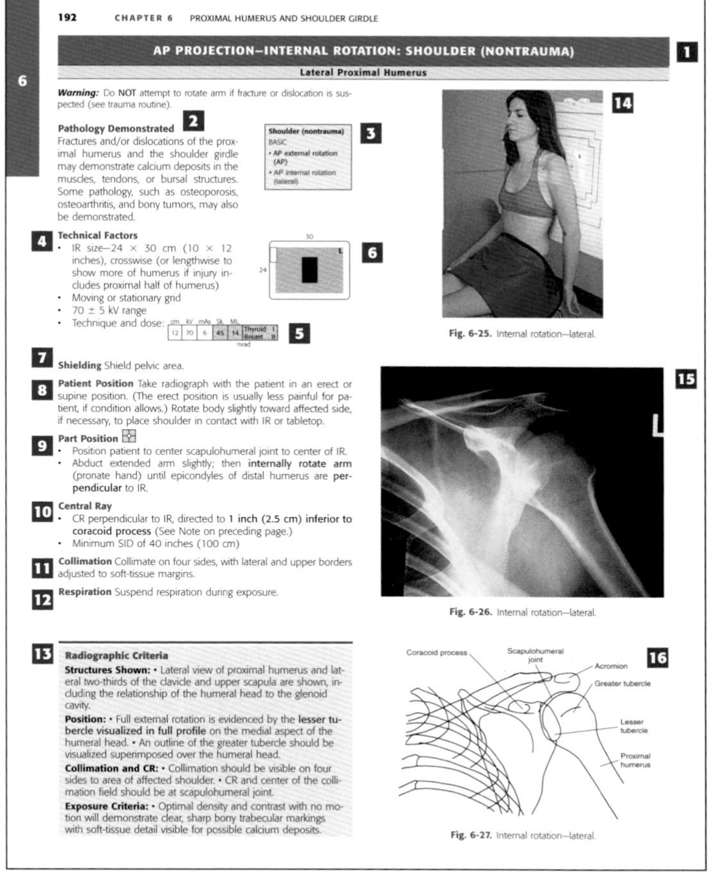
192 CHAPTER 6 PROXIMAL HUMERUS AND SHOULDER GIRDLE

1 **AP PROJECTION—INTERNAL ROTATION: SHOULDER (NONTRAUMA)**

Lateral Proximal Humerus

Warning: Do NOT attempt to rotate arm if fracture or dislocation is suspected (see trauma routine).

2 **Pathology Demonstrated**
Fractures and/or dislocations of the proximal humerus and the shoulder girdle may demonstrate calcium deposits in the muscles, tendons, or bursal structures. Some pathology, such as osteoporosis, osteoarthritis, and bony tumors, may also be demonstrated.

3 **Shoulder (nontrauma)**
BASIC
• AP external rotation (AP)
• AP internal rotation (lateral)

4 **Technical Factors**
• IR size—24 × 30 cm (10 × 12 inches), crosswise (or lengthwise to show more of humerus if injury includes proximal half of humerus)
• Moving or stationary grid
• 70 ± 5 kV range
• Technique and dose: 5

6

7 **Shielding** Shield pelvic area.

8 **Patient Position** Take radiograph with the patient in an erect or supine position. (The erect position is usually less painful for patient, if condition allows.) Rotate body slightly toward affected side, if necessary, to place shoulder in contact with IR or tabletop.

9 **Part Position**
• Position patient to center scapulohumeral joint to center of IR.
• Abduct extended arm slightly; then **internally rotate arm** (pronate hand) until epicondyles of distal humerus are **perpendicular** to IR.

10 **Central Ray**
• CR perpendicular to IR, directed to **1 inch (2.5 cm) inferior to coracoid process** (See Note on preceding page.)
• Minimum SID of 40 inches (100 cm)

11 **Collimation** Collimate on four sides, with lateral and upper borders adjusted to soft-tissue margins.

12 **Respiration** Suspend respiration during exposure.

13 **Radiographic Criteria**
Structures Shown: • Lateral view of proximal humerus and lateral two-thirds of the clavicle and upper scapula are shown, including the relationship of the humeral head to the glenoid cavity.
Position: • Full external rotation is evidenced by the **lesser tubercle visualized in full profile** on the medial aspect of the humeral head. • An outline of the greater tubercle should be visualized superimposed over the humeral head.
Collimation and CR: • Collimation should be visible on four sides to area of affected shoulder. • CR and center of the collimation field should be at scapulohumeral joint.
Exposure Criteria: • Optimal density and contrast with no motion will demonstrate clear, sharp bony trabecular markings with soft-tissue detail visible for possible calcium deposits.

14

Fig. 6-25. Internal rotation—lateral.

15

Fig. 6-26. Internal rotation—lateral.

16

Fig. 6-27. Internal rotation—lateral.

1 **PROJECTION TITLE BAR** The projection title bar describes the specific position/projection to be radiographed, including the proper name of the position, if such applies.

2 **PATHOLOGY DEMONSTRATED** The pathology demonstrated section gives a summary of conditions or pathologies that may be demonstrated by the exam and/or projection. This summary helps the technologist understand the purpose of the exam and which structures or tissues should be most clearly demonstrated.

3 **PROJECTION SUMMARY BOX** The projection summary box lists all the specific **basic** or **special projections** most commonly performed for that body part. The projection highlighted in blue is the projection described on that page.

4 **TECHNICAL FACTORS** The technical factors section lists the technical factors for the projection. Technical factors include the **image receptor (IR) size** recommended for the average adult; whether the IR should be placed **crosswise** or **lengthwise** in relation to the patient; a **grid,** if one is needed; and the **kV range** for the projection.

5 **TECHNIQUE AND DOSE BAR** The technique and dose bar summarizes a suggested starting technique for the projection for an average adult and the **approximate patient dose** for the exposure and the size of the exposure field. This is given in millirads of skin dose, midline dose, and specific radiosensitive organ dose. See Chapter 2, p. 73, for a more complete discussion of patient dosages.

6 **IMAGE RECEPTOR ICON** The image receptor icon gives a visual display of the **IR relative size (cm) and orientation (crosswise or lengthwise), patient ID blocker location, relative collimated field size, location of R and L markers,** and **the recommended AEC cell location** if AEC is used.

7 **SHIELDING** The shielding section describes shielding that should be used for the projection. See Chapter 2, p. 71, for more information on specific area shielding.

8 **PATIENT POSITION** The patient position section indicates the **general body position** required for the projection.

9 **PART POSITION** The part position section gives a clear, **step-by-step description** of how the body part should be positioned in relation to the IR and/or tabletop. The **CR icon,** ⊕, is included for all those projections in which the **CR is of primary importance** to remind the technologist to pay special attention to the CR during the positioning process for that projection.

10 **CENTRAL RAY** The central ray section provides a description of the **precise location of the CR** in relation to both the IR and the body part. The **minimum SID** (source-to-image receptor distance) is listed. See Chapter 2, p. 48, for the advantages of increasing the SID from 40 inches (100 cm) to 44 or 48 inches (110 to 120 cm) for general tabletop procedures.

11 **COLLIMATION** The collimation section describes the collimation of the x-ray field recommended for that projection.

12 **RESPIRATION** The respiration section lists the breathing requirements for that projection.

13 **RADIOGRAPHIC CRITERIA BOX** The radiographic criteria box describes the four-step evaluation/critique process that should be completed for each processed radiographic image. This process is divided into four categories of information as related to the following: (1) **structures that should be shown;** (2) **evidence of correct positioning;** (3) **correct collimation and CR location;** and (4) **acceptable exposure factors.**

14 **POSITIONING PHOTOGRAPH** The positioning photograph demonstrates the correct patient and part position in relation to the CR and IR.

15 **RADIOGRAPHIC IMAGE** The radiographic image demonstrates a correctly positioned and correctly exposed radiographic image of the featured projection.

16 **ANATOMY LINE DRAWING** The anatomy line drawing indicates and interprets the specific anatomic parts visible on the radiographic image shown on the page.

CHAPTER 1

General Anatomy, Terminology, and Positioning Principles

CONTRIBUTORS TO PAST EDITIONS Cindy Murphy, RT R, ACR, BHSc, Kathy M. Martensen, BS, RT(R), Barry T. Anthony, RT(R)

CONTENTS

GENERAL, SYSTEMIC, AND SKELETAL ANATOMY AND ARTHROLOGY

General Anatomy

Anatomy is the science of the structure of the human body, whereas **physiology** deals with functions of the body, or how the body parts work. In the living subject, it is almost impossible to study anatomy without also studying some physiology. Radiographic study of the human body, however, is primarily a study of the anatomy of the various systems with lesser emphasis on the physiology. Consequently, anatomy of the human system will be emphasized in this radiographic anatomy and positioning textbook.

Note: Phonetic respelling* of anatomic and positioning terms is included throughout this text to aid in correct pronunciation of those terms commonly used in medical radiography.

STRUCTURAL ORGANIZATION

Several levels of structural organization comprise the human body. The lowest level of organization is the **chemical level.** All the chemicals necessary for maintaining life are composed of **atoms,** joined in various ways to form **molecules.** Various chemicals in the form of molecules are organized to form **cells.**

Cells

The cell is the basic structural and functional unit of the entire human being. Every single part of the body, whether muscle, bone, cartilage, fat, nerve, skin, or blood, is composed of cells.

Tissues

Tissues are groups of similar cells that, together with their intercellular material, perform a specific function. The four basic types of tissues are as follows:

1. ***Epithelial*** *(ep'i-the'le-al):* Tissues that cover internal and external surfaces of the body, including lining of vessels and organs, such as the stomach and intestines
2. ***Connective:*** Tissues that bind together and support the various structures
3. ***Muscular:*** Tissues that make up the substance of a muscle
4. ***Nervous:*** Tissues that make up the substance of nerves and nerve centers

Organs

When various tissues are joined to perform a specific function, the result is an organ. Organs usually have a specific shape. Examples of organs of the human body are the kidneys, heart, liver, lungs, stomach, and brain.

System

A system consists of a group or an association of organs that have a similar or common function. The urinary system, consisting of the kidneys, ureters, bladder, and urethra, is an example of a body system. There are **10 individual body systems** comprising the total body.

Organism

The 10 systems of the body functioning together constitute the total organism—one living being.

*Dorland's illustrated medical dictionary, ed 28, Philadelphia, 1994, WB Saunders.

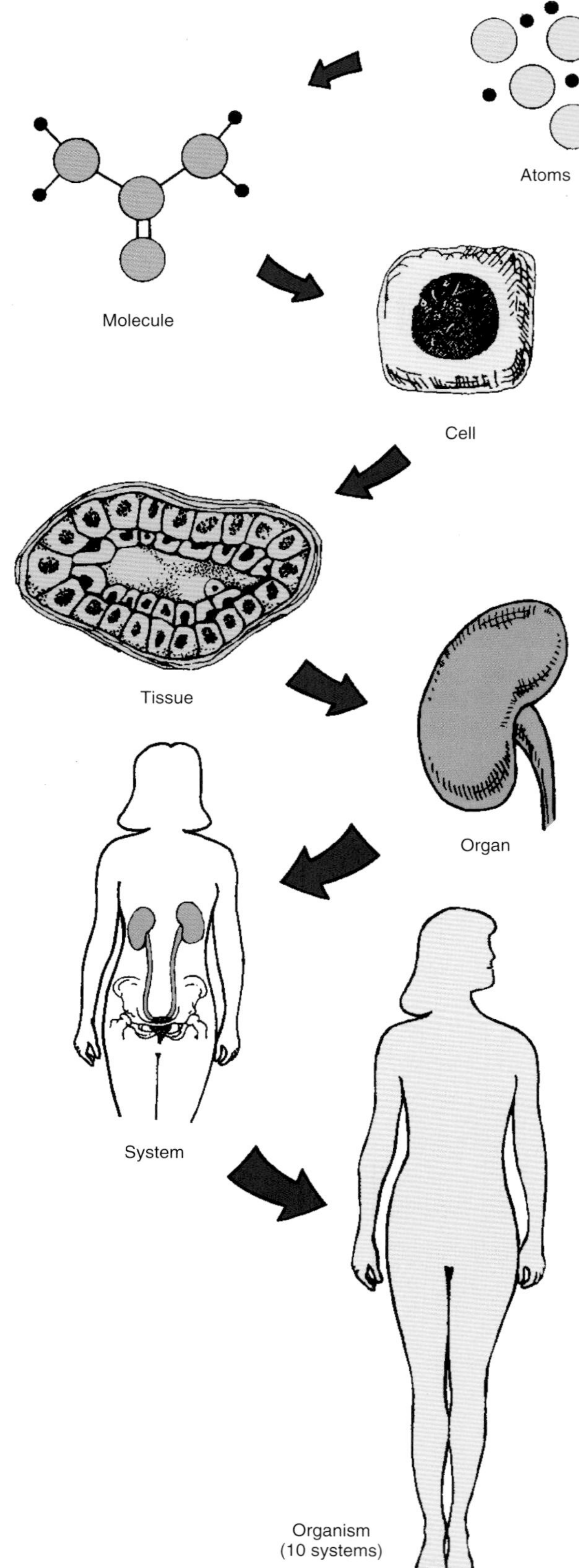

Fig. 1-1. Levels of human structural organization.

Systemic Anatomy

BODY SYSTEMS

The human body is a structural and functional unit made up of 10 lesser units termed *systems.* These 10 systems are (1) skeletal, (2) circulatory, (3) digestive, (4) respiratory, (5) urinary, (6) reproductive, (7) nervous, (8) muscular, (9) endocrine, and (10) integumentary *(in-teg-u-men'tar-e).*

Skeletal System

The skeletal system is an important system for the technologist to study. The skeletal system includes the **206 separate bones** of the body and their associated cartilages and joints. The study of bones is termed **osteology,** whereas the study of joints is termed **arthrology.**

The four functions of the skeletal system are as follows:

1. To support and protect the body
2. To allow movement by interacting with the muscles to form levers
3. To produce blood cells
4. To store calcium

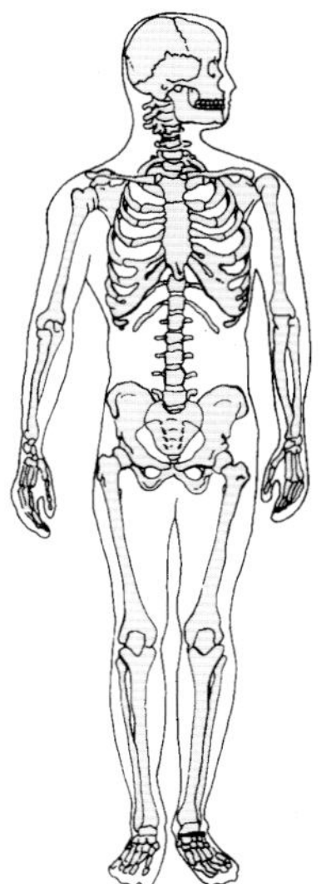

Fig. 1-2. Skeletal system.

Circulatory System

The circulatory system is composed of the following:

- The **cardiovascular organs**—heart, blood, and blood vessels
- The **lymphatic system**—lymph nodes, lymph vessels, lymph glands, and spleen

The six functions of the circulatory system are as follows:

1. To distribute oxygen and nutrients to the cells of the body
2. To carry cell waste and carbon dioxide from the cells
3. To transport water, electrolytes, hormones, and enzymes
4. To protect against disease
5. To prevent hemorrhage by forming blood clots
6. To help regulate body temperature

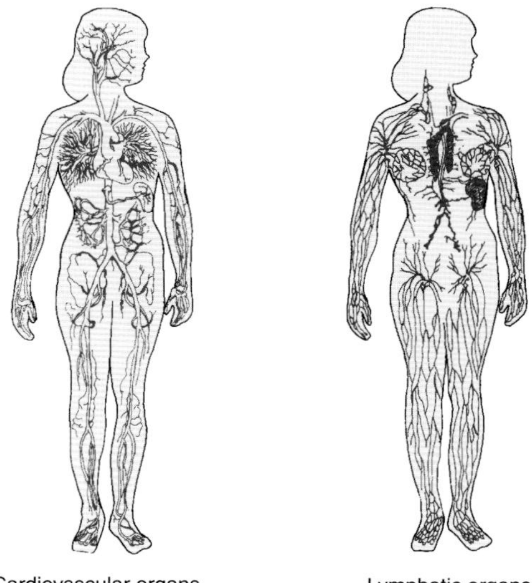

Fig. 1-3. Circulatory system.

Digestive System

The digestive system includes the alimentary canal and certain accessory organs. The alimentary canal is made up of the mouth, pharynx, esophagus, stomach, small intestine, large intestine, and anus. Accessory organs of digestion include the salivary glands, liver, gallbladder, and pancreas.

The twofold function of the digestive system is as follows:

1. To prepare food for absorption by the cells through numerous physical and chemical breakdown processes
2. To eliminate solid wastes from the body

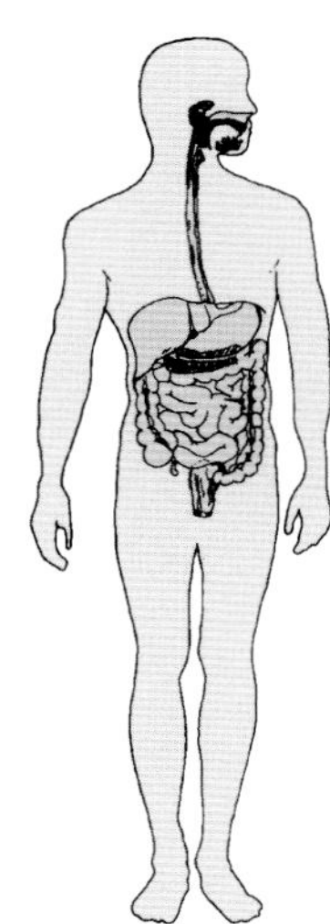

Fig. 1-4. Digestive system.

Respiratory System

The respiratory system is composed of two lungs and a series of passages connecting the lungs to the outside atmosphere. The structures making up the passageway from the exterior to the alveoli of the lung interior are the nose, mouth, pharynx, larynx, trachea, and bronchial tree.

The three functions of the respiratory system are as follows:

1. To supply oxygen to the blood and eventually to the cells
2. To eliminate carbon dioxide from the blood
3. To assist in regulating the acid-base balance of the blood

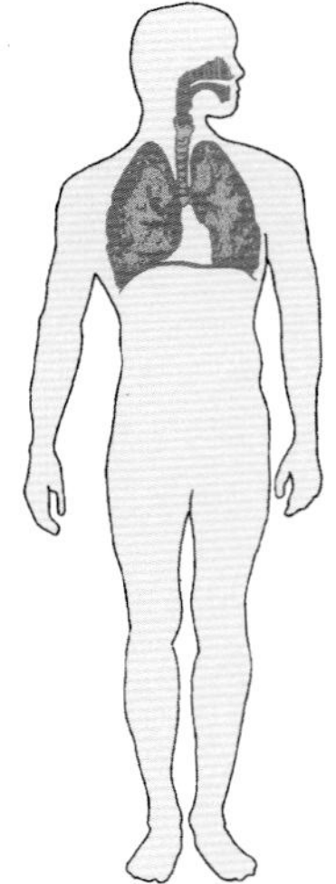

Fig. 1-5. Respiratory system.

Urinary System

The urinary system includes those organs that produce, collect, and eliminate urine. The organs of the urinary system are the kidneys, ureters, bladder, and urethra.

The four functions of the urinary system are as follows:

1. To regulate the chemical composition of the blood
2. To eliminate many waste products
3. To regulate fluid and electrolyte balance and volume
4. To maintain the acid-base balance of the body

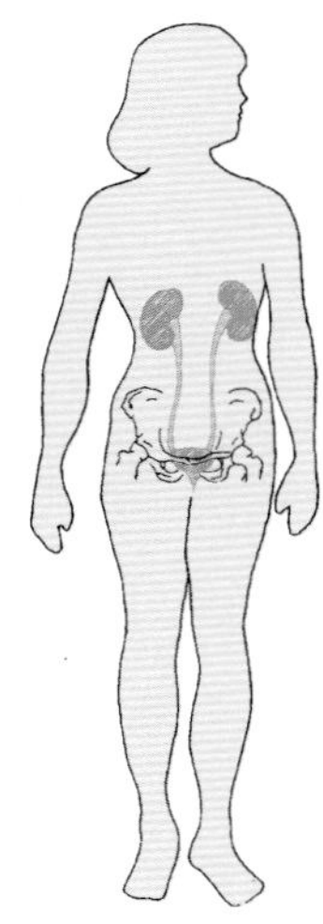

Fig. 1-6. Urinary system.

Reproductive System

The reproductive system includes those organs that produce, transport, and store the germ cells. The testes in the male and the ovaries in the female produce mature germ cells. Transport and storage organs of the male include the vas deferens, prostate gland, and penis. The organs of reproduction in the female are the uterine tubes, uterus, and vagina.

The function of the reproductive system is to reproduce the organism.

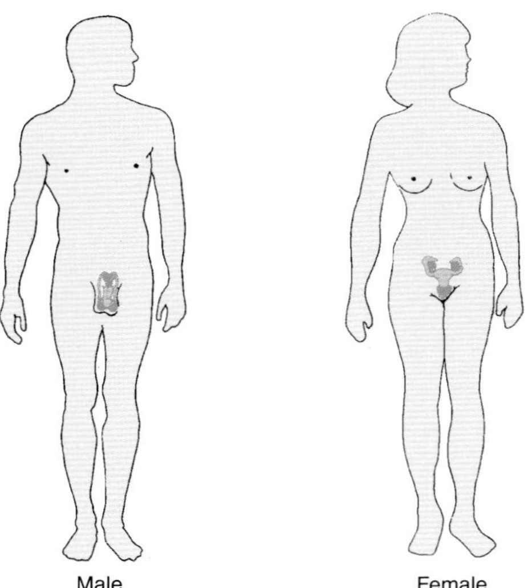

Fig. 1-7. Reproductive system.

Nervous System

The nervous system is composed of the brain, spinal cord, nerves, ganglia, and special sense organs such as the eyes and ears.

The function of the nervous system is to regulate body activities with electrical impulses traveling along various nerves.

Muscular System

The muscular system includes all muscle tissues of the body and is subdivided into three types: (1) skeletal, (2) visceral, and (3) cardiac.

Most of the muscle mass of the body is skeletal muscle, which is striated and under voluntary control. The voluntary muscles act in conjunction with the skeleton to allow body movement. About 43% of the weight of the human body is composed of voluntary or striated skeletal muscle.

Visceral muscle, which is smooth and involuntary, is located in the walls of hollow internal organs such as blood vessels, the stomach, and intestines. These muscles are termed *involuntary* because their contraction is usually not under voluntary or conscious control.

Cardiac muscle is found only in the walls of the heart and is involuntary but striated.

The three functions of muscle tissue are as follows:

1. To allow movement, such as locomotion of the body or movement of substances through the alimentary canal
2. To maintain posture
3. To produce heat

Endocrine System

The endocrine system includes all the ductless glands of the body. These glands include the testes, ovaries, pancreas, adrenals, thymus, thyroid, parathyroids, pineal, and pituitary. The placenta acts as a temporary endocrine gland.

Hormones, which are the secretions of the endocrine glands, are released directly into the bloodstream.

The function of the endocrine system is to regulate bodily activities through the various hormones carried by the cardiovascular system.

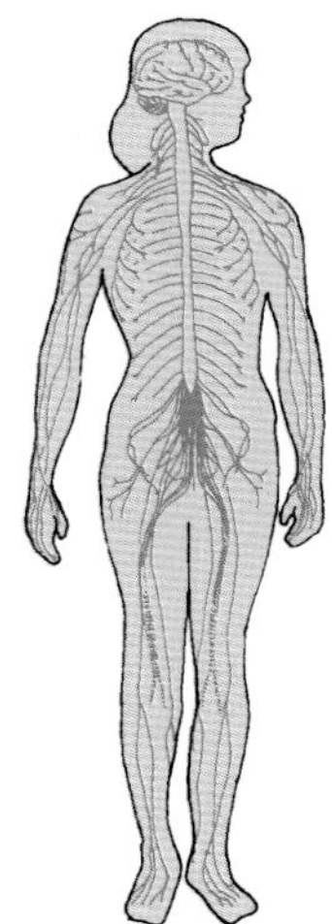

Fig. 1-8. Nervous system.

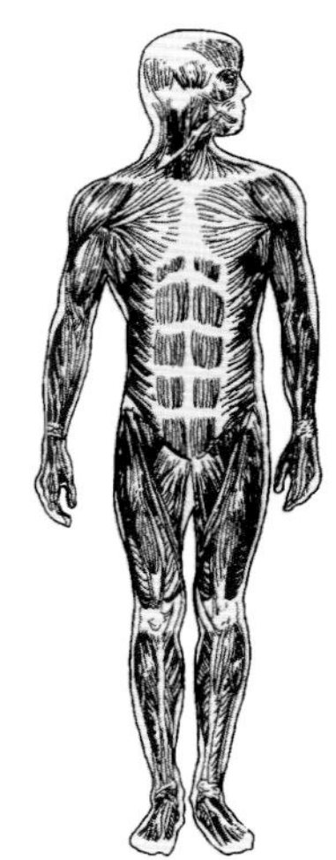

Fig. 1-9. Muscular system.

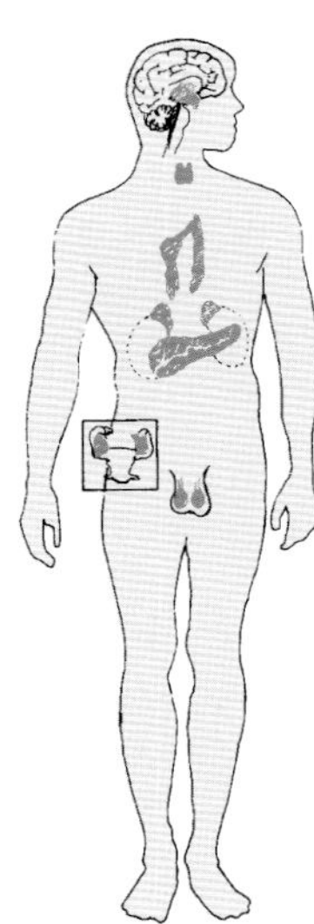

Fig. 1-10. Endocrine system.

Integumentary System

The tenth and final body system is the **integumentary** *(in-teg-u-men'tar-e)* system, which is composed of the skin and all structures derived from the skin. These derived structures include hair, nails, and sweat and oil glands.

The skin is an organ that is essential to life. In fact, the skin is the largest organ of the body, covering a surface area of approximately 7620 square centimeters in the average adult.

The four functions of the integumentary system are as follows:

1. To regulate body temperature
2. To protect the body
3. To eliminate waste products through perspiration
4. To receive certain stimuli such as temperature, pressure, and pain

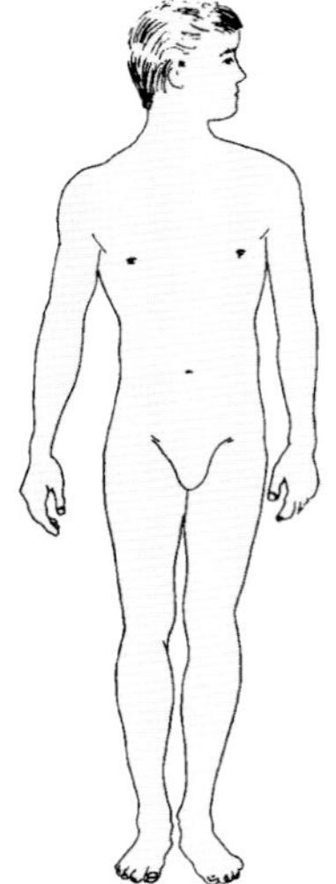

Fig. 1-11. Integumentary system.

Skeletal Anatomy

Because a large part of general diagnostic radiography involves examinations of the bones and joints, **osteology** *(os'te-ol'o-je)* (the study of bones) and **arthrology** *(ar-throl'o-je)* (the study of joints) are important subjects for the technologist.

OSTEOLOGY

The adult skeletal system is composed of **206 separate bones,** forming the framework of the entire body. Certain cartilages, such as at the ends of long bones, are included in the skeletal system. These bones and cartilages are united by ligaments and provide surfaces to which the muscles attach. Because muscles and bones must combine to allow body movement, these two systems are sometimes collectively referred to as the *locomotor system.*

The adult human skeleton is divided into either the **axial skeleton** or the **appendicular skeleton.**

Axial Skeleton

The **axial** *(ak'se-al)* **skeleton** includes all bones that lie on or near the central axis of the body. The adult axial skeleton consists of **80 bones** and includes the skull, vertebral column, ribs, and sternum (the darker-colored regions of the body skeleton in Fig. 1-12).

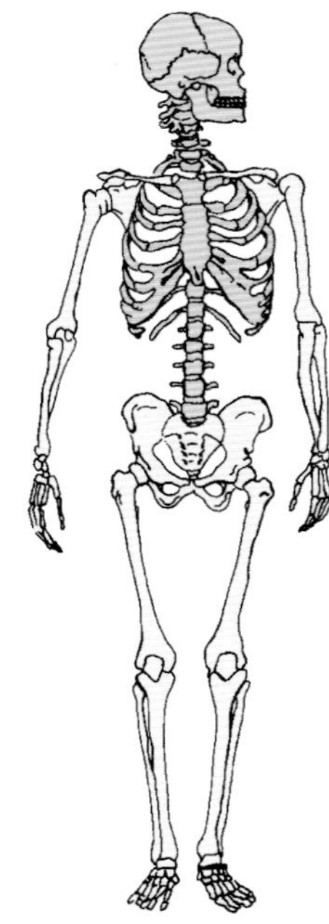

Fig. 1-12. Axial skeleton—80 bones.

ADULT AXIAL SKELETON		
Skull	Cranium	8
	Facial bones	14
Hyoid		1
Auditory ossicles (small bones in each ear)		6
Vertebral column	Cervical	7
	Thoracic	12
	Lumbar	5
	Sacrum	1
	Coccyx	1
Thorax	Sternum	1
	Ribs	24
TOTAL BONES IN ADULT AXIAL SKELETON		80

Appendicular Skeleton

The second division of the skeleton is the **appendicular** *(ap'en-dik'u-lar)* portion. This division consists of all bones of the upper and lower limbs (extremities) and the shoulder and pelvic girdles (the darker-colored regions in Fig. 1-13). There are **126 separate bones** in the adult appendicular skeleton.

ADULT APPENDICULAR SKELETON		
Shoulder girdles	Clavicles	2
	Scapula (scapulae)	2
Upper limbs	Humerus (humeri)	2
	Ulna (ulnae)	2
	Radius (radii)	2
	Carpals	16
	Metacarpals	10
	Phalanges	28
Pelvic girdle	Hip bones	2
Lower limbs	Femur (femora)	2
	Tibias	2
	Fibula (fibulae)	2
	Patella (patellae)	2
	Tarsals	14
	Metatarsals	10
	Phalanges	28
TOTAL BONES IN ADULT APPENDICULAR SKELETON		126
Entire adult skeleton—**206 separate bones.**		
(This includes 2 sesamoid bones of lower limb at the knee, patellae.)		

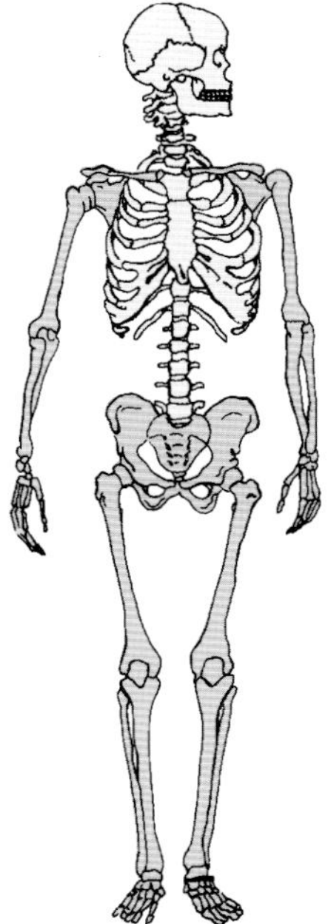

Fig. 1-13. Appendicular skeleton—126 bones.

Sesamoid Bones

Sesamoid bones are a special type of small, oval-shaped bone found in the tendons (mostly near joints). Although sesamoid bones are present even in a developing fetus, they are not counted as part of the normal axial or appendicular skeleton, except for the two patellae, the largest sesamoid bones. The other most common sesamoid bones are located in the posterior foot at the base of the first toe (Figs. 1-14 and 1-15).

In the upper limb, sesamoid bones are most commonly found in tendons near the palmar surface of the hand at the base of the thumb. Others may be found in tendons of other upper or lower limb joints.

Any sesamoid bone can be fractured by trauma and may need to be demonstrated radiographically.

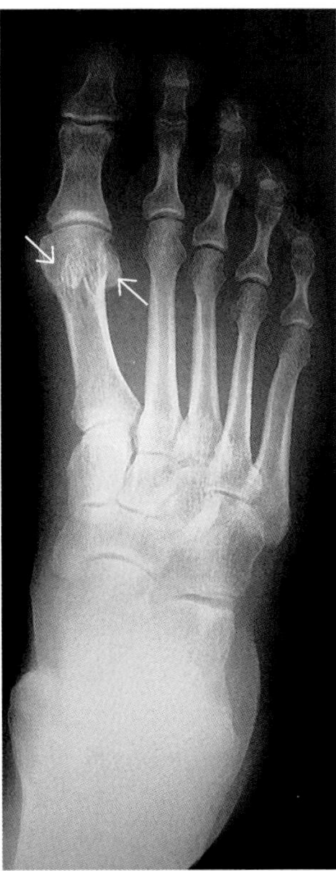

Fig. 1-14. Sesamoid bones on the posterior base of first toe.

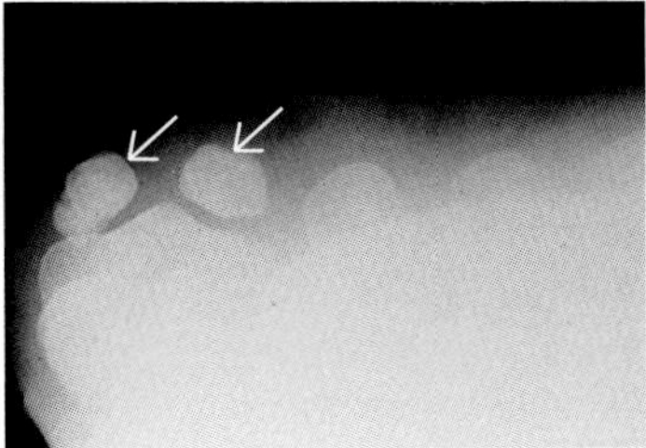

Fig. 1-15. Sesamoid bones. Tangential projection (base of first toe).

CLASSIFICATION OF BONES

Each of the 206 bones of the body can be classified according to shape as follows:

- Long bones
- Short bones
- Flat bones
- Irregular bones

Long Bones

Long bones consist of a **body** and **two ends** or **extremities.** Long bones are found only in the appendicular skeleton. (Fig. 1-16 is a radiograph of a humerus, a typical long bone of the upper arm.)

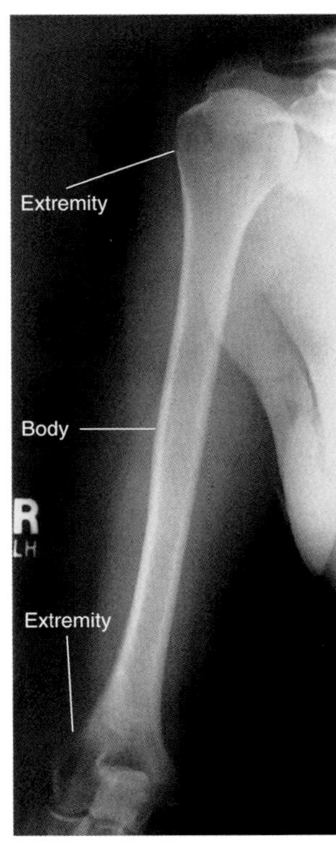

Fig. 1-16. Long bone (humerus).

Composition: The outer shell of most bones is composed of hard or dense bone tissue known as **compact bone,** or **cortex,** meaning an external layer. Compact bone has few intercellular empty spaces and serves to protect and support the entire bone.

The **body** (older term is **shaft**) contains a thicker layer of compact bone than the ends to help resist the stress of the weight placed on them.

Inside the shell of compact bone and especially at both ends of each long bone is found **spongy,** or **cancellous, bone.** Cancellous bone is highly porous and usually contains red bone marrow, which is responsible for the production of red blood cells.

The body of a long bone is hollow. This hollow portion is known as the **medullary** *(med'u-lar"e)* **cavity.** In the adult the medullary cavity usually contains fatty yellow marrow. A dense fibrous membrane, the **periosteum** *(per"e-os'te-am),* covers bone except at the articulating surfaces. The articulating surfaces are covered with a layer of **hyaline cartilage.**

Hyaline *(hi'ah-lin),* meaning glassy or clear, is a common type of cartilage or connecting tissue, also known as "gristle." Its name comes from the fact that it is not visible with ordinary staining techniques, thus appearing as "clear" or glassy in lab studies. It is present in many places, including the covering over ends of bones, where it is called **articular cartilage.**

The **periosteum** is essential for bone growth, repair, and nutrition. Bones are richly supplied with blood vessels that pass into them from the periosteum. Near the center of the body of long bones, a **nutrient artery** passes obliquely through the compact bone via a **nutrient foramen** into the medullary cavity.

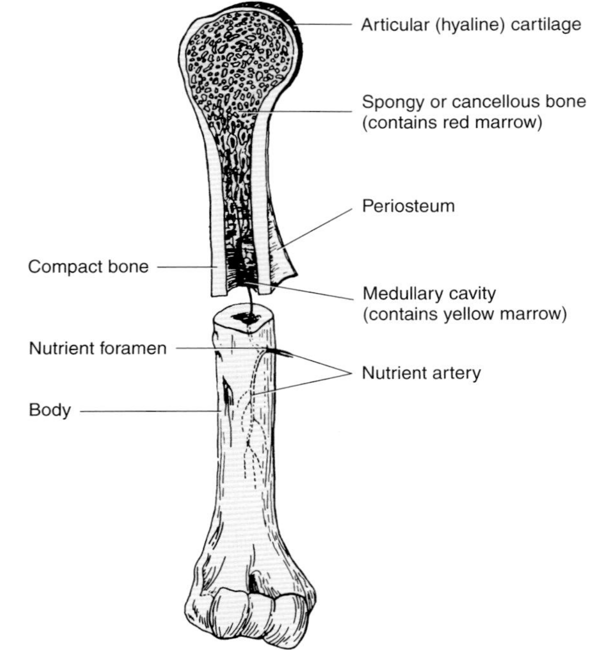

Fig. 1-17. Long bone.

Short Bones

Short bones are roughly cuboidal and are found only in the wrists and ankles. Short bones consist mainly of cancellous tissue with a thin outer covering of compact bone. The eight **carpal bones** of each wrist and the seven **tarsal bones** of each foot are all short bones.

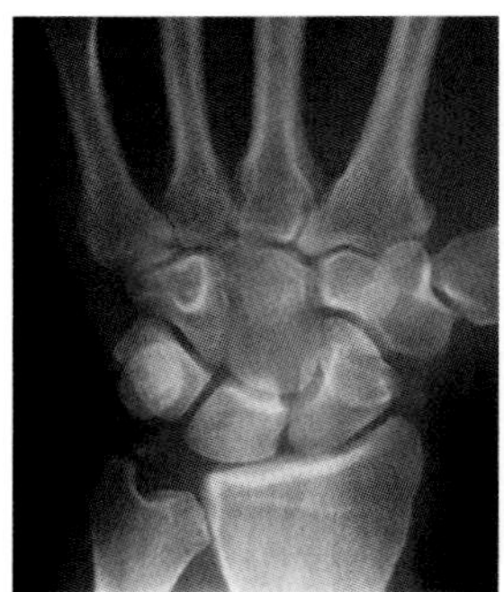

Fig. 1-18. Short bones (carpals).

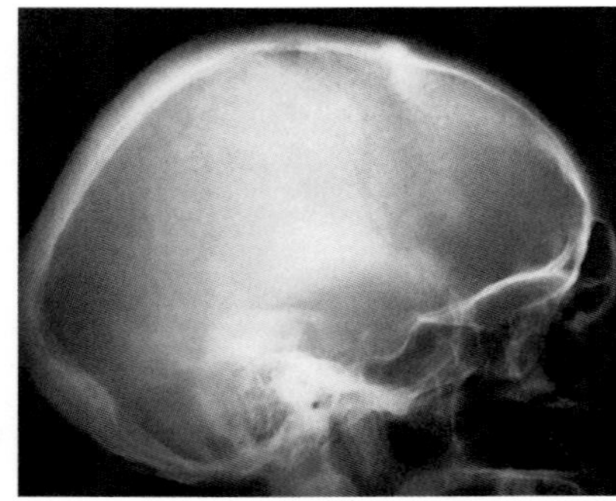

Fig. 1-19. Flat bones (calvarium).

Flat Bones

Flat bones consist of two plates of compact bone with cancellous bone and marrow between them. Examples of flat bones are the bones making up the **calvarium** (skull cap), **sternum, ribs,** and **scapulae.**

The narrow space between the inner and the outer table of flat bones in the cranium is known as **diploe** *(dip'lo-e).* Flat bones provide protection for interior contents and broad surfaces for muscle attachment.

Irregular Bones

Bones that have peculiar shapes are lumped into one final category—irregular bones. **Vertebrae, facial bones, bones of the base of the cranium,** and **bones of the pelvis** are examples of irregular bones.

Blood Cell Production

In adults, **red blood cells (RBCs)** are produced by the red bone marrow of certain flat and irregular bones such as the **sternum, ribs, vertebrae,** and **pelvis,** as well as the ends of the long bones.

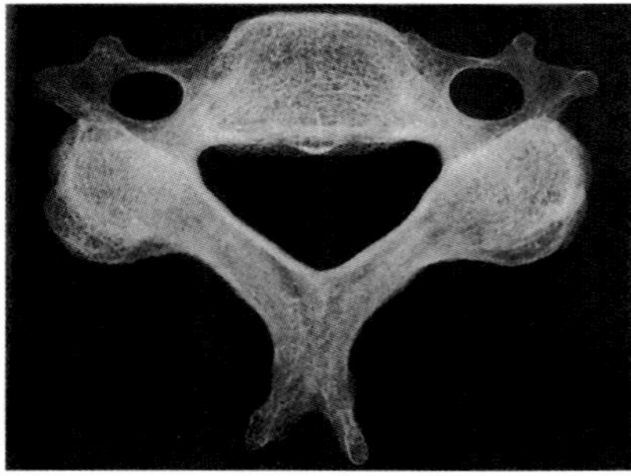

Fig. 1-20. Irregular bone (vertebra).

DEVELOPMENT OF BONES

The process by which bones form in the body is known as **ossification** *(os″i-fi-ka′shun).* The embryonic skeleton is composed of fibrous membranes and hyaline cartilage. Ossification begins about the sixth embryonic week and continues until adulthood.

Bone Formation

Two kinds of bone formation are known. When bone replaces membranes, the ossification is termed **intramembranous** *(in″trah-mem′brah-nus).* When bone replaces cartilage, the result is **endochondral** *(en″do-kon′dral)* (intracartilaginous) ossification.

Intramembranous ossification Intramembranous ossification occurs rapidly and takes place in bones that are needed for protection, such as sutures of the flat bones of the skullcap, which are centers of growth in early bone development.

Endochondral ossification Endochondral ossification occurs much slower than intramembranous ossification and occurs in most parts of the skeleton, especially in the long bones.

Primary and Secondary Centers of Endochondral Ossification

The first center of ossification is termed the **primary center** and occurs in the midbody area. This primary center of ossification in growing bones is called the **diaphysis** *(di-af′i-sis).* This becomes the **body** in a fully developed bone.

Secondary centers of ossification appear near the ends or extremities of long bones. Most secondary centers appear after birth, whereas most primary centers appear before birth. Each secondary center of ossification is termed an **epiphysis** *(e-pif′i-sis).* Epiphyses of the distal femur and the proximal tibia are the first to appear and may be present at birth in the term newborn. Cartilaginous plates, termed **epiphyseal plates,** are found between the diaphysis and each epiphysis until skeletal growth is complete.

Growth in the length of bones results from a longitudinal increase in these epiphyseal cartilaginous plates. This is followed by progressive ossification through endochondral bone development until all the cartilage has been replaced by bone, at which time growth to the skeleton is complete. This process of epiphyseal fusion of the long bones occurs progressively from the age of puberty to **full maturity,** which is **about 25 years.** However, the time for each bone to complete growth varies for different regions of the body. In addition, the female skeleton usually matures more quickly than the male skeleton. Extensive charts that list the normal growth patterns of the skeleton are available.

Radiograph Demonstrating Bone Growth

Fig. 1-22 shows a radiograph of the knee region of a 6-year-old child. Primary and secondary centers of endochondral ossification or bone growth are well demonstrated and labeled.

Primary centers The primary centers of bone growth show well-developed bone and include the **diaphysis** (body) area.

Secondary centers The secondary centers of bone growth are the **epiphyses,** which are shown at the distal end of the femur and the proximal end of the tibia and fibula. These epiphyses are separated from the main bone by a space or joint called an **epiphyseal plate.** These are made up of cartilage that does not visualize on radiographs because there is no calcium in these areas at this stage of growth. Therefore these epiphyseal plates disappear completely as they are replaced with calcium when growth is completed.

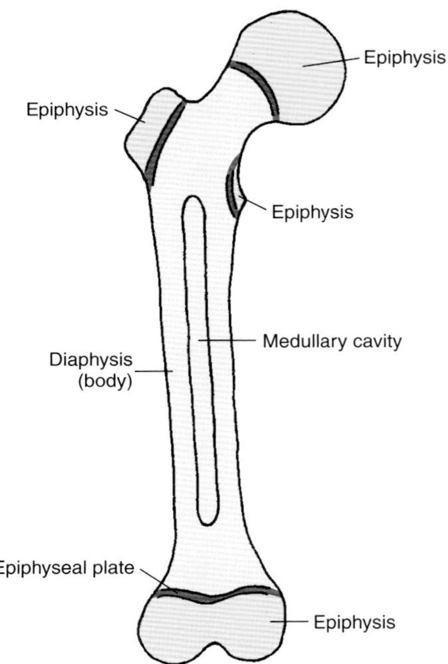

Fig. 1-21. Endochondral ossification (femur).

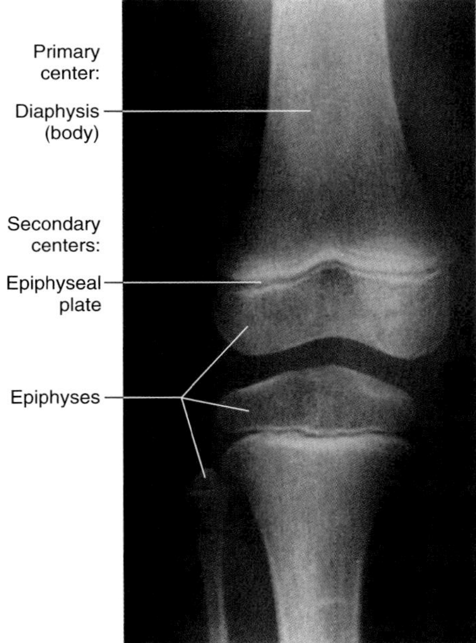

Fig. 1-22. Knee region (6-year-old child).

1

Arthrology (Joints)

The study of joints or articulations is called **arthrology.** It is important to understand that movement does not occur in all joints. Indeed, the first two types of joints to be described are immovable or only slightly movable joints held together by several fibrous layers, or cartilage. These are joints adapted for growth rather than for movement.

CLASSIFICATION OF JOINTS

Functional

Joints classified according to their function in relation to their mobility or lack of mobility are as follows:

- **Synarthrosis** *(sin"ar-thro'sis*—Immovable joint
- **Amphiarthrosis** *(am"fe-ar-thro'sis)*—Joint with limited movement
- **Diarthrosis** *(di"ar-thro'sis)*—Freely movable joint

Structural

Sometimes all joints or articulations of the body are grouped or classified according to the above three functional classes. However, the primary classification system of joints, which is recognized by *NOMINA ANATOMICA* and used in this textbook, **is a structural classification** based on the **three types of tissue that separate the ends of bones** in the different joints. These three classifications by tissue types, along with their subclasses, are as follows:

- **Fibrous** *(fi'brus)* **joints**
  1. Syndesmosis *(sin"des-mo'sis)*
  2. Suture *(su'tur)*
  3. Gomphosis *(gom-fo'sis)*
- **Cartilaginous** *(kar"ti-laj'i-nus)* **joints**
  1. Symphysis *(sim'fi-sis)*
  2. Synchondrosis *(sin"kon-dro'sis)*
- **Synovial** *(si-no've-al)* **joints**

Fibrous Joints

Fibrous joints lack a joint cavity. The adjoining bones, which are nearly in direct contact with each other, are **held together by fibrous connective tissue.** Three types of fibrous joints are **syndesmoses,** which are slightly movable; **sutures,** which are immovable; and **gomphoses,** a unique type of joint with only very limited movement (Fig. 1-23).

1. Syndesmoses

The only true syndesmosis joint in the body (as classified by *NOMINA ANATOMICA*) is the **distal tibiofibular joint.*** Fibrous ligaments hold the distal tibia and fibula together at this joint, which is only **slightly movable,** or **amphiarthrodial.**

2. Sutures

Sutures are found between bones in the skull. These bones make contact with one another along interlocking or serrated edges and are held together by layers of fibrous tissue, or ligaments. Therefore movement is very limited at these articulations, and in adults, they are considered **immovable,** or **synarthrodial joints.**

*Clemente CD: Gray's anatomy, ed 13, Philadelphia, 1985, Lea & Febiger (p 332).

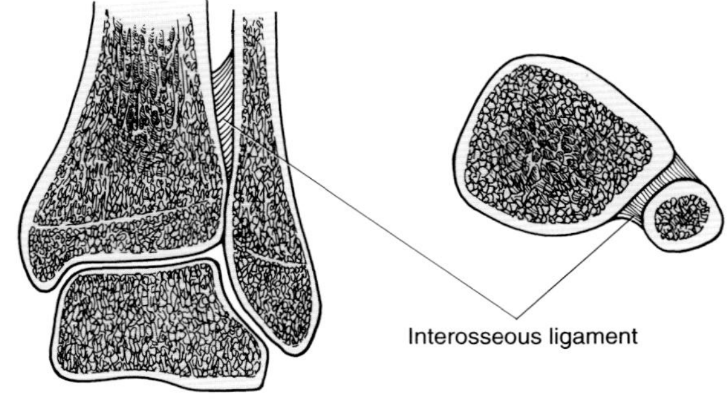

Distal tibiofibular joint–Only true syndesmosis joint*
1. **Syndesmosis**–Amphiarthrodial (slightly movable)

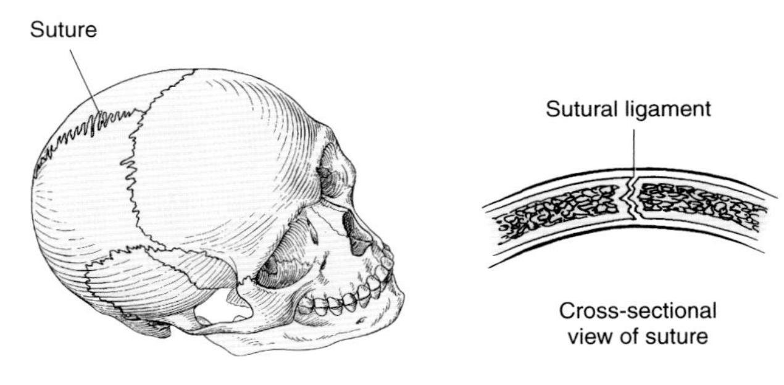

Skull suture.
2. **Suture**–Synarthrodial (immovable)

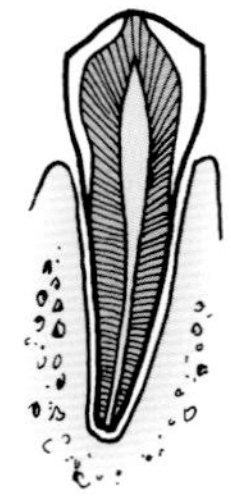

Roots of teeth

3. **Gomphosis**–Amphiarthrodial (only limited movement)

Fig. 1-23. Fibrous joints—three types.

Some limited expansion-compression type movement at these sutures can occur in the infant skull, such as during the birthing process, but at adulthood active bone deposition partially or completely obliterates these suture lines.

3. Gomphoses

A **gomphosis** joint is a third unique type of fibrous joint, in which a conical process is inserted into a socketlike portion of bone. This joint or fibrous union, which strictly speaking does not occur between bones but between the roots of the teeth and the alveoli of the mandible and maxillae, is a specialized type of articulation allowing only very limited movement.

Cartilaginous Joints

Cartilaginous joints also lack a joint cavity, and the articulating bones are **held tightly together by cartilage.** Like fibrous joints, they allow little or no movement. Therefore these joints are either synarthrodial or amphiarthrodial and are held together by two types of cartilage, symphyses and synchondroses.

1. Symphyses

The essential feature of a symphysis is **the presence of a broad, flattened disk of fibrocartilage** between two contiguous bony surfaces. These fibrocartilage disks form relatively thick pads that are capable of being compressed or displaced, thereby allowing some movement of these bones, which makes these joints **amphiarthrodial** (slightly movable).

Examples of such symphyses are the intervertebral disks (between bodies of the vertebrae) and the symphysis pubis (between the two pubic bones of the pelvis).

2. Synchondroses

A typical synchondrosis is a **temporary form of joint** wherein the connecting **hyaline cartilage** (which on long bones is called an *epiphyseal plate*) is converted into bone at adulthood. These temporary types of growth joints are considered **synarthrodial** or immovable.

Examples of such joints are the epiphyseal plates between the epiphyses and the diaphyses (bodies) of long bones and at the three-part union of the pelvis, which forms a cup-shaped acetabulum for the hip joint.

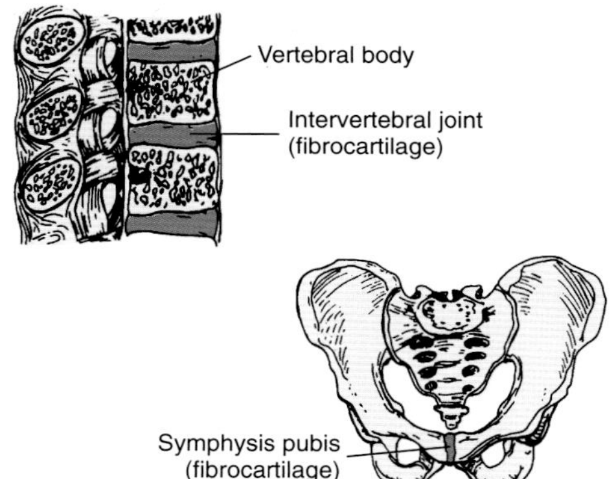

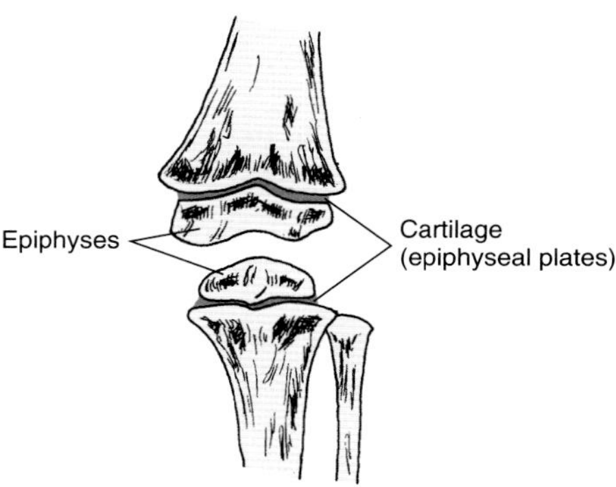

1. Symphyses—Amphiarthrodial (slightly movable)

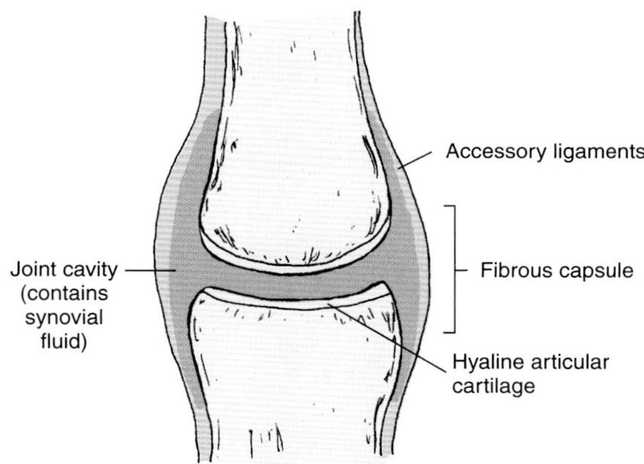

2. Synchondroses—Synarthrodial (immovable)

Fig. 1-24. Cartilaginous joints—two types.

Synovial Joints

Synovial joints are those freely movable joints, mostly of the upper and lower limbs, characterized by a **fibrous capsule containing synovial fluid.** The ends of the bones making up a synovial joint may make contact but are completely separate and contain a joint space or cavity, which allows for the wide range of movement at these joints. Synovial joints are generally **diarthrodial,** or freely movable. (Exceptions to this are the sacroiliac joints of the pelvis, which are amphiarthrodial or slightly movable.)

The exposed ends of these bones contain thin protective coverings of **hyaline articular cartilage.** The **joint cavity,** which contains a viscous lubricating **synovial fluid,** is enclosed and surrounded by a **fibrous capsule** reinforced by strengthening **accessory ligaments.** These ligaments limit motion in undesirable directions. The inner surface of this fibrous capsule is thought to secrete the lubricating synovial fluid.

Fig. 1-25. Synovial joints—diarthrodial (freely movable).

Movement Types of Synovial Joints

Synovial joints occur in considerable number and variety, and they are grouped according to the **six types of movements** they permit. These are listed in order from the least to the greatest permitted movement.

Note: The preferred name is listed first, followed by older term or synonym in parentheses. (This practice is followed throughout this textbook.)

1. Plane (gliding) joints

This type of synovial joint permits the least movement, which as the name implies, is **a sliding or gliding motion between the articulating surfaces.**

Examples of such joints are the **intermetacarpal, carpometacarpal,** and **intercarpal** joints of the hand and wrist. The right and left lateral **atlantoaxial joints** between C1 and C2 vertebrae are also classified as plane, or gliding, joints. which permits some rotational movement between these vertebrae as described in Chapter 9 on the cervical spine.

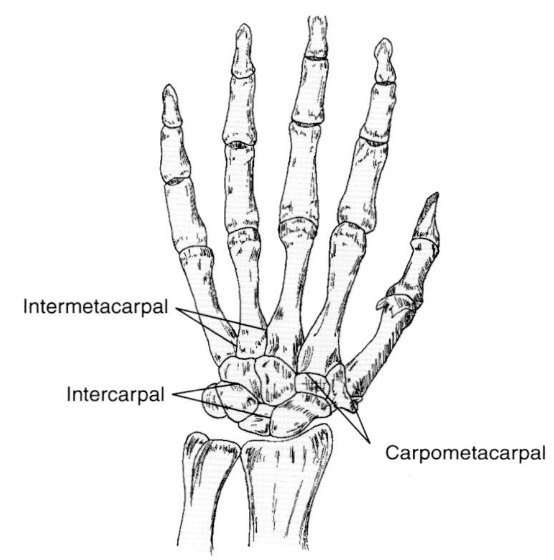

Fig. 1-26. Plane (gliding) joints.

2. Ginglymus (hinge) joints

The articular surfaces of a ginglymus *(jin'gli-mus),* or hinge, joint are molded to each other in such a way to permit **flexion and extension movements** only. The articular fibrous capsule on this type of joint is thin on those surfaces where bending takes place, but strong collateral ligaments firmly secure the bones at the lateral margins of the fibrous capsule.

Examples of such joints are the **interphalangeal joints** of both fingers and toes, the **knee joint,** the **elbow joint,** and the **ankle joint.**

3. Trochoid (pivot) joints

The trochoid *(tro'koid)* joint is formed by a bony, pivotlike process that is surrounded by a ring of ligaments and/or bony structure. This allows **rotational movements** around a single axis.

Examples of such joints are the **proximal** and **distal radioulnar joints** of the forearm, which demonstrate this pivot movement during rotation of the hand and wrist.

Another example is the joint **between the first and second cervical vertebrae.** The dens of the axis (C2) forms the pivot, and the anterior arch of the atlas (C1), combined with posterior ligaments, forms the ring.

4. Ellipsoid (condyloid) joints

In the ellipsoid *(e-lip' soid),* or condyloid, joint movement occurs primarily in one plane, combined with a slight degree of rotation at an axis at right angles to the primary plane of movement. The rotational movement is somewhat limited by associated ligaments and tendons.

This type of joint therefore allows primarily four directional movements: **flexion and extension** and **abduction and adduction. Circumduction** movement also occurs, which results from conelike sequential movements of flexion, abduction, extension, and adduction.

Examples of ellipsoid joints are the **second through fifth metacarpophalangeal joints of fingers,** the **wrist joint,** and the **metatarsophalangeal joints of the toes.**

5. Sellar (saddle) joints

The term *sellar (sel'ar),* or saddle, describes this joint structure well in that the ends of the bones are shaped concave-convex and positioned opposite to each other (Fig. 1-30). (Two saddlelike structures fit into each other.)

Movements of this biaxial-type sellar joint are the same as for ellipsoidal joints, namely **flexion, extension, adduction, abduction,** and **circumduction.**

The best example of a true sellar joint is the **first carpometacarpal joint** of the thumb.

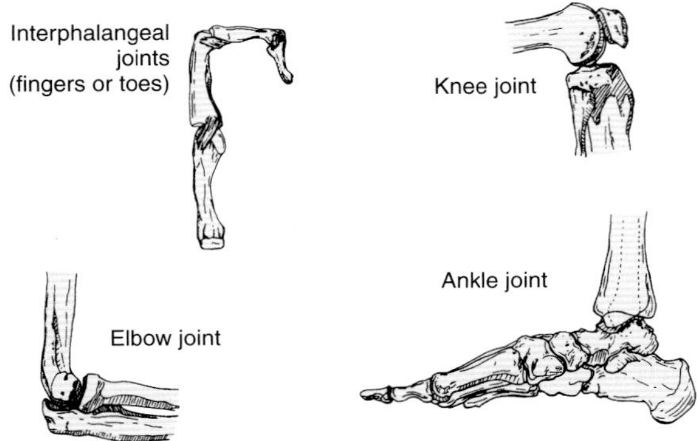

Fig. 1-27. Ginglymus (hinge) joints.

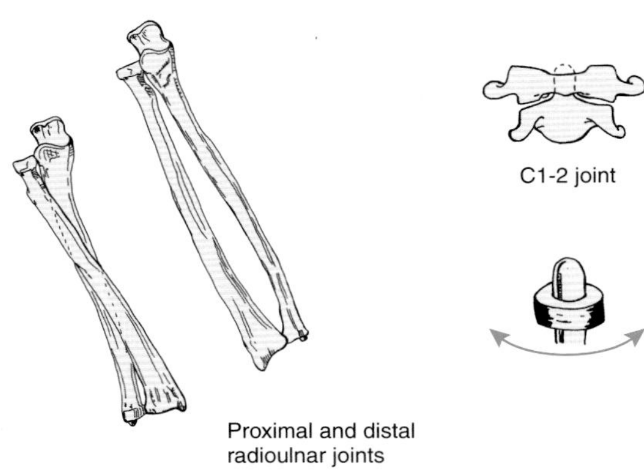

Fig. 1-28. Trochoid (pivot) joints.

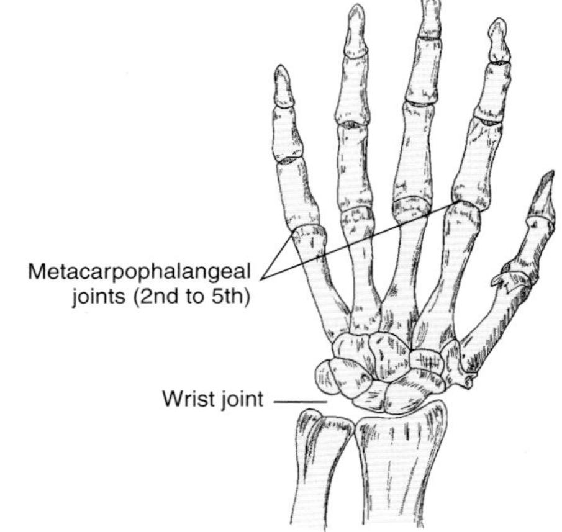

Fig. 1-29. Ellipsoid (condyloid) joints.

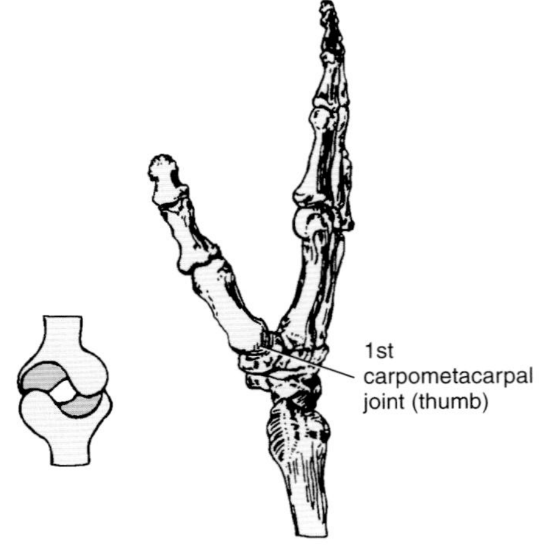

Fig. 1-30. Sellar (saddle) joints.

6. Spheroid (ball and socket) joints

The spheroid *(sfe'roid)*, or ball and socket, joint allows the greatest freedom of motion. The distal bone making up the joint is capable of motion around an almost indefinite number of axes, with one common center.

The greater the depth of the socket, the more limited the movement. The deeper joint, however, is stronger and more stable. For example, the hip joint is a much stronger and more stable joint than the shoulder joint, but the range of movement is more limited in the hip.

Movements of spheroid joints are **flexion, extension, abduction, adduction, circumduction,** and **medial** and **lateral rotation.**

The two examples of ball and socket joints are the **hip joint** and the **shoulder joint.**

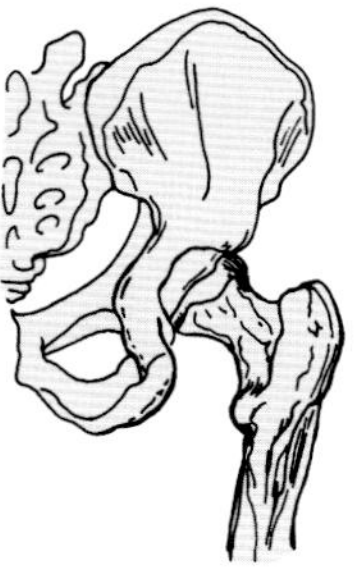

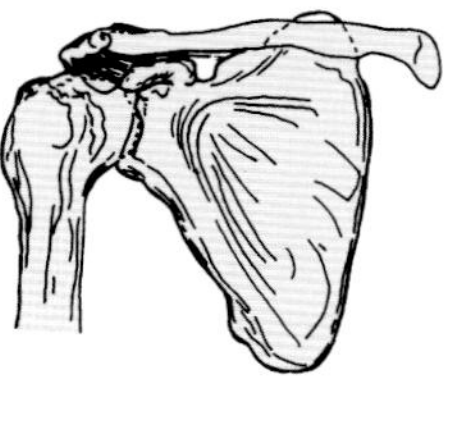

Fig. 1-31. Spheroid (ball and socket) joints.

SUMMARY OF JOINT CLASSIFICATION

JOINT CLASSIFICATION	MOBILITY CLASSIFICATION	MOVEMENT TYPES	MOVEMENT DESCRIPTION	EXAMPLES
Fibrous Joints				
Syndesmoses	Amphiarthrodial (slightly movable)	—	—	Distal tibiofibular joint
Sutures	Synarthrodial (immovable)	—	—	Skull sutures
Gomphoses	Very limited movement	—	—	Areas around roots of teeth
Cartilaginous Joints				
Symphyses	Amphiarthrodial (slightly movable)	—	—	Intervertebral disks Symphysis pubis
Synchondroses	Synarthrodial (immovable)	—	—	Ephiphyseal plates of long bones and between the three parts of the pelvis
Synovial Joints	Diarthrodial (freely movable), with exceptions of the sacroiliac joints (synovial joints with only very limited motion [amphiarthrodial])	Plane (gliding)	Sliding or gliding	Intermetacarpal, intercarpal, and carpometacarpal joints, C1 on C2 vertebrae
		Ginglymus (hinge)	Flexion and extension	Interphalangeal joints of fingers and toes and knee, ankle, and elbow joints
		Trochoid (pivot)	Rotational	Proximal and distal radioulnar and between C1 and C2 vertebrae
		Ellipsoid (condyloid)	Flexion and extension Abduction and adduction Circumduction	2nd to 5th metacarpophalangeal and wrist joints
		Sellar (saddle)	Flexion and extension Abduction and adduction Circumduction	First carpometacarpal joint (thumb)
		Spheroid (ball and socket)	Flexion and extension Abduction and adduction Circumduction Medial and lateral rotation	Hip and shoulder joints

Note: Arthrology, or the study of joints, continues throughout this text as specific anatomy, including all joints of the human body, is studied in more detail in following chapters.

POSITIONING TERMINOLOGY

Radiographic positioning refers to the study of patient positioning to **radiographically demonstrate or visualize specific body parts on image receptors (IRs).** Each person planning to work as a radiologic technologist must clearly understand the correct use of positioning terminology. This section lists, describes, and illustrates those commonly used terms consistent with the positioning and projection terminology as approved and published by *The American Registry of Radiologic Technologists* (ARRT).*

These terms are also generally consistent with those used in Canada, according to the Canadian Association of Medical Radiation Technologists *(CAMRT),* with the exception of the term "view." (See summary of potentially misused terms at the end of this section.)

Throughout this text the use of named positions (proper names of the person first describing a specific position or procedure) are referred to as a **method,** such as the Towne, Waters, and Caldwell methods. Both the ARRT and the CAMRT concur with the use of the name method in parentheses after the projection or position term.

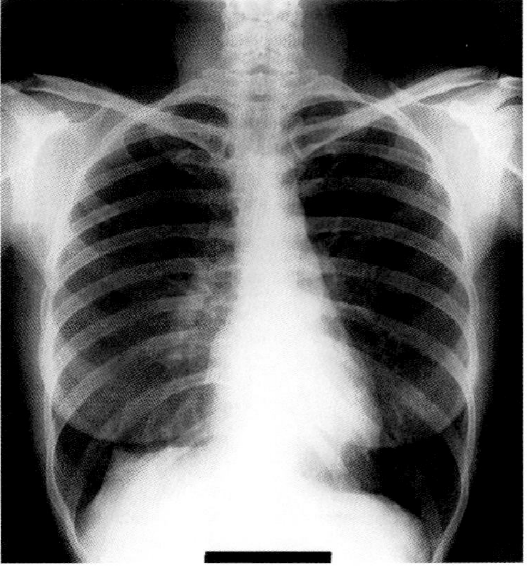

Fig. 1-32. Chest radiograph.

General Terms

Radiograph *(ra'de-o-graf):* A radiograph is a film or other base material containing a processed image of an anatomic part of a patient as produced by action of x-rays on an IR.

Radiography *(ra"de-og'rah-fe):* The production of radiographs or other forms of radiographic images.

Radiograph vs. x-ray film: In practice, the terms **radiograph** and **x-ray film** (or just film) are often used interchangeably. However, the x-ray film specifically refers to the physical piece of material on which a radiographic image is exposed. The term *radiograph* includes the film **and** the image.

Radiographic images: Radiographic images are a representation of the patient's anatomic structures. They can be obtained, viewed as hardcopy **(radiographs)** using film-screen techniques with chemical processing, or they can be obtained as digital images that can be manipulated, viewed, transported, and stored digitally.

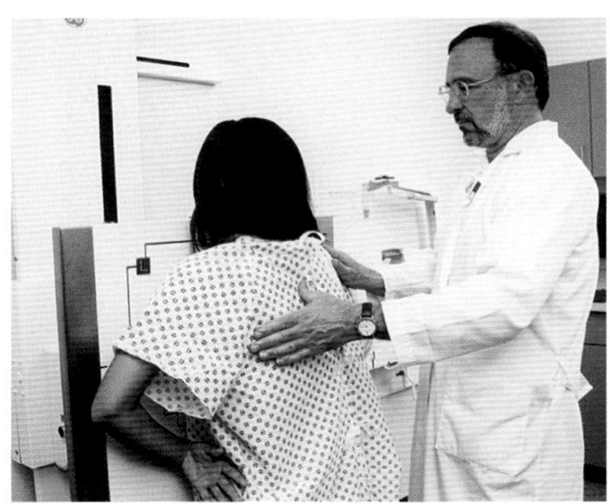

Fig. 1-33. Radiographic examination.

Radiographic examination or procedure

A radiologic technologist is shown positioning the patient for a routine chest examination or procedure (Fig. 1-33). A radiographic examination includes five general functions:

1. Positioning of the body part and central ray (CR) alignment
2. Selection of radiation protection measures
3. Selection of exposure factors (radiographic technique) on the control panel (generator)
4. Patient instructions relating to respiration (breathing) and initiation (or "making") of the exposure
5. Processing of the IR

Anatomic (an"ah-tom'ik) position

The anatomic position is an **upright position, arms adducted** (down), **palms forward, head and feet directed straight ahead.** This specific body position is used as a reference for other positioning terms (Fig. 1-34).

Note: When referring to one part of the body in relationship to other parts, the radiographer must always think of the person as **standing erect in the anatomic position,** even when describing parts of a patient who is lying down; otherwise, confusion as to the meaning of the description may result.

Viewing radiographs: A general rule in viewing radiographs is to display them so that **the patient is facing the viewer,** with the patient in the **anatomic position.** This is described in more detail later in this chapter.

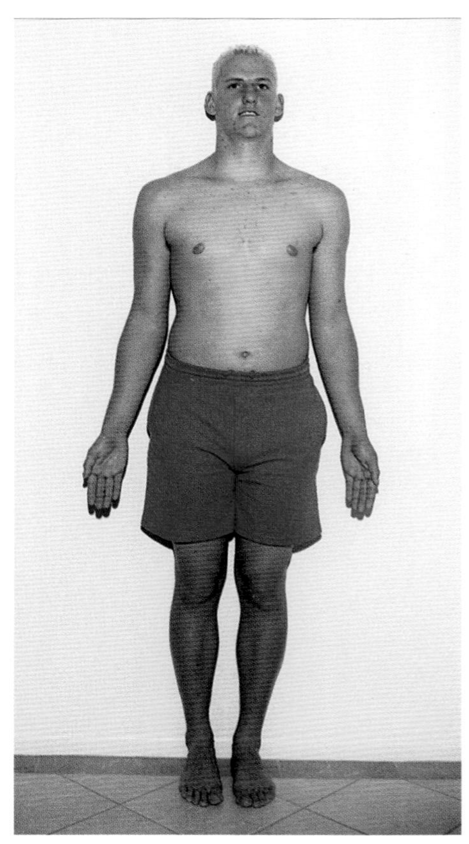

Fig. 1-34. Anatomic position.

*ARRT educator's handbook, ed 3, St. Paul, 1990, The American Registry of Radiologic Technologists, and personal communication and correspondence with ARRT, November 1999.

Body Planes, Sections, and Lines

Positioning terms describing CR angles or relationships between body parts are often related to **imaginary planes** passing through the body in the **anatomic position.** The study of CT (computed tomography) and MRI (magnetic resonance imaging) emphasizes sectional anatomy, which also involves the primary body planes and sections as described below.

PLANE: STRAIGHT LINE SURFACE CONNECTING TWO POINTS

Four common planes as used in radiography are as follows:

Sagittal (saj'i-tal) plane

A sagittal plane is any **longitudinal** plane dividing the body into **right and left parts.**

The **mid sagittal plane,** sometimes called the **median plane,** is a midline sagittal plane dividing the body into **equal right and left parts.** It passes approximately through the sagittal suture of the skull. Any plane parallel to the midsagittal or median plane is called a **sagittal plane.**

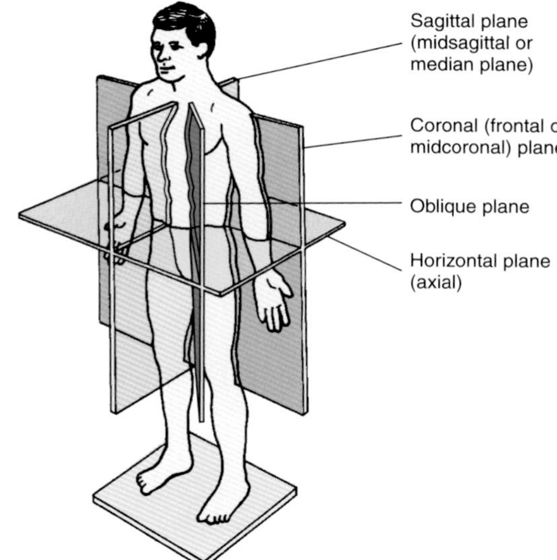

Fig. 1-35. Sagittal, coronal, oblique, and horizontal body planes.

Coronal (ko-ro'nal) plane

A coronal plane is any **longitudinal** plane dividing the body into **anterior and posterior parts.**

The **mid coronal plane** divides the body into approximately **equal anterior and posterior parts.** It is called a coronal plane because it passes approximately through the coronal suture of the skull. Any plane parallel to the midcoronal or frontal plane is called a **coronal plane.**

Horizontal (axial) plane

A horizontal (axial) plane is any **transverse** plane passing though the body at **right angles to the longitudinal plane,** dividing the body into superior and inferior portions.

Oblique plane

An oblique plane is a **longitudinal** or **transverse** plane that is at an angle or slant and **not parallel** to the sagittal, coronal, or horizontal planes.

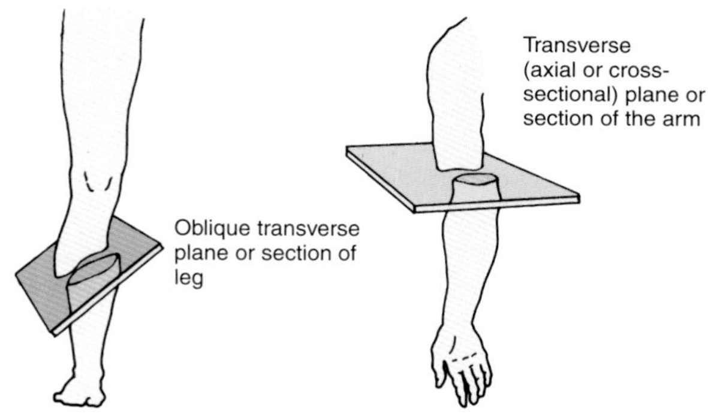

Fig. 1-36. Transverse and oblique sections of body parts.

SECTION: "CUT" OR "SLICE" IMAGE OF BODY PART

Longitudinal sections—sagittal, coronal, and oblique

These sections or images run **lengthwise** in the direction of the long axis of the body or any of its parts, regardless of the position of the body (erect or recumbent).

Longitudinal sections or images may be taken in the **sagittal, coronal,** or **oblique planes.**

Transverse or axial sections (cross-sections)

Sectional images are at **right angles along any point of the longitudinal axis** of the body or its parts.

Sagittal, coronal, and axial images: CT and MRI images are obtained in these three common orientations or views. (MRI sectional images are shown in Figs. 1-37 through 1-39.)

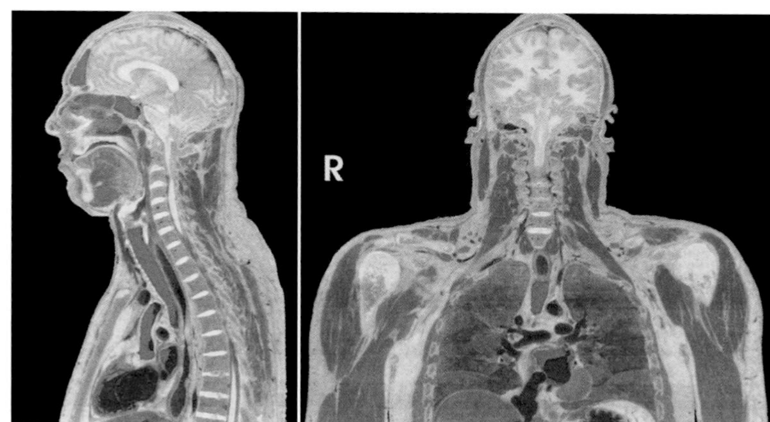

Fig. 1-37. Sagittal image. **Fig. 1-38.** Coronal image.

Longitudinal MRI images.

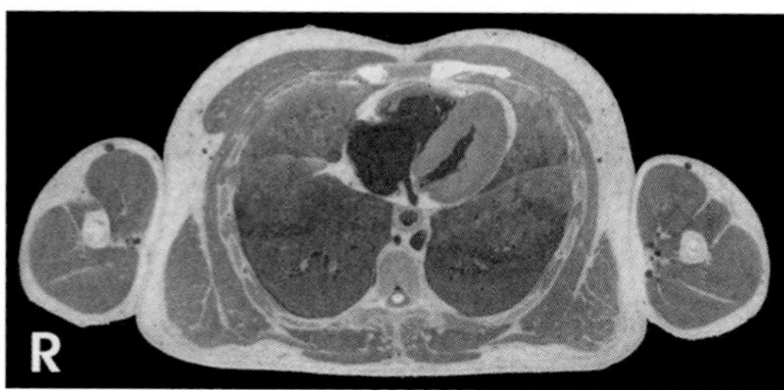

Fig. 1-39. Axial (cross-sectional) MRI image—midthorax.

1

PLANES OF THE SKULL

Base plane of skull

This precise transverse plane is formed by connecting the lines from the infraorbital margins (inferior edge of bony orbits) to the superior margins of the external auditory meatus (EAM), the external opening of the ear. This is also sometimes called the **anthropologic plane** or the **Frankfort horizontal plane** as used in orthodontics and cranial topography to measure and locate specific cranial points or structures.

Occlusal plane

This horizontal plane is formed by the biting surfaces of the upper and lower teeth with jaws closed (used as a reference plane of the head for dental and skull radiography).

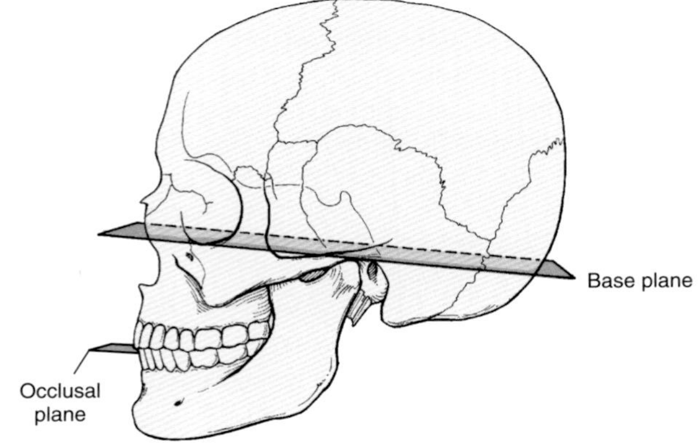

Fig. 1-40. Planes of skull.

Body Surfaces and Parts

TERMS FOR THE BACK AND FRONT PORTIONS OF THE BODY

Posterior *(pos-te're-or)* ***or dorsal*** *(dor'sal)*

Refers to the **back half** of the patient, or that part of the body seen when viewing the person from the back; includes the bottom of feet and the back of hands as seen in the anatomic position.

Anterior *(an-te're-or)* ***or ventral*** *(ven'tral)*

Refers to **front half** of patient, or that part seen when viewed from the front; includes the tops of feet and the fronts or palms of hands in the anatomic position.

TERMS FOR SURFACES OF THE HANDS AND FEET

Three terms used in radiography to describe specific surfaces of the upper and lower limbs are as follows:

Plantar *(plan'tar)*

Refers to the **sole** or **posterior** surface of the foot.

Dorsal *(dor'sal)*

Foot: Refers to the **top** or **anterio**r surface of the foot (dorsum pedis).

Hand: Refers to the **back** or **posterior** aspect of the hand (dorsum manus).

Note: The term **dorsum** (or **dorsal**) in general refers to the vertebral or posterior part of the body. However, when used in relationship with the foot, dorsum (dorsum pedis) specifically refers to the **upper surface,** or **anterior aspect,** of the foot opposite the sole, whereas for the hand (dorsum manus), it refers to the back or posterior surface opposite the palm.*†

Palmar *(pal'mar)*

Refers to the **palm of the hand;** in the anatomic position, the same as the **anterior or ventral** surface of the hand.

*Dorland's illustrated medical dictionary, ed 28, Philadelphia, 1994, WB Saunders.
†Mosby's medical, nursing & allied health dictionary, ed 5, St. Louis, 1998, Mosby.

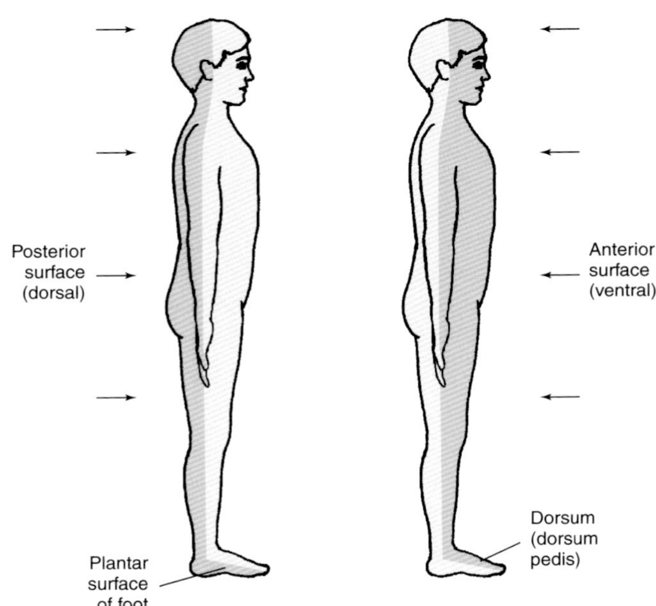

Fig. 1-41. Posterior vs. anterior.

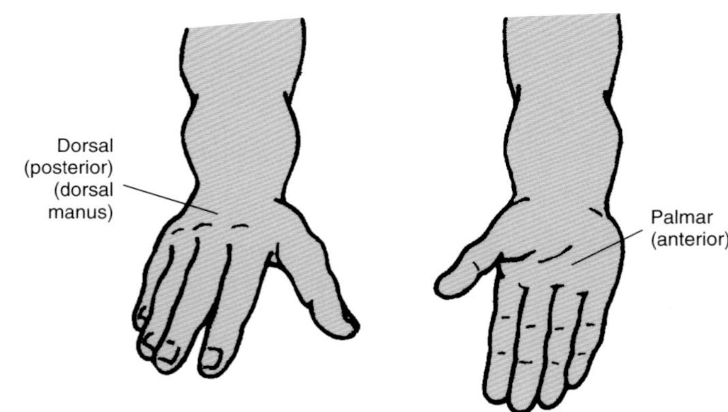

Fig. 1-42. Dorsal and palmar surfaces of hand.

Radiographic Projections

Projection is a positioning term that describes the **direction or path of the CR of the x-ray beam** as it passes through the patient, projecting an image onto the IR.

COMMON PROJECTION TERMS

Posteroanterior *(pos"ter-o-an-te're-or)* ***(PA) projection***

A projection of the CR from **posterior to anterior.**

Combines these two terms, posterior and anterior, into one word, abbreviated as PA. The CR enters at the posterior surface and exits at the anterior surface (PA projection).

Assumes a **true PA** without intentional rotation, which requires the CR to be perpendicular to the coronal body plane and parallel to the sagittal plane, unless some qualifying oblique or rotational term is used to indicate otherwise.

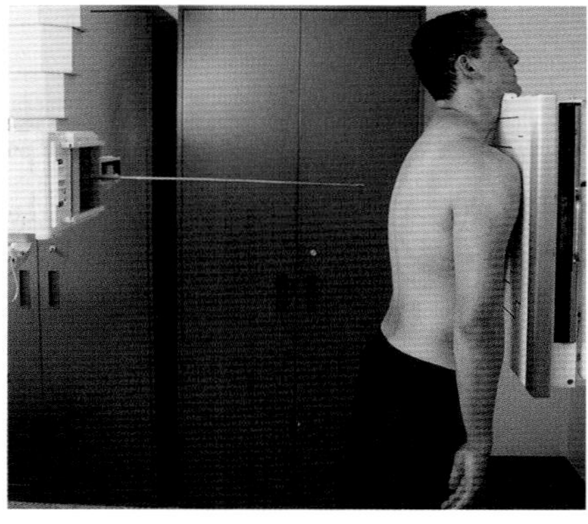

Fig. 1-43. PA projection.

Anteroposterior *(an"ter-o-pos-te're-or)* ***(AP) projection***

A projection of CR from **anterior to posterior,** the opposite of PA.

Combines these two terms, anterior and posterior, into one word.

Describes the direction of travel of the CR, which enters at an anterior surface and exits at a posterior surface (AP projection).

Assumes a **true AP** without rotation unless a qualifier term is also used, indicating it to be an oblique projection.

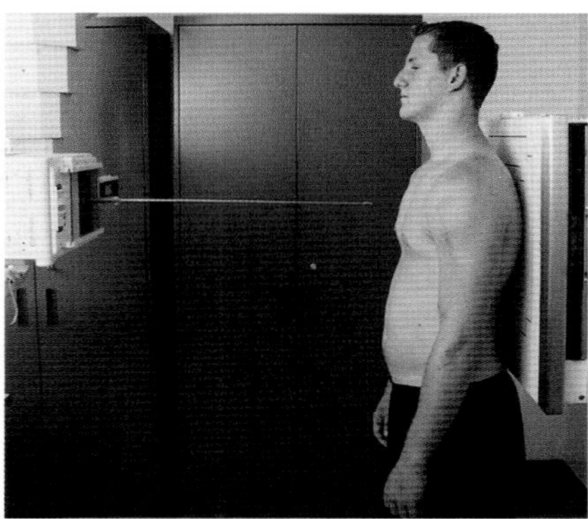

Fig. 1-44. AP projection.

AP oblique projection

An AP projection of the upper or lower limb that is obliqued or rotated. Thus it is not a true AP and **must also include a qualifying term** indicating which way it is rotated, such as medial or lateral rotation (Fig. 1-45). (For obliques of the whole body, see oblique ***position*** descriptions later in this chapter.)

PA oblique projection

A PA projection of the upper limb with lateral rotation (from PA) is shown in Fig. 1-46. (This is applicable to both upper and lower limbs.) Must also include a qualifying term indicating which way it is rotated.

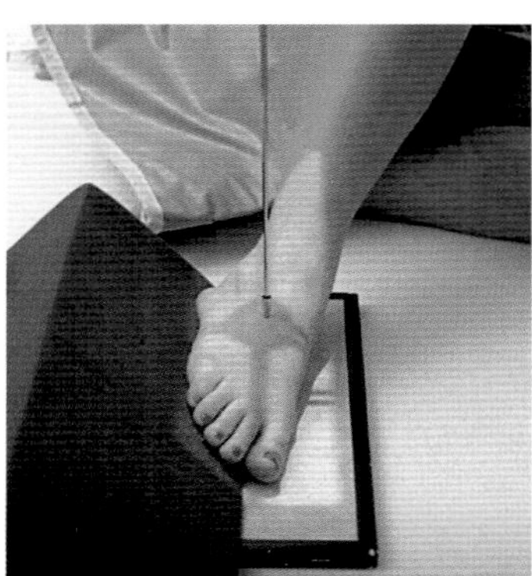

Fig. 1-45. AP oblique projection—medial rotation (from AP).

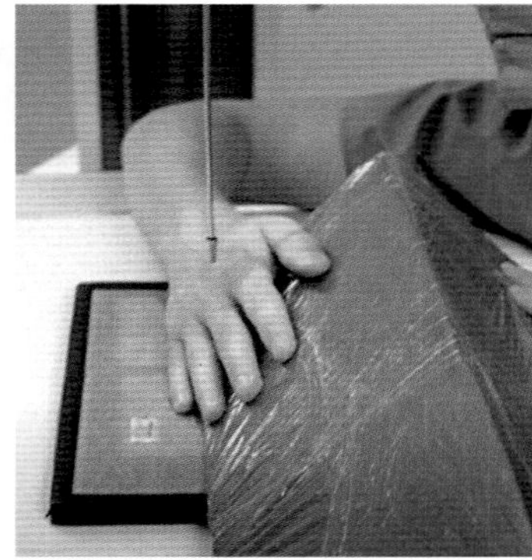

Fig. 1-46. PA oblique projection—lateral rotation (from PA).

Mediolateral and lateromedial projections

A **lateral** projection described by the **path of the CR.** Two examples are the **mediolateral** projection of the ankle (Fig. 1-47) and the **lateromedial** projection of the wrist (Fig. 1-48). Determining the medial and lateral sides is again based on the patient in the anatomic position.

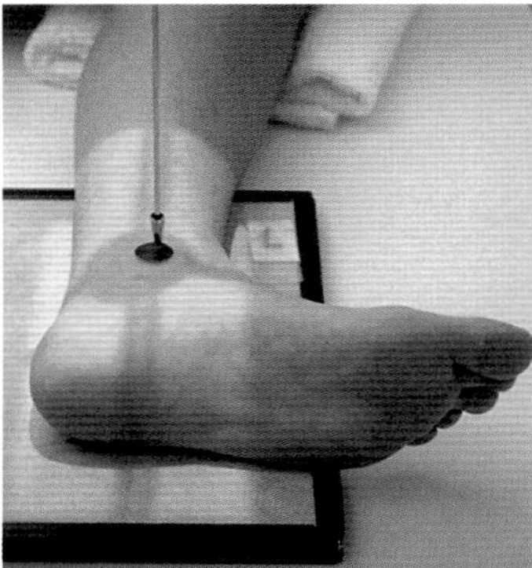

Fig. 1-47. Mediolateral projection (ankle).

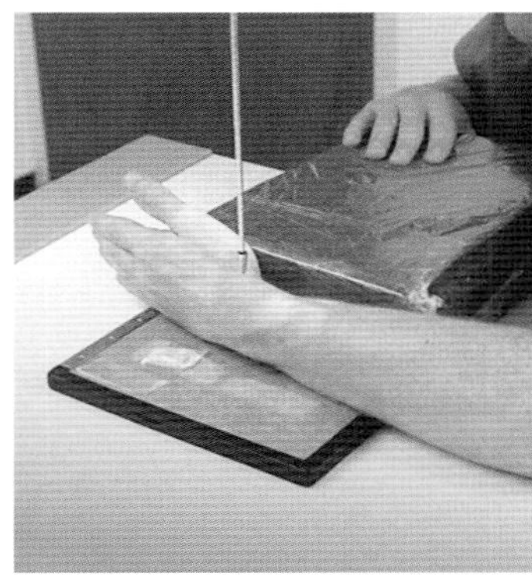

Fig. 1-48. Lateromedial projection (wrist).

1

Body Positions

In radiography, the term ***position*** is used in two ways, first as **general body positions** described below; and second as **specific body positions,** which are described in the pages that follow.

GENERAL BODY POSITIONS

The eight most commonly used general body positions in radiography are as follows:

1. ***Supine*** *(soo'pine)*
   Lying on back, facing upward.

2. ***Prone*** *(pro-n)*
   Lying on abdomen, facing downward (head may be turned to one side).

3. ***Erect*** *(e'reckt') (upright)*
   An **upright position,** to stand or sit erect.

4. ***Recumbent*** *(re-kum'bent) (reclining)*
   Lying down in any position (prone, supine, on side, and so on).
   - **Dorsal recumbent:** Lying on back (supine).
   - **Ventral recumbent:** Lying face down (prone).
   - **Lateral recumbent:** Lying on side (right or left lateral).

5. ***Trendelenburg**** *(tren-del'en-berg)*
   A recumbent position with the whole body tilted so that the **head is lower than the feet.**

6. ***Fowler's***† *(fow'lerz)* ***position***
   A recumbent position with the body tilted so that the **head is higher than the feet.**

7. ***Sim's position*** *(semiprone position)*
   A recumbent oblique position with the patient lying on the **left anterior side,** with the right knee and thigh flexed and with the left arm extended down behind the back. A modified Sim's position as used for insertion of the rectal tube for barium enema is shown in Fig. 1-53 (demonstrated in Chapter 15, Lower GI System).

8. ***Lithotomy*** *(li-thot'o-me)* ***position***
   A **recumbent** (supine) position with knees and hip flexed and thighs abducted and rotated externally, supported by ankle supports.

*Friedrich *Trendelenburg,* a surgeon in Leipzig, 1844-1924.
†George Ryerson *Fowler,* an American surgeon, 1848-1906.

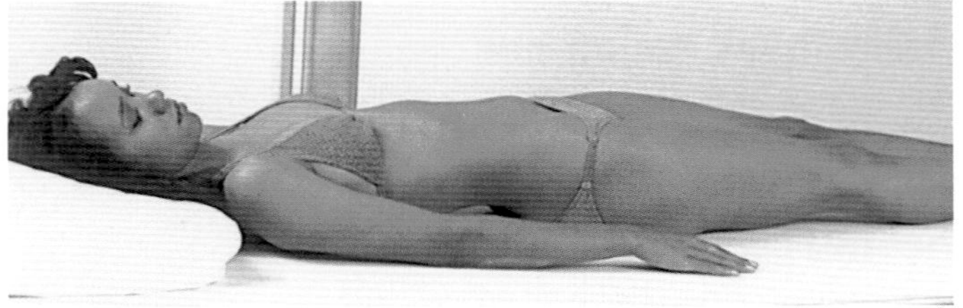

Fig. 1-49. Supine position.

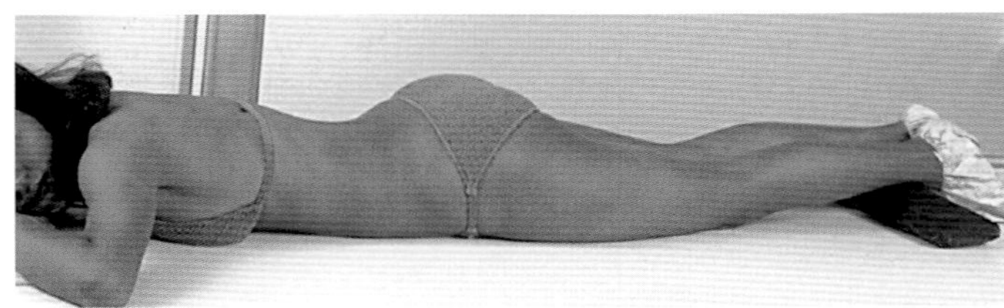

Fig. 1-50. Prone position.

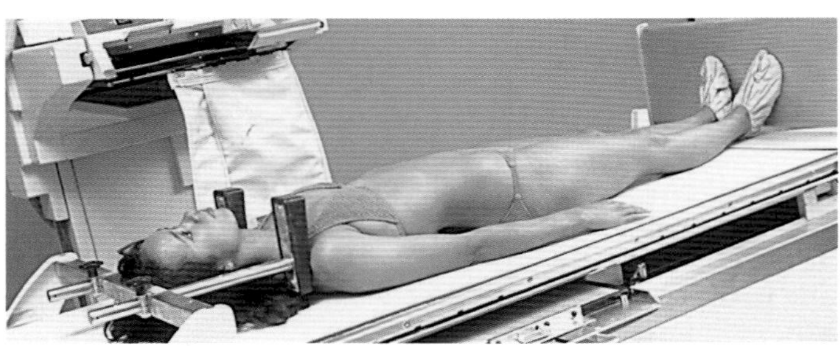

Fig. 1-51. Trendelenburg position—head lower than feet.

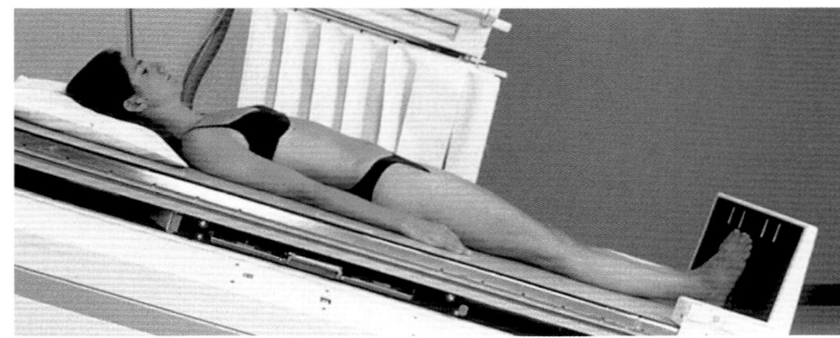

Fig. 1-52. Fowler's position—feet lower than head.

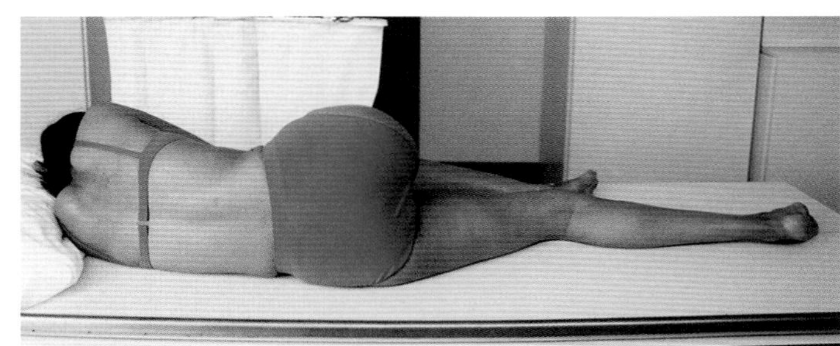

Fig. 1-53. Modified Sim's position.

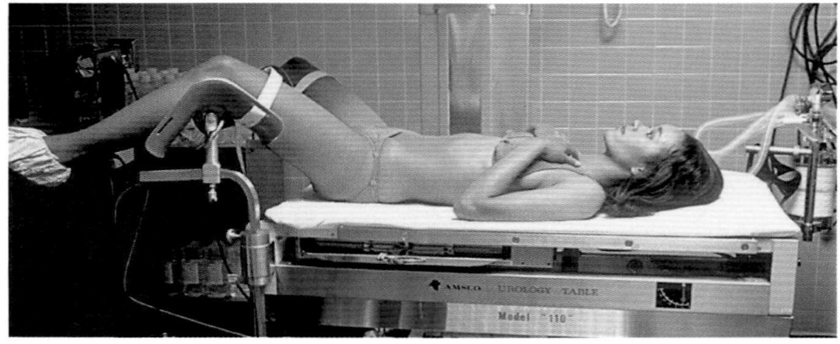

Fig. 1-54. Modified lithotomy position (for retrograde urography).

SPECIFIC BODY POSITIONS

In addition to a general body position, the second way the term ***position*** is used in radiography is to refer to a specific body position described by the body part closest to the IR (obliques and laterals) or by the surface on which the patient is lying (decubitus).

Lateral *(lat'er-al)* ***position***

Refers to the side of, or a side view.

Specific lateral positions described by the **part closest to the IR,** or **that body part from which the CR exits** (Figs. 1-55 and 1-56).

A true lateral position will always be 90°, or perpendicular, or at a right angle, to a true AP or PA projection. If it is not a true lateral, it is an oblique position.

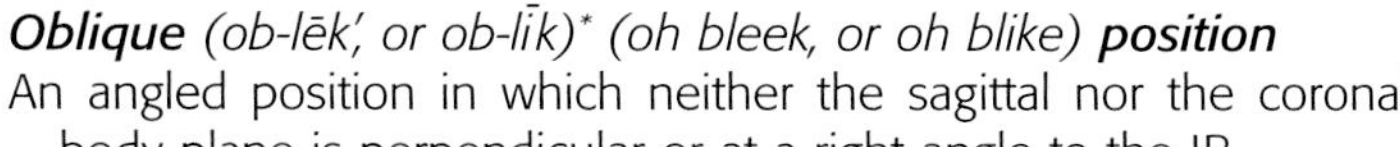

Oblique *(ob-lēk', or ob-līk)* (oh bleek, or oh blike)* ***position***

An angled position in which neither the sagittal nor the coronal body plane is perpendicular or at a right angle to the IR.

Oblique body positions of the thorax, abdomen, or pelvis are described by the **part closest to the IR,** or that **body part from which the CR exits.**

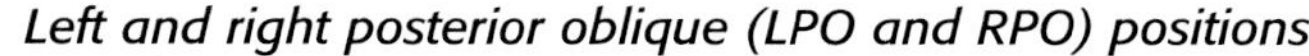

Left and right posterior oblique (LPO and RPO) positions

Describes that specific oblique position in which the **left or right posterior** aspect of the body is closest to the IR (Figs. 1-57 and 1-58).

Exit of the CR from the left or right posterior aspect of the body.

Note: These can also be referred to as **AP oblique projections** because the CR enters an anterior surface and exits posteriorly. This, however, **is not a complete description** and also requires a specific position clarifier such as **LPO or RPO position.** Therefore throughout this text these body obliques will be referred to as **positions** and not projections.

Obliques of upper and lower limbs, however, are correctly described as AP or PA obliques but use either **medial** or **lateral rotation** as a qualifier (see Figs. 1-45 and 1-46).

Right and left anterior oblique (RAO and LAO) positions

Refers to those oblique positions in which the **right or left anterior** aspect of the body is closest to the IR and can be erect or recumbent general body positions (Figs. 1-59 and 1-60).

Note: These can also be described as **PA oblique projections** if a position clarifier is added, such as an RAO or LAO **position.**

It is **not** correct to use these oblique terms or abbreviations LPO, RPO, RAO, or LAO as projections because they do not describe the direction or path of the CR; rather these are **positions.**

**Ob-lēk'* is the preferred pronunciation according to Dorland's Illustrated Medical Dictionary (ed 28), Webster's New World Dictionary (ed 3), and the American College Dictionary. *Ob-līk'* is the second pronunciation, as especially used in the military.

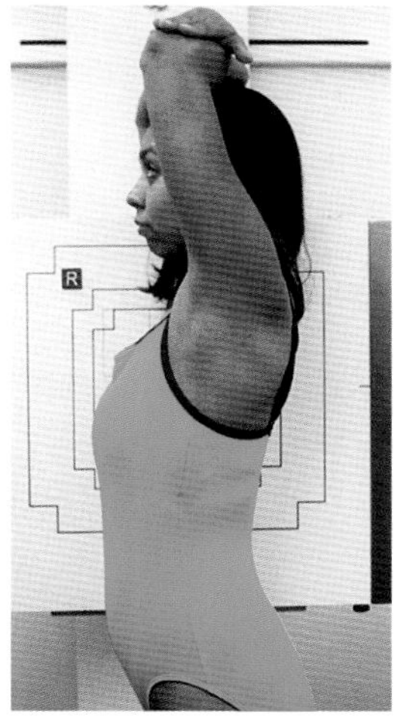

Fig. 1-55. Erect R lateral position.

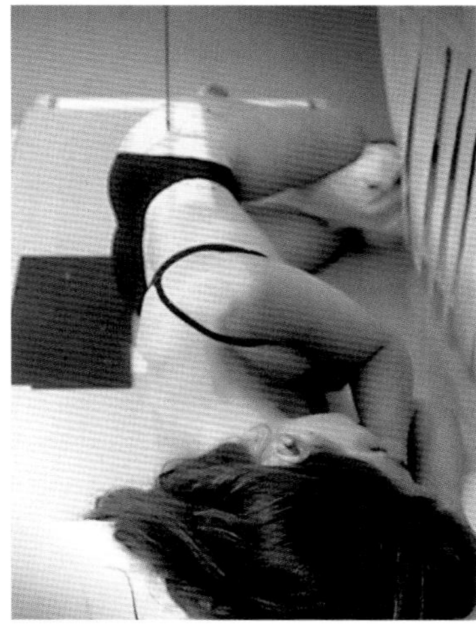

Fig. 1-56. Recumbent R lateral position.

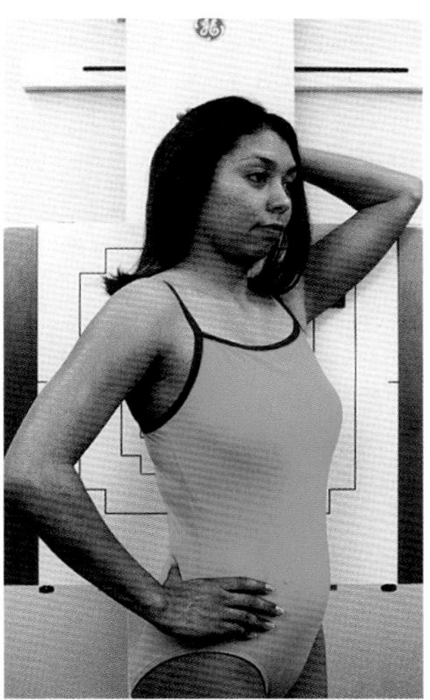

Fig. 1-57. Erect LPO position.

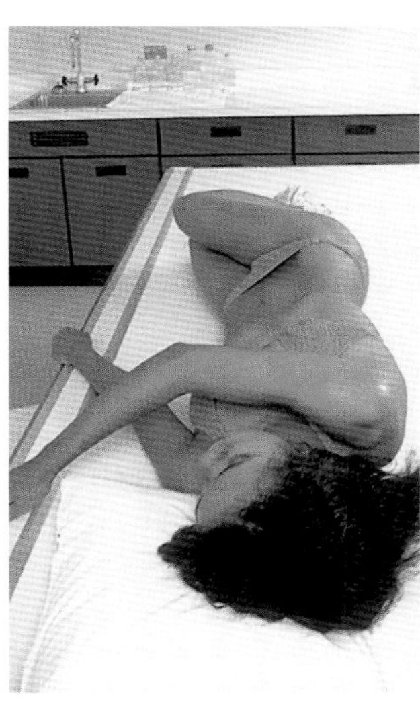

Fig. 1-58. Recumbent LPO position.

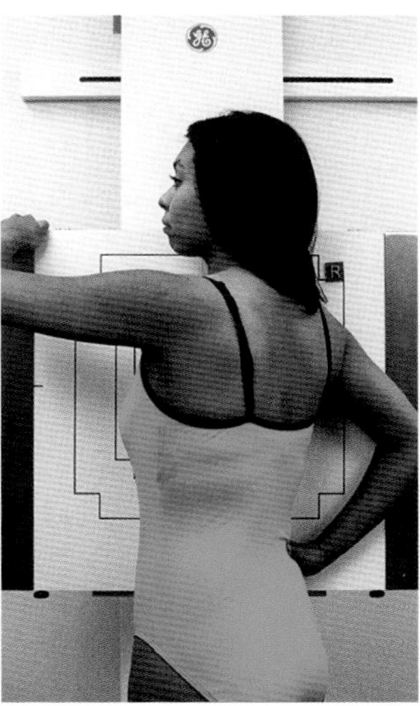

Fig. 1-59. Erect RAO position.

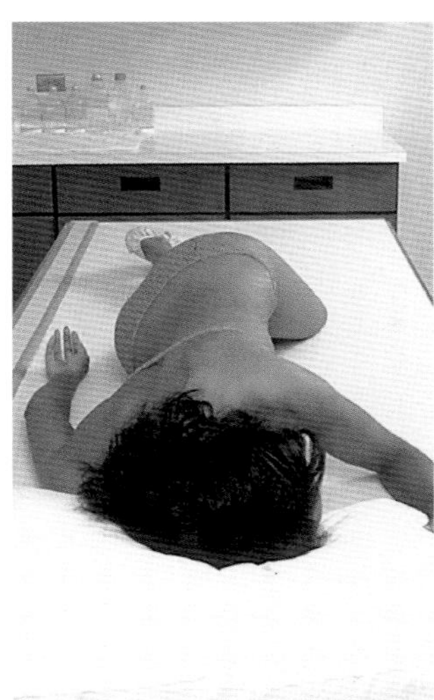

Fig. 1-60. Recumbent RAO position.

1

Decubitus (de-ku'bi-tus) (decub) position

The word decubitus literally means to "lie down," or the position assumed in "lying down."*

This body position, meaning to **lie on a horizontal surface,** is designated according to **that surface on which the body is resting.** This therefore refers to the patient lying on one of the following body surfaces: **back** (dorsal), **front** (ventral), or **side** (right or left lateral).

In radiographic positioning, decubitus is **always used with a horizontal x-ray beam.**

Decubitus positions are essential to detect air-fluid levels or free air in a body cavity such as in the chest or abdomen, where the air rises to the uppermost part of the body cavity.

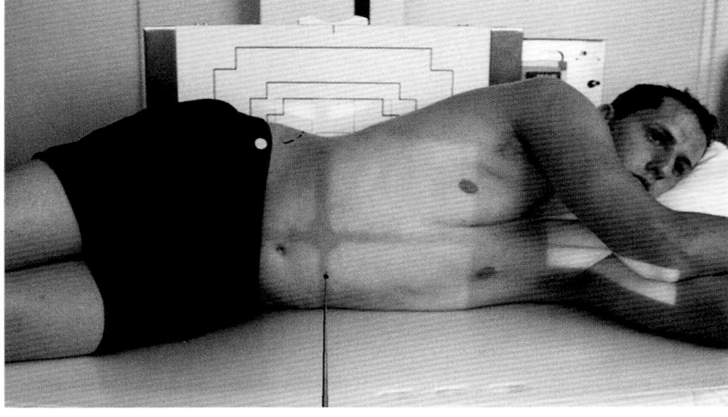

Fig. 1-61. Left lateral decubitus position (AP projection).

Right or left lateral decubitus position—AP or PA projection

In this position the patient **lies on the side** and the **x-ray beam is directed horizontally** from **anterior to posterior (AP)** (Fig. 1-61) or **posterior to anterior (PA)** (Fig. 1-62).

The AP or PA projection is important as a qualifying term with decubitus positions to denote the direction of the CR.

This position is either a **left lateral decub** (Fig. 1-61) or **right lateral decub** (Fig. 1-62). It is named according to the dependent side (side down) and the AP or PA projection indication.

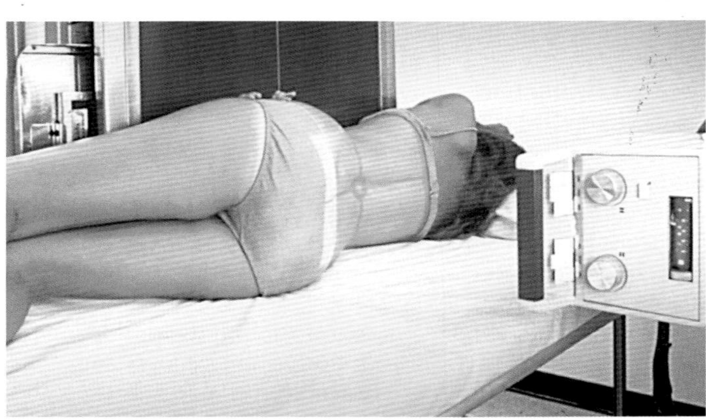

Fig. 1-62. Right lateral decubitus position (PA projection).

Dorsal decubitus position—left or right lateral

In this position the patient is **lying on the dorsal** (posterior) surface with **the x-ray beam directed horizontally,** exiting from the side closest to the IR (Fig. 1-63).

The position is named according to the surface on which the patient is lying (dorsal or ventral) and by the side closest to the IR (right or left).

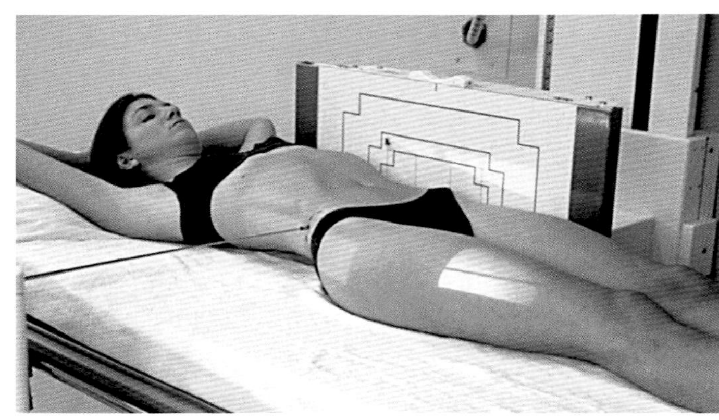

Fig. 1-63. Dorsal decubitus position (L lat.).

Ventral decubitus position—right or left lateral

In this position the patient is **lying on the ventral (anterior) surface** with the **x-ray beam directed horizontally,** exiting from the side closest to the IR (Fig. 1-64).

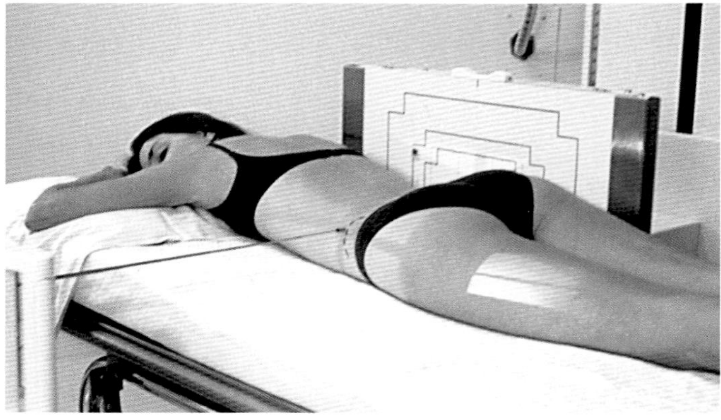

Fig. 1-64. Ventral decubitus position (R lat.).

*Dorland's illustrated medical dictionary, ed 28, Philadelphia, 1994, WB Saunders.

Additional Special Use Projection Terms

Following are some additional terms commonly used to describe **projections.** These terms, as shown by their definitions, also refer to the path or projection of the CR and are therefore projections rather than positions.

Axial (ak'se-al) projection

Axial refers to the **long axis** of a structure or part (around which a rotating body turns or is arranged).

Special application—AP or PA axial: In radiographic positioning, the term *axial* has been used to describe **any angle of the CR more than 10 degrees along the long axis of the body.*** It should be noted, however, that in a true sense an axial projection would be directed along, or parallel to, the long axis of the body or part. The term *semiaxial,* or "partly" axial, more accurately describes any angle along the axis that is not truly along or parallel to the long axis. However, for the sake of consistency with other references, the term *axial projection* will be used throughout this text to describe both axial and semiaxial projections as defined above and as illustrated in Figs. 1-65 through 1-67.

Inferosuperior and superoinferior axial projections

Inferosuperior projections are frequently performed for the shoulder and hip, where the CR enters below or inferiorly and exits above or superiorly (Fig. 1-67).

The opposite of this is the **superoinferior** projection, such as a special nasal bones projection (Fig. 1-65).

Tangential (tan"jen'shal) projection

Tangential means **touching a curve or surface at only one point.**

This is a special use of the term *projection* to describe a projection that merely skims a body part to project that part into profile and away from other body structures

Examples: Following are three examples or applications of the term *tangential projection* as defined above:

- Zygomatic arch projection (Fig. 1-68)
- Trauma skull projection for demonstrating depressed skull fracture (Fig. 1-69)
- Special projection of patella (Fig. 1-70)

AP axial projection—lordotic position

This is a **specific AP chest projection** for demonstrating the apices of the lungs. It is also sometimes called the **apical lordotic projection.** In this case the long axis of the body is angled rather than the CR.

The term **lordotic** comes from **lordosis,** a term denoting curvature of the cervical and lumbar spine (see Figs. 1-84 and 1-85). As the patient assumes this position (Fig. 1-71), the lumbar lordotic curvature is exaggerated, making this a descriptive term for this special chest projection.

*Ballinger PW, Frank ED: Merrill's atlas of radiographic positions and radiologic procedures, ed 10, vol 1, St. Louis, 2003, Mosby.

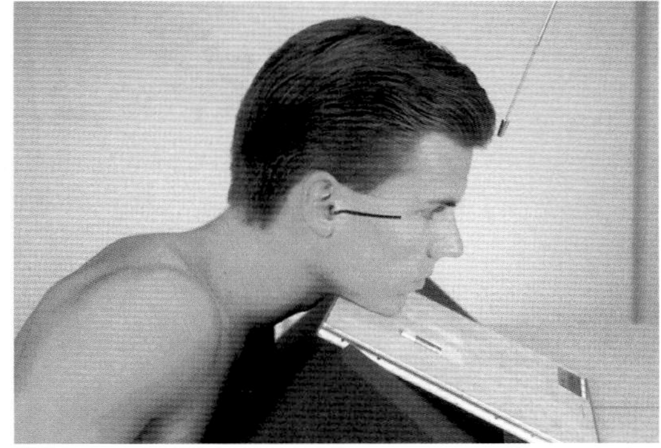

Fig. 1-65. Axial (superoinferior) projection.

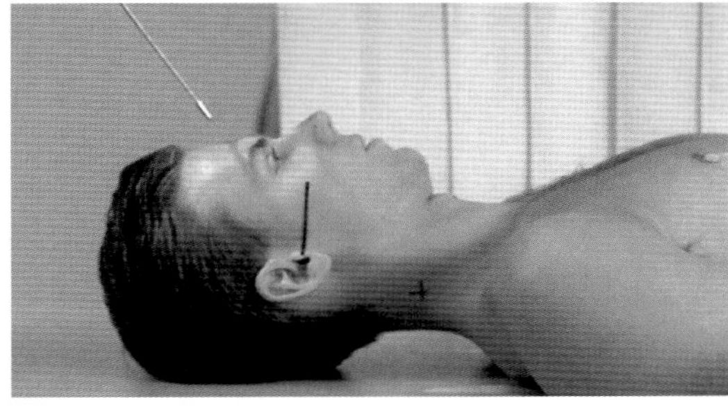

Fig. 1-66. AP axial (semiaxial) projection (CR 30 degrees caudal).

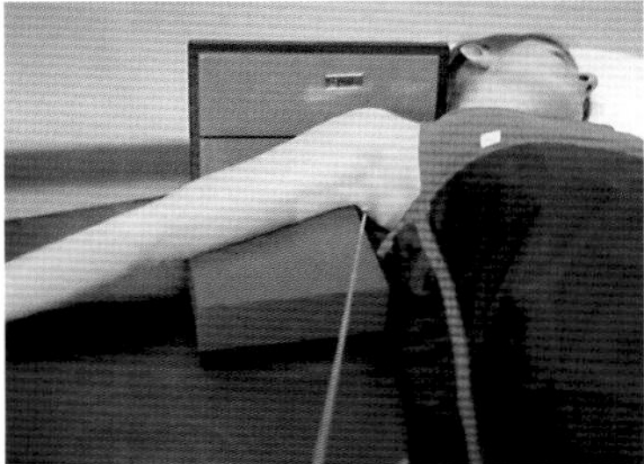

Fig. 1-67. Inferosuperior axial projection.

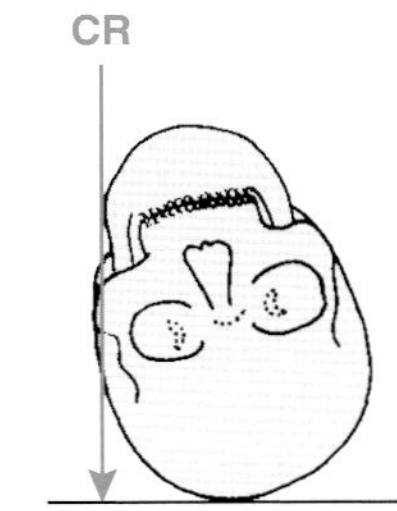

Fig. 1-68. Tangential projection (zygomatic arch).

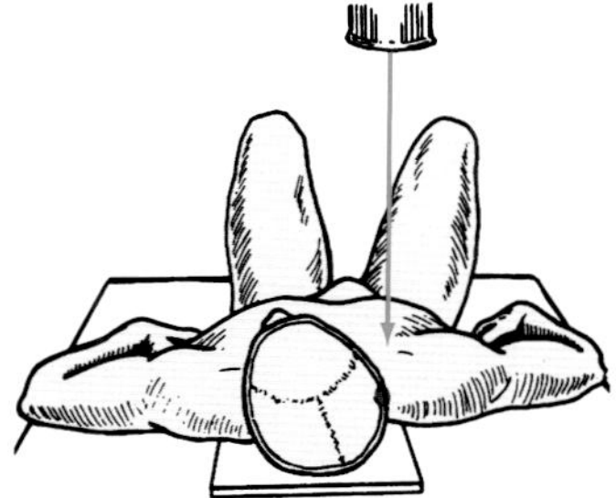

Fig. 1-69. Tangential projection (skull fracture).

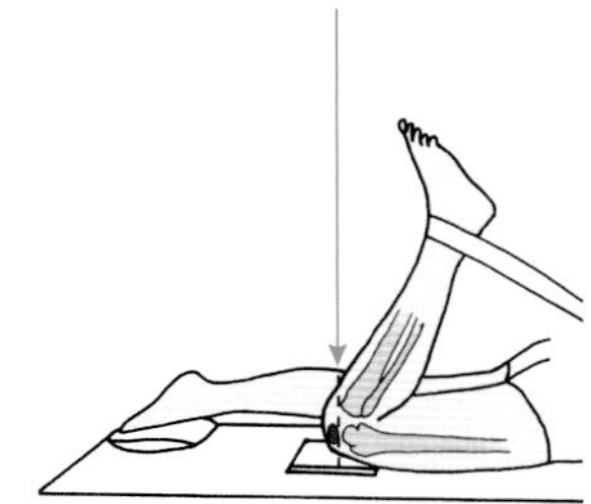

Fig. 1-70. Tangential projection (patella).

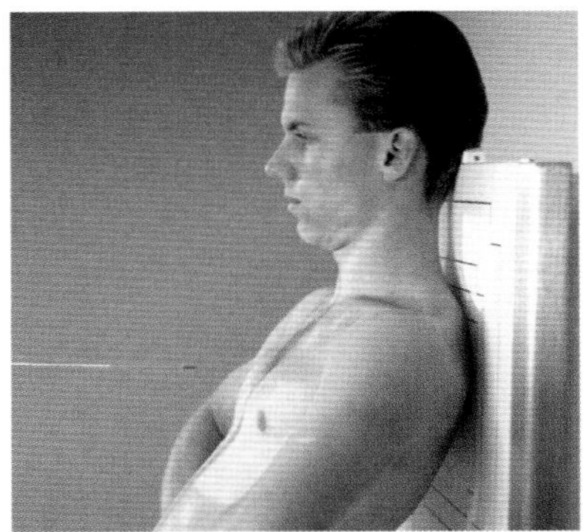

Fig. 1-71. AP axial chest lordotic projection.

Transthoracic lateral projection (right lateral position)

A **lateral projection through the thorax.**

Requires a qualifying positioning term (right or left lateral position) to indicate which shoulder.

Note: This is a special adaptation of the projection term, meaning the CR passes through the thorax even though it does not include an entrance or exit site. In practice this is a common lateral shoulder projection and is referred to as a **right** or **left transthoracic lateral shoulder.**

Dorsoplantar and plantodorsal projections

These are secondary terms for AP or PA projections of the foot.

Dorsoplantar (DP) describes the path of the CR from the **dorsal** (anterior) surface to the **plantar** (posterior) surface of the foot (Fig. 1-73).

A special plantodorsal projection of the heel bone (calcaneus) is called an **axial plantodorsal projection** (PD) because the angled CR enters the plantar surface of the foot and exits the dorsum surface (Fig. 1-74).

Note: Remember, the term **dorsum** for the **foot** refers to the anterior surface, dorsum pedis (Fig. 1-41).

Parietoacanthial and acanthioparietal projections

The CR enters at the cranial **parietal** bone and exits at the **acanthion** (junction of nose and upper lip) for the **parietoacanthial projection** (Fig. 1-75).

The opposite CR direction would describe the **acanthioparietal projection** (Fig. 1-76).

These are also known as **PA Waters** and **AP reverse Waters** methods to visualize the facial bones.

Submentovertex (SMV) and verticosubmental (VSM) projections

These projections are for the **skull** and **mandible.**

CR enters below the chin, or mentum, and exits at the vertex or top of the skull for the **submentovertex (SMV) projection** (Fig. 1-77).

The less common opposite projection of this would be the **verticosubmental (VSM) projection,** entering at top of the skull and exiting below the mandible (not shown).

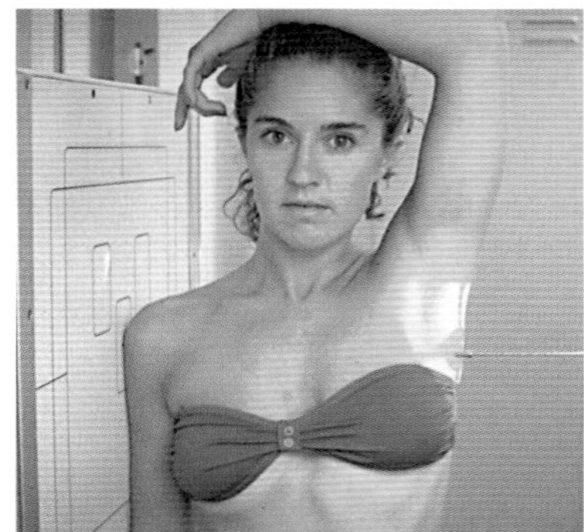

Fig. 1-72. Transthoracic lateral shoulder projection (R lateral shoulder position).

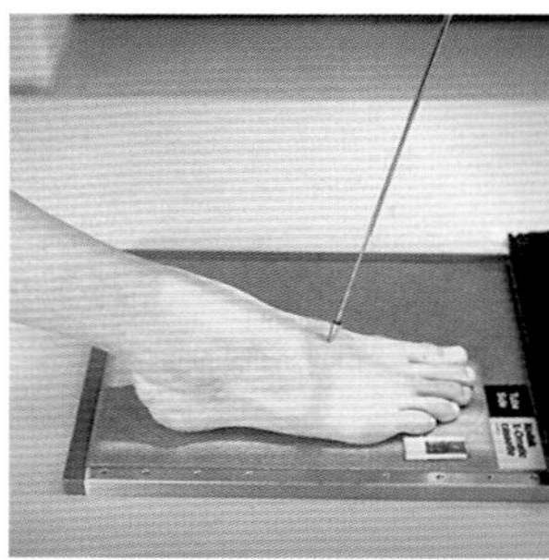

Fig. 1-73. AP or dorsoplantar (DP) projection of foot.

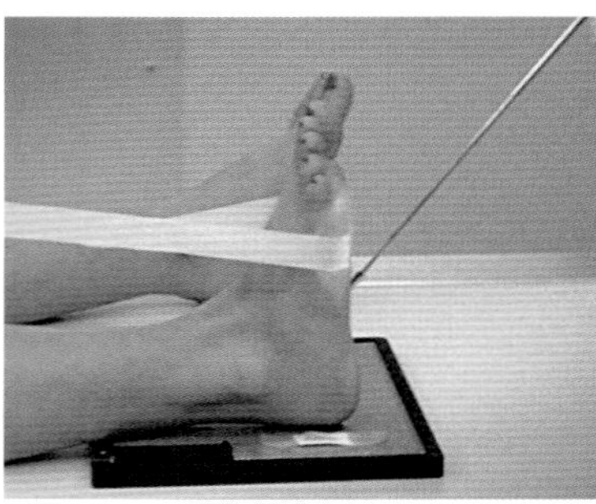

Fig. 1-74. Axial plantodorsal (PD) projection of calcaneus.

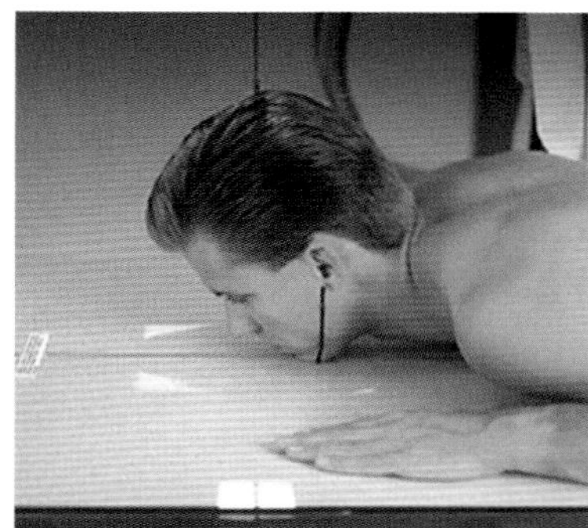

Fig. 1-75. Parietoacanthial projection (PA Waters).

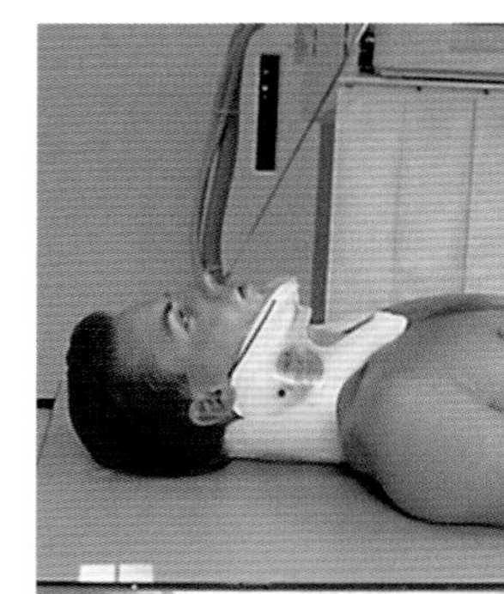

Fig. 1-76. Acanthioparietal projection (reverse Waters).

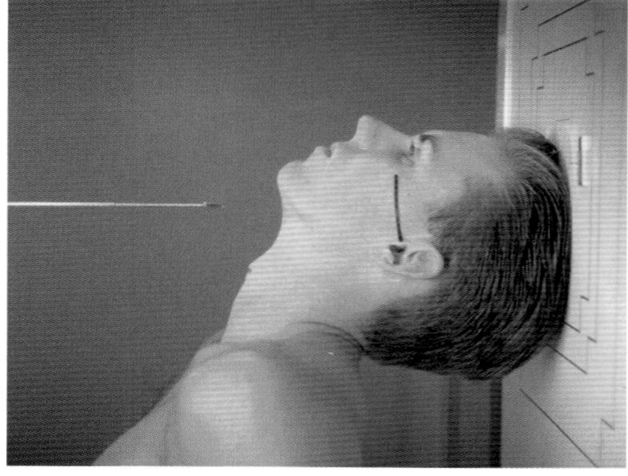

Fig. 1-77. Submentovertex (SMV) projection.

Relationship Terms

Following are paired positioning and/or anatomic terms describing relationships to parts of the body with opposite meanings:

Medial (me'de-al) vs. lateral

Toward vs. **away from the center,** or **median plane.**

In the anatomic position the **medial** aspect of any body part is the "inside" part **closest to the median plane,** and the lateral part is away from the center, or **away from median plane or midline of body.**

Examples: In the anatomic position the thumb is on the lateral aspect of the hand. The lateral part of the abdomen and thorax is that part away from the median plane.

Proximal (prok'si-mal) vs. distal (dis'tal)

Proximal is **near the source** or beginning, and **distal** is **away from.** In regard to the upper and lower limbs, proximal and distal would be that part closest to or away from the trunk, the source or beginning of that limb.

Examples: The elbow is proximal to the wrist. The finger joint closest to the palm of the hand is called the *proximal interphalangeal (PIP) joint,* and the joint near the distal end of the finger is the *distal interphalangeal (DIP) joint* (see Chapter 5).

Cephalad (sef'ah-lad) vs. caudad (kaw'dad)

Cephalad means **toward,** whereas **caudad** means **away from,** the head end of the body.

A **cephalad angle** is any angle toward the head end of the body (Figs. 1-79 and 1-81). (*Cephalad,* or *cephalic,* literally means "head" or "toward the head.")

A **caudad angle** is any angle toward the feet or away from the head end (Fig. 1-80). (*Caudad* or *caudal* comes from *cauda,* literally meaning "tail.")

In human anatomy, cephalad and caudad can also be described as **superior** (toward the head) or **inferior** (toward the feet).

Note: As shown in Figs 1-79, 1-80, and 1-81, these terms are correctly used to describe the direction of CR angle for all axial projections along the entire length of the body, not just projections of the head.

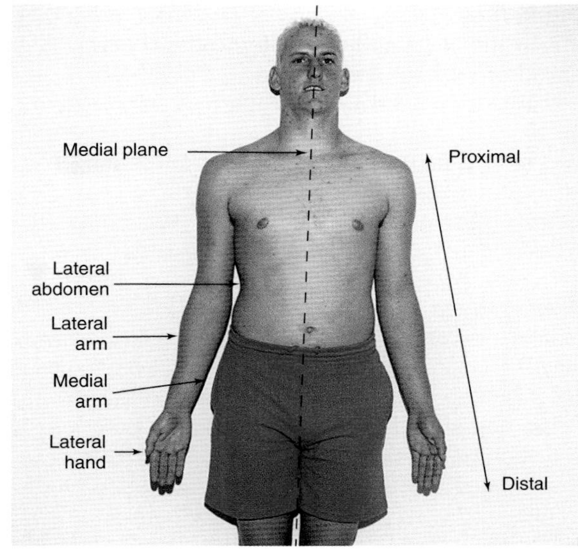

Fig. 1-78. Medial vs. lateral, proximal vs. distal.

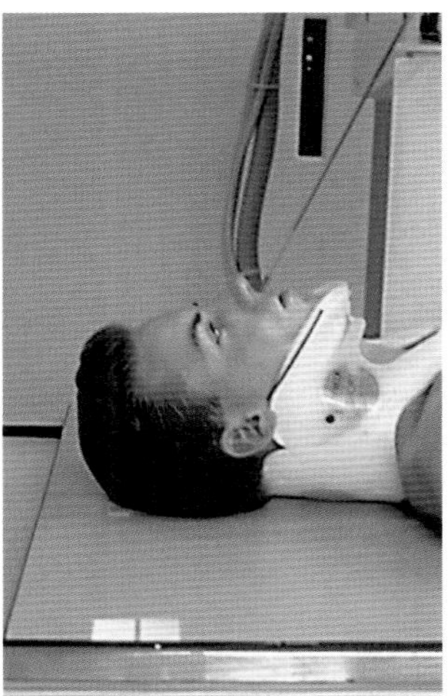

Fig. 1-79. Cephalad CR angle (superior).

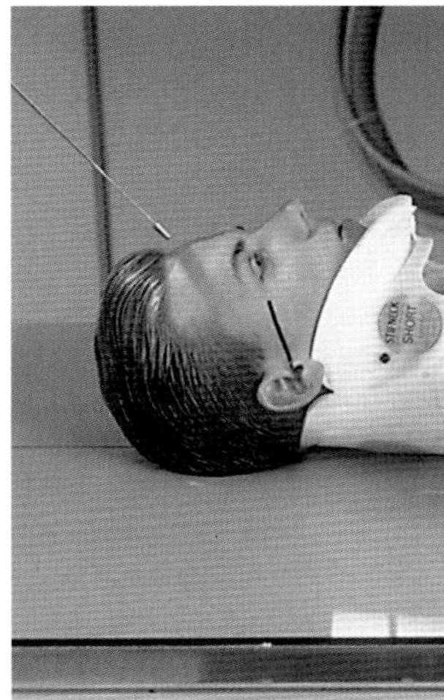

Fig. 1-80. Caudad CR angle (inferior).

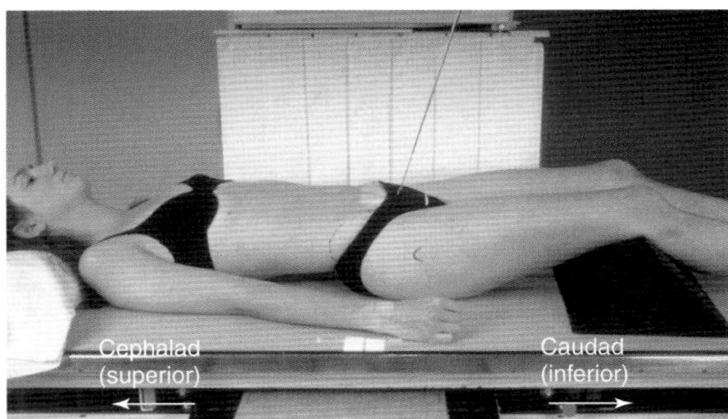

Fig. 1-81. Cephalic angle (AP axial projection of sacrum).

1

Interior (internal, inside) vs. *exterior (external, outer)*

Interior is inside of something, **nearer to the center,** and **exterior** is situated **on or near the outside.**

The prefix **intra** means **within** or **inside** (e.g., intravenous: inside a vein).

The prefix **inter** means situated **between something** (e.g., intercostal: located between the ribs).

The prefix **exo** means **outside** or **outward** (e.g., exocardial: something developing or situated outside the heart).

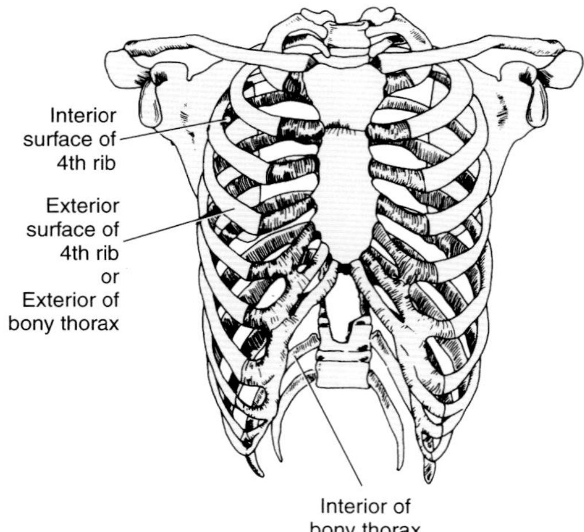

Fig. 1-82. Bony thorax.

Superficial vs. *deep*

Superficial is **nearer** the skin surface; **deep** is **farther away.**

Example: The cross-sectional drawing in Fig. 1-83 shows that the humerus is deep compared with the skin of the arm.

Another example would be a superficial tumor or lesion, which is located near the surface, compared with a deep tumor or lesion, which is located deeper within the body or part.

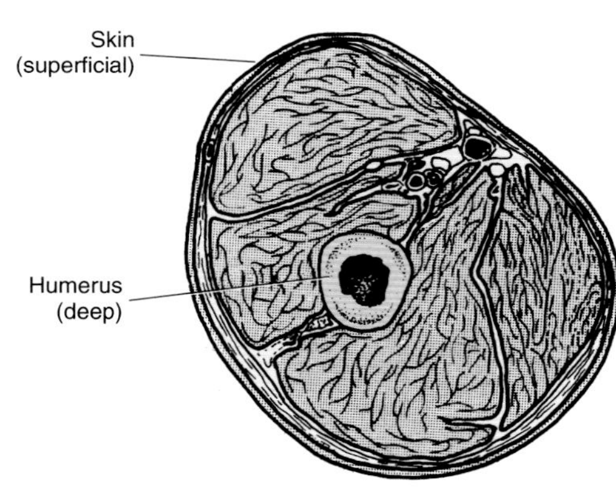

Fig. 1-83. Cross-section of arm.

Ipsilateral *(ip"si-lat'er-al)* vs. ***contralateral*** *(kon"trah-lat'er-al)*

Ipsilateral is on the **same side** of the body or part; **contralateral** is on the **opposite side.**

Example: The right thumb and the right great toe are ipsilateral; the right knee and the left hand are contralateral.

Terms Describing Curvature of the Spine

Lordosis (lor-do'sis) vs. ***kyphosis*** *(ki-fo'sis)*

These terms both describe a **front-to-back,** or **anterior-to-posterior, curvature** of the spine.

Lordosis is a **"swayback"** type of curvature, most commonly of the lumbar spine region.

Kyphosis is a **"humpback"** type of curvature, usually of the thoracic spine region.

Scoliosis (sko"le-o'sis)

Scoliosis is a lateral, or **side-to-side, curvature** of the spine. (See Chapter 9 on the Vertebral Column for more information on these terms.)

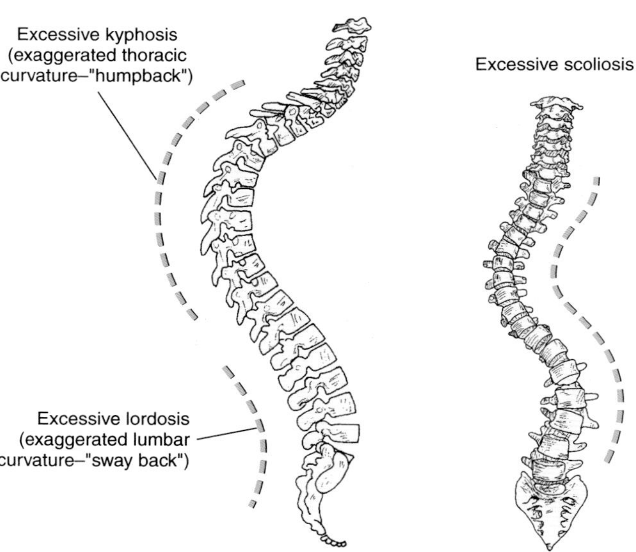

Fig. 1-84. Lordosis and kyphosis.

Fig. 1-85. Scoliosis.

Terms Related to Movements

The final group of positioning and related terms that every technologist should know relates to various movements. Most of these are listed as paired terms describing movements in opposite directions.

Flexion vs. extension

In flexing or extending a joint, **the angle** between parts **is decreased** or **increased.**

Flexion decreases the angle of the joint (see examples of knee, elbow, and wrist flexions in Fig. 1-86).

Extension increases the angle as the body part moves from a flexed to a straightened position. This is true for the knee, elbow, and wrist joints, as shown.

Hyperextension

Extending a joint **beyond the straight or neutral position.**

Abnormal hyperextension: A hyperextended elbow or knee results when the joint is extended beyond the straightened or neutral position. This is not a natural movement for these two joints and results in injury or trauma.

Normal flexion and hyperextension of spine: Flexion is bending forward, and extension is returning to the straight or neutral position. A backward bending **beyond the neutral position** is **hyperextension.** In practice, however, the terms *flexion* and *extension* are commonly used for these two extreme flexion and hyperextension projections of the spine (Fig. 1-87).

Normal hyperextension of wrist: A second example of a special use of the term *hyperextension* is that of the wrist, where the carpal canal or carpal tunnel view of the carpals is visualized by a special **hyperextended wrist movement** in which the wrist is extended beyond the neutral position. This specific wrist movement is also called **dorsiflexion** (backward or posterior flexion) (Fig. 1-88, *left*).

Acute flexion of wrist: An acute or full flexion of the wrist is required for a special tangential projection for a carpal bridge view of the posterior aspect of the wrist (Fig. 1-88, *right*).

Ulnar deviation vs. radial deviation of wrist

Deviation literally means "to turn aside" or "to turn away from the standard or course."*

Ulnar deviation is to turn or bend the hand and wrist from the natural position toward the ulnar side, and **radial deviation** is toward the radial side of the wrist.

Note: Earlier editions of this textbook, as well as other positioning references, have defined these wrist movements as ulnar and radial flexion movements because they describe specific flexion movements toward either the ulna or the radius.† However, because practitioners in the medical community, including orthopedic physicians, commonly use the terms *ulnar* and *radial deviation* for these wrist movements, this text has also changed its terminology to *ulnar* and *radial deviation movements* to prevent confusion and ensure consistency with other medical references.

*Dorland's illustrated medical dictionary, ed 28, Philadelphia, 1994, WB Saunders.
†Frank ED, Ballinger PW, Bontrager KL: Two terms, one meaning, Radiologic Technology 69:517, 1998.

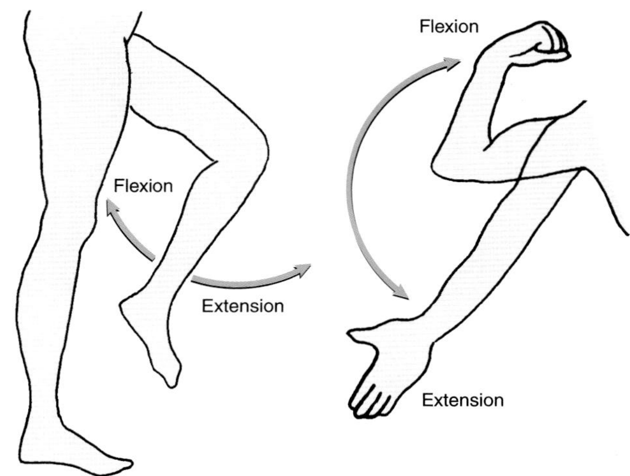

Fig. 1-86. Flexion vs. extension.

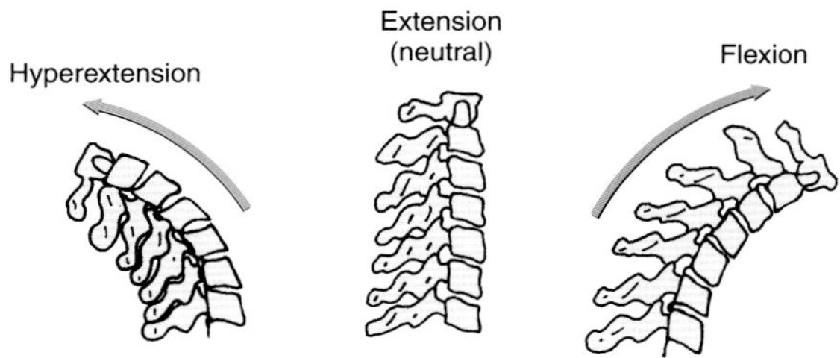

Fig. 1-87. Hyperextension, extension, and flexion of spine.

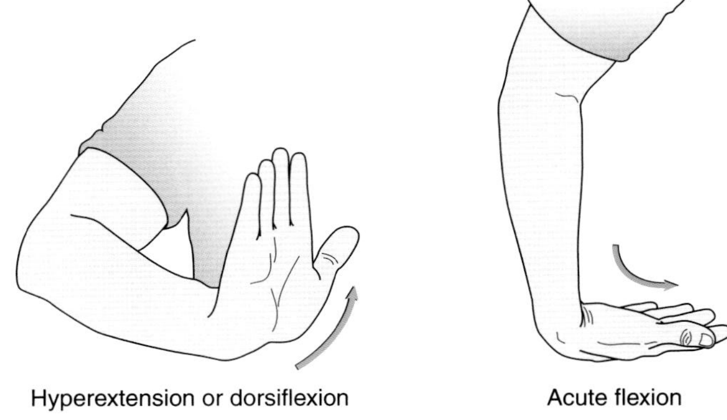

Fig. 1-88. Wrist hyperextension and flexion movements.

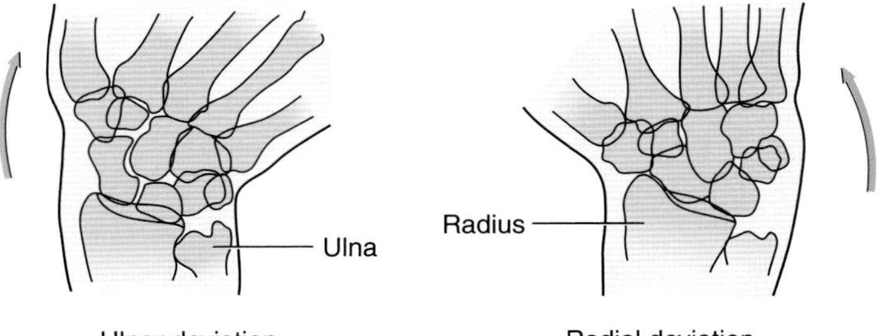

Fig. 1-89. Ulnar vs. radial deviation wrist movements.

*Dorsiflexion vs. **plantar flexion of foot***

Dorsiflexion of foot: to **decrease the angle** (flex) between the dorsum (top of foot) and the lower leg, moving foot and toes upward.

Plantar flexion of foot: extending the ankle joint, moving foot and toes downward from the normal position; flexing or decreasing the angle toward the plantar (posterior) surface of the foot.

Note: See preceding page for dorsiflexion of the wrist (Fig. 1-88) compared with dorsiflexion of the foot (Fig. 1-90).

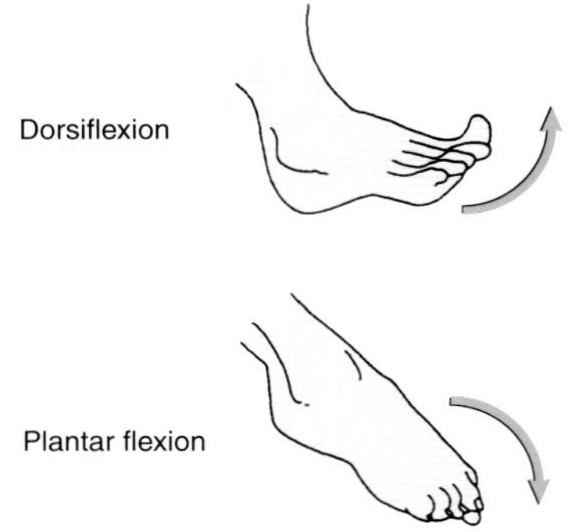

Fig. 1-90. Movements of ankle and foot.

*Eversion (e-ver'zhun) vs. **inversion** (in-ver'zhun)*

Eversion is an **outward stress movement** of the foot at the ankle joint.

Inversion is **inward stress** movement of the foot as applied to the foot without rotation of the leg.

The plantar surface (sole) of the foot is turned or rotated away from the median plane of the body (the sole faces in a more lateral direction) for eversion and toward the median plane for inversion (Figs. 1-91 and 1-92).

The leg does not rotate, and stress is applied to the medial and lateral aspects of the ankle joint for evaluation of possible widening of the joint space (ankle mortise).

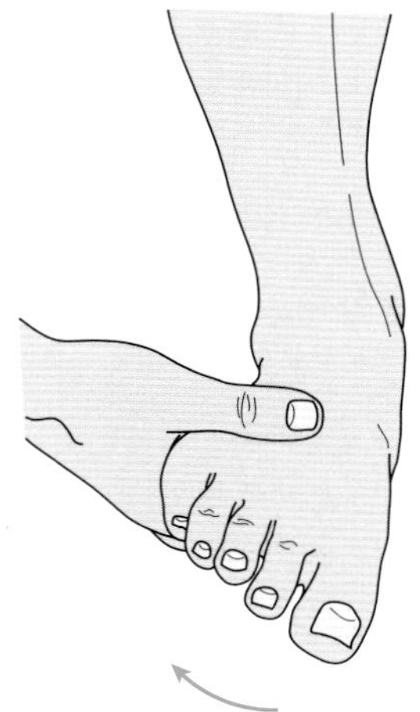

Fig. 1-91. Eversion (valgus stress).

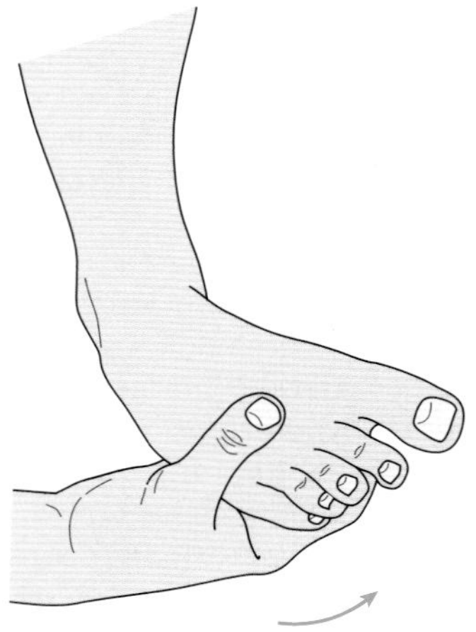

Fig. 1-92. Inversion (varus stress).

*Valgus (val'gus) vs. **varus** (va'rus)*

Valgus describes the bending of the part **outward** or **away from the midline** of the body. *Valgus* is sometimes used to describe **eversion stress** of the ankle joint.

Varus, meaning "knock-kneed," describes the bending of a part **inward** or **toward the midline.** The term *varus stress* is sometimes also used to describe **inversion stress** applied at the ankle joint.

Note: The terms *valgus* and *varus* are also used to describe the loss of alignment of bone fragments. (See Fracture Terms, Chapter 19.)

*Medial (internal) rotation vs. **lateral (external) rotation***

Medial rotation is a rotation or turning of a body part, moving the **anterior** aspect of the part **toward the inside,** or median, plane.

Lateral rotation is a rotation of an **anterior** body part **toward the outside,** or away from the median plane.

Note: Remember, in radiographic positioning these terms describe the movement of the **anterior** aspect of the part being rotated. Thus in the forearm movements (Fig. 1-93), the anterior aspect of the forearm moves medially or internally on medial rotation and laterally or externally on lateral rotation. Another example is the medial and lateral obliques of the knee, in which the **anterior** part of the knee is rotated medially and laterally in **either AP** or **PA** projections (see Chapter 7).

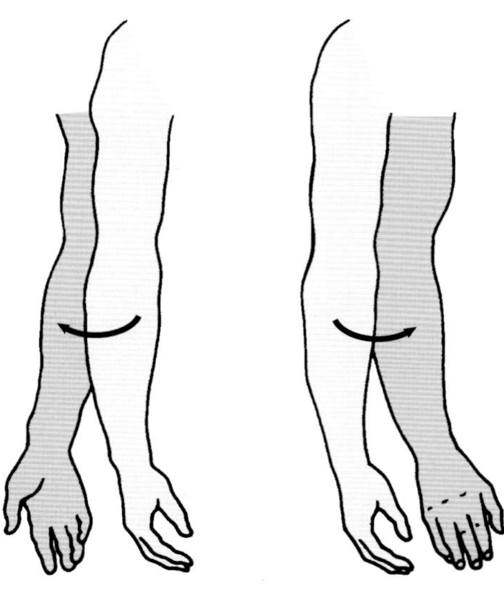

Fig. 1-93. Rotational movements of upper limb. **A,** Lateral (external) rotation. **B,** Medial (internal) rotation.

Abduction *(ab-duk'shun) vs.* ***adduction*** *(ah-duk'shun)*

Abduction is the lateral movement of the arm or leg **away** from the body.

Another application of this term is the abduction of the fingers or toes, which means spreading them apart.

Adduction is a movement of arm or leg **toward** the body, to draw toward a center or medial line.

Adduction of the fingers or toes means moving them together or toward each other.

Note: A memory aid is to associate the *d* in towar<u>d</u> with the *d* in a<u>d</u>duction.

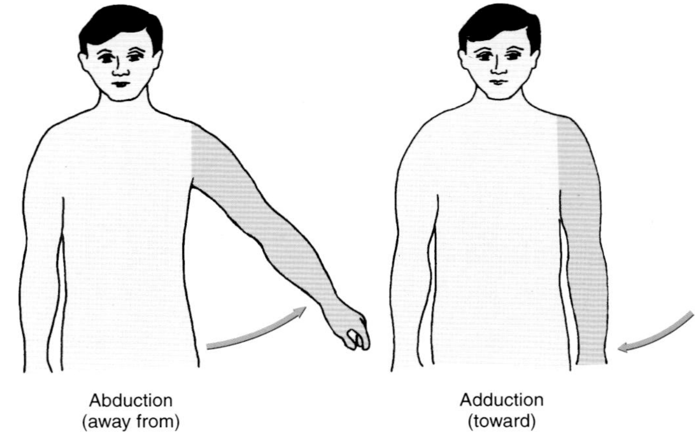

Fig. 1-94. Movements of upper limb.

Supination *(su"pi-na'shun) vs.* ***pronation*** *(pro-na'shun)*

Supination is a rotational movement of the hand into the anatomic position (palm up in supine position or forward in erect position).

This movement rotates the radius of the forearm laterally along its long axis.

Pronation is a rotation of the hand into the opposite of the anatomic position (palm down or back).

Note: To help remember these terms, relate them to the body positions of supine and prone. *Supine* or *supination* means face up or palm up, and *prone* or *pronation* means face down or palm down.

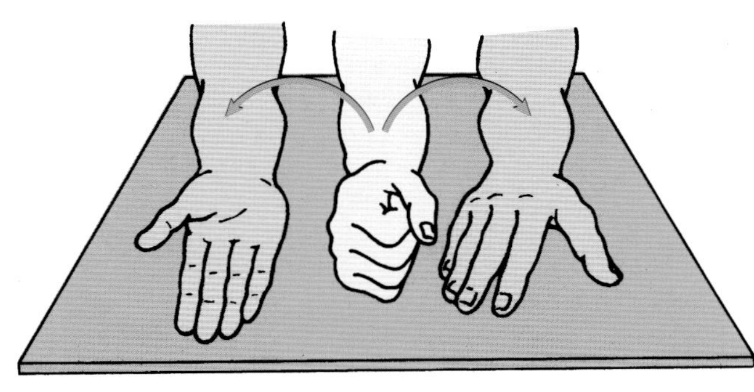

Fig. 1-95. Movements of hand.

Protraction *(pro-trak'shun) vs.* ***retraction*** *(re-trak'shun)*

Protraction is a **movement forward** from a normal position.

Retraction is a **movement backward** or the condition of being drawn back.

Example: Protraction is moving the jaw forward (sticking the chin out) or drawing the shoulders forward. Retraction is the opposite of this, moving the jaw backward or squaring the shoulders, as in a military stance.

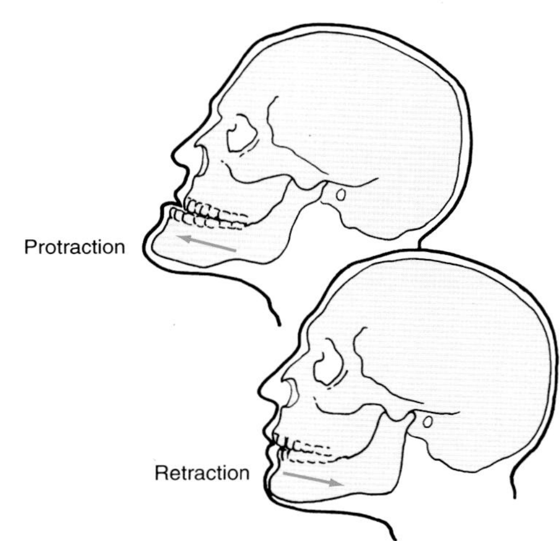

Fig. 1-96. Movements of protraction and retraction.

1

Elevation vs. depression

Elevation is a **lifting, raising,** or **moving of a part superiorly.**

Depression is a **letting down, lowering,** or **moving of a part inferiorly.**

Example: Shoulders are elevated when they are raised, as when shrugging the shoulders. Depressing the shoulders is lowering them.

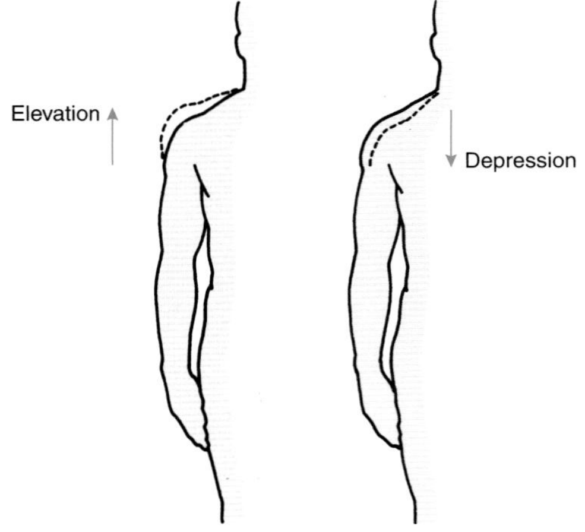

Fig. 1-97. Elevation and depression movements of shoulders.

Circumduction (ser"kum-duk'shun)

Circumduction means **to move around in the form of a circle.** This term describes sequential movements of flexion, abduction, extension, and adduction, resulting in a cone-type movement at any joint where the four movements are possible (e.g., fingers, wrist, arm, leg).

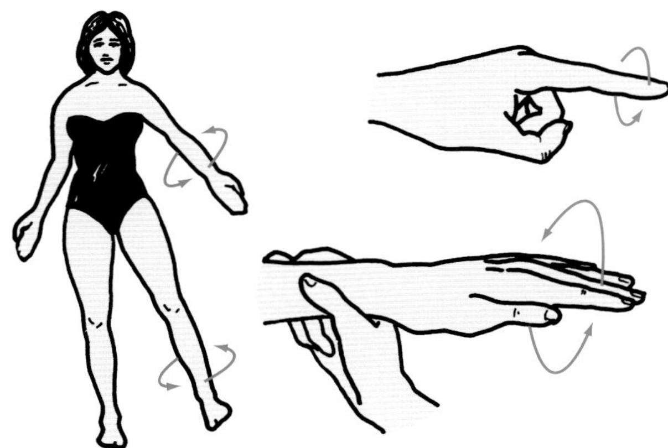

Fig. 1-98. Circumduction movements.

Rotation vs. Tilt

Rotation is to turn or rotate a body part on its axis.

In Fig. 1-99 the midsagittal plane of the entire body, including the head, is **rotated.**

Tilt is a slanting or tilting movement with respect to the long axis.

Fig. 1-100 demonstrates no rotation of the head but a **tilting** (slanting) of the midsagittal plane of the head, which therefore is not parallel to the tabletop.

Understanding the difference between these two terms becomes important in skull and facial bone positioning (see Chapters 12 and 13).

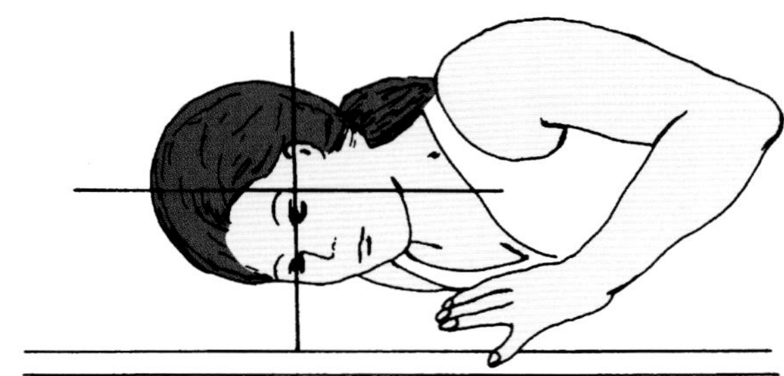

Fig. 1-99. Rotation—midsagittal plane rotated.

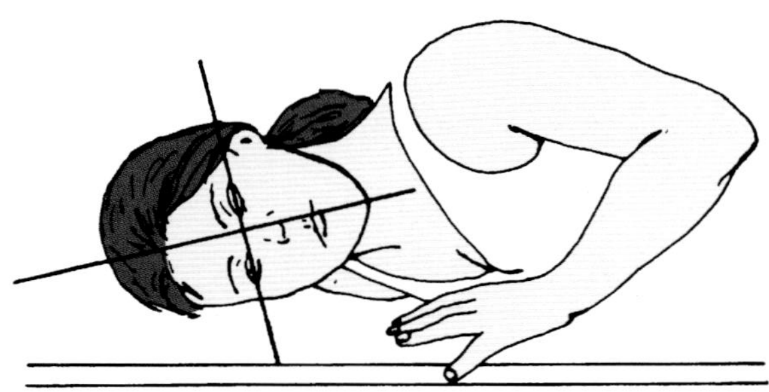

Fig. 1-100. Tilt—midsagittal plane of head tilted.

Summary of Potentially Misused Positioning Terms

The three terms **position, projection,** and **view** are sometimes confusing and used incorrectly in practice. These terms should be understood and used correctly as follows:

Position

Position is a term used to indicate the patient's **general physical position,** such as **supine, prone, recumbent,** or **erect.**

Position is also used to describe **specific body positions** by that body part closest to the IR, such as **laterals** and **obliques.**

The term **position** should be **"restricted to the discussion of the patient's physical position."***

Projection

Projection is a correct positioning term describing or referring to the **path or direction of the central ray** (CR) projecting an image onto an image receptor (IR).

The term **projection** should be **"restricted to the discussion of the path of the central ray."***

View

View is **not** a correct positioning term in the United States.

View describes the **radiographic image** as seen from the vantage of the image receptor.

The term **view** should be **"restricted to the discussion of a radiograph or image."***

Canadian terminology: The following information is printed on the front of the CAMRT certification exam.†

Position: *"The placement of the body."*

Projection: *"The surfaces of the body that the central ray transverses as it leaves the x-ray tube, passes through the patient, and strikes the film"* (image receptor).

View: *"The surface of the body closest to the film"* (image receptor).

Note: In Canada the term *view* is commonly used interchangeably with *position* (i.e., *lateral view* and *lateral position* would mean essentially the same thing, one referring to what is seen on the image and one describing how the patient is positioned).†

*ARRT Educators Handbook, ed 3, St. Paul, 1990, ARRT.
†Personal communication and correspondence with the Council of Education for Radiological Technology (CAMRT), November 1999.

SUMMARY OF PROJECTIONS AND POSITIONS

Projections (Path of CR)	General Body Positions	Specific Body Positions (That Part Closest to IR)
Posteroanterior (PA)	Anatomic	R or L lateral
Anteroposterior (AP)	Supine	Obliques
Mediolateral	Prone	• Left posterior, LPO
Lateromedial	Erect (upright)	• Right posterior, RPO
AP or PA oblique	Recumbent	• Left anterior, LAO
AP or PA axial	Trendelenburg	• Right anterior, RAO
Tangential	Sim's	Decubitus
Transthoracic	Fowler's	• Left lateral
Dorsoplantar (DP)	Lithotomy	• Right lateral
Plantodorsal (PD)		• Ventral
Inferosuperior axial		• Dorsal
Superoinferior axial		• Lordotic
Axiolateral		
Submentovertex (SMV)		
Verticosubmental (VSM)		
Parietoacanthial		
Acanthoparietal		
Craniocaudal		

SUMMARY OF POSITIONING-RELATED TERMS

Body Planes, Sections, and Lines

Longitudinal planes or sections
- Sagittal
- Coronal
- Oblique

Transverse planes or sections
- Horizontal, axial, or cross-sections
- Oblique

Base plane
Occlusal plane
Infraorbitomeatal line (IOML)

Body Surfaces

Posterior
Anterior
Plantar
Dorsum
Palmar

Relationship Terms

Medial vs. lateral
Proximal vs. distal
Cephalad vs. caudad
Ipsilateral vs. contralateral
Internal vs. external
Superficial vs. deep
Lordosis vs. kyphosis (scoliosis)

Movement Terms

Flexion vs. extension (acute flexion vs. hyperextension)
Ulnar vs. radial deviation
Dorsiflexion vs. plantar flexion
Eversion vs. inversion
Valgus vs. varus
Medial vs. lateral rotation
Abduction vs. adduction
Supination vs. pronation
Protraction vs. retraction
Elevation vs. depression
Tilt vs. rotation
Circumduction

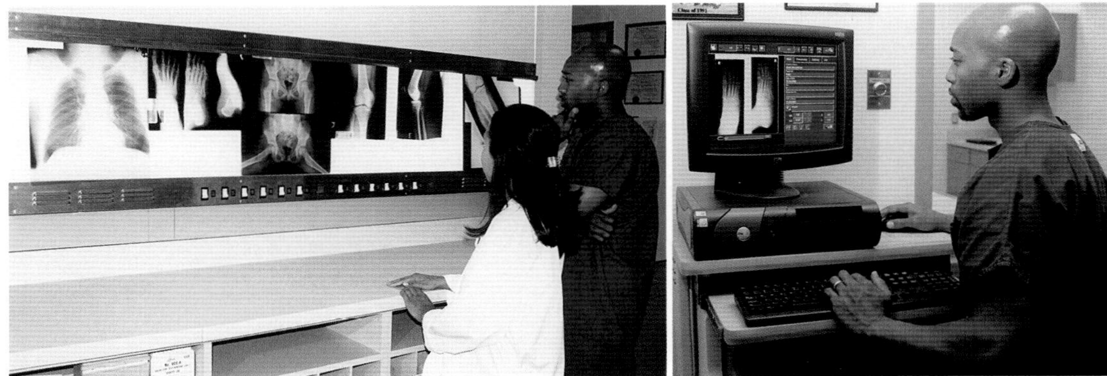

Fig. 1-101. Viewing radiographs and digital radiographic images.

POSITIONING PRINCIPLES

1

Radiographic Criteria

The goal of every technologist should be to take not just a "passable" radiograph but rather an optimal one that can be evaluated by a **definable standard,** as described under **radiographic criteria**.

An example of a five-part radiographic technique as used in this text for a lateral forearm is shown on the right. The positioning photo and the resulting optimal radiograph (Figs. 1-102 and 1-103) are also shown below for this lateral forearm as described in Chapter 5.

RADIOGRAPHIC CRITERIA FORMAT

The technologist should review and compare the radiograph with this standard to determine how close to an optimal image was achieved. A systematic method of learning how to critique radiographs is to break the critique down into these **five parts.**

1. ***Structures shown:*** Describes precisely what anatomic parts and structures should be clearly visualized on that radiograph.
2. ***Position:*** Generally describes two things: (1) placement of body part in relationship to the IR and (2) positioning factors that are important for the projection.

   For example, the key positioning factors for a correctly positioned lateral forearm are (1) ulna/radius aligned to long axis of IR, (2) elbow flexed 90°, and (3) no rotation from a true lateral position. (Evidence as to how rotation can be determined is then described.)
3. ***Collimation and CR:*** Describes two factors: (1) where the collimation borders should be in relation to that body part and (2) the location of the central ray (CR).

   A correct central ray location is especially important whenever automatic exposure control (AEC) is used. It is also important for all upper and lower limbs, where the joints are the primary interest area; the CR must be accurately centered to the joint to prevent image distortion.

   The small icon box ⌖ is included in the positioning description on each positioning page where the CR is of primary importance. This is not the case for this lateral forearm, so the CR is described as the "midpoint of radius and ulna" rather than a precise anatomic location.

   Critiquing the radiographic image for correct CR location is easily done by imagining a large X extending from the four corners of the collimation field, the center of which is the precise CR location.
4. ***Exposure criteria:*** Describes how exposure factors or technique (kV, mA, and time) can be evaluated for optimum exposure for that body part. **No motion** is a first priority, and a description of how the presence or absence of motion can be determined is listed. (Motion is included with exposure criteria because exposure time is the primary controlling factor for motion.)
5. ***Image markers:*** A fifth area of critique involves image markers. Patient ID markers, R or L side marker, and/or patient position or time markers should be correctly placed so that they are not superimposed over essential anatomy.

   Note: This part of radiographic criteria on image markers is not listed on each positioning page throughout the text because it is essentially the same for **all** projections. However, it should **always be included** in clinical practice when evaluating and critiquing radiographic images.

SAMPLE LATERAL FOREARM CRITERIA

Radiographic Criteria

Structures Shown: • Lateral projection of entire radius and ulna; proximal row of carpals, elbow, and distal end of humerus; and pertinent soft tissues such as fat pads and stripes of wrist and elbow joints.

Position: • Long axis of forearm aligned with long axis of IR • Elbow flexed 90° • No rotation from true lateral as evidenced by the following: • Head of the ulna should be superimposed over the radius. • Humeral epicondyles should be superimposed. • Radial head should superimpose the coronoid process with radial tuberosity seen in profile.

Collimation and CR: • Collimation borders visible at skin margins along length of forearm with only minimal collimation at both ends to ensure that essential joint anatomy is included. • CR and center of collimation field to midpoint of radius and ulna.

Exposure Criteria: • Optimum density and contrast with no motion will visualize sharp cortical margins and clear, bony trabecular markings and fat pads and stripes of the wrist and elbow joints.

Image Markers: • Patient ID markers, R or L side marker, and/or patient position or time markers should be placed so that they are not superimposed over essential anatomy.

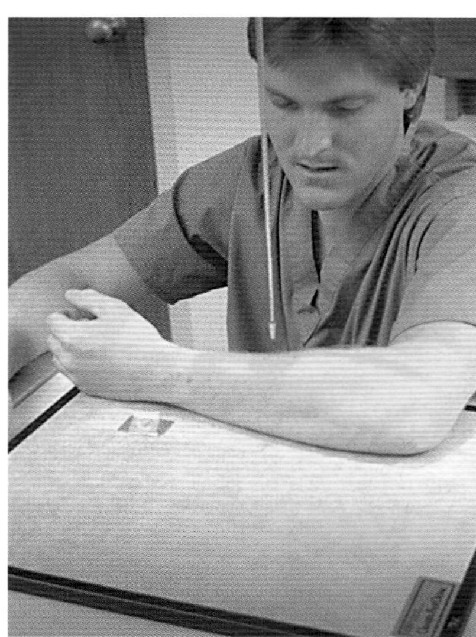

Fig. 1-102. Accurate positioning for lateral forearm.

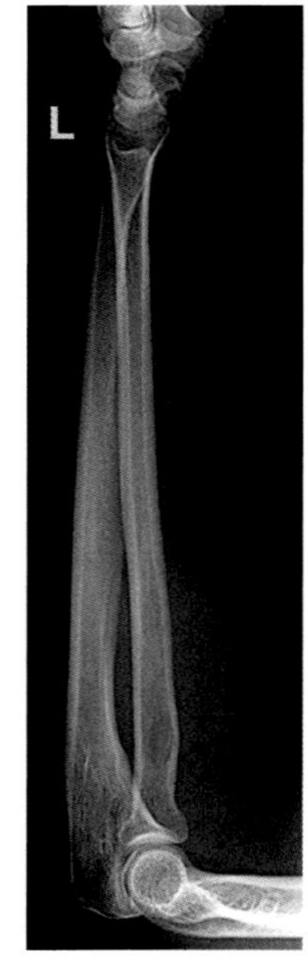

Fig. 1-103. Lateral forearm.

Image Markers and Patient Identification

A **minimum** of two types of markers should be imprinted on **every** radiographic image. These are (1) **patient identification and date** and (2) **anatomic side markers.**

PATIENT IDENTIFICATION AND DATE (CONVENTIONAL FILM-SCREEN CASSETTE SYSTEMS)

Generally this patient information, which includes data such as name, date, case number, and institution, is provided on an index card then photoflashed on the film in the space provided by a lead block in the film holder. Each cassette or film holder should have a marker on the exterior indicating this area where the patient ID, including the date, will be flashed (Fig. 1-104). Care must be taken so that this area does not obscure the essential anatomy being demonstrated.

Throughout this text the preferred location of this patient ID marker is shown in relation to the body part. A general rule for chests and abdomens is to place the patient ID information at the top margin of the IR on chests, and on the lower margin on abdomens (see small arrows on Fig. 1-105). This marker should always be placed where it is least likely to cover essential anatomy.

ANATOMIC SIDE MARKER

A right or left radiopaque marker must also appear on every radiographic image, correctly indicating the patient's right or left side or which limb is being radiographed, the right or left. This may be either the word "Right" or "Left" or just the initials "R" or "L." This side marker should preferably be placed directly on the IR inside the lateral portion of the collimated border of the side being identified with the placement such that the marker will not be superimposed over essential anatomy.

Remember, these are radiopaque markers and thus must be placed just within the collimation field so that they will be exposed by the x-ray beam and included on the image.

The two markers, the patient ID and the anatomic side marker, must be correctly placed on **ALL** radiographic images. Generally, it is not an acceptable practice to write this information on the image after it is processed because of legal and liability problems from potential mismarkings. A **radiograph taken without these two markers may need to be repeated,** which obviously results in unnecessary radiation to the patient, making this a serious error.

ADDITIONAL MARKERS OR IDENTIFICATION

Certain other markers or identifiers may also be used, such as **technologist initials,** which are generally placed on the R or L marker to identify the specific technologist responsible for that exam. Sometimes the exam room number is also included.

Time indicators are also commonly used, noting the minutes of elapsed time in a series, such as the 1 min., 5 min., 15 min., and 20 min. series of radiographs taken in an intravenous urogram (IVU) procedure.

Another important marker on all decubitus positions is a decub marker or some type of indicator such as an **arrow identifying which side is up.** An **"upright"** or **"erect"** marker must also be used to identify erect chest or abdomen positions compared with recumbent, in addition to an arrow indicating which side is up.

Inspiration (INSP) and **expiration** (EXP) markers are used for special comparison PA projections of the chest. **Internal** (INT) and **external** (EXT) markers may be used for rotation projections such as for the proximal humerus and shoulder. Sample markers are shown in Fig. 1-106.

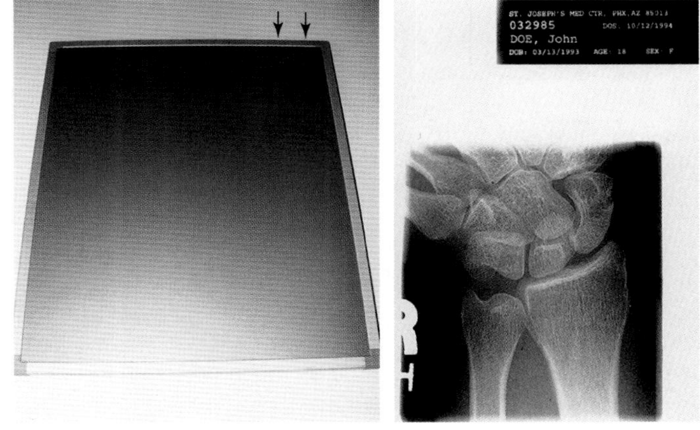

Fig. 1-104. Patient ID information.

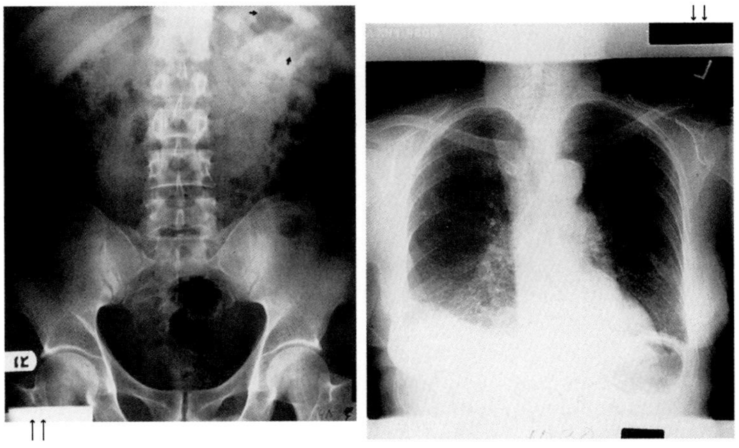

Fig. 1-105. Correctly placed side markers and patient ID marker (patient's right to viewer's left).

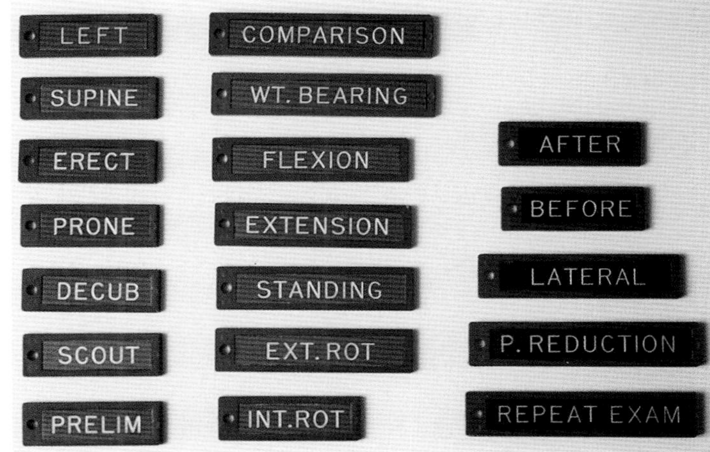

Fig. 1-106. Sample markers.

Professional Ethics and Patient Care

The radiologic technologist is an important member of the health care team responsible in general for radiologic examination of patients. This includes being responsible for one's actions under a specific **code of ethics.**

Code of ethics describes the **rules of acceptable conduct toward others,** as defined within that profession.

CAMRT Code of Ethics*

The Association recognizes its obligation to identify and promote exemplary professional standards of practice, conduct, and performance. Adherence to these standards is the personal and professional responsibility of each member. This Code of Ethics requires that every member of the Association shall:

- provide service with dignity and respect to all people regardless of race, national or ethnic origin, colour, gender, sexual orientation, religious affiliation, age, type of illness, or mental or physical challenge;
- earn the trust and confidence of the public through exemplary professional competence and conduct;
- conduct all procedures and examinations in keeping with current radiation safety standards where these standards shall apply;
- practice only those procedures for which the member is qualified or has been properly delegated by appropriate authority, provided that the member has received training to an acceptable level of competence in such delegated acts;
- practice only those disciplines of medical radiation technology in which the member is certified by the Association and is currently competent;
- recognize that, while patients must seek diagnostic information from their physician, an opinion expressed to another health care professional with regard to the appearances of a procedure or examination may assist in diagnosis or treatment;
- recognize and protect the confidential nature of all information acquired during contact with each patient, except where disclosure of such information is required by law or necessary to the treatment of the patient;
- cooperate with other health care professions;
- advance the art and science of medical radiation technology; and
- participate in the affairs of the Association in a responsible and professional way.

June 1997

*Code of Ethics as adopted by Canadian Association of Medical Radiation Technologists, June 1997.

ARRT Code of Ethics*

The Code of Ethics forms the first part of the *Standards of Ethics.* The Code of Ethics shall serve as a guide by which Registered Technologists and Candidates may evaluate their professional conduct as it relates to patients, health care, consumers, employers, colleagues and other members of the health care team. The Code of Ethics is intended to assist Registered Technologists and Candidates in maintaining a high level of ethical conduct and in providing for the protection, safety and comfort of patients. The Code of Ethics is aspirational.

1. The radiologic technologist conducts herself or himself in a professional manner, responds to patient needs, and supports colleagues and associates in providing quality patient care.
2. The radiologic technologist acts to advance the principle objective of the profession to provide services to humanity with full respect for the dignity of mankind.
3. The radiologic technologist delivers patient care and service unrestricted by concerns of personal attributes or the nature of the disease or illness, and without discrimination on the basis of sex, race, creed, religion, or socioeconomic status.
4. The radiologic technologist practices technology founded upon theoretical knowledge and concepts, uses equipment and accessories consistent with the purposes for which they were designed, and employs procedures and techniques appropriately.
5. The radiologic technologist assesses situations; exercises care, discretion, and judgment; assumes responsibility for professional decisions; and acts in the best interest of the patient.
6. The radiologic technologist acts as an agent through observation and communication to obtain pertinent information for the physician to aid in the diagnosis and treatment of the patient and recognizes that interpretation and diagnosis are outside the scope of practice for the profession.
7. The radiologic technologist uses equipment and accessories, employs techniques and procedures, performs services in accordance with an accepted standard of practice, and demonstrates expertise in minimizing the radiation exposure to the patient, self, and other members of the health care team.
8. The radiologic technologist practices ethical conduct appropriate to the profession and protects the patient's right to quality radiologic technology care.
9. The radiologic technologist respects confidences entrusted in the course of professional practice, respects the patient's right to privacy, and reveals confidential information only as required by law or to protect the welfare of the individual or the community.
10. The radiologic technologist continually strives to improve knowledge and skills by participating in continuing education and professional activities, sharing knowledge with colleagues, and investigating new aspects of professional practice.

*Code of ethics of the American Registry of Radiologic Technologists, effective July 2002.

Protocol and Order for General Diagnostic Radiographic Procedures

Each radiology department should establish an agreed-on protocol and order by which all general diagnostic radiographic procedures are performed. This is necessary for an orderly and effective working system whereby all technologists (students or graduate technologists) follow the same order and procedure.

Following are sample protocols for general diagnostic **film-screen** and **digital imaging** radiographic procedures as established and used by a Midwestern university hospital.*

FILM-SCREEN IMAGING

1. Read and assess requisition. Pay special attention to reason for exam to determine how positioning or technique may require adjusting.
2. Determine the film-screen combination and the size and number of cassettes you will need.
3. Stock passbox/cassette cabinet with needed cassettes.
4. Prepare radiographic room.
5. Correctly identify the patient. (Check arm band or have patient repeat full name.)
6. Dress patient correctly.
7. Explain to the patient what you will be doing and what is expected.
8. Place cassette in cassette holder or on tabletop in correct LW/CW direction.
9. Assist patients to position and place you want them for the first radiograph.
10. Measure the anatomic part to be radiographed.
11. Use a grid if part measures over 12 cm.
12. Determine the mAs and kV to be used and set it on the generator.
13. Accurately position the patient.
14. Identify right and left side of patient with the proper lead marker.
15. Restrain the patient if needed.
16. Use lead gonadal shielding on anyone under 50 years of age.
17. Provide lead aprons and gloves, if necessary, for everyone assisting with restraint in the room.
18. Give patient proper breathing instructions as required.
19. Take exposure, while watching patient through window.
20. Repeat steps 8 through 18 for each radiographic view needed.
21. Patient is not to be left alone in the radiographic room unless restrained and holding a call pull cord.
22. Explain that you are going to develop and view the radiographs you have taken to determine if optimal radiographs have been obtained.
23. Fog each exposed cassette with the patient's identification card.
24. Process the radiographs by running them through the processor.
25. Record the date, time, number of films, name, room number, technique used, and patient history on the requisition.
26. Properly evaluate radiographs. If no radiographs require repeating, place radiographs in proper slot or send with patient if indicated.
27. Place a correct patient exam card in the designated computer terminal completed box, including the time, room number, number of radiographs, and rejects.
28. Assist the patient from table to wheel chair, cart, or walking position.
29. Open door for the patient.
30. Explain to outpatients where they are to go next. Take inpatients to the proper holding area and place a "To Go" card in the transaide area.
31. Straighten up radiographic room, change linens, and clean table off with alcohol.
32. Wash your hands.

DIGITAL IMAGING

1. Read and assess requisition. Pay special attention to reason for exam to determine how positioning or technique may require adjusting.
2. Determine the type, size, and number of image plates (IP) you will need. Choose the smallest possible size of cassette. If the IPs have not been used within 48 hours, erase them before using.
3. Stock passbox/cassette cabinet with needed cassettes.
4. Prepare radiographic room.
5. Correctly identify the patient. (Check arm band or have patient repeat full name.)
6. Dress the patient correctly.
7. Explain to the patient what you will be doing and what is expected.
8. Position cassette in cassette holder or on tabletop so the purple corner is oriented caudally or to the patient's left side and the green strip is oriented cephalically or to the patient's right side.
9. Assist the patient in assuming the desired position and place for the first image. Make certain the part of interest is placed in the center of the cassette. When doing extremity work, keep views close together and use lead strips to mask areas not in exposure.
10. Measure the anatomic part to be radiographed.
11. Use a grid if part measures over 12 cm.
12. Determine the mAs and kv to be used and set it on the generator.
13. Accurately position the patient.
14. Identify right and left side of patient with the proper lead marker.
15. Restrain the patient if needed.
16. Use lead gonadal shielding on anyone under 50 years of age.
17. Provide lead aprons and gloves, if necessary, for everyone assisting with restraint in the room.
18. Give patient proper breathing instructions as required.
19. Take exposure, while watching patient through window.
20. Repeat steps 8 through 18 for each radiographic view needed.
21. Patient is not to be left alone in the radiographic room unless restrained and holding a call pull cord.
22. Explain that you are going to develop and view the images you have taken to determine if optimal radiographs have been obtained.
23. Insert cassette into plate reader with purple corners going first and white side up.
24. Enter patient identification information into image processor.
25. Pick exam and mode under which image should be processed.
26. Wait for image reader to indicate that the image has been processed and the imaging plate erased, and then remove plate from reader.
27. Record the date, time, number of films, name, room number, technique used, and patient history on the requisition.
28. Properly evaluate images. Adjust technical quality as needed. If no images require repeating, send images to reading station and create hard copies when required.
29. Place a correct patient exam card in the designated computer terminal completed box, including the time, room number, number of radiographs, and rejects.
30. Assist the patient from table to wheel chair, cart, or walking position.
31. Open the door for the patient.
32. Explain to outpatients where they are to go next. Take inpatients to the proper holding area and place a "To Go" card in the transaide area.
33. Straighten up the radiographic room, change linens, and clean table off with alcohol.
34. Wash your hands.

*Submitted by Kathy Martensen, BS, RT (R), University of Iowa Hospitals and Clinics, Iowa City, Iowa.

1

Room and Exam Preparation

After preparing the room (protocol steps 1 to 4 on previous page), identifying and greeting the patient, and carefully explaining the procedure (protocol steps 5 to 8), the technologist begins the patient positioning process.

Positioning Methods and Steps

Much of a general diagnostic technologist's work involves steps 9 to 19 of the sample protocols. This includes careful and accurate positioning of the patient in such a way as to demonstrate correctly on image receptors certain body parts as requested by a physician for diagnostic purposes. For the student technologist, radiographic positioning skills become a central or core function or skill that every technologist must learn and master.

FIXED VS. FLOATING TABLETOP

Factors influencing the positioning process or steps include the type of equipment being used. One example is the specific type of x-ray table, namely the economical **fixed tabletop** type (more common in physicians' offices or clinics), versus the **floating tabletop** type commonly used in radiology departments.

Most modern x-ray tables have a floating tabletop, which allows the technologist to easily move both the patient and tabletop together in any direction without having to physically slide or move the patient with the sheet as is required on a fixed tabletop. Some floating tabletops are moved manually by activating a release hand switch that allows the tabletop to be manually moved either lengthwise or crosswise. Other table types, when used in combination with fluoroscopy, have motor-driven features that electrically move the tabletop either crosswise or lengthwise when these switches are pressed. These switches or controls are on the front of the table or on the fluoroscopy unit controls (see technologist's left hand in Fig. 1-108).

Cassette Tray and Bucky Grid Each of these table types has a pullout cassette tray under the table, which includes a Bucky-type moving grid.

In general, the specific positioning method and steps as described in this text are the same with film-screen imaging or with digital imaging. Positioning is also similar with either the floating tabletop and separate movable Bucky tray or the fixed tabletop and movable Bucky tray combination.

BEAM-RESTRICTING DEVICES

All modern equipment includes an **illuminated adjustable collimator,** which allows careful and accurate restriction of the x-ray beam field-size in each of the four dimensions. Most adjustable collimators also include positive beam limitation (PBL) features that automatically collimate to the cassette size in the Bucky tray. All x-ray equipment built between 1974 and 1993 in the United States and Canada is required to include PBL features. (See Radiation Protection in Chapter 2 for more information on PBL systems and requirements.)

These adjustable collimators include a projected light field and central ray (CR) location as visible on the patient's left knee and on the partially pulled out Bucky tray and cassette as shown in Fig. 1-109. This allows for accurate visualization of the size and location of the actual projected x-ray beam in relation to the specific part or area of the patient being radiographed. The lighted exposure field from the collimator also contains centering lines and a central circle or cross indicating the location of the CR on the specific body part.

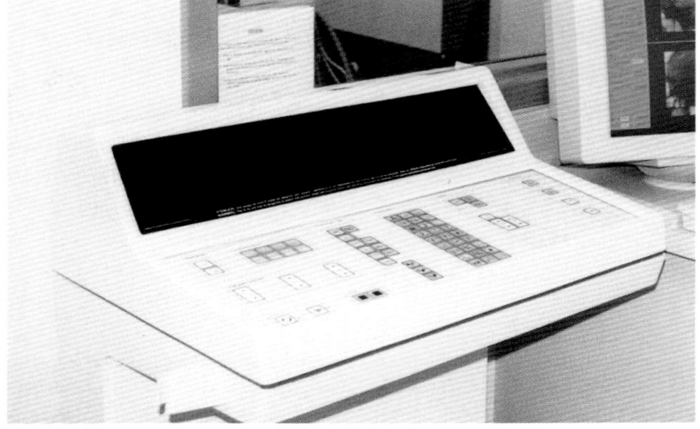

Fig. 1-107. Control panel, includes three exposure variables—kV, mA, and time(s) in seconds.

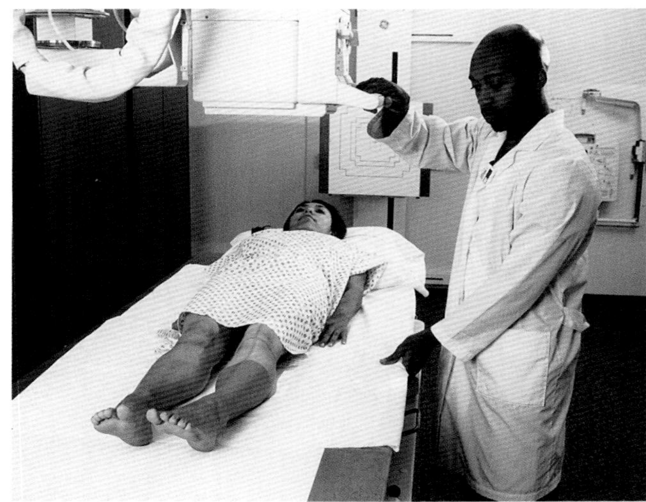

Fig. 1-108. Floating tabletop and movable Bucky tray (patient and tabletop move together).

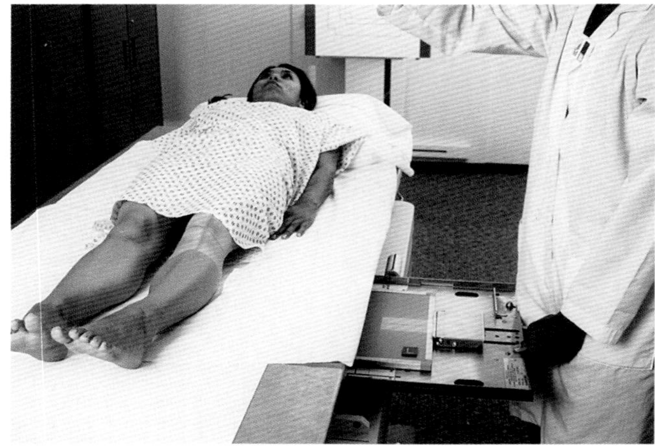

Fig. 1-109. Adjustable collimator (x-ray beam limitation device). Includes illuminated exposure field containing center area CR lines and a CR indicator light projected onto the Bucky tray.

POSITIONING SEQUENCE AND ROUTINE (PROTOCOLS 9-19)

With time and experience, each technologist develops a sequence or positioning routine that works best with the specific equipment being used. However, for the student initially learning the steps and principles of radiographic positioning, an orderly and systemized step-by-step procedure for the positioning parts of the protocol is described below. This prevents the development of careless and inaccurate habits that may result in inconsistent and sloppy work.

Step 1. General Patient Positioning (Protocol 9)

For an exam performed on the x-ray table, the positioning process begins by assisting the patient onto the x-ray table and into one of the following body positions: supine, prone, lateral, or oblique (Fig. 1-110).

The correct size cassette should be placed in the Bucky tray either lengthwise or crosswise or under the part being radiographed for tabletop exams.

Note: The x-ray tube should have been checked to ensure that the central ray (CR) of the collimator light is centered to the center line of the table when the table is in the center "notched" position. (This should be done before the patient is placed on the x-ray table.) This ensures that the CR and x-ray beam, when used for part centering, will be aligned correctly with the IR when the cassette in the Bucky tray is pushed in all the way.

Step 2. Measuring Part Thickness (Protocol 10)

The body part being radiographed is then measured, and the correct exposure factors (technique) are set on the control panel (protocol 12). Part measurement is not required if AEC (automatic exposure control) is used.

Step 3. Part Positioning (Protocol 13)

For most projections the specific body part being examined is first positioned in relation to the central ray (CR). This means that for these projections the **CR is first, or primary, in the positioning process.** The patient is turned and moved as needed to center the body part to the CR. In this example (Fig. 1-112), the patient and tabletop (with floating-type tabletop) is moved to align the correct body part (knee) to the CR as indicated by the "+" in the light field.

Step 4. Image Receptor (IR) Centering (Protocols 14-19)

After the part has been centered to the CR, the **IR is also centered to the CR.** The image receptor (IR) may be the traditional film-screen cassette or an image plate with computed radiography systems. For table Bucky procedures, this centering is done by moving the IR in the Bucky tray longitudinally to center the IR to the projected center light of the CR (Fig. 1-113).

Central Ray (CR) Icon ⌖ This icon is included on each positioning page in this textbook for those projections in which the **CR is of primary importance,** reminding the technologist to pay special attention to the CR during the positioning process.

Accurate CR centering is especially important for upper and lower limbs, wherein joints are the primary interest area and the CR must be accurately directed to the mid-joint region. This is also important when using AEC and for digital receptors, wherein correct CR centering is essential for correctly exposed images.

Collimation The collimator light borders are then adjusted or closed as needed to include only the essential anatomy.

Markers The R or L marker is placed correctly to be in the exposure field without covering essential anatomy (protocol 14).

Final Positioning Step A final check for correct gonadal shield placement should be done (protocol 16) before making the exposure, with breathing instructions as needed (protocols 18 and 19).

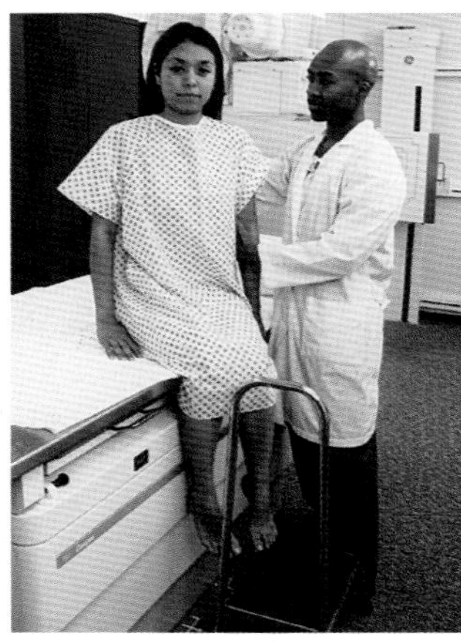

Fig. 1-110. Step 1: Patient positioning (onto x-ray table).

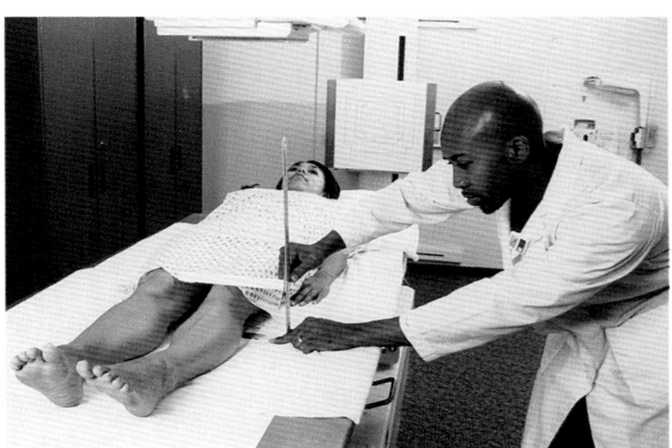

Fig. 1-111. Step 2: Part measured.

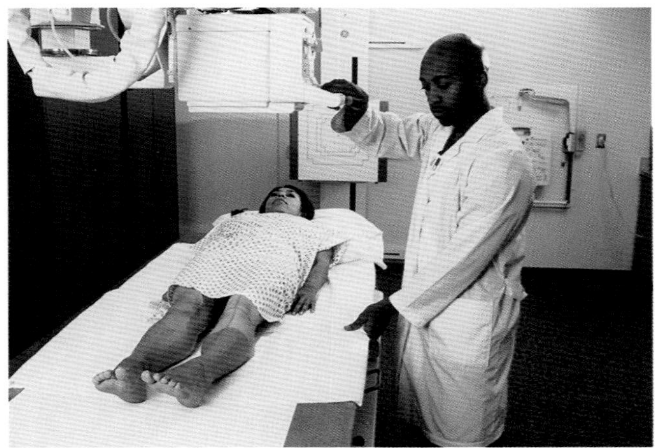

Fig. 1-112. Step 3: Part positioning. ⌖ Part centered to CR (knee is being aligned to CR with floating tabletop).

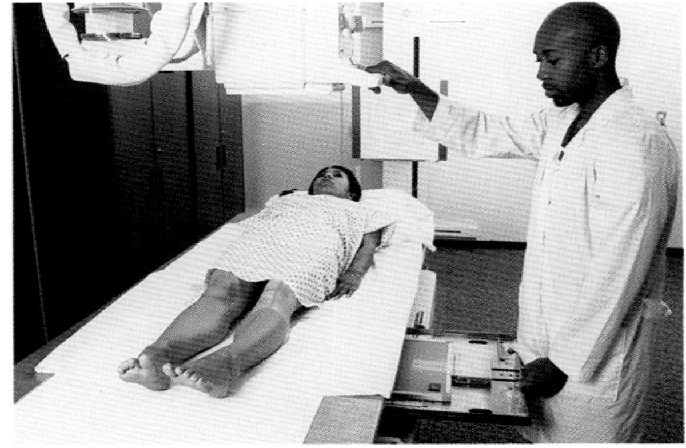

Fig. 1-113. Step 4: IR positioning. ⌖ IR centered to CR (cassette in Bucky tray is aligned lengthwise to CR).

Essential Projections

ROUTINE (BASIC) PROJECTIONS

Certain routine or basic projections are listed and described in this text for each radiographic examination or procedure commonly performed throughout the United States and Canada. Routine or basic projections are defined as **those projections commonly taken on all average patients who can cooperate fully.** This, of course, varies depending on the radiologist's preference and geographical differences.

SPECIAL (ALTERNATE) PROJECTIONS

In addition to the routine or basic projections, certain special or alternative projections are also included for each examination or procedure described in this text. These are defined as **those projections most commonly taken to better demonstrate specific anatomic parts or certain pathologic conditions or those that may be necessary for patients who cannot cooperate fully.**

This author recommends (on the basis of recent survey results) that all students learn and demonstrate proficiency for all essential projections as listed in this text. This includes all routine (basic) projections, as well as all special (alternative) projections, as listed and described in each chapter. An example of these basic and special projection boxes for Chapter 3 (Chest) are shown on the right. Knowing all of these projections ensures that students are prepared to function as imaging technologists in any part of the country.

Principles for Determining Positioning Routines

Two general rules or principles are helpful in remembering and understanding the reasons that certain minimum projections are routine or basic for various radiographic examinations.

A MINIMUM OF TWO PROJECTIONS (90° FROM EACH OTHER)

The first general rule in diagnostic radiology suggests that a **minimum of two projections** taken as near 90° from each other as possible are required for most radiographic procedures. Exceptions include an AP mobile (portable) chest, a single AP abdomen (called a KUB—kidneys, ureter, and bladder), or an AP of the pelvis, in which only one projection provides ample initial information.

Three reasons for this general rule of a minimum of two projections are as follows:

1. Superimposition of Anatomic Structures Certain pathologic conditions (such as some fractures, small tumors) may not be visualized on one projection only.

2. Localization of Lesions or Foreign Bodies A minimum of two projections, taken at 90° or as near right angles from each other as possible, are essential in determining the location of any lesion or foreign body (Fig. 1-114).

Example: Foreign bodies (the white densities are metallic fragments) embedded in tissues of the hand. Note that both the PA and lateral projections are necessary to determine the exact location of these metallic fragments in two dimensions.

3. Determination of Alignment of Fractures All fractures require a minimum of two projections, taken at 90° or as near right angles as possible, both to visualize fully the fracture site and to determine alignment of the fractured parts (Figs. 1-115 and 1-116).

Chest
BASIC
- PA 96
- Lateral 98

Upper Airway
BASIC
- Lateral 105
- AP 106

Chest
SPECIAL
- AP supine or semierect 100
- Lateral decubitus 101
- AP lordotic 100
- Anterior obliques 103
- Posterior obliques 104

Sample basic and special routines boxes for Chapter 3, Chest.

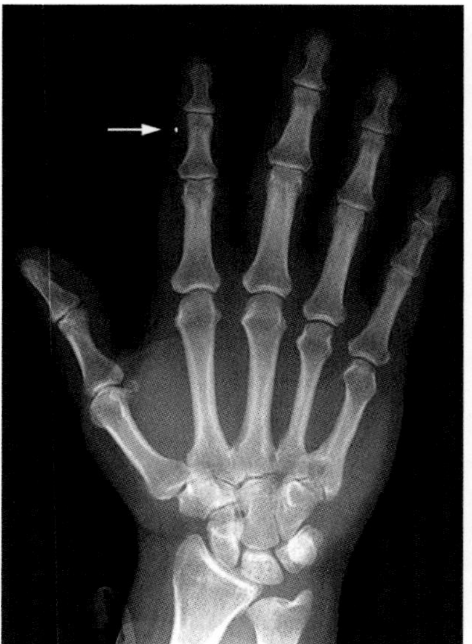
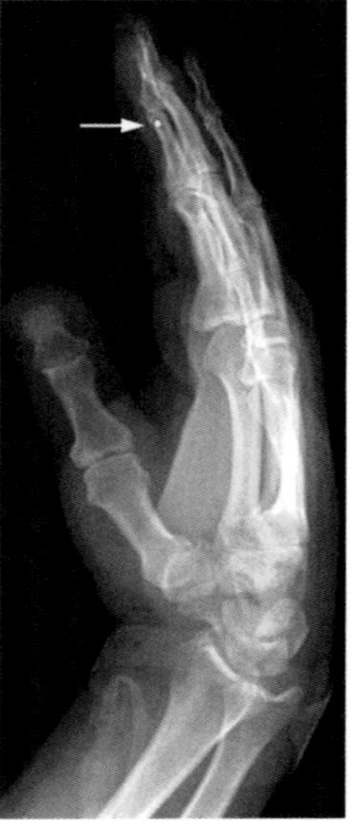

Fig. 1-114. Foreign bodies (metallic fragment in soft tissue).

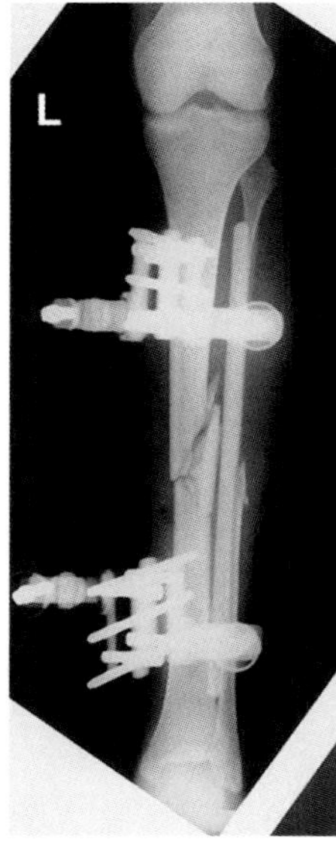

Fig. 1-115. AP for fracture alignment.

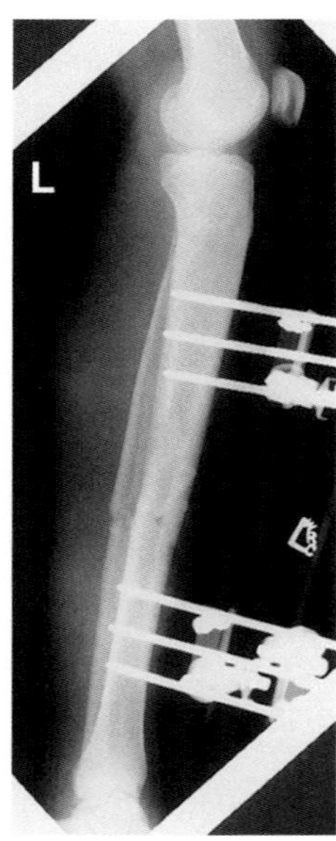

Fig. 1-116. Lateral for fracture alignment.

A MINIMUM OF THREE PROJECTIONS WHEN JOINTS ARE IN INTEREST AREA

This second general rule or principle suggests that all radiographic procedures of the skeletal system involving joints require a minimum of **three** projections rather than only two. These are **AP** or **PA, lateral,** and **oblique.**

The reason for this rule is that more information is needed than can be provided on only two projections. For example, with the multiple surfaces and angles of the bones making up the joint, a small oblique chip fracture or other abnormality within the joint space may not be visualized on either the frontal or the lateral views but may be well demonstrated in the oblique position.

Examples of exams generally requiring **three** projections as routine or basic (joint is in prime interest area):

- Fingers
- Hand
- Elbow
- Foot
- Toes
- Wrist
- Ankle
- Knee

Examples of exams requiring **two** projections as routine or basic:

- Forearm
- Hips
- Postreduction upper and lower limbs (only two projections for alignment purposes, even if joint is in prime interest area)
- Humerus
- Tibia-fibula
- Femur
- Chest

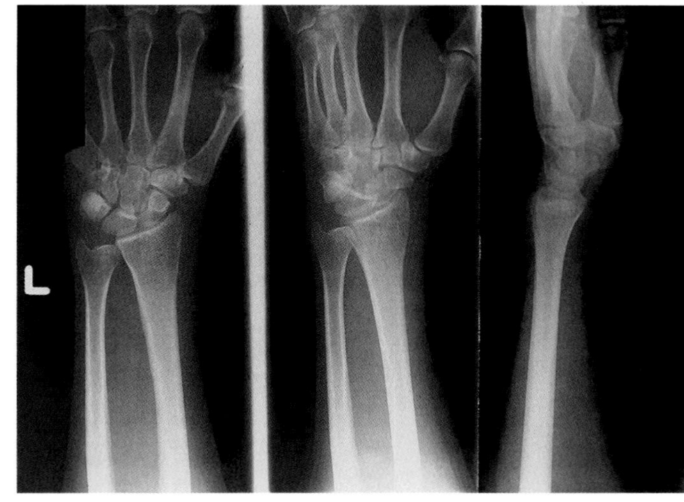

Fig. 1-117. Wrist—requires three projections.

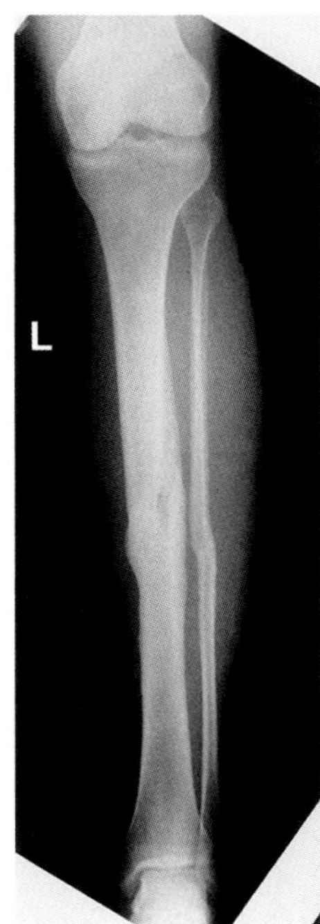

Fig. 1-118.

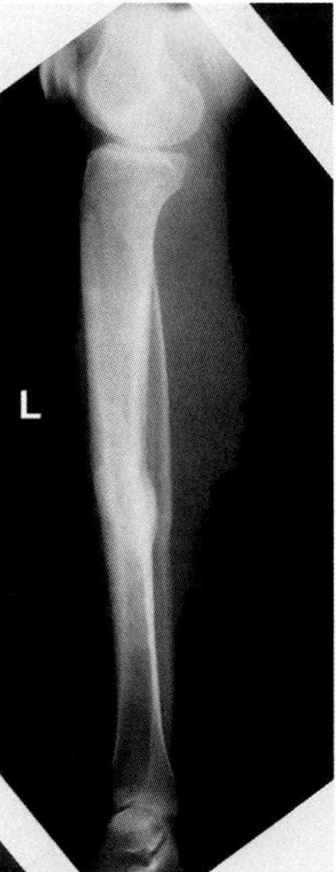

Fig. 1-119.

Lower leg—requires two projections/positions.
Note: This is the same patient as in Figs. 1-115 and 1-116 on preceding page, now demonstrating the healed fractures correctly aligned.

IMAGE RECEPTOR (FILM) SIZES

Use of metric (SI) units for all film-screen cassettes (or image plates with computed radiography) is increasingly common throughout the world, including the United States. However, several sizes of image receptors are still available in both English (traditional) and metric (System Internationale) sizes as indicated below:

TABLE OF COMMONLY AVAILABLE IR SIZES

METRIC (SI)	TRADITIONAL (ENGLISH)	USE
18 × 24 cm	(7.1 × 9.5 inches)	Mammography
(20.3 × 25.4 cm)	***8 × 10 inches***	General
24 × 24 cm	(9.5 × 9.5 inches)	Fluoro & general
(25.4 × 30.5 cm)	***10 × 12 inches***	Grid cassettes
24 × 30 cm	(9.5 × 11.8 inches)	General & mammo
18 × 43 cm	(7.1 × 16.9 inches)	Upper & lower limbs
(17.8 × 43.2 cm)	7 × 17 inches	Upper & lower limbs
30 × 35 cm	(11.8 × 13.8 inches)	General
35 × 35 cm	(13.8 × 13.8 inches)	General
35 × 43 cm	(13.8 × 16.9 inches)	General
(35.6 × 43.2 cm)	14 × 17 inches	General
(35.6 × 91.4 cm)	***14 × 36 inches***	Erect spine
(35.6 × 129.6 cm)	***14 × 51 inches***	Full lower limb
(12.7 × 30.5 cm)	***5 × 12 inches***	Mandible
(22.9 × 30.5 cm)	***9 × 12 inches***	(Panorama)
Image Plates With Computed Radiography (CR)		
18 × 24 cm or	**8 × 10 inches**	General
24 × 30 cm or	**10 × 12 inches**	General
35 × 35 cm	(13.8 × 13.8 inches)	General
35 × 43 cm	(13.8 × 16.9 inches)	General
Direct Conversion Digital Detectors With Digital Radiography (DR)		
Maximum—**43 × 49 cm**	(17 × 19 inches)	Chest unit
Maximum—**41 × 41 cm**	(16 × 16 inches)	Chest unit
Maximum—**43 × 43 cm**	(17 × 17 inches)	Table Bucky unit
Maximum—**19 × 23 cm**	(7.5 × 9 inches)	Mammography

*Film sizes most commonly available (in bold).

(In the table above, sizes marked * in the original are shown as ***bold italic***.)

CONVERSION TABLES

English—Metric Conversions

1 inch = 2.54 cm
1 cm = 0.3937 inch

SID Conversions

40 inches = 101.60 or **100** cm, or 1 meter*
44 inches = 111.76 or **110** cm*
48 inches = 121.92 or **120** cm*
72 inches = 182.88 or **180** cm*

*In practice, 40 inches SID is commonly equated to an even 100 cm (1 meter), 44 inches to 110 cm, 48 inches to 120 cm, and 72 inches to 180 cm.

Topographic Positioning Landmarks

Radiographic positioning requires the location of specific structures or organs within the body, many of which are not visible to the human eye from the exterior. Therefore certain landmarks that are parts of the bony skeleton as shown on these drawings can be located by gentle palpation and used to locate internal structures or organs.

Palpation: **Palpation** refers to the process of applying light pressure with the fingertips directly on the patient to locate these positioning landmarks. **This must be done gently** because the area being palpated may be painful or sensitive for the patient. Also, **the patient should always be informed of the purpose of this palpation before beginning this process, and their permission should be obtained.**

POSITIONING AND BONY LANDMARKS

Throughout this textbook bony landmarks are used as guides for radiographic positioning. On actual patients, most of these landmarks are not visible under clothing or hospital gowns, and palpation is required to locate them for accurate positioning.

Note: Palpation of certain of these landmarks, such as the ischial tuberosity (10) and/or symphysis pubis (9), may be embarrassing for the patient, and technologists should use other related landmarks as described in later chapters.

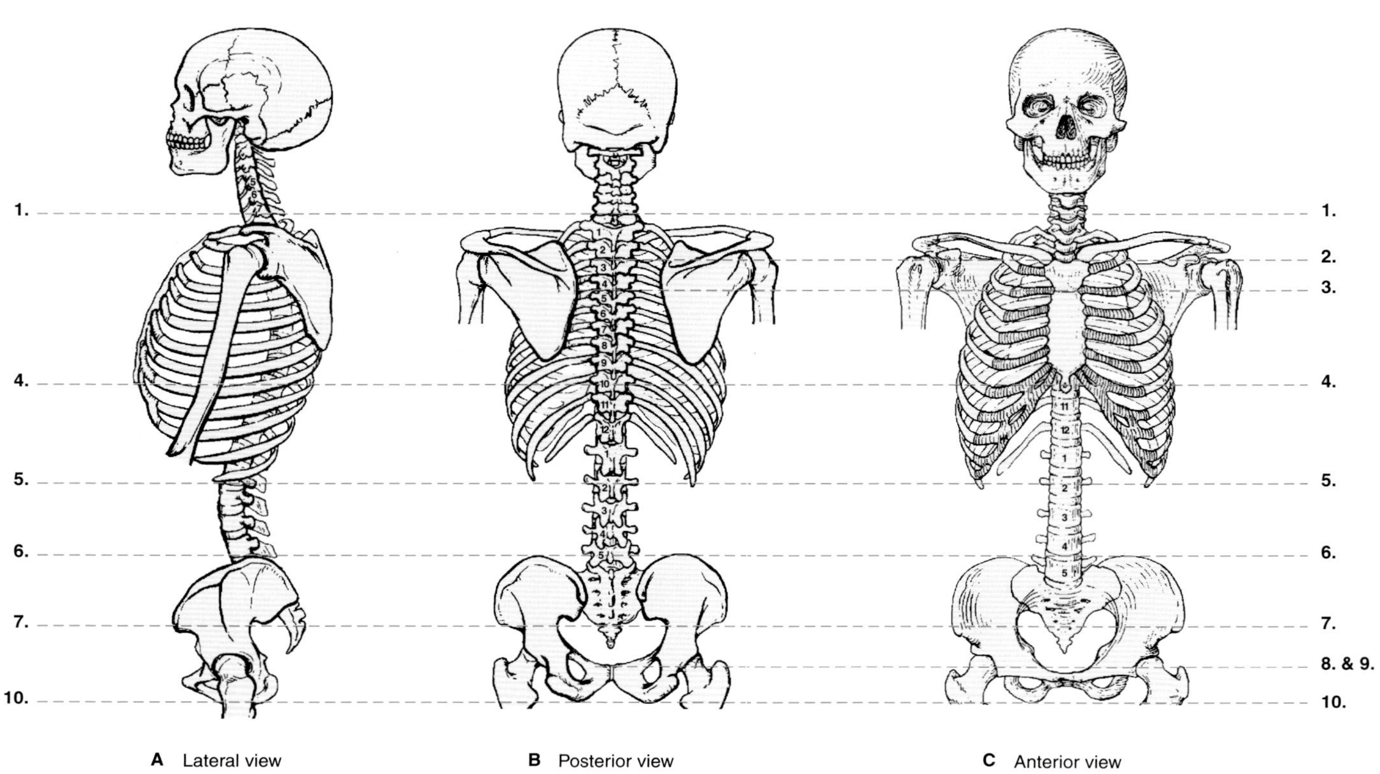

Fig. 1-120. Positioning landmarks. **A,** Lateral view. **B,** Posterior view. **C,** Anterior view.

BONY LANDMARKS

LANDMARK	USED FOR POSITIONING THESE BODY PARTS	CORRESPONDING LEVEL OF VERTEBRAL COLUMN
1. **Vertebra prominens** (long spinous process of C7)	Upper margin of chest, C- or T-spine	C7–T1
2. **Jugular notch** (superior margin of sternum)	Chest, sternum, clavicle, T-spine	T2-3
3. **Sternal angle** (raised area of junction of manubrium and body of sternum)	Chest, sternum	T4–5
4. **Xiphoid process** (distal portion of sternum)	Sternum, stomach, gallbladder, T-spine, upper margin of abdomen	T9-10
5. **Inferior costal (rib) margin** (lateral inferior border of rib cage)	Stomach, gallbladder, ribs	L2–3
6. **Iliac crest** (uppermost margin of curved border of ilium portion of pelvis)	Midabdomen, stomach, gallbladder, colon, L-spine, sacrum	L4-5 interspace
7. **Anterior superior iliac spine (ASIS)** (prominent anterior border of iliac crest)	Hips, pelvis, sacrum	S1–2
8. **Greater trochanter** (bony process of proximal femur; to locate requires firm palpation while rotating leg and femur)	Abdomen, pelvis, hip	Distal coccyx or slightly inferior to
9. **Symphysis pubis** (anterior junction of pubic bones of pelvis)	Lower margin of abdomen, pelvis, hip, sacrum, coccyx	≈ 1 inch (2.5 cm) inferior to distal coccyx
10. **Ischial tuberosity** (lowermost, posteriorly located bony process of pelvis)	Prone abdomen, colon, coccyx	1 to 2 inches (2.5 to 5 cm) inferior to distal coccyx

Body Habitus

Radiographic positioning requires an understanding of the common variations in body form or shape (habitus). This variation in form or shape of the body has a significant effect on the shape and location of internal body organs. Therefore each technologist must learn to recognize these body types and know the effect on internal organs as described in each chapter pertaining to the positioning of these organ systems.

The four common body types are illustrated by the drawings below, with appropriate percentages of the general population represented by each type.

Hypersthenic: This "stocky," massive build body type represents only 5% of the population. The thoracic cavity is wide and deep from front to back with a short vertical dimension, indicating a high diaphragm. This also makes the upper abdomen very wide, affecting the location of organs such as the gallbladder, stomach, and colon as seen in this drawing and as described in later chapters.

Sthenic: This represents the nearer average but slightly heavy-set and frequently more muscular-type persons. The chest and abdominal organs are nearer average in shape and location but tend toward the hypersthenic, massive body type as seen on the drawing below.

Hyposthenic: This represents the nearer average but more slender and sometimes taller body type. The gallbladder and stomach are lower and nearer the centerline, with the colon also located somewhat lower in the abdomen.

Asthenic: This is the more extreme slender body type (10%) with a thoracic cavity that is narrow and shallow but with a long vertical dimension, indicating a low diaphragm. The upper abdomen is also narrower on top and wider at its lower dimension, placing most of the abdominal organs low in the abdomen.

General population and body types: The photographs below represent examples of the more common body types found among the general population.

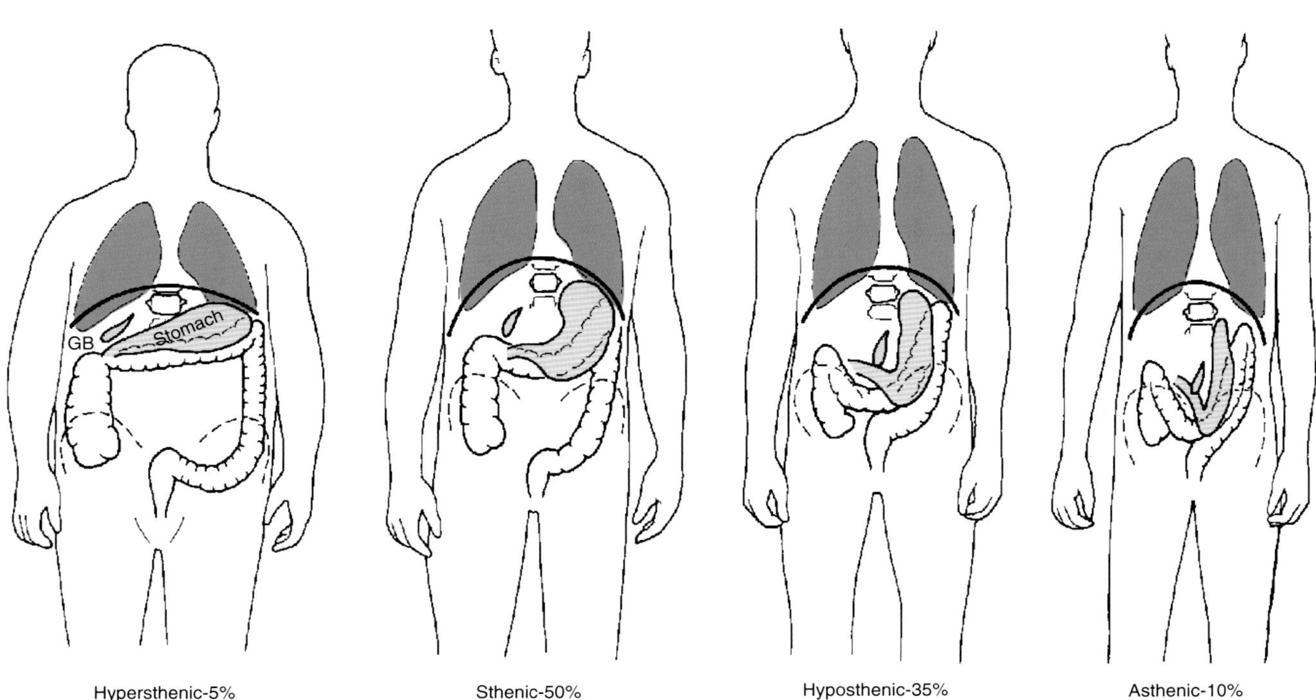

Fig. 1-121. Body habitus types.

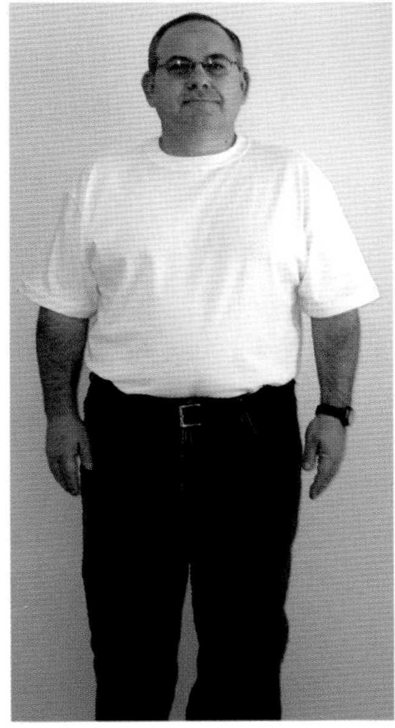

Fig. 1-122. Hypersthenic/sthenic.

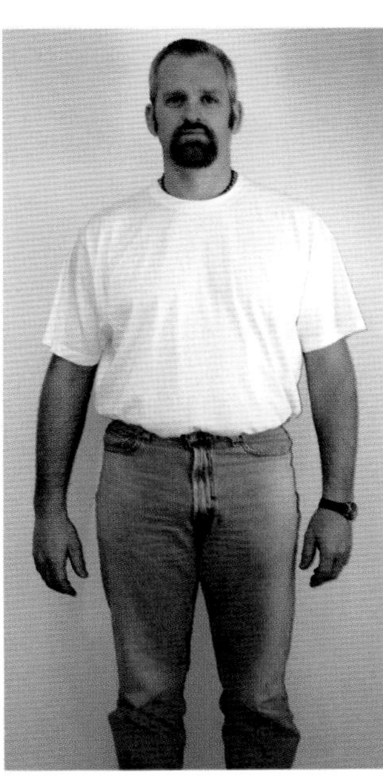

Fig. 1-123. Sthenic.

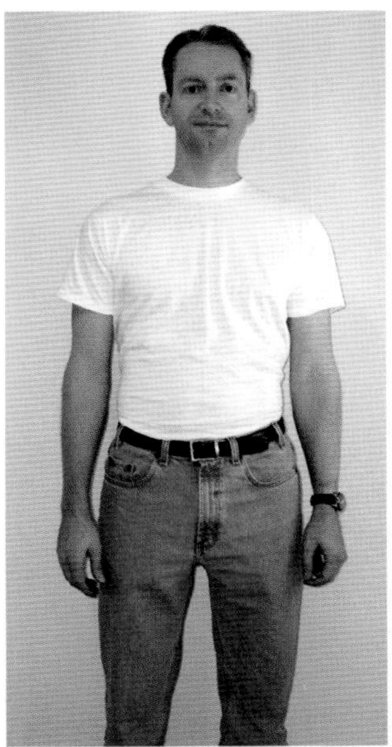

Fig. 1-124. Hyposthenic/asthenic.

Viewing Radiographic Images

The way **PA** and **AP projection** radiographic images are placed for viewing depends on the radiologist's preference and the most common practice in that part of the country. However, in the United States and Canada a common and accepted way to place radiographic images for viewing is to display them **so that the patient is facing the viewer,** with the patient in the anatomic position. **This always places the patient's left to the viewer's right.** This is true for **either AP or PA projections.**

Lateral positions are marked R or L by the side of the patient closest to the IR. The placement of lateral radiographic images for viewing varies depending on the radiologist's preference. One common method is to place the image so that the viewer is seeing the image from the same perspective as the x-ray tube. Thus if the left marker is placed anteriorly to the patient, the L would be on the viewer's right (Fig. 1-129). Some radiologists, however, prefer to view laterals turned 90° and viewed so that the anteriorly placed L marker is on the viewer's left. Technologists should determine the preferred method for viewing laterals in their department.

PA or AP oblique projections are placed for viewing the same as a PA or AP projection, with the patient's right to the viewer's left.

Decubitus chests and abdomens are generally viewed the way the x-ray tube "sees" them, placed crosswise with the upside of the patient also on the upper part of the view box (Fig. 1-128).

Upper and lower limbs are viewed as projected by the x-ray beam onto the IR; the R or L lead marker appears right-side-up if it has been placed on the IR correctly.

Images including the digits (hands and feet) are generally placed with the **digits up.** Other images of the limbs, however, are viewed in the anatomic position with the **limbs hanging down** (Fig. 1-131).

Viewing CT or MRI Images

The generally accepted way of viewing all CT and MRI axial images is similar to that for conventional radiographs even though the image represents a thin "slice" or sectional view of anatomic structures. In general, these images are again placed **so the patient's right is to the viewer's left** (Fig. 1-130).

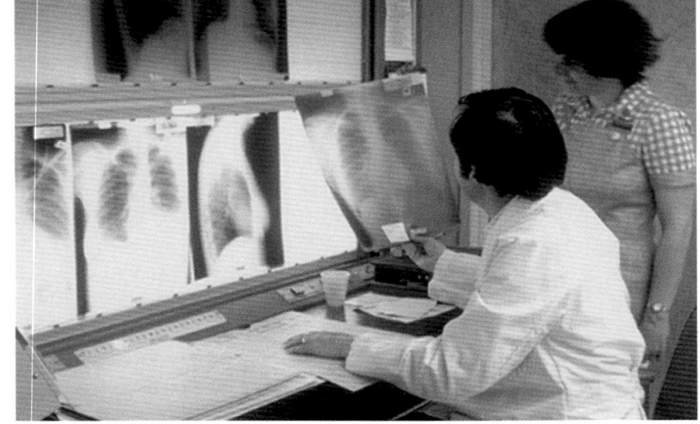

Fig. 1-125. Viewing chest radiographs (patient's right always to viewer's left, both PA and AP).

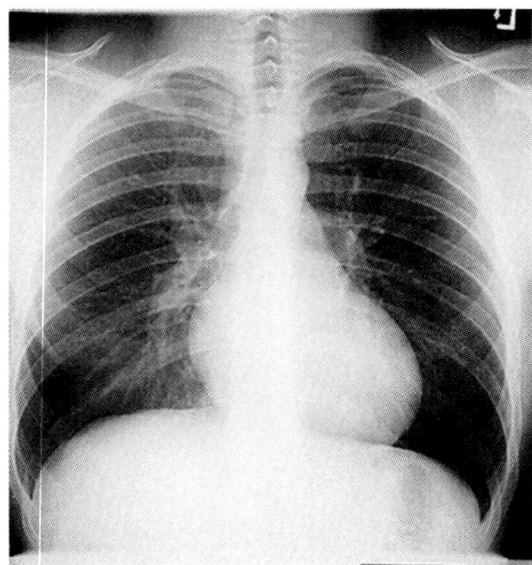

Fig. 1-126. PA chest (L appears reversed).

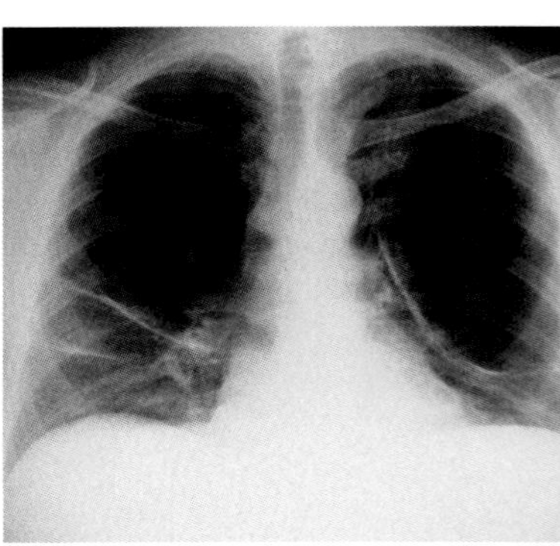

Fig. 1-127. AP chest (L appears right-side-up).

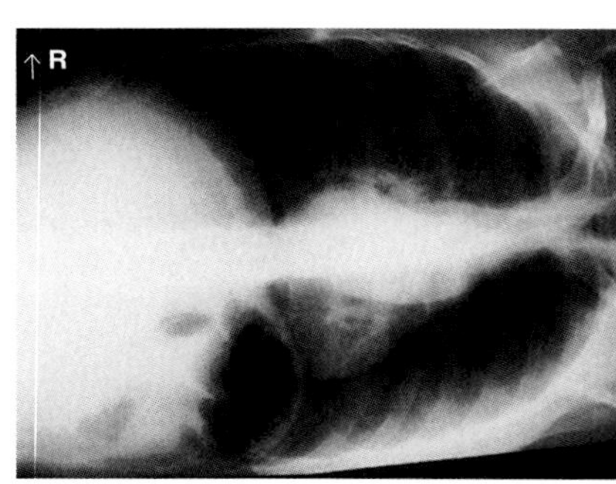

Fig. 1-128. Left lateral decubitus chest.

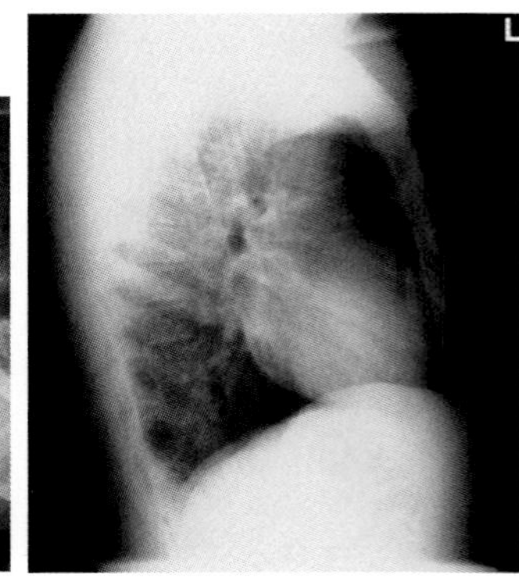

Fig. 1-129. Left lateral chest.

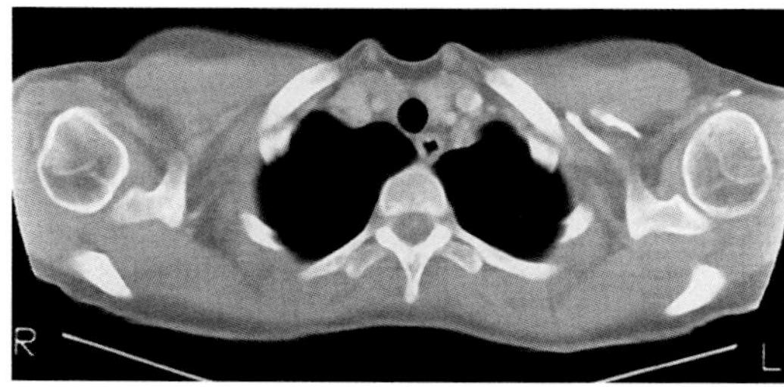

Fig. 1-130. Axial (cross-sectional) image (upper thorax—level of T3); patient's right to viewer's left.

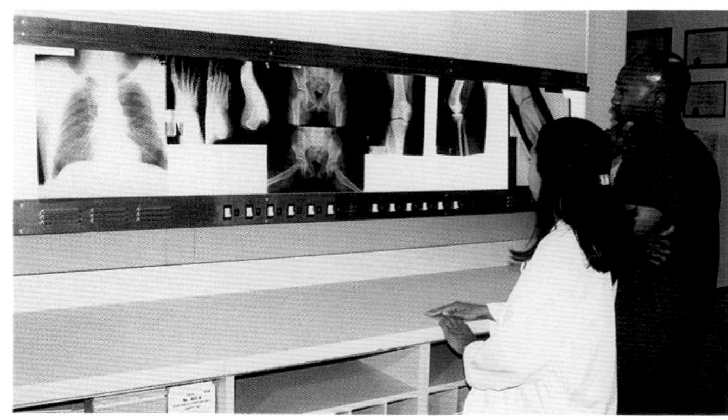

Fig. 1-131. Viewing upper or lower limb radiographs (hands and feet, digits up).

CHAPTER 2

Image Quality, Digital Technology, and Radiation Protection

CONTRIBUTIONS BY **Cindy Murphy,** RT R, ACR, BHSC, **Joseph Popovitch,** RT R, ACR, DHSA, **Richard Geise,** PhD, FACR, FAAPM

CONTRIBUTORS TO PAST EDITIONS Kathy M. Martensen, BS, RT(R), E. Russel Ritenour, PhD, Barry T. Anthony, RT(R)

CONTENTS

IMAGE QUALITY IN FILM-SCREEN IMAGING

Introduction

Since the discovery of x-rays in 1895, methods of acquiring and storing x-ray images have evolved. Conventional film-screen technology with the associated chemical processing and film libraries is rapidly being replaced by digital technology. Digital technology utilizes computers and detectors to acquire and process images; specialized digital communication networks are used to transmit and store the x-ray images.

This period of technological transition necessitates that students have an understanding of all image acquisition technologies because they will find themselves working in imaging departments that acquire images using only digital technology, only film-screen technology, or a combination of both. Although the pace and degree of technological change require ongoing curriculum revisions in some subjects, other aspects of radiologic technology will not change. Examples of this are radiographic anatomy, positioning, patient care, and radiation protection principles. These remain constant, and radiologic technologists who are already certified can keep current with the technological advances, such as those in digital imaging, through professional continuing education.

Chapter 2 provides an introduction to radiographic technique and image quality for both film-screen imaging and digital imaging. This study of radiographic technique and image quality includes factors that determine the accuracy with which the structures being imaged are reproduced in the image. Each of these factors has a specific effect on the final image, and the technologist must strive to maximize these factors to produce the best image possible.

Chapter 2 also describes methods of digital image acquisition, discusses the application of digital imaging, and provides an introduction to the important principles of radiation safety.

Film Images

Film images (defined as radiographs) provide a two-dimensional image of anatomic structures. The exposed film must undergo chemical processing (developing, fixing, washing, and drying) for the image to be visible. The film image, which is actually composed of a deposit of metallic silver on a polyester base, is permanent; it cannot be altered. The various shades of gray displayed on the image are representative of the densities and atomic numbers of the tissues being examined. The film image or radiograph is often referred to as a "hard-copy."

Exposure Factors for Film-Screen Imaging

The radiographer must select *exposure factors* on the control panel of the imaging equipment each time a radiographic image is to be produced. The exposure factors required for each examination will be determined by numerous variables, including the density/atomic number and thickness of the anatomic part, the speed of the film-screen system, and any pathology present.

Exposure factors, sometimes referred to as *technique factors,* include:

- **Kilovoltage** (kV)—controls the energy (penetrating power) of the x-ray beam
- **Milliamperage** (mA)—controls the quantity or number of x-rays produced
- **Exposure time** (ms)—controls the duration of the exposure, usually expressed in milliseconds

Each of these exposure factors has a specific effect on the quality of the radiographic image. When performing radiographic procedures, technologists must apply their knowledge of exposure factors and imaging principles to ensure the images obtained are of the **highest quality possible,** while exposing the patients to the **lowest radiation dose possible.**

Notes:

1. ***kV (kVp)***—*In the past kVp (kilovoltage peak) was used to indicate the peak voltage with single-phase generators, which are seldom used today. With current three-phase high-frequency generators, the peak kV and average kV are essentially the same. Therefore in this text* ***kV*** *will be used rather than kVp.*
2. ***mAs***—*The factors milliamperage (mA) and time (s) are expressed as the product of mA multiplied by time, which equals milliampere seconds (mAs).*
3. ***AEC***—*Many units are equipped with automatic exposure control (AEC). These systems provide automatic termination of exposure time when sufficient radiation (exposure) is received by the selected ionization chamber cell.*

Image Quality Factors

Film-based radiographic images are evaluated on **four quality factors.** These four primary image quality factors are:

- Density
- Contrast
- Resolution
- Distortion

Each of these four factors has specific parameters by which it is controlled.

DENSITY

Definition

Radiographic density is defined as the **amount of "blackness" on the processed film image.** When a film image (radiograph) with high density is viewed, less light is transmitted through the image.

Controlling Factors

The **primary controlling factor** of film density is **mAs.** mAs controls density by controlling the quantity of x-rays emitted from the x-ray tube and the duration of the exposure. The relationship for our purpose can be described as linear; doubling the mAs will double the quantity/duration of x-rays emitted, thus doubling the density on the film.

The distance of the x-ray source from the image receptor, or **Source Image Receptor Distance (SID),** also has an effect on radiographic density according to the inverse square law. If the SID is doubled, the intensity of the x-ray beam will be reduced to one-fourth, which then reduces radiographic density to one-fourth. A standard SID is generally used to reduce this variable.

Other factors that influence the density on a film image include kV, part thickness, chemical development time/temperature, grid ratio, and film-screen speed.

Adjusting Film Image Density

When film images (using manual technique settings) are under or overexposed, a general rule states that a minimum change in mAs of 25% to 30% is required to make a visible difference in the radiographic density on the repeat film image (radiograph). Some incorrectly exposed images may require a greater change, frequently 50% to 100%, or sometimes even greater. The radiograph of the hand obtained using 2 mAs in Fig. 2-2 was underexposed; the repeat radiograph was obtained using 4 mAs (Fig. 2-3). Doubling the mAs in this example resulted in doubling the density on the film image. kV should not require an adjustment, providing the optimal kV for the part thickness was used. SID also should not require adjustment; it is a constant.

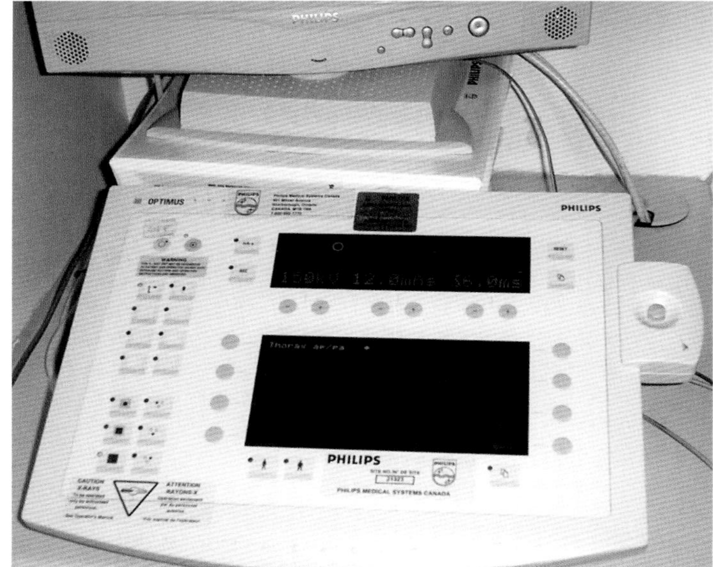

Fig. 2-1. kV, mA, and time (s) controls.

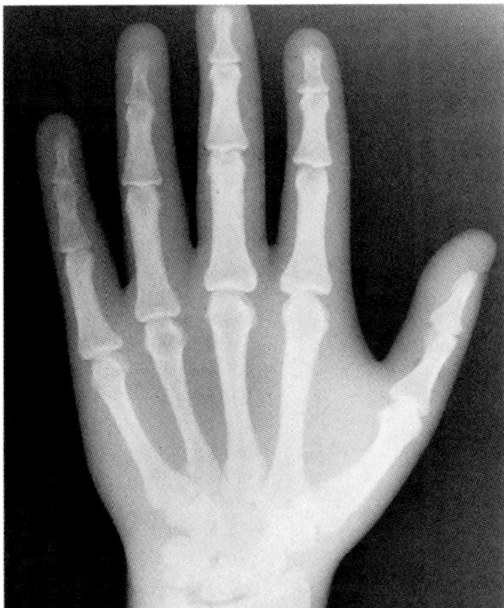

Fig. 2-2. 2 mAs (60 kV)—underexposed.

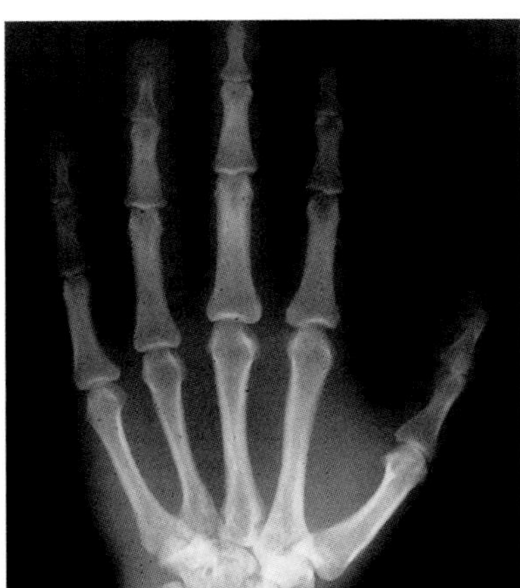

Fig. 2-3. 4 mAs (60 kV)—repeated, double mAs.

Density and the Anode Heel Effect

The intensity of the radiation emitted from the cathode end of the x-ray tube is greater than that at the anode end; this phenomenon is known as the *anode heel effect.* There is greater attenuation or absorption of the x-rays at the anode end because of the angle of the anode; the x-rays emitted from deeper within the anode must travel through more anode material before exiting; thus they are attenuated more.

Studies show that the difference in intensity from the cathode to the anode end of the x-ray field when using a 17-inch (43-cm) image receptor (IR) at 40-inch (100-cm) SID can vary from 30% to 50%, depending on the anode angle* (Fig. 2-4). The anode heel effect is more pronounced when using a shorter SID and a large field size.

Applying the anode heel effect to clinical practice will assist in obtaining quality images of body parts that have a significant variation in thickness along the longitudinal axis of the x-ray field. The patient should be positioned so that the **thicker portion of the part is at the cathode end** of the x-ray tube and the **thinner part is under the anode** (the cathode and anode ends of the x-ray tube are usually marked on the protective housing). The abdomen, thoracic spine, and long bones of the limbs (such as the femur and tibia/fibula) are examples of structures that vary enough in thickness to warrant correct use of the anode heel effect.

On the lower right is a summary chart of body parts and projections for which the anode heel effect can be applied; this is also noted in the positioning pages for each of these projections throughout the text. In practice, the most common use of the anode heel effect is for anteroposterior (AP) projections of the thoracic spine.

It should be noted that it may not always be practical or even possible to take advantage of the anode heel effect; this will depend on the patient's condition or the arrangement of specific x-ray equipment in a room.

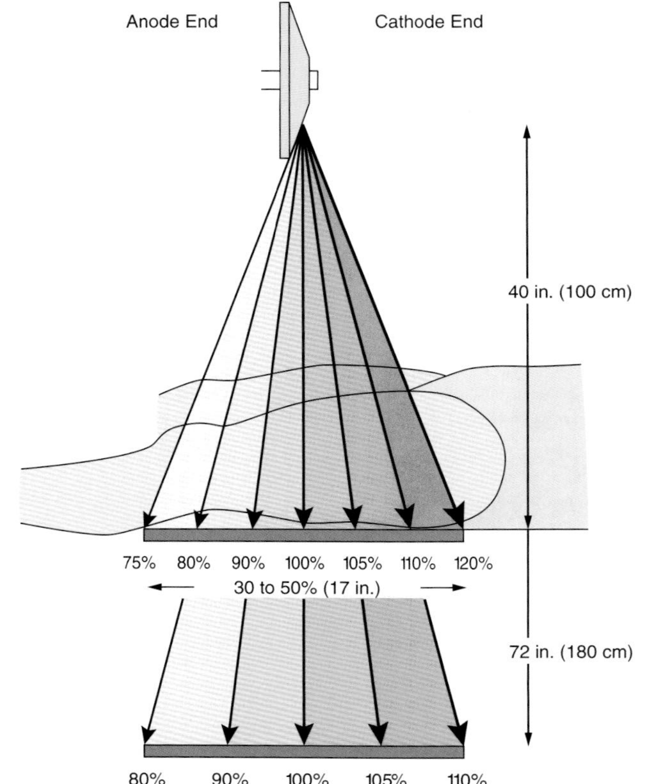

Fig. 2-4. Anode heel effect.

SUMMARY OF ANODE HEEL EFFECT APPLICATIONS		
PROJECTION	**ANODE END**	**CATHODE END**
Thoracic spine • AP	Head	Feet
Femur • AP and lateral (Fig. 2-4)	Feet	Head
Humerus • AP and lateral	Elbow	Shoulder
Leg (tibia/fibula) • AP and lateral	Ankle	Knee
Forearm • AP and lateral	Wrist	Elbow

Compensating Filters

Compensating filters such as wedge filters are sometimes used to filter out a portion of the primary beam toward the thin or less dense part of the body being imaged. This has the same general effect as the correct use of the anode heel effect and in most cases will be much more effective in producing a nearer uniform film density for those body parts with the greatest variation in thickness or tissue density along the length of the image receptor. For example, when a wedge filter is being used on an AP thoracic spine projection, the thicker part of the filter should be placed at the head end of the patient, where the part thickness is less.

Summary of density factors Adequate density, as **primarily controlled by mAs,** must be visible on the processed film to accurately demonstrate the structures being radiographed. Too little density (underexposed) or too much density (overexposed) will not adequately demonstrate the required structures. Correct use of the anode heel effect and/or compensating filters helps to demonstrate optimal film density on anatomic parts that vary significantly in thickness.

*Gratale P, Wright DL, Daughtry L: Using the anode heel effect for extremity radiography, Radiologic Technology (61)3:195, 1990.

CONTRAST

Definition

Radiographic contrast is defined as **the difference in density on adjacent areas of a radiographic image.** The greater this difference, the higher the contrast; the less the density differences, the lower the contrast. This is demonstrated by the step wedge and the chest radiograph in Fig. 2-5, which shows greater differences in densities between adjacent areas; thus this would be **high contrast.** Fig. 2-6 demonstrates **low contrast** with less difference in density on adjacent areas of the step wedge and the associated radiograph.

Contrast can also be described as **long-scale** or **short-scale contrast,** referring to the total range of all optical densities from the lightest to the darkest parts of the radiographic image. This is also demonstrated in Fig. 2-5, which shows short-scale/high-contrast (greater differences in adjacent densities and fewer visible density steps) compared with Fig. 2-6, which illustrates long-scale/low-contrast.

Contrast allows the anatomic detail on a radiographic image to be visualized. Optimum radiographic contrast is therefore important, and an understanding of contrast is essential in evaluating image quality.

Low or high contrast is not necessarily good or bad by itself. For example, low contrast (long-scale contrast) is desirable on radiographic images of the chest. Many shades of gray are required to visualize the fine lung markings, as illustrated by the two chest radiographs in Figs. 2-5 and 2-6. The low-contrast (long-scale contrast) image in Fig. 2-6 demonstrates more shades of gray, as evident by the faint outlines of the vertebrae visible through the heart and mediastinal structures. The shades of gray that outline the vertebrae are less visible through the heart and mediastinum on the high-contrast chest radiograph in Fig. 2-5.

Controlling Factors

The **primary controlling factor** for contrast in film-based imaging is kilovoltage, or **kV.** kV controls the energy or penetrating power of the primary x-ray beam. The higher the kV, the greater the energy and the more uniformly the x-ray beam penetrates the various mass densities of all tissues. Therefore **higher kV** produces less variation in attenuation (differential absorption), resulting in **lower contrast.**

Kilovoltage (kV) is also a **secondary controlling factor** of density. Higher kV, resulting in both more x-rays and greater energy x-rays, will cause more x-ray energy to reach the image receptor (IR) with a corresponding increase in overall density. A general rule of thumb states that a **15% increase in kV will increase film density, similar to doubling the mAs.** Thus in the lower kV range, such as 50 to 70 kV, an 8- to 10-kV increase will double the density (equivalent to doubling the mAs). In the 80- to 100-kV range, a 12- to 15-kV increase is required to double the density. The importance of this relates to radiation protection, because as kV is increased, mAs can be significantly reduced, resulting in less radiation being absorbed by the patient.

There are other factors that affect radiographic contrast. The amount of *scatter* radiation the film-screen receives influences the radiographic contrast. Scatter radiation is radiation that has been changed in direction and intensity as a result of interaction with patient tissue. The amount of scatter produced is dependent on the intensity of the x-ray beam, the amount of tissue irradiated, and the type/thickness of the tissue. Close collimation of the x-ray field reduces the amount of tissue irradiated, thus reducing the amount of scatter produced, thus increasing contrast. Close collimation also reduces the radiation dose to the patient and the technologist.

Irradiation of thick body parts produces a considerable amount of scatter radiation, which will decrease image contrast. A device called a *grid* is used to absorb much of the scatter radiation before it hits the IR. A general rule of thumb is that grids should be used for any body part that measures over 10 cm. Chapter 19 provides rules for correct use of grids.

Summary of contrast factors Selection of the appropriate kV is a balance between optimal image contrast and lowest possible patient dose. A general rule states that the **highest kV and lowest mAs that yield sufficient diagnostic information should be used on each radiographic examination.*** Close collimation and correct use of grids also ensure that the processed radiographic image displays optimal contrast.

*Statkiewicz-Sherer MA, Visconti PJ, Ritenour ER: Radiation protection in medical radiography, ed 3, St. Louis, 1998, Mosby.

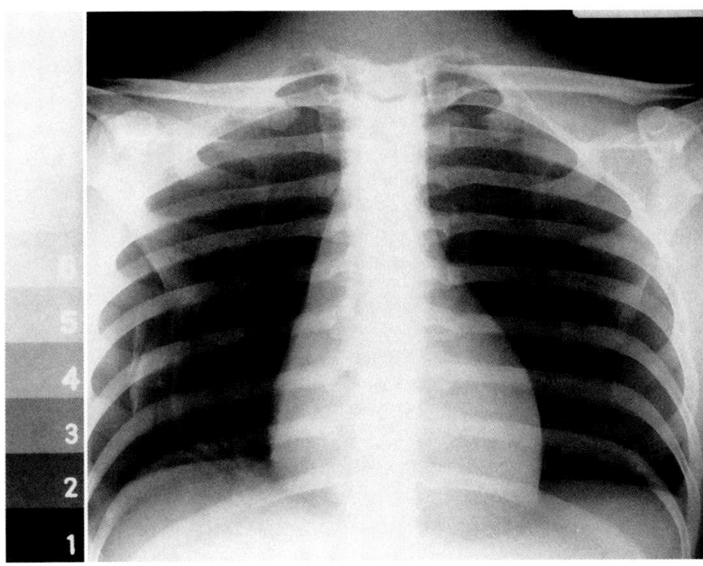

Fig. 2-5. High-contrast, short-scale 50 kV, 800 mAs.

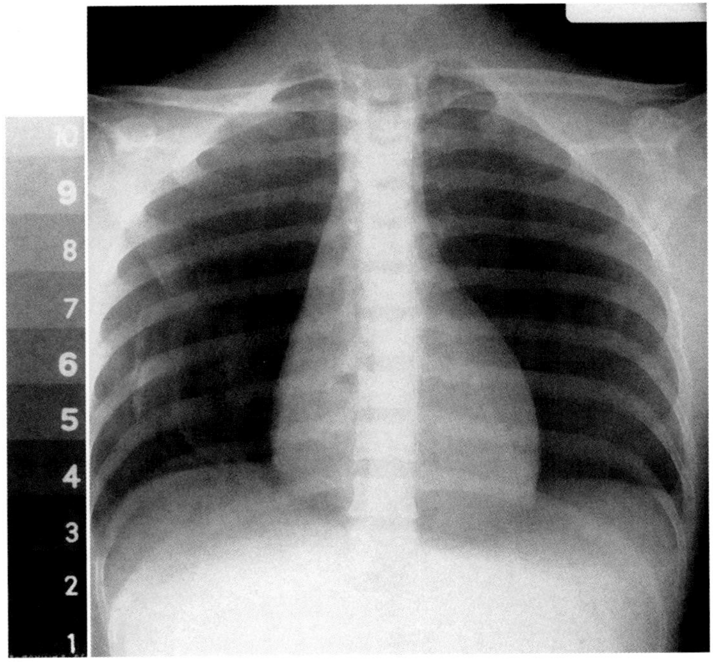

Fig. 2-6. Low-contrast, long-scale 110 kV, 10 mAs.

2

2

RESOLUTION

Definition

Resolution is defined as the **recorded sharpness of structures on the image.** Resolution on a radiographic image is demonstrated by the clarity or sharpness of fine structural lines and borders of tissues or structures on the image. Resolution is also known as **detail, recorded detail, image sharpness,** or **definition.** Resolution of film-screen images is generally measured and expressed as line pairs per millimeter (lp/mm), typically 5 to 6 lp/mm. Lack of visible sharpness or resolution is known as **blur** or **unsharpness.**

Controlling Factors

The optimal radiograph displays a sharp image, as listed under "Radiographic Criteria" for each position in this text. Resolution with film-screen imaging is controlled by **geometric factors, film-screen system,** and **motion.**

Geometric Factors Geometric factors that control/influence resolution are **focal spot size, SID,** and **OID** (Object Image receptor Distance). The effect of OID is explained and illustrated on p. 48, Fig. 2-12.

The use of the **small focal spot** results in **less geometric unsharpness** (see Fig. 2-7). To illustrate, a point source is commonly used as the source of x-rays in the x-ray tube; however, the actual source of x-rays is an area on the anode known as the *focal spot.* Most x-ray tubes are dual focus, that is, they have two focal spots: large and small. Use of the small focal spot results in less unsharpness of the image, or an image with a decreased *penumbra.* Penumbra is the **unsharp edges of the projected image.** However, even with the use of the small focal spot, some penumbra is present.

Film-Screen System With film-screen imaging systems, the *film-screen speed* used for an exam affects the detail visualized on the resultant film. A faster film-screen system allows shorter exposure times, which are helpful in preventing patient motion and reducing dose; however, the image is less sharp than if a slower system were used.

Motion The greatest deterrent to image sharpness as related to positioning is *motion.* Two types of motion influence radiographic detail: **voluntary** and **involuntary.**

Voluntary motion is that which the patient can control. Motion from breathing or movement of body parts during the exposure can be prevented or at least minimized by **controlled breathing** and **patient immobilization.** The use of support blocks, sandbags, or other immobilization devices can be used to effectively reduce motion. These devices are most effective for examinations of upper or lower limbs, as will be demonstrated throughout this text.

Involuntary motion cannot be controlled by the patient at will. Therefore involuntary motion, such as peristaltic action of abdominal organs, tremors, or chills, is more difficult, if not impossible, to control.

If motion unsharpness is present on the image, the technologist must determine whether this blurring or unsharpness is due to voluntary or involuntary motion. This determination is important because there are different ways to control these two types of motion.

Difference between voluntary and involuntary motion
Voluntary motion is visualized as **generalized blurring of linked structures,** such as the blurring of the diaphragm and upper abdominal organs as evident in Fig. 2-8. Voluntary motion can be minimized through the use of high mA and short exposure times. Increased patient cooperation is also a factor in decreasing voluntary motion; a thorough explanation of the procedure and clear breathing instructions are helpful.

Involuntary motion is identified by **localized unsharpness or blurring.** This type of motion is less obvious but can be visualized on abdominal images as localized blurring of the edges of the bowel, with other bowel outlines appearing sharp (gas in the bowel appears as dark areas). Study Fig. 2-9 carefully to see this slight blurring in the left upper abdomen, indicated by small black arrows. The remaining edges of the bowel throughout the abdomen appear sharp. Fig. 2-8, by comparison, demonstrates overall blurring through the abdomen of both the diaphragm and bowel patterns.

A clear explanation of the procedure by the technologist will aid in reducing voluntary motion; however, a decrease in exposure time with an associated increase in mA is the best and sometimes only way to minimize motion unsharpness due to involuntary motion.

Summary of resolution factors Use of a **small focal spot,** an **increase in SID,** and a **decrease in OID** result in less geometric unsharpness and increased resolution. Patient motion also affects image quality; **short exposure times** and **increased patient cooperation** help minimize voluntary motion unsharpness. Involuntary motion unsharpness is controlled only by short exposure times.

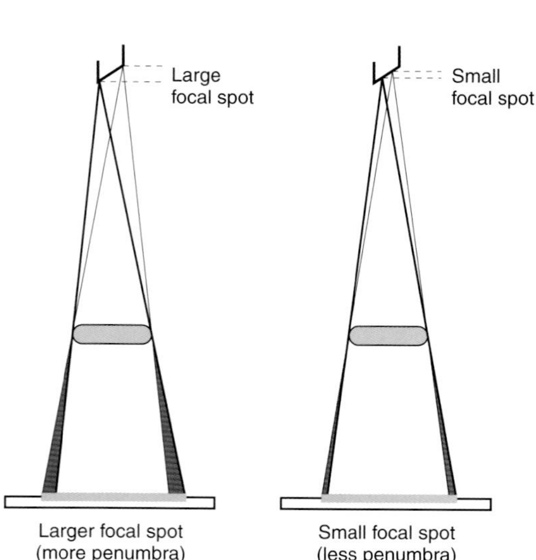

Fig. 2-7. Effect of focal spot size.

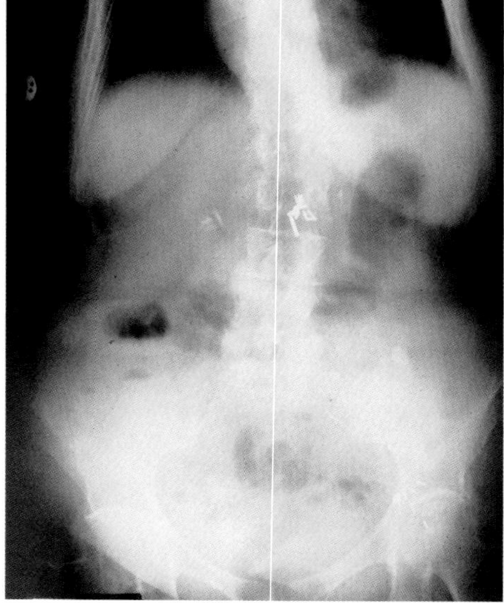

Fig. 2-8. Voluntary motion (breathing motion)—blurring of diaphragm and overall unsharpness.

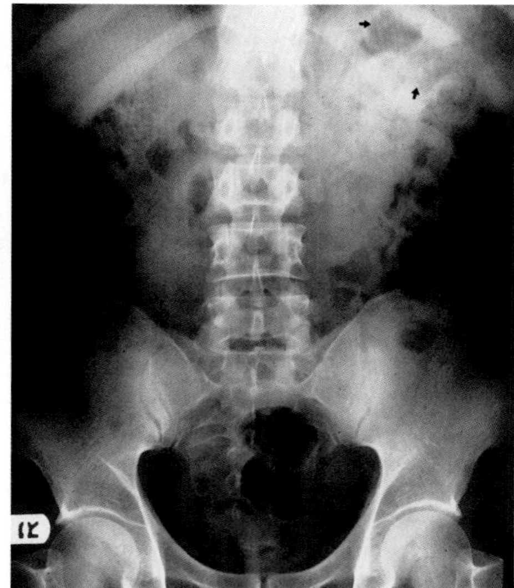

Fig. 2-9. Involuntary motion (from peristaltic action)—localized blurring in upper left abdomen (see *arrows*).

DISTORTION

Definition

The fourth and final image quality factor is *distortion,* which is defined as the **misrepresentation of object size or shape** as projected onto radiographic recording media. There are two types of distortion: size distortion (magnification) and shape distortion.

It is important to note that no radiographic image reproduces the exact size of the body part being radiographed. This is impossible, because a degree of magnification and/or distortion always exists as a result of OID and the divergence of the x-ray beam. Nevertheless, distortion can be minimized and controlled by following some basic principles.

X-Ray Beam Divergence

X-ray beam divergence is a basic but important concept in the study of radiographic positioning. It occurs because x-rays originate from a small source in the x-ray tube (the focal spot) and diverge as they travel to the image receptor (IR) (Fig. 2-10). The field size of the x-ray beam is limited by a collimator consisting of adjustable lead collimators. The collimator and shutters absorb the x-rays on the periphery, thereby controlling the size of the x-ray beam.

When using perpendicular rays, the **center point of the x-ray beam,** which strikes the IR 90° to the plane of the IR, is called the *central ray (CR).* This part of the beam theoretically has no divergence; therefore the **least amount of distortion** is at this point on the image. All other aspects of the x-ray beam strike the IR at some angle other than 90°, with the angle of divergence increasing to the outermost portions of the x-ray beam. In instances in which the x-ray field is large and the SID is short, the angle of divergence of x-rays at the outer margins is greater. The potential for distortion at these outer margins is increased.

Fig. 2-10 demonstrates three points on a body part (marked *A, B,* and *C*) projected onto the IR. More magnification is demonstrated at the periphery (*A* and *B*) than at the point of the central ray (*C*). Because of the effect of the divergent x-ray beam, combined with at least some OID, this type of size distortion is inevitable. It is important for technologists to closely control and minimize distortion as much as possible.

Controlling Factors

Four primary controlling factors of distortion are:

- Source image receptor distance (SID)
- Object image receptor distance (OID)
- Object image receptor alignment
- Central ray alignment/centering

1. SID The first controlling factor for distortion is SID. The effect of SID on size distortion (magnification) is demonstrated in Fig. 2-11. Note that **at a greater SID, less magnification occurs than at a shorter SID.** This is the reason chest radiographs are obtained at a minimum SID of 72 inches (180 cm) rather than the 40 to 48 inches (100 to 122 cm) commonly used for most other examinations. A 72-inch (180-cm) SID results in less magnification of the heart and other structures within the thorax.

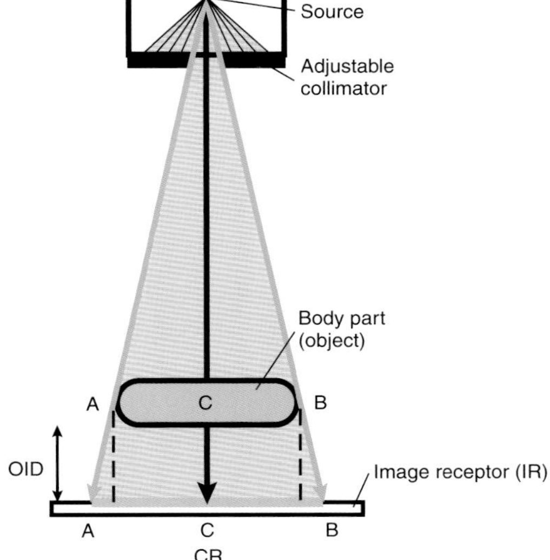

Fig. 2-10. X-ray beam divergence.

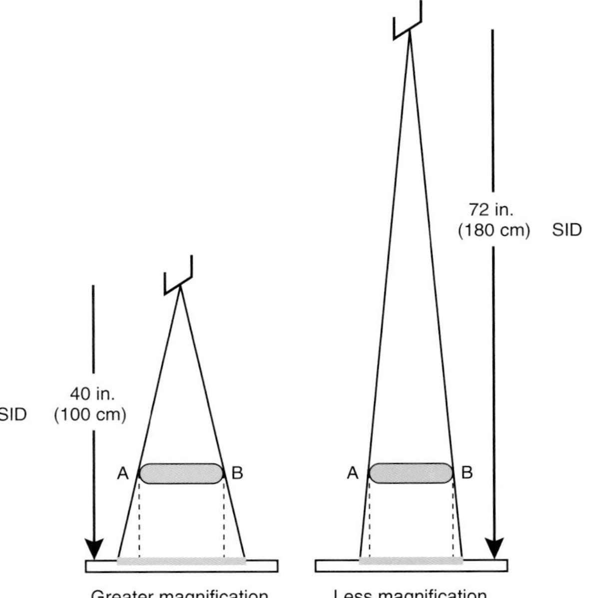

Fig. 2-11. Effect of SID.

2

Minimum 40-inch (or 100-cm) SID It has been a long-standing common practice to use 40 inches (rounded to 100-102 cm) as the standard SID for most radiographic exams. However, in the interest of improving image resolution or recorded detail by decreasing magnification and distortion and also reducing anode heel effect, it is becoming more common to increase the standard SID to 44 or 48 inches (112 or 122 cm). As an added benefit, certain studies have shown that increasing the SID from 40 to 48 inches also reduces the entrance or skin dose by 12% or 13%, even considering the increased mAs required.* (Increasing SID from 40 to 48 inches requires an increase in mAs of approximately 40%.) The increase in the entrance or skin dose is due to the higher degree of skin dose received with less SID.

In this textbook the suggested SID listed on each positioning page is a **minimum of 40 inches,** with 44 or 48 inches recommended if the equipment and room arrangement allow. Some newer x-ray tubes with steep anode angles and smaller focal spots also require a greater than 40-inch SID for sufficient field coverage for the larger IRs. However, increasing the SID to a total of 48 inches may make it difficult for shorter technologists to reach the tube and collimator controls. Therefore it is suggested that 44 inches (112 cm) may be the most practical and effective SID for general diagnostic radiography. However, each technologist must determine the departmental protocol regarding appropriate SID for the technique chart exposure guidelines for that department.

2. OID The second controlling factor for distortion is OID (Object Image receptor Distance). The effect of OID on magnification or size distortion is clearly illustrated in Fig. 2-12. **The closer the object being radiographed is to the image receptor, the less the magnification and shape distortion and the better the detail or resolution.**

This factor is the basis of one advantage in acquiring images of the upper and lower limbs on the tabletop rather than using the Bucky grid. In the tabletop method, the cassette is placed under the patient on top of the table rather than in the Bucky tray, thus decreasing the OID, since the Bucky tray in most floating-type tabletops is from 3 to 4 inches (8 to 10 cm) below the tabletop. This decrease in OID reduces magnification and distortion, thus increasing image sharpness.

3. Object Image Receptor Alignment A third important controlling factor of distortion related to positioning is *object IR alignment.* This refers to the **alignment or plane of the object being radiographed in relation to the plane of the image receptor.** If the object plane is not parallel to the plane of the image receptor, distortion occurs. The greater the angle of inclination of the object or the IR, the greater the amount of distortion.

The effect of improper object alignment is most obvious at the **joints or ends of bony structures.** This is best demonstrated on joints involving the upper and lower limbs. For example, if a finger being radiographed is not parallel to the IR, the joint spaces between the phalanges will not be open because of the overlapping of the bones, as demonstrated in Fig. 2-13.

This is also demonstrated by the two oblique hand positions in Figs. 2-14 and 2-15.

*Kebart RC, Jame CC: Benefits of increasing focal film distance, Radiologic Technology 62(6):434, 1991.

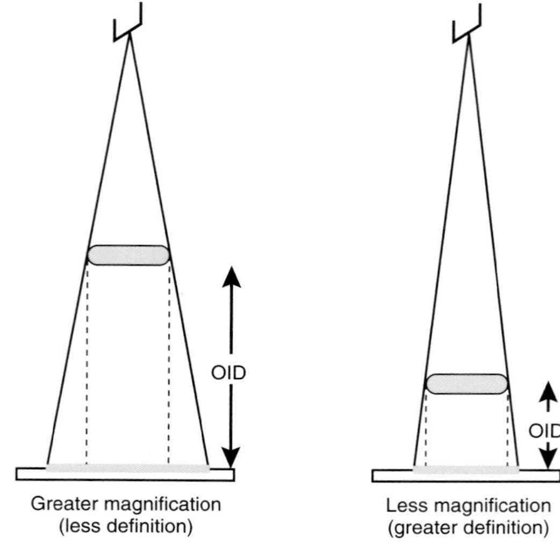

Fig. 2-12. Effect of OID.

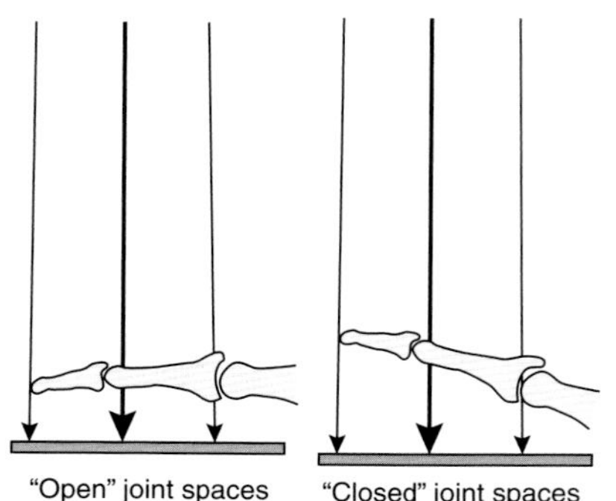

Fig. 2-13. Object alignment and distortion.

Effect of improper object IR alignment In Fig. 2-14 the digits (fingers) are supported and aligned **parallel to the image receptor,** resulting in open interphalangeal joints and undistorted phalanges.

In Fig. 2-15, where the digits are not parallel to the IR, the interphalangeal joints of the digits are not open and possible pathology within these joint regions may not be visible. Note the open joints of the digits on Fig. 2-16 compared with Fig. 2-17 (see *arrows*). Additionally, the phalanges will be either foreshortened or elongated.

These examples demonstrate the important principle of correct object IR alignment. **The plane of the body part being imaged must be as near parallel to the plane of the IR as possible** to produce an image of minimal distortion.

4. Central Ray Alignment The fourth and final controlling factor for distortion is *central ray alignment* (centering), an important principle in positioning. As previously stated, only the center of the x-ray beam, the central ray (CR), has no divergence, because it projects that part of the object at 90°, or perpendicular, to the plane of the IR. Therefore the **least possible distortion occurs at the central ray.** Distortion increases as the angle of divergence increases from the center of the x-ray beam to the outer edges. For this reason, correct centering or correct central ray alignment and placement is important in minimizing image distortion.

An example of correct central ray placement for an AP knee is shown in Fig. 2-18. The CR passes through the knee joint space with minimal distortion, and the joint space should appear open.

Fig. 2-19 demonstrates correct centering for an AP femur, in which the CR is correctly directed perpendicular to the IR and centered to the area of the midfemur. The knee joint, however, is now exposed to divergent rays (as shown by *arrow*), which will create distortion of the knee joint. The knee joint space will therefore not appear open on the AP femur projection, and a second AP knee projection with the CR centered to the knee joint will be required to optimally visualize the knee joint.

Central ray angle For most projections the CR is aligned **perpendicular,** or 90°, to the plane of the IR. For certain body parts, however, a specific angle of the CR is required, as indicated in the positioning descriptions in this text as *central ray angle.* This means the CR is angled from the vertical in a cephalic or caudad direction to utilize distortion intentionally and not superimpose anatomic structures.

Summary of distortion factors Using the correct SID, **minimizing OID,** ensuring the **object and IR are aligned,** and correctly **aligning or centering the CR and the part** can control distortion in a radiographic image.

SUMMARY OF IMAGE QUALITY AND PRIMARY CONTROLLING FACTORS

QUALITY FACTOR	PRIMARY CONTROLLING FACTORS
1. Density	mAs (mA and time)
2. Contrast	kV
3. Resolution	Geometric factors • Focal spot size • SID • OID Motion (voluntary and involuntary) Film-screen speed
4. Distortion	• SID • OID • Object IR alignment • CR alignment or centering

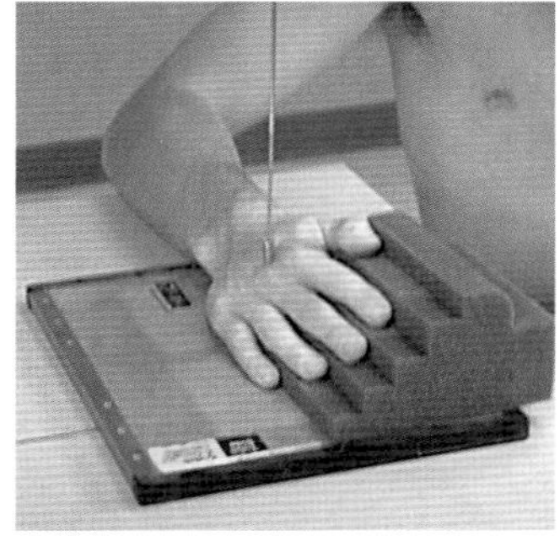

Fig. 2-14. Digits parallel to IR—joints open.

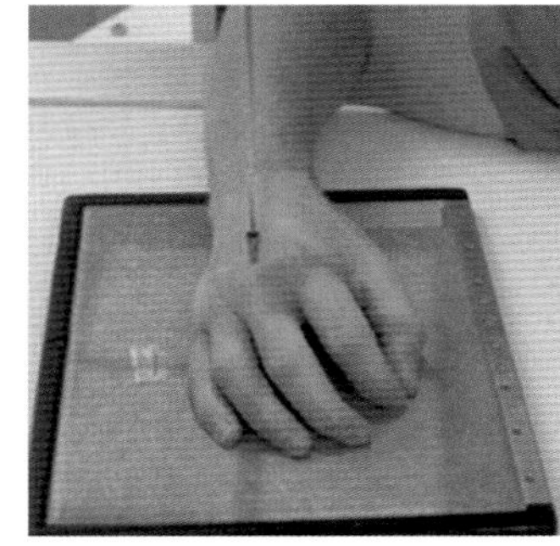

Fig. 2-15. Digits not parallel—joints not open.

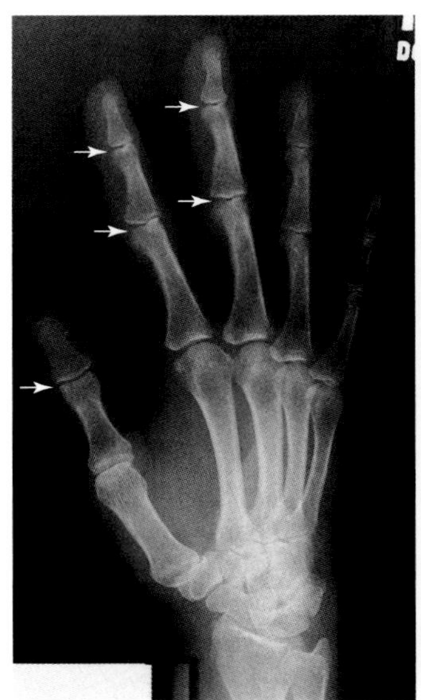

Fig. 2-16. Digits parallel—joints open.

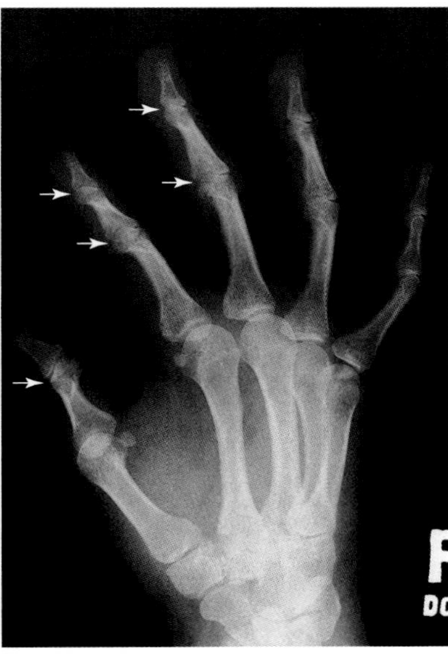

Fig. 2-17. Digits not parallel—joints not open.

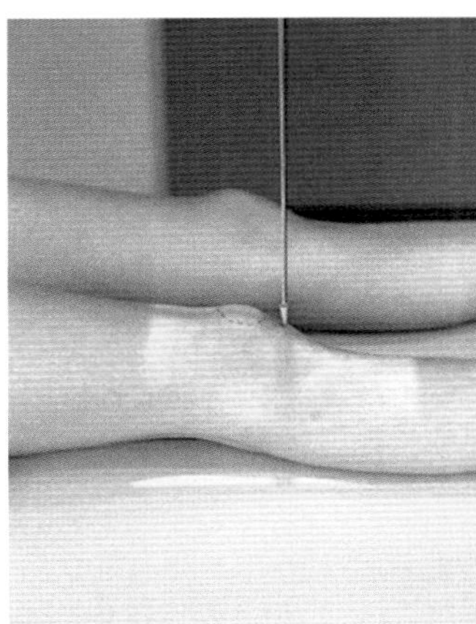

Fig. 2-18. Correct CR centering for AP knee.

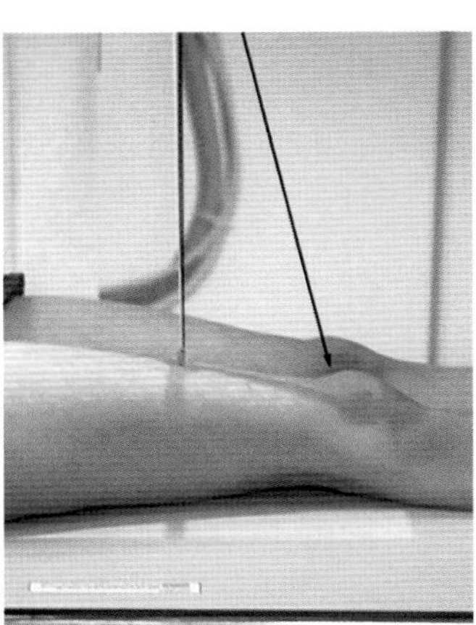

Fig. 2-19. Correct CR centering for AP femur (distortion occurs at knee).

IMAGE QUALITY IN DIGITAL RADIOGRAPHY

Digital imaging in radiologic technology involves application of analog-to-digital conversion theory, and computer software and hardware. Although digital imaging differs from film-screen imaging in the method of image acquisition, factors affecting x-ray production, attenuation, and geometry of the x-ray beam still apply. This section is intended as a brief practical introduction to a very sophisticated topic.

Digital Images

Digital images in radiologic technology are **a numeric representation of the x-ray intensities that are transmitted through the patient.** They are viewed on a computer monitor and are referred to as **soft-copy images.** Each digital image is two-dimensional and is formed by a *matrix* of picture elements called *pixels* (see Fig. 2-20). In diagnostic imaging each pixel represents one extremely small portion of the original information. For illustrative purposes, consider a sheet of graph paper. The series of squares on the sheet can be compared to the matrix, and each individual square can be compared to a pixel.

Digital imaging is unique in the type of processing required to visualize the images. Digital images require computer hardware and software applications to process images (Fig. 2-21), whereas film-based images use chemical processing to visualize the anatomic structures. Digital processing involves the **systematic application of highly complex mathematical formulas** called *algorithms.* A number of mathematical manipulations are performed on image data to enhance image appearance and optimize quality. Algorithms are applied by the computer to every dataset obtained before the technologist sees the image.

Display matrix

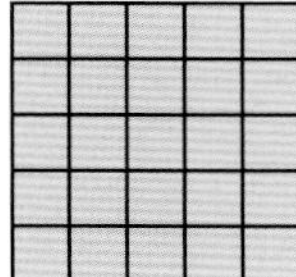

Pixel

Fig. 2-20. Two-dimensional matrix display—pixel.

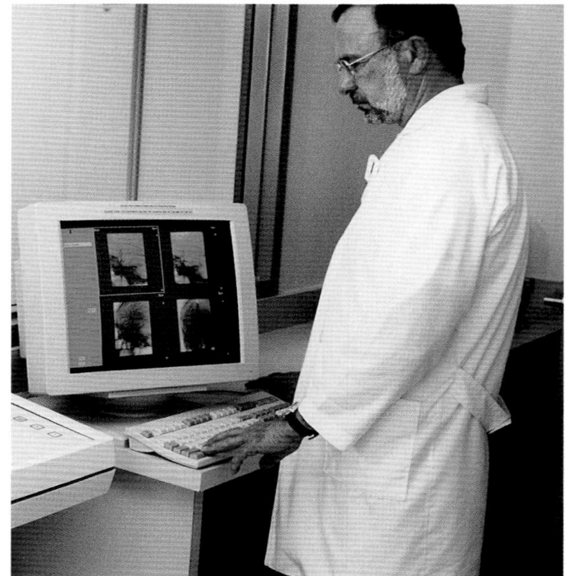

Fig. 2-21. Processing digital image.

Exposure Factors for Digital Imaging

Although kV and mA and time (mAs) must be selected to digitally acquire radiographic images (Fig. 2-22), they do not have the same direct effect on image quality as in film-screen imaging. It must be remembered, however, that the kV and mAs used for the exposure will still affect patient dose.

Milliamperage (mA) controls the number of x-rays produced, and **mAs** controls the number of x-rays times the duration of the exposure. Digital processing of the image allows for correction of inaccurate mAs selection; an image of optimal quality can thus be obtained with a range of mAs values as described under "Wide latitude."

Kilovoltage (kV) controls the penetrating power of the x-rays with all radiographic imaging, digital or film-screen systems. The kV appropriate for the part thickness and lowest practical patient dose must be selected by the technologist. Compared with film-screen imaging, changes in kV can have less of a direct effect on final digital image contrast because the resultant contrast is also a function of the digital processing. However, changes in kV, as well as in mAs, will still affect patient dose.

Wide latitude Depending on the technology, a digital detector can require fewer x-rays to optimally digitize and represent the anatomic information, compared with film imaging, where the acceptable range of exposures to produce a diagnostic image is restricted. This **wide range of acceptance of exposure factors to produce an acceptable image** is called *wide latitude.* The wide latitude of the digital imaging systems results in fewer repeats, increased efficiency, and cost reduction.

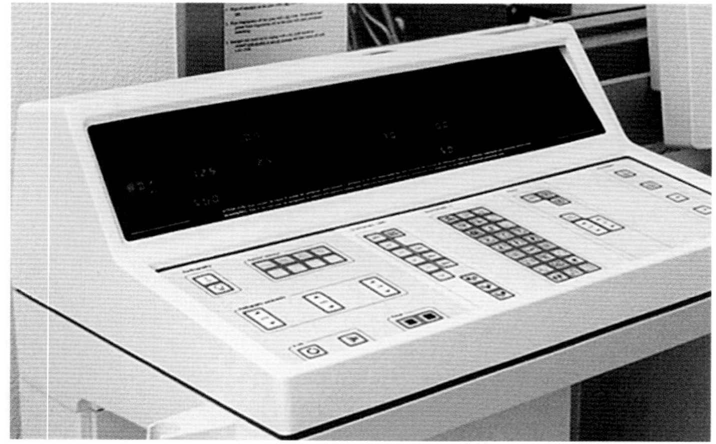

Fig. 2-22. Exposure controls—kV, mA, and time.

Image Quality Factors

The factors used to evaluate digital image quality include:

- **Brightness**
- **Contrast**
- **Resolution**
- **Distortion**
- **Exposure index**
- **Noise**

BRIGHTNESS

Definition

Brightness is defined as **the intensity of light that represents the individual pixels in the image on the monitor.** In digital imaging the term *brightness* replaces the film-based term *density* (Figs. 2-23 and 2-24).

Controlling Factors

Digital imaging systems are designed to electronically display the optimal image brightness under a wide range of exposure factors. Brightness is under the control of the processing software through the application of predetermined digital processing algorithms. Thus, unlike the linear relationship between mAs and density in film-screen imaging, changes in mAs will not have a controlling effect on digital image brightness. It is important to note that although the density of a film image cannot be altered once it is exposed and chemically processed, the user can adjust the brightness of the digital image after exposure (see Post-Processing later in this chapter).

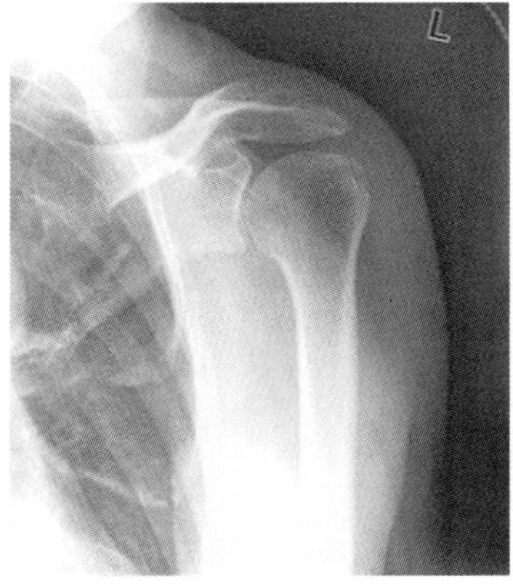

Fig. 2-23. AP shoulder—high brightness (light).

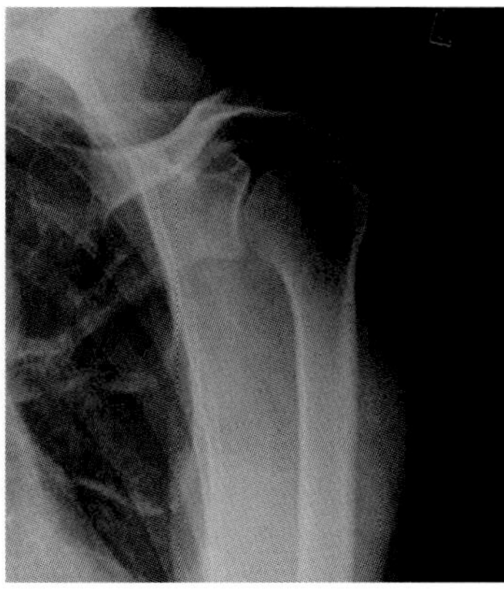

Fig. 2-24. AP shoulder—less brightness (dark).

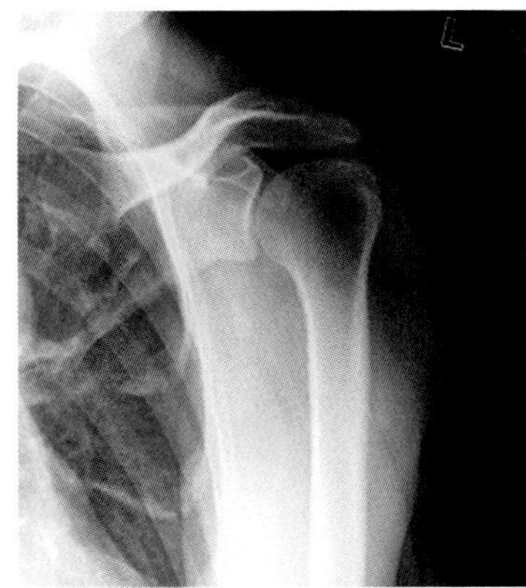

Fig. 2-25. AP shoulder—higher contrast.

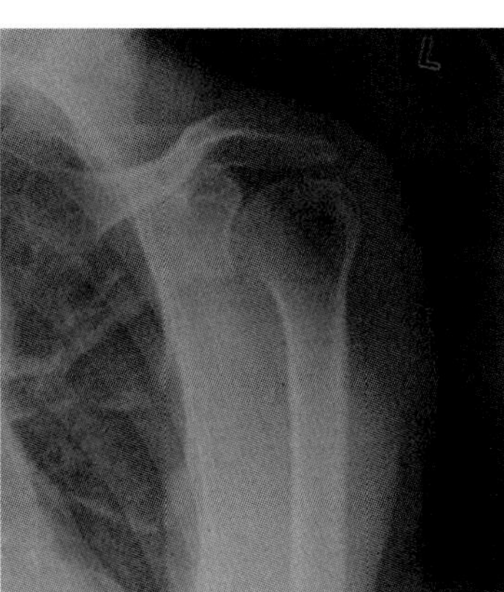

Fig. 2-26. AP shoulder—lower contrast.

CONTRAST

Definition

In digital imaging *contrast* is defined as **the difference in brightness between light and dark areas of an image.** This definition is similar to that used in film-based imaging, where contrast is the difference in density of adjacent areas on the film (see Figs. 2-25 and 2-26, which show several examples of different contrast images). *Contrast resolution* refers to an imaging system's ability to distinguish between similar tissues.

Controlling Factors

Digital imaging systems are designed to electronically display optimal image contrast, under a wide range of exposure factors. Radiographic contrast is affected by the digital processing computer through the application of predetermined algorithms, unlike film-screen imaging, in which kV is the controlling factor for image contrast. It is important to note that although the contrast of a film image cannot be altered after exposure and processing, the user can manipulate the contrast of the digital image (see Post-Processing later in this chapter).

Pixels and bit depth Each pixel demonstrates a single shade of gray when viewed on a monitor; it is representative of the physical properties of the anatomic structure. The range of possible shades of gray demonstrated is related to the pixel's *bit depth,* which is determined by the manufacturer. Although a comprehensive description of bit depth is beyond the scope of this text, it is important to note that the **greater the bit depth of a system,** the **greater the contrast resolution.**

Since computer theory is based on the binary system, a 14-bit system, for example, is represented as 2^{14}; the 14-bit-deep pixel could represent any one of 16,384 possible shades of gray, from black to white. Bit depth is determined by the manufacturer's system design and is closely related to the imaging procedures the equipment is designed for. The most common bit depths available are 10, 12, and 16. For example, a digital system for chest imaging should have a bit depth in excess of 10 bits (2^{10}) in order to capture all the required information; the x-ray beam exiting a patient having a chest x-ray can have a range of over 1024 intensities.

Pixel sizes There are two pixel sizes in medical imaging. These are *acquisition pixel size,* which is the minimum size that is inherent to the acquisition system, and *display pixel size,* which is the minimum pixel size that can be displayed by a monitor. A general radiography acquisition matrix may be as high as 3000 × 3000 pixels—over 9 million pixels (9 megapixels) in a 17- × 17-inch (43- × 43-cm) image.

Scatter radiation control Since digital detectors are more sensitive to low-energy radiation, controlling scatter radiation is an important factor in obtaining the appropriate image contrast. This is accomplished through correct use of grids, close collimation, and selection of the optimal kV.

RESOLUTION

Definition

Resolution in digital imaging is defined as **the recorded sharpness or detail of structures on the image,** the same as described for film-screen imaging.

Resolution in a digital image is a combination of the traditional factors explained previously for film-screen imaging (focal spot size, geometric factors, and motion) and, just as important, **the acquisition pixel size.** This pixel size is inherent to the digital imaging detector. Minimum resolution size in digital imaging is typically measured in microns rather than line pairs. The current range for digital general radiographic imaging is from 100 to 200 microns (approximately 5 to 2.5 line pairs per mm).

Controlling Factors

In addition to **pixel size,** resolution is also controlled by the **display matrix.** The perceived resolution of the image is dependent on the display capabilities of the monitor.

DISTORTION

Definition and Controlling Factors

Distortion is defined as **the misrepresentation of object size or shape as projected onto radiographic recording media,** just as for film-screen imaging. The factors that affect distortion (SID, OID, and central ray alignment) are therefore the same for film-screen imaging and digital imaging. Refer to the previous section of this chapter; minimizing distortion is an important image quality factor.

EXPOSURE INDEX

Definition

Exposure index in digital imaging is **a numeric value that is representative of the exposure the image receptor received.** Depending on the manufacturer of the system, the exposure index may also be called the *sensitivity (S) number.*

Controlling Factors

The exposure index is dependent on the intensity of the radiation striking the detector. It is a calculated value from the effect of mAs, kV, total detector area irradiated, and objects exposed (e.g., air, metal implants, patient anatomy). Depending on the manufacturer and the technique used to calculate this value, the exposure index displayed for each exposure is directly or indirectly proportional to the radiation striking the IR.

An **"S" number,** as used by certain manufacturers, is **inversely proportional** to the radiation striking the detector. For example, if the range for an acceptable "S" number for certain exams is 150 to 250, an "S" value higher than 250 would indicate underexposure, and a value lower than 150 would indicate overexposure.

An **exposure index,** however, as used by other manufacturers is **directly proportional** to the radiation striking the IR as determined through logarithmic calculations. For example, if an acceptable exposure index is typically 2.0 to 2.4, an index value lower than 2.0 would indicate underexposure, whereas an index value higher than 2.4 would indicate overexposure.

This text will use the term **exposure index** rather than "S" number when referring to this variable.

It has been stated previously that digital imaging systems are able to display quality images that have been obtained through use of a wide range of exposure factors. Despite this wide latitude, there are limitations and the technologist must ensure that the exposure factors used were adequate (similar to reviewing a film image to confirm adequate contrast and density are present). Checking the exposure index is key in verifying that **optimal quality digital radiographic images were obtained with the least possible dose to the patient.**

If the exposure index is outside the recommended range for the digital system, the image may still appear acceptable when viewed on the monitor of the technologist's workstation. It is important to remember that the monitor the technologist uses to view the image is typically of lower resolution than the radiologist's reporting workstation. The technologist's workstation is intended to allow verification of positioning and general image quality; however, this image is not of diagnostic quality. The monitor of a radiologist's reporting workstation typically provides superior spatial and contrast resolution due to increased display matrix with smaller pixels and superior brightness characteristics.

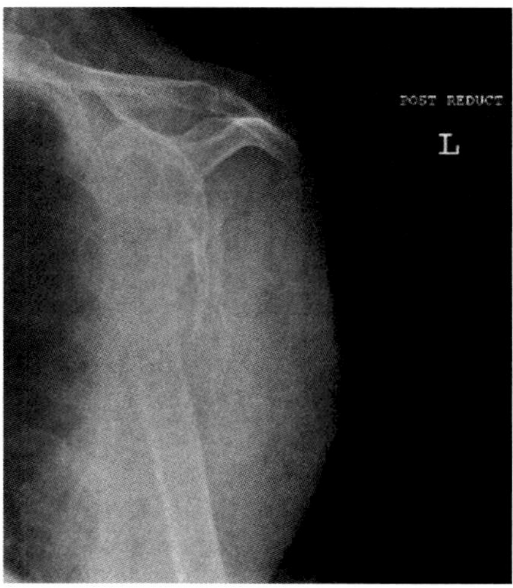

Fig. 2-27. Low exposure index (high "S" number) indicates **underexposure** with "noisy" undesirable image.

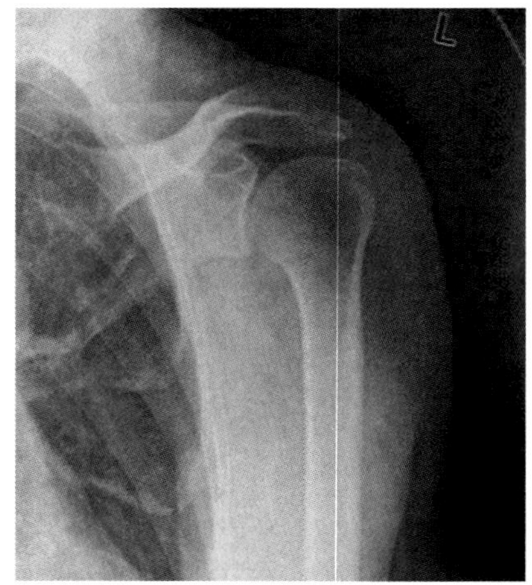

Fig. 2-28. Example of desirable exposure with acceptable exposure index or "S" number.

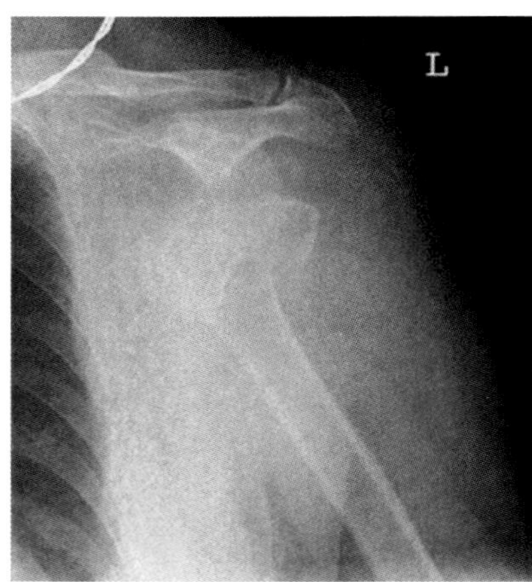

Fig. 2-29. High exposure index (low "S" number) indicates **overexposure** with "noisy" undesirable image.

NOISE

Definition

Noise is defined as **a random disturbance that obscures or reduces clarity.** In a radiographic image this translates into a grainy or mottled appearance of the image.

Signal-to-Noise Ratio (SNR)

One way to describe noise in digital image acquisition is the concept of *signal-to-noise ratio* (SNR). The number of x-ray photons that strike the detector (mAs) can be considered the *"signal."* Other factors that negatively affect the final image are classified as *"noise."* **A high SNR is desirable** in imaging, where the signal (mAs) is greater than the noise in order to demonstrate low-contrast soft-tissue structures. **A low SNR is undesirable;** a low signal (low mAs) with the accompanying high noise obscures soft-tissue detail and demonstrates a grainy or mottled image.

High SNR Although a high SNR is favorable (Fig. 2-30), technologists must ensure that exposure factors used are not beyond what is required for the projection so as not to overexpose the patient needlessly. Overexposed images are not readily evident with digital processing and display, so checking the exposure index as described on the previous page is the best way to determine this.

Low SNR When insufficient mAs is selected for a projection, the detector does not receive the appropriate amount of radiation, resulting in a low SNR and a *noisy* image (Fig. 2-31). This mottle may not be readily visible on the lower-resolution monitor of the technologist's workstation, but the exposure index, as checked for each projection, can aid in determining this.

Scatter radiation is a potential source of noise that can be controlled by the use of grids and correct collimation as described previously.

A secondary factor concerning noise in a radiographic image is *electronic noise*. Although a comprehensive discussion on electronic noise is beyond the scope of this text, electronic noise typically results from inherent noise in the electronic system, nonuniformity of the image receptor, or power fluctuations.

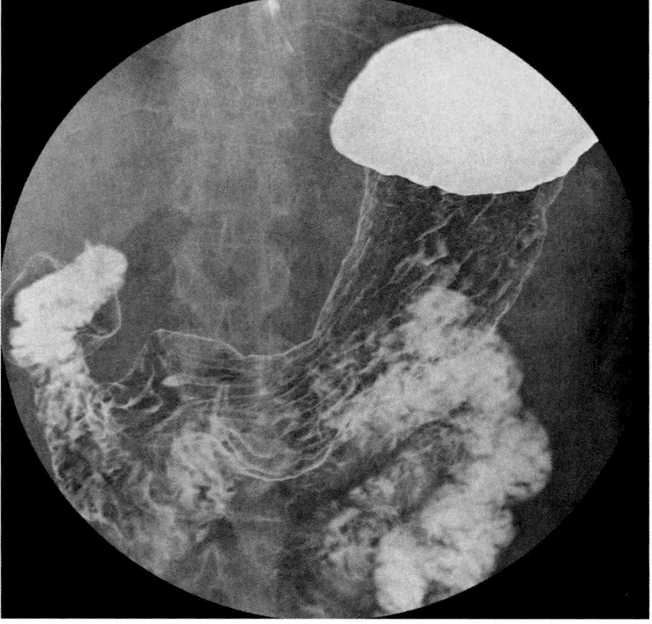

Fig. 2-30. Good quality image—**acceptable SNR.**

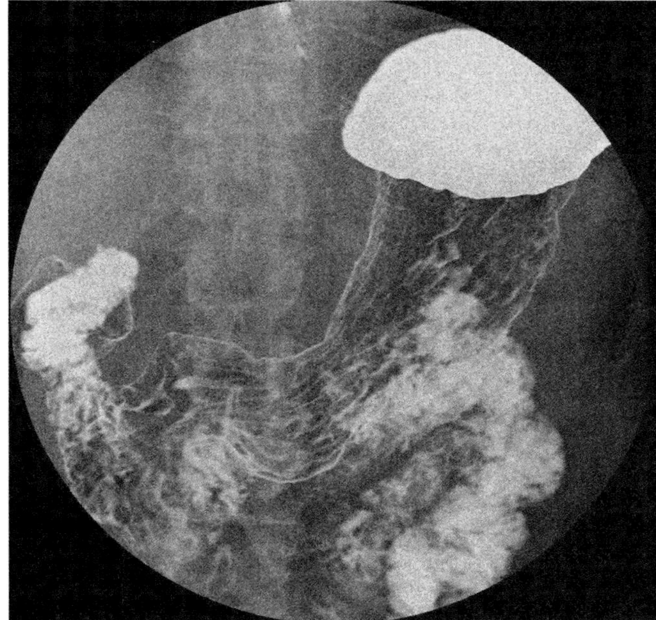

Fig. 2-31. Poor quality image, "noisy" (grainy)—**low SNR.**

2

Post-Processing

One of the advantages of digital imaging technology over film-screen technology is the ability to *post-process* the image. Post-processing refers to **changing or enhancing the electronic image in order to improve its diagnostic quality.** To post-process, algorithms are applied to the image to modify pixel values. Once viewed, the changes made may be saved, or the image default settings may be reapplied to enhance the diagnostic quality of the image.

Post-processing and exposure index range Once an acceptable exposure index range for the system has been determined, then what is important is whether the image is inside or outside this range. If the exposure index is below this range (indicating low SNR), post-processing will then not be effective in minimizing noise; more "signal" cannot be created with post-processing. Theoretically, if the algorithms are correct, the image should have optimal contrast and brightness. However, even if the algorithms used are correct and exposure factors are within an acceptable range as indicated by the exposure index values, certain post-processing options may still be applied for specific image effects.

Post-processing options There are a variety of post-processing options available in medical imaging (see Figs 2-32 through 2-35). The most common ones include the following:

Windowing: The user can adjust image contrast and brightness on the monitor. There are two types of adjustments possible: *window width,* which controls the **contrast** of the image (within a certain range), and *window level,* which controls the **brightness** of the image, also within a certain range.

Smoothing: Brightness values of adjacent pixels can be brought closer together.

Magnification: All or part of an image can be magnified.

Edge enhancement: Brightness can be increased along the edges of structures to increase the visibility of the edges.

Subtraction: Background anatomy can be removed to allow visualization of contrast media–filled vessels (used in angiography).

Image reversal: The dark and light pixel values of an image are reversed—the x-ray image reverses from a negative to a positive.

Annotation: Text may be added to images.

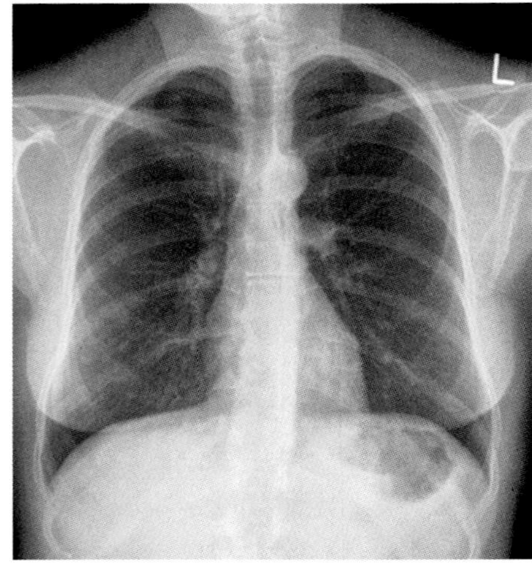

Fig. 2-32. Chest without any post-processing options applied.

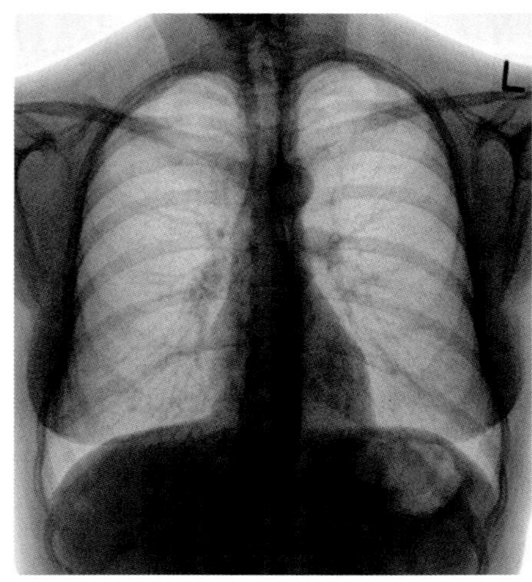

Fig. 2-33. Chest image with reversal option.

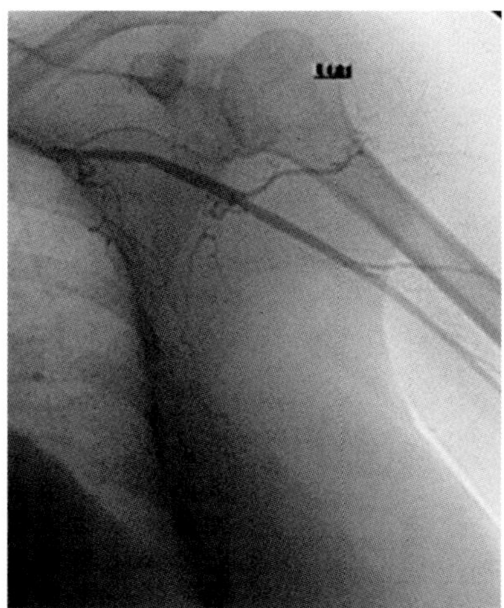

Fig. 2-34. Subtracted AP shoulder angiogram image.

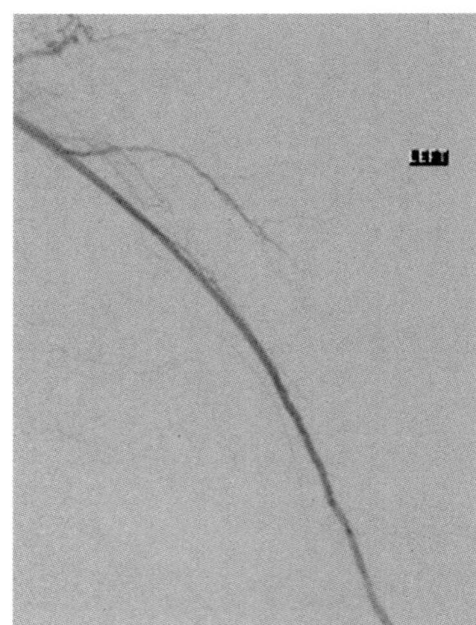

Fig. 2-35. Subtracted and magnified option of shoulder angiogram.

APPLICATIONS OF DIGITAL TECHNOLOGY

Advances in computer technology have changed the way radiologic images are acquired and the way the images are managed. Computer technology has also affected the way patient information is managed in health care in general. These changes will continue at an increasing rate as film-screen imaging and chemical processing become obsolete and the various forms of digital imaging evolve.

This section introduces and describes four types of digital imaging technologies in use today: (1) *computed tomography (CT),* (2) *digital fluoroscopy (DF)* (two types), (3) *computed radiography (CR),* and (4) *direct digital radiography (DR).* Also included in this section are some related digital health care applications.

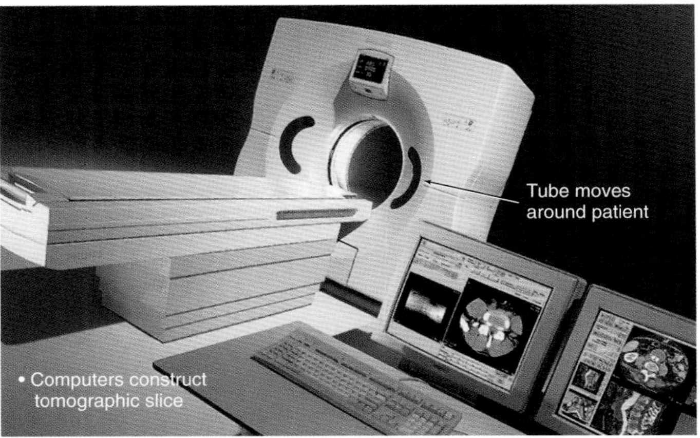
Tube moves around patient
• Computers construct tomographic slice

Fig. 2-36. Computed tomography (CT). (Courtesy Philips Medical Systems.)

Computed Tomography (CT)

Computed tomography (CT) was one of the first applications of computers to radiologic technology. CT was first developed in the late 1970s and early 1980s and utilizes a complex computer and mechanical system (Fig. 2-36). It acquires sectional anatomic images primarily in the axial plane, but the data can also be reconstructed in the sagittal and coronal planes, as well as into three-dimensional images. The concept may be simplified by comparing the procedure to imaging a loaf of bread; plain radiography captures images of the loaf as a whole, whereas CT images the loaf in individual slices (also called sections or cuts), which are viewed independently.

A portion of the radiation for each CT slice is attenuated by the patient, and the remnant radiation is measured by detectors. Low-density structures (lungs/air-filled structures) will attenuate very little of the x-ray beam, whereas higher-density structures (bones, contrast media) attenuate all or nearly all of the x-ray beam. The attenuation information exits the detectors in analog form, and the analog signal is converted to a digital signal. A computer performs a series of high-level mathematical calculations (algorithms) to reconstruct an image based on the attenuation values. Various algorithms are available in the software for different body areas and applications.

Advantages of CT CT has several advantages over conventional radiography, including the following: (1) contrast resolution is superior, (2) structures are visualized without superimposition, and (3) acquired data may be viewed in alternative planes.

Refer to Chapter 22 for more complete information on CT.

2

Digital Fluoroscopy (DF)

Fluoroscopy provides dynamic (moving) imaging of structures, compared with plain radiography, which provides static images. Fluoroscopy has an application in gastrointestinal procedures, intraoperative imaging, and angiography/interventional procedures. X-radiation and a complex series of components commonly referred to as the imaging chain are required to produce and display the image in real time.

Currently there are **two types** of technology being used in digital fluoroscopic (DF) systems. First is **the analog-to-digital conversion.** This more common system uses an image intensifier and a television system to first produce an analog or visible image. This visible image from the output side of the image intensifier is then recorded by a high-resolution video camera and converted to a digital format (Fig. 2-37).

A second type of a DF system utilizes the latest technology consisting of **direct digital conversion,** sometimes referred to as "flat detectors." Currently, this type of technology is used primarily in cardiac and vascular applications (Fig. 2-38). With this newer system, the digital detector replaces the image intensifier, the video camera, and the digital conversion system (compare the two systems in Fig. 2-39).

Advantages of the flat detector technology include the following:

- Image quality is improved because of smaller pixel size and a higher detection quantum efficiency (DQE) (more x-rays are converted into visible light).
- Contrast resolution is greater.
- Smaller size allows health professionals more room to maneuver during the procedure.

The primary disadvantage of the flat panel x-ray detector is that it is more expensive than image intensification technology.

During the fluoroscopic procedure static (still) images, as well as dynamic (moving) images, may be obtained with both of these systems. These static images can be viewed and post-processed as required. They are then saved to the digital archive or may be printed to film with a laser printer.

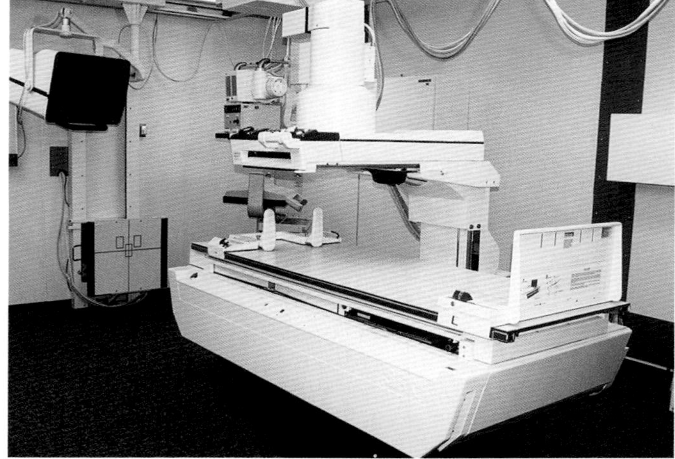

Fig. 2-37. Digital fluoroscopy—analog-to-digital type with image intensifier.

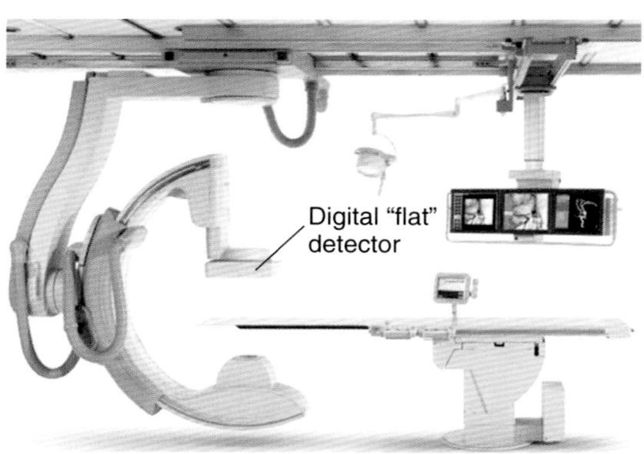

Fig. 2-38. Direct digital conversion—C-arm type with flat detector. (Courtesy Philips Medical Systems.)

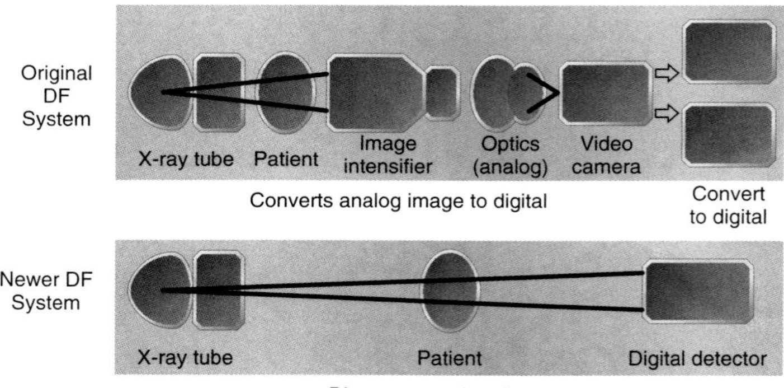

Fig. 2-39. Comparison of DF systems. (Modified from illustrations by GE Medical Systems.)

Computed Radiography (CR)

Computed radiography (CR) is a method of digital image acquisition for general diagnostic radiography. Exposure factors required for CR are similar to those for conventional film-screen techniques (including AEC). As explained in the previous section, CR digital imaging systems have wide exposure latitude, which reduces the number of repeats caused by incorrect exposure factor selection. Accuracy of exposure factors selected is confirmed by checking the exposure index, available after the image is digitally processed.

*The main components of a CR system include the **image plates (IP)**, the **IP reader**, and the **technologist workstation.***

Image plates (IP) As can be seen in Fig. 2-40, the CR system uses the typical general diagnostic x-ray tube and table, but an imaging plate/cassette replaces the film-screen cassette in the Bucky tray. This IP records an invisible (latent) image in a similar way that a latent image is formed on the x-ray film when struck by the x-rays passing through the patient. The image plates recording the latent image are composed of photostimulable phosphors.

Unlike film, the IP can be used repeatedly, does not need to be "light tight," and can even be opened briefly in the light without the loss of the latent image because it does not contain light-sensitive film. Imaging plate cassettes are available in standard sizes as listed on page 37 of Chapter 1.

Patient information is linked to the CR image electronically using a bar code reader or by manual input on the keyboard at the reader; therefore the usual lead blocker found on conventional film cassettes is not present.

Image plate reader (Fig. 2-41) After the exposure is made on the IP and the patient ID is linked, the plate is placed into the IP reader. Inside the reader, the IP is removed from the cassette and the recorded image is read line by line by the laser scanner. As the laser scans the image, the IP phosphors release electrons that emit light equal to their stored energy. This light output is converted to an electrical signal and then to a digital format for manipulation, enhancement, viewing, and printing if desired. The IP is then erased by a bright light inside the reader, reloaded into the cassette, and returned ready for the next exposure. This entire process takes about 20 seconds.

Technologist workstation The workstation includes a bar code reader (optional), a monitor for image display, and a keyboard with a mouse or trackball for entering commands for any post-processing. The technologist verifies the patient position and checks the exposure index at this workstation.

Image archiving After the image quality has been verified and any adjustments have been made, the image can then be transmitted to the digital archive for viewing and reading by the referring physician or radiologist. Images may also be printed onto film by a laser printer.

Refer to Fig. 2-47 on page 60 for an illustration of the steps in CR image acquisition. Comparing CR to the steps in film-screen image acquisition demonstrates that many of the steps are similar because both CR and film-screen imaging use cassettes.

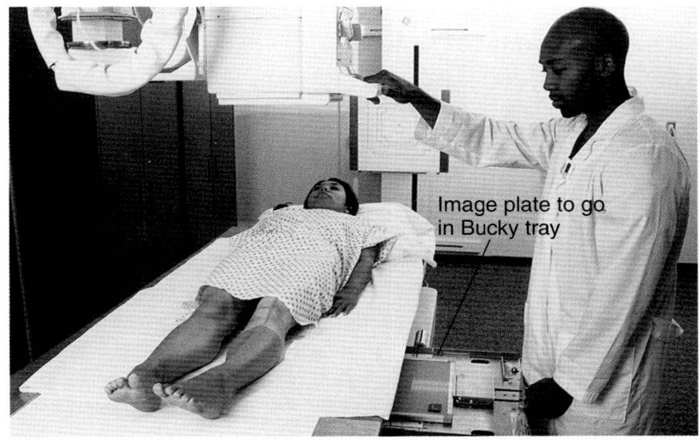

Fig. 2-40. Computed radiography (CR), used with conventional x-ray unit, except cassette with image plates replaces film-screen cassette in Bucky tray.

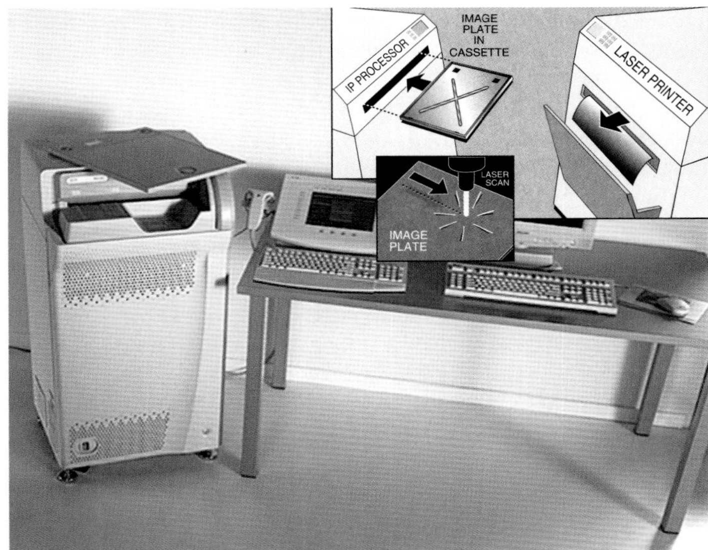

Fig. 2-41. Image plate reader/processor and computer workstation. (Modified from Philips Medical Systems photo.)

2

Practical Application of CR

Regardless of the technology used to acquire radiographic images, accurate positioning and attention to technical details are important. When using digital technology, however, attention to these details becomes additionally important because of the following factors:

Collimation In addition to the obvious benefit of reducing radiation dose to the patient, collimation that is closely restricted to the part being examined is key to ensuring optimal image quality. The software processes the entire x-ray field as a data set; therefore any unattenuated beam is included in the calculations for brightness and contrast. If the collimation is not closely restricted, the exposure index will be misrepresented and the image may exhibit lower contrast.

30% rule A minimum of 30% of the IR must be exposed for an accurate exposure index. If collimation is less than 30% of the IR, the exposure index is no longer accurate. The technologist must then ensure that appropriate exposure factors for the body part being examined were used.

Accurate centering of part and IR Because of the way the IP reader scans the exposed imaging plate, the body part and CR should be centered to the IR.

Use of lead masks Use of lead masks (lead blockers) for multiple images on one IR is recommended when using CR (Fig. 2-42). This is due to the hypersensitivity of the image plate phosphors to lower energy scatter radiation; even small amounts may affect the image.

Use of grids Use of grids for parts over 10 cm is especially important when acquiring images using CR because of the hypersensitivity of the image plate phosphors to scatter radiation.

Exposure factors Because of their wide exposure latitude, CR systems are able to process an acceptable image from a broad range of exposure factors (kV, mAs). It is important to remember, however, that the ALARA principle (exposure to patient As Low As Reasonably Achievable) must be followed, and the lowest exposure factors required to obtain a diagnostic image must be used. Once the image is available for viewing, the technologist must check the exposure index to verify that the exposure factors used are consistent with a diagnostic image.

Evaluation of exposure index values As soon as the image is available for viewing at the workstation, it is critiqued for positioning and exposure accuracy. The technologist must then check the exposure index to verify that the exposure factors used were in the correct range for optimum quality with the lowest radiation dose to the patient.

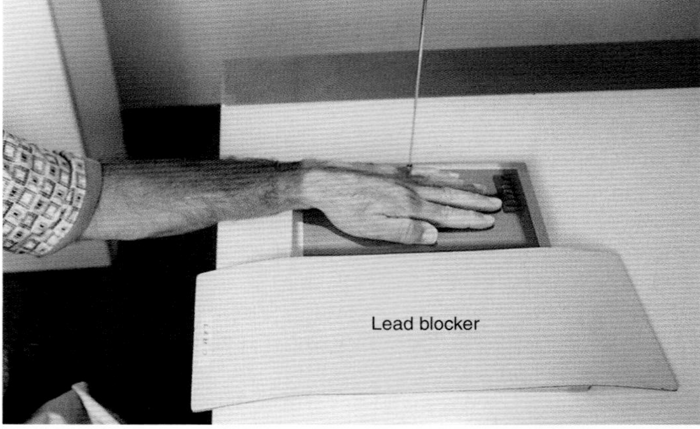

Fig. 2-42. Lead blockers on cassette and close collimation are important with use of IP cassettes.

Direct Digital Radiography (DR)

In addition to CR (computed radiography) a second more recently developed method of digital image acquisition in radiography is *direct digital radiography (DR)* (Fig. 2-43). DR involves a direct conversion method, wherein a digital detector detects the radiation intensities transmitted through the patient, which are then converted to a digital format. The data are then processed, and an image is displayed. This digital detector replaces the IP/cassette and image reader used in CR.

Advantages of DR Several significant advantages of DR over CR and film-screen imaging are: (1) DR eliminates the handling of cassettes, which translates into a significant timesaving feature for the technologist, (2) DR systems increase efficiency because the time for image processing is shorter, generally seconds, and (3) exposure factors for DR may be reduced when compared with exposure factors for CR and film-screen. This is due to the higher DQE of the detector.

DR and CR both have the advantage of the technologist being able to view a *preview image* to evaluate for positioning errors and confirm the exposure index. The projection may be repeated immediately if necessary. Also the operator is able to post-process and manipulate the image.

As with CR and film-screen acquisition, DR can be used for both grid and non-grid examinations. In reality, however, when using DR for traditional non-grid exams, the grid is often not removed for practical reasons: it is expensive, fragile, and may be easily damaged. Because of the high DQE of the detector, the increase in exposure as required when using a grid is less of an issue, although the exception to this would be pediatric examinations (because of the increased sensitivity of pediatric patients to radiation exposure).

Flow chart comparisons Refer to Fig. 2-48, which illustrates the steps in DR image acquisition. When compared with the steps in CR (see Fig. 2-47) and film-screen image acquisition (see Fig. 2-46), DR is obviously more time-efficient because the steps of cassette handling are eliminated.

DR chest imaging system There are dedicated DR systems available for chest imaging (Fig. 2-44). This is advantageous because large numbers of patients are imaged more efficiently without handling of cassettes or any chemical processing. Detector sizes for DR chest units vary depending on the manufacturer, from 41 × 41 cm (16 × 16 inches) to 43 × 43 cm (17 × 17 inches).

Digital mammography Mammography images may be obtained using CR or DR technology (Fig. 2-45). An advantage of digital acquisition in mammography is high-contrast resolution with possible reductions in patient dose, which is especially important for mammography. Post-processing capabilities provide the opportunity for image manipulation to improve visibility of fine microcalcifications. (See Chapter 18 for more information on digital mammography.)

Practical Application of DR

Regardless of the digital technology used to acquire radiographic images, accurate positioning and attention to certain technical details is important, as described for CR on the preceding page. For DR these details include **careful collimation** (the 30% rule does not apply for DR because of its method of image acquisition), correct use of **grids,** and careful attention to **exposure factors and evaluation of exposure index values,** remembering the ALARA principle. When using either CR or DR technology, attention to these details is essential.

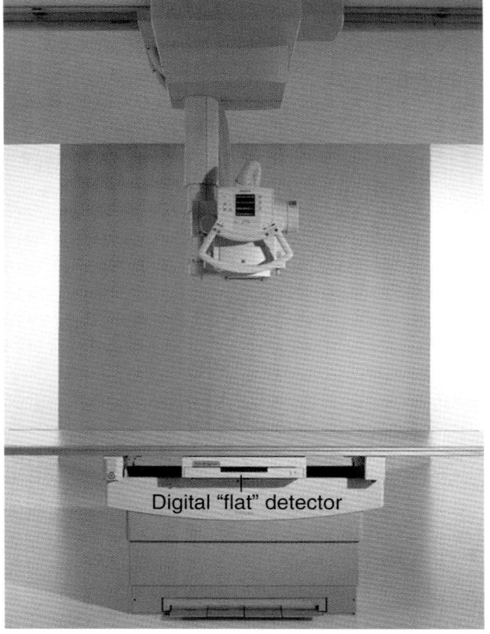

Fig. 2-43. Direct digital radiography (DR) unit. (Courtesy Philips Medical Systems.)

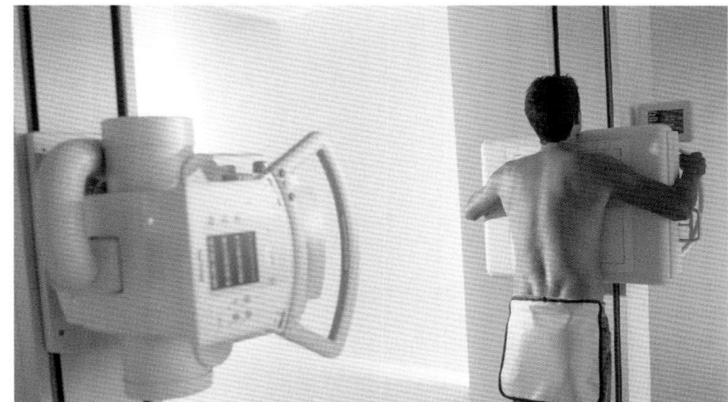

Fig. 2-44. DR chest imaging system. (Courtesy Philips Medical Systems.)

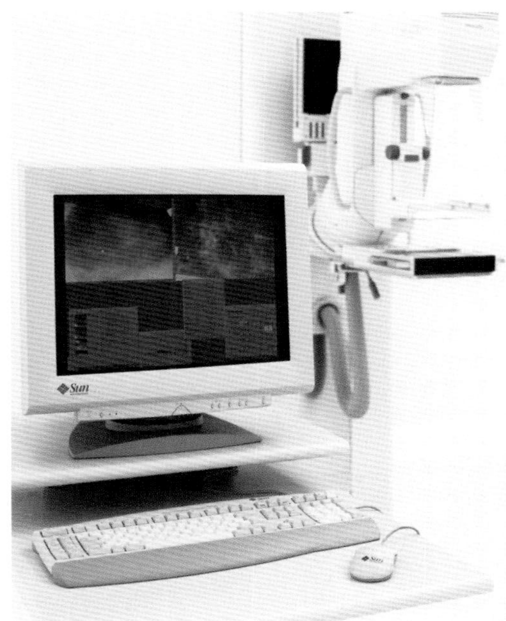

Fig. 2-45. CR mammography unit. (Courtesy Philips Medical Systems.)

2

Flow Chart Comparisons—Steps of Image Production

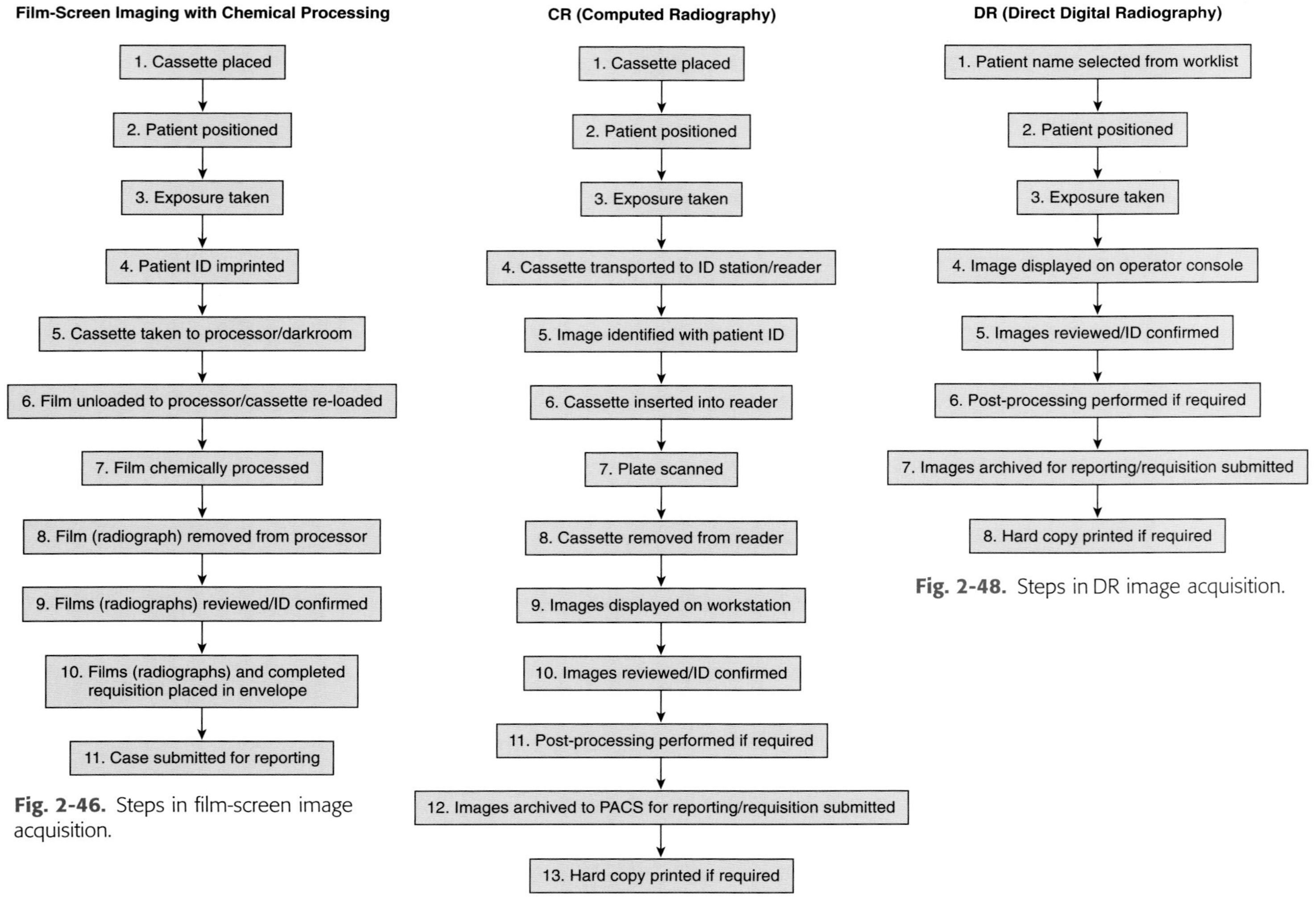
Film-Screen Imaging with Chemical Processing
1. Cassette placed
2. Patient positioned
3. Exposure taken
4. Patient ID imprinted
5. Cassette taken to processor/darkroom
6. Film unloaded to processor/cassette re-loaded
7. Film chemically processed
8. Film (radiograph) removed from processor
9. Films (radiographs) reviewed/ID confirmed
10. Films (radiographs) and completed requisition placed in envelope
11. Case submitted for reporting
CR (Computed Radiography)
1. Cassette placed
2. Patient positioned
3. Exposure taken
4. Cassette transported to ID station/reader
5. Image identified with patient ID
6. Cassette inserted into reader
7. Plate scanned
8. Cassette removed from reader
9. Images displayed on workstation
10. Images reviewed/ID confirmed
11. Post-processing performed if required
12. Images archived to PACS for reporting/requisition submitted
13. Hard copy printed if required
DR (Direct Digital Radiography)
1. Patient name selected from worklist
2. Patient positioned
3. Exposure taken
4. Image displayed on operator console
5. Images reviewed/ID confirmed
6. Post-processing performed if required
7. Images archived for reporting/requisition submitted
8. Hard copy printed if required

Fig. 2-46. Steps in film-screen image acquisition.

Fig. 2-47. Steps in CR image acquisition.

Fig. 2-48. Steps in DR image acquisition.

Picture Archiving and Communication Systems (PACS)

As imaging departments move from film-based acquisition and archiving (hard-copy film and document storage) to digital acquisition and archiving (soft-copy storage), a complex computer network has been created to manage images. The network is called *Picture Archiving and Communication Systems (PACS)* and can be likened to a "virtual film library."

PACS is a sophisticated array of hardware and software that can connect all modalities with digital output (nuclear medicine, ultrasound, computed tomography, magnetic resonance imaging, angiography, mammography, and radiography), as illustrated in Fig. 2-49. The acronym PACS can be best explained as:

P—Picture: the digital medical image(s)

A—Archiving: the "electronic" storage of the images

C—Communication: the routing (retrieval/sending) and displaying of the images

S—System: the specialized computer network that manages the complete system

The connection of various equipment types and modalities to a PACS is complex. Standards have been developed to ensure that all manufacturers and types of equipment are able to communicate and effectively transmit images and information. Current standards include **DICOM** (Digital Imaging Communications in Medicine) and **HL7** (Health care Level 7). Although standards may not always provide for an instantaneous functionality between devices, they do allow for resolution of connectivity problems.

For optimum efficiency the PACS should be integrated with the *Radiology Information System* **(RIS)** or the *Hospital Information System* **(HIS).** Since these information systems support the operations of an imaging department through exam scheduling, patient registration, report archiving, and film tracking, integration with PACS maintains integrity of patient data and records and promotes overall efficiency.

When using a PACS, instead of having hard-copy radiographs to process, handle, view, transport, and store, the soft-copy digital images are processed using a computer, viewed on a monitor, and stored electronically. Most PACS use web browsers to enable easy access to the images by users from any location. Physicians may view these radiologic images from a personal computer at virtually any location, including their home.

Advantages of PACS Some of the identified advantages of PACS include:

- Elimination of less efficient traditional film libraries and their inherent problem of physical space requirements for hard-copy images
- Convenient search for and retrieval of images
- Rapid (electronic) transfer of images within the hospital (e.g., clinics, operating rooms, treatment units)
- Ease in consulting outside specialists—teleradiology
- Simultaneous viewing of images at multiple locations
- Elimination of misplaced, damaged, or missing films
- Increase in efficiency of reporting exams with soft-copy images (compared with hard-copy images)
- Reduction of the health and environmental impact associated with chemical processing, as a result of decreased use

The growth of computer applications in radiologic technology has led to new career paths for radiologic technologists. The *PACS Administrator* and the *Diagnostic Imaging Information Technologist* are new positions that many radiologic technologists are pursuing.

Telemedicine and Teleradiology

Telemedicine is a general term for the **delivery of health care using telecommunications and computer technology.**

Advantages of telemedicine Telemedicine is advantageous because:

- Specialists are more easily consulted from remote areas, which increases efficiency/effectiveness of health care.
- Health care costs are lowered since the expertise from the large medical centers can serve multiple sites, reducing the number of physicians required and/or the cost of travel by physicians and patients.
- Hard-copy patient information (images, reports etc.) does not get lost in the traditional mail system.

Telemedicine is subdivided into specific specialties—for example, telecardiology, teledermatology, and (of interest to radiologic technologists) teleradiology.

Teleradiology is defined as the **electronic transmission of diagnostic imaging studies from one location to another for the purposes of interpretation and/or consultation.** With the increase of PACS and web-based viewing, the line between PACS and teleradiology has become blurred.

Applications The applications of teleradiology may be broadly classified as:

- *On-call systems*—Refers to the transmission of images after hours to a radiologist who is on call. The images are typically sent to the radiologist's home.
- *Off-site systems*—Refers to coverage for remote areas that may not have a radiologist on site.
- *In-hospital systems*—Refers to the transmission of images from the imaging department to an in-hospital unit or clinic (e.g., ICU, ortho clinic, OR).

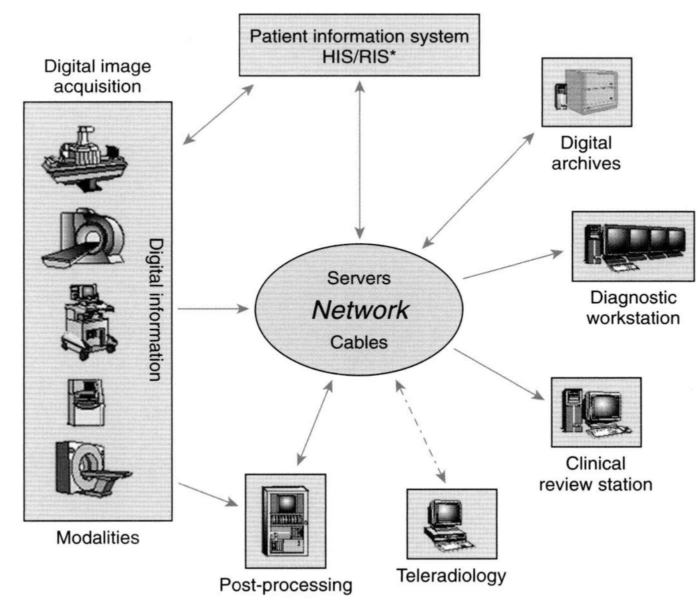

Fig. 2-49. A full PACS network that includes digital acquisition, communication, reporting, and archiving. **HIS,* Hospital Information System; *RIS,* Radiology Information System. (Modification of diagram from Philips Medical Systems.)

Computer-Assisted Detection (CAD)

Computer-assisted detection (CAD) was initially introduced for use in mammography to provide a "second look" at the radiographic image and is now being studied for use with chest radiographs. The overall goals were to enhance radiologist performance by increasing diagnostic accuracy and to increase confidence in reporting. The CAD systems use **computerized detection algorithms, pattern recognition, neural networks, and artificial intelligence to analyze digital images for various suspicious lesions.**

The typical procedure when using CAD is for the radiologist to perform the initial read and then have the image interpreted by the CAD device. If the image has not been acquired digitally, the hard-copy image must be digitized to provide suitable data for the computer.

Highly complex algorithms that result in approximately a billion operations per image process the digital images. Systems will provide a laser printout of the image (on paper), or a digital display when any suspicious lesions or masses are identified. The radiologist can then use this information as an alternative perspective in formulating the final diagnostic report. Some published studies have shown that CAD increases a radiologist's performance by 10%.

Another benefit to CAD is the lack of intra-observer variation; that is, the detection by the computer is reproducible. In addition, computers are not subject to the limitations of human observers, such as distraction, fatigue, or the effects of a heavy workload.

Integrated Health care Enterprise (IHE)

In many cases imaging departments within a health care institution use their own computerized information system; for example, the *Radiology Information System* **(RIS)** serves only the diagnostic imaging department. Although it is desirable to integrate all patient records, to do so presents a huge technical challenge.

A broader *integrated health care enterprise* **(IHE)** is the next step in health care record management. Patients' digital image files will be integrated with their medical records into an *electronic patient record (EPR);* radiology, pathology, laboratory results, and medical records will exist in the same digital file.

All the patient information (test results, medical images, scheduled exams, and patient progress) should ideally be digitally available to health care providers worldwide. It will be no small chore to orchestrate this; communication and transmission standards between each medical department will need to be clearly established. Technical infrastructure must be in place and health professionals will need to be trained/retrained on the IHE system. Also, a financial commitment will be required to upgrade and/or interface existing systems, and there must be an acceptance to change the way records are currently maintained. Concerns regarding security of records and privacy of information have been addressed by the *Health and Insurance Portability and Accountability Act* **(HIPPA),** and policies governing data transmission, use, and storage have been implemented.

With this future direction in mind there is discussion that the term PACS may not be appropriate. One suggested replacement is **IMAC**—*Image and Information Management and Communication*—which would more accurately reflect the future of a totally integrated healthcare enterprise.

Digital Imaging–Glossary of Terms

ALARA: The principle that radiation exposure should be kept as low as reasonably achievable.

Algorithms: Highly complex mathematical formulas that are systematically applied to a data set for digital processing.

Attenuation: A reduction in intensity of the x-ray beam due to absorption and scattering.

Bit-depth: Representative of the number of shades of gray that can be demonstrated by each pixel. Bit depth is determined by the manufacturer based on the imaging procedures the equipment is required for.

Brightness: The intensity of light that represents the individual pixels in the image on the monitor.

Central ray (CR): The center point of the x-ray beam (point of least distortion of projected image).

Computer-assisted detection (CAD): Use of computerized functions to analyze digital images for suspicious lesions or abnormalities.

Computed radiography (CR): A method of acquiring radiographic images digitally. The main components of a CR system include photostimulable phosphor image plates, an image plate reader, and a workstation.

Contrast: The density difference on adjacent areas of a radiographic image.

Contrast resolution: An imaging system's ability to distinguish between similar tissues.

Density: The amount of blackness on a film image.

Digital archive: A digital storage and image management system; in essence, a sophisticated computer system for storage of patient files and images.

Direct digital radiography (DR): A method of acquiring radiographic images digitally. The DR detector replaces the film-screen system and the CR imaging plate as the image receptor, utilizing a more direct approach to image capture.

Display matrix: Series of "boxes" that give form to the image.

Display pixel size: Pixel size of the monitor, related to the display matrix.

Distortion: Misrepresentation of object size or shape as projected onto radiographic recording media.

Edge enhancement: A post-processing technique that increases brightness along the edges of structures on an image to increase the visibility of the edges.

Exposure index: A numeric value that is representative of the exposure the image receptor received in digital radiography.

Exposure latitude: Range of exposure factors that will produce an acceptable image.

Exposure level: A term used by certain equipment manufacturers to indicate exposure index. The value is directly proportional to the exposure and is calculated logarithmically.

Hard-copy radiograph: A film-based radiographic image.

Hospital Information System (HIS): Computer system designed to support and integrate the operations of the entire hospital.

Image plate (IP): With computed radiography the image plate records the latent images, similar to the film in a film-screen cassette used in film-screen imaging systems.

Kilovoltage: The energy of the x-ray photon.

Milliamperage: The quantity or numbers of x-ray photons.

Milliampere-seconds: The quantity of x-ray photons and the duration of the exposure.

Noise: Random disturbance that obscures or reduces clarity. In a radiographic image this translates into a grainy or mottled appearance of the image.

Penumbra: The unsharp edges of the projected image.

Pixel: Picture element; an individual component of the image matrix.

Post-processing: Changing or enhancing the electronic image in order to view it from a different perspective or improve its diagnostic quality.

Radiology Information System (RIS): A computer system that supports the operations of a radiology department. Typical functions include exam order processing, exam scheduling, patient registration, report archiving, film tracking, and billing.

Resolution: The recorded sharpness of structures on the image; may also be called detail, sharpness, or definition.

Sensitivity "S" number: A term used by some equipment manufacturers to indicate exposure index. The S number is inversely proportional to the radiation striking the detector.

Smoothing: A post-processing technique that adjusts brightness values of adjacent pixels closer together.

Soft-copy radiograph: A radiographic image viewed on a computer monitor.

Telemedicine: The delivery of health care services using telecommunications and computer technology.

Teleradiology: The electronic transmission of diagnostic imaging studies from one location to another for the purposes of interpretation and/or consultation.

Unsharpness: Decreased sharpness or resolution on an image.

Windowing: The user adjusting the window level and window width (image contrast and brightness).

Window level: Controls the brightness of a digital image (within a certain range).

Window width: Controls the range of gray levels of an image (the contrast).

Workstation: A computer that serves as a digital post-processing station and/or an image review station.

Glossary of Acronyms

AEC: Automatic exposure control
ALARA: As low as reasonably achievable
CAD: Computer-assisted detection
CR: Computed radiography and/or central ray
CT: Computed tomography
DICOM: Digital Imaging Communications in Medicine
DR: Direct digital radiography
DQE: Detection quantum efficiency
HIPAA: Health and Insurance Portability and Accountability Act
HIS: Hospital Information System
HL7: Health care Level 7
IHE: Integrated health care enterprise
IMAC: Image and Information Management and Communication
IR: Image receptor
kV: Kilovoltage
mA: Milliampere
mAs: Milliampere seconds
OID: Object image receptor distance
PACS: Picture Archiving and Communication System
RIS: Radiology Information System
SID: Source image receptor distance
SNR: Signal-to-noise ratio

REFERENCES

Baxes GA: Digital image processing, New York, 1994, John Wiley & Sons.

Bushong S: Radiologic science for technologists, ed 6, St. Louis, 2001, Mosby.

Carlton R, Adler AM: Principles of radiographic imaging, ed 3, New York, 2001, Delmar Publishers.

Dreyer KJ, Mehta A, Thrall JH: PACS picture archiving and communication systems: a guide to the digital revolution, New York, 2002, Springer-Verlag.

Englebardt SP, Nelson R: Health care informatics: an interdisciplinary approach, St. Louis, 2002, Mosby.

Furlow B: Digital medical image management, Radiol Technol 70(5):434-448, 1999.

Huang HK: PACS: basic principles and applications, New York, 1999, Wiley-Liss Inc.

Neitzel U: Integrated digital radiography with a flat electronic detector, Medicamundi 41(2):14-19, 1997.

Page D: Computed radiography offers easy entry to the world of PACS, Diagn Imaging, August, 1999.

Papp J: Quality management in the imaging sciences, St. Louis, 2002, Mosby.

Shepherd CT: Radiographic image production and manipulation, New York, 2003, McGraw-Hill.

Willis CE: 10 Fallacies about CR: decisions in imaging economics, The Journal of Imaging Technology Management, December 2002.

RADIATION PROTECTION

With Richard Geise, PhD

As professionals, technologists have the important responsibility of protecting their patients, themselves, and fellow workers from excessive radiation. A complete understanding of radiation protection is essential for every technologist but is beyond the scope of this anatomy and positioning text. However, the basic principles and applied aspects of radiation protection, as described below, should be an essential part of a course in radiographic positioning. It is the responsibility of every technologist to **always ensure that the radiation dose to both the patient and the technologist is kept *as low as reasonably achievable* (ALARA).**

Units of Radiation

UNITS OF RADIATION EXPOSURE–ROENTGEN (R)

Roentgen is a measurement of **radiation exposure in air,** measured by the amount of ionization in a given unit of air.

UNITS OF RADIATION DOSE–RAD AND REM

Rad and rem are units of **dose** (ionization within tissue, also described as energy absorbed by tissue). In diagnostic radiology using x-ray energy, the three units can be considered equivalent (1 R = 1 rad = 1 rem). **Rads** are used primarily for **patient doses,** and **rem** are used for **radiation protection** purposes, such as in reporting worker doses with film badges.

Traditional vs. SI units The SI (System Internationale, commonly known as the metric system) is the national standard for units of radiation measurement since 1958. However, just as the United States is slow in converting to the metric system for other measurements, conventional units of radiation measurements such as the **roentgen, rad,** and **rem** are still in common use in the U.S. In this section, both traditional and SI units will be used in describing various dose limits. Tables are provided on the right to facilitate conversions between traditional and SI systems and to convert among units within the SI system.

Technologist Protection

In January 1994 the Nuclear Regulatory Commission (NRC) changed some of the standards concerning maximum permissible doses. The correct term now for maximum permissible dose is **dose-limiting recommendations.**

Annual dose limit The dose-limiting recommendation for occupationally exposed workers is **5 rem (50 mSv) of whole-body effective dose (ED) per year.** This 5 rem, or 50 mSv, is also sometimes referred to as the **annual effective dose limit** for whole-body occupational exposure.

The ED for the **general public** is **0.1 rem (1 mSv) per year** for continuous or frequent exposure and **0.5 rem (5 mSv) per year** for infrequent exposure.*

Cumulative dose limit The cumulative lifetime ED limit for an occupationally exposed worker is **1 rem (10 mSv) times the years of age.** For example, a 50-year-old technologist has a maximum allowable accumulated dose of 50 rem (500 mSv). However, because of the small risk of long-term effects of low-level radiation, technologists must limit their exposure to the **least amount possible,** or even less than the allowable 5 rem (50 mSv) per year.

*NCRP Reprint 116, Limits of exposure to ionizing radiation, National Council of Radiologic Protection and Measurements, 1993.

Exposure should be monitored for each occupationally exposed worker. If **0.1 rem (1 mSv)** or more of exposure could potentially be received per year, the area should be supervised by a qualified radiation protection officer.

Minors **Individuals under 18 years of age** should not be employed in situations in which they are occupationally exposed. The ED limit for minors is that of the general public, 0.1 rem (1 mSv) per year for continuous or **frequent exposure.**

CONVERSION TABLE–TRADITIONAL TO SI UNITS

TO CONVERT FROM (TRADITIONAL UNITS)	TO (SI UNITS)	MULTIPLY BY
Roentgen (R)	**C/kg** (Coulombs/kg of air)	**2.58×10^{-4} (.000258)**
Rad (radiation absorbed dose)	**Gray** (Gy)	10^{-2} (.01) (1 rad = .01 Gy)
Rem (radiation equivalent man)	**Seivert** (SV)	10^{-2} (.01) (1 rem = .01 Sv)

Note: Patient doses throughout this textbook are given in mrads (1 mrad = 10^{-2} (.01) or .01 mGy, and 1 mGy = 100 mrad)
Dose limits are given in rem (Seivert, Sv)
(1 rem = 0.01 Sv or 10 mSv, and 1 mSv = 0.1 rem)

SI PREFIXES AND CONVERSIONS

PREFIX	SYMBOL	EXPONENTIAL EXPRESSION	MULTIPLICATION FACTOR
giga	G	10^9	1,000,000,000
mega	M	10^6	1,000,000
kilo	k	10^3	1,000
hecto	h	10^2	100
deca	da	10^1	10
BASE UNIT		10^1	1
deci	d	10^{-1}	0.1
centi	c	10^{-2}	0.01
milli	m	10^{-3}	0.001
micro	μ	10^{-6}	0.000,001
nano	n	10^{-9}	0.000,000,001

SUMMARY OF DOSE-LIMITING RECOMMENDATIONS

Occupational Workers: (Whole-Body Effective Dose–ED)
Annual = 5 rem (50 mSv)
Lifetime accumulation = 1 rem (10 mSv) × years of age

General Population:
Annual = 0.1 rem (1 mSv) for frequent exposure
= 0.5 (5 mSv) for infrequent exposure

Individuals Under 18: Same as general population dose for infrequent exposure (should not be employed in situations with frequent or occupational exposure)

Pregnant Technologists: (Requires a second film badge under lead apron)
.05 rem (0.5 mSv) during any 1 month
0.5 rem (5 mSv) for gestation period

2

Pregnant technologists The pregnant occupationally exposed worker should take all precautions possible to keep exposure to the embryo or fetus as low as possible. The recommended maximum equivalent dose to the fetus is 0.05 rem, or **50 mrem (0.5 mSv), during any 1 month** and **0.5 rem, or 500 mrem (5 mSv),** for the **gestation period.**

Also, pregnant technologists should wear a second film badge or other monitoring device at the abdomen area **under the lead apron.** These monitoring devices must be clearly marked to distinguish the badge worn under the apron at the abdomen from that worn at the collar area.

Personnel monitoring **Film badges** or **TLD** (thermoluminescent dosimetry) **badges** must always be worn by all personnel who have the potential of receiving more than one-fourth the recommended dose limit. They must be worn **at the waist or chest level,** except in **fluoroscopy,** where they should be worn at the **collar area outside the lead apron.** Film badges need to be changed and read every month, and TLD badges at least every 3 months.

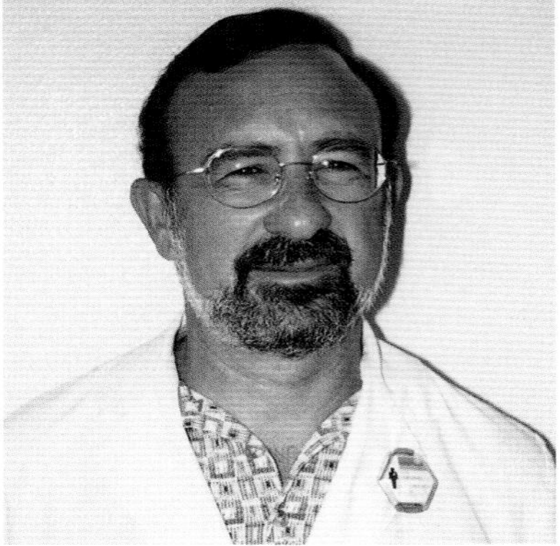

Fig. 2-50. Technologist wearing a TLD.

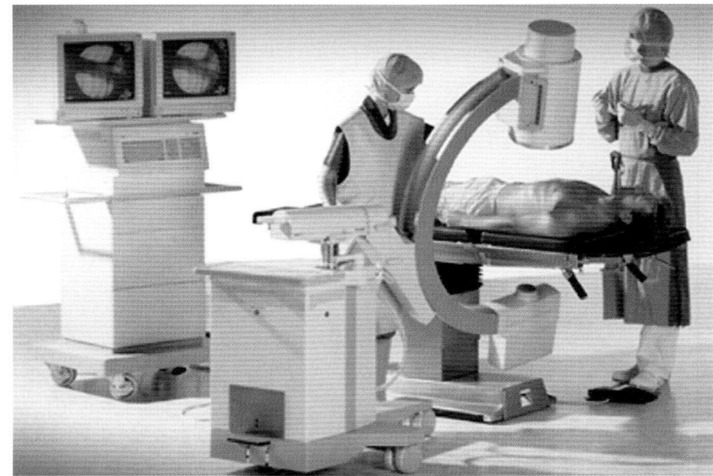

Fig. 2-51. C-arm mobile digital fluoroscopy unit. (Courtesy Phillips Medical Systems.)

ALARA Principles

The protection principle called **ALARA** goes much further in protecting the worker than the ED level. This principle states that occupational exposure should be kept **"*A*s *L*ow *A*s *R*easonably *A*chievable."** This is an important principle that all technologists should strive for. Following is a summary of four important ways ALARA can be achieved:

1. **Always wear a film badge or other monitoring device.** Although the badge doesn't lower exposure of the wearer, long-term accurate records of badge readings are important for determining protection practices.
2. **Restraint devices** or retention bands should be used whenever possible, and only as a last resort should anyone stay in the room to restrain patients—this should **never** be radiology personnel. If restraining patients is necessary, this should be done by **a person other than an occupationally exposed worker.** This person should never stand in the primary or useful beam and should always wear protective aprons and gloves.
3. Practice the use of close **collimation, filtration of primary beam, optimum kV techniques, high-speed screens and film, and minimum repeat exams.** Exposure of the technologist is due primarily to scattered radiation from the patient and other sources. Therefore reduction in patient exposure results in reduced exposure of the technologist as well.
4. Follow the **three-part cardinal rule** of radiation protection: the **time, distance,** and **shielding** principle. The technologist should minimize **time** in an exposure field, stand **as far away** from the source as possible, and use **lead shielding** when in an exposure field.

This is important in trauma and mobile radiography, especially with **C-arm fluoroscopy units** (Fig. 2-51). These are used with orthopedic or biliary tract surgery, foreign body localization, pacemaker insertion, and interventional vascular procedures. Protection from scatter is important for mobile fluoroscopy units such as the C-arm because of the potential for increased patient and worker doses, as described in detail in Chapter 19 in the discussion of trauma and mobile radiography.

Patient Doses

GENERAL DIAGNOSTIC PROCEDURES

Skin Entrance Exposure (SEE) For a particular x-ray examination, it is possible to refer to several different "doses" to the patient. The number most often quoted is the exposure to the skin in the region where the radiation first strikes the body, commonly called the **skin entrance exposure,** or **SEE.** This exposure is approximately the skin dose. The skin dose has the highest numeric value of all the doses, but in radiography it has the least biologic significance. As the radiation passes through the body on the way to the image receptor, its intensity drops as much as several hundred times. The average doses to specific organs are useful for estimating the likelihood that those organs will develop cancer from radiation.

Effective Dose The effective dose (**ED,** sometimes referred to as just **E**) takes into account the dose to all organs and their relative risk of becoming cancerous (or in the case of the gonads, the risk of genetic damage). The ED is the quantity that can be used to **compare average radiation to the whole body from a radiologic procedure with that received from natural background radiation.**

The patient dose chart on the next page shows the **SEE, specific organ doses,** and the **ED** for an average-size patient for a sampling of common radiographic projections.

The chart demonstrates the effects of using different kV and compares doses of AP versus posteroanterior (PA) projections. It also shows the effect of gonadal shielding and the total ED values for male and female.

This chart also reveals that for **males** the highest ED for these sample projections is #10, the **AP unshielded hip** (ED = 84 mrem). This is primarily due to the high testes dose, which can be greatly reduced with gonadal shielding (ED is reduced to 14).

For the **female** the highest ED is #4, the **AP thoracic spine on a 35- × 43-cm film without breast shields** (ED = 63). This is primarily due to the high breast dose, which can be reduced by breast shielding or collimation to a 18- × 43-cm size (ED reduced to 35).

PATIENT DOSE CHART—FILM-SCREEN IMAGING

					Organ Doses Rounded to the Nearest mrad						ED (mrem)	
COMPARISONS	PROJECTION	KV	MAS	SEE (MR)	TESTES	OVARIES	THYROID	MARROW	LUNG	BREAST	MALE	FEMALE
1. AP	AP chest (72″ SID)	120	2	12	0	0	4	1	7	10	2	5
vs. PA	PA chest (72″ SID)	120	2	12	0	0	1	2	7	1	2	2
2. AP	AP skull (10″ × 12″)	80	25	302	0	0	92	4	1	1	3	5
vs. PA	PA skull (10″ × 12″)	80	25	302	0	0	8	10	0	0	3	3
3. AP	AP esophagram	110	6	142	0	0	48	9	66	124	15	54
vs. PA	PA esophagram	110	6	142	0	0	9	16	69	10	16	20
4. 14 × 17	AP thoracic spine	75	20	209	0	0	23	8	72	158	15	<u>63</u>
vs. 7 × 17	AP thoracic spine	80	20	241	0	0	26	5	34	94	6	35
5. 7 × 17	AP lumbar spine	80	40	483	2	74	0	10	16	4	10	29
vs. 14 × 17	AP lumbar spine	75	40	418	2	92	0	17	33	8	17	42
vs. 14 × 17 shielded	AP lumbar spine	75	40	418	1	92	0	17	33	8	17	42
6. AP	AP upper GI	110	15	356	0	26	2	21	99	13	26	37
vs. PA	PA upper GI	110	15	356	0	14	2	43	90	9	28	34
vs. Lateral	Lateral upper GI	110	30	1100	1	18	5	33	147	20	42	53
7. 80 kV	AP abdomen	80	22	266	6	68	0	13	4	1	10	26
vs. 70 kV	AP abdomen	70	41	365	6	80	0	13	4	1	13	31
vs. 70 kV shielded	AP abdomen	70	41	365	2	80	0	13	4	1	11	31
8. AP	AP barium enema	110	10	237	8	89	0	22	6	1	12	32
vs. PA	PA barium enema	110	10	237	5	78	0	51	5	1	15	34
vs. PA shielded	PA barium enema	110	10	237	1	78	0	51	5	1	14	34
9. AP	AP pelvis	80	40	483	45	100	0	23	1	0	26	39
vs. AP shielded	AP pelvis	80	40	483	6	100	0	23	1	0	16	39
10. AP	AP hip (one 10″ × 12″)	80	40	483	322	59	0	9	0	0	<u>84</u>	18
vs. AP shielded	AP hip (one 10″ × 12″)	80	40	483	42	14	0	9	0	0	14	7

Notes: SID = 40 in (100 cm) unless specified. **Film size** = 14 × 17 in (35 × 43 cm) unless specified. **Film-screen speed** = 400. **"Shielded"** refers to male or female gonadal shield in place: —male gonadal shield, —female gonadal shield. **Patient thickness** = 20 cm AP or PA and 34 cm laterally. **The effective dose (ED)** can be compared with the U.S. average yearly background of 300 mrem. Organ dose estimates based on tables in Keriakes JG, Rosenstein M: Handbook of radiation doses in nuclear medicine and diagnostic x-ray, Boca Raton, 1980, CRC Press. Breast doses and ED estimates by authors.

FLUOROSCOPIC PROCEDURES

Typical patient exposures during several gastrointestinal (GI) fluoroscopy procedures are shown in the dose chart on the right, which includes approximate skin entrance exposures (SEE) during fluoroscopy and spot filming. This does not include doses from overhead films for those exams that can be determined from the dose chart above. Fluoroscopic procedures generally involve **much higher patient doses** than conventional "overhead tube" diagnostic exams because of the need to penetrate the barium or iodine contrast media and the time required to manipulate the media in the patient. Fortunately, however, the volume of tissue exposed during fluoroscopy and spot filming is fairly small.

Using magnification mode in fluoroscopy generally increases the dose rate but decreases the volume of tissue exposed. Pulsed fluoroscopy may be used to reduce dose in proportion to the number of pulses used per second. Spot film doses also can be reduced by using photospot cameras or digital fluoroscopy as described in Chapter 14 on the upper GI system.

DOSE CHART FOR FLUOROSCOPY—FILM-SCREEN IMAGING

Typical Upper GI

Overall	Maximum in one location
17 spot films, no overheads	5 spot films at 400 mR each
5 minutes of fluoroscopy	$1\frac{1}{2}$ minutes of fluoroscopy at 3 R/minute

Total maximum skin exposure (SEE): *6.5 R (6500 mR)*

Typical Double-Contrast Barium Enema

Overall	Maximum in one location
11 spot films, no overheads	3 spot films at 233 mR each
7 minutes of fluoroscopy	$1\frac{1}{2}$ minutes of fluoroscopy at 4 R/minute

Total maximum skin entrance exposure (SEE): *6.7 R (6700 mR)*

Worker Protection During Fluoroscopy

EXPOSURE PATTERNS AND WORKER PROTECTION

During routine fluoroscopy of the gastrointestinal tract, personnel are exposed to radiation scattered by the patient and other objects being irradiated. Exposure to this scatter radiation drops dramatically as the workers move away from the patient and table. This is demonstrated in Fig. 2-52, which shows estimated scatter radiation exposure fields directly beside the intensifier tower without tower drape shielding in place.

The intensifier tower, tower lead drapes, Bucky slot shield, x-ray table, patient foot rest (if present), and even the radiologist all provide a source of shielding for the technologist.

The important Bucky slot shield closes the 2- or 3-inch space under the tabletop when the Bucky is all the way to the end of the tabletop. Note that zone F, the area behind the radiologist and away from the patient and table (Fig. 2-53), has the lowest exposure rate of less than 25 mR per hour.

When the intensifier tower is lowered as close as possible to the patient, much of the scatter to the worker's eyes and neck region is eliminated. The vertical and lateral dimensions of the exposure field move in dramatically as the distance between the patient and the intensifier tower is reduced.

WORKER PROTECTION PRACTICES

Even with correct shielding in place and the intensifier tower as close to the patient as possible, a certain amount of scatter radiation is present during routine fluoroscopy (Fig. 2-53).

Scatter is greatest in the immediate region of the patient close to the table on each side of the radiologist, who has the leaded tower drapes between his or her body and the patient. Therefore technologists and/or other workers in the room can reduce their exposure by not standing close to the table on either side of the radiologist but instead staying out of the higher scatter fields as much as possible.

Everyone involved in a fluoroscopic procedure must wear a lead apron as a protective measure. A 0.5-mm lead equivalent apron reduces the scattered radiation to the majority of the body by typically 10 or more times. This is usually enough to reduce risks to a reasonable level well below recommended dose limits. Typical doses behind aprons are less than 10 mrem per month (immeasurable by film badges) in low-use departments and are almost never above 20 mrem per month for technologists involved in only GI fluoroscopy. At these levels it may not be necessary to reassign a pregnant technologist to keep fetal exposure from fluoroscopy below recommended dose limits. Reassignment, however, should be considered on an individual basis in light of the ALARA principle.

Personnel should be cautious if using "lightweight" aprons or ones that have large cutouts around the arms and low necklines. These allow more exposure to dose-sensitive organs such as the thyroid, lungs, and even breasts at certain angles.

Many older aprons do not have specific thyroid shields. These can be separate collar-type shields, which can be worn with the neck cutout-type apron (Fig. 2-54), or they can be the newer type aprons, which include a raised collar-type extension for thyroid protection (Fig. 2-55).

Wearing thyroid shields when available is consistent with the ALARA principle, but the overall reduction in effective dose and risk provided by thyroid shields is small. Also, additional lead protection provided by gloves and lead glasses is generally not needed by technologists during routine GI fluoroscopic duties if recommended practices are followed.

Fluoroscopy Exposure Rate Limits Because of the potential higher patient and worker doses during fluoroscopy, federal standards set limits of exposure rates of intensified fluoroscopy units at 10 R/min. With most modern equipment, however, the average fluoroscopy rate is between 3 and 4 R/min.

EXPOSURE LEVELS

ZONE	MR/HR	MR/MIN
A.	>400	>6.7
B.	400	6.7
	▼	▼
	200	3.3
C.	200	3.3
	▼	▼
	100	1.7
D.	100	1.7
	▼	▼
	50	0.8
E.	50	0.8
	▼	▼
	25	0.4
F.	<25	<0.4

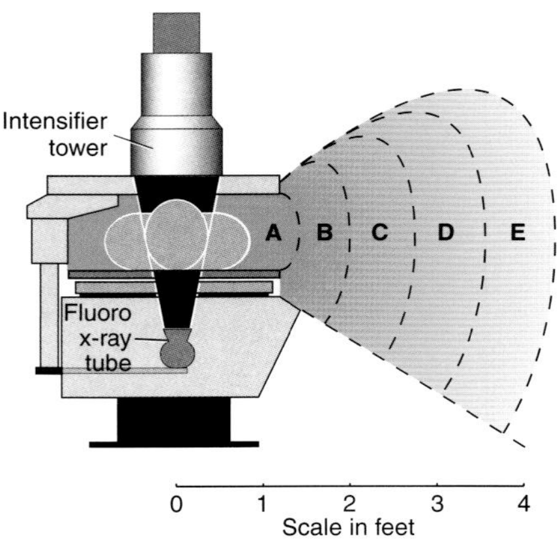

Fig. 2-52. Fluoroscopy exposure patterns **without tower drape shields in place.**

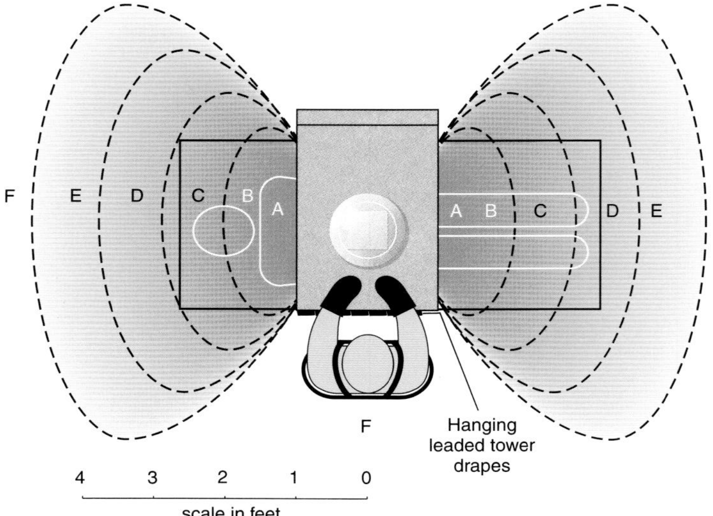

Fig. 2-53. Fluoroscopy exposure patterns during fluoroscopy **with tower drape shields in place** and with intensifier tower close to patient.

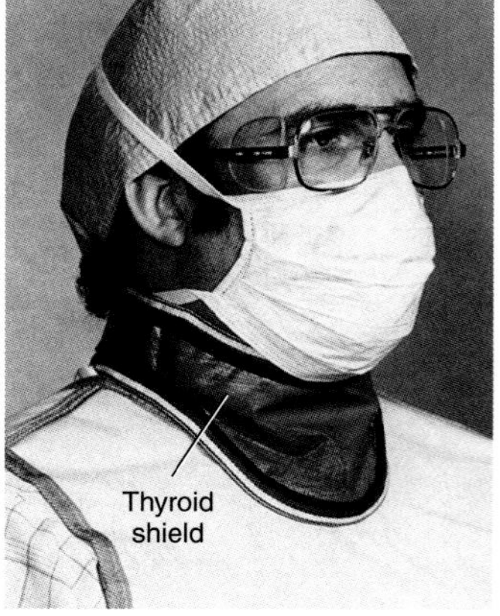

Fig. 5-54. Thyroid shields with regular neck cutout apron. (Courtesy Nuclear Association, Carle, N.Y.)

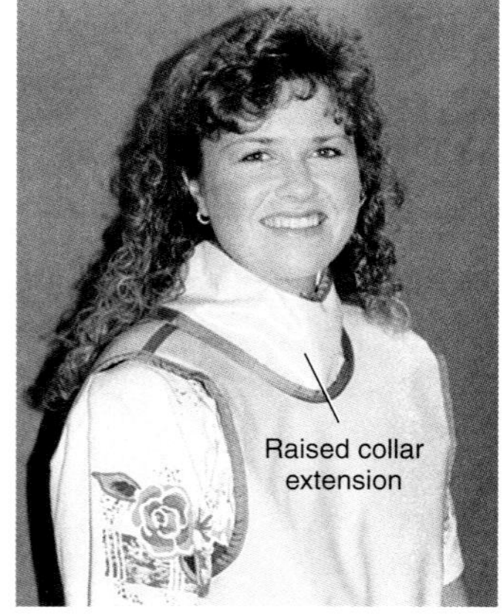

Fig. 2-55. Apron with raised collar extensions. (Courtesy Shielding International, Inc., Madras, Ore.)

Patient Protection

Professional radiologic technologists subscribe to a code of ethics that includes responsibility for controlling and limiting the radiation exposure to all patients under their care. This is a serious responsibility, and each of the following seven ways of reducing patient exposure must be understood and consistently put into practice as described on the following pages.

1. Minimum repeat radiographs
2. Correct filtration
3. Accurate collimation
4. Specific area shielding (gonadal and female breast shielding)
5. Protection for pregnancies
6. Use of high-speed film-screen combinations (not applicable for digital imaging)
7. Minimal patient exposure through selecting projections and exposure factors with the least patient dose—for example:
    - Use of higher kV, lower mAs techniques (see Chapter 8, AP pelvis)
    - Use of PA rather than AP projections to reduce dose to anterior upper thoracic region (thyroid or neck area and female breasts) (see Chapter 10, spine scoliosis series)
    - Use of techniques consistent with the system speed for digital radiography as confirmed by exposure index values

Note: Eye dose is not considered in effective dose determination. Larger doses than those normally received in diagnostic radiology are required to cause cataract formation.

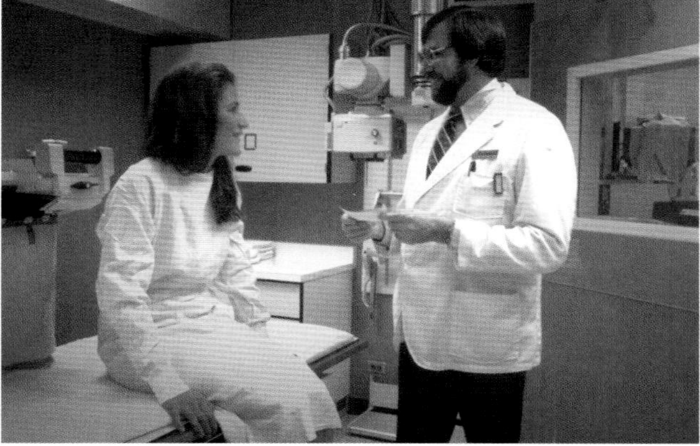

Fig. 2-56 Clear, precise instructions help relieve patient anxieties and prevent unnecessary repeats.

1. MINIMUM REPEAT RADIOGRAPHS

The first basic and most important way to prevent unnecessary radiation is to **prevent unnecessary repeat radiographs.** One of the primary causes for repeat radiographs is **poor communication** between the technologist and the patient. Unclear and misunderstood breathing instructions are one of the common causes of motion and the need to repeat radiographs.

When procedures are not clearly explained, the patient can have added anxiety and nervousness because of the fear of the unknown. This stress from uncertainty and fear often increases the patient's state of mental confusion and ability to cooperate fully. To prevent this, the technologist must take the necessary time, even with heavy schedules and full work loads, to **carefully and fully explain the breathing instructions, as well as the procedure in general, in simple terms that the patient can understand.**

Patients must be forewarned of any movements or strange noises by the equipment during the exposure. Also, any burning sensation or other possible effects from injections during exposures should be explained to the patient.

Carelessness in positioning and selection of incorrect exposure factors are also common causes for repeats and should be prevented.

Correct and accurate positioning requires a good knowledge and understanding of anatomy, because this allows the technologist to visualize the size, shapes, and locations of structures being radiographed. This is the reason for combining the anatomy with positioning in every chapter of this text.

2. CORRECT FILTRATION

Filtration of the primary x-ray beam reduces exposure to the patient by absorbing most of those lower-energy "unusable" x-rays, which primarily expose the patient's skin and superficial tissue. The net effect of filtration is a "hardening" of the x-ray beam, resulting in an increase in the effective energy or penetrability of the x-ray beam.

Filtration is described in two ways. First is **inherent** or built-in filtration from the structures making up the x-ray tube itself. For most x-ray tubes, this is approximately 0.5-mm aluminum (Al) equivalent.

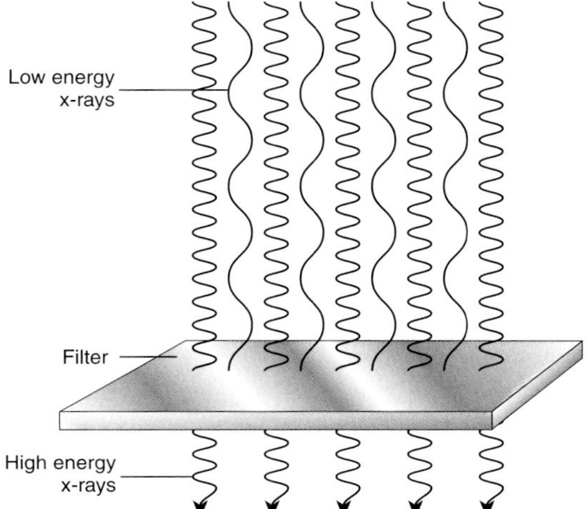

Fig. 2-57 Filtration removes low-energy x-rays (which are not useful) from the beam by absorbing them while permitting higher-energy x-rays to pass through.

Second, and more important to technologists, is **added filtration,** which is the amount of filtration added between the x-ray tube and the collimator and within the collimator itself.

Minimum total filtration (inherent plus added) is **2.5-mm Al equivalent** for equipment producing 70 kV or greater.

Aluminum (Al) is the metal most commonly used for filters in diagnostic radiology, with molybdenum (Mo) often used in mammography. The amount of required added filtration as established by federal laws depends on the operating kV range of the equipment. The manufacturers of x-ray equipment are required to meet these standards.

Periodic Checking of Filtration The filtration of diagnostic imaging equipment should be checked yearly and after a major equipment service, such as replacement of the tube or collimator. This should be done by qualified personnel, such as a medical physicist. The responsibility of the technologist is to ensure that the proper filter material for each tube is checked when needed and that it remains in place.

3. ACCURATE COLLIMATION

Accurate collimation is an essential way to reduce patient exposure by **limiting the size and shape of the x-ray beam to only the area of clinical interest** or that area to be visualized on the image receptor. Careful and accurate collimation is emphasized and demonstrated throughout this textbook.

The adjustable collimator is commonly used for general diagnostic radiographic equipment. The illuminated light field defines the x-ray beam field on accurately calibrated equipment and can be used effectively to determine the tissue area being irradiated. Safety standards require that collimators be accurate to within **2% of the SID.**

The concept of divergence of the x-ray beam must be considered in accurate collimation. Therefore the illuminated field size as it appears on the skin surface of the patient will appear smaller than the actual size of the anatomic area to which one is collimating. This is most evident on an exam such as a lateral thoracic or lumbar spine (Fig. 2-58), in which there is considerable distance from the skin surface to the IR in the Bucky tray. In such cases the light field, when collimated correctly to the area of interest, will appear much too small unless one considers the divergence of the x-ray beam.

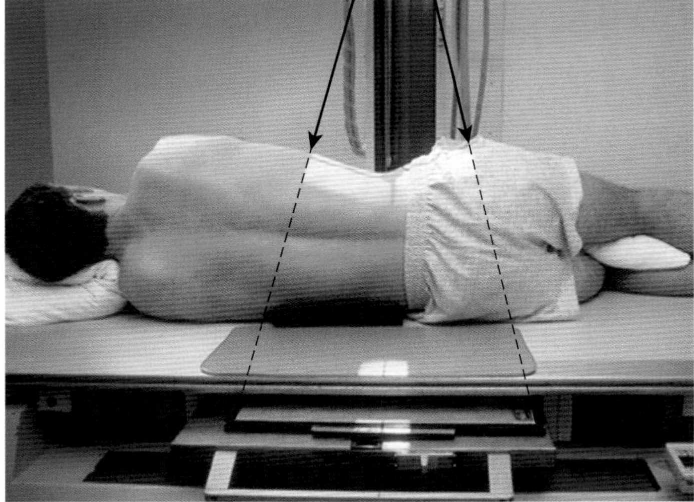

Fig. 2-58. Close four-sided collimation. (Collimation field may appear too small because of divergence of x-rays.)

Collimation and Tissue Dose Accurate and close collimation to the area of interest results in a dramatic drop-off in tissue dosage as one moves away from the border of the collimated x-ray field. For example, the dose at **3 cm** from the edge of the exposure field will be about **10%** of that received in the field. At a distance of **12 cm** the dose will be only about **1%** of that within the field.*

Positive Beam Limitation (PBL) All general purpose x-ray equipment built between 1974 and 1993 in the United States and Canada requires collimators with PBL features that automatically collimate the useful x-ray beam to the film size. (This requirement became optional after May 3, 1993, as a result of a change in FDA regulations.) The PBL feature consists of sensors in the film cassette holder that, when activated by placing a cassette in the cassette holder (Bucky tray), automatically signal the collimator to adjust the x-ray beam to that film or IR size.

The PBL device can be deactivated or overridden with a key, but this should be done only under special conditions in which larger collimation by manual control is needed. A red warning light automatically comes on as a reminder that the PBL system has been deactivated, and regulations require that the key cannot be removed while the system is being overridden (Fig. 2-59).

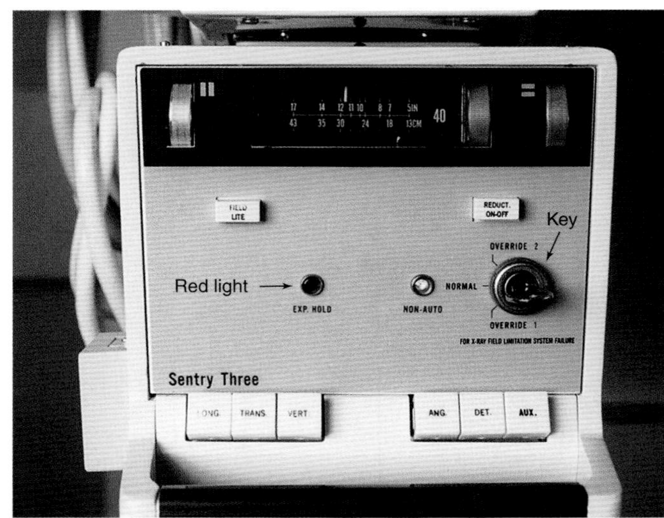

Fig. 2-59. Automatic collimation (PBL).

Manual Collimation Even with automatic collimation (PBL), the operator can also manually reduce the collimation field size even further. This should be done for all exams in which the IR is larger than the critical area being radiographed. Accurate manual collimation also is required for exams of the upper and lower limbs taken tabletop wherein the PBL device is not activated. Throughout the positioning pages of this textbook, collimation guidelines are provided to maximize patient protection by careful and accurate collimation.

This practice of close collimation to only the area of interest reduces patient exposure in **two ways.** First, it **reduces the volume of tissue directly irradiated,** and second, it **reduces the accompanying scatter radiation.** This scatter radiation resulting from lack of accurate collimation or other shielding not only adds unnecessary increased patient exposure but also results in decreased image quality by the "fogging" effect of scatter radiation. (This is especially true in high-volume tissue areas such as the abdomen or chest.)

*Keriakes JG, Rosenstein M: Handbook of radiation doses in nuclear medicine and diagnostic x-ray, Boca Raton, 1980, CRC Press.

Three Reasons for Four-Sided Collimation In addition to (1) reducing patient exposure and (2) improving image quality, a third reason for this general rule of at least some visible collimation on all four sides is that it acts as (3) a **check system to ensure that maximum collimation did occur.** If there is no collimation border visible on the radiograph on any one or more sides on exams taken tabletop where there is no automatic collimation, then no evidence exists that the primary beam was restricted at all.

An added benefit for at least some collimation on all four sides, if possible, is the ability to check the final radiograph for **correct central ray location.** As described previously in Chapter 1, this is done by imagining a large X ending from the four corners of the collimation field, the center of which is the CR location.

Collimation rule A general rule followed throughout this text indicates that collimation should **limit the exposure field to only the area of interest,** and **collimation borders should be visible on the IR on all four sides** if the IR size is large enough to allow this without "cutting off" essential anatomy.

4. SPECIFIC AREA SHIELDING

Specific area shielding is required when radiosensitive tissue or organs such as the thyroid gland, breasts, and gonads are in or near the useful beam. Examples of this type of area shielding are **breast** and **gonadal** shields, which can be used over female breasts and male or female gonads for examinations such as a scoliosis spine series.

The most common and most important area shielding is **gonadal shielding,** used to protect the reproductive organs from irradiation when they are in or near the primary beam. The two general types of specific area shielding are **shadow shields** and **contact shields.**

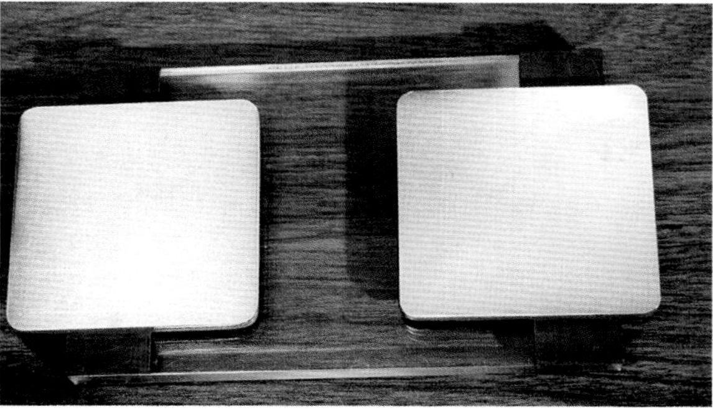

Fig. 2-60. Breast shadow shields to be attached to collimator exit surface with Velcro.

Shadow Shields As the name implies, shadow shields, which are attached to the collimator, are devices placed between the x-ray tube and the patient, thus casting a shadow of the shield over the specific areas being shielded. One such type of shield is shown in Fig. 2-60, where the shields are attached to the collimator exit surface with Velcro. These shields can be adjusted to cast a shadow from the collimator light over the areas being shielded.

Another type of shadow shield is shown in Fig. 2-61, where individual breast and gonad shields are attached with magnets directly to the bottom of the collimator. These may also be combined with clear lead compensating filters to provide a more uniform exposure for body parts that are not uniform in thickness or density, such as for a thoracic and lumbar spine scoliosis radiograph (Fig. 2-62).

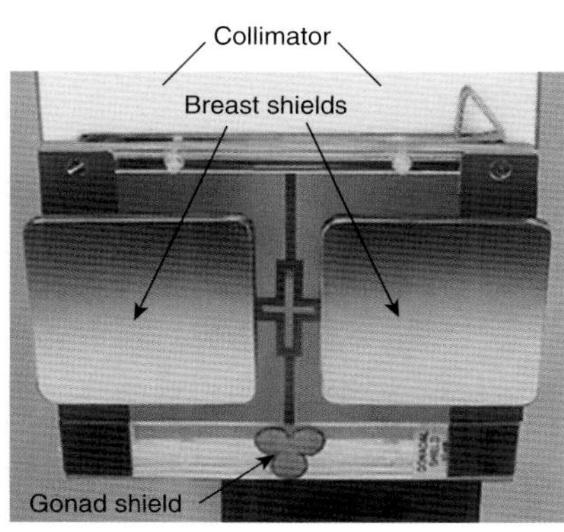

Fig. 2-61. Shadow shields in place under collimator (attached with magnets). (Courtesy Nuclear Associates, Carle, N.Y.)

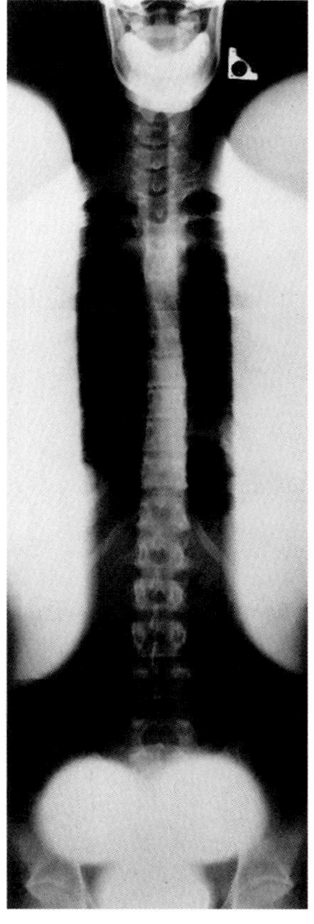

Fig. 2-62. AP spine for scoliosis with compensating filter and breast and gonad shields in place. (Courtesy Nuclear Associates, Carle, NY.)

Gonadal Contact Shields Flat contact gonadal shields are most commonly used for patients in recumbent positions. Larger vinyl-covered lead shields of **0.5-mm lead equivalent** placed over the gonadal area in general may be used to **absorb scatter and/or leakage radiation** (Fig. 2-63). These shields are usually made from the same lead-impregnated vinyl materials used for lead aprons.

Gonadal contact shields, which absorb 95% to 99% of primary rays in the 50- to 100-kV range, require a **minimum of 1-mm lead equivalent when placed in the primary x-ray field.** Examples of these may be smaller vinyl-covered lead material cut into various shapes to be placed directly over the reproductive organs, as shown in Figs. 2-64 and 2-65.

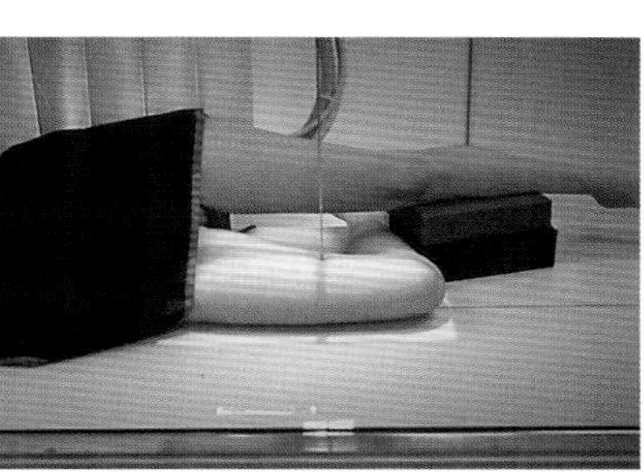

Fig. 2-63. Vinyl-covered lead shield in place over pelvis for lateral mid- and distal femur.

Male Gonadal shields for males should be placed distally to the symphysis pubis, covering the area of the testes and scrotum (Fig. 2-64). The upper margin of the shield should be at the symphysis pubis. Smaller sizes should be used for smaller males or children. These are slightly tapered at the top and wider at the bottom to better shield the testes and scrotum without obscuring pelvic and hip structures.

Female Placement of gonadal shielding on females to cover the area of the ovaries, fallopian tubes, and uterus may be more difficult to determine. A general guideline for female adults is to shield an area $4\frac{1}{2}$ to 5 inches (11 to 13 cm) proximal or superior to the symphysis pubis and 3 to $3\frac{1}{2}$ inches (8 to 9 cm) each way from the pelvic midline. The lower border of the shield should be at or slightly above the symphysis pubis, with the upper border extending just above the level of the ASIS (anterior superior iliac spines) (Fig. 2-65).

Various-shaped female ovarian shields may be used, but they should be wider in the upper region to cover the area of the ovaries and narrower towards the bottom to offer less obstruction of pelvic or hip structures. The shielded area would be proportionally smaller on children. For example, a 1-year-old female would require a shield only about $2\frac{1}{2}$ to 3 inches (6 to 7 cm) wide and 2 inches (5 cm) in height placed directly superior to the symphysis pubis.*

Gonadal shields, if placed correctly, will reduce the gonadal dose **50% to 90%** if the gonads are in the primary x-ray field.

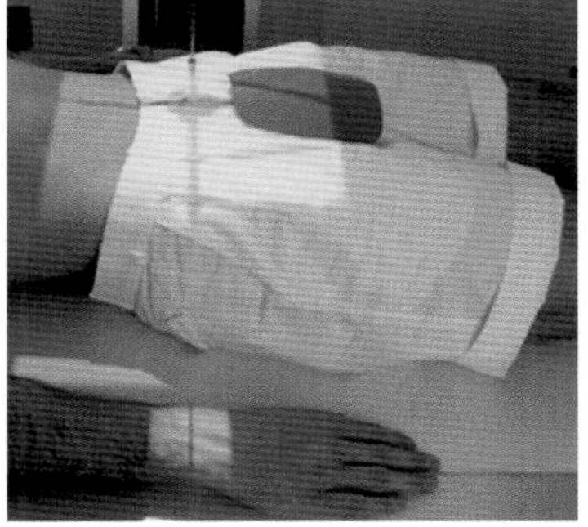

Fig. 2-64. AP pelvis. Flat contact shield (1-mm lead equivalent).

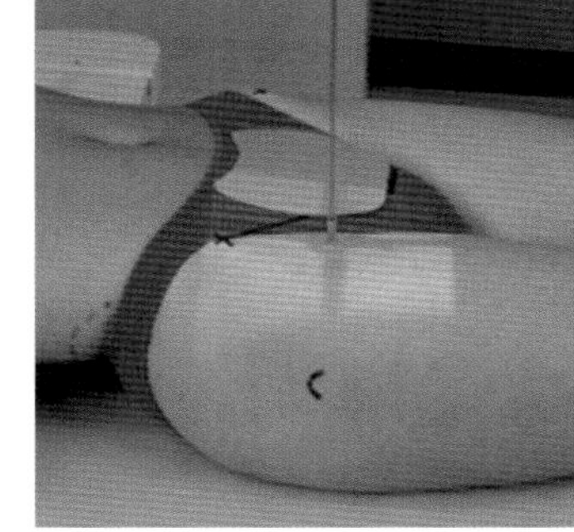

Fig. 2-65. AP right hip. Flat contact shield (1-mm lead equivalent).

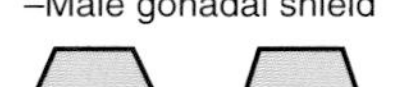

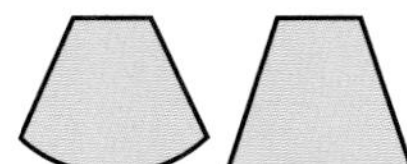

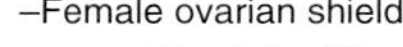

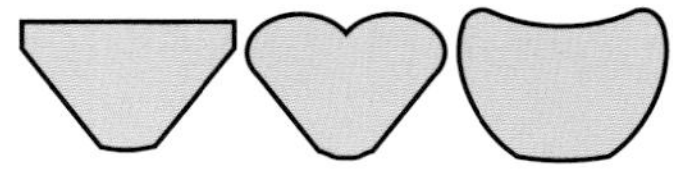

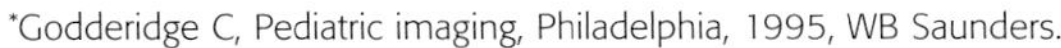

*Godderidge C, Pediatric imaging, Philadelphia, 1995, WB Saunders.

Summary Rules for Specific Area Shielding Consistent and correct use of specific area shielding is a challenge for each technologist because of the added time and equipment required. The importance, however, of protecting radiation-sensitive organs and the gonads of children and adults of reproductive age from unnecessary radiation exposure should be sufficient motivation to consistently practice the following three rules for gonadal shielding:

1. **It should be used on all potentially reproductive-age patients.** A common departmental policy is to include specific area shielding for all children and those adults of reproductive age. (A good policy followed in many departments is to shield gonads for all patients when possible.)
2. **It should be used when the radiation-sensitive areas lie within or near** (2 inches or 5 cm) **the primary beam unless such shielding obscures essential diagnostic information.**
3. **Accurate beam collimation** and careful positioning must accompany the use of such shielding. Specific area shielding is important, but this should always be a **secondary** protective measure and **not** a substitute for accurate collimation.

5. PROTECTION FOR PREGNANCIES

Pregnancies and potential pregnancies require special consideration for all women of childbearing age because of the evidence that the developing embryo is especially sensitive to radiation. This concern is particularly critical during the first 2 months of pregnancy, when the fetus is most sensitive to radiation exposure and the mother is usually not yet aware of the pregnancy.

In the past the **10-day** or **LMP rule** (last menstrual period), as stated by the ICRP (International Commission on Radiation Protection), was used as a safeguard for potential early pregnancies. This rule stated that all radiologic examinations involving the pelvis and lower abdomen should be scheduled during the first 10 days following the onset of menstruation because no conception will have occurred during this time.

More recently, this rule is being abandoned as reported in various documents by both the ICRP and the American College of Radiology because of the potential harm of canceling essential x-ray procedures during this 10-day period. Studies have shown that if x-ray exams are clinically indicated, they should be performed, even during this period. Exceptions to this are those higher dose exams of the pelvic area or fluoroscopy procedures that can be delayed a few weeks without compromising the health of the patient. However, posters or signs (Figs. 2-66 and 2-67) should be posted in examination rooms and waiting room areas, reminding the patient to inform someone of their known pregnancy or potential pregnancy.

If x-ray procedures are performed during this period of potential pregnancy, it is important to use all those radiation protection practices already described, especially careful collimation.

For **known pregnancies,** the following exams result in higher doses to the fetus and embryo and should require confirmation from the referring physician and the radiologist that the exam is indicated:

- Lumbar spine
- Sacrum and coccyx
- Intravenous urogram (IVU)
- Fluoroscopic procedures (abdomen)
- Pelvis
- Proximal femur and hip
- Computed tomography

6. OPTIMUM-SPEED FILM-SCREEN COMBINATIONS (NOT APPLICABLE WITH DIGITAL IMAGING)

The sixth protection practice involves the use of high-speed film-screen combinations, which reduces patient dose dramatically. For all film-screen combinations, over 99% of the radiographic image results from light emitted by the intensifying screens, and less than 1% from the primary rays themselves. Therefore the speed of the intensifying screens has a great effect on the required x-ray exposure to the patient in producing radiographs.

IF YOU ARE PREGNANT
PLEASE TELL THE TECHNOLOGIST

SENORAS-SI ESTAN EMBARAZADAS FAVOR
DE NOTIFICAR A LOS TECHNOLOGISTAS

Fig. 2-66. Warning sign. (Courtesy St. Joseph's Hospital, Phoenix, Ariz.)

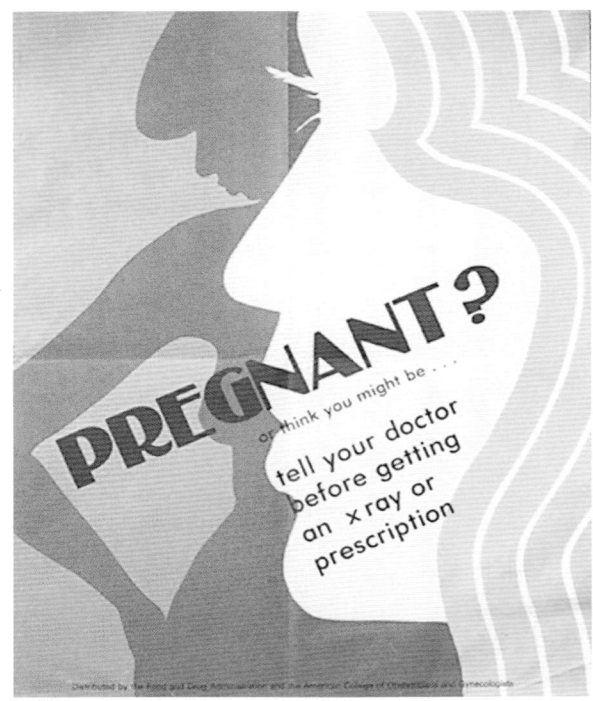

Fig. 2-67. Warning poster.

Certain rare earth high-speed screens in common use today have speeds that are four or more times faster than those of the more commonly used 100-speed (par-speed) screens. Therefore the patient exposure can be reduced to one-quarter or less.

Some films with thicker emulsion or with different chemical dyes are also faster or more sensitive, thus reducing the amount of exposure required. The use of higher-speed screens and films, however, does result in some loss of image definition or sharpness of detail, and the radiologist must balance the reduction in patient exposure with the potential loss of detail in the resultant image. A common practice is to use slower 100-speed (detail) screens with tabletop procedures, such as upper and lower limbs, when a grid is not used and optimum detail is important.

Faster-speed screens are commonly used for larger body parts when grids and higher exposure techniques are required.

Film-Screen Rule Use the highest speed film-screen combination that results in diagnostically acceptable radiographs.

Note: Departmental protocol or routine generally indicates which speed film-screen combinations should be used for which types of procedures. This is not a decision usually made by individual technologists.

7. MINIMIZE PATIENT EXPOSURE BY SELECTING PROJECTIONS AND EXPOSURE FACTORS WITH THE LEAST PATIENT DOSE

The seventh and final way technologists can reduce patient exposure, as described in this text, requires an understanding and awareness of the amount of radiation the patient receives with each exposure. For example, technologists should know the effect of various exposure combinations on patient dose. They should also know the dose differences to the thyroid and female breasts on AP compared with PA projections for the head, neck, and upper thorax region. In the same way that a good understanding of anatomy is important in learning positioning, some knowledge of **patient dose ranges** is also important for each projection or radiographic procedure.

When a repeat is necessary because of a positioning or technique error, approximately how much additional dose is being given to the patient? What is the effect on dosage when the kV is increased and mAs decreased? How much can the ovarian dose be reduced for certain projections, such as a female hip, if a correctly placed ovarian shield is used? How much more dose to the testes does a male receive on an axiolateral or inferosuperior lateral hip, compared with other lateral hip projections?

To answer these questions for technologists, sample patient doses are included with each projection described in this textbook in a small icon box format, as shown on the upper right and as described below:

DOSE CALCULATIONS

Skin Dose (Sk) Skin entrance dose was determined by using certain adjustment factors with source-skin distance and backscatter considerations. Thus the exposure in roentgens (R) as emitted from the x-ray tube is converted to absorbed dose units at the skin as measured in millirad (mrad).

Midline Dose (ML) Midline doses are similar to specific organ doses located in midbody regions. All doses, as listed, assume accurate collimation to the region of interest.

Gonadal Dose (Gon) Gonadal doses, as listed for male (M) and female (F), assume no specific gonadal shields were used. These doses would be 50% to 90% less than those listed if correctly placed gonadal shields were used as described under gonadal contact shields on p. 71.

These gonadal doses are given without shielding to remind the technologist of the extreme importance of gonadal shielding whenever possible when the gonads are in or near the primary exposure field if such shielding does not cover essential anatomy.

Gonadal doses for certain upper and lower limb procedures and procedures of the head and neck region are indicated as NDC (no detectable contribution). This indicates that the contribution to the gonadal dose was insignificant.

Thyroid and/or Breast Doses Certain projections of the head, neck, and thorax include significant primary and/or scatter dose to the thyroid gland and/or female breasts, which are radiosensitive organs that should be shielded if possible. These doses will replace the gonadal doses where available to emphasize the need to shield these regions or to take PA rather than AP projections when possible.

SAMPLE EXPOSURE AND DOSE ICON BOXES—AP LUMBAR SPINE, CHAPTER 10.

Technique and Dose–AP

	cm	kV	mAs	Sk.	ML.	Gon.
@80 kV:	17	80	15	242	62	M 1 F 27
@92 kV:	17	92	8	176	51	M 1 F 21
				mrad		

Measurement and Techniques (Exposure Factors):

cm (17) –AP lumbar measurement for this model "patient" (see Note 1)
kV (80 or 92) –Kilovoltage required for this "patient"
mAs (15 or 8) –mAs required at specified kV

Patient Doses in mrad @ 80 kV, 15 mAs and @ 92 kV, 8 mAs:

Sk Skin entrance dose
ML Midline dose
Gon. Gonadal doses for the male (M) and female (F) with accurate collimation as indicated, assuming no specific gonadal shields were used

(Thyroid and/or breast doses when available will be substituted for gonadal doses for projections involving the upper body where these doses become significant and gonadal doses are insignificant.)

Additional Factors:

- 40-inch (100-cm) SID
- Kodak 100-speed screens for tabletop procedures
- Kodak 400-speed screens used with grids
- 12:1 Bucky grid and 6:1 portable grids

Note 1: Some of the models as demonstrated in this textbook are smaller than the average adult patient, indicating that the kV or mAs would be higher on larger patients, with corresponding **higher doses.**

Note 2: Exposure factors (kV and mAs) are listed only to indicate the basis for the associated patient doses and are not recommended technique factors that can be used in any department. Variables such as screen and film speed, grid ratio, film processing, SID, filters, and equipment calibration will determine the technique required for specific equipment.

Note 3: All doses as calculated for this textbook are based on an output at 1 meter SID (100 cm or about 40 inches) of 6 mR/mAs at 80 kV. This is for a three-phase generator with a half value layer of 3-mm aluminum at 80 kV.

Note 4: Doses were calculated in part using tables in Keriakes JG, Rosenstein M: Handbook of radiation doses in nuclear medicine and diagnostic x-ray, Boca Raton, 1980, CRC Press.

Specific organ doses were calculated based on a "Computer Program for Tissue Doses in Diagnostic Radiology (CD13)" from the Center for Devices and Radiological Health, Rockville, Md.

CHAPTER 3

Chest

CONTRIBUTIONS BY **Nancy Johnson,** BA, RT(R)(CV)(CT)(QM)

CONTRIBUTORS TO PAST EDITIONS Karen Brown, RT(R), Kathy M. Martensen, BS, RT(R)

CONTENTS

RADIOGRAPHIC ANATOMY

Chest

Chest radiographic examinations are the most common of all radiographic procedures. Student radiographers typically begin their clinical experience taking chest radiographs. Before beginning such clinical experience, however, it is important to learn and understand chest anatomy, including relative relationships of all anatomy within the chest cavity.

The **chest,** or **thorax,** is the upper part of the trunk between the neck and the abdomen. Radiographic **anatomy of the chest is divided into three sections:** the **bony thorax,** the **respiratory system proper,** and the **mediastinum.**

BONY THORAX

The **bony thorax** is that part of the skeletal system providing a protective framework for the parts of the chest involved with breathing and blood circulation. **Thoracic viscera** is the term used to describe these parts of the chest consisting of the lungs and the remaining thoracic organs contained in the mediastinum.

Anteriorly, the bony thorax consists of the **sternum** (breastbone), which is made up of three divisions. The superior portion is the **manubrium** *(mah-nu'bre-um),* the large center portion is the **body,** and the smaller inferior portion is the **xiphoid process.**

Superiorly, the bony thorax consists of the **two clavicles** (collarbones) connecting the sternum to the **two scapulae** (shoulder blades), the **twelve pairs of ribs** circling the thorax, and the **twelve thoracic vertebrae** posteriorly. A detailed description of all parts of the bony thorax is presented in Chapter 11.

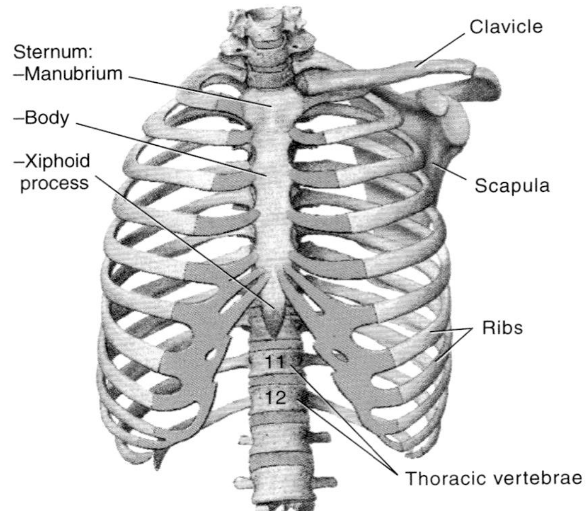

Fig. 3-1. Bony thorax.

Topographic Positioning Landmarks

Accurate and consistent radiographic positioning requires certain landmarks, or reference points, to center the image receptor (IR) correctly to ensure that all essential anatomy is included on that specific projection. These topographic landmarks need to be parts of the body that are easily and consistently located on patients, such as parts of the bony thorax. For chest positioning, two of these landmarks are the **vertebra prominens** and the **jugular notch.**

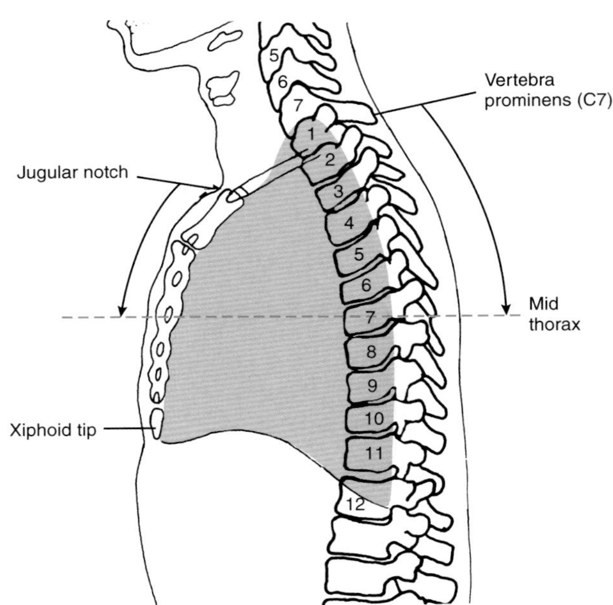

Fig. 3-2. Topographic landmarks.

Vertebra prominens (seventh cervical vertebra)

The vertebra prominens can be an important landmark for determining the central ray location on a posteroanterior (PA) chest projection. It can be readily palpated on most patients by applying light pressure with the fingertips at the base of the neck. The vertebra prominens is the first prominent process felt as you gently but firmly palpate down the back of the neck with the head dropped forward. With a little practice this landmark can be readily located on most patients, especially if the head and neck are flexed forward.

Jugular notch (manubrial or suprasternal notch)

The jugular notch is an important landmark for determining the central ray placement on anteroposterior (AP) chest projections. This is easily palpated as a deep notch or depression on the superior portion of the sternum below the thyroid cartilage (commonly known as *Adam's apple).*

The midthorax, at the level of T7 (seventh thoracic vertebra), can easily be located from these two landmarks, as described later in this chapter.

Xiphoid tip The inferior tip of the sternum, the **xiphoid tip,** which corresponds to the level of T9 or T10 (ninth or tenth thoracic vertebra), can also be palpated. This corresponds to the approximate level of the anterior portion of the diaphragm, which separates the chest cavity from the abdominal cavity. However, this is not a reliable landmark for positioning the chest because of body habitus variations and the variable lower position of the posterior lungs, which may extend as far as T11 or T12 on inspiration, as shown in Fig. 3-2.

RESPIRATORY SYSTEM

Respiration is the exchange of gaseous substances between the air we breathe and the bloodstream. The respiratory system consists of those parts of the body through which air passes as it travels from the nose and mouth into the lungs. Four general divisions of the respiratory system shown in Fig. 3-3 are the **pharynx, trachea, bronchi,** and **lungs.**

An important structure of the respiratory system is the dome-shaped **diaphragm,** which is the chief muscle of inspiration. Each half of the diaphragm is termed a **hemidiaphragm** (*hemi-* meaning "half"). As the dome of the diaphragm moves downward, it **increases** the volume of the thoracic cavity. This, along with certain other dimensional movements of the thorax described later in this chapter, **decreases** the intrathoracic pressure, creating a "sucking" action or negative pressure effect, resulting in air being drawn into the lungs through the nose and mouth, pharynx, larynx, trachea, and bronchi.

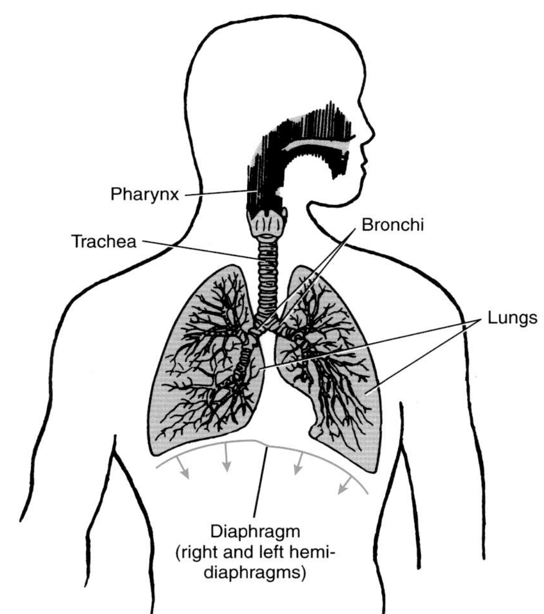

Fig. 3-3. Respiratory system.

Pharynx

The **pharynx** *(far'inks)* (upper airway) is a structure or passageway important to the respiratory system because air must pass through it before entering the respiratory system proper, which begins with the larynx, or voice box. The pharynx, also referred to as the *upper airway* or the *upper respiratory tract,* is that posterior area between the nose and mouth above, and the larynx and the esophagus below. This is the area that serves as **a passageway for both food and fluids, as well as air, thus making it common to both the digestive and respiratory systems.** For this reason the pharynx is **not** considered part of the respiratory system proper.

The pharynx has three divisions, as shown in Fig. 3-4: the **nasopharynx** *(na"zo-far'inks),* **oropharynx** *(o"ro-far'inks),* and **laryngopharynx** *(lah-ring"go-far'inks).* The interior of the pharynx communicates posteriorly with certain cavities, the nose above (nasopharynx), the mouth (oropharynx), and the larynx below (laryngopharynx), as well as the esophagus. The **hard palate** and **soft palate** make up the roof of the oral cavity. The lower posterior aspect of the soft palate is called the **uvula** *(u'vu-lah),* which marks the boundary between the nasopharynx and the oropharynx.

The laryngopharynx lies above and posterior to the larynx and extends from the upper border of the **epiglottis** *(ep"i-glot'is)* to where the laryngopharynx narrows to join the esophagus.

The upper portion of the epiglottis projects upward behind the tongue and acts as a lid for the slanted opening of the larynx. During the act of swallowing, the epiglottis flips down and covers the laryngeal opening, which prevents food and fluid from entering the larynx and bronchi.

Additional structures shown on this sectional lateral drawing are the **hyoid bone,** the **thyroid cartilage** of the larynx (Adam's apple), the **thyroid gland,** and the **trachea,** which are described in more detail in the next sections on the larynx and trachea.

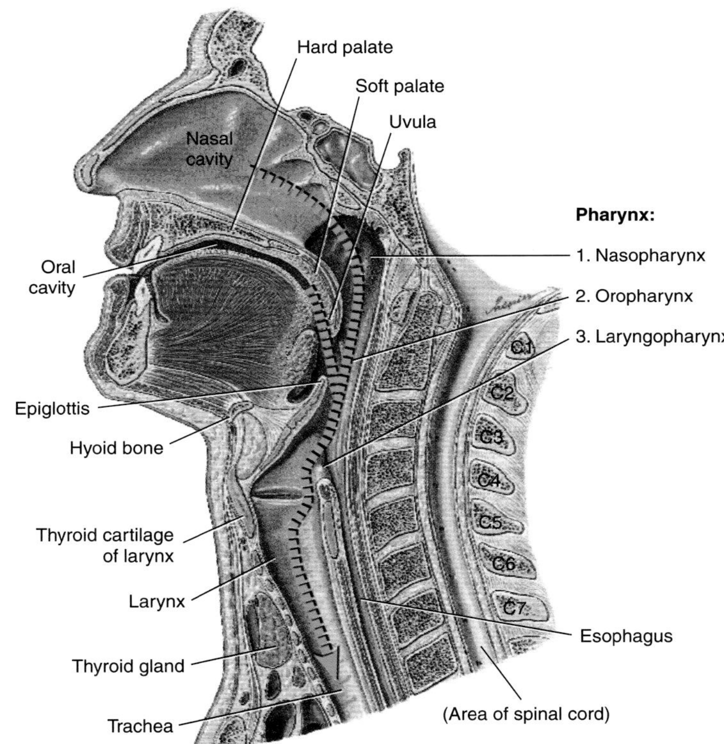

Fig. 3-4. Pharynx, upper airway (midsagittal section).

Air pathway The dotted blue lines in Fig. 3-4 indicate the pathway that air may take from the external environment to the trachea and eventually to the lungs. Note that air passing through either the nose or mouth must pass through at least some portion of the pharynx.

Esophagus

The **esophagus** is the part of the digestive system that connects the pharynx with the stomach. Note the relationship of the esophagus to both the pharynx and the larynx. It begins at the distal end of the laryngopharynx and continues downward to the stomach, **posterior to the larynx and trachea.** (Chapter 14 describes the esophagus in detail along with the upper digestive system.)

Four Parts of Respiratory System

The four parts of the respiratory system proper important in chest radiography are as follows:

1. **Larynx** *(lar'inks)* (voice box)
2. **Trachea** *(tra'ke-ah)*
3. **Right** and **left bronchi** *(bron'chi)*
4. **Lungs**

The larynx, trachea, and bronchi form a continuous, tubular structure through which air can pass from the nose and mouth into the lungs, as shown in Figs. 3-3 and 3-4 on the preceding page.

Note: Remember the pharynx serves as a passage for both air and food and thus is not considered part of the respiratory system proper.

Larynx (voice box)

The **larynx,** or voice box, is a cagelike, cartilaginous structure approximately 1½ to 2 inches (4 to 5 cm) in length in an adult. The larynx is in the anterior portion of the neck, suspended from a small bone called the **hyoid** (Fig. 3-5). The hyoid bone is found in the upper neck just below the tongue or floor of the mouth (Fig. 3-4). The hyoid bone is **not** part of the larynx.

The larynx serves as the organ of voice. Sounds are made as air passes between the **vocal cords** located within the larynx (Fig. 3-6). The upper margin of the larynx is at the approximate level of **C3.** Its lower margin, where the larynx junctions with the trachea, is at the level of **C6.**

The framework of the larynx consists of cartilages, connected by ligaments and moved by numerous muscles that assist in the complex sound-making or voice process. The largest and least mobile of these cartilages is the **thyroid cartilage,** which consists of two fused platelike structures that form the anterior wall of the larynx. The prominent anterior projection of the thyroid cartilage is easily palpated and is known as the **laryngeal prominence,** or Adam's apple. This prominent structure is an important positioning landmark because it is easy to locate. The laryngeal prominence of the thyroid cartilage located at approximately the level of **C5** is an excellent topographic reference for locating specific skeletal structures in this region.

The **cricoid** *(kri'koid)* **cartilage** is a ring of cartilage forming the inferior and posterior wall of the larynx. It is attached to the first ring of cartilage of the trachea.

One of the cartilages making up the larynx is the uniquely shaped **epiglottis,** which resembles a leaf with the narrow distal stem portion attached to a part of the thyroid cartilage. As described on the preceding page, the epiglottis flips down and covers the trachea during the act of swallowing (see *arrows,* Fig. 3-6).

Axial (cross-sectional) image of larynx Because of the wide acceptance of CT (computed tomography) and MRI (magnetic resonance imaging), the technologist must recognize anatomic structures in cross-section. Fig. 3-7 shows an axial (also called *cross-sectional*) view of the midportion of the larynx at the level of C5. Only major structures are labeled in this section. A more detailed study of the cross-sectional anatomy of the chest is found in Chapter 22.

Note: Conventional CT images such as seen here are commonly viewed as though one were facing the patient. Thus the patient's right is to the viewer's left. This is the same way conventional radiographs are placed for viewing (see Chapter 1, p. 40).

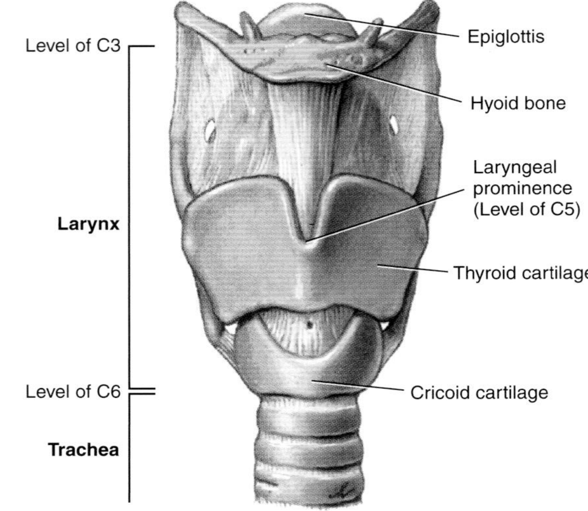

Fig. 3-5. Larynx (frontal view).

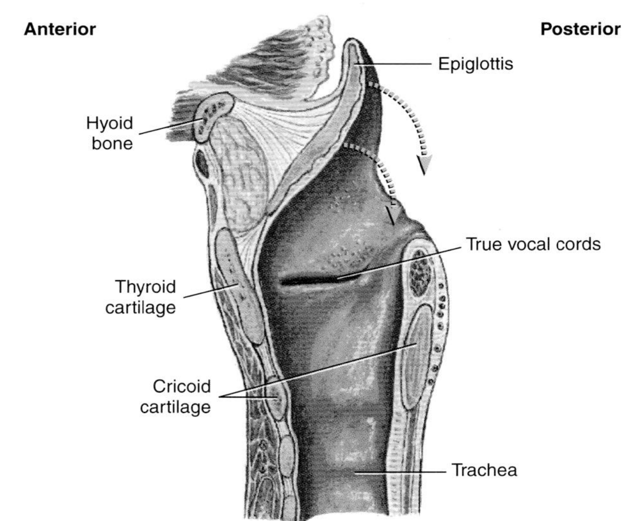

Fig. 3-6. Larynx (lateral view).

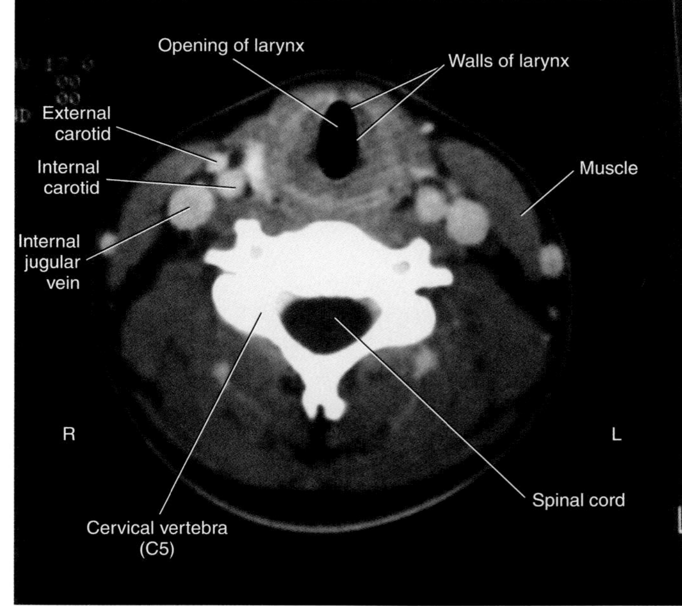

Fig. 3-7. CT image of neck through larynx—axial (cross) section at level of C5.

Trachea

Continuing from the larynx downward, the second division of the respiratory system proper is the **trachea,** or windpipe. It is a fibrous muscular tube about $\frac{3}{4}$ inch (2 cm) in diameter and $4\frac{1}{2}$ inches (11 cm) long. Approximately 20 C-shaped rings of cartilage are embedded in its walls. These rigid rings keep the airway open by preventing the trachea from collapsing during inspiration.

The trachea, located just anterior to the esophagus, extends from its junction with the larynx at the level of **C6** (sixth cervical vertebra) downward to the level of **T4** or **T5** (fourth or fifth thoracic vertebra), where it divides into right and left primary bronchi.

Certain glands located near the respiratory system are the **thyroid, parathyroid,** and the **thymus glands.**

Thyroid gland The thyroid gland is a vascular organ located anteriorly in the neck region just below the larynx with its right and left lateral lobes lying on each side and distal to the proximal trachea (Fig. 3-8). In the adult it weighs 25 to 30 g (approximately 1 ounce) and has a rich blood supply. As with other such glandular organs, the thyroid gland is more radiosensitive than many other body structures or organs. Therefore knowing the relative size and location of this gland is important for radiographers to be able to reduce exposures to these regions as much as possible by shielding and by collimation of the x-ray beam.

One of the unique features of the thyroid gland is its ability to store certain hormones, then slowly release them to aid in the regulation of body metabolism. These hormones also help regulate body growth and development, as well as activity of the nervous system, especially in children.

Parathyroid glands Parathyroid glands are small, rounded glands embedded on the posterior surfaces of the lateral lobes of the thyroid gland. Usually two parathyroids are attached to each lateral thyroid lobe, as shown in Fig. 3-8. They store and secrete certain hormones that aid in specific blood functions, including blood calcium levels.

Thymus gland The thymus gland is located just distal to the thyroid gland (see Fig. 3-8) and is demonstrated and described later in this chapter as part of mediastinal structures (see Fig. 3-22).

Radiographs

The AP and lateral radiographs of the upper airway visualize the air-filled trachea and larynx. This AP radiograph (Fig. 3-9) demonstrates a column of air primarily in the upper trachea region, as seen in the lower half of the radiograph (darkened area, *arrows*). Certain enlargements or other abnormalities of the thymus or thyroid glands may be demonstrated on such radiographs, as well as pathology within the airway system itself.

The lateral radiograph (Fig. 3-10) demonstrates the air-filled trachea and larynx *(A)* and the region of the esophagus *(B)* and shows the locations relative to each other. Note that the esophagus is located more posteriorly and the trachea anteriorly. The general locations of the thyroid gland *(C)* and the thymus gland *(D)* are also demonstrated.

Axial (Cross-Sectional) Image of Trachea

Fig. 3-11 is a CT image through the upper chest at the approximate level of T3. Observe again that the trachea is located anteriorly to the esophagus, both of which are anterior to the thoracic vertebrae. The upper lungs are located to each side of the trachea and the thoracic vertebrae.

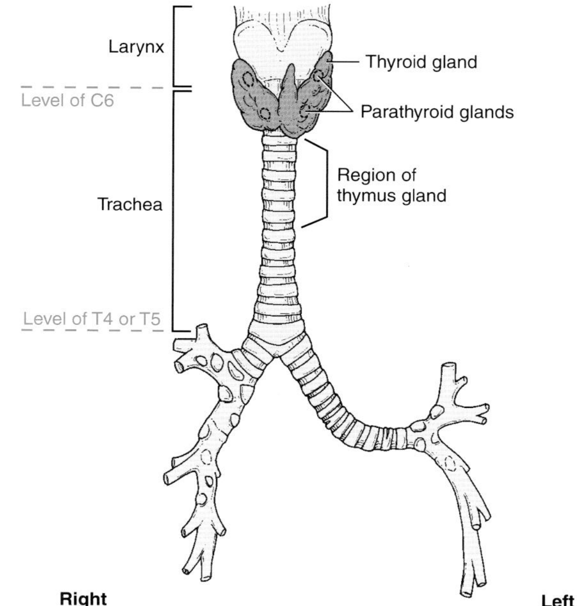

Fig. 3-8. Trachea.

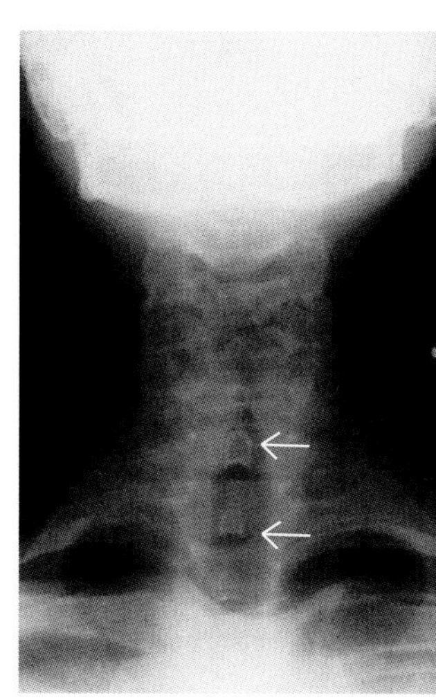

Fig. 3-9. AP upper airway.

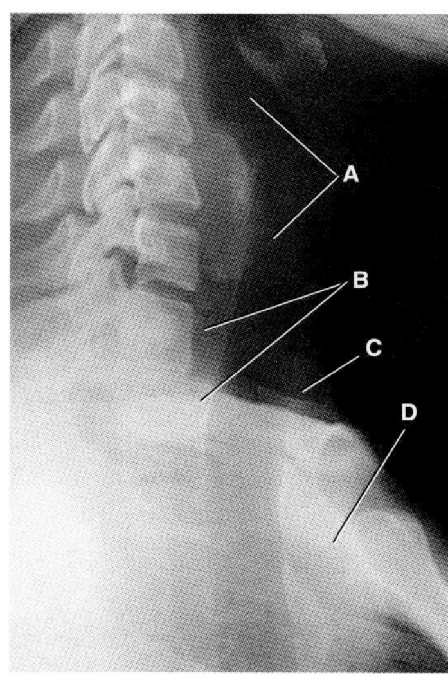

Fig. 3-10. Lateral upper airway. **A,** Air-filled trachea and larynx; **B,** Esophagus; **C,** Region of the thyroid gland; **D,** Region of the thymus gland.

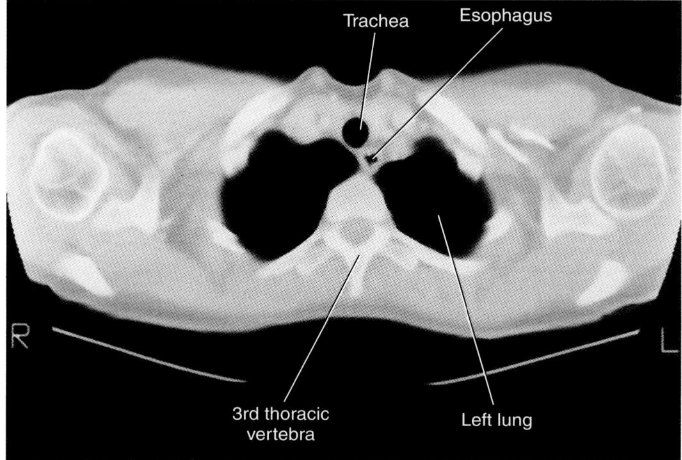

Fig. 3-11. Axial (cross) section at level of T3.

Right and left bronchi

The third part of the respiratory system consists of the **right** and **left primary bronchi,** also known as the right and left main stem bronchi.

The **right primary bronchus** is **wider** and **shorter** than the left bronchus. The right primary bronchus is also more vertical; therefore the angle of divergence from the distal trachea is less abrupt for the right bronchus than for the left. This **difference in size and shape** between the two primary bronchi is important because food particles or other foreign objects that happen to enter the respiratory system are more likely to enter and lodge in the **right** bronchus.

The **right bronchus** is about 2.5 cm long and 1.3 cm in diameter. The angle of divergence of the right bronchus is only about 25°.

The **left bronchu**s is smaller in diameter (1.1 cm) than the right, but about twice as long (5 cm). The divergent angle of the left bronchus is approximately 37°. This increased angle and the smaller diameter make food particles or other foreign matter less likely to enter the left bronchus compared with the right.

The **carina** *(kah-ri'nah)* is a specific prominence, or ridge, of the lowest tracheal cartilage, as seen at the bottom and inside portion of the trachea, where it divides into right and left bronchi. As viewed from above through a bronchoscope, the carina is to the left of the midline, and the right bronchus appears more open than the left, which clearly demonstrates why particles coming down the trachea are more likely to enter the right bronchus.

The position of the carina, as shown in Fig. 3-12, is at the lower level of the division into the right and left primary bronchi. This is at the approximate level of T5 and is used as a specific reference point or level for CT of the thorax, as described in Chapter 22.

Secondary Bronchi, Lobes, and Alveoli

In addition to the difference in size and shape between the right and left bronchi, another important difference is that the **right** bronchus divides into **three** secondary bronchi, but the **left** divides into only **two,** with each entering individual lobes of the lungs. Thus the **right lung** contains **three lobes** and the **left** contains **two lobes,** as demonstrated in Figs. 3-13, 3-14, and 3-15. These secondary bronchi continue to subdivide into smaller branches, termed **bronchioles,** that spread to all parts of each lobe.

Each of these small **terminal bronchioles** terminates in very small air sacs called **alveoli.** The two lungs contain from 500 to 700 million alveoli. Here oxygen and carbon dioxide are exchanged in the blood through the thin walls of the alveoli.

Axial (Cross-Sectional) Image of Bronchi and Lungs

Fig. 3-14 represents an axial (cross-sectional) image through the heart at the approximate level of T7.

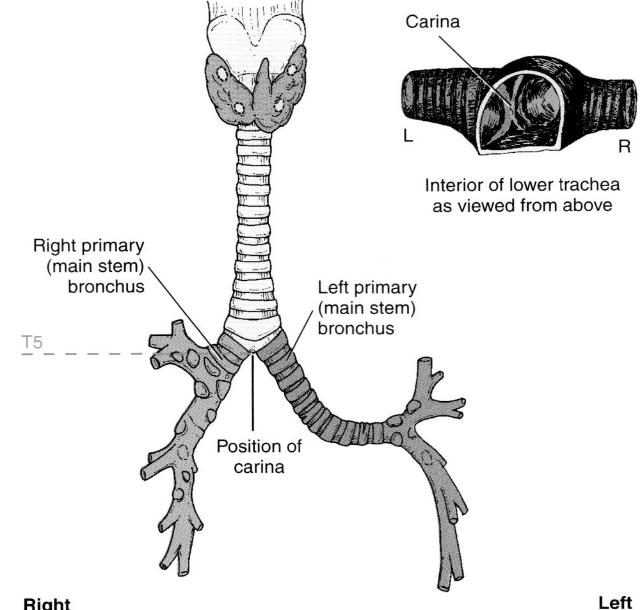

Fig. 3-12. Bronchi.

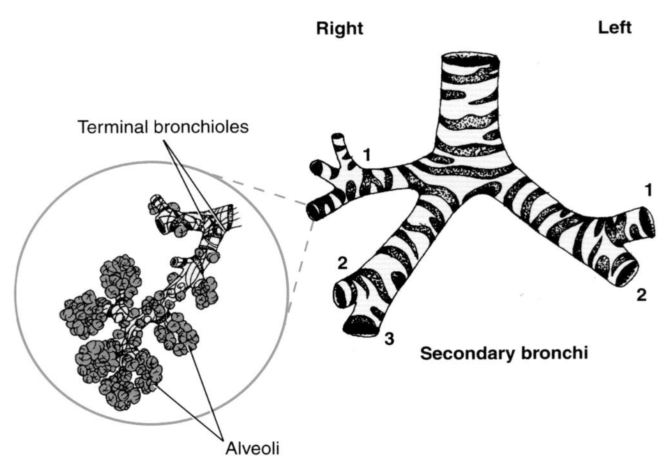

Fig. 3-13. Secondary bronchi and alveoli.

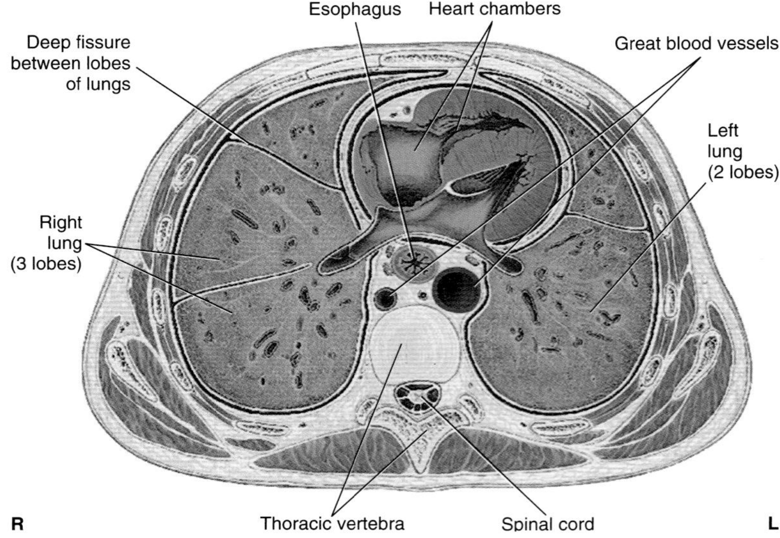

Fig. 3-14. Axial (cross-sectional) image of lungs and heart, level of T7.

3

Lungs

The fourth and last division of the respiratory system is made up of the two large, spongy **lungs,** located on each side of the thoracic cavity. The lungs fill all of the space not occupied by other structures. Remember that the right lung is made up of **three** lobes, the **superior** (upper), **middle,** and **inferior** (lower) lobes, divided by **two deep fissures.** The left lung has only **two** lobes, the **superior** (upper) and **inferior** (lower), separated by a **single deep oblique fissure.**

The lungs are made up of a light, spongy, but highly elastic substance called **parenchyma** *(pah-reng'ki-mah).* This allows for the breathing mechanism responsible for expansion and contraction of the lungs, which brings oxygen in and removes the carbon dioxide from the blood through the thin walls of the alveoli.

Each lung is contained in a delicate double-walled sac, or membrane, called the **pleura,** visualized in both the frontal (Fig. 3-15) and the cross-sectional (Fig. 3-16) drawings. The outer layer of this pleural sac lines the inner surface of the chest wall and diaphragm and is called the **parietal pleura.** The inner layer covering the surface of the lungs, also dipping into the fissures between the lobes, is called the **pulmonary** or **visceral pleura** (Fig. 3-16).

The potential space between the double-walled pleura is called the **pleural cavity,** which contains a lubricating fluid allowing movement of one or the other during breathing. When a lung collapses or when air or fluid collects between these two layers, this space may be visualized radiographically. Air or gas present in this pleural cavity results in a condition called a **pneumothorax,** wherein the air or gas pressure in the pleural cavity may cause the lung to collapse.

Accumulation of fluid in the pleural cavity (pleural effusion) creates a condition called a **hemothorax.**

Cross-Section of Lungs and Heart

Fig. 3-16 demonstrates a cross-sectional view through the lower third of the mediastinum and lungs. Clearly demonstrated is the double-walled membrane, the **pleura,** which completely encloses the lungs, including around the heart. The outer membrane, the **parietal pleura,** and the inner membrane, the **pulmonary** (or **visceral**) **pleura,** are clearly visible, as is the potential space between them, the **pleural cavity.**

The double-walled **pericardial sac,** which surrounds the heart, is also identified. This drawing demonstrates the relationship of the pericardial sac surrounding the heart with the pleural sac surrounding the lungs. The pleural and pericardial spaces or cavities are exaggerated on this drawing to better demonstrate these parts. Normally no space exists between the double walls of the pericardial sac or between the parietal and visceral pleura unless pathology is present.

CT Cross-Sectional Image

The CT image in Fig. 3-17 at the approximate level of T10 shows the relationship and relative size of the heart, descending aorta, esophagus, and lungs. The heart is located more to the **left,** as can also be seen on a PA chest radiograph. The heart is also shown to be located in the anterior portion of the chest cavity directly behind the sternum and left anterior ribs. The esophagus is posterior to the heart, with the descending aorta between the esophagus and the thoracic vertebrae.

Note that the right hemidiaphragm and upper liver are shown within the right lung region, indicating this is a lower thoracic level image.

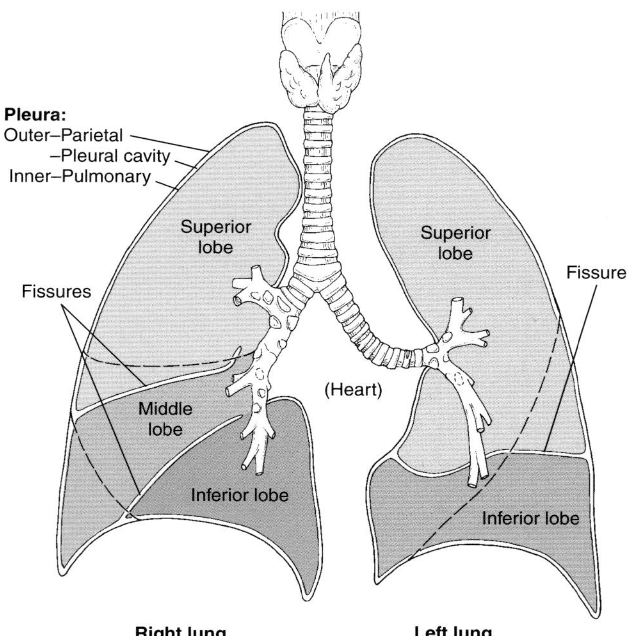

Fig. 3-15. Lungs.

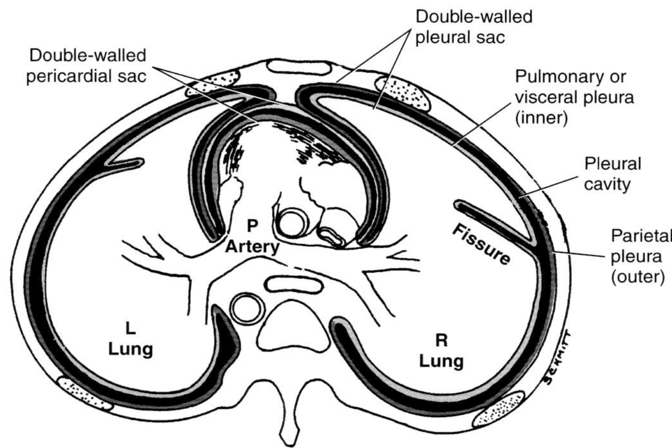

Fig. 3-16. Cross-section of lower mediastinum and lungs.

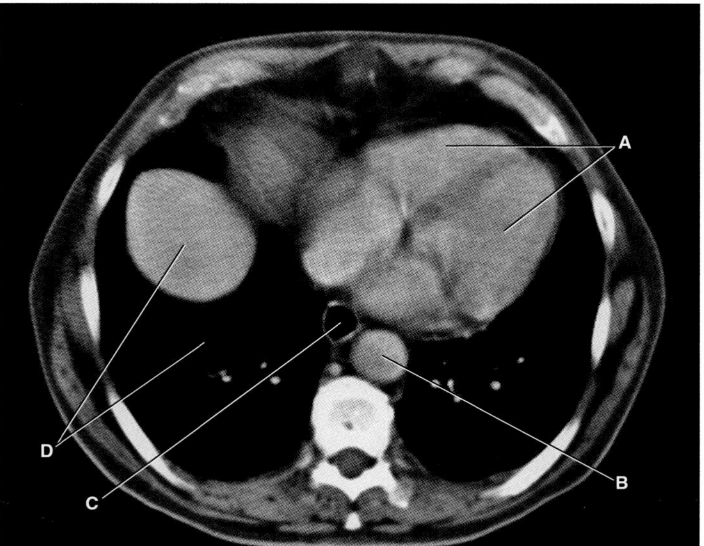

Fig. 3-17. CT image of lower thorax (level of T10). **A,** Heart; **B,** Descending aorta; **C,** Esophagus; **D,** Right lung, hemidiaphragm, and upper liver.

3

PA Chest Radiograph

Enormous amounts of medical information can be obtained from a properly exposed and carefully positioned PA chest radiograph. Although the technical factors are designed to optimally visualize the lungs and other soft tissues, the bony thorax can also be seen. The clavicles, scapulae, and ribs can be identified by carefully studying the chest radiograph in Fig. 3-18. The sternum and thoracic vertebrae are superimposed along with mediastinal structures, such as the heart and great vessels; therefore the sternum and vertebrae are not well visualized on a PA chest radiograph.

The **lungs** and **trachea** (see Fig. 3-18, *dotted outline, A*) of the respiratory system are well shown, although usually the bronchi are not easily seen. The first portion of the respiratory system, the larynx, is usually above the top border of the radiograph and cannot be seen. The heart, the large blood vessels, and the diaphragm are also well visualized.

The labeled parts on the radiograph are also demonstrated in Fig. 3-19, a frontal view of the thorax with the bony structures removed. The thyroid gland, large blood vessels, and thymus gland are also demonstrated in their relationship to the lungs and heart.

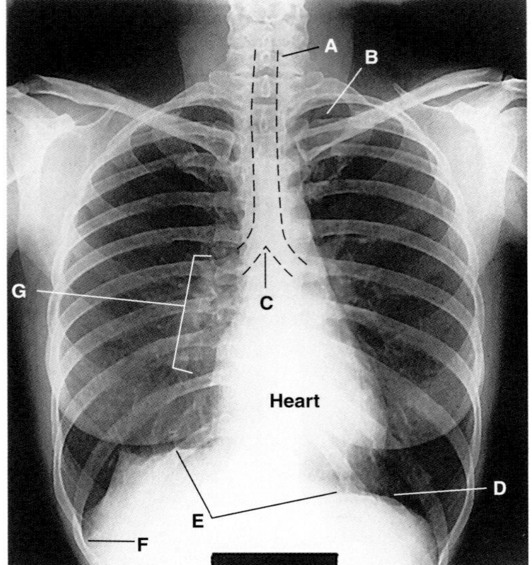

Fig. 3-18. PA chest radiograph.

Parts of Lungs

Radiographically important parts of the lungs (Figs. 3-18 and 3-19) are as follows:

The **apex** *(B)* of each lung is that **rounded upper area above the level of the clavicles.** The apices of the lungs extend up into the lower neck area to the level of T1 (first thoracic vertebra). This important part of the lungs must be included on chest radiographs.

The **carina** *(C)* is shown as the point of bifurcation, the lowest margin of the separation of the trachea into the right and left bronchi.

The **base** *(D)* of each lung is the lower concave area of each lung that rests on the **diaphragm** *(E).* The diaphragm is a muscular partition separating the thoracic and abdominal cavities.

3

The **costophrenic angle** *(F)* refers to the extreme outermost lower corner of each lung, where the diaphragm meets the ribs. In positioning for chest radiographs, know the relative locations of the uppermost and lowermost parts of the lungs, namely, the apices and the costophrenic angles, respectively, to ensure that these regions are included on every chest radiograph. Pathology, such as a small amount of fluid collection, would be evident at these costophrenic angles in the erect position.

The **hilum** (hilus) *(G),* also known as the **root** region, is the central area of each lung, where the bronchi, blood vessels, lymph vessels, and nerves enter and leave the lungs.

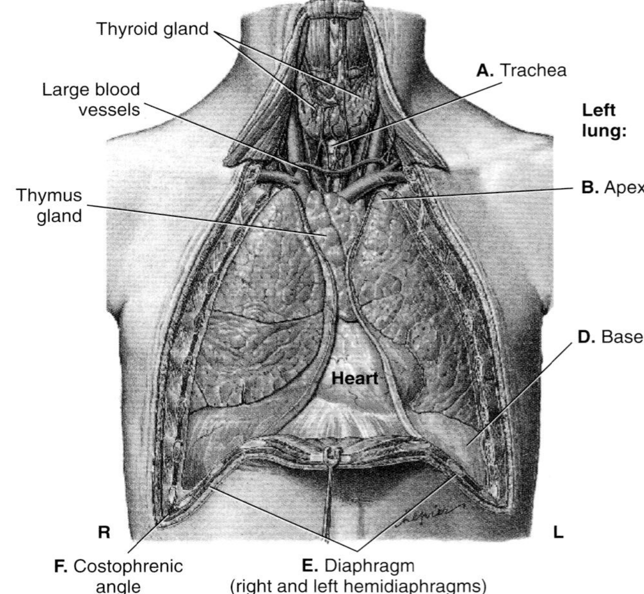

Fig. 3-19. Lungs.

Lateral Chest View

The lateral chest radiograph (Fig. 3-20) is marked to demonstrate the same parts as labeled in the adjoining drawing (Fig. 3-21). This drawing shows the left lung as seen from the medial aspect. Because this is the left lung, only two lobes are seen. Note that some of the **lower lobe** *(D)* extends above the level of the **hilum** *(C)* posteriorly, whereas some of the **upper lobe** *(B)* extends below the hilum anteriorly. The posterior part of the **diaphragm** is the most inferior part of the diaphragm. The single deep **oblique fissure** dividing the two lobes of the left lung is again shown, as is the end-on view of a bronchus in the hilar region.

The right lung is usually about 1 inch shorter than the left lung. The reason for this difference is the large space-occupying liver located in the right upper abdomen, which pushes up on the **right hemidiaphragm.** The right and left hemidiaphragms *(F)* are seen on the lateral chest radiograph in Fig. 3-20. The more superior of the two is the right hemidiaphragm, as also seen on the PA chest radiograph (Fig. 3-18).

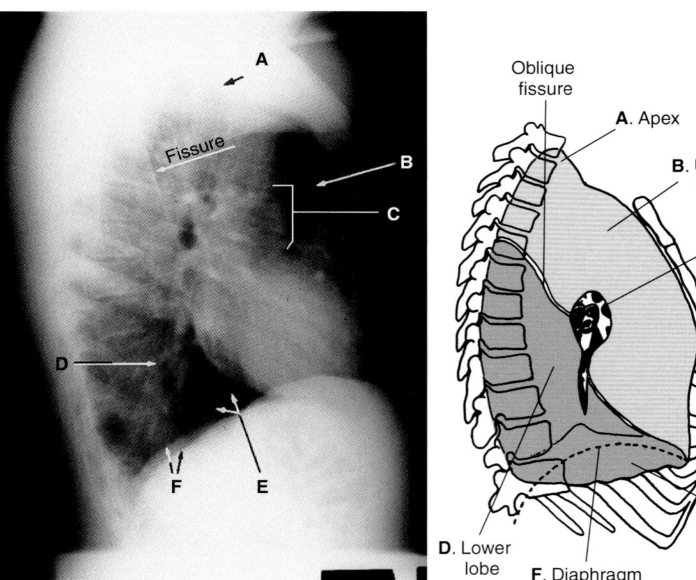

Fig. 3-20. Lateral chest radiograph.

Fig. 3-21. Medial left lung.

MEDIASTINUM

The medial portion of the thoracic cavity between the lungs is called the **mediastinum.** The thyroid and parathyroid glands, as described earlier in this chapter, are **not** considered mediastinal structures, because they are located more superiorly and are not within the mediastinum. The thymus gland, however, is located within the mediastinum, inferior to the thyroid gland and anterior to the trachea and esophagus (Fig. 3-22).

Four radiographically important structures located in the mediastinum are the (1) **thymus gland,** (2) **heart and great vessels,** (3) **trachea,** and (4) **esophagus.**

Thymus Gland

The **thymus gland,** located behind the upper sternum, is said to be a temporary organ because it is very prominent in an infant and reaches its maximum size of about 40 g at puberty, then gradually decreases until it almost disappears in the adult. At its maximum size it would appear much larger than shown in Fig. 3-22. It may be visualized on chest radiographs of children but generally will not for adults because the denser lymphatic tissue has been replaced by less dense fat. At its maximum development, the thymus gland lies above and anterior to the heart and pericardium.

The thymus gland functions primarily during childhood and puberty to aid with the functioning of certain body immune systems that help the body in its resistance to diseases. It is believed to contribute to the ability of the body to produce antibodies, which serve in rejecting foreign tissue and cells.

Heart and Great Vessels

The **heart** and the roots of the **great vessels** are enclosed in a double-walled sac called the pericardial sac, as demonstrated in an earlier drawing (Fig. 3-16). The heart is located posterior to the body of the sternum and anterior to the fifth to eighth thoracic vertebrae. It lies obliquely in the mediastinal space, and approximately two-thirds of the heart lies to the left of the median plane.

The **great vessels** in the mediastinum are the inferior and superior vena cava, aorta, and large pulmonary arteries and veins. The **superior vena cava** is a large vein that returns blood to the heart from the upper half of the body (Fig. 3-22). The **inferior vena cava** is a large vein returning blood from the lower half of the body.

The **aorta** is the largest artery in the body (1 to 2 inches, or 2 to 5 cm, in diameter in an average adult). It carries blood to all parts of the body through its various branches. The aorta is divided into three parts: the **ascending aorta** (coming up out of the heart), the **arch of the aorta,** and the **descending aorta,** which passes through the diaphragm into the abdomen, where it becomes the abdominal aorta.

Various **pulmonary arteries and veins** present in the mediastinum are shown in Figs. 3-23 and 3-24. These supply blood and return blood to and from all segments of the lungs. The arterial network surrounds the small air sacs, or alveoli, where oxygen and carbon dioxide are exchanged with the blood.

See Chapter 21 for more complete drawings of the heart and great vessels as part of the total body circulatory system.

Trachea and Esophagus

The trachea, within the mediastinum, separates into the right and left primary and secondary bronchi, as shown in Fig. 3-23.

The proximal esophagus is located posterior to the trachea and continues down through the mediastinum **anterior to the descending aorta** until it passes through the diaphragm into the stomach.

Note also in Fig. 3-24 that the heart is located in the very **anterior** aspect of the thoracic cavity, directly behind the sternum.

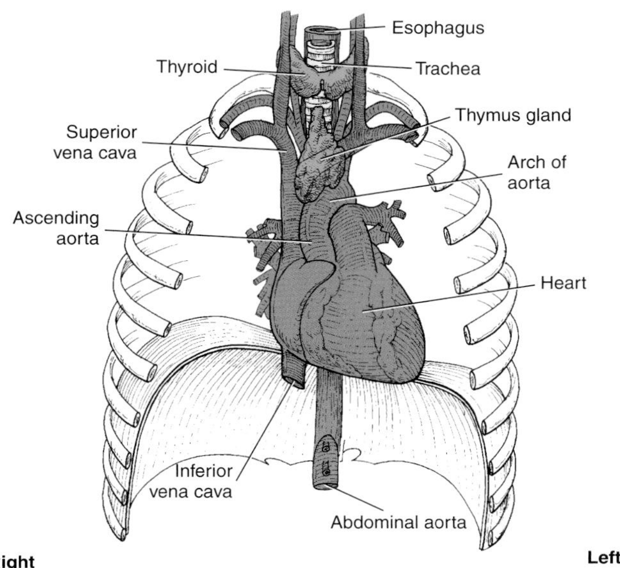

Fig. 3-22. Structures within mediastinum (anterior view).

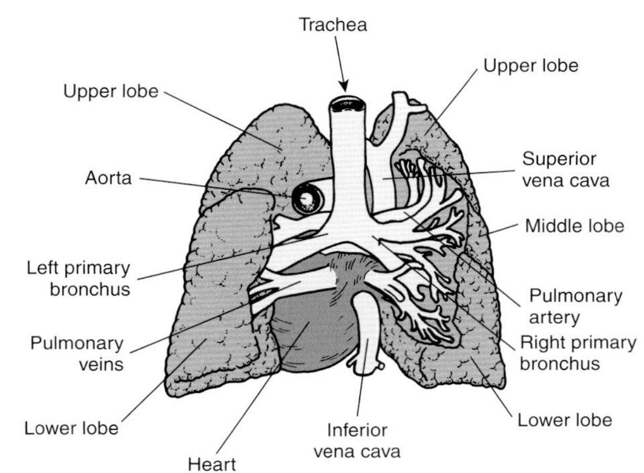

Fig. 3-23. Lungs and structures within mediastinum (posterior view).

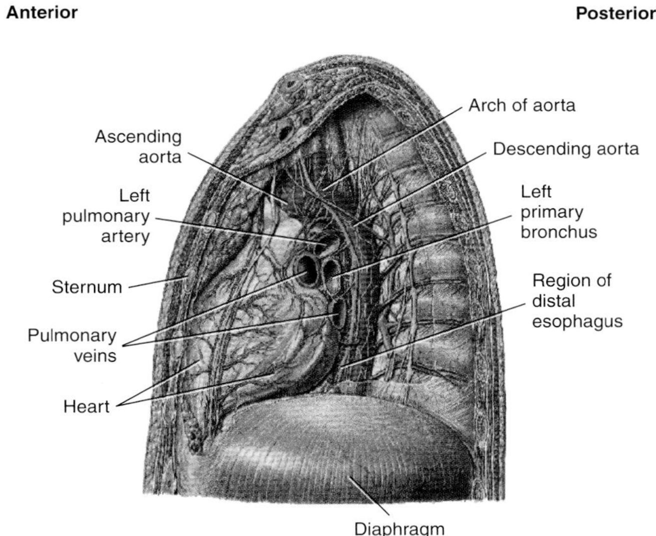

Fig. 3-24. Mediastinal relationships on left side with lung removal.

3

RADIOGRAPHIC POSITIONING

Body Habitus

Body habitus requires special consideration in chest radiography. For example, the massively built **hypersthenic** patient has a thorax that is very **broad** and very **deep** from front to back but is **shallow** in vertical dimension, as shown with the PA radiograph in Fig. 3-26. Therefore care must be taken that the sides or the costophrenic angles are not cut off on a PA chest, which must be taken with the IR placed crosswise. Careful centering is also required on the lateral projection to ensure that the anterior or posterior margins are included on the radiograph.

The other extreme is the slender **asthenic** patient. In this build, the thorax is **narrow** in width and **shallow** from front to back but is very **long** in its vertical dimension. Therefore in positioning for such a chest, the technologist must ensure that the IR is long enough to include both the upper apex areas, which extend well above the clavicles, and the lower costophrenic angles. A nearer average **hyposthenic** chest PA radiograph is shown in Fig. 3-27. Care in vertical collimation for such patients must also be exercised so that the costophrenic angles are not cut off on the lower margin.

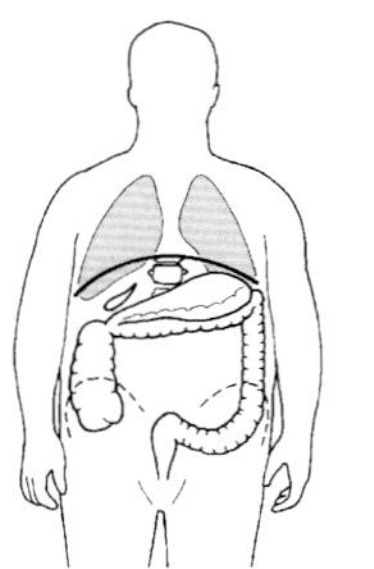
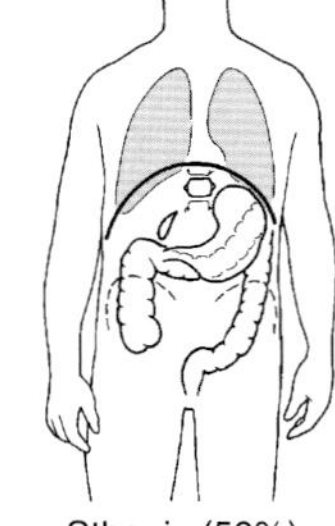
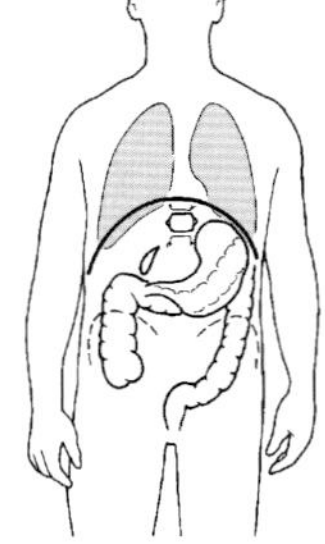
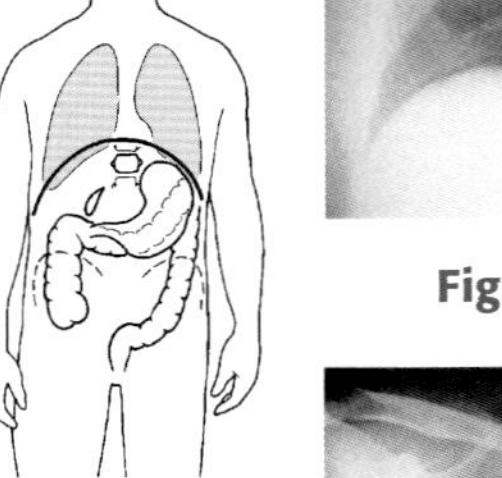

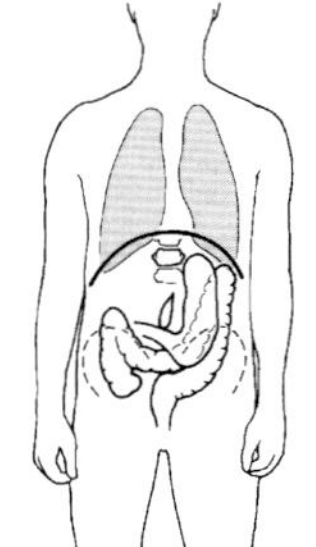
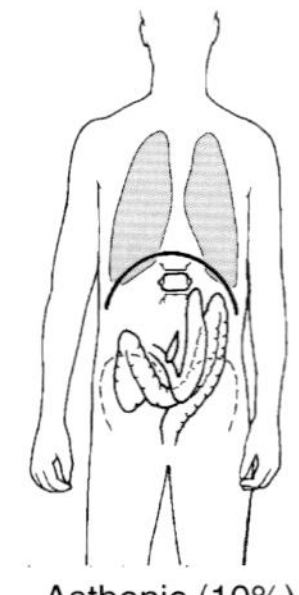
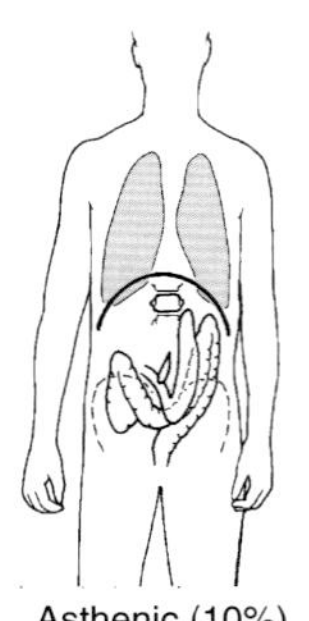

Fig. 3-25. Body habitus.

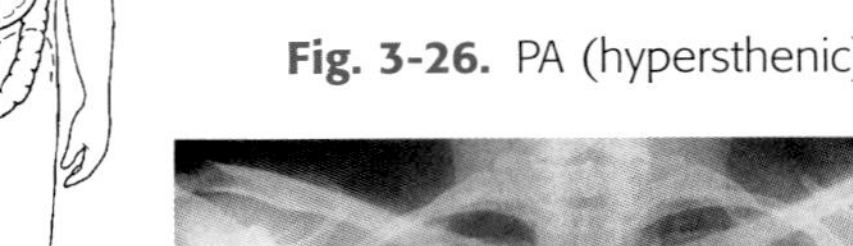

Fig. 3-26. PA (hypersthenic).

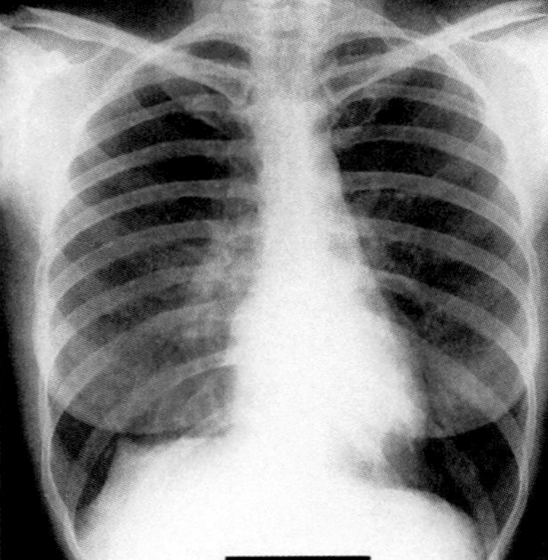

Fig. 3-27. PA (hyposthenic).

Breathing Movements

Movements of the bony thorax during inspiration (taking air in) and expiration (expelling air) greatly change the dimensions of the thorax, and thus the thoracic volume. To increase the volume of the chest during inspiration, the thoracic cavity increases in diameter in **three dimensions.**

The first of these is the **vertical diameter,** which is increased primarily by the diaphragm contracting and moving downward, thereby increasing the thoracic volume.

The **transverse diameter** is the second dimension increased during inspiration. The ribs swing outward and upward, which increases the transverse diameter of the thorax.

The third dimension is the **anteroposterior diameter,** also increased during inspiration by the raising of the ribs, especially the second through the sixth ribs.

During expiration the elastic recoil of the lungs, along with the weight of the thoracic walls, causes the three diameters of the thorax to return to normal.

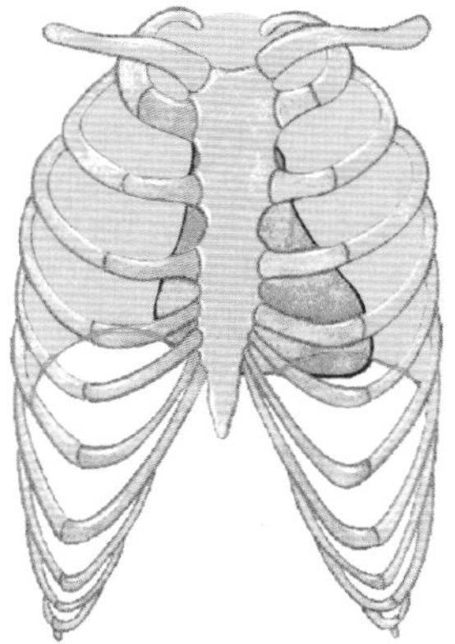
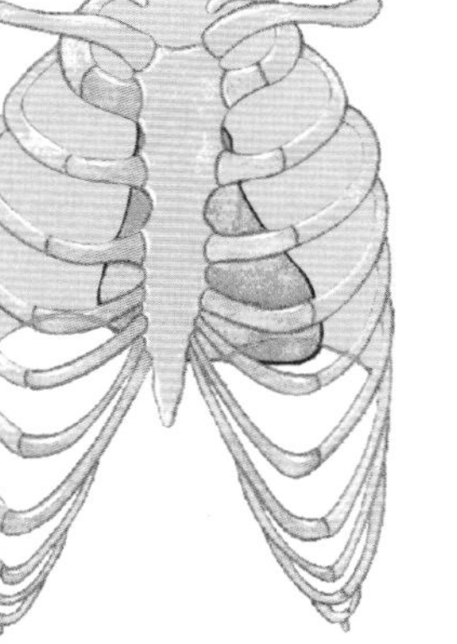

Fig. 3-28. Expiration.

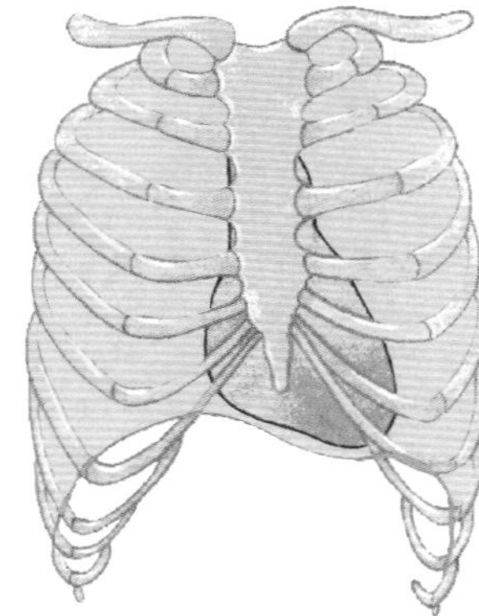

Fig. 3-29. Inspiration.

Degree of Inspiration

To determine the degree of inspiration in chest radiography, one should be able to identify and count the rib pairs on a chest radiograph. The first and second pairs are the most difficult to locate. When a chest radiograph is taken, the patient should take as deep a breath as possible and then hold it to fully aerate the lungs. Taking a second deep breath before holding it allows for a deeper inspiration.

The best way to determine the degree of inspiration is to observe how far down the diaphragm has moved by counting the pairs of ribs in the lung area above the diaphragm. A general rule for average adult patients is to "show" a **minimum of ten** on a good PA chest radiograph. To determine this, start at the top with the first rib and count down to the **tenth** or **eleventh** rib posteriorly. The posterior part of each rib, where it joins a thoracic vertebra, is the most superior part of the rib. The diaphragm should always be checked to see that it is below the level of at least the tenth rib. (Fig. 3-30 shows eleven posterior ribs, which can be expected in many healthy patients.)

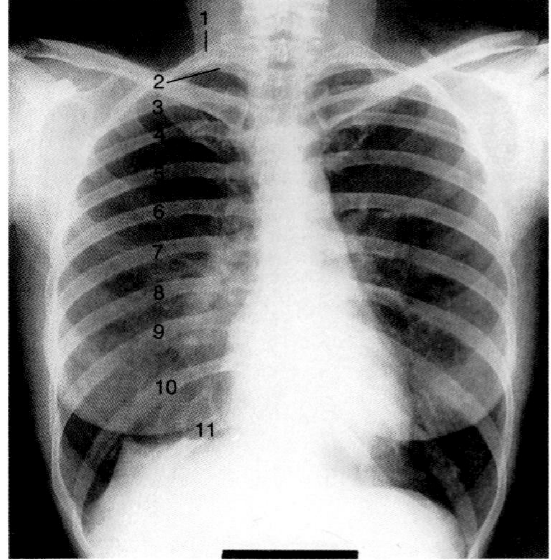

Fig. 3-30. Posterior ribs.

Positioning Considerations

Patient preparation for chest radiography includes the removal of all opaque objects from the chest and neck regions, including clothes with buttons, snaps, hooks, or any objects that would be visualized on the radiograph as a shadow. To ensure that all such objects are removed from the chest region, the usual procedure is to ask the patient to remove all clothing, including bras, necklaces, or other objects around the neck. The patient then puts on a hospital gown, which commonly has the opening in the back.

Long hair braided or tied together in bunches with rubber bands or other fasteners may cause suspicious shadows on the radiograph if left superimposing the chest area. Oxygen lines or electrocardiogram (ECG) monitor leads should be carefully moved to the side of the chest if possible.

RADIATION PROTECTION

Patients should be protected from unnecessary radiation for all diagnostic radiographic examinations, especially for chest radiographs because these are the most common of all radiographic examinations.

Repeat Exposures Even though chest radiographic exams are often considered the simplest of all radiographic procedures, they also are the exam with the highest number of repeats in many radiology departments. Therefore minimize unnecessary radiation exposure from repeat exposures by taking extra care in positioning, central ray (CR) centering, and selecting correct exposure factors if automatic exposure control (AEC) systems are not used. Reduce patient dose as much as possible through the use of correct radiation protection practices by close collimation and gonadal shielding.

Collimation Careful collimation is important in chest radiography. Restricting the primary x-ray beam by collimation not only reduces patient dose by reducing the volume of tissue irradiated but also improves image quality by reducing scatter radiation.

Gonadal Shielding In addition to careful collimation, a leaded gonadal shield should be used for the abdominal area below the lungs. This is especially important for children, pregnant women, and all those of childbearing age. A minimal rule is that **gonadal shielding should be used on all patients of reproductive age.** Many departments, however, have a general policy of gonadal shielding for all patients in chest radiography.

A common type of gonadal shield for chest radiography is some type of freestanding, adjustable mobile shield placed between the patient and the x-ray tube. A vinyl-covered lead shield that ties around the waist can also be used. Both of these types of shields should provide shielding from the level of the iliac crests or slightly higher, to the midthigh area.

Back Scatter Protection To protect the gonads from scatter and secondary radiation from the cassette or IR holder device and the wall behind it, some references suggest a freestanding shield or a wraparound shield also be placed over the gonads between the patient and the IR.

TECHNICAL FACTORS

Kilovoltage (kV) Generally, kV should be high enough to result in sufficient contrast to demonstrate the many shades of gray needed to visualize the finer lung markings. Thus in general, chest radiography uses **low contrast,** described as a **long-scale contrast,** with more shades of gray. This requires high kV of 110 to 125.

Lower kV, yielding high contrast, will not provide sufficient penetration to visualize well the fine lung markings in the areas behind the heart and the lung bases. Too high contrast is evident when the heart and other mediastinal structures appear underexposed, even though the lung fields are sufficiently penetrated.

As a general rule, in chest radiography, the use of high kV (above 100) **requires the use of grids.** Either moving grids or fine-line focused fixed grids can be used.

Exceptions to this are some mobile chests taken with equipment that is limited to 80 to 90 kV, for which IRs without grids may be used, but this is not recommended.

Exposure Time and Milliamperage (mAs—milliampere seconds) Generally, chest radiography requires the use of high mA and short exposure times to minimize the chance of motion and resultant loss of sharpness.

Sufficient mAs should be used to provide for optimum density of lungs and mediastinal structures. A determining factor for this on PA chest radiographs is to be able to **see faint outlines of at least the mid- and upper vertebrae and posterior ribs through the heart and other mediastinal structures.**

Placement of Image Markers Throughout the positioning sections of this text, the correct or best placement of patient ID information and image markers is indicated. The top portion of each positioning page includes a drawing that demonstrates the correct image receptor size and placement (lengthwise or crosswise) and indicates the best location for patient ID blocker and the location and type of image marker used for that specific projection or position.

PEDIATRIC APPLICATIONS

Supine vs. Erect Generally, with newborns and small infants, for whom head support is required, chest radiographs are taken AP supine. Laterals also may be taken supine with a horizontal beam to demonstrate fluid levels (dorsal decubitus). However, erect PA and laterals are preferred whenever possible, using immobilization devices such as the **Pigg-O-Stat** (described in Chapter 20 on Pediatric Radiography).

Technical Factors **Lower kV** (60 to 70) and **less mAs** are required for pediatric patients with the **shortest exposure time possible** (to prevent motion). Higher-speed imaging systems or receptors are generally used with pediatric patients for two reasons: (1) to reduce the chance of motion and (2) to reduce patient exposure dose. (Important because of the sensitivity of young tissue to radiation exposure.) See Chapter 20 for more detailed information on special positioning considerations required with pediatric patients.

3

GERIATRIC APPLICATIONS

CR Centering Frequently, older patients have less inhalation capability with resulting "more shallow" lung fields, which requires a **higher CR location** (CR to T6-7, see p. 89).

Technical Factors Certain pathologic conditions are more common in geriatric patients, such as **pneumonia** or **emphysema,** which may require different exposure factor adjustments as described under **Pathologic Indications,** p. 91.

Instructions and Patient Handling More care, time, and patience are frequently required in explaining breathing and positioning requirements for geriatric patients. Helping and supporting these patients in the positioning process are important. Arm supports for keeping arms raised high for the lateral position are essential for many older patients.

Breathing Instructions

Breathing instructions are very important in chest radiography because any chest or lung movement occurring during the exposure will result in "blurring" of the radiographic image. Chest radiographs must be taken on **full** inspiration to demonstrate the lungs as they appear fully expanded.

HOLD BREATH ON SECOND INSPIRATION

More air can be inhaled without too much strain on the **second** breath compared with the first. Therefore the patient should be asked to **hold the second full inspiration** rather than the first. However, the full inspiration should not be forced to the point of strain, causing unsteadiness. This needs to be explained to the patient before the exposure as the patient is being positioned.

INSPIRATION AND EXPIRATION

Occasionally, exceptions exist to taking chest radiographs on full inspiration only. For certain conditions, comparison radiographs are taken on both **full inspiration** and **full expiration.** Indicators for this include a possible small **pneumothorax** (air or gas in the pleural cavity), fixation or lack of normal movement of the diaphragm, the presence of a foreign body, or to distinguish between an opacity in the rib or in the lung. When such comparison radiographs are taken, they should be labeled "inspiration" and "expiration."

Note the pneumothorax of the upper right lung on expiration demonstrated in the chest radiograph in Fig. 3-32 *(arrows).* This is not evident on the inspiration radiograph of the same patient taken during the same exam in Fig. 3-31.

Note also the number of ribs showing above the diaphragm, indicating the degree of inspiration (10 ribs) and expiration (8 ribs).

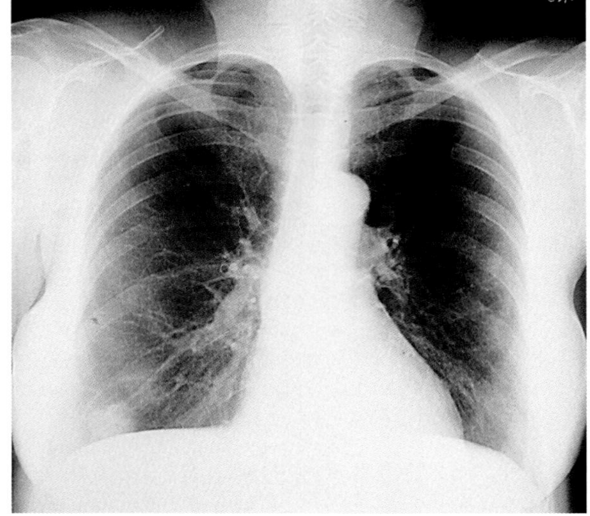

Fig. 3-31. Inspiration. (Courtesy Llori Lundh.)

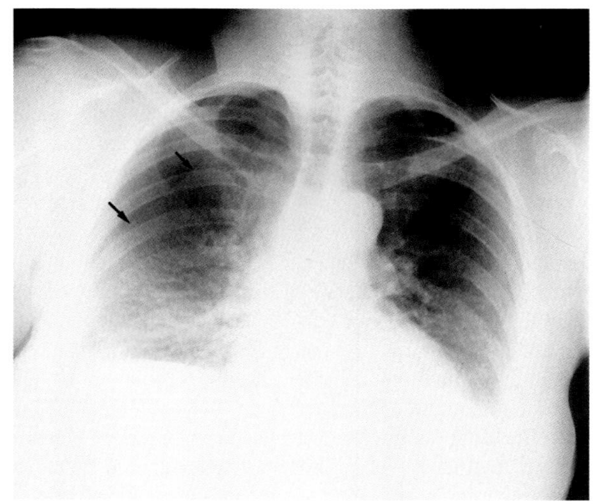

Fig. 3-32. Expiration. (Courtesy Llori Lundh.)

ERECT CHEST RADIOGRAPHS

All chest radiographs should be taken in an erect position if the patient's condition allows. Three reasons for this are as follows:

1. Allows the Diaphragm to Move Down Farther

An erect position causes the liver and other abdominal organs to drop, allowing the diaphragm to move farther down on full inspiration, thus allowing the lungs to fully aerate.

2. Visualizes Possible Air and Fluid Levels in Chest

If both air and fluid are present within a lung or within the pleural space, the heavier fluid, such as blood or pleural fluid resulting from infection or trauma, will gravitate to the lowest position, whereas the air will rise. In the recumbent position, a pleural effusion will spread out over the posterior surface of the lung, resulting in a hazy appearance of the entire lung. In the upright position, fluid will locate near the base of the lung. The partially erect chest radiograph (Fig. 3-33) shows some fluid in the right lower thoracic cavity. The supine radiograph of the same patient (Fig. 3-34) shows a generalized hazy appearance of the entire right lung resulting from the presence of fluid now spread throughout the right thorax.

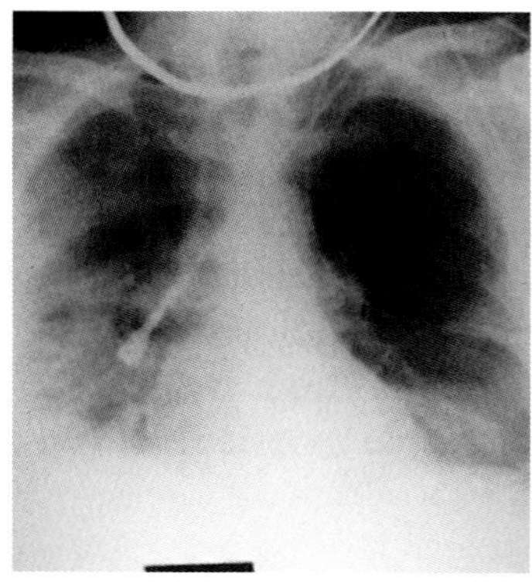

Fig. 3-33. Partially erect, some fluid evident in right lower lung.

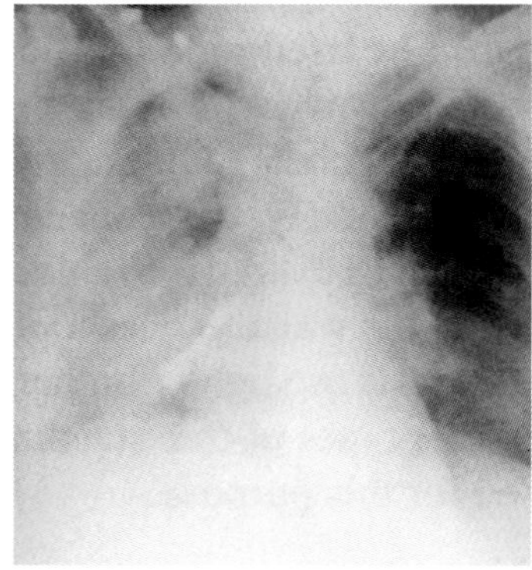

Fig. 3-34. Supine, 40 inches (same patient as Fig. 3-33; shows fluid throughout right lung).

3. Prevents Engorgement and Hyperemia of Pulmonary Vessels

The term **engorgement** literally means "distended or swollen with fluid."* **Hyperemia** *(hy"per-e'me-ah)* is an excess of blood partially resulting from a relaxation of the distal small blood vessels or arterioles.*

In general, an erect position tends to minimize engorgement and hyperemia of pulmonary vessels, whereas a supine position will increase these, which can change the radiographic appearance of these vessels and the lungs in general.

PA 72-inch (180-cm) SID (Source Image Receptor Distance)

Chest radiographs taken AP rather than PA at 72 inches (180 cm) will cause **increased magnification of the heart shadow,** which complicates the diagnosis of possible cardiac enlargement. The reason for this is the **anterior location** of the heart within the mediastinum, placing it closer to the IR on the PA, thus resulting in less magnification. A longer SID, such as 72 inches, or 180 cm, magnifies less because the x-ray beam has less divergence.

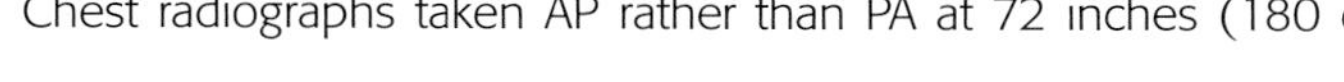

*Dorland's illustrated medical dictionary, ed 28, Philadelphia, 1994, WB Saunders.

Radiographic Criteria

The description for each chest projection or position in this chapter includes a radiographic criteria section. This section lists and describes specific criteria by which one can evaluate the resultant radiograph. The goal of every technologist should be to take the "optimal" radiograph. These criteria provide a **definable standard** by which every chest radiographic image can be evaluated to determine where improvements can be made.

Certain important radiographic criteria for all routine PA and lateral chest radiographs are as follows:

PA CHEST POSITIONING

True PA, No Rotation Even a slight amount of rotation on a PA chest projection will result in distortion of size and shape of the heart shadow, because the heart is located anteriorly in the thorax. Therefore it is important that there be **NO rotation.** To prevent rotation, ensure that the patient is standing evenly on both feet with both shoulders rolled forward and downward. Also, check the posterior aspect of the shoulders, as well as the lower posterior rib cage and the pelvis to ensure no rotation. **Scoliosis** and excessive **kyphosis** make it more difficult to prevent rotation. Scoliosis is lateral, or side-to-side, curvature of the spine, which is frequently combined with excessive kyphosis, a "hump back" curvature. Together these spinal curvatures frequently result in some "twisting" deformity of the bony thorax, making a true PA without some rotation more difficult or impossible.

Rotation on PA chest radiographs can be determined by examining both sternal ends of the clavicles for a symmetric appearance in relationship to the spine. On a true PA chest without any rotation, both the **right and left sternal ends of the clavicles will be the same distance from the center line of the spine.** Note the rotation evident in Fig. 3-36 by the difference in distance between the center of the spinal column and the sternal end of the right clavicle as compared with the left.

The direction of rotation can be determined by which sternal end of the clavicle is closest to the spine. For example, in Fig. 3-36 the left side of the thorax is moved toward the IR (right side moved away from IR), which creates a slight left anterior oblique (LAO) that will decrease the distance of the left clavicle from the spine.

Extending the Chin Sufficient extension of the patient's neck will ensure that the chin and neck are not covering up or superimposing the uppermost lung regions, the apices of the lungs. This is demonstrated by the two radiographs in Figs. 3-37 and 3-38. Also, be sure the upper collimation border is high enough so that the apices are not cut off.

Minimizing Breast Shadows The patient with large pendulous breasts should be asked to lift them up and outward and then remove her hands as she leans against the chest board (image receptor) to keep them in this position. This will lessen the effect of breast shadows over the lower lung fields. Remember, however, that depending on the size and density of the breasts, breast shadows over the lower lateral lung fields cannot be totally eliminated (Fig. 3-39).

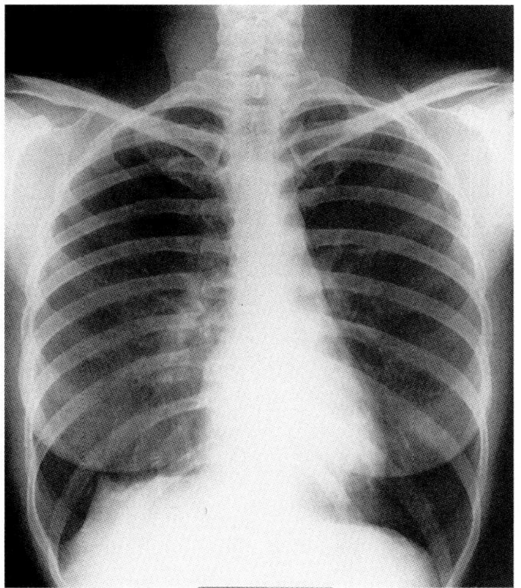

Fig. 3-35. Without rotation.

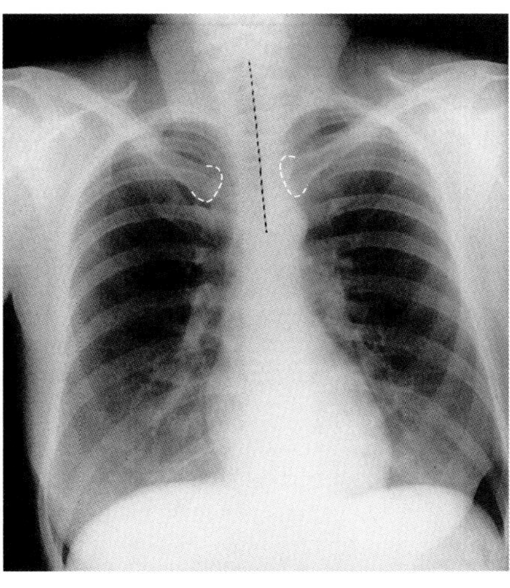

Fig. 3-36. With rotation (slight LAO).

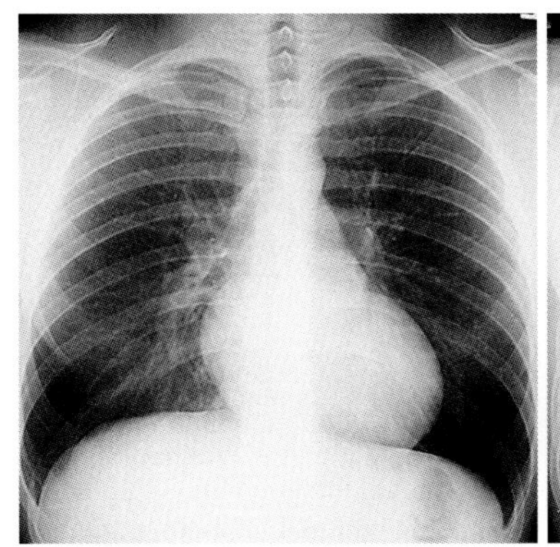

Fig. 3-37. Chin up.

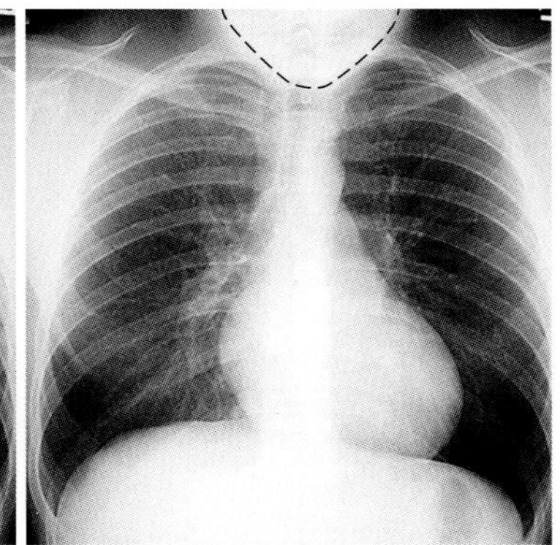

Fig. 3-38. Chin down.

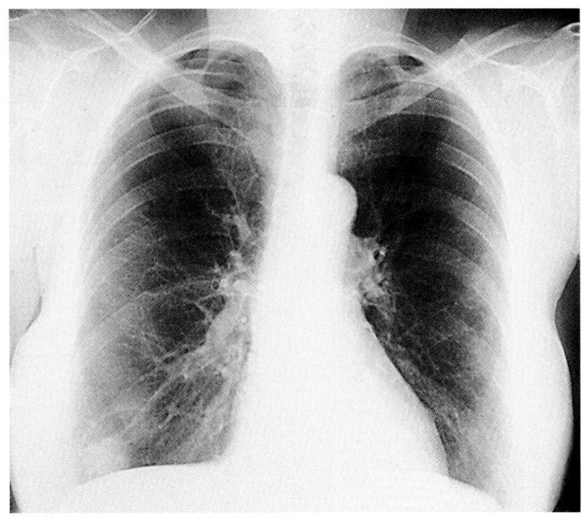

Fig. 3-39. Breast shadows evident.

3

LATERAL CHEST POSITIONING

Side Closest to IR The patient's side closest to the IR is best demonstrated on the finished radiograph. A **left lateral** should be done unless departmental protocol indicates otherwise, or unless certain pathology in the right lung indicates the need for a right lateral. A left lateral will better demonstrate the heart region because the heart is located primarily in the left thoracic cavity.

True Lateral, NO Rotation or Tilt Ensure that the patient is standing straight with weight evenly distributed on both feet with arms raised. As a check against rotation, confirm that the posterior surfaces of the shoulder and the pelvis are directly superimposed and perpendicular to the IR. Because of the divergent x-ray beam, the posterior ribs on the side farthest away from the IR will be magnified slightly and also will be projected slightly posterior compared with the side closest to the IR on a true lateral chest. This will be more noticeable on a broad-shouldered patient. However, this separation of posterior ribs resulting from divergence of the x-ray beam at the commonly used 72-inch (180-cm) SID **should only be ¼ to ½ inches, or about 1 cm.** Any more separation than this indicates rotation of the thorax from a true lateral position.*

Note: Some references suggest an intentional slight anterior rotation of the side away from the IR so that the posterior ribs will be directly superimposed. This may be preferred in some departments, but because the heart and most lung structures are near midline structures and thus not affected by the beam divergence, a straight lateral with respect to the IR is more common, which will cause a slight separation of the posterior ribs and costophrenic angles as described above.

Fig. 3-41 demonstrates a lateral chest with **excessive rotation,** as indicated by **the amount of separation of the right and left posterior ribs,** and **separation of the two costophrenic angles.** This represents a positioning error and would generally require a repeat.

3

Direction of Rotation The direction of rotation on a lateral chest is sometimes difficult to determine on a radiograph. Frequently, however, this can be determined by identifying the left hemidiaphragm by the gastric air bubble in the stomach or by the inferior border of the heart shadow, both of which are associated with the left hemidiaphragm.*

No Tilt There also should be **no tilt** or leaning "sideways." The **midsagittal plane must be parallel to the IR.** This means that if the patient's shoulders are firmly against the chest board (IR) on a lateral chest, the lower lateral thorax and/or hips may be an inch or two away. This is especially true on broad-shouldered patients. Tilt, if present, may be evident by closed disk spaces of thoracic vertebra.

Arms Raised High Ensure that the patient raises both arms sufficiently high to prevent superimposition on the upper chest field. Patients who are weak or unstable may need to grasp a support (Fig. 3-42).

When the patient's arms are not raised sufficiently, the soft tissues of the upper arm will superimpose portions of the lung field, as demonstrated in Fig. 3-43. *Arrows* demonstrate margins of soft tissues of the arms overlying upper lung fields. This would require a repeat and should be avoided.

*Martensen K: Radiographic critique, Philadelphia, 1996, WB Saunders.

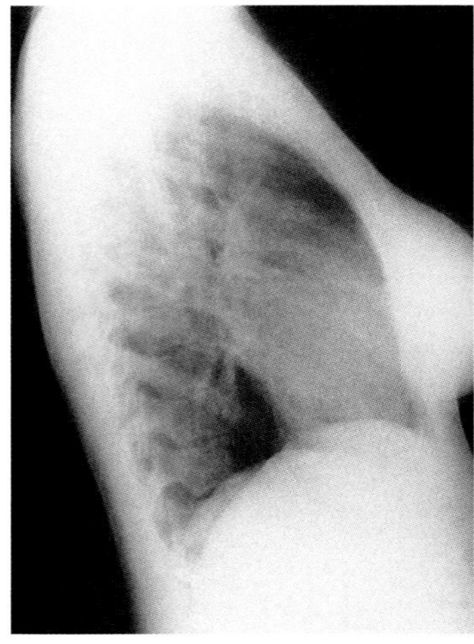

Fig. 3-40. Without excessive rotation (ribs superimposed).

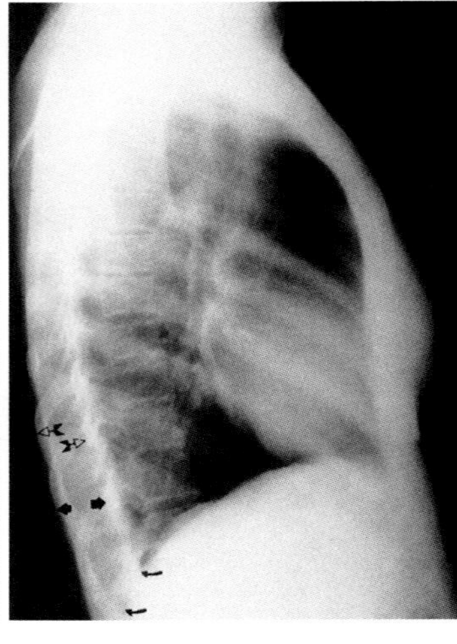

Fig. 3-41. Excessive rotation—**positioning error** (ribs **not** superimposed).

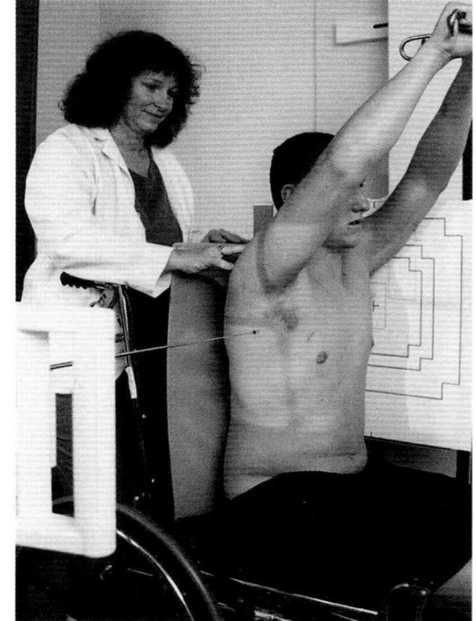

Fig. 3-42. Arms raised high.

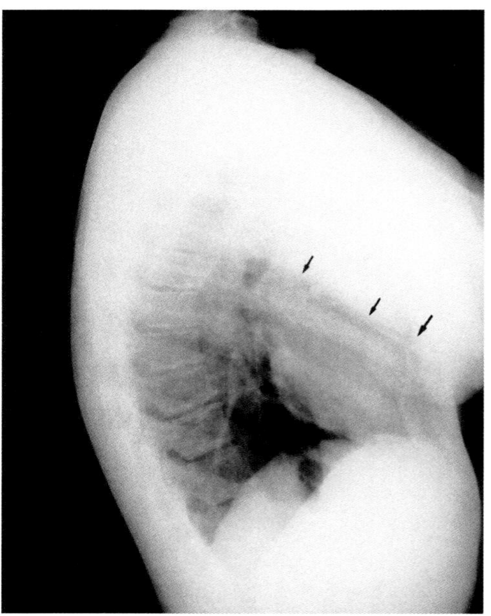

Fig. 3-43. Arms not raised—**positioning error.**

Central Ray Location

The top of the shoulder has traditionally been used for chest positioning. This method includes placing the top of the cassette or other IR $1\frac{1}{2}$ to 2 inches (5 cm) above the shoulders and centering the CR to the center of the IR. However, this positioning method is inconsistent, considering variations in lung field dimensions due to differences in body habitus, as demonstrated by comparing Figs. 3-44 and 3-45. The small circle indicates where the CR was placed on these two patients. The center of the lungs (indicated by *X*) is shown to be near the center of the IR for the male in Fig. 3-44 but is above center on the small and older female in Fig. 3-45. This centering error unnecessarily exposes a large portion of the upper abdomen.

These variations demonstrate the importance of a chest positioning method that **consistently centers the central ray to the center of the lung fields on all types of patients with accurate collimation on *both* top and bottom.**

CENTRAL RAY CHEST-POSITIONING METHOD

Bony topographic landmarks are consistent and reliable as a means of determining CR locations. Landmarks for locating the center of the lung fields are as follows:

Vertebra Prominens (PA Chest) The vertebra prominens corresponds to the level of T1 and the uppermost margin of the apex of the lungs. This landmark, which can be palpated at the base of the neck, is the preferred landmark for locating the CR on a PA chest (Figs. 3-46 and 3-47). For the average female, this is down about 7 inches (18 cm); for the male, about 8 inches (20 cm).

One way of determining this distance is by an average hand spread as shown. Most hands can reach 7 inches (18 cm). The 8-inch (20-cm) distance can be determined by estimating an additional inch. If the hand spread method is used, practice with a ruler to consistently determine these distances.

These differences between male and female are true for near-average body types in the general population, with crossover exceptions in which certain larger athletic females may have longer lung fields and some males may have shorter lungs. However, for purposes of chest positioning for the general population, the average measurements of **7 inches (18 cm) for a female** and **8 inches (20 cm) for a male** can be used as reliable guidelines.

Exceptions Other noteworthy exceptions in centering involve variations in body types. For example, the author found that 15% to 20% of the general male population were the well-developed athletic sthenic/hyposthenic type, which requires centering to nearer T8, or 9 inches (20 to 25 cm) down from the vertebra prominens. About 5% to 10% of the population are the hypersthenic type, which requires only from 6 to 7 inches (15 to 18 cm) down.

Note: For most patients this CR level for PA chests is also near the level of the **inferior angle of the scapula,** which corresponds to the level of T7 on an average patient.

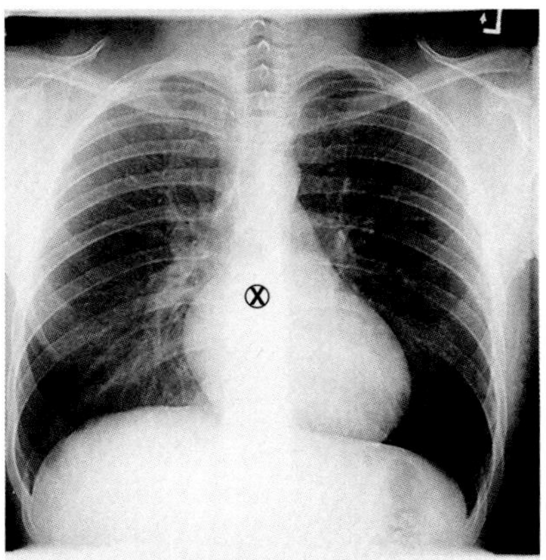

Fig. 3-44. Average sthenic/hyposthenic male (correct CR and collimation).

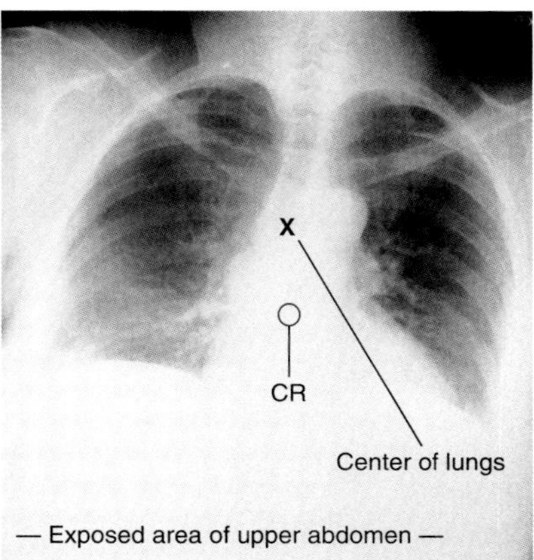

Fig. 3-45. Small and older female (incorrect CR and collimation).

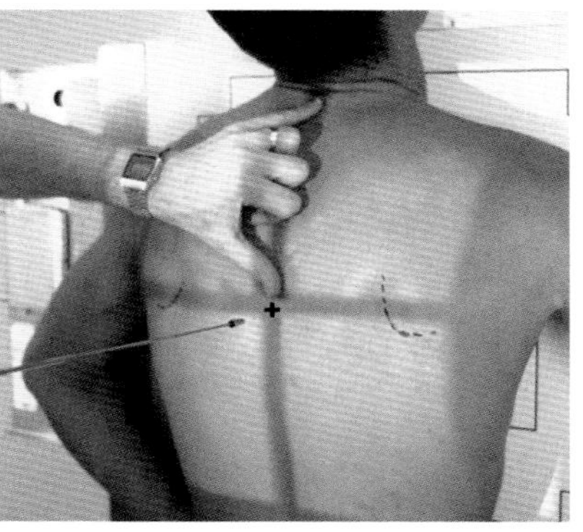

Fig. 3-46. Correct CR using vertebra prominens. Distance on average male is 8 inches, or 20 cm.

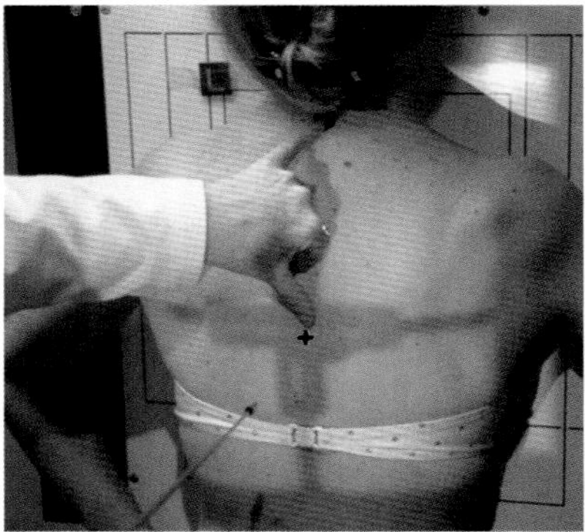

Fig. 3-47. Correct CR utilizing vertebra prominens. Distance on average female is 7 inches, or 18 cm.

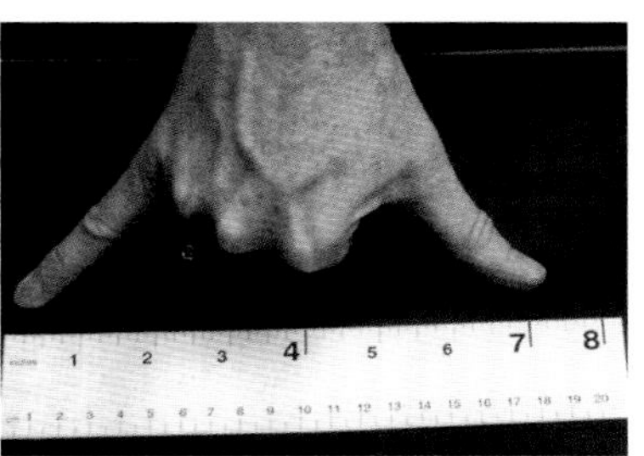

Fig. 3-48. Hand spread method—7 or 8 inches (18-20 cm).

3

Jugular Notch (AP Chest) The easily palpated jugular notch is the recommended landmark for location of the CR for AP chest radiographs. The level of T7 on an average adult is 3 to 4 inches (8 to 10 cm) below the jugular notch. For most older or hypersthenic patients, this is approximately **3 inches (8 cm).** For younger and/or sthenic/hyposthenic athletic types, this is nearer **4 or even 5 inches (10 to 12 cm).**

This distance can also be determined by the technologist's hand width. The average-sized hand width with the fingers together is approximately 3 inches (8 cm). See Fig. 3-50.

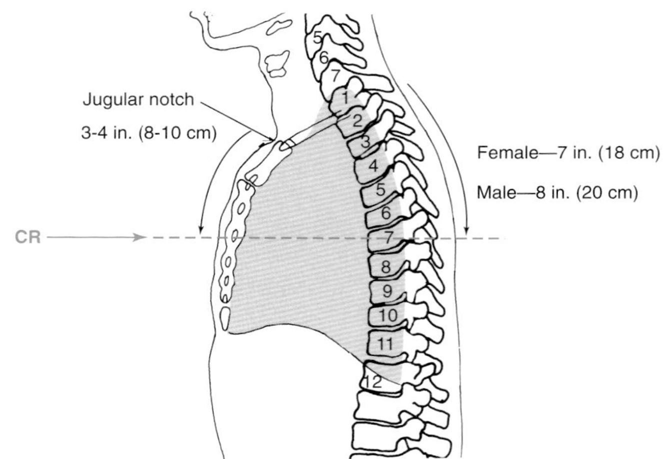

Fig. 3-49. Topographic landmark for AP chest.

LUNG DIMENSIONS AND FILM HOLDER (IR) PLACEMENT

PA or AP chest radiographs are most commonly taken with the cassette film holder or IR placed lengthwise. However, contrary to common belief, **the width or horizontal dimension of the average PA or AP chest is greater than the vertical dimension.**

A study performed by the author also shows that the width or horizontal dimension on a PA or AP chest exceeds 13 inches (33 cm) on 15% to 20% of patients. This requires that the 14- × 17-inch (35- × 43-cm) film holder or IR be placed **crosswise** so as not to cut off lateral lung margins on these patients.

PA Chest Most erect PA chests are done with dedicated chest units, which may not allow for this crosswise placement of the IR. However, cassettes with portable stationary grids can be placed crosswise for this purpose.

As the patient is standing and facing the chest IR, one can determine whether to place the IR crosswise on larger patients by standing behind the patient and placing one's hands squarely on each side of the chest. If there is any doubt that both sides of the chest can be included, the IR should be placed **crosswise,** remembering that the height of the average lung field is less than the width.

Note: Newer digital chest units may include larger image receptors such as 43 × 49 cm (17 × 19 inches), which eliminates this concern (see Chapter 1, p. 37).

AP Chest For recumbent AP chest radiographs (usually taken at less than 72 inches, or 180 cm, with an accompanying increase in divergence of the x-ray beam), the chance of the side borders of the lungs being cut off increases if the IR is placed lengthwise. Therefore it is recommended that for most AP chest radiographs, the 14- × 17-inch (35- × 43-cm) IR be placed **crosswise.** The IR and CR should be centered to a point 3 to 4 inches (8 to 10 cm) below the jugular notch (Fig. 3-50).

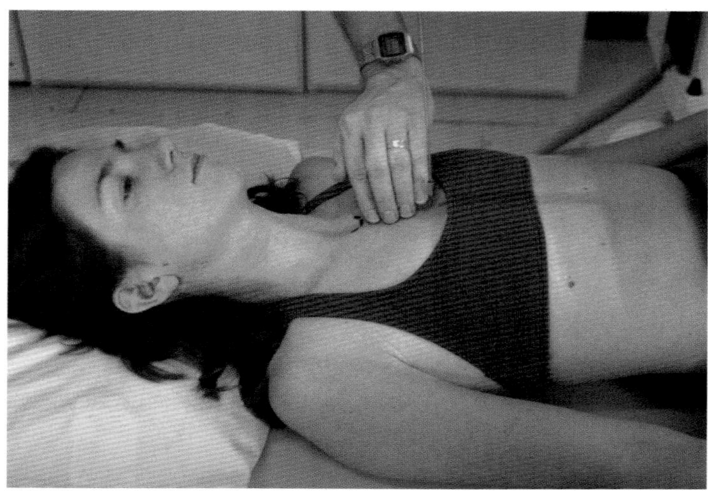

Fig. 3-50. Film crosswise, CR 3 to 4 inches (8 to 11 cm) below jugular.

COLLIMATION GUIDELINES

Side collimation borders can easily be determined by adjusting the illuminated field margins to the **outer skin margins** on each side of the posterior chest surface (remembering that lungs expand during deep inspiration). The upper and lower collimation borders, however, are more difficult to determine because these lung margins are not visible externally.

A reliable method for upper and lower chest collimation is to adjust the upper border of the illuminated light field to the **vertebra prominens,** which (with the divergent rays) will result in an upper collimation margin on the IR of about 1½ inches, or 4 cm, above the vertebra prominens (Fig. 3-51). This will then also result in a lower collimation border of 1 to 2 inches (3 to 5 cm) below the costophrenic angles, if the CR was correctly centered. These distances above and below the lungs allow for some margin of error in CR placement without cutting off upper or lower lungs.

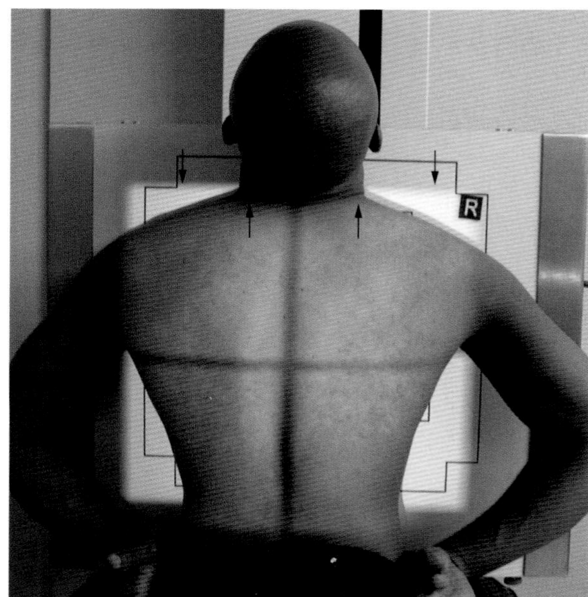

Fig. 3-51. Collimation guidelines, PA chest: CR–T7 or T8; sides–outer skin margins; upper–level of vertebra prominens.

3

Digital Imaging Considerations

The following guidelines should be followed when chest images are acquired using digital imaging technology. (See Chapter 2 on application of digital technology.)

1. Collimination In addition to the obvious benefit of reducing radiation dose to the patient, collimation that is closely restricted to the part being examined is key in ensuring the image processed by the computer will be of optimal quality. This close collimation also improves image quality by reducing secondary and scatter radiation from surrounding areas (such as the dense abdomen below) from reaching the highly sensitive CR or DR image receptors. This also allows the computer to provide accurate information regarding the exposure index number.

2. Accurate centering Because of the technique used by the CR or DR image receptor, it is important that the body part and central ray be accurately centered to the IR. In chest imaging this includes centering the central ray to the center of the lung fields as described in preceding pages of this chapter.

3. Exposure factors Digital imaging systems are known for their wide exposure latitude; they are able to process an acceptable image from a broad range of exposure factors (kV and mAs). It is important to remember, however, that the ALARA principle must still be followed and the lowest exposure factors required to obtain a diagnostic image must be used. This includes using the highest possible kV and the lowest mAs consistent with good image quality.

4. Post-processing evaluation of exposure index values Once the image is available for viewing, the image will be critiqued for positioning and exposure accuracy. The technologist must then also **check the exposure index number** to verify that the exposure factors used were in the correct range to ensure optimum quality with the least radiation to the patient.

Alternative Modalities or Procedures

CONVENTIONAL AND COMPUTED TOMOGRAPHY

Tomography is a conventional radiographic procedure commonly performed to examine and identify masses or other pathology in either the mediastinum or in the lung. **Computed tomography (CT)** is most frequently used for such purposes. Conventional or plain film tomography is rarely performed any more for chest imaging.

Spiral/helical CT provides much faster scanning, which is especially advantageous in the thorax region. When nonspiral CT is used for imaging small thoracic masses, problems occur with nonuniform breath holds (patient not holding breath in the same position for each exposure). (See Chapter 22 for more information on spiral/helical CT.)

BRONCHOGRAPHY

Bronchograms were commonly performed in the past to examine the bronchial tree and lungs after introduction of a catheter and positive contrast media into the bronchi. PA, lateral, and frequently, obliques were then taken to rule out pathologies such as obstructions, fistulas, carcinoma, bronchitis, or bronchiectasis. **CT** has replaced bronchography as the preferred study for such purposes today.

SONOGRAPHY (ULTRASOUND)

Ultrasound may be used to detect **pleural effusion** (fluid within pleura space) or for guidance when inserting a needle to aspirate the fluid (thoracentesis).

Echocardiogram is an ultrasound exam using sound waves to create an image of the heart. (Note that this is not the same as an electrocardiogram, which is a totally different type of exam that examines the electrical activity of the heart.)

NUCLEAR MEDICINE

Certain nuclear medicine procedures involving radionuclides can be used to evaluate and diagnose pulmonary diffusion conditions or pulmonary emboli.

MAGNETIC RESONANCE IMAGING

Cardiovascular MRI procedures can be used to demonstrate and evaluate certain pathology, such as congenital heart disorders, graft patency, cardiac tumors, thrombi, pericardial masses, and aortic dissection and aneurysms.

MRI is unlikely to replace echocardiography for cardiac evaluation. MRI, however, can be used as an adjunct to CT to provide multiplanar views of tumors and masses and to further assess mediastinal pathology and to evaluate aortic dissection and aneurysm.

Pathologic Indications

INTRODUCTION

The **pathologic indications,** as listed below and in each chapter of this textbook, are not intended to be inclusive of all diseases or pathologic conditions that technologists should know or that may be covered in a separate pathology course. They do, however, represent those conditions more commonly encountered, and the knowledge and understanding of these pathologic indications should be considered **basic** and **essential** for all technologists.

Patient histories with these pathologic indications noted will help the technologist select the optimum exposure factors and ensure that the necessary projections or body positions are being utilized.

This is also important information for understanding and being prepared to respond to the patient's needs and reactions during the radiographic procedure. For the chest, these pathologic indications are numerous and complex. The more common of these for youth and adults are listed alphabetically as follows (see Chapter 20 for infants and children):

INDICATIONS

Aspiration *(as-pi-ra'shun)* (mechanical obstruction) is most common in small children, when **foreign objects** are swallowed or aspirated into the air passages of the bronchial tree. In adults it may also occur with food particles, creating coughing and gagging (relieved by Heimlich maneuver). Aspiration may be demonstrated in lower airways on frontal and lateral chest radiographs or AP and lateral radiographs of the upper airway.

Atelectasis *(at"e-lek-tah-sis)* is a condition rather than a disease, in which collapse of all or a portion of a lung occurs as a result of an obstruction of the bronchus or a puncture or "blowout" of an air passageway. With less air in the lung than normal, this region appears more radiodense and may cause the trachea and heart to shift to the affected side.

Bronchiectasis *(brong"ke-ek'tah-sis)* is an irreversible dilation or widening of bronchi or bronchioles resulting from repeated pulmonary infection or obstruction. Areas of bronchial walls are destroyed and chronically inflamed, resulting in increased mucus production, causing chronic cough and expectoration (coughing up sputum). Pus can collect in dilated regions, resulting in an increase in regional radiodensity because of less air in these regions (most common in lower lobes).

Bronchitis *(brong-ki'tis)* is an acute (short-term) or chronic (long-term) condition in which excessive mucus is secreted into the bronchi, creating cough and shortness of breath. The chief cause is cigarette smoking. Infectious bronchitis is caused by viruses or bacteria. Bronchitis generally involves lower lobes as demonstrated on radiographs by hyperinflation and more dominant lung markings.

Chronic obstructive pulmonary disease (COPD) is a form of persistent obstruction of airway as caused by either emphysema or chronic bronchitis (smoking is the predominant cause of COPD). Mild cases of COPD are usually not detectable on chest radiographs, but more severe conditions are clearly demonstrated. (See **emphysema** below.)

Cystic fibrosis *(sis'tik fi-bro'sis)* is the most common of inherited diseases, in which secretions of heavy mucus cause progressive "clogging" of bronchi and bronchioles. This may be demonstrated on chest radiographs as increased radiodensities in specific lung regions, along with hyperinflation.

Dyspnea *(disp'ne-ah)* is a condition of shortness of breath, which creates a sensation of difficulty in breathing, most common in older persons. Although generally caused by physical exertion, it may also be caused by restrictive or obstructive defects within the lungs or airways.

Dyspnea may also be caused by pulmonary edema related to cardiac conditions. PA and lateral chest radiographs are commonly taken as an initial procedure followed by other exams to make a diagnosis.

Emphysema *(em"fi-se'-mah)* is an irreversible and chronic lung disease in which alveoli air spaces become greatly enlarged as a result of alveolar wall destruction and loss of alveolar elasticity. Air tends not to be expelled during expiration, resulting in very labored breathing with serious impedance of gas exchange within the lungs. Causes include smoking or long-term dust inhalation. Emphysema is evident on chest radiographs by **increased lung dimensions,** barrel chest with depressed and flattened diaphragm obscuring costophrenic angles, and an elongated heart shadow. Lung fields appear very **radiolucent,** requiring a significant **decrease** in exposure factors from a normal chest, even with the increased chest dimensions.

Epiglottitis *(ep"i-glo-ti'tis)* is most common in children ages 2 to 5. See Chapter 20 for more information on this serious, **life-threatening condition, which can develop very rapidly.** Soft tissue lateral of upper airway may demonstrate edema or swelling at the point of the epiglottis.

3

Lung neoplasia

Neoplasm refers to a growth or tumor. Neoplasms may be benign or malignant.

Benign: A **hamartoma** *(ham"ahr-to'ma)* is the most common benign pulmonary mass generally found in peripheral regions of the lungs. These are seen on chest radiographs as small radiodense masses with rather sharp outlines.

Malignant: Many types of lung cancers exist, with more than 90% starting in the bronchi (bronchogenic carcinoma). Less common is alveolar cell carcinoma, which originates in the alveoli of the lungs. Also, many cancers start elsewhere in the body, such as the breast, colon, prostate, and other parts, before spreading to the lungs. Studies have shown that smoking is the primary cause in about 90% of all lung cancer in men and 70% in women.

Lung cancer may be demonstrated on chest radiographs as slight shadows in the early stages, or as more sharply defined larger radiopaque masses in more advanced cases. Malignant lung tumors, however, rarely calcify; therefore calcified radiopaque masses or nodules are generally benign.

CT scans may demonstrate small nodules that are not yet seen on chest radiographs. Biopsies, however, are usually required to determine whether these shadows are results of inflammation or are cancerous.

Pleural effusion (an older, outdated term is "hydrothorax") is a condition of abnormal accumulation of fluid in the pleural cavity.

Types of pleural effusion

Empyema *(em"pi-e'mah)* exists if the fluid is pus. Empyema causes include chest wounds, obstruction of bronchi, or ruptured lung abscess. It may develop when pneumonia or a lung abscess spreads into the pleural space.

Hemothorax *(he"mo-thor'aks)* exists if the fluid is blood. A common cause of right-side or bilateral pleural effusion is congestive heart failure. Causes of left-side effusion include trauma, pulmonary infarct, pancreatitis, and subphrenic abscess.

Any type of pleural effusion is demonstrated by **fluid levels** with horizontal beam chest radiographs. Small amounts are best shown by a lateral decubitus position with **affected side down** or with **erect position.**

Pleurisy *(ploor'i-se)* is characterized by inflammation (usually caused by a virus or bacterium) of the pleura surrounding lungs. The cause is visceral and parietal pleura "rubbing" during respiration, resulting in severe pain. It frequently follows pneumonia or trauma to the chest. Pleurisy may be demonstrated radiographically by associated pleural effusion. A condition called "dry pleurisy," however, does not include fluid accumulation and thus is generally not visible on radiographs.

Pneumonia *(noo-mon'ya)* (pneumonitis) is an inflammation of the lungs resulting in **accumulation of fluid** within certain sections of the lungs, creating increased radiodensities in these regions. The most common initial diagnostic exam includes PA and lateral erect horizontal beam radiographs. Types of pneumonia are derived from the location and cause of the inflammation. Normal exposure factors are generally used initially. The radiologist may request secondary images with increased density to see through the area of interest to rule out a lesion in the same anatomic region if film-screen imaging methods are being employed.

Types of pneumonia

Aspiration pneumonia is caused by aspiration of a foreign object or food into the lungs, which irritates the bronchi, resulting in edema.

Bronchopneumonia is a bronchitis of both lungs most commonly caused by *Streptococcus* or *Staphylococcus* bacteria.

Lobar pneumonia is generally confined to one or two lobes of the lungs.

Viral (interstitial) pneumonia causes inflammation of the alveoli and connecting lung structures. It is most commonly evident by increased radiodensities in the region surrounding the hila.

Pneumothorax *(noo"mo-thor'aks)* is an accumulation of air in pleural space, causing partial or complete collapse of that lung and resulting in immediate and severe shortness of breath and chest pain. It may be caused by trauma or a pathologic condition that causes spontaneous rupture of a weakened area of lung.

Radiographically, the affected lung can be seen displaced away from the chest wall. Most evident on chest radiographs is the fact that **no lung markings** are seen in the region of the collapsed lung. Care should be taken to identify the lung edge or boundary. Chest radiographs for pneumothorax should be taken **erect.** If the patient cannot assume an erect position, a horizontal beam **lateral decubitus** position with the **affected side up** should be taken (not down as with pleural effusion).

Erect PA inspiration/expiration radiographs are commonly taken to demonstrate a small pneumothorax, which is best seen at the apex of an erect PA radiograph with maximum expiration.

Pulmonary edema is a condition of excess fluid within the lung, most frequently caused by a backup in pulmonary circulation commonly associated with congestive heart failure (CHF). A common cause is coronary artery disease, in which blood flow to the heart muscle is restricted. This weakens the heart and results in inadequate pulmonary circulation, causing a backup of blood in the lungs. This is seen on chest radiographs by a diffuse increase in radiodensity in the hilar regions fading toward the periphery of the lung and air-fluid levels with horizontal beam projections for more severe conditions.

Pulmonary emboli is a sudden blocking of an artery of the lung. Large clots can cause sudden death, but usually other arteries compensate and supply blood to affected areas to prevent tissue death (pulmonary infarct). Chest radiographs rarely demonstrate this condition. Occasionally, a wedge-shaped opacity (Hampton's hump) may be seen, suggesting pulmonary infarct (tissue necrosis or death).

Diagnosis involves high-resolution CT scans or nuclear medicine perfusion scans outlining the blood supply (perfusion) to the affected region, demonstrating which lung segment is not receiving blood.

Respiratory distress syndrome (RDS), (commonly called **hyaline membrane disease [HMD],** in infants and **adult respiratory distress syndrome [ARDS],** in adults) is an emergency condition, in which the alveoli and capillaries of the lung are injured or infected, resulting in leakage of fluid and blood into the spaces between alveoli or into the alveoli themselves with formation of hyaline membranes. (HMD results from a lack of lung development, in which the alveoli collapse due to a lack of internal tension.)

This can be detected radiographically by increased density throughout the lungs in a granular pattern as the normal air-filled spaces are filled with fluid. The most common radiographic sign is an "air bronchogram."

Tuberculosis *(too-ber"ku-lo'sis),* or TB, is a contagious disease (potentially fatal) caused by airborne bacteria. At one time TB resulted in more than 30% of all deaths, but development of vaccines and antibiotics such as streptomycin in the 1940s and 1950s nearly eliminated the threat of this disease. However, its occurrence has begun to rise again with the increased incidence of acquired immunodeficiency syndrome (AIDS) and in the presence of urban overcrowding and unsanitary conditions.

Primary tuberculosis refers to tuberculosis that occurs in persons who have never had the disease before. Hilar enlargement, along with enlarged mediastinal lymph nodes, is an important sign of primary tuberculosis. Small focal spot lesions may be found anywhere in the lungs, and unilateral pleural effusion is common, especially in adults.

Reactivation (secondary) tuberculosis usually develops in adults and is generally first evident on radiograph bilaterally in upper lobes as irregular calcifications that are mottled in appearance. An upward retraction of the hila is frequently evident. As healing occurs, fibrous tissue develops with calcification surrounding the region and leaving a type of cavity, which can be seen on tomograms of this region. **AP lordotic projections** are also frequently requested to demonstrate the calcifications and cavitations of the apices and upper lobes.

Occupational lung disease (forms of pneumoconiosis)

Anthracosis *(an-thre-ko'sis),* also called **black lung pneumoconiosis,** is caused by deposits of coal dust. With long-term inhalation (10 years or more), it spreads throughout the lungs and is demonstrated on chest radiographs as small opaque spots or conglomerate masses.

Asbestosis *(as"bes-to'sis)* is caused by inhalation of asbestos dust (fibers), resulting in pulmonary fibrosis. It may develop into lung cancer, especially in those who smoke.

Silicosis *(sil"i-ko'sis)* is a permanent condition of the lungs caused by inhaling silica (quartz) dust, a form of sand dust. Occupationally exposed patients include certain mine workers, sandblasters, and those who work in similar professions. Chest x-rays show distinctive patterns of nodules and scarring densities. Patients with silicosis are three times more likely to develop tuberculosis than are persons without silicosis.*

*Berkow R, Beer M, Fletcher A: The Merck manual of medical information, Whitehouse Station, NJ, 1997, Merck Research Laboratories.

SUMMARY OF PATHOLOGIC INDICATIONS

CONDITION OR DISEASE	MOST COMMON RADIOGRAPHIC EXAM	POSSIBLE RADIOGRAPHIC APPEARANCE	EXPOSURE FACTOR ADJUSTMENT*
Aspiration (mechanical obstruction)	PA and lat chest and lat upper airway	Radiodense or radiopaque outline	Soft-tissue technique for upper airway (−)
Atelectasis (collapse of all or portion of lung)	PA and lat chest and PA inspiration/expiration	Radiodense lung regions with shift of heart and trachea in severe cases	Increase (+)
Bronchiectasis	PA and lat chest with bronchogram or CT	Radiodense lower lungs	Generally none
Bronchitis	PA and lat chest	Hyperinflation (general radiolucency) and dominant lung markings of lower lungs	Generally none
Chronic obstructive pulmonary disease (COPD)	PA and lat chest	Appears as emphysema in severe cases	Decrease (−)
Cystic fibrosis	PA and lat chest	Increased radiodensities in specific lung regions	Increase with severe condition (+)
Dyspnea (difficult breathing)	PA and lat chest	Dependent on cause of dyspnea	Dependent on cause
Emphysema	PA and lat chest	Increased lung dimensions, barrel-chested, flattened diaphragm, radiolucent lungs	Significant decrease, dependent on severity (−)
Epiglottitis	Soft-tissue lateral upper airway	Narrowing of upper airway at epiglottic region	Soft-tissue lateral technique (−)
Lung neoplasm			
• Benign (hamartoma)	PA and lat chest	Radiodensities with sharp outlines; mass may be calcified (radiopaque)	Generally none
• Malignant types	PA and lat chest, CT scans	Slight shadows in early stages, larger defined radiopaque masses in advanced stages	Generally none
Pleural effusion (hydrothorax) (fluid in pleural cavity) • Empyema (fluid is pus) • Hemothorax (fluid is blood)	Erect PA and lat chest or horizontal beam lateral decub with **affected side down**	Increased radiodensity, air-fluid levels, possible mediastinal shift (see Atelectasis)	Increase (+)
Pleurisy	PA and lat chest	Possible air-fluid levels, or none with "dry" pleurisy	Generally none
Pneumonia (pneumonitis) • Aspiration pneumonia • Bronchopneumonia • Lobar (pneumococcal) • Viral (interstitial)	PA and lat chest	Patchy infiltrate with increased radiodensity	Increase (+)
Pneumothorax	Erect PA and lat chest or lat decub **affected side up**, PA inspiration/expiration for small pneumothorax	Lung seen displaced from chest wall, no lung markings	Generally none
Pulmonary edema (fluid within lungs)	PA and lat chest; horizontal beam projection for air-fluid levels	Increased diffuse radiodensity in hilar regions; air-fluid levels	Increase (+)
Pulmonary emboli (sudden blockage of artery in lung)	PA and lat chest and perfusion scans (nuclear medicine)	Rarely demonstrated on chest radiographs except for possible wedge-shaped opacity (Hampton's hump)	Generally none
Respiratory distress syndrome (RDS)—commonly called *hyaline membrane disease* (HMD) in children	PA and lat erect chest	Granular pattern of increased radiodensity throughout lungs, possible air-fluid levels	Increase (+)
Tuberculosis			
• Primary tuberculosis	PA and lat chest	Small opaque spots throughout lungs; enlargement of hilar region in early stages	Generally none
• Reactivation (secondary) tuberculosis	PA and lat chest and AP lordotic chest, tomograms	Calcification regions with cavitations, frequently in area of upper lobes and apices with upward retraction of hila	None or slight increase (+)
Occupational lung diseases (forms of pneumoconiosis)			
• Anthracosis (black lung)	PA and lat chest	Small opaque spots throughout lungs	Generally none
• Asbestosis	PA and lat chest	Calcifications (radiodensities) involving the pleura	Generally none
• Silicosis	PA and lat chest	Distinctive pattern of scarring and dense nodules	Generally none

*Automatic exposure control (AEC) systems are designed to correct exposure density automatically for patient size variances and for these pathologic conditions; if they are calibrated correctly and used as intended, manual adjustments generally are not needed when AEC is used. However, these exposure adjustments may be needed for more extreme cases, or for repeats, even with AEC. Manual exposure adjustments are also important when setting manual exposure techniques such as for tabletop or mobile exams when AEC is not used.

3

Survey Information (See Appendix A)

CHEST

Basic projections: PA and **lateral** were the two most common **basic projections** throughout the United States and Canada as expected, followed by AP supine.

Special projections/positions: The most common **special projections/positions** in order of preference were the **AP lordotic, lateral decubitus, anterior obliques,** and **posterior obliques.** These results were consistent throughout all regions of the United States and Canada.

Basic (Routine) and Special Projections

Certain basic and special projections for the chest are demonstrated and described on the following pages as suggested standard or basic projections and as special departmental procedures that all student technologists should master.

BASIC PROJECTIONS

Standard or basic projections, also sometimes referred to as "routines," are those projections commonly taken on average patients who are helpful and can cooperate in performing the procedure.

SPECIAL PROJECTIONS

Special projections are those more common projections taken as extra or additional projections to better demonstrate certain pathologic conditions or specific body parts or when the patient is not able to cooperate fully.

BASIC AND SPECIAL PROJECTIONS

Chest
BASIC
- PA 96
- Lateral 98

Chest
SPECIAL
- AP supine or semi-erect 100
- Lateral decubitus 101
- AP lordotic 102
- Anterior oblique 103
- Posterior oblique 104

Upper airway
BASIC
- Lateral 105
- AP 106

PA PROJECTION: CHEST

Ambulatory Patient

Pathology Demonstrated

When performed erect, PA demonstrates pleural effusions, pneumothorax, atelectasis, and signs of infection.

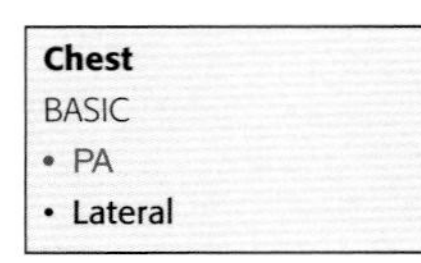
Chest
BASIC
• PA
• Lateral

Technical Factors

- IR size—35 × 43 cm (14 × 17 inches), lengthwise or crosswise (see Note below).
- Moving or stationary grid
- 110-125 kV range
- Technique and dose:

cm	kV	mAs	Sk.	ML.	
22	110	3	17	5	Thyroid 1 Breast 1
			mrad		

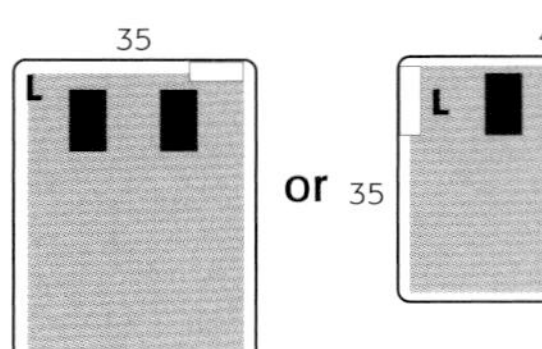

Dark boxes indicate AEC chamber selections.

Shielding Secure lead shield around waist or use an adjustable mobile shield on a stand behind patient.

Patient Position

- Patient erect, feet spread slightly, weight equally distributed on both feet
- Chin raised, resting against IR
- Hands on lower hips, palms out, elbows partially flexed
- Shoulders rotated forward against IR to allow scapulae to move laterally clear of lung fields; shoulders depressed downward to move clavicles below the apices

Part Position

- Align midsagittal plane to CR and to midline of IR with equal margins between lateral thorax and sides of IR.
- Ensure **no rotation** of thorax.
- Raise or lower CR and IR as needed to the level of T7 for average patient. (Top of IR will be 1½ to 2 inches, or 4 to 5 cm, above shoulders on most average patients.)

Central Ray

- CR perpendicular to IR and centered to **midsagittal plane at level of T7** (7 to 8 inches, or 18 to 20 cm, below vertebra prominens, or to inferior angle of scapula)
- IR centered to CR
- SID of 72 inches (180 cm)

Collimation Collimate on four sides to area of lung fields. (Top border of illuminated field should be to level of vertebra prominens, and lateral borders to outer skin margins.)

Respiration Exposure made at end of **second full inspiration.**

Note: With 35 × 43 cm (14 × 17 inch) film-screen grid cassette systems, place cassette crosswise for hypersthenic-type patients.

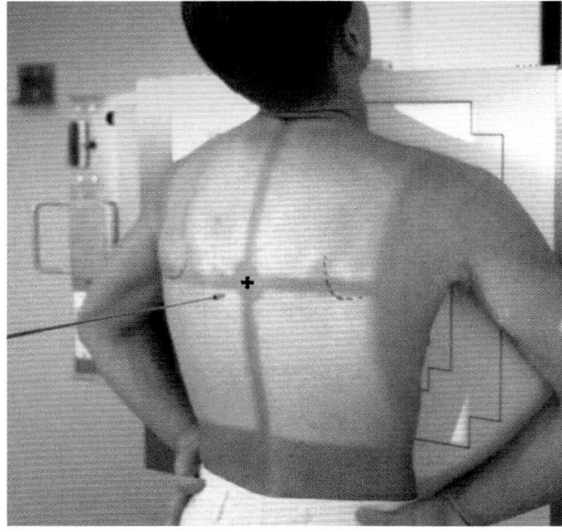

Fig. 3-52. PA chest.

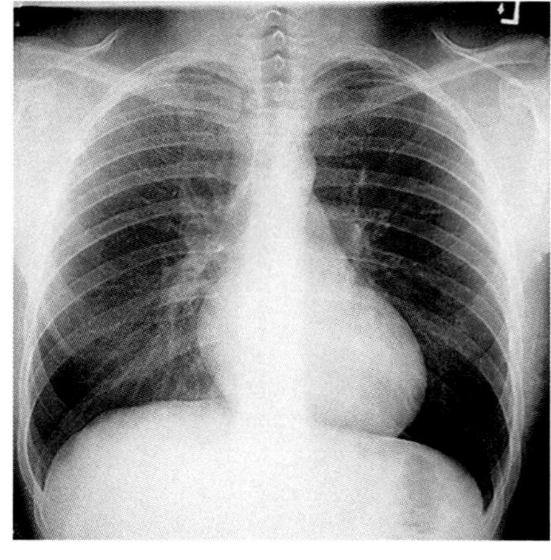

Fig. 3-53. PA chest.

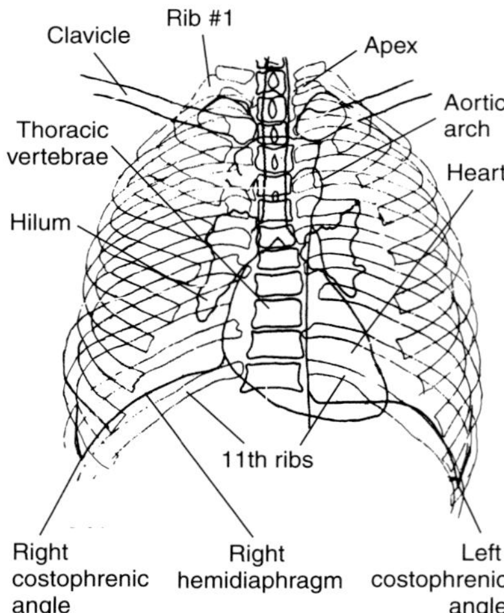

Fig. 3-54. PA chest.

Radiographic Criteria

Structures Shown: • Included are both lungs from apices to costophrenic angles and the air-filled trachea from T1 down. Hilum region markings, heart, great vessels, and bony thorax are demonstrated.

Position: • Chin sufficiently elevated to prevent superimposing apices • Sufficient forward shoulder rotation to prevent superimposition of scapulae over lung fields • Larger breast shadows (if present) primarily lateral to lung fields • **No Rotation:** Both sternoclavicular joints the same distance from center line of spine • Distance from lateral rib margins to vertebral column the same on each side from upper to lower rib cage.

Note: Scoliosis and kyphosis may also cause asymmetry of sternoclavicular joints and rib cage margins as evident by R to L spinal curvature.

Collimation and CR: • Collimation margins near equal on top and bottom with center of collimation field (CR) to T7 region on most patients • **Full Inspiration with No Motion** • Visualizes a minimum of 10 posterior ribs above diaphragm (11 on many patients) • **No motion** evident by sharp outlines of rib margins, diaphragm, and heart borders, as well as sharp lung markings in hilum region and throughout lungs.

Exposure Criteria: • Sufficient long-scale contrast to visualize fine vascular markings within lungs • Faint outlines of at least mid- and upper thoracic vertebrae and posterior ribs visible through heart and mediastinal structures.

PA PROJECTION: CHEST

On Stretcher If Patient Cannot Stand

Pathology Demonstrated
When performed erect, PA demonstrates pleural effusions, pneumothorax, atelectasis, and signs of infection.

Chest
BASIC
• PA
• Lateral

Technical Factors
- IR size—35 × 43 cm (14 × 17 inches), lengthwise or crosswise
- Moving or stationary grid
- 110-125 kV range
- Technique and dose:

cm	kV	mAs	Sk.	ML.	
22	110	3	17	5	Thyroid 1 Breast 1
			mrad		

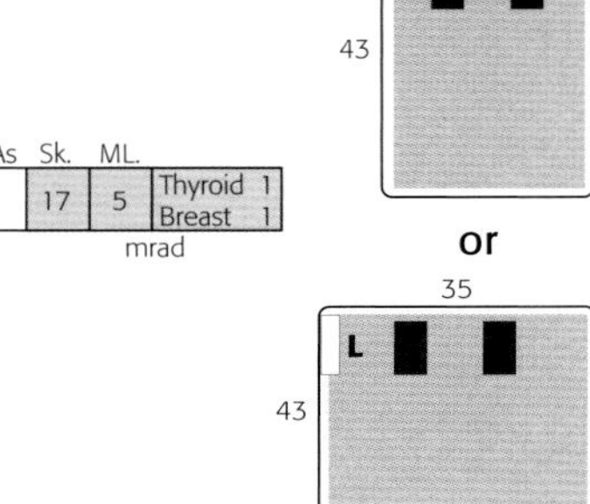

Shielding Secure lead shield around waist to shield gonads.

Patient Position
- Patient erect, seated on cart, legs over the edge
- Arms around cassette unless a chest IR device is used, then position as for an ambulatory patient
- Shoulders rotated forward and downward
- **No rotation** of thorax

Part Position
- Adjust the height of IR so top of receptor is about 1½ to 2 inches (4 to 5 cm) above top of shoulders and CR is at T7.
- If portable cassette is used because patient cannot be placed up against chest board, place pillow or padding on lap to raise and support cassette as shown, but keep cassette against chest for minimum OID (Fig. 3-56).

Central Ray
- CR perpendicular to the IR and centered to the **midsagittal plane at the level of T7** (7 to 8 inches, or 18 to 20 cm, below vertebra prominens to inferior angle of scapula)
- Cassette centered to level of CR (if portable film-screen grid cassette is used)
- SID of 72 inches (180 cm)

Collimation Collimate to area of lung fields. Upper border of illuminated field should be **to level of vertebra prominens,** which with divergent rays, will result in upper collimation border on IR to about 1½ inches, or 4 cm, above apex of lungs.

Respiration Make exposure on **second full inspiration.**

Note: Use compression band or other means to ensure that patient is stable and will not waver or move during exposure.

Radiographic Criteria
Radiograph should appear similar to ambulatory PA chest as described on preceding page.

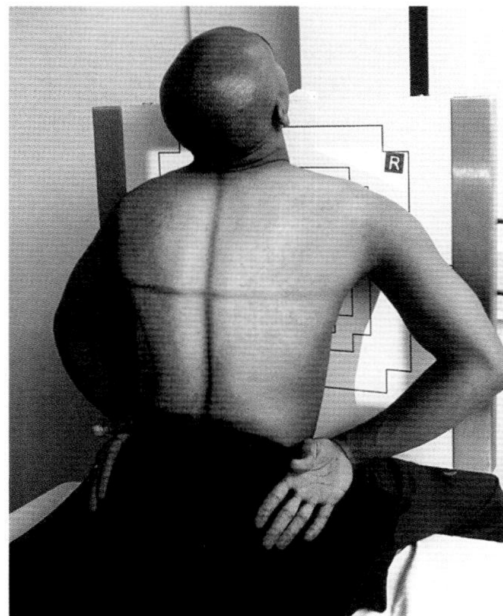

Fig. 3-55. PA chest (patient seated, chest against chest board).

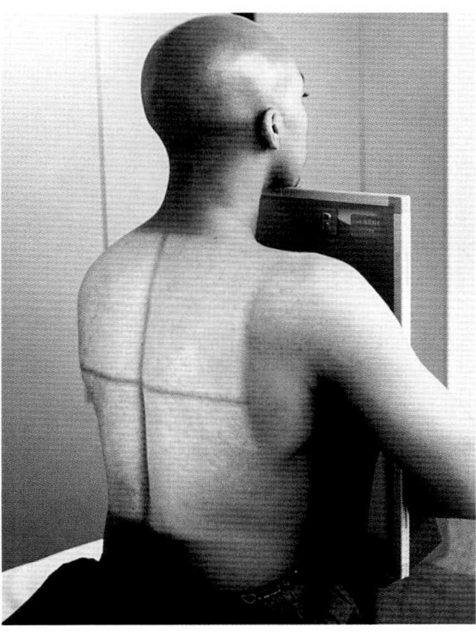

Fig. 3-56. PA chest (patient seated, holding cassette).

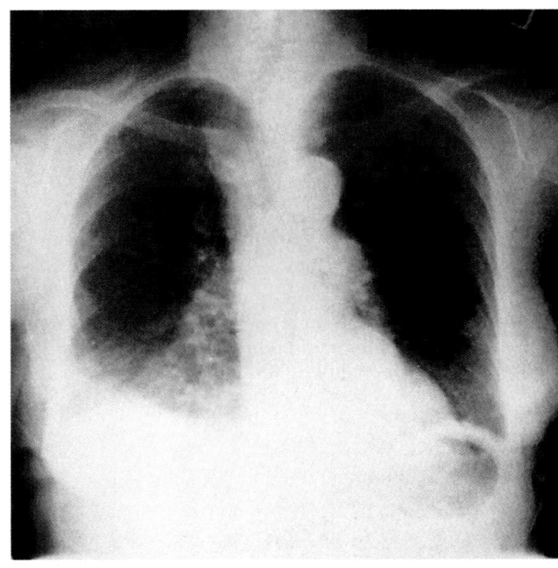

Fig. 3-57. PA chest.

LATERAL POSITION: CHEST

Ambulatory Patient

Chest
BASIC
• PA
• Lateral

Pathology Demonstrated

A 90° perspective from PA may demonstrate pathology situated posterior to the heart, great vessels, and sternum.

Technical Factors

- IR size—35 × 43 cm (14 × 17 inches), lengthwise
- Moving or stationary grid
- 110-125 kV
- Technique and dose:

cm	kV	mAs	Sk.	ML.	mrad
30	125	6	40	35	Thyroid 3 Breast 9

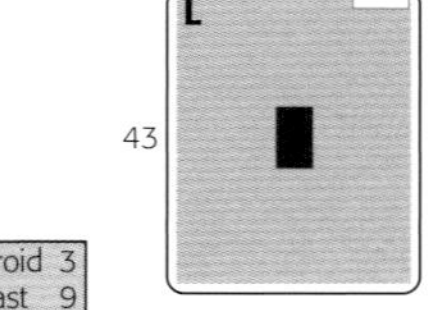

Shielding Secure lead shield around waist or use mobile lead shield to protect gonads.

Patient Position

- Patient erect, **left side** against IR unless patient's complaint is on right side (in that case, do a right lateral if departmental protocol includes this option)
- Weight evenly distributed on both feet
- Arms raised above head, chin up

Part Position

- Center patient to CR and to IR anteriorly and posteriorly.
- Position in a **true lateral** position (coronal plane is perpendicular, and sagittal plane is parallel to IR; see Note 1 below).
- Lower CR and IR slightly from PA if needed (see Note 2 below).

Central Ray

- CR perpendicular, directed to **midthorax at level of T7** (3 to 4 inches or 8 to 10 cm below level of jugular notch)
- SID of 72 inches (180 cm)

Collimation Collimate on four sides to area of lung fields (top border of light field to level of vertebra prominens).

Respiration Make exposure at end of **second full inspiration.**

Note 1: Ensure that **midsagittal plane** is **parallel to IR,** which for slender but broader-shouldered patients will result in hips and lower thorax **not** being against IR.

Note 2: This increase in OID of the lower chest will also result in the costophrenic angles of the lungs being projected lower because of the divergence of the x-ray beam. Therefore **the CR and IR need to be lowered a minimum of 1 inch, or 2 cm, from the PA** on this type of patient to prevent cutoff of costophrenic angles.

Radiographic Criteria

Structures Shown: • Included are the entire lungs from apices to the costophrenic angles and from the sternum anteriorly to posterior ribs and thorax posteriorly.

Position: • Chin and arms elevated sufficiently to prevent excessive soft tissues from superimposing apices • **No rotation:** posterior ribs and costophrenic angle on side away from IR projected slightly (¼ to ½ inch or 1 to 2 cm) posterior because of divergent rays.
Note: For direction of rotation, see p. 88 and critique radiographs on p. 107.

Collimation and CR: • Collimation margins are near equal on top and bottom. • The hilum region should be in the approximate center of the IR.

Exposure Criteria: • No motion evident by sharp outlines of the diaphragm and lung markings • Should have sufficient exposure and long-scale contrast to **visualize rib outlines and lung markings through the heart shadow and upper lung areas** without overexposing other regions of the lungs.

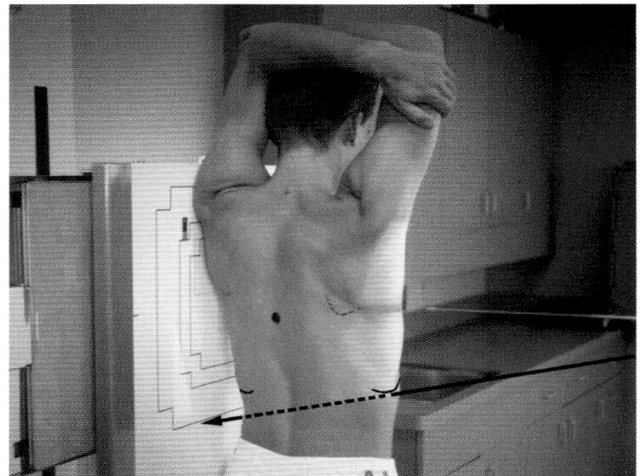

Fig. 3-58. Left lateral chest position.

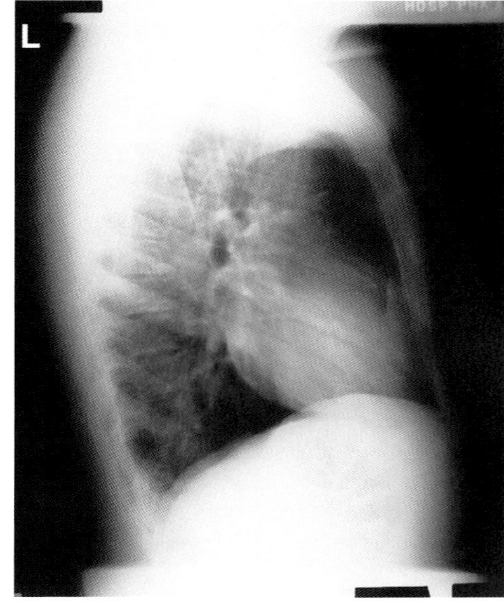

Fig. 3-59. Lateral chest.

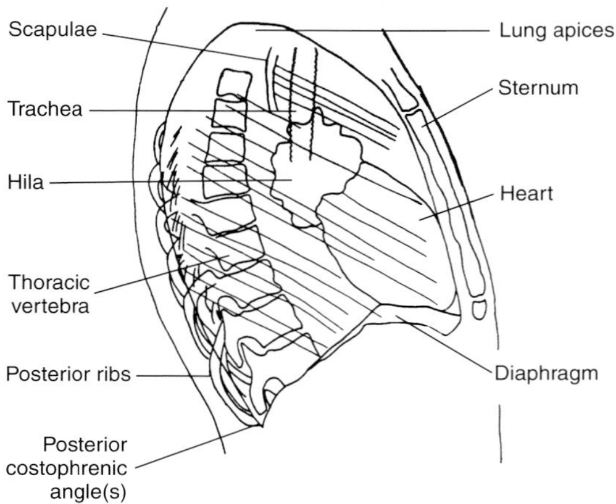

Fig. 3-60. Lateral chest.

LATERAL POSITION: CHEST

With Wheelchair or Cart If Patient Cannot Stand

Chest
BASIC
- **PA**
- Lateral

Pathology Demonstrated

A 90° perspective from PA may demonstrate pathology situated posterior to the heart, great vessels, and sternum.

Technical Factors

- IR size—35 × 43 cm (14 × 17 inches), lengthwise
- Moving or stationary grid
- 110-125 kV
- Technique and dose:

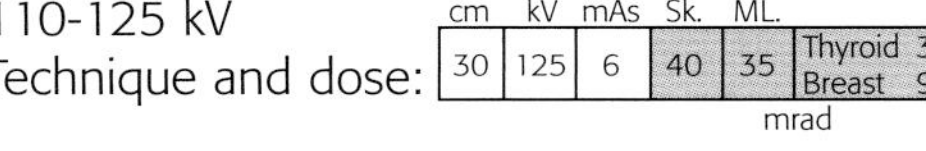

cm	kV	mAs	Sk.	ML.	mrad
30	125	6	40	35	Thyroid 3 Breast 9

35 L 43

Shielding Secure lead shielding around waist to protect gonads.

Patient Position on Cart

- Patient seated on cart; legs over the edge if this is easier for patient (ensure that cart does not move)
- Arms crossed above head, or hold on to arm support
- Chin kept up

Patient Position in Wheelchair

- Remove armrests, if possible, or place pillow or other support under smaller patients so that armrests of wheelchair do not superimpose lower lungs.
- Turn patient in wheelchair to lateral position as close to IR as possible.
- Have patient lean forward and place support blocks behind back; raise arms above head and have patient hold on to support bar—**keeping arms high.**

Part Position

- Center patient to CR and to IR by checking anterior and posterior aspects of thorax; adjust CR and IR to level of T7.
- Ensure **no rotation** by viewing patient from tube position.

Central Ray

- CR perpendicular, directed to **level of T7** (3 to 4 inches, or 8 to 10 cm, below level of jugular notch)
- SID of 72 inches (180 cm)
- Top of IR about 1 inch (2.5 cm) above vertebra prominens

Collimation Collimate on four sides to area of lung fields.

Respiration Make exposure at end of **second full inspiration.**

Note: Always attempt to have patient sit completely erect in wheelchair or on cart if possible. However, if the patient's condition does not allow this, the head end of the cart can be raised as nearly erect as possible using a radiolucent support behind back (Fig. 3-63). All attempts should be made to get patient as nearly erect as possible.

Radiographic Criteria

Radiograph should appear similar to ambulatory lateral position as described under radiographic criteria on preceding page.

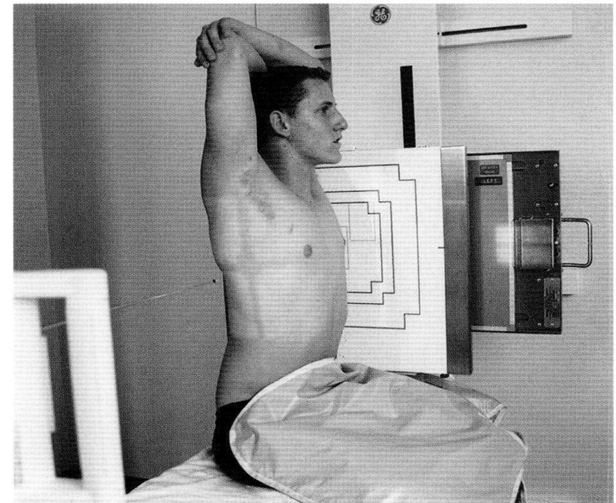

Fig. 3-61. Left lateral chest position on cart.

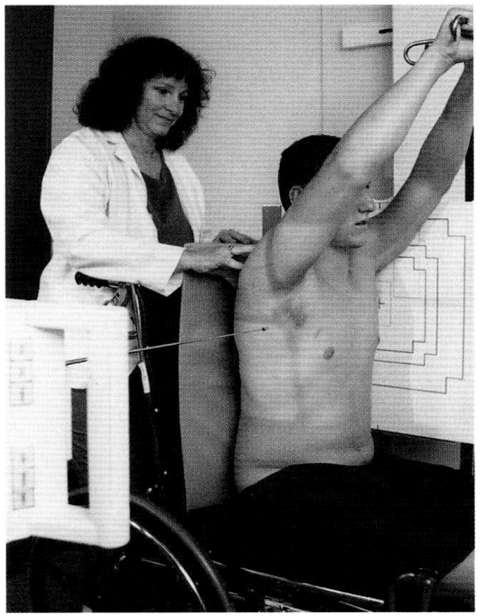

Fig. 3-62. Left lateral position in wheelchair (arms up, support behind back).

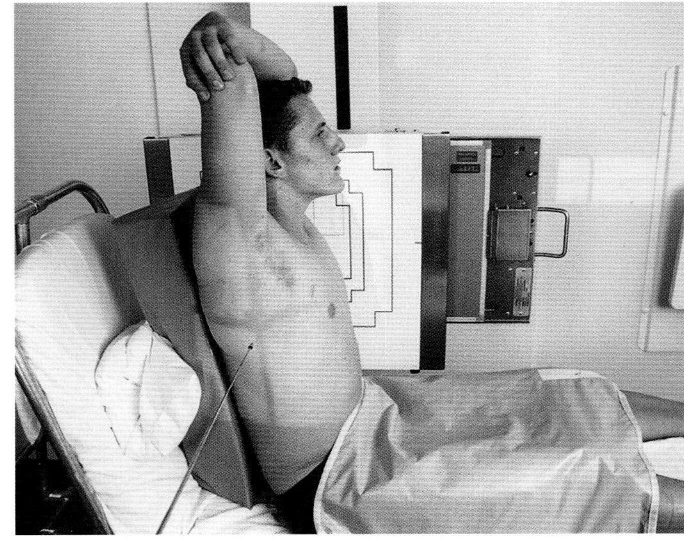

Fig. 3-63. Erect, supported left lateral position.

3

AP PROJECTION: CHEST

Supine or Semierect (in Department or as Bedside Portable)

Chest
SPECIAL
- AP supine or semierect

Pathology Demonstrated

This projection demonstrates pathology involving the lungs, diaphragm, and mediastinum. Determining air-fluid levels (pleural effusion) requires a completely erect position with a horizontal CR as in a PA or decubitus chest projection.

Technical Factors

- IR size—35 × 43 cm (14 × 17 inches) crosswise (average to large)
- Screens or stationary grid (screens commonly used with portables at 70-80 kV)
- 80-100 kV range with grid (large patient)
- Technique and dose:

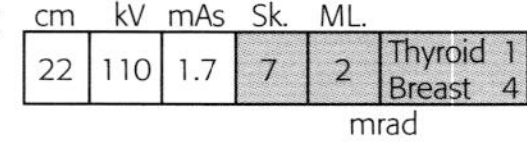

cm	kV	mAs	Sk.	ML.	
22	110	1.7	7	2	Thyroid 1 Breast 4

mrad

Shielding Place lead shield to shield gonads.

Patient Position

- Patient is supine on cart; if possible, the head end of the cart or bed should be raised into a semierect position (see Notes below).
- Roll patient's shoulders forward by rotating arms medially or internally.

Part Position

- Place IR under or behind patient; align center of IR to CR (top of IR about 1½ inches, or 4 to 5 cm, above shoulders).
- Center patient to CR and to IR; check by viewing patient from the top, near the tube position.

Central Ray

- CR angled **caudad to be perpendicular to long axis of sternum** (generally requires ±5° caudad angle, to prevent clavicles from obscuring the apices)
- CR to **level of T7,** 3 to 4 inches (8 to 10 cm) below jugular notch
- Minimum SID of 40 inches (100 cm) for supine (see Notes)

Collimation Collimate to area of lung fields.

Respiration Make exposure at end of **second full inspiration.**

Notes: Crosswise IR placement is recommended for large or hypersthenic type patients to minimize chance of lateral cutoff. This requires **accurate CR alignment to center of IR** with only minimal caudal angle to prevent grid cutoff if grid is used.

For **semierect position,** use 72 inches (180 cm) SID if this is possible. Always indicate the SID used; also indicate those projections obtained, such as AP supine or AP semierect.

Radiographic Criteria

- Criteria for chest radiographs taken in supine or semierect positions should be similar to those for a PA projection described on a preceding page, with three exceptions:
  1. The heart will appear larger as a result of increased magnification from a shorter SID and increased OID of the heart.
  2. Possible pleural effusion for this type of patient will often obscure vascular lung markings when compared with a fully erect PA chest projection.
  3. Usually there will not be as full an inspiration, with only eight or nine posterior ribs visualized above diaphragm. Thus the lungs will appear more dense because the lungs are not as fully aerated.
- Correct CR angle: Three posterior ribs should be seen above clavicles, indicating unobscured apical region.

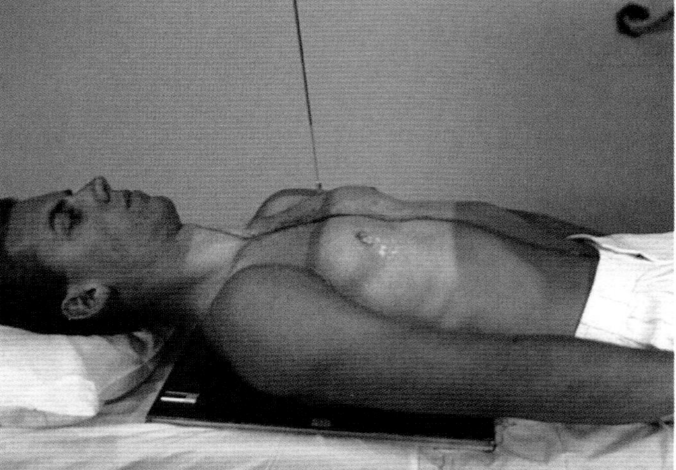

Fig. 3-64. AP supine.

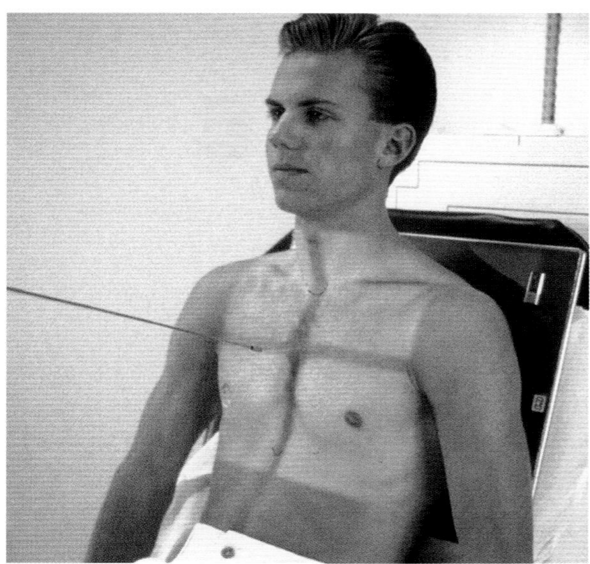

Fig. 3-65. AP semierect.

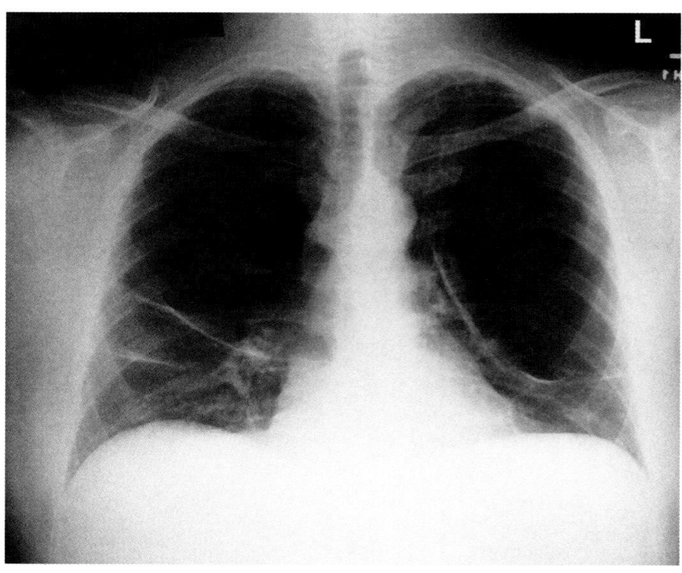

Fig. 3-66. AP.

LATERAL DECUBITUS POSITION (AP PROJECTION): CHEST

Chest
Special
- AP supine or semierect
- Lateral decubitus (AP)

Pathology Demonstrated
Small **pleural effusions** are demonstrated by air-fluid levels in pleural space; or **small amounts of air** in pleural cavity demonstrate a possible pneumothorax (see Notes below).

Technical Factors
- IR size—35 × 43 cm (14 × 17 inches), **crosswise** (crosswise with respect to patient)
- Moving or stationary grid
- 110-125 kV range
- **Use decub marker (or arrow)**
- Technique and dose:

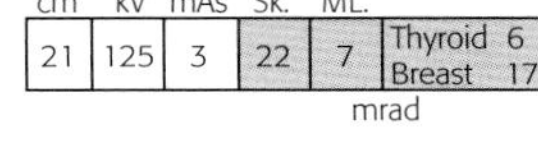

cm	kV	mAs	Sk.	ML.	mrad
21	125	3	22	7	Thyroid 6 Breast 17

Shielding Place lead shield to shield gonads.

Patient Position
- Cardiac board on the cart or radiolucent pad under patient
- Patient lying on right side for right lateral decubitus and on left side for left lateral decubitus (see Notes below)
- Patient's chin and both arms raised above head to clear lung field; back of patient firmly against IR; cart secured to prevent patient from moving forward and possibly falling; pillow under patient's head
- Knees flexed slightly and coronal plane parallel to IR with **no body rotation**

Part Position
- Adjust height of IR to center thorax to IR (see Notes below).
- Adjust patient and cart to center midsagittal plane and T7 to CR (top of IR is about 1 inch, or 2.5 cm, above vertebra prominens).

Central Ray
- CR horizontal, directed to center of IR, to **level of T7,** 3 to 4 inches (8 to 10 cm) inferior to level of jugular notch. A **horizontal beam must be used** to show air-fluid level or pneumothorax.
- SID of 72 inches (180 cm)

Collimation Collimate to area of lung fields (see Notes below).

Respiration Make exposure at end of **second full inspiration.**

Alternate Positioning Some prefer that the head be 10° lower than the hips to reduce the apical lift caused by the shoulder, thereby allowing the entire chest to remain horizontal (requires support under hips).

Notes: Place appropriate marker to indicate which side of chest is up.

Radiograph may be taken as a right or left lateral decubitus. For **possible fluid** in pleural cavity (pleural effusion), the suspected side should be **down.** Do **not** cut off that side of the chest.

For possible **small amounts of air** in pleural cavity (pneumothorax), the affected side should be **up** and care must be taken **not** to cut off this side of the chest.

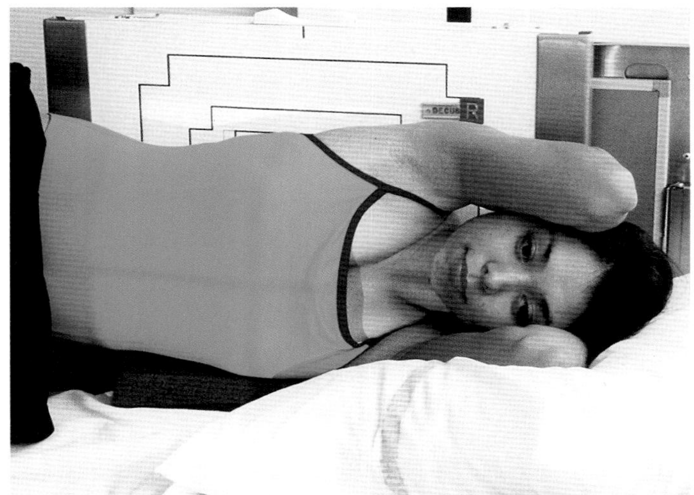

Fig. 3-67. Left lateral decubitus position (AP projection).

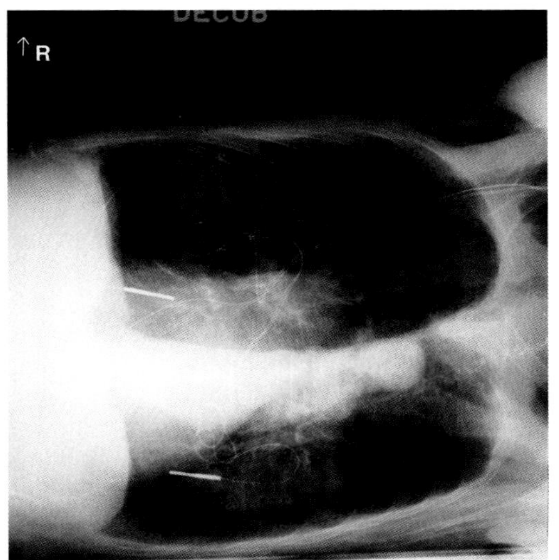

Fig. 3-68. Left lateral decubitus.

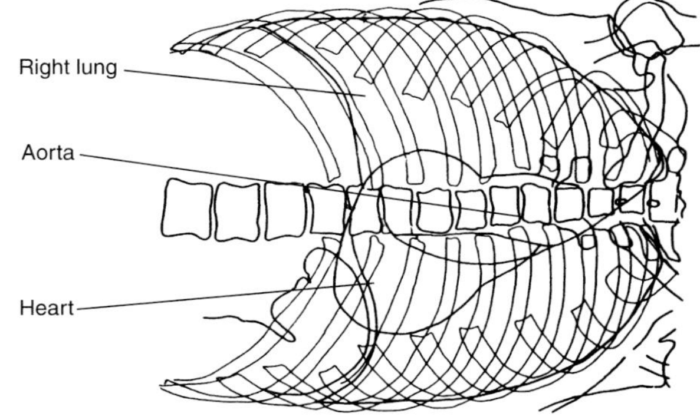

Fig. 3-69. Left lateral decubitus.

Radiographic Criteria

Structures Shown: • Entire lungs including apices and both costophrenic angles and both lateral borders of ribs should be included.

Position: • **No rotation** should show equal distance from vertebral column to the lateral borders of ribs on both sides; sternoclavicular joints should be same distance from the vertebral column. • Arms should not superimpose upper lungs.

Collimation and CR: • Center of collimation field (CR) should be to area of T7 on average-sized patients.

Exposure Criteria: • **No motion;** diaphragm, ribs and heart borders, and lung markings should appear sharp. • Optimal contrast scale and exposure should result in **faint visualization of vertebrae and ribs through heart shadow.**

AP LORDOTIC PROJECTION: CHEST

Chest
Special
- AP supine or semierect
- Lateral decubitus (AP)
- AP lordotic
- Anterior oblique
- Posterior oblique

Pathology Demonstrated
Projection is performed primarily to rule out calcifications and masses beneath the clavicles.

Technical Factors
- IR size—35 × 43 cm (14 × 17 inches), lengthwise
- Moving or stationary grid
- 110-125 kV range
- Technique and dose:

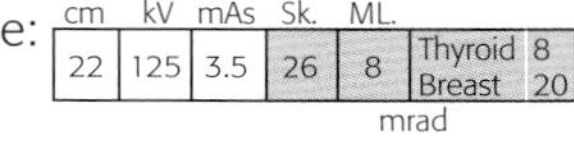

cm	kV	mAs	Sk.	ML.		
22	125	3.5	26	8	Thyroid	8
					Breast	20

mrad

35
43

Shielding Secure lead shield around waist to shield gonads.

Patient Position
- Patient standing about 1 foot (30 cm) away from IR and leaning back with shoulders, neck, and back of head against IR
- Both patient's hands on hips, palms out; shoulders rolled forward

Part Position
- Center midsagittal plane to CR and to centerline of IR.
- Center cassette to CR. (Top of IR should be about 3 inches, or 7 to 8 cm, above shoulders on average patient.)

Central Ray
- CR **perpendicular** to IR, centered to **midsternum** (3 to 4 inches, or 9 cm, below jugular notch)
- SID of 72 inches (180 cm)

Collimation Collimate to area of lungs of interest.

Respiration Make exposure at end of **second full inspiration.**

Exception (Fig. 3-71) If patient is weak and unstable and/or is not able to assume the erect lordotic position, an **AP semiaxial projection** may be taken with the patient in a supine position. Shoulders are rolled forward and arms positioned as for lordotic position.

The **CR** is directed **15° to 20° cephalad,** to the midsternum.

3

Radiographic Criteria

Structures Shown: • Entire lung fields and clavicles should be included.

Position: • Clavicles should appear nearly horizontal and **above or superior to apices** with medial aspects of clavicles superimposed by first ribs. • Ribs appear distorted, with posterior ribs appearing nearly horizontal superimposing anterior ribs. • **No rotation,** sternal ends of the clavicles should be the same distance from vertebral column on each side. The lateral borders of the ribs on both sides should appear to be near equal distances from the vertebral column.

Collimation and CR: • Center of collimation field (CR) should be mid sternum with collimation visible on top and bottom.

Exposure Criteria: • **No motion;** diaphragm, heart, and rib outlines should appear sharp. • Optimal contrast scale and exposure should **visualize the faint vascular markings of lungs, especially in area of apices and upper lungs.**

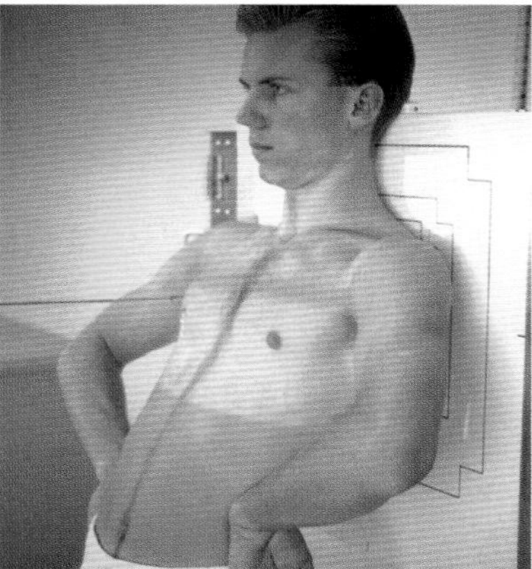

Fig. 3-70. AP lordotic.

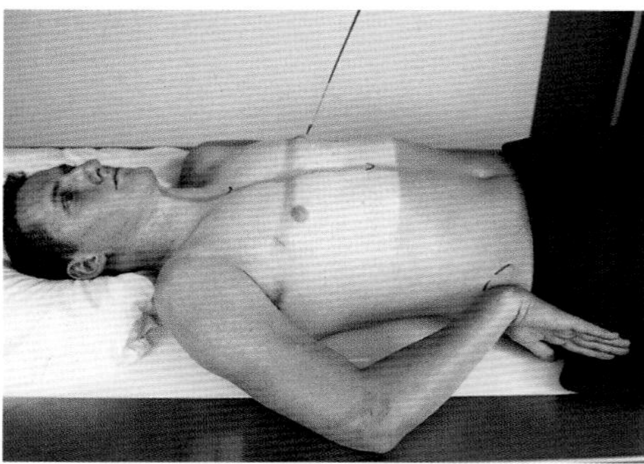

Fig. 3-71. Exception: semi-axial AP.

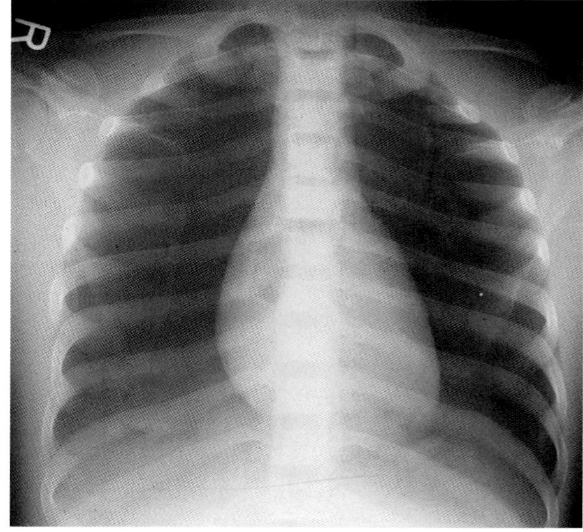

Fig. 3-72. AP lordotic.

ANTERIOR OBLIQUE POSITIONS—RAO & LAO: CHEST

Chest
Special
- AP supine or semierect
- Lateral decubitus (AP)
- AP lordotic
- Anterior oblique

Pathology Demonstrated

Pathology involves the lung fields, trachea, and mediastinal structures, including the size and contours of the heart and great vessels.

Technical Factors

- IR size—35 × 43 cm (14 × 17 inches), lengthwise
- Moving or stationary grid
- 110-125 kV range
- Technique and dose:

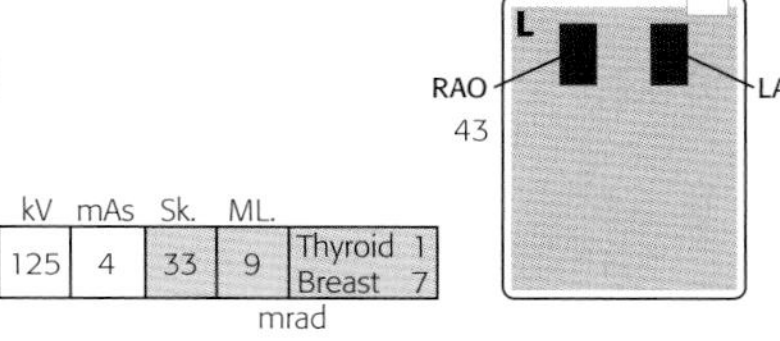

cm	kV	mAs	Sk.	ML.	
23	125	4	33	9	Thyroid 1 Breast 7

mrad

Shielding Secure lead shield around waist to shield gonads.

Patient Position
- Patient erect, rotated 45° with left anterior shoulder against IR for the LAO; and 45° with right anterior shoulder against IR for the RAO (see Notes below for 60° LAO)
- Patient's arm flexed nearest IR and hand placed on hip, palm out
- Opposite arm raised to clear lung field and hand rested on head or on chest unit for support, keeping arm raised as high as possible
- Patient looking straight ahead; chin raised

Part Position
As viewed from the x-ray tube, center the patient to CR and to IR, with top of IR about 1 inch (2.5 cm) above vertebra prominens.

Central Ray
- CR perpendicular, directed **to level of T7** (7 to 8 inches, or 8 to 10 cm, below level of vertebra prominens)
- SID of 72 inches (180 cm)

Collimation Collimate to area of lungs.

Respiration Make exposure at end of **second full inspiration.**

Notes: For **anterior** obliques, the side of interest is generally the side **farthest** from the IR. Thus the **RAO** will best visualize the **left** lung.

Certain positions for studies of the **heart** require an **LAO** with an increase in rotation to 60°.

Less rotation (15° to 20°) may be of value for better visualization of the various areas of the lungs for possible pulmonary diseases.

Exception Either erect or recumbent posterior obliques can be taken if patient cannot assume an erect position for anterior obliques or if supplementary projections are required.

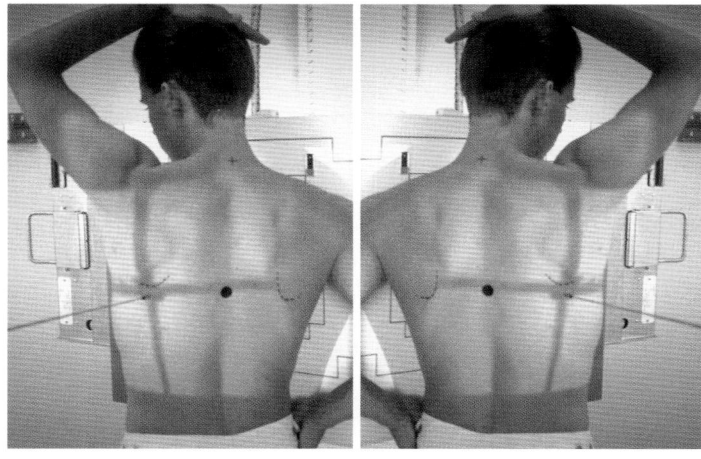

Fig. 3-73. 45° RAO position. **Fig. 3-74.** 45° LAO position.

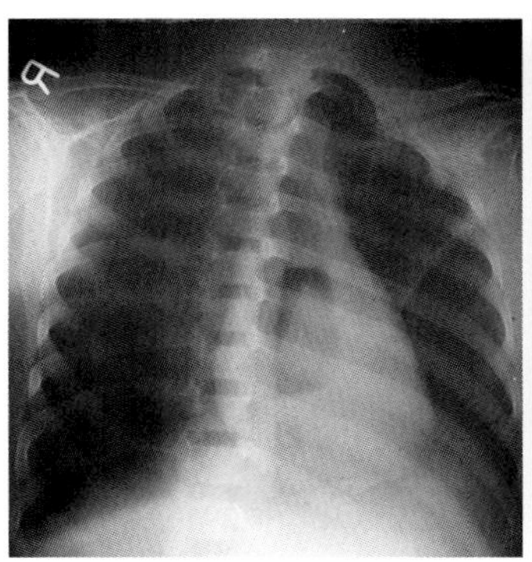

Fig. 3-75. 45° RAO position.

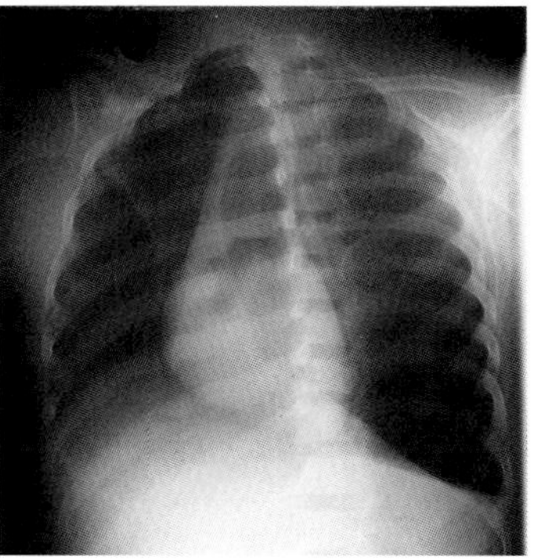

Fig. 3-76. 45° LAO position.

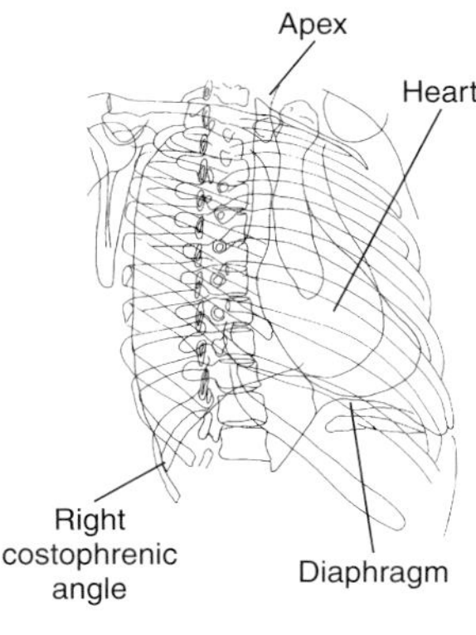

Fig. 3-77. 45° RAO position.

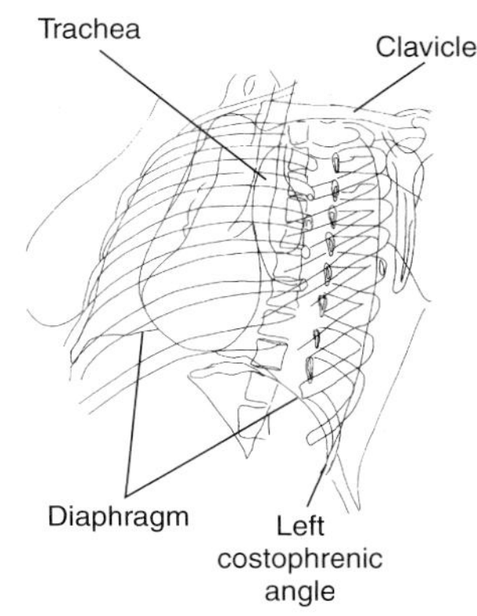

Fig. 3-78. 45° LAO position.

Radiographic Criteria

Structures Shown: • Both lungs from the apices to the costophrenic angles should be included. • The air-filled trachea, great vessels, and heart outlines are best visualized on a 60° LAO. (A 45° RAO will also visualize these structures.)

Position: • To evaluate for a 45° rotation, the distance from the outer margin of the ribs to the vertebral column on the side farthest from the IR should be approximately two times the distance of the side closest to the IR.

Collimation and CR: • Collimation borders on top and bottom should be near equal with CR at level of T7.

Exposure Criteria: • **No motion;** the outline of the diaphragm and heart should appear sharp. • Optimal exposure and contrast visualize vascular markings throughout lungs and rib outlines except through the most dense regions of the heart.

POSTERIOR OBLIQUE POSITIONS—RPO & LPO: CHEST

Chest
Special
- AP supine or semierect
- Lateral decubitus (AP)
- AP lordotic
- Anterior oblique
- Posterior oblique

Pathology Demonstrated
Pathology involves the lung fields, trachea, and mediastinal structures, including the size and contours of the heart and great vessels.

Technical Factors
- IR size—35 × 43 cm (14 × 17 inches), lengthwise
- Moving or stationary grid
- 110-125 kV range
- Technique and dose:

cm	kV	mAs	Sk.	ML.	
22	125	3	35	10	Thyroid 10 Breast 20

mrad

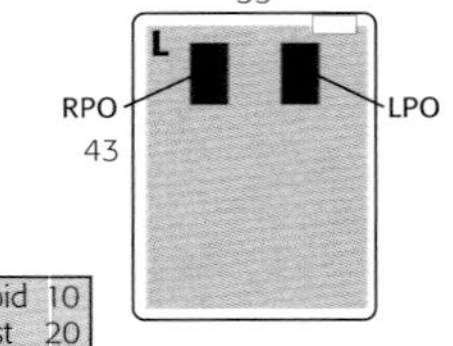

Shielding Secure lead shield around waist to shield gonads.

Patient Position (Erect)
- Patient erect, rotated 45° with right posterior shoulder against IR for RPO, and 45° with left posterior shoulder against IR for LPO
- Arm closest to the IR raised and head supported; other arm placed on hip with palm out
- Patient looking straight ahead

Patient Position (Recumbent)
- If patient cannot stand or sit, take posterior obliques on table.
- Place supports under patient's head and under elevated hip and shoulder.

Part Position
- Top of IR about 1 inch (2 cm) above vertebra prominens, or about 5 inches (12 cm) above level of jugular notch (2 inches or 5 cm above shoulders)
- Thorax centered to CR and to IR

Central Ray
- CR perpendicular, to the **level of T7**
- SID of 72 inches (180 cm)

Collimation Collimate to area of lungs.

Respiration Exposure made after **second full inspiration.**

Note: **Posterior** obliques best visualize the side **closest** to the IR.
Posterior positions show the same anatomy as the opposite anterior oblique. Thus the LPO position corresponds to the RAO, and the RPO to the LAO.

Radiographic Criteria
Radiographic criteria are similar to those of anterior obliques described on previous page. However, because of increased magnification of anterior diaphragm, lung fields usually appear shorter on posterior obliques compared with anterior obliques. The heart and great vessels also appear larger on posterior obliques because they are farther from the IR.

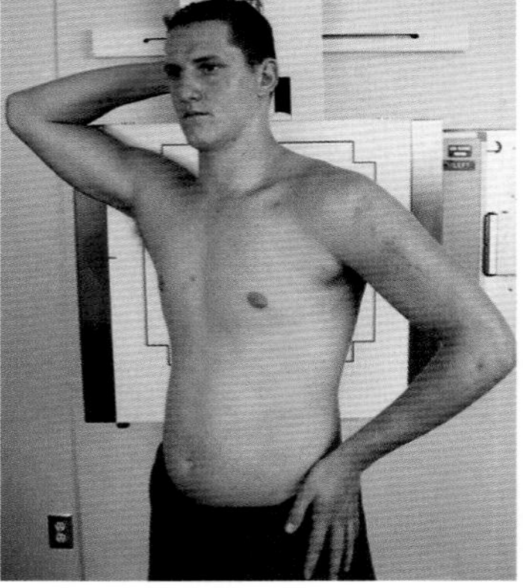

Fig. 3-79. 45° RPO position.

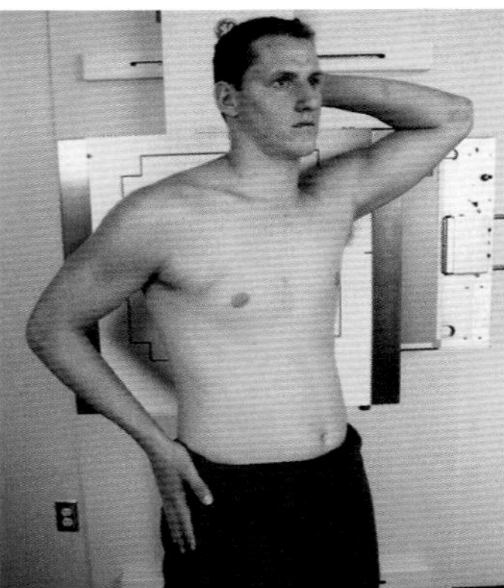

Fig. 3-80. 45° LPO position.

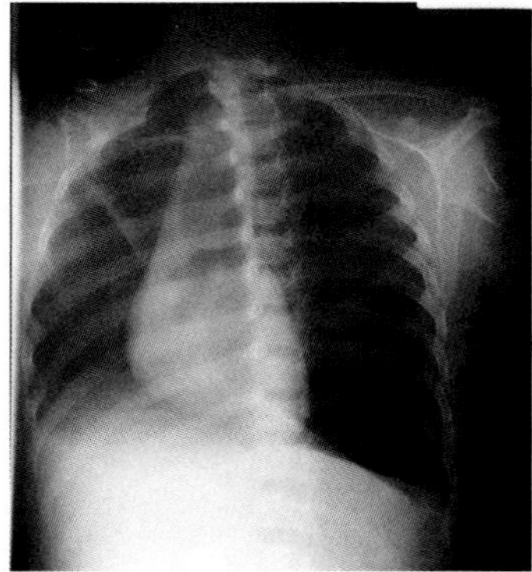

Fig. 3-81. 45° RPO position.

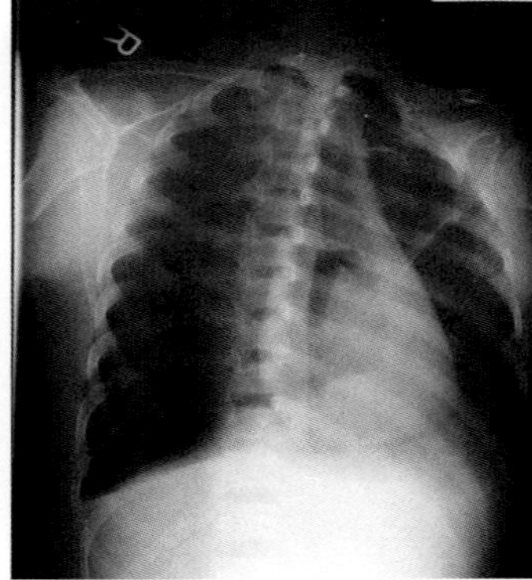

Fig. 3-82. 45° LPO position.

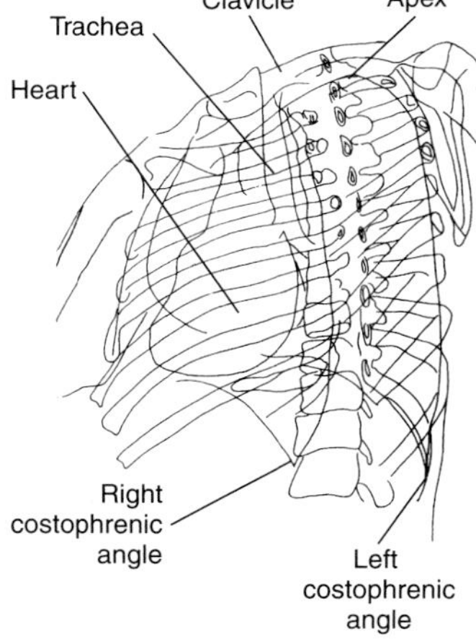

Fig. 3-83. 45° RPO position.

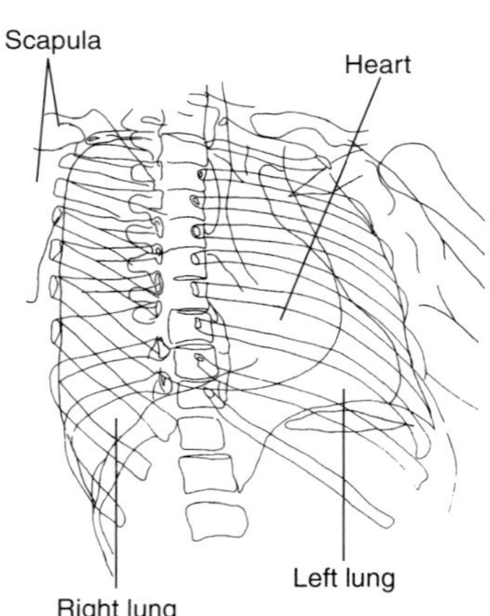

Fig. 3-84. 45° LPO position.

LATERAL POSITION: UPPER AIRWAY

Upper Airway
Basic
- Lateral
- AP

Pathology Demonstrated
Pathology is of the air-filled larynx and trachea, including the region of thyroid and thymus glands and upper esophagus if object is opaque or if contrast media is present. Soft-tissue lateral is frequently taken to rule out **epiglottitis,** which may be life-threatening for a young child.

Technical Factors
- IR size—24 × 30 cm (10 × 12 inches), lengthwise
- Moving or stationary grid
- 80 ± 6 kV range (see Note below).
- Technique and dose:

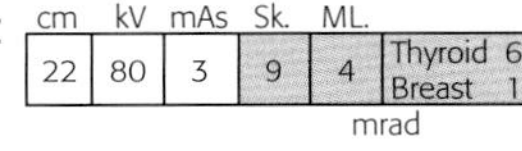

cm	kV	mAs	Sk.	ML.	
22	80	3	9	4	Thyroid 6 Breast 1

mrad

Shielding Secure lead shield around waist to shield gonads.

Patient Position Patient should be upright if possible, seated or standing in a lateral position (may be taken in R or L lateral and may be taken recumbent tabletop if necessary).

Part Position
- Position patient to center upper airway to CR and to center of IR (larynx and trachea lie anterior to cervical and thoracic vertebrae).
- Rotate shoulders posteriorly with arms hanging down, clasping hands behind back.
- Raise chin slightly and have patient look directly ahead.
- Adjust IR height to place top of IR at level of EAM (external auditory meatus), which is the opening of the external ear canal. (See below if area of primary interest is the trachea rather than the larynx.)

Central Ray
- CR perpendicular to center of IR **at level of C6 or C7,** midway between the laryngeal prominence of the thyroid cartilage and the jugular notch
- SID of 72 inches (180 cm), if possible, to minimize magnification

Collimation Collimate to area of interest.

Respiration Make exposure **during a slow, deep inspiration** to ensure filling trachea and upper airway with air.

Note on centering and exposure for neck region: Centering should be to laryngeal prominence (C5), with exposure factors for a soft-tissue lateral neck if the area of interest is primarily the larynx and upper trachea.

Centering and exposure for distal larynx and trachea region: If the distal larynx and upper and midtrachea are the primary areas of interest, the IR and CR should be lowered to place the CR at the upper jugular notch (T1) with exposure factors approximately those for a lateral chest.

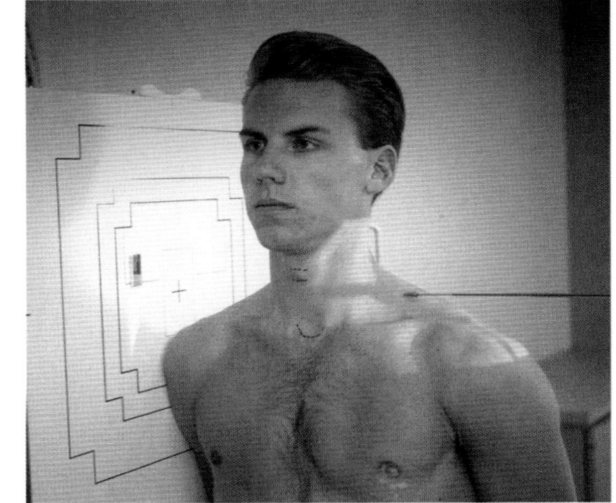

Fig. 3-85. Right lateral position—upper airway.

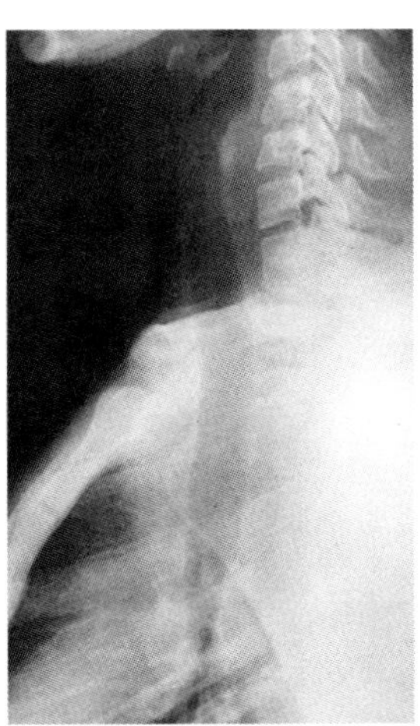

Fig. 3-86. Lateral—upper airway (for distal larynx and trachea region).

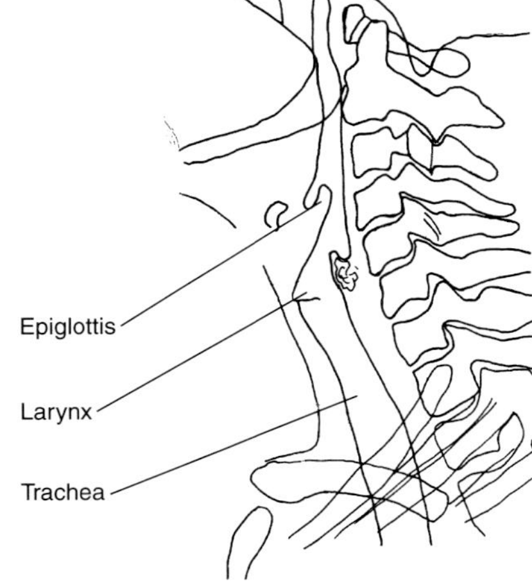

Fig. 3-87. Lateral—upper airway.

Radiographic Criteria

Structures Shown: • The larynx and trachea should be filled with air and well visualized.

Position: • Centering for the **neck region** (larynx and proximal trachea) should include the EAM at the upper border of the image and T2 or T3 on the lower border. If the **distal larynx and trachea** is the primary area of interest, the centering should be lower to include the area from C3 to T4 or T5 on the image. • The shadows of the shoulders should be primarily posterior to and not superimpose the area of the trachea.

Collimation and CR: • Collimation borders should appear on both sides with ideally only minimal (¼ inch or less) borders on top and bottom. The center of the collimation field should be to the CR location as described above.

Exposure Criteria: • Optimal exposure includes a soft-tissue technique wherein the air-filled larynx and upper trachea are not overexposed. The cervical vertebrae will appear underexposed.

AP PROJECTION: UPPER AIRWAY

Upper Airway
Basic
- Lateral
- AP

Pathology Demonstrated
Pathology is of the air-filled larynx and trachea, including the region of thyroid and thymus glands and upper esophagus if object is opacified or if contrast media is present.

Technical Factors
- IR size—24 × 30 cm (10 × 12 inches), lengthwise
- Moving or stationary grid
- 75-80 kV range
- Technique and dose:

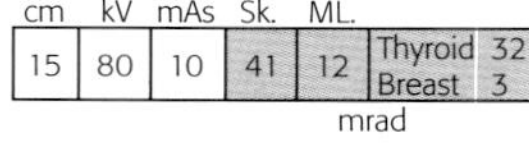

cm	kV	mAs	Sk.	ML.		
15	80	10	41	12	Thyroid	32
					Breast	3

mrad

Shielding Secure lead shield around waist to protect gonads.

Patient Position Patient should be upright if possible, seated or standing with back of head and shoulders against IR (may be taken recumbent tabletop if necessary).

Part Position
- Align midsagittal plane to CR and to midline of grid or table.
- Raise chin so that **acanthiomeatal line is perpendicular to the IR** (line from the acanthion or area directly under the nose and the meatus or EAM); have patient look directly ahead.
- Adjust the IR height to place top of IR about 1 or 1½ inches (3 to 4 cm) below EAM. (See Note below for explanation of centering.)

Central Ray
- CR perpendicular to center of IR **at level of T1-2,** about 1 inch (2.5 cm) above the jugular notch
- Minimum SID of 40 inches (102 cm)

Collimation Collimate to area of interest.

Respiration Make exposure **during a slow, deep inspiration** to ensure filling of trachea and upper airway with air.

Note on exposure: Exposure for this AP projection should be approximately that of an AP of the cervical and/or thoracic spine.

Centering for upper airway and trachea: Centering for this AP projection is similar to that of the lateral distal larynx and upper trachea position described on the previous page, because the most proximal larynx area is not visualized on the AP as a result of the superimposed base of skull and mandible. Therefore more of the trachea can be visualized.

Radiographic Criteria

Structures Shown: • The larynx and trachea from C3 to T4 should be filled with air and visualized through the spine. The area of the proximal cervical vertebrae (the lower margin of the shadow of the superimposed mandible and base of skull) to the midthoracic region should be included.

Position (See Notes above) • **No rotation** should occur, as evidenced by the symmetric appearance of the sternoclavicular joints. • The mandible should superimpose the base of the skull with spine aligned to center of film.

Collimation and CR: • Collimation borders should appear on both sides with ideally only minimal (¼ inch or less) borders on top and bottom. • The center of collimation field (CR) should be to area of T1-2.

Exposure Criteria: • Optimal exposure should be just dark enough to visualize the air-filled trachea through the cervical and thoracic vertebrae.

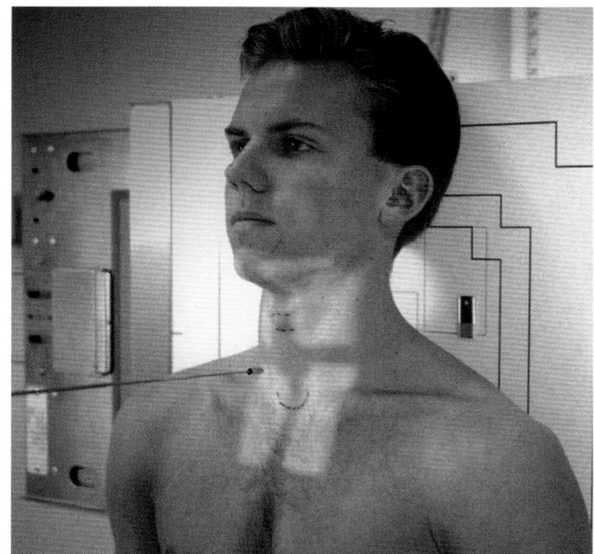

Fig. 3-88. AP—upper airway.

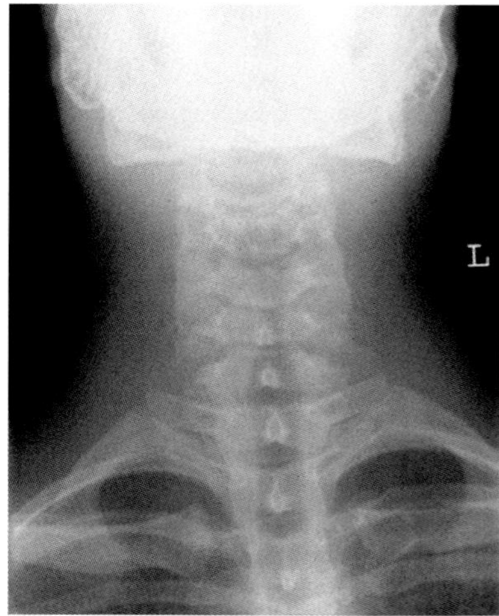

Fig. 3-89. AP—Upper airway.

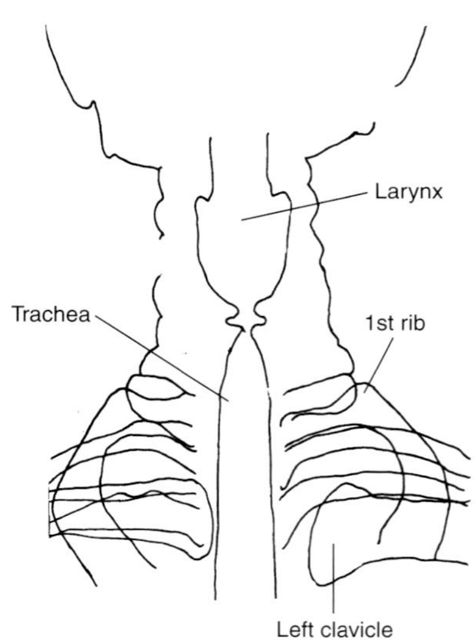

Fig. 3-90. AP—upper airway.

RADIOGRAPHS FOR CRITIQUE

Each of the chest radiographs below demonstrates certain errors that required a repeat. These, as well as additional chest radiographs for critique, are also available as part of the accompanying audiovisuals and instructor's manual.

Critique these five radiographs for errors in one or more of the five categories as described in the textbook and as outlined on the right. As a starting critique exercise, place a check in each category that demonstrates a **repeatable error** for that radiograph.

Student workbooks provide more space for writing comments and complete critique answers for each of these radiographs. Answers are provided in Appendix B at the end of this textbook and in the workbooks.

	RADIOGRAPHS				
	A	B	C	D	E
1. Structures shown	____	____	____	____	____
2. Positioning	____	____	____	____	____
3. Collimation and CR	____	____	____	____	____
4. Exposure criteria	____	____	____	____	____
5. Markers	____	____	____	____	____

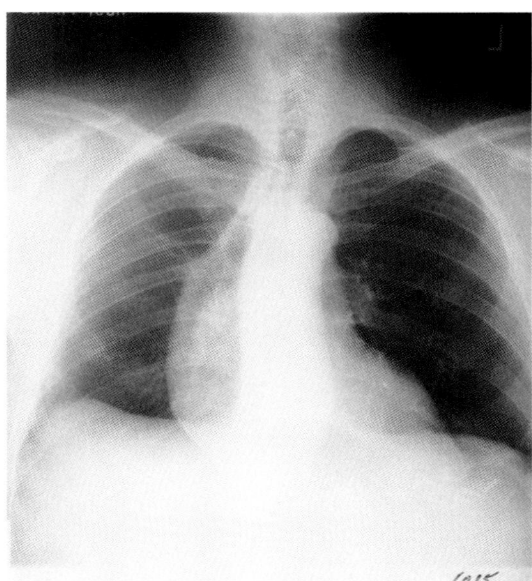

Fig. C3-91. PA chest, 43-year-old male. A

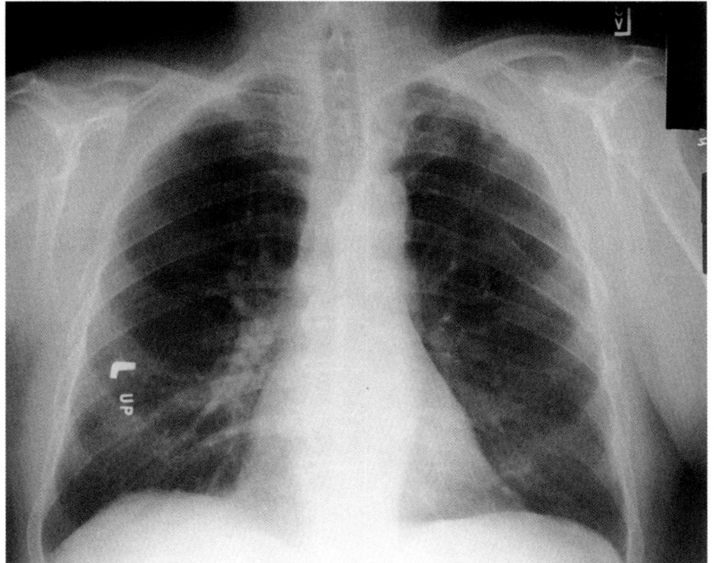

Fig. C3-92. PA chest, 74-year-old male. B

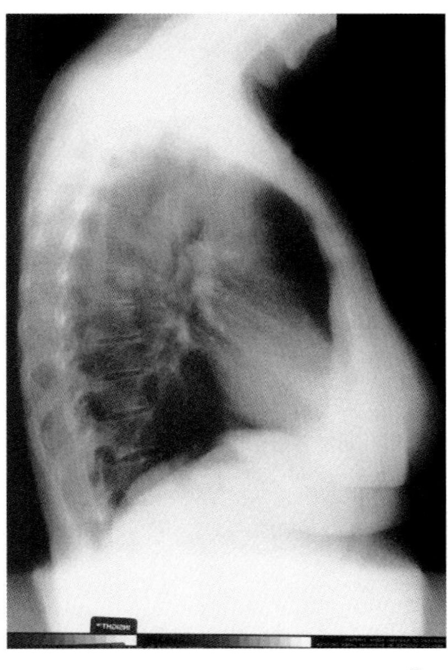

Fig. C3-93. Lateral chest, female. C

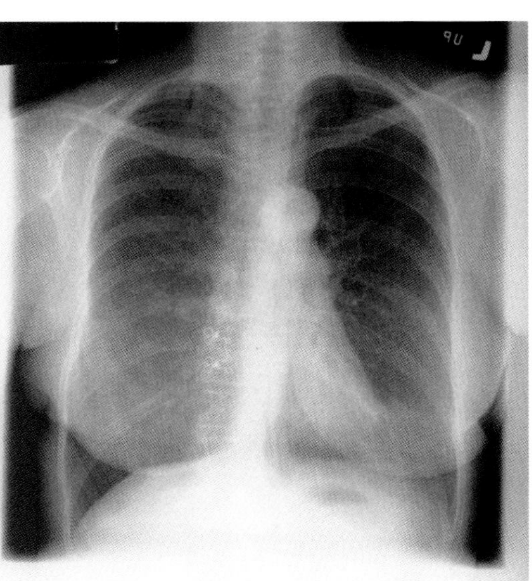

Fig. C3-94. PA chest, 73-year-old female. D

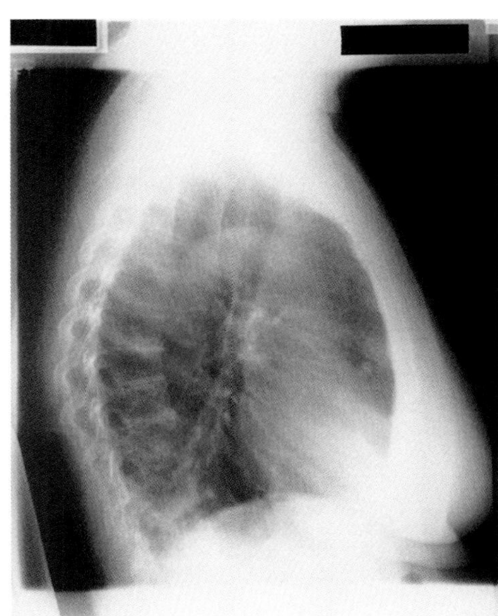

Fig. C3-95. Lateral chest, taken in wheelchair. E

CHAPTER 4

Abdomen

CONTRIBUTORS TO PAST EDITIONS John P. Lampignano, MEd, RT(R)(CT), Kathy M. Martensen, BS, RT(R), Barry T. Anthony, RT(R)

CONTENTS

RADIOGRAPHIC ANATOMY

Abdominal Radiography

This chapter covers the anatomy and positioning for what are sometimes called "plain films" (images) of the abdomen. The most common is an AP supine abdomen, also sometimes called a *KUB* (*k*idneys, *u*reters, and *b*ladder). These are taken without the use of contrast media.

Plain radiographs of the abdomen (KUB) are commonly taken before performing abdominal examinations using contrast media to rule out certain pathologies.

Acute abdominal series: Certain acute or emergency conditions of the abdomen may develop from conditions such as bowel obstruction, perforations involving free intraperitoneal air (air outside the digestive tract), excessive fluid in the abdomen, or a possible intraabdominal mass. These acute or emergency conditions require what is commonly called an "acute abdominal series," or a "two-way" or "three-way abdomen" series, wherein several abdominal radiographs are taken in different positions to demonstrate air-fluid levels and/or free air within the abdominal cavity.

Abdominal radiography requires an understanding of anatomy and relationships of the organs and structures within the abdominopelvic cavity.

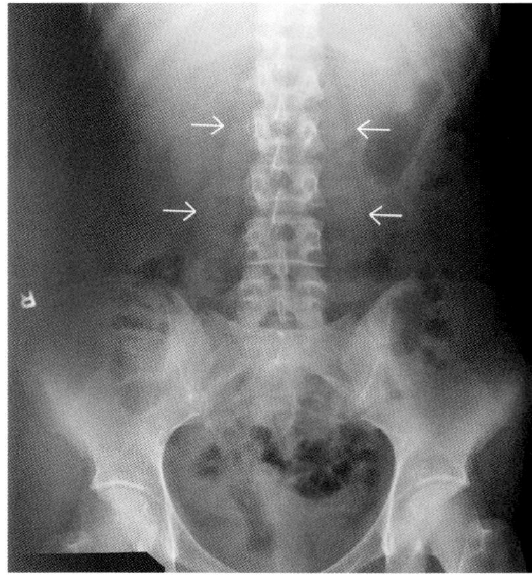

Fig. 4-1. AP abdomen (KUB). Arrows indicate psoas muscles.

ABDOMINAL MUSCLES

Many muscles are associated with the abdominopelvic cavity. The three that are the most important in abdominal radiography are the diaphragm and the right and left psoas *(so'es)* major.

The **diaphragm** is an umbrella-shaped muscle separating the abdominal cavity from the thoracic cavity. The diaphragm must be perfectly motionless during radiography of either the abdomen or the chest. Motion of the patient's diaphragm can be stopped by providing appropriate breathing instructions.

The two **psoas major** muscles are located on either side of the lumbar vertebral column. The lateral borders of these two muscles should be faintly visible on a diagnostic abdominal radiograph of a small to average-sized patient when correct exposure factors are used (see *arrows,* Fig. 4-1).

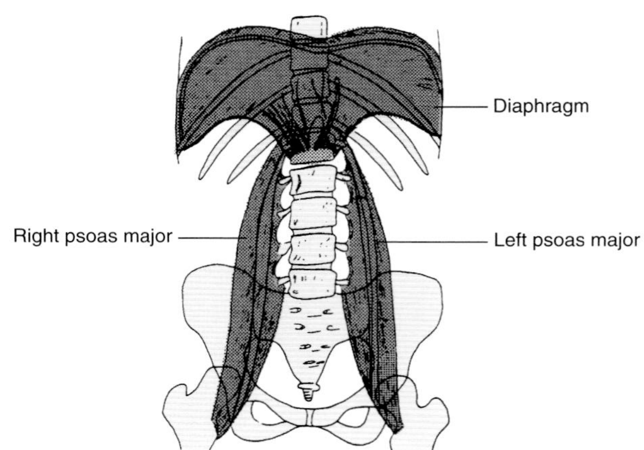

Fig. 4-2. Abdominal muscles.

Abdominal Organ Systems

The various organ systems found within the abdominopelvic cavity are presented briefly in this chapter. Each of these systems is described in greater detail in later chapters devoted to those specific systems.

DIGESTIVE SYSTEM

4

The **digestive system,** along with its accessory organs, the **liver, gallbladder,** and **pancreas,** fills much of the abdominal cavity. The pancreas is located posterior to the stomach and is not well visualized on this drawing.

The **spleen** (part of the lymphatic system) is also partially visible in the left upper abdomen posterior to the stomach. The six organs of the digestive system are as follows:

1. Oral cavity
2. Pharynx
3. Esophagus
4. Stomach
5. Small intestine
6. Large intestine

Oral Cavity, Pharynx, and Esophagus The **oral cavity** (mouth) and the pharynx (oropharynx and laryngopharynx) are common to both the respiratory system and the digestive system, as described in Fig. 3-4 of Chapter 3. The **esophagus** is located in the mediastinum of the thoracic cavity.

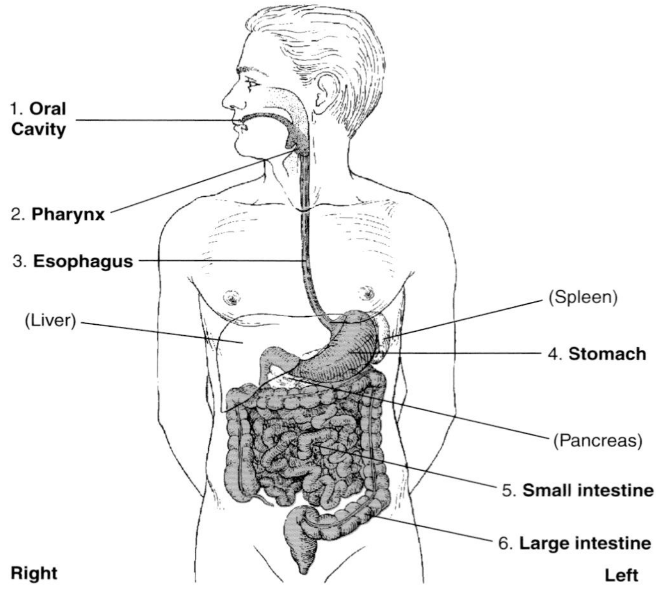

Fig. 4-3. Digestive tract.

Stomach and Small and Large Intestines The three digestive organs within the abdominal cavity are the **stomach** and **small** and **large intestines.**

Stomach

The stomach is the first organ of the digestive system located within the abdominal cavity. The stomach is an expandable reservoir for swallowed food and fluids. The size and shape of the stomach are highly variable depending on the volume of its contents and on the body habitus.

Gastro is a common term for stomach (the Greek word *gaster* means "stomach"). Thus the term *gastrointestinal (GI) tract* or *system* describes the entire digestive system, starting with the stomach and continuing through the small and large intestines.

Small intestine

The small intestine continues from the stomach as a long, tubelike convoluted structure about 4.5 to 5.5 meters (15 to 18 feet) in length. The three parts of the small intestine as labeled in Figs. 4-4 and 4-5 are as follows:

A. Duodenum *(doo"o-de'num)*
B. Jejunum *(je-joo'num)*
C. Ileum *(il'eum)*

Duodenum (A): The first portion of the small intestine, the duodenum, is the shortest but the widest in diameter of the three segments. It is about 25 cm, or 10 inches, in length. When filled with contrast medium, the duodenum looks like the letter *C.* The proximal portion of the duodenum is called the *duodenal bulb,* or *cap.* It has a certain characteristic shape, usually well seen on barium studies of the upper GI tract. Ducts from the liver, gallbladder, and pancreas drain into the duodenum.

Jejunum and ileum (B and C): The remainder of the small bowel lies in the central and lower abdomen. The first two-fifths following the duodenum is termed the **jejunum,** and the distal three-fifths is called the **ileum.** The orifice (valve) between the distal ileum and the cecum portion of the large intestine is the **ileocecal valve.**

Radiograph of stomach and small intestine (Fig. 4-5)

Air is seldom seen filling the entire stomach or small intestine on a plain abdominal radiograph of a healthy, ambulatory adult. This radiograph visualizes the stomach, small intestine, and proximal large intestine, because they are filled with radiopaque barium sulfate. Note the duodenal bulb and the long convoluted loops of the three labeled parts of the small intestine located in the mid- and lower abdomen.

Large intestine

The sixth and last organ of digestion is the large intestine, which begins in the right lower quadrant at the junction with the small intestine at the **ileocecal valve.** The portion of the large intestine below the ileocecal valve is a saclike area termed the **cecum.** The **appendix (vermiform appendix)** is attached to the posteromedial aspect of the cecum.

The vertical portion of the large bowel above the cecum is the **ascending colon,** which joins the **transverse colon** at the **right colic** (*kol'ik,* referring to colon) **flexure.** The transverse colon joins the **descending colon** at the **left colic flexure.** Alternate secondary names for the two colic flexures are **hepatic** and **splenic flexures** based on their proximity to the liver and spleen, respectively.

The descending colon continues as the S-shaped **sigmoid colon** in the lower left abdomen. The **rectum** is the final 15 cm (6 inches) of the large intestine. The rectum ends at the **anus,** the sphincter muscle at the terminal opening of the large intestine.

As will be seen in body habitus drawings, the shape and location of the large intestine vary greatly, with the transverse colon located high on wide hypersthenic types, and low in the abdomen on slender hyposthenic and asthenic types. This is demonstrated in Chapters 14 and 15, the upper and lower GI systems.

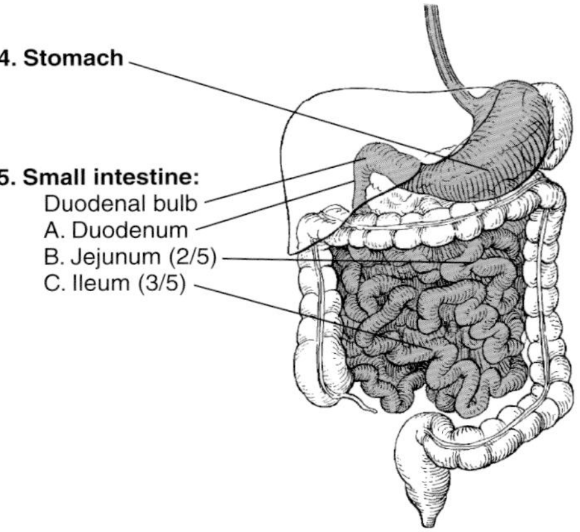

Fig. 4-4. Stomach and small intestine.

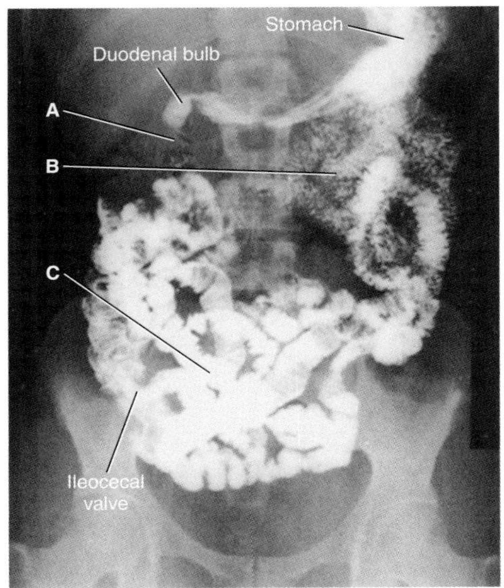

Fig. 4-5. Stomach and small intestine radiograph.

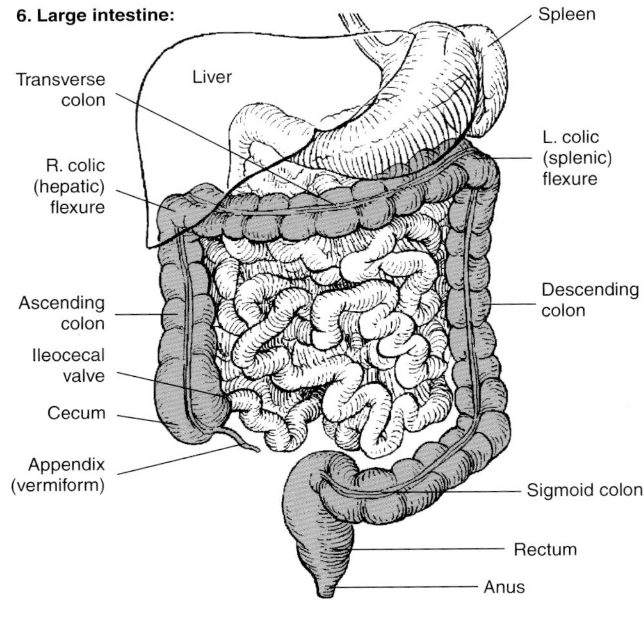

Fig. 4-6. Large intestine.

4

SPLEEN

The spleen is part of the **lymphatic system,** which along with the heart and blood vessels, is part of the circulatory system. It is an important abdominal organ and occupies a space posterior and to the left of the stomach in the **left upper quadrant,** as shown in Fig. 4-7.

The spleen may be visualized faintly on plain abdominal radiographs, particularly if the organ is enlarged. It is a fragile organ and is sometimes lacerated during trauma to the lower left posterior rib cage.

ACCESSORY DIGESTIVE ORGANS

Three accessory organs of digestion, also located in the abdominal cavity, are the (1) pancreas, (2) liver, and (3) gallbladder.

Pancreas The pancreas, which is not seen on a plain abdominal radiograph, is an elongated gland located **posterior to the stomach** and near the posterior abdominal wall, between the duodenum and the spleen. The average length is about 12.5 cm (6 inches). Its head is nestled in the C-loop of the duodenum, and the body and tail of the pancreas extend toward the upper left abdomen. This relationship of the duodenum and head of the pancreas is sometimes referred to as "the romance of the abdomen."

The pancreas is part of the **endocrine** (internal) secretion system and also part of the **exocrine** (external) secretion system. The endocrine portion of the pancreas produces certain essential hormones, such as insulin, which aids in controlling the blood sugar level of the body. As part of its exocrine functions, the pancreas produces large amounts (up to 1½ quart, or 1500 ml, daily) of digestive juices that move to the duodenum through a main pancreatic duct as needed for digestion.

Liver The liver is the largest solid organ in the body, occupying most of the **right upper quadrant.** One of its numerous functions is the production of bile, which assists in the digestion of fats. If bile is not needed for digestion, it is stored and concentrated for future use in the gallbladder.

Gallbladder The gallbladder is a pear-shaped sac located below the liver. The primary functions of the gallbladder are to store and concentrate bile and to contract and release bile when stimulated by an appropriate hormone. The gallbladder in most cases cannot be visualized with conventional radiographic techniques without contrast media. The gallbladder and biliary ducts are described in detail in Chapter 16.

COMPUTED TOMOGRAPHY CROSS-SECTIONAL IMAGES

Cross-sectional (axial) CT images through various levels of the abdomen demonstrate anatomic relationships of the digestive organs and their accessory organs, as well as the spleen.

Fig. 4-8 demonstrates a sectional view of the upper abdomen at the level of T10 or T11 (thoracic vertebrae 10 or 11) just below the diaphragm. Note the proportionally large size of the **liver** at this level in the right upper abdomen and a cross-sectional view through the **stomach** to the left of the liver. The **spleen** is clearly shown posterior to the stomach in the left upper abdomen.

Fig. 4-9 demonstrates a little lower cross-sectional image through the upper third of the abdomen at the level of L1 or L2 (lumbar vertebrae 1 or 2). The **pancreas** is now seen adjacent to a portion of the duodenal loop posterior to the distal part of the **stomach.** Note the air-fluid level in the stomach with the heavy barium fluid mixture (white) in the posterior stomach. The dark air-filled portion of the stomach is on top (anteriorly), indicating that the patient was lying in a supine position for this CT scan.

A small inferior part of the **spleen** is seen in the left posterior abdomen just lateral to the **left kidney.** The major blood vessels of the abdomen, the **inferior vena cava,** and the **aorta** are seen clearly.

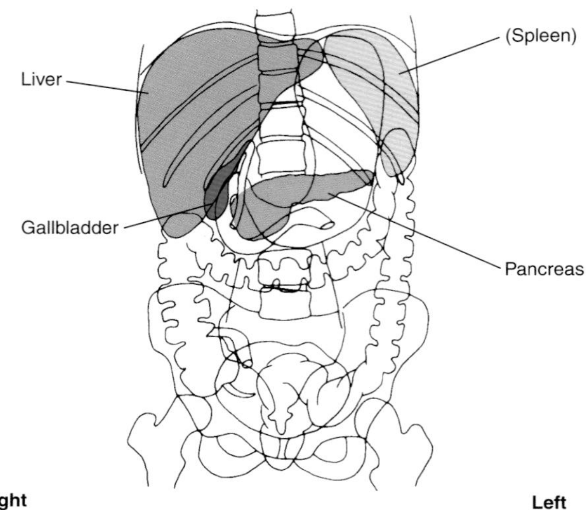

Fig. 4-7. Spleen and accessory organs of digestion—pancreas, liver, and gallbladder.

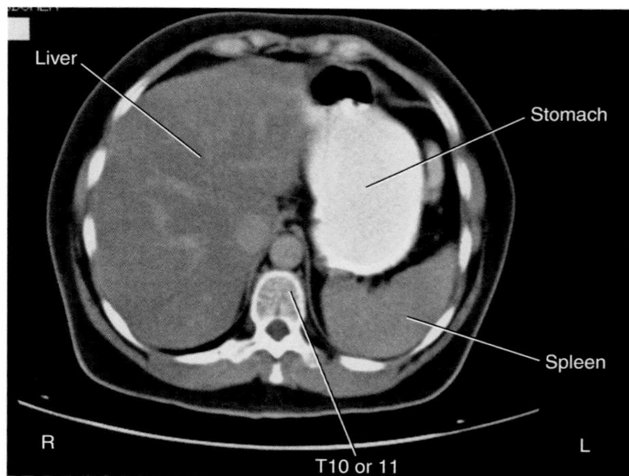

Fig. 4-8. CT image of upper abdomen (level of T10 or T11).

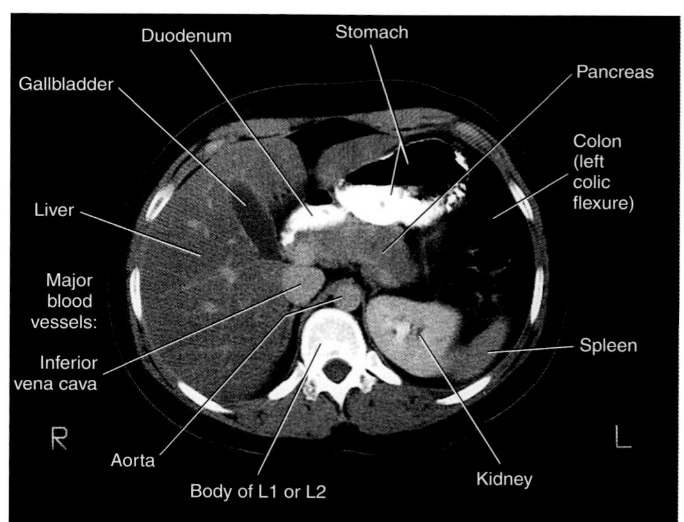

Fig. 4-9. CT image of abdomen demonstrating stomach, liver, gallbladder, pancreas, and spleen (level of L1 or L2).

Note: It is not certain from this one scan why at least the upper part of the right kidney is not visible at this level.

4

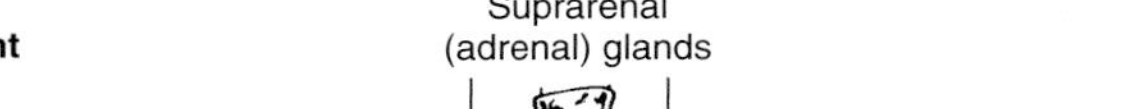

Urinary System

The urinary system is another important abdominal system. Although this system is introduced in this chapter, it is covered in detail in Chapter 17.

The urinary system is composed of the following:

- Two kidneys
- Two ureters *(u-re'ters)** or *(yoo-re–t'ers)*†
- One urinary bladder
- One urethra *(u-re'thrah)** or *(yoo-re'thra)*†

Each **kidney** drains by way of its own **ureter** to the single **urinary bladder.** The bladder, situated above and behind the symphysis pubis, serves to store urine. Under voluntary control, the stored urine passes to the exterior via the **urethra.** The two **suprarenal** (adrenal) **glands** of the endocrine system are located at the superomedial portion of each kidney. The bean-shaped kidneys are located on either side of the lumbar vertebral column. The right kidney is usually situated a little lower than the left one because of the presence of the large liver on the right.

Waste materials and excess water are eliminated from the blood by the kidneys and are transported through the ureters to the urinary bladder.

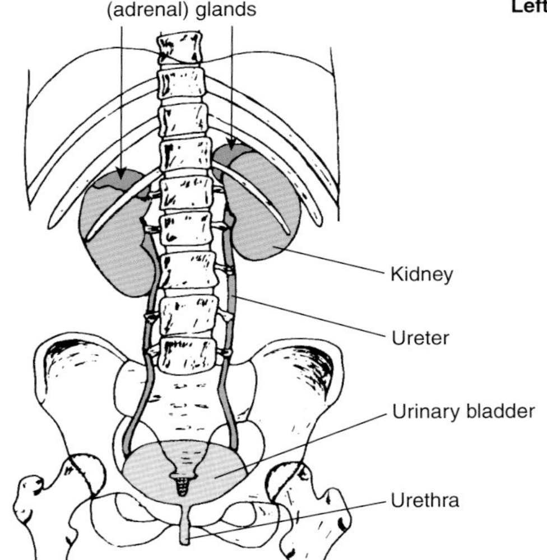

Fig. 4-10. Urinary system.

EXCRETORY OR INTRAVENOUS UROGRAM (IVU)

The kidneys are usually faintly seen on a plain abdominal radiograph because of a fatty capsule that surrounds each kidney. The contrast medium examination shown in Fig. 4-11 is an **excretory** or **intravenous urogram** (IVU), which is a radiographic examination of the urinary system, wherein the contrast media is injected intravenously. During this examination the hollow organs of this system are visualized by means of the contrast media that has been filtered from the blood flow by the kidneys. The organs as labeled are (A) **left kidney,** (B) **left proximal ureter,** (C) **left distal ureter** before emptying into the urinary bladder, and (D) **the area of the right suprarenal** (adrenal) **gland,** just above the right kidney.

Note: The term **intravenous pyelogram (IVP)** has often been used in the past for this examination. However, this is **not** an accurate term for this exam because *pyelo* refers to the renal pelvis of the kidney, and the excretory or intravenous urogram includes a study of the entire urinary tract, which includes the total collecting system. (The terms *excretory urogram* [EU] and *intravenous urogram* [IVU] are both current and correct terms, but **intravenous urogram** [IVU] is the term most commonly used.)

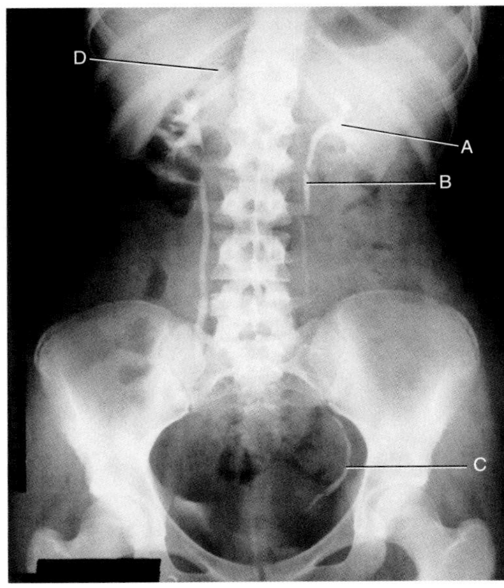

Fig. 4-11. Intravenous urogram (IVU). **A,** Left kidney. **B,** Left proximal ureter. **C,** Left distal ureter. **D,** Right suprarenal gland.

Sectional Image

This sectional CT image (Fig. 4-12) may appear confusing at first because of the numerous small odd-shaped cross-sectional images visualized. However, as you study the relationships between these structures and imagine a thin "slice" view through the level of about L2-L3 of the drawings (Fig. 4-10) and on the previous page (Fig. 4-7), you should be able to identify each of these structures as labeled in Fig. 4-12. See how many of the structures labeled A-J you can identify without looking at the answers below.

A. Inferior lobe of liver	F. L2-L3 vertebra
B. Ascending colon	G. Left kidney
C. Right kidney	H. Left ureter
D. Right ureter	I. Descending colon
E. Right psoas major muscle	J. Loops of small intestines (jejunum)

Two major blood vessels of the abdomen are also seen labeled as K and L. K is the large abdominal aorta, and L the inferior vena cava.

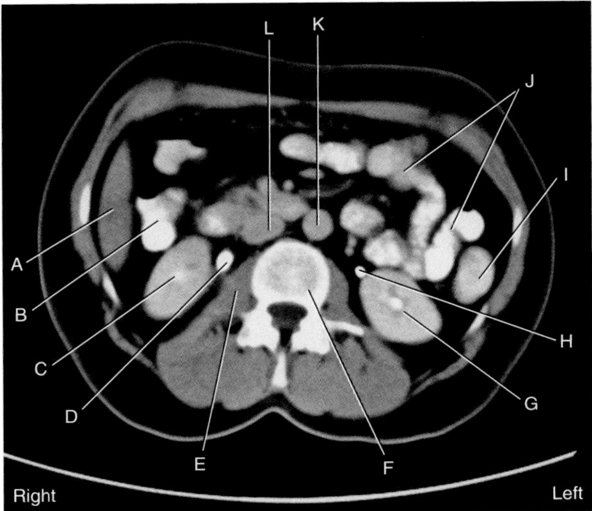

Fig. 4-12. CT image of abdomen, level of kidneys, and proximal ureters.

*Dorland's illustrated medical dictionary, ed 28, Philadelphia, 1994, WB Saunders.
†Webster's new world dictionary, ed 3 (College).

Abdominal Cavity

Four important terms describing anatomy of the abdominal cavity are demonstrated on the drawings to the right and described below. These four terms are as follows:

1. **Peritoneum** *(per″i-to-ne′um)*
2. **Mesentery** *(mes′en-ter″e)*
3. **Omentum** *(o-men′tum)*
4. **Mesocolon** *(mez′o-ko″lon)*

PERITONEUM

Most of the abdominal structures and organs, as well as the wall of the abdominal cavity in which they are contained, are covered to varying degrees by a large serous, double-walled, saclike membrane termed the **peritoneum.** In fact, the total surface area of the peritoneum is about equal to the total surface area of the skin covering the entire body.

A greatly simplified cross-section of the abdominal cavity is shown in Fig. 4-13. Two types of peritoneum exist: the parietal and the visceral. The two-layered peritoneum adhering to the cavity wall is termed **parietal peritoneum,** whereas that portion covering an organ is termed **visceral peritoneum.** The space or cavity between the parietal and visceral portions of the peritoneum is called the **peritoneal cavity.** This space is really only a potential cavity, because normally it is filled with various organs. If all the loops of bowel and the other organs of the abdominal cavity were included in the drawing, little actual space would be left in the peritoneal cavity. This cavity contains some serous lubricating-type fluid, which allows organs to move against each other without friction. An abnormal accumulation of this serous fluid constitutes a condition called **ascites.** (See Pathologic Indications, p. 119.)

Note that a layer of visceral peritoneum only **partially** covers certain organs that are more closely attached to the posterior abdominal wall (Fig. 4-13). At this level, the ascending and descending colon, the aorta, and the inferior vena cava are only partially covered; therefore this lining would **not** be considered mesentery, and these structures and organs are called **retroperitoneal,** as described on the following page.

MESENTERY

The peritoneum forms large folds that bind the abdominal organs to each other and to the walls of the abdomen. Blood and lymph vessels and the nerves that supply these abdominal organs are contained within these folds of peritoneum. One of these double folds holding the small intestine in place is called the **mesentery.** Mesentery is that **double fold of peritoneum** extending anteriorly from the posterior abdominal wall completely enveloping a loop of **small bowel.** The specific term for a double fold of peritoneum loosely connecting the small intestine to the posterior abdominal wall is **mesentery** (Fig. 4-14).

OMENTUM

A specific type of double-fold peritoneum extending from the **stomach** to another organ is called **omentum** (Fig. 4-14). The **lesser omentum** extends superiorly from the lesser curvature of the stomach to portions of the liver. The **greater omentum** connects the transverse colon to the greater curvature of the stomach inferiorly. The greater omentum drapes down over the small bowel then folds back on itself to form an apron along the anterior abdominal wall.

If one entered the abdomen through the midanterior wall, the first structure encountered beneath the parietal peritoneum would be the greater omentum. Varying amounts of fat are deposited in the greater omentum, which serves as a layer of insulation between the abdominal cavity and the exterior. This is sometimes called the "fatty apron" because of its location and the amount of fat contained therein (Fig. 4-15).

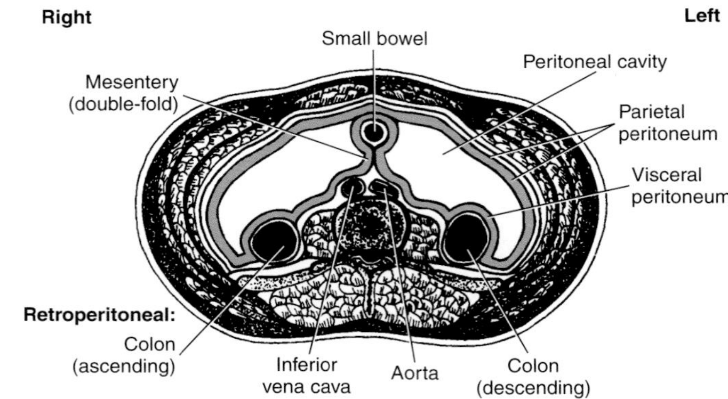

Fig. 4-13. Cross section—abdominal cavity (demonstrates peritoneum, mesentery, and retroperitoneal structures).

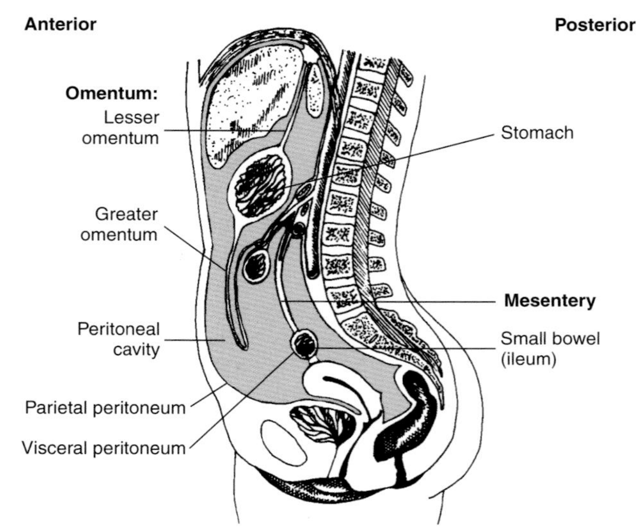

Fig. 4-14. Midsagittal section—abdominal cavity (demonstrates peritoneum, mesentery, and omentum).

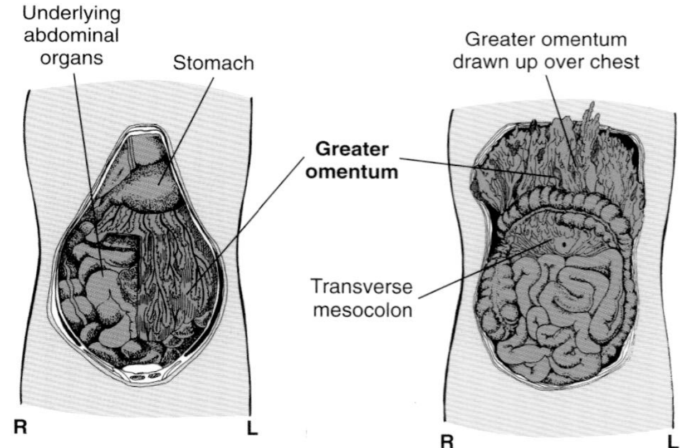

Fig. 4-15. Greater omentum (part of omentum removed and lifted up, exposing small bowel and the transverse mesocolon connected to transverse colon).

MESOCOLON

The peritoneum that attaches the **colon** to the posterior abdominal wall is the **mesocolon.** Four forms of mesocolon exist, each named according to that portion of the colon to which it is attached—the ascending, transverse, descending, and sigmoid or pelvic. The **transverse mesocolon** is shown in Fig. 4-15 as that visceral peritoneum loosely connecting the transverse colon to the posterior abdominal wall.

4

GREATER AND LESSER SAC

The drawing in Fig. 4-16 shows the two parts of the peritoneal cavity. The major portion of the peritoneal cavity is termed the **greater sac,** commonly referred to as simply the **peritoneal cavity.**

A smaller portion of the upper posterior peritoneal cavity located posterior to the stomach is termed the **lesser sac.** This sac has a special name, the **omentum bursa.**

This drawing again shows the **mesentery** connecting one loop of **small intestine** (ileum) to the posterior abdominal wall. A full drawing of a normal abdomen would, of course, have many loops of small bowel connected to the posterior wall by mesentery.

Mesentery-type folds, from which other abdominal organs are suspended, use the prefix *meso-,* such as the **transverse mesocolon,** again shown to be connecting the transverse colon to the posterior abdominal wall.

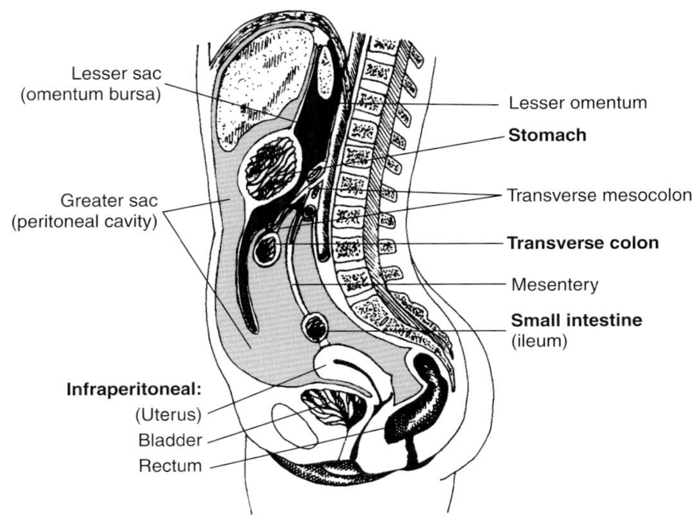

Fig. 4-16. Sagittal section—abdominal cavity (demonstrates greater and lesser sacs, transverse mesocolon, and infraperitoneal structures).

RETROPERITONEAL AND INFRAPERITONEAL ORGANS

The organs shown in drawing Fig. 4-17 are considered either **retroperitoneal** (*retro,* meaning "backward" or "behind") or **infraperitoneal** (*infra,* meaning "under" or "beneath").

Retroperitoneal Organs Structures closely attached to the posterior abdominal wall that are retroperitoneal as shown on this drawing are the **kidneys** and **ureters, adrenal glands, pancreas, duodenum, ascending** and **descending colon, upper rectum, abdominal aorta,** and **inferior vena cava.**

Remember that these retroperitoneal structures are less mobile and move around less within the abdomen than other intraperitoneal organs. Fig. 4-16 demonstrates, for example, that the **stomach, small intestine,** and **transverse colon** are only loosely attached to the abdominal wall by long loops of different types of peritoneum and thus change or vary greatly in their position within the abdomen compared with the retroperitoneal or infraperitoneal structures. (This is an important consideration in GI positioning.)

Infraperitoneal Pelvic Organs Located under or beneath the peritoneum in the true pelvis are the **lower rectum, urinary bladder,** and **reproductive organs.**

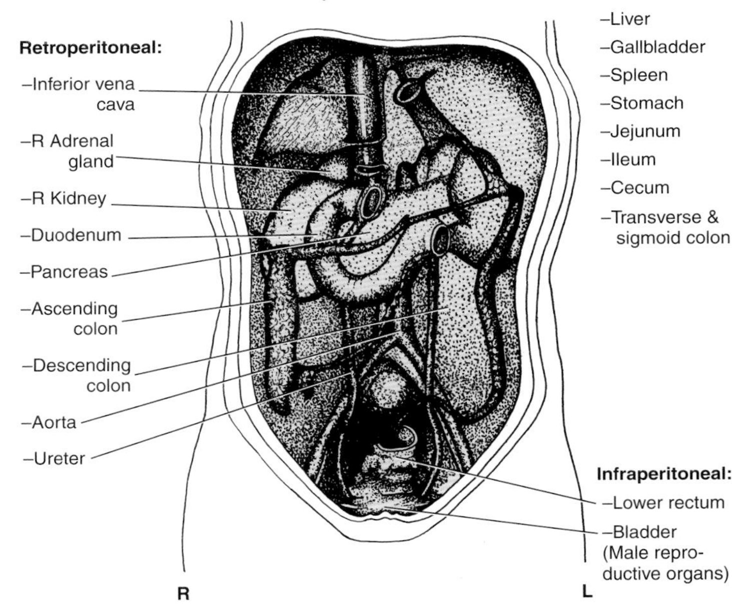

Fig. 4-17. Retroperitoneal and infraperitoneal organs.

MALE VS. FEMALE PERITONEAL ENCLOSURES

One significant difference exists between the male and female peritoneal enclosures. The lower aspect of the peritoneum is a **closed sac in the male** and **not in the female.** In the male the lower peritoneal sac lies above the urinary bladder, totally separating the reproductive organs from those within the peritoneal cavity. On the female, however, the uterus, uterine (Fallopian) tubes, and ovaries pass directly into the peritoneal cavity (see Fig. 4-16).

INTRAPERITONEAL ORGANS

Organs within the abdominal cavity that are either partially or completely covered by some type of visceral peritoneum but are not retro- or infraperitoneal may be called intraperitoneal (*intra,* meaning "within"). These organs, which have been removed from the drawing in Fig. 4-17, are the **liver, gallbladder, spleen, stomach, jejunum, ileum, cecum,** and **transverse** and **sigmoid colon.**

SUMMARY OF ABDOMINAL ORGANS IN RELATIONSHIP TO THE PERITONEAL CAVITY

Intraperitoneal Organs	Retroperitoneal Organs	Infraperitoneal (Pelvic) Organs
Liver	Kidneys	Lower rectum
Gallbladder	Ureters	Urinary bladder
Spleen	Adrenal glands	Reproductive organs
Stomach	Pancreas	Male—closed sac
Jejunum	Duodenum	Female—open sac (the female uterus, tubes, and ovaries, extending into the peritoneal cavity)
Ileum	Ascending and descending colon	
Cecum	Upper rectum	
Transverse colon	Major abdominal blood vessels (aorta and inferior vena cava)	
Sigmoid colon		

4

Quadrants and Regions

To help describe the locations of various organs or other structures within the abdominopelvic cavity, the abdomen may be divided into either **four quadrants** or **nine regions.**

FOUR ABDOMINAL QUADRANTS

If two imaginary perpendicular planes (at right angles) were passed through the abdomen at the umbilicus (or navel), they would divide the abdomen into four quadrants. One plane would be transverse through the abdomen at the **level of the umbilicus,** which on most people is at the level of the **intervertebral disk between L4 and L5** (fourth and fifth lumbar vertebrae), which is about at the level of the iliac crests on a female.

The vertical plane would coincide with the **midsagittal plane** or midline of the abdomen and would pass through both the umbilicus and the symphysis pubis. These two planes would divide the abdominopelvic cavity into four quadrants: the **right upper quadrant** (RUQ), the **left upper quadrant** (LUQ), the **right lower quadrant** (RLQ), and the **left lower quadrant** (LLQ).

Note: The four-quadrant system is most frequently used in radiography in localizing a particular organ or for describing the location of abdominal pain or other symptoms.

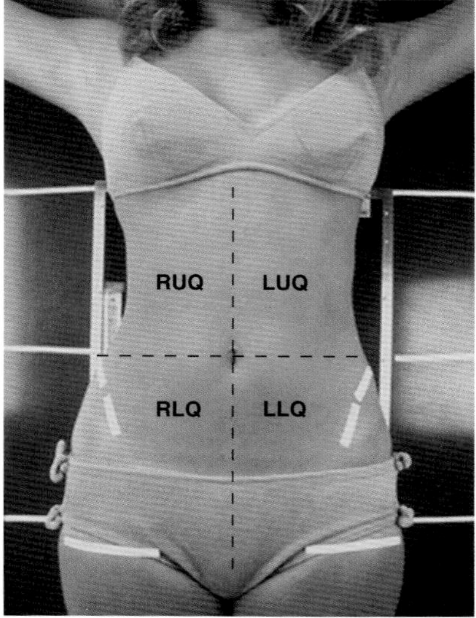

Fig. 4-18. Four abdominal quadrants.

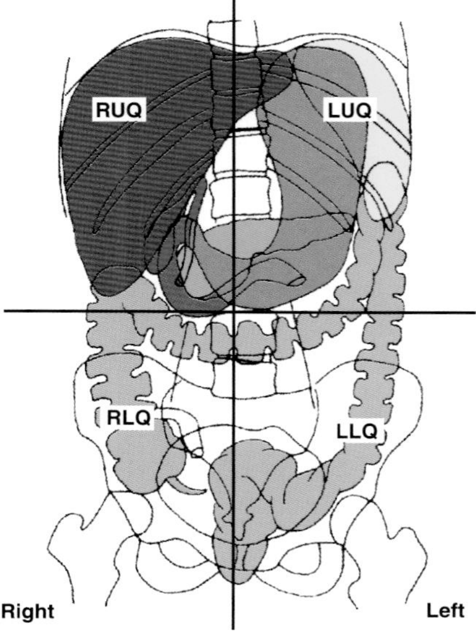

Fig. 4-19. Four quadrants with certain abdominal structures.

ANATOMY SUMMARY CHART—FOUR QUADRANT ABDOMEN*

RUQ	LUQ	RLQ	LLQ
Liver	Spleen	Ascending colon	Descending colon
Gallbladder	Stomach	Appendix (vermiform)	Sigmoid colon
Right colic (hepatic) flexure	Left colic (splenic) flexure	Cecum	$^2/_3$ of jejunum
Duodenum	Tail of pancreas	$^2/_3$ of ileum	
Head of pancreas	Left kidney	Ileocecal valve	
Right kidney	Left suprarenal gland		
Right suprarenal gland			

*Quadrant locations of structures and organs (primary location on average adult).

NINE ABDOMINAL REGIONS

The abdominopelvic cavity can also be divided into nine regions by using two horizontal or transverse planes and two vertical planes. The two transverse/horizontal planes are the **transpyloric plane** and the **transtubercular plane.** The two vertical planes are the **right** and **left lateral planes** (Fig. 4-20).

The transpyloric plane is at the level of the lower border of L1 (first lumbar vertebra), and the transtubercular plane is at the level of L5 (the fifth lumbar vertebra). The right and left lateral planes are parallel to the midsagittal plane and are located midway between it and each anterior superior iliac spine (ASIS).

Names of Regions The names of these nine regions are identified below. Technologists should be familiar with the locations and names of these nine regions. However, generally locating most structures and organs within the four-quadrant system is sufficient for radiographic purposes because of variables that affect specific locations of organs, such as body habitus, body position, and age (see organ outlines in Fig. 4-20 for general locations of organs within these nine regions).

1. Right hypochondriac
2. Epigastric
3. Left hypochondriac
4. Right lateral (lumbar)
5. Umbilical
6. Left lateral (lumbar)
7. Right inguinal (iliac)
8. Pubic (hypogastric)
9. Left inguinal (iliac)

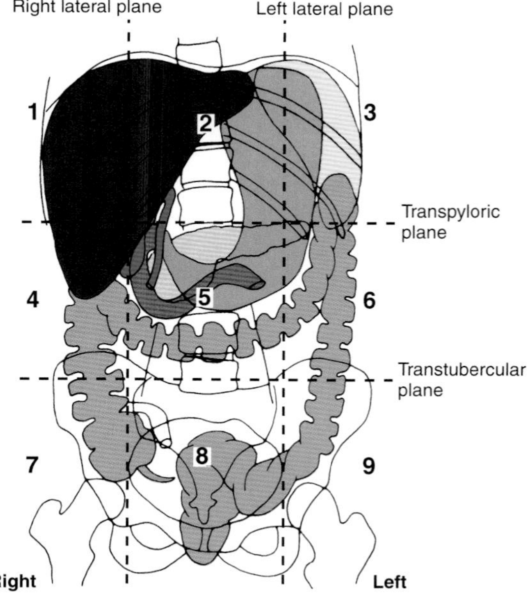

Fig. 4-20. Nine regions with certain abdominal structures.

TOPOGRAPHIC LANDMARKS

Abdominal borders and organs within the abdomen are not visible from the exterior, and because these soft tissue organs cannot be palpated directly, certain bony landmarks are used for this purpose.

Note: Remember that palpation must be done gently because the patient may have painful or sensitive areas within the abdomen and pelvis. Also, be sure that the patient is informed of the purpose of this palpation before beginning.

SEVEN LANDMARKS OF THE ABDOMEN

The following seven palpable landmarks are important in positioning the abdomen or for locating organs within the abdomen. It is suggested that one should practice finding these bony landmarks on oneself before attempting to locate them on another person or on a patient the first time.

Positioning for abdominal radiographs in either anteroposterior (AP) or posteroanterior (PA) projections requires a quick but accurate location of these landmarks on thin patients, as well as on heavy-set or muscular patients, who will require more firm palpation.

1. **Xiphoid tip (level of T9-T10):** The tip of the xiphoid process is the most distal or inferior process of the sternum. This can best be palpated by first gently pressing on the soft abdomen below the distal sternum, then moving upward carefully against the firm, distal margin of the xiphoid process.

This landmark approximates the superior anterior portion of the diaphragm, which is also the **superior margin of the abdomen.** This, however, is not a primary landmark for positioning the abdomen because of variations in body types and the importance of including all of the lower abdomen on most abdomen radiographic images.

2. **Inferior costal (rib) margin (level of L2-L3):** This landmark is used to locate upper abdominal organs, such as the gallbladder and/or stomach.

3. **Iliac crest (level of L4-L5 vertebral interspace):** The crest of the ilium is the uppermost portion of the curved border of the ilium. The iliac crest can be easily palpated by pressing inward and downward along the midlateral margin of the abdomen. The uppermost or most superior portion of this crest is the **most commonly used abdominal landmark** and corresponds approximately to the level of the **midabdomen,** which is also at or just slightly below the level of the umbilicus on most persons. If the center of the cassette or image receptor (IR) is centered to this level, the lower abdomen area will generally be included on the lower margin of the IR.

Note: To ensure that all of the upper abdomen including the diaphragm is included on the IR requires centering about 5 cm (2 inches) above the level of the crest for most patients, which will usually cut off some of the important lower abdomen. This then would require a second IR centered lower to include this lower region.

4. **Anterior superior iliac spine (ASIS):** The ASIS can be found by locating the iliac crest, then palpating anteriorly and inferiorly until a prominent projection or "bump" is felt (more prominent on females). This is a commonly used landmark for positioning of pelvic and vertebral structures but can also be a secondary landmark for general abdominal positioning.

5. **Greater trochanter:** This landmark is more easily palpated on thin patients. Gentle but very firm palpation is generally required to feel the movement of the trochanter with one hand while rotating the leg internally and externally at the knee area with the other hand. This is not as precise a landmark as other bony landmarks of the pelvis, but the uppermost margin of the trochanter generally lies slightly superior (3 to 4 cm, or 1 to 1½ inches) to the level of the symphysis pubis. With practice this can also be used as a secondary landmark for abdomen positioning.

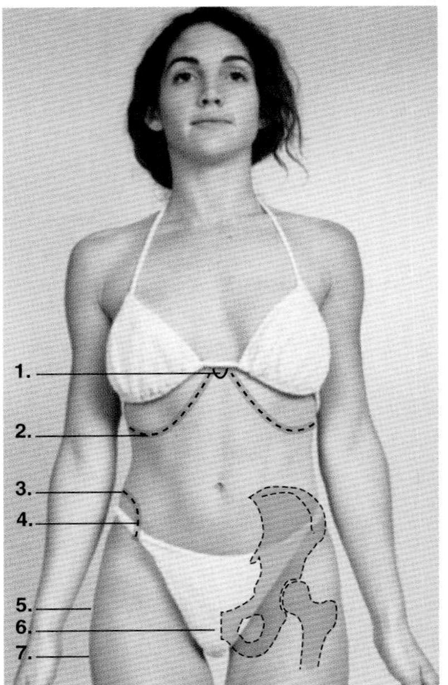

Fig. 4-21. Topographic landmarks.

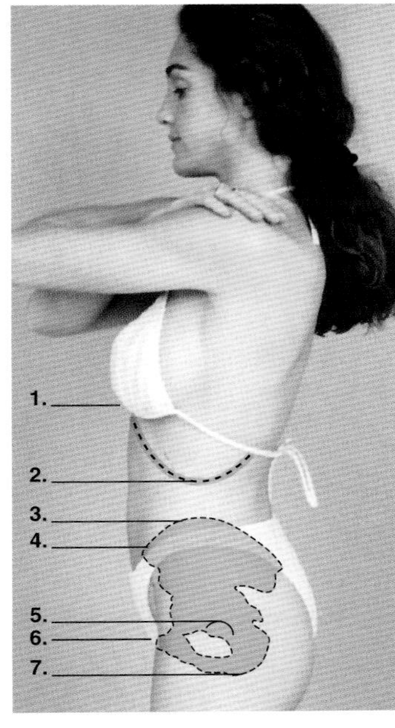

Fig. 4-22. Topographic landmarks.

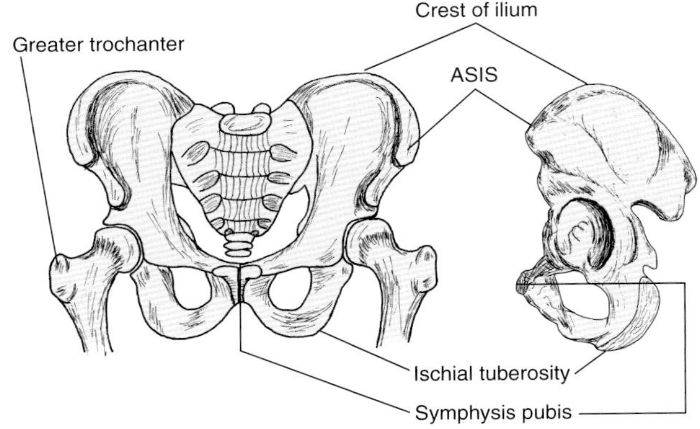

Fig. 4-23. Topographic landmarks of pelvis.

6. **Symphysis pubis:** The symphysis pubis is the anterior junction (joint) of the two pelvic bones. The most superior anterior portion of the pubis can be palpated when the patient is in a supine position. This landmark corresponds to the **inferior margin of the abdomen.** Palpation of this area, however, may be embarrassing to some patients. With practice, the level of the symphysis pubis or the lower margin of the abdomen can be identified by palpating the greater trochanter or in reference to the iliac crest as being at the level of the center of the cassette or IR. This then places the lower margin of the IR at the symphysis pubis.

7. **Ischial tuberosity:** This can be used to determine the lower margin on a PA abdomen with the patient in a **prone position.** These two bony prominences, which can be most easily palpated on thin patients, bear most of the weight of the trunk when one is seated. The lower margins of the ischial tuberosities are about 1 to 4 cm (1½ inches) below or distal to the symphysis pubis. This landmark may be used for positioning a PA projection of the colon when the rectal area is to be included on the IR. This, however, may also be uncomfortable and embarrassing for the patient, and other landmarks can and should be used when possible.

RADIOGRAPHIC POSITIONING

Patient Preparation

Patient preparation for abdominal radiography includes removal of all clothing and any opaque objects in the area to be radiographed. The patient should wear a hospital gown with the opening and ties in the back (if this type of gown is used). Shoes and socks may remain on the feet. Generally no pre-exam patient instructions are required unless barium studies are scheduled also.

General Positioning Considerations

Make patients as comfortable as possible on the radiographic table. A pillow under the head and support under the knees will enhance comfort for a supine abdomen. Place clean linen on the table and cover patients to keep them warm and to protect their modesty.

Breathing Instructions

One of the key factors in good abdominal radiography is the prevention of motion. Motion may result from either **voluntary** movements, such as breathing, or from **involuntary** movements, such as peristaltic action of the bowel. The difference between these two types of motion is illustrated in Chapter 1. However, what is important to remember in preventing any potential motion in abdominal radiography is to use the **shortest exposure time possible.**

A second way to prevent voluntary motion is by providing **careful breathing instructions** to the patient. Most abdominal radiographs are taken on expiration; the patient is instructed to "take in a deep breath—let it all out and hold it—don't breathe." Before making the exposure, make sure that the patient is following instructions and that sufficient time has been allowed for all breathing movements to cease.

Abdominal radiographs are exposed on **expiration,** with the diaphragm in a superior position to better visualize abdominal structures.

Image Markers

Markers, such as patient ID information, should be clear and legible. Correctly placed R and L markers and "up side" markers, such as short arrows, are used for erect and decubitus projections and should be visible without superimposing abdominal structures.

Radiation Protection

Good radiation protection practices are especially important in abdominal radiography because of the proximity of the radiation-sensitive gonadal organs.

4

Repeat exposures: Careful positioning and selection of correct exposure factors are ways of reducing unnecessary exposure from repeat examinations. Providing clear breathing instructions also assists in eliminating repeats that often result from motion caused by breathing during the exposure.

Collimation: For abdominal radiographs of small patients, some side collimation to skin borders is possible if it does not cut off abdominal anatomy.

Collimation on the top and bottom for adults should be adjusted directly to the margins of the IR or film holder, allowing for divergence of the x-ray beam. Essential anatomy will be cut off on average-sized adults if extra collimation margins are shown on the top and bottom borders of a typical 35 × 43 cm (14 × 17 inch) abdominal image.

Gonadal shielding: For abdominal radiographs, **gonadal shields should be used for males,** with the upper edge of the shield carefully placed at the pubic symphysis (Fig. 4-24). For females, gonadal shields should be **used only when such shields do not obscure essential anatomy** in the lower abdominopelvic region. Generally, the decision to shield female gonads on abdominal radiographs should be made by a physician to determine whether essential anatomy will be obscured. The top of an ovarian shield should be at or slightly above the level of ASIS and the lower border at the symphysis pubis.

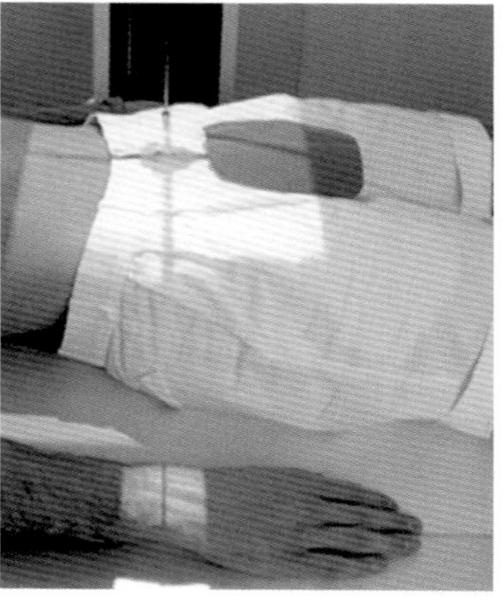

Fig. 4-24. Gonadal shielding—male.

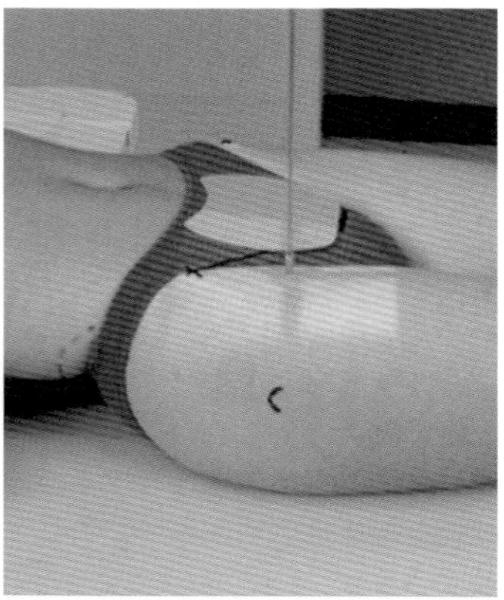

Fig. 4-25. Gonadal shielding—female (only use if shielding does not obscure essential anatomy).

Pregnancy protection: See Chapter 2, p. 72, describing the 10-day or LMP rule (last menstrual period), concerning safeguards for potential early pregnancies with abdomen or pelvic projections.

Exposure Factors

The principal exposure factors for abdominal radiographs are as follows:

1. Medium kV (70-80)
2. Short exposure time
3. Adequate mAs for sufficient density

Correctly exposed abdominal radiographs on an average-sized patient should faintly visualize the lateral borders of the psoas muscles, lower liver margin, kidney outlines, and lumbar vertebrae transverse processes. This requires moderate contrast using medium kV exposure to allow for visualization of various abdominal structures, including possible small semiopaque stones in the gallbladder or kidneys.

Pediatric Applications

Acute abdomen routines for pediatrics generally include only a supine and one horizontal beam projection to show air-fluid levels. For patients under 2 or 3 years of age, the lateral decubitus may be difficult to obtain, and an AP erect abdomen using an immobilization device such as a Pigg-O-Stat is preferred (see Chapter 20).

Motion prevention is of utmost importance in pediatrics, and short exposure time in addition to higher-speed film and screens are essential. Children under 12 or 13 years of age require a significant reduction in kV and mAs. Confirmed technique factors for children of various sizes and ages for the equipment being used should always be available to minimize repeats due to exposure errors.

Geriatric Applications

Older patients often require extra care and patience in explaining what is expected of them. Careful breathing instructions are essential, as is assistance in helping patients move into the position required. Extra radiolucent padding under the back and buttocks for thin patients and blankets to keep patients warm add greatly to their comfort on supine abdomen radiographic procedures.

Digital Imaging Considerations

The following summary reviews the guidelines that should be followed with digital imaging (CR and DR) of the abdomen as described in this chapter:

1. **Close collimation** Close collimation to the body part being imaged and **accurate centering** are most important in digital imaging for the abdomen.

2. **Exposure factors** It is important that the ALARA principle be followed and the **lowest exposure factors required to obtain a diagnostic image** be used. This includes the highest kV and the lowest mAs that will result in desirable image quality. For digital imaging, this may require some increase in kV compared with film-screen imaging.

3. **Postprocessing evaluation of exposure index values** The exposure index number on the final processed image must be checked to verify that the exposure factors used were in the correct range to ensure optimum quality with the least radiation to the patient.

Alternative Modalities

COMPUTED TOMOGRAPHY AND MAGNETIC RESONANCE IMAGING

Computed tomography (CT) and magnetic resonance imaging (MRI) are very useful in the evaluation and early diagnosis of small neoplasms involving abdominal organs such as the liver and pancreas. With the use of IV contrast media, CT is also able to discriminate between a simple cyst and a solid neoplasm.

Both CT and MRI also provide valuable information in assessing the extent that neoplasms have spread to surrounding tissues or organs. MRI, for example, may be able to demonstrate blood vessels within neoplasms and assess their relationship and involvement with surrounding organs without the need for contrast media injection.

MRI is also being used to visualize the biliary and pancreatic ducts in addition to the ERCP procedure (endoscopic retrograde cholangiopancreatogram), a fluoroscopic procedure using a contrast media injected endoscopically (described in Chapter 16).

SONOGRAPHY (ULTRASOUND)

Ultrasound has become the method of choice when imaging the **gallbladder** for detection of gallstones (in the gallbladder or bile ducts). It is of limited use in the evaluation of the hollow viscus of the gastrointestinal (GI) tract for bowel obstruction or perforation, but along with CT, it is very useful in detecting and evaluating lesions or inflammation of soft-tissue organs such as the liver or pancreas. Ultrasound is also widely used, along with CT, for demonstrating abscesses, cysts, or tumors involving the kidneys, ureters, or bladder.

Ultrasound with compression, in combination with clinical evaluation, can be used successfully to diagnose **acute appendicitis.**

NUCLEAR MEDICINE

Nuclear medicine is useful as a noninvasive means of evaluating GI motility and reflux as related to possible bowel obstruction. It is also useful for evaluation of lower GI bleeding.

With the injection of specific radionuclides, nuclear medicine imaging can be used to demonstrate the entire liver and the major bile ducts and gallbladder.

Pathologic Indications

A plain **AP supine radiograph** of the abdomen (**KUB**) is generally taken before contrast medium is introduced into the various abdominal organ systems to evaluate and diagnose diseases and conditions involving these systems. Pathologic indications and terms specifically related to each of these systems are provided in Chapters 14 through 17.

The **acute abdomen series,** however, as described in this chapter, is performed most commonly to evaluate and diagnose conditions or diseases related to **bowel obstruction and/or perforation.** This requires demonstrating air-fluid levels and possible intraperitoneal "free" air using horizontal beam erect or decubitus body positions. Following are terms and pathologic diseases or conditions as related to the acute abdominal series exam:

Ascites *(ah-si'tez)* is an abnormal accumulation of fluid in the peritoneal cavity of the abdomen. It is generally caused by long-standing (chronic) conditions such as cirrhosis of the liver or by metastatic disease to the peritoneal cavity.

Pneumoperitoneum refers to free air or gas in the peritoneal cavity. This is a serious condition requiring surgery when caused by perforation of a gas-containing viscus, such as by a gastric or duodenal ulcer. It can also be caused by trauma penetrating the abdominal wall.

Small amounts of residual air may be evident radiographically up to 2 or 3 weeks following abdominal surgery. It is best demonstrated with a horizontal beam erect abdomen or chest radiograph, where even a small amount of free air can be seen as it rises to the highest position under the diaphragm.

Mechanical bowel obstruction is complete or nearly complete blockage of the flow of intestinal contents. Its causes are as follows:

- **Fibrous adhesions:** The most common cause of mechanical-based obstruction, in which a fibrous band of tissue interrelates with intestine, creating a blockage.
- **Crohn's disease** *(Krōnz)*: A chronic inflammation of the intestinal wall that results in bowel obstruction in at least half of those afflicted. The cause is unknown. Crohn's disease is most common in young adults and is characterized by loops of small bowel joined by fistulas or connected openings with adjacent loops of intestine.
- **Intussusception:** The telescoping of a section of bowel into another loop, creating an obstruction. Intussusception is most common in the distal small bowel region (ileus), and it is more common in children than in adults. This condition requires treatment within 48 hours to prevent necrosis (tissue death).
- **Volvulus:** The twisting of a loop of intestine, creating an obstruction. Volvulus may require surgery to correct.

Ileus–nonmechanical bowel obstruction is categorized as *adynamic* (without power or force) ileus and is most frequently caused by peritonitis, or *paralytic* (paralysis) ileus, which is caused by a lack of intestinal motility. It occurs frequently in postoperative patients, usually 24 to 72 hours after abdominal surgery. Unlike mechanical obstructions, it rarely leads to perforation, and the radiographic appearance is characterized by a large amount of air and fluid with air-fluid levels visible in a greatly dilated small and large bowel with no distinct point of obstruction visible (unlike a mechanical obstruction).

Ulcerative colitis is a chronic disease involving inflammation of the colon that occurs primarily in young adults and most frequently involves the rectosigmoid region. In some cases, it becomes a very severe acute process, causing serious complications, such as a toxic megacolon (extreme dilation of a segment of colon) with potential perforation into the peritoneal cavity. **Barium enema is strongly contraindicated** with symptoms of toxic megacolon.

SUMMARY OF PATHOLOGIC INDICATIONS

CONDITION OR DISEASE	MOST COMMON RADIOGRAPHIC EXAM	POSSIBLE RADIOGRAPHIC APPEARANCE	EXPOSURE FACTOR ADJUSTMENT*
Ascites	Acute abdomen series	General abdominal haziness	Increase, depending on severity (+ or ++)
Pneumoperitoneum (air in peritoneal cavity)	Acute abdomen series—erect chest or abdomen	Thin crest-shaped radiolucency under dome of right hemidiaphragm on erect	Decrease (−)
Mechanical bowel obstruction			
Fibrous adhesions	Acute abdomen series	Distended loops of air-filled small bowel	Decrease, depending on severity of distention (− or − −)
Crohn's disease	Acute abdomen series	Distended loops of air-filled small bowel	Decrease, depending on severity of distention (− or − −)
Intussusception (most common in children)	Acute abdomen series	Air-filled "coiled spring" appearance	Decrease (−)
Volvulus (most common in sigmoid colon)	Acute abdomen series	Large amounts of air in sigmoid with tapered narrowing at site of volvulus	Slight decrease (−)
Ileus (nonmechanical obstruction)	Acute abdomen series	Large amounts of air in entire dilated small and large bowel with air-fluid levels visualized	Decrease, depending on severity of distention (− or − −)
Adynamic or paralytic			
Ulcerative colitis	Plain AP abdomen	Deep air-filled mucosal protrusions of colon wall, usually in rectosigmoid region	Decrease (−)
Severe case may lead to toxic megacolon and bowel perforation	Acute abdomen series for possible free air **(BE contraindicated)**	Dilated loop of colon	Decrease (−)

*Automatic exposure control (AEC) systems are designed to correct exposure density automatically for patient size variances and for these pathologic conditions. If they are calibrated correctly and used as intended, manual adjustments generally are not needed when AEC is used. However, these exposure adjustments may be needed for more extreme cases, or for repeats, even with AEC. They are also important when setting manual exposure techniques, such as for tabletop or mobile exams when AEC is not used.

Survey Information

ABDOMEN—BASIC AND SPECIAL

The common **basic** abdomen projections in the latest survey (see Appendix A) continue to be the **AP supine** (99%), **AP erect** (78%), and **lateral decubitus** (60%).

The **dorsal decubitus** is a consistent special projection throughout both the U.S. and Canada, with about 48% indicating it as a **special** projection in their departments in the U.S. and 32% in Canada.

The **lateral abdomen** is also a special position as indicated by 41% of the total survey respondents in the 1999 survey. It is sometimes taken as part of a survey study of the abdomen for elderly patients to demonstrate the prevertebral region for calcification or potential aneurysm of the aorta.

ACUTE ABDOMEN ROUTINE

In addition to the supine and erect or decubitus abdomen, the **PA chest** was indicated to be part of a three-way acute abdomen series by an increasing percentage in the U.S.—75% in 1999, 68% in 1995, and 60% in 1989. Therefore the three-way acute abdomen series (AP and erect abdomen plus PA chest) is presented as basic or routine. However, acute abdomen routines will vary depending on the institution. Students and technologists should determine the routine for their departments.

One reason the PA chest is commonly included in the three-way acute abdomen series is that the erect chest best visualizes free intraperitoneal air under the diaphragm. The erect abdomen will also visualize free air if the IR is centered high enough to include the diaphragm; however, the exposure technique for the chest best visualizes small amounts of this air if present.

BASIC AND SPECIAL PROJECTIONS

The most common basic and special projections for the abdomen are demonstrated and described on the following pages.

Abdomen (KUB)
BASIC
- **AP supine** 121

SPECIAL
- **PA prone** 122
- **Lateral decubitus (AP)** 123
- **AP erect** 124
- **Dorsal decubitus (lateral)** 125
- **Lateral** 126

Acute abdomen (three-way, with PA chest)
BASIC
- **AP supine** 127
- **AP erect** 127
- **PA chest erect** 127

SPECIAL
- **Left lateral decubitus (AP)** 127

4

AP PROJECTION—SUPINE POSITION: ABDOMEN

KUB

Abdomen
BASIC
• AP supine (KUB)

35

43

R

Pathology Demonstrated

Pathology of abdomen, including bowel obstruction, neoplasms, calcifications, ascites, and scout for contrast media studies of abdomen.

Technical Factors

- IR size—35 × 43 cm (14 × 17 inches), lengthwise
- Moving or stationary grid
- 70-80 kV range
- Technique and dose:

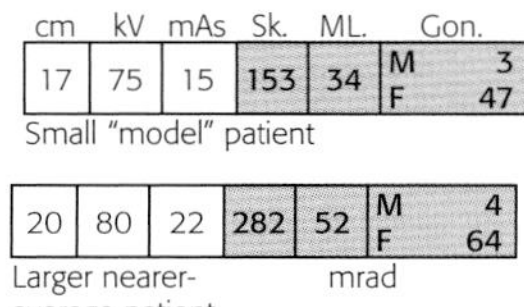

cm	kV	mAs	Sk.	ML.	Gon.
17	75	15	153	34	M 3 / F 47

Small "model" patient

cm	kV	mAs	Sk.	ML.	Gon.
20	80	22	282	52	M 4 / F 64

Larger nearer-average patient — mrad

Shielding Use gonadal shields on males (also on females of reproductive age, only if such shielding does not obscure essential anatomy as determined by a physician).

Patient Position

- Supine with midsagittal plane centered to midline of table and/or cassette
- Arms placed at patient's sides, away from body
- Legs extended with support under knees if this is more comfortable

Part Position

- Center of cassette to **level of iliac crests,** with bottom margin at symphysis pubis (see Notes below)
- **No rotation** of pelvis or shoulders (check that both ASISs are the same distance from table-top)

Central Ray

- CR perpendicular to and directed to **center of IR** (to level of iliac crest)
- Minimum SID of 40 inches (100 cm)

Collimation Collimate closely on sides to skin margins and on top and bottom to IR borders.

Respiration Make exposure at end of **expiration** (allow about 1 second delay after expiration to cause involuntary motion of bowel to cease).

Notes: A tall hyposthenic- or asthenic-type patient may require **two images lengthwise,** one centered lower to include the symphysis pubis and the second centered high to include the upper abdomen and diaphragm.

A broad hypersthenic-type patient may also require two 35 × 43 cm (14 × 17 inches) images placed **crosswise,** one centered lower to include the symphysis pubis and the second for the upper abdomen, with a minimum of 3 to 5 cm (1 to 2 inches) overlap.

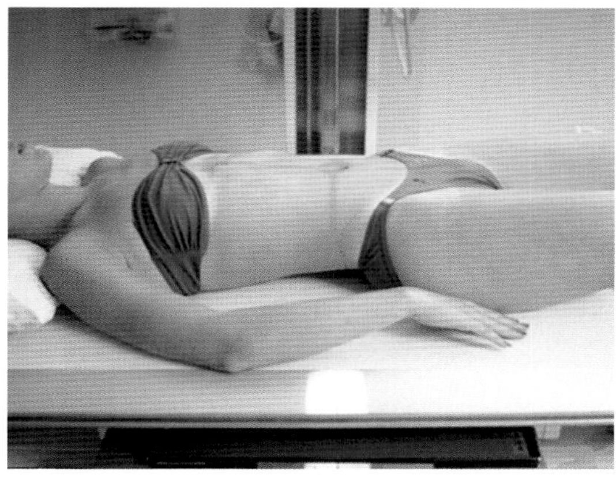

Fig. 4-26. AP abdomen.

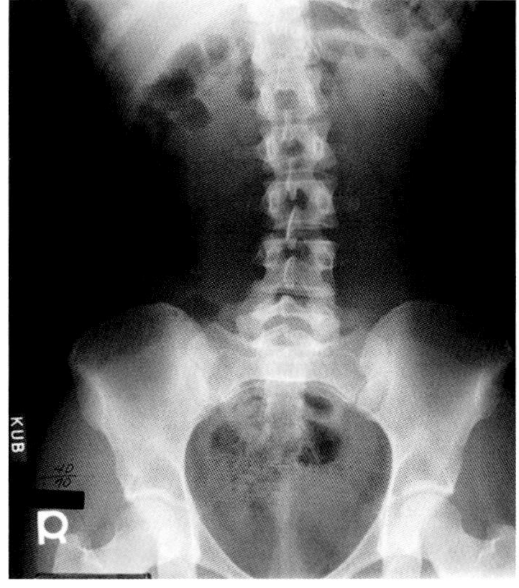

Fig. 4-27. AP abdomen.

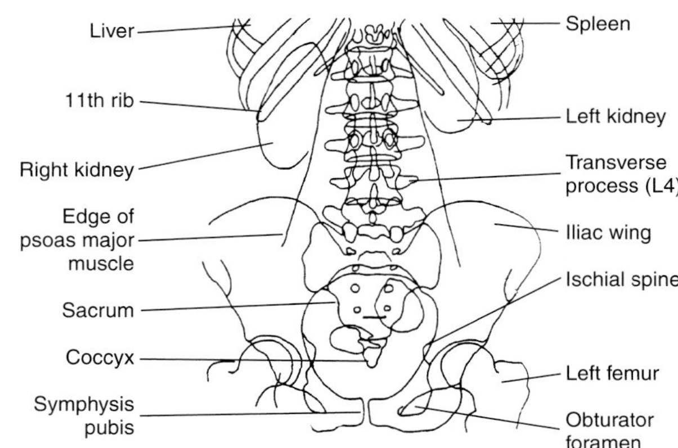

Fig. 4-28. AP abdomen.

Radiographic Criteria

Structures Shown: • Outline of liver, spleen, kidneys, and air-filled stomach and bowel segments and the arch of the symphysis pubis for the urinary bladder region.

Position: • No rotation: Iliac wings, obturator foramina (if visible), and ischial spines appear symmetric, and outer lower rib margins are the same distance from spine (elongation of iliac wing indicates rotation in that direction).

Collimation and CR: • Collimation border to film margins on top and bottom to prevent cutoff of essential anatomy. • Center of IR (CR) at level of iliac crest. • See note about possible two films.

Exposure Criteria: • No motion: Ribs and all gas bubble margins appear sharp. • Sufficient exposure (mAs) and long-scale contrast (kV) visualize psoas muscle outlines, lumbar transverse processes, and ribs. • Margins of liver and kidneys should be visible on smaller to average-sized patients.

PA PROJECTION—PRONE POSITION: ABDOMEN

Abdomen
SPECIAL
- PA prone
- Lateral decubitus (AP)
- AP erect
- Dorsal decubitus (lateral)
- Lateral

Pathology Demonstrated
Pathology of abdomen, including bowel obstruction, neoplasms, calcifications, ascites, and scout for contrast media studies of abdomen.

Note: This projection is **less desirable** than the AP if the kidneys are of primary interest because of **the increased OID.**

Technical Factors
- IR size—35 × 43 cm (14 × 17 inches), lengthwise
- Moving or stationary grid
- 70-80 kV range
- Technique and dose:

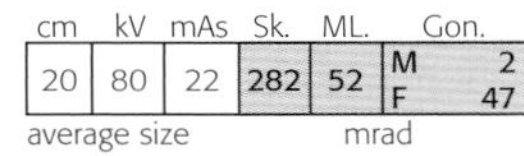

cm	kV	mAs	Sk.	ML.	Gon.
20	80	22	282	52	M 2 F 47

average size — mrad

Shielding Use gonadal shields on males (also on females of reproductive age, only if such shielding does not obscure essential anatomy as determined by a physician).

Patient Position
- Prone with midsagittal plane of body centered to midline of table and/or IR
- Legs extended with support under ankles
- Arms up beside head; clean pillow provided

Part Position
- No rotation of pelvis or shoulders and thorax
- Center of IR to **iliac crest**

Central Ray
- CR perpendicular to and directed to **center of IR** (to level of iliac crest)
- Minimum SID of 40 inches (100 cm)

Collimation Collimate closely on all sides to skin margins and on top and bottom to IR borders.

Respiration Make exposure at end of **expiration.**

Note: Tall, asthenic-type patients may require two images lengthwise; broad hypersthenic types may also require two images placed crosswise.

Fig. 4-29. PA abdomen.

Fig. 4-30. PA abdomen.

Radiographic Criteria

Structures Shown: • Outline of liver, spleen, kidneys, and air-filled stomach and bowel segments and the arch of the symphysis pubis for the urinary bladder region.

Position: • **No rotation:** Iliac wings appear symmetric, and sacroiliac joints and outer lower rib margins (if visible) should be the same distance from spine.

Collimation and CR: • Collimation borders to IR margins on top and bottom to prevent cutoff of essential anatomy. • Center of IR (CR) at level of iliac crest (see note about possible two images).

Exposure Criteria: • No motion: Ribs and all gas bubble margins appear sharp. • Exposure (mAs) and long-scale contrast (kV) are sufficient to visualize psoas muscle outlines, lumbar transverse processes, and ribs. • Margins of liver and kidneys should be visible on smaller to average-sized patients.

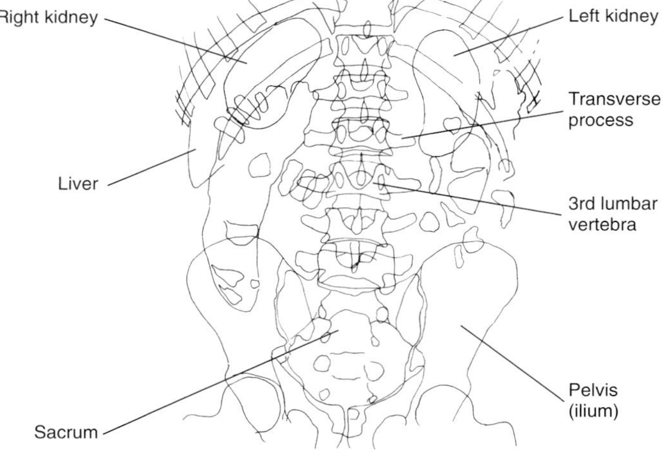

Fig. 4-31. PA abdomen.

LATERAL DECUBITUS POSITION (AP PROJECTION): ABDOMEN

Abdomen
SPECIAL
- PA prone
- Lateral decubitus (AP)
- AP erect
- Dorsal decubitus (lateral)
- Lateral

Pathology Demonstrated
Abdominal masses, air-fluid levels, and possible accumulations of intraperitoneal air are demonstrated. (Small amounts of free intraperitoneal air are best demonstrated with chest technique on erect PA chest.)

Important: Patient should be on side **a minimum of 5 minutes** before exposure (to allow air to rise or abnormal fluids to accumulate); **10 to 20 minutes is preferred,** if possible, to best demonstrate potential small amounts of intraperitoneal air.

Left lateral decubitus best visualizes free intraperitoneal air in the area of the liver in the right upper abdomen away from the gastric bubble.

Technical Factors
- IR size—35 × 43 cm (14 × 17 inches), crosswise to the table (lengthwise with the patient)
- Moving or stationary grid
- 70-80 kV range
- Technique and dose:

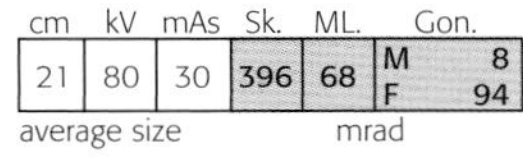

cm	kV	mAs	Sk.	ML.	Gon.	
21	80	30	396	68	M	8
					F	94
average size			mrad			

Marker: Place arrow or other appropriate marker to indicate "up" side.

Shielding Use gonadal shield on males.

Patient Position
- Lateral recumbent on radiolucent pad, firmly against table or vertical grid device (with wheels on cart locked so as not to move away from table)
- Patient on firm surface, such as a cardiac or back board, positioned under the sheet to prevent sagging and anatomy cutoff
- Knees partially flexed, one on top of the other to stabilize patient
- Arms up near head; clean pillow provided

Part Position
- Adjust patient and cart so that center of IR and CR are about **2 inches (5 cm) above level of iliac crests** (to include diaphragm). Proximal margin of cassette will be approximately at level of axilla.
- Ensure no rotation of pelvis or shoulders.
- Adjust height of cassette to center midsagittal plane of patient to center of IR, but ensure that **upside of abdomen is clearly included on the IR.**

Central Ray
- CR **horizontal,** directed to **center of IR,** at about 2 inches (or 5 cm) above level of iliac crest; use of a horizontal beam to show air-fluid levels and free intraperitoneal air
- Minimum SID of 40 inches (100 cm)

Collimation Collimate on four sides; **do not cut off upper abdomen.**

Respiration Make exposure at end of **expiration.**

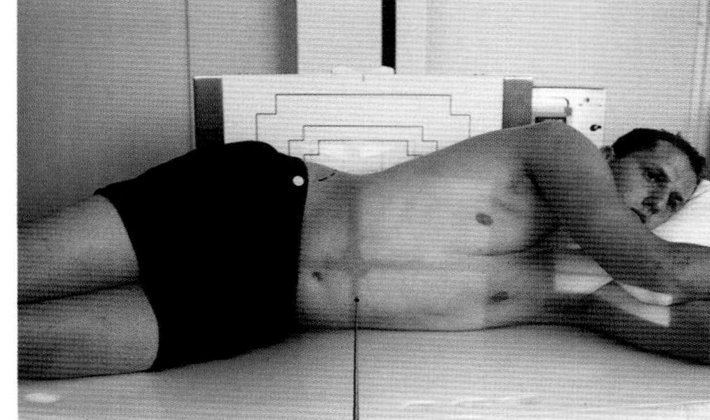

Fig. 4-32. Left lateral decubitus position (AP).

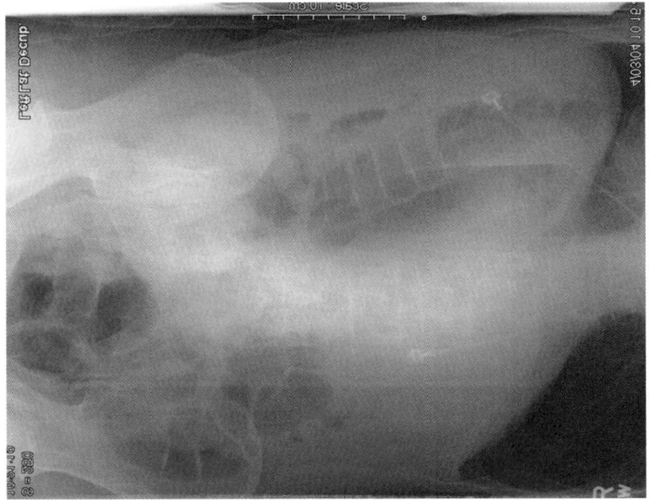

Fig. 4-33. Left lateral decubitus (AP).

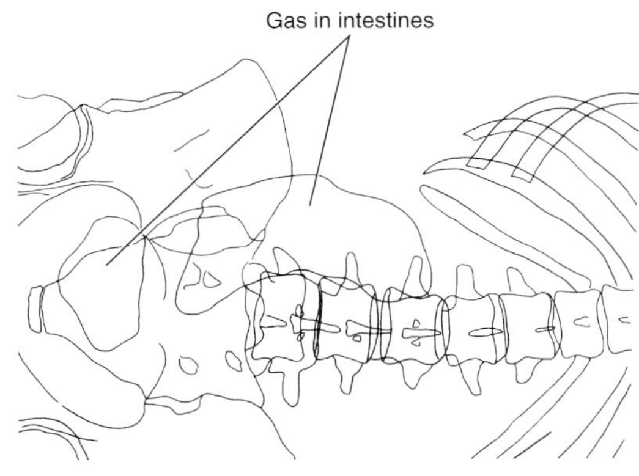

Fig. 4-34. Left lateral decubitus (AP).

Radiographic Criteria

Structures Shown: • Air-filled stomach and loops of bowel and air-fluid levels where present. • Should include bilateral diaphragm.

Position: • No rotation: Iliac wings appear symmetric, and outer rib margins are the same distance from spine. • Spine should be straight (unless scoliosis is present), aligned to center of IR.

Collimation and CR: • Collimation borders to IR margins to prevent cutoff of essential anatomy. • CR about 2 inches (5 cm) above level of iliac crest.

Exposure Criteria: • No motion: Ribs and all gas bubble margins sharp. • Exposure sufficient to visualize spine and ribs and soft tissue but not to overexpose possible intraperitoneal air in upper abdomen. • Slightly less overall density than supine abdomen.

AP PROJECTION—ERECT POSITION: ABDOMEN

Abdomen
SPECIAL
• PA prone
• Lateral decubitus (AP)
• AP erect
• Dorsal decubitus (lateral)
• Lateral

Pathology Demonstrated

Abnormal masses, air-fluid levels, and accumulations of intraperitoneal air under diaphragm are demonstrated.

Take erect radiograph first if patient comes to department ambulatory or in wheelchair in an erect position.

Technical Factors

- IR size—35 × 43 cm (14 × 17 inches), lengthwise
- Moving or stationary grid (use erect markers)
- 70-80 kV range
- Technique and dose:

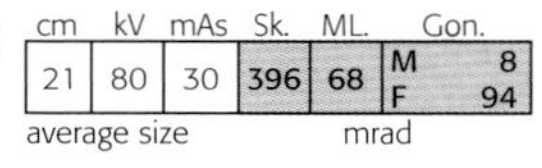

cm	kV	mAs	Sk.	ML.	Gon.
21	80	30	396	68	M 8, F 94

average size — mrad

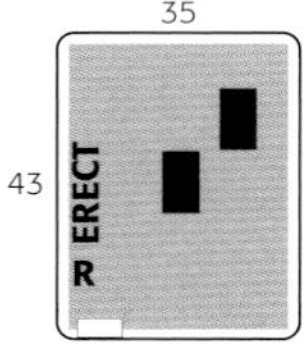

Marker: Include erect marker on IR.

Shielding

- Use gonadal shields on males. An adjustable freestanding mobile shield can be used as for chests.

Patient Position

- Upright, legs slightly spread, back against table or grid device (see Note below for weak or unsteady patients)
- Arms at sides away from body
- Midsagittal plane of body centered to midline of table or erect Bucky

Part Position

- Do not rotate pelvis or shoulders.
- Adjust height of IR so the center is about **2 inches (5 cm) above iliac crest** (to include diaphragm), which for the average patient will place the **top of the IR approximately at the level of the axilla.**

Central Ray

- CR **horizontal,** to **center of IR**
- Minimum SID of 40 inches (100 cm)

Collimation Collimate closely on all four sides; do **NOT** cut off upper abdomen.

Respiration Exposure should be made at end of **expiration.**

Note: Patient should be upright a minimum of **5 minutes,** but **10 to 20 minutes** is desirable, if possible, before exposure for visualizing small amounts of intraperitoneal air. If a patient is too weak to maintain an erect position, a lateral decubitus should be taken.

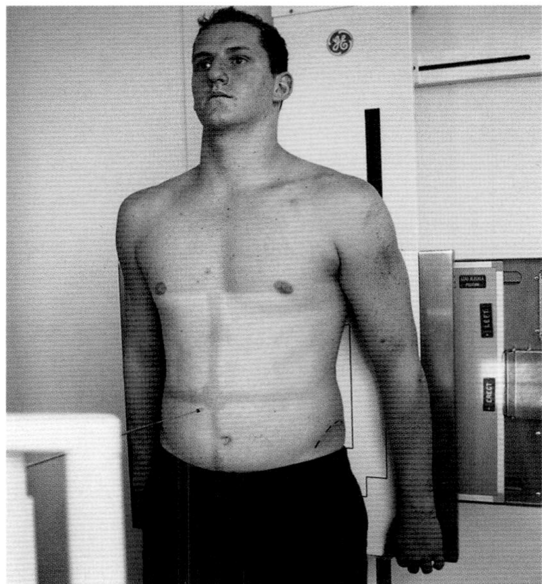

Fig. 4-35. Erect AP—to include diaphragm.

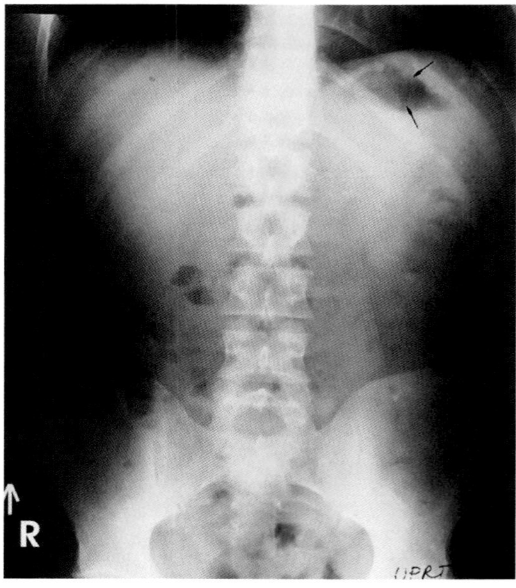

Fig. 4-36. Erect AP—to include diaphragm.

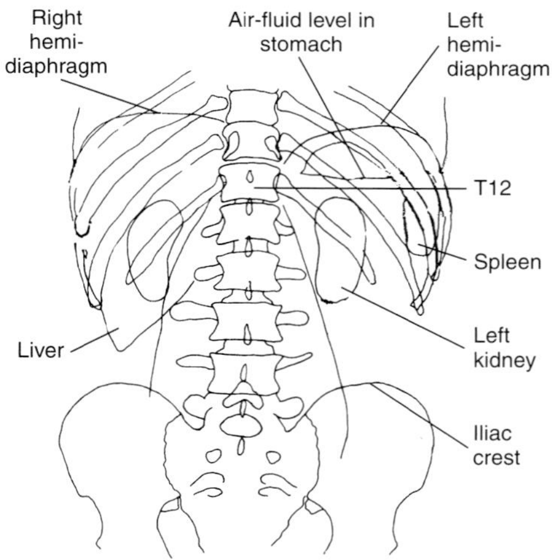

Fig. 4-37. Erect AP.

Radiographic Criteria

Structures Shown: • Air-filled stomach and loops of bowel and air-fluid levels where present. • Should include **bilateral diaphragm** and as much of lower abdomen as possible. • Small free, intraperitoneal crescent-shaped air bubble if present seen under **right** hemidiaphragm, away from gas in stomach *(small black arrows).*

Position: • **No rotation:** Iliac wings appear symmetric, and outer rib margins are the same distance from spine. Spine should be straight (unless scoliosis is present), aligned to center of IR.

Collimation and CR: • Collimation borders to top and bottom margins of IR to prevent cutoff of essential anatomy. • CR about 5 cm (2 inches) above level of iliac crest.

Exposure Criteria: • No motion: Ribs and all gas bubble margins appear sharp. • Exposure is sufficient to visualize spine and ribs and soft tissue but not to overexpose possible intraperitoneal air in upper abdomen. Slightly less overall density than supine abdomen is preferred.

DORSAL DECUBITUS POSITION (RIGHT OR LEFT LATERAL): ABDOMEN

Abdomen
SPECIAL
- PA prone
- Lateral decubitus (AP)
- AP erect
- Dorsal decubitus (lateral)

Pathology Demonstrated
Abnormal masses, accumulations of gas, air-fluid levels, **aneurysms** (a widening or dilation of the wall of an artery, vein, or the heart), **calcification of aorta or other vessels,** and **umbilical hernias.**

Technical Factors
- IR size—35 × 43 cm (14 × 17 inches), crosswise
- Moving or stationary grid
- 70-80 kV range
- Technique and dose:

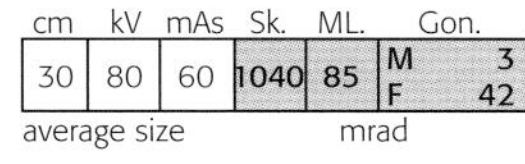

cm	kV	mAs	Sk.	ML.	Gon.
30	80	60	1040	85	M 3 F 42

average size mrad

Shielding
- Use gonadal shields on males.

Patient Position
- Supine on radiolucent pad, side against table or vertical grid device; secure cart so that it does not move away from table or grid device.
- Pillow under head, arms up beside head; support under partially flexed knees may be more comfortable for the patient.

Part Position
- Adjust patient and cart so that center of IR and CR is **2 inches (5 cm) above level of iliac crest** (to include diaphragm).
- Ensure that **no rotation** of pelvis or shoulders exists (both ASISs should be the same distance from table-top).
- Adjust height of IR to align midcoronal plane to centerline of IR.

Central Ray
- CR **horizontal,** to **center of IR** 2 inches (5 cm) above iliac crest, and to midcoronal plane
- Minimum SID of 40 inches (100 cm)

Collimation Collimate to upper and lower abdomen soft tissue borders. **Close collimation is important** because of increased scatter from higher kV and need for soft tissue visibility.

Respiration Exposure is made at end of **expiration.**

Note: This may be taken as a right or left lateral; appropriate R or L lateral marker should be used, indicating which side is closest to IR.

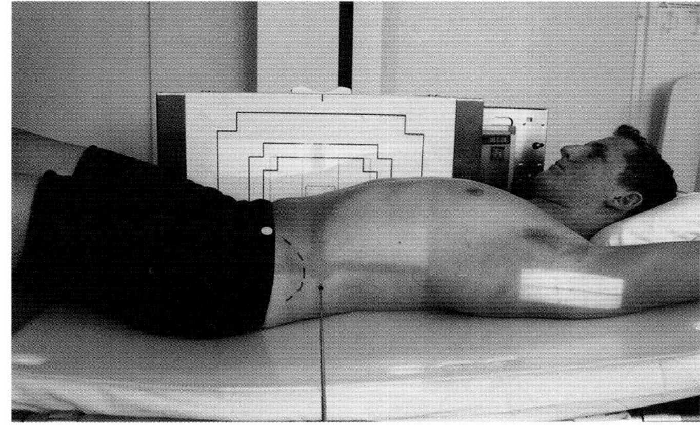

Fig. 4-38. Dorsal decubitus—right lateral position.

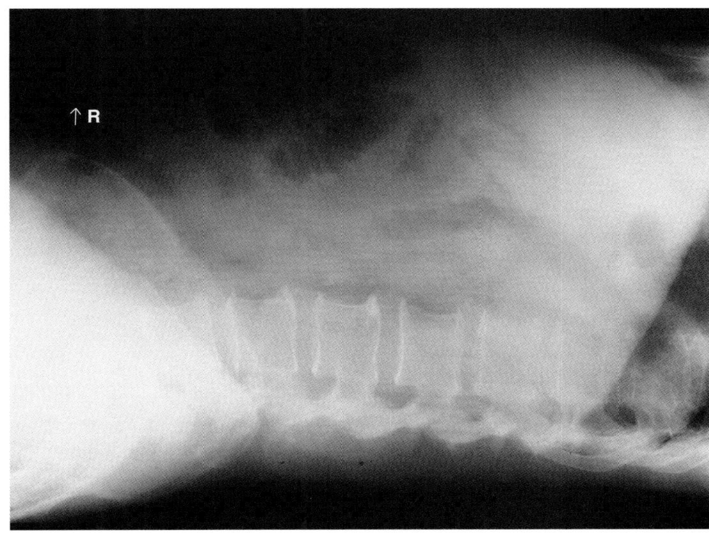

Fig. 4-39. Dorsal decubitus—right lateral position.

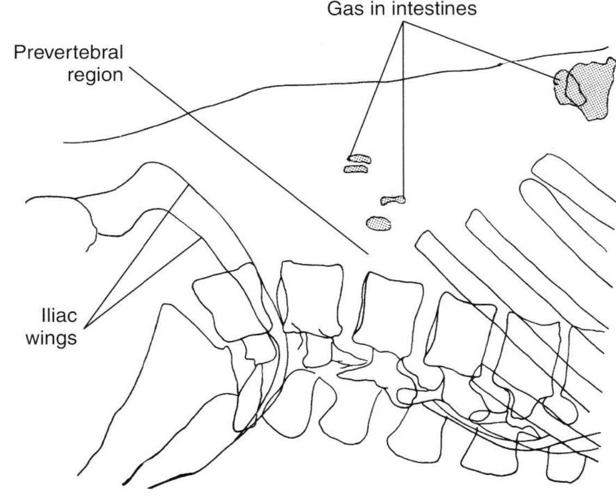

Fig. 4-40. Dorsal decubitus—right lateral position.

Radiographic Criteria
Structures Shown: • Diaphragm and as much of lower abdomen as possible should be included. • Air-filled loops of bowel in abdomen with soft tissue detail should be visible in anterior abdomen and in prevertebral regions.

Position: • **No rotation** as evident by superimposition of posterior ribs and posterior borders of iliac wings and bilateral ASISs.

Collimation and CR: • Collimation borders to tissue margins of anterior and posterior abdomen. • Center of collimation field (CR) to prevertebral region about 2 inches (5 cm) above level of iliac crest.

Exposure Criteria: • No motion: Rib and gas bubble margins appear sharp. • Lumbar vertebrae may appear about 50% underexposed with soft tissue detail visible in anterior abdomen and in prevertebral region of lower lumbar vertebra.

4

LATERAL POSITION: ABDOMEN

Abdomen
SPECIAL
- PA prone
- Lateral decubitus (AP)
- AP erect
- Dorsal decubitus (lateral)
- Lateral

Pathology Demonstrated
Abnormal soft-tissue masses, umbilical hernia, prevertebral region for possible aneurysms of aorta or calcifications.

Technical Factors
- IR size—35 × 43 cm (14 × 17 inches), lengthwise to table
- Moving or stationary grid
- 80-85 kV range
- Lead blocker placed on tabletop behind patient to reduce scatter
- Technique and dose:

cm	kV	mAs	Sk.	ML.	Gon.
30	80	60	1040	85	M 3 F 42
average size				mrad	

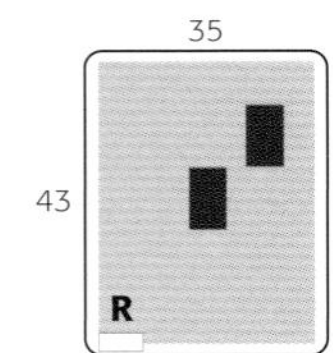

Shielding
- Use gonadal shields on males.

Patient Position
- Patient in lateral recumbent position on right or left side, pillow for head
- Elbows flexed, arms up, knees and hips partially flexed, pillow between knees to maintain a lateral position

Part Position
- Align midcoronal plane to CR and midline of table.
- Ensure pelvis and thorax are **not rotated** but in a true lateral position.

Central Ray
- CR perpendicular to table, centered **about 2 inches (5 cm) above level of iliac crest** to midcoronal plane
- IR centered to CR
- Minimum SID of 40 inches (100 cm)

Collimation Collimate closely to upper and lower IR borders and to anterior and posterior skin borders to minimize scatter.

Respiration Suspend breathing on **expiration.**

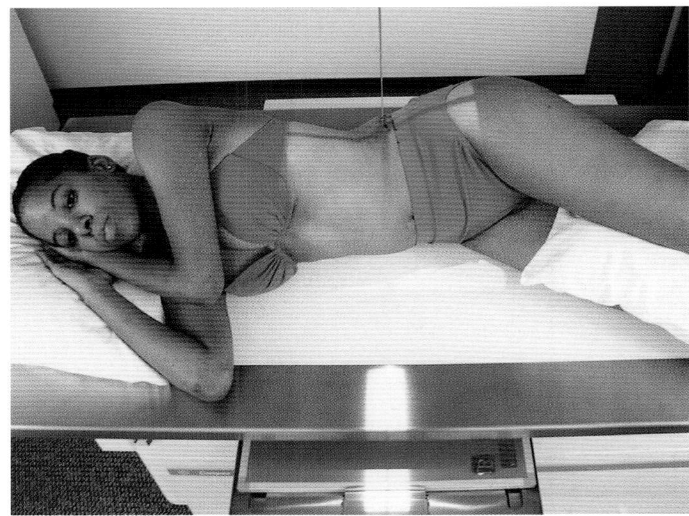

Fig. 4-41. Right lateral abdomen.

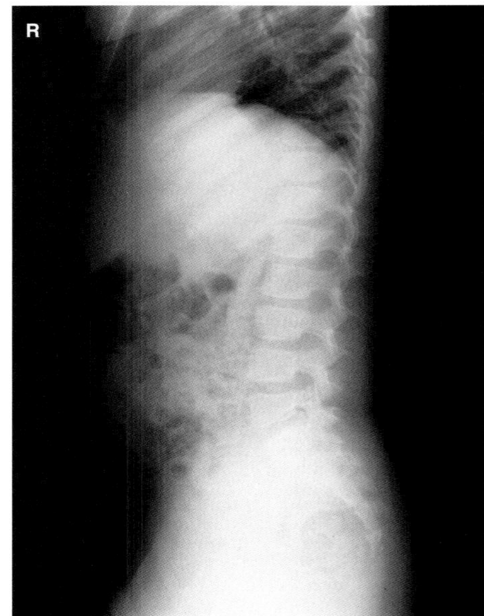

Fig. 4-42. Right lateral abdomen.

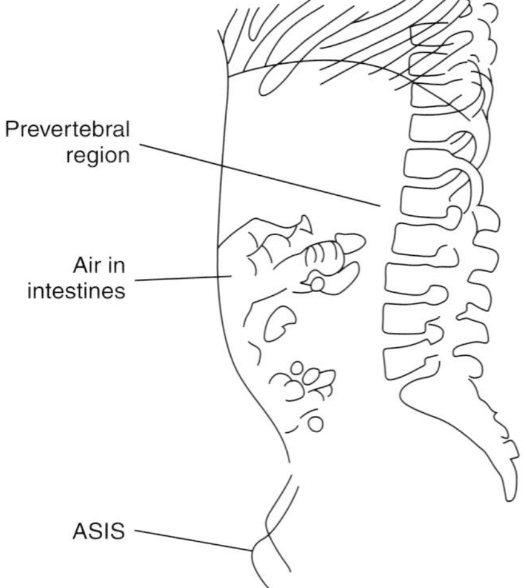

Fig. 4-43. Right lateral abdomen.

Radiographic Criteria
Structures Shown: • Diaphragm and as much of lower abdomen as possible should be included. • Air-filled loops of bowel in abdomen with soft tissue detail should be visible in prevertebral and anterior abdomen regions.

Position: • **No rotation** as evident by superimposition of posterior ribs and posterior borders of iliac wings and bilateral ASISs.

Collimation and CR: • Collimation borders to tissue margins of anterior and posterior abdomen. • Center of collimation field (CR) to prevertebral region about 2 inches (5 cm) above level of iliac crest.

Exposure Criteria: • No motion: Rib and gas bubble margins appear sharp. • Lumbar vertebrae may appear about 50% underexposed with soft tissue detail visible in anterior abdomen and in prevertebral region of lower lumbar vertebra.

ACUTE ABDOMINAL SERIES: ACUTE ABDOMEN

Three-Way Abdomen: (1) AP Supine (2) Erect (or Lateral Decubitus) Abdomen (3) PA Chest

Departmental routine: Determine whether departmental protocol includes an erect PA chest as part of acute abdomen series routine. Minimum positions must include at least one erect or decubitus horizontal beam projection abdomen in addition to AP supine.

Acute abdomen (three-way)
BASIC
- AP supine
- AP erect
- PA chest

SPECIAL
- Left lateral decubitus

Specific Clinical Indications for Acute Abdominal Series

1. **Ileus** (nonmechanical small bowel obstruction) or mechanical ileus (obstruction of bowel from hernia, adhesions, etc.)
2. **Ascites** (abnormal fluid accumulation in abdomen)
3. **Perforated hollow viscus** (such as bowel or stomach, evident by free intraperitoneal air)
4. **Intraabdominal mass** (neoplasms—benign or malignant)
5. **Post-op** (abdominal surgery)

Remember to **take erect images first** if patient comes to the department in an erect position.

Image Receptor, Collimation, and Shielding 35 × 43 cm (14 ×17 inches), moving or stationary grids; collimation and shielding the same as described on preceding pages

Patient and Part Positioning Note that most department routines for the erect abdomen include centering high to demonstrate possible free intraperitoneal air under the diaphragm even if a PA chest is included in the series.

Breathing Instructions Chest is taken on full inspiration; abdomen is taken on expiration.

Central Ray CR to level of iliac crest on supine, and about 5 cm (2 inches) above level of crest to include diaphragm on erect or decubitus.

Notes:
- **Left lateral decubitus** replaces erect position if the patient is too ill to stand.
- **Horizontal beam** is necessary to visualize air-fluid levels.
- Erect PA chest or AP erect abdomen best visualizes **free air under diaphragm.**
- For decubitus, patient should be upright or on the side for a minimum of **5 minutes** before exposure, **with 10 to 20 minutes** preferred to demonstrate potential small amounts of intraperitoneal air.

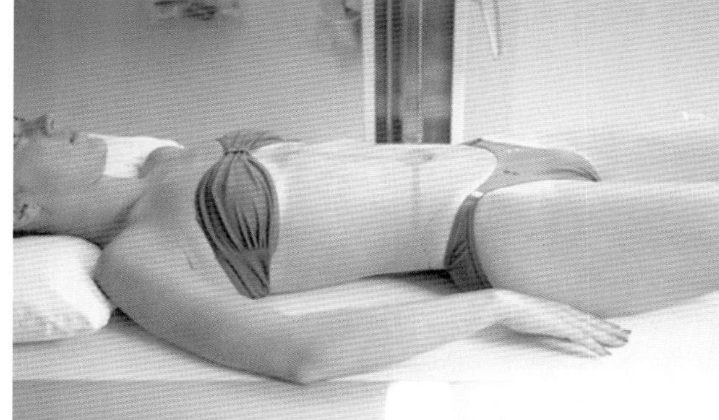

Fig. 4-44. AP supine.

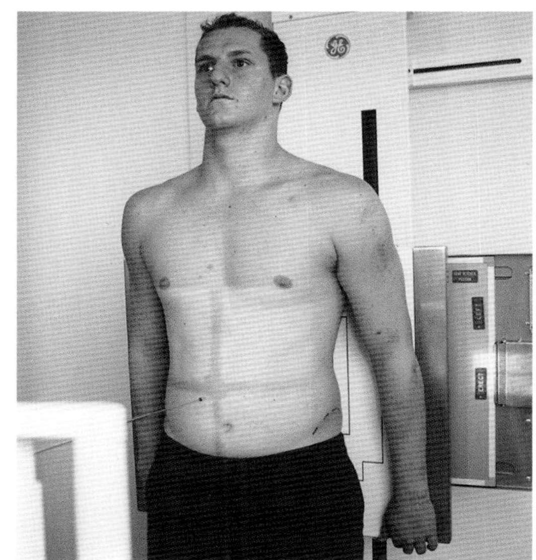

Fig. 4-45. AP erect.

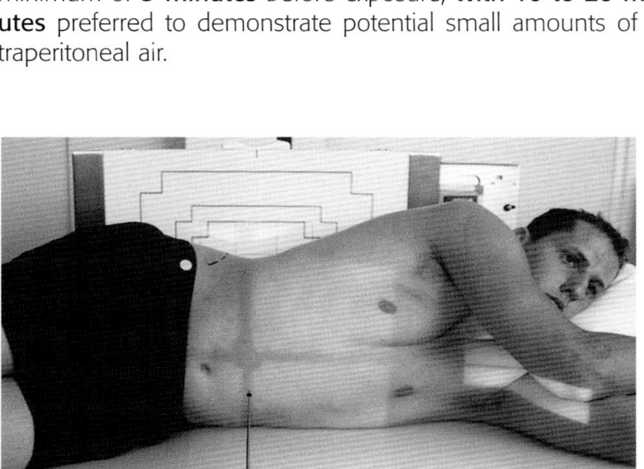

Fig. 4-46. Left lateral decubitus (special projection, if patient cannot stand for AP erect abdomen).

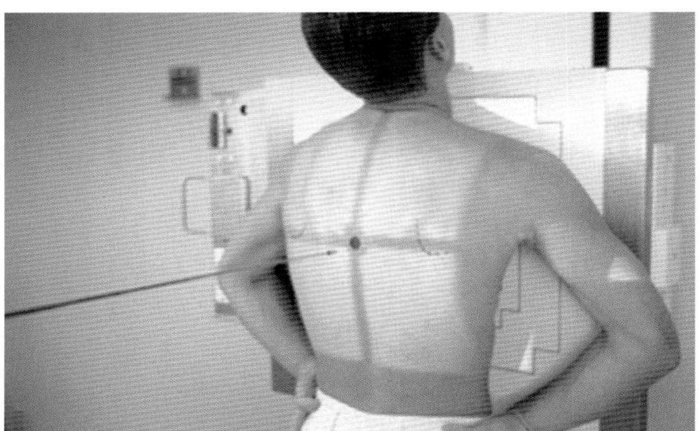

Fig. 4-47. PA chest erect.

RADIOGRAPHS FOR CRITIQUE

Each of the abdominal radiographs below demonstrates at least **one repeatable error.** These, as well as other radiographs for critique, are available as part of the accompanying audiovisuals. Together, these tools will provide a basis for classroom and/or positioning lab discussion on radiographic critique.

See whether you can critique each of these four radiographs below based on the categories as described in the textbook and as outlined on the right. As a starting critique exercise, place a check in each category that demonstrates a **repeatable error** for that radiograph.

Student workbooks provide more space for writing comments and complete critique answers for each of these radiographs. Answers are provided in Appendix B.

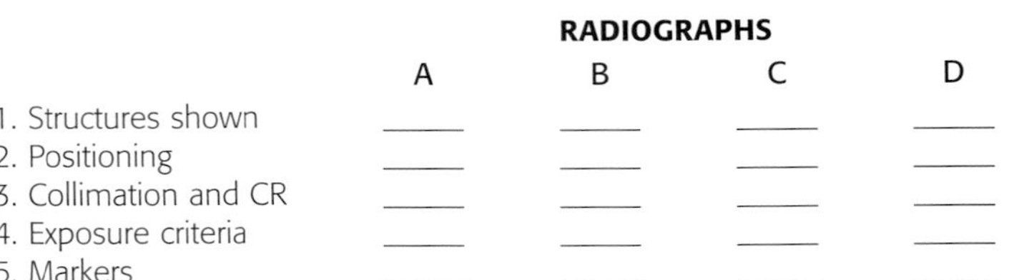

	RADIOGRAPHS			
	A	B	C	D
1. Structures shown	____	____	____	____
2. Positioning	____	____	____	____
3. Collimation and CR	____	____	____	____
4. Exposure criteria	____	____	____	____
5. Markers	____	____	____	____

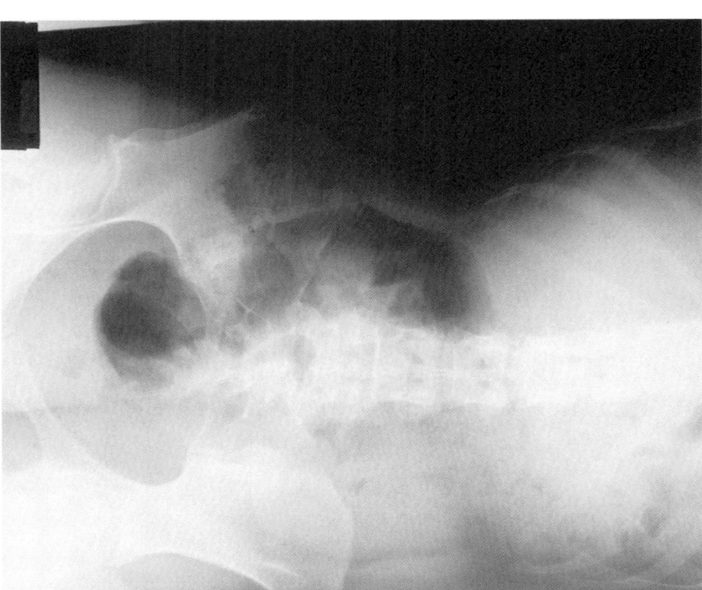

Fig. C4-48. Left lateral decubitus abdomen. A

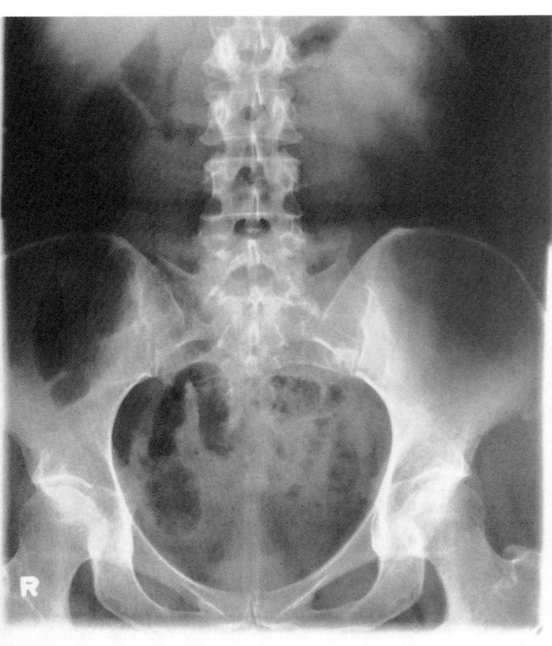

Fig. C4-49. AP supine abdomen—KUB. B

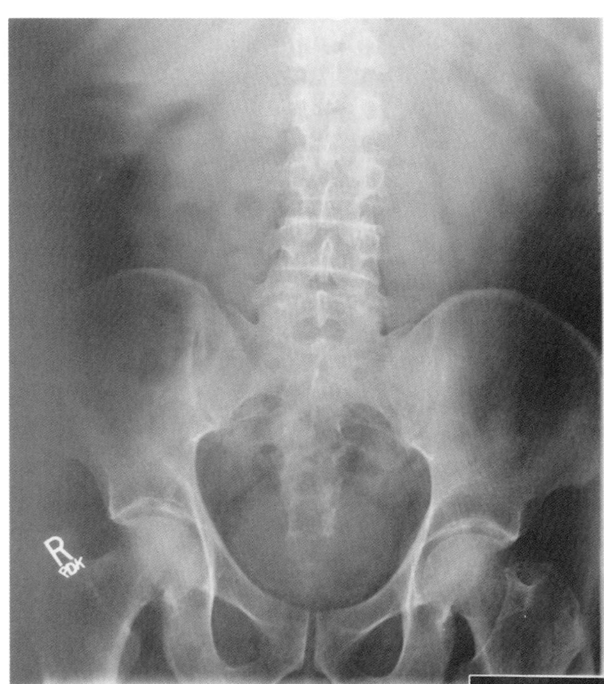

Fig. C4-50. AP supine abdomen. C

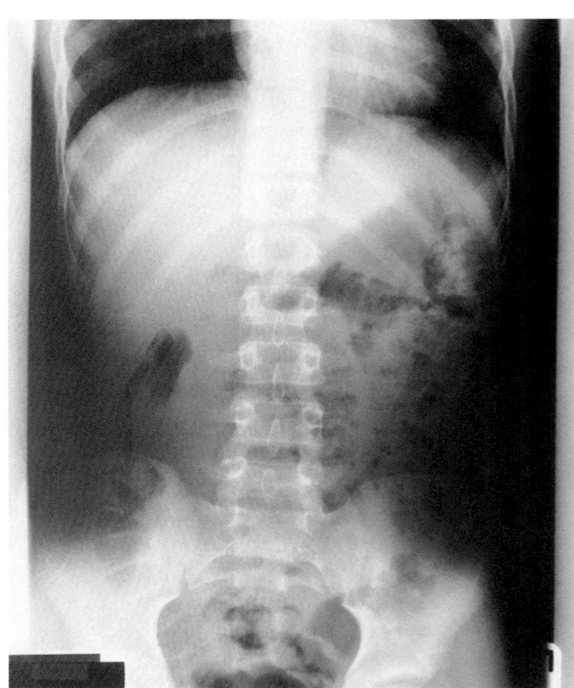

Fig. C4-51. AP erect abdomen. D

CHAPTER 5

Upper Limb

CONTRIBUTIONS BY **Nancy Johnson,** BA, RT(R)(CV)(CT)(QM)

CONTRIBUTORS TO PAST EDITIONS John P. Lampignano, MEd, RT(R)(CT), Kathy M. Martensen, BS, RT(R), Donna Davis, MEd, RT(R)(CV), Linda S. Lingar, MEd, RT(R)(M)

CONTENTS

RADIOGRAPHIC ANATOMY

Upper Limb (Extremity)

The bones of the upper limb can be divided into four main groups: (1) **hand and wrist,** (2) **forearm,** (3) **arm** (humerus), and (4) **shoulder girdle.** The first three groups are discussed in this chapter. The important wrist and elbow joints are included, but the shoulder joint and the proximal humerus are discussed in Chapter 6 with the shoulder girdle.

The shape and structure of each of the bones and the articulations, or joints, of the upper limb must be thoroughly understood by technologists so that each part can be identified and demonstrated on radiographs.

HAND AND WRIST

The 27 bones on each hand and wrist are divided into the following three groups:

1. Phalanges (fingers and thumb)	14
2. Metacarpals (palm)	5
3. Carpals (wrist)	8
TOTAL	27

The most distal bones of the hand are the **phalanges** *(fa-lan'-jez),* which comprise the digits (fingers and thumb). The second group of bones is the **metacarpals** *(met'ah-kar'pals);* these bones comprise the palm of each hand. The third group of bones, the **carpals** *(kar'pals),* consists of the bones of the wrist.

Phalanges—Fingers and Thumb (Digits)

Each finger and thumb is called a *digit,* and each digit consists of two or three separate small bones called *phalanges* (singular, **phalanx** *[fa'lanks]*). The digits are numbered, starting with the thumb as (1) one, and ending with the little finger as (5) five.

Each of the four fingers (digits two, three, four, and five) are composed of three phalanges: the **proximal, middle,** and **distal.** The thumb, or first digit, has just two phalanges: the **proximal** and **distal.**

Each phalanx consists of three parts: a distal rounded **head,** a **body** (shaft), and an expanded **base,** similar to that of the metacarpals.

Metacarpals (Palm)

The second group of bones of the hand, making up the palm, consists of the five **metacarpals.** These bones are numbered the same as the digits, with the first metacarpal being on the thumb, or lateral, side when the hand is in the anatomic position.

Each metacarpal is composed of three parts, similar to the phalanges. Distally the rounded portion is the **head.** The **body** (shaft) is the long curved portion; the anterior part is concave in shape, and the posterior, or dorsal, portion is convex. The **base** is the expanded proximal end, which articulates with associated carpals.

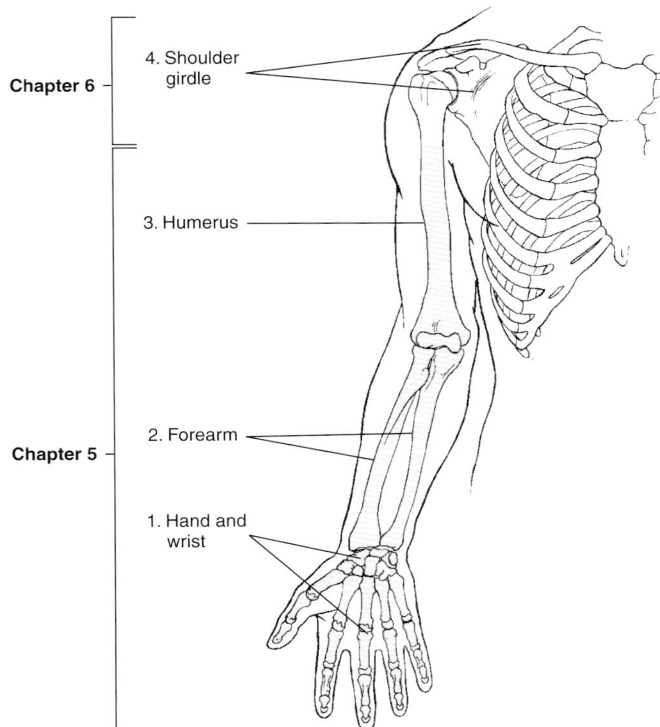

Fig. 5-1. Right upper limb (anterior view).

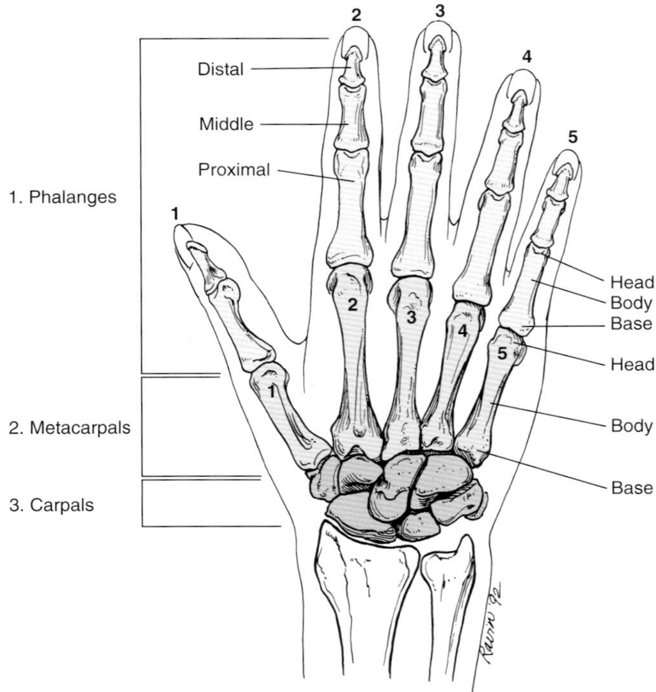

Fig. 5-2. Right hand and wrist (posterior view).

Joints of the Hand

The joints, or articulations, between the individual bones of the upper limb are important in radiology because small chip fractures may occur near the joint spaces. Therefore accurate identification of all joints of the phalanges and metacarpals of the hand is required.

Thumb (first digit) The thumb has only two phalanges, so the joint between them is called the **interphalangeal,** or **IP, joint.** The joint between the first metacarpal and the proximal phalanx of the thumb is called the **first metacarpophalangeal,** or **MCP, joint**. The name of this joint consists of the names of the two bones making up this joint. The proximal bone is named first, followed by the distal bone.

For radiographic purposes the first metacarpal is considered part of the thumb and must be included in its entirety in a radiograph of the thumb, **from the distal phalanx to the base of the first metacarpal.** This inclusion is not the case with the fingers, which for positioning purposes only include the three phalanges: the distal, middle, and proximal.

Fingers (second through fifth digits) The second through fifth digits each have three phalanges; therefore they also have three joints each. Starting from the most distal portion of each digit, the joints are the **distal interphalangeal,** or **DIP joint,** followed by the **proximal interphalangeal,** or **PIP, joint,** and most proximally, the **metacarpophalangeal,** or **MCP, joint.**

Metacarpals The metacarpals articulate with the phalanges at their distal ends and are called **metacarpophalangeal,** or **MCP, joints.** At the proximal end the metacarpals articulate with the respective carpals and are called **carpometacarpal,** or **CMC, joints.** The five metacarpals (MCs) articulate with specific carpals as follows:

- First MC with trapezium
- Second MC with trapezoid
- Third MC with capitate
- Fourth and 5th MC with hamate

REVIEW EXERCISE WITH RADIOGRAPH

In identifying joints and phalanges of the hand, it is important to remember that the specific digit and hand must be included in descriptions. A radiograph of a hand (Fig. 5-4) demonstrates the phalanges and metacarpals, as well as the joints described previously. A good review exercise is to cover up the answers listed below and identify each part labeled A through R on Fig. 5-4. Then check your answers against the following:

A. First carpometacarpal joint of right hand
B. First metacarpal of right hand
C. First metacarpophalangeal joint of right hand
D. Proximal phalanx of the first digit (or thumb) of right hand
E. Interphalangeal joint of first digit (or thumb) of right hand
F. Distal phalanx of first digit (or thumb) of right hand
G. Second metacarpophalangeal joint of right hand
H. Proximal phalanx of second digit of right hand
I. Proximal interphalangeal joint of second digit of right hand
J. Middle phalanx of second digit of right hand
K. Distal interphalangeal joint of second digit of right hand
L. Distal phalanx of second digit of right hand
M. Middle phalanx of fourth digit of right hand
N. Distal interphalangeal joint of fifth digit of right hand
O. Proximal phalanx of third digit of right hand
P. Fifth metacarpophalangeal joint of right hand
Q. Fourth metacarpal of right hand
R. Fifth carpometacarpal joint of right hand

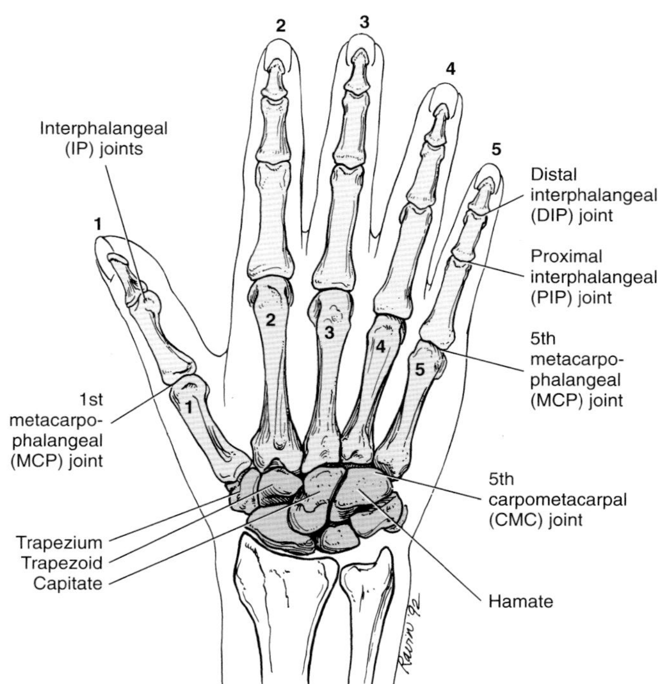

Fig. 5-3. Joints of right hand and wrist.

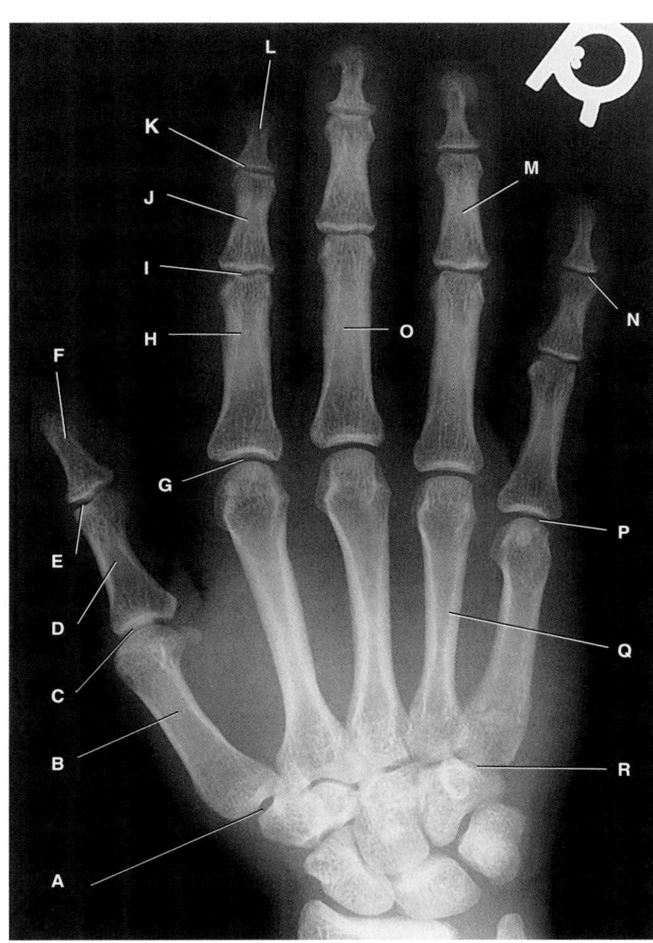

Fig. 5-4. PA radiograph of right hand.

5

Carpals (Wrist)

The third group of bones of the hand and wrist are the **carpals,** the bones of the wrist. Learning the names of the eight carpals is easiest when they are divided into two rows of four each.

Proximal row Beginning on the lateral, or thumb, side is the **scaphoid** *(skaf'oid),* sometimes referred to as the *navicular.* One of the tarsal bones of the foot is also sometimes called the *navicular* or *scaphoid.* However, the correct term for the tarsal bone of the **foot** is the **navicular,** and the carpal bone of the **wrist** is the **scaphoid.**

The scaphoid, a boat-shaped bone, is the largest bone in the proximal row and **articulates with the radius proximally.** Its location and articulation with the forearm make it important radiographically because it is **the most frequently fractured carpal bone.**

The **lunate** (moon-shaped) is the second carpal in the proximal row and **also articulates with the radius.** It is distinguished by the deep concavity on its distal surface, where it articulates with the capitate of the distal row of carpals (best seen on anterior view; see Fig. 5-6).

The **third** carpal is the **triquetrum** *(tri-kwe'trum),* which has three articular surfaces and is distinguished by its pyramidal shape and anterior articulation with the small pisiform.

The **pisiform** *(pi'si-form)* (pea-shaped) is the smallest of the carpal bones and is located anterior to the triquetrum, most evident in the carpal sulcus view (Fig. 5-7).

Distal row The second, more distal row of the four carpals articulates with the five metacarpal bones. Starting again on the lateral, or thumb, side is the **trapezium** *(trah-pe'ze-um),* a four-sided, somewhat irregularly shaped bone located between the scaphoid medially and the first metacarpal distally. The wedge-shaped **trapezoid** *(trap'e-zoid),* also four-sided, is the smallest bone in the distal row. This bone is followed by the largest of the carpal bones, the **capitate** *(kap'i-tat),* or *os magnum,* meaning "large bone." It also is identified by its large rounded head that fits proximally into a concavity formed by the scaphoid and lunate bones.

The last carpal in the distal row is the **hamate** *(ham'ate),* which is easily distinguished by the hooklike process called the **hamulus** *(ham'u-lus),* or hamular process, projecting from its palmar surface (see Fig. 5-7).

Carpal Sulcus (Canal or Tunnel View)

Fig. 5-7 is a drawing of the carpals as they would appear in a tangential view down the wrist and arm from the palm or volar side of a hyperextended wrist. This view demonstrates the carpal sulcus formed by the concave anterior or palmar aspect of the carpals. The anteriorly located pisiform and the hamulus process of the hamate are visualized best on this view. This concave area or groove is called the *carpal sulcus (carpal tunnel* or *canal),* through which major nerves and tendons pass.

The term *hamate* means hooked, describing the shape of the hamate in the illustration. The trapezium and its relationship to the thumb and trapezoid are well demonstrated.

Summary Chart of Carpal Terminology

The preferred terms as listed in the summary chart on the right are used throughout this text. Secondary terms listed as synonyms in the box are terms commonly used in earlier literature.

The names of these eight carpals may be remembered more easily by using a mnemonic (in which a sentence or phrase is formed using the first letter of each carpal). Two mnemonic samples are provided in the summary chart.

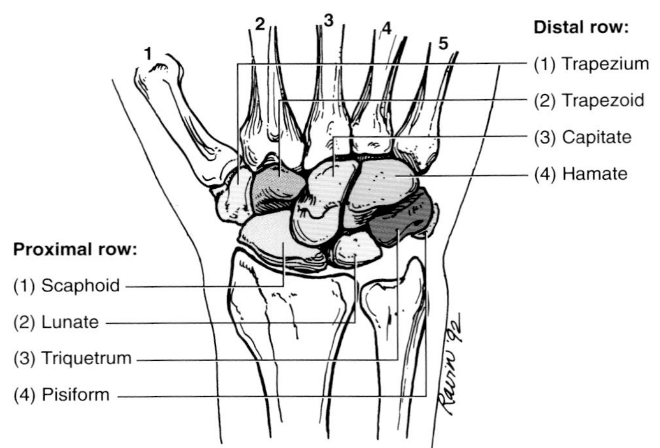

Fig. 5-5. Right carpals (dorsal or posterior view).

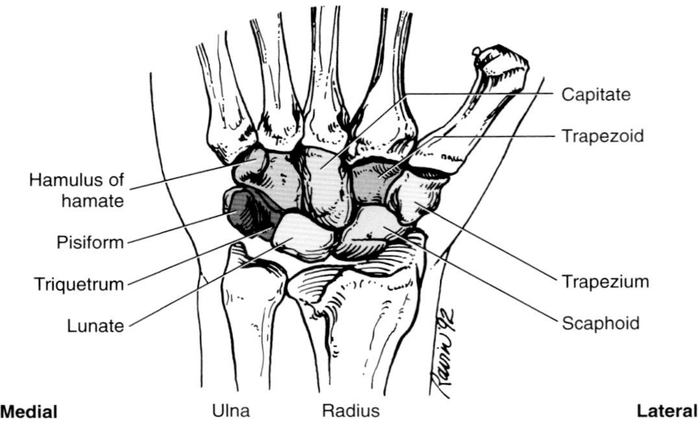

Fig. 5-6. Right carpals (palmar or anterior view).

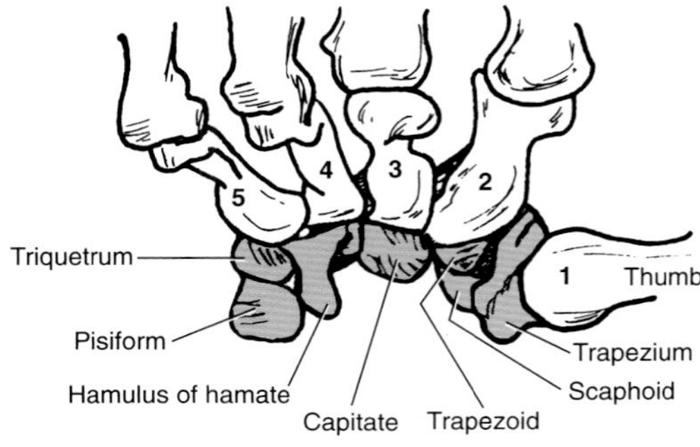

Fig. 5-7. Carpal sulcus (canal or tunnel view).

MNEMONICS, PREFERRED TERMS, AND SYNONYMS

MNEMONIC			PREFERRED TERM	SYNONYM
Send	or	Steve	Scaphoid	(Navicular)
Letter		Left	Lunate	(Semilunar)
To		The	Triquetrum	(Triangular or cuneiform)
Peter		Party	Pisiform	(None)
To		To	Trapezium	(Greater multangular)
Tell' em (to)		Take	Trapezoid	(Lesser multangular)
Come		Carol	Capitate	(Os magnum)
Home		Home	Hamate	(Unciform)

REVIEW EXERCISE WITH RADIOGRAPHS

Five projections for the wrist are shown in Figs. 5-8 through 5-12. A good review exercise is to cover the answers that follow and identify each carpal bone as labeled. Check your answers against those listed.

Note in the lateral position (see Fig. 5-12) that the trapezium *(E)* and scaphoid *(A)* are located more anteriorly. Note also that the ulnar deviation projection (Fig. 5-10) best demonstrates the scaphoid without the foreshortening and overlapping as seen on the PA (Fig. 5-8).

The radial deviation projection (Fig. 5-9) best demonstrates the interspaces and the carpals on the ulnar (lateral) side of the wrist, namely, the hamate *(H)*, triquetrum *(C)*, pisiform *(D)*, and lunate *(B)*. The outline of the end-on view of the hamulus process of the hamate *(h)* also can be seen on this radial deviation radiograph. The hamulus process also is demonstrated well on the carpal canal projection of Fig. 5-11, as is the hooklike process of *D* on the pisiform. Answers are as follows:

A. Scaphoid
B. Lunate
C. Triquetrum
D. Pisiform
E. Trapezium
F. Trapezoid
G. Capitate
H. Hamate
h. Hamulus (hamular process of hamate)

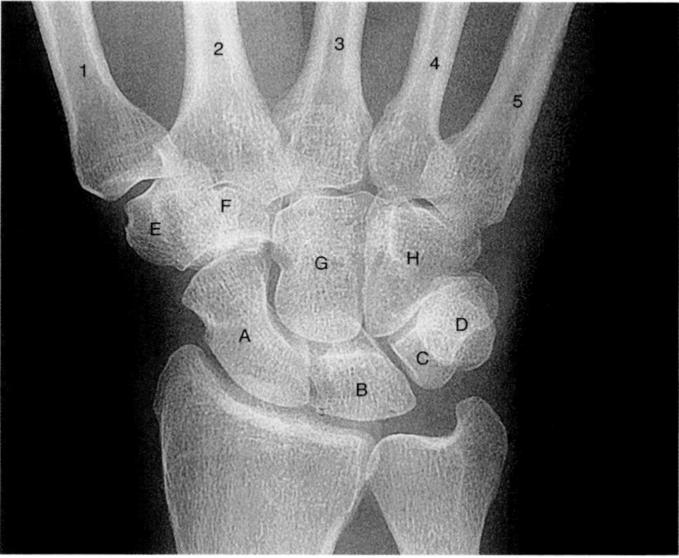

Fig. 5-8. PA wrist.

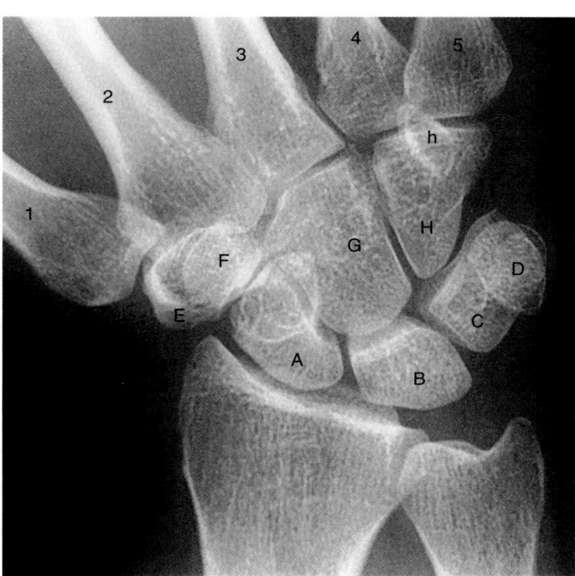

Fig. 5-9. Radial deviation.

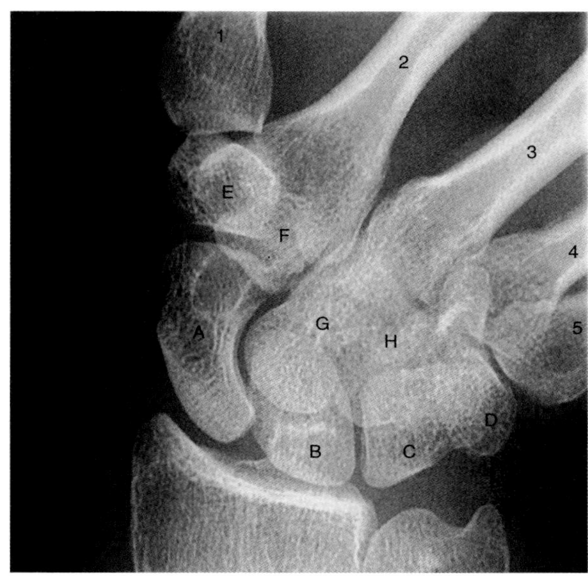

Fig. 5-10. Ulnar deviation (for scaphoid).

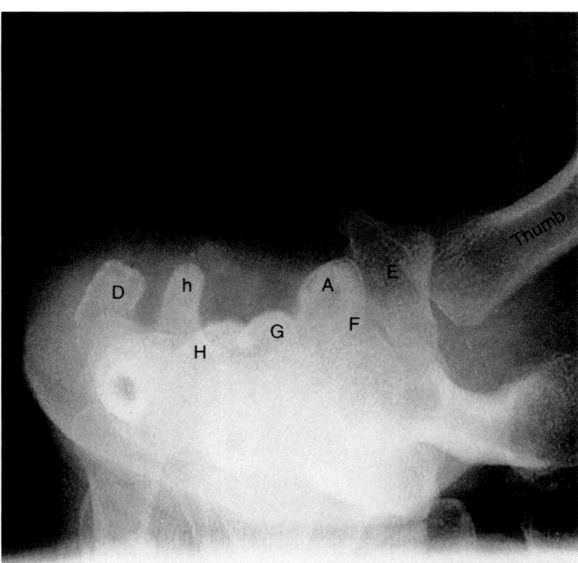

Fig. 5-11. Carpal canal. The scaphoid (A) is partially superimposed with the trapezoid (F) on this projection.

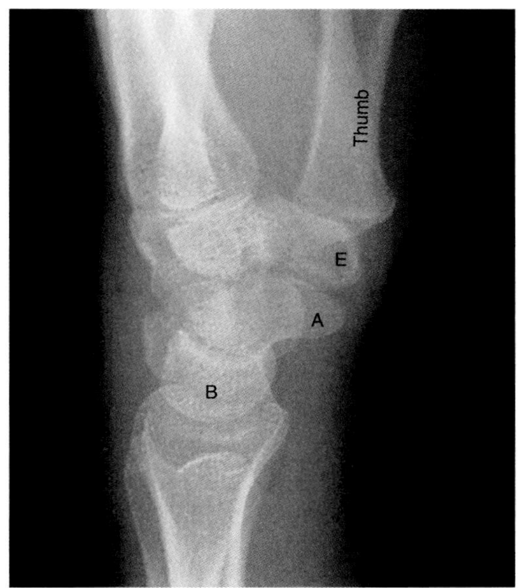

Fig. 5-12. Lateral.

5

FOREARM—RADIUS AND ULNA

The second group of upper-limb bones are those of the forearm, namely, the **radius** on the lateral or thumb side and the **ulna** on the medial side (Fig. 5-13).

The radius and ulna articulate with each other at the **proximal radioulnar joint** and at the **distal radioulnar joint,** as shown in Fig. 5-14. These two joints allow for the rotational movement of the wrist and hand, as described later in this chapter.

Radius and Ulna (Fig. 5-14)

Small conical projections, called **styloid processes,** are located at the extreme distal ends of both the radius and ulna. The radial styloid process can be palpated on the thumb side of the wrist joint. The radial styloid process extends more distally than does the ulnar styloid process.

The **ulnar notch** is a small depression on the medial aspect of the distal radius. The head of the ulna fits into the ulnar notch.

The **head of the ulna** is located near the wrist at the **distal** end of the ulna. When the hand is pronated, the ulnar head and styloid process are easily felt and seen on the "little finger" side of the distal forearm.

The **head of the radius** is located at the **proximal** end of the radius near the elbow joint. The long midportion of both the radius and the ulna is called the **body** *(shaft).*

The radius is the shorter of the two bones of the forearm and the only one of the two directly involved in the wrist joint. During the act of pronation the radius is the bone that rotates around the more stationary ulna.

The proximal radius demonstrates the round disklike **head** and the **neck** of the radius, a tapered constricted area directly below the head. The rough oval process on the medial and anterior side of the radius, just distal to the neck, is the **radial tuberosity.**

Proximal Ulna

The ulna is the longer of the two bones of the forearm and is primarily involved in the formation of the elbow joint. The two beaklike processes of the proximal ulna are called the **olecranon** and **coronoid processes** (Figs. 5-14 and 5-15). The olecranon process can be palpated easily on the posterior aspect of the elbow joint.

The medial margin of the coronoid process opposite the radial notch *(lateral)* is commonly referred to as the **coronoid tubercle** (see Fig. 5-14 and AP elbow radiograph in 5-19).

The large concave depression, or notch, articulating with the distal humerus is the **trochlear** *(trok'le-ar)* **notch** (semilunar notch). The small shallow depression located on the lateral aspect of the proximal ulna is the **radial** *(ra'de-al)* **notch.** The head of the radius articulates with the ulna at the radial notch. This joint, or articulation, is the proximal radioulnar joint that combines with the distal radioulnar joint to allow rotation of the forearm during pronation. During the act of pronation, the radius crosses over the ulna near the upper third of the forearm (see Fig. 5-25)

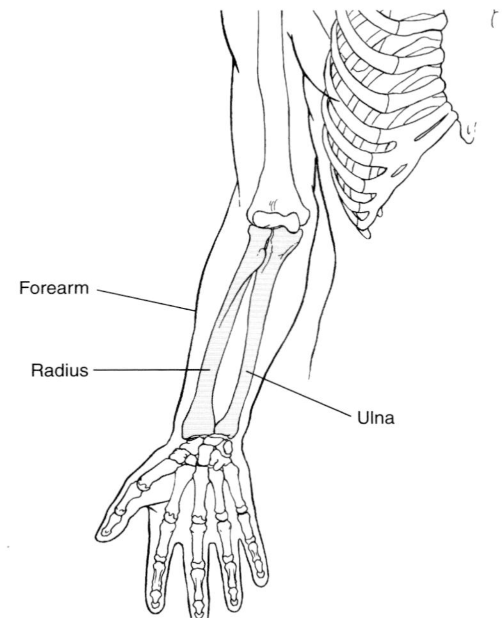

Fig. 5-13. Right upper limb (anterior view).

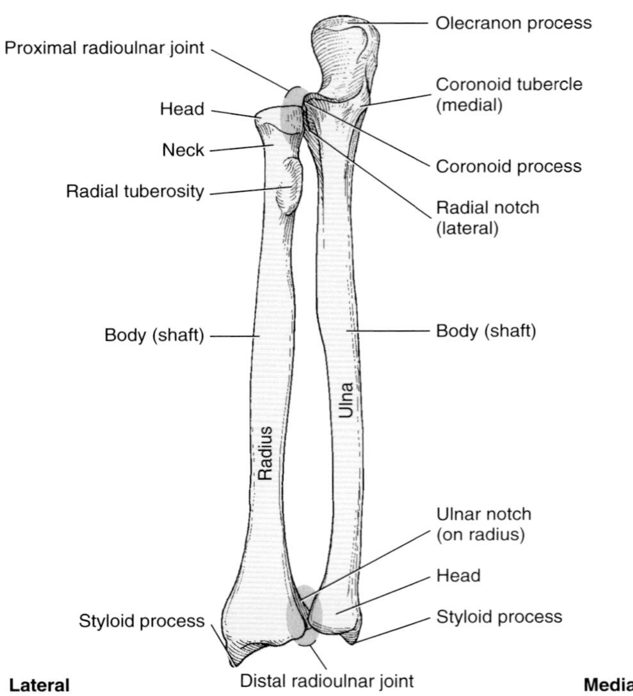

Fig. 5-14. Right radius and ulna (anterior view).

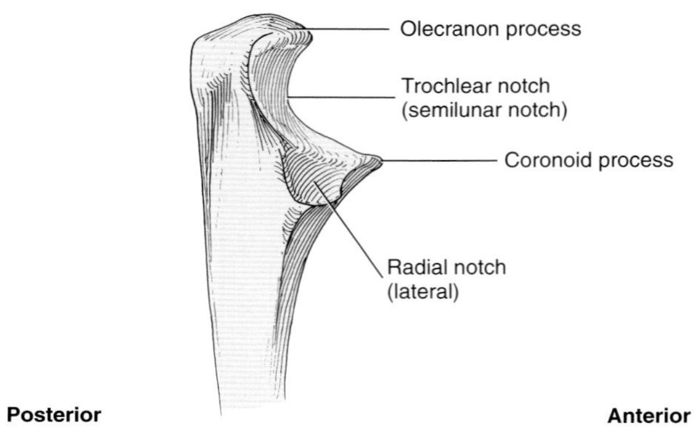

Fig. 5-15. Left proximal ulna (lateral view).

Distal Humerus

The parts of the proximal humerus are discussed in Chapter 6 with the shoulder girdle. However, the midhumerus and distal humerus are included in this chapter as part of the elbow joint.

The **body** (shaft) of the humerus is the long center section, and the expanded distal end of the humerus is the **humeral condyle.** The articular portion of the humeral condyle is divided into two parts: the **trochlea** *(trok'le-ah)* and the **capitulum** *(kah-pit'u-lum).*

The **trochlea** (meaning "pulley") is shaped like a pulley or spool, with two rimlike outer margins and a smooth depressed center portion called the **trochlear sulcus,** or *groove.* This depression of the trochlea, which continues inferiorly and posteriorly, appears circular on a lateral end-on view; on a lateral elbow radiograph, it appears as a less dense (more radiolucent) area (Figs. 5-17 and 5-20). The **trochlea** is located more medially and articulates with the **ulna.**

The **capitulum,** meaning "little head," is located on the lateral aspect and articulates with the head of the **radius.** (A memory aid is to associate the capitulum, "cap," with the "head" of the radius.) In earlier literature, the capitulum was called **capitellum** *(kap"i-tel'um).*

The articular surface making up the rounded articular margin of the capitulum is just slightly smaller than that of the trochlea (see Fig. 5-18). This structure becomes significant in evaluating for a true lateral position of the elbow, as does the direct superimposition of the two **epicondyles** *(ep"e-kon'dils).*

The **lateral epicondyle** is the small projection on the lateral aspect of the distal humerus above the capitulum. The **medial epicondyle** is larger and more prominent than the lateral and is located on the medial edge of the distal humerus. In a true lateral position the directly superimposed epicondyles (which are difficult to recognize) are seen as proximal to the circular appearance of the trochlear sulcus (Fig. 5-17).

The distal humerus has specific **depressions** on both the anterior and the posterior surfaces. The two shallow **anterior depressions** are the **coronoid fossa** and the **radial fossa** (Figs. 5-16 and 5-17). As the elbow is completely flexed, the coronoid process and the radial head are received by these respective fossae, as the names indicate.

The deep **posterior depression** of the distal humerus is the **olecranon fossa** (not specifically shown on these illustrations). The olecranon process of the ulna fits into this depression when the arm is fully extended. Soft-tissue detail by way of specific fat pads located within the deep olecranon fossa is important in trauma diagnosis of the elbow joint.

The lateral view of the elbow (Fig. 5-17) clearly demonstrates specific parts of the proximal radius and ulna. The **head** and **neck** of the radius are well demonstrated, as are the **radial tuberosity** (partially seen on the proximal radius) and the large concave **trochlear (semilunar) notch.**

True lateral elbow Specific positions, such as an **accurate lateral** with **90° flexion,** with possible associated visualization of fat pads, are essential for evaluation of joint pathology for the elbow.

A good criterion by which to evaluate a true lateral position of the elbow when it is flexed 90° is the appearance of the three concentric arcs, as labeled in Fig. 5-18. The first and smallest arc is the **trochlear sulcus.** The second, intermediate arc appears double-lined as the outer ridges or rounded edges of the **capitulum** and **trochlea.*** (The smaller is the capitulum, and the larger is the medial ridge of the trochlea.) The **trochlear notch of the ulna** appears as a third arc of a true lateral elbow. If the elbow is rotated even slightly from a **true** lateral, the arcs do not appear symmetrically aligned in this way, and the elbow joint space is not as open.

*Berquist TH: Imaging of orthopedic trauma and surgery, Philadelphia, 1986, WB Saunders (pp 583-584).

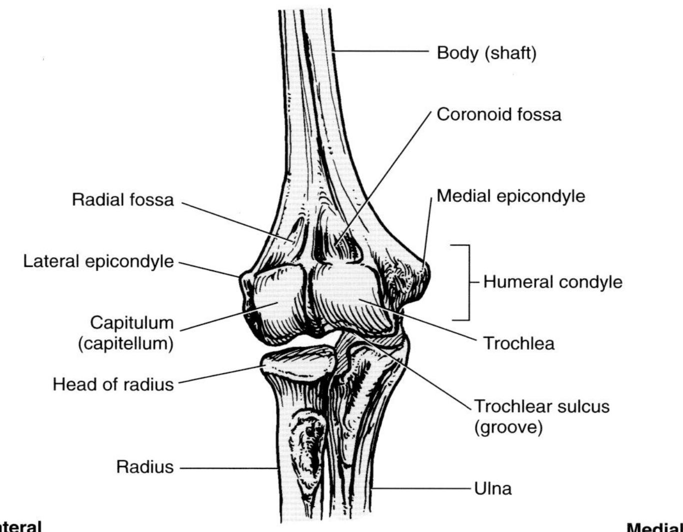

Fig. 5-16. Distal humerus (anterior view).

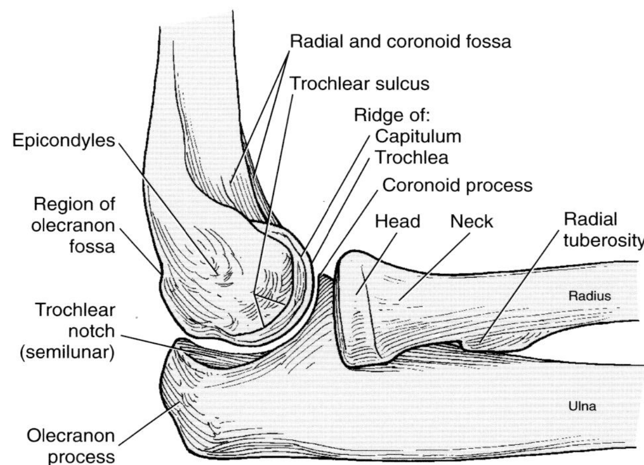

Fig. 5-17. Lateral elbow.

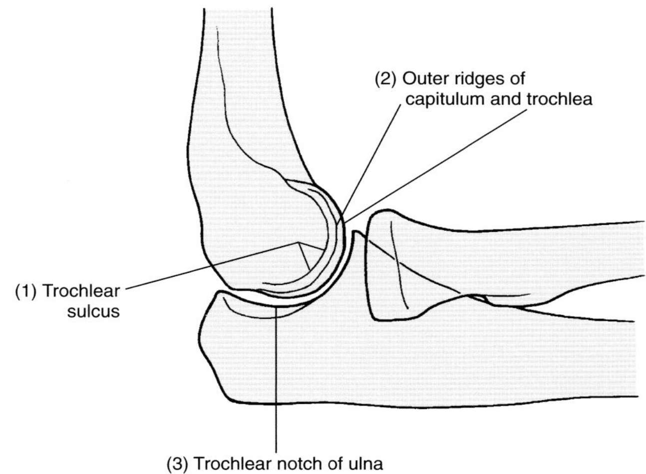

Fig. 5-18. True lateral elbow—three concentric arcs.

5

REVIEW EXERCISE WITH RADIOGRAPHS

These AP and lateral radiographs of the elbow provide a review of anatomy and demonstrate the three concentric arcs as evidence of a true lateral position (Figs. 5-19 and 5-20). Answers to the labels are as follows:

A. Medial epicondyle
B. Trochlea (medial aspect)
C. Coronoid tubercle
D. Radial head
E. Capitulum
F. Lateral epicondyle
G. Superimposed epicondyles of humerus
H. Olecranon process
I. Trochlear sulcus
J. Trochlear notch
K. Double outer ridges of capitulum and trochlea (capitulum being the smaller of the two areas and trochlea the larger)
L. Coronoid process of ulna
M. Radial head
N. Radial neck
O. Radial tuberosity

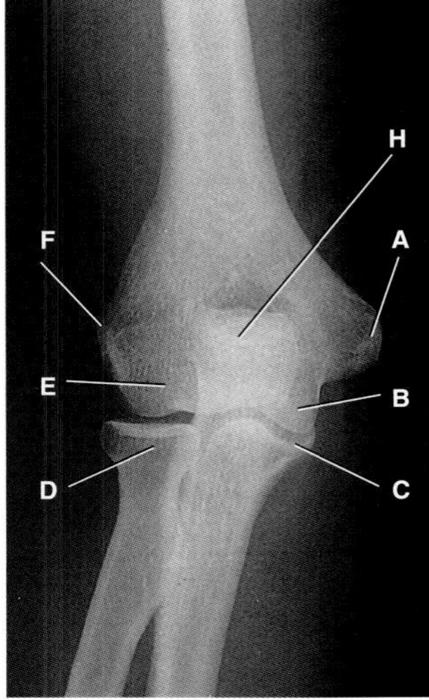

Fig. 5-19. AP.

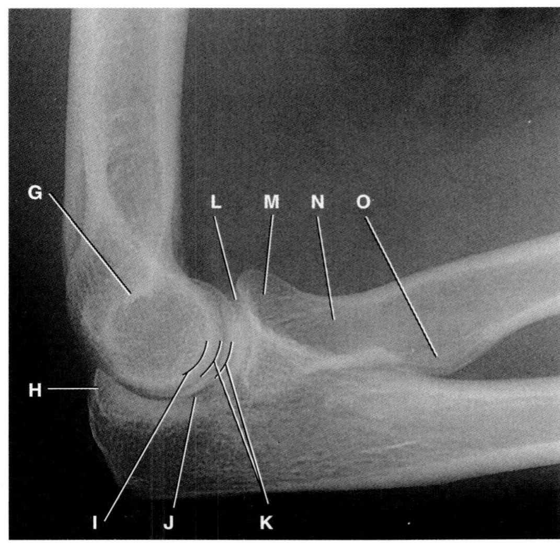

Fig. 5-20. Lateral.

CLASSIFICATION OF JOINTS

A general description of joints or articulations with the various classifications and movement types is provided in Chapter 1. These classifications are reviewed and described here more specifically, for each joint of the hand, wrist, forearm, and elbow.

All joints of the upper limb as described in this chapter are classified as **synovial** and therefore are freely movable, or **diarthrodial.** Only the movement types differ.

Hand and Wrist (Fig. 5-21)

Interphalangeal (IP) joints Beginning distally with the phalanges, all IP joints are **ginglymus,** or **hinge-type,** joints with movements in two directions only—**flexion** and **extension.** This movement is in one plane only, around the transverse axis. This includes the single IP joint of the thumb (first digit) and the distal and proximal IP joints of the fingers (second to fifth digits).

Metacarpophalangeal (MCP) joints The MCP joints are **ellipsoidal,** or **condyloid-type,** joints that allow movement in four directions: **flexion, extension, abduction,** and **adduction. Circumduction** movement also occurs at these joints, which is a conelike sequential movement in these four directions.

The first MCP joint (thumb) is also generally classified as an ellipsoidal or condyloid joint, although it has very limited abduction and adduction movements due to the wider and less-rounded head of the first metacarpal.

Carpometacarpal (CMC) joints The first CMC joint of the thumb is a **sellar,** or **saddle-type,** joint. This joint best demonstrates the shape and movements of a saddle joint, which allows a great range of movement, including **flexion, extension, abduction, adduction, circumduction, opposition,** and some degree of **rotation.**

The second through fifth CMC joints are **plane,** or **gliding-type,** joints, which allow the least amount of movement of the synovial class joints. The joint surfaces are flat or slightly curved, with movement limited by a tight fibrous capsule.

Intercarpal joints The intercarpal joints between the various carpals also only have a **plane,** or **gliding-type,** movement.

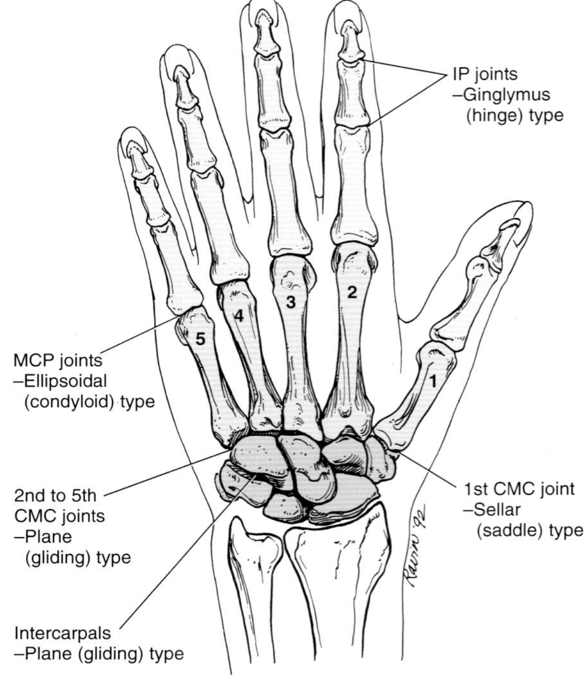

Fig. 5-21. Joints of left hand and wrist (posterior view).

5

Wrist Joint

The wrist joint is an **ellipsoidal,** or **condyloid-type,** joint and is freely movable, or **diarthrodial,** of the **synovial classification.** Of the two bones of the forearm, only the radius articulates directly with two carpal bones, the **scaphoid** and **lunate.** This wrist joint is called the ***radiocarpal joint.***

The **triquetral** bone, however, is also part of the wrist joint in that it is opposite the **articular disk.** The articular disk is part of the total wrist articulation, including a joint between the distal radius and ulna of the forearm, called the ***distal radioulnar joint.***

The articular surface of the distal radius, along with the total articular disk, forms a smooth, concave-shaped articulation with the three carpals to form the complete wrist joint.

The total wrist joint is enclosed by an articular synovial capsule strengthened by ligaments that allow movements in four directions, plus circumduction.

The synovial membrane lines the inner surfaces of these four wrist ligaments in addition to lining the distal end of the radius and the articular surfaces of the adjoining carpal bones.

Wrist ligaments The wrist has numerous important ligaments that stabilize the wrist joint. Two of these are shown in the drawing in Fig. 5-22. The **ulnar collateral ligament** is attached to the styloid process of the ulna and fans out to attach to the triquetrum and the pisiform. The **radial collateral ligament** extends from the styloid process of the radius primarily to the lateral side of the scaphoid, but it also has attachments to the trapezium.

Five additional ligaments not shown on this drawing are crucial to the stability of the wrist joint and are often damaged during trauma. These five ligaments are commonly imaged with conventional arthrography or MRI:

- Dorsal radiocarpal ligament
- Palmar radiocarpal ligament
- Triangular fibrocartilage complex (TFCC)
- Scapholunate ligament
- Lunotriquetral ligament

Elbow Joint

The elbow joint is also of the **synovial classification** and is thus freely movable, or **diarthrodial.** The elbow joint is generally considered a **ginglymus** (hinge) type of joint with flexion and extension movements between the humerus and the ulna and radius. The complete elbow joint, however, includes three joints enclosed in one articular capsule. In addition to the hinge joints between the humerus and ulna and the humerus and radius, the **proximal radioulnar joint** (trochoidal, or pivot-type) also is considered part of the elbow joint.

The following pages in this chapter discuss the importance of accurate lateral positioning of the elbow for visualization of certain fat pads within the elbow joint.

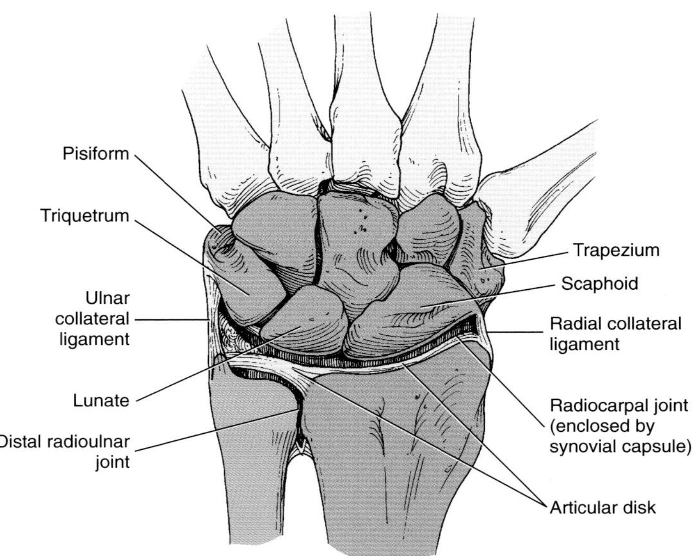

Fig. 5-22. Left wrist joint with articular disk (posterior view).

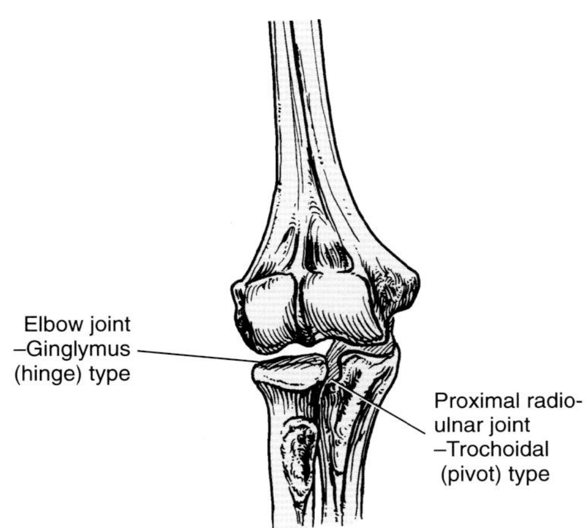

Fig. 5-23. Elbow joint.

SUMMARY OF HAND, WRIST, FOREARM, AND ELBOW JOINTS

Classification: *Synovial* (articular capsule containing synovial fluid)

Mobility Type: *Diarthrodial* **(freely movable)**

Movement Type:

1. Interphalangeal joints	-***Ginglymus*** (hinge)
2. Metacarpophalangeal joints	-***Ellipsoidal*** (condyloid)
3. Carpometacarpal joints:	
First digit (thumb)	-***Sellar*** (saddle)
Second–fifth digits	-***Plane*** (gliding)
4. Intercarpal joints	-***Plane*** (gliding)
5. Wrist (radiocarpal) joint	-***Ellipsoidal*** (condyloid)
6. Proximal: radioulnar joint	-***Trochoidal*** (pivot)
7. Elbow joint:	
Humeroulnar and humeroradial	-***Ginglymus*** (hinge)
Proximal radioulnar	-***Trochoidal*** (pivot)

WRIST JOINT MOVEMENT TERMINOLOGY

Certain terminology involving movements of the wrist joint may be confusing but must be understood by technologists, because special projections of the wrist are described by these movements.

These terms were described in Chapter 1 as turning or bending the hand and wrist from its natural position toward the ulna side for **ulnar deviation** and toward the radius for **radial deviation.**

Ulnar deviation (special **scaphoid** projection): The ulnar deviation movement of the wrist "opens up" and best demonstrates the carpals on the opposite side (the radial side) of the wrist, namely, the scaphoid, trapezium, and trapezoid. Because the scaphoid is the most frequently fractured carpal bone, this ulnar-deviation projection is commonly known as a *special scaphoid projection* or *view.*

Radial deviation*:* A less frequent PA wrist projection involves the radial-deviation movement that opens and best demonstrates the carpals on the opposite, or the ulnar side, of the wrist, namely, the hamate, pisiform, triquetrum, and lunate.

Note: See Chapter 1, p. 25, for additional explanations of these terms that traditionally in positioning reference books, including some previous editions of this textbook, were called *ulnar flexion* and *radial flexion,* respectively.

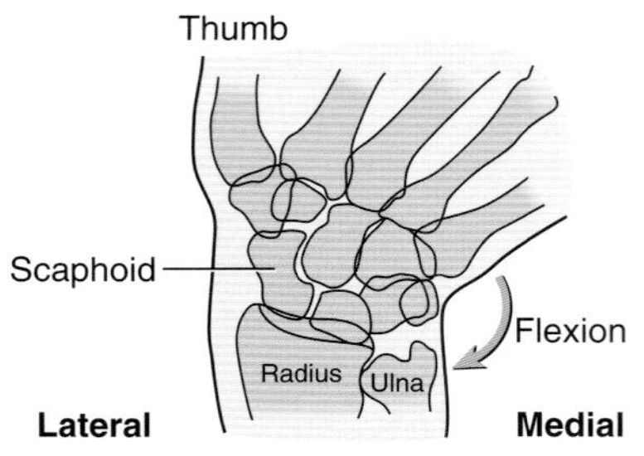

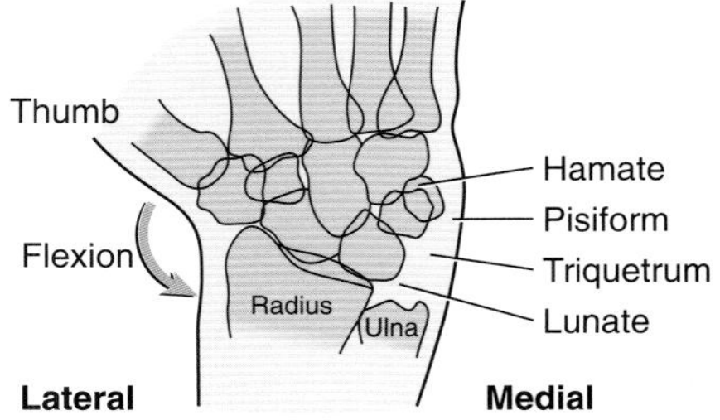

Fig. 5-24. Wrist movements.

FOREARM ROTATIONAL MOVEMENTS

The radioulnar joints of the forearm also involve some special rotational movements that must be understood in radiographing the forearm. For example, the **forearm generally should not be radiographed in a pronated position (a PA projection),** which may appear to be the most natural position for the forearm and hand. The forearm routinely should be radiographed in an **AP projection** with the hand **supinated,** or palm up. The reason becomes clear in studying the "cross-over" position of the radius and ulna when the hand is pronated (Fig. 5-25). This cross-over results from the unique pivot-type rotational movements of the forearm involving both the proximal and the distal radioulnar joints.

Summary: To prevent superimposition of the radius and ulna resulting from these pivot-type rotational movements, the forearm is radiographed with the **hand supinated** for an **AP projection.**

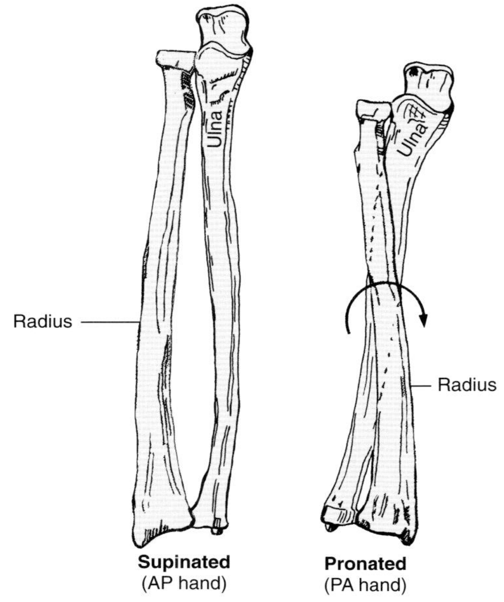

Fig. 5-25. Forearm rotational movements.

ELBOW ROTATIONAL MOVEMENTS

The appearance of the proximal radius and ulna changes as the elbow and distal humerus is rotated or obliqued either medially or laterally as shown with these radiographs. Note that on the AP radiograph with no rotation, the proximal radius is superimposed only slightly by the ulna (Fig. 5-26).

The radius and ulna can be separated with lateral rotation of the elbow, as shown on Fig. 5-27, whereas medial rotation completely superimposes them, as seen in Fig. 5-28. This relationship is crucial in critiques of AP projections of the elbow; **lateral rotation separates** the radius and ulna and **medial rotation superimposes.** (This concept is demonstrated further with the oblique elbow projections on pp. 170 and 171.)

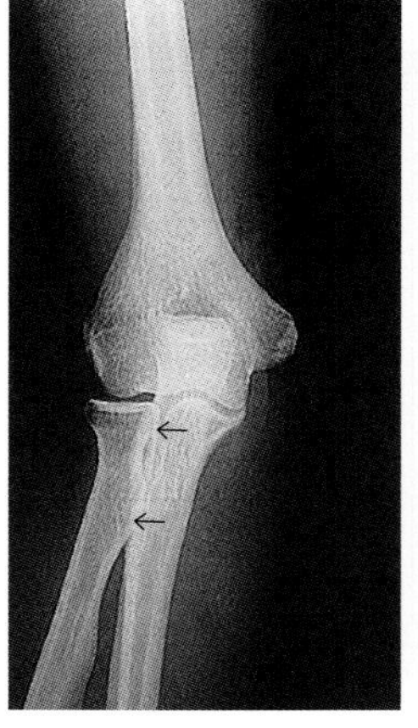

Fig. 5-26. AP, **no rotation**—radius and ulna partially superimposed.

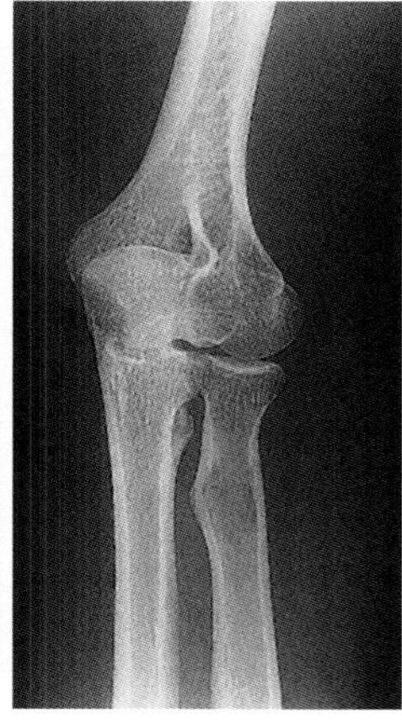

Fig. 5-27. AP, **lateral rotation**—separation of radius and ulna.

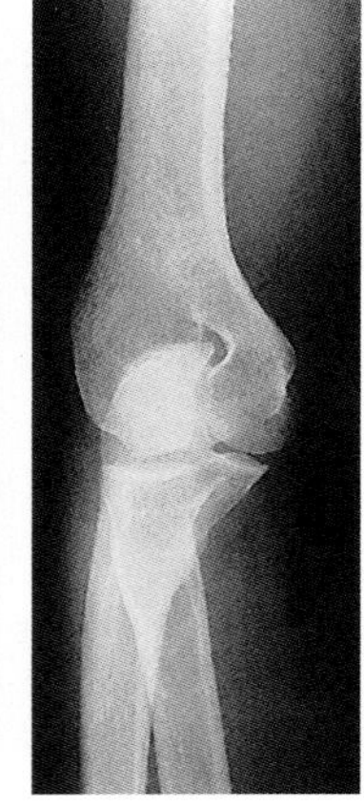

Fig. 5-28. AP, **medial rotation**—superimposed radius and ulna.

5

IMPORTANCE OF VISUALIZING FAT PADS

Radiographs of the upper and lower limbs are taken not only to evaluate for disease or trauma to bony structures but also to evaluate associated soft tissues, such as certain accumulations of fat called ***fat pads, fat bands,*** or ***stripes.*** In some cases the displacement of an adjoining fat pad or band may be the only indication of disease or significant injury or fracture within a joint region.

For diagnostic purposes the most important fat pads or bands are those located around certain joints of the upper and lower limbs. These fat pads are extrasynovial (outside the synovial sac) but are located within the joint capsule. Therefore any changes within the capsule itself alter the normal position and shape of the fat pads. Most often such changes are a result of fluid accumulation (effusion) within the joint, indicating the presence of an injury involving that joint.

The radiolucent fat pads are seen as densities that are slightly more lucent than surrounding structures. Fat pads and their surrounding soft tissue are of only slightly different density, making them difficult to visualize on radiographs. This visualization requires long-scale contrast techniques with optimum exposure or density to visualize these soft-tissue structures. (They generally are not visible on printed radiographs without enhancement, as shown on the illustrations on this page.)

Wrist Joint*

The wrist joint includes two important fat stripes. First, a **scaphoid fat stripe (A)** is visualized on the PA and the oblique views. It is elongated and slightly convex in shape and is located between the radial collateral ligament and adjoining muscle tendons immediately lateral to the scaphoid (Fig. 5-29). The absence or displacement of this fat stripe may be the only indicator of a fracture on the radial aspect of the wrist.

A second fat stripe is visualized on the lateral view of the wrist. This **pronator fat stripe (B)** is normally visualized approximately 1 centimeter ($^4/_{10}$ inch) from the anterior surface of the radius (Fig. 5-31). Subtle fractures of the distal radius can be indicated by the displacement or obliteration of the plane of this fat stripe.

Elbow Joint*†

The three significant fat pads or stripes of the elbow are visualized only on the lateral projection. They are not seen on the AP because of their superimposition over the bony structures. On the lateral view the **anterior fat pad (C),** which is formed by the superimposed coronoid and radial pads, is seen as slightly radiolucent teardrop shapes located just anterior to the distal humerus (Fig. 5-32). Trauma or infection can cause the anterior fat pad to be elevated and more visible and distorted in shape. This is visible only on a lateral elbow flexed 90°.

The **posterior fat pad (D)** is located deep within the olecranon fossa and is normally **not visible** on a negative elbow exam. The visualization of this fat pad, on a 90° flexed lateral elbow radiograph, indicates that a change within the joint has caused its position to change, suggesting the presence of a joint pathologic process.

To ensure an accurate diagnosis, the elbow **must be flexed 90°** on the lateral view. If the elbow is extended beyond the 90° flexed position, the olecranon slides into the olecranon fossa, elevates the posterior fat pad, and causes it to appear. In this situation the pad is visible whether the exam is negative or positive. Generally, visualization of the posterior fat pad is considered more reliable than that of the anterior fat pads.

The **supinator fat stripe (E)** is a long thin stripe just anterior to the proximal radius. It can be used to indicate the diagnosis of nonobvious radial head or neck fractures.

In summary, for the anterior and posterior fat pads to be useful diagnostic indicators on the lateral elbow, the elbow must be (1) **flexed 90°,** (2) in a **true lateral position,** and (3) **optimum exposure techniques,** including soft tissue detail to visualize fat pads, must be used.

*McQuillen-Martensen K: Radiographic critique, Philadelphia, 1996, WB Saunders.
†Griswold R: Elbow fat pads: a radiography perspective, Radiol Technol 53:303-307, 1982.

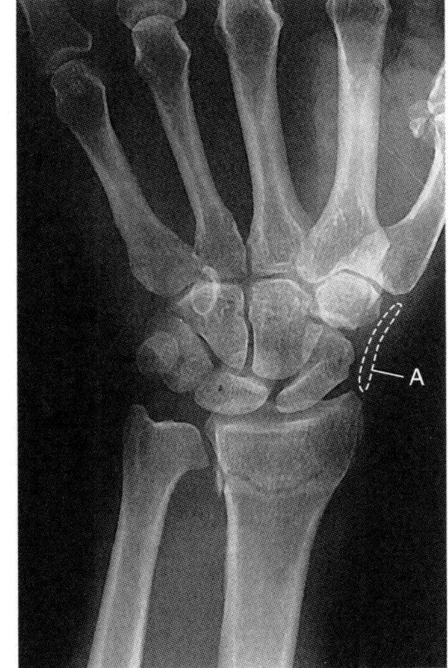

Fig. 5-29. PA wrist—**scaphoid fat band (A).**

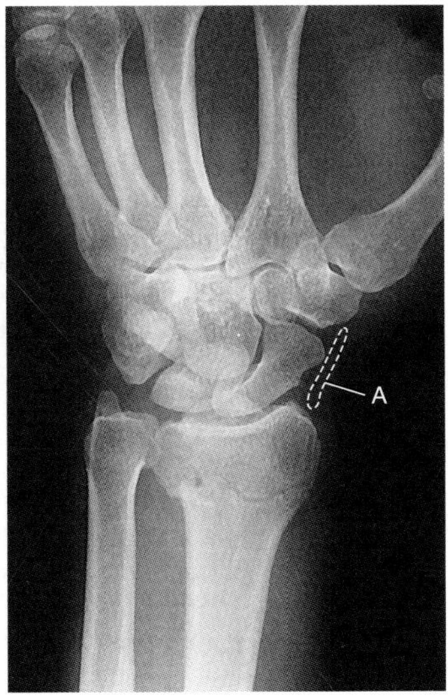

Fig. 5-30. Oblique wrist—**scaphoid fat band (A).**

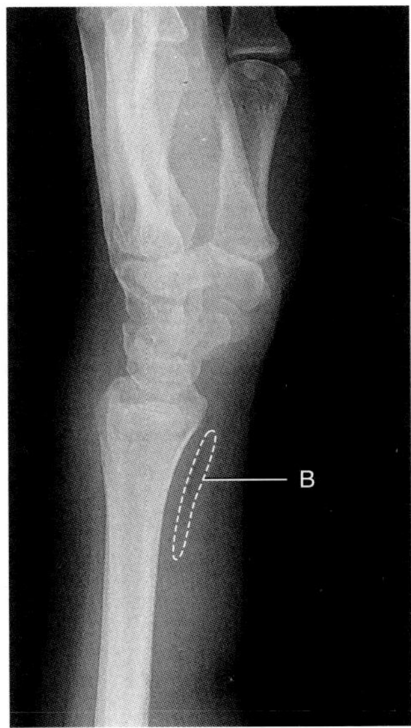

Fig. 5-31. Lateral wrist view—**pronator fat stripe (B).**

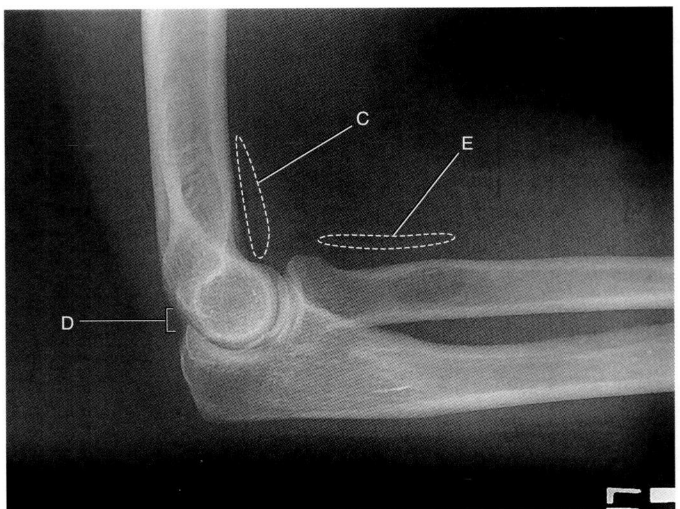

Fig. 5-32. Lateral elbow (anterior and posterior fat pads), as follows:
- **Anterior fat pad (C)**
- **Posterior fat pad (D),** not visible
- **Supinator fat stripe (E)**

RADIOGRAPHIC POSITIONING

General Positioning Considerations

Radiographic examinations involving the upper limb on ambulatory patients are generally done with the patient seated sideways at the end of the table in a position that is neither strained nor uncomfortable (Fig. 5-33). An extended tabletop may make this position more comfortable, especially if the patient is in a wheelchair. The patient also should be moved away from the x-ray beam from the region of scatter radiation as much as possible. The height of the tabletop should be near shoulder height so that the arm can be fully supported, as shown.

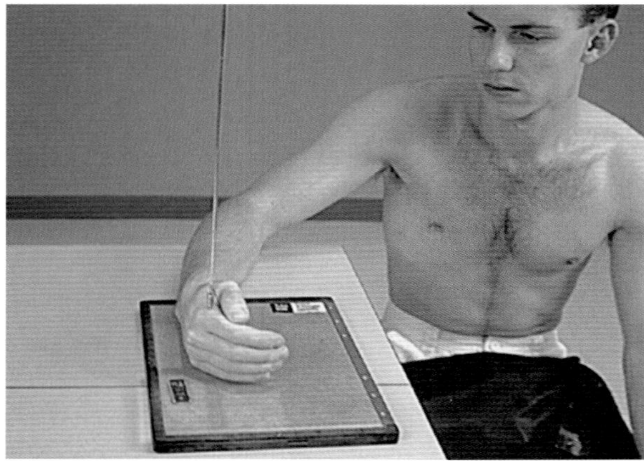

Fig. 5-33. Ambulatory patient—lateral hand (lead shield across lap covering gonads).

Gonadal Shielding

Gonadal shielding is important for exams of the upper limb because of the proximity of the gonads to the divergent x-ray beam and scatter radiation, a risk for those patients seated at the end of the table, as well as for trauma patients taken on a cart. Therefore a lead, vinyl-covered shield should be draped over the patient's lap or gonadal area. Even though the gonadal rule states that this action should be done on patients of reproductive age when the gonads lie within or close to the primary field, a good practice is to provide gonadal shielding for all patients.

Distance

A common minimum source image receptor distance (SID) is 40 inches, or 100 cm. When radiographs are taken with IRs directly on the tabletop, to maintain a constant SID, the tube height must be increased as compared with radiographs taken with the IR in the Bucky tray. This difference is generally 3 to 4 inches (8 to 10 cm) for floating-type tabletops.

Trauma Patients

Trauma patients can be radiographed on the table or taken directly on the cart, as shown in Fig. 5-34. The patient should be moved to one side to provide the necessary space on the cart for the cassette.

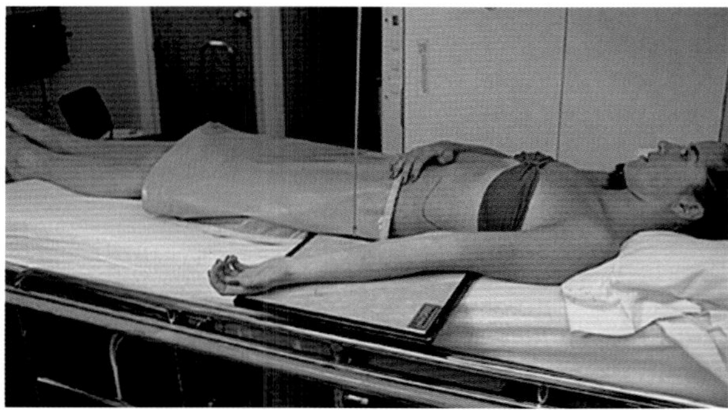

Fig. 5-34. Trauma patient—AP forearm.

Pediatric Patients

Patient motion plays an important role in pediatric radiography. Immobilization is needed in many cases to assist children in maintaining the proper position. Sponges and tape are useful, but sandbags should be used with caution because of their weight. Parents are frequently asked to assist with the radiographic examinations of their children. If parents are permitted in the radiography room during the exposure, proper shielding must be provided.

Also important is for the technologist to speak to the child in a soothing manner and with language the child can readily understand to ensure maximal cooperation. (See Chapter 20 for more detailed explanations regarding upper-limb radiography of young pediatric patients.)

Geriatric Patients

Providing **clear and complete instructions** with elderly patients is essential. Routine upper-limb examinations may need to be altered to accommodate the older patient's physical condition. Geriatric patients may have more difficulty in holding some of the strenuous positions required, so ensure that adequate immobilization is used to prevent movement during the exposure. Radiographic exposure technique may need to be reduced because of certain destructive pathologies commonly seen in the elderly, such as osteoporosis.

Exposure Factors

The principal exposure factors for images of the upper limbs are as follows:

1. Lower to medium kV (50-70)
2. Short exposure time
3. Small focal spot
4. Adequate mAs for sufficient density

Correctly exposed images of the upper limbs should demonstrate soft-tissue margins for fat pad visualization and fine trabecular markings of all bones being radiographed.

Cassettes

With conventional film-screen imaging, cassettes with detail-intensifying screens are generally used for adult extremities to achieve optimal recorded detail. Grids are not used for the upper limbs unless the body part (such as the shoulder) measures more than 10 cm. (Some references suggest a grid for more than 13 cm.)

Increase Exposure With Cast

An upper limb with a cast requires an increase in exposure. The increase depends on the thickness and type of cast, as outlined in the following table:

CAST CONVERSION CHART

TYPE OF CAST	INCREASE IN EXPOSURE
Small to medium plaster cast	Increase mAs 50%-60% or +5-7 kV
Large plaster cast	Increase mAs 100% or +8-10 kV
Fiberglass cast	Increase mAs 25%-30% or +3-4 kV

5

Collimation, General Positioning, and Markers

Again, the collimation rule should be followed: **collimation borders should be visible on all four sides if the IR is large enough to allow it without cutting off essential anatomy.**

A general rule concerning IR size is to use the smallest receptor size possible for the specific part being imaged. Four-sided collimation is generally possible, however, even with a minimal size IR for most, if not all, radiographic exams of the upper limb.

Two or more projections may be taken on one IR, but this requires close collimation. **Lead masks** placed on top of the IR are also recommended to help prevent exposure from scatter and secondary radiation from the adjacent exposure.

A general positioning rule especially applicable to the upper limbs is to **always place the long axis of the part being imaged parallel to the long axis of that portion of the IR being exposed.** Also, **all body parts should be oriented in the same direction** when two or more projections are taken on the same IR.

Patient ID information and side markers within the collimation borders must be demonstrated on each image. The patient ID blocker on the cassette should always be placed in the **corner least likely to superimpose essential anatomy.**

Correct Centering

Accurate centering and alignment of the body part to the receptor and central ray are important for exams of the upper limb, where shape and size distortion must be avoided and the narrow joint spaces clearly demonstrated. Therefore the following three positioning principles should be remembered for upper limb exams:

1. Part should be **parallel to plane of IR.**
2. CR should be **90° or perpendicular to part and IR,** unless a specific CR angle is indicated.
3. CR should be directed to **correct centering point.**

Digital Imaging Considerations

The following guidelines should be followed when upper limb images are acquired using digital imaging technology (CR or DR).

1. **Collimation:** In addition to the obvious benefit of reducing radiation dose to the patient, collimation that is closely restricted to the part being examined is key in ensuring that the image processed by the computer is of optimal quality. Close collimation also allows the computer to provide accurate information regarding the exposure index number.
2. **30% rule:** Most CR systems require that at least 30% of the image plate be exposed to obtain an accurate exposure index value. Images smaller than this can still be obtained, but the exposure index value is not meaningful. However, the image quality can still be evaluated by magnifying a small part of the image to assess for image graininess.
3. **Lead masking:** Generally, most CR systems allow multiple projections on one image plate if both accurate collimation and lead masking are used to prevent secondary and scatter exposure from the adjacent image.
4. **Accurate centering:** Because of the way the image plate reader scans the exposed imaging plate, it is important in digital imaging, as with all radiographic imaging, that the body part and central ray be accurately centered to the IR.
5. **Grid use with DR:** As already mentioned, grids are generally not used with film-screen imaging for body parts measuring 10 cm or less. This is also true for CR using image plates. However, with DR (direct digital radiography), grids may be used if the grid is an integral part of the image receptor mechanism. In such cases, because it may be impractical and difficult to remove the grid, it may be left in place, even for smaller body parts such as for upper and lower limb exams.
6. **Evaluation of exposure index values:** After the image is processed and ready for viewing, the image will be critiqued for exposure accuracy. It must then be checked for an acceptable exposure index or "S" number to verify that the exposure factors used were in the correct range to ensure an optimum quality image with the least possible radiation dose to the patient.

EXPOSURE FACTORS

Digital imaging systems are known for their wide exposure latitude; they are able to process an acceptable image from a broad range of exposure factors (kV and mAs). It is still important, however, that the ALARA principle be followed; thus the **lowest exposure factors that will produce an optimal image should be used.** This includes using the highest possible kV and the lowest mAs consistent with desirable image quality as viewed on a radiologist type interpretation monitor. Insufficient mAs results in a noisy (grainy) image on an interpretation monitor, even though it may appear satisfactory on a workstation monitor.

Generally **60 kV** is the lowest factor used for any CR or DR procedure (with the exception of mammography).

Alternative Modalities or Procedures

ARTHROGRAPHY

Arthrography is commonly used to image tendinous, ligamentous, and capsular pathology associated with diarthrodial joints, such as the wrist, elbow, shoulder, and ankle. This procedure requires the use of a radiographic contrast medium injected into the joint capsule under sterile conditions (see Chapter 21).

COMPUTED TOMOGRAPHY AND MAGNETIC RESONANCE IMAGING

Computed tomography (CT) and magnetic resonance imaging (MRI) are often used on upper limbs to evaluate soft-tissue and skeletal involvement of lesions, as well as soft-tissue injuries. The cross-sectional computed tomography images are also excellent for determination of displacement and alignment relationships with certain fractures that may be difficult to visualize with conventional radiographs.

NUCLEAR MEDICINE

Nuclear medicine bone scans are useful to demonstrate osteomyelitis, metastatic bone lesions, stress fractures, and cellulitis. Nuclear medicine scans demonstrate the pathologic process within 24 hours of onset. Nuclear medicine is more sensitive than radiography because it assesses the **physiologic aspect** instead of the anatomic aspect.

Pathologic Indications

The pathologic indications that all technologists should be most familiar with in relation to the upper limb include the following (not an inclusive list):

Bone metastases: The transfer of disease or cancerous lesions from one organ or part not directly connected. All malignant tumors have the ability to metastasize, or transfer malignant cells from one body part to another, through the blood stream, lymphatic vessels, or direct extension. Metastases are the most common of malignant bone tumors.

Bursitis *(ber-si'tis):* Inflammation of the bursae or fluid-filled sacs enclosing the joints; generally involves the formation of calcification in associated tendons, causing pain and limitation of joint movement.

Carpal tunnel syndrome *(kar'pal):* A common painful disorder of the **wrist and hand** resulting from compression of the median nerve as it passes through the center of the wrist; most commonly found in middle-aged women.

Fracture *(frak'chur):* A break in the structure of bone caused by a force (direct or indirect). There are numerous types of fractures; they are named by the extent of the fracture, direction of fracture lines, alignment of bone fragments, and integrity of overlying tissue (see Chapter 19 for additional trauma and fracture terminology). Some of the more common examples are as follows:

- **Barton's fracture:** Fracture and dislocation of the **posterior lip of the distal radius** involving the wrist joint
- **Bennett's fracture:** Fracture of the **base of the first metacarpal bone,** extending into the carpometacarpal joint, complicated by subluxation with some posterior displacement
- **Boxer's fracture:** A transverse fracture extending through the **metacarpal neck;** most commonly seen in the **fifth metacarpal**
- **Colles' fracture:** A transverse fracture of the **distal radius** with the distal fragment being **displaced posteriorly;** an associated ulnar styloid fracture seen in 50% to 60% of cases
- **Smith's fracture:** Reverse of the Colles' fracture, or a transverse fracture of the **distal radius** with the distal fragment displaced **anteriorly**

Joint effusion: Accumulated fluid (synovial or hemorrhagic) in the joint cavity. It is a sign of an underlying condition, such as a fracture, dislocation, soft-tissue damage, or inflammation.

Osteoarthritis *(os"te-o-ar-thri'tis):* Also known as ***degenerative joint disease*** **(DJD)*;*** a noninflammatory joint disease characterized by gradual deterioration of the articular cartilage with hypertrophic (enlargement or overgrown) bone formation. This is the most common type of arthritis. It is considered a normal part of the aging process.

Osteomyelitis *(os"te-o-mi"e-li'tis):* Local or generalized **infection of bone or bone marrow** that may be caused by bacteria introduced by trauma or surgery. However, it is more commonly the result of an infection from a contiguous source, such as a diabetic foot ulcer.

Osteopetrosis *(os"te-o-pe-tro'sis):* A hereditary disease marked by **abnormally dense bone.** It commonly occurs as a result of fractures of affected bone and may lead to obliteration of the marrow space. Also known as *marble bone.*

Osteoporosis *(os"te-o-po-ro'sis):* A **reduction in the quantity of bone** or **atrophy** of skeletal tissue. It occurs in postmenopausal women and elderly men, resulting in bone trabeculae that are scanty and thin. Most fractures sustained by women over the age of 50 are secondary to osteoporosis.

Paget's disease *(osteitis deformans):* One of the more common chronic skeletal diseases; a destructive bone disease followed by a reparative process of overproduction of very dense yet soft bones that tend to fracture easily. It is most common in men over age 40. The cause is unknown, but some evidence suggests involvement of a viral infection. Paget's disease can occur in any bone but most commonly affects the pelvis, femur, skull, vertebrae, clavicle, and humerus.

Rheumatoid arthritis (RA) *(ru'ma-toyd):* A chronic systemic disease with inflammatory changes occurring throughout the body's connective tissues, the earliest change being soft-tissue swelling, most prevalent around the ulnar styloid of the wrist. Early bone erosions also typically occur first at the second and third MCP joints or the third PIP joint. RA is three times more common in women than men.

"Skier's thumb": A sprain or tear of the **ulnar collateral ligament of the thumb,** near the MCP joint of the hyperextended thumb. It results from an injury such as falling on an outstretched arm and hand, causing the thumb to be bent back toward the arm. (An older term, "gamekeeper's thumb," referred to the action of holding game by the neck between thumb and index fingers.) The PA stress projection of bilateral thumbs (Folio method) best demonstrates this condition.

Tumors (bone tumors or neoplasms): Tumors are most often benign (noncancerous) but may be malignant (cancerous). CT and MRI are helpful in determining the type and exact location and size of the tumor. Specific types of tumors are listed on p. 143.

5

Malignant bone tumors

- **Multiple myelomas:** These are the most common of the **primary cancerous bone tumors.** Multiple myelomas generally affect persons between the ages of 40 to 70 years. As the name implies, these tumors occur in various parts of the body, arising from bone marrow or marrow plasma cells. Therefore these are not truly exclusive bony tumors. They are highly malignant and usually fatal within a few years. The typical radiographic appearance is multiple "punched-out" osteolytic (loss of calcium in bone) lesions scattered throughout the affected bones.
- **Osteogenic sarcomas (osteosarcomas):** The second most common type of **primary cancerous bone tumor,** these generally affect persons ages 10 to 20 years but can occur at any age. They may develop in older persons with Paget's disease.
- **Ewing's sarcoma:** A common primary **malignant bone tumor** in children and young adults, Ewing's sarcoma arises from bone marrow. Symptoms are similar to osteomyelitis with low-grade fever and pain. Stratified new bone formation results in an "onion peel" appearance on radiographs. Prognosis is poor by the time this sarcoma is evident on radiographs.
- **Chondrosarcoma:** A slow-growing **malignant tumor of the cartilage.** Appearance is similar to other malignant tumors but often also contains dense calcifications within cartilaginous mass.

Benign bone or cartilaginous tumors (chondromas)

- **Enchondroma:** Slow-growing **benign cartilaginous tumor** most often found in small bones of hands and feet of adolescents and young adults. Generally, enchondromas are well-defined, radiolucent-appearing tumors with thin cortex, often leading to pathologic fractures with only minimal trauma.
- **Osteochondromas** (exostosis): The most common type of **benign bone tumor,** usually occurring in persons ages 10 to 20 years. Osteochondromas arise from the outer cortex with the tumor growing parallel to the bone, pointing away from the adjacent joint. They are most common at the knee but also occur on the pelvis and scapula of children or young adults.

SUMMARY OF PATHOLOGIC INDICATIONS

CONDITION OR DISEASE	MOST COMMON RADIOGRAPHIC EXAM	POSSIBLE RADIOGRAPHIC APPEARANCE	MANUAL EXPOSURE FACTOR ADJUSTMENT*
Bursitis	AP and lat joint	Fluid-filled joint space with possible calcification	None
Carpal tunnel syndrome	PA and lat wrist; Gaynor-Hart method	Possible calcification in the carpal sulcus	None
Fractures	AP and lat of long bones; AP, lat, and oblique if joint involved	Disruption in bony cortex with soft-tissue swelling	None
Joint effusion	AP and lat joint	Fluid-filled joint cavity	None
Osteoarthritis (DJD)	AP and lat affected area	Narrowing of joint space with periosteal growths on the joint margins	None or decrease (−)
Osteomyelitis	AP and lat affected bone; nuclear medicine bone scan	Soft-tissue swelling and loss of fat-pad detail visibility	Decrease (−) (for soft tissue− −)
Osteopetrosis (marble bone)	AP and lat long bone	Chalky white or opaque appearance with a lack of distinction between the bony cortex and trabeculae	Increase (+)
Osteoporosis	AP and lat affected area	Best visibility in distal extremities and joints as a decrease in bone density; long bones demonstrating a thin cortex	Decrease (−)
Paget's disease	AP and lat affected area	Mixed areas of sclerotic and cortical thickening along with radiolucent lesions, a "cotton wool" appearance	May require increase (+)
Rheumatoid arthritis	AP and lat hand/wrist	Closed joint spaces with subluxation of the MCP joints	Decrease (−)
"Skier's thumb"	PA bilateral stress projection thumbs (Folio method)	Widening of inner MCP joint space of thumb and increase in degrees of angle of MCP line.	None
Tumors (neoplasms) —malignant and benign	AP and lat affected area	Appearance dependent on type and stage of tumor	None

AP, anteroposterior; *lat,* lateral; *DJD,* degenerative joint disease; *MCP,* metacarpophalangeal.
*Dependent on stage or severity of disease or condition.

Survey Information

Knowing the routines and special projections being performed most commonly in various parts of the country helps students understand why it is important to learn every projection, even if it is not commonly performed in their own department. In this way, students are prepared to function anywhere they may choose for employment.

SUMMARY OF SURVEY RESULTS

Thumb The common basic projections continue to be **AP, lateral,** and **oblique.**

Robert's method This special projection, **AP with 10° CR angle,** was first added to the 5th (previous) edition of this textbook. This projection is performed to visualize the base of the first metacarpal, such as for a possible Bennett's fracture.

Folio method ("skier's thumb") This **PA bilateral stress thumbs** projection has been added to this 6th edition because of its increasingly common use for ruling out ulnar collateral ligament tears or sprains to the MCP joint region of the thumb resulting from falls on an outstretched hand, hyperextending the thumb.

Hand The common basic projections continue to be **PA, oblique,** and **fan lateral.** In the U.S., 88% of the facilities (and 79% in Canada) indicated the fan lateral to be a basic projection, whereas 38% in the U.S. and 26% in Canada indicated the lateral hand in extension as a basic projection.

Norgaard method An **AP bilateral oblique hand projection** ("ball-catcher," Norgaard method) is included as a special projection for evaluation of early arthritic changes at the joints of the hands and fingers, especially at the base of the phalanges. In the U.S., 45% of facilities (and 57% in Canada) indicated this was being performed as a special projection in 1999.

Wrist The common basic wrist projections are **PA, oblique,** and **lateral.** The **ulnar deviation** for the **scaphoid** also was indicated as basic for 43% of facilities in the U.S. and 67% in Canada. The **Stecher method** for the scaphoid was special for 51% in the U.S. in 1999 compared with only 40% in 1995.

The **carpal canal projection** was the highest percentage special projection in the U.S. at 59%, but only 31% in Canada.

The **carpal bridge tangential projection** was indicated as a special projection in both 1995 and 1999 by 37% in the U.S. and in 1999 by 21% in Canada.

Forearm AP and **lateral** are the common basic projections as indicated by 99% to 100% of facilities in the U.S. and Canada.

Elbow The **AP** and **lateral** were basic for 99% of facilities in the U.S. and Canada. The **obliques** showed a range of differences, with the highest percentage indicating both **internal** and **external obliques** as basic, 54% in the U.S. and 36% in Canada. The next-highest basic was the **external only oblique,** with 30% in the U.S. and 34% in Canada. The **internal only oblique** was basic for 25% in the U.S. and 14% in Canada.

Humerus The routine for nontrauma humerus continues to be an **AP** (98%) and **rotational lateral,** with the most common being **lateromedial,** patient **AP** (91% in U.S., 71% in Canada), and less frequently the **mediolateral** with patient **PA** (25% in U.S. and 51% in Canada). (See Chapter 6 for trauma proximal humerus and shoulder routines.)

Standard and Special Operating Procedures

Certain basic and special projections for the hand, wrist, forearm, elbow, and humerus are demonstrated and described on the following pages as suggested standard basic and special departmental routines or procedures.

BASIC PROJECTIONS

Standard, or basic, projections (also sometimes referred to as *routine projections* or *departmental routines*) are those projections commonly performed on average patients who are helpful and can cooperate in performing the procedure.

SPECIAL PROJECTIONS

Special projections are those more common projections taken as extra or additional projections to better demonstrate certain pathologic conditions or specific body parts.

BASIC AND SPECIAL PROJECTIONS

Proximal humerus, scapular Y, and transthoracic lateral—see Chapter 6.

5

PA PROJECTION: FINGERS

Fingers
BASIC
- PA
- PA oblique
- Lateral

Pathology Demonstrated

Fractures and/or dislocations of the distal, middle, and proximal phalanges; distal metacarpal; and associated joints are demonstrated. Some pathologic processes, such as osteoporosis and osteoarthritis, also may be demonstrated.

24
18
R

Technical Factors

- IR size—18 × 24 cm (8 × 10 inches)
- Division in thirds crosswise
- Detail screen, tabletop
- Digital IR (use lead masking)
- 50-60 kV range
- Technique and dose:

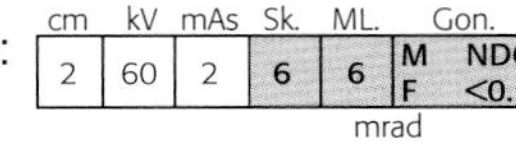

cm	kV	mAs	Sk.	ML.	Gon.
2	60	2	6	6	M NDC F <0.1
				mrad	

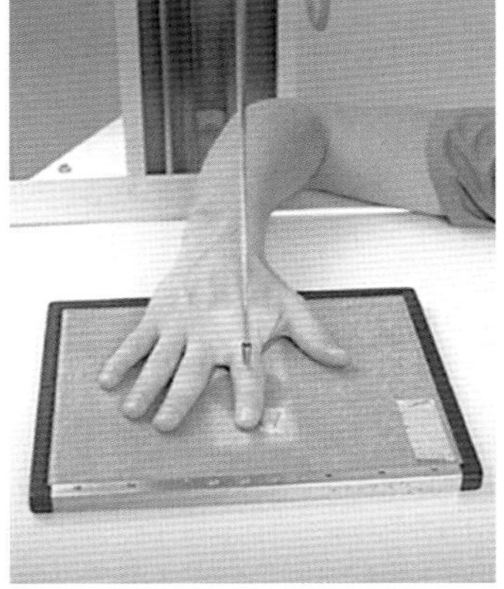

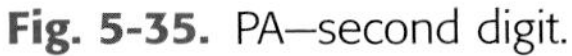

Fig. 5-35. PA—second digit.

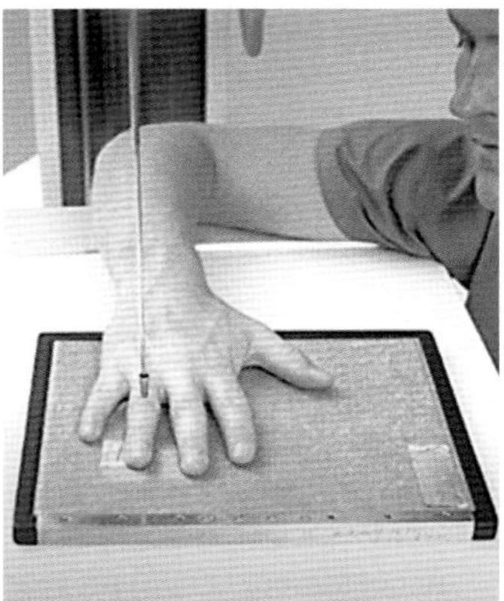

Fig. 5-36. PA—fourth digit.

Note: A possible alternate routine includes a larger IR to include the entire hand for the PA projection of the finger for possible secondary trauma or pathology to other aspects of the hand and wrist. Then oblique and lateral projections of affected finger only would be taken.

Shielding Place lead shield over patient's lap.

Patient Position Seat patient at end of table, with elbow flexed about 90° with hand and forearm resting on table.

Part Position

- Pronate hand with fingers extended.
- Center and align long axis of affected finger to long axis of portion of IR being exposed.
- Separate adjoining fingers from affected finger.

Central Ray

- CR perpendicular to IR, directed to **PIP joint**
- Minimum SID of 40 inches (100 cm)

Collimation Collimate on four sides to area of affected finger.

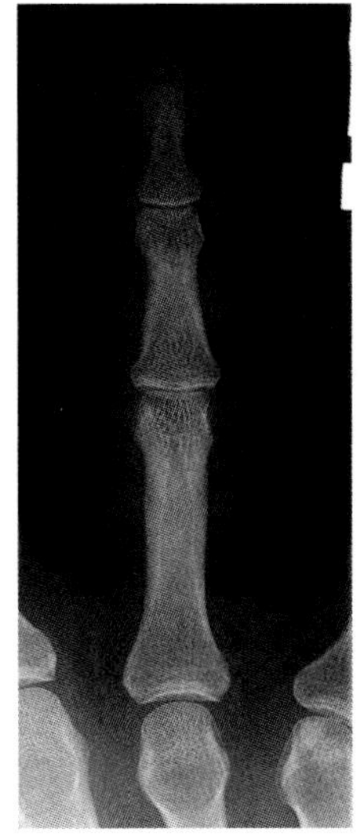

Fig. 5-37. PA—fourth digit.

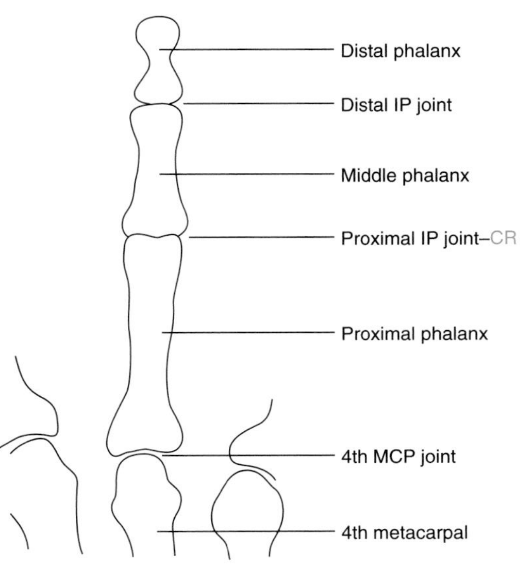

Fig. 5-38. PA—fourth digit.

Radiographic Criteria

Structures Shown: • Distal, middle, and proximal phalanges; distal metacarpal; and associated joints.

Position: • Long axis of finger should be aligned with and parallel to side border of IR. • **No rotation** of fingers is evidenced by symmetric appearance of both sides or concavities of the shafts of the phalanges and distal metacarpals. • The amount of tissue on each side of the phalanges should appear equal. • Fingers should be separated with no overlapping of soft tissues. • Interphalangeal joints should appear open, indicating hand was fully pronated.

Collimation and CR: • Collimation should be visible on four sides to area of affected finger. • CR and midpoint of collimation field should be to the PIP joint.

Exposure Criteria: • Optimal density and contrast with no motion demonstrate soft-tissue margins and clear, sharp bony trabecular markings.

PA OBLIQUE PROJECTION—MEDIAL OR LATERAL ROTATION: FINGERS

Fingers
BASIC
• PA
• PA oblique
• Lateral

Pathology Demonstrated
Fractures and or dislocations of the distal, middle, and proximal phalanges; distal metacarpal; and associated joints are visible. Some pathologies such as osteoporosis and osteoarthritis may also be demonstrated.

Technical Factors
- IR size—18 × 24 cm (8 × 10 inches)
- Tabletop, divided in thirds crosswise
- Detail screen, tabletop
- Digital IR (use lead masking)
- 50-60 kV range
- **Accessories:** 45° foam wedge block or step wedge
- Technique and dose:

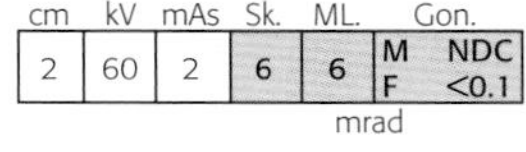

cm	kV	mAs	Sk.	ML.	Gon.
2	60	2	6	6	M NDC F <0.1

mrad

Shielding Place lead shield over patient's lap to shield gonads.

Patient Position Seat patient at end of table, with elbow flexed about 90° with hand and wrist resting on cassette and fingers extended.

Part Position
- Place hand with fingers extended against 45° foam wedge block, placing hand in a 45° lateral oblique (thumb side up).
- Position hand on cassette so that the long axis of finger is aligned with long axis of the one-third of IR being exposed.
- Separate fingers and carefully place finger being examined against block so that it is supported in a 45° oblique and **parallel to IR.**

Central Ray
- CR perpendicular to IR, to **PIP joint**
- Minimum SID of 40 inches (100 cm)

Collimation Collimate on four sides to affected finger.

Optional medial oblique (Fig. 5-39): Second digit also may be taken in a 45° medial oblique (thumb side down) with thumb and other fingers flexed to prevent superimposition. This position places the part closer to IR for improved definition but also may be more painful for patient.

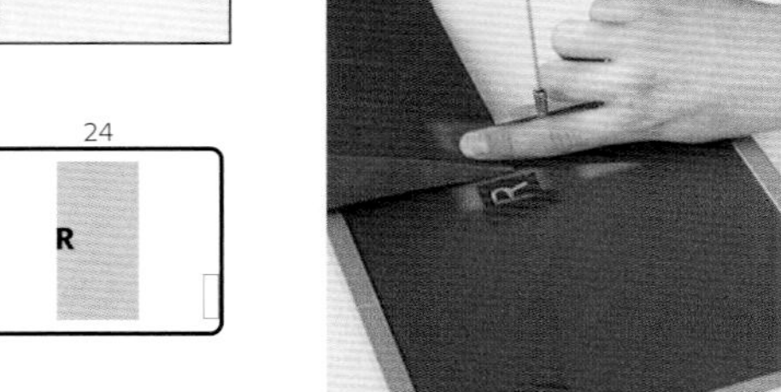

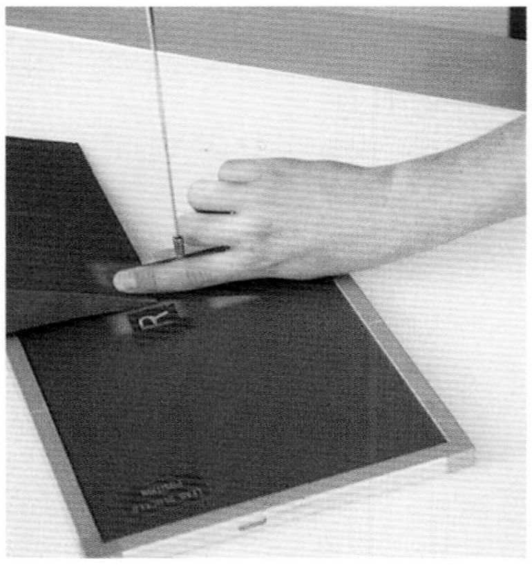

Fig. 5-39. Second digit (medial rotation).

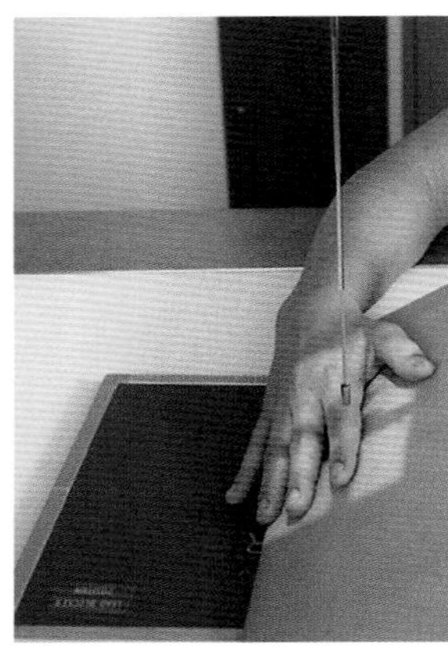

Fig. 5-40. Second digit (optional lateral rotation).

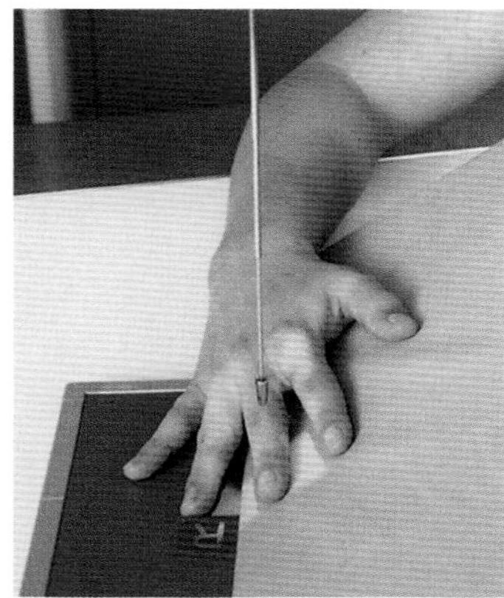

Fig. 5-41. Third digit (lateral rotation).

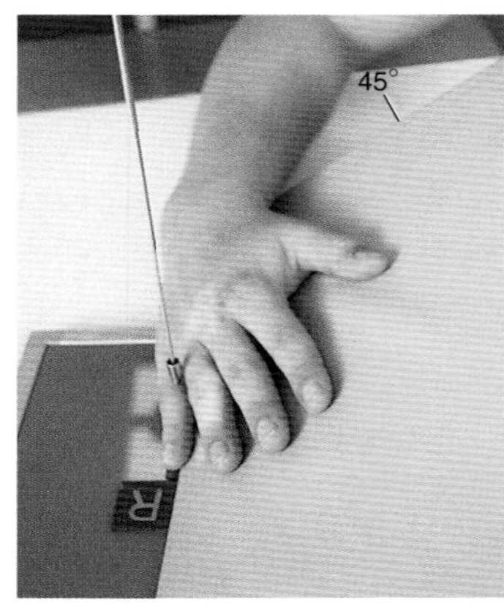

Fig. 5-42. Fifth digit (lateral rotation).

Radiographic Criteria

Structures Shown: • 45° oblique view of the distal, middle, and proximal phalanges; distal metacarpal; and associated joints.

Position: • Interphalangeal and metacarpophalangeal joint spaces should be open, indicating correct central ray location and that the phalanges are parallel to the IR. • Long axis of finger should be aligned to side border of IR. • View of finger being examined should be 45° oblique • No superimposition of adjacent fingers should occur.

Collimation and CR: • Collimation should be visible on four sides to area of affected finger. • CR and center of collimation field should be to the PIP joint.

Exposure Criteria: • Optimal density and contrast with no motion demonstrate soft-tissue margins and clear, sharp bony trabecular markings.

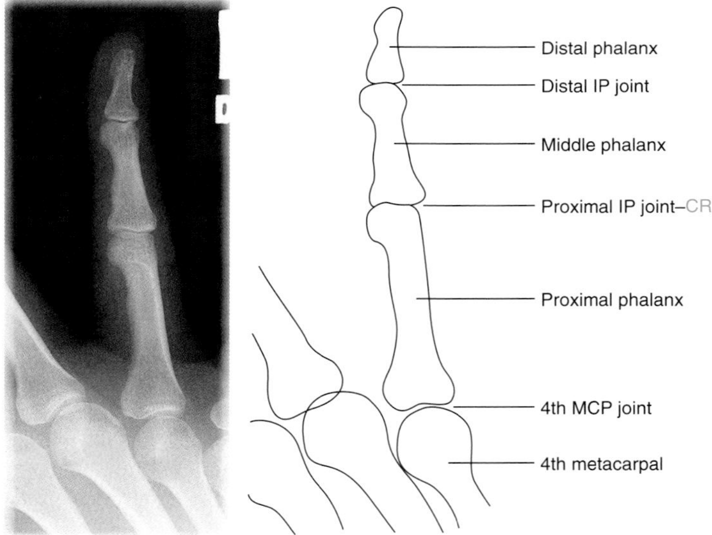

Fig. 5-43. Fourth digit.

Fig. 5-44. Fourth digit.

LATERAL—LATEROMEDIAL OR MEDIOLATERAL PROJECTIONS: FINGERS

Fingers
BASIC
• PA
• PA oblique
• Lateral

Pathology Demonstrated

Fractures and/or dislocations of the distal, middle, and proximal phalanges; distal metacarpal; and associated joints are shown. Some pathologic processes, such as osteoporosis and osteoarthritis, also may be demonstrated.

24

18 R

Technical Factors

- IR size—18 × 24 cm (8 × 10 inches)
- Division in thirds crosswise
- Detail screen, tabletop
- Digital IR (use lead masking)
- 50-60 kV range
- **Accessories:** Sponge support block
- Technique and dose:

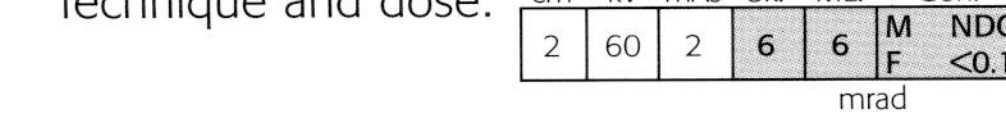
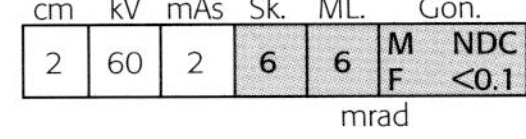

cm	kV	mAs	Sk.	ML.	Gon.
2	60	2	6	6	M NDC F <0.1
				mrad	

Shielding Place lead shield over patient's lap to shield gonads.

Patient Position Seat patient at end of table, with elbow flexed about 90° with hand and wrist resting on cassette and fingers extended.

Part Position

- Place hand in lateral position (thumb side up) with finger to be examined fully extended and centered to portion of IR being exposed (see note for second digit lateral).
- Align and center finger to long axis of portion of IR being exposed and to CR.
- Use sponge block or other radiolucent device to support finger and prevent motion. Flex unaffected fingers.
- Ensure that long axis of finger is **parallel to IR.**

Central Ray

- CR perpendicular to IR, directed to **PIP joint**
- Minimum SID of 40 inches (100 cm)

Collimation Collimate on four sides to affected finger.

Note: For second digit a mediolateral is advised (Fig. 5-45) if patient can assume this position. Place the second digit in contact with cassette. (Definition is improved with less OID.)

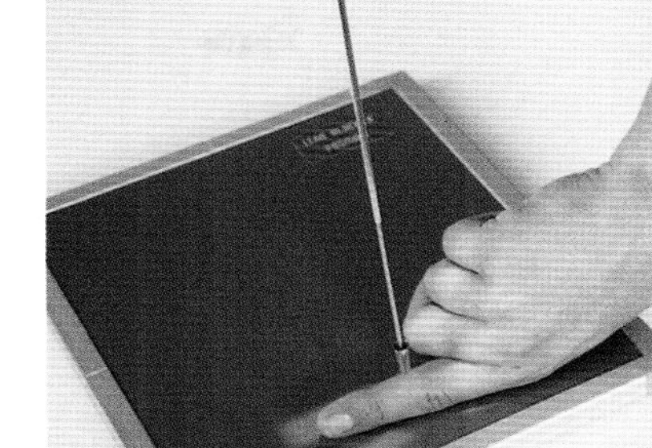

Fig. 5-45. Second digit (mediolateral).

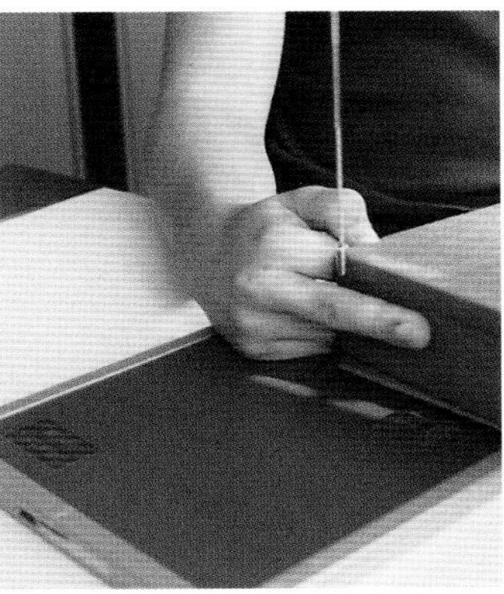

Fig. 5-46. Third digit (lateromedial).

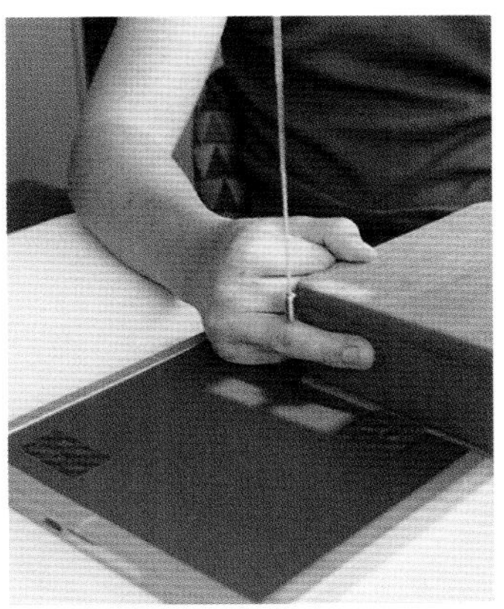

Fig. 5-47. Fourth digit (lateromedial).

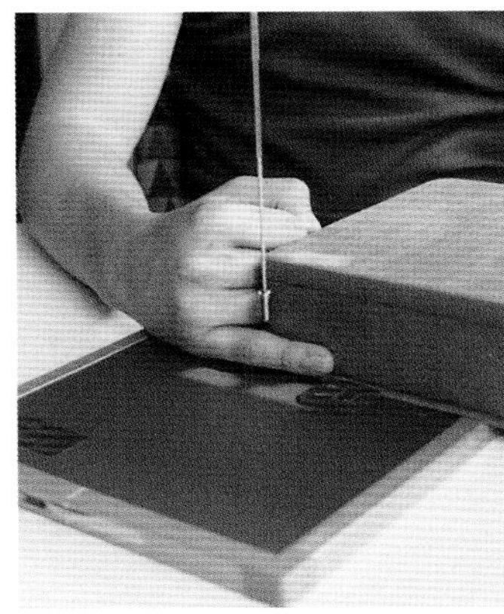

Fig. 5-48. Fifth digit (lateromedial).

Radiographic Criteria

Structures Shown: • Lateral view of the distal, middle, and proximal phalanges; distal metacarpal; and associated joint are visible.

Position: • Interphalangeal and metacarpophalangeal joint spaces should be open, indicating correct central ray location and that the phalanges are parallel to the IR. • Long axis of finger should be aligned to the side border of IR. • Finger should be in **true lateral position,** as indicated by the concave appearance of the anterior surface of the shaft of the phalanges.

Collimation and CR: • Collimation should be visible on four sides to area of affected finger. • CR and center of collimation field should be to the **PIP joint.**

Exposure Criteria: • Optimal density and contrast with no motion demonstrate soft-tissue margins and clear, sharp bony trabecular markings.

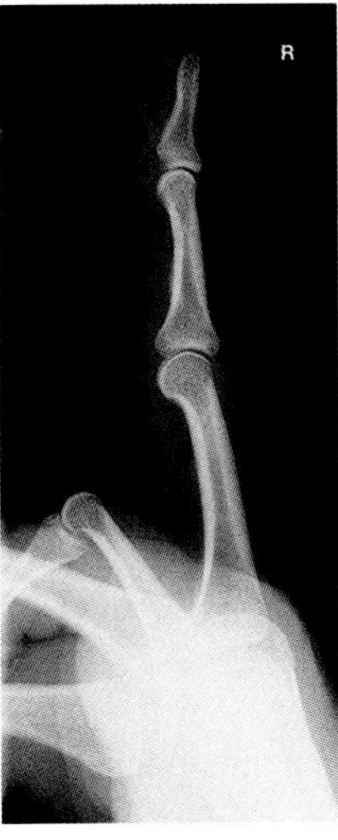

Fig. 5-49. Fourth digit.

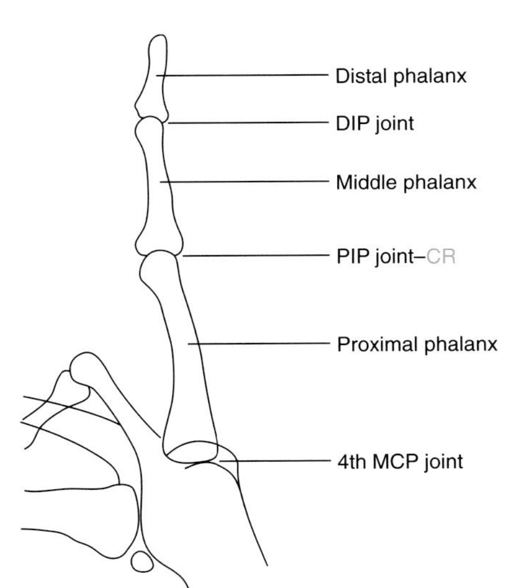

Fig. 5-50. Fourth digit.

AP PROJECTION: THUMB

Pathology Demonstrated

Fractures and/or dislocations of the distal and proximal phalanges, distal metacarpal, and associated joints are demonstrated. Some pathologic processes, such as osteoporosis and osteoarthritis, also may be demonstrated. (See special AP Robert's projection for Bennett's fracture at base of first metacarpal.)

Thumb
BASIC
• AP
• PA oblique
• Lateral

Technical Factors

- IR size—18 × 24 cm (8 × 10 inches)
- Division in thirds crosswise
- Detail screen, tabletop
- Digital IR (use lead masking)
- 50-60 kV range
- Technique and dose:

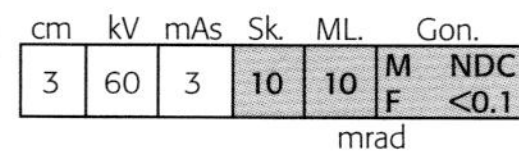

cm	kV	mAs	Sk.	ML.	Gon.
3	60	3	10	10	M NDC F <0.1

mrad

Shielding Place lead shield over patient's lap to shield gonads.

Patient Position—AP Seat patient facing table, arms extended in front, with hand rotated internally to supinate thumb for AP projection (Fig. 5-51).

Part Position—AP

First demonstrate this awkward position on yourself so that the patient can see how it is done and better understand what is expected.

- Internally rotate hand with fingers extended until posterior surface of thumb is in contact with IR (may need to hold fingers back with other hand as shown).
- Align thumb to long axis of portion of IR being exposed.
- Center **first MCP joint** to CR and to center of portion of IR being exposed. (Remember, first metacarpal is considered part of thumb.)

Exception—PA (only if patient cannot position for previous AP)

- Place hand in near-lateral position and rest thumb on sponge support block that is high enough so that thumb is not rotated but in position for a **true PA projection.**

Note: As a rule, the PA is **not** advisable because it results in a loss of definition due to increased OID.

Central Ray

- CR perpendicular to IR, to **first MCP joint**
- Minimum SID of 40 inches (100 cm)

Collimation Collimate on four sides to area of thumb, remembering that **thumb includes entire first metacarpal.**

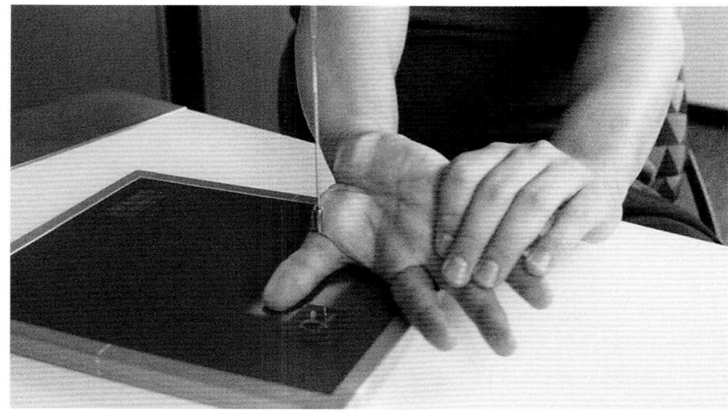

Fig. 5-51. AP thumb—CR to first MCP joint.

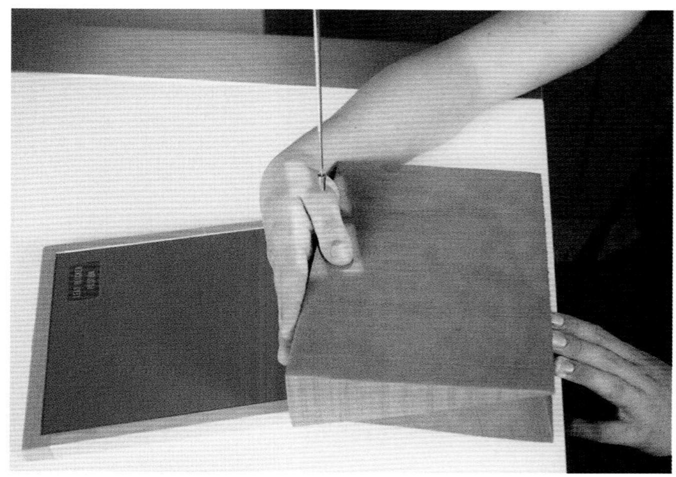

Fig. 5-52. PA (exception).

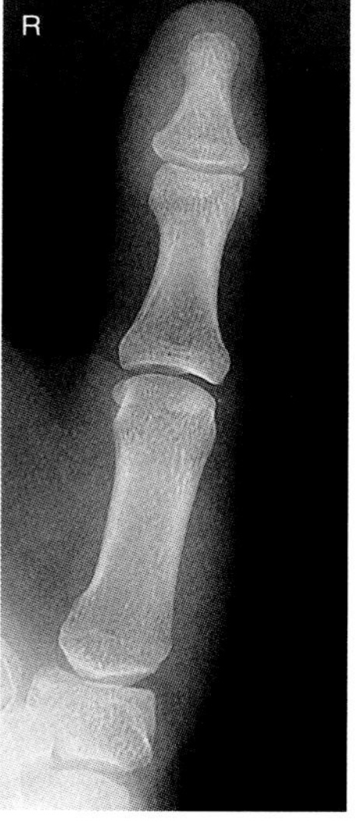

Fig. 5-53. AP thumb.

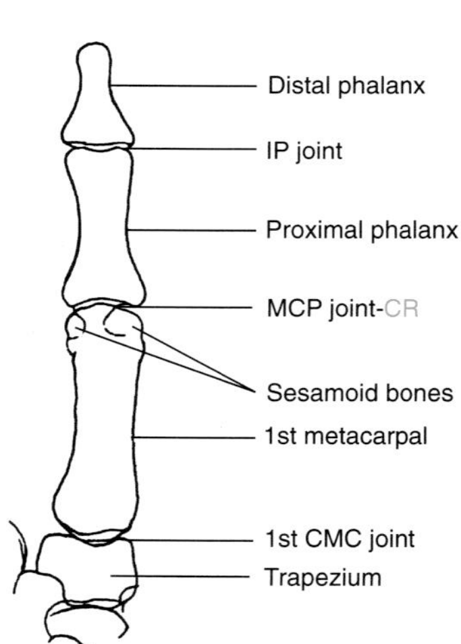

Fig. 5-54. AP thumb.

Radiographic Criteria

Structures Shown: • Distal and proximal phalanges, first metacarpal, trapezium, and associated joints are visible. • Interphalangeal and metacarpophalangeal joints should appear open.

Position: • Long axis of thumb should be aligned to side border of IR. • **No rotation,** as evidenced by the concave sides of the phalanges and by equal amounts of soft tissue appearing on each side of the phalanges, should be present.

Collimation and CR: • Collimation should be visible on four sides to area of thumb. • CR and center of the collimation field should be at the **first MCP joint.**

Exposure Criteria: • Optimal density and contrast with no motion demonstrate soft-tissue margins and clear, sharp bony trabecular markings.

PA OBLIQUE PROJECTION—MEDIAL ROTATION: THUMB

Thumb
BASIC
- AP
- PA oblique
- Lateral

Pathology Demonstrated

Fractures and/or dislocations of the distal and proximal phalanges, distal metacarpal, and associated joints are shown. Some pathologic processes, such as osteoporosis and osteoarthritis, also may be demonstrated.

Technical Factors

- IR size—18 × 24 cm (8 × 10 inches)
- Division in thirds crosswise
- Detail screen, tabletop
- Digital IR (use lead masking)
- 50-60 kV range
- Technique and dose:

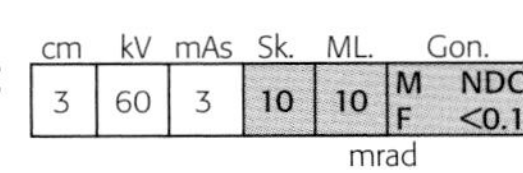

cm	kV	mAs	Sk.	ML.	Gon.
3	60	3	10	10	M NDC F <0.1
			mrad		

Shielding Place lead shield over patient's lap to shield gonads.

Patient Position Seat patient at end of table, with elbow flexed about 90° with hand resting on cassette.

Part Position

- Abduct thumb slightly with palmar surface of hand in contact with cassette. (This action naturally places thumb in a 45° oblique position.)
- Align long axis of thumb to long axis of third of IR being exposed.
- Center **first MCP joint** to CR and to center of portion of IR being exposed.

Central Ray

- CR perpendicular to IR, directed to **first MCP joint**
- Minimum SID of 40 inches (100 cm)

Collimation Collimate on four sides to thumb, ensuring that **all of first metacarpal is included.**

Radiographic Criteria

Structures Shown: • Distal and proximal phalanges, first metacarpal, trapezium, and associated joints are visualized in a 45° oblique position. • Interphalangeal and metacarpophalangeal joints should appear open.

Position: • Long axis of thumb should be aligned with side border of IR.

Collimation and CR: • Collimation should be visible on four sides to area of affected thumb. • CR and center of collimation field should be at **first MCP joint.**

Exposure Criteria: • Optimal density and contrast with no motion demonstrate soft-tissue margins and clear, sharp bony trabecular markings.

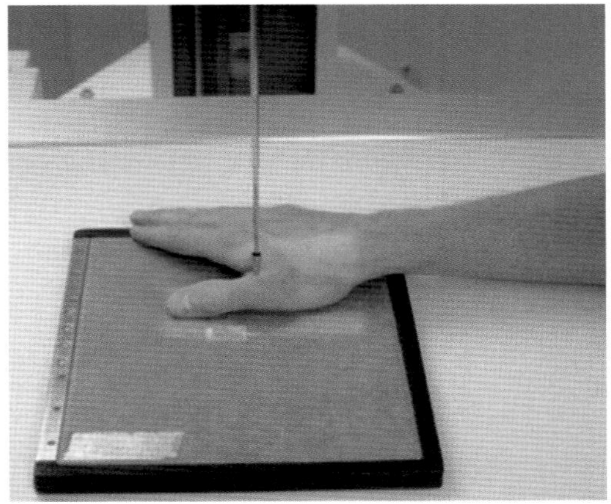

Fig. 5-55. Oblique thumb—CR to first MCP joint.

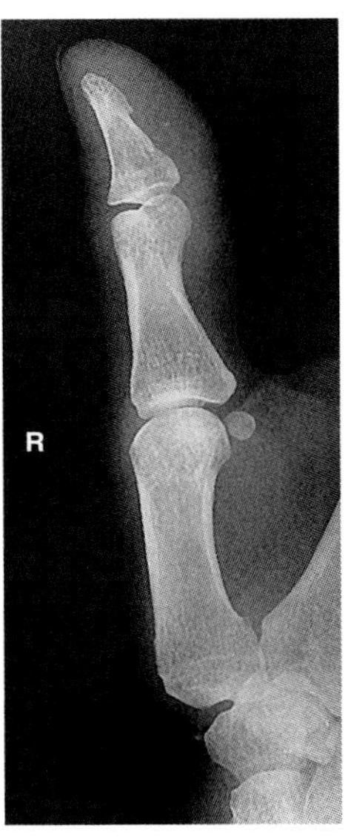

Fig. 5-56. Oblique thumb.

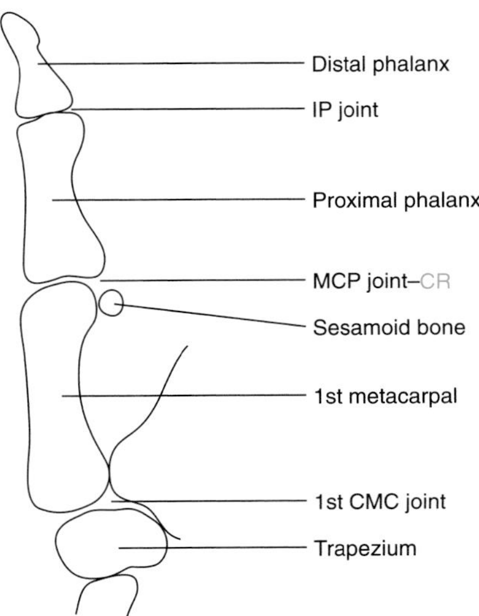

Fig. 5-57. Oblique thumb.

5

LATERAL POSITION: THUMB

Thumb
BASIC
- AP
- PA oblique
- Lateral

24
R
18

Pathology Demonstrated

Fractures and/or dislocations of the distal and proximal phalanges, distal metacarpal, and associated joints are shown. Some pathologic processes, such as osteoporosis and osteoarthritis, also may be demonstrated.

Technical Factors

- IR size—18 × 24 cm (8 × 10 inches)
- Division in thirds crosswise
- Detail screen, tabletop
- Digital IR (use lead masking)
- 50-60 kV range
- Technique and dose:

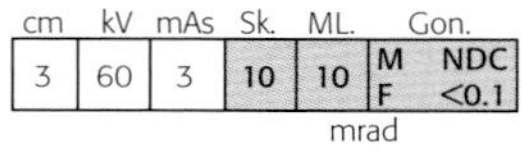

cm	kV	mAs	Sk.	ML.	Gon.
3	60	3	10	10	M NDC F <0.1
			mrad		

Shielding Place lead shield over patient's lap to shield gonads.

Patient Position Seat patient at end of table, with elbow flexed about 90° with hand resting on cassette, palm down.

Part Position

- Start with hand pronated and thumb abducted, with fingers and hand slightly arched; then rotate hand slightly medial until thumb is in a **true lateral position.** (May need to provide sponge or other support under lateral portion of hand.)
- Align long axis of thumb to long axis of portion of IR being exposed.
- Center **first MCP joint** to CR and to center of portion of IR being exposed.
- Entire lateral aspect of thumb should be in direct contact with cassette.

Central Ray

- CR perpendicular to IR, directed to **first MCP joint**
- Minimum SID of 40 inches (100 cm)

Collimation Collimate on four sides to thumb area. (Remember that thumb includes **entire first metacarpal.**)

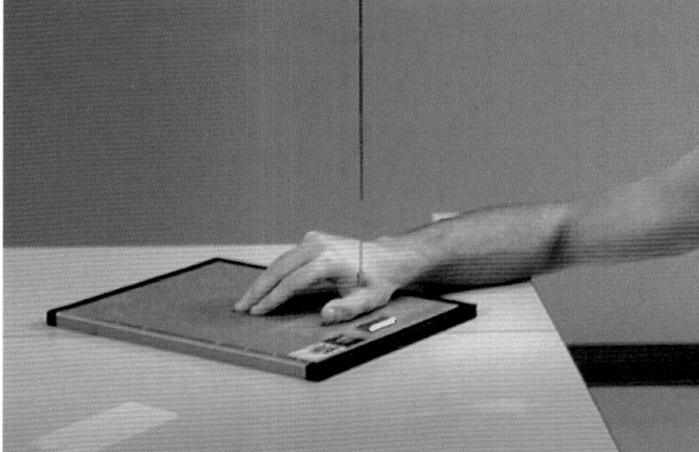

Fig. 5-58. Patient position—lateral thumb.

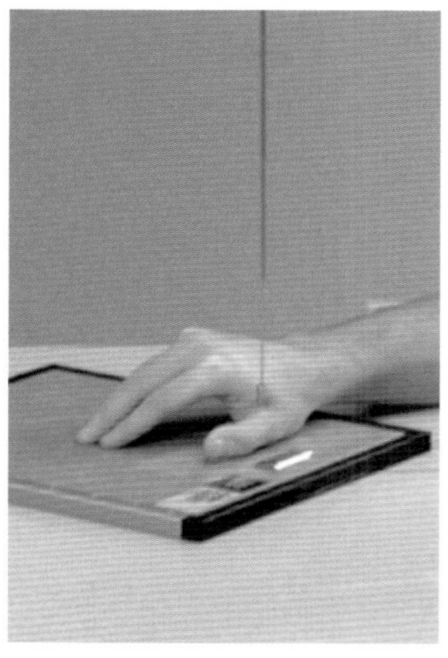

Fig. 5-59. Part position—lateral thumb; CR to first MCP joint.

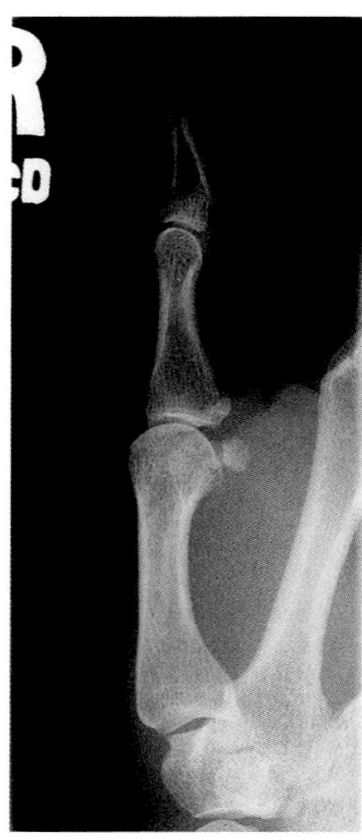

Fig. 5-60. Lateral thumb.

Radiographic Criteria

Structures Shown: • Distal and proximal phalanges, first metacarpal, trapezium (superimposed), and associated joints are visualized in the lateral position. • Interphalangeal and metacarpophalangeal joints should appear open.

Position: • Long axis of thumb should be aligned to side border of IR. • Thumb should be in a **true lateral position,** evidenced by the concave-shaped anterior surface of the proximal phalanx and first metacarpal and the relatively straight posterior surfaces.

Collimation and CR: • Collimation should be visible on four sides to area of affected thumb. • CR and center of collimation field should be at the **first MCP joint.**

Exposure Criteria: • Optimal density and contrast with no motion demonstrate soft-tissue margins and clear, sharp bony trabecular markings.

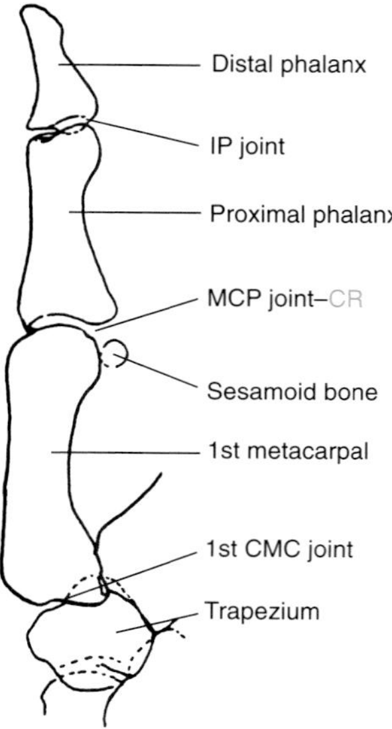

Fig. 5-61. Lateral thumb.

5

AP PROJECTION (MODIFIED ROBERT'S METHOD)*: THUMB

Pathology Demonstrated

This special projection demonstrates fractures and/or dislocations of the **first CMC joint.** Some pathologic processes such as osteoarthritis, may be demonstrated.

Base of first metacarpal is demonstrated for ruling out **Bennett's fracture.**

Thumb
BASIC
• PA
• PA oblique
• Lateral
SPECIAL
• AP, Robert's
• PA stress (Folio method)

Technical Factors

- IR size—18 × 24 cm (8 × 10 inches)
- Detail screen, tabletop
- Digital IR—(use lead masking)
- 50-60 kV range
- Technique and dose:

cm	kV	mAs	Sk.	ML.	Gon.
3	60	3	10	10	M NDC F <0.1
				mrad	

24

R

18

Shielding Place lead shield over patient's lap to shield gonads.

Patient Position Seat patient parallel to end of table, with hand and arm fully extended.

Part Position

- Rotate arm internally until posterior aspect of thumb is resting on cassette.
- Place thumb in center of the IR, parallel to side border of cassette.
- Extend fingers so that soft tissue does not superimpose first CMC joint.
- Advise patient to hold fingers with the other hand, if necessary.

Central Ray

- CR directed **15° proximally** (toward wrist), entering at the **first CMC joint**
- Minimum SID of 40 inches (100 cm)

Collimation Collimate on four sides to area of thumb and first CMC joint.

Radiographic Criteria

Structures Shown: • An AP projection of the thumb and first CMC joint are visible without superimposition. • Base of first metacarpal and trapezium should be well visualized.

Position: • Long axis of the thumb should be aligned to side border of IR. • **No rotation,** as evidenced by the symmetric appearance of both concave sides of the phalanges and by the equal amounts of soft tissue appearing on each side of the phalanges, should exist. • First CMC and MCP joints should appear open.

Collimation and CR: • Collimation should be visible on four sides to area of affected thumb. • CR and center of collimation field should be at **first CMC joint.**

Exposure Criteria: • Optimal density and contrast with no motion demonstrate soft-tissue margins and clear, sharp bony trabecular markings.

*Long B, Rafert J: Orthopaedic radiography, Philadelphia, 1995, WB Saunders.

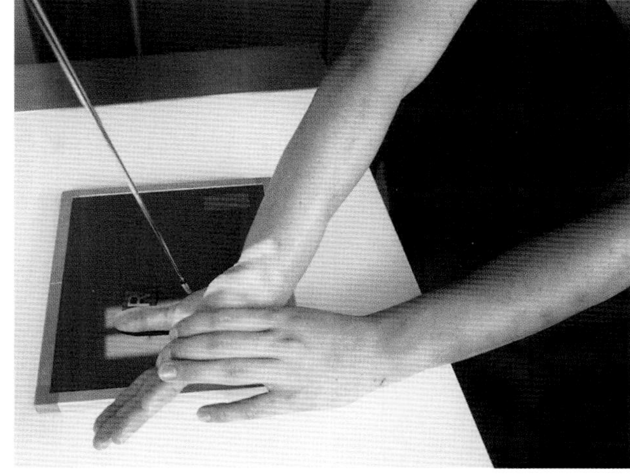

Fig. 5-62. AP projection—modified Robert's method; CR 15° to first CMC joint.

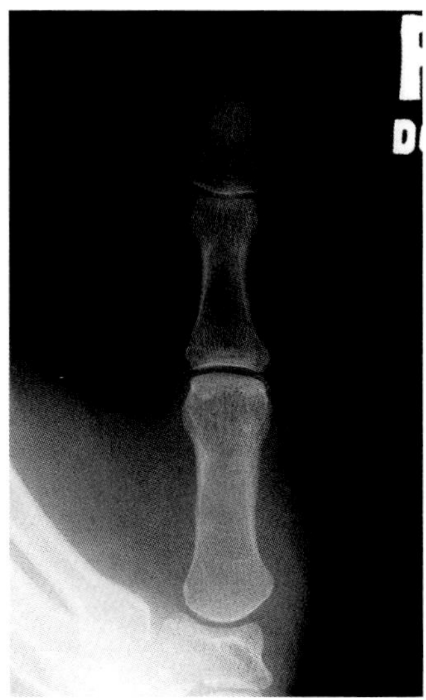

Fig. 5-63. AP projection—modified Robert's method.

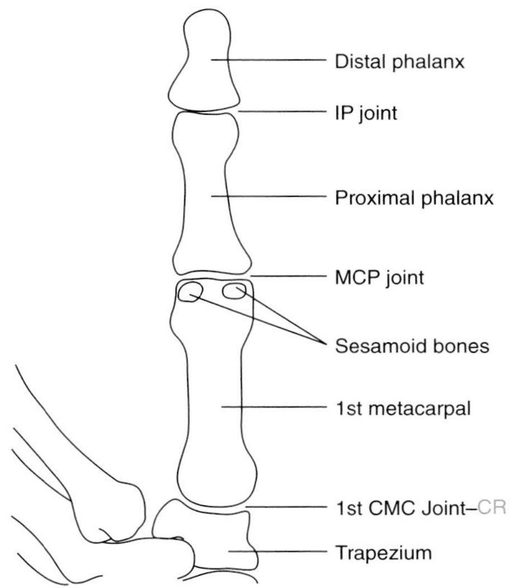

Fig. 5-64. AP projection—modified Robert's method.

PA STRESS "SKIER'S THUMB" PROJECTION

Folio Method*

Pathology Demonstrated

Sprain or tearing of ulnar collateral ligament of thumb at the MCP joint, result of acute hyperextension of thumb.

Thumb
BASIC
• **PA**
• **PA oblique**
• Lateral
SPECIAL
• **AP, Robert's**
• PA stress (Folio method)

Technical Factors

- IR size–18 × 24 cm (8 × 10 inches) crosswise
- Detail screen or digital IR, tabletop
- 50-60 kV range
- Technique and dose:

cm	kV	mAs	Sk.	ML.	Gon.
3	60	3	10	10	M NDC F <0.1

mrad

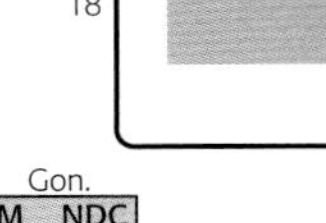

Shielding Place lead shield over patient's lap to shield gonads.

Patient Position Seat patient at end of table with both hands extended and pronated on IR.

Part Position

- Position both hands side by side to center of cassette, rotated laterally into ± 45° oblique position, resulting in true PA projection of both thumbs.
- Place supports as needed under both wrist and proximal thumb regions to prevent motion. Ensure that hands are rotated enough to place thumbs parallel to IR (cassette) for **true PA projection** of both thumbs.
- Place round spacer, such as a roll of medical tape, between proximal thumb regions; wrap rubber bands around distal thumbs as shown.
- Immediately before exposure, ask patient to firmly pull thumbs apart and hold.

Note: Explain procedure carefully to patient and observe patient applying tension on rubber band without motion before initiating exposure. Work quickly because this can be painful for patient.

Central Ray

- CR **perpendicular** to IR directed to **midway between MCP joints**
- Minimum SID of 40 inches (100 cm)

Collimation Collimate on four sides to include second metacarpals and entire thumbs, from CMC joints proximally to distal phalanges distally.

Radiographic Criteria

Structures Shown: • Entire thumbs from 1st metacarpals to distal phalanges. Demonstrates **metacarpophalangeal** angles, and joint spaces at **MCP joints.**

Position: • Metacarpophlangeal (MCP) and interphalangeal (IP) joints should appear open, indicating thumbs were parallel to IR and perpendicular to CR. • **No rotation** of thumbs as evidenced by symmetrical appearance of concavities of shafts of first metacarpals and phalanges. • Distal phalanges should appear to be pulled together indicating that tension was applied.

Collimation and CR: • Collimation should be visible on four sides. • CR and center of collimation field should be **midway** between the two MCP joints.

Exposure Criteria: • Optimal density and contrast with **no motion** demonstrates soft-tissue margins and clear, sharp bony edges and trabecular markings.

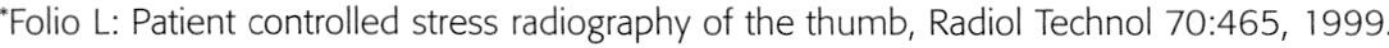

*Folio L: Patient controlled stress radiography of the thumb, Radiol Technol 70:465, 1999.

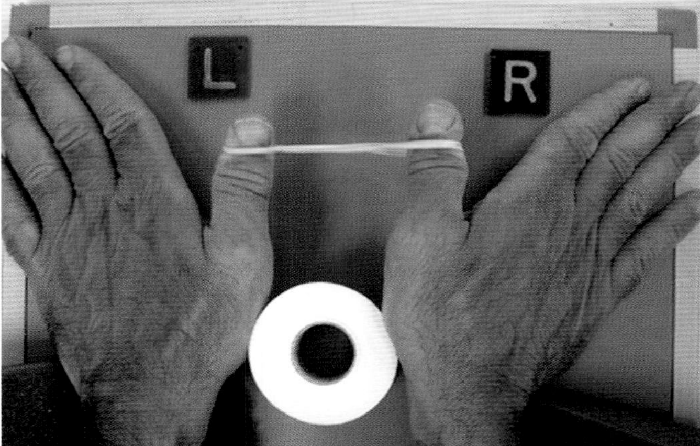

Fig. 5-65. PA stress projection of bilateral thumbs; CR perpendicular to midway between MCP joints, firm tension applied.

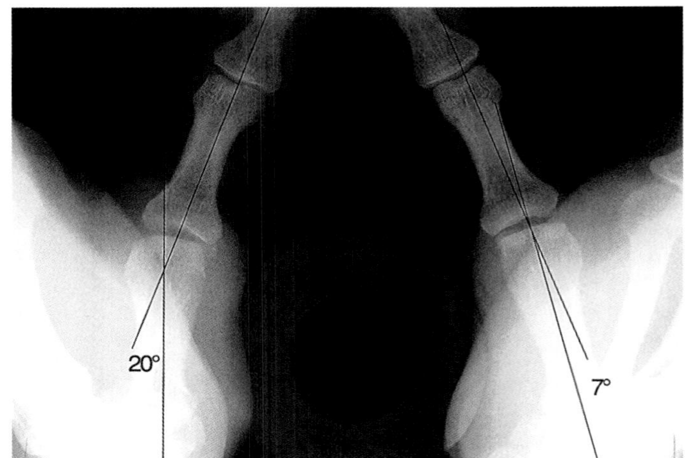

Fig. 5-66. PA stress projection of bilateral thumbs with tension applied. 20° MCP angle on left indicating sprain or torn ulnar collateral ligament. (From Ballinger PW, Frank ED: Merrill's atlas of radiographic positions and radiologic procedures, ed 10, St. Louis, 2003, Mosby.)

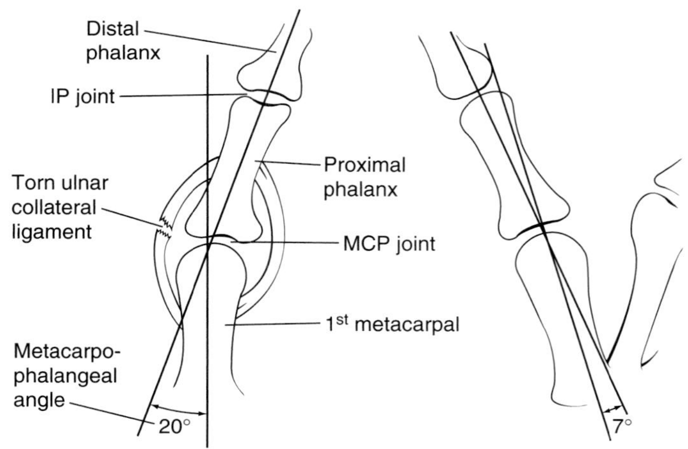

Fig. 5-67. PA stress projection of bilateral thumbs with tension applied (demonstrates torn ulnar collateral ligament on left).

5

PA PROJECTION: HAND

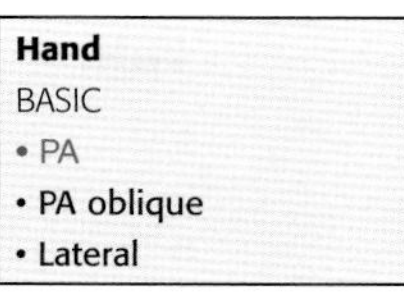

Pathology Demonstrated
Fractures, dislocations, or foreign bodies of the phalanges, metacarpals, and all joints of the hand are shown. Pathologic processes such as osteoporosis and osteoarthritis also may be demonstrated.

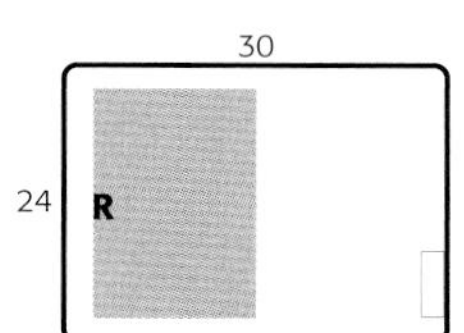

Technical Factors
- IR size—24 × 30 cm (10 × 12 inches)
- Division of IR in half crosswise or for large hand—18 × 24 cm (8 × 10 inches) lengthwise
- Digital IR (use lead masking)
- Detail screen, tabletop
- 50-60 kV range
- Technique and dose:

cm	kV	mAs	Sk.	ML.	Gon.
4	62	3	11	11	M NDC F <0.1

mrad

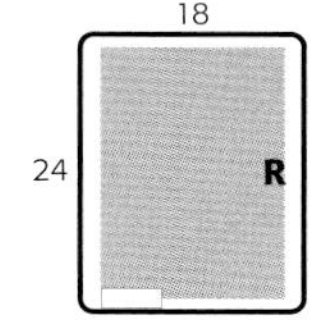

Shielding Place lead shield over patient's lap to shield gonads.

Patient Position Seat patient at end of table with elbow flexed about 90° and hand and forearm resting on table.

Part Position
- Pronate hand with palmar surface in contact with cassette; spread fingers slightly.
- Align long axis of hand and forearm with long axis of portion of IR being exposed.
- Center hand and wrist to unmasked half of IR.

Central Ray
- CR perpendicular to IR, directed to **third MCP joint**
- Minimum SID of 40 inches (100 cm)

Collimation Collimate on four sides to outer margins of hand and wrist.

Note: If exams of both hands and/or wrists are requested, generally the body parts should be positioned and exposed separately for correct CR placement.

Radiographic Criteria

Structures Shown: • PA projection of entire hand and wrist and about 1 inch (2.5 cm) of distal forearm are visible. Note that PA projection of hand demonstrates oblique view of the thumb.

Position: • Metacarpophalangeal and interphalangeal joints should appear open, indicating correct CR location and that hand was fully pronated. • Long axis of hand and wrist aligned to long axis of IR. • **No rotation** of hand, as evidenced by the following: the symmetric appearance of both sides or concavities of shafts of metacarpals and phalanges of digits 2 through 5; the amount of soft tissue on each side of phalanges 2 through 5 appearing equal. • Digits should be separated slightly with soft tissues not overlapping.

Collimation and CR: • Collimation should be visible on four sides. • CR and center of collimation field should be to **third MCP joint.**

Exposure Criteria: • Optimal density and contrast with no motion demonstrate soft-tissue margins and clear, sharp bony trabecular markings.

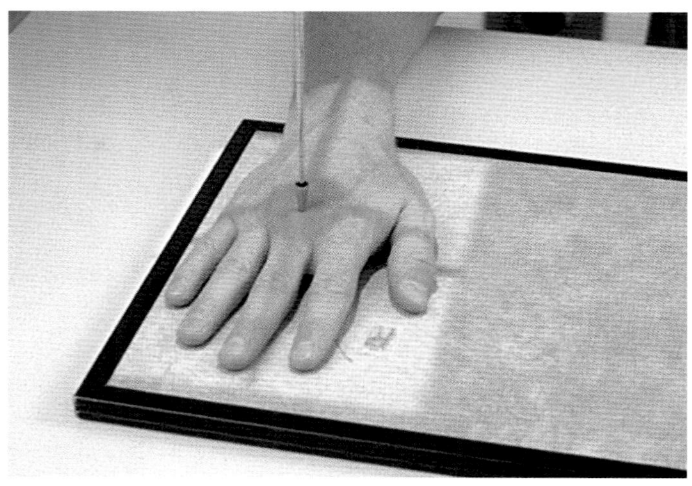

Fig. 5-68. PA hand, CR to third MCP joint.

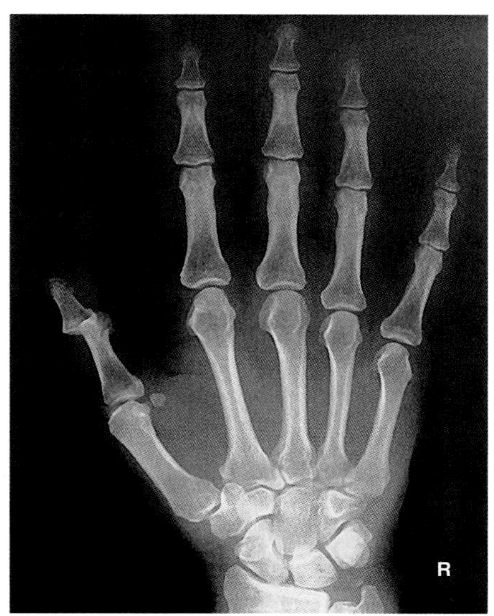

Fig. 5-69. PA hand.

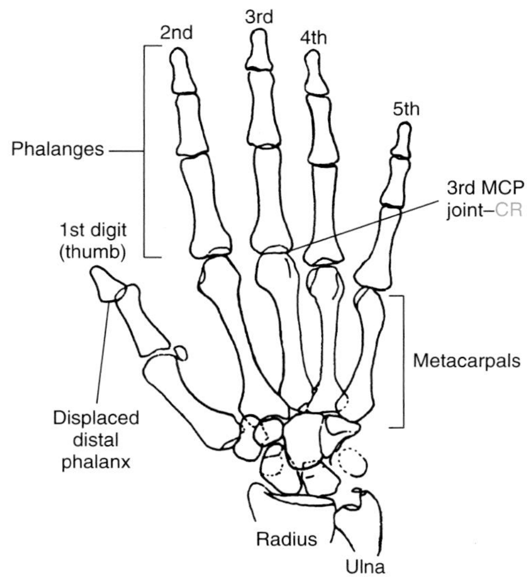

Fig. 5-70. PA hand.

PA OBLIQUE PROJECTION: HAND

Hand
BASIC
- PA
- PA oblique
- Lateral

Pathology Demonstrated

Fractures and/or dislocations of the phalanges, metacarpals, and all joints of the hand are shown. Pathologic processes, such as osteoporosis and osteoarthritis, also may be demonstrated.

Technical Factors

- IR size—24 × 30 cm (10 × 12 inches)
- Division of IR in half crosswise
- Digital IR—using lead masking
- Detail screen, tabletop
- 55-65 kV range
- Technique and dose:

cm	kV	mAs	Sk.	ML.	Gon.
4	64	3	12	12	M NDC F <0.1

mrad

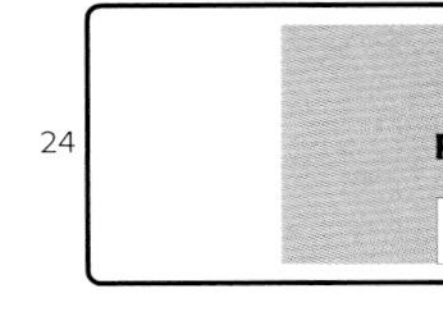

Shielding Place lead shield over patient's lap to shield gonads.

Patient Position Seat patient at end of table with elbow flexed about 90° and hand and forearm resting on table.

Part Position

- Pronate hand on cassette; center and align long axis of hand to long axis of portion of IR being exposed.
- Rotate entire hand and wrist laterally 45° and support with radiolucent wedge or step block, as shown, so that all digits are separated and **parallel to IR** (see Exception below).

Central Ray

- CR perpendicular to IR, directed to **third MCP joint**
- Minimum SID of 40 inches (100 cm)

Collimation Collimate on four sides to hand and wrist.

Exception: For a routine oblique hand, use a support block to place digits parallel to IR (Fig. 5-71). This block prevents foreshortening of phalanges and obscuring of interphalangeal joints. If the **metacarpals only** are of interest, the image can be taken with thumb and finger tips touching cassette (Fig. 5-72).

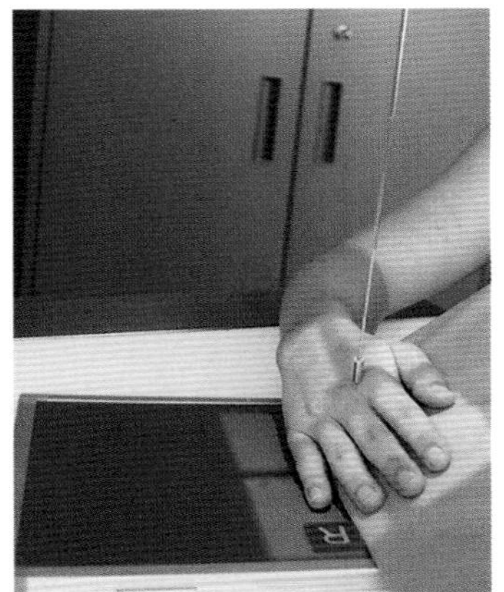

Fig. 5-71. Routine oblique hand (digits parallel).

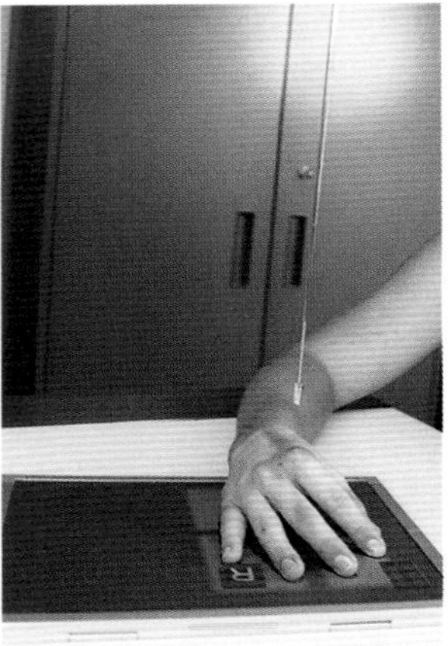

Fig. 5-72. Exception: Oblique hand for metacarpals (digits not parallel)—not recommended for digits.

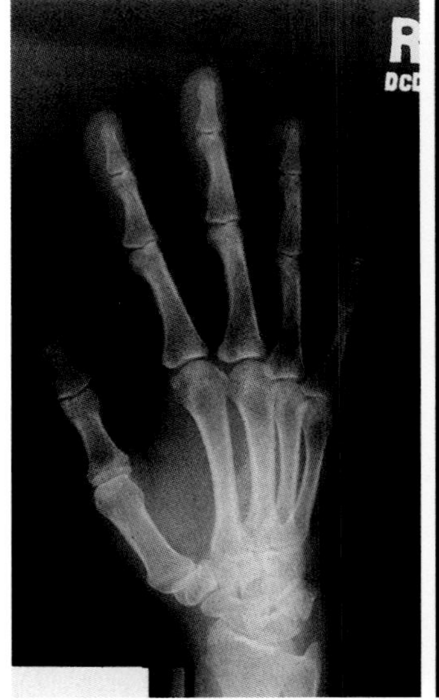

Fig. 5-73. Oblique hand (digits parallel).

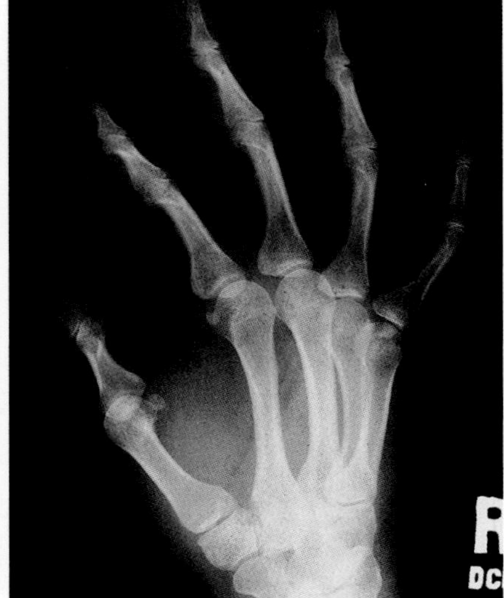

Fig. 5-74. Oblique hand (digits not parallel)—joint spaces not open.

Radiographic Criteria

Structures Shown: • Oblique projection of the entire hand and wrist and about 2.4 cm (1 inch) of distal forearm are visible.

Position: • Metacarpophalangeal and interphalangeal joints are open without foreshortening of midphalanges or distal phalanges, indicating fingers are parallel to IR. • Long axis of hand and wrist should be aligned with IR. • 45° oblique is evidenced by the following: Midshafts of third, fourth, and fifth metacarpals should not overlap; some overlap of distal heads of third, fourth, and fifth metacarpals but no overlap of distal second and third metacarpals should occur; excessive overlap of metacarpals indicates overrotation, and too much separation indicates underrotation.

Collimation and CR: • Collimation should be visible on four sides to area of affected hand. • CR and center of collimation field should be at **third MCP joint.**

Exposure Criteria: • Optimal density and contrast with no motion demonstrate soft-tissue margins and clear, sharp bony trabecular markings.

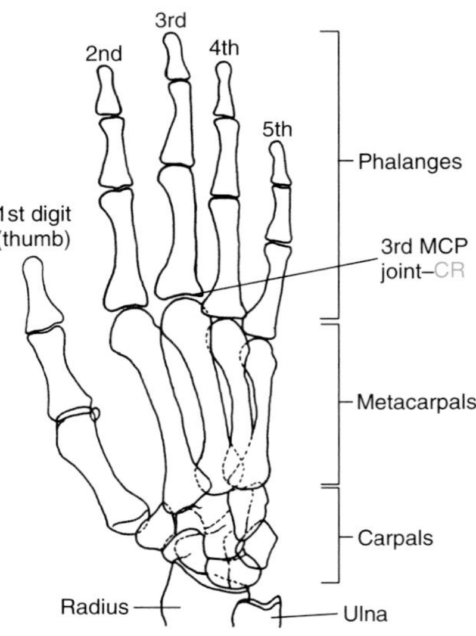

Fig. 5-75. Oblique hand (digits parallel).

"FAN" LATERAL—LATEROMEDIAL PROJECTION: HAND

Hand
BASIC
- PA
- PA oblique
- Lateral

18 × 24, R

Pathology Demonstrated

Fractures and dislocations of the phalanges, anterior/posterior displaced fractures, and dislocations of the metacarpals are shown. Some pathologic processes, such as osteoporosis and osteoarthritis, also may be demonstrated in the phalanges.

Technical Factors

- IR size—18 × 24 cm (8 × 10 inches) lengthwise
- Detail screen, tabletop
- 55-65 kV range
- Accessories—45° foam step support
- Technique and dose:

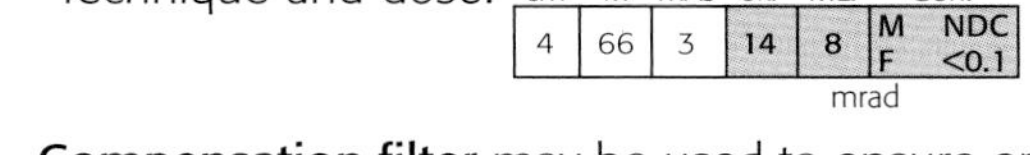

cm	kV	mAs	Sk.	ML.	Gon.
4	66	3	14	8	M NDC F <0.1

mrad

Compensation filter may be used to ensure optimum exposure of phalanges and metacarpals because of thickness difference.

Shielding Place lead shield over patient's lap to shield gonads.

Patient Position Seat patient at end of table with elbow flexed about 90° and hand and forearm resting on table.

Part Position

- Align long axis of hand to long axis of IR.
- Rotate hand and wrist into lateral position with thumb side up.
- Spread fingers and thumb into a "fan" position and support each digit on radiolucent step block as shown. Ensure that all digits, including the thumb, are separated and **parallel to IR** and that the metacarpals are **not** rotated but remain in a true lateral position.

Central Ray

- CR perpendicular to IR, directed to **second MCP joint**
- Minimum SID of 40 inches (100 cm)

Collimation Collimate on four sides to outer margins of hand and wrist.

Note: The "fan" lateral position is the preferred lateral for the hand if phalanges are area of interest. (See next page for alternative projections.)

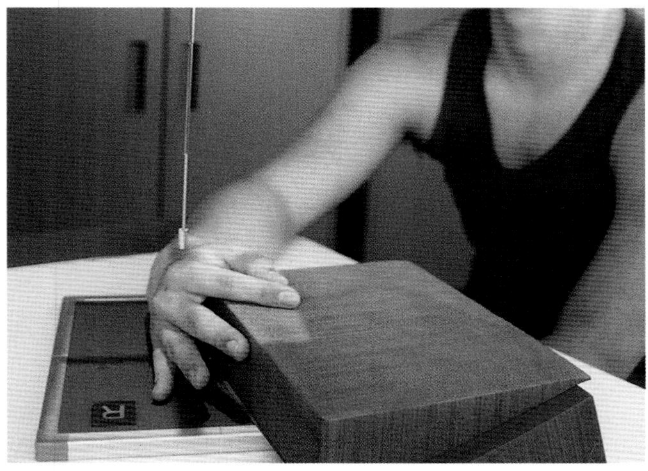

Fig. 5-76. Patient position—fan lateral hand (digits kept separated and parallel to IR); CR to second MCP joint.

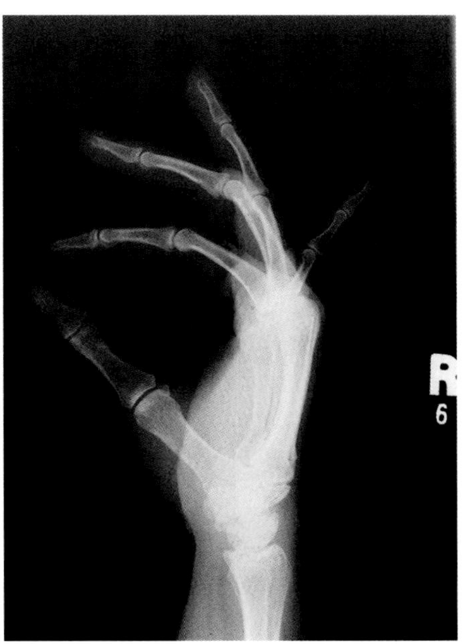

Fig. 5-77. Fan lateral.

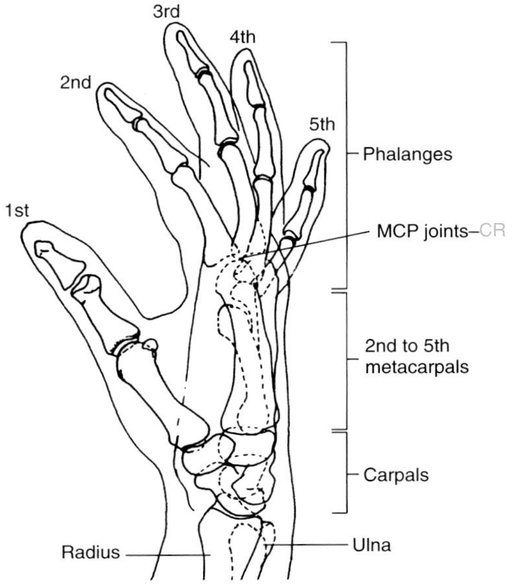

Fig. 5-78. Fan lateral.

Radiographic Criteria

Structures Shown: • Entire hand and wrist and about 2.5 cm (1 inch) of distal forearm are visible.

Position: • Fingers should appear equally separated, with phalanges in the lateral position and joint spaces open, indicating fingers were parallel to IR. • Thumb should appear in a slightly obliqued position completely free of superimposition, with joint spaces open. • Long axis of hand and wrist should be aligned to long axis of IR. • Hand and wrist should be in a true lateral position, as evidenced by the following: Distal radius and ulna are superimposed; metacarpals are superimposed.

Collimation and CR: • Collimation should be visible on four sides to area of affected hand. • CR and center of collimation field should be at **second MCP joint.**

Exposure Criteria: • Optimal density and contrast with no motion demonstrate soft-tissue margins and clear, sharp bony trabecular markings. • Outlines of individual metacarpals demonstrated are superimposed. • Midphalanges and distal phalanges of both thumb and fingers should appear sharp but may be slightly overexposed.

5

LATERAL IN EXTENSION AND FLEXION—LATEROMEDIAL PROJECTIONS: HAND

(Alternatives to Fan Lateral)

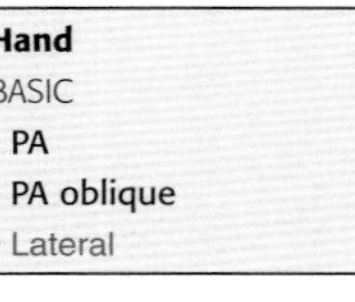

Hand
BASIC
• PA
• PA oblique
• Lateral

Pathology Demonstrated

The lateral in either extension or flexion is an alternative to the fan lateral for localization of foreign bodies of the hand and fingers and also demonstrates anterior or posterior displaced fractures of the metacarpals.

The lateral in a natural flexed position may be less painful for the patient.

Technical Factors

- IR size—18 × 24 cm (8 × 10 inches) lengthwise
- Detail screen, tabletop
- 55-65 kV range
- Technique and dose:

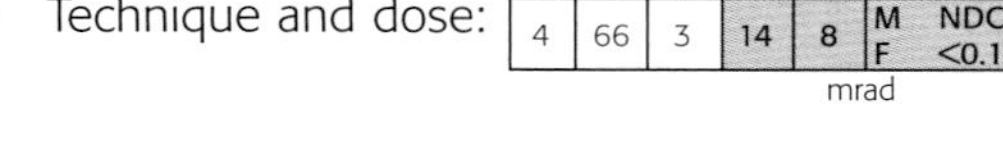

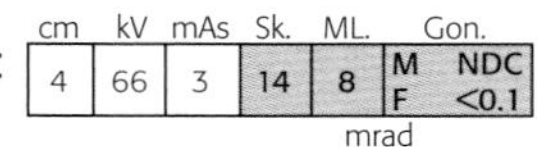

cm	kV	mAs	Sk.	ML.	Gon.
4	66	3	14	8	M NDC F <0.1

mrad

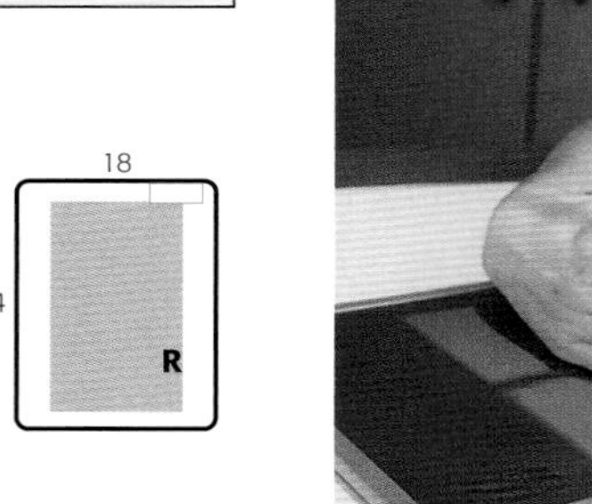

Fig. 5-79. Lateral in extension.

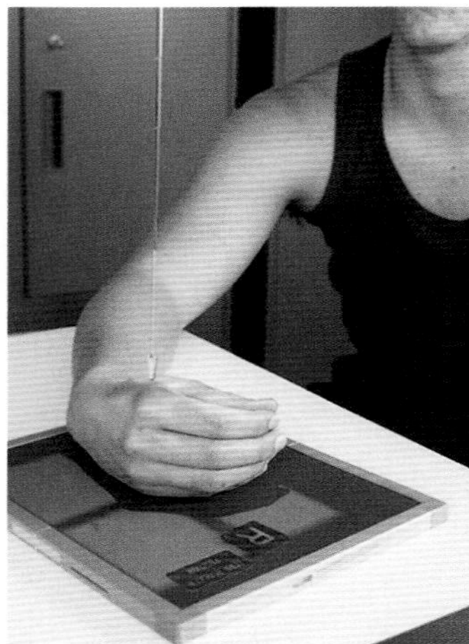

Fig. 5-80. Lateral in flexion.

Shielding Place lead shield over patient's lap to shield gonads.

Patient Position Seat patient at end of table with elbow flexed about 90° and hand and forearm resting on table.

Part Position

Rotate hand and wrist, with thumb side up, into a **true lateral position,** with second to fifth MCP joints centered to IR and CR.

- ***Lateral in extension:*** Extend fingers and thumb and support against a radiolucent support block. Ensure that all fingers are directly superimposed for a true lateral position.
- ***Lateral in flexion:*** Flex fingers into a natural flexed position, with thumb lightly touching the first finger; maintain true lateral position.

Central Ray

- CR perpendicular to IR, directed to the **second to fifth MCP joints**
- Minimum SID of 40 inches (100 cm)

Collimation Collimate to outer margins of hand and wrist.

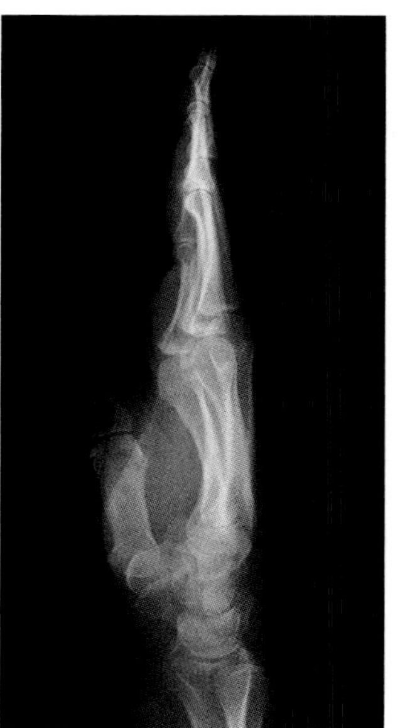

Fig. 5-81. Lateral in extension.

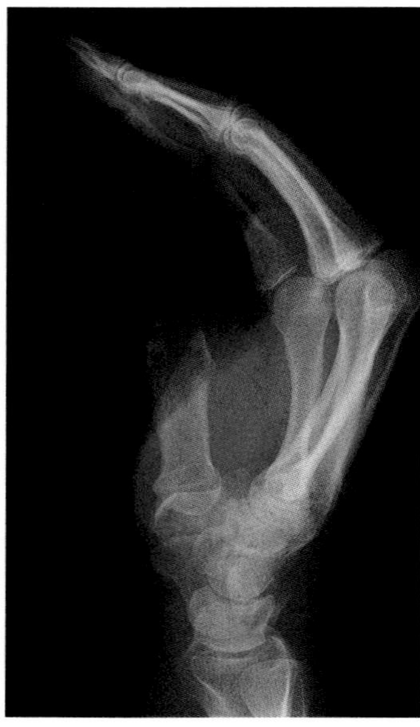

Fig. 5-82. Lateral in flexion.

Radiographic Criteria

Structures Shown: • Entire hand and wrist and about 2.5 cm (1 inch) of distal forearm are visible. • Thumb should appear slightly obliqued and free of superimposition with joint spaces open.

Position: • Long axis of the hand and the wrist are aligned with long axis of the IR. • Hand and wrist should be in a **true lateral position,** as evidenced by the following: Distal radius and ulna are superimposed; metacarpals and phalanges are superimposed.

Collimation and CR: • Collimation should be visible on four sides to area of affected hand. • CR and center of collimation field should be at **second to fifth MCP joints.**

Exposure Criteria: • Optimal density and contrast with no motion demonstrate soft-tissue margins and clear, sharp bony trabecular markings. • Margins of individual metacarpals and phalanges are visible but mostly superimposed.

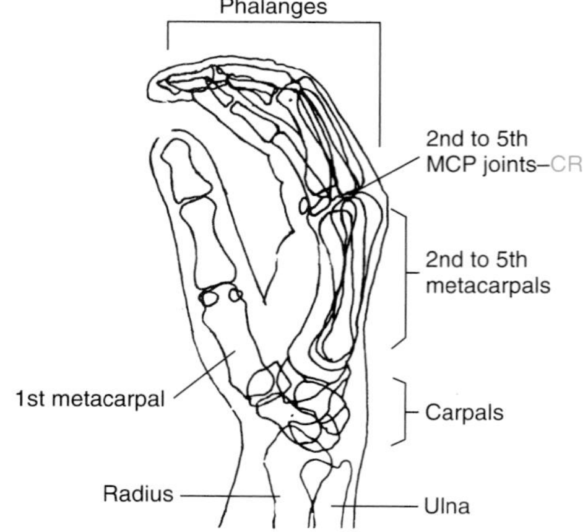

Fig. 5-83. Lateral in flexion.

5

AP OBLIQUE BILATERAL PROJECTION: HAND

Norgaard Method, or "Ball-Catcher's Position"

Hand
SPECIAL
• AP oblique bilateral

Pathology Demonstrated

This position is performed commonly to evaluate for early evidence of rheumatoid arthritis at the second through fifth proximal phalanges and MCP joints. It also may demonstrate fractures of the base of the fifth metacarpal.

Both hands are generally taken with one exposure for bony structure comparison of both hands.

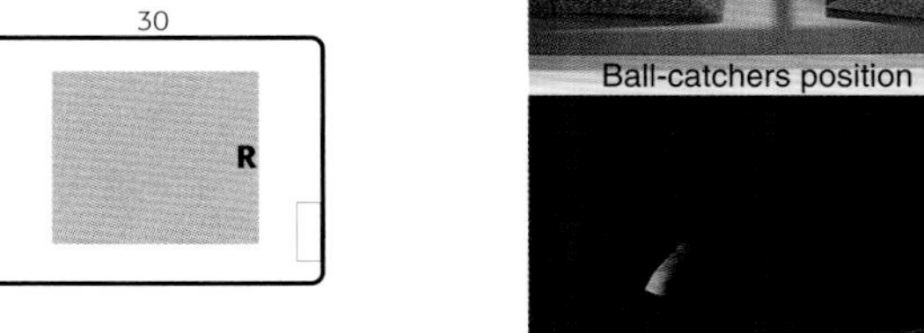

Technical Factors

- IR size—24 × 30 cm (10 × 12 inches) crosswise
- Detail screen, tabletop
- 55-65 kV range
- Technique and dose:

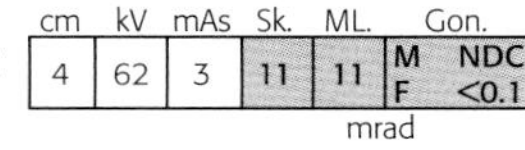

cm	kV	mAs	Sk.	ML.	Gon.
4	62	3	11	11	M NDC / F <0.1
			mrad		

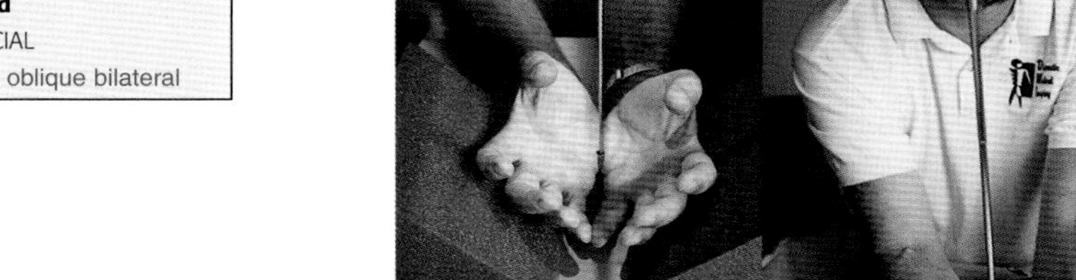

Fig. 5-84. AP bilateral 45° oblique. CR between fifth MCP joints.

Shielding Place lead shield over patient's lap to shield gonads.

Patient Position Seat patient at end of table with both hands extended.

Part Position

- Supinate hands and place medial aspect of both hands together at center of IR.
- From this position, internally rotate hands 45° and support posterior aspect of hands on 45° radiolucent blocks (Fig. 5-84).
- Extend fingers and ensure that they are relaxed, slightly separated but parallel to IR.
- Abduct both thumbs to avoid superimposition.

Central Ray

- CR perpendicular, directed to midpoint between both hands at **level of fifth MCP joints**
- Minimum SID of 40 inches (100 cm)

Collimation Collimate on four sides to outer margins of hands and wrists.

Note: A modification of the Norgaard method is the ball-catcher's position with the fingers partially flexed, which distorts the interphalangeal joints but visualizes the MCP joints equally well.

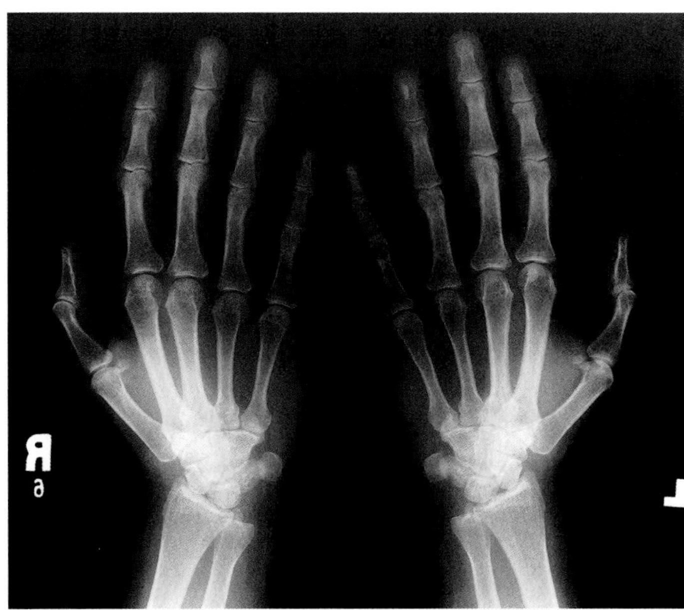

Fig. 5-85. AP 45° bilateral oblique.

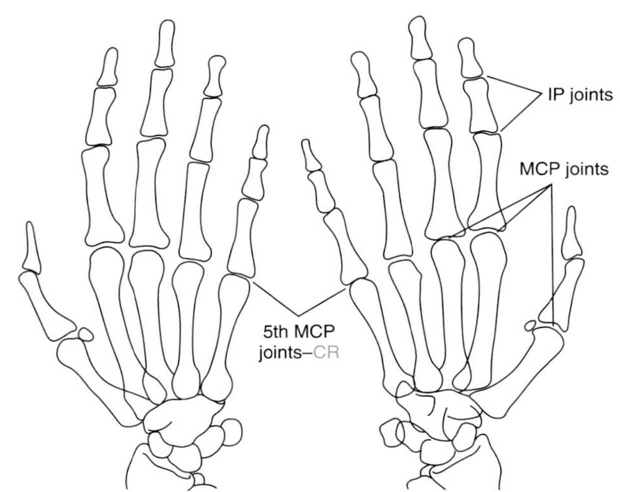

Fig. 5-86. AP 45° bilateral oblique.

Radiographic Criteria

Structures Shown: • Both hands from the carpal area to tips of digits in 45° oblique position are visible.

Position: • 45° oblique evidenced by the following: Midshafts of second through fifth metacarpals and base of phalanges should not overlap; MCP joints should be open; no superimposition of the thumb and second digit should occur.

Collimation and CR: • Collimation should be visible on four sides to outer margins of hands and wrists. • CR and center of collimation field to midway between both hands at **level of fifth MCP joints.**

Exposure Criteria: • Optimal density and contrast with no motion are demonstrated by clear, sharp bony trabecular markings and joint space margins of MCP joints.

5

PA (AP) PROJECTION: WRIST

Wrist
BASIC
• PA
• PA oblique
• Lateral

Pathology Demonstrated

Fractures of distal radius or ulna or isolated fractures of radial or ulnar styloid processes, as well as fractures of individual carpal bones, are demonstrated. Some pathologic processes, such as osteomyelitis and arthritis, also may be demonstrated.

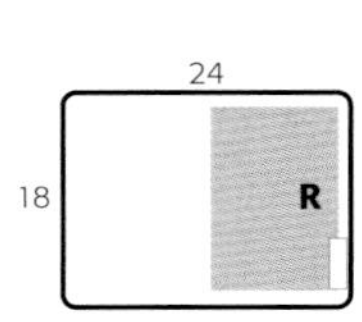

Technical Factors

- IR size—18 × 24 cm (8 × 10 inches)
- Division in half, crosswise
- Detail screen, tabletop
- Digital IR (use lead masking)
- 60 ± 6 kV range
- Technique and dose:

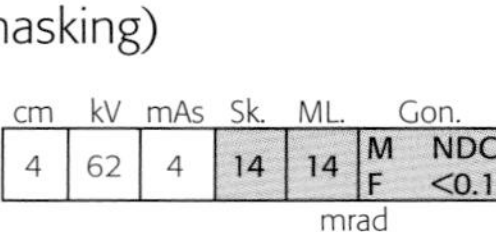

cm	kV	mAs	Sk.	ML.	Gon.	
4	62	4	14	14	M	NDC
					F	<0.1
			mrad			

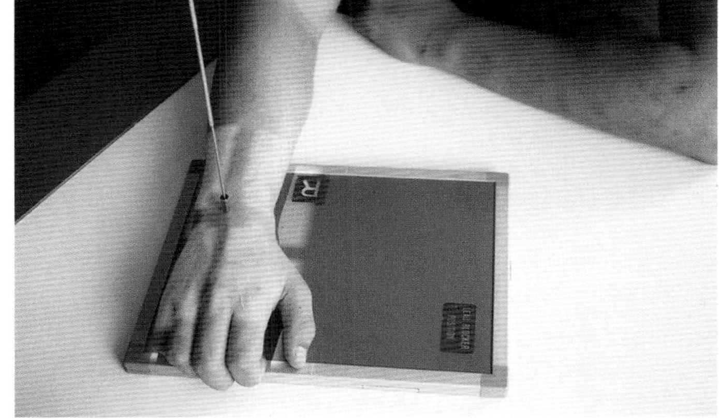

Fig. 5-87. PA wrist.

Shielding Place lead shield over patient's lap to shield gonads.

Patient Position Seat patient at end of table with elbow flexed about 90° and hand and wrist resting on cassette, palm down. Drop shoulder so that shoulder, elbow, and wrist are on same horizontal plane.

Part Position

- Align and center long axis of hand and wrist to portion of IR being exposed, with carpal area centered to CR.
- With hand pronated, arch hand slightly **to place wrist and carpal area in close contact with cassette.**

Central Ray

- CR perpendicular to IR, directed to **midcarpal area**
- Minimum SID of 40 inches (100 cm)

Collimation Collimate to wrist on all four sides; include distal radius and ulna and midmetacarpal area.

Alternative AP: To better demonstrate intercarpal spaces and wrist joint, an AP wrist may be taken, with hand slightly arched to place **wrist and carpals in close contact with cassette** and because the intercarpal spaces are more parallel to the divergent rays (Fig. 5-88). This wrist projection is good for visualizing the carpals if the patient can assume this position easily.

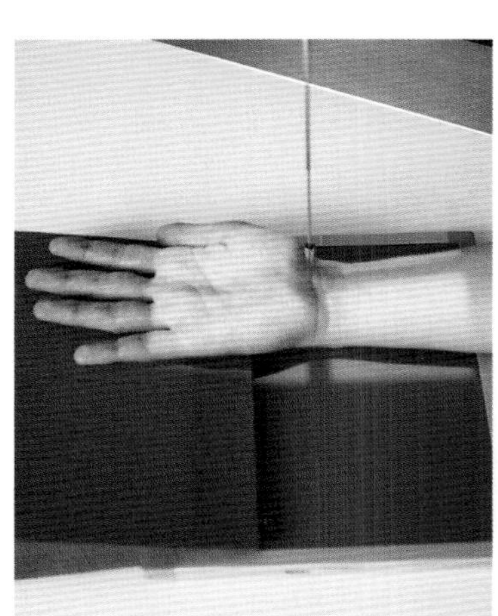

Fig. 5-88. Alternate AP wrist.

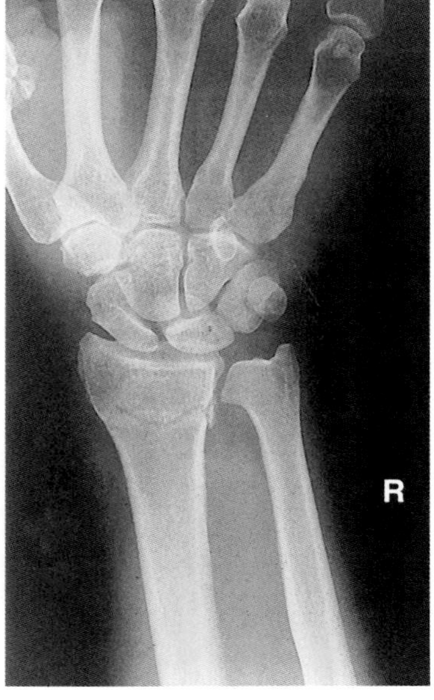

Fig. 5-89. PA wrist.

Radiographic Criteria

Structures Shown: • Midmetacarpals and proximal metacarpals; carpals; distal radius, ulna, and associated joints; and pertinent soft tissues of the wrist joint, such as fat pads and fat stripes, are visible. • The intercarpal spaces do not all appear open because of irregular shapes that result in overlapping.

Position: • Long axis of the hand, wrist, and forearm is aligned with IR. • True PA is evidenced by the following: Equal concavity shapes are on each side of the shafts of the proximal metacarpals; near equal distances exist among the proximal metacarpals; separation of the distal radius and ulna is present, except for possible minimal superimposition at the distal radioulnar joint.

Collimation and CR: • Collimation should be visible on four sides to area of affected wrist. • CR and center of collimation field should be to the **midcarpal area.**

Exposure Criteria: • Optimal density and contrast with no motion should visualize soft tissue, such as pertinent fat pads, and sharp, bony margins of the carpals and clear trabecular markings.

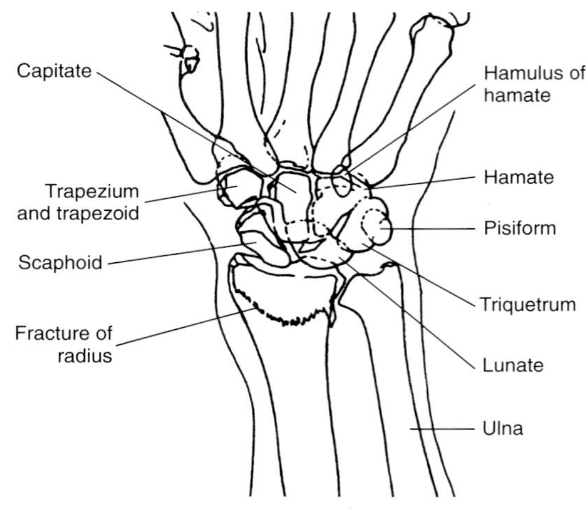

Fig. 5-90. PA wrist.

PA OBLIQUE PROJECTION—LATERAL ROTATION: WRIST

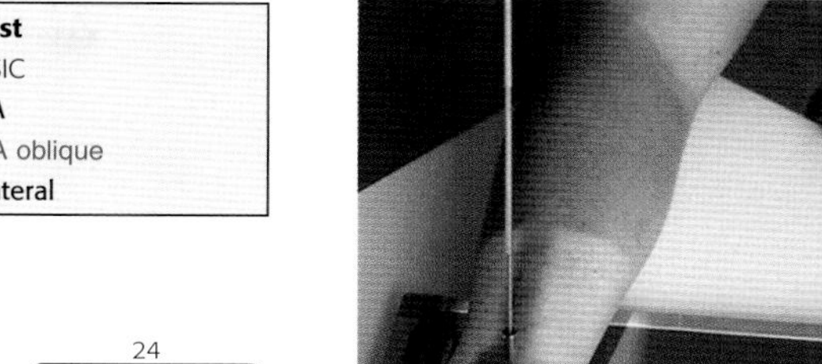

Pathology Demonstrated
Fractures of distal radius or ulna or isolated fractures of radial or ulnar styloid processes, as well as fractures of individual carpal bones, are demonstrated. Some pathologic processes, such as osteomyelitis and arthritis, also may be demonstrated.

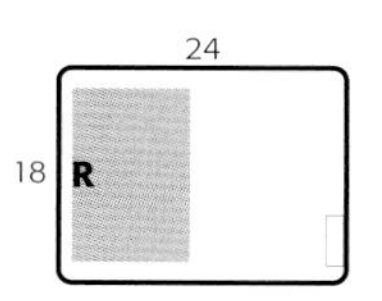

Technical Factors
- IR size—18 × 24 cm (8 × 10 inches)
- Division in half, crosswise
- Digital IR (use lead masking)
- Detail screen, tabletop
- 60 ± 6 kV range
- Technique and dose:

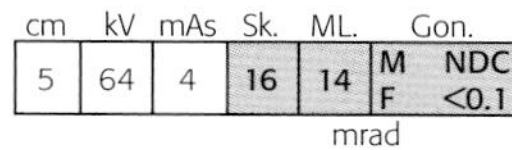

cm	kV	mAs	Sk.	ML.	Gon.
5	64	4	16	14	M NDC / F <0.1
			mrad		

Shielding Place lead shield over patient's lap to shield gonads.

Patient Position Seat patient at end of table, with elbow flexed about 90° and hand and wrist resting on cassette, palm down.

Part Position
- Align and center hand and wrist to portion of IR being exposed.
- From pronated position, rotate wrist and hand laterally 45°.
- For stability, place a 45° support under thumb side of hand to support hand and wrist in a 45° oblique position (Fig. 5-92), or partially flex fingers to arch hand so that fingertips rest lightly on cassette (Fig. 5-91).

Central Ray
- CR perpendicular to IR, directed to **midcarpal area**
- Minimum SID of 40 inches (100 cm)

Collimation Collimate to wrist on four sides and include distal radius and ulna and the midmetacarpal area, at least.

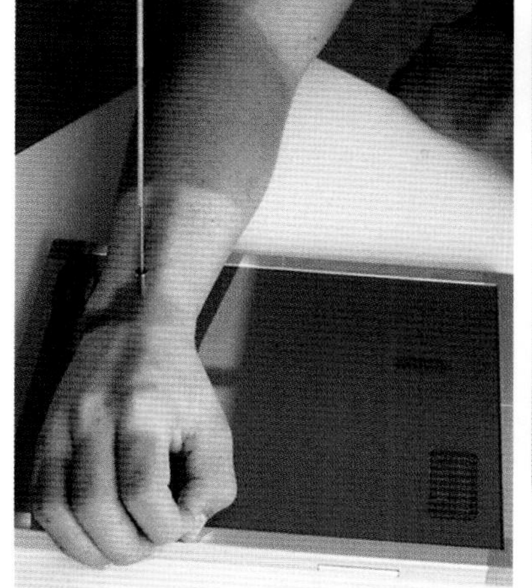

Fig. 5-91. Oblique wrist.

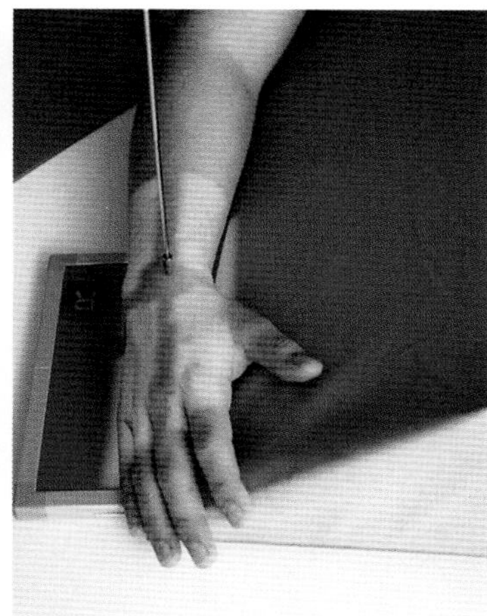

Fig. 5-92. Oblique wrist (with 45° support).

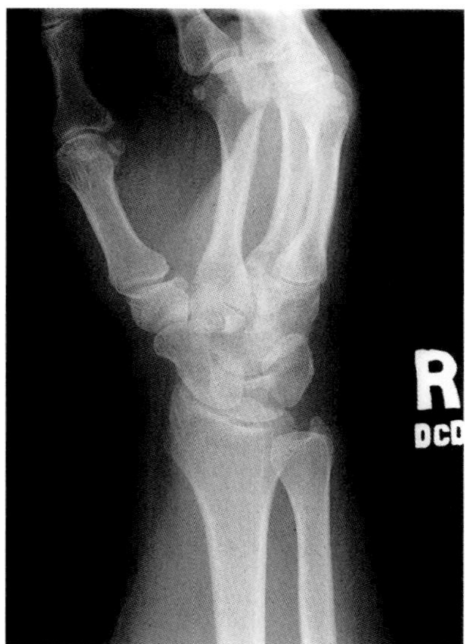

Fig. 5-93. Oblique wrist.

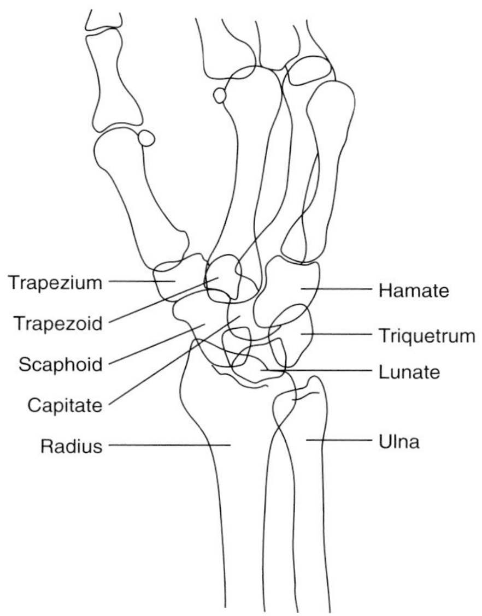

Fig. 5-94. Oblique wrist.

Radiographic Criteria

Structures Shown: • Distal radius, ulna, carpals, and at least to midmetacarpal area are visible. • The trapezium and scaphoid should be well visualized, with only slight superimposition of other carpals on their medial aspects.

Position: • Long axis of the hand, wrist, and forearm should be aligned with IR. • 45° oblique of the wrist should be evident by ulnar head being partially superimposed by distal radius. • The proximal third, fourth, and fifth metacarpals should appear mostly superimposed.

Collimation and CR: • Collimation should be visible on four sides to area of affected wrist. • CR and center of collimation field should be to midcarpal area.

Exposure Criteria: • Optimal density and contrast with no motion demonstrate the carpals and their overlapping borders, soft-tissue margins, and clear, sharp bony trabecular markings.

LATERAL–LATEROMEDIAL PROJECTION: WRIST

Wrist
BASIC
- PA
- PA oblique
- Lateral

Pathology Demonstrated
Fractures or dislocations of the distal radius or ulna, specifically anteroposterior dislocations of **Barton's, Colles', or Smith's type fracture,** are shown. Osteoarthritis also may be demonstrated primarily in the trapezium and first CMC joint.

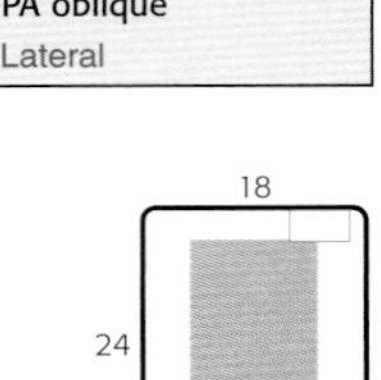

Technical Factors
- IR size—18 × 24 cm (8 × 10 inches) lengthwise
- Detail screen, tabletop
- Digital IR—(use lead masking)
- 64 ± 6 kV range; increased kV (±4) from PA and oblique
- Technique and dose:

cm	kV	mAs	Sk.	ML.	Gon.
7	66	5	22	16	M NDC F <0.1
			mrad		

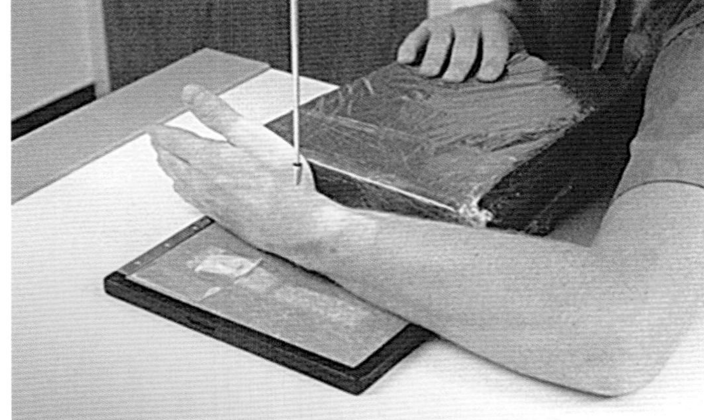

Fig. 5-95. Patient position—lateral wrist.

Shielding Place lead shield over patient's lap to shield gonads.

Patient Position Seat patient at end of table, with both arm and forearm resting on the table and elbow flexed about 90°. Place wrist and hand on cassette in thumb-up lateral position. Shoulder, elbow, and wrist should be on same horizontal plane.

Part Position
- Align and center hand and wrist to long axis of IR.
- Adjust hand and wrist into a **true lateral** position, with fingers comfortably flexed; or if support is needed to prevent motion, use a radiolucent support block and sandbag and place block against extended hand and fingers as shown.

Central Ray
- CR perpendicular to IR, directed to **midcarpal area**
- Minimum SID of 40 inches (100 cm)

Collimation Collimate on four sides, including distal radius and ulna and the metacarpal area.

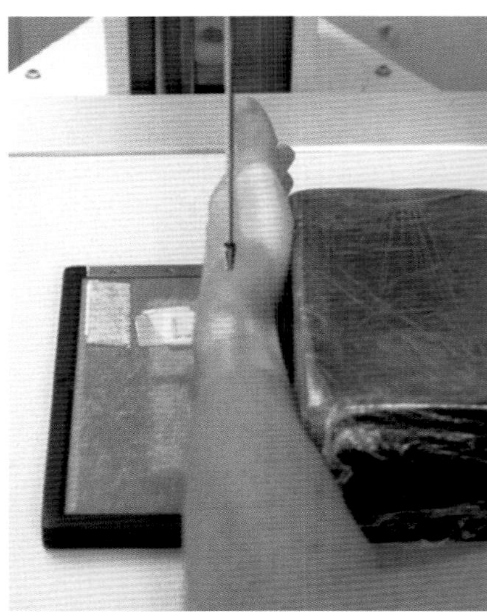

Fig. 5-96. Part position—lateral wrist.

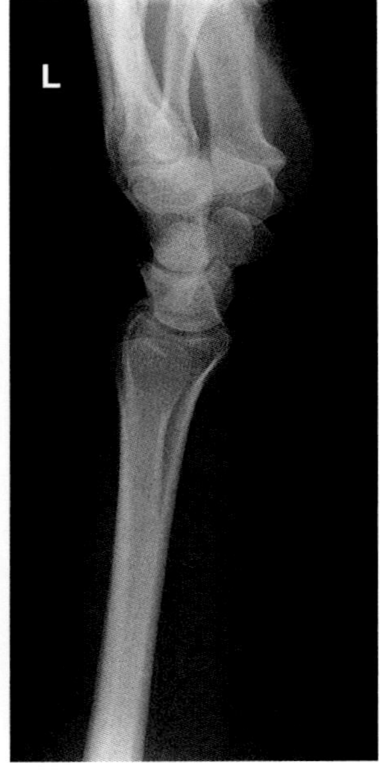

Fig. 5-97. Lateral wrist.

Radiographic Criteria

Structures Shown: • Distal radius and ulna, carpals, and at least the midmetacarpal area are visible.

Position: • Long axis of the hand, wrist, and forearm should be aligned with long axis of IR. • **True lateral** position is evidenced by the following: Ulnar head should be superimposed over distal radius; proximal second through fifth metacarpals all should appear aligned and superimposed.

Collimation and CR: • Collimation should be visible on four sides to area of affected wrist. • CR and center of collimation field should be to **midcarpal region.**

Exposure Criteria: • Optimal density and contrast with no motion demonstrate clear, sharp bony trabecular markings and soft tissue, such as margins of pertinent fat pads of the wrist and borders of the distal ulna, seen through the superimposed radius.

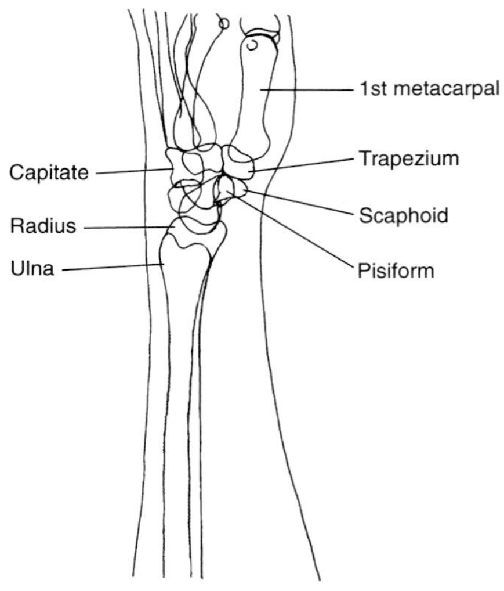

Fig. 5-98. Lateral wrist.

PA SCAPHOID—WITH CR ANGLE AND ULNAR DEVIATION: WRIST

Wrist
SPECIAL
• Scaphoid views: CR angle, ulnar deviation

Warning: If patient has possible wrist trauma, do **not** attempt this position before routine wrist series has been completed to rule out possible fractures of distal forearm and/or wrist.

Pathology Demonstrated
Fractures of the **scaphoid** are demonstrated.

Technical Factors
- IR size—18 × 24 cm (8 × 10 inches)
- Division in half, crosswise
- Detail screen, tabletop
- Digital IR (use lead masking)
- 60 ± 6 kV range
- Technique and dose:

cm	kV	mAs	Sk.	ML.	Gon.	
4	64	4	16	16	M	NDC
					F	<0.1
				mrad		

Shielding Place lead shield over patient's lap to shield gonads.

Patient Position Seat patient at end of table, with wrist and hand on cassette, palm down, and shoulder, elbow, and wrist on same horizontal plane.

Part Position
- Position wrist as for a PA projection—palm down and hand and wrist aligned to center of long axis of portion of IR being exposed, with scaphoid centered to CR.
- Without moving forearm, gently evert hand (move toward ulnar side) as far as patient can tolerate without lifting or rotating distal forearm.

Central Ray
- Angle CR **10° to 15° proximally,** along long axis of forearm and toward elbow. (CR angle should be perpendicular to long axis of scaphoid.)
- Center CR to **scaphoid.** (Locate scaphoid at a point 2 cm or ¾ inch distal and medial to radial styloid process.)
- Minimum SID is 40 inches (100 cm).

Collimation Collimate on four sides to carpal region.

Note: Obscure fractures of the scaphoid may require several projections taken with different CR angles, such as a four-projection series with the CR angled proximally 0°, 10°, 20°, and 30°.*

Radiographic Criteria

Structures Shown: • Distal radius and ulna, carpals, and proximal metacarpals are visible. • Scaphoid should be demonstrated clearly without foreshortening, with adjacent carpal interspaces open (evidence of CR angle).

Position: • Long axis of wrist and forearm should be aligned with side border of IR. • Ulnar deviation should be evident by the angle of the long axis of the metacarpals to that of the radius and ulna. • **No rotation** of wrist is evidenced by appearance of distal radius and ulna, with minimal superimposition of distal radioulnar joint.

Collimation and CR: • Collimation should be visible on four sides to area of affected wrist. • CR and center of collimation field should be to the **scaphoid.**

Exposure Criteria: • Optimal density and contrast with no motion visualize the scaphoid borders and clear, sharp bony trabecular markings.

*Rafert JA, Long BW: Technique for diagnosis of scaphoid fractures, Radiol Technol 63(1):16-21, 1991.

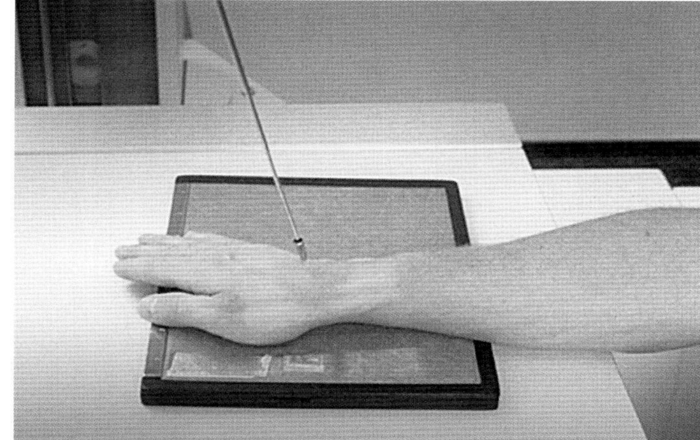

Fig. 5-99. PA wrist (scaphoid)—ulnar deviation with 15° CR angle.

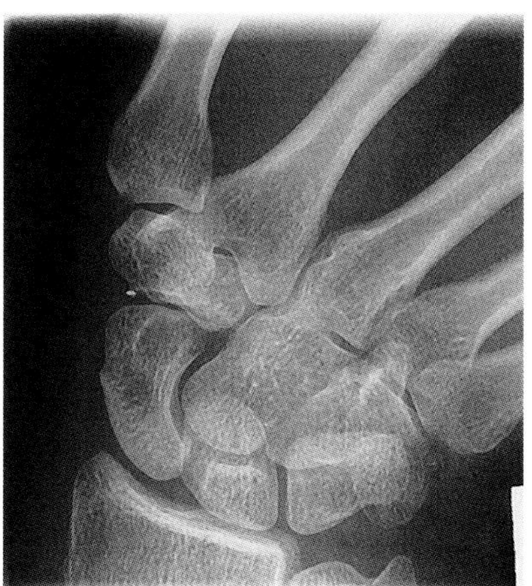

Fig. 5-100. 15° CR angle.

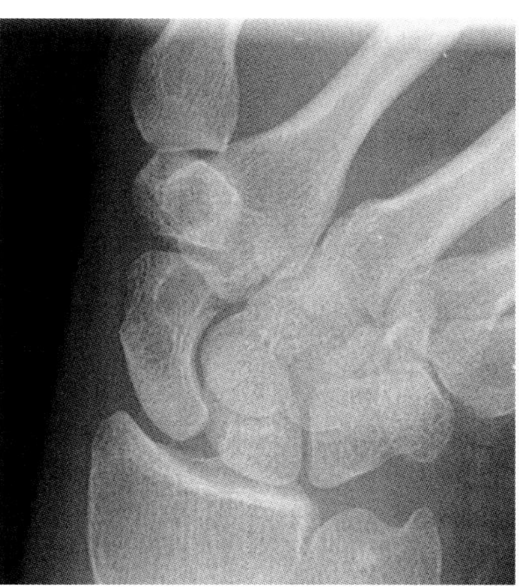

Fig. 5-101. 25° CR angle.

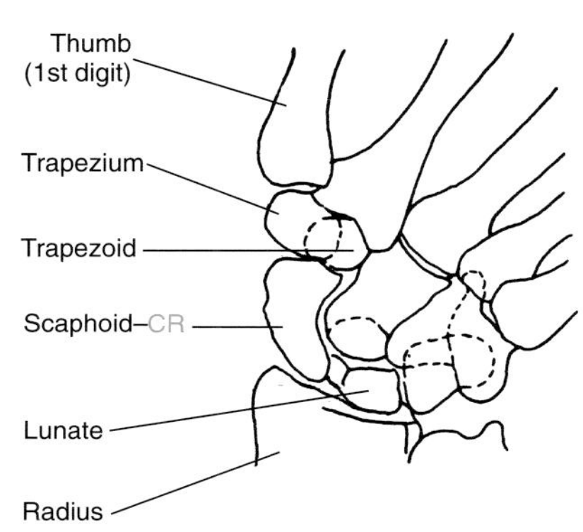

Fig. 5-102. 15° angle.

5

PA SCAPHOID—HAND ELEVATED AND ULNAR DEVIATION: WRIST

Modified Stecher Method*

Warning: If patient has possible wrist trauma, do **not** attempt this position before routine wrist series has been completed to rule out possible fractures of distal forearm and/or wrist.

Wrist
SPECIAL
- Scaphoid views: CR angle, ulnar deviation, modified Stecher method

24
18
R

Pathology Demonstrated

Fractures of the **scaphoid** are shown. This is an alternative projection to the CR angle ulnar deviation method demonstrated on the preceding page.

Technical Factors

- IR size—18 × 24 cm (8 × 10 inches)
- Division in half, crosswise
- Detail screen, tabletop
- Digital IR (use lead masking)
- 60 ± 6 kV range
- Technique and dose:

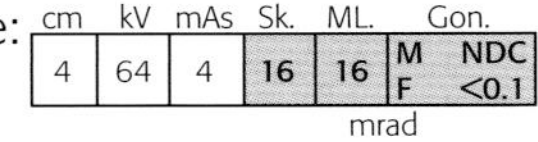

cm	kV	mAs	Sk.	ML.	Gon.
4	64	4	16	16	M NDC F <0.1
			mrad		

Shielding Place lead shield over lap to shield gonads.

Patient Position Seat patient at end of table, with elbow flexed and resting on table, wrist and hand on cassette, palm down, with shoulder, elbow, and wrist on same horizontal plane.

Part Position

- Place hand and wrist palm down on cassette with **hand elevated on 20° angle sponge.**
- Ensure that wrist is in direct contact with cassette.
- Gently evert or turn hand outward (toward ulnar side) unless contraindicated because of severe injury (Fig. 5-104).

Alternate method: Have patient clench the fist along with ulnar deviation to obtain a similar position of the scaphoid.

Central Ray

- CR **perpendicular to IR,** directed to **scaphoid** (2 cm, or ¾ inch, proximal and 2 cm, or ¾ inch, lateral to first CMC joint)
- Minimum SID of 40 inches (100 cm)

Collimation Collimate on four sides to carpal region.

Note: Stecher* indicated that elevation of the hand 20° rather than angling of the CR places the scaphoid parallel to the IR. Stecher also suggested that clenching of the fist is an alternative to elevation of the hand or angling of the CR. Bridgman† recommended ulnar deviation in addition to the hand elevation for less scaphoid superimposition.

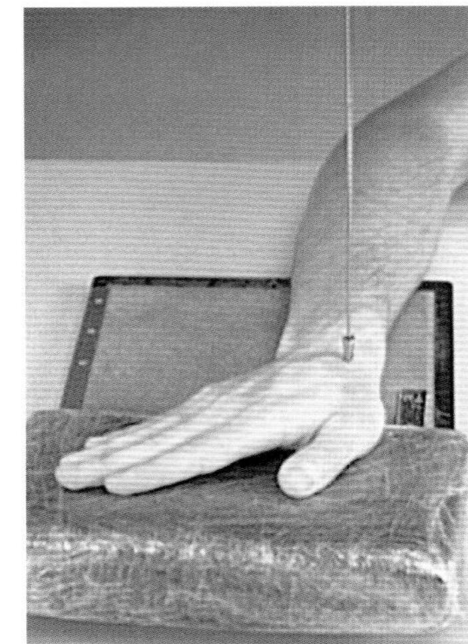

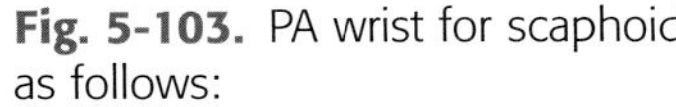

Fig. 5-103. PA wrist for scaphoid as follows:
- Hand elevated 20°
- Ulnar deviation if possible
- No CR angle

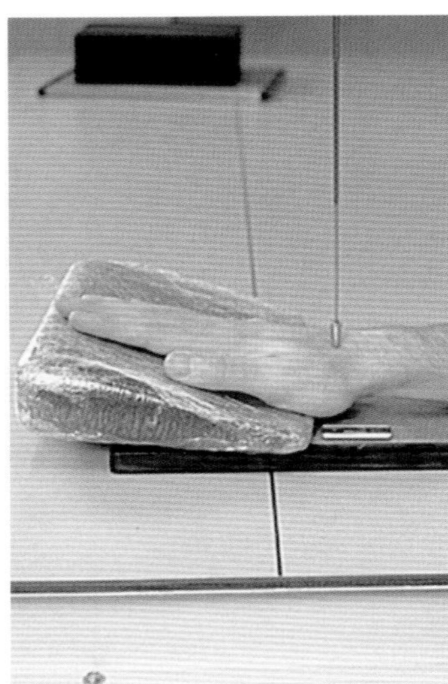

Fig. 5-104. Severe pain as follows:
- Hand elevated 20°
- **No** ulnar deviation
- No CR angle

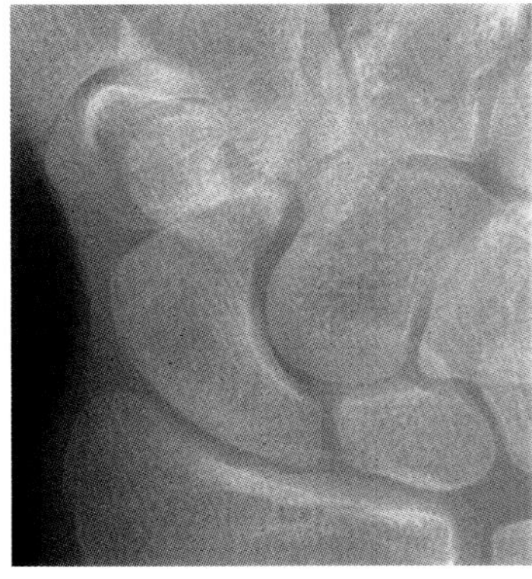

Fig. 5-105. Hand elevated, ulnar deviation, and no CR angle.

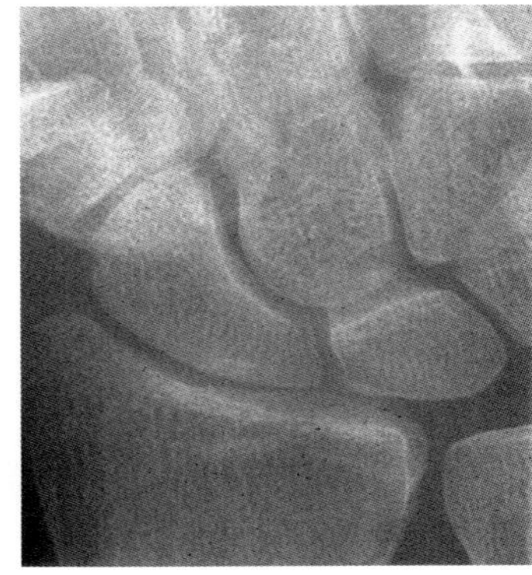

Fig. 5-106. Hand elevated, no ulnar deviation, or CR angle.

Radiographic Criteria

Structures Shown: • The distal radius and ulna, carpals, and proximal metacarpals are visible. • The carpals are visible, with adjacent interspaces more open on the lateral (radial) side of the wrist. • Scaphoid is shown, without foreshortening or superimposition of adjoining carpals.

Position: • Long axis of wrist and forearm should be aligned with side border of IR. • Ulnar deviation is evidenced by only minimal if any superimposition of distal scaphoid. • **No rotation** of wrist is evidenced by the appearance of distal radius and ulna with no or only minimal superimposition of distal radioulnar joint.

Collimation and CR: • Collimation should be visible on four sides to area of affected wrist. • CR and center of collimation field should be to **scaphoid.**

Exposure Criteria: • Optimal density and contrast with no motion visualize the scaphoid borders and clear, sharp bony trabecular markings.

5

*Stecher WR: Roentgenography of the carpal navicular bone, AJR 37:704-705, 1937.
†Bridgman CF: Radiography of the carpal navicular bone, Med Radiog Photog 25:104-105, 1949.

PA PROJECTION—RADIAL DEVIATION: WRIST

Warning: If patient has possible wrist trauma, do **not** attempt this position before routine wrist series has been completed to rule out possible fractures of distal forearm and/or wrist.

Wrist
SPECIAL
- **Scaphoid views: CR angle, ulnar deviation, modified Stecher method**
- Radial deviation

24
18 **R**

Pathology Demonstrated

Fractures of the carpal bones on the ulnar side of the wrist, especially the lunate, triquetrum, pisiform, and hamate, are shown.

Technical Factors

- IR size—18 × 24 cm (8 × 10 inches)
- Division in half, crosswise
- Detail screen, tabletop
- Digital IR—(use lead masking)
- 60 ± 6 kV range
- Technique and dose:

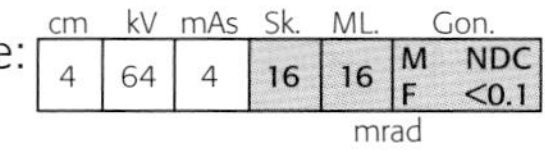

cm	kV	mAs	Sk.	ML.	Gon.
4	64	4	16	16	M NDC F <0.1
				mrad	

Shielding Place lead shield over patient's lap to shield gonads.

Patient Position Seat patient at end of table, with elbow flexed at 90° and resting on table, wrist and hand on cassette, palm down, with shoulder, elbow, and wrist on same horizontal plane.

Part Position

- Position wrist as for a PA projection—palm down with wrist and hand aligned to center of long axis of portion of IR being exposed.
- Without moving forearm, gently invert the hand (move medially toward thumb side) as far as patient can tolerate without lifting or rotating distal forearm.

Central Ray

- CR **perpendicular to IR,** directed to **midcarpal area**
- Minimum SID of 40 inches (100 cm)

Collimation Collimate on four sides to carpal region.

Radiographic Criteria

Structures Shown: • The distal radius and ulna, the carpals, and the proximal metacarpals are visible. • The carpals are visible, with adjacent interspaces more open on the medial (ulnar) side of the wrist.

Position: • The long axis of forearm is aligned to the side border of the IR • Extreme radial deviation is evidenced by the angle of the long axis of the metacarpals to that of the radius and ulna and the space between the triquetrum/pisiform and the styloid process of the radius. • **No rotation** of the wrist is evidenced by the appearance of the distal radius and ulna.

Collimation and CR: • Collimation should be visible on four sides to the area of the affected wrist. • CR and center of the collimation field should be to the **midcarpal area.**

Exposure Criteria: • Optimal density and contrast with no motion visualize the carpal borders and clear, sharp bony trabecular markings.

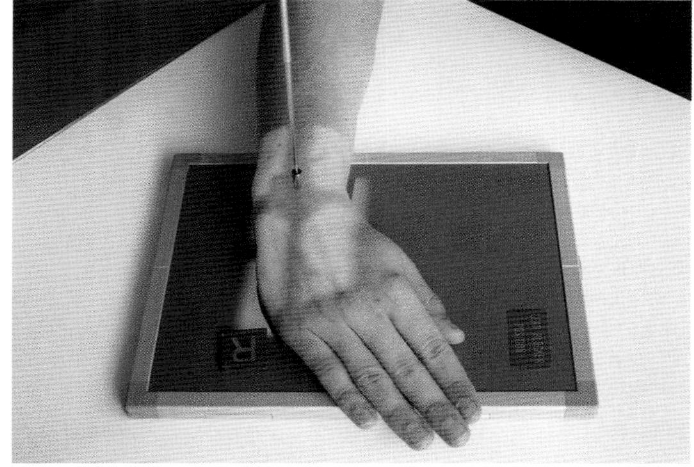

Fig. 5-107. PA wrist-radial deviation.

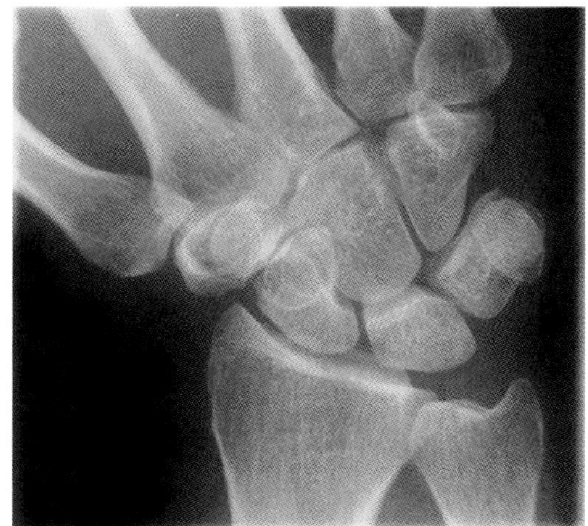

Fig. 5-108. Radial deviation.

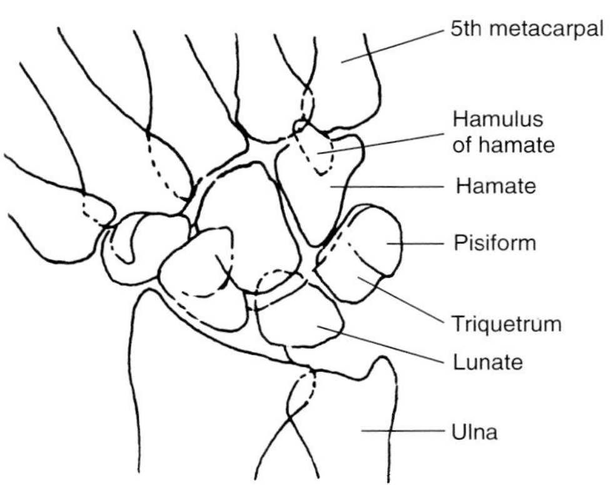

Fig. 5-109. Radial deviation.

CARPAL CANAL (TUNNEL)—TANGENTIAL, INFEROSUPERIOR PROJECTION: WRIST

Gaynor-Hart Method

Warning: If patient has possible wrist trauma, do **not** attempt this position before routine wrist series has been completed to rule out possible fractures of distal forearm and/or wrist.

Wrist
SPECIAL
- **Scaphoid views: CR angle, ulnar deviation, modified Stecher method**
- **Radial deviation**
- Carpal canal

Pathology Demonstrated

This projection is performed most commonly to rule out abnormal calcification and bony changes in the carpal sulcus that may impinge on the **median nerve,** as with **carpal tunnel syndrome.**

It also visualizes fractures of the hamulus process of the hamate, pisiform, and trapezium.

24

18 R

Technical Factors

- IR size—18 × 24 cm (8 × 10 inches)
- Detail screen, tabletop
- 64 ± 6 kV range
- Technique and dose:

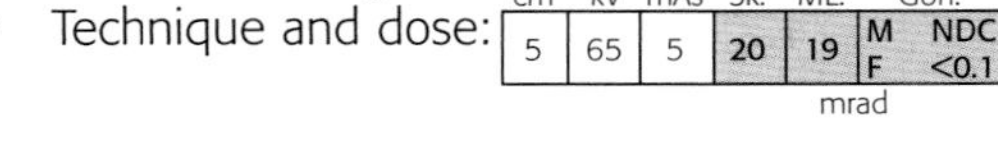
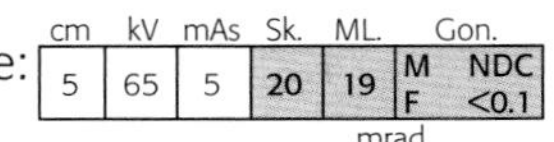

cm	kV	mAs	Sk.	ML.	Gon.
5	65	5	20	19	M NDC F <0.1
				mrad	

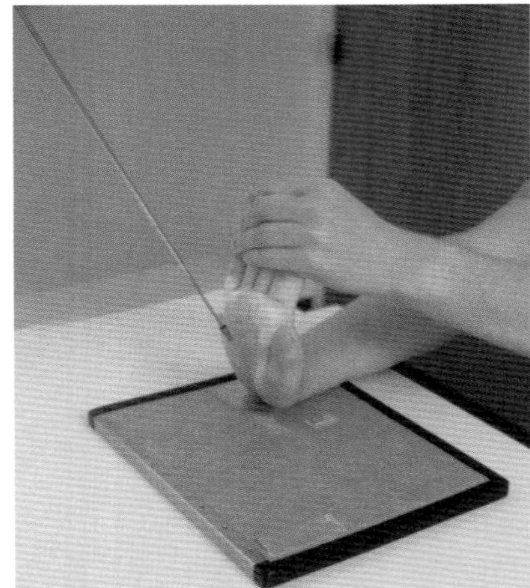

Fig. 5-110. Tangential projection. CR 25° to 30° to long axis of hand.

Shielding Place lead shield over patient's lap to shield gonads.

Patient Position Seat patient at end of table, with wrist and hand on cassette and palm down (pronated).

Part Position

- Align hand and wrist to long axis of portion of IR being exposed.
- Ask patient to hyperextend wrist (dorsiflex) as far as possible by grasping the fingers with other hand and gently but firmly hyperextending the wrist until the long axis of the metacarpals and the fingers are as near vertical (90° to forearm) as possible (without lifting the wrist and forearm from the cassette).
- Rotate entire hand and wrist about **10° internally** (toward radial side) to prevent superimposition of pisiform and hamate.

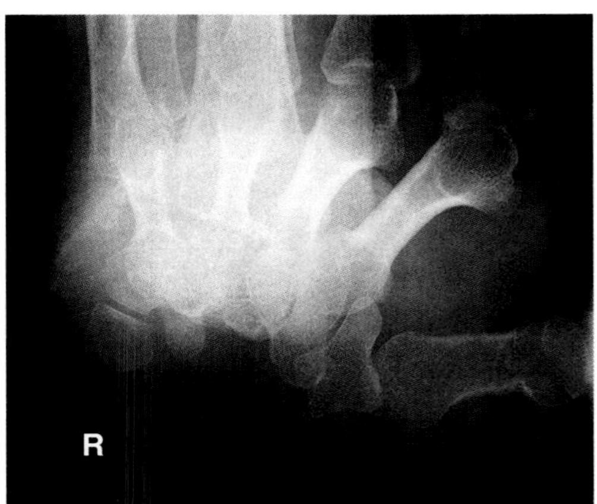

Fig. 5-111. Tangential projection.

Central Ray

- Angle CR **25° to 30° to the long axis of the hand.** (The total CR angle in relationship to the IR must be increased if patient cannot hyperextend wrist as far as indicated.)
- Direct CR to a point **2 to 3 cm (1 inch) distal to the base of third metacarpal** (center of palm of hand).
- Minimum SID is 40 inches (100 cm).

Collimation Collimate on four sides to area of interest.

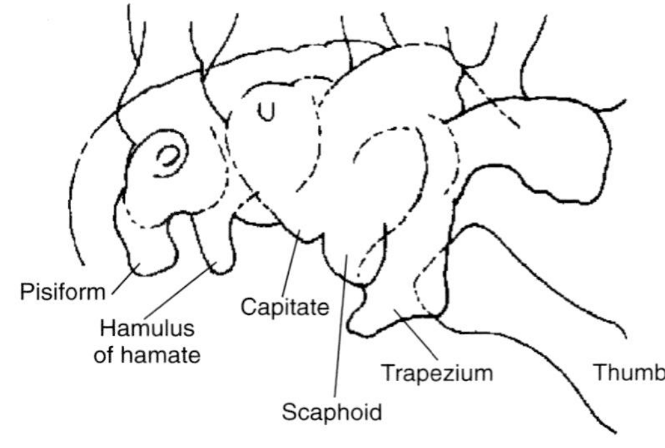

Fig. 5-112. Tangential projection.

Radiographic Criteria

Structures Shown: • The carpals are demonstrated in a tunnel-like, arched arrangement.

Position: • The pisiform and the hamulus process should be separated and visible in profile without superimposition. • The rounded palmar aspects of the capitate and the scaphoid should be visualized in profile, as well as that aspect of the trapezium that articulates with the first metacarpal.

Collimation and CR: • Collimation should be visible on four sides to area of affected wrist. • CR and center of collimation field should be to **midpoint of the carpal canal.**

Exposure Criteria: • Optimal density and contrast should visualize soft tissues and possible calcifications in carpal canal region, and outlines of superimposed carpals should be visible without overexposure of these carpals in profile. Trabecular markings and bony margins should appear clear and sharp, indicating no motion.

5

CARPAL BRIDGE—TANGENTIAL PROJECTION: WRIST

Warning: If patient has possible wrist trauma, do **not** attempt this position before routine wrist series has been completed to rule out possible fractures of distal forearm and/or wrist.

Wrist
SPECIAL
- **Scaphoid views: CR angle, ulnar deviation, modified Stecher method**
- **Radial deviation**
- **Carpal canal**
- Carpal bridge

Pathology Demonstrated

Calcifications or other pathology of the dorsal aspect of the carpal bones are shown.

Technical Factors

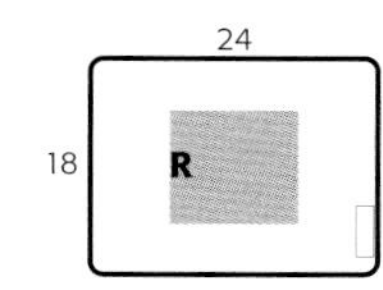

- IR size—18 × 24 cm (8 × 10 inches)
- Detail screen, tabletop
- 64 ± 6 kV range
- Technique and dose:

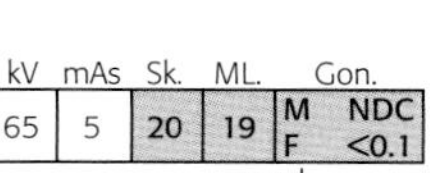

cm	kV	mAs	Sk.	ML.	Gon.
5	65	5	20	19	M NDC F <0.1

mrad

Shielding Secure lead shield around waist to shield gonads.

Patient Position Have patient stand or sit at end of the table and then lean over and place dorsal surface of hand, **palm upward,** on cassette.

Part Position

- Center dorsal aspect of carpals to IR.
- Gently flex wrist as far as patient can tolerate or until the hand and forearm form as near a 90° (right angle) as possible.

Central Ray

- Angle the CR **45° to the large axis of the forearm.**
- Direct the CR to a **midpoint of the distal forearm about 4 cm (1½ inches) proximal to the wrist joint.**
- Minimum SID is 40 inches (100 cm).

Collimation Collimate all four sides to area of interest.

Fig. 5-113. Carpal bridge—tangential projection; central ray 45° to forearm.

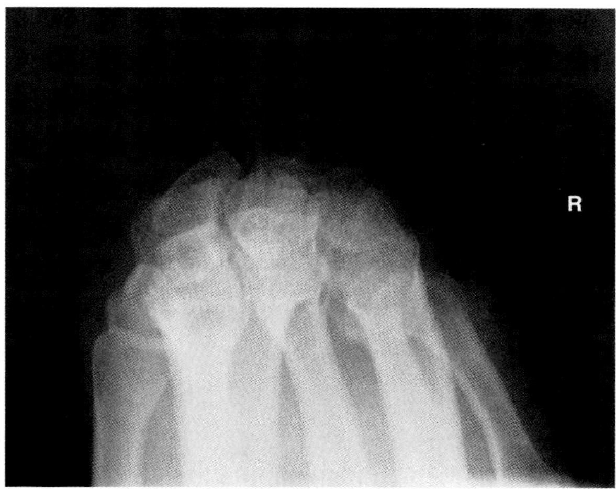

Fig. 5-114. Carpal bridge.

Radiographic Criteria

Structures Shown: • A tangential view of the dorsal aspect of the scaphoid, lunate, and triquetrum is visible. • An outline of the capitate and trapezium superimposed is visible.

Position: • Dorsal aspect of the carpal bones should be visualized clear of superimposition and centered to IR.

Collimation and CR: • Collimation should be visible on four sides to area of affected wrist. • CR and center of the collimation field should be to the area of the **dorsal carpal bones.**

Exposure Criteria: • Optimal density and contrast with no motion should demonstrate the dorsal aspect of the carpal bones, with sharp borders and clear, sharp bony trabecular markings. • Outlines of the proximal metacarpals should be visualized through superimposed structures without overexposure of the dorsal aspects of carpals seen in profile.

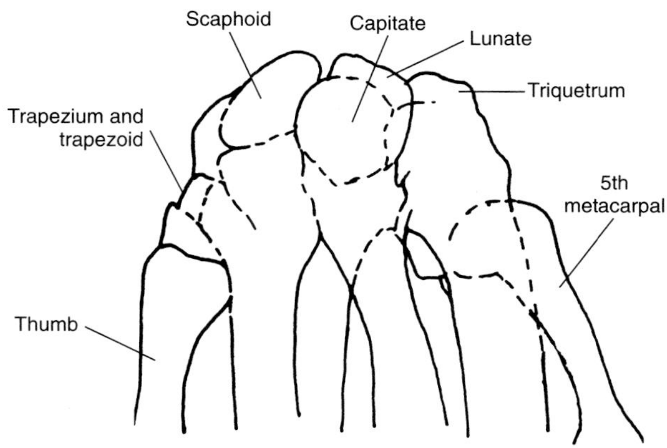

Fig. 5-115. Carpal bridge.

AP PROJECTION: FOREARM

Forearm
BASIC
- **AP**
- Lateral

Pathology Demonstrated
Fractures and dislocations of the radius or ulna and pathologic processes, such as osteomyelitis or arthritis, are demonstrated.

Technical Factors
- IR size—30 × 35 cm (11 × 14 inches) for smaller patients; 35 × 43 cm (14 × 17 inches) for large patients
- Division in half, lengthwise
- Detail screen, tabletop
- Digital IR (use lead masking)
- 60 ± 6 kV range
- Technique and dose:

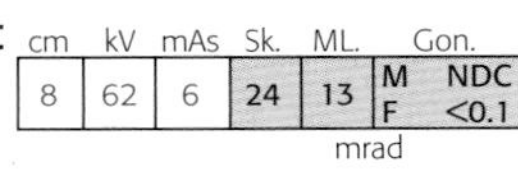

cm	kV	mAs	Sk.	ML.	Gon.
8	62	6	24	13	M NDC F <0.1

mrad

30 (35)
35 (43)
R

Shielding Place lead shield over patient's lap to shield gonads.

Patient Position Seat patient at end of table, with hand and arm fully extended and **palm up (supinated).**

Part Position
- Drop shoulder to place entire upper limb on same horizontal plane.
- Align and center forearm to long axis of IR, ensuring that both wrist and elbow joints are included. (Use as large an IR as necessary.)
- Instruct patient to lean laterally as necessary to place entire wrist, forearm, and elbow in as near a true frontal position as possible. (Medial and lateral epicondyles should be the same distance from IR.)

Central Ray
- CR perpendicular to IR, directed to **midforearm**
- Minimum SID of 40 inches (100 cm)

Collimation Collimate lateral borders to the actual forearm area with minimal collimation at both ends to avoid cutting off anatomy at either joint. Considering divergence of the x-ray beam, ensure that a **minimum** of 3 to 4 cm (1 to 1½ inches) distal to wrist and elbow joints is included on the IR.

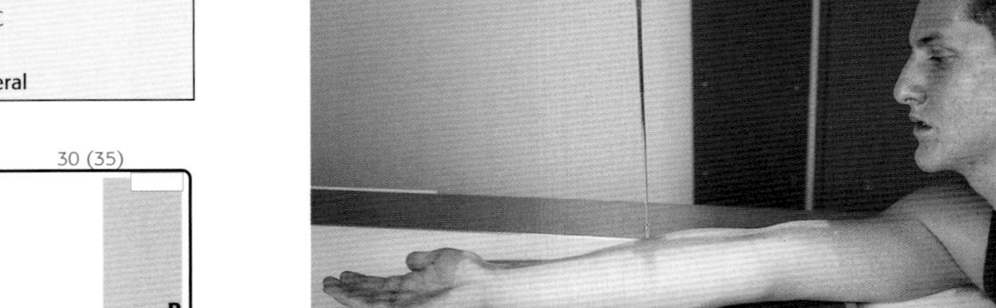

Fig. 5-116. AP forearm (including both joints).

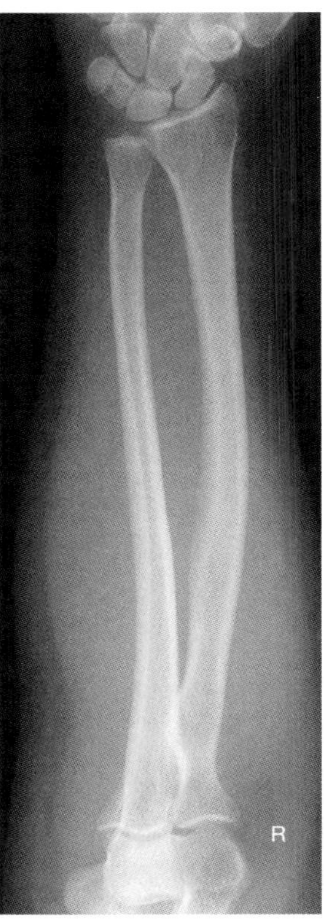

Fig. 5-117. AP (both joints).

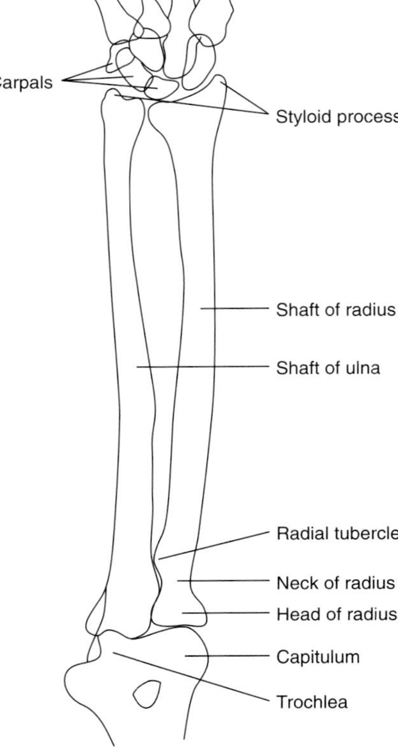

Fig. 5-118. AP (both joints).

Radiographic Criteria
Structures Shown: • AP projection of the entire radius and ulna is shown, with a minimum of proximal row carpals and distal humerus, as well as pertinent soft tissues, such as fat pads and stripes of the wrist and elbow joints.

Position: • Long axis of forearm should be aligned to long axis of IR. • **No rotation** is evidenced by humeral epicondyles visualized in profile, with the radial head, neck, and tuberosity slightly superimposed by the ulna. • Wrist and elbow joints spaces are open only partially because of beam divergence.

Collimation and CR: • Collimation borders are visible at the skin margins along the length of the forearm, with only minimal collimation at both ends to ensure that essential joint anatomy is included. • CR and center of the collimation field should be to the approximate midpoint of the radius and ulna.

Exposure Criteria: • Optimal density and contrast with no motion should visualize soft tissue and sharp, cortical margins and clear, bony trabecular markings.

5

LATERAL—LATEROMEDIAL PROJECTION: FOREARM

Forearm
BASIC
- **AP**
- Lateral

Pathology Demonstrated

Fractures and dislocations of the radius or ulna and pathologic processes, such as osteomyelitis or arthritis, are shown.

Technical Factors

- IR size—30 × 35 cm (11 × 14 inches) or 35 × 43 cm (14 × 17 inches)
- Division in half, lengthwise
- Detail screen, tabletop
- Digital IR (use lead masking)
- 64 ± 6 kV range (+4 kV from AP)
- To make best use of the anode-heel effect, placement of elbow at cathode end of x-ray beam
- Technique and dose:

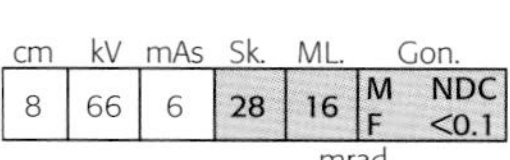

cm	kV	mAs	Sk.	ML.	Gon.
8	66	6	28	16	M NDC F <0.1
			mrad		

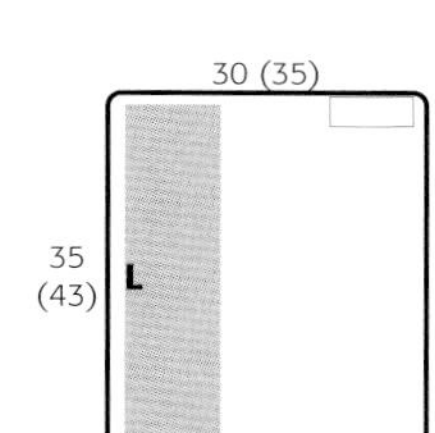

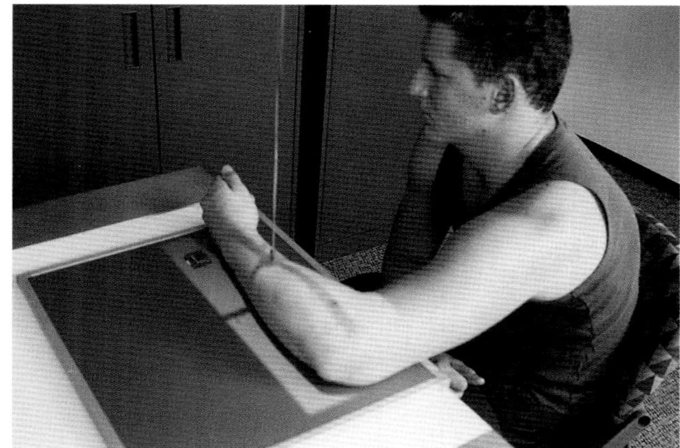

Fig. 5-119. Lateral forearm (including both joints).

Shielding Place lead shield over patient's lap to shield gonads.

Patient Position Seat patient at end of table, with elbow flexed 90°.

Part Position

- Drop shoulder to place entire upper limb on same horizontal plane.
- Align and center forearm to long axis of IR; ensure that both wrist and elbow joints are included on IR.
- Rotate hand and wrist into **true lateral position** and support hand to prevent motion, if needed. (Ensure that distal radius and ulna are directly superimposed.)
- For heavy muscular forearms, place support under hand and wrist as needed to place radius and ulna parallel to IR.

Central Ray

- CR perpendicular to IR, directed to **midforearm**
- Minimum SID of 40 inches (100 cm)

Collimation Collimate both lateral borders to the actual forearm area. Also, collimate at both ends to avoid cutting off anatomy at either joint. Considering divergence of the x-ray beam, ensure that a **minimum** of 3 to 4 cm (1 to 1½ inches) distal to wrist and elbow joints is included on the IR.

Radiographic Criteria

Structures Shown: • Lateral projection of the entire radius and ulna, proximal row of carpal bones, elbow, and distal end of the humerus are visible, as well as pertinent soft tissue, such as fat pads and stripes of the wrist and elbow joints.

Position: • Long axis of forearm should be aligned with long axis of IR. • Elbow should be flexed 90°. • **No rotation** should occur. The head of the ulna should be superimposed over the radius, and humeral epicondyles should be superimposed. • Radial head should superimpose coronoid process, with radial tuberosity seen in profile.

Collimation and CR: • Collimation borders should be visible at skin margins along the length of the forearm, with minimal collimation at both ends to ensure that essential joint anatomy is included. • CR and center of the collimation field should be to the midpoint of the radius and ulna.

Exposure Criteria: • Optimal density and contrast with no motion should visualize sharp cortical margins and clear, sharp bony trabecular markings, as well as fat pads and stripes of the wrist and elbow joints.

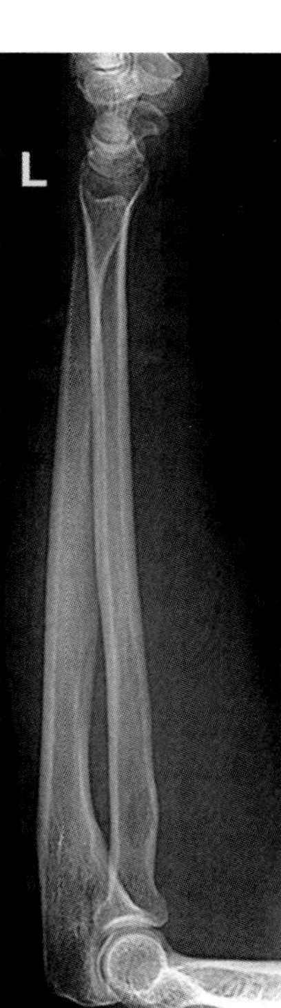

Fig. 5-120. Lateral (both joints).

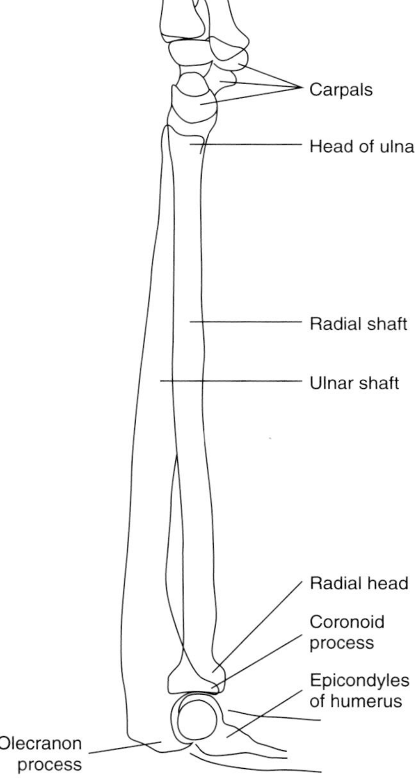

Fig. 5-121. Lateral (both joints).

5

AP PROJECTION: ELBOW

(Elbow Fully Extended)

Pathology Demonstrated
Fractures and dislocations of the elbow and pathologic processes, such as osteomyelitis and arthritis, are demonstrated.

Elbow
BASIC
- AP
- Oblique:
  Lateral (external)
  Medial (internal)
- Lateral

Technical Factors
- IR size—24 × 30 cm (10 × 12 inches)
- Division in half, crosswise
- Detail screen, tabletop
- Digital IR (use lead masking)
- 60 ± 6 kV range
- Technique and dose:

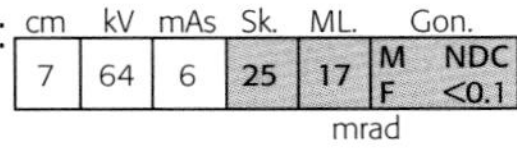

cm	kV	mAs	Sk.	ML.	Gon.
7	64	6	25	17	M NDC F <0.1

mrad

Shielding Place lead shield over pelvic area.

Patient Position Seat patient at end of table, with elbow fully extended, if possible. (See following page if patient cannot fully extend elbow.)

Part Position
- Extend elbow, supinate hand, and align arm and forearm to long axis of portion of IR being exposed.
- Center elbow joint to center of portion of IR being exposed.
- Ask patient to lean laterally as necessary for **true AP projection.** (Palpate epicondyles to ensure that they are parallel to the IR.)
- Support hand as needed to prevent motion.

Central Ray
- CR perpendicular to IR, directed to **midelbow joint,** which is approximately 2 cm (¾ inch) distal to midpoint of a line between epicondyles
- Minimum SID of 40 inches (100 cm)

Collimation Collimate on four sides to area of interest.

Radiographic Criteria

Structures Shown: • Distal humerus, elbow joint space, and proximal radius and ulna are visible.

Position: • Long axis of arm should be aligned with long axis of IR. • **No rotation** is evidenced by the following: appearance of bilateral epicondyles seen in profile; radial head, neck, and tubercles separated or only slightly superimposed by ulna • Elbow joint space appears open with fully extended arm.

Collimation and CR: • Collimation should be visible on four sides to area of affected elbow. • CR and center of the collimation field should be to the **midelbow joint.**

Exposure Criteria: • Optimal density and contrast with no motion should visualize soft-tissue detail and sharp, bony cortical margins and clear, bony trabecular markings.

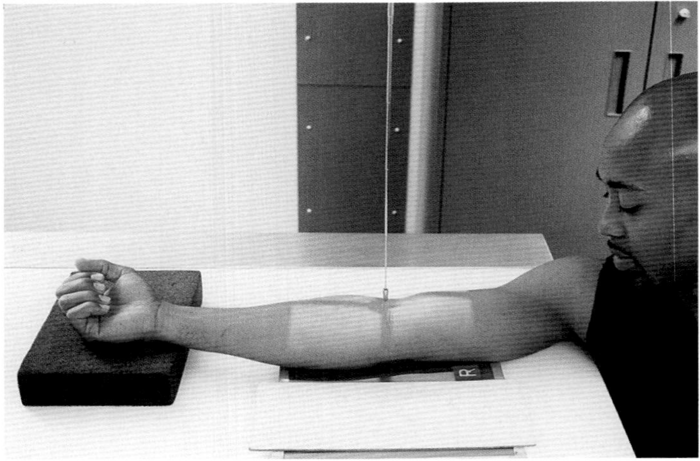

Fig. 5-122. AP elbow (fully extended).

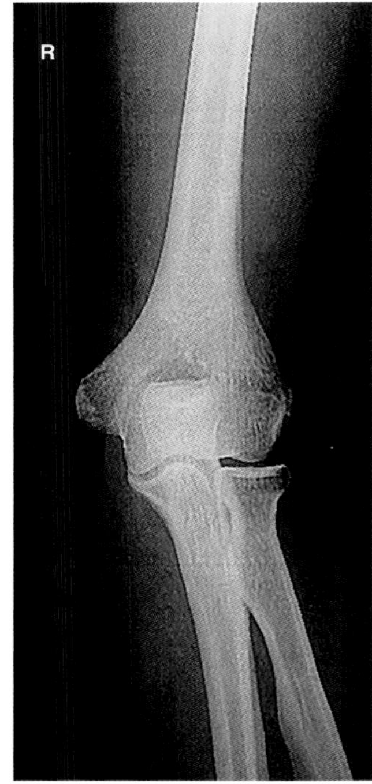

Fig. 5-123. AP (extended).

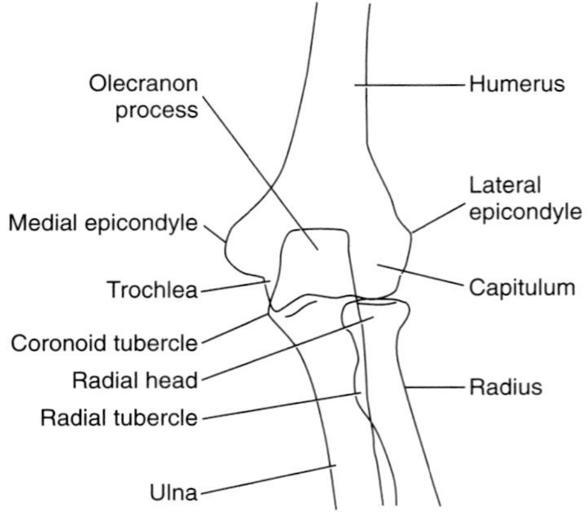

Fig. 5-124. AP (extended).

AP PROJECTION: ELBOW

(When Elbow Cannot Be Fully Extended)

Pathology Demonstrated
Fractures and dislocations of the elbow and pathologic processes, such as osteomyelitis and arthritis, are demonstrated.

Elbow
BASIC
- AP
- Oblique:
  Lateral (external)
  Medial (internal)
- Lateral

Technical Factors
- IR size—24 × 30 cm (10 × 12 inches)
- Division in half, crosswise
- Detail screen, tabletop
- Digital IR (use lead masking)
- 64 ± 6 kV range; exposure increased 4 to 6 kV because of increased part thickness due to partial flexion
- Technique and dose:

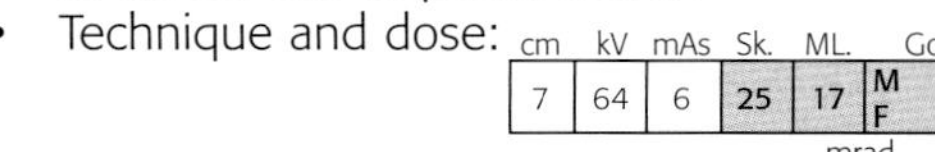

cm	kV	mAs	Sk.	ML.	Gon.
7	64	6	25	17	M NDC F <0.1

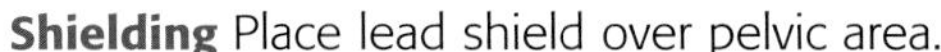
mrad

Shielding Place lead shield over pelvic area.

Patient Position Seat patient at end of table, with elbow partially flexed.

Part Position
- Obtain **two** AP projections—one with **forearm parallel** to IR and one with **humerus parallel** to IR.
- Place support under wrist and forearm for projection with humerus parallel to IR, if needed to prevent motion.

Central Ray
- CR **perpendicular** to IR, directed to **midelbow joint,** which is approximately 2 cm (3/4 inch) distal to midpoint of a line between epicondyles
- Minimum SID of 40 inches (100 cm)

Collimation Collimate on four sides to area of interest.

Note: If patient cannot partially extend elbow as shown (Fig. 5-125) and elbow remains **flexed near 90°**, take the two AP projections as described, but **angle the CR 10° to 15°** into elbow joint, or if flexed **more than 90°**, use the **Jones method** (see p. 173).

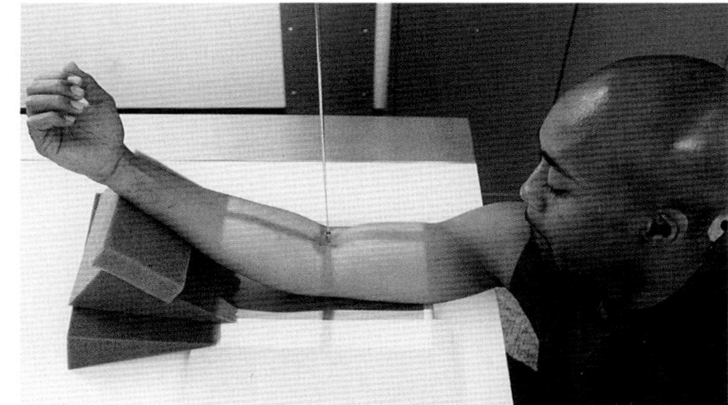

Fig. 5-125. AP elbow (partially flexed); humerus parallel to IR.

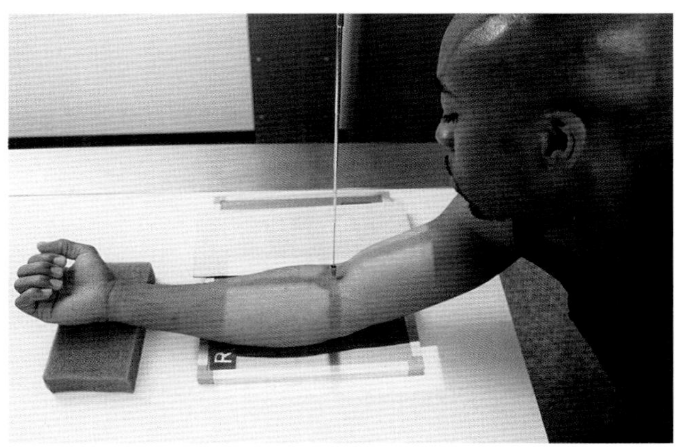

Fig. 5-126. AP elbow (partially flexed); forearm parallel to IR.

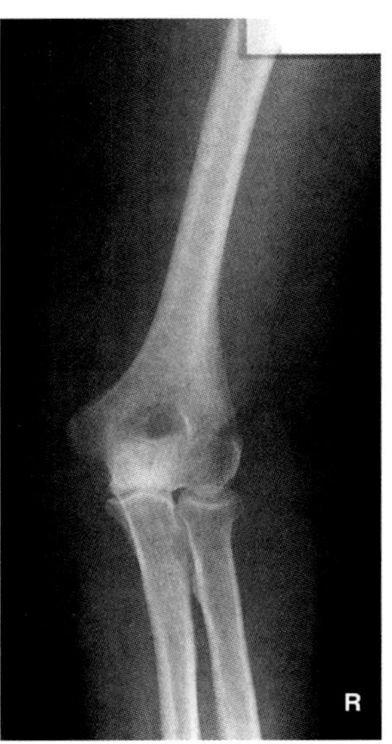

Fig. 5-127. Humerus parallel.

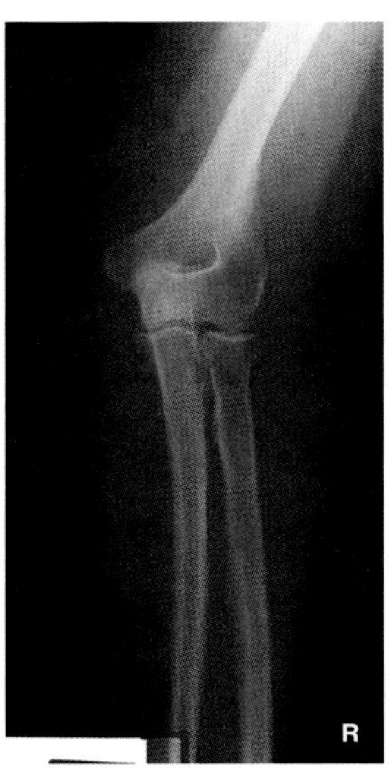

Fig. 5-128. Forearm parallel.

Radiographic Criteria

Structures Shown: • Distal humerus is best visualized on "humerus parallel" projection, and proximal radius and ulna on "forearm parallel" projection. **Note:** Structures in elbow joint region are partially obscured, depending on the amount of elbow flexion possible.

Position: • Long axis of arm should be aligned with side border of IR. • No rotation is evidenced by the following: Epicondyles seen in profile; radial head and neck separated or only slightly superimposed over ulna on forearm parallel projection.

Collimation and CR: • Collimation should be visible on four sides to area of affected elbow. • CR and center of the collimation field should be to the **midelbow joint.**

Exposure Criteria: • Optimal density and contrast with no motion should visualize soft-tissue detail and sharp, bony cortical margins and clear, bony trabecular markings. • Distal humerus, including epicondyles, should be demonstrated with sufficient density on "humerus parallel" projection. • On "forearm parallel" projection the proximal radius and ulna should be well visualized with density so as to visualize both soft tissue and bony detail.

AP OBLIQUE PROJECTION—LATERAL (EXTERNAL) ROTATION: ELBOW

Pathology Demonstrated
Fractures and dislocations of the elbow, primarily the radial head and neck, and some pathologic processes, such as osteomyelitis and arthritis, are demonstrated.

Elbow
BASIC
- AP
- Oblique:
  - Lateral (external)
  - Medial (internal)
- Lateral

External oblique: Best visualizes **radial head** and **neck** and **capitulum** of humerus

30
24
R

Technical Factors
- IR size—24 × 30 cm (10 × 12 inches)
- Division in half, crosswise
- Detail screen, tabletop
- Digital IR (use lead masking)
- 60 ± 6 kV range
- Technique and dose:

cm	kV	mAs	Sk.	ML.	Gon.
7	64	6	25	17	M NDC F <0.1

mrad

Shielding Place lead shield over patient's lap to protect gonads.

Patient Position Seat patient at end of table, with arm fully extended and shoulder and elbow on same horizontal plane (lowering shoulder as needed).

Part Position
- Align arm and forearm to long axis of portion of IR being exposed.
- Center elbow joint to CR and to portion of IR being exposed.
- Supinate hand and **rotate laterally** the entire arm so that the distal humerus and the anterior surface of the elbow joint are approximately 45° to cassette. (Patient must lean laterally for sufficient lateral rotation.) Palpate epicondyles to determine approximately 45° rotation of distal humerus.

Central Ray
- CR perpendicular to IR, directed to **midelbow joint** (a point approximately 2 cm, or ¾ inch, distal to midpoint of line between the epicondyles as viewed from the x-ray tube)
- Minimum SID of 40 inches (100 cm)

Collimation Collimate on four sides to area of interest.

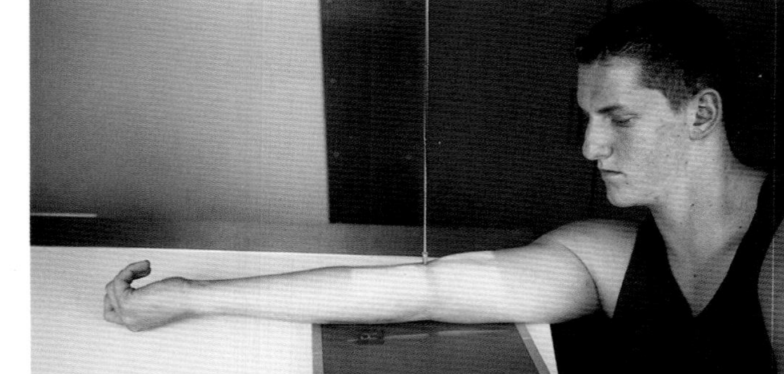

Fig. 5-129. Lateral—external oblique.

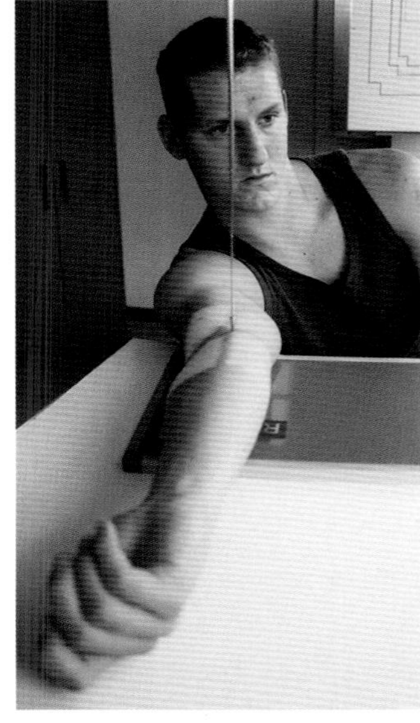

Fig. 5-130. End view, showing 45° lateral rotation.

Radiographic Criteria

Structures Shown: • An oblique view of the distal humerus and proximal radius and ulna is visible.

Position: • Long axis of arm should be aligned with side border of IR. • Correct 45° lateral oblique should visualize the **radial head, neck,** and **tuberosity,** free of superimposition by ulna. • The lateral epicondyle and capitulum should appear elongated and in profile.

Collimation and CR: • Collimation should be visible on four sides to area of affected elbow. • CR and center of collimation field should be to **midelbow joint.**

Exposure Criteria: • Optimal density and contrast with no motion should visualize soft-tissue detail and sharp, bony cortical margins with clear, bony trabecular markings.

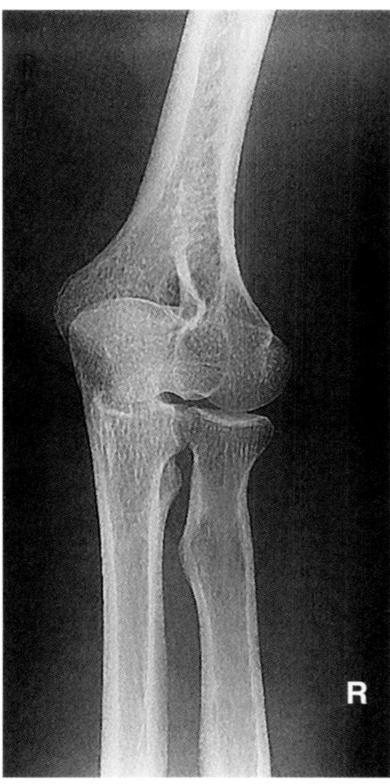

Fig. 5-131. Lateral rotation—external oblique.

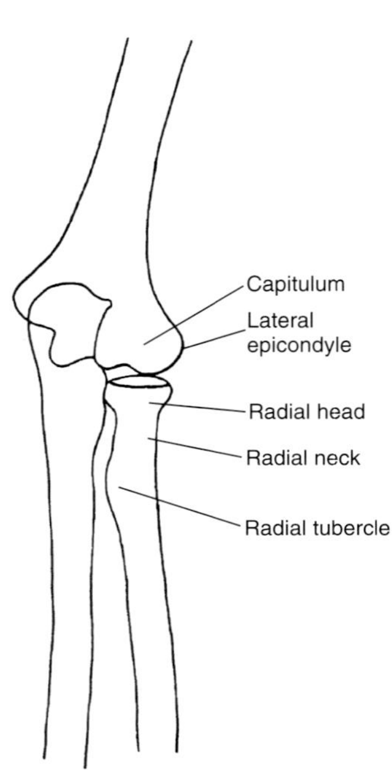

Fig. 5-132. Lateral—external oblique.

AP OBLIQUE PROJECTION—MEDIAL (INTERNAL) ROTATION: ELBOW

Elbow
BASIC
• AP
• Oblique:
Lateral (external)
Medial (internal)
• **Lateral**

Pathology Demonstrated

Fractures and dislocations of the elbow, primarily the coronoid process, and some pathologic processes, such as osteoporosis and arthritis, are shown.

Internal oblique: Best visualizes **coronoid process** of ulna and trochlea in profile

Technical Factors

30

24 **R**

- IR size—24 × 30 cm (10 × 12 inches)
- Division in half, crosswise
- Detail screen, tabletop
- Digital IR (use lead masking)
- 60 ± 6 kV range
- Technique and dose:

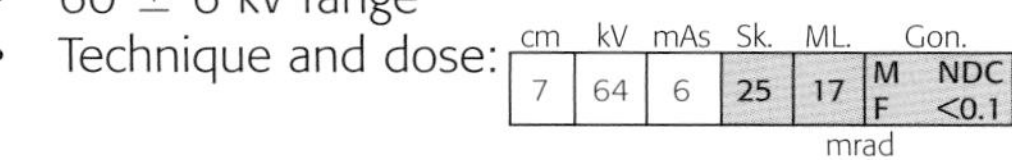

cm	kV	mAs	Sk.	ML.	Gon.
7	64	6	25	17	M NDC F <0.1
			mrad		

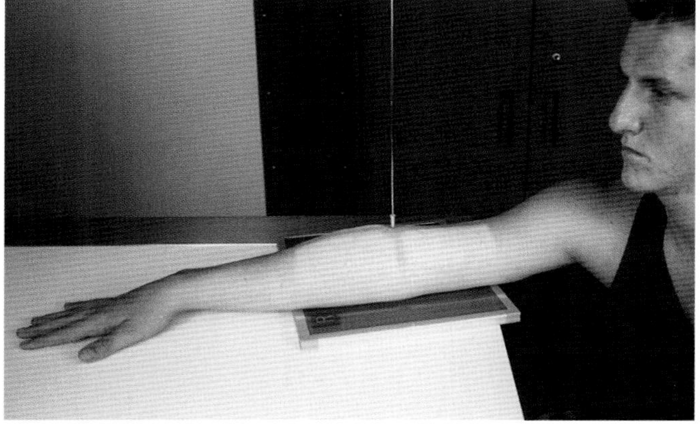

Fig. 5-133. Medial (internal) oblique.

Shielding Place lead shield over patient's lap to protect gonads.

Patient Position Seat patient at end of table, with arm fully extended and shoulder and elbow on same horizontal plane.

Part Position

- Align arm and forearm to long axis of portion of IR being exposed. Center elbow joint to CR and to portion of IR being exposed.
- Pronate hand into a natural palm-down position and rotate arm as needed until distal humerus and anterior surface of elbow are rotated **45°** (palpating epicondyles to determine a **45°** rotation of distal humerus).

Central Ray

- CR perpendicular to IR, directed to **midelbow joint** (approximately 2 cm, or ¾ inch, distal to midpoint of line between epicondyles as viewed from the x-ray tube)
- Minimum SID of 40 inches (100 cm)

Collimation Collimate on four sides to area of interest.

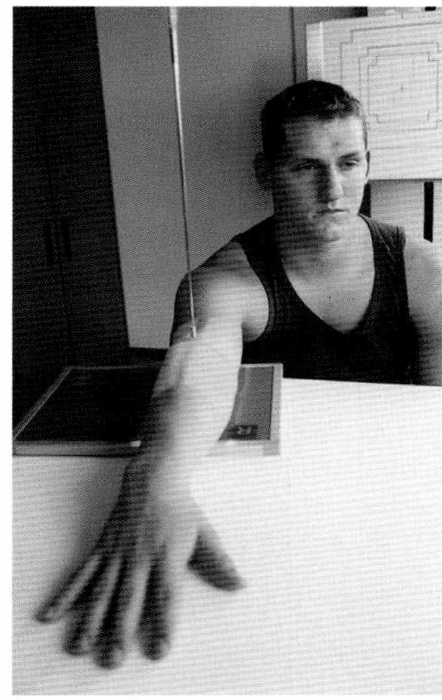

Fig. 5-134. End view, showing 45° internal oblique.

Radiographic Criteria

Structures Shown: • Oblique view of the distal humerus and proximal radius and ulna is visible.

Position: • Long axis of arm should be aligned with side border of IR. • A correct 45° medial oblique should visualize the coronoid process of the ulna in profile. • The medial epicondyle and the trochlea should appear elongated and in partial profile. • The olecranon process should appear seated in the olecranon fossa and the trochlear notch partially open and visualized. • Radial head and neck should be superimposed and centered over the proximal ulna.

Collimation and CR: • Collimation should be visible on four sides to area of affected elbow. • CR and center of collimation field should be at **midelbow joint.**

Exposure Criteria: • Optimal density and contrast with no motion should visualize soft-tissue detail and bony cortical margins and clear, bony trabecular markings.

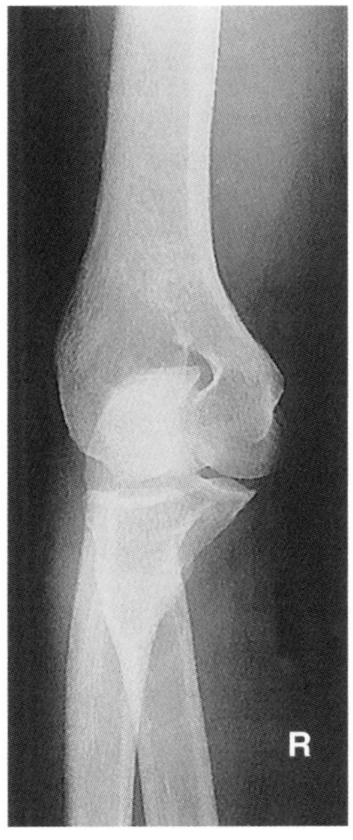

Fig. 5-135. Medial—internal oblique.

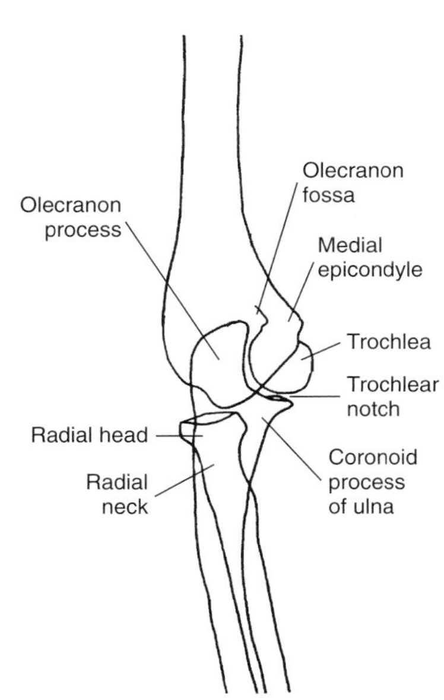

Fig. 5-136. Medial—internal oblique.

5

LATERAL—LATEROMEDIAL PROJECTION: ELBOW

Elbow
BASIC
• AP
• Oblique:
Lateral (external)
Medial (internal)
• Lateral

Pathology Demonstrated
Fractures and dislocations of the elbow and some bony pathologic processes, such as osteomyelitis and arthritis, are shown. Elevated or displaced fat pads of the elbow joint may be visualized.

Technical Factors
- IR size—18 × 24 cm (8 × 10 inches), crosswise
- Detail screen, tabletop
- 60 ± 6 kV range
- Technique and dose:

cm	kV	mAs	Sk.	ML.	Gon.
7	64	6	25	17	M NDC / F <0.1

mrad

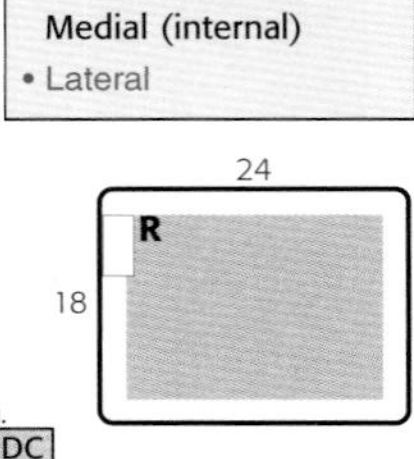

Shielding Place lead shield over patient's lap to protect gonads.

Patient Position Seat patient at end of table, with elbow flexed 90° (see Note below).

Part Position
- Align long axis of forearm to long axis of cassette.
- Center elbow joint to CR and to center of IR.
- Drop shoulder so that humerus and forearm are on same horizontal plane.
- Rotate hand and wrist into true lateral position, thumb side up.
- Place support under hand and wrist to elevate hand and distal forearm as needed for heavy muscular forearm so that forearm is parallel to IR for true lateral elbow.

Central Ray
- CR perpendicular to IR, directed to **midelbow joint** (a point approximately 4 cm, or 1½ inches, medial to easily palpated posterior surface of olecranon process)
- Minimum SID of 40 inches (100 cm)

Collimation Collimate on four sides to area of interest.

Note: Diagnosis of certain important joint pathologic processes (such as possible visualization of the posterior fat pad) depends on 90° flexion of the elbow joint.*

Exception: Certain soft-tissue diagnoses require less flexion (only 30° to 35°), but these views should be taken only when specifically indicated.

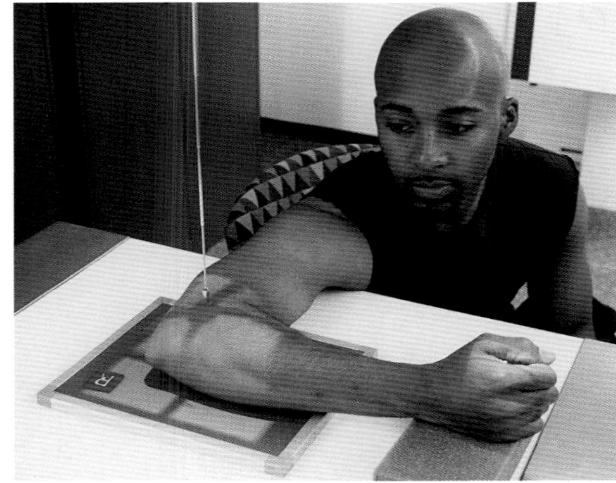

Fig. 5-137. Lateral—elbow flexed 90° (forearm parallel to IR).

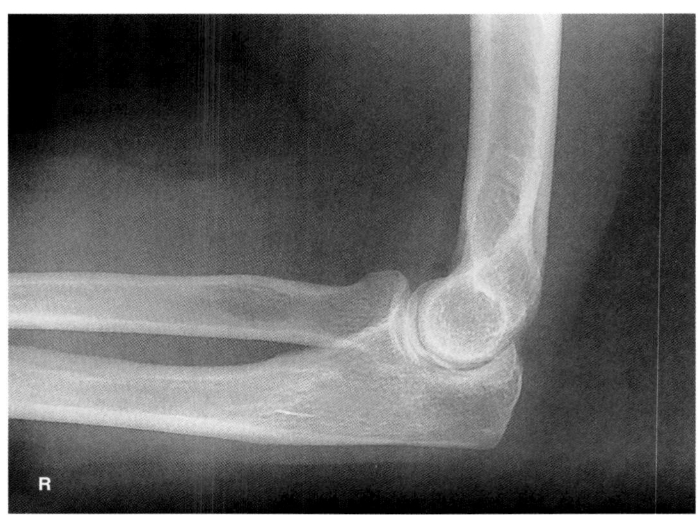

Fig. 5-138. Lateral elbow.

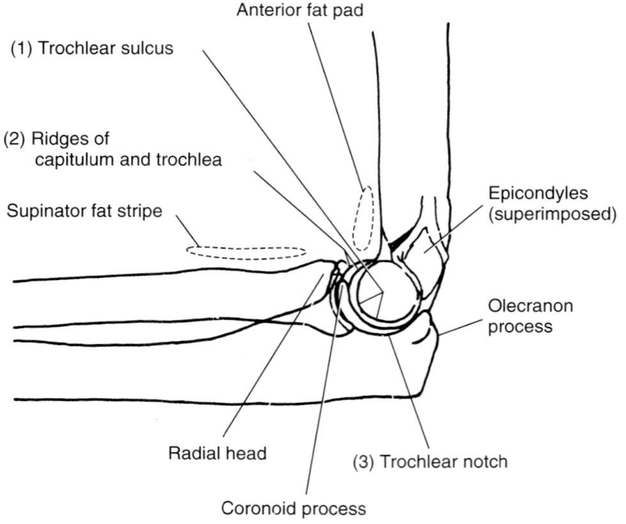

Fig. 5-139. Lateral elbow.

Radiographic Criteria

Structures Shown: • A lateral projection of the distal humerus and proximal forearm, the olecranon process, and the soft tissues and fat pads of the elbow joint are visible.

Position: • Long axis of the arm should be aligned with the long axis of the IR, with the elbow joint flexed 90°. • About one-half of the radial head should be superimposed by the coronoid process, and the olecranon process should be visualized in profile. • A true lateral view is indicated by three concentric arcs of the trochlear sulcus, double ridges of the capitulum and trochlea, and the trochlear notch of the ulna. In addition, superimposition of the humeral epicondyles occurs.

Collimation and CR: • Collimation should be visible on four sides to area of affected elbow. • CR and center of collimation field should be **midpoint of the elbow joint.**

Exposure Criteria: • No motion and optimal density and contrast should visualize sharp cortical margins and clear trabecular markings, as well as soft-tissue margins of the anterior and posterior fat pads.

*Griswold R: Elbow fat pads: a radiography perspective, Radiol Technol 53:303-307, 1982.

ACUTE FLEXION PROJECTIONS: ELBOW

Jones Method (AP projections of elbow in acute flexion)

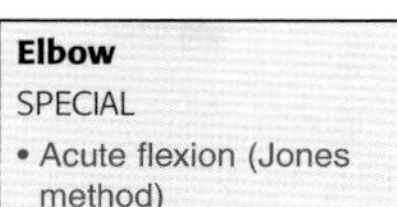

Pathology Demonstrated
Fractures and moderate dislocations of the elbow in acute flexion are demonstrated.

Note: To visualize both the distal humerus and the proximal radius and ulna, **two** projections are required—one with the **CR perpendicular to the humerus** and one with the CR angled so that it is **perpendicular to the forearm.**

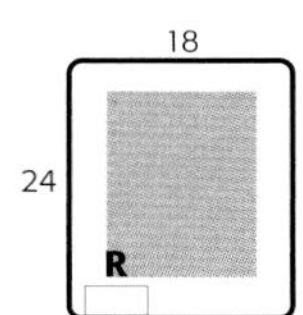

Technical Factors
- IR size—18 × 24 cm (8 × 10 inches) lengthwise (or divide in half, crosswise, for two projections)
- Detail screen, tabletop
- 64 ± 6 kV range (increase 4 to 6 kV for proximal forearm)

Shielding Place lead shield over patient's lap to shield gonads.

Patient Position Seat patient at end of table, with acutely flexed arm resting on cassette.

Part Position
- Align and center humerus to long axis of IR, with forearm acutely flexed and fingertips resting on shoulder.
- Adjust cassette to center elbow-joint region to center of IR.
- Palpate epicondyles and ensure they are equal distances from cassette for **no rotation.**

Central Ray
- ***Distal humerus:*** CR **perpendicular to IR and humerus,** directed to **a point midway between epicondyles**
- ***Proximal forearm:*** CR **perpendicular to forearm** (angling CR as needed), directed to a point approximately **2 inches (5 cm) proximal or superior to olecranon process**
- Minimum SID of 40 inches (100 cm)

Collimation Collimate on four sides to area of interest.

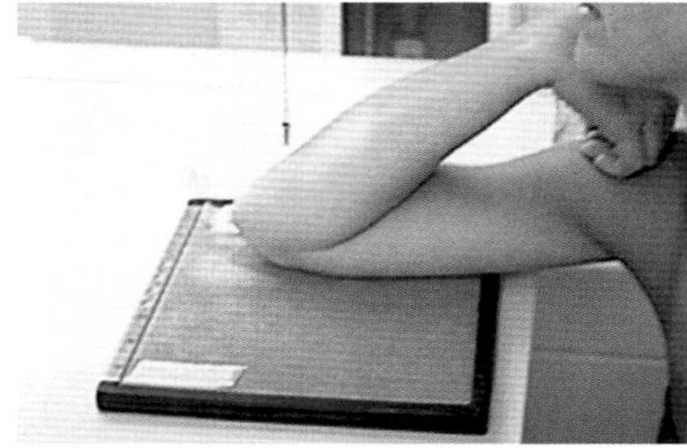

Fig. 5-140. For distal humerus—central ray perpendicular to **humerus.**

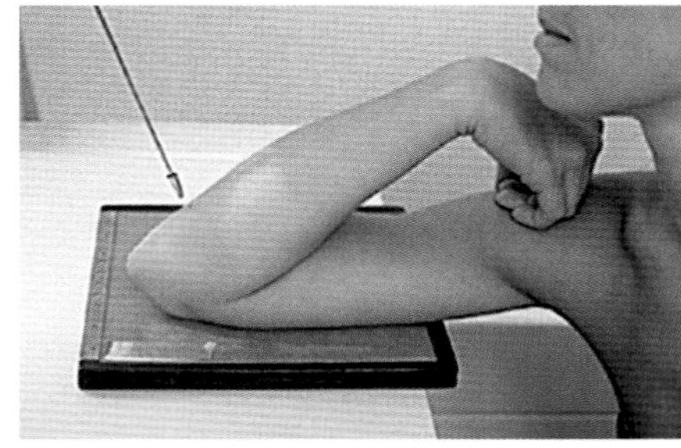

Fig. 5-141. For proximal forearm—central ray perpendicular to **forearm.**

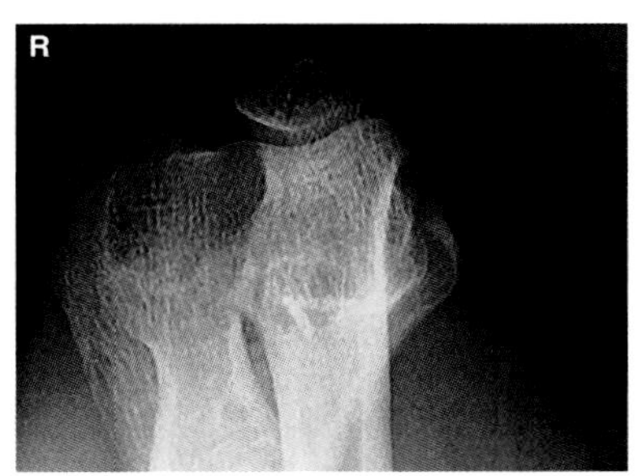

Fig. 5-142. Distal humerus.

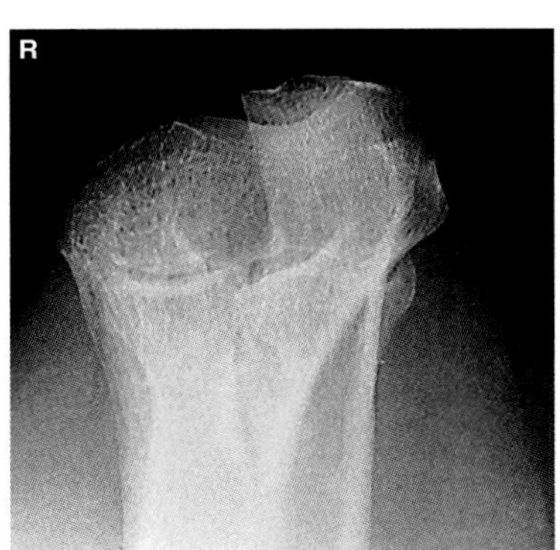

Fig. 5-143. Proximal forearm.

Radiographic Criteria for Specific Projections
• Four-sided collimation borders should be visible with CR and center of collimation field midway between epicondyles.
Proximal Humerus: • Forearm and humerus should be directly superimposed. • Medial and lateral epicondyles and parts of trochlea, capitulum, and olecranon process all should be seen in profile. • Optimal exposure should visualize distal humerus and olecranon process through superimposed structures. Soft-tissue detail is not readily visible on either projection.
Distal Forearm: • Proximal ulna and radius, including outline of radial head and neck, should be visible through superimposed distal humerus. • Optimal exposure visualizes outlines of proximal ulna and radius superimposed over humerus.

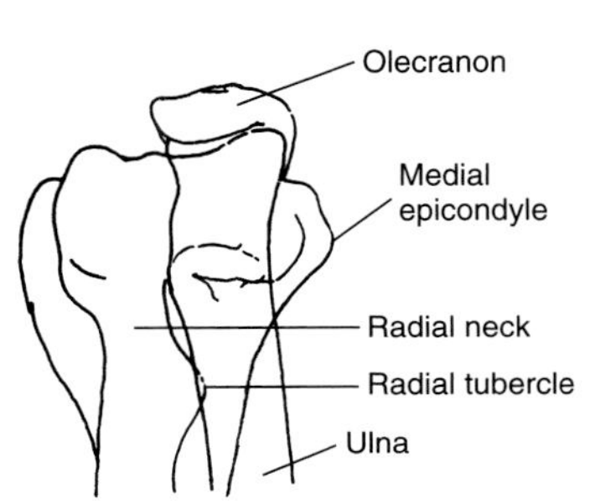

Fig. 5-144. Distal humerus.

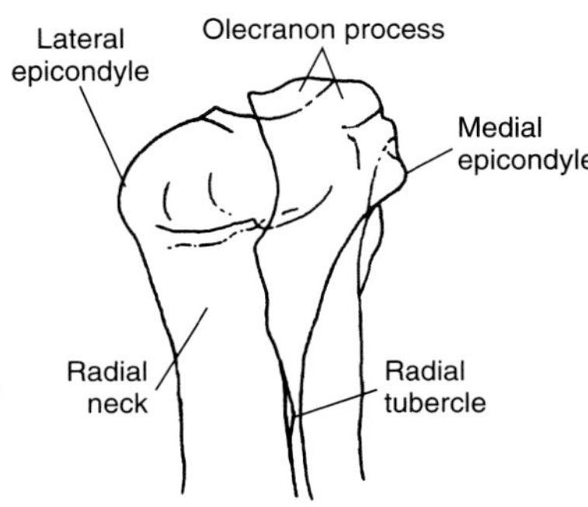

Fig. 5-145. Proximal forearm.

TRAUMA AXIAL LATERALS—AXIAL LATEROMEDIAL PROJECTIONS: ELBOW

Coyle Method*

These are special projections taken for pathologic processes or trauma to the area of the radial head and/or the coronoid process of ulna. These are effective projections when patient cannot extend elbow fully for medial or lateral obliques of the elbow.

Elbow
SPECIAL
- Acute flexion (Jones method)
- Trauma axial laterals (Coyle method)

Pathology Demonstrated

Fractures and dislocations of the elbow, particularly the radial head (Part Position 1) and coronoid process (Part Position 2), are shown.

Technical Factors

- IR size—18 × 24 cm (8 × 10 inches) crosswise
- Detail screen, tabletop
- 70 ± 6 kV range (see Note below)
- Technique and dose:

cm	kV	mAs	Sk.	ML.	Gon.
8	68	6	29	18	M NDC F <0.1

mrad per projection

Shielding Place lead shield over gonadal area.

Patient Position Seat patient in a supine or erect position, at the end of the table.

Part Position 1—Radial Head

- Elbow flexed 90° if possible; **hand pronated**
- CR directed at a **45° angle toward shoulder,** centered to radial head (midelbow joint)
- Minimum SID of 40 inches (100 cm)

Part Position 2—Coronoid Process

- Elbow flexed **only 80°** from extended position (because more than 80° may obscure coronoid process) and hand pronated
- CR angled **45° from shoulder,** into midelbow joint
- Minimum SID of 40 inches (100 cm)

Collimation Collimate on four sides to area of interest.

Note: Increase exposure factors by 4 to 6 kV from lateral elbow because of angled CR. These projections are effective with or without a splint.

Radiographic Criteria for Specific Anatomy

For Radial Head: • The joint space between radial head and capitulum should be open and clear. • The radial head, neck, and tuberosity should be in profile and free of superimposition, except for a small part of the coronoid process. • The distal humerus and epicondyles appear distorted because of the 45° angle.

For Coronoid Process: • The distal portion of the coronoid appears elongated but in profile. • The joint space between coronoid process and trochlea should be open and clear. • The radial head and neck should be superimposed by ulna. • Optimal exposure factors should visualize clearly the coronoid process in profile. Bony margins of superimposed radial head and neck should be visualized faintly through the proximal ulna.

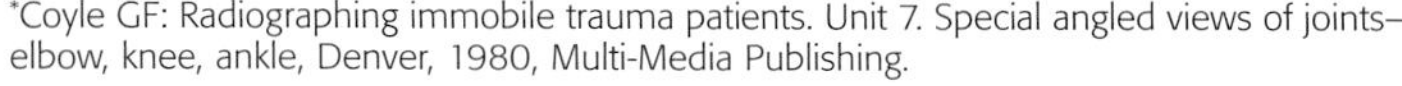

*Coyle GF: Radiographing immobile trauma patients. Unit 7. Special angled views of joints—elbow, knee, ankle, Denver, 1980, Multi-Media Publishing.

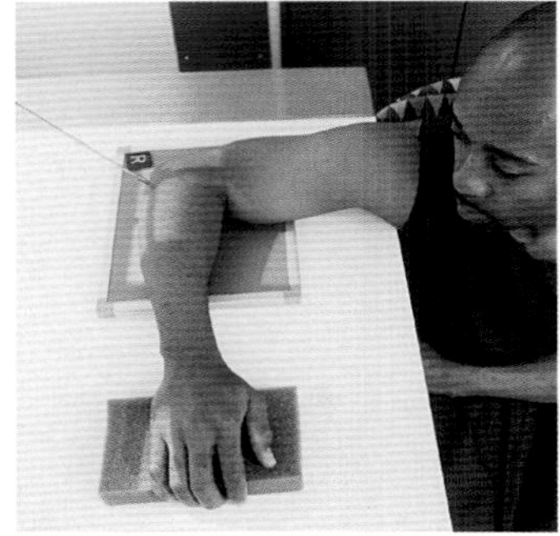

Fig. 5-146. Erect for **radial head**—flexed **90°**.

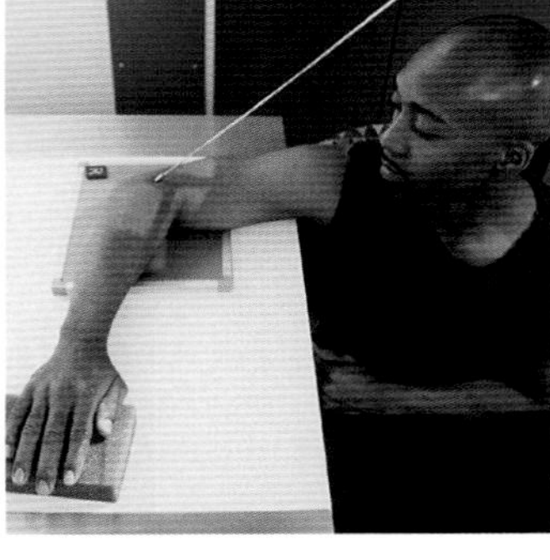

Fig. 5-147. Erect for **coronoid process**—flexed **80°**.

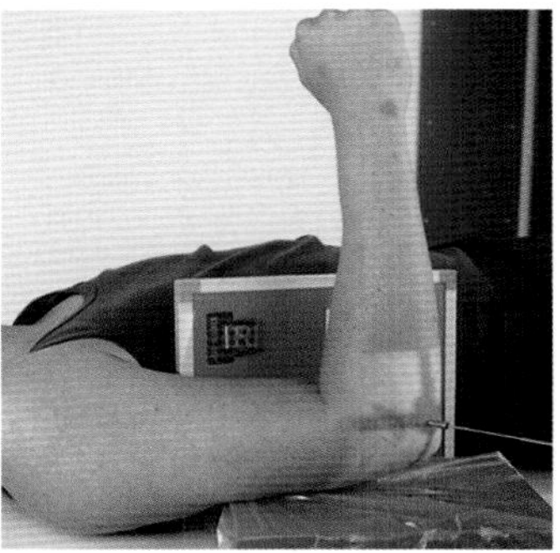

Fig. 5-148. Supine, angled 45° for **radial head**—flexed **90°**.

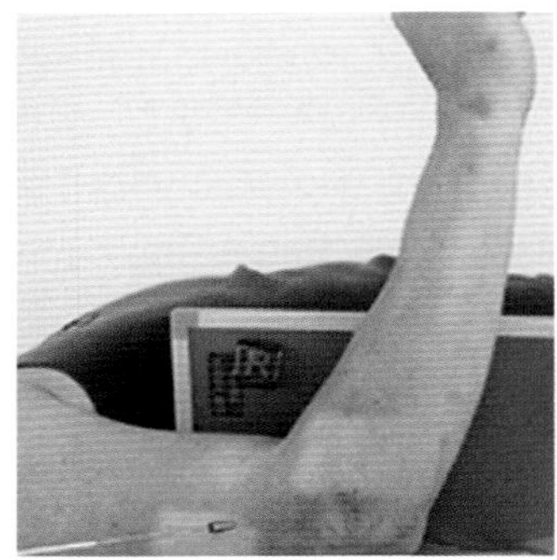

Fig. 5-149. Supine, angled 45° for **coronoid process**—flexed **80°**.

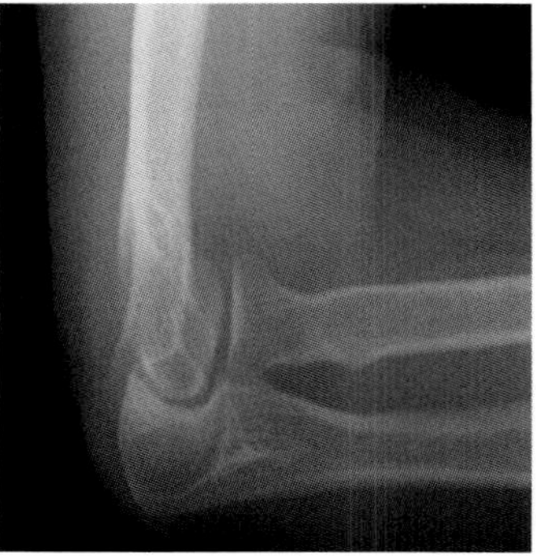

Fig. 5-150. For radial head.

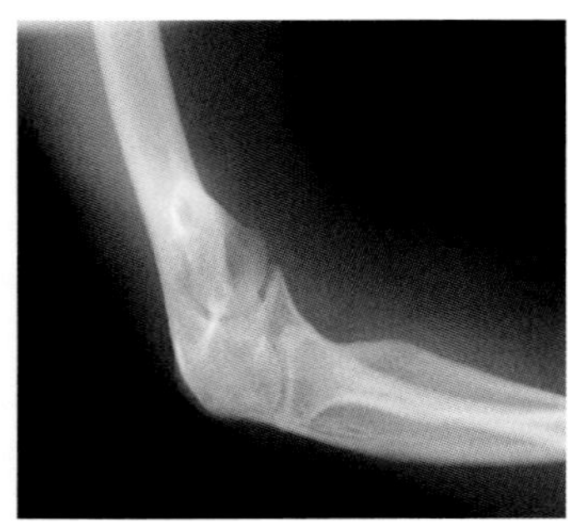

Fig. 5-151. For coronoid process.

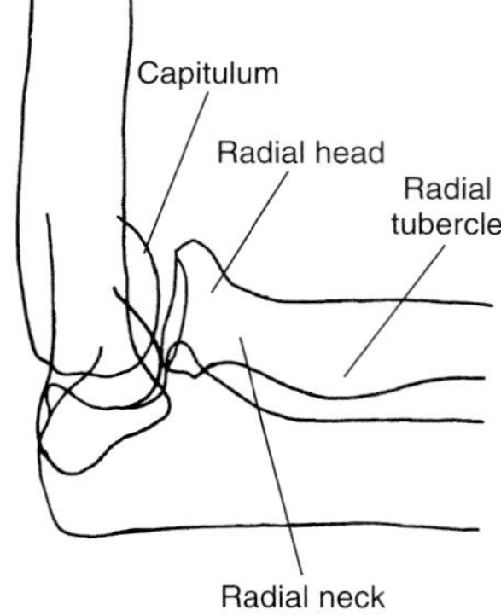

Fig. 5-152. For radial head.

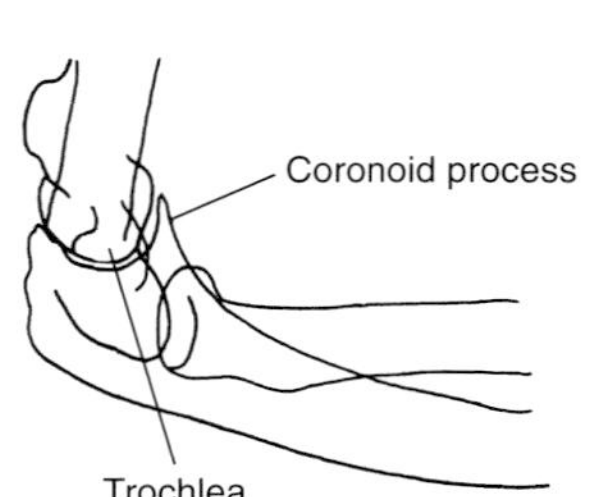

Fig. 5-153. For coronoid process.

RADIAL HEAD LATERALS—LATEROMEDIAL PROJECTIONS: ELBOW

Elbow
SPECIAL
- Acute flexion (Jones method)
- Trauma axial laterals (Coyle method)
- Radial head projections

Pathology Demonstrated
Occult fractures of the radial head and/or neck are demonstrated.

Technical Factors
- IR size—18 × 24 cm (8 × 10 inches)
- Division in half, crosswise
- Detail screen, tabletop
- Digital IR (use lead masking)
- 60 ± 6 kV range
- Technique and dose:

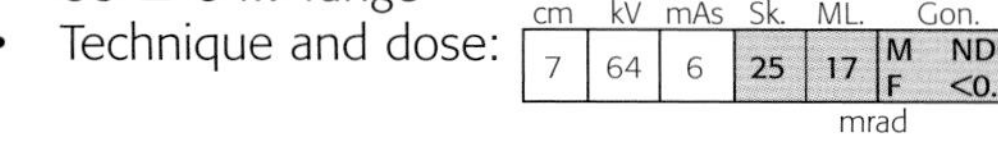
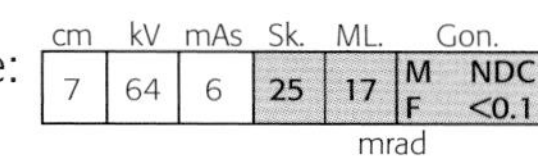

cm	kV	mAs	Sk.	ML.	Gon.
7	64	6	25	17	M NDC F <0.1
			mrad		

Shielding Place lead shield over patient's lap to shield gonads.

Patient Position Seat patient at end of table, arm **flexed 90°** and resting on cassette with humerus, forearm, and hand on same horizontal plane. Place support under hand and wrist if needed.

Part Position
- Center radial head area to center of the portion of film being exposed, positioned so that distal humerus and proximal forearm are placed "square" with, or parallel with, the borders of the cassette.
- Center radial head region to CR.
- Take **four projections,** the only difference among the four being the rotation of the hand and wrist from (1) maximum external rotation to (4) maximum internal rotation, demonstrating different parts of the radial head projected clear of the coronoid process. Near-complete rotation of radial head occurs in these four projections, as follows:
  1. Supinate hand (palm up) and externally rotate as far as patient can tolerate.
  2. Place hand in true lateral position (thumb up).
  3. Pronate hand (palm down).
  4. Internally rotate hand (thumb down) as far as patient can tolerate.

Central Ray
- CR perpendicular to IR, directed to **radial head** (approximately 2 to 3 cm, or 1 inch, distal to lateral epicondyle)
- Minimum SID of 40 inches (100 cm)

Collimation Collimate on four sides to area of interest (including at least 10 cm [3 to 4 inches] of proximal forearm, as well as distal portion of humerus).

Radiographic Criteria for Specific Anatomy
- Elbow should be flexed 90° in true lateral position, as evidenced by direct superimposition of epicondyles.
- Radial head and neck should be partially superimposed by ulna but completely visualized in profile in the various projections.
- **Radial tuberosity** should be visualized in various positions and degrees of profile as follows (see small *arrows*): (1) Fig. 5-155, slightly anterior; (2) Fig. 5-157, not in profile, superimposed over radial shaft; (3) Fig. 5-159, slightly posterior; (4) Fig. 5-160, seen posteriorly, adjacent to ulna when hand and wrist are at maximum internal rotation.
- Optimal exposure with no motion should clearly visualize sharp, bony margins and clear trabecular markings of the radial head and neck area.

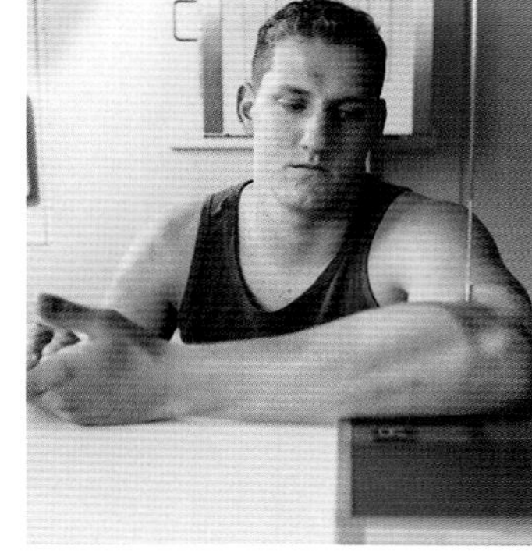
Fig. 5-154. 1. Hand supinated (maximum external rotation).

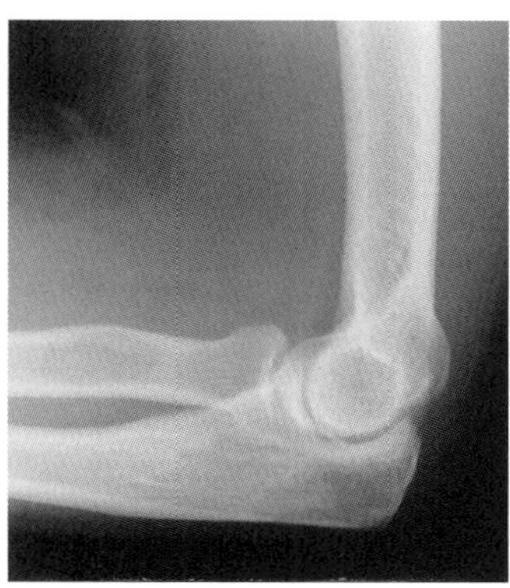
Fig. 5-155. Hand supinated (maximum external rotation).

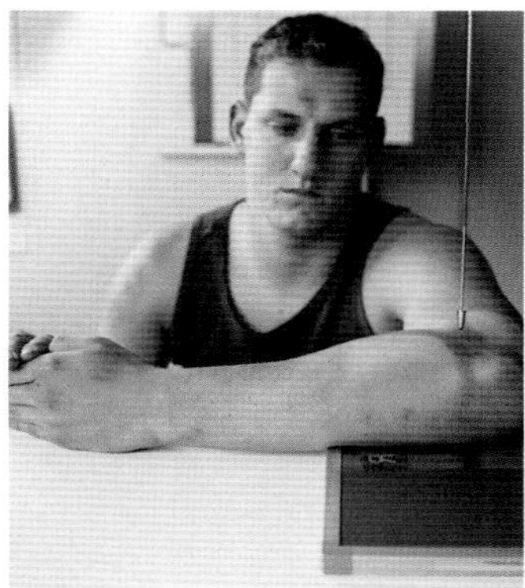
Fig. 5-156. 2. Hand lateral.

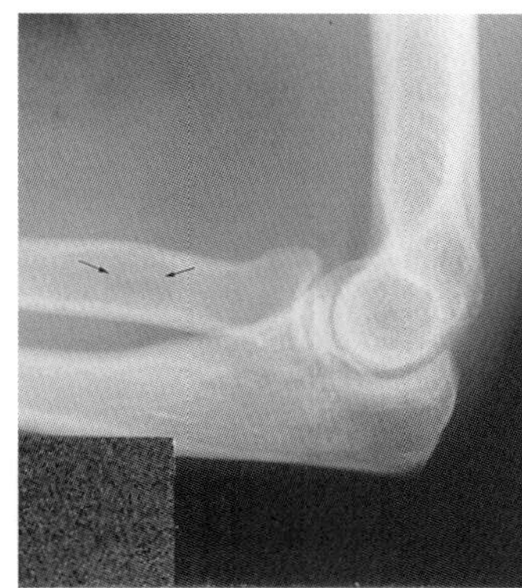
Fig. 5-157. Hand lateral.

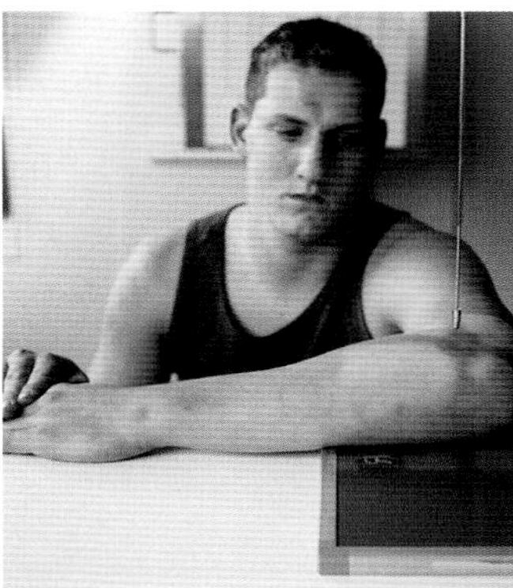
Fig. 5-158. 3. Hand pronated.

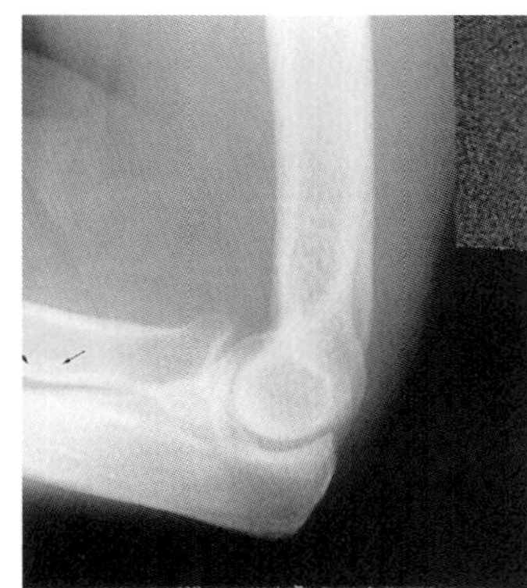
Fig. 5-159. Hand pronated.

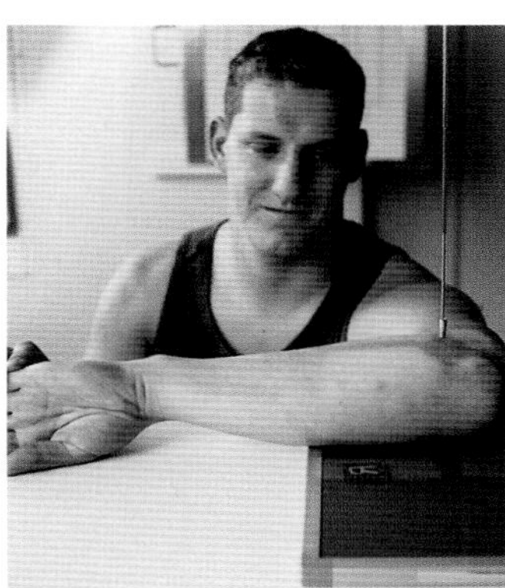
Fig. 5-160. 4. Hand with maximum internal rotation.

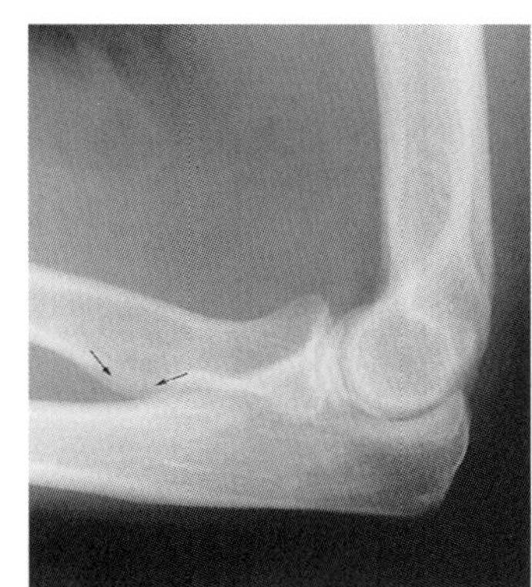
Fig. 5-161. Hand with maximum internal rotation.

AP PROJECTION: HUMERUS

Warning: Do **not** attempt to rotate arm if fracture or dislocation is suspected.

Humerus
BASIC
- AP
- Rotational lateral
- Horizontal beam lateral

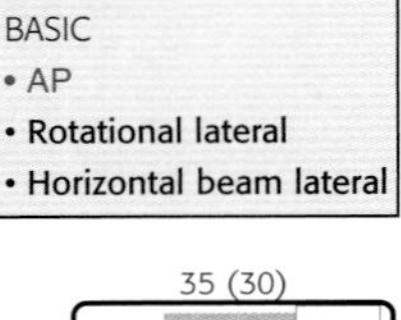

Pathology Demonstrated

Fractures and dislocation of the humerus, and other pathologic processes, such as osteoporosis and arthritis, are demonstrated.

Technical Factors

- IR size—lengthwise (large enough to include entire humerus)
  - —For larger patient, 35 × 43 cm (14 × 17 inches); may need to place cassette diagonally to include both joints
  - —For smaller patient, 30 × 35 cm (11 × 14 inches)
- Moving or stationary grid (nongrid, detail screen for smaller patient)
- 70 ± 6 kV range
- Technique and dose:

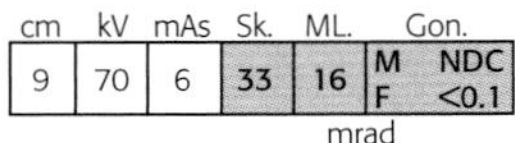

cm	kV	mAs	Sk.	ML.	Gon.
9	70	6	33	16	M NDC F <0.1

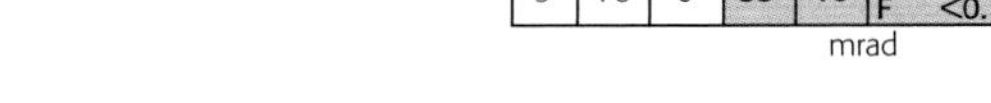

Shielding Secure or place lead shield over pelvic area.

Patient Position Position patient erect or supine. Adjust height of cassette so that shoulder and elbow joints are equidistant from ends of IR.

Part Position

- Rotate body toward affected side as needed to bring shoulder and proximal humerus in contact with cassette.
- Align humerus to long axis of IR, unless diagonal placement is needed to include both shoulder and elbow joints.
- Extend hand and forearm as far as patient can tolerate.
- Abduct arm slightly and gently supinate hand so that **epicondyles of elbow are equidistant** from IR.

Central Ray

- CR perpendicular to IR, directed to **midpoint of humerus**
- Minimum SID of 40 inches (100 cm)

Collimation Collimate on sides to soft-tissue borders of humerus and shoulder. (Lower margin of collimation field should include the elbow joint and about 2.5 cm, or 1 inch, minimum of proximal forearm.)

Respiration Suspend respiration during exposure.

Radiographic Criteria

Structures Shown: • AP projection of the entire humerus, including the shoulder and elbow joints, is visible.

Position: • Long axis of humerus should be aligned to long axis of IR. • **True AP** projection is evidenced at proximal humerus by the following: Greater tubercle is seen in profile laterally; humeral head is partially seen in profile medially, with minimal superimposition of the glenoid cavity. • Distal humerus: Lateral and medial epicondyles are both visualized in profile.

Collimation and CR: • Collimation borders are visible at the skin margins along the length of the humerus, with minimal collimation at both ends to ensure that essential joint anatomy is included. • CR and center of the collimation field should be to the approximate midpoint of the humerus.

Exposure Criteria: • Optimal density and contrast with no motion visualize sharp cortical margins and clear, bony trabecular markings at both the proximal and the distal portions of the humerus.

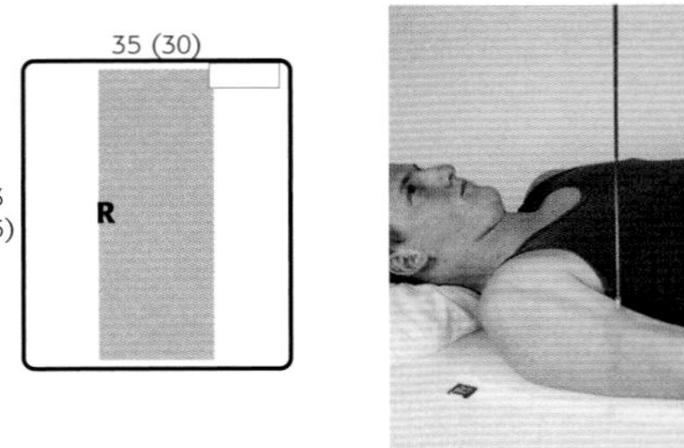

Fig. 5-162. Anteroposterior supine.

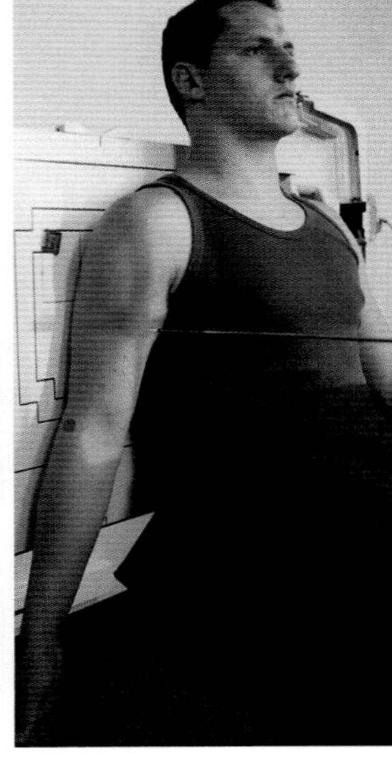

Fig. 5-163. Anteroposterior erect.

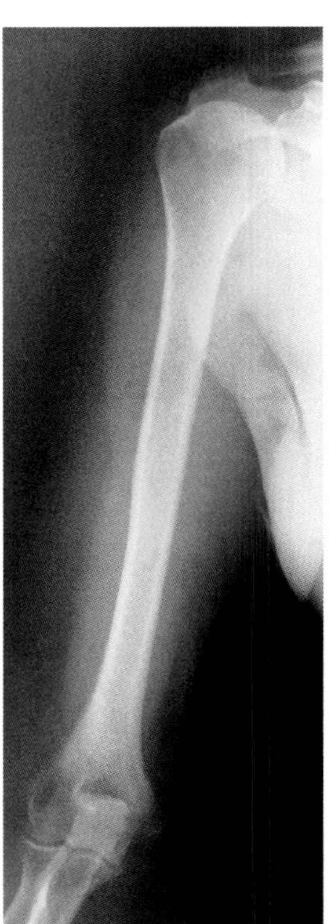

Fig. 5-164. Anteroposterior.

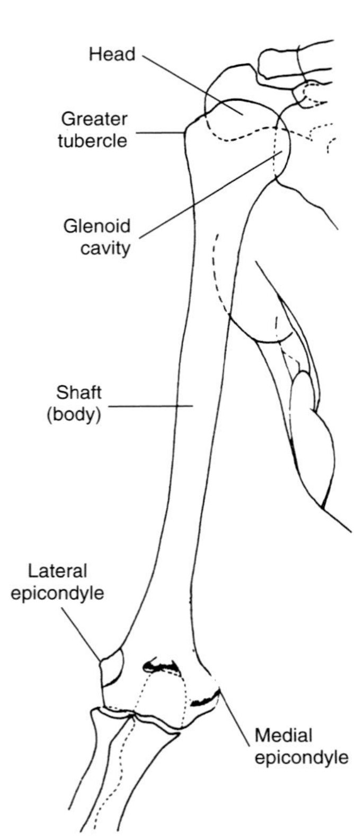

Fig. 5-165. Anteroposterior.

ROTATIONAL LATERAL—LATEROMEDIAL OR MEDIOLATERAL PROJECTIONS: HUMERUS

Warning: Do **not** attempt to rotate arm if fracture or dislocation is suspected (see Trauma Horizontal Beam Lateral on p. 178).

Humerus
BASIC
- AP
- Rotational lateral
- **Horizontal beam lateral**

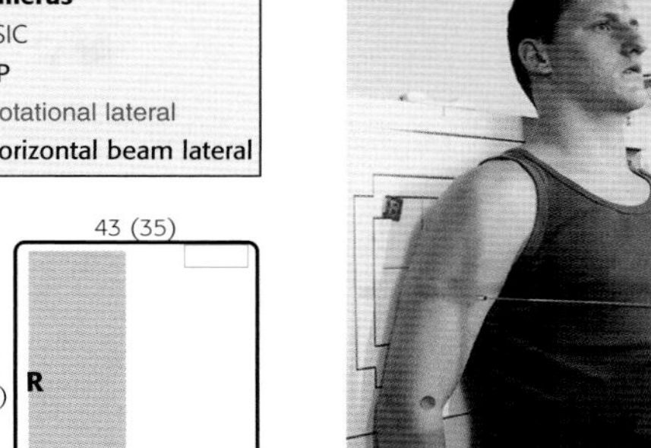

Pathology Demonstrated

Fractures and dislocation of the humerus and pathologic processes, such as osteoporosis and arthritis, are demonstrated.

Technical Factors

- IR size—lengthwise (large enough to include entire humerus)
  —For larger patient, 35 × 43 cm (14 × 17 inches)
  —For smaller patient, 30 × 35 cm (11 × 14 inches)
- Moving or stationary grid (nongrid, detail screen for smaller patient)
- 70 ± 6 kV range
- Technique and dose:

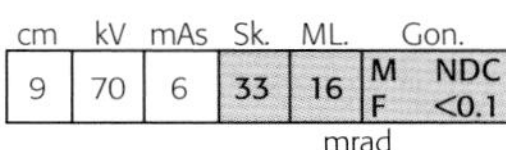

cm	kV	mAs	Sk.	ML.	Gon.
9	70	6	33	16	M NDC F <0.1
				mrad	

Shielding Secure or place lead shield over pelvic area.

Patient and Part Position

- Position patient erect or supine, as either lateromedial or mediolateral projection.
- *Lateromedial:* Position patient erect with back to IR and elbow partially flexed, with body rotated toward affected side as needed to bring humerus and shoulder in contact with cassette. **Internally rotate arm** as needed for lateral position; **epicondyles are perpendicular** to IR.
- *Mediolateral:* Face patient toward IR (Fig. 5-167) and oblique as needed (20° to 30° from PA) to allow close contact of humerus to IR; flex elbow 90° as shown.
- Adjust cassette height so that shoulders and elbow joints are equidistant from ends of cassette.

Central Ray

- CR perpendicular to IR, centered to **midpoint of humerus**
- Minimum SID of 40 inches (100 cm)

Collimation Collimate on four sides to soft-tissue border of humerus, ensuring that all of shoulder and elbow joints are included.

Respiration Suspend respiration during exposure.

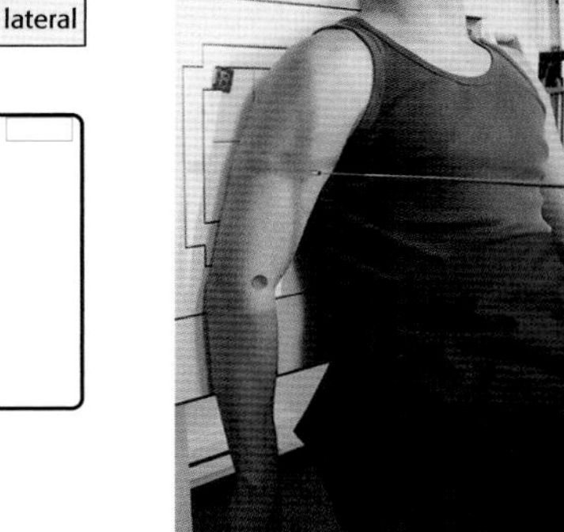

Fig. 5-166. Erect lateral—lateromedial, back to IR.

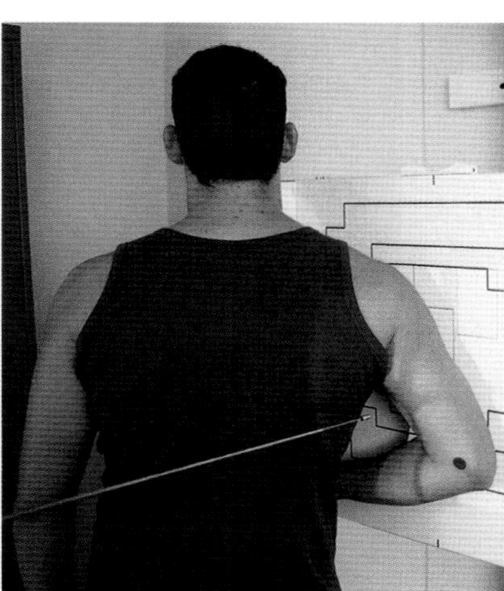

Fig. 5-167. Erect lateral—mediolateral, facing IR.

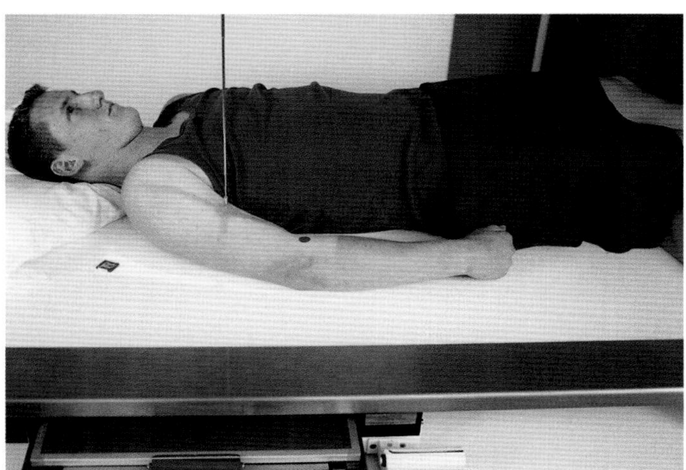

Fig. 5-168. Supine lateromedial projection.

Radiographic Criteria

Structures Shown: • A lateral projection of the entire humerus, including elbow and shoulder joints, is visible.

Position: • True lateral projection is evidenced by the following: Epicondyles are directly superimposed; lesser tubercle is shown in profile medially, partially superimposed by lower portion of glenoid cavity.

Collimation and CR: • Collimation borders should be visible at the skin margins along the length of the humerus, with minimal collimation at both ends to ensure that essential joint anatomy is included. • CR and center of collimation field should be to the approximate midpoint of the humerus.

Exposure Criteria: • Optimal density and contrast with no motion visualize clear, sharp bony trabecular markings of entire humerus.

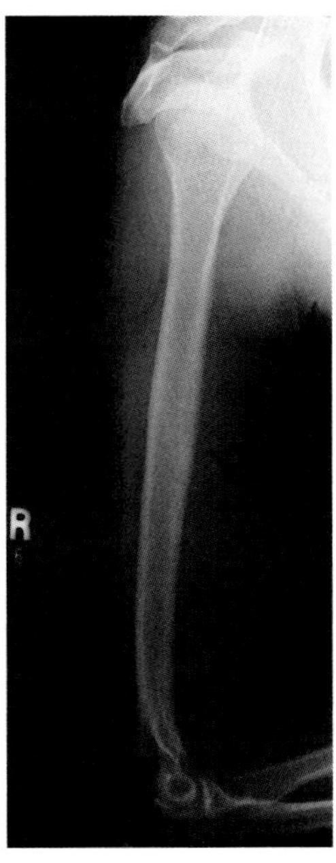

Fig. 5-169. Erect mediolateral.

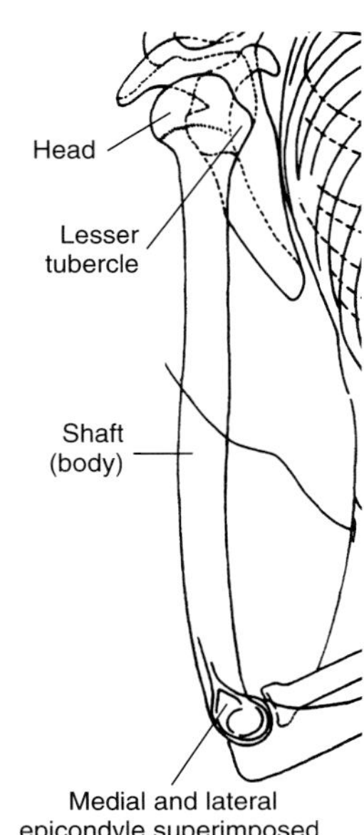

Fig. 5-170. Lateral.

5

TRAUMA HORIZONTAL BEAM LATERAL—LATEROMEDIAL PROJECTION: HUMERUS

Warning: Do **not** attempt to rotate arm if fracture or dislocation is suspected.

Proximal Humerus: See Transthoracic Lateral or Scapular Y in Chapter 6.

Humerus
BASIC
- AP
- Rotational lateral
- Horizontal beam lateral

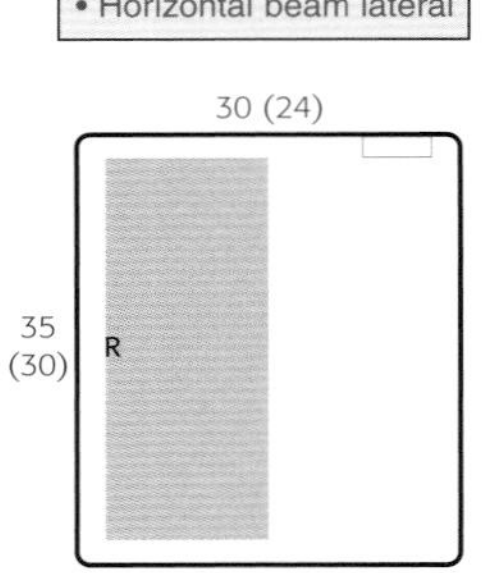

Pathology Demonstrated

Fractures and dislocations of the mid- and distal humerus and other pathologic processes, such as osteoporosis and arthritis, are demonstrated.

Technical Factors

- IR size—30 × 35 cm (11 × 14 inches); for smaller patient, 24 × 30 cm (10 × 12 inches)
- Detail screen, nongrid with film-screen imaging.
- 64 ± 6 kV range
- Technique and dose:

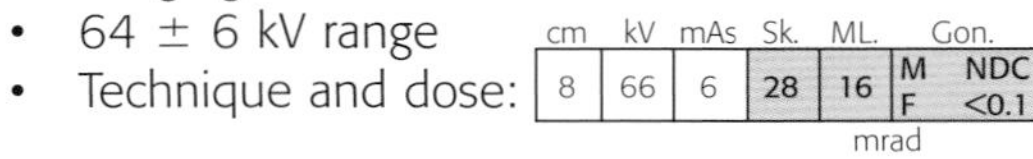

cm	kV	mAs	Sk.	ML.	Gon.
8	66	6	28	16	M NDC
					F <0.1

mrad

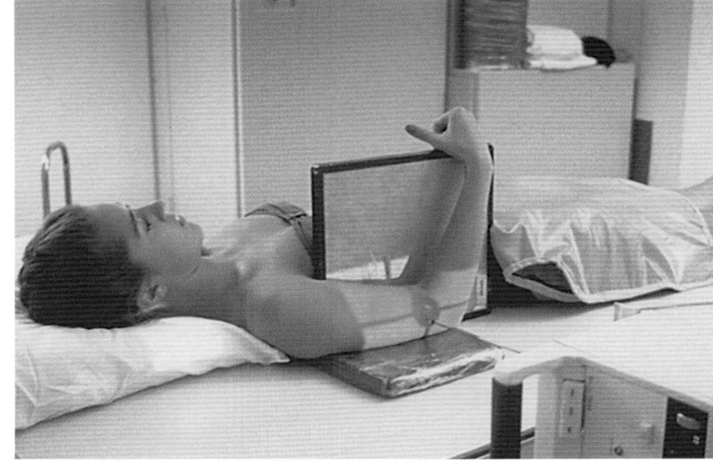

Fig. 5-171. Horizontal beam lateral (mid- and distal humerus).

Shielding Place lead shield **over thorax and pelvis,** between the cassette and patient.

Patient and Part Position

- With patient recumbent, take image as a horizontal beam lateral, placing support under arm.
- Flex elbow if possible, but do not attempt to rotate arm; projection should be 90° from AP.
- Gently place cassette between arm and thorax (top of IR to axilla).

Central Ray

- CR perpendicular to **midpoint of distal two-thirds of humerus**
- Minimum SID of 40 inches (100 cm)

Collimation Collimate to soft-tissue margins.

Respiration **Suspend respiration** during exposure. (This step is important to prevent movement of cassette during the exposure.)

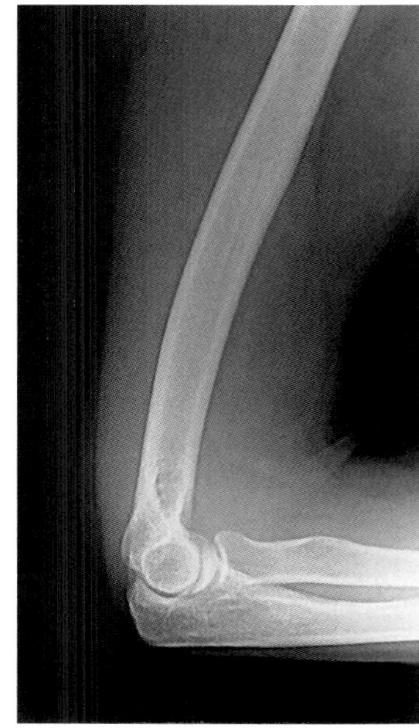

Fig. 5-172. Lateral (mid- and distal humerus).

Radiographic Criteria

Structures Shown: • A lateral projection of the mid- and distal humerus, including the elbow joint, is visible. • The distal two-thirds of the humerus should be well visualized.

Position: • The long axis of the humerus should be aligned with the long axis of the IR. • The elbow is flexed 90°.

Collimation and CR: • Collimation borders should be visible at the skin margins along the length of the humerus. • CR and center of the collimation field should be to the approximate midpoint of the distal two thirds of the humerus.

Exposure Criteria: • Optimal density and contrast with no motion should visualize sharp cortical borders and clear, sharp bony trabecular markings.

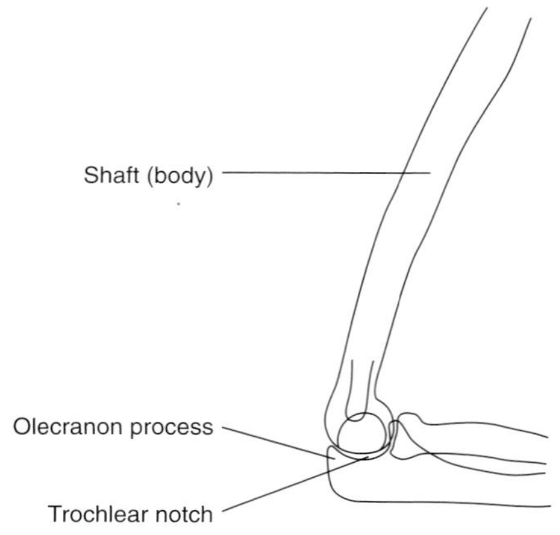

Fig. 5-173. Lateral (mid- and distal humerus).

5

RADIOGRAPHS FOR CRITIQUE

Each of these upper-limb radiographs demonstrates some error in positioning that requires a repeat. These, along with accompanying lecture slides of radiographs, provide a basis for classroom and/or positioning laboratory discussion.

Critique these radiographs for errors in one or more of the five categories, as described in this textbook and as outlined on the right. As a starting critique exercise, place a check in each category that demonstrates a **repeatable error** for that radiograph.

Student workbooks provide more space for writing comments and complete critique answers for each radiograph. Answers are provided in Appendix B, at the end of this textbook and in the workbooks.

	RADIOGRAPHS					
	A	B	C	D	E	F
1. Structures shown	____	____	____	____	____	____
2. Positioning	____	____	____	____	____	____
3. Collimation and CR	____	____	____	____	____	____
4. Exposure criteria	____	____	____	____	____	____
5. Markers	____	____	____	____	____	____

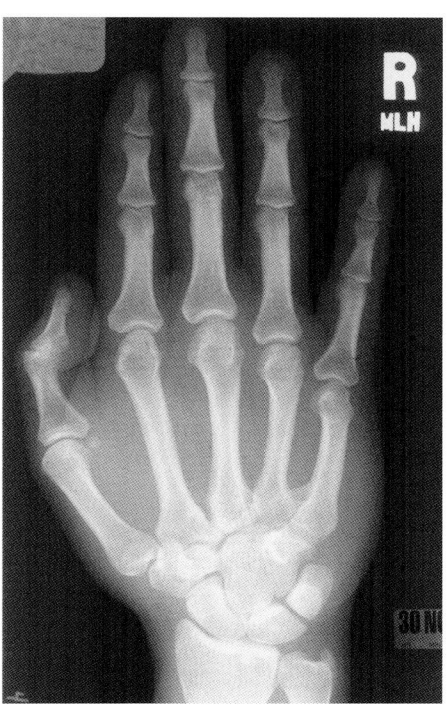

Fig. C5-174. PA hand. A

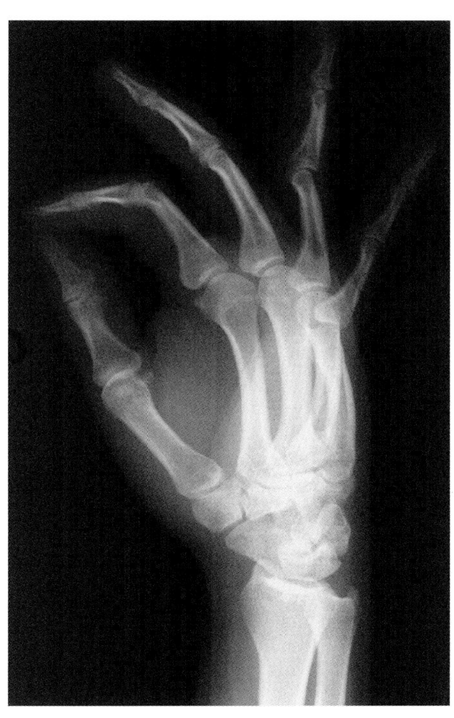

Fig. C5-175. Lateral hand. B

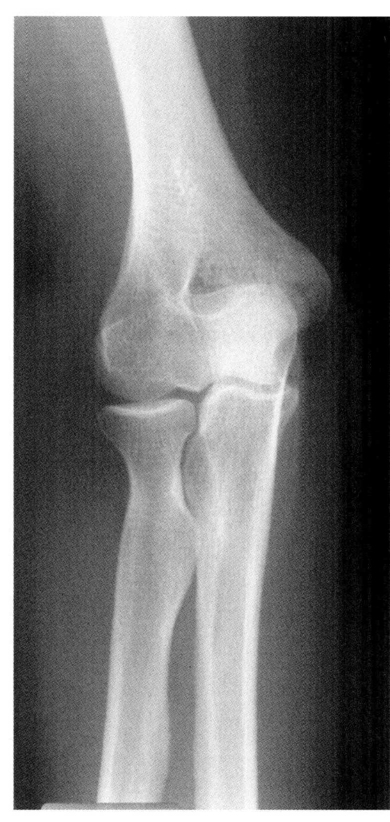

Fig. C5-176. AP oblique elbow. C

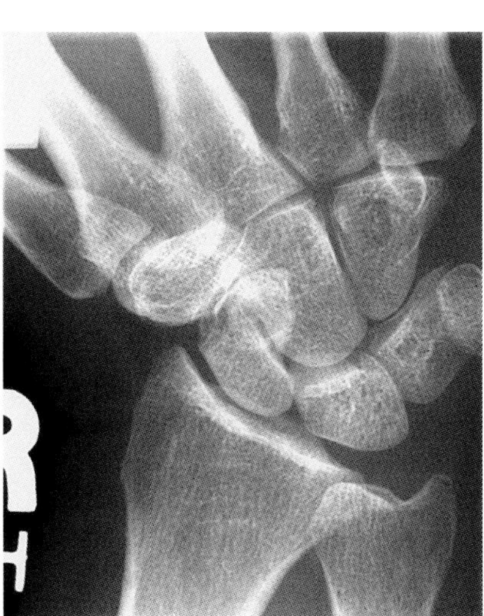

Fig. C5-177. PA wrist. D

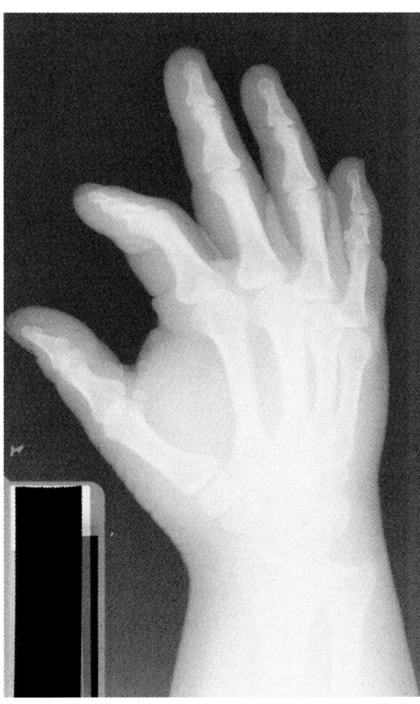

Fig. C5-178. PA oblique hand. E

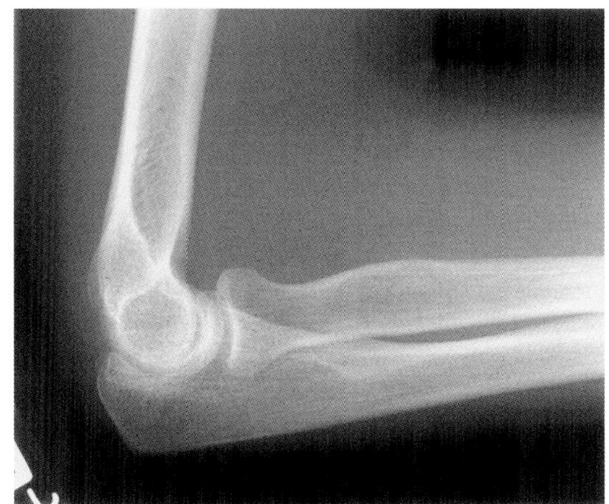

Fig. C5-179. Lateral elbow. F

CHAPTER 6

Proximal Humerus and Shoulder Girdle

CONTRIBUTORS TO PAST EDITIONS Linda S. Lingar, MEd, RT(R)(M), Donna Davis, MEd, RT(R)(CV)

CONTENTS

RADIOGRAPHIC ANATOMY

Upper Limb (Extremity)

The hand, wrist, and mid- and distal humerus of the upper limb were described in Chapter 5. The **proximal humerus** is covered in this chapter, along with the shoulder girdle, which includes the **clavicle** and **scapula.**

HUMERUS

The **humerus** is the largest and longest bone of the upper limb. Its length on an adult equals approximately one-fifth of the body height. The humerus articulates with the **scapula** (shoulder blade) at the shoulder joint.

Proximal Humerus

The proximal humerus is the part of the upper arm that articulates with the scapula, making up the shoulder joint. The most proximal part is the rounded **head** of the humerus. The slightly constricted area directly below and lateral to the head is the **anatomic neck,** which appears as a line of demarcation between the rounded head and the adjoining greater and lesser tubercles.

The process directly below the anatomic neck on the anterior surface is the **lesser tubercle** *(tu'ber-k'l)* (tuberosity in earlier literature). The larger lateral process is the **greater tubercle,** to which the pectoralis major and supraspinatus muscles attach. The deep groove between these two tubercles is the **intertubercular** *(in"ter-tu-ber'ku-lar)* **groove** (bicipital groove). The tapered area below the head and tubercles is the **surgical neck,** and distal to the surgical neck is the long **body** (shaft) of the humerus.

The surgical neck gets its name because it is the site of frequent fractures requiring surgery. Fractures at the thick anatomic neck are rarer.

The **deltoid tuberosity** is the roughened raised triangular elevation along the anterolateral surface of the body (shaft) to which the deltoid muscle is attached.

Anatomy of Proximal Humerus on Radiograph

Fig. 6-3 is an AP radiograph of the shoulder taken with **external rotation,** which places the humerus in a **true AP** or frontal position. Fig. 6-2 represents a neutral rotation (natural position of arm without internal or external rotation). This places the humerus in an oblique position midway between an AP (external rotation) and a lateral (internal rotation).

Some anatomic parts are more difficult to visualize on radiographs than on drawings. However, a good understanding of the location and relationship between various parts helps in this identification. The following parts are shown in Fig. 6-3.

A. Head of humerus
B. Greater tubercle
C. Intertubercular groove
D. Lesser tubercle
E. Anatomic neck
F. Surgical neck
G. Body

The relative location of the greater and lesser tubercles is significant in determining a true frontal view or a true AP projection of the proximal humerus. Note that the **lesser tubercle is located anteriorly and the greater tubercle is located laterally** in a true AP projection.

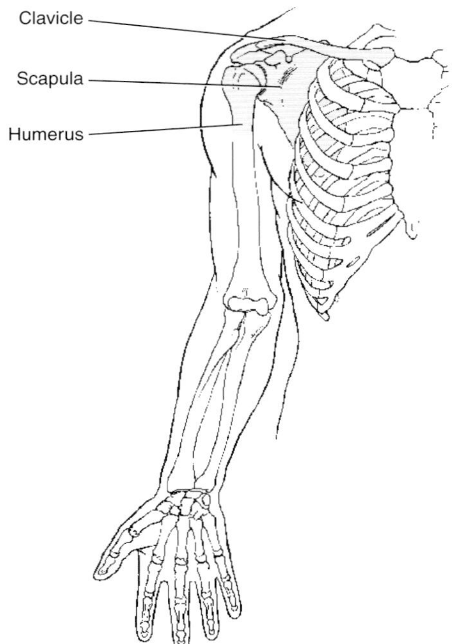

Fig. 6-1. Shoulder girdle.

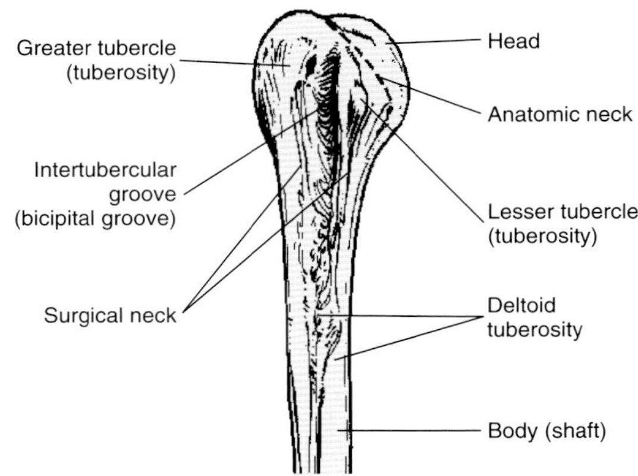

Fig. 6-2. Frontal view of proximal humerus—neutral rotation (oblique position).

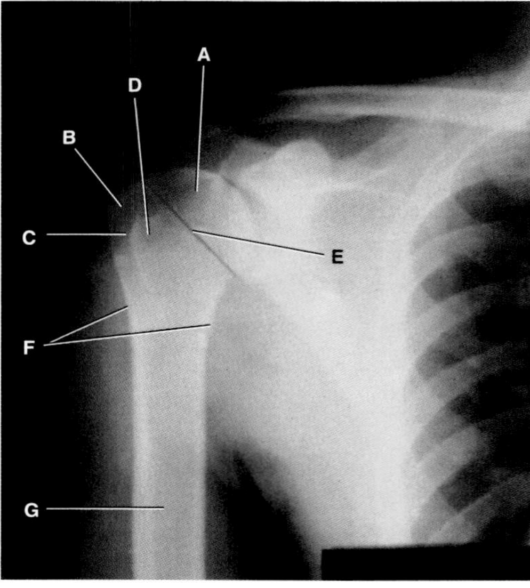

Fig. 6-3. AP shoulder—external rotation.

SHOULDER GIRDLE

The shoulder girdle consists of two bones: the **clavicle** and the **scapula.** The function of the clavicle and scapula is to connect each upper limb to the trunk or axial skeleton. Anteriorly the shoulder girdle connects to the trunk at the upper sternum, but posteriorly the connection to the trunk is incomplete because the scapula is connected to the trunk by muscles only.

Each shoulder girdle and upper limb connect at the shoulder joint between the scapula and the humerus. Each clavicle is located over the upper, anterior rib cage. Each scapula is situated over the upper, posterior rib cage.

The upper margin of the scapula is at the level of the **second posterior rib,** and the lower margin is at the level of the **seventh posterior rib** (T7). Note that the lower margin of the scapula corresponds to T7, also used as a landmark for location of the central ray for chest positioning (see Chapter 3).

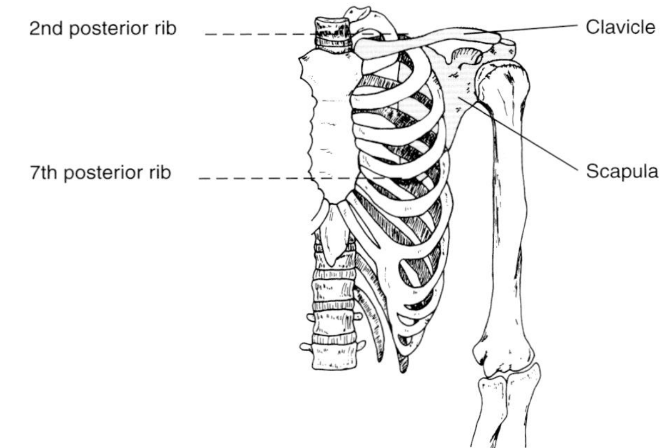

Fig. 6-4. Shoulder girdle.

Clavicle

The clavicle (collar bone) is a long bone with a double curvature having three main parts: the two ends and the long central portion. The lateral or **acromial** *(ah-kro'me-al)* **extremity** (end) of the clavicle articulates with the acromion of the scapula. This joint or articulation is termed the **acromioclavicular** *(ah-kro"me-o-klah-vik'u-lar)* **joint** and can generally be readily palpated.

The medial or **sternal extremity** (end) articulates with the manubrium, which is the upper part of the sternum. This articulation is termed the **sternoclavicular** *(ster"no-klah-vik'u-lar)* **joint.** This joint is also easily palpated, and the combination of the sternoclavicular joints on either side of the manubrium helps form an important positioning landmark called the **jugular** *(jug'u-lar)* **notch,** also called the *suprasternal* or *manubrial notch* in earlier literature.

The **body** (shaft) of the clavicle is the elongated portion between the two extremities.

The acromial end of the clavicle is flattened and has a downward curvature at its attachment with the acromion. The sternal end is more triangular in shape and is also directed downward to articulate with the sternum.

In general, a difference in size and shape of the clavicle exists between males and females. The **female clavicle** is usually **shorter** and **less curved** than the male clavicle. The clavicle in the male tends to be thicker and more curved, usually being most curved in heavily muscled males.

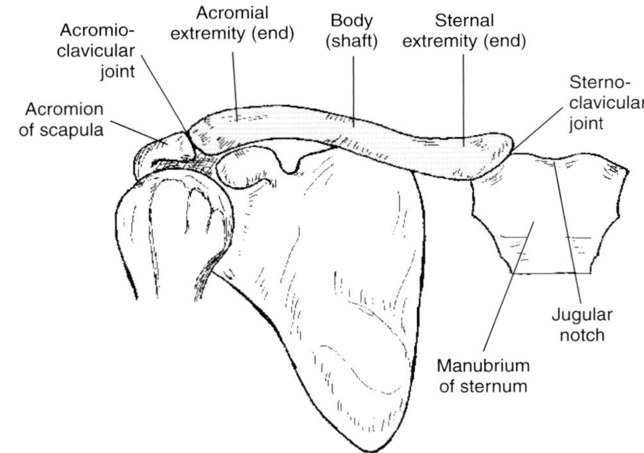

Fig. 6-5. Clavicle.

Radiograph of the clavicle

The AP radiograph of the clavicle in Fig. 6-6 identifies the two joints and the three parts of the clavicle as follows:

A. Sternoclavicular joint
B. Sternal extremity
C. Body
D. Acromial extremity
E. Acromioclavicular joint

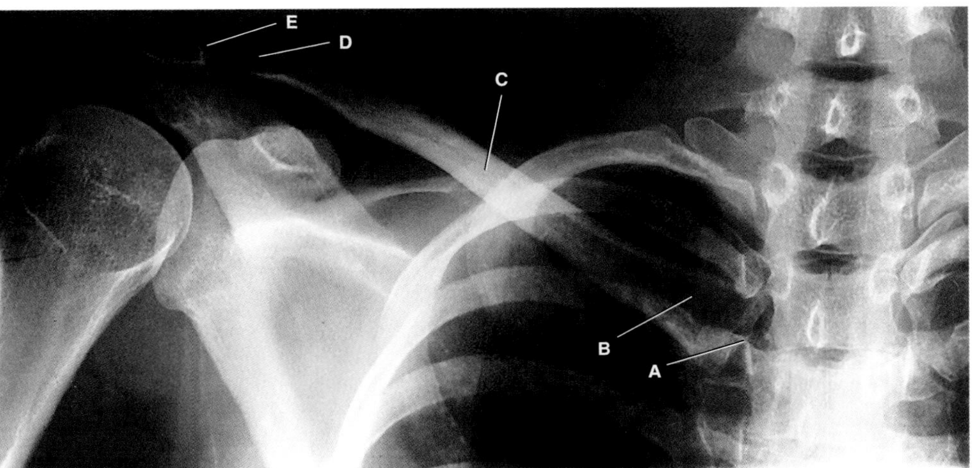

Fig. 6-6. AP radiograph of clavicle.

6

Scapula

The scapula (shoulder blade), which forms the posterior part of the shoulder girdle, is a flat triangular bone with three borders, three angles, and two surfaces. The three borders include the **medial** (vertebral) **border,** which is the long edge or border near the vertebrae; the **superior border,** or the uppermost margin of the scapula; and the **lateral** (axillary) **border,** or the border nearest the axilla *(ak-sil'ah)* (Fig. 6-7). *Axilla* is the medical term for the armpit.

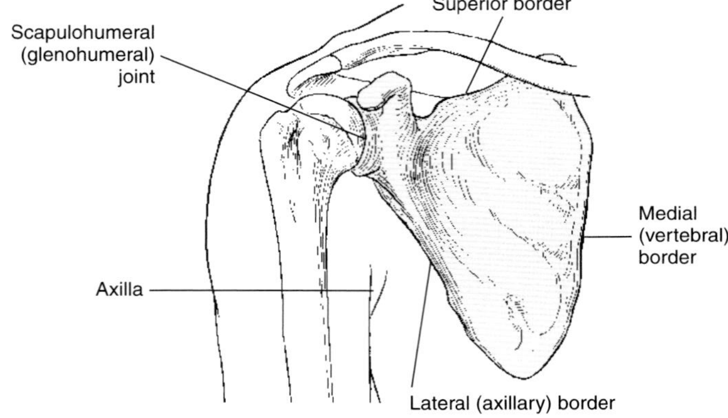

Fig. 6-7. Scapula—three borders and scapulohumeral (glenohumeral) joint.

Anterior view The three corners of the triangular-shaped scapula are called *angles* (Fig. 6-8). The **lateral angle,** sometimes called the *head of the scapula,* is the thickest part and ends laterally in a shallow depression called the *glenoid cavity* (fossa).

The humeral head articulates with the glenoid cavity of the scapula to form the **scapulohumeral** *(skap'u-lo-hu'mer-al)* **joint,** also known as the *glenohumeral joint,* or *shoulder joint.*

The constricted area between the head and the body of the scapula is the **neck.** The **superior** and **inferior angles** refer to the upper and lower ends of the medial or vertebral border. The **body** (blade) of the scapula is arched for greater strength. The thin, flat, lower part of the body is sometimes referred to as the *wing* or ala of the scapula, although these are not preferred anatomic terms.

The anterior surface of the scapula is termed the **costal** *(kos'tal)* **surface** because of the proximity to the ribs (*costa,* literally meaning "rib"). The mid area of the costal surface presents a large concavity or depression, the **subscapular fossa.**

The **acromion** is a long, curved process extending laterally over the head of the humerus. The **coracoid process** is a thick, beaklike process projecting anteriorly beneath the clavicle. The **scapular notch** is a notch on the superior border partially formed by the base of the coracoid process.

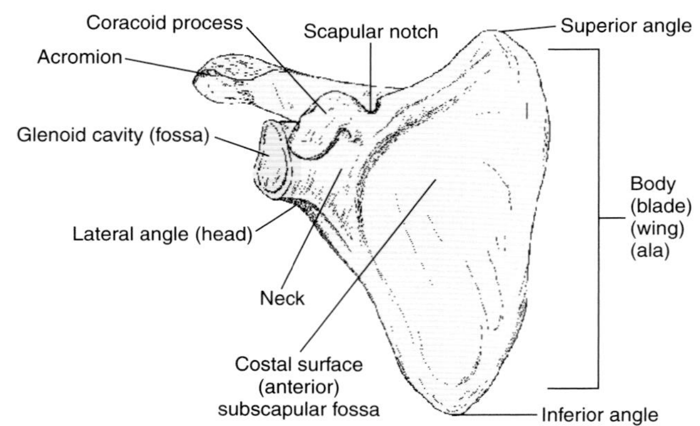

Fig. 6-8. Scapula—anterior view.

Posterior view Fig. 6-9 shows a prominent structure on the dorsal or posterior surface of the scapula, called the **spine.** The elevated spine of the scapula starts at the vertebral border as a smooth triangular area and continues laterally to end at the **acromion.** The acromion overhangs the shoulder joint posteriorly.

The posterior border or ridge of the spine is somewhat thickened and is termed the **crest** of the spine. The spine separates the posterior surface into an **infraspinous** *(in"frah-spi'nus)* **fossa** and a **supraspinous fossa.** (Older terms for these fossae are "infraspinatus" and "supraspinatus," respectively.) Both of these fossae serve as surfaces of attachment for shoulder muscles. The names of these muscles are associated with the respective fossae.

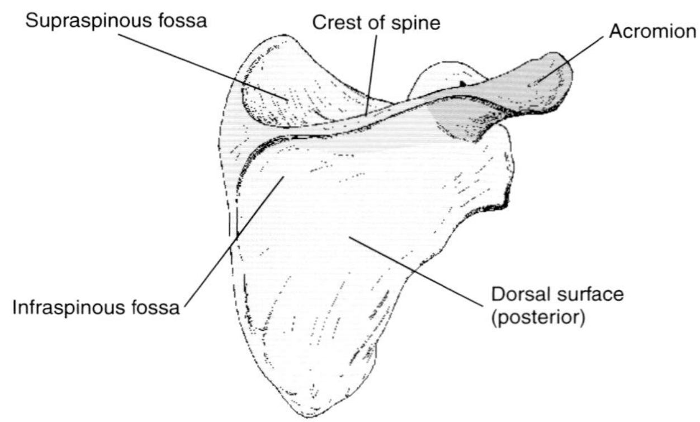

Fig. 6-9. Scapula—posterior view.

Lateral view The lateral view of the scapula demonstrates relative positions of the various parts of the scapula (Fig. 6-10). The thin scapula looks like the letter Y in this position. The upper parts of the Y are the acromion and coracoid process. The **acromion** is the expanded distal end of the spine extending superiorly and posteriorly to the glenoid cavity (fossa). The **coracoid process** is located more anteriorly in relationship to the glenoid cavity or shoulder joint.

The bottom leg of the Y is the body of the scapula. The posterior surface or back portion of the thin body portion of the scapula is the **dorsal surface.** The **spine** extends from the dorsal surface at its upper margin. The anterior surface of the body is the **ventral** (costal) **surface.** The **lateral** (axillary) **border** is a thicker edge or border extending from the **glenoid cavity** to the **inferior angle,** as shown on this lateral view.

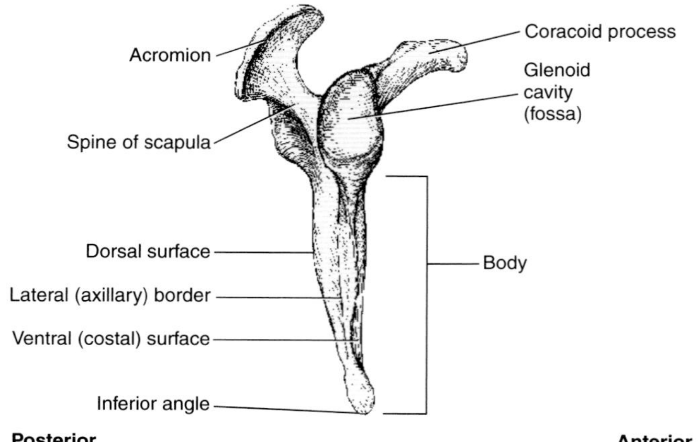

Fig. 6-10. Scapula—lateral view.

REVIEW EXERCISE WITH RADIOGRAPHS OF SCAPULA

AP projection: Fig. 6-11 is an AP projection of the scapula taken with the arm abducted so as not to superimpose the scapula. Knowing shapes and relationships of anatomic parts should help in identifying each of the following parts:

A. Acromion
B. Neck of scapula (about 1 inch below the coracoid process)
C. Scapular notch
D. Superior angle
E. Medial (vertebral) border
F. Inferior angle
G. Lateral (axillary) border
H. Glenoid cavity (fossa) or scapulohumeral joint

Lateral projection: This scapular Y lateral projection of the scapula is taken with the patient in an anterior oblique position with the upper body rotated until the scapula is separated from the rib cage in a true end-on or lateral projection (Fig. 6-12).

Note that this lateral view of the scapula results in a Y shape, wherein the acromion and the coracoid process make up the upper legs of the Y and the body makes up the long lower leg.

The scapular Y position gets its name from this Y shape, resulting from a true lateral view of the scapula. The labeled parts as seen on this view are as follows:

A. Acromion
B. Coracoid process
C. Inferior angle
D. Spine of scapula
E. Body of scapula

Proximal Humerus and Scapula

Inferosuperior (axiolateral) projection: This projection (as illustrated in Fig. 6-14) results in a lateral view of the head and neck of the humerus. It also demonstrates the relationship of the humerus to the glenoid cavity, which makes up the scapulohumeral (shoulder) joint.

Anatomy of the scapula may appear confusing in this position, but understanding relationships between the various parts will help in identification.

Part ***A*** of Fig. 6-13 is the tip of the **coracoid process,** which is located anterior to the shoulder joint and would therefore be located superiorly with the patient lying on her back, as shown in Fig. 6-14.

Part ***B*** is the **glenoid cavity,** which is the articulating surface of the **lateral angle** or **head** of the scapula.

Part ***C*** is the **spine** of the scapula, which is located posteriorly with the patient lying on her back, as shown in Fig. 6-14.

Part ***D*** is the **acromion,** which is the extended portion of the spine superimposed over the humerus in this position.

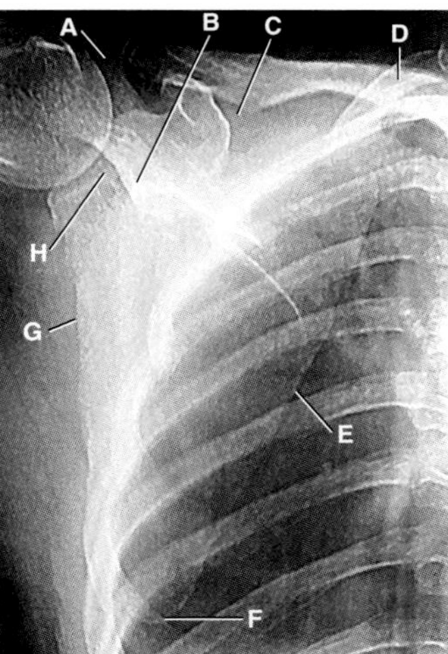

Fig. 6-11. AP projection.

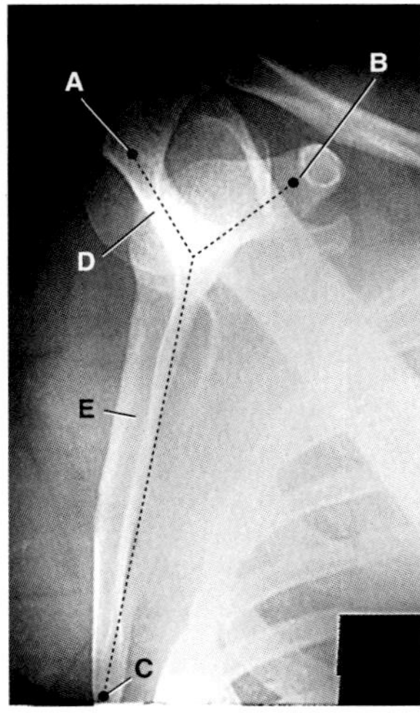

Fig. 6-12. Lateral (scapular Y) position.

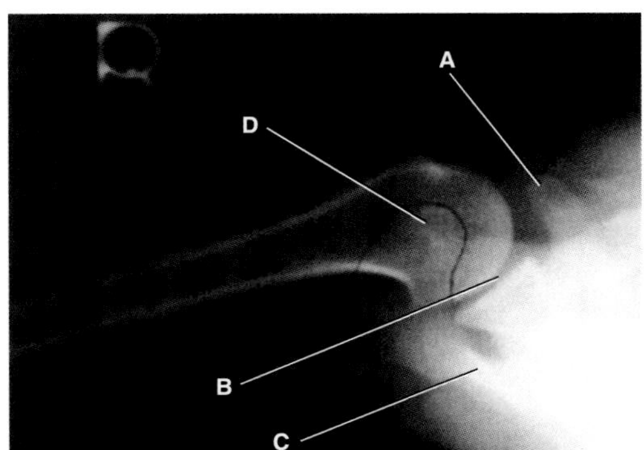

Fig. 6-13. Inferosuperior axial projection.

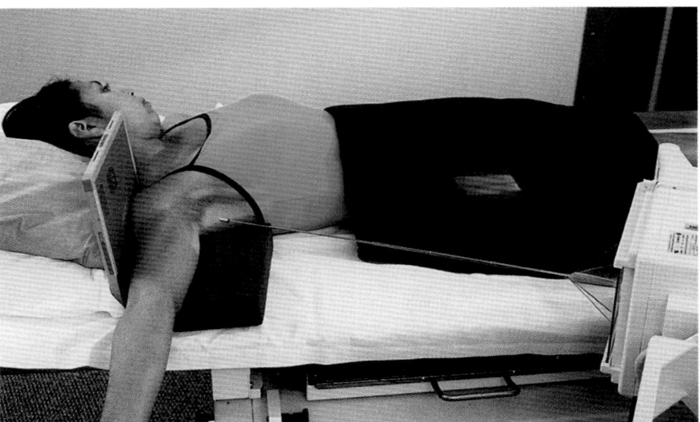

Fig. 6-14. Inferosuperior axial projection.

6

CLASSIFICATION OF JOINTS

There are three joints or articulations involved in the shoulder girdle: the **sternoclavicular joint,** the **acromioclavicular joint,** and the **scapulohumeral joint** (glenohumeral or shoulder joint, Fig. 6-15).

Classification

The three shoulder girdle joints (articulations) are classified as **synovial joints,** characterized by a fibrous capsule containing synovial fluid.

Mobility Type

The mobility type of all three of these joints is **freely movable,** or **diarthrodial.** All synovial joints are by nature of their structure freely movable. Therefore the only difference between these three joints is their movement type.

Movement Type

The **scapulohumeral** (glenohumeral) or shoulder joint involves articulation between the head of the humerus and the glenoid cavity of the scapula. The movement type is a **spheroidal** (or **ball and socket) joint,** which allows great freedom of movement. These movements are **flexion, extension, abduction, adduction, circumduction, medial** (internal), and **lateral** (external) **rotation.**

The glenoid cavity is very shallow, allowing the greatest freedom in mobility of any joint in the human body, but at some expense to its strength and stability. Strong ligaments, tendons, and muscles surround the joint, providing stability. However, stretching of the muscles and tendons can cause separation or dislocation of the humeral head from the glenoid cavity. Dislocations at the shoulder joint occur more frequently than at any other joint in the body, requiring the need for frequent radiographic shoulder exams to evaluate for structural damage. The shoulder girdle also includes two joints involving both ends of the clavicle, called the *sternoclavicular* and *acromioclavicular joints.*

The **sternoclavicular joint** is a **double plane,** or **gliding, joint** because the sternal end of the clavicle articulates with the manubrium or upper portion of the sternum and the cartilage of the first rib. This allows a limited amount of gliding motion in nearly every direction.

The **acromioclavicular joint** is also a small synovial joint of the **plane,** or **gliding, movement type** between the acromial end of the clavicle and the medial aspect of the acromion of the scapula. Two types of movement occur at this joint. The primary movement is a gliding action between the end of the clavicle and the acromion. Some secondary rotary movement also occurs as the scapula moves forward and backward with the clavicle. This allows the scapula to adjust its position as it remains in close contact with the posterior chest wall. The rotary type movement, however, is limited, and this joint is generally termed a *plane,* or *gliding-type, joint.*

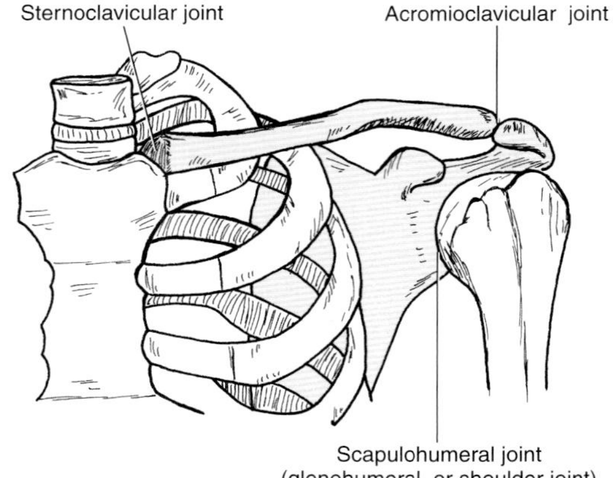

Fig. 6-15. Joints of shoulder girdle.

SUMMARY OF SHOULDER GIRDLE JOINTS

Classification:	*Synovial* (articular capsule containing synovial fluid)
Mobility type:	*Diarthrodial* (freely movable)
Movement types:	
1. Scapulohumeral (glenohumeral) joint	*Spheroidal* or *ball and socket*
2. Sternoclavicular joint	*Plane* or *gliding*
3. Acromioclavicular joint	*Plane* or *gliding*

RADIOGRAPHIC POSITIONING

Proximal Humerus Rotation

RADIOGRAPHS OF PROXIMAL HUMERUS

Rotational views of the proximal humerus or shoulder girdle are commonly taken on nontrauma patients when gross fractures or dislocations of the humerus have been ruled out. These AP rotational projections demonstrate the scapulohumeral joint (shoulder joint) well for possible calcium deposits or other pathology. Note specifically the location and shapes of the **greater tubercle** *(A)* and the **lesser tubercle** *(B)* on these external, internal, and neutral rotation radiographs (Figs. 6-17, 6-19, and 6-21).

By studying the position and relationships of the greater and lesser tubercles on a radiograph of the shoulder, you can determine the rotational position of the arm. This understanding enables you to know which rotational view is necessary to visualize specific parts of the proximal humerus.

External rotation: The external rotation position represents a true **AP projection** of the humerus in the anatomic position, as determined by the epicondyles of the distal humerus. Positioning requires supination of the hand and external rotation of the elbow so that the interepicondylar line is **parallel to the IR** (Fig. 6-16).

Note: You can check this on yourself by dropping your arm at your side and externally rotating your hand and arm while palpating the epicondyles of your distal humerus.

On the external rotation view (Fig. 6-17), the **greater tubercle** *(A),* which is located anteriorly in a neutral position, is now seen in **profile laterally.** The **lesser tubercle** *(B)* is now located **anteriorly,** just medial to the greater tubercle.

Internal rotation: For the internal rotation position, the hand and arm are rotated internally until the epicondyles of the distal humerus are **perpendicular to the IR,** thus placing the humerus in a **true lateral position.** The hand must be pronated and the elbow adjusted to place the epicondyles **perpendicular to the IR** (Fig. 6-18).

The AP projection of the shoulder taken in the internal rotation position is therefore a lateral position of the humerus in which the **greater tubercle** *(A)* is now rotated around to the anterior and medial aspect of the proximal humerus. The **lesser tubercle** *(B)* is seen in profile medially.

Neutral rotation: Neutral rotation is appropriate for a trauma patient when rotation of the part is unacceptable. The epicondyles of the distal humerus will appear at an **approximate 45° angle to the IR.** This results in a 45° oblique position of the humerus when the **palm of the hand is facing inward** against the thigh. The neutral position then is about midway between the external and internal positions and places the greater tubercle anteriorly but still lateral to the lesser tubercle, as seen on the radiograph in Fig. 6-21.

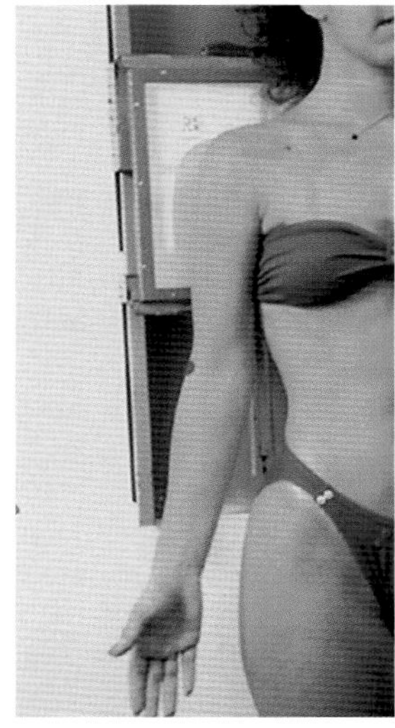

Fig. 6-16. External rotation (AP projection of humerus).

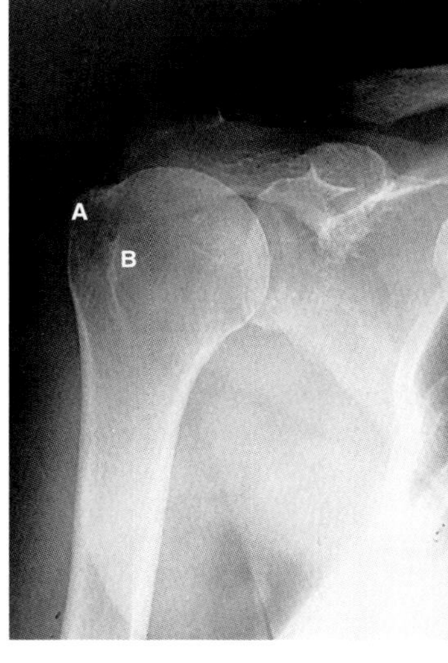

Fig. 6-17. External rotation (AP projection of humerus).

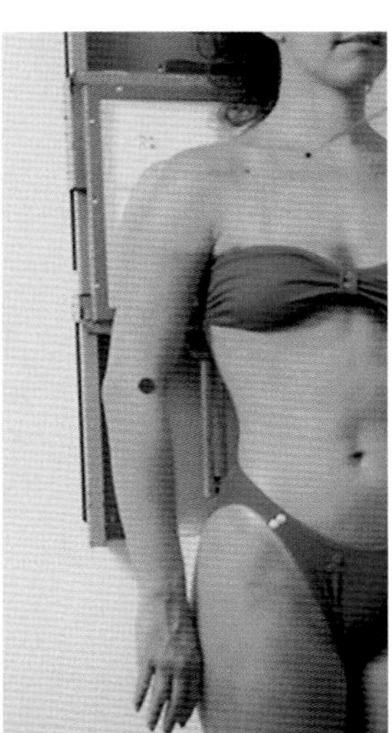

Fig. 6-18. Internal rotation (lateral projection of humerus).

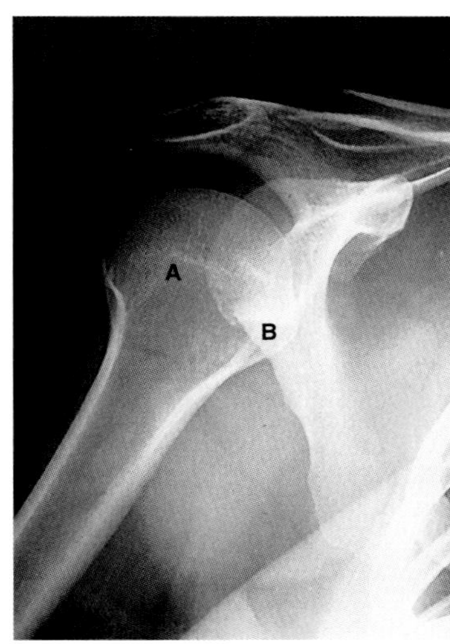

Fig. 6-19. Internal rotation (lateral projection of humerus).

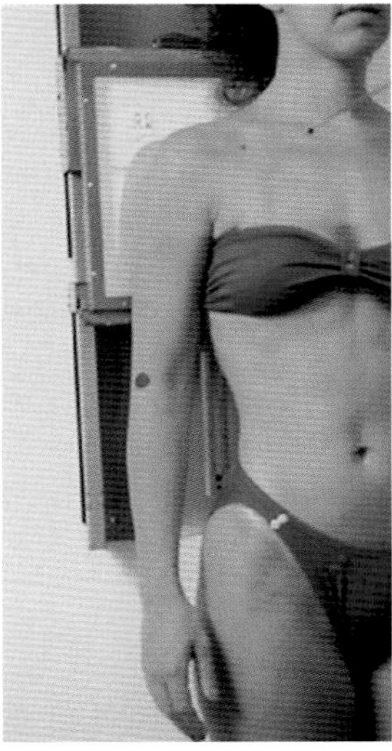

Fig. 6-20. Neutral rotation (oblique projection of humerus).

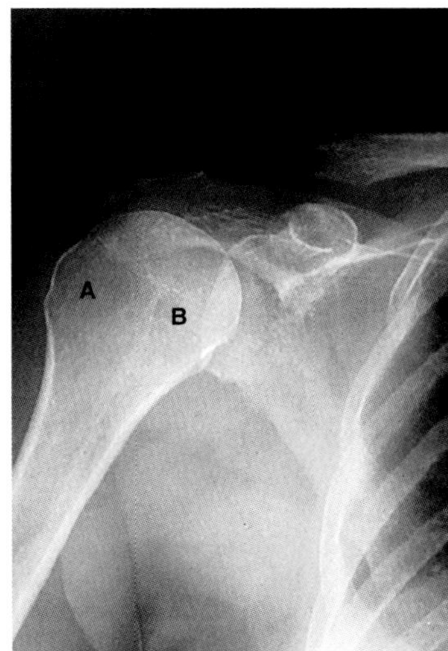

Fig. 6-21. Neutral rotation (oblique projection of humerus).

Positioning and Exposure Considerations

General positioning considerations for the proximal humerus and shoulder girdle (clavicle and scapula) are similar to other upper and lower limb procedures.

Technique Considerations

Adult shoulders generally measure from 10 to 15 cm, which requires the use of a grid and other technical consideration as listed below. Children and thin, asthenic adults may measure less than 10 cm, requiring exposure factor adjustments without the use of grids. AC joints also generally measure less than 10 cm, thus requiring less kV (65-70) without grids.

Average adult shoulder

1. Medium kV, 70-80 with grids if over 10 cm (if less than 10 cm, 65-70 kV without grids)
2. Higher mA with short exposure times
3. Small focal spot
4. Center cell for AEC if used (manual techniques may be recommended with certain projections)
5. Adequate mAs for sufficient density (to visualize soft tissues, bone margins, and trabecular markings of all bones)
6. 400-speed (high-speed) film-screen combination recommended with grid techniques
7. 40 to 44 inches (100 to 110 cm) SID, except for AC joints, which require a 72-inch (180-cm) SID for less beam divergence

Shielding

Gonads Generally, gonadal shielding is important for upper limb radiography because of the proximity of parts of the upper limb, such as the hand or wrists, to the gonads when radiographed in a supine position. The relationship of the divergent x-ray beam to the pelvic region when a patient is in an erect seated position also necessitates gonadal protection. Of course, covering the pelvic region whenever possible on all procedures is good practice and reassures the patient.

Thyroid, lungs, and breasts Radiography of the shoulder region may provide potentially significant doses to the thyroid and lung regions and to the breasts, which are all weighted radiosensitive organs having relative risk of becoming cancerous as compared with whole-body effective doses (see Chapter 2, p. 67). Therefore **close collimation** to the area of interest is very important, in addition to providing **contact shields** over that portion of the lungs, breast, and thyroid regions that do not obscure the area of interest.

Pediatric Applications

In general, the routines for shoulder girdle radiographic examinations do not vary significantly from adult to pediatric patients, although it is essential to decrease exposure technique to compensate for the decrease in tissue quantity and density. **Patient motion** plays an important role in pediatric radiography. Immobilization is often necessary to assist the child in maintaining the proper position. Sponges and tape are very useful, but caution is necessary when using sandbags because of their weight.

Parents are frequently asked to assist with the radiographic examinations of their children. If parents are permitted in the radiography room during the exposure, proper shielding must be provided. To ensure maximum cooperation, the technologist should speak to the child in a soothing manner and use words the child can easily understand.

Geriatric Applications

It is essential to provide clear and complete instructions so that the older patient understands. Routine shoulder girdle examinations may need to be altered to accommodate the older patient's physical condition. Reduction in radiographic technique may be necessary as a result of destructive pathologies commonly seen in geriatric patients.

Digital Imaging Considerations

The following guidelines should be followed when using digital imaging systems (CR or DR) for imaging the proximal humerus and shoulder girdle. These were described in more detail in Chapter 5 for the upper limb and are again summarized as follows:

1. **Collimation:** Close collimation is important to ensure that the final image after processing is of optimal quality.
2. **Accurate centering:** Because of the way the digital image plate reader scans the exposed imaging plate, it is important that the body part and central ray be accurately centered to the IR.
3. **Exposure factors:** It is important that the ALARA principle be followed: that is, the lowest exposure factors required to obtain a diagnostic image should be used. This includes using the highest kV and the lowest mAs that will still result in a final image of diagnostic quality.
4. **Postprocessing evaluation of exposure index values:** After the image is processed and ready for viewing, it must also be checked for an acceptable exposure index value to verify that the exposure factors used were in the correct range to ensure an optimum quality image with the least possible radiation dose to the patient.

Alternative Modalities or Procedures

ARTHROGRAPHY

Arthrography is commonly used to image soft-tissue pathologies such as rotator cuff tears associated with the shoulder girdle. This procedure, which is described in more detail in Chapter 21, requires the use of a radiographic contrast medium injected into the joint capsule under fluoroscopy and sterile conditions.

COMPUTED TOMOGRAPHY AND MAGNETIC RESONANCE IMAGING

Computed tomography (CT) and magnetic resonance imaging (MRI) are often used on the shoulder to evaluate soft-tissue and skeletal involvement of lesions and soft-tissue injuries. The cross-sectional CT images are also excellent for determining the extent of fractures. MRI is useful in the diagnosis of rotator cuff tears, with or without the use of a contrast agent.

NUCLEAR MEDICINE

Nuclear medicine bone scans are useful in demonstrating osteomyelitis, metastatic bone lesions, and cellulitis. Nuclear medicine scans will demonstrate pathology within 24 hours of onset. Nuclear medicine is more sensitive than radiography because it assesses the physiologic aspect instead of the anatomic aspect.

SONOGRAPHY (ULTRASOUND)

Ultrasound is useful for musculoskeletal imaging of joints such as the shoulder to evaluate soft tissues within the joint for possible rotator cuff tears, bursa injuries, or disruption and damage to nerves, tendons, or ligaments. These studies can be used as an adjunct to more expensive MRI studies. Ultrasound also allows for dynamic evaluation during joint movements.

Pathologic Indications

Pathologic indications involving the shoulder girdle that all technologists should be familiar with include the following:

AC joint separation: Trauma to the upper shoulder region resulting in a partial or complete tear of the acromioclavicular (AC) and/or coracoclavicular (CC) ligaments.

Acromioclavicular (AC) dislocation *(ah-kro"mi-o-klah-vik'u-lar):* The distal clavicle is usually displaced superiorly. This injury is most commonly caused by a fall.

Bankart lesion is a fracture of the anteroinferior glenoid rim.

Bursitis *(ber-si'tis)* is an inflammation of the bursa, or fluid-filled sacs enclosing the joints. It generally involves the formation of calcification in associated tendons, causing pain and limitation of joint movement.

Hill-Sachs defect is a compression fracture of the articular surface of the humeral head often associated with an anterior dislocation of the humeral head.

Idiopathic chronic adhesive capsulitis (frozen shoulder) is a disability of the shoulder joint caused by chronic inflammation in and around the joint. It is characterized by pain and limitation of motion. (*Idiopathic* means "of unknown cause.")

Impingement syndrome is impingement of the greater tuberosity and soft tissues on the coracoacromial ligamentous and osseous arch, generally during abduction of the arm.*

*Manaster BJ: *Handbooks in radiology,* ed 2, Chicago, 1997, Year Book Medical Publishers, Inc.

Osteoarthritis: As described in Chapter 4, osteoarthritis is also known as **degenerative joint disease** (DJD), a noninflammatory joint disease characterized by gradual deterioration of the articular cartilage with hypertrophic bone formation. DJD is the most common type of arthritis and is considered to be a normal part of the aging process. It generally occurs in persons over age 50, chronically obese persons, and athletes.

Osteoporosis *(os"te-o-po-ro'sis)* and resultant fractures result from a reduction in the quantity of bone or atrophy of skeletal tissue. Osteoporosis occurs in postmenopausal women and elderly men, resulting in bony trabeculae that are scanty and thin. Most fractures sustained by women over the age of 50 are secondary to osteoporosis.

Rheumatoid *(ru'ma-toyd)* **arthritis** is a chronic systemic disease characterized by inflammatory changes occurring throughout the body's connective tissues.

Rotator cuff tear is a traumatic injury to one or more of the muscles that make up the rotator cuff—teres minor, supraspinous, infraspinous, and subscapularis. Rotator cuff tears limit the range of motion of the shoulder.

Shoulder dislocation: Traumatic removal of humeral head from glenoid cavity. 95% of shoulder dislocations are anterior in which the humeral head is projected anterior to the glenoid cavity.

Tendonitis *(ten"deni'tis)* is an inflammatory condition of the tendon, usually resulting from a strain.

SUMMARY OF PATHOLOGIC INDICATIONS

CONDITION OR DISEASE	MOST COMMON RADIOGRAPHIC EXAM	POSSIBLE RADIOGRAPHIC APPEARANCE	MANUAL EXPOSURE FACTOR ADJUSTMENT*
AC dislocation	Bilateral erect AC joints	Widening of the AC joint space	None
AC joint separation	Bilateral, erect AC joints (with and without weights)	Asymmetric widening of AC joint compared to opposite side (>3mm)	None
Bankart lesion	AP internal rotation, scapular Y, West Point, or Grashey	Fracture involving the glenoid rim	None
Bursitis	AP and lateral shoulder	Fluid-filled joint space with possible calcification	None
Hill-Sachs defect	AP internal rotation, exaggerated external rotation, axillary lateral, or West Point	Compression fracture and possible anterior dislocation of humeral head	None
Idiopathic chronic adhesive capsulitis (frozen shoulder)	AP and lateral shoulder	Possible calcification or other joint space abnormalities	None
Impingement syndrome	Scapular Y Neer method	Subacromial spurs	None
Osteoarthritis	AP and lateral shoulder	Narrowing of the joint space	Decrease (−)
Osteoporosis (resultant fractures)	AP and lateral shoulder	Thin bony cortex	Decrease (−)
Rheumatoid arthritis	AP and lateral shoulder	Closed joint space	Decrease (−)
Rotator cuff tear	Arthrogram and/or MRI	Tear in the musculature	None
Shoulder dislocation	Scapular Y, transthoracic lateral or Garth method	Separation between humeral head and glenoid cavity	None
Tendonitis	Neer method and/or MRI	Calcified tendons	None

*Depends on stage or severity of disease or condition.

6

Survey Information

Knowing both the more common and the newer routines and special projections being performed in various parts of the country helps students understand the need for learning these projections or positions, even though they may not be performed at their facility. In this way, students are prepared to function anywhere they may choose for employment. For example, the **apical oblique** and the **inferosuperior West Point** shoulder are both about twice as frequently performed in the East and Midwest U.S. as they are in either the Western U.S. or Canada as indicated by the 2000 survey.

SUMMARY OF SURVEY RESULTS

Shoulder: The nonacute trauma routine shoulder projection continues to be the **AP** in **internal** and **external** rotation throughout the U.S. and Canada. The second most common routine nontrauma shoulder was the posterior **oblique for glenoid cavity (Grashey method),** which nearly half reported as routine and half reported as a special projection. This was consistent in all regions of the U.S. and Canada.

The **bicipital groove tangential (Fisk method)** was consistently the most common special shoulder projection.

The acute trauma shoulder routine includes the **AP neutral rotation,** with the **scapular Y lateral** a little more common than the **transthoracic lateral** throughout the U.S. and much more common in Canada. This trend of increased use of the scapular Y lateral as part of a trauma shoulder lateral routine has continued throughout the U.S. (2000—78%, 1995—62%, 1989—41%).

Clavicle: The clavicle routine continues to be both a **0° AP** and a **15°-to-30° cephalad AP.** The PA 0° and the 15°-to-30° caudal projections are routine for only 18% in U.S. and 5% in Canada.

Scapula: The most common scapula routine is the **AP** and the **erect anterior oblique lateral.**

AC joints: The **AP bilateral erect, with and without weights,** continues to be routine, with the "patient holding on to weights" method most common (57% in the United States, 62% in Canada). Surprisingly, the alternate method of tying weights to wrists with arms and hands relaxed (recommended method—see p. 204) is routine for only 9% in U.S. and 4% in Canada. (This may be the result of a misunderstanding of the survey question by respondents.)

Standard and Special Operating Procedures

Certain basic and special projections for the shoulder, clavicle, AC joints, and scapula are demonstrated and described on the following pages as suggested standard basic and special departmental routines or procedures.

BASIC PROJECTIONS

Standard or basic projections, also sometimes referred to as *routine projections* or *departmental routines,* are those projections commonly taken on average patients who are helpful and can cooperate in performing the procedure.

SPECIAL PROJECTIONS

Special projections are those more common projections taken as extra or additional projections to better demonstrate certain pathologic conditions or specific body parts.

BASIC AND SPECIAL PROJECTIONS

AP PROJECTION—EXTERNAL ROTATION: SHOULDER (NONTRAUMA)

AP Proximal Humerus

Warning: Do **NOT** attempt to rotate arm if fracture or dislocation is suspected (see trauma routine).

Shoulder (nontrauma)
BASIC
- AP external rotation (AP)
- **AP internal rotation (lateral)**

Pathology Demonstrated

Fractures and/or dislocations of the proximal humerus and shoulder girdle are demonstrated. This projection may demonstrate calcium deposits in the muscles, tendons, or bursal structures. Some pathologies, such as osteoporosis and osteoarthritis, may also be demonstrated.

Technical Factors

- IR size—24 × 30 cm (10 × 12 inches), crosswise (or lengthwise to show more of humerus if injury includes proximal half of humerus)
- Moving or stationary grid
- 70 ± 5 kV range
- Technique and dose:

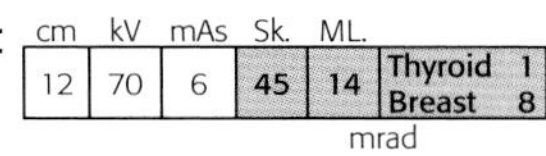

cm	kV	mAs	Sk.	ML.	mrad
12	70	6	45	14	Thyroid 1 Breast 8

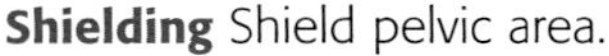

Shielding Shield pelvic area.

Patient Position Take radiograph with the patient in an erect or supine position. (The erect position is usually less painful for patient, if condition allows.) Rotate body slightly toward affected side if necessary to place shoulder in contact with IR or tabletop.

Part Position
- Position patient to center scapulohumeral joint to center of IR.
- Abduct extended arm slightly; then **externally rotate arm** (supinate hand) until epicondyles of distal humerus are **parallel** to IR.

Central Ray
- CR **perpendicular** to IR, directed to **1 inch (2.5 cm) inferior to coracoid process** (See Note below.)
- Minimum SID of 40 inches (100 cm)

Collimation Collimate on four sides, with lateral and upper borders adjusted to soft-tissue margins.

Respiration Suspend respiration during exposure.

Note: The coracoid process may be difficult to palpate directly on most patients, but it can be approximated by knowing that it is about $^{3}/_{4}$ inches (2 cm) inferior to the lateral portion of the more readily palpated clavicle.

Radiographic Criteria

Structures Shown: • AP projection of proximal humerus and lateral two-thirds of the clavicle and upper scapula are shown, including the relationship of the humeral head to the glenoid cavity.

Position: • Full external rotation is evidenced by the **greater tubercle visualized** in **full profile** on the lateral aspect of the proximal humerus. Lesser tubercle is superimposed over humeral head.

Collimation and CR: • Collimation should be visible on four sides to the area of the affected shoulder. • CR and center of the collimation field should be at scapulohumeral joint.

Exposure Criteria: • Optimum density and contrast with no motion will demonstrate clear, sharp bony trabecular markings with soft-tissue detail visible for possible calcium deposits.

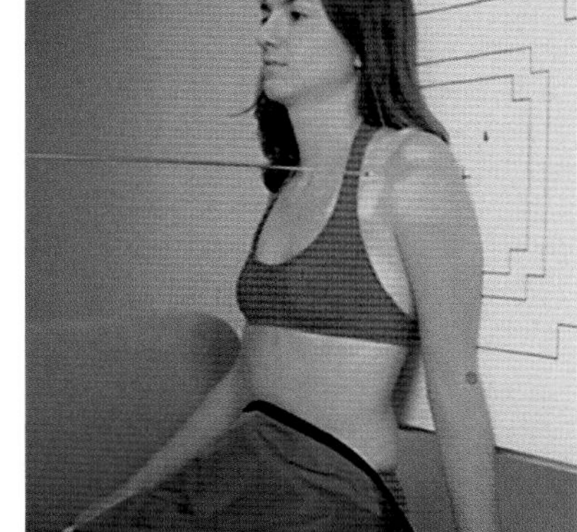

Fig. 6-22. External rotation—AP.

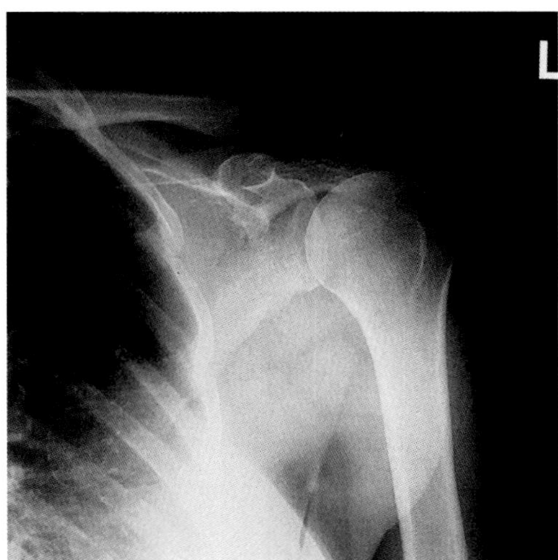

Fig. 6-23. External rotation.

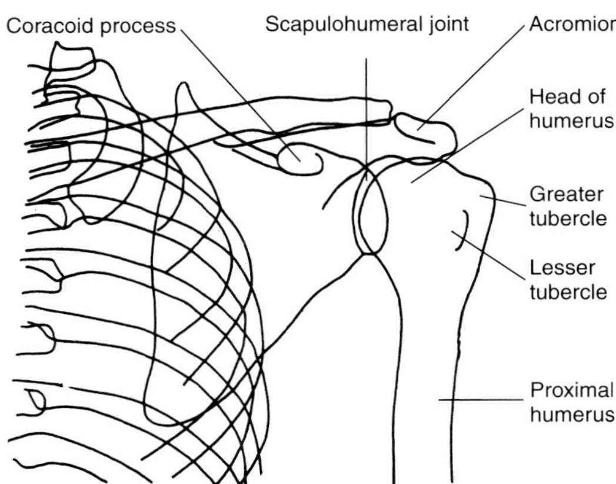

Fig. 6-24. External rotation.

6

AP PROJECTION—INTERNAL ROTATION: SHOULDER (NONTRAUMA)

Lateral Proximal Humerus

Warning: Do **NOT** attempt to rotate arm if fracture or dislocation is suspected (see trauma routine).

Shoulder (nontrauma)
BASIC
• AP external rotation (AP)
• AP internal rotation (lateral)

Pathology Demonstrated
Fractures and/or dislocations of the proximal humerus and the shoulder girdle may demonstrate calcium deposits in the muscles, tendons, or bursal structures. Some pathology, such as osteoporosis, osteoarthritis, and bony tumors, may also be demonstrated.

Technical Factors

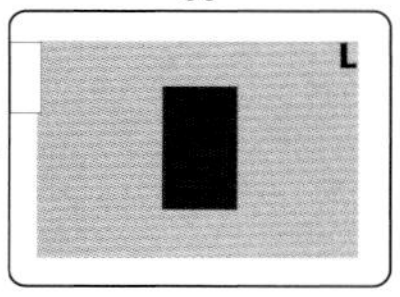

- IR size—24 × 30 cm (10 × 12 inches), crosswise (or lengthwise to show more of humerus if injury includes proximal half of humerus)
- Moving or stationary grid
- 70 ± 5 kV range
- Technique and dose:

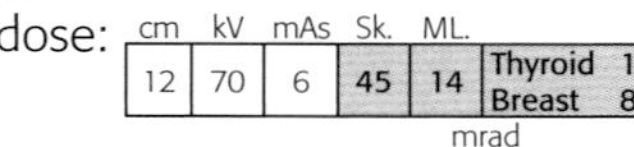
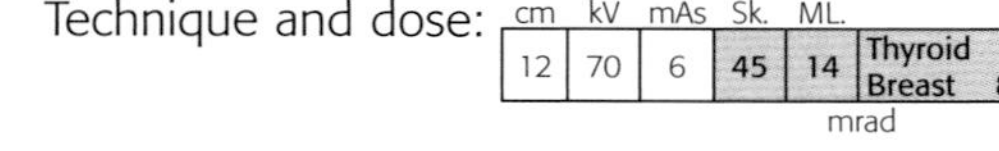

cm	kV	mAs	Sk.	ML.	
12	70	6	45	14	Thyroid 1 Breast 8

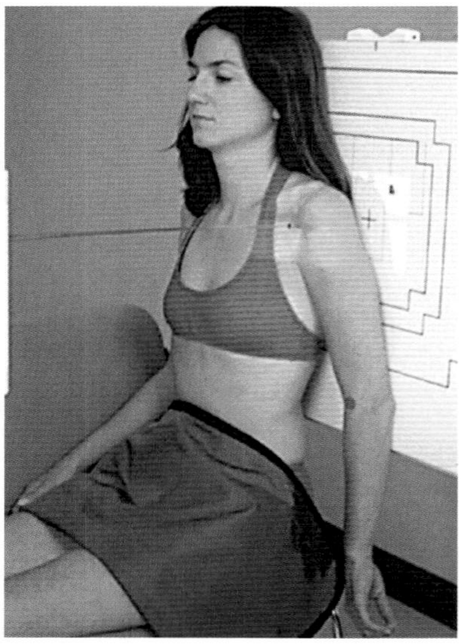

mrad

30

24

L

Fig. 6-25. Internal rotation—lateral.

Shielding Shield pelvic area.

Patient Position Take radiograph with the patient in an erect or supine position. (The erect position is usually less painful for patient, if condition allows.) Rotate body slightly toward affected side, if necessary, to place shoulder in contact with IR or tabletop.

Part Position

- Position patient to center scapulohumeral joint to center of IR.
- Abduct extended arm slightly; then **internally rotate arm** (pronate hand) until epicondyles of distal humerus are **perpendicular** to IR.

Central Ray

- CR perpendicular to IR, directed to **1 inch (2.5 cm) inferior to coracoid process** (See Note on preceding page.)
- Minimum SID of 40 inches (100 cm)

Collimation Collimate on four sides, with lateral and upper borders adjusted to soft-tissue margins.

Respiration Suspend respiration during exposure.

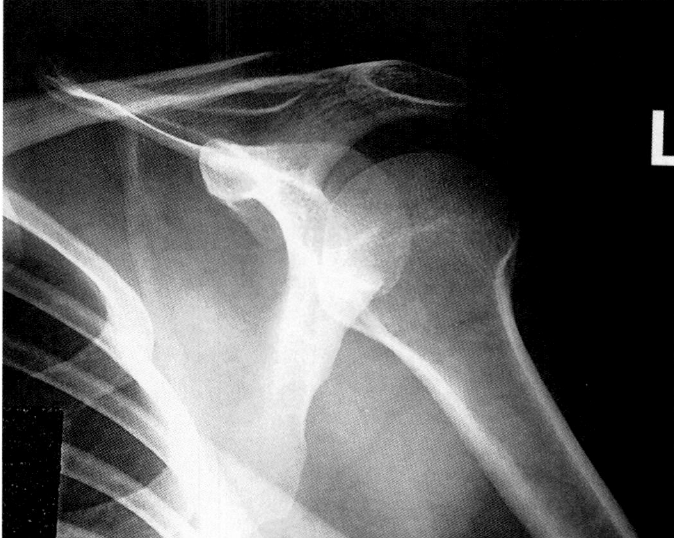

Fig. 6-26. Internal rotation—lateral.

Radiographic Criteria

Structures Shown: • Lateral view of proximal humerus and lateral two-thirds of the clavicle and upper scapula are shown, including the relationship of the humeral head to the glenoid cavity.

Position: • Full external rotation is evidenced by the **lesser tubercle visualized in full profile** on the medial aspect of the humeral head. • An outline of the greater tubercle should be visualized superimposed over the humeral head.

Collimation and CR: • Collimation should be visible on four sides to area of affected shoulder. • CR and center of the collimation field should be at scapulohumeral joint.

Exposure Criteria: • Optimal density and contrast with no motion will demonstrate clear, sharp bony trabecular markings with soft-tissue detail visible for possible calcium deposits.

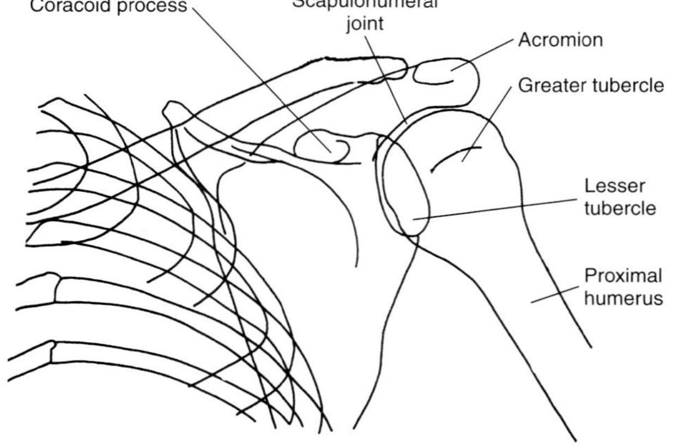

Fig. 6-27. Internal rotation—lateral.

INFEROSUPERIOR AXIAL PROJECTION: SHOULDER (NONTRAUMA)

Lawrence Method

Warning: Do **NOT** attempt to rotate arm or force abduction if fracture or dislocation is suspected.

Shoulder (nontrauma)
SPECIAL
- **Inferosuperior axial (Lawrence method)**

Pathology Demonstrated

Fractures and/or dislocations of the proximal humerus are shown. Osteoporosis, osteoarthritis, and the Hill-Sachs defect with exaggerated rotation may also be demonstrated.

Technical Factors

- IR size—18 × 24 cm (8 × 10 inches), crosswise.
- Stationary grid (CR to centerline of grid, crosswise to prevent grid cutoff because of CR angle)
- 70 ± 5 kV range
- Technique and dose:

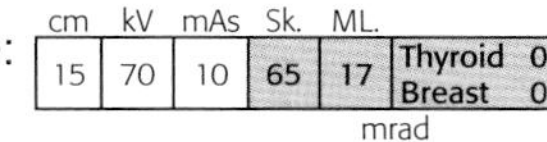

cm	kV	mAs	Sk.	ML.	
15	70	10	65	17	Thyroid 0 Breast 0
			mrad		

Shielding Place lead shield over pelvis and radiosensitive regions.

Patient Position Position patient supine with shoulder raised about 2 inches (5 cm) from tabletop by placing support under arm and shoulder to place body part near center of IR.

Part Position

- Move patient toward the front edge of tabletop and place a cart or other arm support against front edge of table to support abducted arm.
- Rotate head toward opposite side, place vertical cassette on table as close to neck as possible, and support with sand bags.
- Abduct arm 90° from body if possible; keep in **external rotation,** palm up, with support under arm and hand.

Central Ray

- Direct CR **medially 25° to 30°**, centered **horizontally to axilla and humeral head.** If abduction of arm is less than 90°, the CR medial angle should also be decreased to 15° to 20° if possible.
- Minimum SID is 40 inches (100 cm).

Collimation Collimate closely on four sides.

Respiration Suspend respiration during exposure.

An **alternative position** is exaggerated **external** rotation.* An anterior dislocation of the humeral head may result in a compression fracture of the articular surface of the humeral head, called the *Hills-Sachs defect.* This is best demonstrated with exaggerated external rotation, wherein the thumb is pointed down and posteriorly about 45°.

Radiographic Criteria

Structures Shown: • Lateral view of proximal humerus in relationship to the scapulohumeral cavity is shown. • Coracoid process of scapula and lesser tubercle of humerus will be seen in profile. • The spine of the scapula will be seen on edge below the scapulohumeral joint.

Position: • Arm is seen to be abducted about 90° from the body. • The superior and inferior borders of the glenoid cavity should be directly superimposed, indicating correct CR angle.

Collimation and CR: • Collimation should be visible on four sides to the affected shoulder. • CR and center of the collimation field should be at the axilla and humeral head.

Exposure Criteria: • Optimal density and contrast with no motion will demonstrate clear, sharp bony trabecular markings. • The bony margins of the acromion and distal clavicle will be visible through the humeral head.

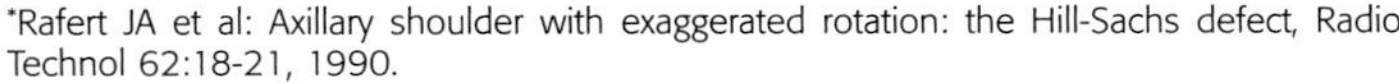

*Rafert JA et al: Axillary shoulder with exaggerated rotation: the Hill-Sachs defect, Radiol Technol 62:18-21, 1990.

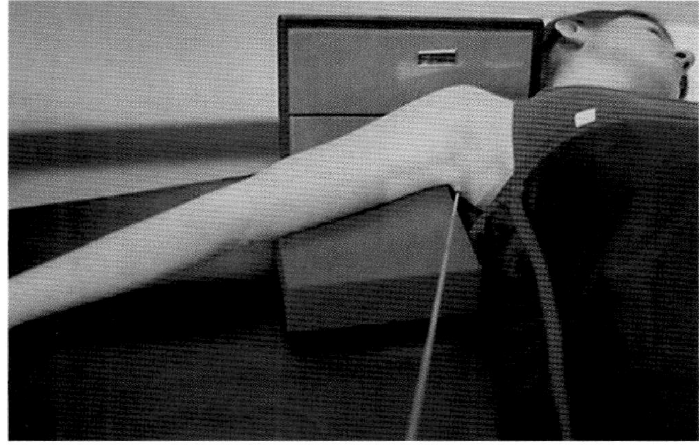

Fig. 6-28. Inferosuperior axial.

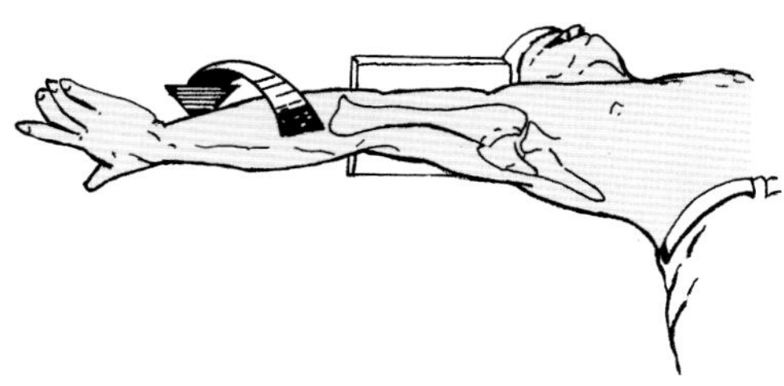

Fig. 6-29. Alternate position—exaggerated rotation.

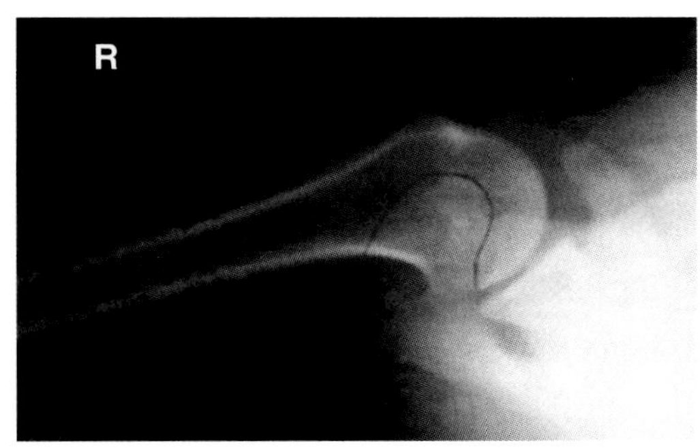

Fig. 6-30. Inferosuperior axiolateral.

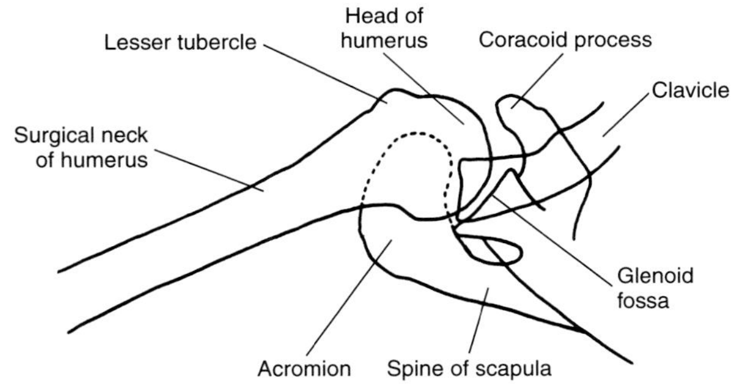

Fig. 6-31. Inferosuperior axiolateral.

INFEROSUPERIOR AXIAL PROJECTION: SHOULDER (NONTRAUMA)

West Point Method

Warning: Do **NOT** attempt to rotate arm or force full abduction if fracture or dislocation is suspected.

Shoulder (nontrauma)
Special
• **Inferosuperior axial (Lawrence method)**
• Inferosuperior axial (West Point method)

Pathology Demonstrated

Performed for specific pathology such as Hill-Sachs defects and Bankart fractures.

Technical Factors

- IR size—18 × 24 cm (8 × 10 inches), crosswise
- Vertical cassette holder (grid cannot be used because of double CR angle)
- 70 ± 5 kV range
- Technique and dose:

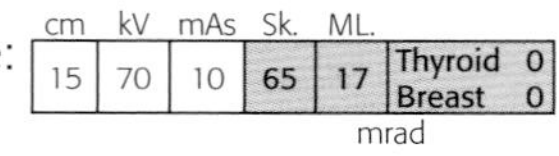

cm	kV	mAs	Sk.	ML.	
15	70	10	65	17	Thyroid 0 Breast 0
			mrad		

24

18 R

Shielding Shield pelvic area.

Patient Position Position patient prone on the table with the affected shoulder elevated approximately 3 inches (7.5 cm) from tabletop.

Part Position

- Abduct affected arm 90°, with elbow flexed to allow forearm to hang freely over the side of the table.
- Rotate head away from affected side and place IR in vertical cassette holder and secure against the superior surface of the shoulder.

Central Ray

- CR directed **25° anterior** (**down** from horizontal) and **25° medial,** passing through the **midscapulohumeral joint**
- Minimum SID of 40 inches (100 cm)

Collimation Collimate on four sides to area of affected shoulder.

Respiration Suspend respiration during exposure.

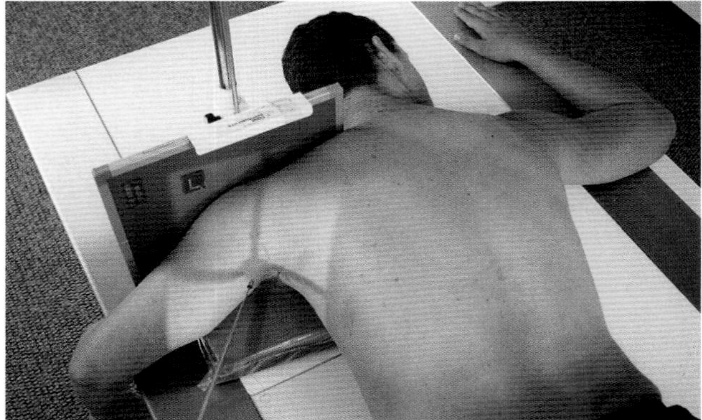

Fig. 6-32. Inferosuperior axial—West Point method.

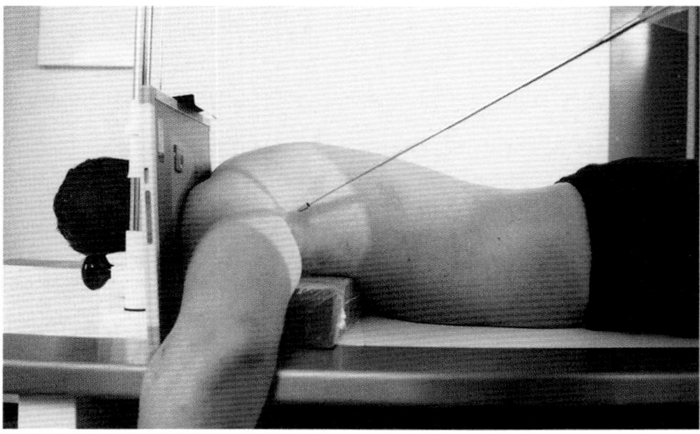

Fig. 6-33. Inferosuperior axial—West Point method.

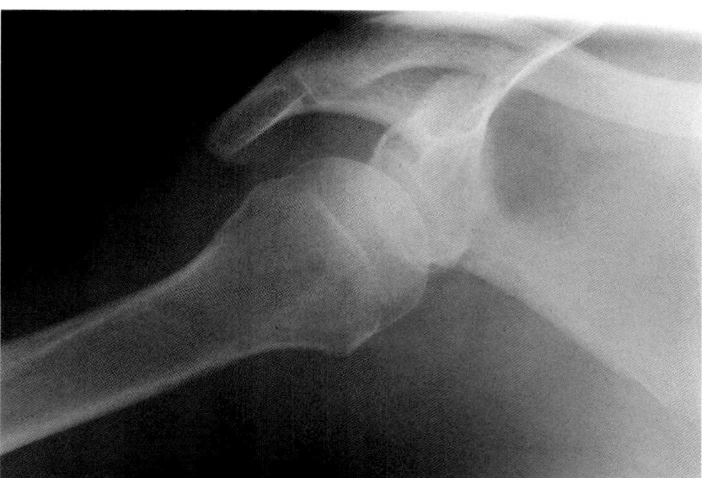

Fig. 6-34. Inferosuperior axial—West Point method.

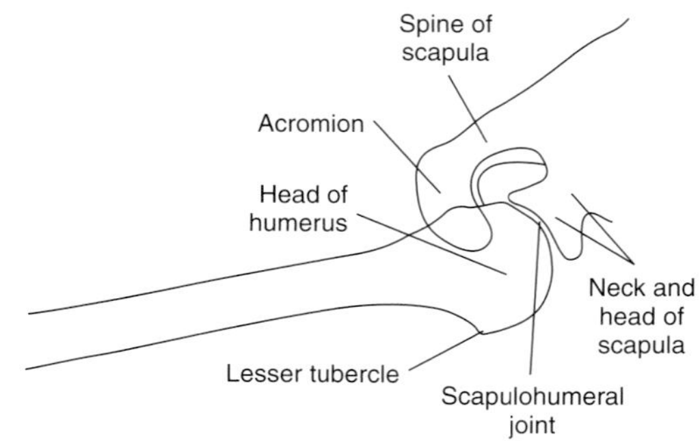

Fig. 6-35. Inferosuperior axial—West Point method.

Radiographic Criteria

Structures Shown: • An axial view of the shoulder girdle is shown. • The anteroinferior aspect of glenoid rim is well demonstrated. • The humeral head is seen free of coracoid superimposition.

Position: • With elbow flexed and forearm hanging down, the patient's arm should be in natural internal rotation. • Lesser tubercle will be seen in profile anteriorly.

Collimation and CR: • Collimation should be visible on four sides to area of affected shoulder. • CR and center of the collimation field should be at the glenohumeral joint.

Exposure Criteria: • Optimal density and contrast with no motion will demonstrate soft tissue and clear, sharp bony trabecular markings.

POSTERIOR OBLIQUE POSITION—GLENOID CAVITY: SHOULDER (NONTRAUMA)

Grashey Method

Shoulder (nontrauma)
SPECIAL
- Inferosuperior axial (Lawrence method)
- Inferosuperior axial (West Point method)
- Posterior oblique (Grashey method)

Pathology Demonstrated

Fractures and/or dislocations of the proximal humerus and fractures of the glenoid labrum or brim are demonstrated; may demonstrate a Bankart fracture and the integrity of the scapulohumeral joint; may also demonstrate certain pathologies, such as osteoporosis and osteoarthritis.

Technical Factors

24
18 R

- IR size—18 × 24 cm (8 × 10 inches), crosswise
- Moving or stationary grid
- 75 ± 5 kV range
- Technique and dose:

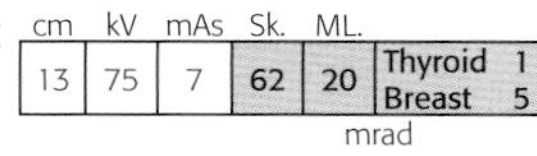

cm	kV	mAs	Sk.	ML.	
13	75	7	62	20	Thyroid 1 Breast 5
				mrad	

Shielding Place gonadal shielding over pelvic area.

Patient Position Take radiograph with the patient in an erect or supine position. (The erect position is usually less painful for patient, if condition allows.)

Part Position

- Rotate body **35° to 45°** toward affected side (see Note below). If the radiograph is done with the patient in the supine position, place supports under elevated shoulder and hip to maintain this position.
- Center midscapulohumeral joint to CR and to center of IR.
- Adjust cassette so that top of IR is about 2 inches (5 cm) above shoulder and side of IR is about 2 inches (5 cm) from lateral border of humerus.
- Abduct arm slightly with arm in neutral rotation.

Central Ray

- CR **perpendicular** to IR, **centered to scapulohumeral joint,** which is approximately **2 inches (5 cm) inferior and medial to superolateral border** of shoulder
- Minimum SID of 40 inches (100 cm)

Collimation Collimate so that upper and lateral borders of the light field are to the soft-tissue margins.

Respiration Suspend respiration during exposure.

Note: The degree of rotation varies depending on how flat- or round-shouldered the patient is. Having a rounded or curved shoulder and back requires more rotation to place body of scapula parallel to IR.

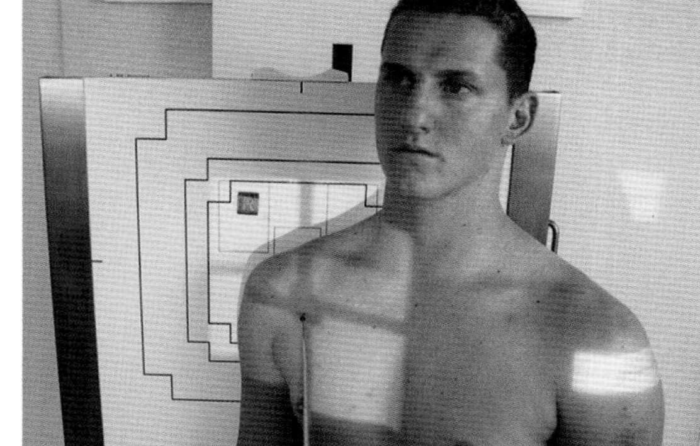

Fig. 6-36. Posterior oblique—RPO.

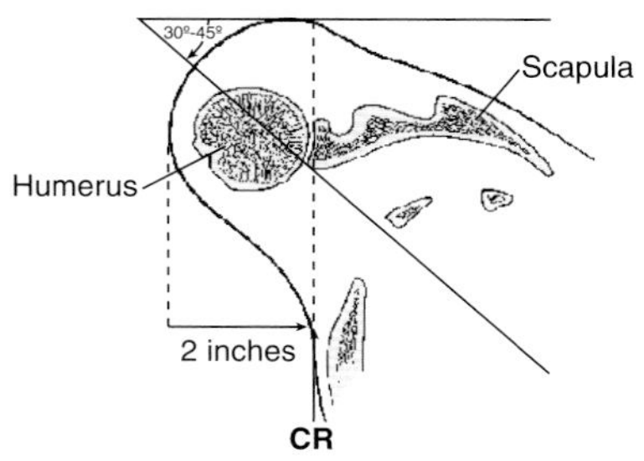

Fig. 6-37. Top view of posterior oblique.

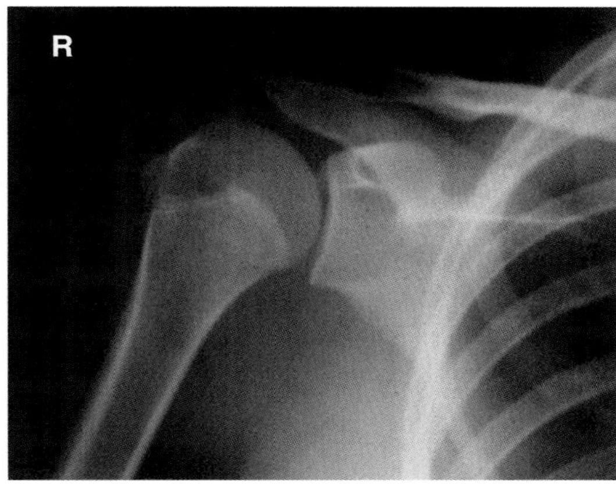

Fig. 6-38. Posterior oblique.

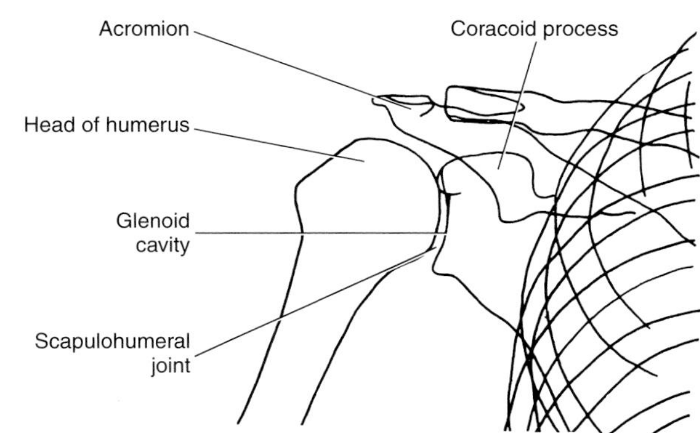

Fig. 6-39. Posterior oblique.

Radiographic Criteria

Structures Shown: • Glenoid cavity should be seen in profile without superimposition of humeral head.

Position: • The scapulohumeral joint space should be open. Anterior and posterior rims of glenoid cavity are superimposed.

Collimation and CR: • Collimation should be visible on four sides to area of affected shoulder. • CR and center of the collimation field should be at the midglenohumeral joint.

Exposure Criteria: • Optimal density and contrast with no motion will visualize soft-tissue margins and clear, sharp bony trabecular markings. • Soft-tissue detail of the joint space and axilla should be visualized.

TANGENTIAL PROJECTION—INTERTUBERCULAR (BICIPITAL) GROOVE: SHOULDER (NONTRAUMA)

Fisk Method

Shoulder (nontrauma)
SPECIAL
- Inferosuperior axial (Lawrence method)
- Inferosuperior axial (West Point method)
- Posterior oblique (Grashey method)
- Tangential projection (Fisk method)

Pathology Demonstrated

Pathologies of the intertubercular groove, such as bony projections of the humeral tubercles, are demonstrated.

Technical Factors

- IR size—18 × 24 cm (8 × 10 inches), crosswise
- Detail screen cassette, nongrid
- 60 ± 5 kV range
- Technique and dose:

	cm	kV	mAs	Sk.	ML.	Thyroid	Breast
Erect	–	65	4	31	10	0	0
Supine	–	65	3	14	5	0	0

mrad

24
18
R

Shielding Place lead shield over pelvic area.

Patient Position and Central Ray

Erect (Fisk method)

- Patient standing, leaning over end of table with elbow flexed and posterior surface of forearm resting on table, hand supinated holding cassette, head turned away from affected side (lead shield placed between back of IR and forearm reduces backscatter to IR)
- Patient leaning forward slightly to place humerus **10° to 15°** from vertical
- CR perpendicular to IR, directed to groove area at midanterior margin of humeral head (groove can be located by careful palpation)

Supine

- Patient supine, arm at side, hand supinated
- Vertical cassette placed on table against top of shoulder and against neck (head turned away from affected side)
- CR **10° to 15° posterior from horizontal,** directed to groove at midanterior margin of humeral head
- Minimum SID of 40 inches (100 cm)

Collimation Collimate closely on four sides to area of anterior humeral head.

Respiration Suspend respiration during exposure.

Radiographic Criteria

Structures Shown: • The anterior margin of the humeral head is seen in profile. • The humeral tubercles and intertubercular groove are seen in profile.

Position: • A correct CR angle of 10° to 15° to the long axis of the humerus will demonstrate the intertubercular groove and the tubercles in profile without superimposition of acromion process.

Collimation and CR: • Collimation should be visible on four sides to area of affected shoulder. • CR and center of the collimation field should be at the intertubercular groove.

Exposure Criteria: • Optimal density and contrast with no motion will visualize sharp borders and sharp bony trabecular markings and will demonstrate the complete intertubercular groove seen through soft tissue without excessive density or burnout.

Fig. 6-40. Erect superoinferior tangential projection.

Fig. 6-41. Supine inferosuperior tangential projection.

Fig. 6-42. Erect tangential.

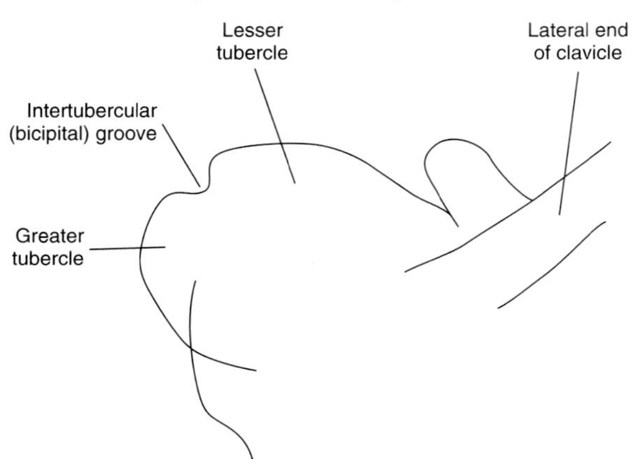

Fig. 6-43. Tangential.

AP PROJECTION—NEUTRAL ROTATION: SHOULDER (TRAUMA)

Warning: Do **NOT** attempt to rotate arm if fracture or dislocation is suspected; take as is in neutral rotation, which generally places humerus in an oblique position.

Shoulder (trauma)
BASIC
• AP (neutral rotation)
• Transthoracic lateral or
• Scapular Y lateral

Pathology Demonstrated
Fractures and/or dislocations of the proximal humerus and the shoulder girdle are demonstrated. Calcium deposits in the muscles, tendons, or bursal structures may be demonstrated. Some pathologies, such as osteoporosis and osteoarthritis, may also be demonstrated.

Technical Factors
- IR size—24 × 30 cm (10 × 12 inches), crosswise (or lengthwise to show more of humerus if injury includes proximal half of humerus)
- Moving or stationary grid
- 70 ± 5 kV range
- Technique and dose:

30

24 R

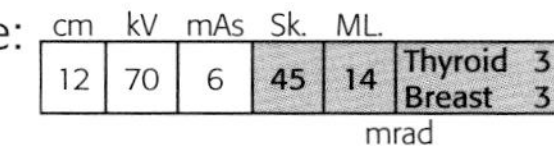

cm	kV	mAs	Sk.	ML.	mrad
12	70	6	45	14	Thyroid 3
					Breast 3

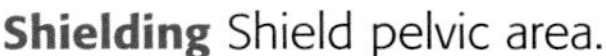

Shielding Shield pelvic area.

Patient Position Take radiograph with the patient in an erect or supine position. (The erect position is usually less painful for patient if condition allows.) Rotate body slightly toward affected side if necessary to place shoulder in contact with IR or tabletop.

Part Position
- Position patient to center scapulohumeral joint to IR.
- Place patient's arm at side in "as is" neutral rotation. (Epicondyles are generally approximately 45° to plane of IR.)

Central Ray
- CR **perpendicular** to IR, directed to **midscapulohumeral joint,** which is approximately ¾ inches (2 cm) inferior and slightly lateral to the coracoid process (See Note below.)
- Minimum SID of 40 inches (100 cm)

Collimation Collimate on four sides, with lateral and upper borders adjusted to soft-tissue margins.

Respiration Suspend respiration during exposure.

Note: The coracoid process may be difficult to palpate directly on most patients, but it can be approximated by knowing that it is about ¾ inches (2 cm) inferior to the lateral portion of the readily palpated clavicle. Also, the scapulohumeral joint is generally found at the base or pit of the concave-like depression just medial to the humeral head.

Radiographic Criteria

Structures Shown: • The proximal one-third of the humerus, upper scapula, and lateral two-thirds of the clavicle are shown, including the relationship of the humeral head to the glenoid cavity.

Position: • With neutral rotation both the greater and lesser tubercles will be mostly superimposed by humeral head.

Collimation and CR: • Collimation should be visible on four sides to the affected shoulder. • CR and center of the collimation field should be at the midscapulohumeral joint.

Exposure Criteria: • Optimal density and contrast with no motion will visualize sharp bony trabecular markings. • The outline of the medial aspect of the humeral head will be visible through the glenoid cavity and soft-tissue detail should be visible to show possible calcium deposits.

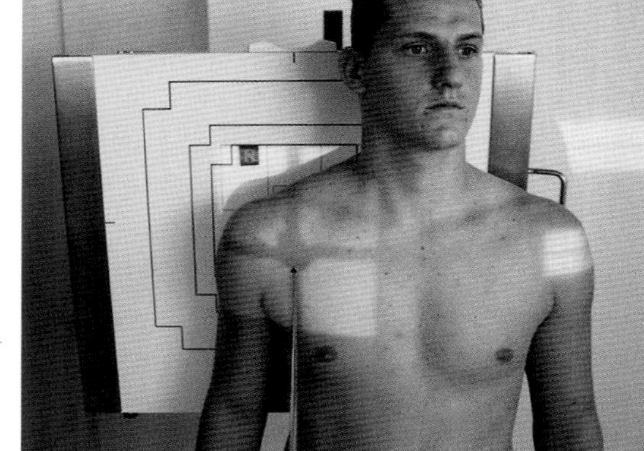

Fig. 6-44. AP erect—neutral rotation.

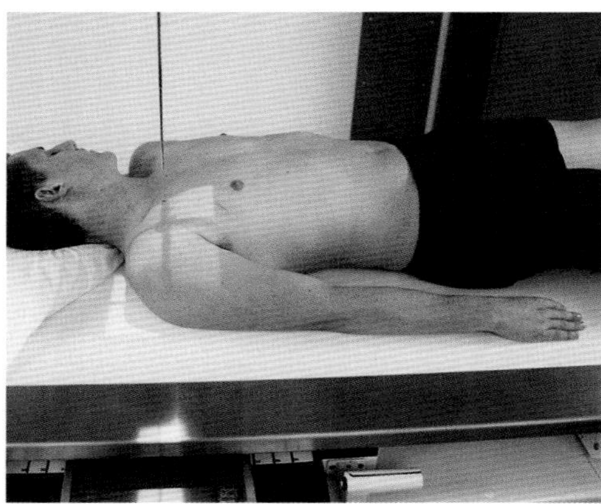

Fig. 6-45. AP supine—neutral rotation.

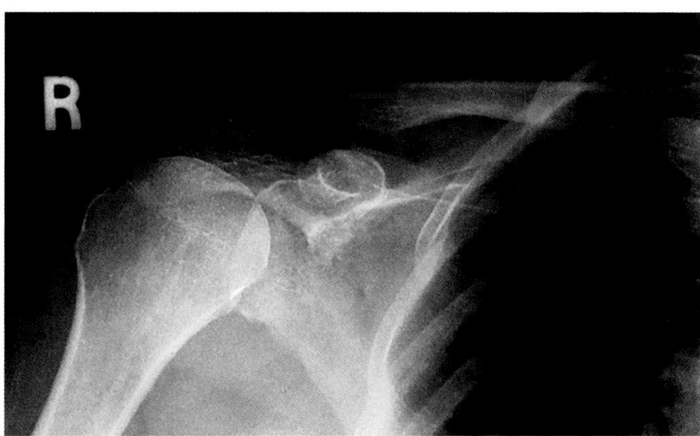

Fig. 6-46. AP projection—neutral rotation.

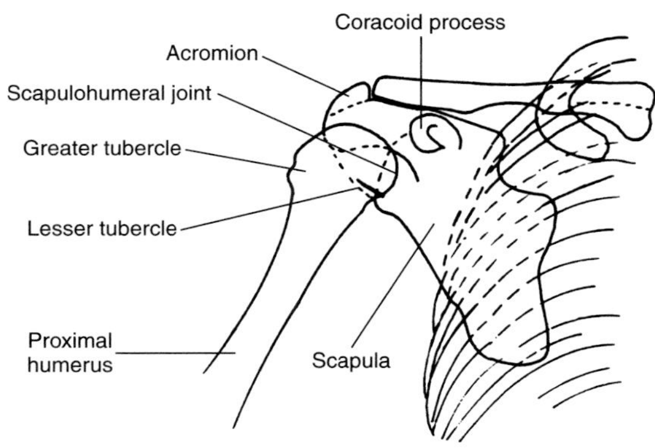

Fig. 6-47. AP projection—neutral rotation.

TRANSTHORACIC LATERAL PROJECTION: SHOULDER (TRAUMA)

Lawrence Method

Shoulder (trauma)
BASIC
- AP (neutral rotation)
- Transthoracic lateral

or

- Scapular Y lateral

Pathology Demonstrated
Fractures and/or dislocation of the proximal humerus are demonstrated.

Technical Factors
- IR size—24 × 30 cm (10 × 12 inches), lengthwise
- Moving or stationary grid, vertical, CR to centerline
- 75 ± 5 kV range
- Minimum of 3 seconds exposure time with breathing technique (4 or 5 seconds is desirable)
- Technique and dose:

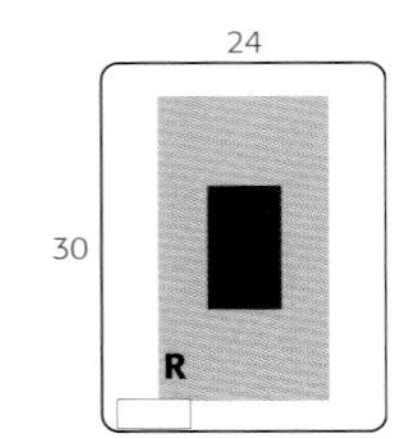

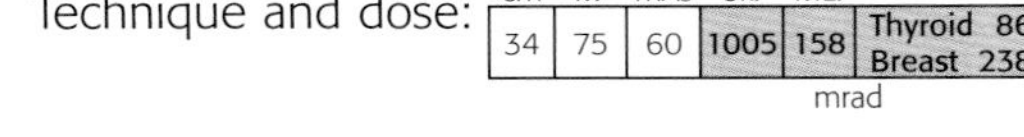

cm	kV	mAs	Sk.	ML.	mrad
34	75	60	1005	158	Thyroid 86 Breast 238

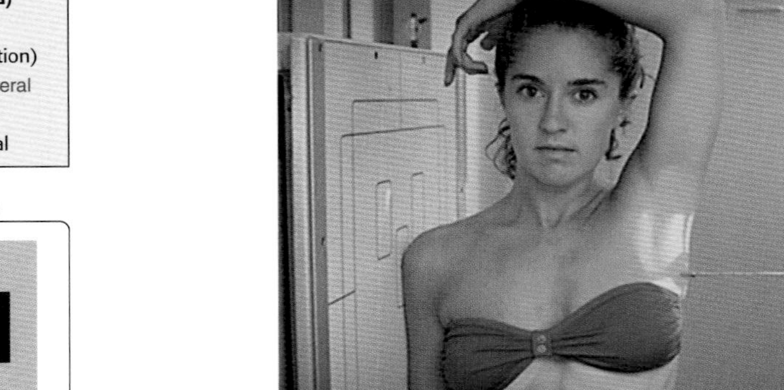

Fig. 6-48. Erect transthoracic lateral projection (R lateral).

Shielding Shield pelvic area.

Patient Position Take radiograph with the patient in an erect or supine position. (The erect position is preferred, which may also be more comfortable for patient.) Place patient in lateral position with side of interest against IR. With patient supine, place grid lines **vertically** and **center CR to centerline** to prevent grid cutoff.

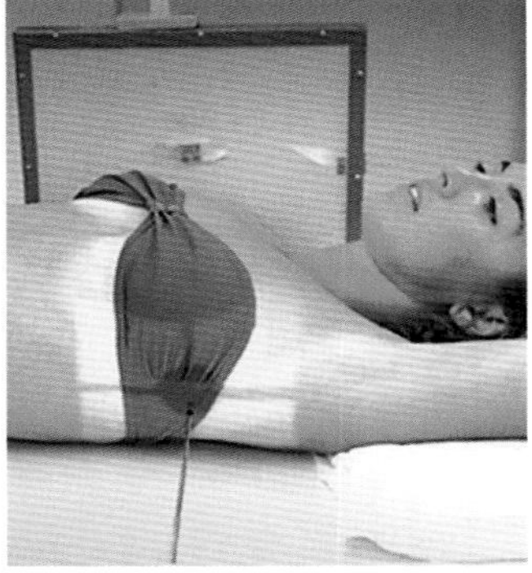

Fig. 6-49. Supine transthoracic lateral projection (R lateral).

Part Position
- Place affected arm at patient's side in **neutral rotation;** drop shoulder if possible.
- Raise opposite arm and place hand over top of head; elevate shoulder as much as possible to prevent superimposing affected shoulder.
- Center surgical neck and center of IR to CR as projected through thorax.
- Ensure that thorax is in a true lateral position, or with slight anterior rotation of unaffected shoulder to minimize superimposition of humerus by thoracic vertebrae.

Central Ray
- CR perpendicular to IR, directed through thorax to **surgical neck** (See Note below.)
- Minimum SID of 40 inches (100 cm)

Collimation Collimate on four sides to area of interest.

Respiration **Breathing technique is preferred** if patient can cooperate. Patient should be asked to gently breathe short, shallow breaths without moving affected arm or shoulder. (This will best visualize proximal humerus by blurring out ribs and lung structures.)

Note: If patient is in too much pain to drop injured shoulder and elevate uninjured arm and shoulder high enough to prevent superimposition of shoulders, **angle CR 10° to 15° cephalad.**

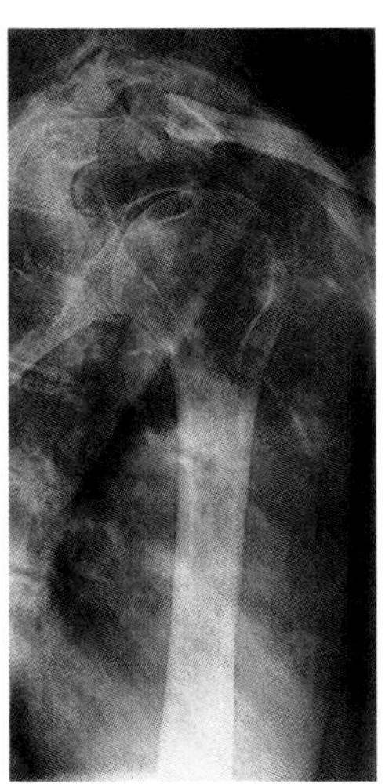

Fig. 6-50. Transthoracic lateral.

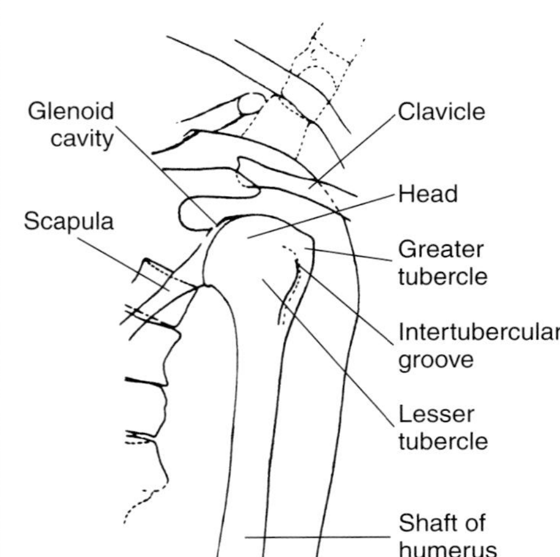

Fig. 6-51. Transthoracic lateral.

Radiographic Criteria

Structures Shown: • Lateral view of the proximal half of the humerus and glenohumeral joint should be visualized through the thorax without superimposition of the opposite shoulder.

Position: • The outline of the shaft of the proximal humerus should be clearly visualized anterior to the thoracic vertebrae. • The relationship of the humeral head and the glenoid cavity should be demonstrated.

Collimation and CR: • Collimation should be visible on four sides to area of affected shoulder. • CR and center of collimation field should be at the surgical neck of the affected humerus.

Exposure Criteria: • Optimal density and contrast will demonstrate the entire outline of the humeral head and the proximal half of the humerus. • Overlying ribs and lung markings should appear blurred because of breathing technique, but bony outlines of the humerus should appear sharp, indicating no motion of the arm during the exposure.

SCAPULAR Y LATERAL—ANTERIOR OBLIQUE POSITION: SHOULDER (TRAUMA)

Warning: Do NOT attempt to rotate arm if fracture or dislocation is suspected.

Pathology Demonstrated

Fractures and/or dislocations of the proximal humerus and scapula are demonstrated. The humeral head will be demonstrated inferior to the coracoid process with anterior dislocations, and for less common posterior dislocations the humeral head will be demonstrated inferior to the acromion process.

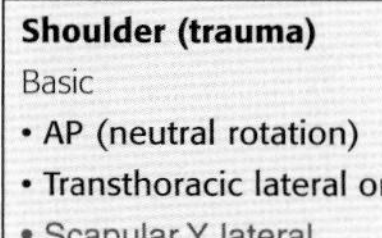

Shoulder (trauma)
Basic
- AP (neutral rotation)
- Transthoracic lateral or
- Scapular Y lateral

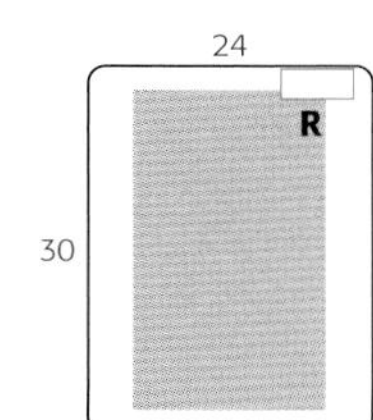

Technical Factors

- IR size—24 × 30 cm (10 × 12 inches), lengthwise
- Moving or stationary grid
- AEC not recommended
- Digital IR—very close collimation required
- 75 ± 5 kV range
- Technique and dose:

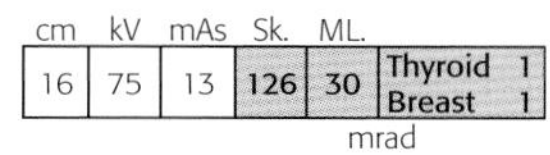

cm	kV	mAs	Sk.	ML.	
16	75	13	126	30	Thyroid 1 Breast 1

mrad

Shielding Shield pelvic area.

Patient Position Take radiograph with the patient in an erect or recumbent position. (The erect position is usually more comfortable for patient.)

Part Position

- Rotate into an anterior oblique position as for a lateral scapula with patient facing the IR. Average patient will be in a 45° to 60° anterior oblique position. Palpate scapular borders to determine correct rotation for a true lateral position of scapula.
- Center scapulohumeral joint to CR and to center of IR.
- Abduct arm slightly if possible so as to not superimpose proximal humerus over ribs; do **not** attempt to rotate arm.

Central Ray

- CR perpendicular to IR, directed to the **scapulohumeral joint** (2 or 2½ inches (5 or 6 cm) below top of shoulder) (See Note below.)
- Minimum SID of 40 inches (100 cm)

Collimation Collimate on four sides to area of interest.

Respiration Suspend respiration during exposure.

Note: If patient's condition requires it, this scapular Y lateral may be taken recumbent in the opposite posterior oblique position with injured shoulder elevated. (See p. 207, for lateral scapula recumbent.)

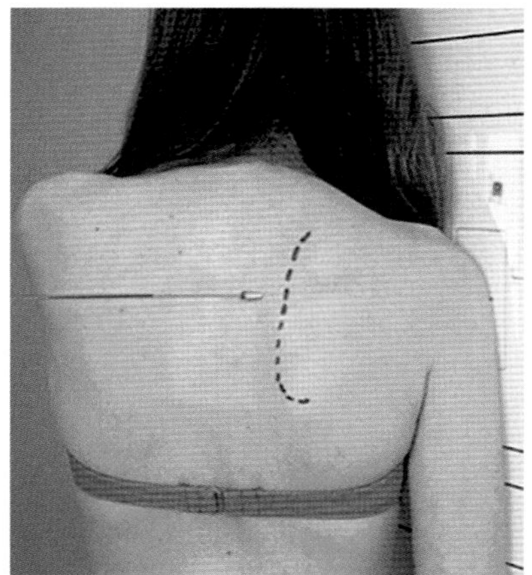

Fig. 6-52. Scapular Y lateral with CR perpendicular.

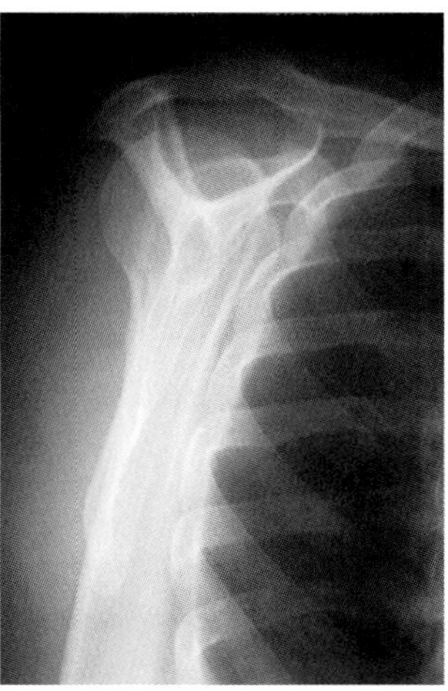

Fig. 6-53. Scapular Y lateral with no dislocation.

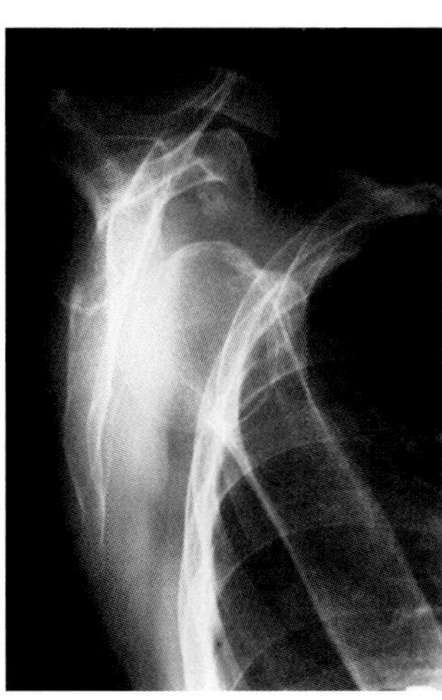

Fig. 6-54. Scapular Y lateral with anterior dislocation.

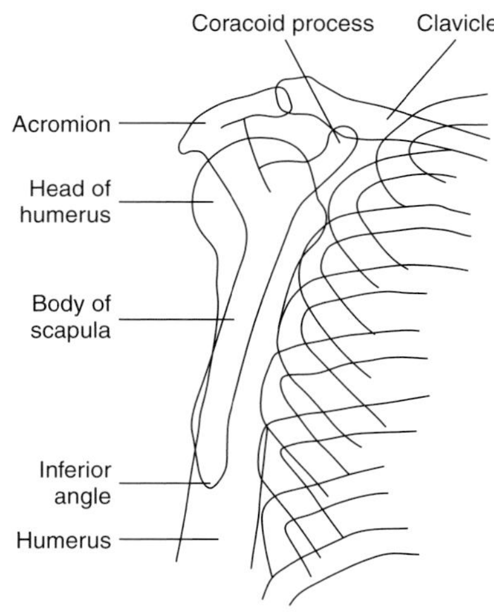

Fig. 6-55. Scapular Y lateral.

Radiographic Criteria

Structures Shown: • A true lateral view of the scapula, proximal humerus, and scapulohumeral joint.

Position: • The thin body of the scapula should be seen on end without rib superimposition. • The acromion and coracoid processes should appear as nearly symmetric upper limbs of the Y. • The humeral head should appear superimposed over the base of the Y if the humerus is not dislocated.

Collimation and CR: • Collimation is visible on four sides to area of affected shoulder. • CR and center of the collimation field should be at the humeral head and surgical neck region.

Exposure Criteria: • Optimal density and contrast with no motion will visualize sharp bony borders and the outline of body of scapula through the proximal humerus.

TANGENTIAL PROJECTION—SUPRASPINATUS OUTLET: SHOULDER (TRAUMA)

Neer Method

6

Warning: Do **NOT** attempt to rotate arm if fracture or dislocation is suspected.

Pathology Demonstrated

Fractures and/or dislocations of the proximal humerus and scapula are visualized. Specifically demonstrates the **coracoacromial arch** for the **supraspinatus outlet** region for possible **shoulder impingement.***†

Shoulder (trauma)
SPECIAL
• Supraspinatus outlet (Neer method)

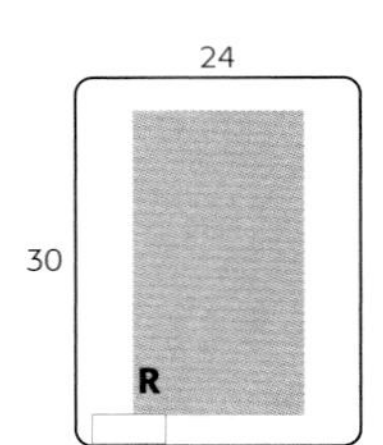

Technical Factors

- IR size—24 × 30 cm (10 × 12 inches), lengthwise
- Moving or stationary grid
- 75 ± 5 kV range
- AEC not recommended
- Technique and dose:

cm	kV	mAs	Sk.	ML.	
16	75	13	126	30	Thyroid 1 Breast 1
			mrad		

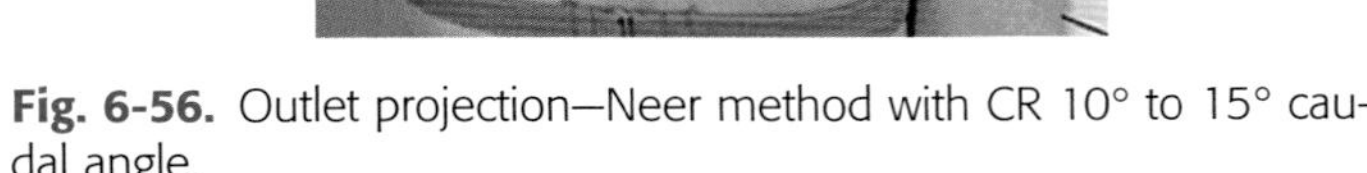

Fig. 6-56. Outlet projection—Neer method with CR 10° to 15° caudal angle.

Shielding Shield pelvic area.

Patient Position Take radiograph with the patient in an erect or recumbent position. (The erect position is usually more comfortable for patient.)

Part Position

- With patient facing the IR, rotate into an anterior oblique position as for a lateral scapula.
- Average patient will be in a 45° to 60° anterior oblique position. Palpate scapular borders to determine correct rotation.
- Center scapulohumeral joint to CR and to center of IR.
- Abduct arm slightly so as not to superimpose proximal humerus over ribs; do not attempt to rotate arm.

Central Ray

- Requires a **10° to 15° CR caudal angle,** centered posteriorly to pass through the superior margin of humeral head
- Minimum SID of 40 inches (100 cm)

Collimation Collimate on four sides to area of interest.

Respiration Suspend respiration during exposure.

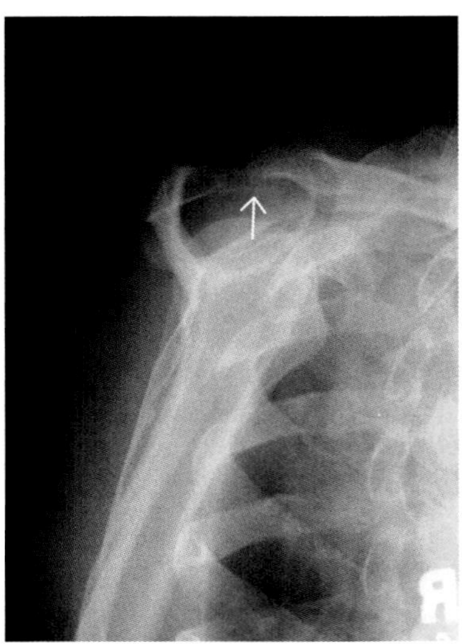

Fig. 6-57. Outlet projection—Neer method.

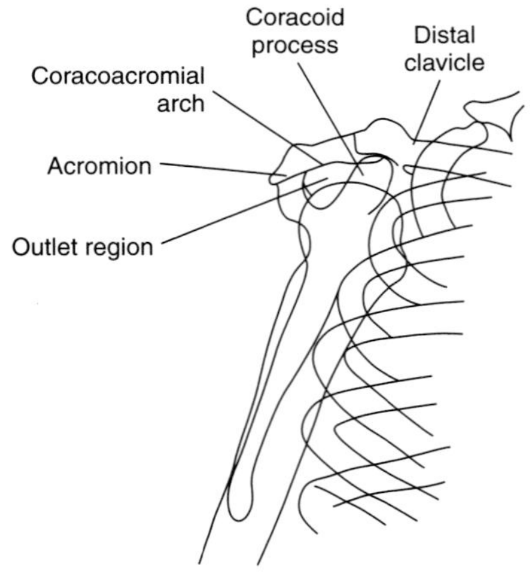

Fig. 6-58. Outlet projection—Neer method.

Radiographic Criteria

Structures Shown: • Proximal humerus will be superimposed over thin body of the scapula, which should be seen on end without rib superimposition

Position: • The acromion and coracoid processes should appear as nearly symmetric upper limbs of the Y. • The humeral head should appear superimposed and centered to the glenoid fossa just below the supraspinatus outlet region. • The supraspinatus outlet region will appear open, free of superimposition by humeral head (see small arrow in Fig. 6-57).

Collimation and CR: • Collimation is visible on four sides to area of affected shoulder. • CR and center of collimation field to supraspinatus outlet region.

Exposure Criteria: • Optimal density and contrast will demonstrate the Y appearance of the upper lateral scapula superimposed by humeral head with outline of body of scapula visible through humerus. • Bony margins will appear clear and sharp, indicating no motion.

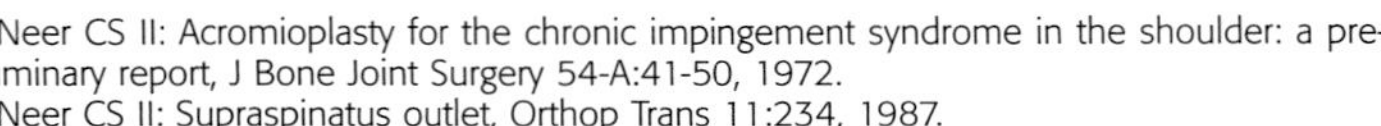

*Neer CS II: Acromioplasty for the chronic impingement syndrome in the shoulder: a preliminary report, J Bone Joint Surgery 54-A:41-50, 1972.

†Neer CS II: Supraspinatus outlet, Orthop Trans 11:234, 1987.

AP APICAL OBLIQUE AXIAL PROJECTION: SHOULDER (TRAUMA)

Garth Method

Shoulder (trauma)
SPECIAL
- **Supraspinatus outlet (Neer method)**
- Apical oblique (Garth method)

Pathology Demonstrated

A good trauma projection for possible scapulohumeral dislocations (especially posterior dislocations), glenoid fractures, Hill-Sachs lesions, and soft-tissue calcifications.*†

18
24
R

Technical Factors

- IR size—18 × 24 cm (8 × 10 inches), lengthwise
- Moving or stationary grid
- Digital IR—very close collimation required
- 75 ± 5 kV range
- Technique and dose:

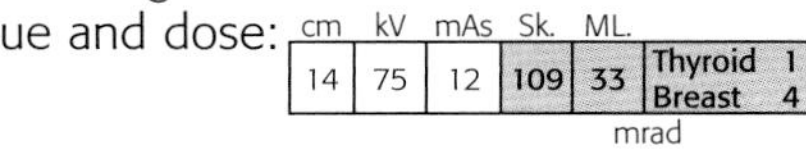

cm	kV	mAs	Sk.	ML.	mrad
14	75	12	109	33	Thyroid 1, Breast 4

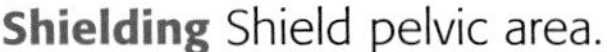

Shielding Shield pelvic area.

Patient Position Take radiograph with the patient in an erect or supine position. (The erect position is usually less painful, if patient's condition allows.) Rotate body 45° toward affected side (posterior surface of affected shoulder against IR).

Part Position

- Center scapulohumeral joint to CR and mid-IR.
- Adjust IR so that the 45°-angled CR will project the scapulohumeral joint to the center of the IR.
- Flex elbow and place arm across chest, or with trauma, arm at side as is.

Central Ray

- CR **45° caudad,** centered to the **scapulohumeral joint**
- Minimum SID of 40 inches (100 cm)

Collimation Collimate closely to area of interest.

Respiration Suspend respiration during exposure.

Radiographic Criteria

Structures Shown: • The humeral head, glenoid cavity, and neck and head of the scapula are well demonstrated free of superimposition.

Position: • The coracoid process is projected over part of humeral head, which appears elongated. • The acromion and AC joint are projected superior to the humeral head.

Collimation and CR: • Collimation should be visible on four sides to area of affected shoulder. • CR and center of collimation field should be at the scapulohumeral joint.

Exposure Criteria: • Optimal density and contrast with no motion will demonstrate clear, sharp bony trabecular markings and soft-tissue detail for possible calcifications.

*Sloth C, Lundgren JS: The apical oblique radiograph in examination of acute shoulder trauma, Europ J Radiol 9:147-151, 1989.

†Garth WP Jr, Slappey CE, Ochs CW: Roentgenographic demonstration of instability of the shoulder: the apical oblique projection, J Bone Joint Surg 66-A:1450-1453, 1984.

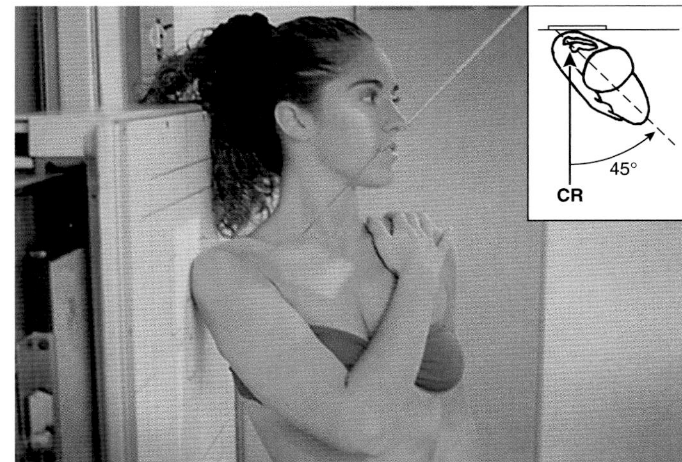

Fig. 6-59. Erect apical oblique axial projection—45° posterior oblique, CR 45° caudad.

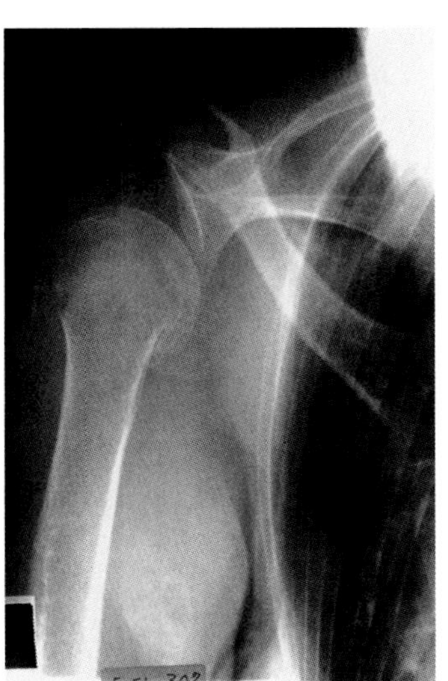

Fig. 6-60. Apical oblique projection. (Note impacted fracture of humeral head but no major scapulohumeral dislocation.)

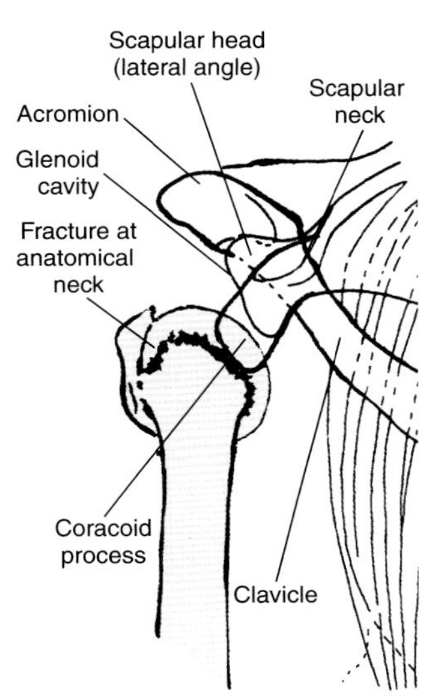

Fig. 6-61. Apical oblique projection. (Note impacted fracture of humeral head but no major scapulohumeral dislocation.)

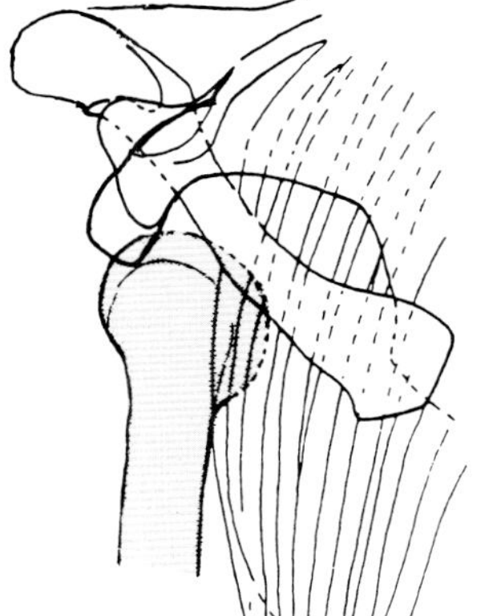

Fig. 6-62. Appearance of humerus if a dislocation has occurred. Anterior dislocation (most common), humerus projected inferiorly.

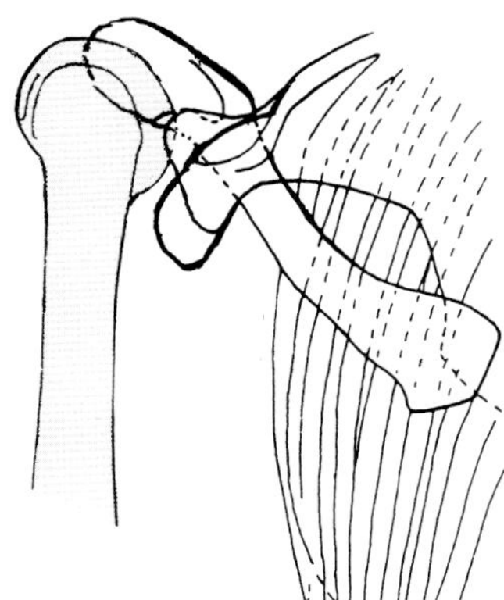

Fig. 6-63. Posterior dislocation, humerus projected superiorly.

AP AND AP AXIAL PROJECTIONS: CLAVICLE

6

Clavicle
BASIC
• AP and AP axial

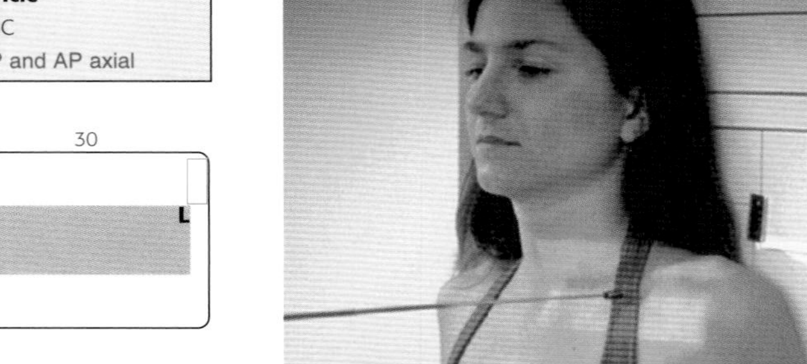

Pathology Demonstrated
Fractures and/or dislocations of the clavicle are demonstrated.

Departmental routines commonly include both AP and AP axial projections.

Technical Factors
- IR size—24 × 30 cm (10 × 12 inches), crosswise
- Moving or stationary grid
- AEC not recommended
- Digital IR—requires very close collimation
- 70 ± 5 kV range
- Technique and dose:

cm	kV	mAs	Sk.	ML.	
14	70	8	134	34	Thyroid 60 Breast 2

mrad (2 projections)

Shielding Shield pelvic area.

Patient Position Take radiograph with the patient in an erect or supine position with arms at sides, chin raised, looking straight ahead. Posterior shoulder should be in contact with IR or tabletop, without rotation of body.

Part Position
- Center clavicle and IR to CR. (Clavicle can readily be palpated with medial aspect at jugular notch and lateral portion at AC joint above shoulder.)

Central Ray
AP
- CR **perpendicular** to **midclavicle**

AP Axial
- CR **15° to 30° cephalad** to **midclavicle** (See Note below.)
- Minimum SID of 40 inches (100 cm)

Collimation Collimate to area of clavicle. (Ensure that both AC and sternoclavicular joints are included.)

Respiration Suspend respiration at end of inhalation (helps to elevate clavicles).

Alternate PA: The radiograph may also be taken as a PA projection and/or a PA axial with 15° to 20° caudal angle.

Note: Thin (asthenic) patients require 10° to 15° more angle than patients with thick shoulders and chest (hypersthenic).

Radiographic Criteria
AP 0°: • Collimation borders should be visible with entire clavicle visualized, including both AC and sternoclavicular joints.
AP Axial: • Correct angulation of CR will project most of the clavicle above the scapula and ribs. •Only the medial portion of clavicle will be superimposed by the first and second ribs. • Optimal exposure will demonstrate the distal clavicle and AC joint without excessive density. • The bony margins and trabecular marking should appear sharp, indicating no motion, and the medial clavicle and sternoclavicular joint should also be visualized through the thorax.

Fig. 6-64. AP—CR 0°.

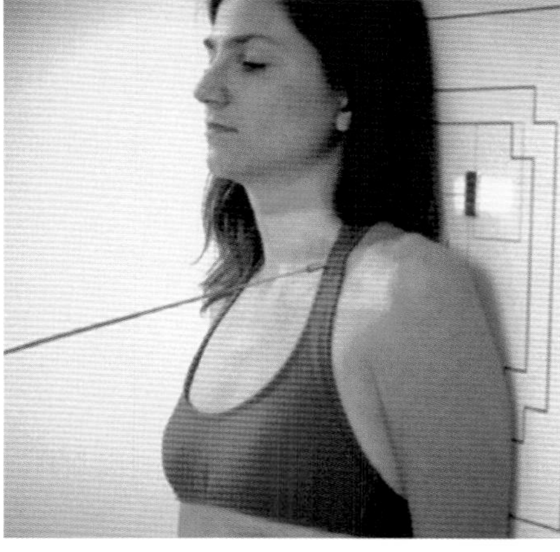

Fig. 6-65. AP axial—CR 15° to 30° cephalad.

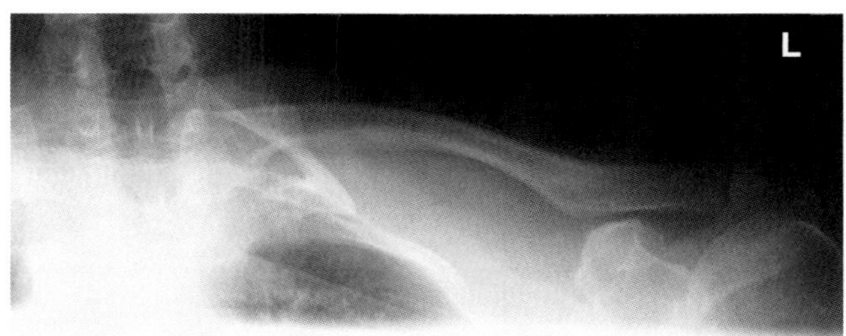

AP axial—CR 30° cephalad.

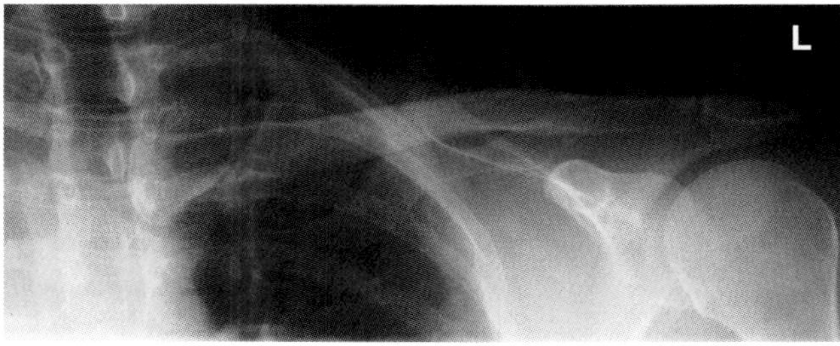

Fig. 6-66. AP clavicle—CR 0°.

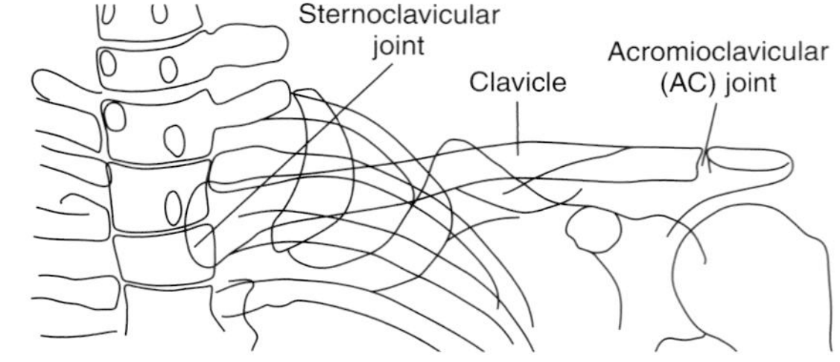

Fig. 6-67. AP clavicle—CR 0°.

AP PROJECTION: AC JOINTS

Bilateral With and Without Weights

Warning: Shoulder and/or clavicle projections should be completed first to rule out fractures, or this radiograph may be taken without weights first and checked before taking with weights.

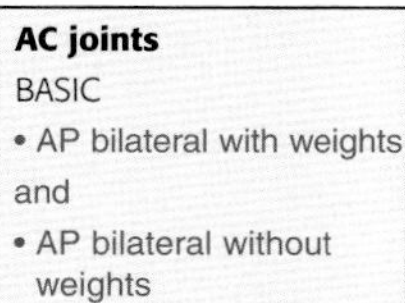
AC joints
BASIC
- AP bilateral with weights
and
- AP bilateral without weights

Pathology Demonstrated
AC joint separation is demonstrated. A widening of one joint space, as compared with the other view with weights, usually indicates an AC joint separation.

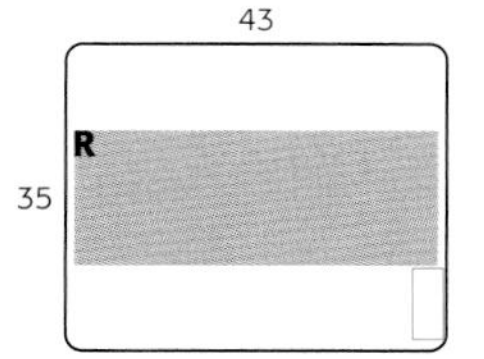

or

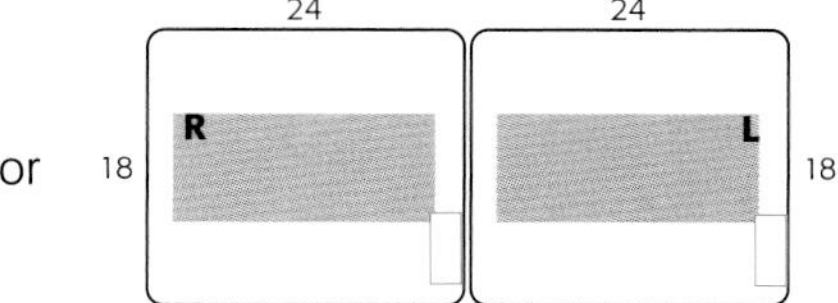

Technical Factors
- IR size—35 × 43 cm (14 × 17 inches), crosswise, or 7 × 17 inches (14 × 43 cm), if available
- "With weight" and "without weight" markers
- Nongrid
- AEC not recommended
- 65 ± 5 kV with screen; 65-70 kV with grid on larger patients
- For broad-shouldered patients, **two 18- × 24-cm** (8- × 10-inch) **cassettes crosswise** placed side by side and exposed simultaneously to include both AC joints on one exposure
- Technique and dose:

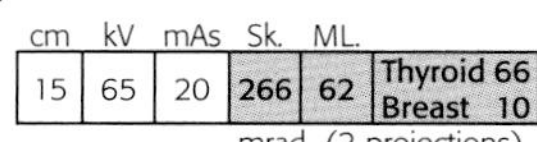

cm	kV	mAs	Sk.	ML.	
15	65	20	**266**	**62**	Thyroid 66 Breast 10

mrad (2 projections)

Shielding Secure gonadal shield around waist.

Patient Position Take radiograph with the patient in an erect position, posterior shoulders against cassette with equal weight on both feet; arms at side; no rotation of shoulders or pelvis; looking straight ahead. (May be taken seated if patent's condition requires.) **Two sets** of bilateral AC joints are taken in the same position, one **without weights** and one **stress view with weights.**

Part Position
- Position patient to direct CR to midway between AC joints.
- Center midline of IR(s) to CR (top of IR should be <2 inch, or 5 cm, above shoulders).

Central Ray
- CR perpendicular to a **midpoint between AC joints,** 1 inch (2.5 cm) above jugular notch (See Note below.)
- Minimum SID of **72 inches (180 cm)**

Collimation Collimate with a long, narrow light field to area of interest; upper light border should be to upper shoulder soft-tissue margins.

Respiration Suspend respiration during exposure.

Weights After the first exposure is made without weights and the cassette(s) has (have) been changed, for large adult patients strap 8- to 10-pound weights to each wrist and, with shoulders relaxed, **gently** allow weights to hang from wrists pulling down on each arm and shoulder. The same amount of weight must be used on each wrist. Less weight (5 to 8 pounds per limb) may be used for smaller or asthenic patients, and more weight for larger or hypersthenic patients. (Check department protocol for the amount of applied weights.)

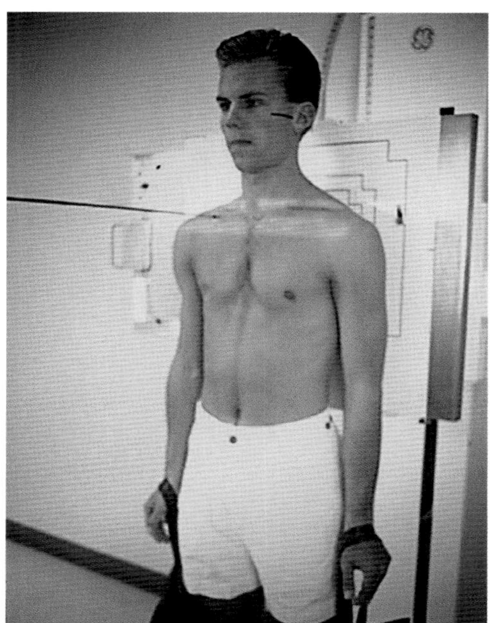

Fig. 6-68. Stress view with weights (weights tied to wrists). Male, 8 to 10 pounds per limb, two cassettes side-by-side.

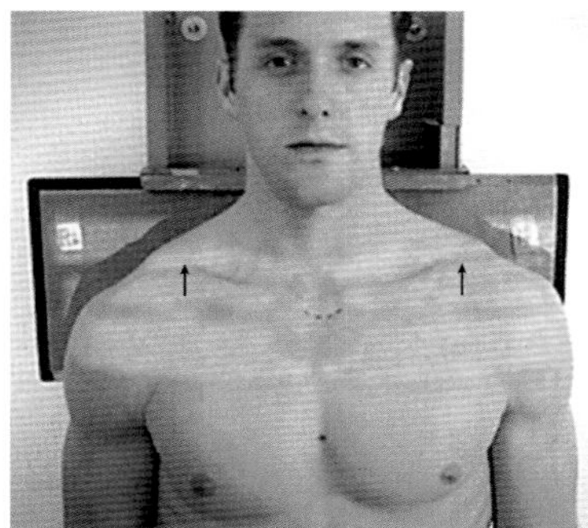

Fig. 6-69. AC joints marked by *arrows.*

Note: Patients should **NOT** be asked to hold on to the weights with their hands; rather the **weights should be attached to the wrists so that the hands, arms, and shoulders are relaxed** to determine possible AC joint separation. Holding on to weights may result in false-negative radiographs because they will tend to pull on the weights, resulting in contraction rather than relaxation of the shoulder muscles.

AP PROJECTION: AC JOINTS—cont'd

Bilateral With and Without Weights

Alternate AP axial projection: A 15° cephalic angle centered at the level of the AC joints projects the AC joint superior to the acromion, providing optimal visualization.

Alternate supine position: If patient's condition requires, the radiograph may be taken supine by tying both ends of a long strip of gauze to patient's wrists and placing around patient's feet with knees partially flexed, then **slowly** and **gently** straightening legs and pulling down on shoulders. May also be done by an assistant **gently** pulling down on arms and shoulders.

Warning: This method should only be done by experienced and qualified personnel to prevent additional injury.

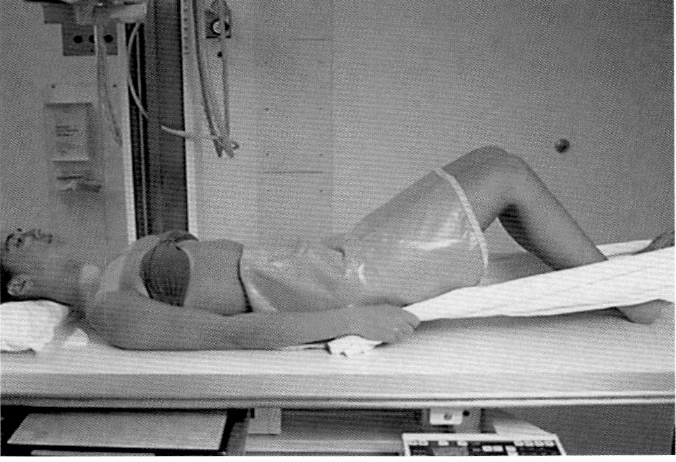

Fig. 6-70. Alternate supine position.

Radiographic Criteria

Structures Shown: • Both AC joints, as well as the entire clavicles and SC joints, are demonstrated.

Position: • Both AC joints are on the same horizontal plane. • **No rotation,** as evidenced by symmetric appearance of the SC joints on each side of the vertebral column.

Collimation and CR: • Collimation should be visible on four sides, remembering to include both AC joints. • CR and center of the collimation field should be at the midpoint between the AC joints.

Exposure Criteria and Markers: • Optimal density and contrast will clearly demonstrate the AC joints and soft tissue without excessive density. Bony margins and trabecular marking will appear sharp, indicating no motion. • **Right and left markers,** as well as markers indicating **with** and **without weights,** should be visible without superimposing essential anatomy.

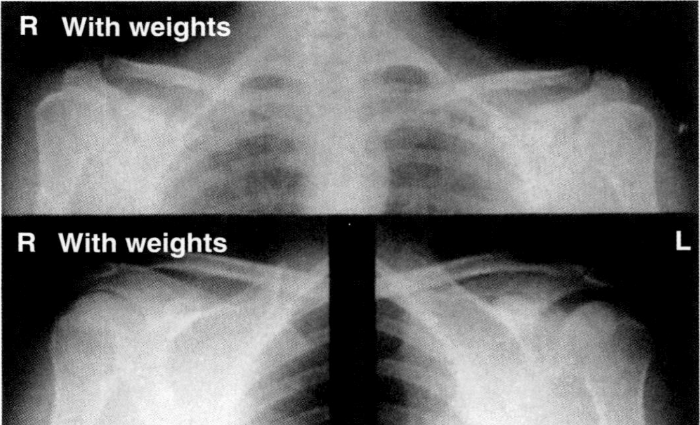

Fig. 6-71. AP acromioclavicular joints with weights (single image and two images exposed simultaneously).

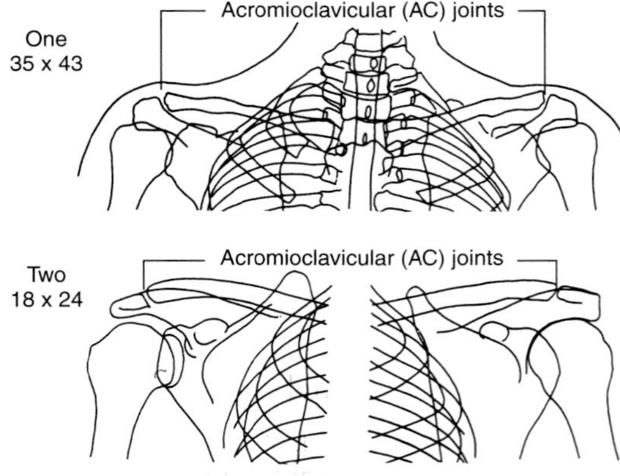

Fig. 6-72. AC joints.

AP PROJECTION: SCAPULA

Pathology Demonstrated
Fractures of the scapula are demonstrated.

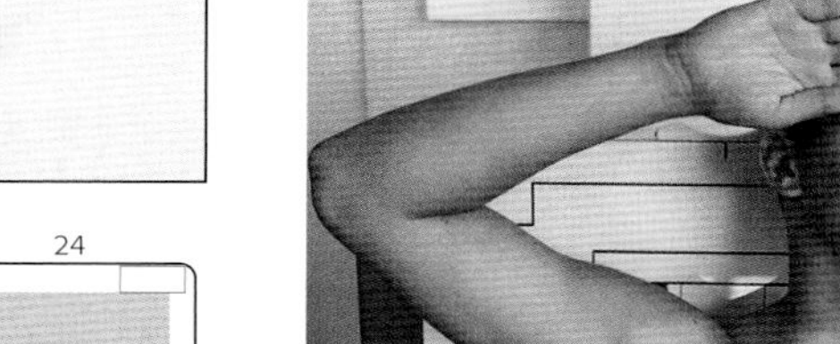
Scapula
BASIC
- AP
- Lateral

Technical Factors
- IR size—24 × 30 cm (10 × 12 inches), lengthwise
- Moving or stationary grid
- 75 ± 5 kV range
- Minimum of 3 seconds exposure time with breathing technique (4 or 5 seconds is desirable); no AEC
- Technique and dose:

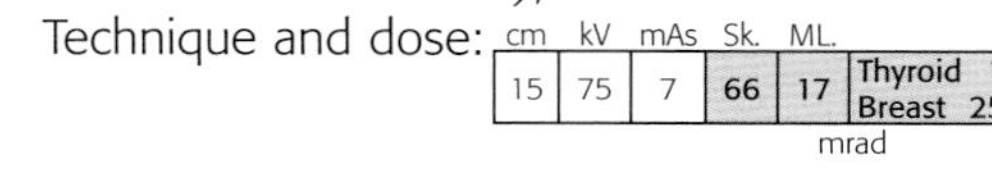

cm	kV	mAs	Sk.	ML.	
15	75	7	66	17	Thyroid 1 Breast 25

mrad

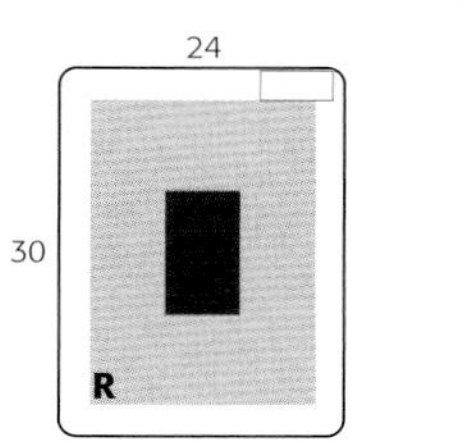

Shielding Place gonadal shield over pelvic area.

Patient Position Take radiograph with the patient in an erect or supine position. (The erect position may be more comfortable for patient.) Posterior surface of shoulder is in direct contact with tabletop or IR without rotation of thorax. (Rotation toward affected side would place scapula into a truer posterior position, but it would also result in greater superimposition of rib cage.)

Part Position
- Position patient so that midscapula area is centered to CR.
- Adjust cassette to center to CR. Top of IR should be about 2 inches, or 5 cm, above shoulder, and lateral border of IR should be about 2 inches, or 5 cm, from lateral margin of rib cage.
- Gently **abduct arm 90°** and supinate hand. (Abduction will move scapula laterally to clear more of thoracic structures.)

Central Ray
- CR perpendicular **to midscapula, 2 inches (5 cm) inferior to coracoid process,** or to **level of axilla, and approximately 2 inches (5 cm) medial from lateral border of patient**
- Minimum SID of 40 inches (100 cm)

Collimation Collimate on four sides to area of scapula.

Respiration **Breathing technique** is preferred if patient can cooperate. Ask patient to breathe gently without moving affected shoulder or arm.

Radiographic Criteria

Structures Shown: • The lateral portion of the scapula is free of superimposition. • The medial portion of the scapula is seen through the thoracic structures.

Position: • Affected arm seen to be abducted 90° and hand supinated, as evidenced by the lateral border of the scapula free of superimposition.

Collimation and CR: • Collimation should be visible on four sides to the area of the affected scapula. • CR and center of the collimation field should be at midscapula area.

Exposure Criteria: • Optimal density and contrast with no motion will demonstrate clear, sharp bony trabecular markings of the lateral portion of the scapula. Ribs and lung structures will appear blurred with proper breathing technique.

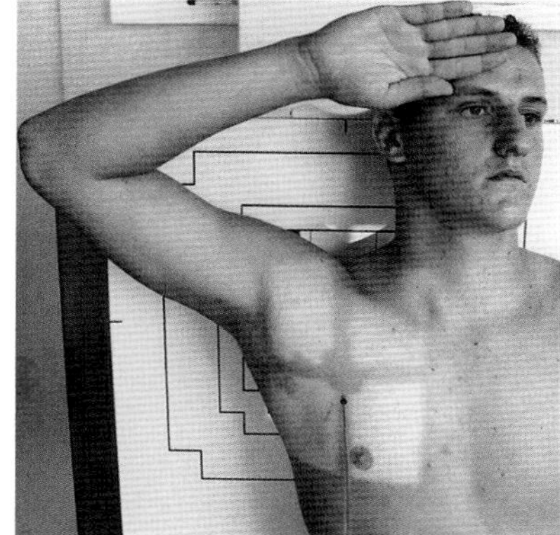

Fig. 6-73. AP erect.

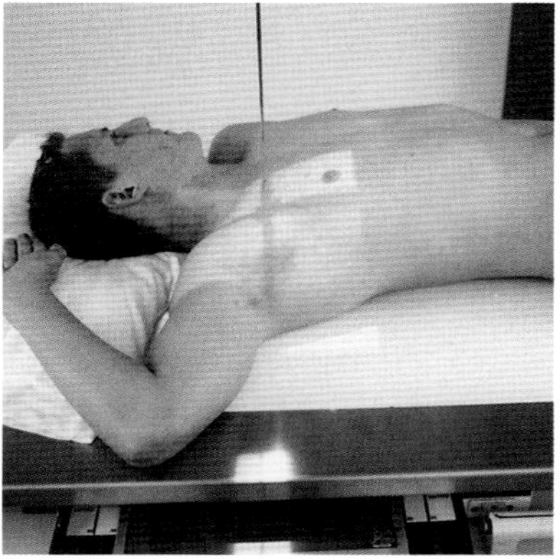

Fig. 6-74. AP supine.

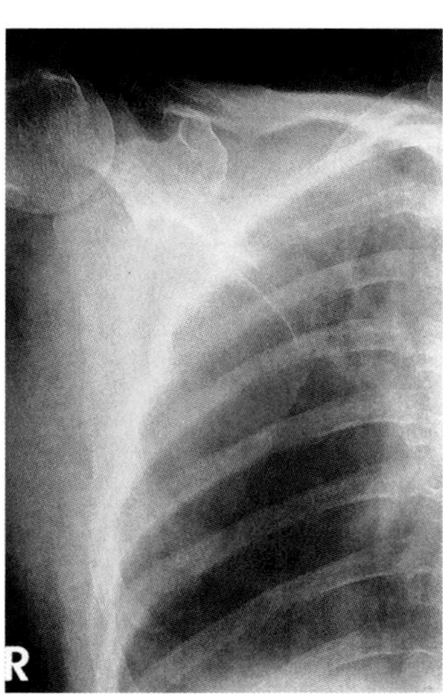

Fig. 6-75. AP scapula.

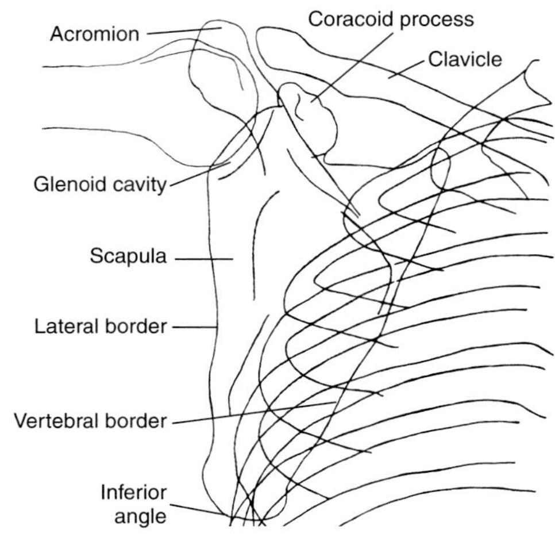

Fig. 6-76. AP scapula.

LATERAL POSITION—RAO OR LAO: SCAPULA

Patient Erect—See p. 207 for Patient Recumbent

Scapula
BASIC
- AP
- Lateral
  - –Erect
  - **–Recumbent**

Pathology Demonstrated

Horizontal fractures of the scapula are demonstrated. Arm placement should be determined by scapular area of interest.

Technical Factors

- IR size—24 × 30 cm (10 × 12 inches), lengthwise
- Moving or stationary grid
- AEC not recommended
- Digital IR—requires very close collimation
- 75 ± 5 kV range
- Technique and dose:

cm	kV	mAs	Sk.	ML.	
16	75	13	131	38	Thyroid 0 Breast 0
			mrad		

24 × 30 L

Shielding Secure gonadal shield around waist.

Patient Position Take radiograph with the patient in an erect or recumbent position. (The erect position is preferred if patient's condition allows.) Face patient toward IR in an anterior oblique position.

Part Position (Erect)

- Have patient reach across front of chest and grasp opposite shoulder. This best demonstrates **body** of scapula (Figs. 6-77 and 6-78).

  or
- Have patient drop affected arm, flex elbow, and place arm behind lower back with arm partially abducted, or just let arm hang down at patient's side. This best demonstrates **acromion and coracoid processes** (Figs. 6-79 and 6-80).
- **Palpate borders of scapula** and rotate patient until the scapula is in a **true lateral position.** The average patient will be rotated 30° to 45° from the lateral position, which results in a 45° to 60° anterior oblique position. The position of humerus (down at side or up across anterior chest) has an effect on the amount of body rotation required. Less rotation is required with arm up across anterior chest. (The flat posterior surface of body of scapula should be perpendicular to IR.)
- Align patient to center midvertebral border to CR and to IR.

Central Ray

- CR to **midvertebral border of scapula**
- Minimum 40 inches (100 cm) SID

Collimation Collimate to area of scapula.

Respiration Suspend respiration during exposure.

Radiographic Criteria

Structures Shown and Position: • Entire scapula should be visualized in a lateral position, as evidenced by direct superimposition of vertebral and lateral borders. • True lateral is shown by direct superimposition of vertebral and lateral borders. • Body of scapula should be in profile, free of superimposition by ribs. • As much as possible, the humerus should not superimpose area of interest of the scapula.

Collimation and CR: • Collimation should be visualized on four sides to area of scapula. • CR and center of collimation field to lateral border of midscapula.

Exposure Criteria: • Optimal exposure with no motion will demonstrate sharp bony borders and trabecular marking without excessive density in area of inferior angle. • Bony borders of both the acromion and coracoid processes should be seen through the head of the humerus.

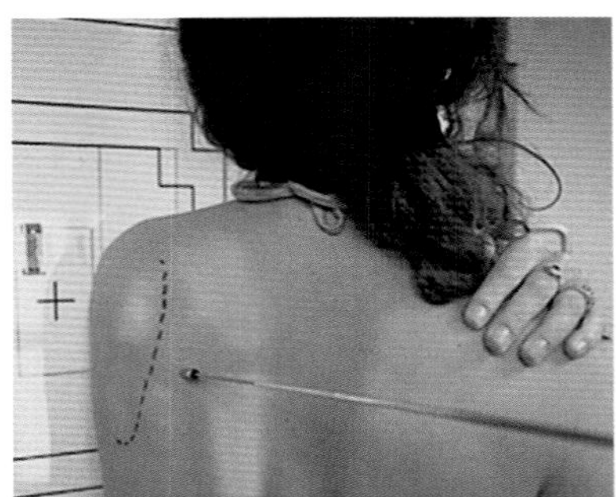

Fig. 6-77. Lateral for body of scapula (≈45° LAO).

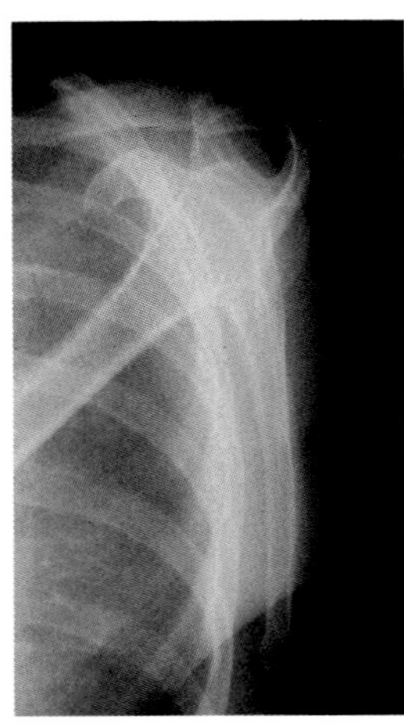

Fig. 6-78. Lateral for body of scapula (≈45° LAO).

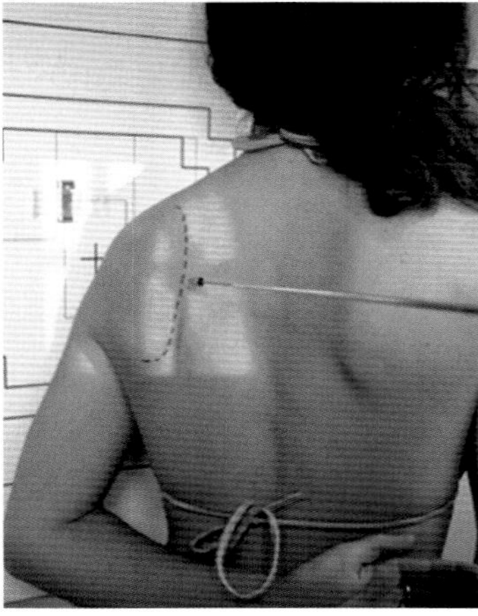

Fig. 6-79. Lateral for **acromion or coracoid process** (≈60° LAO).

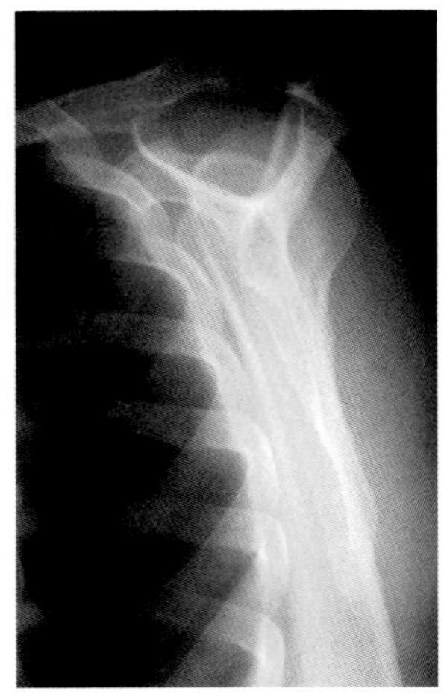

Fig. 6-80. Lateral for **acromion or coracoid process** (≈60° LAO).

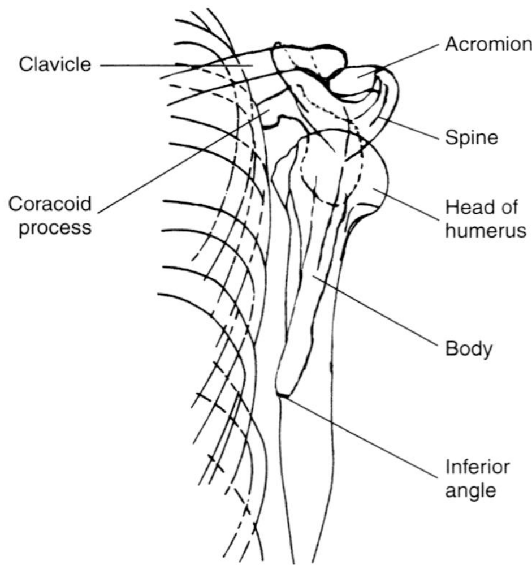

Fig. 6-81. Lateral scapula.

LATERAL POSITION—LPO OR RPO: SCAPULA

Patient Recumbent—**See p. 206 for Patient Erect**

Scapula
BASIC
• **AP**
• Lateral

Pathology Demonstrated

Fractures of the scapula are demonstrated.

Note: This position results in a magnified image because of increased OID.

Technical Factors

- IR size—24 × 30 cm (10 × 12 inches), lengthwise
- Moving or stationary grid
- AEC not recommended
- Digital IR—requires very close collimation
- 75 ± 5 kV range
- Technique and dose:

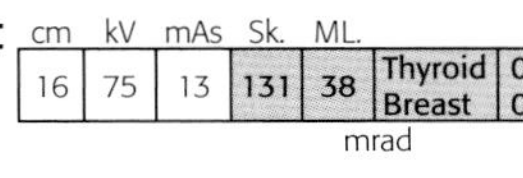

cm	kV	mAs	Sk.	ML.		
16	75	13	131	38	Thyroid	0
					Breast	0
			mrad			

24

30

R

Shielding Place lead shield over pelvic area.

Patient Position Take radiograph with the patient in a supine position, and place affected arm across chest. Then rotate entire body about 30° or as needed to elevate affected shoulder until body of scapula is in a true lateral position. Flex knee of affected side to help patient maintain this oblique body position.

Part Position

- Palpate borders of scapula by grasping medial and lateral borders of body of scapula with fingers and thumb (Fig. 6-82, *inset*). Carefully adjust body rotation as needed to bring the plane of scapular body **perpendicular to IR.**
- Align patient on tabletop so that the center of the midlateral (axillary) border of scapula is centered to CR and to center of IR.

Central Ray

- CR to **midscapula lateral border**
- Minimum 40 inches (100 cm) SID

Collimation Collimate to area of scapula.

Respiration Suspend respiration during exposure.

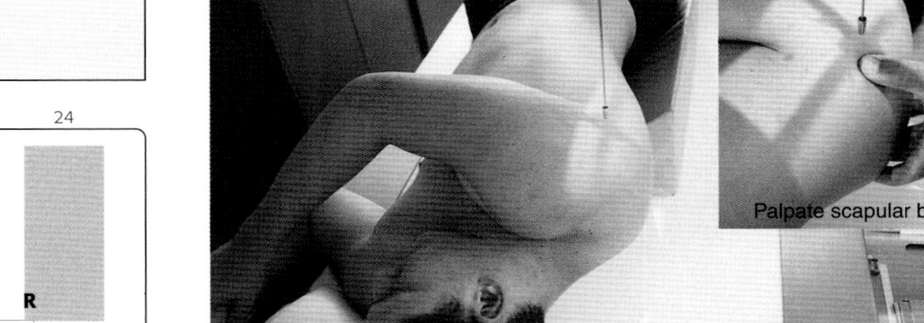

Fig. 6-82. Lateral scapula position.

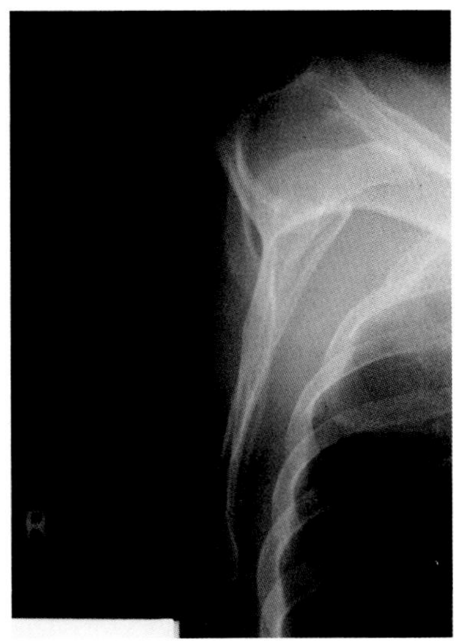

Fig. 6-83. Lateral scapula.

Radiographic Criteria

Structures Shown: • Entire scapula should be visualized in a lateral position.

Position: • True lateral is shown by direct superimposition of vertebral and lateral borders. • Body of scapula should be seen in profile, free of superimposition by ribs. • As much as possible, the humerus should not superimpose area of interest of the scapula.

Collimation and CR: • Collimation should be visualized on four sides to area of scapula. • CR and center of collimation field to lateral border of midscapula.

Exposure Criteria: • Optimal exposure with no motion will demonstrate sharp bony borders and trabecular markings. • Entire scapula should be visualized without excessive density in area of inferior angle. • Bony borders of both the acromion and coracoid processes should be seen through the head of the humerus.

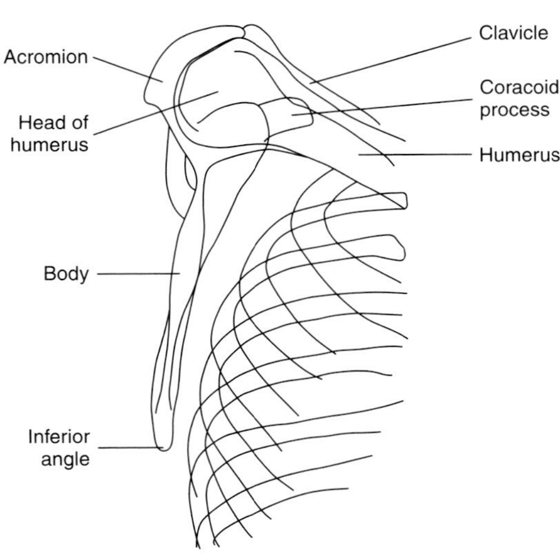

Fig. 6-84. Lateral scapula.

RADIOGRAPHS FOR CRITIQUE

6

Critique each of these four radiographs based on the categories described in the textbook and outlined on the right. As a starting critique exercise, place a check in each category that demonstrates a **repeatable error** for that radiograph.

Student workbooks provide more space for writing comments and complete critique answers for each of these radiographs. Answers are provided in Appendix B (at the end of this textbook) and in the workbooks.

	RADIOGRAPHS			
	A	B	C	D
1. Structures shown	____	____	____	____
2. Positioning	____	____	____	____
3. Collimation and CR	____	____	____	____
4. Exposure criteria	____	____	____	____
5. Markers	____	____	____	____

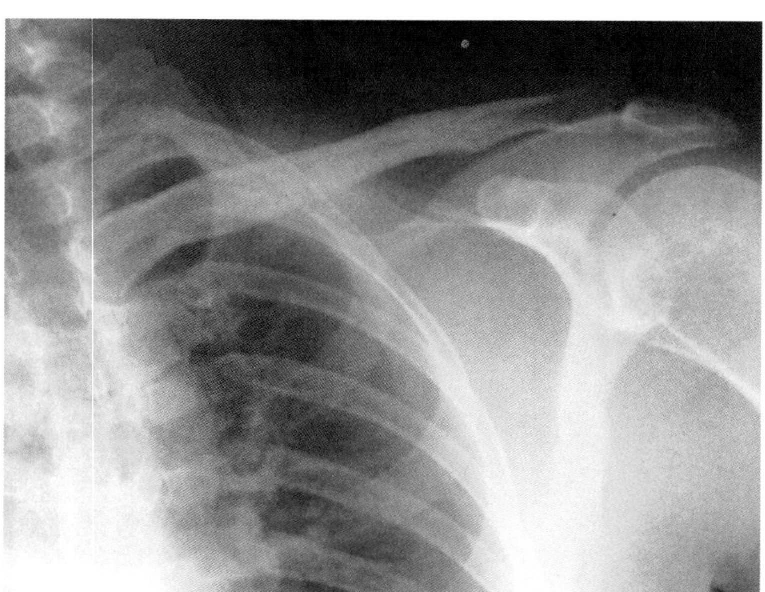

Fig. C6-85. AP clavicle. A

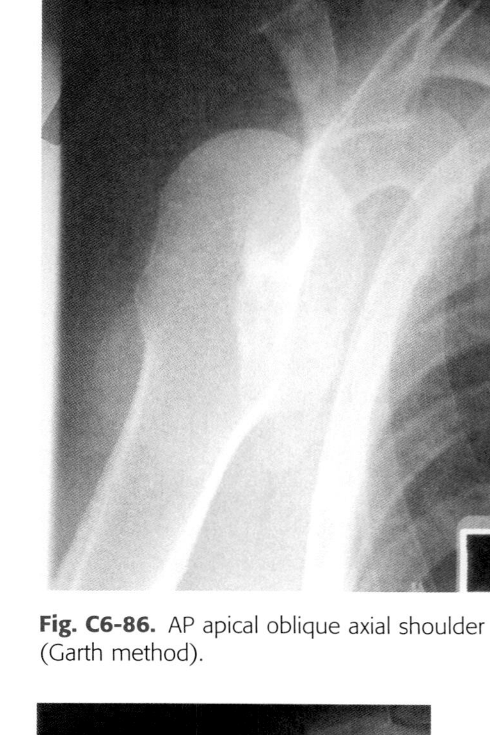

Fig. C6-86. AP apical oblique axial shoulder (Garth method). B

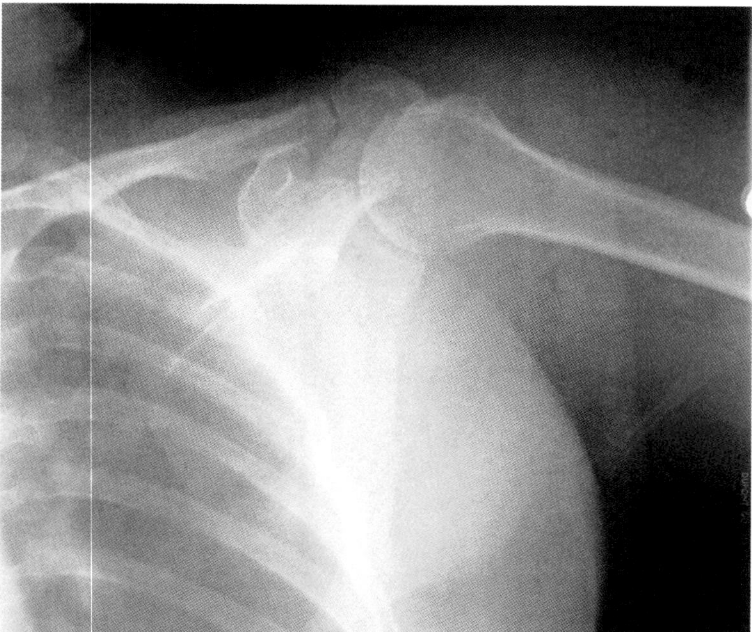

Fig. C6-87. AP scapula. C

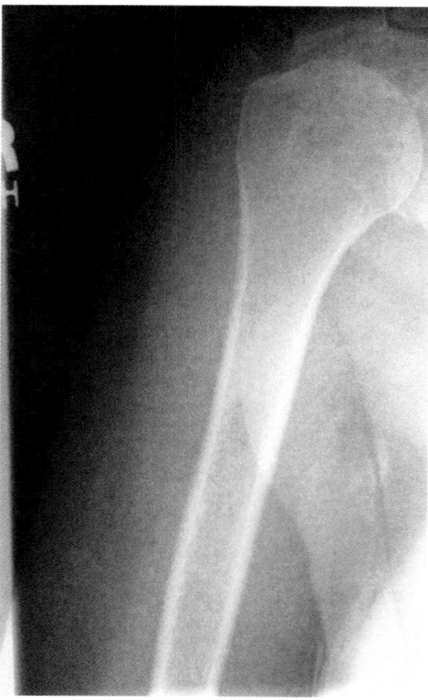

Fig. C6-88. AP shoulder and proximal humerus. D

CHAPTER 7

Lower Limb

CONTRIBUTIONS BY **Beth L. Vealé,** MEd, RT(R)(QM)
CONTRIBUTOR TO PAST EDITIONS Jeannean Hall-Rollins, MRC, BS, RT(R)(CV)

CONTENTS

RADIOGRAPHIC ANATOMY

7

Lower Limb

The bones of the lower limb are divided into four main groups: (1) the foot, (2) leg, (3) femur, and (4) hip. This chapter includes a thorough study of the anatomy and positioning for the first three groups: the **foot, leg,** and **mid** and **distal femur.** The **ankle** and **knee joints** are also included in this study.

FOOT

The bones of the foot are fundamentally similar to the bones of the hand and wrist studied in Chapter 5.

The 26 bones of one foot are divided into three groups:

1. Phalanges (toes/or digits)	14
2. Metatarsals (instep)	5
3. Tarsals	7
Total	26

Phalanges—Toes (Digits)

The most distal bones of the foot are the **phalanges,** which make up the toes, or digits. The five digits of each foot are numbered one through five starting on the medial or big toe side of the foot. Note that the large toe, or first digit, has only two phalanges, similar to those of the thumb. These are the **proximal phalanx** and the **distal phalanx.** Each of the second, third, fourth, and fifth digits has a **middle phalanx** in addition to a proximal and a distal phalanx. Because the first digit has two phalanges, and digits two through five have three apiece, there are **14 phalanges** in each foot.

The similarities to the hand are obvious because there are also 14 phalanges in each hand. However, two noticeable differences exist in that the phalanges of the foot are smaller and their movements are more limited than those of the hand.

When any of the bones or joints of the foot are described, the specific digit and foot should also be identified. For example, referring to the "distal phalanx of the first digit of the right foot" would leave no doubt as to which bone is in question.

The distal phalanges of the second through fifth toes are very small and may be difficult to identify as separate bones on a radiograph.

Metatarsals

The five bones of the instep are the **metatarsal** bones. These are numbered along with the digits, with number one on the medial side and number five on the lateral side.

Each of the metatarsals comprises three parts. The small, rounded distal part of each metatarsal is the **head.** The centrally located, long, slender portion is termed the **body** (shaft). The expanded, proximal end of each metatarsal is the **base.**

The **base of the fifth metatarsal** is expanded laterally into a prominent rough **tuberosity,** which provides for the attachment of a tendon. The proximal portion of the fifth metatarsal, including this tuberosity, is readily visible on radiographs and is **a common trauma site** for the foot; therefore this area must be well visualized on radiographs.

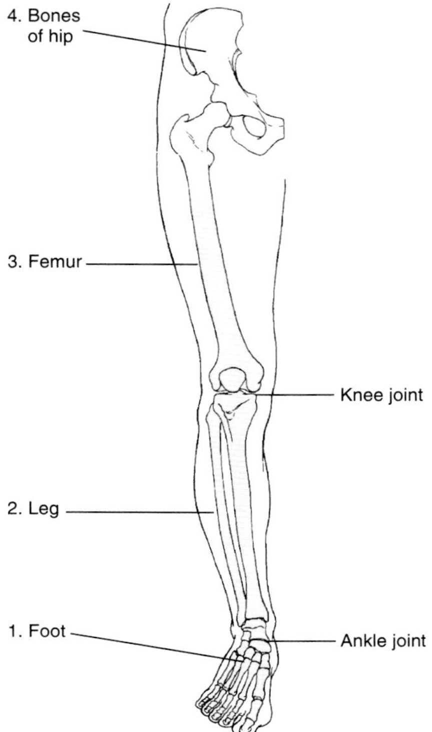

Fig. 7-1. Lower limb.

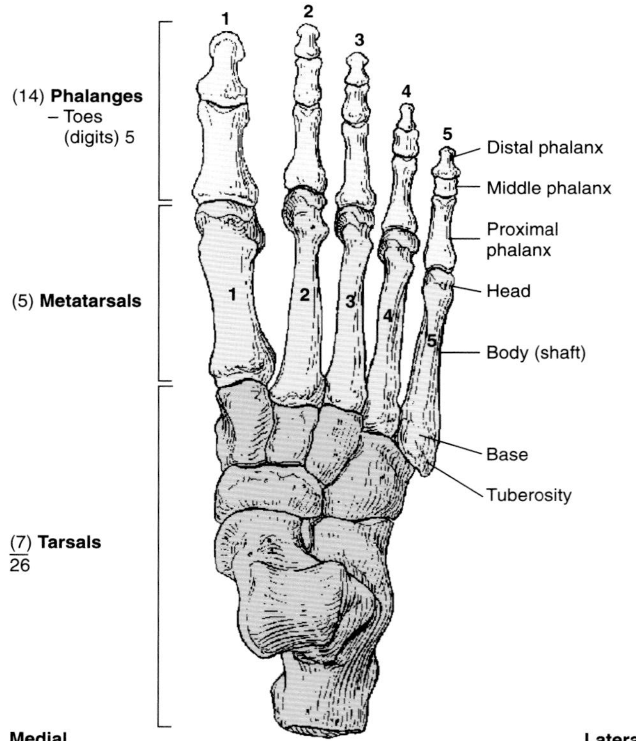

Fig. 7-2. Bones of foot.

Joints of Phalanges (Digits) and Metatarsals

Joints of digits The joints or articulations of the digits of the foot are important to identify because fractures may involve the joint surfaces. Each joint of the foot has a name derived from the two bones on either side of that joint. Between the proximal and distal phalanges of the first digit is the **interphalangeal (IP) joint.**

Because digits two through five are composed of three bones each, these digits also have two joints each. Between the middle and distal phalanges is the **distal interphalangeal joint,** or **DIP joint.** Between the proximal and middle phalanges is the **proximal interphalangeal joint,** or **PIP** joint.

Joints of metatarsals Each of the joints at the head of the metatarsal is a **metatarsophalangeal joint,** or **MTP joint,** and each of the joints at the base of the metatarsal is a **tarsometatarsal joint,** or **TMT joint.** The base of the third metatarsal or the third tarsometatarsal joint is important because this is the centering point or the central ray (CR) location for an AP and oblique foot.

When joints of the foot are described, it is important to state the name of the joint first, then include which digit or metatarsal and which foot. For example, an injury or fracture may be described as near the distal interphalangeal joint of the fifth digit of the left foot.

Sesamoid Bones

Several small detached bones, called **sesamoid** bones, are often found in the feet and hands. These extra bones, which are embedded in certain tendons, are often present near various joints. In the upper limbs, sesamoid bones are quite small and are most often found on the palmar surface near the metacarpophalangeal joints, or occasionally at the interphalangeal joint of the thumb.

In the **lower limbs,** sesamoid bones tend to be larger and more significant radiographically. The largest sesamoid bone in the body is the *patella,* or *knee cap,* as described later in this chapter. Also, the sesamoid bones illustrated in Figs. 7-3 and 7-4 are almost always present on the posterior or **plantar surface at the head of the first metatarsal** near the first MTP joint. Sesamoid bones may also be found near other joints of the foot. Sesamoid bones are important radiographically, because fracturing these small bones is possible. Because of their plantar location, they can be quite painful and cause discomfort when weight is placed on that foot. Special tangential projections may be necessary to demonstrate a fracture of a sesamoid bone, as will be demonstrated later in this chapter (p. 231).

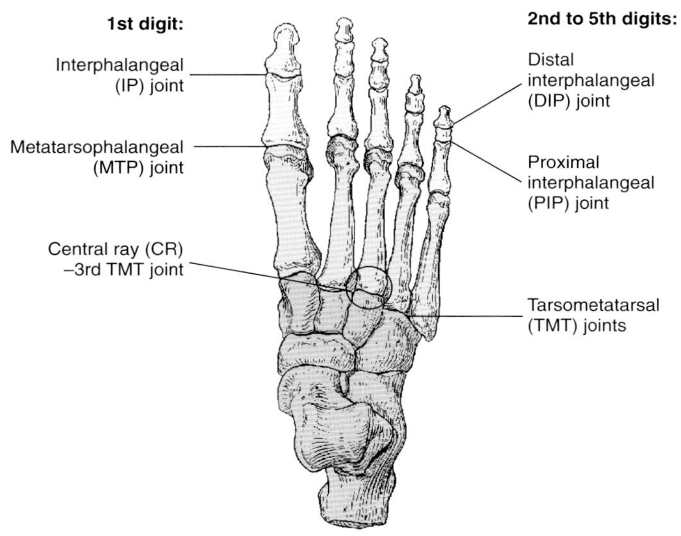

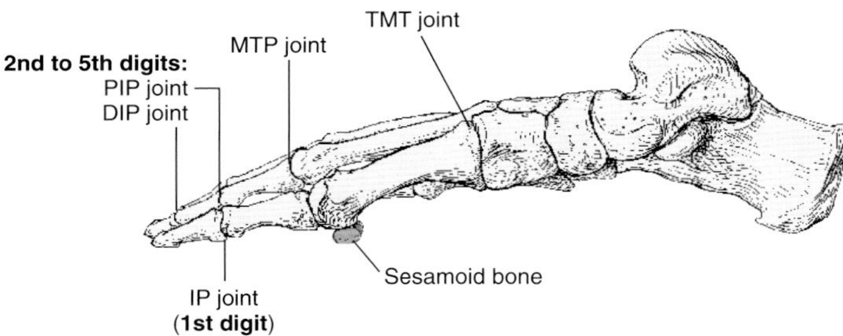

Fig. 7-3. Joints of right foot.

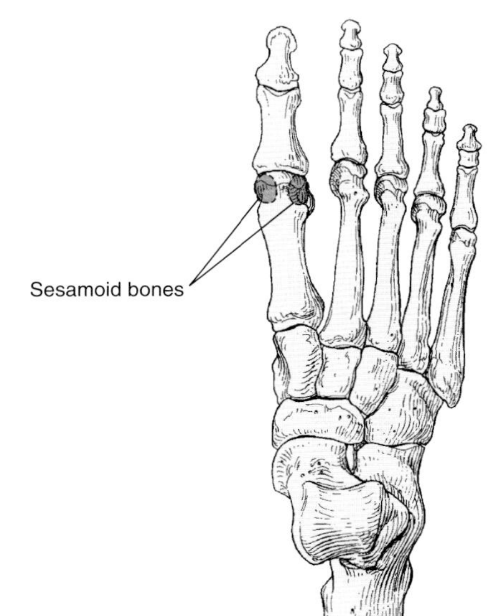

Fig. 7-4. Sesamoid bones.

7

TARSALS

The seven large bones of the proximal foot are termed *tarsal bones.* The names of the tarsals can be remembered with the aid of a mnemonic: **C**ome **t**o **C**olorado (the) **n**ext **3 C**hristmases.

(1) **C**ome	–**C**alcaneus (os calcis)
(2) **T**o	–**T**alus (astragalus)
(3) **C**olorado	–**C**uboid
(4) **N**ext	–**N**avicular (scaphoid)
(5-6-7) **3 C**hristmases	–**First, second,** and **third** cuneiforms

Note above that the calcaneus, talus, and navicular bones are also sometimes known by alternative names, the *os calcis, astragalus,* and *scaphoid,* respectively. Correct usage, however, dictates that the tarsal bone of the foot should be called the *navicular,* and the carpal bone of the wrist, which has a similar shape, should be called the *scaphoid.* (The carpal bone, unfortunately, has more often been called the *navicular* rather than the preferred *scaphoid.*)

Similarities to the upper limb are less obvious with the tarsals in that only **seven tarsal bones** are compared with the **eight carpal bones** of the wrist. Also, the tarsals are larger and less mobile because they provide a basis of support for the body in an erect position, compared with the more mobile carpals of the hand and wrist.

The seven tarsal bones are sometimes referred to as the *ankle bones,* although only one of the tarsals, the talus, is directly involved in the ankle joint. Each of these tarsals will be studied individually along with a list of the bones with which they articulate.

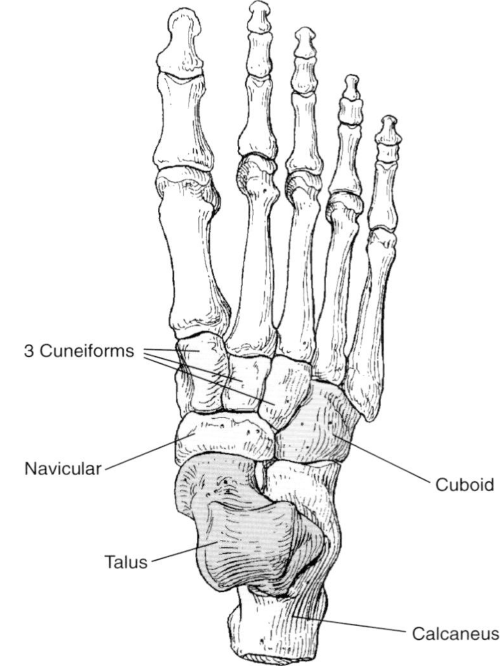

Fig. 7-5. Tarsals (7).

Calcaneus

The largest and strongest bone of the foot is the *calcaneus (kal-ka'ne-us).* The posterior portion is often called the *heel bone.* The most posterior-inferior part of the calcaneus contains a process called the **tuberosity.** Certain large tendons are attached to this rough and striated process, which at its widest points has two small rounded processes. The largest of these is labeled as the **lateral process.** The **medial process** is smaller and less pronounced.

Another ridge of bone that varies in size and shape and is visualized laterally on an axial projection is the **peroneal trochlea** *(per"o-ne'al trok'le-ah).* Sometimes, in general, this is also called the **trochlear process.** On the medial proximal aspect is a larger more prominent bony process called the **sustentaculum tali** *(sus"ten-tak'u-lum),* literally meaning a support for the talus.

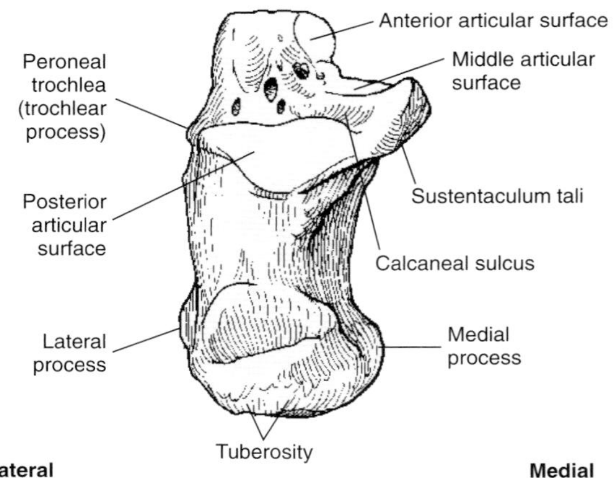

Fig. 7-6. Left calcaneus (superior or proximal surface).

Articulations The calcaneus articulates with **two** bones: anteriorly with the **cuboid** and superiorly with the **talus.** The superior articulation with the talus forms the important **subtalar** (talocalcaneal) joint. Three specific articular facets appear at this joint with the talus through which the weight of the body is transmitted to the ground in an erect position. These are the larger **posterior articular facet** and the smaller **anterior** and **middle articular facets.**

Note that the middle articular facet is the upper portion of the prominent sustentaculum tali, which provides the medial support for this important weight-bearing joint.

The deep depression between posterior and middle articular facets is called the **calcaneal sulcus** (Fig. 7-6). This, combined with a similar groove or depression of the talus, forms an opening for certain ligaments to pass through. This opening in the middle of the subtalar joint is the **sinus tarsi** or tarsal sinus (Fig. 7-7).

Talus

The talus is the second largest tarsal bone and is located between the lower leg and the calcaneus. Therefore the weight of the body is transmitted by this bone through the important ankle and talocalcaneal joints.

Articulations The talus articulates with **four** bones: superiorly with the **tibia** and **fibula,** inferiorly with the **calcaneus,** and anteriorly with the **navicular.**

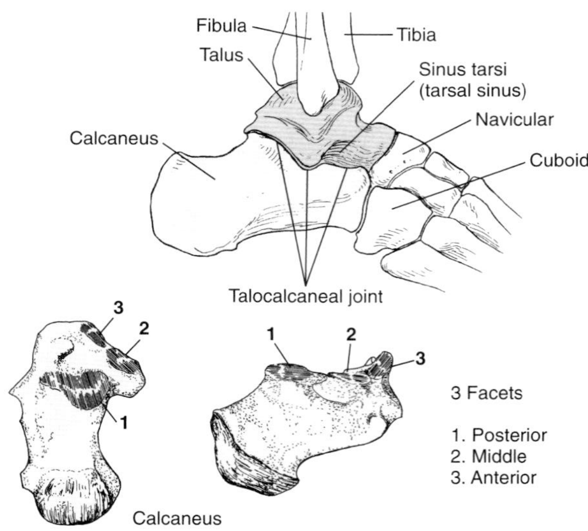

Fig. 7-7. Calcaneus and talus (with ankle and subtalar joints).

Navicular

The navicular is a flattened, oval-shaped bone located on the medial side of the foot between the talus and the three cuneiforms.

Articulations The **navicular** articulates with **four** bones: posteriorly with the talus and anteriorly with the three cuneiforms.

Cuneiforms (3)

The three cuneiforms (meaning *wedge-shaped*) are located on the medial and midaspects of the foot between the first three metatarsals distally and the navicular proximally. The largest cuneiform, articulating with the first metatarsal, is the **medial** (first) cuneiform. The **intermediate** (second) cuneiform, which articulates with the second metatarsal, is the smallest of the cuneiforms. The **lateral** (third) cuneiform articulates with the third metatarsal distally and with the cuboid laterally. All three cuneiforms articulate with the navicular proximally.

Articulations The **medial cuneiform** articulates with **four** bones: the navicular proximally, the first and second metatarsals distally, and the intermediate laterally.

The **intermediate cuneiform** also articulates with **four** bones: the navicular proximally, the second metatarsal distally, and the medial and lateral cuneiforms on each side.

The **lateral cuneiform** articulates with **six** bones: the navicular proximally, the second, third, and fourth metatarsals distally, the intermediate cuneiform medially, and the cuboid laterally.

Cuboid

The cuboid is located on the lateral aspect of the foot, distal to the calcaneus and proximal to the fourth and fifth metatarsals.

Articulations The **cuboid** articulates with **four** bones: the calcaneus proximally, the lateral cuneiform medially, and the fourth and fifth metatarsals distally. (Occasionally, it will also articulate with a fifth bone, the *navicular.*)

Arches

Longitudinal arch The bones of the foot are arranged in **longitudinal** and **transverse arches** providing a strong, shock-absorbing support for the weight of the body. The springy, longitudinal arch comprises a medial and a lateral component with most of the arch on the medial and midaspects of the foot.

Transverse arch The transverse arch is located primarily along the plantar surface of the distal tarsals and the tarsometatarsal joints. The transverse arch is primarily made up by the wedge-shaped cuneiforms, especially the smaller second and third cuneiforms in combination with the larger first cuneiform and the cuboid (Fig. 7-9).

SUMMARY OF TARSALS AND ARTICULATING BONES

1. **Calcaneus (2)**
   Cuboid
   Talus
2. **Talus (4)**
   Tibia and fibula
   Calcaneus
   Navicular
3. **Navicular (4)**
   Talus
   Three cuneiforms
4. **Medial cuneiform (4)**
   Navicular
   First and second metatarsals
   Intermediate cuneiform
5. **Intermediate cuneiform (4)**
   Navicular
   Second metatarsal
   Medial and lateral cuneiforms
6. **Lateral cuneiform (6)**
   Navicular
   Second, third, and fourth metatarsals
   Intermediate cuneiform
   Cuboid
7. **Cuboid (4)**
   Calcaneus
   Lateral cuneiform
   Fourth and fifth metatarsals

The numbers in parentheses indicate the total number of bones with which each of these tarsals articulates.

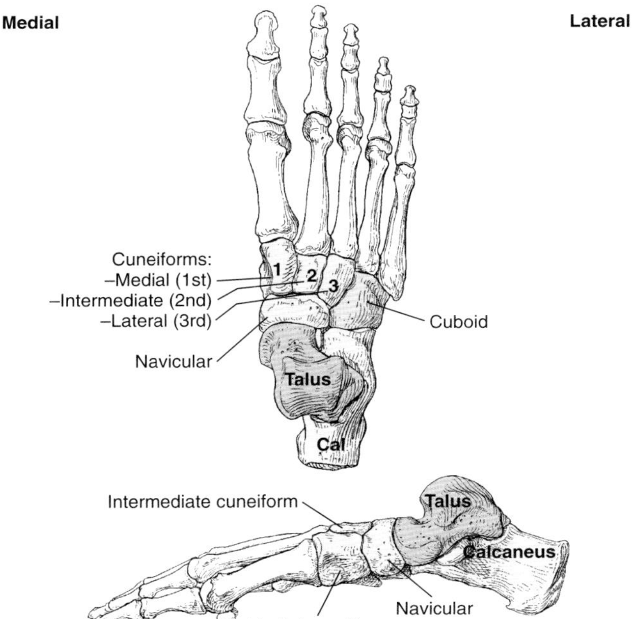

Fig. 7-8. Navicular, cuneiforms (3), and cuboid.

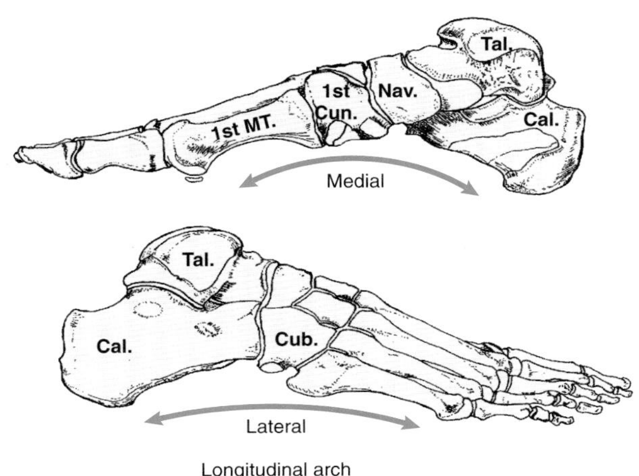

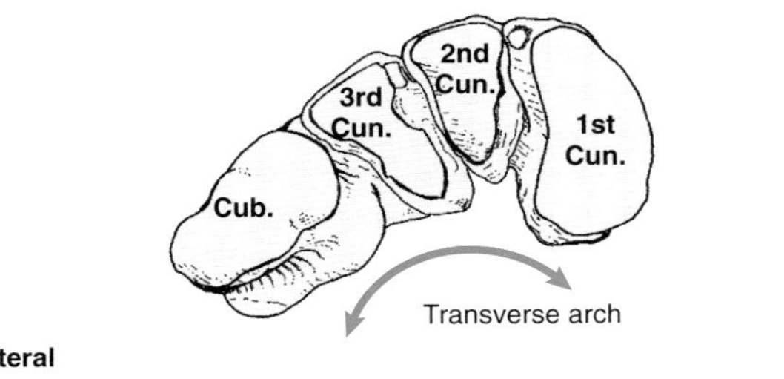

Fig. 7-9. Arches and tarsal relationships.

ANKLE JOINT

Frontal View

The **ankle joint** is formed by three bones, the two long bones of the lower leg, the **tibia** and **fibula,** and one tarsal bone, the **talus.** The expanded distal end of the slender fibula, which extends well down alongside the talus, is termed the **lateral malleolus.**

The distal end of the larger and stronger tibia has a broad articular surface for articulation with the similarly shaped broad upper surface of the talus. The medial elongated process of the tibia that extends down alongside the medial talus is termed the **medial malleolus.**

The inferior portions of the tibia and fibula form a deep "socket" or three-sided opening called a **mortise** into which the upper talus fits. The entire three-part joint space of the ankle mortise, however, is **not seen** on a true frontal view (AP projection) because of overlapping of portions of the distal fibula and tibia by the talus. This is caused by the more posterior position of the distal fibula, as shown on these drawings. A 15° internally rotated AP projection, called the **mortise position,*** will be demonstrated later (Fig. 7-15) to visualize this mortise joint that should have an even space over the entire talar surface.

The **anterior tubercle** is an expanded process at the distal anterior and lateral tibia, shown to articulate with the superolateral talus and partially overlapping the fibula anteriorly (Figs. 7-10 and 7-11).

The **distal tibial joint surface** forming the roof of the ankle mortise joint is called the **tibial plafond** (ceiling). Certain types of fractures of the ankle in children and youth involve the distal tibial epiphysis and the tibial plafond.

Lateral View

The ankle joint, seen in a true lateral position in Fig. 7-11, demonstrates that the **distal fibula is located about 1 cm or nearly ½ inch posterior in relationship to the distal tibia.** This relationship becomes important in evaluation for a **true lateral** radiograph of the leg, ankle, or foot. A common mistake in positioning a lateral ankle is to rotate the ankle slightly so that the medial and lateral malleoli are directly superimposed. However, this will result in a partially oblique ankle, as these drawings illustrate. Therefore a true lateral requires the **lateral malleolus** to be about **1 cm (½ inch) posterior** to the medial malleolus. Note also that the lateral malleolus extends about **1 cm, or nearly ½ inch, more distal** than its counterpart, the medial malleolus (best seen on frontal view, Fig. 7-10).

Axial View

An axial view of the inferior margin of the distal tibia and fibula is shown in Fig. 7-12. This visualizes an "end-on" view of the ankle joint looking from the bottom up, demonstrating the concave inferior surface of the tibia (tibial plafond). Also demonstrated are the relative positions of the **lateral** and **medial malleoli** of the fibula and tibia, respectively. The smaller **fibula** is shown to be **more posterior.** A line drawn through the midportions of the two malleoli will be approximately **15° to 20°** from the coronal plane (the true side-to-side plane of the body). Therefore the lower leg and ankle must be rotated 15° to 20° to bring the intermalleolar line parallel to the coronal plane. This relationship of the distal tibia and fibula becomes important in positioning for various views of the ankle joint or ankle mortise as described in the positioning sections of this chapter.

Ankle Joint

The ankle joint is a **synovial joint** of the **ginglymus,** or **hinge, type** with flexion and extension (dorsiflexion and plantar flexion) movements only. This requires strong collateral ligaments extending from the medial and lateral malleoli to the calcaneus and talus. Lateral stress can result in a "sprained" ankle with stretched or torn collateral ligaments and torn muscle tendons resulting in an increase in parts of the mortise joint space.

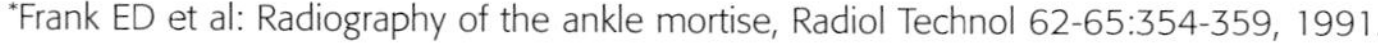

*Frank ED et al: Radiography of the ankle mortise, Radiol Technol 62-65:354-359, 1991.

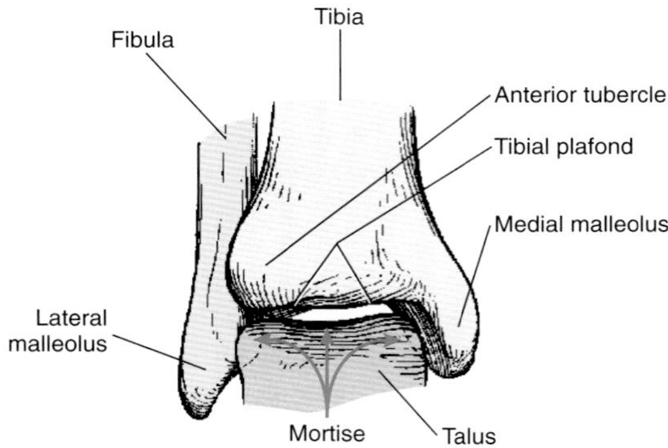

Fig. 7-10. Right ankle joint—frontal view.

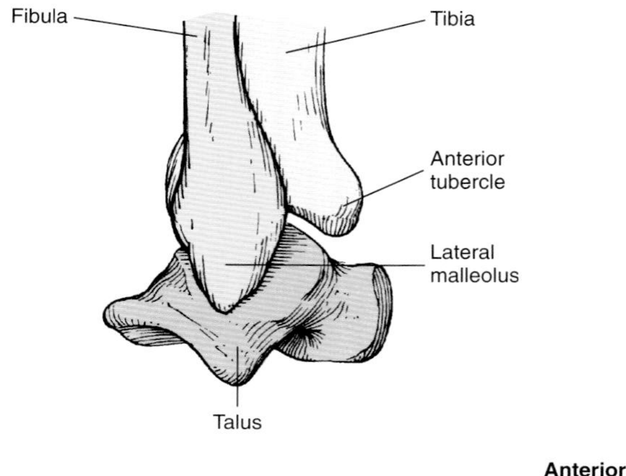

Fig. 7-11. Right ankle joint—true lateral view.

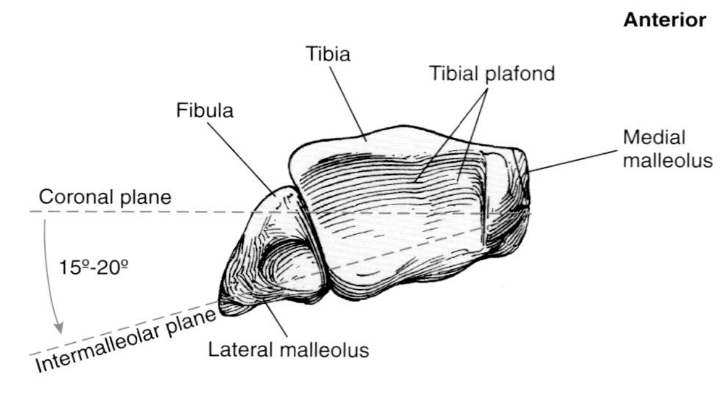

Fig. 7-12. Ankle joint—axial view. (Figs. 7-10 to 7-12 Courtesy Mayo Foundation.)

REVIEW EXERCISE WITH RADIOGRAPHS

Three common projections of the foot and ankle are shown with labels for an anatomy review of the bones and joints. A good review exercise is to cover up the answers (listed below) and identify all the labeled parts before checking the answers.

Lateral Left Foot (Fig. 7-13)

A. Tibia
B. Calcaneus
C. Tuberosity of calcaneus
D. Cuboid
E. Fifth metatarsal tuberosity
F. Superimposed cuneiforms
G. Navicular
H. Subtalar joint
I. Talus

Oblique Right Foot (Fig. 7-14)

A. Interphalangeal joint of first digit of right foot
B. Proximal phalanx of first digit of right foot
C. Metatarsophalangeal (MTP) joint of first digit of right foot
D. Head of first metatarsal
E. Body of first metatarsal
F. Base of first metatarsal
G. Second or intermediate cuneiform (partially superimposed over first or medial cuneiform)
H. Navicular
I. Talus
J. Tuberosity of calcaneus
K. Third or lateral cuneiform
L. Cuboid
M. Tuberosity of the base of the fifth metatarsal
N. Fifth metatarsophalangeal (MTP) joint of right foot
O. Proximal phalanx of fifth digit of right foot

AP Mortise View Right Ankle (Fig. 7-15)

A. Fibula
B. Lateral malleolus
C. "Open" mortise joint of ankle
D. Talus
E. Medial malleolus
F. Tibial epiphyseal plate (epiphyseal fusion site)

Lateral Ankle (Fig. 7-16)

A. Fibula
B. Calcaneus
C. Cuboid
D. Tuberosity at base of fifth metatarsal
E. Navicular
F. Talus
G. Sinus tarsi
H. Anterior tubercle
I. Tibia

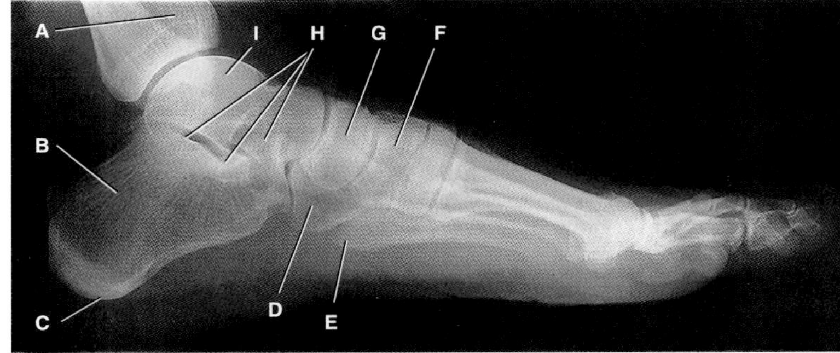

Fig. 7-13. Lateral left foot.

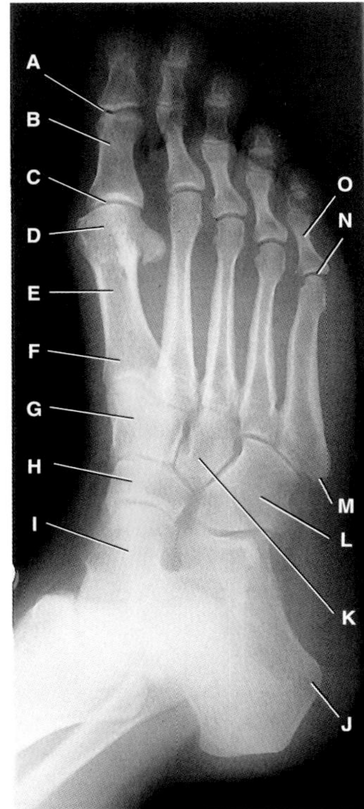

Fig. 7-14. Oblique right foot.

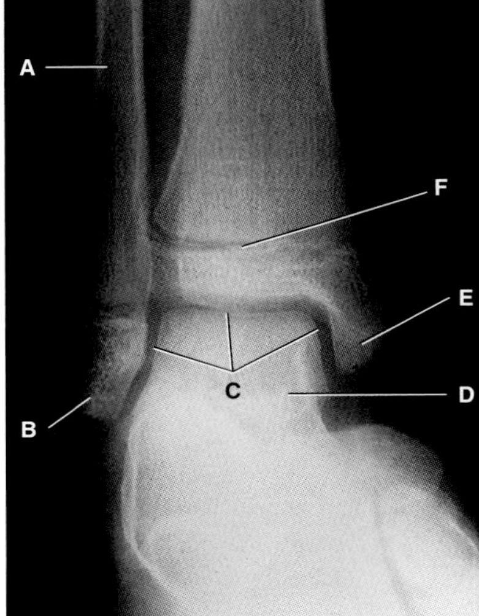

Fig. 7-15. AP right ankle (mortise view—15° medial oblique).

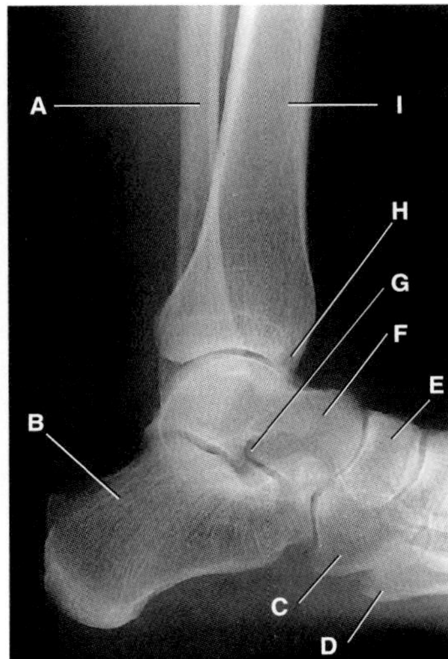

Fig. 7-16. Lateral ankle.

7

LEG—TIBIA AND FIBULA

The second group of bones of the lower limb to be studied in this chapter are the two bones of the lower leg: the **tibia** and **fibula.**

Tibia

The tibia, as one of the larger bones of the body, is the weight-bearing bone of the lower leg. The tibia can easily be felt through the skin in the anteromedial part of the leg. It is made up of three parts: the central **body** (shaft) and **two extremities.**

Proximal extremity The **medial** and **lateral condyles** are the two large processes making up the medial and lateral aspects of the proximal tibia.

The **intercondylar eminence** includes two small pointed prominences, called the **medial and lateral intercondylar tubercles,** located on the superior surface of the tibial head between the two condyles.

The upper articular surface of the condyles includes two smooth concave **articular facets,** commonly called the **tibial plateau,** which articulate with the femur. As seen on the lateral view, **the articular facets making up the tibial plateau slope posteriorly from 10° to 20°** in relationship to the long axis of the tibia (Fig. 7-18).* This is an important anatomic consideration because when you position an AP knee, the central ray must be angled as needed in relationship to the IR and tabletop to be parallel to the tibial plateau. This CR angle is essential to demonstrate an "open" joint space on an AP knee projection.

The **tibial tuberosity** on the proximal extremity of the tibia is a rough-textured prominence located on the midanterior surface of the tibia just distal to the condyles. This tuberosity is the distal attachment of the patellar tendon, which connects to the large muscle of the anterior thigh. Sometimes in young persons, the tibial tuberosity separates from the body of the tibia, a condition known as *Osgood-Schlatter disease* (see Pathologic Indications, p. 225).

The **body** (shaft) is the long portion of the tibia between the two extremities. Along the anterior surface of the body, extending from the tibial tuberosity to the medial malleolus, is a sharp ridge called the **anterior crest** or **border.** This sharp anterior crest is just under the skin surface and is often referred to as the *shin* or *shin bone.*

Distal extremity The distal extremity of the tibia is smaller than the proximal and ends in a short pyramid-shaped process called the **medial malleolus,** which is easily palpated on the medial aspect of the ankle.

The lateral aspect of the distal extremity of the tibia forms a flattened, triangular-shaped **fibular notch** for articulation with the distal fibula.

Fibula

The smaller fibula can be seen to be located **laterally** and **posteriorly** to the larger tibia. The fibula articulates with the tibia proximally and the tibia and talus distally. The proximal extremity of the fibula is expanded into a **head,** which articulates with the lateral aspect of the posteroinferior surface of the lateral condyle of the tibia. The extreme proximal aspect of the head is pointed and is known as the **apex** of the head of the fibula. The tapered area just below the head is the **neck** of the fibula.

The **body** (shaft) is the long, slender portion of the fibula between the two extremities. The enlarged distal end of the fibula can be felt as a distinct bump on the lateral aspect of the ankle joint and as described earlier is called the **lateral malleolus.**

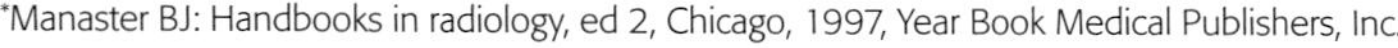

*Manaster BJ: Handbooks in radiology, ed 2, Chicago, 1997, Year Book Medical Publishers, Inc.

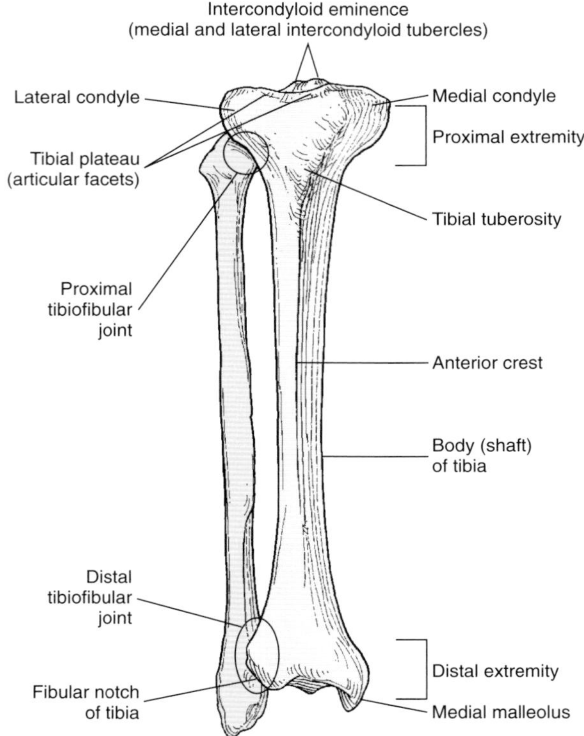

Fig. 7-17. Tibia—anterior view.

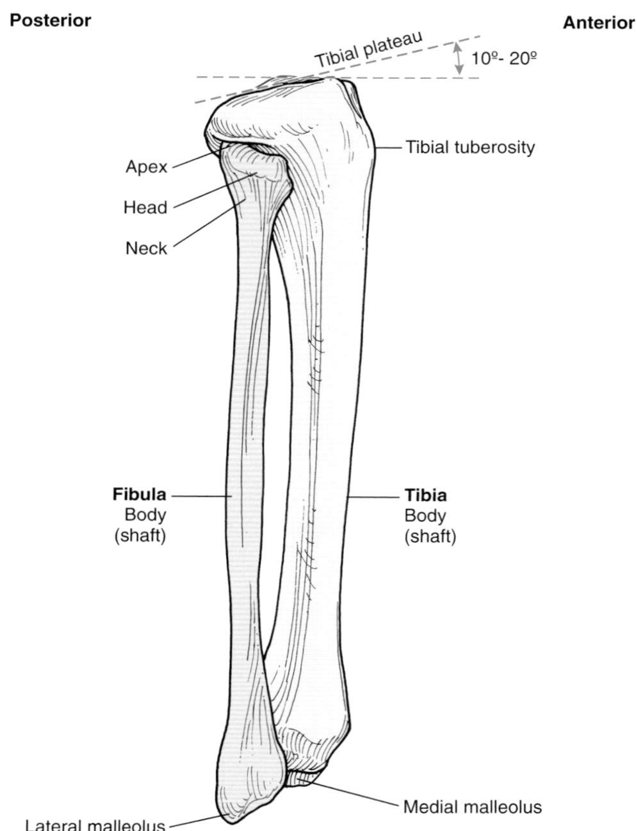

Fig. 7-18. Tibia and fibula—lateral view.

FEMUR

The **femur,** or thigh bone, is the longest and strongest bone in the entire body. The femur is the only long bone between the **hip joint** and the **knee joint.**

Key parts of the proximal femur are shown in Fig. 7-20 and will be described in detail in Chapter 8, along with the hip and pelvis.

Mid- and Distal Femur—Anterior View (Fig. 7-19)

Similar to all long bones, the body or shaft of the femur is the slender, elongated portion of the bone. The distal femur viewed anteriorly demonstrates the position of the patella or knee cap. The **patella,** which is the largest sesamoid bone in the body, is located anteriorly to the distal femur. Note that the most distal part of the patella is **above** or **proximal** to the actual knee joint by approximately ½ inch (1.25 cm) in this position with the lower leg fully extended. This relationship becomes important in positioning for the knee joint.

The **patellar surface** is the smooth and shallow, triangular-shaped depression at the distal portion of the anterior femur extending up under the lower part of the patella as seen in Fig. 7-19. This depression is also sometimes termed the **intercondylar sulcus.** (*Sulcus* means a groove or depression.) Some literature also refers to this depression as the **trochlear groove.** (*Trochlea* means pulley or pulley-shaped structure in reference to the medial and lateral condyles.) All three of these terms should be recognized as referring to this smooth, shallow depression.

Note that the patella itself is mostly superior to the patellar surface with the leg fully extended. However, as the leg is flexed, the patella, which is attached to large muscle tendons, moves distally or downward over the patellar surface. This is best shown on the lateral knee drawing (Fig. 7-21) on p. 218.

Mid- and Distal Femur—Posterior View (Fig. 7-20)

The posterior view of the distal femur best demonstrates the two large rounded condyles separated distally and posteriorly by the deep **intercondylar fossa** or notch, above which is the popliteal surface (see p. 218).

The rounded distal portions of the **medial** and **lateral condyles** contain smooth articular surfaces for articulation with the tibia. The **medial condyle extends lower or more distally** than the lateral when the femoral shaft is vertical, as in Fig. 7-20. This explains why the **CR must be angled 5° to 7° cephalad for a lateral knee** to cause the two condyles to be directly superimposed when the femur is parallel to the IR. The explanation for this is also seen in Fig. 7-19, which demonstrates that in an erect anatomic position, wherein the distal femoral condyles are parallel to the floor at the knee joint, the femoral shaft is at an angle of approximately 10° from vertical for an average adult. The range is 5° to 15°.* This angle would be greater on a short person with a wider pelvis and less on a tall person with a narrow pelvis. Therefore in general, this angle is greater on a woman than on a man.

A distinguishing difference between the medial and lateral condyles is the presence of the **adductor tubercle,** a slightly raised area that receives the tendon of an adductor muscle. This tubercle is present on the **posterolateral aspect of the medial condyle.** It is best seen on a slightly rotated lateral view of the distal femur and knee. The presence of this adductor tubercle on the medial condyle is important in critiquing a lateral knee for rotation in that it allows the viewer to determine if the knee is underrotated or overrotated to correct a positioning error when the knee is not in a true lateral position. This is shown on the radiograph in Fig. 7-33 (p. 220).

The **medial** and **lateral epicondyles,** which can be palpated, are rough prominences for attachments of ligaments and are located on the outermost portions of the condyles. The medial epicondyle, along with the adductor tubercle, is the more prominent of the two.

*Keats TE et al: Radiology 87:904, 1966.

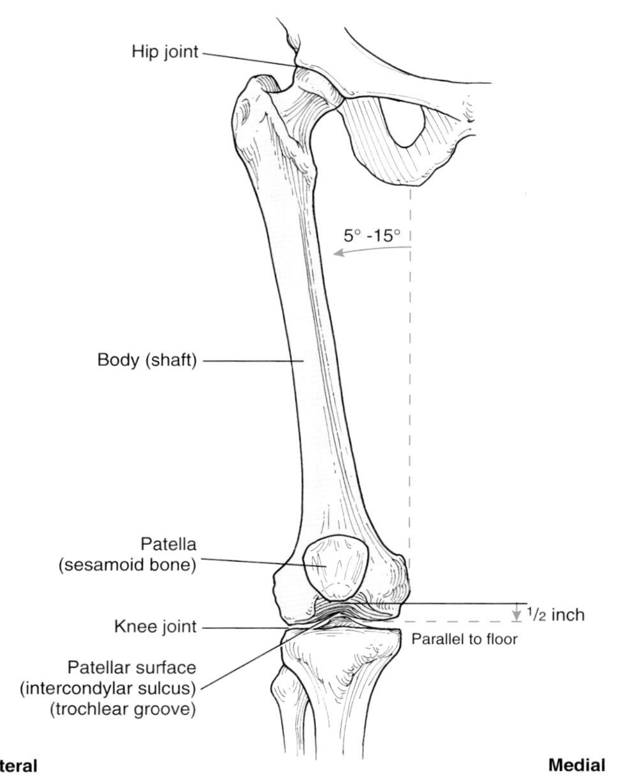

Fig. 7-19. Femur—anterior view.

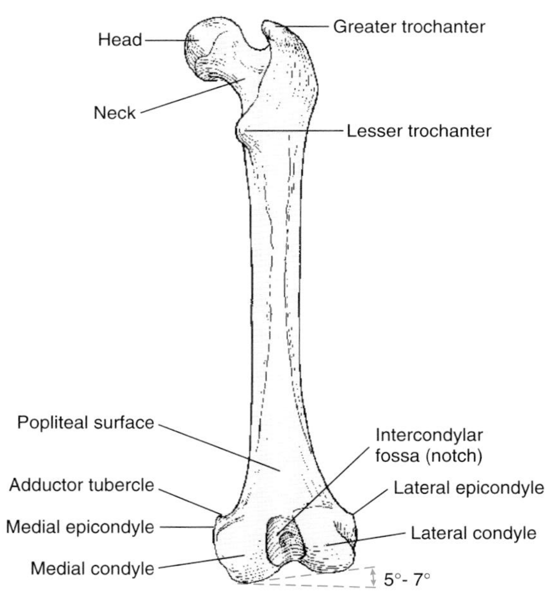

Fig. 7-20. Femur—posterior view.

7

Distal Femur and Patella (Lateral View)

The lateral view in Fig. 7-21 demonstrates the relationship of the patella to the **patellar surface** of the distal femur. The patella, as a large sesamoid bone, is embedded in the tendon of the large quadriceps femoris muscle. Therefore as the lower leg is flexed, the patella moves downward and is drawn inward into the intercondylar groove or sulcus. A partial flexion of near 45°, as shown in this drawing, shows the patella being pulled only partially downward, but with 90° flexion, the patella would move down farther over the distal portion of the femur. This movement and the relationship of the patella to the distal femur becomes important in positioning for the knee joint and for the tangential projection of the femoropatellar joint (articulation between patella and distal femur).

The posterior surface of the distal femur just proximal to the intercondylar fossa is called the **popliteal surface** over which popliteal blood vessels and nerves pass.

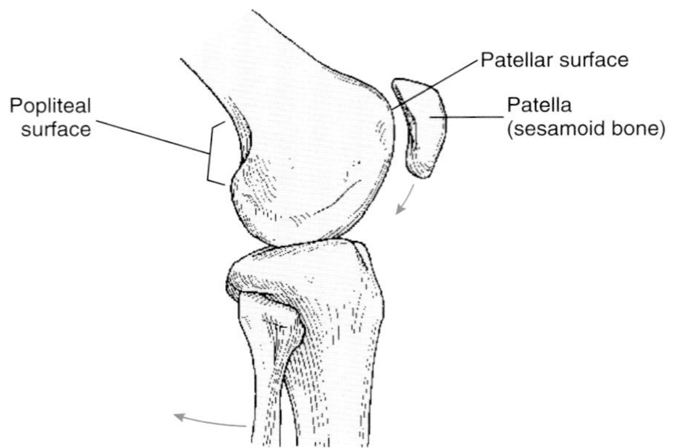

Fig. 7-21. Distal femur and patella—lateral view.

Distal Femur and Patella (Axial View)

The axial or end-on view of the distal femur again demonstrates the relationship of the patella to the **patellar surface** (intercondylar sulcus or trochlear groove) of the distal femur. The femoropatellar joint space is visualized in this axial view (Fig. 7-22). Other parts of the distal femur are also well visualized.

The **intercondylar fossa** (notch) is shown to be very deep on the posterior aspect of the femur. The **epicondyles** are seen as rough prominences on the outermost tips of the large **medial** and **lateral condyles.**

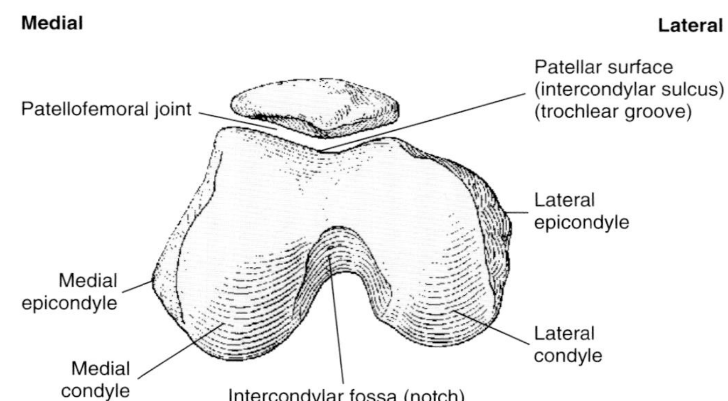

Fig. 7-22. Distal femur and patella—axial view.

Patella

The **patella** (knee cap) is a flat triangular bone about 2 inches, or 5 cm, in diameter. The patella appears to be upside down because its pointed **apex** is located along the **inferior border** and its **base** is the **superior** or **upper border.** The outer or **anterior surface** is convex and rough, and the inner **posterior surface** is smooth and oval-shaped for articulation with the femur. The patella serves to protect the anterior aspect of the knee joint and acts as a pivot to increase the leverage of the large quadriceps femoris muscle, the tendon of which attaches to the tibial tuberosity of the lower leg. The patella is somewhat loose and movable in its more superior position when the leg is extended and the quadriceps muscles are relaxed. However, as the leg is flexed and the muscles tighten, it moves distally and becomes locked into position. It should be noted that the patella articulates only with the femur, not with the tibia.

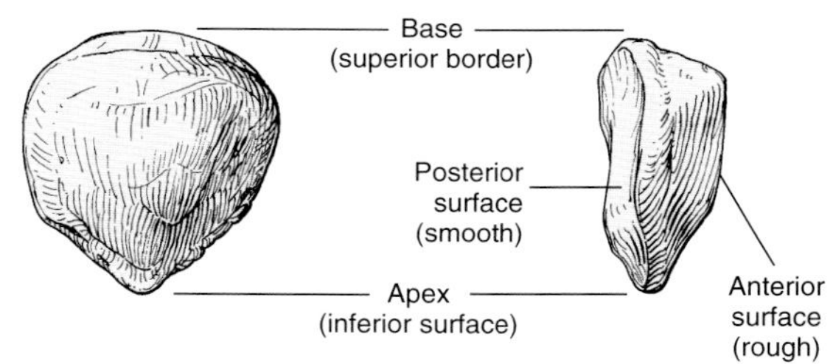

Fig. 7-23. Patella.

KNEE JOINT

The knee joint proper is a large complex joint primarily involving the **femorotibial joint** between the two condyles of the **femur** and the corresponding condyles of the **tibia.** The **patellofemoral joint** is also part of the knee joint, wherein the patella articulates with the anterior surface of the distal femur.

Proximal Tibiofibular Joint and Major Knee Ligaments

The proximal fibula is not part of the knee joint because it does not articulate with any aspect of the femur, even though the **fibular lateral collateral ligament (LCL)** extends from the femur to the lateral proximal fibula as shown in Fig. 7-24. The head of the fibula, however, does articulate with the lateral condyle of the tibia, to which it is attached by this ligament.

Additional major knee ligaments shown on this posterior view are the **tibial (medial) collateral ligament (MCL),** located medially, and the major **posterior** and **anterior cruciate** *(kroo'she-at)* **ligaments** (PCL and ACL), located within the knee joint capsule. (Note that the abbreviations **ACL, PCL, LCL,** and **MCL** are commonly used to refer to these four ligaments.*) The knee joint is highly dependent on these two important pairs of major ligaments for stability.

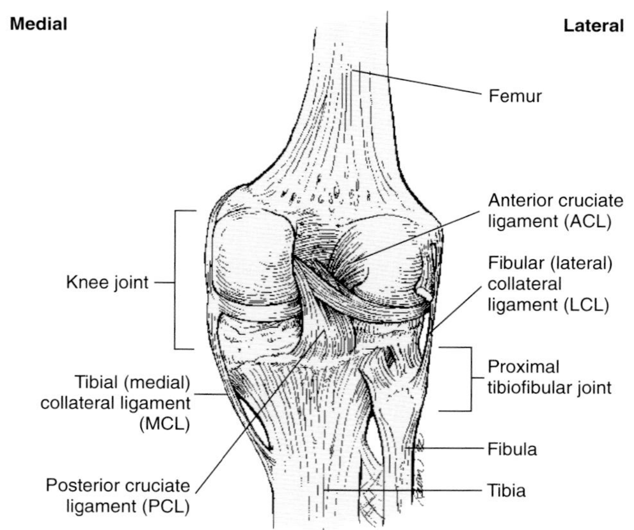

Fig. 7-24. Knee joint and proximal tibiofibular joint—posterior view.

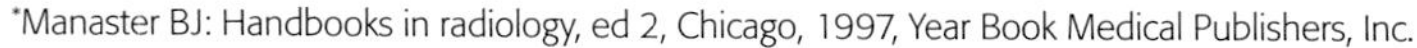

*Manaster BJ: Handbooks in radiology, ed 2, Chicago, 1997, Year Book Medical Publishers, Inc.

KNEE JOINT—Cont'd

The two **collateral ligaments** are strong bands at the sides of the knee that **prevent adduction and abduction** movements at the knee. The two **cruciate ligaments** are strong, rounded cords that cross each other as they attach to the respective anterior and posterior aspects of the intercondylar eminence of the tibia. They stabilize the knee joint by **preventing anterior or posterior movement** within the knee joint.

In addition to these two major pair of ligaments, an anteriorly located **patellar ligament** and various minor ligaments exist that help in maintaining the integrity of the knee joint (Fig. 7-26). The patellar ligament is shown as part of the tendon of insertion of the large quadriceps femoris muscle extending over the patella to the tibial tuberosity. The **infrapatellar fat pad** is posterior to this ligament, which aids in protecting the anterior aspect of the knee joint.

Synovial Membrane and Cavity

The articular cavity of the knee joint is the largest joint space of the human body. The total knee joint is a synovial type enclosed in an **articular capsule,** or **bursa.** It is a complex saclike structure filled with a lubricating-type synovial fluid. This is demonstrated in the arthrogram radiograph, wherein a combination of negative and positive contrast media has been injected into the articular capsule or bursa (Fig. 7-28).

The articular cavity, or bursa, of the knee joint extends upwards under and superior to the patella, identified as the **suprapatellar bursa** (Fig. 7-26). Distal to the patella, the **infrapatellar bursa** is separated by a large **infrapatellar fat pad,** which can be identified on radiographs. The spaces posterior and distal to the femur can also be seen and are filled with negative contrast media on the lateral arthrogram radiograph.

Menisci (Articular Disks)

The **medial** and **lateral menisci** *(me-nis'ci)* are fibrocartilage disks between the articular facets of the tibia (tibial plateau) and the femoral condyles (Fig. 7-27). They are crescent-shaped and are thicker at their external margins and taper to a very thin center portion. They act as shock absorbers to reduce some of the direct impact and stress occurring at the knee joint. Along with the synovial membrane, the menisci are also believed to function in producing synovial fluid, which acts as a lubricant for the articulating ends of the femur and tibia that are covered with a tough, slick hyaline membrane.

Knee Trauma

The knee has great potential for traumatic injury, especially in activities such as skiing or snowboarding, or in contact sports such as football or basketball. For example, a tear of the tibial (medial) collateral ligament (MCL) is frequently associated with a tear of the anterior cruciate ligament (ACL) and a tear of the medial meniscus. Patients with these injuries typically come to the imaging department for either an MRI (magnetic resonance imaging) exam to visualize these soft-tissue structures of the knee or a knee arthrogram.

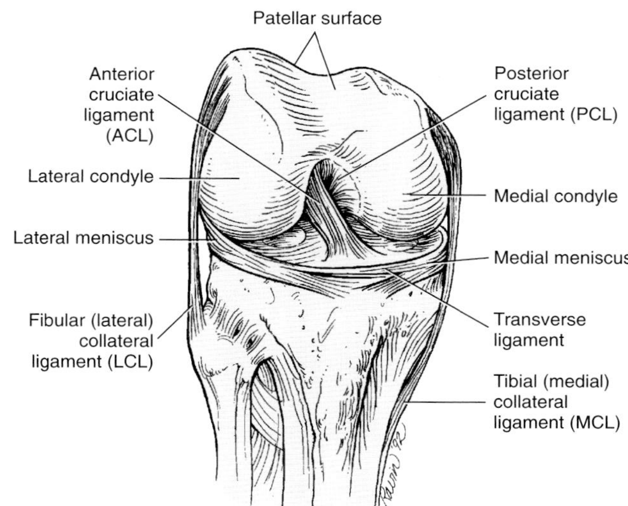

Fig. 7-25. Right knee joint (flexed)—**anterior** view.

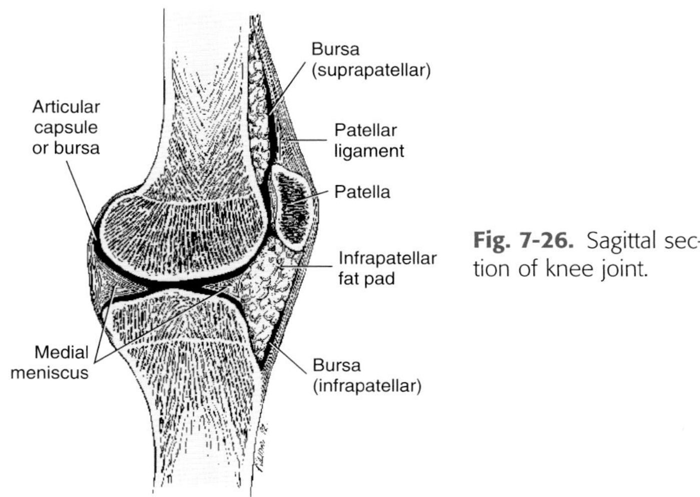

Fig. 7-26. Sagittal section of knee joint.

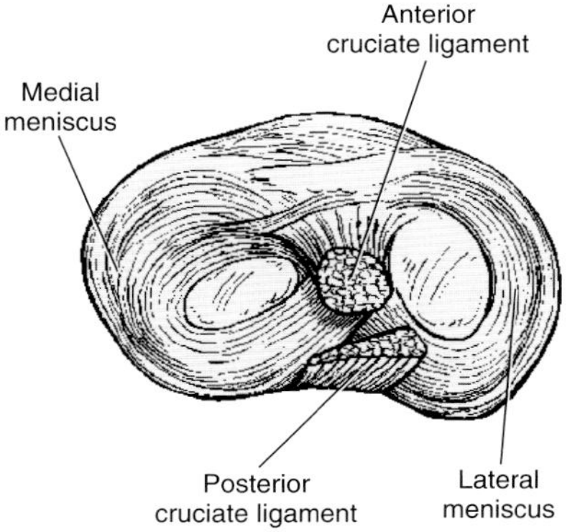

Fig. 7-27. Superior view of articular surface of tibia (shows menisci and cruciate ligament attachments).

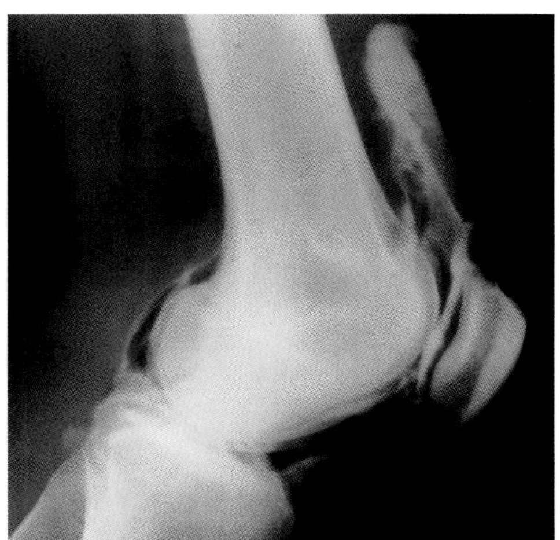

Fig. 7-28. Lateral knee arthrogram radiograph (demonstrates articular capsule or bursa as outlined by a combination of negative and positive contrast media).

REVIEW EXERCISE WITH RADIOGRAPHS

Common projections of the leg, knee, and patella are shown with labels for an anatomy review.

AP Leg (Fig. 7-29)
A. Medial condyle of the tibia
B. Body or shaft of tibia
C. Medial malleolus
D. Lateral malleolus
E. Body or shaft of fibula
F. Neck of fibula
G. Head of fibula
H. Apex (styloid process) of head of fibula
I. Lateral condyle of tibia
J. Intercondylar eminence (tibial spine)

Lateral Leg (Fig. 7-30)
A. Intercondylar eminence (tibial spine)
B. Tibial tuberosity
C. Body or shaft of tibia
D. Body or shaft of fibula
E. Medial malleolus
F. Lateral malleolus

AP Knee (Fig. 7-31)
A. Medial and lateral intercondylar tubercles; extensions of intercondylar eminence (tibial spine)
B. Lateral epicondyle of femur
C. Lateral condyle of femur
D. Lateral condyle of tibia
E. Articular facets of tibia (tibial plateau)
F. Medial condyle of tibia
G. Medial condyle of femur
H. Medial epicondyle of femur
I. Patella (seen through femur)

Lateral Knee (Fig. 7-32)
A. Base of patella
B. Apex of patella
C. Tibial tuberosity
D. Neck of fibula
E. Head of fibula
F. Apex (styloid process) of head of fibula
G. Superimposed medial and lateral condyles
H. Patellar surface (intercondylar sulcus or trochlear groove)

Lateral Knee (Fig. 7-33)
(Demonstrating some rotation)
I. Adductor tubercle
J. Lateral condyle
K. Medial condyle

Tangential Projection (Femoropatellar Joint) (Fig. 7-34)
A. Patella
B. Femoropatellar joint
C. Lateral condyle
D. Patellar surface (intercondylar sulcus, trochlear groove)
E. Medial condyle

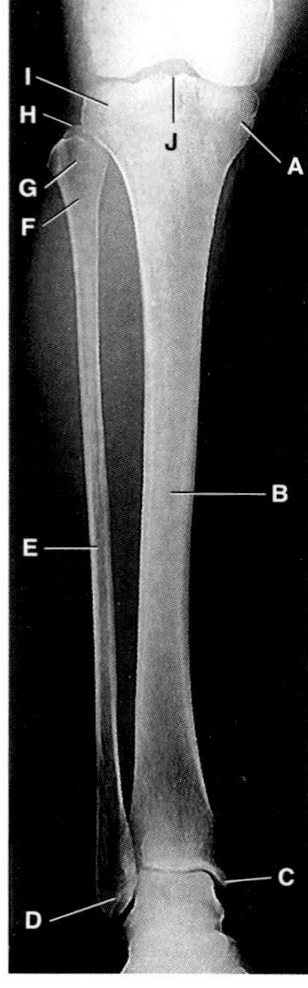

Fig. 7-29. AP leg.

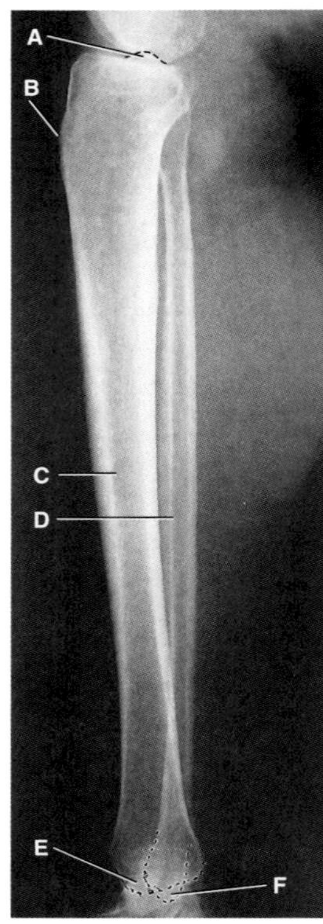

Fig. 7-30. Lateral leg.

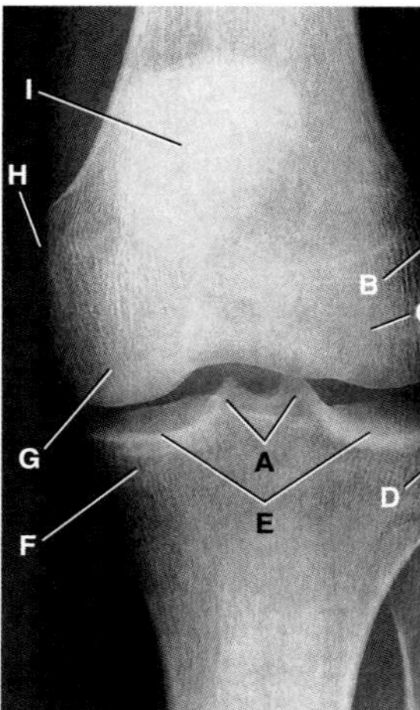

Fig. 7-31. AP knee.

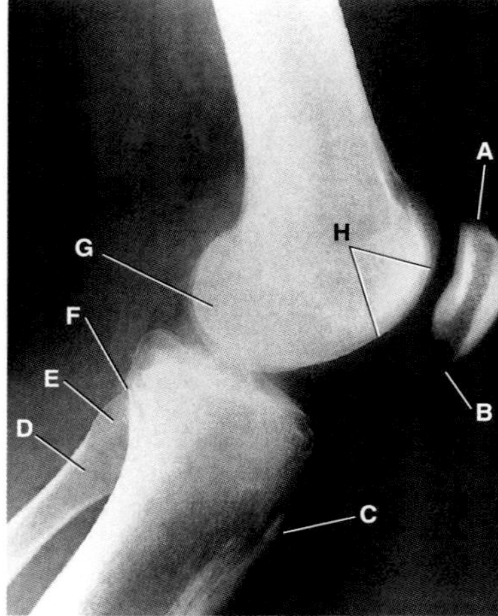

Fig. 7-32. Lateral knee—true lateral.

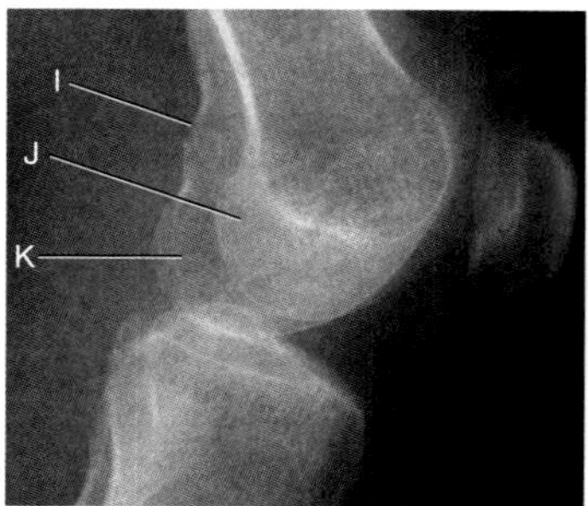

Fig. 7-33. Slightly rotated lateral knee (medial condyle more posterior).

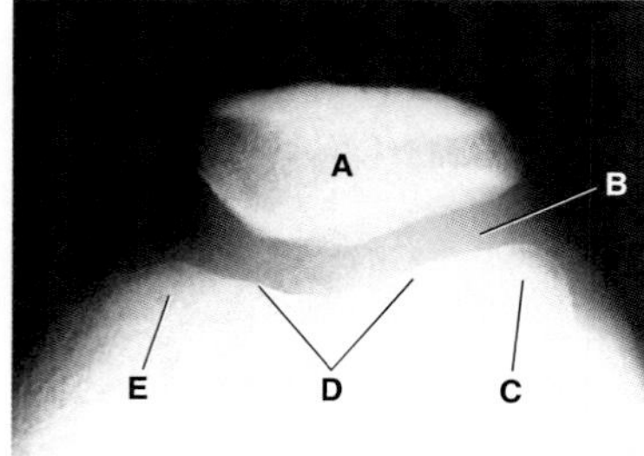

Fig. 7-34. Tangential projection (femoropatellar joint).

CLASSIFICATION OF JOINTS

The joints or articulations of the lower limb are (with one exception) all classified as **synovial joints,** characterized by a fibrous-type capsule containing synovial fluid. Therefore they also are (with the one exception) **diarthrodial,** or freely movable.

The one exception to the synovial joint is the **distal tibiofibular joint,** which is classified as a **fibrous joint** with fibrous interconnections between the surfaces of the tibia and fibula. It is of the **syndesmosis type** and is only slightly **movable,** or **amphiarthrodial.** The most distal part of this joint, however, is smooth and lined with a synovial membrane that is continuous with the ankle joint.

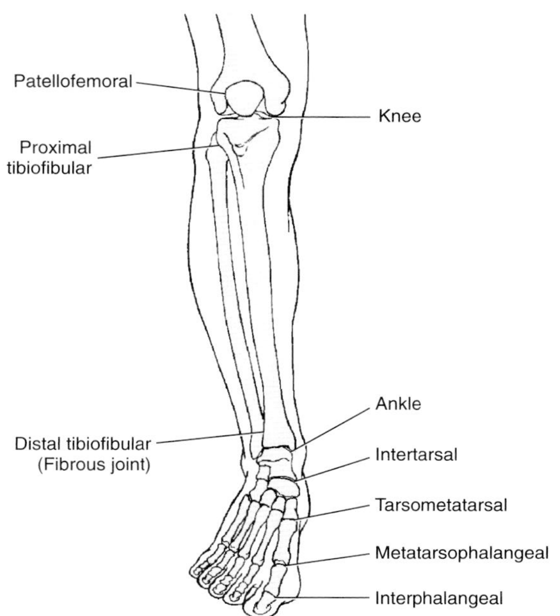

Fig. 7-35. Joints of lower limb.

7

SUMMARY OF FOOT, ANKLE, LEG, AND KNEE JOINTS — ALL JOINTS OF LOWER LIMB EXCEPT DISTAL TIBIOFIBULAR

Classification:	*Synovial (articular capsule containing synovial fluid)*
Mobility type:	*Diarthrodial (freely movable)*
Movement type:	
1. Interphalangeal joints	***Ginglymus or hinge:*** Flexion and extension movements
2. Metatarsophalangeal joints	***Modified ellipsoidal or condyloid:*** Flexion, extension, abduction, and adduction (Circumduction similar to the metacarpophalangeal joints of the hand is generally not possible)
3. Tarsometatarsal joints	***Plane or gliding:*** Limited gliding movement
4. Intertarsal joints	***Plane or gliding:*** Subtalar in combination with some other intertarsal joints provides for gliding and rotation; results in inversion and eversion of the foot
5. Ankle joint	***Ginglymus or hinge:*** Dorsiflexion and plantar flexion only (side-to-side movements only occur with stretched or torn ligaments)
6. Knee joint(s):	
Femorotibial	***Special type—ginglymus or hinge:*** Flexion and extension and some gliding and rotational movements when knee is partially flexed
Patellofemoral	***Sellar or saddle:*** Considered a saddle type because of its shape and relationship of the patella to the distal femur
7. Proximal tibiofibular joint	***Plane or gliding:*** Limited gliding movement between lateral condyle and head of fibula
Distal tibiofibular	
Classification:	*Fibrous*
Mobility type:	Amphiarthrodial *(slightly movable) of the* ***syndesmosis*** *type*

SURFACES AND PROJECTIONS OF FOOT

Surfaces: The surfaces of the foot are sometimes confusing because the top or anterior surface of the foot is called the **dorsum.** *Dorsal* usually refers to the posterior part of the body. *Dorsum,* in this case, comes from the term **dorsum pedis**, which refers to the upper surface, or the surface opposite the sole of the foot.

The sole of the foot is the **posterior** surface or **plantar surface.** Using these terms, one can describe the common projections of the foot.

Projections: The **anteroposterior (AP) projection** of the foot is the same as a **dorsoplantar (DP) projection.** The less common **posteroanterior (PA) projection** can also be called a **plantodorsal (PD) projection.** Technologists should be familiar with each of these projection terms and know which projection they represent.

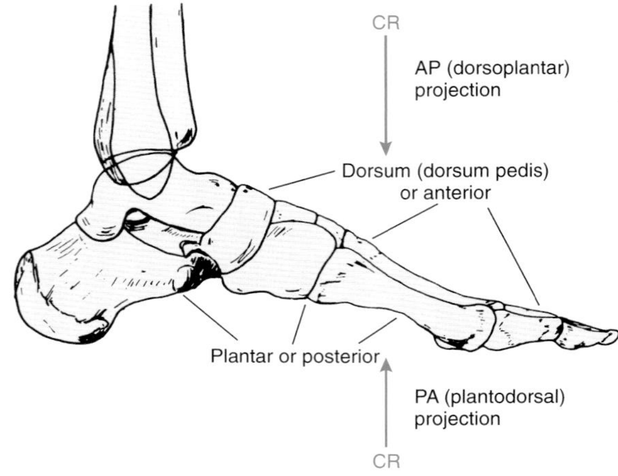

Fig. 7-36. Surfaces and projections of foot.

MOTIONS OF FOOT AND ANKLE

Other potentially confusing terms involving the ankle and intertarsal joints are **dorsiflexion, plantar flexion, inversion,** and **eversion.** To decrease the angle (flex) between the dorsum pedis and the anterior part of the lower leg is to **dorsiflex** at the ankle joint. Extending the ankle joint or pointing the foot and toe downward with respect to the normal position is termed *plantar flexion.*

Inversion, or **varus,** is an inward turning or bending of the ankle and subtalar (talocalcaneal) joints, and **eversion,** or **valgus,** is an outward turning or bending. The lower leg does not rotate during inversion or eversion. Most sprained ankles result from an accidental forced inversion or eversion.

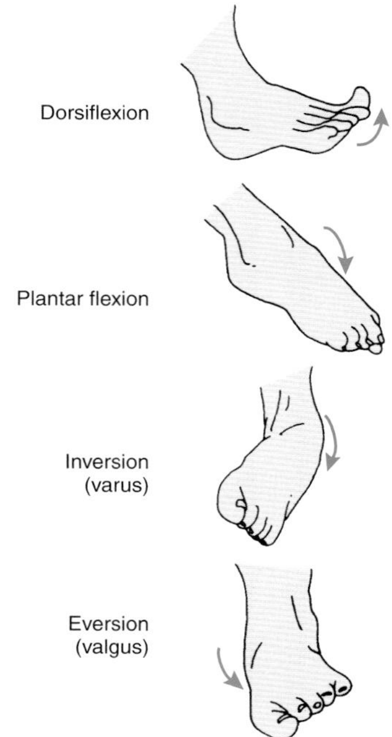

Fig. 7-37. Motions of foot and ankle.

RADIOGRAPHIC POSITIONING

Positioning Considerations

Radiographic examinations involving the lower limb below the knee are generally done on a tabletop as shown in Fig. 7-38. Severe trauma cases or patients who are difficult to move can also be radiographed directly on the cart.

DISTANCE

A common minimum SID (source-image receptor distance) is 40 inches, or 100 cm. When you are radiographing with cassettes directly on the tabletop, to maintain a constant SID, increase the tube height as compared with radiographs taken with the cassette in the Bucky tray. This difference is generally 3 to 4 inches (8 to 10 cm) for floating-type tabletops. The same minimum 40 inches (100 cm) SID should also be used when you are radiographing directly on the cart, unless exposure factors are adjusted to compensate for a change in SID.

GONADAL SHIELDING

Gonadal shielding is important for exams of the lower limb because of the proximity of the gonads to the divergent x-ray beam and scatter radiation. Therefore a lead vinyl-covered shield should be draped over the patient's gonadal area as shown. Even though the gonadal rule states this should be done on patients of reproductive age when the gonads lie within or close to the primary field, providing gonadal shielding for all patients is good practice.

Bucky Tray Out of Exposure Field A good practice for all tabletop exams of the lower limb is to move the Bucky tray, which is not being used, up under the pelvic region and out from under the exposure field to reduce possible scatter and secondary rays from these structures when they are in the x-ray field under the tabletop.

COLLIMATION

The collimation rule should again be followed: namely, that **collimation borders should be visible on all four sides if the IR is large enough to allow this without cutting off essential anatomy.** A general rule concerning IR size is to **use the smallest IR size possible for the specific part being radiographed.** Four-sided collimation is generally possible, however, even with a minimal size IR for most if not all radiographic exams of the lower limb.

Two or more projections may be taken on one IR for some exams such as for the toes, foot, ankle, or lower leg. This requires close collimation of the part being radiographed.

With **digital imaging,** such as with computed radiography (CR), lead masks should be used to cover the parts of the IR not in the collimation field. The reason for this is fogging from scatter radiation because of the hypersensitivity of the image receptor plates.

Four-sided collimation allows for checking radiographs for accuracy of centering and positioning by placing a large imaginary "X" from the four corners of the collimation field. The center point of the "X" indicates the CR location.

GENERAL POSITIONING

A general positioning rule, especially applicable to both the upper and lower limbs, is to **always place the long axis of the part being radiographed parallel to the long axis of the IR.** If more than one projection is taken on the same IR, the part should be parallel to the long axis of the part of the IR being used. Also, **all body parts should be oriented in the same direction,** when two or more projections are taken on the same IR.

An exception to this rule is the lower leg of an adult. This limb generally has to be placed diagonally to include both the knee and the ankle joints as shown in Fig. 7-38.

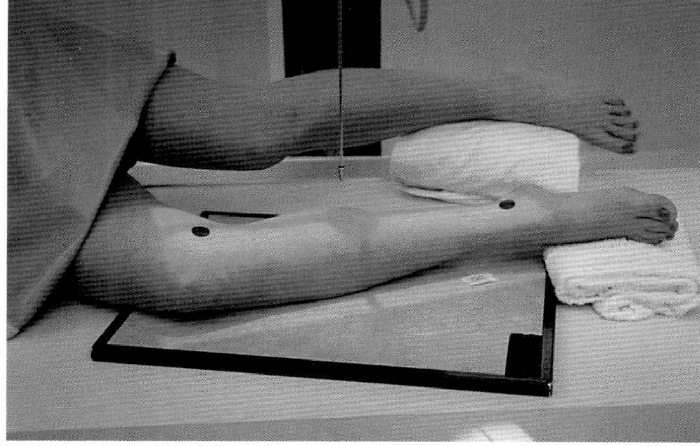

Fig. 7-38. Tabletop mediolateral projection of lower limb demonstrating the following:
- Correct CR location
- Good collimation
- Gonadal shielding
- Diagonal placement of the IR to include both knee and ankle joints

CORRECT CENTERING

Accurate centering and alignment of the body part to the IR and correct central ray location are especially important for exams of the upper and lower limbs, where shape and size distortion must be avoided and the narrow joint spaces clearly demonstrated. Therefore in general, the part being radiographed should **be parallel to the plane of the IR—the central ray should be 90° or perpendicular and should be directed to the correct centering point,** as indicated on each positioning page. (Exceptions to the 90° or perpendicular CR do occur, as indicated in the following pages.)

EXPOSURE FACTORS

The principal exposure factors for radiographs of the lower limbs are as follows:

1. Lower-to-medium kV (50-70)
2. Short exposure time
3. Small focal spot
4. Adequate mAs for sufficient density

Correctly exposed radiographs of the lower limbs should generally visualize both soft-tissue margins and fine bony trabecular markings of bones being radiographed.

Optional Technique for Foot An increase to 70 or 75 kV with accompanying decrease in mAs will increase exposure latitude to result in a more uniform exposure density between the phalanges and the tarsals.

IMAGE RECEPTORS

For exams distal to the knee, image receptors without grids are generally used. With film and screen imaging, detail (extremity) screens are commonly used for adult extremities for better detail.

Grids: A general rule states that grids should be used with body parts measuring more than 10 cm. (Some references suggest a grid for more than 13 cm.) This rule places the average knee (measuring 9 to 13 cm) at a size where either a screen or grid may be used depending on patient size and departmental preferences. This text recommends a screen on smaller patients measuring 10 cm or less and a grid for larger patients measuring more than 10 cm, especially on the AP knee. Anything proximal to the knee such as the mid- or distal femur requires the use of a grid. When grids are used, you may choose either the moving Bucky grid under the tabletop or a fine-lined portable grid.

Positioning Considerations—cont'd

PEDIATRIC APPLICATIONS

Pediatric patients should be addressed in language that they are able to understand. Parents are often helpful in positioning younger children in nontrauma situations. If parents are allowed to stay in the room, they must be provided appropriate shielding. Immobilization will be needed in many cases to assist the child in holding the limb in the proper position. Sponges and tape are very useful, but sandbags should be used with caution because of their weight. Accurate part measurement is critical to setting technical factors.

In general, exposure factors must be decreased because of the decrease in tissue quantity and density. Shorter exposure times, along with the highest mA possible, will help to eliminate motion on the radiograph.

GERIATRIC APPLICATIONS

Older patients must be handled carefully when being moved, and radiography of the lower limbs is no exception. Look for telltale signs of hip fractures (i.e., foot in extreme external rotation position). Routine positioning maneuvers may need to be adjusted to accommodate patients' potential pathology and lack of joint flexibility. Positioning aids and supports should be used to increase patient comfort and assist in immobilizing the limb in the correct position.

Exposure factors may require adjustment because of underlying pathologic conditions such as osteoarthritis or osteoporosis. Shorter exposure time and higher mA are desirable to reduce the possibility of imaging involuntary or voluntary motion.

PLACEMENT OF MARKERS AND PATIENT ID INFORMATION

At the top of each of the following positioning pages is a small rectangular diagram demonstrating the correct IR size and placement (lengthwise or crosswise). A suggested corner placement for the patient ID blocker is shown for each IR. However, this is only a suggested location, because the location of the blocker changes with each manufacturer. The important consideration is to **always place it in the location least likely to superimpose anatomy of interest** for that projection.

The size and location of multiple projections on one receptor are also shown.

When evaluating final radiographs as part of the evaluation criteria, the patient ID information should always be checked to see whether it is legible and not superimposing essential anatomy. Right (R) and left (L) markers should always be visible on the lateral margin of the collimation field **on at least one projection on each IR** without superimposing any anatomy of interest.

INCREASE EXPOSURE WITH CAST

A lower limb with a cast requires an increase in exposure. The thickness of the cast and the body part and the type of cast will affect the increase in exposure required. A recommended conversion guide for casts is as follows:

CAST CONVERSION CHART

TYPE OF CAST	INCREASE IN EXPOSURE
Small-to-medium plaster cast	Increase mAs 50%-60% or +5-7 kV
Large plaster cast	Increase mAs 100% or +8-10 kV
Fiberglas cast	Increase mAs 25%-30% or +3-4 kV

Digital Imaging Considerations

Following is a summary of guidelines that should be followed when using digital imaging technology (CR or DR) for the lower limbs.

1. **Collimination:** Close collimation is important to provide accurate information to the processing computer regarding the exposure index number.
2. **30% rule:** Most CR systems require that at least 30% of the image plate needs to be exposed to obtain an accurate exposure index value
3. **Lead masking:** Generally most CR systems allow multiple projections on one image plate if both accurate collimation and lead masking are used.
4. **Accurate centering:** For accurate post-processing by the image reader, it is important that the body part and central ray be accurately centered to the IR.
5. **Grid use with DR:** Grids are generally used with DR imaging. With these systems it may be impractical and difficult to remove the grid. Therefore it is commonly left in place even for smaller body parts measuring 10 cm or less, such as for some upper and lower limb exams.
6. **Exposure factors:** It is important that the ALARA principle be followed and the lowest exposure factors required to obtain a diagnostic image be used. This includes the highest kV and the lowest mAs that will result in desirable image quality. May need to increase kV over film-screen imaging for larger body parts, with 60 kV as the minimum on any procedure (exception is mammography).
7. **Post-processing evaluation of exposure index values:** The exposure index number on the final processed image must be checked to verify that the exposure factors used were in the correct range to ensure optimum quality with the least radiation to the patient.

Alternative Modalities or Procedures

ARTHROGRAPHY

Arthrography is commonly used to image large diarthrodial joints such as the knee. This procedure requires the use of a contrast medium injected into the joint capsule under sterile conditions. Disease or traumatic damage to the menisci, ligaments, and articular cartilage may be evaluated with arthrography (see Chapter 4).

COMPUTED TOMOGRAPHY

Computed tomography is often used on the lower limbs to evaluate soft-tissue involvement of lesions. The cross-sectional images are also excellent for determining the extent of fractures and evaluation of bone mineralization.

MAGNETIC RESONANCE IMAGING

Magnetic resonance imaging (MRI) may be used to image the lower limbs when soft-tissue injuries are suspected. The knee is the most often evaluated portion of the lower limb, and MRI is invaluable in detecting ligament damage or meniscal tears of the joint capsule. MRI may also be used to evaluate lesions in the skeletal system.

BONE DENSITOMETRY

Bone densitometry may be used to evaluate the loss of bone in geriatric patients or in patients with a lytic (bone-destroying) type of bone disease (see Chapter 23 for more information on bone density measurement procedures).

NUCLEAR MEDICINE

Nuclear medicine uses radioisotopes injected into the bloodstream. These isotopes are absorbed in great concentration in areas where pathologic conditions exist. Nuclear medicine bone scans are particularly useful in demonstrating osteomyelitis and metastatic bone lesions.

Pathologic Indications

Radiographers should be familiar with those more common pathologic indications relating to the lower limb as follows:

Bone cysts are benign, neoplastic bone lesions filled with clear fluid that most often occur near the knee joint in children and adolescents. Generally, these are not detected on radiographs until a pathologic fracture occurs. When bone cysts are detected on radiographs, they appear as lucent areas with a thin cortex and sharp boundaries.

Chondromalacia patellae (commonly known as *runner's knee*) involves a softening of the cartilage under the patella, which results in wearing away of this cartilage, causing pain and tenderness of this area. Cyclists and runners are vulnerable to this condition.

Chondrosarcomas are malignant tumors of the cartilage that usually occur in the pelvis and long bones of men over age 45.

Enchondroma is a slow-growing **benign cartilaginous tumor** most often found in small bones of hands and feet of adolescents and young adults. Generally, these are well-defined, radiolucent-appearing tumors with thin cortex, often leading to pathologic fractures with only minimal trauma.

Ewing's sarcoma is a common **primary malignant bone tumor** in children and young adults, arising from bone marrow. Symptoms are similar to osteomyelitis, with low-grade fever and pain. Bone has stratified new bone formation, resulting in an "onion peel" look on radiographs. Ewing's sarcoma most generally occurs in the diaphysis of long bones. Unfortunately, prognosis is poor by the time it is evident on radiographs.

Exostosis (osteochondroma) is a benign, neoplastic bone lesion caused by a consolidated overproduction of bone at a joint (usually the knee). The tumor grows parallel to the bone and away from the adjacent joint. Tumor growth stops as soon as epiphyseal plates close. Pain is an associated symptom if the tumor is large enough to irritate surrounding soft tissues.

Fractures are breaks in the structure of bone caused by a force (direct or indirect). Several types of fracture exist, named according to the extent of fracture, direction of the fracture lines, alignment of bone fragments, and integrity of the overlying skin (see Chapter 19 for fracture types and descriptions).

Gout is a form of arthritis that may be hereditary in which uric acid appears in excessive quantities in the blood and may be deposited in the joints and other tissue; common initial attacks occur in the **first MTP joint** of the foot. Later attacks may also occur in other joints, such as the first MCP joint of the hand, but generally these are not seen radiographically until more advanced conditions develop. Most cases occur in men, and first attacks rarely occur before age 30.

Joint effusions are accumulated fluid (synovial or hemorrhagic) in the joint cavity. This is a sign of an underlying condition (i.e., fracture, dislocation, or soft-tissue damage).

Multiple myeloma is the most common type of **primary cancerous bone tumor.** Generally, these tumors affect persons between the ages of 40 to 70 years. As the name implies, they occur in various parts of the body. Because this tumor arises from bone marrow or marrow plasma cells, it is not a truly exclusive bony tumor. Multiple myelomas are highly malignant and usually fatal within a few years. The typical radiographic appearance is multiple "punched-out" osteolytic (loss of calcium in bone) lesions scatted throughout the affected bones.

Osgood Schlatter disease is an inflammation of the bone and cartilage involving the anterior proximal tibia and is most common in boys ages 10 to 15. The cause is believed to be an injury that occurs when the large patellar tendon detaches part of the **tibial tuberosity** to which it is attached. Severe cases may require immobilization by a plaster cast.

Osteoarthritis, also called *degenerative joint disease (DJD),* is a noninflammatory joint disease characterized by gradual deterioration of the articular cartilage with hypertrophic (enlargement or overgrown) bone formation. This is the most common type of arthritis; it is considered a normal part of the aging process

Osteoclastomas (giant cell tumors) are benign lesions that typically occur in long bones of young adults; they usually occur in the proximal tibia or distal femur after epiphyseal closure. These tumors appear on radiographs as large "bubbles" separated by thin stripes of bone.

Osteogenic sarcomas (osteosarcomas) are **highly malignant primary bone tumors** that occur during childhood to young adulthood (peak age, 20). The neoplasm usually occurs in long bones and may cause gross destruction of bone.

Osteoid osteomas are **benign bone lesions** that usually occur in teenagers or young adults. Symptoms include localized pain that typically worsens at night but is relieved by over-the-counter antiinflammatory or pain medications. The tibia and the femur are the most likely locations of these lesions.

Osteomalacia (rickets) literally means *bone softening.* This disease is caused by a lack of bone mineralization because of a deficiency of calcium, phosphorus, and/or vitamin D in the diet or an inability to absorb these minerals. Because of the softness of the bones, bowing defects in weight-bearing parts often result. This disease is known as *rickets* in children and commonly results in bowing of the tibia.

Paget's disease (osteitis deformans) is one of the most common diseases of the skeleton. It is most common in midlife and is twice as common in men than in women. It is a nonneoplastic bone disease that disrupts new bone growth, resulting in an overproduction of very dense, yet soft bone. Bone destruction creates lytic or lucent areas followed by reconstruction of bone, creating sclerotic or dense areas. The result is a very characteristic radiographic appearance that is sometimes described as *cotton wool.* Lesions typically occur in the skull, pelvis, femurs, tibias, vertebrae, clavicles, and ribs. Long bones generally bow and/or fracture because of the softening of the bone, and the associated joint may develop arthritic changes. The **pelvis** is the most common initial site of this disease.

Reiter syndrome affects the sacroiliac joints and lower limbs of young men, with the radiographic hallmark being a specific area of bony erosion at the Achilles tendon insertion on the **posterosuperior margin of the calcaneus.** Involvement is usually bilateral, and arthritis, urethritis, and conjunctivitis are characteristic of this syndrome. This syndrome is caused by a previous infection of the GI tract, such as salmonella, or by a sexually transmitted infection.

7

SUMMARY OF PATHOLOGIC INDICATIONS

CONDITION OR DISEASE	MOST COMMON RADIOGRAPHIC EXAM	POSSIBLE RADIOGRAPHIC APPEARANCE	EXPOSURE FACTOR ADJUSTMENT*
Bone cyst	AP & lat of affected limb	Well-circumscribed lucency	None
Chondromalacia patellae	AP & lat knee, tangential (axial) of femoropatellar joint	Pathology of femoropatellar joint space, possible misalignment of patella	None
Chondrosarcoma	AP & lat of affected limb, CT, MRI	Bone destruction with calcifications in the cartilaginous tumor	None
Enchondroma (benign cartilaginous tumor)	AP & lat of affected limb	Well-defined radiolucent tumor with thin cortex (often results in pathologic fracture with minimal trauma)	None
Ewing sarcoma (malignant bone tumor)	AP & lat of affected limb, CT, MRI	Ill-defined area of bone destruction with surrounding "onion peel" (layers of periosteal reaction)	None
Exostosis (osteochondroma)	AP & lat of affected limb	A projection of bone with cartilaginous cap; grows parallel to shaft and away from nearest joint	None
Gout (a form of arthritis)	AP (oblique) & lat of affected part (most common initially in MTP joint of foot)	Uric acid deposits in joint space; destruction of joint space	None
Multiple myeloma (most common primary cancerous bone tumor)	AP & lat of affected part	Multiple "punched-out" osteolyte lesions throughout affected bone	None
Osgood-Schlatter disease	AP & lat knee	Fragmentation and/or detachment of tibial tuberosity by patellar tendon	None
Osteoarthritis (DJD, degenerative joint disease)	AP, oblique, & lat of affected part	Narrowed, irregular joint spaces with sclerotic articular surfaces and spurs	Advanced stage may require slight decrease (−)
Osteoclastoma (giant cell tumor)	AP & lat of affected part	Large radiolucent lesions with thin strips of bone between	None
Osteogenic sarcoma (primary bone tumor)	AP & lat of affected part, CT, MRI	Extensively destructive lesion with irregular periosteal reaction; classic appearance is *sunburst* pattern that is diffuse periosteal reaction	None
Osteoid osteoma (benign bone lesions)	AP & lat of affected part	Small, round-oval density with lucent center	None
Osteomalacia (rickets)	AP & lat of affected limb	Decreased bone density, bowing deformity in weight-bearing limbs	Loss of bone matrix requires decrease (−)
Paget's disease (osteitis deformans)	AP & lat of affected part(s)	Mixed areas of sclerotic and cortical thickening and lytic or radiolucent lesions; *cotton wool* appearance	Extensive sclerotic areas may require increase (+)
Reiter syndrome	AP & lat of affected part	Asymmetric erosion of joint spaces; calcaneus erosion, usually bilateral	None

*Dependent on stage or severity of disease or condition.

Survey Information

Knowing the routines and special projections being performed most commonly in various parts of the country will help students understand the need to learn each of these projections, even if they are not common in their facility. In this way, students will be prepared to function anywhere they may choose for employment.

Summary of Survey Results

Toes: The common basic projections continue to be **AP** (DP), **oblique,** and **lateral.** The survey indicates that **62% in United States** and **92% in Canada** center the AP for **"affected toe only"** routine, and 47% in the U.S. and 13% in Canada include all the toes and metatarsals as routine on the AP projection. This has not changed significantly in the U.S. over the past 10 years.

Foot: The common basic projections continue to be **AP** (DP), **medial oblique,** and **mediolateral.** The **lateromedial** is indicated to be routine by 16% and special by 30% in the U.S; and in Canada, 22% routine and 11% special. (This is a significant increase as a special projection in the U.S. from earlier surveys.)

The **AP** and **lateral weight-bearing, club foot,** and **sesamoid** projections all continue to be indicated as special, with an increase in the frequency of the club foot and sesamoid projections in the U.S. (These two specials are much less common in Canada.)

Ankle: The one significant change in the ankle routine is the **AP mortise** (15°-20° internal oblique) projection, which was indicated to be basic or routine in 2000 by **74% in U.S.** and **76% in Canada** compared with 40% in both 1995 and 1998 U.S. surveys. The 45° internal oblique ankle has decreased as basic in the U.S. to 62% in 2000, 72% in 1995, and 94% in 1989.

Other basic ankle projections continue to be **AP** and **mediolateral,** with the **lateromedial** and **stress views** as special. No significant change has occurred in these.

Knee: The common basic projections continue to be **AP, lateral,** and **oblique.** In the U.S. 52% and 35% in Canada include **both obliques** as basic, with 24% in U.S. and 18% in Canada indicating the medial oblique only and 13% in U.S. and 6% in Canada indicating the lateral oblique as basic. The **PA knee** is more common as basic in Canada, with 44%, and only 9% in U.S.

For the **intercondylar fossa,** the **Camp Coventry method** is most common in the U.S. at 62% and only 33% in Canada. The **kneeling Holmblad method** is basic by 46% in U.S. and 38% in Canada.

The **patella routine** includes the **PA, lateral,** and **supine Merchant tangential** as the most common routine. The Settegast and Hughston prone tangential projections were less common but still performed by over 20%. The PA oblique and axial oblique (Kuchendorf) are performed by less than 20% and have been dropped from previous editions of this text.

Standard and Special Operating Procedures

Certain basic and special projections for the toes, foot, ankle, leg, knee, and mid and distal femur are demonstrated and described on the following pages as suggested standard basic and special departmental routines or procedures.

BASIC PROJECTIONS

Standard or basic projections, also sometimes referred to as *routine projections* or *departmental routines,* are those projections commonly taken on average patients who are helpful and can cooperate in performing the procedure.

SPECIAL PROJECTIONS

Special projections are those more common projections taken as extra or additional projections to better demonstrate certain pathologic conditions or specific body parts.

7

BASIC AND SPECIAL PROJECTIONS

AP PROJECTION: TOES

Toes
BASIC
- AP
- **Oblique**
- **Lateral**

Pathology Demonstrated

Fractures and/or dislocations of the phalanges of the digits in question are demonstrated. Some pathologies, such as osteoarthritis and gouty arthritis (gout), may be evident, especially in the first digit.

Technical Factors

- IR size—18 × 24 cm (8 × 10 inches), crosswise
- Divide in thirds, crosswise
- Detail screen, tabletop
- Digital IR—use lead masking
- 50-60 kV range
- Technique and dose:

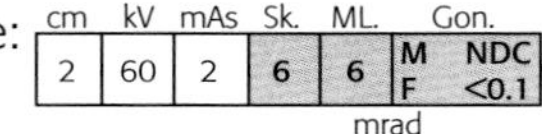

cm	kV	mAs	Sk.	ML.	Gon.
2	60	2	6	6	M NDC F <0.1
				mrad	

Note: Some departmental routines include centering and collimation for the AP toes to include all the toes and distal metatarsals. The majority include centering to the toe of interest with closer collimation to include only one digit on each side of injury. (See survey information, p. 227.)

Shielding Place shield over pelvic region to shield gonads.

Patient Position Take radiograph with patient supine or seated on table; knee should be flexed with plantar surface of foot resting on cassette.

Part Position

- Center and align long axis of digit(s) to CR and long axis of portion of IR being exposed.
- Ensure that MTP joint(s) of digit(s) in question is (are) centered to CR.

Central Ray

- Angle CR **10° to 15° toward calcaneus** (CR perpendicular to phalanges).
- If a **15° wedge** is placed under foot for parallel part-film alignment, then the CR is **perpendicular** to IR (Fig. 7-40).
- Center CR to **MTP joint(s)** in question.
- Minimum SID is 40 inches (100 cm).

Collimation Collimate on four sides to area of interest. On side margins include a minimum of at least part of one digit on each side of digit(s) in question.

CR or DR: Close collimation and lead masking are important over unused portion of image plate to prevent fogging from scatter radiation to the hypersensitive image plate or receptor.

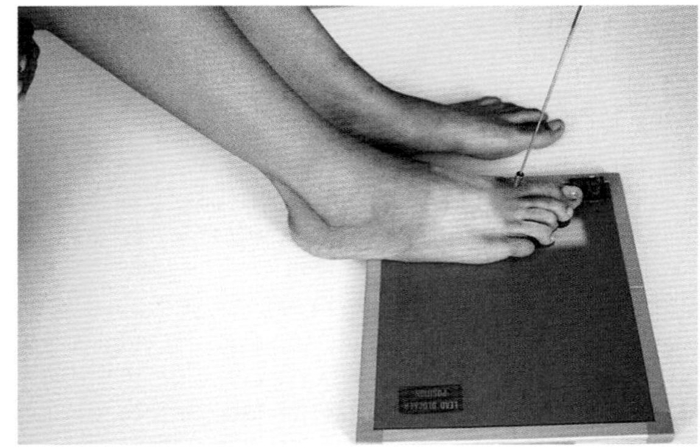

Fig. 7-39. Second digit (CR 10° to 15°).

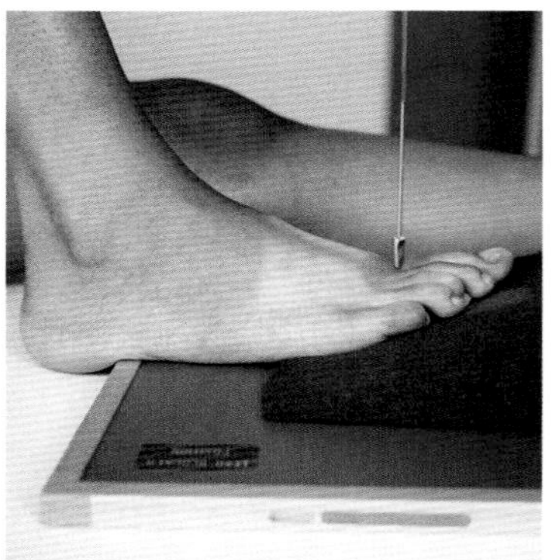

Fig. 7-40. AP first digit with wedge (CR perpendicular).

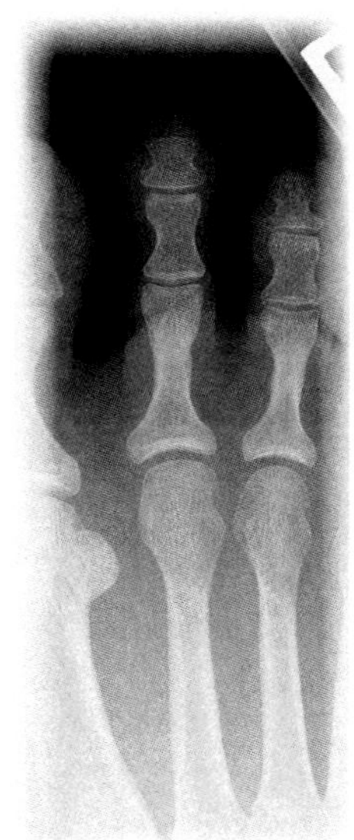

Fig. 7-41. AP second digit.

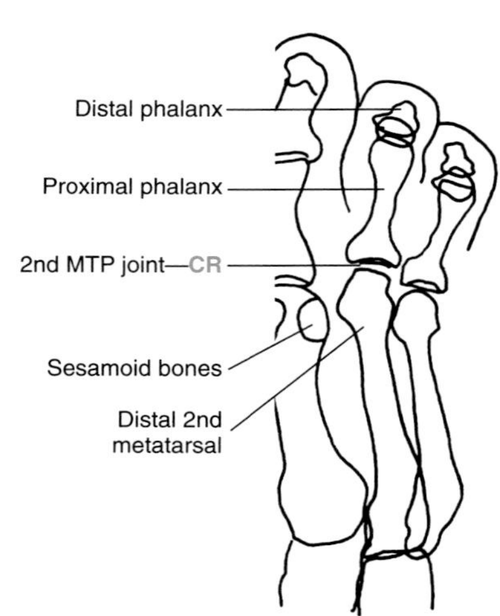

Fig. 7-42. AP second digit.

Radiographic Criteria

Structures Shown: • Digit(s) of interest and a minimum of the distal half of metatarsals should be included.

Position: • Individual digits should be separated with no overlapping of soft tissues. • Long axis of foot aligned to long axis of portion of IR being exposed. • **No rotation** is present if the shafts of the phalanges and distal metatarsals appear equally concave on both sides. Rotation will appear as one side being more concave than the other. The side with increased concavity has been rolled away from the IR.*

Collimation and CR: • Collimation borders should be visible on all four sides with the center (CR) at the **MTP joint(s) of interest** with at least the distal half of metatarsals included.

Exposure Criteria: • No motion as evidenced by sharply defined cortical margins of the bone and detailed bony trabeculae. • Optimal contrast and density will allow visualization of bony cortical margins and trabeculae and soft-tissue structures.

*McQuillen-Martensen K: Radiographic critique, Philadelphia, 1996, WB Saunders.

AP OBLIQUE PROJECTION—MEDIAL OR LATERAL ROTATION: TOES

Toes
BASIC
- AP
- Oblique
- Lateral

Pathology Demonstrated

Fractures and/or dislocations of the phalanges of the digits in question are demonstrated. Some pathologies such as osteoarthritis and gouty arthritis (gout) may be evident, especially in the first digit.

24

18 R

Technical Factors

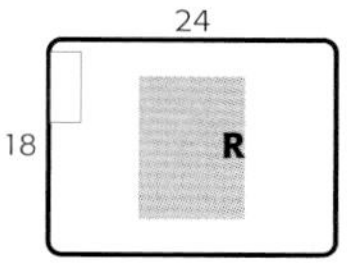

- IR size—18 × 24 cm (8 × 10 inches), crosswise
- Divide in thirds, crosswise
- Detail screen, tabletop
- Digital IR—use lead masking
- 50-60 kV range
- Technique and dose:

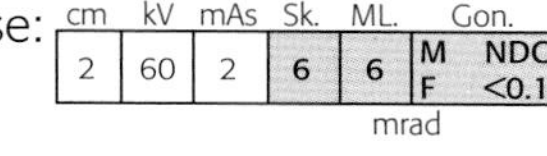

cm	kV	mAs	Sk.	ML.	Gon.
2	60	2	6	6	M NDC F <0.1
				mrad	

Shielding Place lead shield over pelvic area to shield gonads.

Patient Position Take radiograph with patient supine or seated on table; knee should be flexed with plantar surface of foot resting on cassette.

Part Position

- Center and align long axis of digit(s) to CR and long axis of portion of IR being exposed.
- Ensure that MTP joint(s) of digit(s) in question is (are) centered to CR.
- Rotate the leg and foot 30° to 45° medially for the first, second, and third digits and laterally for the fourth and fifth digits. (See Oblique Foot for degrees of oblique, p. 233).
- Use 45° radiolucent support under elevated portion of foot to prevent motion.

Central Ray

- CR **perpendicular** to IR, directed to MTP joint(s) in question
- Minimum SID of 40 inches (100 cm)

Collimation Collimate on four sides to include phalanges and a minimum of distal half of metatarsals. On side margins include a minimum of one digit on each side of digit(s) in question.

CR or DR: Close collimation and lead masking are important over unused portion of image plate to prevent fogging from scatter radiation to the hypersensitive image plate or receptor.

Radiographic Criteria

Structures Shown: • Digit(s) in question and distal half of metatarsals should be included without overlap (superimposition).

Position: • Long axis of foot aligned to long axis of portion of IR being exposed. • Correct obliquity should be evident by increased concavity on one side of shafts and by overlapping of soft tissues of digits. Heads of metatarsals should appear directly side by side with no (or only minimal) overlapping.*

Collimation and CR: • Collimation borders should be visible on all four sides with the center (CR) at the MTP joint(s) of interest. • Interphalangeal and **MTP joints of interest** appear open indicating correct CR.

Exposure Criteria: • No motion as evidenced by sharply defined cortical margins of the bone and detailed bony trabeculae. • Optimal contrast and density will allow visualization of bony cortical margins and trabeculae and soft-tissue structures.

*McQuillen-Martensen K: Radiographic critique, Philadelphia, 1996, WB Saunders.

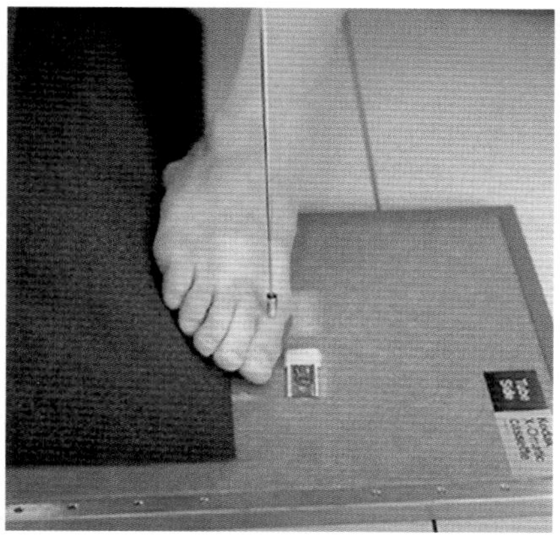

Fig. 7-43. Medial rotation—first digit.

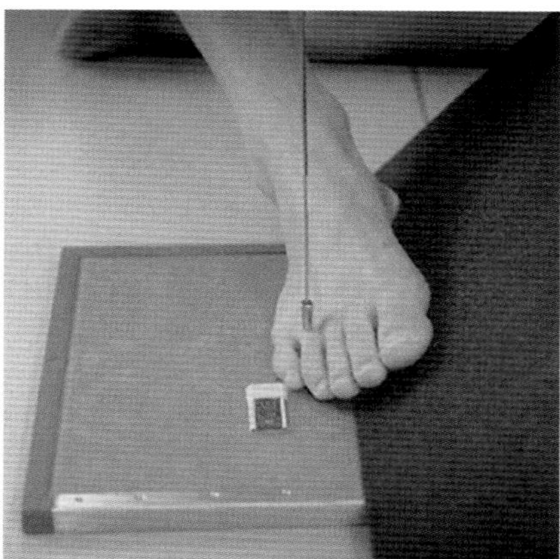

Fig. 7-44. Lateral rotation—fourth digit.

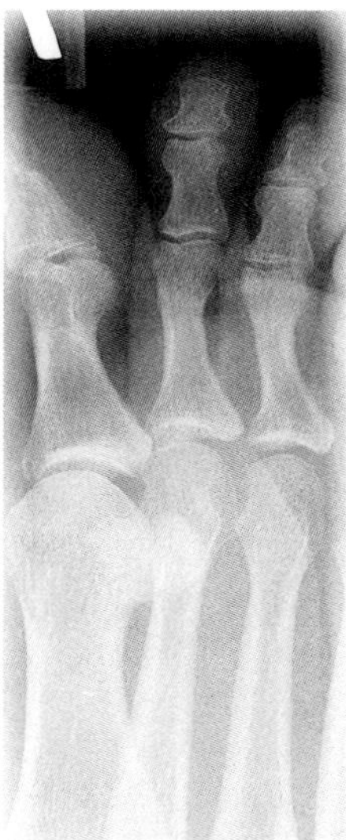

Fig. 7-45. Oblique—second digit.

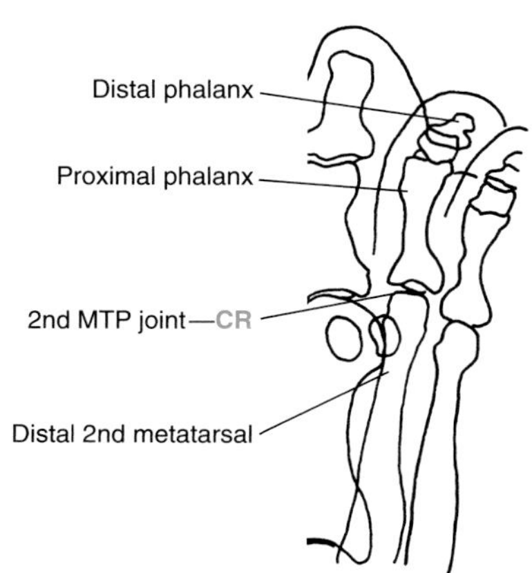

Fig. 7-46. Oblique—second digit.

7

LATERAL—MEDIOLATERAL OR LATEROMEDIAL PROJECTIONS: TOES

Toes
BASIC
- AP
- Oblique
- Lateral

Pathology Demonstrated
Fractures and/or dislocations of the phalanges of the digits in question are demonstrated. Some pathologies such as osteoarthritis and gouty arthritis (gout) may be evident, especially in the first digit.

Technical Factors
- IR size—18 × 24 cm (8 × 10 inches), crosswise
- Divide in thirds, crosswise
- Detail screen, tabletop
- Digital IR—use lead masking
- 50-60 kV range
- Technique and dose:

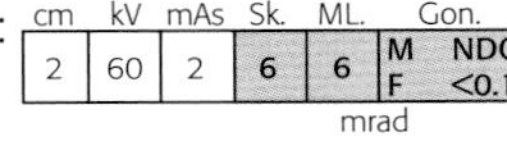

cm	kV	mAs	Sk.	ML.	Gon.
2	60	2	6	6	M NDC / F <0.1

mrad

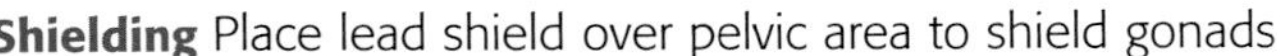

Shielding Place lead shield over pelvic area to shield gonads.

Patient and Part Position
- Rotate affected leg and foot medially (lateromedial) for first, second, and third digits and laterally (mediolateral) for fourth and fifth digits.
- Adjust cassette to center and align long axis of toe in question to CR and to long axis of portion of IR being exposed.
- Ensure that IP joint or PIP joint in question is centered to CR.
- Use tape, gauze, or tongue blade to flex and separate unaffected toes to prevent superimposition.

Central Ray
- CR **perpendicular** to IR
- CR directed to **interphalangeal joint for first digit** and to **proximal interphalangeal joint for second to fifth digits**
- Minimum SID of 40 inches (100 cm)

Collimation Collimate closely on four sides to affected digit.

CR or DR: Close collimation and lead masking are important over unused portion of image plate to prevent fogging from scatter radiation to the hypersensitive image plate or receptor.

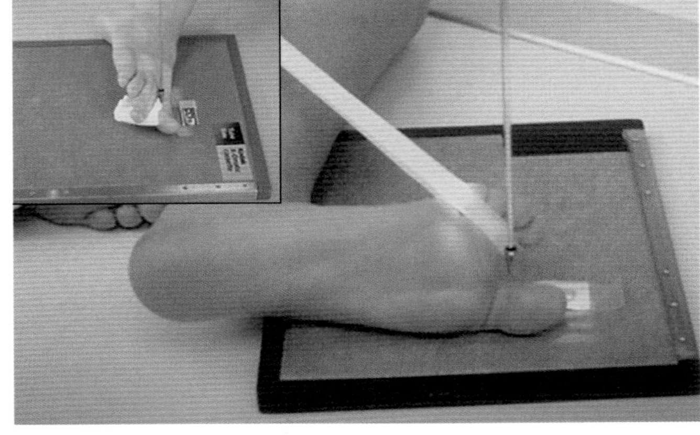

Fig. 7-47. Lateromedial—first digit.

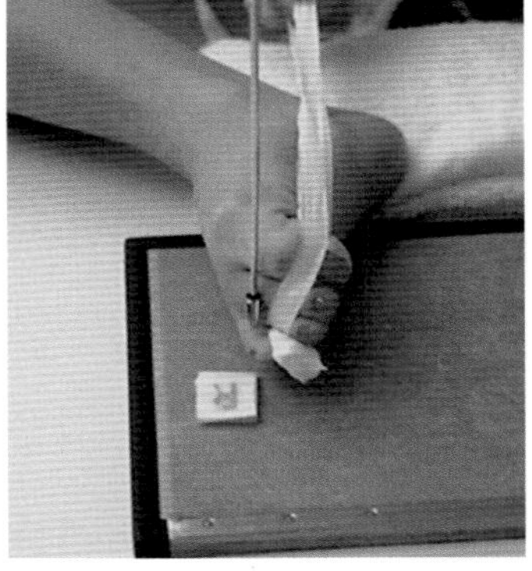

Fig. 7-48. Mediolateral fourth digit.

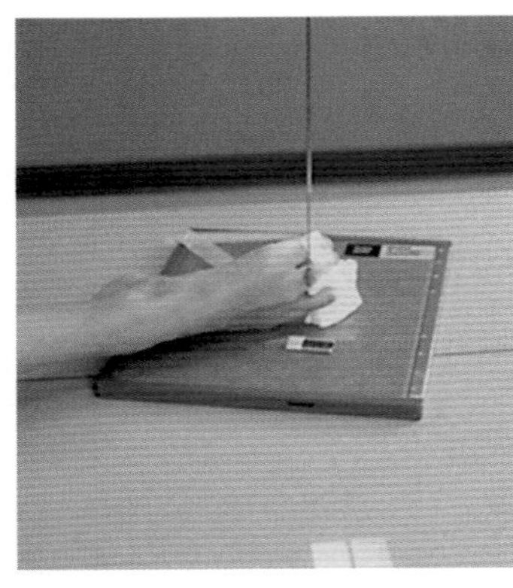

Fig. 7-49. Mediolateral—fourth digit.

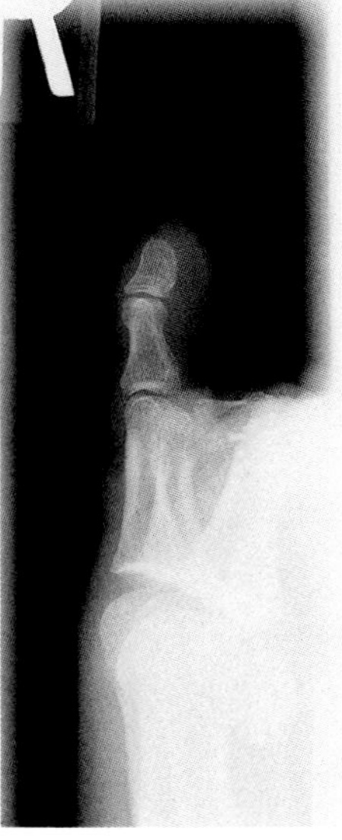

Fig. 7-50. Lateral—second digit.

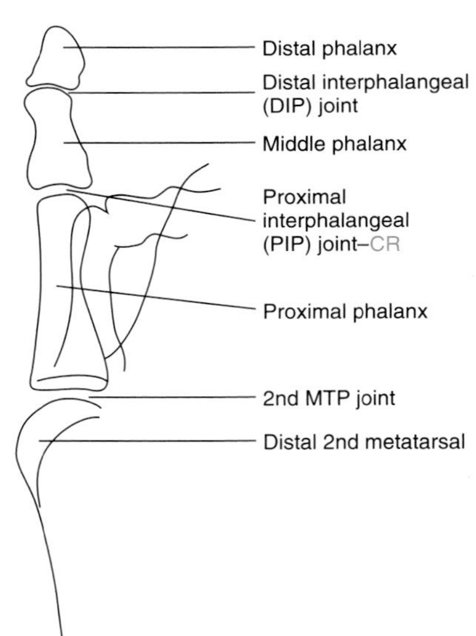

Fig. 7-51. Lateral—second digit.

Radiographic Criteria

Structures Shown: • Phalanges of digit in question should be seen in lateral position free of superimposition by other digits, if possible. (When total separation of toes is not possible, especially third to fifth digits, the distal phalanx at least should be separated and the proximal phalanx visualized through superimposed structures.)

Position: • Long axis of digit is aligned to long axis of portion of IR being used. • True lateral of digit will demonstrate an increased concavity on the anterior surface of the distal phalanx and the posterior surface of the proximal phalanx. Opposing surface of each phalanx will appear straighter.*

Collimation and CR: • Collimation borders should be visible on all four sides with the center (CR) at the appropriate interphalangeal joint. • Interphalangeal joints should appear open and unobstructed. The MTP joint should be visualized even if superimposed.

Exposure Criteria: • No motion as evidenced by sharply defined cortical margins of the bone and detailed bony trabeculae. • Optimal contrast and density will allow visualization of bony cortical margins and trabeculae and soft-tissue structures.

*McQuillen-Martensen K: Radiographic critique, Philadelphia, 1996, WB Saunders.

TANGENTIAL PROJECTION: TOES—SESAMOIDS

Toes
SPECIAL
• Sesamoids (tangential)

Pathology Demonstrated

This projection provides a profile image of the sesamoid bones at the first MTP joint to evaluate extent of injury.

Note: A lateral of first digit in dorsiflexion may also be taken to visualize these sesamoids.

24
18 R

Technical Factors

- IR size—18 × 24 cm (8 × 10 inches), crosswise
- Divide in half if combined with another projection
- Detail screen, tabletop
- Digital IR—use lead masking
- 50-60 kV range
- Technique and dose:

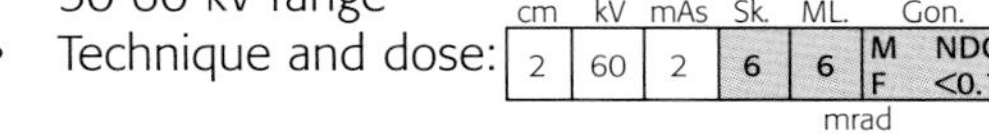

cm	kV	mAs	Sk.	ML.	Gon.
2	60	2	6	6	M NDC F <0.1

mrad

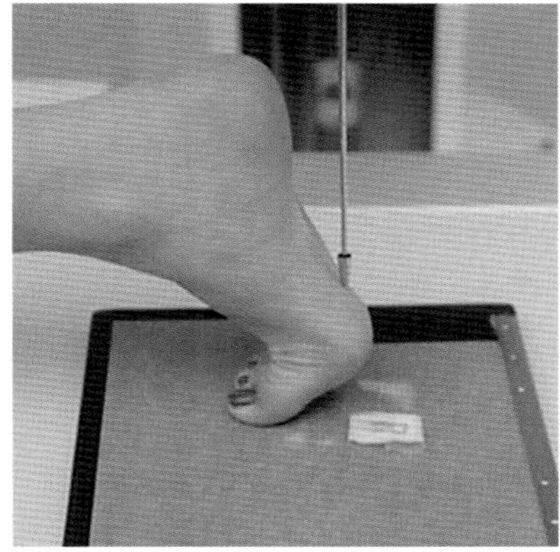

Fig. 7-52. Tangential projection—patient prone.

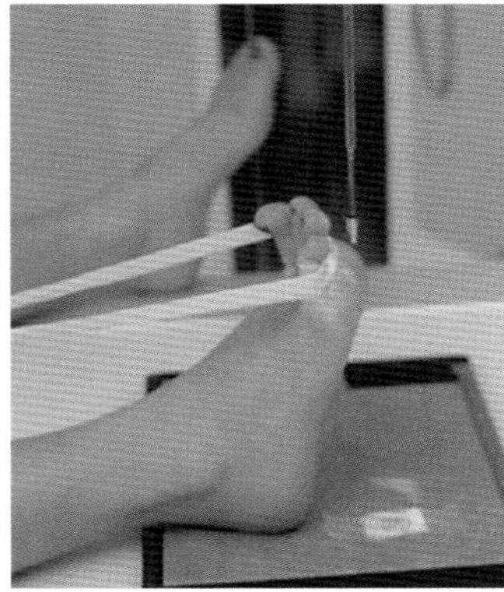

Fig. 7-53. Alternate projection—patient supine.

Shielding Place lead shield over pelvic area to shield gonads.

Patient Position Take radiograph with patient prone; provide pillow for head and small sponge or folded towel under lower leg for patient comfort.

Part Position

- Dorsiflex the foot so that the plantar surface of the foot forms about a **15° to 20° angle** from vertical.
- Dorsiflex the first digit (great toe) and rest on cassette to maintain position.
- Ensure that long axis of foot is not rotated; place sandbags or other support on both sides of foot to prevent movement.

Note: This is an uncomfortable and often painful position; do not keep patient in this position longer than necessary.

Central Ray

- CR **perpendicular** to IR, directed tangentially to posterior aspect of **first MTP joint** (depending on amount of dorsiflexion of foot, may need to angle CR slightly for a true tangential projection)
- Minimum SID of 40 inches (100 cm)

Collimation Collimate closely to area of interest. Include at least the first, second, and third distal metatarsals for possible sesamoids but with CR at first MTP joint.

Alternate projection: If patient cannot tolerate the above prone position, this may be taken in a reverse projection with patient supine by using a long strip of gauze for patient to hold the toes as shown. CR would again be directed tangential to posterior aspect of first MTP joint. Use support to prevent motion. This, however, is not a desirable projection because of the increased OID with accompanying magnification and loss of definition.

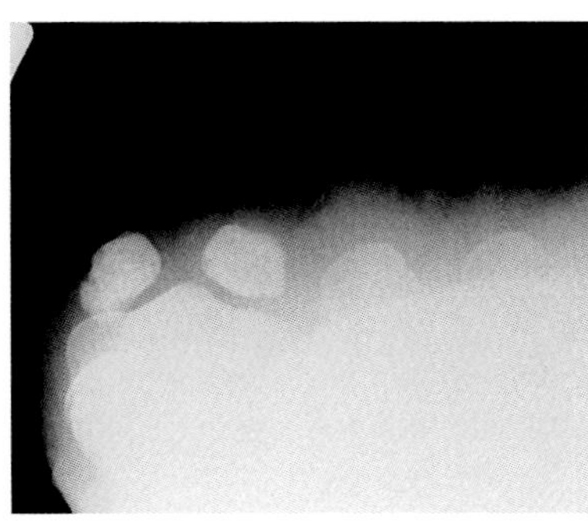

Fig. 7-54. Tangential projection.

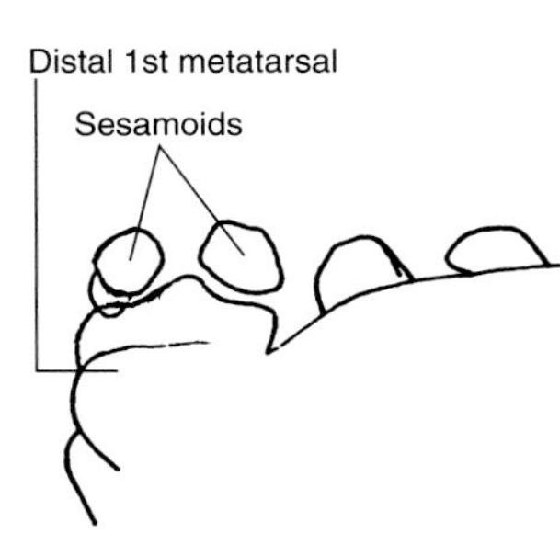

Fig. 7-55. Tangential projection.

Radiographic Criteria

Structures Shown: • Sesamoids should be seen in profile free of superimposition.

Position: • **Borders** of posterior margins of first to third distal metatarsals are seen in profile, indicating correct dorsiflexion of foot.

Collimation and CR: • A minimum of the first three distal metatarsals should be included in collimation field for possible sesamoids, with the center of the four-sided collimation field (CR) at the posterior portion of the first MTP joint. • Centering and angulation are correct if the sesamoids are free of any bony superimposition with open space demonstrated between sesamoids and the first metatarsal.

Exposure Criteria: • No motion as evidenced by sharp bony cortical margins and detailed trabeculae. • Optimal contrast and density will allow visualization of bony cortical margins and trabeculae and soft-tissue structures without the sesamoids appearing overexposed.

AP PROJECTION: FOOT

Dorsoplantar Projection

Pathology Demonstrated

Location and extent of fractures and fragment alignments, joint space abnormalities, soft-tissue effusions, and location of opaque foreign bodies are demonstrated.

Foot
BASIC
• AP
• Oblique
• Lateral

Technical Factors

- IR size—24 × 30 cm (10 × 12 inches), lengthwise
- Divide in half for AP and oblique
- Detail screen, tabletop
- Digital IR—use lead masking
- 60 ± 5 kV range; or 70-75 kV and reduced mAs for increased exposure latitude for more uniform density of phalanges and tarsals
- Technique and dose @ 70 kV:

cm	kV	mAs	Sk.	ML.	Gon.
6	70	2	10	8	M NDC F <0.1
				mrad	

Shielding Place lead shield over pelvic area to shield gonads.

Patient Position Take radiograph with patient supine; give pillow to patient for head; flex knee and place plantar surface (sole) of affected foot flat on cassette (IR).

Part Position

- Extend (plantar flex) foot but maintain plantar surface resting flat and firmly on cassette (IR).
- Align and center long axis of foot to CR and to long axis of portion of IR being exposed. (Use sandbags if necessary to prevent cassette from slipping on tabletop.)
- If immobilization is needed, flex opposite knee also and rest against affected knee for support.

Central Ray

- Angle CR **10° posteriorly** (toward heel), CR perpendicular to metatarsals (see Note below).
- Direct CR to **base of third metatarsal.**
- Minimum SID is 40 inches (100 cm).

Collimation Collimate to outer margins of foot on four sides.

CR or DR: Close collimation and lead masking are important over unused portion of image plate to prevent fogging from scatter radiation to the hypersensitive image plate or receptor.

Note: A high arch requires more angle (15°) and a low arch nearer 5° to be perpendicular to metatarsals. For foreign body, the CR should be perpendicular to IR with no CR angle.

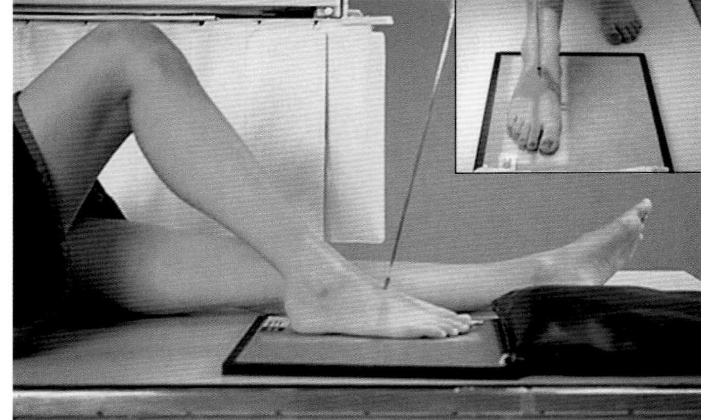

Fig. 7-56. AP foot—CR 10°.

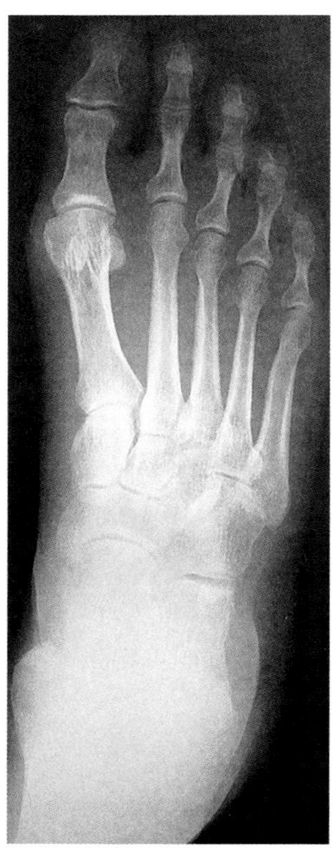

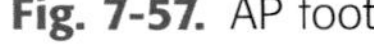

Fig. 7-57. AP foot.

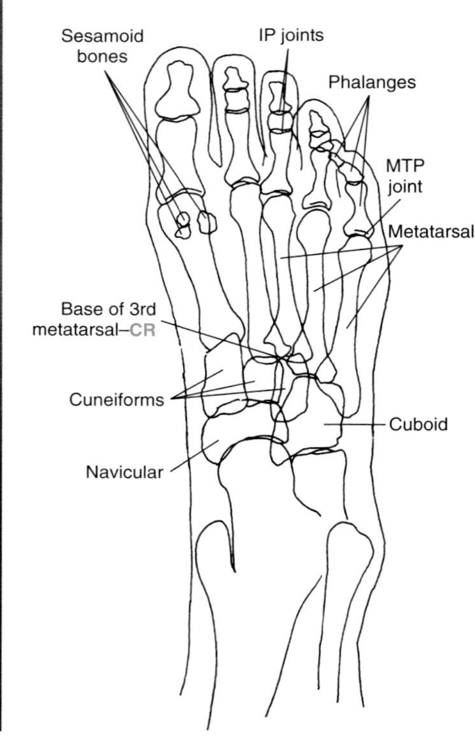

Fig. 7-58. AP foot.

Radiographic Criteria

Structures Shown: • Entire foot should be demonstrated including all phalanges and metatarsals and the navicular, cuneiforms, and cuboids.

Position: • Long axis of foot should be aligned to long axis of portion of IR being exposed. • **No rotation** as evidenced by nearly equal distance between second through fifth metatarsals. Bases of first and second metatarsals are generally separated but bases of second to fifth metatarsals will appear overlapped. • Intertarsal joint space between first and second cuneiforms should be demonstrated.

Collimation and CR: • Center of four-sided collimation field (CR) should be at the **base of third metatarsal,** with collimation borders including the soft tissue surrounding the foot. • The MTP joints should generally appear open. IP joints, however, may appear partially closed because of divergent rays.

Exposure Criteria: • Optimal density and contrast with no motion should visualize sharp borders and trabecular markings of distal phalanges and tarsals distal to talus. (See higher kV technique for more uniform densities between phalanges and tarsals.) • Sesamoid bones (if present) should be seen through head of first metatarsal.

AP OBLIQUE PROJECTION—MEDIAL ROTATION: FOOT

Pathology Demonstrated
Location and extent of fractures and fragment alignments, joint space abnormalities, soft-tissue effusions, and location of opaque foreign bodies are demonstrated.

Foot
BASIC
• AP
• Oblique
• Lateral

Technical Factors
- IR size—24 × 30 cm (10 × 12 inches), lengthwise (divide in half for AP and oblique)
- Detail screen, tabletop
- Digital IR—use lead masking
- 60 ± 5 kV range; or 70-75 kV for increased exposure latitude for more uniform density between phalanges and tarsals
- Technique and dose @70 kV:

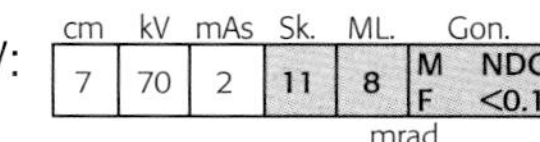

cm	kV	mAs	Sk.	ML.	Gon.
7	70	2	11	8	M NDC F <0.1
			mrad		

Shielding Place lead shield over pelvic area to shield gonads.

Patient Position Take radiograph with patient supine or sitting; flex knee, with plantar surface of foot on table; turn body slightly away from side in question.

Part Position
- Align and center long axis of foot to CR and to long axis of portion of IR being exposed.
- Rotate foot **medially** to place **plantar surface 30° to 40° to plane of IR** (see Note below). The general plane of the dorsum of the foot should be parallel to IR and perpendicular to CR.
- Use 45° radiolucent support block to prevent motion. Use sandbags if necessary to prevent cassette from slipping on tabletop.

Central Ray
- CR **perpendicular** to IR, directed to **base of third metatarsal**
- Minimum SID of 40 inches (100 cm)

Collimation Collimate to outer margins of skin on four sides.

Note: Some references suggest only a 30° oblique routinely. This text recommends more obliquity, nearer 40° to 45°, to best demonstrate tarsals and proximal metatarsals relatively free of superimposition for the foot with an average transverse arch.

Optional Lateral Oblique
- Rotate the foot laterally 30° (less oblique required because of the natural arch of the foot).
- A lateral oblique will best demonstrate the space between first and second metatarsals and between first and second cuneiforms. The navicular will also be well visualized on the lateral oblique.

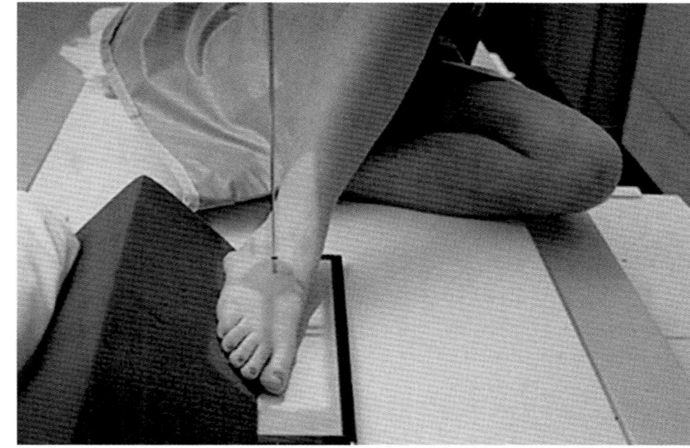

Fig. 7-59. 30° to 40° medial oblique.

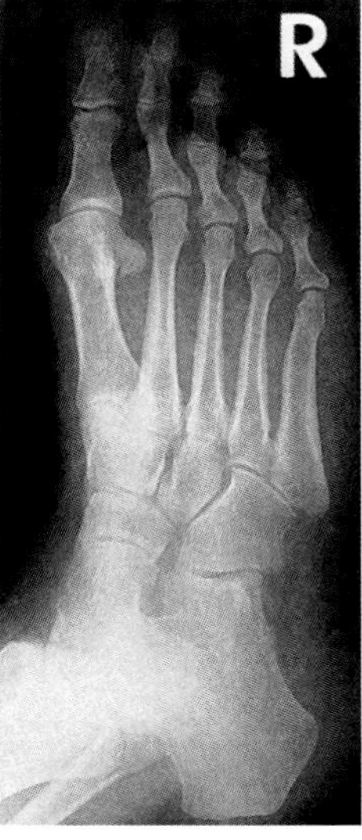

Fig. 7-60. 40° medial oblique.

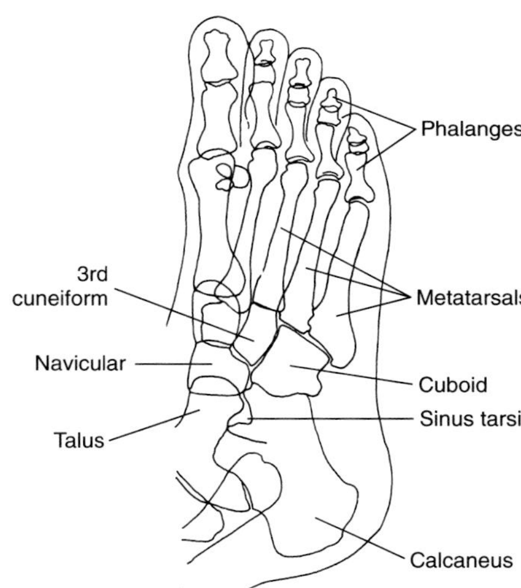

Fig. 7-61. 40° medial oblique.

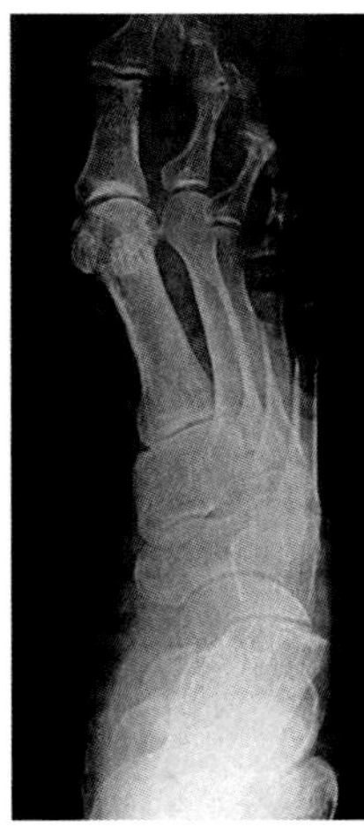

Fig. 7-62. 30° optional lateral oblique.

Radiographic Criteria (medial oblique)

Structures Shown: • Entire foot should be demonstrated from distal phalanges to posterior calcaneus and proximal talus.

Position: • Long axis of foot should be aligned to long axis of IR. • Correct obliquity is demonstrated when third through fifth metatarsals are free of superimposition. First and second metatarsals should also be free of superimposition except for base area. • Tuberosity at base of fifth metatarsal is seen in profile and well visualized. • Joint spaces around cuboid and the sinus tarsi are open and well demonstrated when foot is obliqued correctly.

Collimation and CR: • Center of four-sided collimation (CR) should be to **base of third metatarsal.** • Collimation field should include soft tissue surrounding the foot.

Exposure Criteria: • Optimal density and contrast with no motion should visualize sharp borders and trabecular markings of phalanges, metatarsals, and tarsals.

LATERAL—MEDIOLATERAL OR LATEROMEDIAL PROJECTIONS: FOOT

Foot
BASIC
- **AP**
- **Oblique**
- Lateral

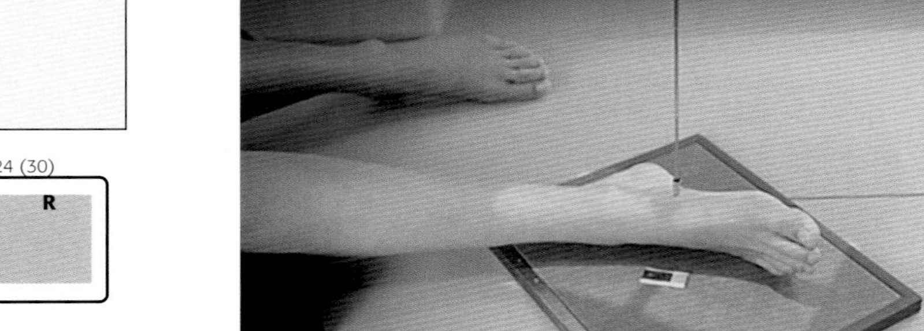

Pathology Demonstrated

Location and degree of anterior or posterior displacement of fracture fragments, or joint abnormalities, soft-tissue effusions, and location of opaque foreign bodies are demonstrated.

Technical Factors

24 (30)
18 (24)
R

- IR size—18 × 24 cm (8 × 10 inches)—smaller foot or 24 × 30 cm (10 × 12 inches)—larger foot
- Detail screen, tabletop
- 60 ± 5 kV range
- Technique and dose:

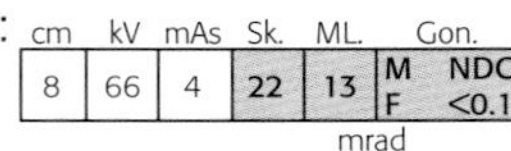

cm	kV	mAs	Sk.	ML.	Gon.
8	66	4	22	13	M NDC F <0.1
			mrad		

Shielding Place lead shield over pelvic area to shield gonads.

Patient Position Take radiograph with patient in lateral recumbent position; provide pillow for head.

Part Position (Mediolateral Projection)

- Flex knee of affected limb about 45°; place opposite leg **behind** the injured limb to prevent overrotation of affected leg.
- Carefully dorsiflex the foot if possible to assist in positioning for a true lateral foot and ankle.
- Place support under leg and knee as needed so that **plantar surface is perpendicular to IR.** Do not **overrotate** foot.
- Align long axis of foot to long axis of IR (unless diagonal placement is needed to include entire foot).
- Center mid area of base of metatarsals to CR.

Central Ray

- CR **perpendicular** to IR, directed to **medial cuneiform** (at level of base of third metatarsal)
- Minimum SID of 40 inches (100 cm)

Collimation Collimate to the outer skin margins of the foot to include about 1 inch or 2 to 3 cm proximal to ankle joint.

CR or DR: Close collimation and lead masking are important over unused portion of image plate to prevent fogging from scatter radiation to the hypersensitive image plate or receptor.

Alternate lateromedial projection: A lateromedial projection may be taken as an alternate lateral. This can be more uncomfortable or painful for patient, but it may be easier to achieve a true lateral in this position.

Fig. 7-63. Mediolateral projection.

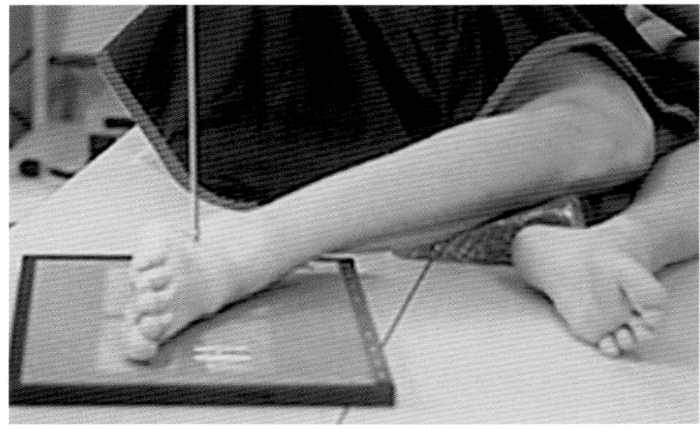

Fig. 7-64. Alternate lateromedial.

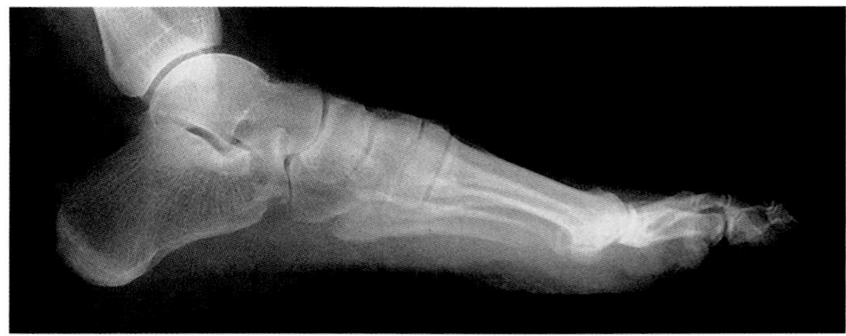

Fig. 7-65. Mediolateral foot.

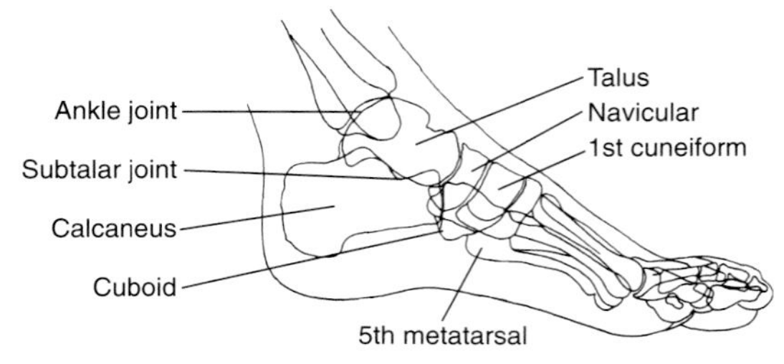

Fig. 7-66. Lateral foot.

Radiographic Criteria

Structures Shown: • Entire foot should be demonstrated and a minimum of 1 inch or 2.5 cm of distal tibia-fibula. • Metatarsals will be nearly superimposed with only the tuberosity of the fifth metatarsal seen in profile.

Position: • The long axis of the foot should be aligned to the long axis of IR. • **True lateral** position is achieved when the tibiotalar joint is open, the distal fibula is superimposed by the posterior tibia, and the distal metatarsals are superimposed.

Collimation and CR: • All soft-tissue structures from phalanges to calcaneus should be included in the center of the four-sided collimated field with the center (CR) to the **medial cuneiform** region.

Exposure Criteria: • Optimal density and contrast should visualize borders of superimposed tarsals and metatarsals. • No motion: Cortical margins and trabecular markings of calcaneus and nonsuperimposed portions of other tarsals should appear sharply defined.

AP AND LATERAL WEIGHT-BEARING PROJECTIONS: FOOT

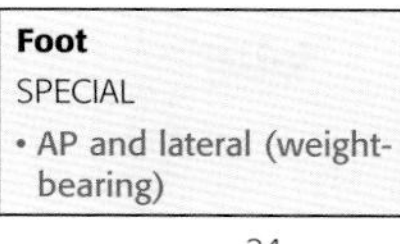
Foot
SPECIAL
- AP and lateral (weight-bearing)

Pathology Demonstrated

These projections are useful in demonstrating the bones of the feet to show the condition of the longitudinal arches under the full weight of body.

Note: Laterals of both feet are usually taken for comparison.

Technical Factors

- IR size 18 × 24 cm (8 × 10 inches) and 24 × 30 cm (10 × 12 inches)
- Detail screen
- 65 ± 5 kV range

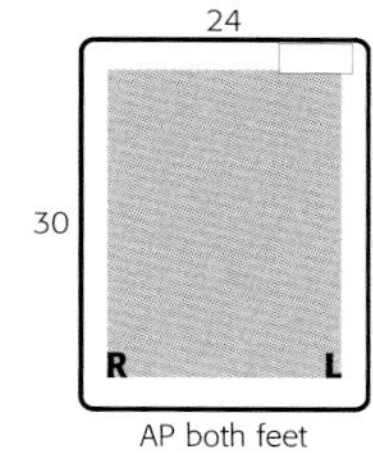

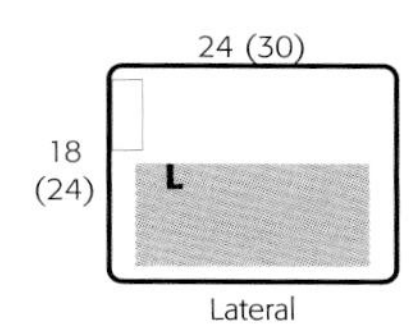

Shielding Shield gonadal area.

Part Position and CR

Note: Some AP routines include separate projections of each foot taken with CR centered to individual foot.

AP:

- Take radiograph with patient standing erect, with full weight evenly distributed on **both** feet. Feet should be directed straight ahead, parallel to each other.
- Angle **CR 15° posteriorly to midpoint between feet at level of base of metatarsals.**

Lateral:

- Have patient stand erect, with weight evenly distributed.
- Have patient stand on wood blocks placed on a step stool or the footrest attached to the table. You may also use a special wood box with a slot for cassette. (It needs to be high enough from floor to get x-ray tube down into a horizontal beam position.)
- Provide some support for patient to hold onto for security.
- Support vertical cassette between feet, with long axis of foot to long axis of IR.
- Change cassettes and turn patient for lateral of other foot for comparison after first lateral is taken.
- Direct **CR horizontally to level of base of third metatarsal.**
- Minimum SID is 40 inches (100 cm).

Collimation Collimate to margins of feet (foot).

Radiographic Criteria

Structures Shown and Position: • For *AP,* projection shows bilateral feet from soft tissue surrounding phalanges to distal portion of talus. • For *lateral,* entire foot should be demonstrated and a minimum of 1 inch, or 2 cm, of distal tibia-fibula. • Distal fibula should be seen superimposed over posterior half of the tibia, and the plantar surfaces of heads of metatarsals should appear directly superimposed if no rotation is present.

Collimation and CR: • *AP,* proper angulation is demonstrated by open tarsometatarsal joint spaces and visualization of the joint between the first and second cuneiforms. • Metatarsal bases should be at the center of the collimated field (CR) with the four-sided collimation including the soft tissue surrounding the feet. • For *lateral,* center of collimated field (CR) should be to level of base of third metatarsal. • Four-sided collimation should include all surrounding soft tissue from the phalanges to the calcaneus and from the dorsum to the plantar surface of the foot with approximately 1 inch, or 2 cm, of the distal tibia-fibula demonstrated.

Exposure Criteria: • Optimal density and contrast should visualize soft tissue and bony borders of superimposed tarsals and metatarsals. Bony trabecular markings should be sharp.

Fig. 7-67. AP—both feet.

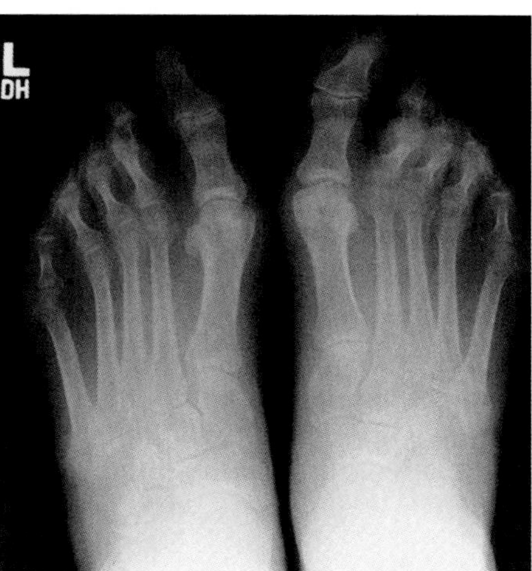

Fig. 7-68. AP– both feet.

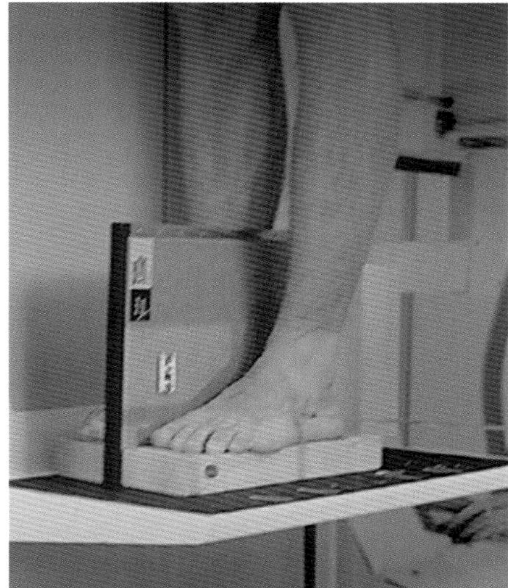

Fig. 7-69. Lateral—left foot.

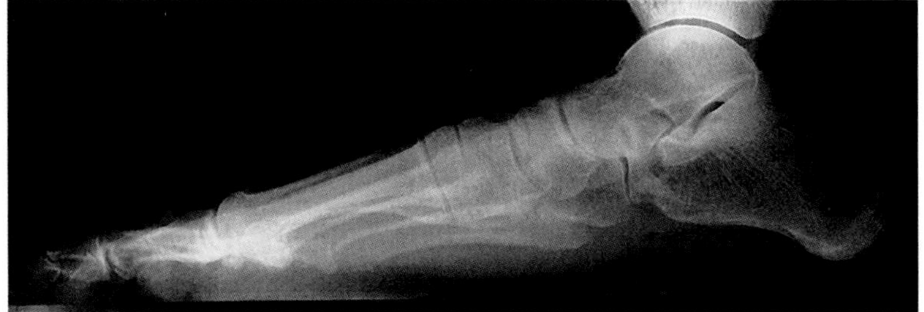

Fig. 7-70. Weight-bearing lateral.

7

PLANTODORSAL (AXIAL) PROJECTION: LOWER LIMB—CALCANEUS

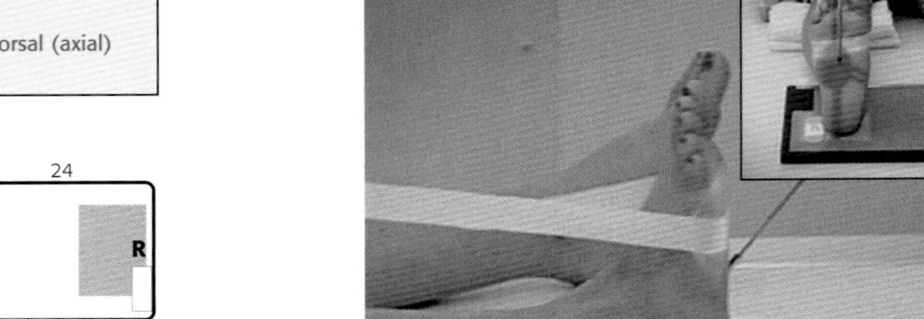

Calcaneus
BASIC
- Plantodorsal (axial)
- **Lateral**

Pathology Demonstrated

Pathologies or fractures with medial or lateral displacement are demonstrated.

Technical Factors

- IR size—18 × 24 cm (8 × 10 inches)
- Divide in half, crosswise
- Detail screen, tabletop
- Digital IR—use lead masking
- 70 ± 5 kV range
- Increase 8-10 kV from other foot projections
- Technique and dose:

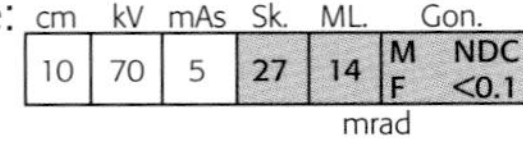

cm	kV	mAs	Sk.	ML.	Gon.
10	70	5	27	14	M NDC F <0.1

mrad

Shielding Place lead shield over pelvic area to shield gonads.

Patient Position Take radiograph with patient supine or seated on table with leg fully extended.

Part Position

- Center and align ankle joint to CR and to portion of IR being exposed.
- Dorsiflex foot so that plantar surface is near perpendicular to IR.
- Loop gauze around foot and ask patient to pull gently but firmly and hold the plantar surface of foot as near perpendicular to IR as possible. (Do **not** keep patient in this position any longer than necessary as this may be very uncomfortable.)

Central Ray

- Direct CR to the **base of third metatarsal** to emerge at a level just distal to lateral malleolus.
- Angle CR **40° cephalad from long axis of foot** (which would also be 40° from vertical **if** long axis of foot is perpendicular to IR). (See Note below.)
- Minimum SID is 40 inches (100 cm).

Collimation Collimate closely to area of calcaneus.

CR or DR: Close collimation and lead masking are important over unused portion of image plate to prevent fogging from scatter radiation to the hypersensitive image plate or receptor.

Note: CR angulation must be increased if long axis of plantar surface of foot is not perpendicular to IR.

Radiographic Criteria

Structures Shown: • Entire calcaneus should be visualized from the tuberosity posteriorly to the talocalcaneal joint anteriorly.

Position: • No rotation; a portion of the sustentaculum tali should appear in profile medially.

Collimation and CR: • CR and center of collimation field should be midway between the distal lateral malleolus and the sustentaculum tali. • With the foot in proper 90° flexion, correct alignment and angulation of the CR are evidenced by an open talocalcaneal joint space and no distortion of the calcaneal tuberosity.

Exposure Criteria: • Optimal density and contrast with no motion will demonstrate sharp bony margins and trabecular markings and will at least faintly visualize the talocalcaneal joint without overexposing the distal tuberosity area.

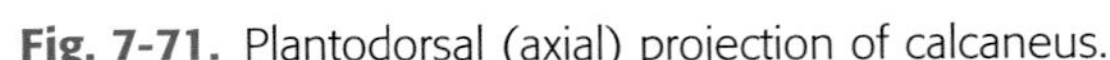

Fig. 7-71. Plantodorsal (axial) projection of calcaneus.

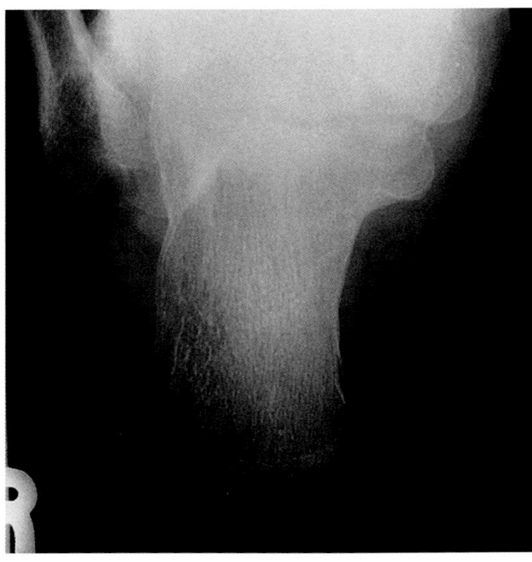

Fig. 7-72. Plantodorsal projection.

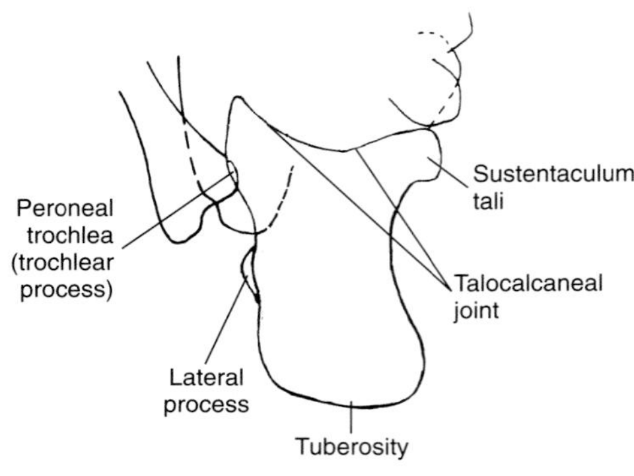

Fig. 7-73. Plantodorsal projection.

LATERAL–MEDIOLATERAL PROJECTION: LOWER LIMB–CALCANEUS

Calcaneus
BASIC
- Plantodorsal
- Lateral

Pathology Demonstrated

Any bony lesions involving the calcaneus, talus, and talocalcaneal joint will be shown and will demonstrate extent and alignment of fractures.

Technical Factors

- IR size—18 × 24 cm (8 × 10 inches)
- Divide in half, crosswise
- Detail screen, tabletop
- Digital IR—use lead masking
- 60 ± 5 kV range
- Technique and dose:

cm	kV	mAs	Sk.	ML.	Gon.
5	65	4	16	16	M NDC F <0.1

mrad

Shielding Place lead shield over pelvic area to shield gonads.

Patient Position Take radiograph with patient in the lateral recumbent position, affected side down. Give the patient a pillow for head. Flex knee of affected limb about 45°; place opposite leg behind the injured limb.

Part Position

- Center calcaneus to CR and to unmasked portion of IR, with long axis of foot parallel to plane of IR.
- Place support under knee and leg as needed to place plantar surface perpendicular to IR.
- Position ankle and foot for a **true lateral,** which places the lateral malleolus about 1 cm posterior to the medial malleolus.
- Dorsiflex foot so that plantar surface is at right angle to leg.

Central Ray

- CR **perpendicular** to IR, directed to a point **1 inch (2.5 cm) inferior to medial malleolus**
- Minimum SID of 40 inches (100 cm)

Collimation Collimate to outer skin margins to include the ankle joint proximally and the entire calcaneus.

CR or DR: Close collimation and lead masking are important over unused portion of image plate to prevent fogging from scatter radiation to the hypersensitive image plate or receptor.

Radiographic Criteria

Structures Shown: • Calcaneus is demonstrated in profile with the talus and distal tibia-fibula demonstrated superiorly, as well as the navicular and the open joint space of the calcaneus and cuboid distally.

Position: • **No rotation** as evidenced by superimposed superior portions of the talus, open talocalcaneal joint, and lateral malleolus superimposed over the posterior half of the tibia and talus. Tarsal sinus and calcaneocuboid joint space should appear open.

Collimation and CR: • CR and the center of the collimation field should be about 1 inch, or 2.5 cm, distal to the tip of the lateral malleolus as seen through the talus. • Four-sided collimation should include ankle joint proximally and talonavicular joint and base of fifth metatarsal anteriorly.

Exposure Criteria: • Optimal exposure will visualize some soft tissue and more dense portions of calcaneus and talus. The outline of the distal fibula should be faintly visible through the talus. Trabecular markings will appear clear and sharp, indicating no motion.

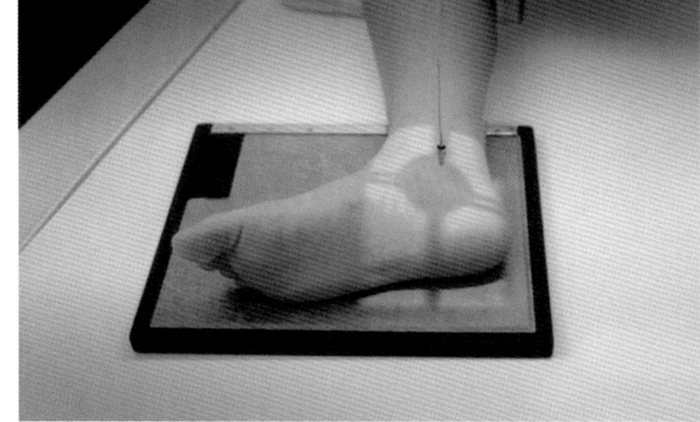

Fig. 7-74. Mediolateral calcaneus.

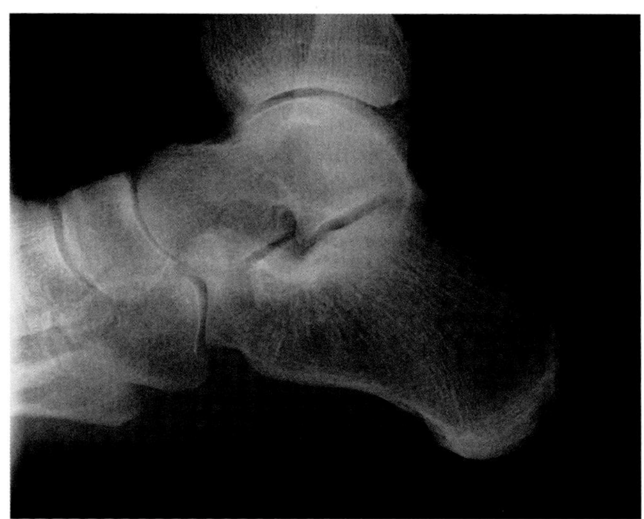

Fig. 7-75. Mediolateral calcaneus.

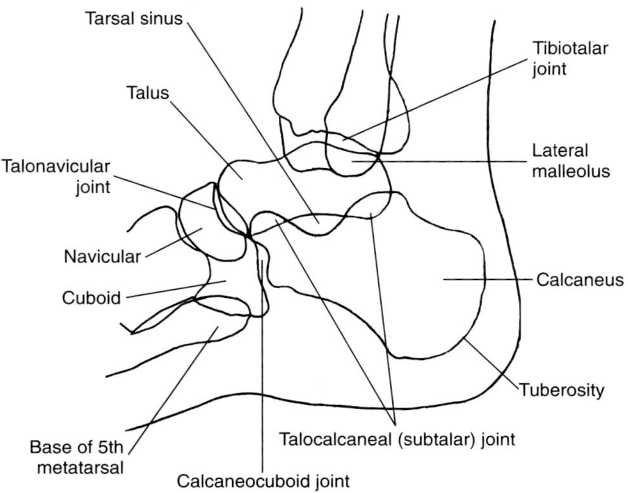

Fig. 7-76. Mediolateral calcaneus.

AP PROJECTION: ANKLE

Pathology Demonstrated
Any bony lesions or diseases involving the ankle joint, distal tibia and fibula, proximal talus, and proximal fifth metatarsal are shown. (The lateral portion of the ankle joint space should not appear open on this projection—see Mortise Projection on p. 239.)

Ankle
BASIC
- AP
- AP mortise (15°)
- Oblique (45°)
- Lateral

Technical Factors
- IR size—24 × 30 cm (10 × 12 inches)
- Divide in half, crosswise
- Detail screen, tabletop
- Digital IR—use lead masking
- 60 ± 5 kV range
- Technique and dose:

cm	kV	mAs	Sk.	ML.	Gon.
8	65	6	27	16	M NDC F <0.1

mrad

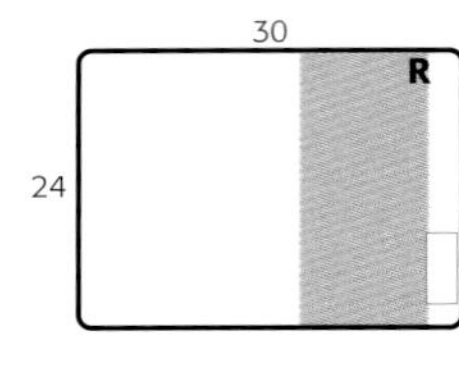

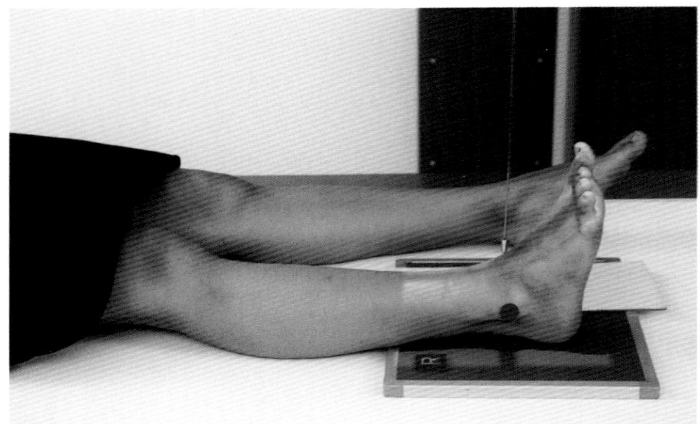
Fig. 7-77. AP ankle.

Shielding Place lead shield over pelvic area to shield gonads.

Patient Position Take radiograph with patient in the supine position; place pillow under head; patient's legs should be fully extended.

Part Position
- Center and align ankle joint to CR and to long axis of portion of IR being exposed.
- Do not force dorsiflexion of the foot but allow it to remain in its natural position (see Note 1 below).
- Adjust the **foot and ankle** for a **true AP projection.** Ensure that the entire lower leg is not rotated. The intermalleolar line will not be parallel to IR (see Note 2 below).

Central Ray
- CR **perpendicular** to IR, directed to **a point midway between malleoli**
- Minimum SID of 40 inches (100 cm)

Collimation Collimate to lateral skin margins, include proximal one half of metatarsals and distal tibia-fibula.

CR or DR: Close collimation and lead masking are important over unused portion of image plate to prevent fogging from scatter radiation to the hypersensitive image plate or receptor.

Note 1: Forced dorsiflexion of the foot can be painful and may cause additional injury.

Note 2: The malleoli will **not** be the same distance from the IR in the anatomic position with a true AP projection. (The lateral malleolus will be about 15° more posterior.) Therefore the lateral portion of the mortise joint should **not** appear open. If this portion of the ankle joint did appear open on a true AP, it may suggest a spread of the ankle mortise from ruptured ligaments.*

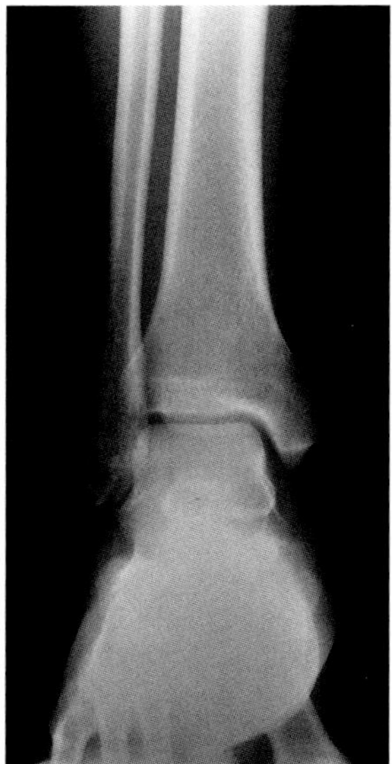
Fig. 7-78. AP ankle. (Courtesy E. Frank, RT (R), FASRT.)

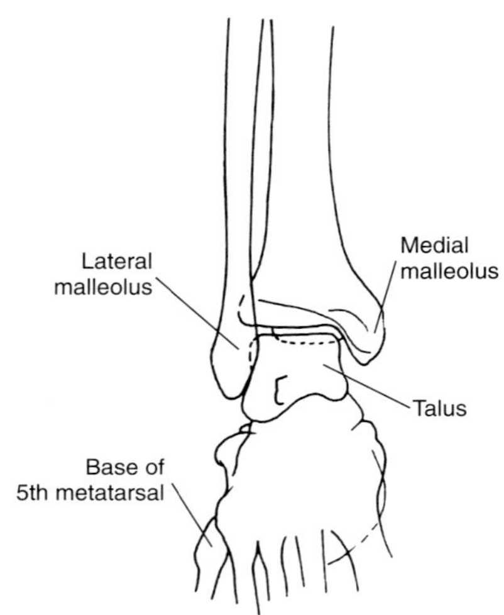

Fig. 7-79. AP ankle.

Radiographic Criteria

Structures Shown: • The distal one-third of the tibia-fibula, the lateral and medial malleoli, and the talus and the proximal half of the metatarsals should be demonstrated.

Position: • The long axis of the leg should be aligned to collimation field and to IR. • No rotation if the medial mortise joint is open and the lateral mortise closed. Some superimposition of the distal fibula by the distal tibia and talus will exist.

Collimation and CR: • CR and the center of the collimation field should be to the tibiotalar joint midway between the medial and lateral malleolus. • The four-sided collimation should include the distal one-third of the lower leg to the proximal half of the metatarsals. All surrounding soft tissue should also be included.

Exposure Criteria: • Optimal exposure with no motion will demonstrate clear bony margins and trabecular markings. • Talus must be penetrated enough to demonstrate the cortical margins and trabeculae of the bone. Soft-tissue structures must also be visible.

*Frank ED et al: Mayo Clinic: Radiography of the ankle mortise, Radiol Technol 62(5):354-359, 1991.

AP MORTISE PROJECTION—15° TO 20° MEDIAL ROTATION: ANKLE

Ankle
BASIC
- **AP**
- AP mortise (15°)
- **Oblique (45°)**
- **Lateral**

Pathology Demonstrated

This projection is particularly useful in evaluating pathology involving the entire ankle mortise* and the proximal fifth metatarsal, a common fracture site.†

Technical Factors

- IR size—24 × 30 cm (10 × 12 inches)
- Divide in half, crosswise
- Detail screen, tabletop
- Digital IR—use lead masking
- 60 ± 5 kV range
- Technique and dose:

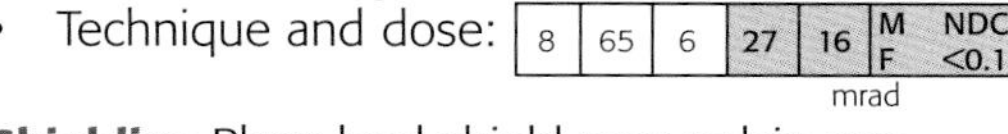

cm	kV	mAs	Sk.	ML.	Gon.
8	65	6	27	16	M NDC F <0.1

mrad

Shielding Place lead shield over pelvic area.

Patient Position Take radiograph with patient in the supine position; place pillow under head; legs should be fully extended.

Part Position

- Center and align ankle joint to CR and to long axis of portion of IR being exposed.
- Do not dorsiflex foot but allow to remain in natural extended (plantar flexed) position (allows for visualization of base of fifth metatarsal, a common fracture site).†
- Internally rotate **entire leg and foot** about **15° to 20°** until the **intermalleolar line is parallel to IR.**
- Place support against foot if needed to prevent motion.

Central Ray

- CR **perpendicular** to IR, directed **midway between malleoli**
- Minimum SID of 40 inches (100 cm)

Collimation Collimate to lateral skin margins, include proximal metatarsals and distal tibia-fibula.

CR or DR: Close collimation and lead masking are important over unused portion of image plate.

Notes: This position should **not** be a substitute for either the AP projection or the oblique ankle position but rather should be a separate projection of the ankle taken routinely when potential trauma or sprains of the ankle joint are involved.*

This is also a common projection taken during open reduction surgery of the ankle.

Radiographic Criteria

Structures Shown: • Distal one-third of the tibia and fibula, the tibial plafond involving the epiphysis if present, the lateral and medial malleoli, the talus, and the proximal half of the metatarsals should be demonstrated. • The entire ankle mortise should be open and well visualized (3-4 mm space over entire talar surface is normal; an extra 2 mm widening is abnormal)†

Position: • Proper obliquity for the mortise joint is evidenced by demonstration of open lateral and medial mortise joints with the malleoli demonstrated in profile. • Only minimal superimposition should exist at the distal tibiofibular joint.

Collimation and CR: • The center of four-sided collimation (CR) should be to midankle joint with the distal one-third of the lower leg to the proximal half of metatarsals included. • All soft-tissue structures should also be demonstrated.

Exposure Criteria: • No motion as demonstrated by sharp bony outlines and trabecular markings. • Optimal exposure should demonstrate soft-tissue structures and also sufficient density for talus and distal tibia and fibula.

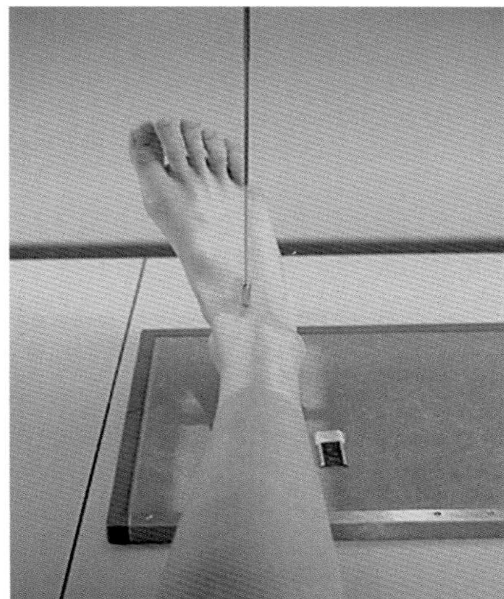

Fig. 7-80. Mortise projection, demonstrating 15° medial rotation of leg and foot.

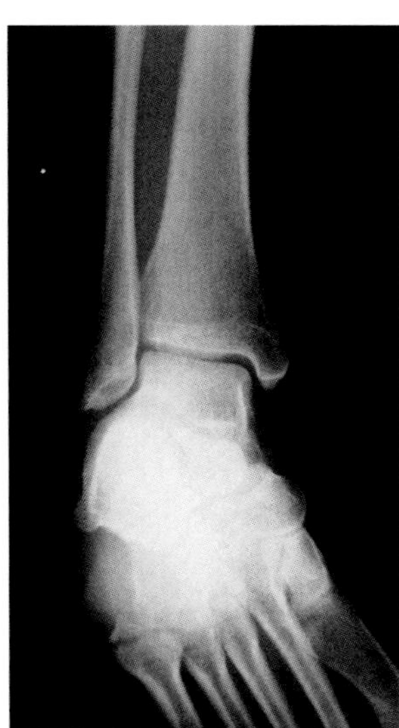

Fig. 7-81. Mortise projection.

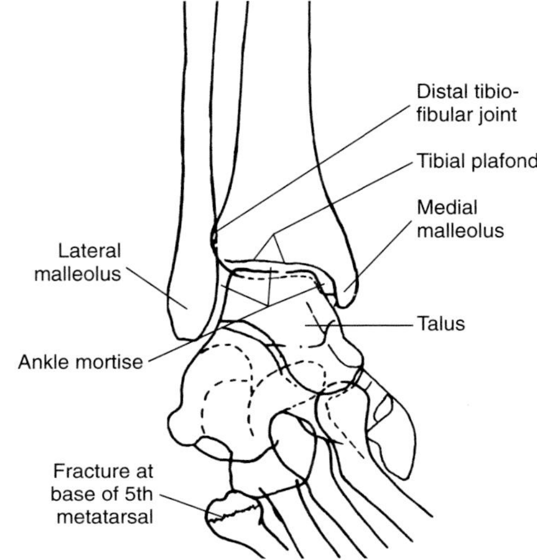

Fig. 7-82. Mortise projection.

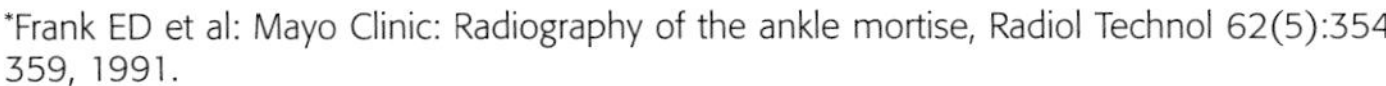

*Frank ED et al: Mayo Clinic: Radiography of the ankle mortise, Radiol Technol 62(5):354-359, 1991.

†Manaster BJ: Handbooks in radiology, skeletal radiology, ed 2, St. Louis, 1997, Year Book.

AP OBLIQUE PROJECTION—45° MEDIAL ROTATION: ANKLE

Ankle
BASIC
- AP
- AP mortise (15°)
- Oblique (45°)
- Lateral

Pathology Demonstrated

Pathologies including possible fractures involving the distal tibiofibular joint, the distal fibula and lateral malleolus, and the base of the fifth metatarsal are demonstrated.

Technical Factors

- IR size—24 × 30 cm (10 × 12 inches)
- Divide in half, crosswise
- Detail screen, tabletop
- Digital IR—use lead masking
- 60 ± 5 kV range
- Technique and dose:

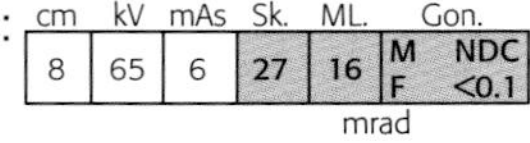

cm	kV	mAs	Sk.	ML.	Gon.
8	65	6	27	16	M NDC F <0.1
			mrad		

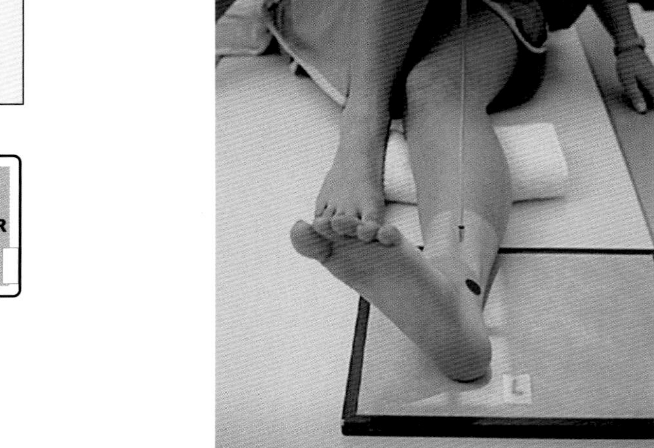

Fig. 7-83. 45° medial oblique.

Shielding Place lead shield over pelvic area to shield gonads.

Patient Position Take radiograph with patient in the supine position; place pillow under head; legs should be fully extended (small sandbag or other support under knee increases comfort of patient).

Part Position

- Center and align ankle joint to CR and to long axis of portion of IR being exposed.
- If patient's condition allows, dorsiflex the foot if needed so that the plantar surface is at least 80° to 85° from the IR (10°-15° from vertical). See Note below.
- **Rotate leg and foot** internally **45°**.

Central Ray

- CR **perpendicular** to IR, directed to a **point midway between malleoli**
- Minimum SID of 40 inches (100 cm)

Collimation Collimate to lateral skin margins; include distal tibia-fibula and proximal metatarsals (see Notes below)

CR or DR: Close collimation and lead masking are important over unused portion of image plate.

Notes: If the foot is extended or plantar flexed more than 10° or 15° from vertical, the calcaneus will be superimposed over the lateral malleolus on this 45° oblique, thus obscuring an important area of interest.

The base of the fifth metatarsal (a common fracture site) will be demonstrated in this projection and should be included in the collimation field. (See p. 239, AP mortise projection.)

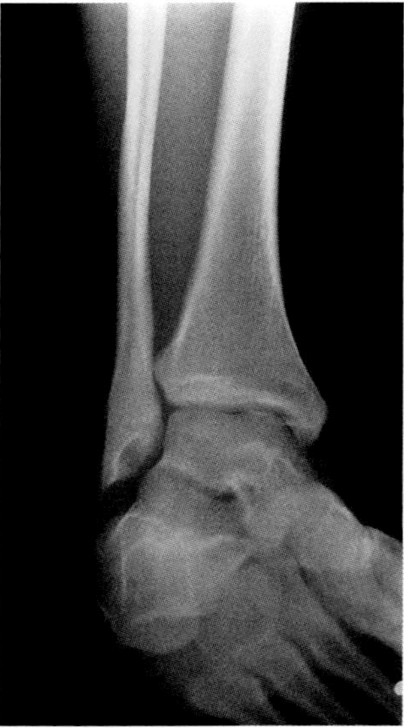

Fig. 7-84. 45° internal oblique. (Courtesy E. Frank, RT (R), FASRT.)

Radiographic Criteria

Structures Shown: • The distal one-third of the lower leg, the malleoli, the talus, and the proximal half of the metatarsals should be seen.

Position: • A 45° medial oblique will demonstrate the distal tibiofibular joint open, with no or only minimal overlap on the average person. • The lateral malleolus and talus joint should show no or only slight superimposition, but the medial malleolus and talus will be partially superimposed.

Collimation and CR: • The ankle joint should be in the center of the four-sided collimated field with the distal one-third of the lower leg to the proximal half of the metatarsals and surrounding soft tissues included.

Exposure Criteria: • The bony cortical margins and trabecular patterns should be sharply defined on the image if no motion is present. • The talus should be sufficiently penetrated to demonstrate the trabeculae, and the soft-tissue structures must also be evident.

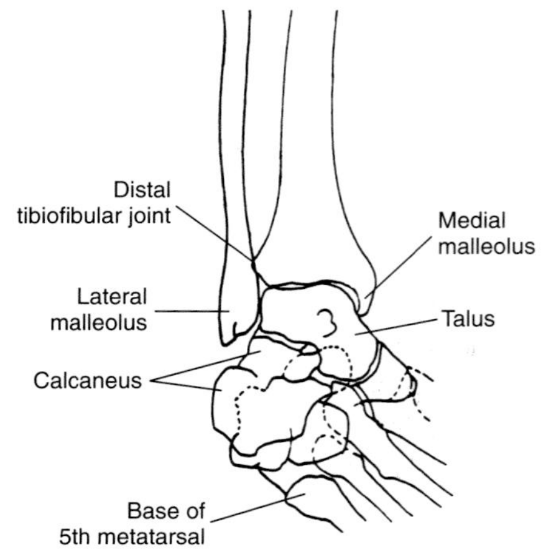

Fig. 7-85. 45° internal oblique.

LATERAL–MEDIOLATERAL (OR LATEROMEDIAL) PROJECTION: ANKLE

Ankle
BASIC
- AP
- AP mortise (15°)
- Oblique (45°)
- Lateral

Pathology Demonstrated

This projection is useful in the evaluation of fractures, dislocations, and joint effusions associated with other joint pathologies.

Technical Factors

- IR size—24 × 30 cm (10 × 12 inches)
- Divide in half, crosswise
- Detail screen, tabletop
- Digital IR—use lead masking
- 60 ± 5 kV range
- Technique and dose:

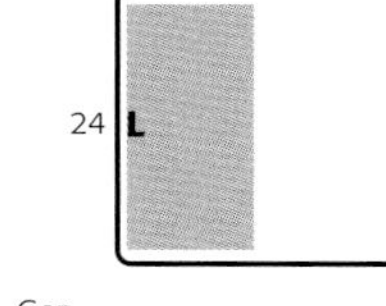

cm	kV	mAs	Sk.	ML.	Gon.
6	65	5	21	16	M NDC F <0.1

mrad

Shielding Place lead shield over pelvic area.

Patient Position Place patient in the lateral recumbent position, affected side down; give pillow for head; flex knee of affected limb about 45°; place opposite leg behind the injured limb to prevent overrotation.

Part Position (Mediolateral Projection)

- Center and align ankle joint to CR and to long axis of portion of IR being exposed.
- Place support under knee as needed to place leg and foot in a **true lateral position.**
- Dorsiflex foot so plantar surface is at a right angle to leg or as far as patient can tolerate; do **not** force. (This will help maintain a true lateral position.)

Central Ray

- CR **perpendicular** to IR, directed to **medial malleolus**
- Minimum SID of 40 inches (100 cm)

Collimation Collimate to include distal tibia and fibula and to midmetatarsal area.

CR or DR: Close collimation and lead masking are important over unused portion of image plate

Alternate lateromedial projection (Fig. 7-87): This lateral may be taken rather than the more commonly preferred mediolateral. (This position is more uncomfortable for patient but may be easier to achieve a true lateral position.)

Radiographic Criteria

Structures Shown: • The distal one-third of the tibia and fibula with the distal fibula superimposed by the distal tibia, the talus, and calcaneus will appear in lateral profile. • The tuberosity of the fifth metatarsal, the navicular, and cuboid will also be visualized.

Position: • **No rotation** is evidenced by the distal fibula being superimposed over **posterior half of tibia.** The tibiotalar joint will be open with uniform joint space.

Collimation and CR: • The center of the four-sided collimation (CR) should be to the midankle joint. The collimation field should include the distal one-third of the lower leg, the calcaneus, the tuberosity of the fifth metatarsal, and surrounding soft-tissue structures.

Exposure Criteria: • No motion, as evidenced by sharp bony margins and trabecular patterns. The lateral malleolus should be seen through the distal tibia and talus, and soft tissue must be demonstrated to evaluate for joint effusion.

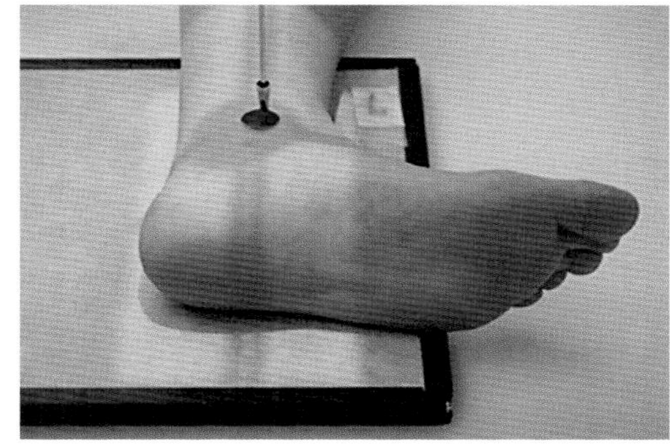

Fig. 7-86. Mediolateral ankle.

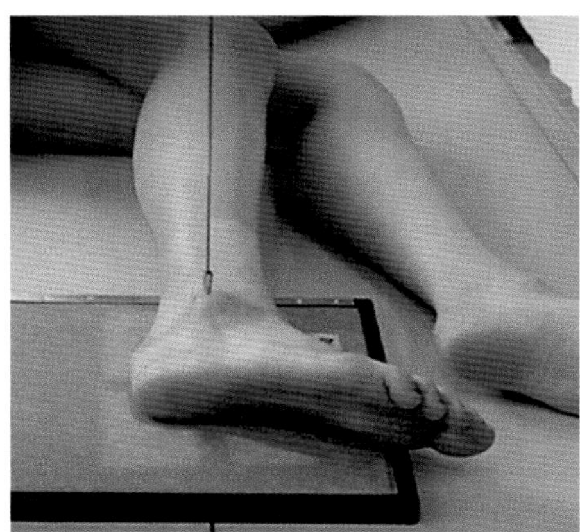

Fig. 7-87. Alternate lateromedial ankle.

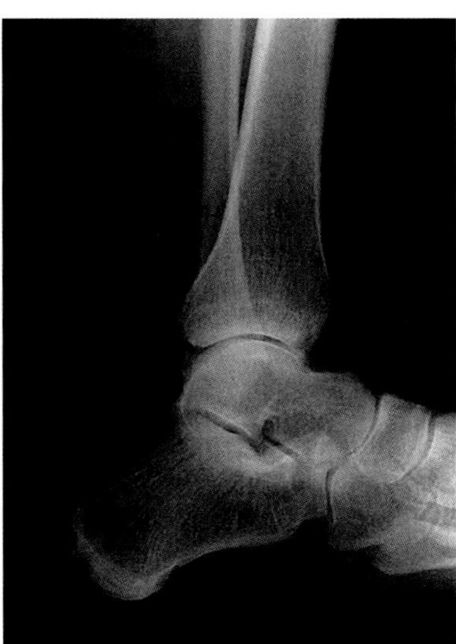

Fig. 7-88. Mediolateral ankle.

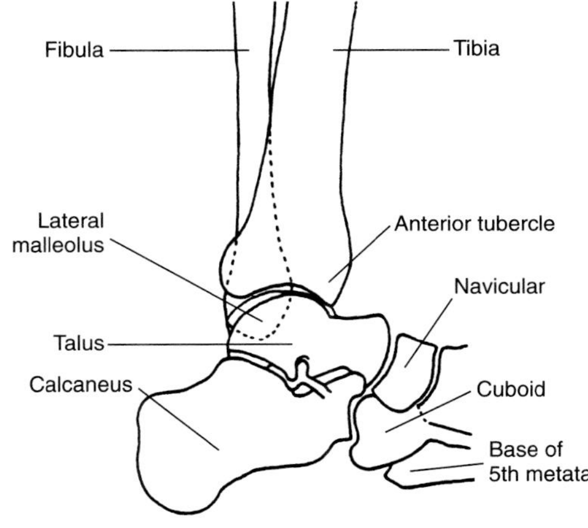

Fig. 7-89. Lateral ankle.

7

AP STRESS PROJECTIONS: ANKLE

Inversion and Eversion Positions

Warning: Proceed with utmost care with injured patient.

Ankle
SPECIAL
• AP stress

Pathology Demonstrated

Pathology involving ankle joint separation due to ligament tear or rupture is demonstrated.

Technical Factors

- IR size—24 × 30 cm (10 × 12 inches)
- Divide in half, crosswise
- Detail screen, tabletop
- Digital IR—use lead masking
- 60 ± 5 kV range
- Technique and dose:

cm	kV	mAs	Sk.	ML.	Gon.
8	65	6	27	16	M NDC F <0.1
			mrad		

30
24 R R
Inversion Eversion

Shielding Place shielding over gonadal area of patient. Supply lead gloves and a lead apron for the individual applying stress if stress positions are handheld during exposures.

Patient Position Take radiograph with patient in the supine position; place pillow under head; leg should be fully extended, support under knee.

Part Position

- Center and align ankle joint to CR and to long axis of portion of IR being exposed.
- Dorsiflex the foot as near the right angle to the leg as possible.
- Stress is applied with leg and ankle in position for a **true AP** with no rotation, wherein the entire plantar surface is turned medially for inversion and laterally for eversion (see Note below).

Central Ray

- CR **perpendicular** to IR, directed to a point **midway between malleoli**
- Minimum SID of 40 inches (100 cm)

Collimation Collimate to lateral skin margins, include proximal metatarsals and distal tibia-fibula.

CR or DR: Close collimation and lead masking are important over unused portion of image plate to prevent fogging from scatter radiation to the hypersensitive image plate or receptor.

Note: A physician or another health professional must be present to either hold the foot and ankle in these stress views (or to strap into position with weights) or to have patient hold this position with long gauze looped around ball of foot. If this is too painful for patient, local anesthesia may be injected by the physician.

Radiographic Criteria

Structures Shown and Position: • Ankle joint for evaluation of joint separation and ligament tear or rupture is shown. The appearance of the joint space may vary greatly depending on the severity of ligament damage.

Collimation and CR: • Midankle joint should be in the center of the collimated field (CR).

Exposure Criteria: • No motion, as evidenced by sharp bony margins and trabecular patterns. Optimal exposure should visualize soft tissue, the lateral and medial malleoli, the talus, and the distal tibia and fibula.

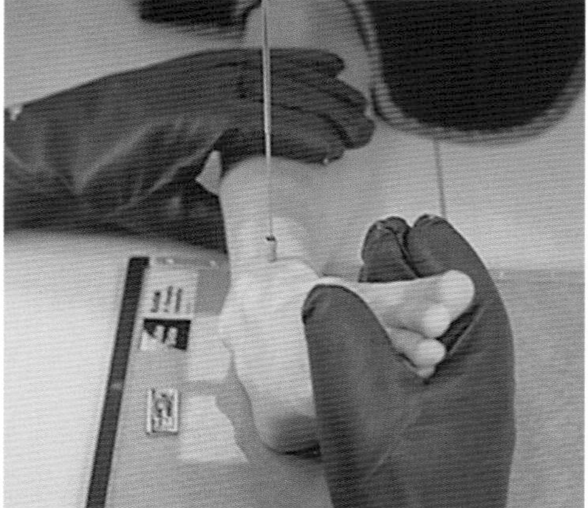

Fig. 7-90. Inversion stress.

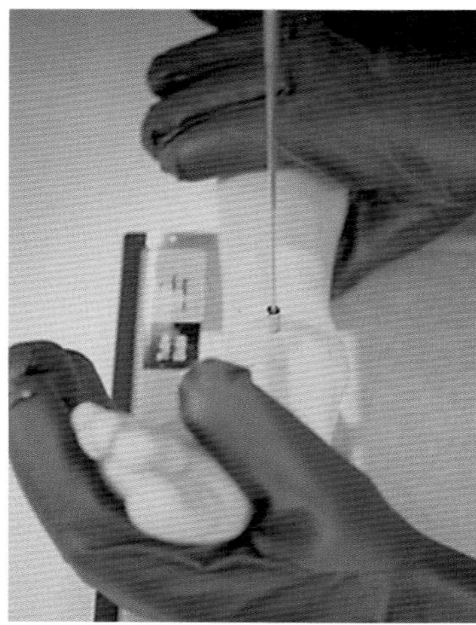

Fig. 7-91. Eversion stress.

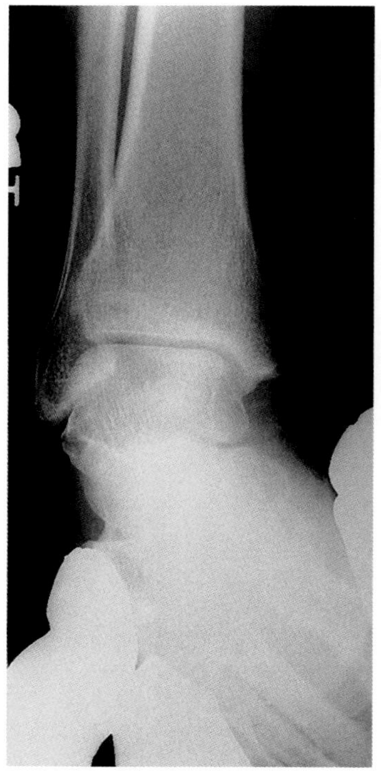

Fig. 7-92. Inversion.

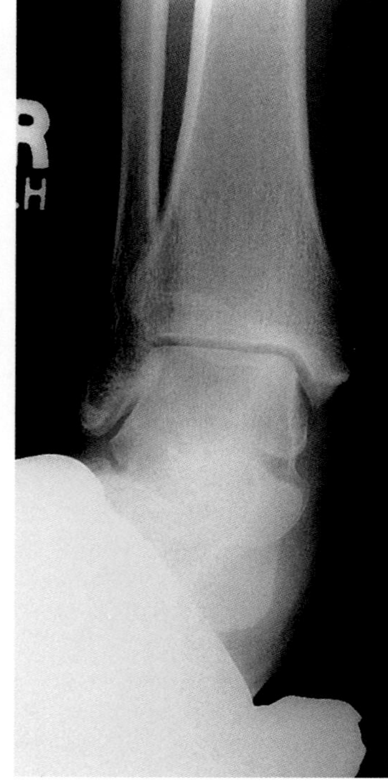

Fig. 7-93. Eversion.

AP PROJECTION: LEG

Leg
- AP
- Lateral

Pathology Demonstrated
Pathologies involving fractures, foreign bodies, or lesions of the bone are demonstrated.

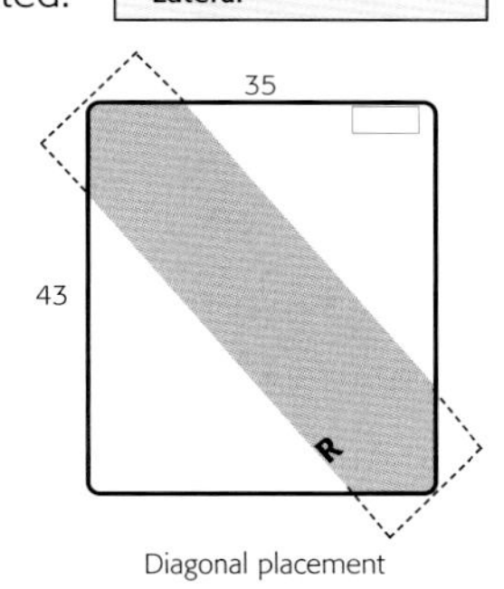

Technical Factors
- IR size—35 × 43 cm (14 × 17 inches) divided in half, lengthwise (or diagonal, which requires 44 inches or 110 cm minimum SID)
- Detail screen, tabletop
- 70 ± 5 kV range
- To make best use of anode-heel effect, place knee at cathode end of x-ray beam
- Technique and dose:

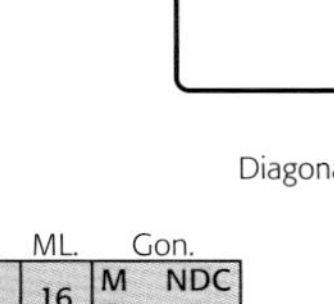

cm	kV	mAs	Sk.	ML.	Gon.
10	70	6	34	16	M NDC F <0.1
			mrad		

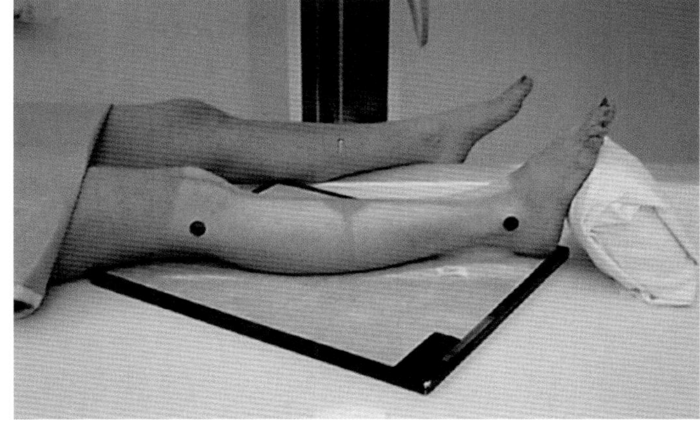

Fig. 7-94. AP leg—Include both joints.

Shielding Place lead shielding over gonadal area.

Patient Position Take radiograph with patient in the supine position; give pillow for head; leg should be fully extended.

Part Position
- Adjust pelvis, knee, and leg into a true AP with no rotation.
- Place sandbag against foot if needed for stabilization, dorsiflex foot to 90° to leg if possible.
- Ensure that both ankle and knee joints are 1 to 2 inches (3 to 5 cm) from ends of IR (so that divergent rays will not project either joint off the IR).
- For most adults the leg must be placed diagonally (corner to corner) on one 35 × 43 cm IR to ensure that both joints are included. (Also, if needed, a second smaller IR may be taken of the joint nearest the injury site.)

Central Ray
- CR **perpendicular** to IR, directed to **midpoint of leg**
- Minimum SID of 40 inches (100 cm); may increase to 44 or 48 inches (110 to 120 cm) to reduce divergence of x-ray beam and to include more of body part (increase mAs accordingly)

Collimation Collimate on both sides to skin margins, with full collimation at ends of IR borders to include maximum knee and ankle joints.

Alternative follow-up exam routine: The routine for follow-up exams of long bones in some departments is to include only the one joint nearest the site of injury and to place this joint a minimum of 2 inches (5 cm) from the end of the IR for better demonstration of this joint. However, for initial exams, it is **important, especially when the injury site is at the distal leg, to also include the proximal tibiofibular joint area** because it is common to have a second fracture at this site. For very large patients, a second AP projection of the knee and proximal leg may be needed on a smaller IR.

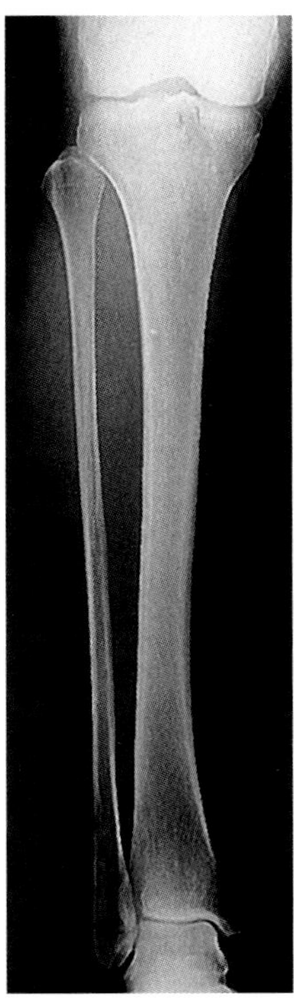

Fig. 7-95. AP leg—both joints. (Courtesy Jim Sanderson, RT.)

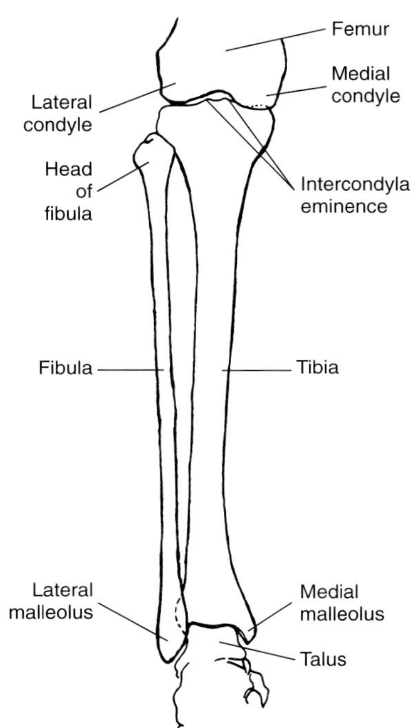

Fig. 7-96. AP leg—both joints.

Radiographic Criteria

Structures Shown: • The entire tibia and fibula should be included with both the ankle and knee joints demonstrated on one (or two if needed) IR(s). (Exception is alternate routine on follow-up exams.)

Position: • **No rotation** as evidenced by demonstration of the femoral and tibial condyles in profile with the intercondylar eminence centered within the intercondylar fossa. • Some overlap of the fibula and tibia will be visible at both the proximal and distal ends.

Collimation and CR: • Close side collimation borders should be visible but only minimal (if any) borders should be visible at the ends to maximize visualization of both joints. • Divergence of the beam will cause the knee and ankle joint spaces to be mostly closed.

Exposure Criteria: • Correct use of the anode-heel effect will result in an image with nearer equal density at both ends of the IR. • No motion is present, evidenced by sharp cortical margins and trabecular patterns. • Contrast should also be sufficient to visualize soft tissue and bony trabecular markings at both ends of tibia.

LATERAL—MEDIOLATERAL PROJECTION: LEG—TIBIA AND FIBULA

Leg
- AP
- Lateral

Pathology Demonstrated
Localization of lesions and foreign bodies and determination of the extent and alignment of fractures are demonstrated.

35

43

R

Diagonal placement

Technical Factors
- IR size—35 × 43 cm (14 × 17 inches) divide in half, lengthwise (or diagonal, which requires 44 inches or 110 cm SID)
- Detail screen, tabletop
- 70 ± 5 kV range
- To make best use of anode-heel effect, place knee at cathode end of x-ray beam
- Technique and dose:

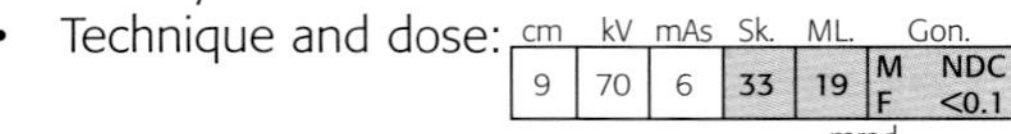

cm	kV	mAs	Sk.	ML.	Gon.
9	70	6	33	19	M NDC F <0.1

mrad

Shielding Place shield over pelvic and gonadal area.

Patient Position Take radiograph with patient in the lateral recumbent position, injured side down; the opposite leg may be placed behind the affected leg and supported with a pillow or sandbags.

Part Position
- Flex knee about 45° and ensure that leg is in a true lateral position. (Plane of patella should be perpendicular to IR.)
- Ensure that both ankle and knee joints are 1 to 2 inches (3 to 5 cm) from ends of IR so that divergent rays will not project either joint off IR.
- For most adults the leg must be placed diagonally (corner to corner) on one 35 × 43 IR to ensure that both joints are included. (Also, if needed a second, smaller IR may be taken of the joint nearest the injury site.)

Central Ray
- CR **perpendicular** to IR, directed to **midleg**
- Minimum SID of 40 inches (100 cm); may increase to 44 or 48 inches (110 to 120 cm) to reduce divergence of x-ray beam to include more of body part (increase mAs accordingly)

Collimation Collimate on both sides to skin margins, with full collimation at ends to include maximum knee and ankle joints.

Alternative follow-up exam routine: The routine for follow-up exams of long bones in some departments is to include only the one joint nearest the site of injury and to place this joint a minimum of 2 inches (5 cm) from the end of the IR for better demonstration of this joint. However, for initial exams it is especially important when the injury site is at the distal leg to include the proximal tibiofibular joint area because it is common to have a second fracture at this site.

Cross-table lateral: If patient cannot be turned, this can be taken cross-table with cassette placed on edge between legs. Place a support under injured leg to center leg to IR, and direct horizontal beam from lateral side of patient.

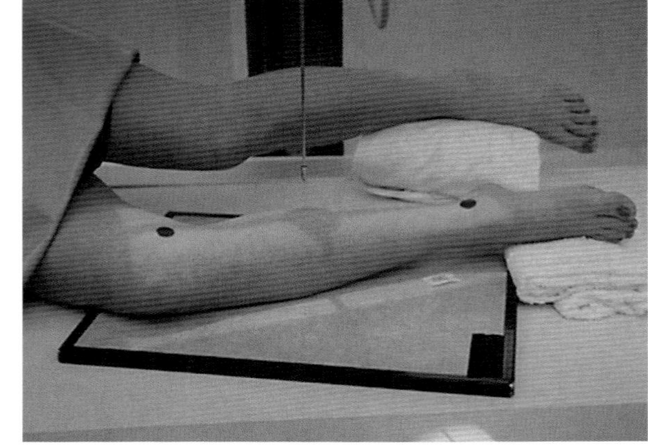

Fig. 7-97. Mediolateral leg—include both joints.

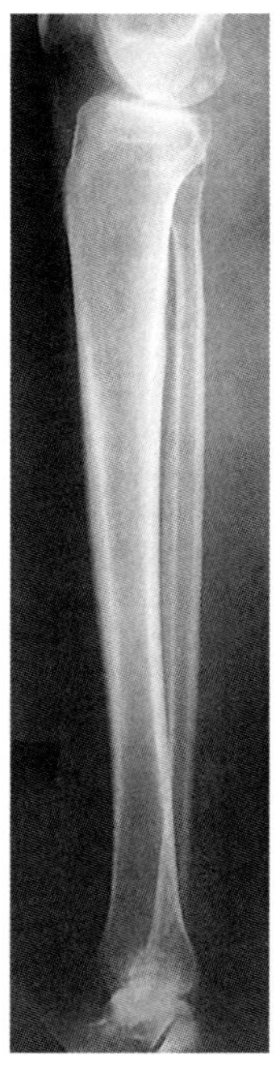

Fig. 7-98. Mediolateral leg. (Courtesy Jim Sanderson, RT.)

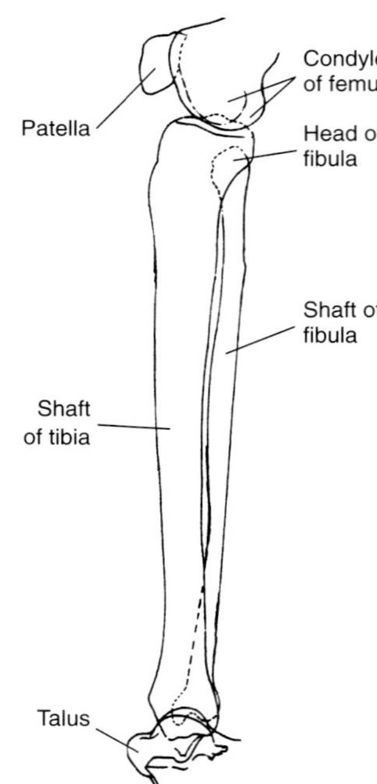

Fig. 7-99. Mediolateral leg.

Radiographic Criteria

Structures Shown: • The entire tibia and fibula should be included with both the ankle and knee joints included on one (or two if needed) IR(s). (Exception is alternate routine on follow-up exams.)

Position: • A true lateral of the tibia and fibula without rotation will demonstrate the tibial tuberosity in profile, a portion of the proximal head of the fibula superimposed by the tibia, and outlines of the distal fibula seen through the posterior half of the tibia. • Posterior borders of femoral condyles should appear superimposed.

Collimation and CR: • Close side collimation borders should be visible, but only minimal, if any, border should be visible at the ends to maximize visualization of both joints.

Exposure Criteria: • Good exposure density without motion will result in visualization of sharp trabecular markings and sharp borders of entire tibia and fibula. • Optimal exposure with correct use of the anode-heel effect will result in near equal density at both ends of the image. • Contrast and density should be sufficient to visualize soft tissue and bony trabecular markings.

AP PROJECTION: KNEE

Knee
BASIC
- AP
- **Oblique (medial & lateral)**
- **Lateral**

Pathology Demonstrated
Any fractures, lesions, or bony changes secondary to degenerative joint disease involving the distal femur, proximal tibia and fibula, patella, and knee joint may be visualized in the AP projection.

Technical Factors
- IR size—18 × 24 cm (8 × 10 inches), lengthwise
- Grid or Bucky, >10 cm (70 ± 5 kV)
- Screen, tabletop, <10 cm (65 ± 5 kV)
- Technique and dose:

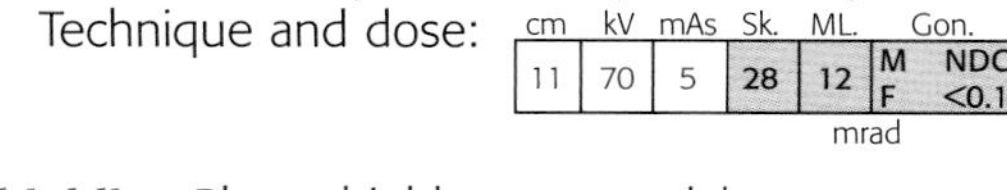
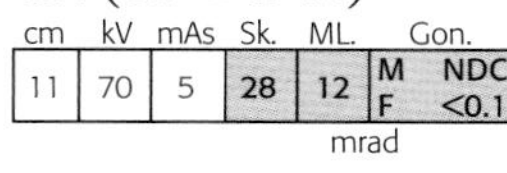

cm	kV	mAs	Sk.	ML.	Gon.	
11	70	5	28	12	M	NDC
					F	<0.1
			mrad			

Shielding Place shield over gonadal area.

Patient Position Take radiograph with patient in the supine position with no rotation of pelvis; give pillow for head; leg should be fully extended.

Part Position
- Align and center leg and knee to CR and to midline of table or IR.
- Rotate leg internally 3° to 5° for a true AP knee (or until **interepicondylar line is parallel** to plane of IR).
- Place sandbags by foot and ankle to stabilize if needed.

Central Ray
- Align CR **parallel to tibial plateau;** for average-size patient, CR is perpendicular to IR (see Note below).
- Direct CR to a point ½ **inch, or 1.25 cm,** distal to apex of patella.
- Minimum SID is 40 inches (100 cm).

Collimation Collimate on both sides to skin margins at ends to IR borders.

Note: A suggested guideline for determining that CR is parallel to tibial plateau for open joint space is to measure distance from ASIS to tabletop to determine CR angle as follows:*
- <19 cm, **3° to 5° caudad** (thin thighs and buttocks)
- 19-24 cm, **0° angle** (average thighs and buttocks)
- >24 cm, **3° to 5° cephalad** (thick thighs and buttocks)

Radiographic Criteria

Structures Shown: • The distal femur and proximal tibia and fibula are shown. • The femorotibial joint space should be open, with the articular facets of the tibia seen on end with only minimal surface area visualized.

Position: • **No rotation** will be evidenced by the symmetric appearance of the femoral and tibial condyles and the joint space. • The approximate medial half of the fibular head should be superimposed by the tibia. • The intercondylar eminence will be seen in the center of the intercondylar fossa.

Collimation and CR: • The collimation field should align with the long axis of the IR. • The center of the collimation field (CR) should be to the midknee joint space.

Exposure Criteria: • Optimal exposure will visualize the outline of the patella through the distal femur, and the fibular head and neck will not appear overexposed. • No motion should exist; trabecular markings of all bones should be visible and appear sharp. Soft-tissue detail should be visible.

*Martensen KM: Alternate AP knee method assures open joint space, Radiol Technol 64(1):19-23, 1992.

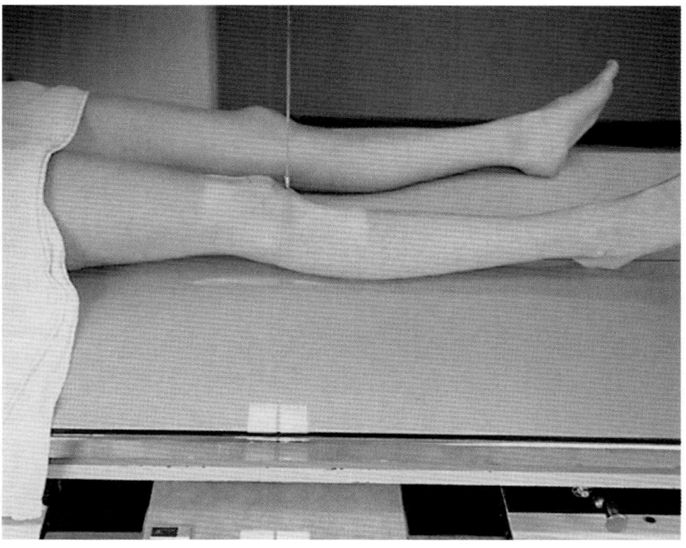

Fig. 7-100. AP knee—CR perpendicular to IR (average patient).

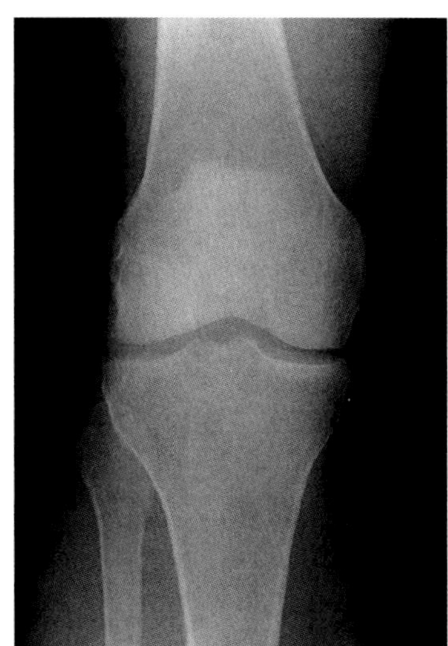

Fig. 7-101. AP knee—0° CR.

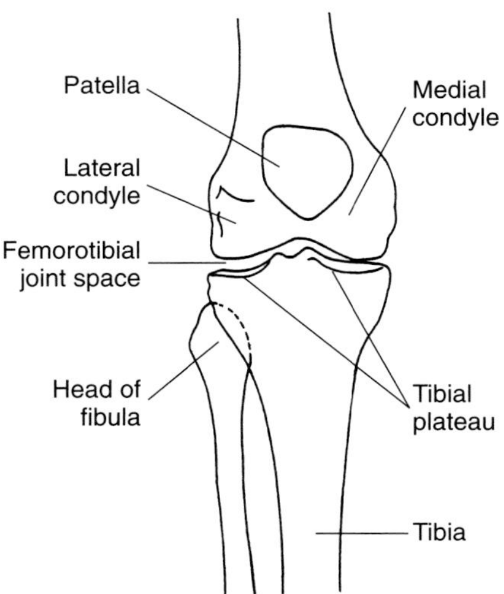

Fig. 7-102. AP knee—0° CR.

7

AP OBLIQUE PROJECTION—MEDIAL (INTERNAL) ROTATION: KNEE

Knee
BASIC
- AP
- Oblique (medial and lateral)
- Lateral

Pathology Demonstrated
Pathology involving the proximal tibiofibular and femorotibial (knee) joint articulations is demonstrated, as well as fractures, lesions, and bony changes secondary to degenerative joint disease, especially on the anterior and medial or posterior and lateral portions of the knee.

Note: A common departmental routine is to include **both** medial and lateral rotation obliques for the knee. If only one oblique is routine, it is most commonly this internal rotation oblique.

Technical Factors
- IR size—18 × 24 cm (8 × 10 inches), lengthwise
- Grid or Bucky, >10 cm (70 ± 5 kV)
- Screen, tabletop, <10 cm (65 ± 5 kV)
- Technique and dose:

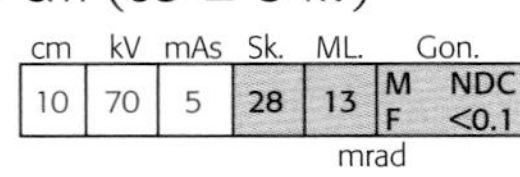

cm	kV	mAs	Sk.	ML.	Gon.	
10	70	5	28	13	M	NDC
					F	<0.1
			mrad			

18 / 24 / R

Shielding Place shield over gonadal area.

Patient Position Take radiograph with patient in the semisupine position with entire body and leg rotated partially away from side of interest; place support under elevated hip; give pillow for head.

Part Position
- Align and center leg and knee to CR and to midline of table or IR.
- Rotate entire leg **internally 45°.** (Interepicondylar line should be 45° to plane of IR.)
- If needed, stabilize foot and ankle in this position with sandbags.

Central Ray
- Angle CR 0° on average patient (see AP Knee, p. 245).
- Direct CR to **midpoint of the knee** at a level ½ **inch (1.25 cm) distal to apex of patella.**
- Minimum SID is 40 inches (100 cm).

Collimation Collimate on both sides to skin margins, with full collimation at ends to IR borders to include maximum femur and tibia/fibula.

Note: The terms *medial (internal) oblique* or *lateral (external) oblique positions* refer to the direction of rotation of the anterior or patella surface of the knee. This is true for descriptions of either AP or PA oblique projections.

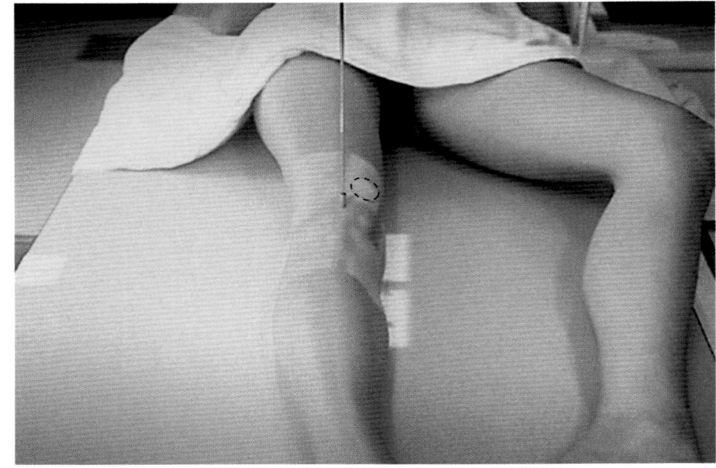

Fig. 7-103. AP medial oblique.

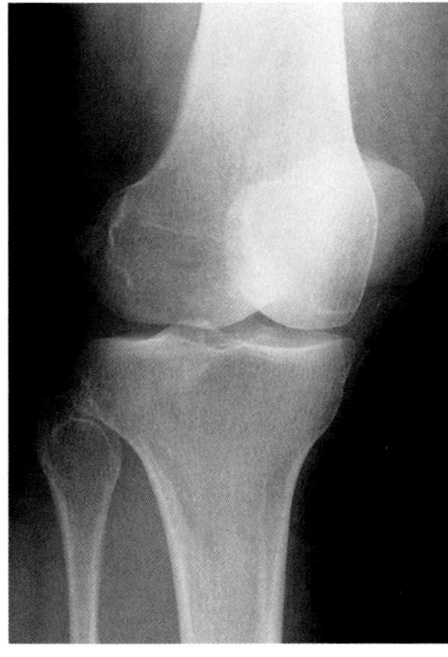

Fig. 7-104. AP medial oblique.

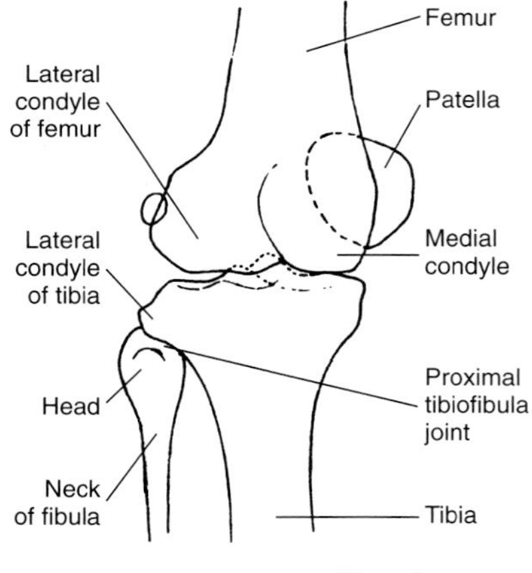

Fig. 7-105. AP medial oblique.

Radiographic Criteria

Structures Shown: • Distal femur and proximal tibia and fibula with the patella superimposing the medial femoral condyle are shown. • The **lateral condyles** of the femur and tibia are well demonstrated, and the medial and lateral knee joint spaces will appear unequal.

Position: • The proper amount of part obliquity will demonstrate the proximal tibiofibular articulation open with the lateral condyles of femur and tibia seen in profile. • The head and neck of fibula will be visualized without superimposition, and approximately half of the patella should be seen free of superimposition by the femur.

Collimation and CR: • CR and center of the collimated field is to the femorotibial (knee) joint space.

Exposure Criteria: • Optimal exposure with no motion should visualize soft tissue in knee joint area, and trabecular markings of all bones should appear clear and sharp. Head and neck area of fibula should not appear overexposed.

AP OBLIQUE PROJECTION—LATERAL (EXTERNAL) ROTATION: KNEE

Knee
BASIC
• AP
• Oblique (medial and lateral)
• Lateral

Pathology Demonstrated

Pathology involving the femorotibial (knee) articulation is demonstrated, as well as fractures, lesions, and bony changes secondary to degenerative joint disease, especially on the anterior and lateral or posterior and medial aspects of the knee.

Note: A common departmental routine is to include **both** medial and lateral rotation obliques for the knee. If only one oblique is routine, it is most commonly the internal rotation oblique (see p. 246).

Technical Factors

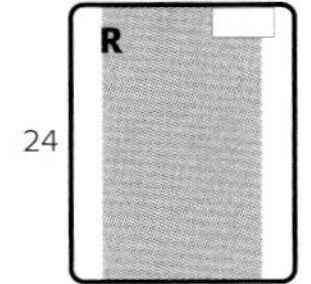

- IR size—18 × 24 cm (8 × 10 inches), lengthwise
- Grid or Bucky, >10 cm (70 ± 5 kV)
- Screen, tabletop, <10 cm (65 ± 5 kV)
- Technique and dose:

cm	kV	mAs	Sk.	ML.	Gon.
10	70	5	28	13	M NDC F <0.1
			mrad		

Shielding Place shield over gonadal area.

Patient Position Take radiograph with patient in the semisupine position, with entire body and leg rotated partially away from side of interest; place support under elevated hip; give pillow for head.

Part Position

- Align and center leg and knee to CR and to midline of table or IR.
- Rotate entire leg **externally 45°.** (Interepicondylar line should be 45° to plane of IR.)
- If needed, stabilize foot and ankle in this position with sandbags.

Central Ray

- Angle CR 0° on average patient (see AP Knee, p. 245).
- Direct CR to **midpoint of the knee** at a level ½ **inch (1.25 cm) distal to apex of patella.**
- Minimum SID is 40 inches (100 cm).

Collimation Collimate on both sides to skin margins, with full collimation at ends to IR borders to include maximum femur and tibia/fibula.

Note: The terms *medial (internal) oblique* or *lateral (external) oblique positions* refer to the direction of rotation of the anterior or patella surface of the knee. This is true for descriptions of either AP or PA oblique projections.

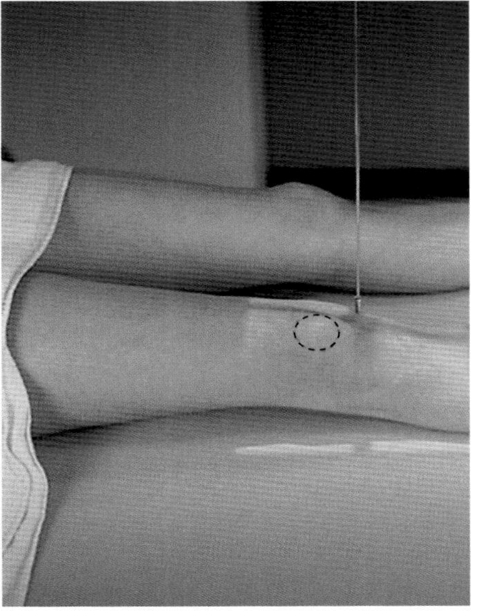

Fig. 7-106. AP lateral oblique.

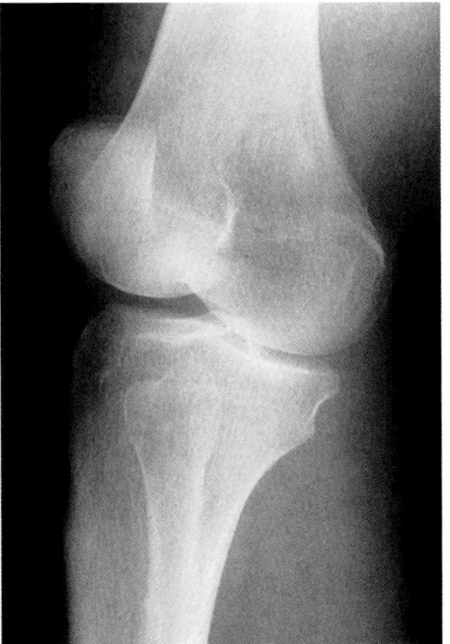

Fig. 7-107. AP lateral oblique.

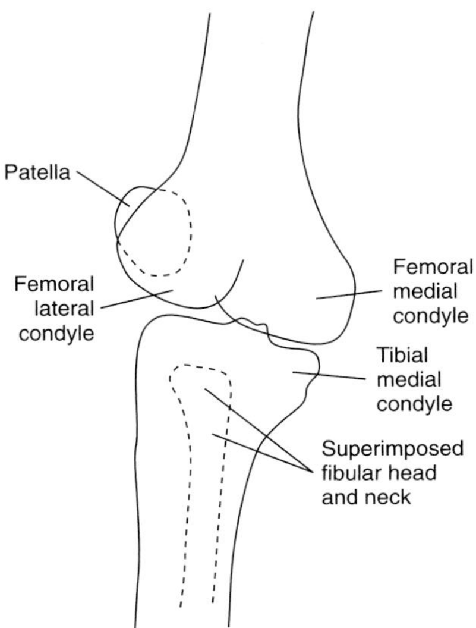

Fig. 7-108. AP lateral oblique.

Radiographic Criteria

Structures Shown: • Distal femur and proximal tibia and fibula, with the patella superimposing the lateral femoral condyle, are shown. • The **medial condyles** of the femur and tibia are demonstrated in profile.

Position: • The proper amount of part obliquity will demonstrate the proximal fibula superimposed by the proximal tibia, the medial condyles of femur, and tibia seen in profile. • Approximately half of the patella should be seen free of superimposition by the femur.

Collimation and CR: • The femorotibial (knee) joint space is the center of the collimated field.

Exposure Criteria: • Optimal exposure should visualize soft tissue in knee joint area, and trabecular markings of all bones should appear clear and sharp, indicating no motion. • Technique should be sufficient to demonstrate the head and neck area of the fibula through the superimposed tibia.

LATERAL—MEDIOLATERAL PROJECTION: KNEE

Knee
BASIC
• AP
• Oblique
• Lateral

Pathology Demonstrated
Fractures, lesions, and joint space abnormalities are demonstrated.

Technical Factors
- IR size—18 × 24 cm (8 × 10 inches), lengthwise
- Grid or Bucky, >10 cm (70 ± 5 kV)
- Screen, tabletop, <10 cm (65 ± 5 kV)
- Technique and dose:

cm	kV	mAs	Sk.	ML.	Gon.
10	70	4	22	11	M NDC F <0.1

mrad

18 (24)
24 (30)
L

Shielding Place shield over gonadal area.

Patient Position Take radiograph with patient in lateral recumbent position, affected side down; give pillow for head; provide support for knee of opposite limb placed behind knee being examined to prevent overrotation.

Part Position
- Adjust rotation of body and leg until knee is in a **true lateral** position (femoral epicondyles directly superimposed and plane of patella perpendicular to plane of IR).
- Flex knee **20° to 30°** (see Note 1 below).
- Align and center leg and knee to CR and to midline of table or IR.

Central Ray
- Angle CR **5° to 7° cephalad** (see Note 2 below).
- Direct CR to a point **1 inch (2.5 cm) distal to** medial epicondyle.
- Minimum SID is 40 inches (100 cm).

Collimation Collimate on both sides to skin margins, with full collimation at ends to IR borders to include maximum femur tibia and fibula.

Cross-table lateral: If patient cannot be turned to the lateral position, use a horizontal beam with IR placed beside knee. Place support under knee to avoid cutting off posterior soft-tissue structures (Fig. 7-109, *inset*).

Note 1: Additional flexion will tighten muscles and tendons that may obscure important diagnostic information in the joint space. The patella will be drawn into the intercondylar sulcus, also obscuring soft-tissue detail from effusion and/or fat pad displacement. Additional flexion may also result in fragment separation of patellar fractures if present.

Note 2: Angle CR 7° to 10° on short patient with wide pelvis and only about 5° on tall, male patient with narrow pelvis (see p. 217).

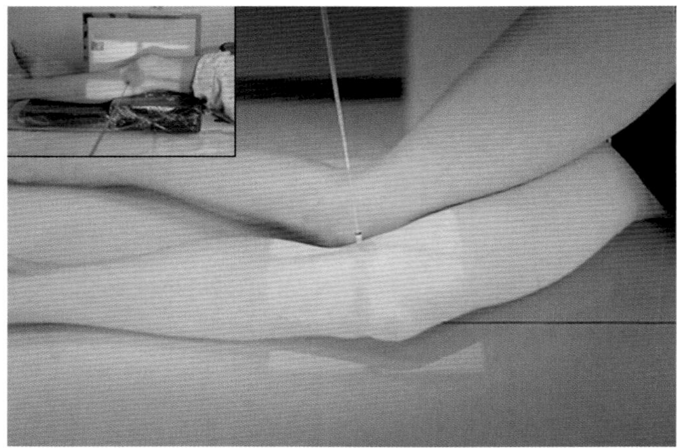

Fig. 7-109. Mediolateral—5° to 7° cephalad. (*Inset*—cross-table lateral.)

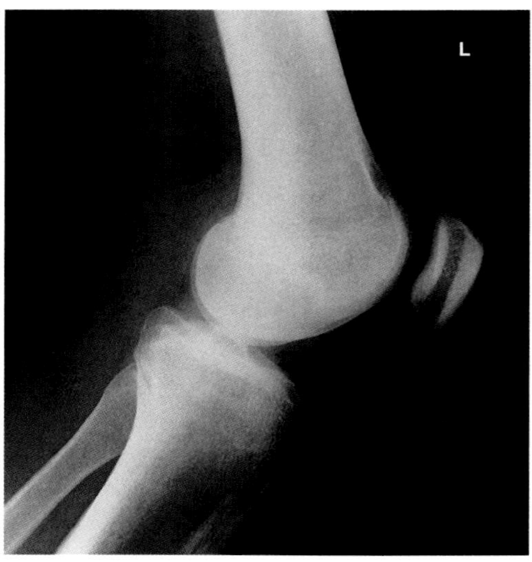

Fig. 7-110. Mediolateral knee.

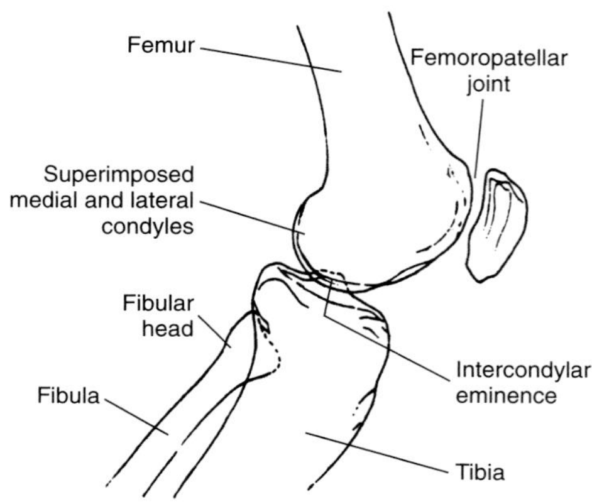

Fig. 7-111. Mediolateral projection.

Radiographic Criteria

Structures Shown: • The distal femur, proximal tibia and fibula, and patella are shown in lateral profile. • Femoropatellar and knee joints should be open.

Position: • Overrotation or underrotation can be determined by identifying the adductor tubercle on medial condyle, if visible (see p. 220, Fig. 7-33) and by the amount of superimposition of fibular head by tibia. (Overrotation, less superimposition of fibular head; underrotation, more superimposition.) • A **true lateral** position of the knee without rotation will demonstrate the **posterior borders** of the femoral condyles directly superimposed. • The patella should be seen in profile with the femoropatellar joint space open.

Collimation and CR: • The 5° to 10° cephalad angle of CR should result in direct superimposition of the **distal borders** of the condyles. • The knee joint is in the center of the collimated field. The top and bottom is collimated minimally. • All surrounding soft-tissue structures should be included.

Exposure Criteria: • Optimal exposure with no motion will visualize important soft-tissue detail, including fat pads anterior to knee joint and sharp trabecular markings.

AP WEIGHT-BEARING BILATERAL KNEE PROJECTION: KNEE

Knee
SPECIAL
• AP bilateral weight-bearing

Pathology Demonstrated
Femorotibial joint spaces of the knees are demonstrated for possible cartilage degeneration or other knee joint pathologies. Both knees are included on same exposure for comparison.

This projection is most commonly taken AP but may be taken PA if requested.

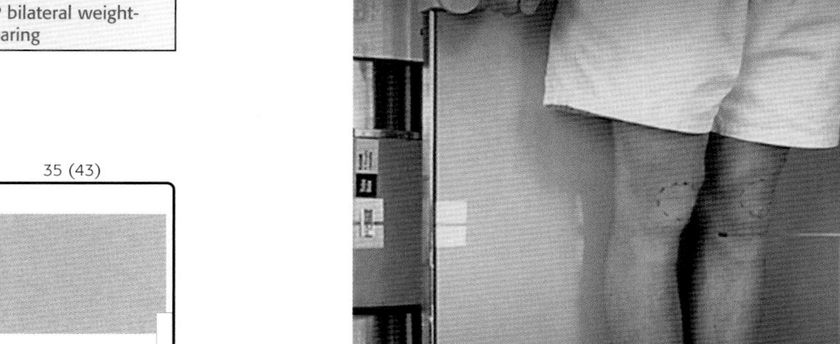

Technical Factors
- IR size—30 × 35 cm (11 × 14 inches) or 35 × 43 cm (14 × 17 inches), crosswise
- Moving or stationary grid
- 70 ± 5 kV range
- Technique and dose:

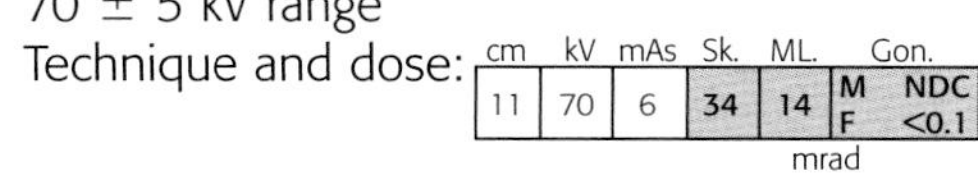

cm	kV	mAs	Sk.	ML.	Gon.
11	70	6	34	14	M NDC F <0.1
				mrad	

Shielding Shield gonadal area.

Patient and Part Position
- Take radiograph with patient erect, standing on attached step or on step stool to place patient high enough for horizontal beam x-ray tube.
- Position feet straight ahead with weight evenly distributed on both feet; provide support handles for patient stability
- Align and center bilateral legs and knees to CR and to midline of table and IR; IR height adjusted to CR.

Central Ray
- CR **perpendicular to IR** (average-sized patient), or **5°** **to 10° caudad** on thin patient, directed to **midpoint between knee joints at level ½ inch (1.25 cm) below apex of patellae**
- Minimum SID of 40 inches (100 cm)

Collimation Collimate to bilateral knee joint region, include some distal femora and proximal tibia for alignment purposes.

Alternate PA: If requested, an alternate PA may be performed with patient facing the table or IR holder, knees flexed at approximately 20°, feet straight ahead, thighs against tabletop or IR holder.

Direct CR **10° caudad** (parallel to tibial plateaus) to **level of knee joints** for PA projection.

Note: The CR angle should be parallel to tibial plateau to best demonstrate "open" knee joint spaces. See AP Knee Projection on p. 245 for correct CR angle.

Fig. 7-112. AP bilateral weight-bearing—CR perpendicular to IR, or 5°-10° caudad on thin patient.

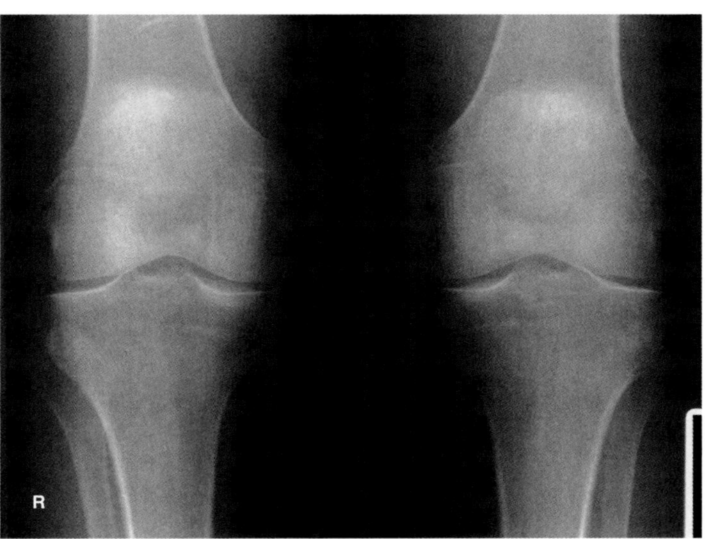

Fig. 7-113. AP bilateral weight-bearing, CR 10° caudad.

Radiographic Criteria

Structures Shown: • The distal femur, proximal tibia, and fibula and femorotibial joint spaces are demonstrated bilaterally.

Position: • **No rotation** of both knees is evident by symmetric appearance of femoral and tibial condyles. • Approximately one-half of proximal fibula will be superimposed by the tibia.

Collimation and CR: • Knee joint spaces should appear open if CR angle was correct (parallel to tibial plateau). • Collimation field should be centered to knee joint spaces and should include sufficient femur and tibia to determine long axis of these long bones for alignment determinations.

Exposure Criteria: • Optimal exposure should visualize faint outlines of patellae through femora. • Soft tissue should be visible, and trabecular markings of all bones should appear clear and sharp, indicating no motion.

7

PA AXIAL PROJECTION—TUNNEL VIEW: KNEE—INTERCONDYLAR FOSSA

(1) Camp Coventry Method and (2) Holmblad Method

Knee—Intercondylar Fossa
BASIC
• PA axial

Pathology Demonstrated

Intercondylar fossa, femoral condyles, tibial plateaus, and the intercondylar eminence are demonstrated and may show evidence of bony or cartilaginous pathology, osteochondral defects, or narrowing of the joint space.

Note: Two methods are described for demonstrating these structures. The prone position (Fig. 7-114) is an easier position for the patient. The Holmblad kneeling method provides another option with a slightly different projection of these structures with an increase in the amount of knee flexion.

Technical Factors

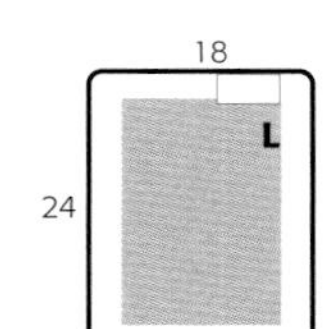

- Film size—18 × 24 cm (8 × 10 inches), lengthwise
- Moving or stationary grid (or screen, <10 cm)
- 75 ± 5 kV range (increase 4-6 kV from PA knee)
- Technique and dose: (with 12:1 Bucky grid)

cm	kV	mAs	Sk.	ML.	Gon.
11	78	5	36	17	M NDC F <0.1
				mrad	

Shielding Place lead shield over gonadal area. Secure around waist in kneeling position and extend shield down to midfemur level.

Patient Position

1. Take radiograph with patient prone; give pillow for head.
2. Have patient kneel on x-ray table.

Part Position

1. Prone:

- Flex knee **40° to 50°;** place support under ankle.
- Center cassette to knee joint considering projection of CR angle.

2. Kneeling:

- With patient kneeling on "all fours," place cassette under affected knee and center IR to popliteal crease.
- Ask patient to support body weight primarily on opposite knee.
- Place padded support under ankle and leg of affected limb to reduce pressure on injured knee.
- Ask patient to slowly **lean forward 20° to 30°** and hold that position. (Results in 60° to 70° knee flexion.)

Central Ray

1. *Prone:* Direct CR **perpendicular to lower leg** (40° to 50° caudad to match degree of flexion).
2. *Kneeling:* Direct CR **perpendicular to IR and lower leg.**

- Direct CR to **midpopliteal crease.**
- Minimum SID is 40 inches (100 cm).

Collimation Collimate on four sides to knee joint area.

Radiographic Criteria

Center of four-sided collimation field should be to midknee joint area. • For this projection the intercondylar fossa should appear in profile, open without superimposition by patella. • **No rotation** will be evidenced by symmetric appearance of the distal posterior femoral condyles and superimposition of approximately half of fibular head by tibia. • Articular facets and intercondylar eminence of tibia should be well visualized without superimposition. • Optimal exposure should visualize soft tissue in the knee joint space and an outline of patella through the femur. • Trabecular markings of femoral condyles and proximal tibia should appear clear and sharp, with no motion.

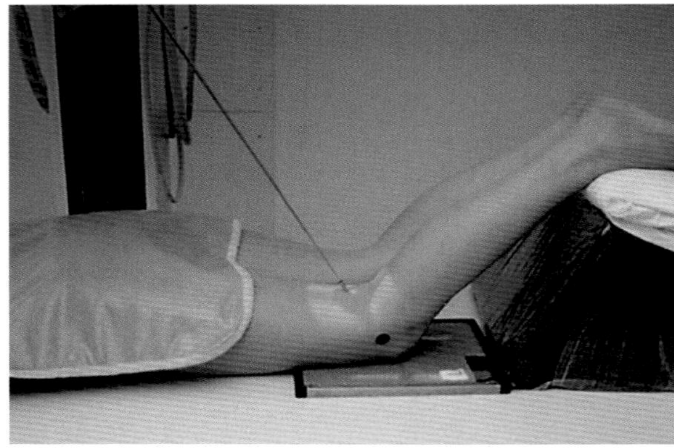

Fig. 7-114. (1) Camp Coventry method—prone position (40° to 50° flexion).

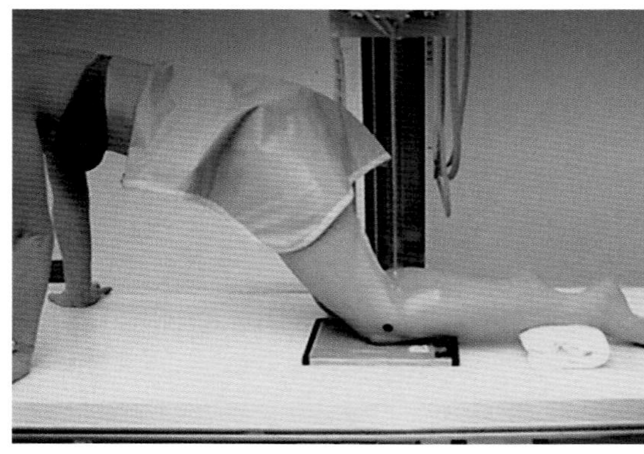

Fig. 7-115. (2) Holmblad method—kneeling position (60° to 70° flexion).

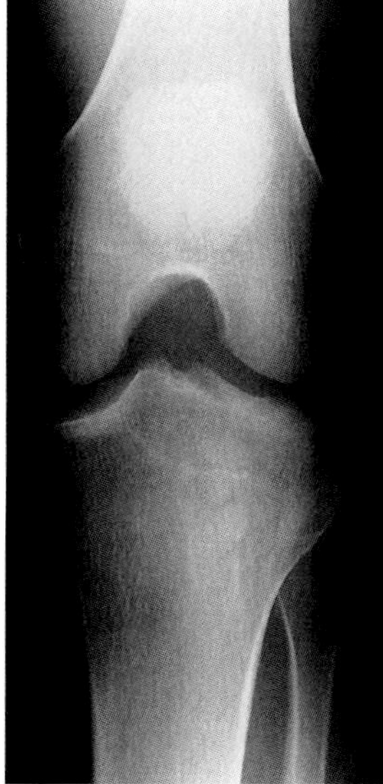

Fig. 7-116. PA axial projection.

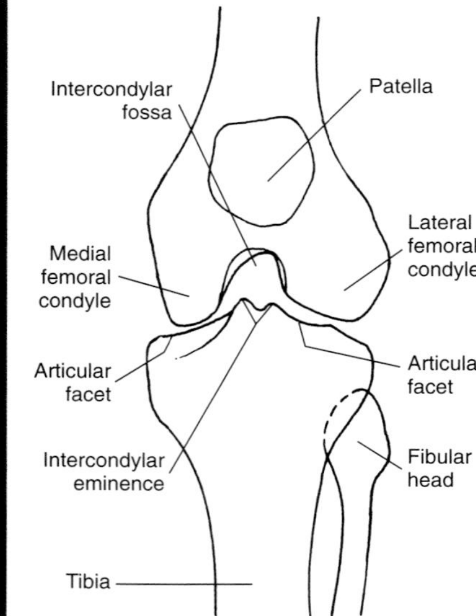

Fig. 7-117. PA axial projection.

AP AXIAL PROJECTION: KNEE—INTERCONDYLAR FOSSA

Knee—Intercondylar Fossa
BASIC
• **PA axial**
SPECIAL
• **AP axial**

Pathology Demonstrated

The intercondylar fossa, femoral condyles, tibial plateaus, and intercondylar eminence are demonstrated for evidence of bony or cartilaginous pathology, osteochondral defects, or narrowing of the joint space.

Note: This is a reversal of the PA axial projection for those who cannot assume the prone position. This, however, is **not** a preferred projection because of the distortion from the CR angle and increased part-IR distance, unless a curved cassette is available. This projection also increases exposure to gonadal region.

Technical Factors

- IR size—18 × 24 cm (8 × 10 inches), crosswise
- Curved cassette preferred if available to reduce part-IR distance.
- Detail screen, small focal spot (65 ± 5 kV range) (grid not needed because of air gap).

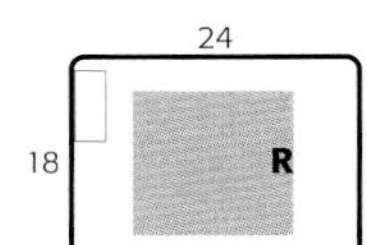

Shielding Place lead shield over pelvic area extending to midfemur.

Patient Position Take radiograph with patient in the supine position. Provide support under partially flexed knee with entire leg in the anatomic position with no rotation.

Part Position

- Flex knee **40° to 45°** and place support under cassette as needed to place cassette firmly against posterior thigh and leg, as shown in Fig. 7-119.
- If curved cassette is available, place under knee, as shown in Fig. 7-120.
- Adjust cassette as needed to center IR to midknee joint area.

Central Ray

- Direct CR **perpendicular to lower leg** (40° to 45° cephalad).
- Direct CR to a point $\frac{1}{2}$ **inch (1.25 cm) distal to apex of patella.**
- Minimum SID is 40 inches (100 cm).

Collimation Collimate on four sides to knee joint area.

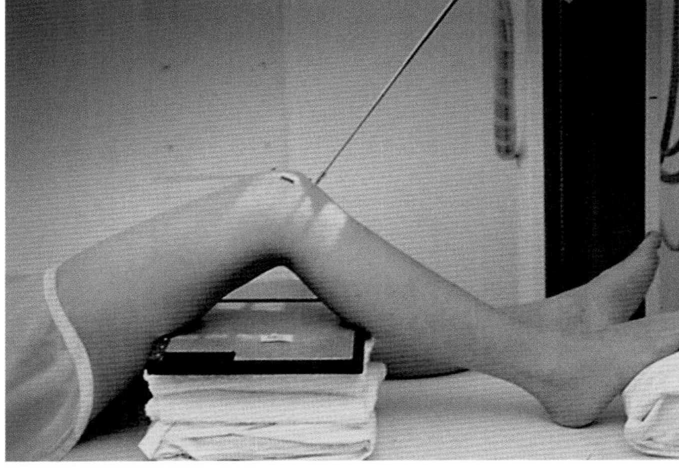

Fig. 7-118. AP axial—18 × 24 cm (8 × 10 inches) cassette crosswise (40° flexion, 40° CR angle).

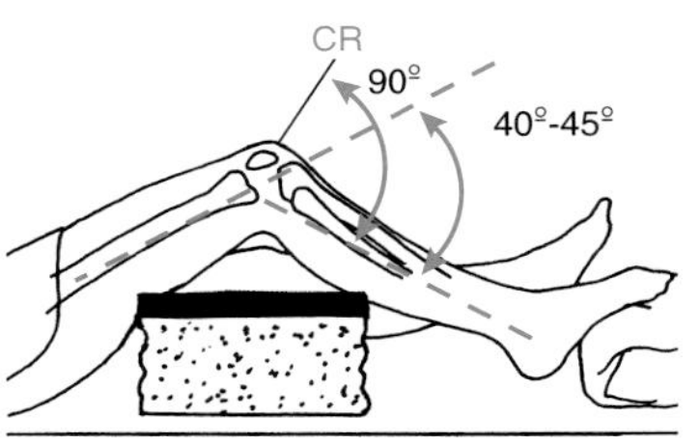

Fig. 7-119. With 18 × 24 cm flat cassette.

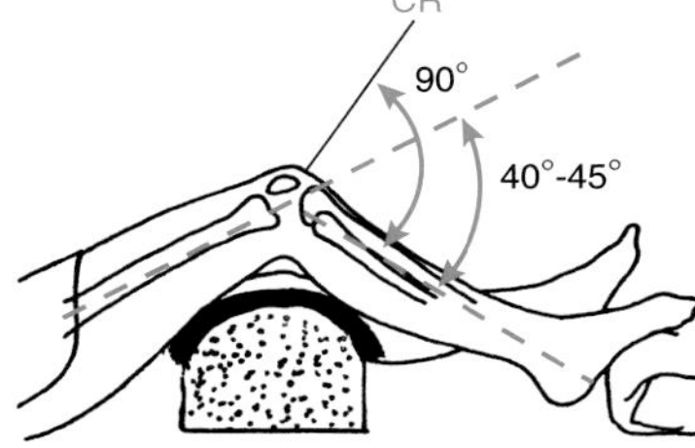

Fig. 7-120. With curved cassette (Béclere method).

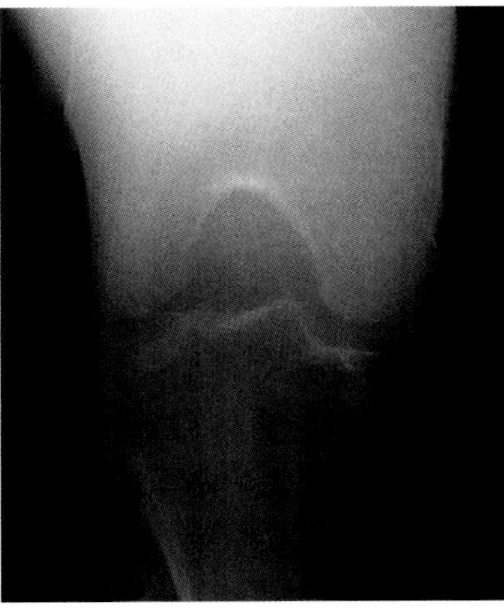

Fig. 7-121. AP axial—40° flexion and CR angle.

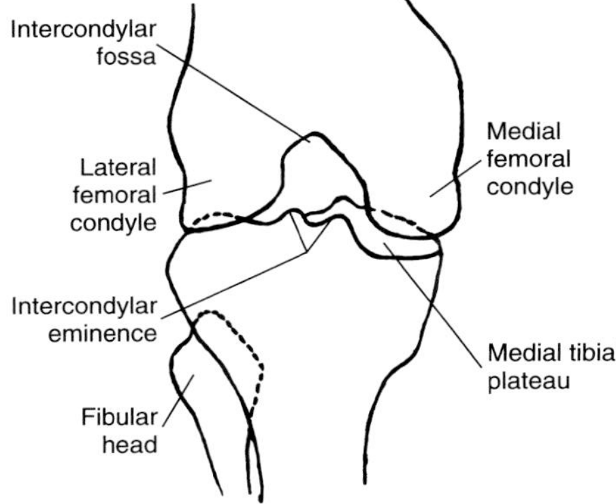

Fig. 7-122. AP axial.

Radiographic Criteria

• Center of four-sided collimation field should be to midknee joint area. • The intercondylar fossa should appear in profile, open without superimposition by patella. The intercondylar eminence and tibial plateau and distal condyles of femur should be clearly visualized. • **No rotation** will be evidenced by symmetric appearance of the distal posterior femoral condyles and superimposition of approximately half of the fibular head by the tibia. • Optimal exposure should visualize soft tissue in the knee joint space and an outline of patella through the femur. • Trabecular markings of femoral condyles and proximal tibia should appear clear and sharp, with no motion.

7

PA PROJECTION: PATELLA

Patella
- PA
- Lateral
- Tangential

Pathology Demonstrated

Patellar fractures are evaluated before flexing the knee joint for other projections.

Technical Factors

- IR size—18 × 24 cm (8 × 10 inches), lengthwise
- Moving or stationary grid (or screen, <10 cm)
- 75 ± 5 kV range (increase 4 to 6 kV from PA knee technique for better patella visualization)
- Technique and dose:

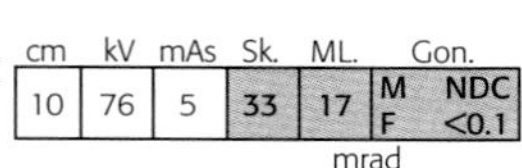

cm	kV	mAs	Sk.	ML.	Gon.
10	76	5	33	17	M NDC F <0.1

mrad

18

24 L

Shielding Place shield over gonadal area.

Patient Position Take radiograph with patient in the prone position, legs extended; give pillow for head; place support under ankle and leg, with smaller support under femur above knee to prevent direct pressure on patella.

Part Position

- Align and center long axis of leg and knee to midline of table or IR.
- **True PA:** Align interepicondylar line parallel to plane of IR. (This usually requires about **5° internal rotation of anterior knee.**)

Central Ray

- CR is **perpendicular** to IR.
- Direct CR to **midpatella area** (which is usually at approximately the midpopliteal crease).
- Minimum SID is 40 inches (100 cm).

Collimation Collimate closely on four sides to include just the area of the patella and knee joint.

Notes: With a potential fracture of patella, extra care should be taken to **not flex knee** and **provide support under thigh** (femur) so as not to put direct pressure on patella area.

The projection may also be taken as an AP projection positioned like an AP knee if patient cannot assume a prone position.

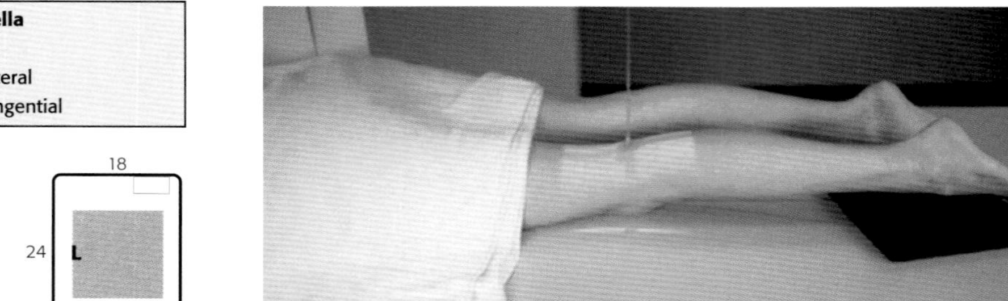
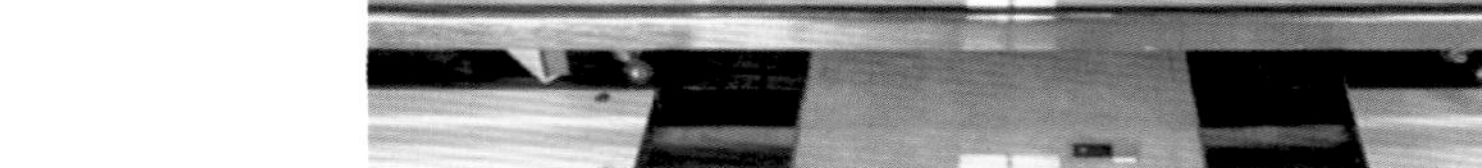

Fig. 7-123. CR 0° to midpatella—PA patella.

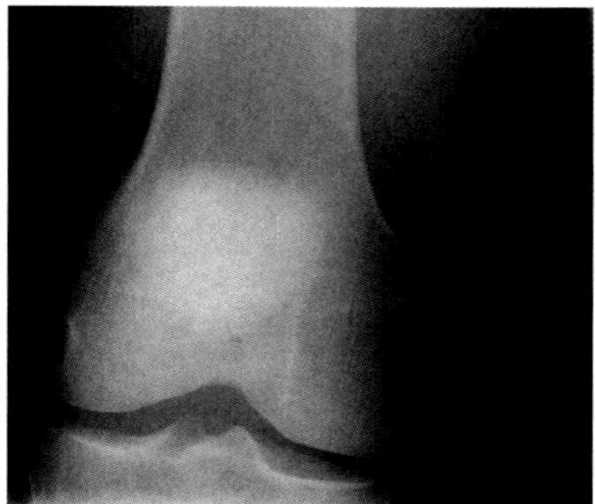

Fig. 7-124. PA patella.

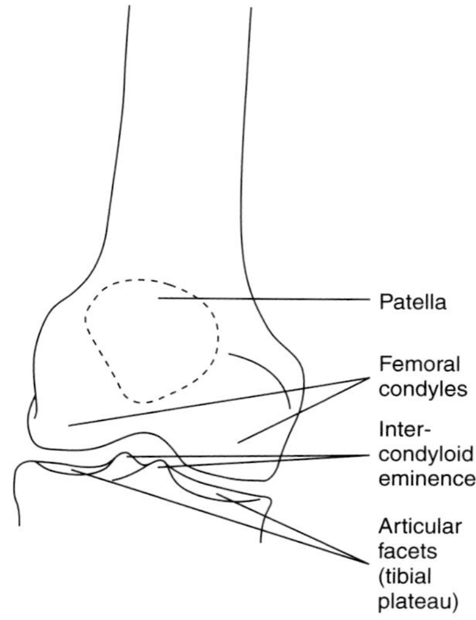

Fig. 7-125. PA patella.

Radiographic Criteria

Structures Shown: • Knee joint and patella are shown, with optimal recorded detail of patella because of decreased OID if taken as a PA projection.

Position: • **No rotation** is present as evidenced by symmetric appearance of the condyles. • The patella will be centered to femur with correct slight internal rotation of anterior knee.

Collimation and CR: • Centering and angulation are correct if the knee joint is open and the patella is in the center of the collimated field.

Exposure Criteria: • Optimal exposure without motion will visualize soft tissue in joint area and also clearly visualize sharp bony trabecular markings and the outline of patella as seen through the distal femur.

LATERAL—MEDIOLATERAL PROJECTION: PATELLA

Patella
- PA
- Lateral
- Tangential

Pathology Demonstrated

In conjunction with the PA, this projection is useful in evaluating patellar fractures as well as abnormalities of the femoropatellar and femorotibial joints.

Technical Factors

- IR size—18 × 24 cm (8 × 10 inches), lengthwise
- Moving or stationary grid, 70 ± 6 kV range or smaller patient <10 cm), screen tabletop, 60 ± 5 kV range (decrease 4-6 kV from lateral knee technique to avoid overexposing the patella)
- Technique and dose:

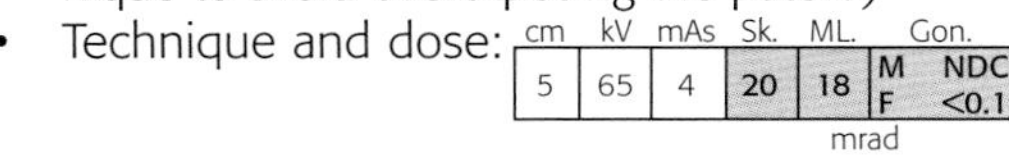

cm	kV	mAs	Sk.	ML.	Gon.
5	65	4	20	18	M NDC / F <0.1

mrad

Shielding Place shield over gonadal area.

Patient Position Take radiograph with patient in lateral recumbent position, affected side down; give pillow for head; provide support for knee of opposite limb placed behind affected knee.

Part Position

- Adjust rotation of body and leg until knee is in a **true lateral** position (femoral epicondyles directly superimposed and plane of patella perpendicular to plane of IR).
- Flex knee **only 5° or 10°**. (Additional flexion may separate fracture fragments if present.)
- Align and center long axis of patella to CR and to centerline of table or IR.

Central Ray

- CR is **perpendicular** to IR.
- Direct CR to the **midfemoropatellar joint.**
- Minimum SID is 40 inches (100 cm).

Collimation Collimate closely on four sides to include just the area of the patella and knee joint.

Note: This can also be taken as a **cross-table lateral** with no knee flexion on a severe trauma patient, as described in Chapter 19 on mobile and trauma radiography.

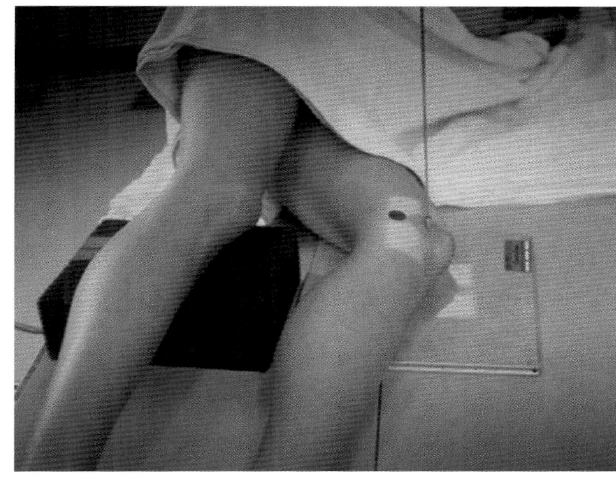

Fig. 7-126. Lateral patella.

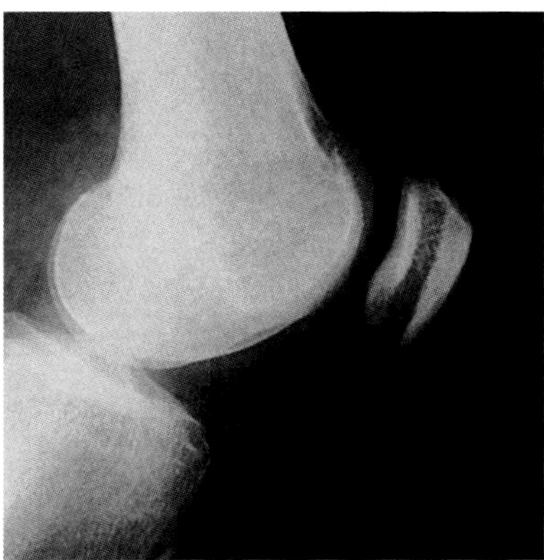

Fig. 7-127. Lateral patella.

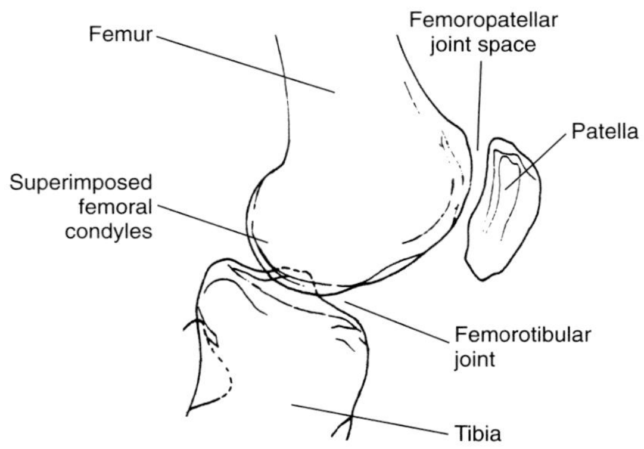

Fig. 7-128. Lateral patella.

Radiographic Criteria

Structures Shown: • A profile image of the patella, the femoropatellar joint, and the femorotibial joint are demonstrated.

Position: • **True lateral:** The anterior and posterior borders of the medial and lateral femoral condyles should be directly superimposed, and the femoropatellar joint space should appear open.

Collimation and CR: • Centering and angulation are correct if the patella is in the center of the film and collimated field with the joint spaces open. • Four-sided collimation should include patella and knee joint with the center to the midfemoropatellar joint space.

Exposure Criteria: • Optimal exposure will visualize soft-tissue detail and the patella well without overexposure. • The trabecular markings of the patella and other bones should appear clear and sharp.

TANGENTIAL (AXIAL OR SUNRISE/SKYLINE) PROJECTIONS: PATELLA

Merchant Bilateral Method

Patella
- PA
- Lateral
- Tangential

Pathology Demonstrated

Subluxation of the patella and other abnormalities of the patella and femoropatellar joint are demonstrated.

Technical Factors

- IR size—24 × 30 cm (10 × 12 inches), crosswise
- Detail screen, small focal spot (grid is not needed because of air gap because of increased OID)
- 65 ± 5 kV range
  Some type of leg support and cassette holder should be used
- Technique and dose:

cm	kV	mAs	Sk.	ML.	Gon.
8	66	11	22	14	M NDC F <0.1
			mrad		

Shielding Place lead shield over entire pelvic area.

Patient Position Take radiograph with patient in the supine position with knees flexed **40°** over the end of the table, resting on a leg support. Patient needs to be comfortable and relaxed for quadriceps muscles to be totally relaxed (see Note below).

Part Position

- Place support under knees to raise distal femora as needed so that they are parallel to tabletop.
- Place knees and feet together and secure legs together below the knees to prevent rotation and to allow patient to be totally relaxed.
- Place cassette on edge against legs about 12 inches (30 cm) below the knees, **perpendicular** to x-ray beam.

Central Ray

- Angle CR caudad, **30° from horizontal** (CR 30° to femora). Adjust CR angle if needed for true tangential projection of femoropatellar joint spaces.
- Direct CR to a point **midway between patellae.**
- SID is 48 inches (120 cm) to 72 inches (180 cm) (increased SID reduces magnification).

Collimation Collimate **tightly** on all sides to patellae.

Note: Patient comfort and total relaxation are essential. The quadriceps femoris muscles must be relaxed to prevent subluxation of patellae, wherein they are pulled into the intercondylar sulcus or groove, which may result in false readings.*

Radiographic Criteria

Structures Shown: • The intercondylar sulcus (trochlear groove) and patella of each distal femur should be visualized in profile with femoropatellar joint space open.

Position: • **No rotation** of the knee is present evidenced by the symmetric appearance of the patella, anterior femoral condyles, and intercondylar sulcus.

Collimation and CR: • Correct CR angle and centering are evidenced by open femoropatellar joint spaces. • Four-sided rectangular collimation field should be limited to area of patellae and anterior femoral condyles.

Exposure Criteria: • Optimal exposure should clearly visualize soft tissue and joint space margins and trabecular markings of patellae. Femoral condyles will appear underexposed with only the anterior margins clearly defined.

*Merchant AC et al: Roentgenographic analysis of patellofemoral congruence, J Bone Joint Surg 56-A:1391-1396, 1974.

Fig. 7-129. Patient position—bilateral tangential, knees flexed 40°.

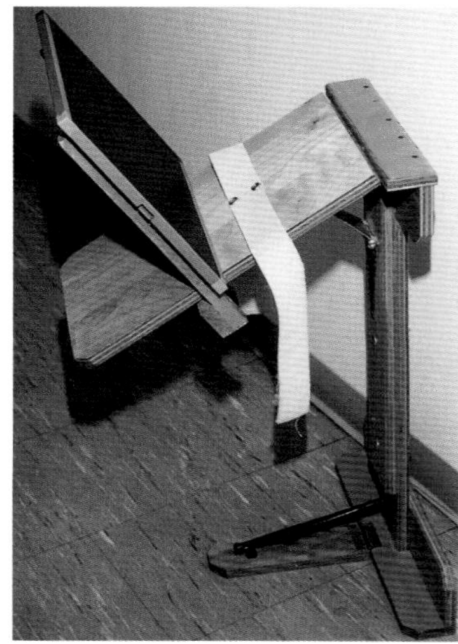

Fig. 7-130. Adjustable type leg support and film holder. (Courtesy St. Joseph's Hospital and Medical Center, Phoenix, AZ.)

Fig. 7-131. Bilateral tangential.

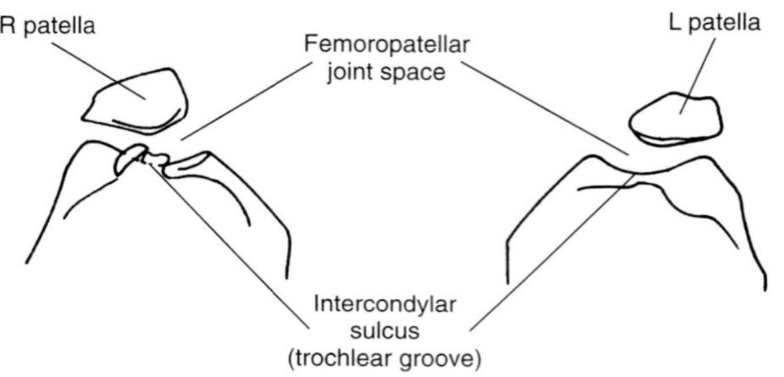

Fig. 7-132. Bilateral tangential.

TANGENTIAL (AXIAL OR SUNRISE/SKYLINE) PROJECTIONS: PATELLA

1. Inferosuperior projection (patient supine, 45° knee flexion)
2. Hughston method (patient prone, 55° knee flexion)
3. Settegast method (patient prone, 90° knee flexion)

Patella
- PA
- Lateral
- Tangential

Summary

Three additional methods for the tangential projections of the patellae and femoropatellar joints are described in a suggested order of preference. Advantages and disadvantages of each are noted. **Both sides** are generally taken for comparison.

Technical Factors

- IR size—24 × 30 cm (10 × 12 inches) or 18 × 24 cm (8 × 10 inches), crosswise
- Detail screen, small focal spot
- 65 ± 5 kV range

30
24
L R

1. Inferosuperior Projection

- Take radiograph with patient in the supine position, legs together with sufficient size support placed under knees for 40° to 45° knee flexion (legs relaxed).
- Ensure no leg rotation.
- Place cassette on edge, resting on midthighs, tilted to be perpendicular to CR. Use sandbags and tape as shown, or other methods to stabilize cassette in this position. It is **not** recommended that patient be asked to sit up to hold cassette in place, because this may place patient's head and neck region into path of x-ray beam.

Central Ray

- Direct CR inferosuperiorly, 10° to 15° angle from lower legs to be **tangential to femoropatellar joint.** Palpate borders of patella to determine specific CR angle required to pass through infrapatellar joint space.
- SID is 40 to 48 inches (100-120 cm).

Note 1: The major advantages to this method are that it does not require special equipment and it is a relatively comfortable position for the patient. Therefore total relaxation can be achieved with 40° to 45° knee flexion if proper-sized support is placed under knees. The only disadvantage is a potential problem holding or supporting the cassette in this position if the patient cannot cooperate fully.

2. Hughston Method* (may be done bilaterally on one IR) Take radiograph with patient in the prone position, with cassette placed under knee; slowly flex knee 45° (see Note 3 below); have patient hold foot with gauze, or rest foot against collimator or other support; place pad between foot and possible **hot** collimator.

Central Ray

- Align CR approximately **15° to 20° from long axis of lower leg** (tangential to femoropatellar joint).
- Direct CR to **midfemoropatellar joint.**
- Minimum SID is 40 inches (100 cm).

Note 2: This is a relatively comfortable position for patient, and relaxation of the quadriceps can be achieved. The major disadvantage is the image distortion caused by the film–body part–beam alignment and the difficulty of less angle knee flexion because of modern equipment and large collimators.

Note 3: Some authors suggest less flexion of only 20° to prevent patella from being drawn into femoropatellar groove, which may prevent detection of subtle abnormalities in alignment.†

*Hughston AC: Subluxation of the patella, J Bone Joint Surg 50-A:1003-1026, 1968.
†Manaster BJ: Handbooks in radiology, skeletal radiol, St. Louis, 1989, Year Book Pub.

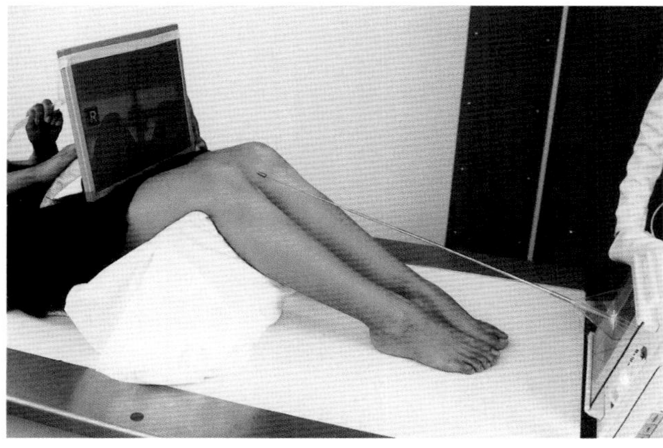

Fig. 7-133. 1. Inferosuperior projection—40° to 45° flexion of knees.

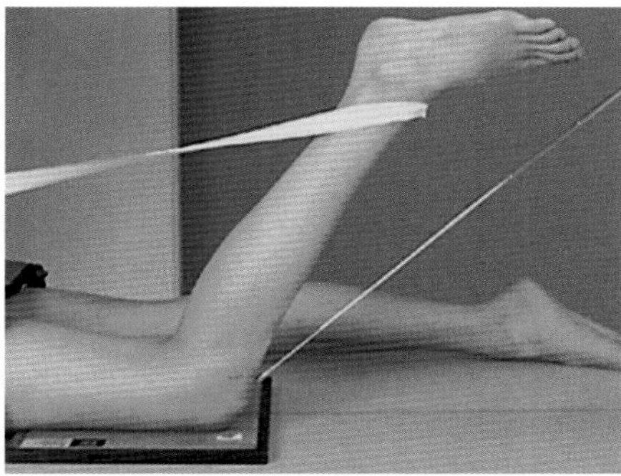

Fig. 7-134. 2. Hughston method*—45° flexion of knee.

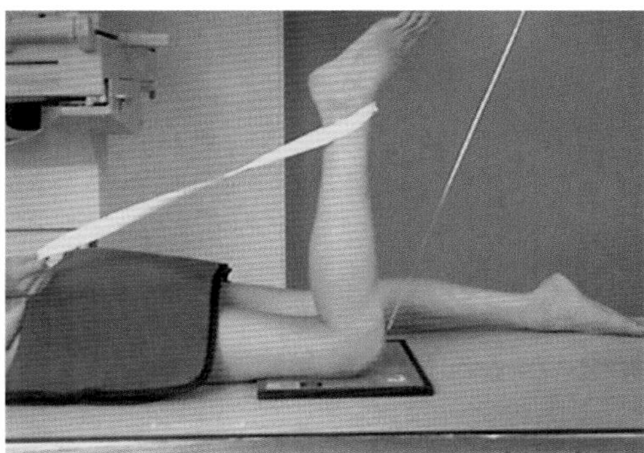

Fig. 7-135. 3. Settegast method—90° flexion of knee (see Note 4 below).

3. Settegast Method

Warning: This acute flexion of knee should **not** be attempted until fracture of patella has been ruled out by other projections.

- Take radiograph with patient in the prone position, with cassette under knee; slowly flex knee to a **minimum of 90°**; have patient hold on to gauze or tape to maintain position.

Central Ray

- Direct CR **tangential to femoropatellar joint space** (15° to 20° from lower leg).
- Minimum SID is 40 inches (100 cm).

Note 4: The major disadvantage to this method is that the acute knee flexion tightens the quadriceps and draws the patella into the intercondylar sulcus, thus reducing the diagnostic value of this projection.*

*Turner GW, Burns CB: Erect position/tangential projection of the patellofemoral joint, Radiol Technol 54(1):11-14, 1982.

7

AP PROJECTION: FEMUR—MID- AND DISTAL

Note: If site of interest is in area of proximal femur, a unilateral hip routine or a pelvis is recommended, as described in Chapter 8.

Femur—Mid- and Distal
BASIC
• AP
• Lateral

Pathology Demonstrated

Mid- and distal femur is demonstrated, including knee joint for detection and evaluation of fractures and/or bone lesions.

Technical Factors

- IR size—35 × 43 cm (14 × 17 inches), lengthwise
- Moving or stationary grid
- 75 ± 5 kV range
- Because of anode-heel effect, place hip or head end of patient at cathode end of x-ray beam
- Technique and dose:

cm	kV	mAs	Sk.	ML.	Gon.
13	75	12	82	25	M 16 F <0.3
				mrad	

35

43

L

Shielding Place lead shield over pelvic area to ensure correct gonadal shielding because of proximity to primary beam.

Patient Position Take radiograph with patient in the supine position, with femur centered to midline of table; give pillow for head. (This projection may also be done on stretcher with portable grid placed under femur.)

Part Position

- Align femur to CR and to midline of table or IR.
- Rotate leg internally about 5° for a true AP as for an AP knee. (For proximal femur, 15° to 20° internal leg rotation is required as for an AP hip.)
- Ensure that knee joint is included on IR, considering the divergence of the x-ray beam. (Lower cassette margin should be about 2 inches or 5 cm below knee joint.)

Central Ray

- CR is **perpendicular** to femur and IR.
- Direct CR to **midpoint of IR.**
- Minimum SID is 40 inches (100 cm).

Collimation Collimate closely on both sides to femur with end collimation to film borders.

Routine to include both joints: Common departmental routines include both joints on all initial femur exams. For a large adult, a second smaller IR should then be used for an AP of either the knee or the hip, ensuring that both hip and knee joints are included. If the hip is included, the leg should be rotated 15° to 20° internally to place the femoral neck in profile.

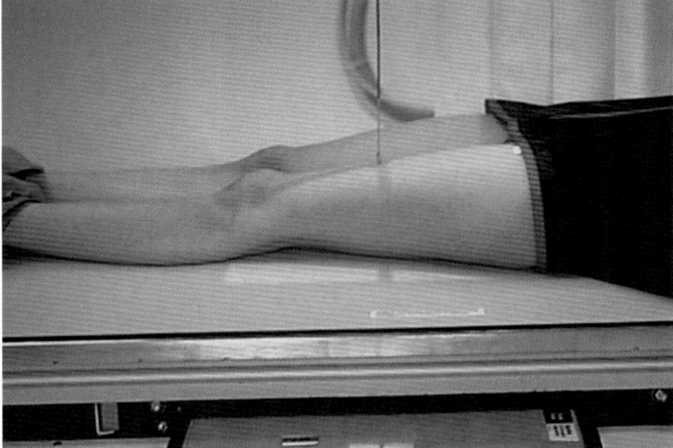

Fig. 7-136. AP—mid- and distal femur (head of cathode end).

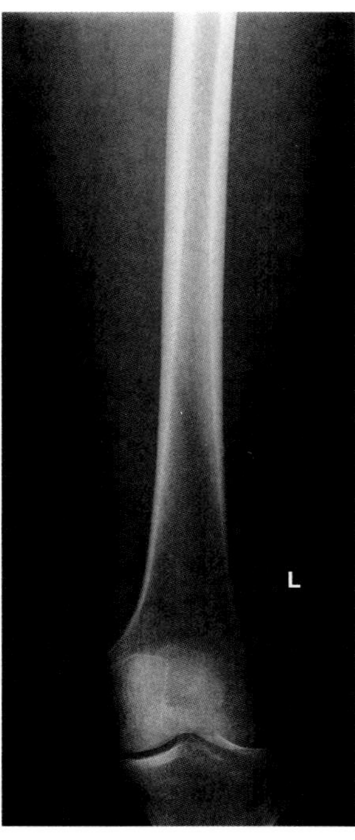

Fig. 7-137. AP—mid- and distal femur.

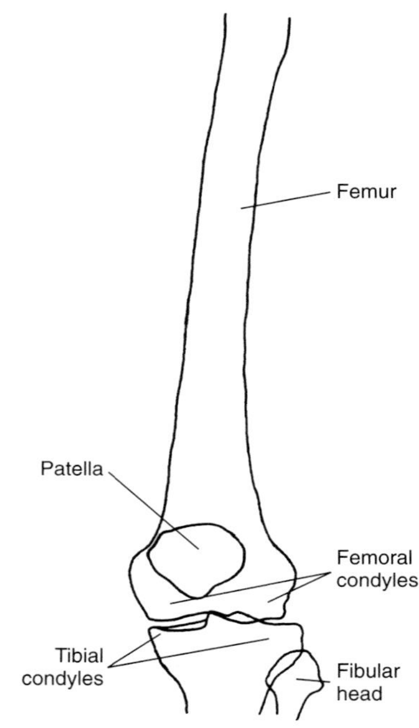

Fig. 7-138. AP—mid- and distal femur.

Radiographic Criteria

Structures Shown: • Distal two-thirds of distal femur, including knee joint, is shown. • Knee joint space will not appear fully open because of divergent x-ray beam.

Position: • **No rotation** is evidenced; femoral and tibial condyles should appear symmetric in size and shape with the outline of patella slightly toward medial side of femur. • The approximate medial half of fibular head should be superimposed by tibia.

Collimation and CR: • Femur should be centered to collimation field and aligned with long axis of IR with knee joint space a minimum of 1 inch (2.5 cm) from distal IR margin. • Minimal collimation borders should be visible on proximal and distal margins of IR.

Exposure Criteria: • Optimal exposure with correct use of anode-heel effect will result in near uniform density of entire femur. • No motion should exist; fine trabecular markings should be clear and sharp throughout length of femur.

LATERAL—MEDIOLATERAL OR LATEROMEDIAL PROJECTIONS: FEMUR—MID AND DISTAL

Note: For possible trauma if site of interest is in area of proximal femur, a unilateral trauma hip routine is recommended, as described in Chapter 8. For nontrauma lateral of mid and proximal femur, see p. 258.

Femur—Mid and Distal
BASIC
• **AP**
• Lateral

Pathology Demonstrated
Mid and distal femur is demonstrated, including knee joint for detection and evaluation of fractures and/or bone lesions.

35
43 L

Technical Factors
- IR size—35 × 43 cm (14 × 17 inches), lengthwise
- Moving or stationary grid
- 75 ± 5 kV range
- Because of anode-heel effect, place the hip of patient at cathode end of x-ray beam
- Technique and dose: (with 12:1 Bucky grid)

cm	kV	mAs	Sk.	ML.	Gon.
11	75	7	47	21	M 9 F <0.2
				mrad	

Shielding Place lead shield over pelvic area to shield gonads.

Patient Position Take radiograph with patient in the lateral recumbent position, or supine for trauma patient.

Part Position
Lateral recumbent (Fig. 7-139):

Warning: Do not attempt this position if patient has severe trauma.

- Flex knee approximately 45° with patient on affected side and align femur to midline of table or IR.
- Place unaffected leg behind affected leg to prevent overrotation.
- Adjust IR to include knee joint (lower IR margin should be about 2 inches, or 5 cm, below knee joint). A second IR to include the proximal femur and hip will generally be required on an adult (see p. 258).

Trauma lateromedial projection (Fig. 7-140):
- Place support under affected leg and knee and support foot and ankle in true AP position.
- Place cassette on edge against medial aspect of thigh to include knee, with horizontal x-ray beam directed from lateral side.

Central Ray
- CR **perpendicular** to femur and IR directed to **midpoint of IR**
- Minimum SID of 40 inches (100 cm)

Collimation Collimate closely on both sides to femur with end collimation to IR borders.

Radiographic Criteria

Structures Shown: • Distal two-thirds of distal femur, including the knee joint, is shown. • Knee joint will not appear open, and distal margins of the femoral condyles will not be superimposed because of divergent x-ray beam.

Position: • **True lateral:** Anterior and posterior margins of medial and lateral femoral condyles should be superimposed and aligned with open femoropatellar joint space.

Collimation and CR: • Femur should be centered to collimation field with knee joint space a minimum of 1 inch (2.5 cm) from distal IR margin. • Minimal collimation borders should be visible on proximal and distal margins of IR.

Exposure Criteria: • Optimal exposure with correct use of anode-heel effect will result in near uniform density of entire femur. • No motion is present; fine trabecular markings should be clear and sharp throughout length of femur.

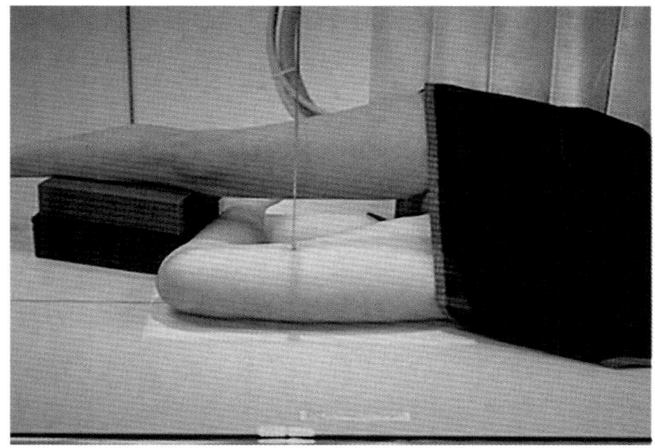

Fig. 7-139. Mediolateral mid and distal femur.

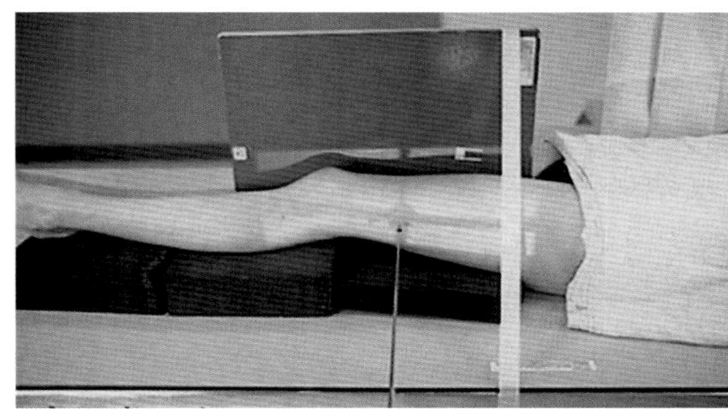

Fig. 7-140. Trauma lateromedial (horizontal beam) projection. Note: When using a grid cassette, care must be taken to prevent grid cut-off.

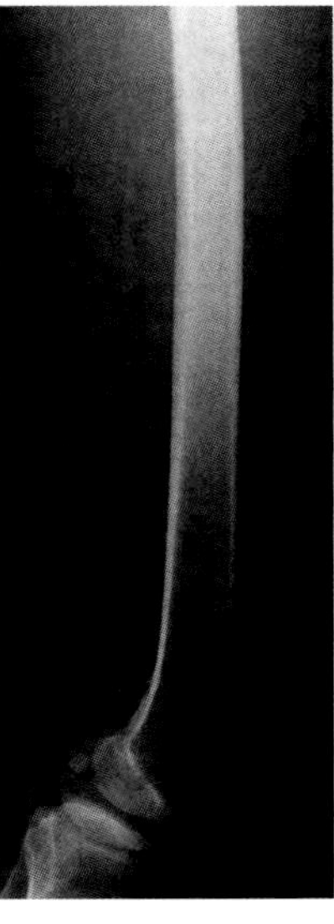

Fig. 7-141. Lateral–mid and distal femur.

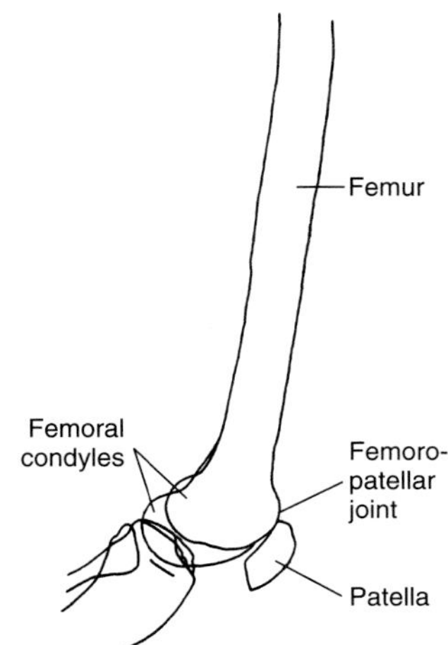

Fig. 7-142. Lateral–mid and distal femur.

7

LATERAL—MEDIOLATERAL PROJECTION: FEMUR—MID AND PROXIMAL

Warning: Do not attempt this position for patient with possible fracture of hip or proximal femur. Refer to trauma lateral hip routine in Chapter 8.

Femur—Mid and Proximal
BASIC
- AP (see AP Hip, Chapter 8)
- Lateral

Pathology Demonstrated

Mid and proximal femur is demonstrated, including lateral hip for detection and evaluation of fractures and bone lesions.

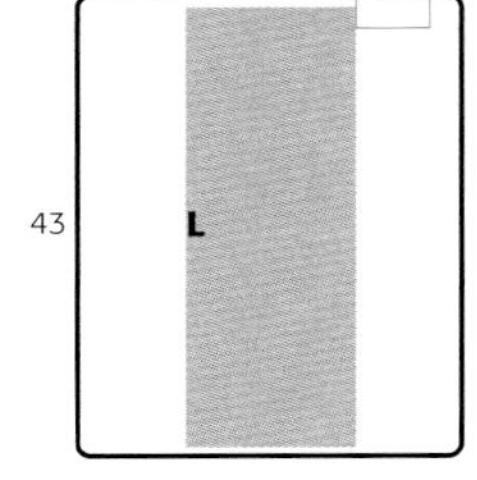

Technical Factors

- IR size—35 × 43 cm (14 × 17 inches), lengthwise
- Moving or stationary grid
- 75 ± 5 kV range
- To make best use of the anode-heel effect, place the hip at cathode end of x-ray beam
- Technique and dose:

cm	kV	mAs	Sk.	ML.	Gon.
14	75	12	81	36	M 62 F 10
				mrad	

Shielding Use of gonadal shielding is generally not possible on this projection without obscuring essential anatomy.

Patient Position Take radiograph with patient in the lateral recumbent position, with affected side down; provide pillow for head.

Part Position

- Flex affected knee about 45° and align femur to midline of table. (Remember the proximal and midportion of the femur is nearer the anterior aspect of the thigh.)
- Extend and support unaffected leg behind affected knee and have patient roll back (posteriorly) about 15° to prevent superimposition of proximal femur and hip joint.
- Adjust IR to include hip joint, considering the divergence of the x-ray beam. (Palpate ASIS and place upper IR margin at the level of this landmark.)

Central Ray

- CR **perpendicular** to femur and IR directed to **midpoint of IR**
- Minimum SID of 40 inches (100 cm)

Collimation Collimate closely on both sides to femur with end collimation to IR borders.

Alternate routine to include both joints: Common departmental routines include both joints on all initial femur exams. On a large adult, this requires a second smaller IR (10 × 12 inches or 24 × 30 cm) of either the hip or knee joint.

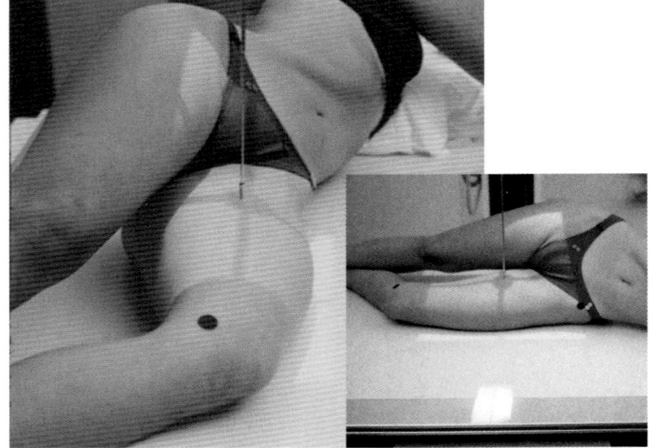

Fig. 7-143. Mediolateral—mid and proximal femur.

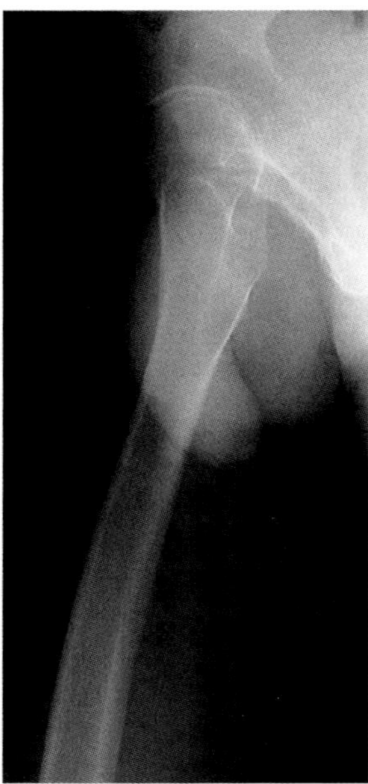

Fig. 7-144. Mediolateral—mid and proximal femur.

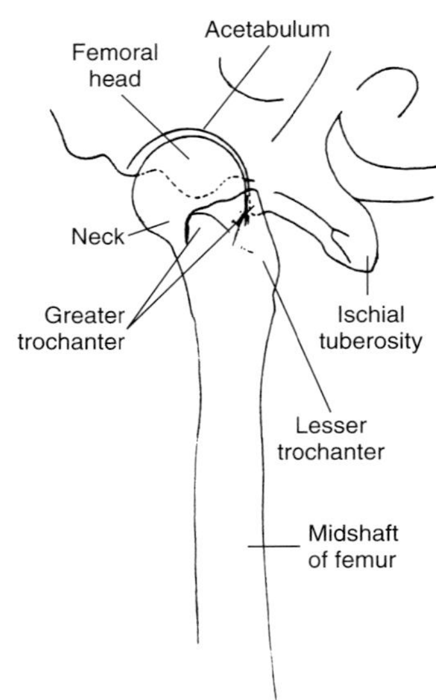

Fig. 7-145. Mediolateral—mid and proximal femur.

Radiographic Criteria

Structures Shown: • Proximal one-half to two-thirds of the proximal femur, including the hip joint, is shown. • Proximal femur and hip joint should not be superimposed by opposite limb.

Position: • **True lateral:** The superimposition of the greater and lesser trochanters by the femur exists, with only a small part of the trochanters visible on medial side. • The greater trochanter should be mostly superimposed by the neck of the femur.

Collimation and CR: • Femur should be centered to collimation field with hip joint a minimum of 1 inch (2.5 cm) from proximal IR margin. • Minimal collimation borders should be on proximal and distal margins of film.

Exposure Criteria: • Optimal exposure with correct use of anode-heel effect will result in near uniform density of entire femur. • No motion is present; fine trabecular markings should be clear and sharp throughout length of femur.

RADIOGRAPHS FOR CRITIQUE

Students should determine whether they can critique each of these six radiographs based on the categories as described in the textbook and as outlined on the right. As a starting critique exercise, place a check in each category that demonstrates a **repeatable error** for that radiograph.

Student workbooks provide more space for writing critique comments and also provide complete critique answers for each of these radiographs. Answers to repeatable errors are provided in Appendix B (at the end of this textbook) and in the workbooks.

	RADIOGRAPHS					
	A	B	C	D	E	F
1. Structures shown	____	____	____	____	____	____
2. Positioning	____	____	____	____	____	____
3. Collimation and CR	____	____	____	____	____	____
4. Exposure criteria	____	____	____	____	____	____
5. Markers	____	____	____	____	____	____

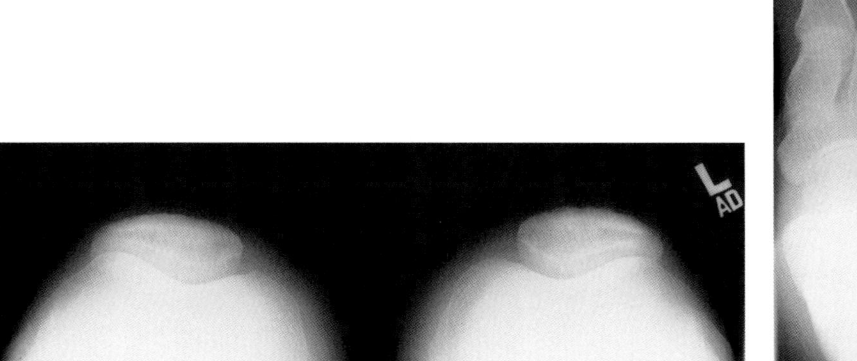

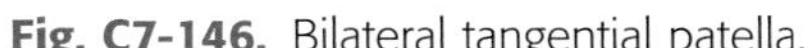

Fig. C7-146. Bilateral tangential patella. A

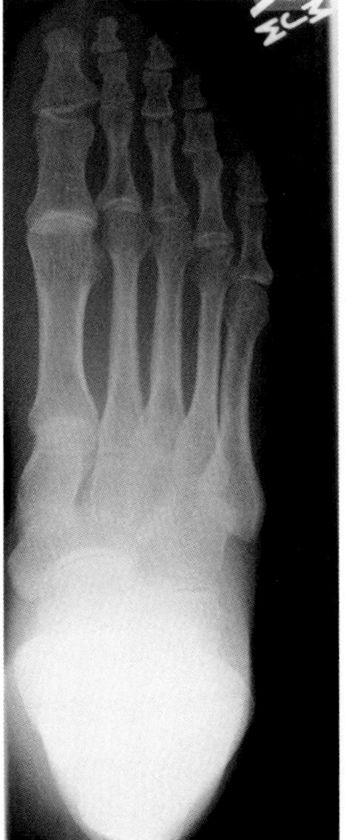

Fig. C7-147. AP foot. B

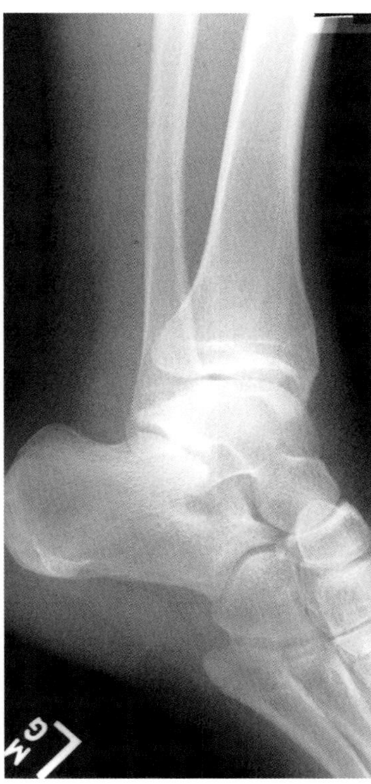

Fig. C7-148. Lateral ankle. C

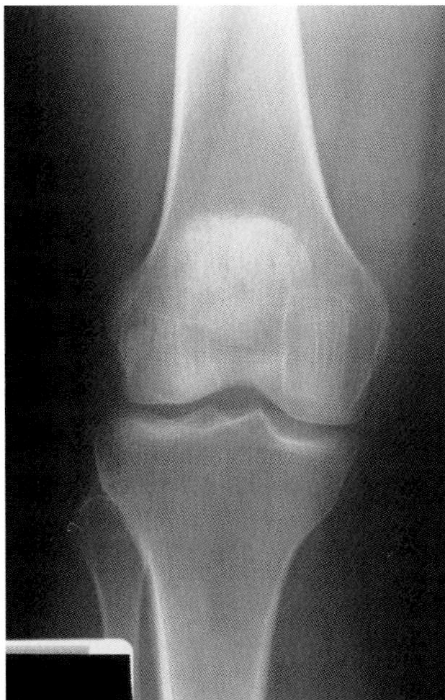

Fig. C7-149. AP knee. D

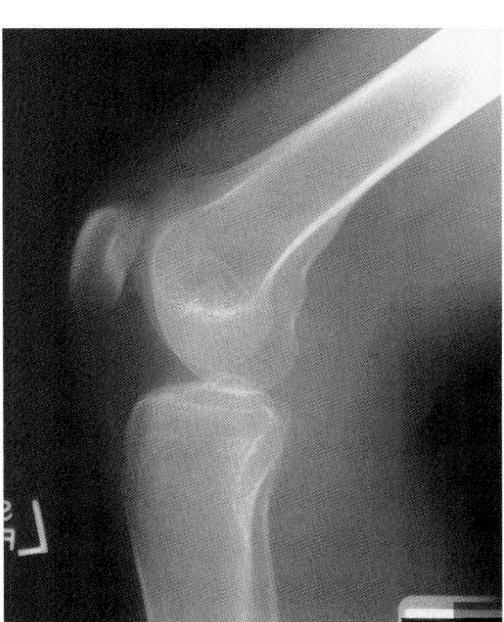

Fig. C7-150. Lateral knee. E

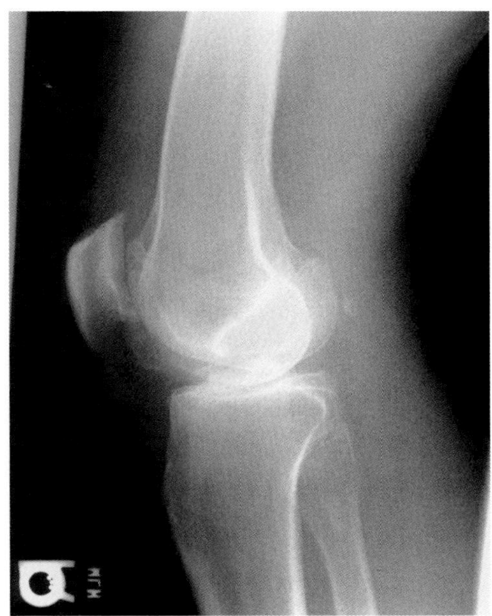

Fig. C7-151. Lateral knee. F

CHAPTER 8

Proximal Femur and Pelvic Girdle

CONTRIBUTIONS BY **Beth L. Vealé,** MEd, RT(R)(QM)
CONTRIBUTOR TO PAST EDITIONS Jeannean Hall-Rollins, MRC, BS, RT(R)(CV)

CONTENTS

RADIOGRAPHIC ANATOMY

Lower Limb (Extremity)

In Chapter 7, three groups of bones of the lower limb—the foot, leg and femur—were described, along with the associated knee and ankle joints.

The lower limb bones discussed in this chapter are the **proximal femur** and the **pelvic girdle.** The joints involving these two groups of bones, also included in this chapter, are the important **hip joint** and the **sacroiliac** and **symphysis pubis** joints of the pelvic girdle.

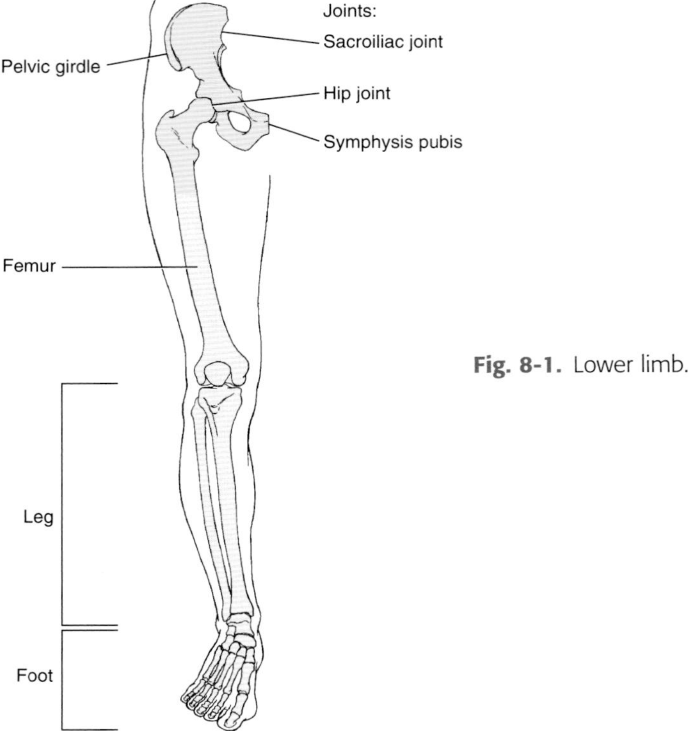

Fig. 8-1. Lower limb.

FEMUR

The **femur** is the longest and strongest bone in the entire body. The entire weight of the body is transferred through this bone and the associated joints at each end. Therefore these joints are a frequent source of pathology when trauma occurs.

Proximal Femur

The proximal femur consists of four essential parts—the (1) head, (2) neck, and (3) greater and (4) lesser trochanters *(tro-kan'ters).*

The **head** of the femur is rounded and smooth for articulation with the hip bones. It contains a depression, or pit, near its center called the ***fovea capitis*** *(fo've-ah cap'i-tis),* wherein a major ligament called the ***ligament of the head of the femur,*** or ***ligament capitis femoris,*** is attached to the head of the femur.

The **neck** of the femur is a strong pyramidal process of bone connecting the head to the body or shaft in the region of the trochanters.

The **greater trochanter** is a large prominence located **superiorly** and **laterally** to the femoral shaft and is palpable as a bony landmark. The **lesser trochanter** is a smaller, blunt, conical eminence that projects **medially** and **posteriorly** from the junction of the neck and shaft of the femur. The trochanters are joined posteriorly by a thick ridge called the **intertrochanteric** *(in"ter-tro"kan-ter'ik)* **crest.** The **body** or **shaft** of the femur is long and almost cylindric.

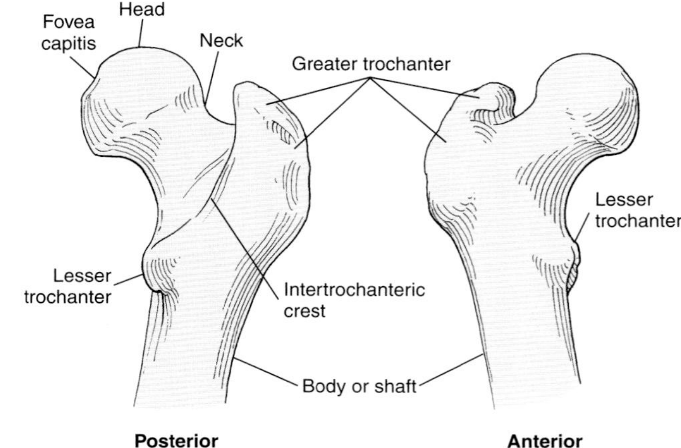

Fig. 8-2. Proximal femur.

Angles of the proximal femur The angle of the neck to the shaft on an average adult is approximately **125°**, with a variance of plus or minus 15° depending on the width of the pelvis and the length of the lower limbs. For instance, in a long-legged person with a narrow pelvis, the femur would be nearer vertical, which would then change the angle of the neck to about 140°. This angle would be less (110° to 115°) for a shorter person with a wider pelvis.

On an average adult in the anatomic position, the longitudinal plane of the femur is about **10° from vertical,** as shown on the left in Fig. 8-3. This vertical angle is nearer 15° on someone with a wide pelvis and shorter limbs and only about 5° on a long-legged person. This angle affects positioning and central ray (CR) angles for a lateral knee, as described in Chapter 7, p. 217, Fig. 7-20.

Another angle of the neck and head of the femur that is important in radiography is the **15° to 20° anterior angle** of the head and neck in relationship to the body of the femur (see right drawing of Fig. 8-3). The head projects somewhat anteriorly or forward as a result of this angle. This angle becomes important in radiographic positioning, wherein the femur and leg must be rotated **15° to 20° internally** to place the femoral neck parallel to the IR for a true AP projection of the proximal femur.

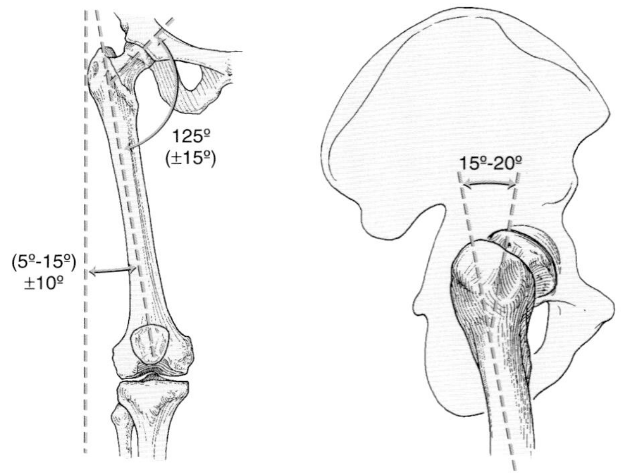

Fig. 8-3. Angles of proximal femur.

Pelvis

The total **pelvis** (meaning a *basin*) serves as the base of the trunk and forms the connection between the vertebral column and the lower limbs. The pelvis consists of four bones—two **hip bones (ossa coxae,** also called **innominate bones**), one **sacrum** *(sa'krum),* and one **coccyx** *(kok'siks).*

Pelvis versus pelvic girdle Sometimes the term *pelvic girdle* is used in reference to the total pelvis. This term, however, is incorrect in that the **pelvic girdle consists only of the two hip** (innominate) **bones,** whereas the term *pelvis* includes **four** bones, the right and **left hip (innominate) bones,** the **sacrum,** and the **coccyx.***

Note: The sacrum and coccyx also are considered parts of the distal vertebral column and in this textbook are discussed in Chapter 10 along with the lumbar spine.

HIP BONE

Each hip bone is composed of three divisions: (1) **ilium** *(il'e-um),* (2) **ischium** *(is'ke-um),* and (3) **pubis** *(pu'bis).* In a child these three divisions are separate bones, but they fuse into one bone during the middle teens. The fusion occurs in the area of the **acetabulum** *(as"e-tab'u-lum).* The acetabulum is a deep, cup-shaped cavity that accepts the head of the femur to form the hip joint.

The ilium is the largest of the three divisions and is located superior to the acetabulum. The ischium is inferior and posterior to the acetabulum, whereas the pubis is inferior and anterior to the acetabulum. Each of these three parts is described in detail in the following sections.

Ilium

Each **ilium** is composed of a **body** and an **ala,** or wing. The body of the ilium is the more inferior portion near the acetabulum and includes the upper two-fifths of the acetabulum. The ala, or wing portion, is the thin and flared upper part of the ilium.

The **crest** of the ilium is the upper margin of the ala and extends from the **anterior superior iliac spine** (ASIS) to the **posterior superior iliac spine** (PSIS). In radiographic positioning the uppermost peak of the crest is often referred to as the **iliac crest,** but it actually extends between the ASIS and PSIS.

Below the ASIS is a less prominent projection referred to as the **anterior inferior iliac spine.** Similarly, inferior to the PSIS is the **posterior inferior iliac spine.**

Positioning landmarks The two important positioning landmarks of these borders and projections are the **iliac crest** and the **ASIS.**

*Gray H: Gray's anatomy, ed 13, Philadelphia, 1985, Lea & Febiger, pp 261, 270.

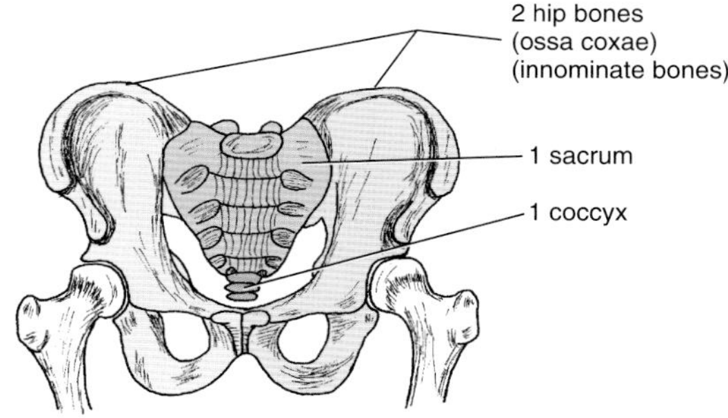

Fig. 8-4. Pelvis—four bones: two hip bones, sacrum, and coccyx.

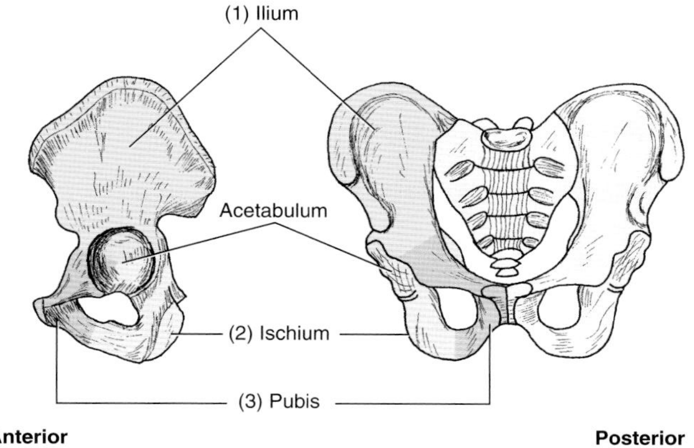

Fig. 8-5. Hip bone—three parts.

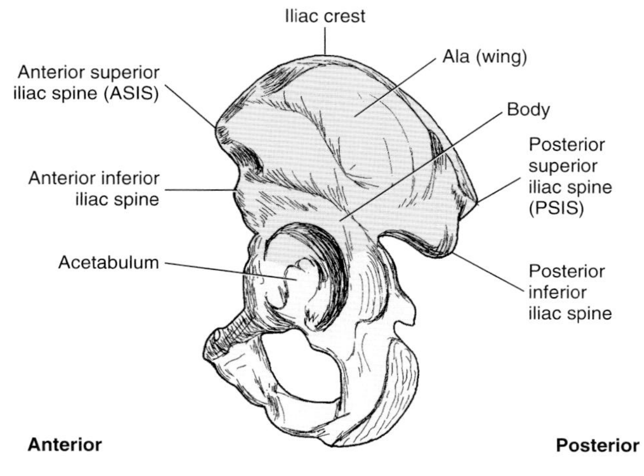

Fig. 8-6. Ilium.

8

Ischium

The **ischium** is that part of the hip bone inferior and posterior to the acetabulum. Each ischium is divided into a **body** and a **ramus.** The upper portion of the body of the ischium makes up the posteroinferior two-fifths of the acetabulum. The lower portion of the body of the ischium (formerly called the *superior ramus*) projects caudally and medially from the acetabulum, ending at the **ischial tuberosity.** Projecting anteriorly from the ischial tuberosity is the **ramus** of the ischium.

The rounded, roughened area near the junction of the lower body and the inferior rami is a landmark termed the **tuberosity** of the ischium, or **ischial** *(is'ke-al)* **tuberosity.**

Posterior to the acetabulum is a bony projection termed the ***ischial spine.*** A small part of the ischial spine also is visible on a frontal view of the pelvis, as shown in Fig. 8-8. (It is also seen in the anatomy review radiograph, Fig. 8-17.)

Directly above the ischial spine is a deep notch termed the **greater sciatic notch.** Below the ischial spine is a smaller notch termed the **lesser sciatic notch.**

Positioning landmark The ischial tuberosities bear most of the weight of the body when an individual sits. They can be palpated through the soft tissues of each buttock in a prone position. However, because of discomfort and possible embarrassment to the patient, this landmark is not as commonly used as are the previously described ASIS and crest of the ilium.

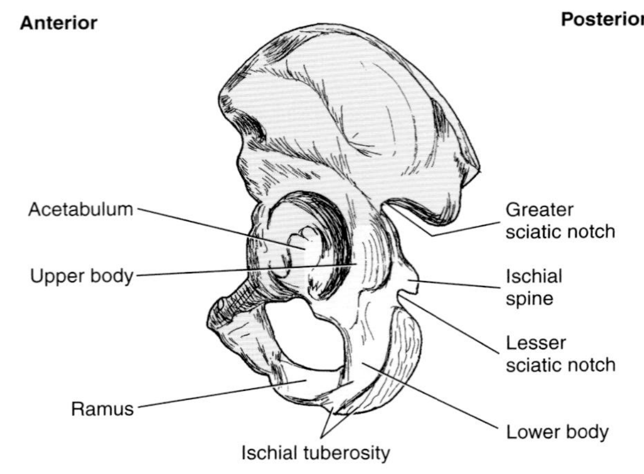

Fig. 8-7. Ischium.

Pubis

The last of the three divisions of one hip bone is the **pubis,** or **pubic bone.** The **body** of the pubis is anterior and inferior to the acetabulum and includes the anteroinferior one-fifth of the acetabulum.

Extending anteriorly and medially from the body of each pubis is a **superior ramus.** The two superior rami meet in the midline to form a slightly movable joint, the **symphysis pubis** *(sim'fi-sis pu'bis),* also correctly called **pubic symphysis.** Each **inferior ramus** passes down and posterior from the symphysis pubis to join the ramus of the respective ischium.

The **obturator foramen** *(ob'tu-ra"tor fo-ra'men)* is a large opening formed by the ramus and body of each ischium and by the pubis. The obturator foramen is the largest foramen in the human skeletal system.

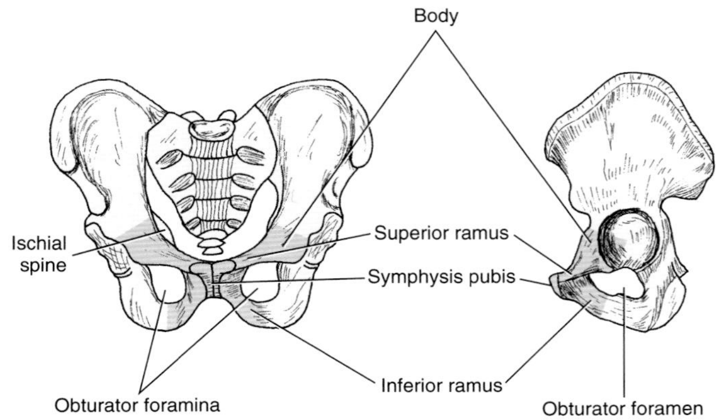

Fig. 8-8. Pubis (pubic bone).

Positioning landmark The crests of the ilium and the ASIS are important positioning landmarks. The superior margin of the symphysis pubis is a possible landmark for pelvis and hip positioning, as well as positioning for the abdomen because it defines the lowermost margin of the abdomen. However, if other associated landmarks are available, the symphysis pubis is generally not used as a palpated landmark because of patient modesty and potential embarrassment.

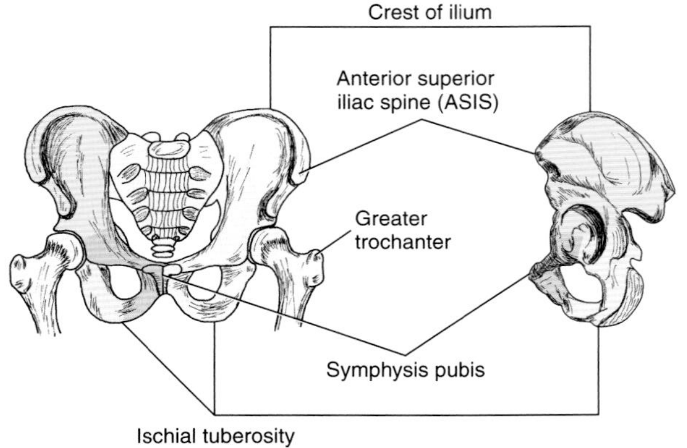

Fig. 8-9. Bony topographic landmarks of the pelvis.

SUMMARY OF TOPOGRAPHIC LANDMARKS

Important positioning landmarks of the pelvis are reviewed in Fig. 8-9. The most superior aspect of the **iliac crest** and the **ASIS** are easily palpated. The ASIS is one of the more frequently used positioning landmarks of the pelvis. It is also most commonly used to check for rotation of the pelvis and/or lower abdomen by determination of whether the distance between the ASIS and tabletop is equal on both sides.

The **greater trochanter** of the femur can be located by firm palpation in the soft tissues of the upper thigh. Note that the prominence of the greater trochanter is about the same level as the upper border of the **symphysis pubis,** whereas the **ischial tuberosity** is $1\frac{1}{2}$ to 2 inches (4 to 5 cm) below the symphysis pubis. These distances vary between a male and female pelvis because of general differences in shape, as described later in this chapter.

TRUE AND FALSE PELVIS

A plane through the **brim** of the pelvis divides the pelvic area into two cavities. The pelvic brim is defined by the upper part of the symphysis pubis anteriorly and the upper, prominent part of the sacrum posteriorly. The general area above or superior to the oblique plane through the pelvic brim is termed the **greater,** or **false, pelvis.** The flared portion of the pelvis formed primarily by the alae, or wings, of the ilia forms the lateral and posterior limits of the false pelvis, whereas the abdominal muscles of the anterior wall define the anterior limits. The lower abdominal organs rest on the floor of the greater pelvis, as well as the fetus within a pregnant uterus.

The area inferior to a plane through the pelvic brim is termed the **lesser,** or **true, pelvis.** The true pelvis is a cavity completely surrounded by bony structures. The size and shape of the true pelvis are of greatest importance during the birth process because the **true pelvis forms the actual birth canal.**

True Pelvis

The oblique plane defined by the brim of the pelvis is termed the **inlet,** or *superior aperture,* of the true pelvis. The **outlet,** or **inferior aperture,** of the true pelvis is defined by the two ischial tuberosities in the tip of the coccyx. The three sides of the triangularly shaped outlet are formed by a line between the ischial tuberosities and a line between each ischial tuberosity and the coccyx. The area between the inlet and outlet of the true pelvis is termed the **cavity** of the true pelvis. During the birth process, the baby must travel through the inlet, cavity, and outlet of the true pelvis.

Birth Canal

During a routine delivery the baby's head first travels through the pelvic inlet, then to the midcavity, and finally through the outlet to exit in a forward direction, as shown in Figs. 8-12 and 8-13.

Because of the sensitivity to radiation by the fetus, radiographs of the pelvis generally are **not** taken during pregnancy. If the dimensions of the birth canal of the pelvis are in question, certain ultrasound procedures can be done to evaluate for potential problems during the birthing process.

Note: In the past certain radiographic procedures called **cephalopelvimetry** *(sef"ah-lo-pel-vim'-e-tre)* **exams** were performed, whereby a specific type of metal ruler (Colcher-Sussman ruler) was placed next to the pelvis for anteroposterior (AP) and lateral projections. In this way the amount of magnification could be determined and actual measurements of the baby's head could be made, as well as inlet and outlet measurements of the mother's pelvis. First and second editions of this textbook described and illustrated this procedure in detail, but these descriptions have been omitted from more recent editions because of advances in sonography (ultrasound), which is now the preferred method to obtain this information. (Ultrasound procedures do not use the ionizing radiation that is potentially hazardous to the fetus as do x-ray exams such as a cephalopelvimetry.)

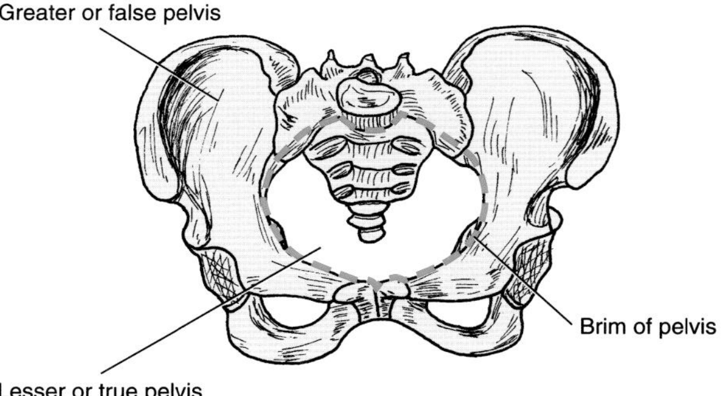

Fig. 8-10. Pelvic cavities.

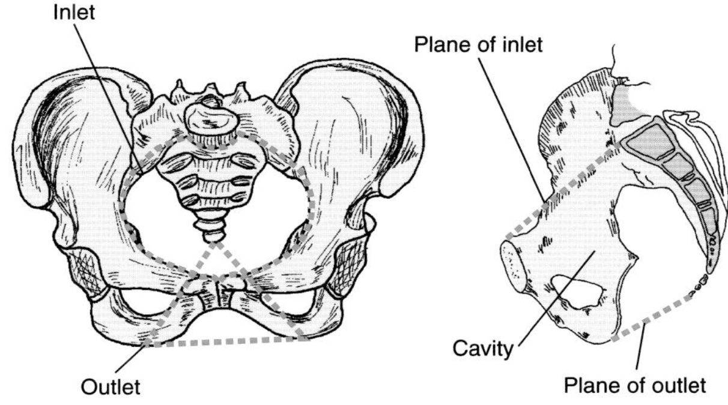

Fig. 8-11. Lesser or true pelvis.

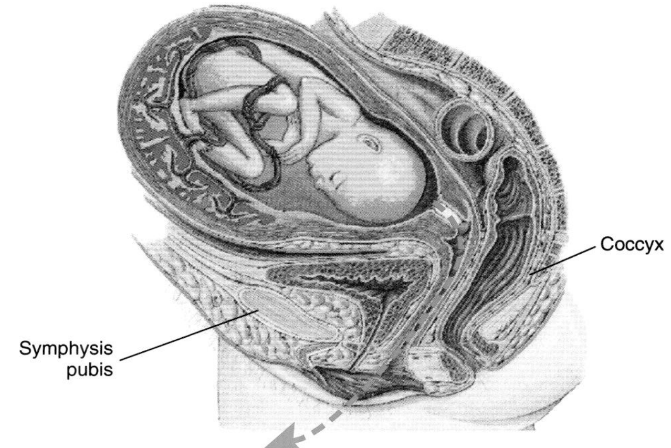

Fig. 8-12. Birth canal—sagittal sectional view.

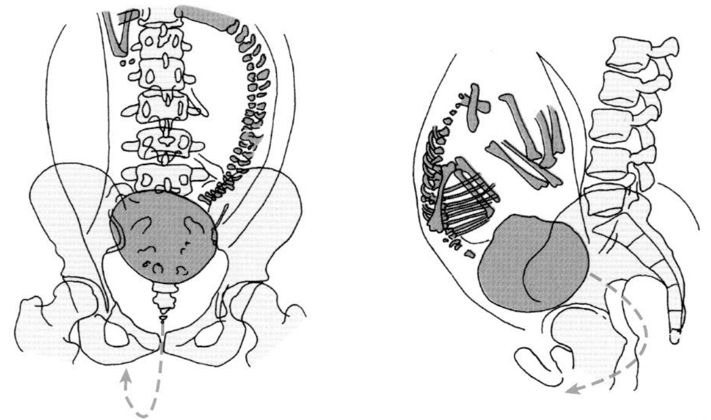

Fig. 8-13. Birth canal—frontal and side views.

8

Male Versus Female Pelvis

The general shape of the female pelvis varies enough from the male pelvis to enable discrimination of one from the other on pelvis radiographic images. In general the **female pelvis** is wider, with the ilia more flared and more shallow from front to back. The **male pelvis** is narrower, deeper, and less flared. In overall appearance on a frontal view, the female pelvis is wider. Therefore the first difference between the male pelvis and the female pelvis is the difference in the **overall general shape** of the entire pelvis.

A second major difference is the **angle of the pubic arch,** formed by the inferior rami of the pubis just below the symphysis pubis. In the female this angle is usually obtuse or greater than 90°, whereas in the male the pubic arch usually forms an acute angle, less than 90°.

A third difference is the **shape of the inlet** or superior aperture. The inlet of the female pelvis is usually larger and more round, whereas in the male it is usually narrower and more oval or heart-shaped. The general shape of the pelvis does vary considerably from one individual to another, so the pelvis of a slender female may resemble a male pelvis. In general, however, the differences are usually obvious enough that the sex of the patient can be determined from a radiographic image of the pelvis.

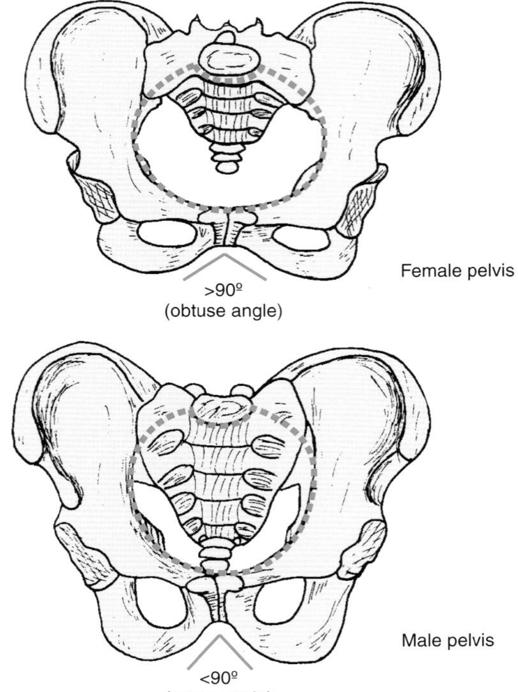

Fig. 8-14. Pelvis—male versus female.

SUMMARY OF MALE AND FEMALE PELVIC CHARACTERISTICS

	MALE	FEMALE
1. General shape	Narrower, deeper, less flared	Wider, more shallow, more flared
2. Angle of pubic arch	Acute angle (<90°)	Obtuse angle (>90°)
3. Shape of inlet	More oval or heart-shaped	More round, larger

Male Versus Female Pelvis Radiographs

Figs. 8-15 and 8-16 are pelvic radiographs of a female subject and male subject, respectively. Note the three differences between typical female pelvis and male pelvis.

First, in overall shape, the male pelvis appears narrower and deeper, with a less-flared appearance of the ilia.

Second, the acute angle of less than 90° of the pubic arch on the male is obvious, as compared with the greater-than-90° angle on the female pelvis. This angle is commonly one of the more noticeable differences.

Third, the shape of the inlet on the male pelvis is not as large or as rounded as that of the female pelvis.

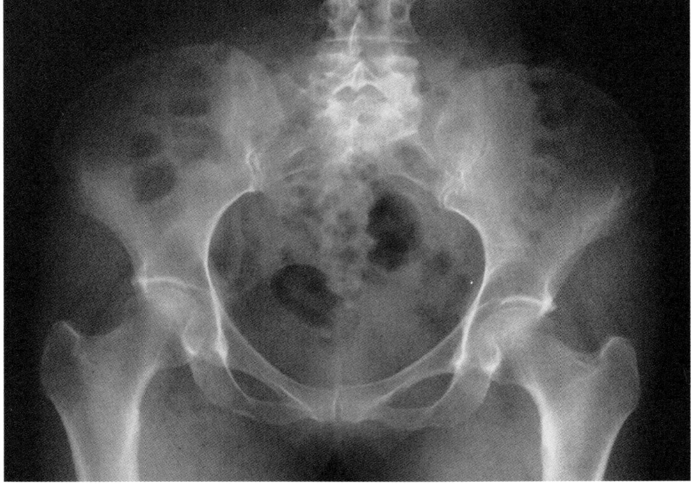

Fig. 8-15. Female pelvis.

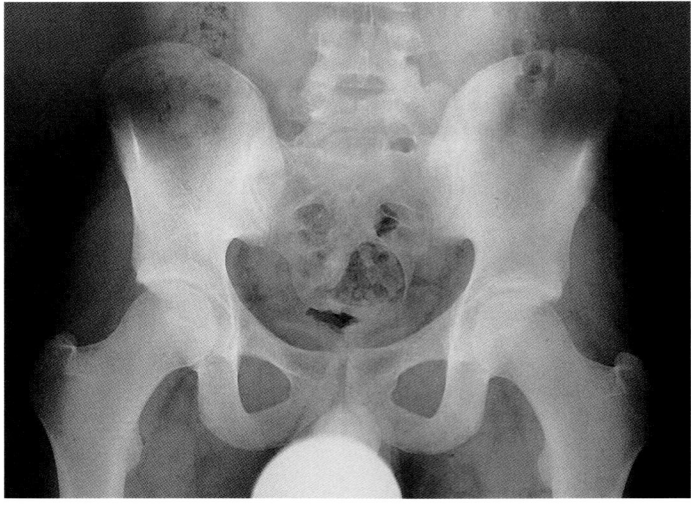

Fig. 8-16. Male pelvis.

REVIEW EXERCISE WITH RADIOGRAPHS

Key pelvic anatomy is labeled on the AP pelvis radiograph of Fig. 8-17. A good review exercise is to cover up the answers (listed below) while identifying the labeled parts.

A. Iliac crest
B. ASIS (anterior end of crest)
C. Body of left ischium
D. Ischial tuberosity
E. Symphysis pubis
F. Inferior ramus of right pubis
G. Superior ramus of right pubis
H. Right ischial spine
I. Acetabulum of right hip
J. Neck of right femur
K. Greater trochanter of right femur
L. Head of right femur
M. Ala, or wing, of right ilium

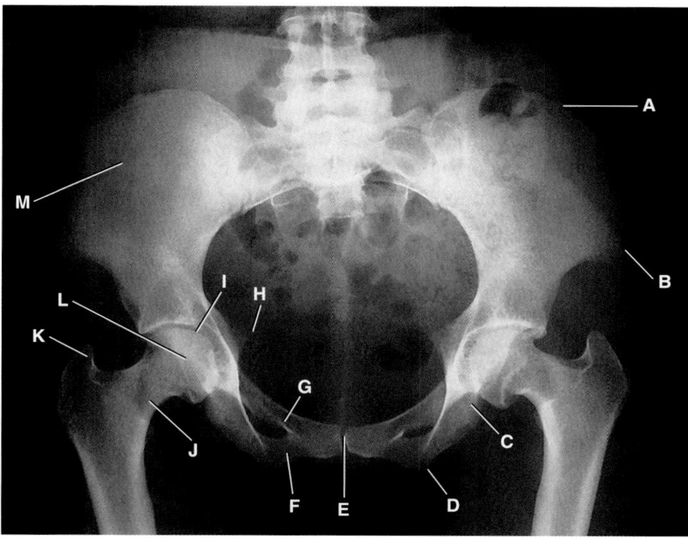

Fig. 8-17. Pelvis—AP.

Lateral Hip

Fig. 8-18 demonstrates a good lateral radiograph of the proximal femur and hip, taken with an inferosuperior projection (horizontal beam lateral) as demonstrated by the positioning of Fig. 8-19. The answers to the labeled parts are as follows:

A. Acetabulum
B. Femoral head
C. Femoral neck
D. Shaft or body
E. Area of lesser trochanter
F. Greater trochanter
G. Ischial tuberosity

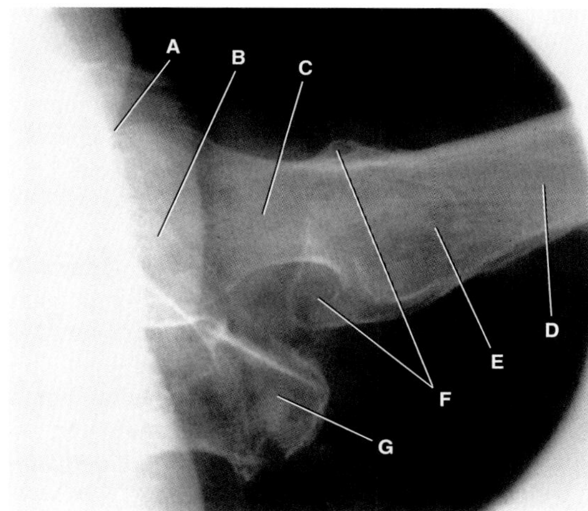

Fig. 8-18. Inferosuperior projection.

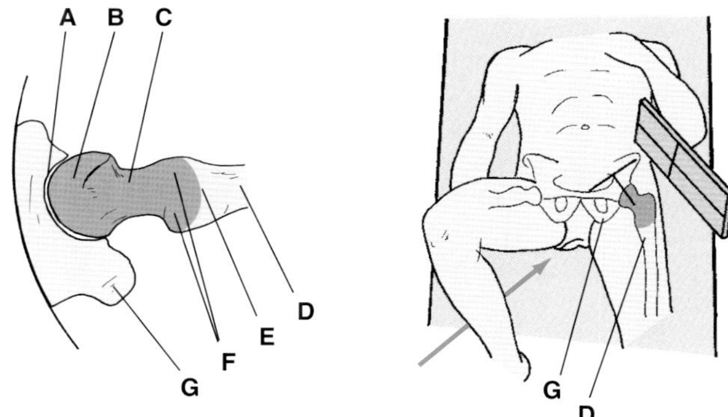

Fig. 8-19. Proximal femur and hip—lateral (inferosuperior projection).

8

CLASSIFICATION OF JOINTS

The number of joints or articulations of the proximal femora and pelvis is limited, with the hip joint being the most obvious. These joints of the pelvic girdle, as listed below, again are described according to their **classification, mobility type,** and **movement type.**

Sacroiliac joints—joints between sacrum and each ilium
Symphysis pubis—structure between right and left pubic bones
Union of acetabulum—a temporary growth joint of each acetabulum that solidifies in midteen years
Hip joints—joints between head of femur and acetabulum of pelvis

Sacroiliac Joints

The sacroiliac joints are wide, flat joints located on each side obliquely between the sacrum and each ilium. These joints are situated at an unusual oblique angle requiring special positioning to visualize the joint spaces radiographically.

The sacroiliac joint is classified as a **synovial joint** in that it is enclosed in a fibrous articular capsule containing synovial fluid. The bones are joined by firm sacroiliac ligaments. Generally, synovial joints by their nature are considered freely movable, or diarthrodial, joints. However, the sacroiliac joint is a special type of synovial joint that permits little movement and is thus **amphiarthrodial.** The reason for this classification is that the joint surfaces are very irregularly shaped and the interconnecting bones are snugly fitted because they serve a weight-bearing function. This shape restricts movement, and the cavity of the joint or the joint space may be reduced in size or even nonexistent in older persons, especially males.

Symphysis Pubis

The symphysis pubic is the articulation of the right and left pubic bones in the midline of the anterior pelvis. The most superior anterior aspect of this joint is palpable and is an important positioning landmark, as described previously.

8

The symphysis pubis is classified as a **cartilaginous joint** of the **symphysis subtype** in that only limited movement is possible **(amphiarthrodial).** The two articular surfaces are separated by a fibrocartilaginous disk and held together by certain ligaments. This interpubic disk of fibrocartilage is a relatively thick pad (thicker in females than males) capable of being compressed or partially displaced, thereby allowing some limited movement of these bones, such as in the case of pelvic trauma or during the birthing process in females.

Union of Acetabulum

The three divisions of each hip bone are separate bones in a child but come together in the acetabulum by fusing during the middle teens to become completely indistinguishable in an adult. Therefore this structure is classified as a **cartilaginous-type** joint of the **synchondrosis subtype,** which is **immovable,** or **synarthrodial,** in an adult. This joint is considered a temporary type of growth joint similar to the joints between the epiphyses and diaphyses of long bones in growing children.

Hip Joint

The hip joint is classified as a **synovial type,** truly characterized by a large fibrous capsule containing synovial fluid. It is a **freely movable,** or **diarthrodial,** joint and is the truest example of a **spheroid** (ball and socket) movement type.

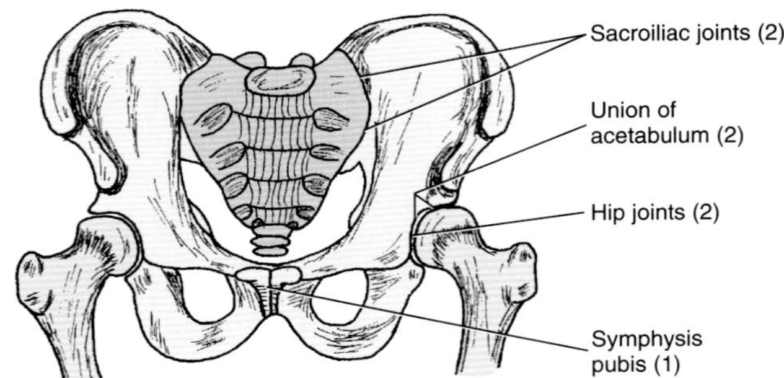

Fig. 8-20. Joints of pelvis.

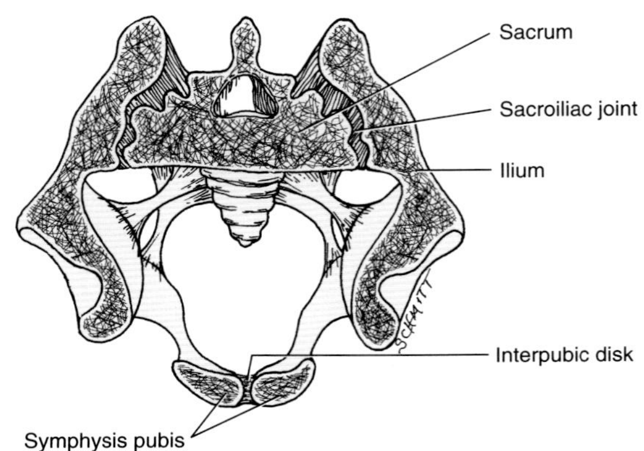

Fig. 8-21. Coronal view of a transverse section showing sacroiliac and symphysis pubis joints.

SUMMARY OF PELVIC JOINTS

JOINTS	CLASSIFICATION	MOBILITY TYPE	MOVEMENT TYPE
Sacroiliac joint	Synovial	Amphiarthrodial	—
Symphysis pubis	Cartilaginous	Amphiarthrodial	—
Union of acetabulum	Cartilaginous	Synarthrodial (for adults)	—
Hip joint	Synovial	Diarthrodial	Spheroidal (ball and socket)

The head of the femur forms more than half a sphere as it fits into the relatively deep, cup-shaped acetabulum. This connection makes the hip joint inherently strong as it supports the weight of the body while still permitting a high degree of mobility. The articular capsule surrounding this joint is strong and dense, with the thickest part being above, as would be expected because it is in line with the weight-bearing function of the hip joints. A series of strong bands of ligaments surround the articular capsule and joint in general, making this joint very strong and stable.

Movements of the hip joint include **flexion** and **extension, abduction** and **adduction, medial** (internal) and **lateral** (external) **rotation,** and **circumduction.**

RADIOGRAPHIC POSITIONING

Positioning Considerations

LOCATION OF HEAD AND NECK

A long-standing traditional method to locate the femoral head and neck is first to determine the midpoint of a line between the ASIS and the symphysis pubis. The **neck** is approximately 2.5 inches (6 to 7 cm), and the **head** 1.5 inches (4 cm) distal and at right angles to the midpoint of this line (Figs. 8-22 and 8-23).

The **greater trochanters** are shown to be located on the same horizontal line as the symphysis pubis. However, the greater trochanters are difficult to palpate accurately on large or obese patients, and palpation of the symphysis pubis can be embarrassing for the patient. Therefore a second method is suggested for location of the femoral head or neck that utilizes only the **ASIS,** which is easily palpated on all types of patients. The level of the symphysis pubis is between 3 and 4 inches (8 to 10 cm) inferior to the level of the ASIS. Therefore the femoral neck can be readily located as being **1 to 2 inches (3 to 5 cm) medial and 3 to 4 inches (8 to 10 cm) distal to the ASIS.** This level also places it on the same horizontal plane as the symphysis pubis and the greater trochanters.

As previously demonstrated, significant differences exist between the male pelvis and female pelvis, but with some practice and allowances for male and female differences, both of these methods work well for location of the femoral head or neck for hip positioning.

APPEARANCE OF PROXIMAL FEMUR IN ANATOMIC POSITION

As described earlier in this chapter under anatomy of the proximal femur, the head and neck of the femur project approximately 15° to 20° anteriorly or forward with respect to the rest of the femur and lower leg. Therefore when the leg is in the true anatomic position, as for a true AP leg, the proximal femur is actually rotated posteriorly by 15° to 20° (Fig. 8-24). Therefore the femoral neck appears shortened and the **lesser trochanter is visible** when the leg and ankle are truly AP, as in a true anatomic position.

INTERNAL ROTATION OF LEG

By **internally rotating the entire leg,** the proximal femur and hip joint are projected in a **true AP** projection. The neck of the femur is now parallel to the imaging surface and will not appear foreshortened.

The **lesser trochanter** is key in the determination of the correct leg and foot position (on a radiographic image). If the entire leg is rotated internally a full 15° to 20°, the outline of the lesser trochanter generally is not visible at all or only slightly visible on some patients when it is obscured by the shaft of the femur. If the leg is straight AP or when externally rotated, then the lesser trochanter is visible (see illustrations on following page).

EVIDENCE OF HIP FRACTURE

The femoral neck is a common fracture site for an older patient who has fallen. The typical physical sign for such a fracture is the **external rotation** of the involved foot, where the lesser trochanter is clearly visualized in profile, as seen on the left hip of Fig. 8-23 and the drawing on the right (Fig. 8-25). This sign is again demonstrated on the following page, Figs. 8-32 and 8-33.

Positioning warning If evidence of a hip fracture is present (external foot rotation), a pelvis radiograph should be taken "as is" **without** attempting to internally rotate the leg as would be necessary for a true AP hip projection.

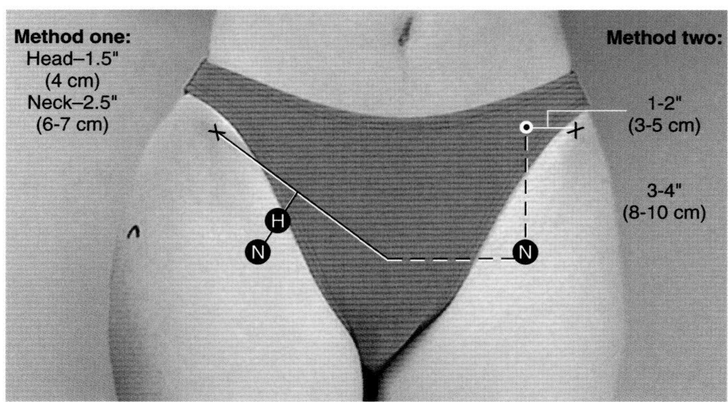

Fig. 8-22. Head (H) or neck (N) localization.

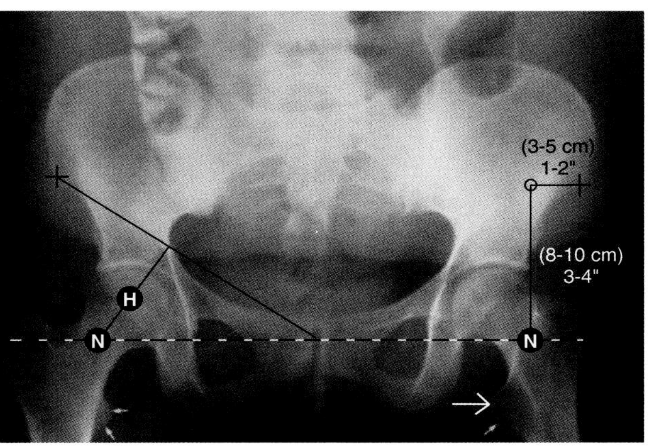

Fig. 8-23. Female pelvis, head (H), and neck (N) location.

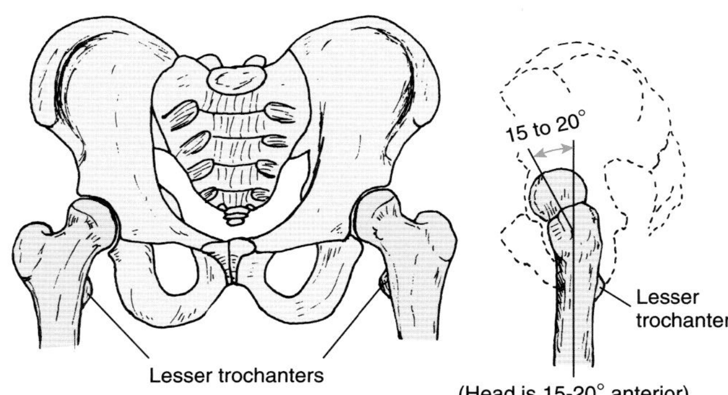

Fig. 8-24. Anatomic position (true AP of knee, leg, and ankle—but not of hip).

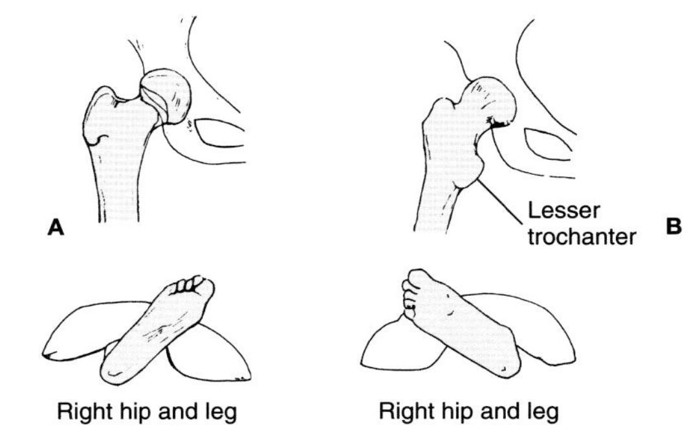

Fig. 8-25. A, Internal rotation (true AP of hip). **B,** External rotation (typical hip fracture position).

8

SUMMARY: EFFECT OF LOWER LIMB ROTATION

The photos and associated pelvis radiographs on this page demonstrate the effect of lower-limb rotation on the appearance of the proximal femora.

1. **Anatomic Position** *(Figs. 8-26 and 8-27):*
   - –Long axes of feet vertical
   - –Femoral necks partially foreshortened
   - –Lesser trochanters **partially visible**

2. **15° to 20° medial rotation** (the desired position to visualize pelvis and hips) *(Figs. 8-28 and 8-29):*
   - –Long axes of feet and lower limbs rotated 15° to 20° internally
   - –Femoral heads and necks in profile
   - –True AP projection of proximal femurs
   - –Less trochanters **not visible** or only slightly visible on some patients

3. **External rotation** *(Figs. 8-30 and 8-31):*
   - –Long axes of feet and lower limbs equally rotated laterally in a normal relaxed position
   - –Femoral necks greatly foreshortened
   - –Lesser trochanters **visible in profile internally**

4. **Typical rotation with hip fracture** *(Figs. 8-32 and 8-33):*
   - –Long axis of left foot externally rotated (on side of hip fracture)
   - –Unaffected right foot and limb in neutral position
   - –Lesser trochanter on externally rotated (left) limb more visible; neck area foreshortened

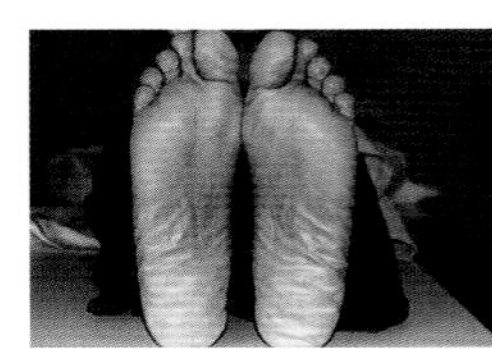

Fig. 8-26.

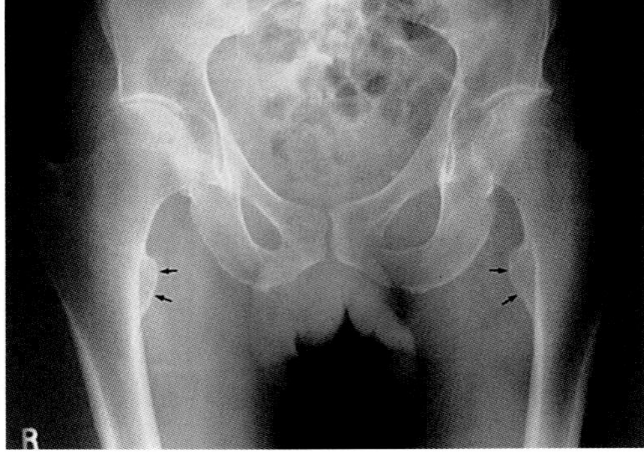

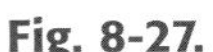

1. Anatomic position. **Fig. 8-27.**

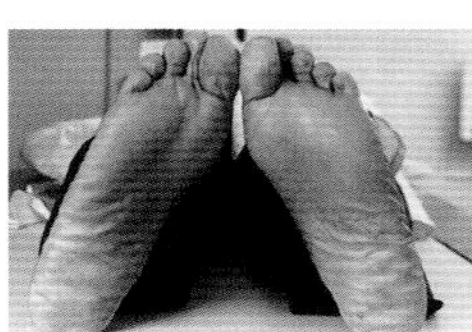

Fig. 8-28.

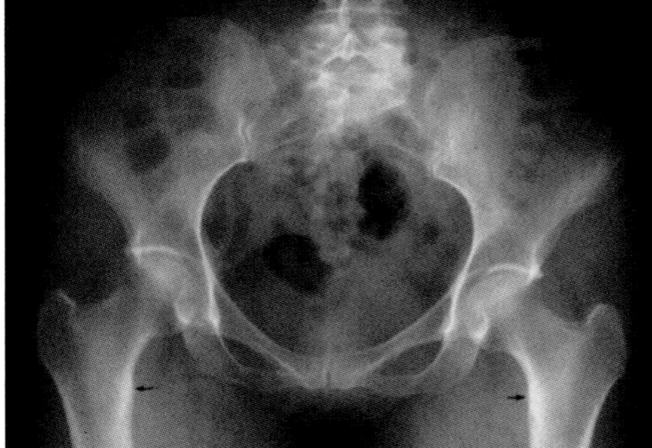

2. 15 to 20° medial rotation. **Fig. 8-29.**

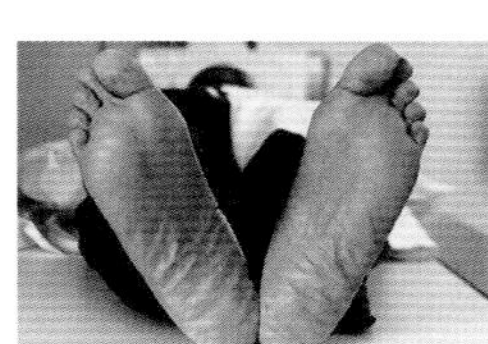

Fig. 8-30.

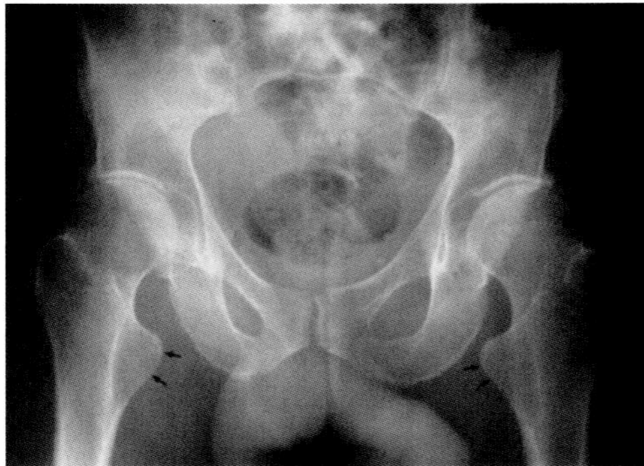

3. External rotation. **Fig. 8-31.**

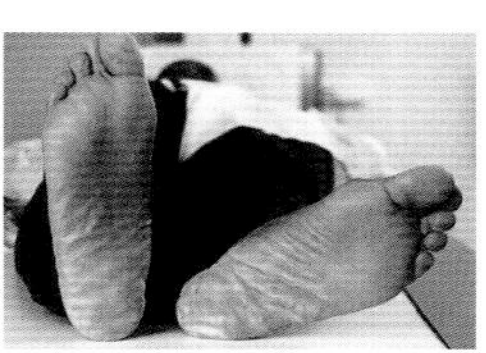

Fig. 8-32.

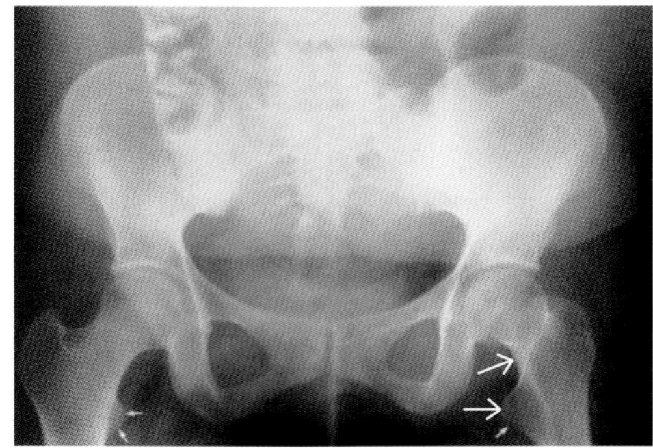

4. Typical rotation with hip fracture. **Fig. 8-33.**

8

SHIELDING GUIDELINES

Accurate gonadal shielding for pelvis and hip exams is especially critical because of the proximity of the radiation-sensitive gonads to the primary rays.

Male Shielding Shielding is easier for males in that small contact shields, such that as shown in Fig. 8-34, can be used on **all males.** The shields are placed over the area of the testes without covering essential anatomy of the pelvis or hips. However, care must be taken for pelvic radiographs that the top of the shield be placed at the **inferior margin of the symphysis pubis** to cover the testes adequately without obscuring the pubic and ischial areas of the pelvis.

Female Shielding Ovarian contact shields for females of child-bearing age or younger, however, require more critical placement to shield the area of the ovaries without covering essential pelvic or hip anatomy. Vinyl-covered lead material cut into various shapes and sizes can be used for this purpose for an AP pelvis or bilateral hip radiograph, as shown in Fig. 8-36 and as described in Chapter 2, p. 71.

For a unilateral hip or proximal femur, larger contact shields can be used to cover the general pelvic area without covering the specific hip being radiographed, as shown in Fig. 8-35. Accurate location of the femoral head and neck makes this type of gonadal shielding possible.

Gonadal shielding may not be possible for females on certain AP pelvic projections in which the entire pelvis, including the sacrum and coccyx, must be demonstrated. Also, gonadal shielding may not be possible on lateral inferosuperior hip projections for males and females because shielding may obscure essential anatomy. However, **gonadal shielding should be used whenever possible for both males and females,** along with **close collimation** for all hip and pelvic projections. General pelvic trauma requiring visualization of the entire pelvis may prohibit ovarian shielding for females. Departmental policy regarding gonadal shielding for pelvic procedures on females should be determined by each technologist.

Exposure Factors and Patient Dose To reduce total radiation dose to the patient, a higher kV range of 90 ± 5 may be used for hip and pelvic exams. This higher kV technique, with lower mAs, results in a lower radiation dose to the patient. Higher kV, however, does decrease contrast and may not be advisable, especially on older patients who may have some loss of bone mass or density due to osteoporosis (see below), thus requiring even lower kV than average.

PEDIATRIC APPLICATIONS

Pelvic and hip radiographic exams are not performed often on children except for newborns with developmental dysplasia of the hip (DDH). Correct shielding is especially important for infants and children because of the repeat radiographic exams frequently required during the growth of the child. If holding of the legs of an infant is required, an individual other than radiology personnel should do this while wearing a lead apron and lead gloves.

The degree and type of immobilization required for older children are dependent on the ability and willingness of the child to cooperate during the procedure. A "mummy wrap" (see Chapter 20) helps prevent the upper limbs from interfering with the anatomy of interest on a challenging patient. At the very least, tape or sandbags may be required to immobilize the legs in the proper degree of internal rotation.

GERIATRIC APPLICATIONS

Geriatric patients are prone to hip fractures resulting from falls and increased incidence of osteoporosis. As noted previously, the position of the patient's foot and leg must be observed in trauma cases.

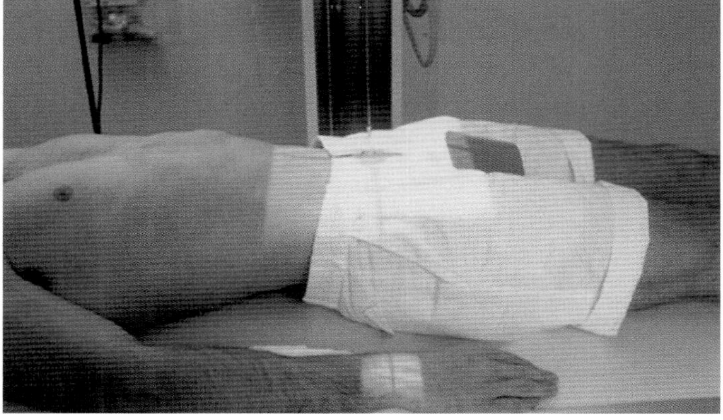

Fig. 8-34. Male gonadal shielding for hips and pelvis.

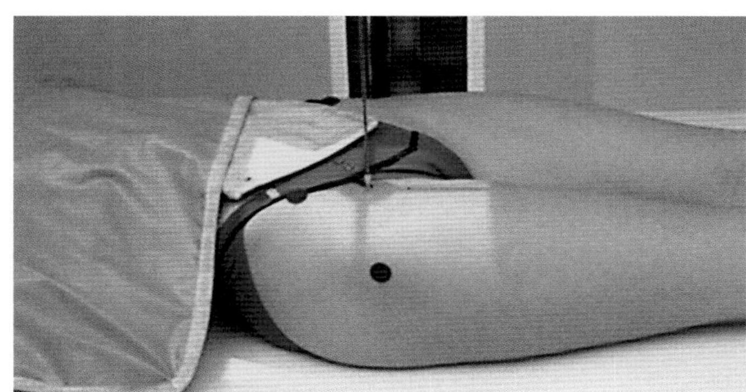

Fig. 8-35. General abdominal and pelvic shielding for proximal femur to include hip.

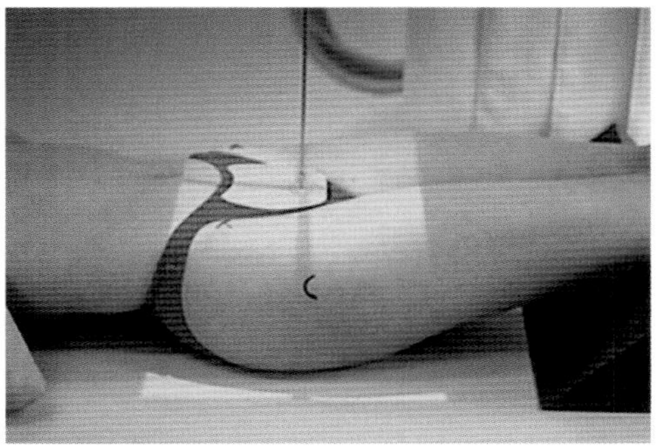

Fig. 8-36. Female gonadal (ovarian) shielding for bilateral hips and proximal femurs.

It is critical that the injured limb not be moved if the leg is externally rotated. An AP projection of both hips for comparison should be taken first, without movement of the affected limb, to check for fractures. This step may then be followed with an inferosuperior (Danelius-Miller) projection of the affected hip.

In nontrauma situations, most geriatric patients require (and appreciate) some immobilization to assist them in holding the feet and legs inverted for the AP pelvis and also to support the limb for the lateral projection.

Patients who have had hip replacement surgery should **not** be placed in the "frog-leg" position for any postsurgical procedures. An inferosuperior lateral is indicated in addition to the AP projection.

8

DIGITAL IMAGING CONSIDERATIONS

The following text reviews a summary of the guidelines that should be followed with digital imaging (CR and DR) of procedures described in this chapter:

1. **Close collimation** to the body part being imaged and **accurate centering** are most important in digital imaging of the hip and pelvis.
2. **Exposure factors:** It is important that the ALARA principle be followed and the **lowest exposure factors required to obtain a diagnostic image be used.** This includes the highest kV and the lowest mAs that will result in desirable image quality. This may require a higher kV than with film-screen imaging.
3. **Postprocessing evaluation of exposure index values:** The exposure index number on the final processed image must be checked to verify that the exposure factors used were in the correct range **to ensure an optimum quality image with the least radiation to the patient.**

Alternative Modalities

COMPUTED TOMOGRAPHY

Computed tomography (CT) is useful in the evaluation of soft-tissue involvement of lesions or the determination of the extent of fractures. CT is also helpful to study the relationship of the femoral head to the acetabulum before hip surgery or for a postreduction study of a developmental hip dislocation.

In general, CT is useful to add to the anatomy or pathologic information already obtained by conventional radiographs. For children the CT exam is useful to examine the relationship of the femoral head to the acetabulum after surgical reduction of a developmental hip dislocation.

MAGNETIC RESONANCE IMAGING

Like CT, magnetic resonance imaging (MRI) can be useful for imaging the lower limb or pelvis when soft-tissue injuries or possible abnormalities related to joints are suspected. In general, depending on clinical history, MRI may be used when additional information not obtained from conventional radiographs is needed.

SONOGRAPHY (ULTRASOUND)

Ultrasound is useful for evaluation of newborns for hip dislocations and assessment of joint stability during movement of the lower limbs. This method is usually done during the first 4 to 6 months of infancy to reduce ionizing radiation exposure.

NUCLEAR MEDICINE

Nuclear medicine bone scans can be useful to provide **early evidence** of certain bony pathologic processes, such as occult fractures, bone infections, metastatic carcinoma, or other metastatic or primary malignancies. Nuclear medicine is more sensitive and generally provides earlier evidence than other modalities because it assesses the physiologic aspect rather than the anatomic aspect of these conditions.

Pathologic Indications

Pathologic indications involving the pelvis and hips that all technologists should be familiar with include the following (not necessarily an inclusive list):

Ankylosing spondylitis: The first effect demonstrated is fusion of the sacroiliac joints. The disease causes extensive calcification of the anterior longitudinal ligament of the spinal column. It is progressive, working up the vertebral column, creating a radiographic characteristic known as "bamboo spine." Males are most often affected.

Avulsion (evulsion) fractures of the pelvis: These fractures cause extreme pain and are difficult to diagnose if not imaged properly. A typical view is the AP pelvis at around 65 kV. The lower kV is required to detect a small avulsion fracture. Fractures occur in adolescent athletes who experience sudden, forceful, or unbalanced contraction of the tendinous and muscular attachments such as might occur while running hurdles. The force of the tendons and muscles sliding over the tuberosities, ASIS, anterior inferior iliac spine (AIIS), superior corner of the symphysis pubis, and the iliac crest may cause avulsion fractures.*

Chondrosarcoma: A malignant tumor of the cartilage, it usually occurs in men over age 45 in the pelvis and long bones. A chondrosarcoma may be completely removed surgically if it does not respond to radiation or chemotherapy.

Developmental dysplasia of the hip (DDH) (older term is "congenital dislocation of the hip [CDH]"): These hip dislocations are caused by conditions present at birth and may require frequent hip radiographs (see Chapter 20).

Legg-Calvé-Perthes disease: Legg-Calvé Perthes disease is the most common type of aseptic or ischemic necrosis. Lesions typically involve only one hip (head and neck of femur). The disease occurs predominantly in 5- to 10-year-old boys, with a limp usually being the first clinical sign. Radiographs demonstrate a flattened femoral head that later can appear fragmented.

Metastatic carcinoma: The malignancy spreads to the bone via the circulatory system, lymphatic system, or direct invasion. Metastatic tumors of the bone are much more common than primary malignancies. Bones containing red bone marrow are the more common metastatic sites (spine, skull, ribs, pelvis, and femurs).

Osteoarthritis: This condition is known as a *degenerative joint disease (DJD),* with degeneration of joint cartilage and adjacent bone causing pain and stiffness. It is the most common type of arthritis and may be considered a normal part of the aging process. It is common in weight-bearing joints such as the hips and provides the first evidence on radiographic images of joints such as the hip on many persons by age 40 before symptoms develop. As the condition worsens, joints become less mobile, and new growths of cartilage and bone are seen as osteophytes (bony outgrowths).

Pelvic ring fractures: Because of the closed ring structure of the pelvis, a severe blow or trauma to one side of the pelvis may result in a fracture site away from the primary trauma, thus requiring clear radiographic visualization of the entire pelvis.

Proximal femur (hip) fractures: These fractures are most common in older adult or geriatric patients with osteoporosis or avascular necrosis. Both osteoporosis (loss of bone mass from metabolic or other factors) and avascular (loss of blood circulation) necrosis (cell death) frequently lead to a weakening or collapse of weight-bearing joints such as the hip joint, and fractures occur with only minimal trauma.

Slipped capital femoral epiphysis (SCFE): This condition usually occurs in 10- to 16-year-olds during rapid growth when even minor trauma can precipitate its development. The epiphysis appears shorter and the epiphyseal plate wider with smaller margins.

*Acute avulsion fractures of the pelvis in adolescent competitive athletes: prevalence, location and sports distribution of 203 cases collected. In Rossi F, Dragoni S: Skeletal Radiol 30(3), 2001.

SUMMARY OF PATHOLOGIC INDICATIONS

CONDITION OR DISEASE	MOST COMMON RADIOGRAPHIC EXAM	POSSIBLE RADIOGRAPHIC APPEARANCE	EXPOSURE FACTOR ADJUSTMENT*
Ankylosing spondylitis	AP pelvis, AP and/or posterior oblique SI joints	Early stage—fusion SI joints; later "bamboo spine" appearance due to calcification of disk spaces of vertebral column	None
Avulsion (evulsion) fractures	AP pelvis (lower kV)	Separation of small fragment of bone at ligament attachments	Decrease (–) kV
Chondrosarcoma	AP pelvis and bilateral "frog-leg," CT, MRI	Lytic (meaning *capable of dissolving*) lesion due to bone destruction; contains scattered calcifications in cartilaginous (radiolucent) tumor	None
Developmental dysplasia of hip–DDH (congenital dislocation of hip–CDH)	AP pelvis and bilateral "frog-leg"	Increased hip joint space and misalignment	None
Legg-Calvé-Perthes disease	AP pelvis and axiolateral of affected hip	Flattened or fragmented femoral head	None
Metastatic carcinoma	AP pelvis, bilateral "frog-leg," CT, MRI	Usually numerous, small lytic lesions	None
Osteoarthritis	AP pelvis and bilateral "frog-leg" or axiolateral, if necessary	Hallmark sign of "spurring" and narrowing of joint space	None or decrease (–)
Pelvic ring fracture	AP, oblique, and lateral of affected part	Bilateral radiolucent lines across bones; misalignment of SI joints, pelvic inlet	None
Proximal femur hip fracture	AP pelvis and axiolateral of affected hip	Radiolucent line(s) crossing bone or radiopaque areas due to overlapping fragments	None
Slipped capital femoral epiphysis (SCFE)	AP pelvis and bilateral "frog-leg"	Epiphysis appearing shorter and epiphyseal plate wider	None

AP, anteroposterior; *SI,* sacroiliac; *CT,* computed tomography; *MRI,* magnetic resonance imaging.
*Dependent on stage or severity of disease or condition.

Summary of Survey Results

Pelvis: In addition to the basic **AP pelvis** projection, the next most common special pelvis projection was the **posterior oblique for the acetabulum** (Judet method), as indicated by 45% in U.S. and 54% in Canada.

Inquiries have been received concerning the question of what is meant by special **"inlet"** and **"outlet" pelvis projections,** which are frequently ordered as such by referring physicians. To clarify this issue, the AP axial for anterior pubic bones (Taylor method) was renamed as an AP axial **outlet projection,** and the AP axial **inlet projection** (modified Lilienfeld method) was added.

Hips and proximal femora: For basic lateral hip positions the most common as indicated by the survey was the **unilateral frog-leg,** 76% in U.S. and 73% in Canada. This projection was followed by the **axiolateral inferosuperior** (Danelius-Miller method) trauma projection, with 75% in U.S. and 55% in Canada.

Sacroiliac (SI) joints: The most common basic SI joint projections were the **AP axial** (69% U.S., 82% Canada), followed by **posterior obliques** (69% U.S., 63% Canada). The anterior obliques were much less common (21% U.S. and Canada) and thus were omitted in the last two editions.

Standard and Special Operating Procedures

Certain basic and special projections or positions for the proximal femora and pelvis are demonstrated and described on the following pages as suggested standard and special departmental procedures.

PELVIS RADIOGRAPHIC GUIDE

The following guide is provided as **a suggested sequence of possible basic and special projections** of the proximal femur and pelvis, as described and illustrated in this textbook. The basic **AP pelvis** is considered the **initial baseline evaluation projection** for either hip or general pelvic pathologic processes or trauma. This projection then is followed by **additional lateral projections for the hip and proximal femur** or additional **special projections of the pelvis** for possible trauma to other parts of the pelvis.

The entire AP pelvis is considered basic for a possible hip fracture even if the side of injury is known so that both hips can be demonstrated for comparison purposes.

AP PELVIS, p. 275
AP projection of entire pelvis
(Bilateral hips)

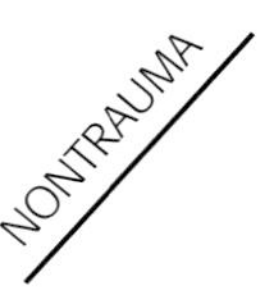

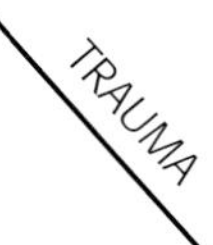

Basic–proximal femur and hip
Lateral
1. Lateral AP bilateral frog-leg **(276)**
or
2. Unilateral frog-leg **(282)**
AP
3. AP unilateral hip **(280)**
(post-op or follow-up exams)

Basic–lateral of proximal femur and hip
1. Axiolateral inferosuperior **(281)**
(Danelius-Miller method)
or

Special–lateral of proximal femur and hip
2. Modified axiolateral hip **(283)**
(Clements-Nakayama method) or
3. Mediolateral projection (Chapter 19)
(Sanderson method)

Special–pelvis
4. AP axial outlet projection **(277)**
(Taylor method)
5. AP axial inlet projection **(278)**
(modified Lilienfeld method)
6. Posterior oblique acetabulum **(279)**
(Judet method)

BASIC PROJECTIONS

Standard or basic projections, at times referred to as *routine projections* or *departmental routines,* are those projections commonly taken on average patients who are helpful and can cooperate in performing the procedure.

SPECIAL PROJECTIONS

Special projections are those more common projections taken as extra or additional projections to demonstrate better certain pathologic conditions or specific body parts.

Pelvis and/or Bilateral Hips
BASIC
- **AP pelvis or bilateral hips** 275
- **AP bilateral frog-leg** 276 **(modified Cleaves method)**

SPECIAL
- **AP axial outlet projections** 277 **(Taylor method)**
- **AP axial inlet projection** 278
- **Posterior oblique acetabulum** 279 **(Judet method)**

Hip and Proximal Femur
BASIC
- **AP unilateral hip** 280

TRAUMA LATERAL
- **Axiolateral inferosuperior (Danelius-Miller method)** 281

SPECIAL NONTRAUMA LATERAL
- **Unilateral frog-leg (modified Cleaves method)** 282

SPECIAL TRAUMA LATERAL
- **Modified axiolateral (Clements-Nakayama method)** 283

Sacroiliac Joints
BASIC
- **AP axial** 284
- **Posterior obliques** 285

AP PELVIS PROJECTION (BILATERAL HIPS): PELVIS

Warning: Do **not** attempt to internally rotate legs if a hip fracture or dislocation is suspected. Take with affected leg "as is."

Pelvis
BASIC
• AP

Pathology Demonstrated

Fractures, joint dislocations, degenerative disease, and bone lesions are demonstrated.

Technical Factors

- IR size—35 × 43 cm (14 × 17 inches), crosswise
- Moving or stationary grid
- 80 ± 5 kV range or 90 ± 5 kV range

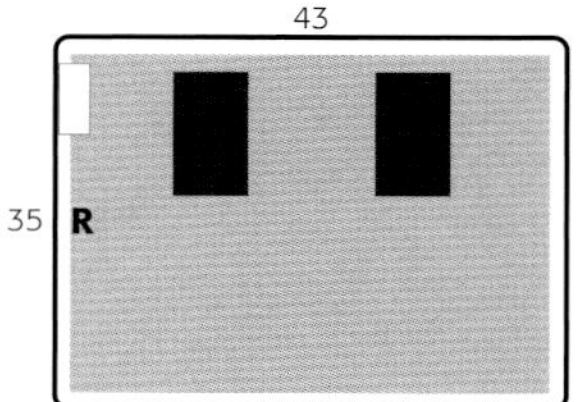

- Technique and dose at 80 kV: or For lower gonadal dose at 90 kV:

	cm	kV	mAs	Sk.	ML.	Gon.
Technique and dose at 80 kV	18	80	12	106	24	M 98 F 36
For lower gonadal dose at 90 kV	18	90	8	76	22	M 68 F 28
						mrad

Shielding Shield gonads on all male patients. Ovarian shielding on females, however, is generally not possible without obscuring of essential pelvis anatomy (unless interest is in area of hips only).

Patient Position With patient supine, place arms at sides or across upper chest; provide pillow for head and support for under knees.

Part Position

- Align midsagittal plane of patient to center line of table and to CR.
- Ensure that pelvis is **not rotated;** distance from tabletop to each ASIS should be equal.
- Separate legs and feet, then **internally rotate** long axes of feet and lower limbs **15° to 20°** (see Warning above). Technologist may need to place sandbag between heels and tape top of feet together or use additional sandbags against feet to retain this position.

Central Ray

- CR is **perpendicular** to IR, directed **midway between level of ASISs and the symphysis pubis.** This is approximately 2 inches (5 cm) inferior to level of ASIS (see Note).
- Center cassette to CR.
- Minimum SID is 40 inches (100 cm).

Collimation Collimate to lateral skin margins and to upper and lower IR borders.

Respiration Suspend respiration during exposure.

Note: If performed as part of a hip routine, centering should be about 2 inches (5 cm) lower to level of midfemoral heads or necks to include more of proximal femora.

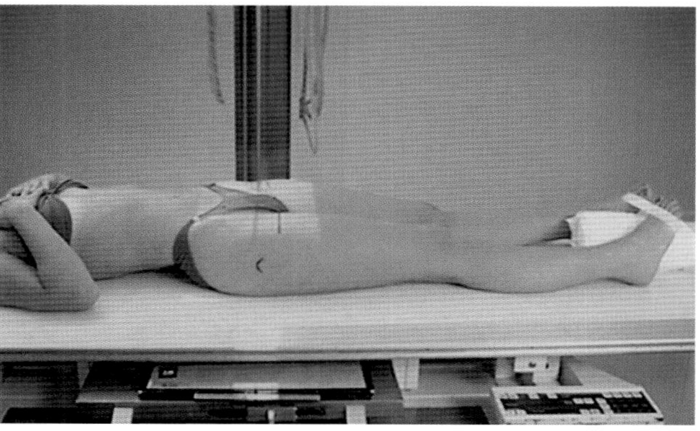

Fig. 8-37. Patient and part position—AP pelvis.

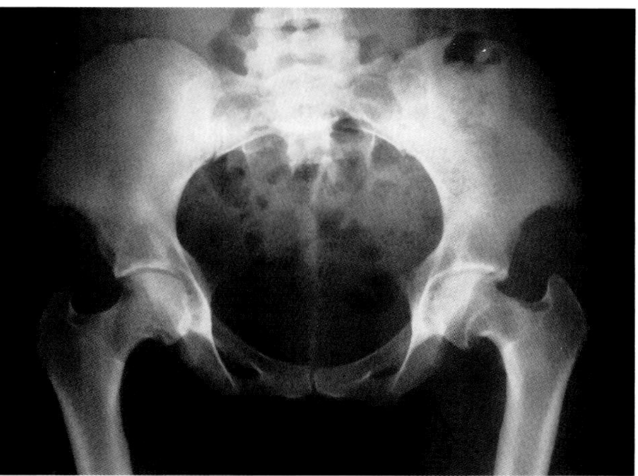

Fig. 8-38. AP pelvis.

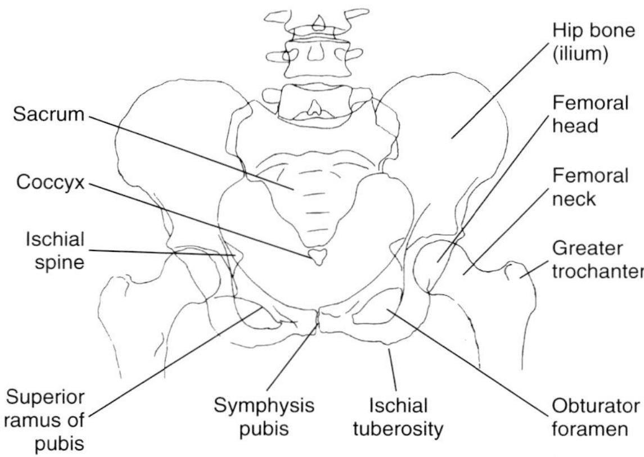

Fig. 8-39. AP pelvis.

Radiographic Criteria

Structures Shown: • Pelvic girdle, L5, sacrum and coccyx, femoral heads and neck, and greater trochanters are visible.

Position: • Lesser trochanters should not be visible at all, or for many patients only the tips are visible. Greater trochanters should appear equal in size and shape. • **No rotation** is evidenced by symmetric appearance of the iliac ala, or wings, the ischial spines, and the two obturator foramina. A foreshortened or closed obturator foramen indicates rotation in that direction. (A closed or narrowed right obturator foramen compared with the left indicates rotation toward the right.) • The right and left ischial spines (if visible) should appear equal in size.

Collimation and CR: • Correct centering evidenced by demonstration of entire pelvis and upper femora without foreshortening in collimated field. • Midsagittal plane of patient should be aligned with central axis of IR. • Collimation borders are minimal on larger patients. Smaller patients should show equal lateral collimation borders just lateral to greater trochanters.

Exposure Criteria: • Optimal exposure visualizes L5 and sacrum area and margins of the femoral heads and acetabula, as seen through overlying pelvic structures, without overexposing the ischium and pubic bones. • Trabecular markings of proximal femora and pelvic structures appear sharp, indicating no motion.

AP BILATERAL "FROG-LEG" PROJECTION: PELVIS

Modified Cleaves Method

Warning: Do **not** attempt this position on patient with destructive hip disease or with potential hip fracture or dislocation.

Pathology Demonstrated
This projection is useful for demonstration of a nontrauma hip or developmental dysplasia of hip (DDH), also known as congenital hip dislocation (CHD).

Pelvis
BASIC
- **AP**
- **AP bilateral frog-leg (modified Cleaves)**

Technical Factors
- IR size—35 × 43 cm (14 × 17 inches), crosswise
- Moving or stationary grid
- 80 ± 5 kV range or 90 ± 5 kV range
- Technique and dose at 80 kV:

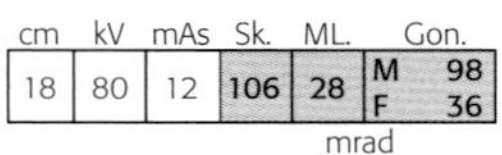

cm	kV	mAs	Sk.	ML.	Gon.
18	80	12	106	28	M 98 F 36

mrad

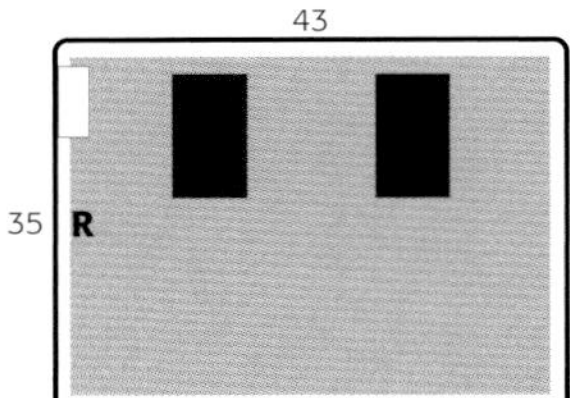

No center AEC cell with shield in place.

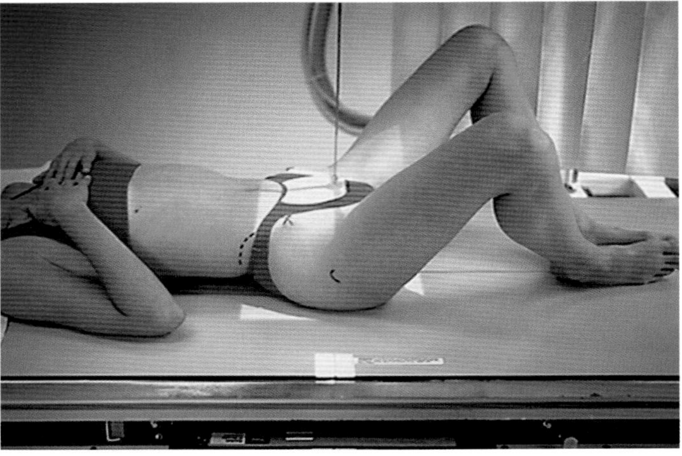

Fig. 8-40. Bilateral frog-leg—femora abducted 40° to 45°.

Shielding Shield gonads for both males and females without obscuring essential anatomy (see Note 1).

Patient Position With patient supine, provide pillow for head and place arms across chest.

Part Position
- Align patient to midline of table and/or IR and to CR.
- Ensure pelvis is **not rotated** (equal distance of ASISs to tabletop).
- Center IR to CR, at level of femoral heads, top of IR approximately at level of iliac crest.
- Flex both knees approximately 90°, as demonstrated.
- Place the plantar surfaces of feet together and **abduct both femurs 40° to 45° from vertical** (see Note 2). Ensure that **both femurs are abducted the same amount** and that pelvis is **not rotated.**
- Place supports under each leg for stabilization if needed.

Central Ray
- CR is **perpendicular** to IR, directed to a point **3 inches (7.5 cm) below level of ASIS** (1 inch, or 2.5 cm, above symphysis pubis).
- Minimum SID is 40 inches (100 cm).

Collimation Collimate to IR borders on four sides.

Respiration Suspend respiration during exposure.

Note 1: This projection is frequently performed for periodic follow-up exams on younger patients, thus **correctly placed gonadal shielding is important for both male and female patients, ensuring that hip joints are not covered.**

Note 2: Less abduction of femurs such as only 20° to 30° from vertical provides for the least foreshortening of femoral necks, but this placement foreshortens the entire proximal femora, which may not be desirable.

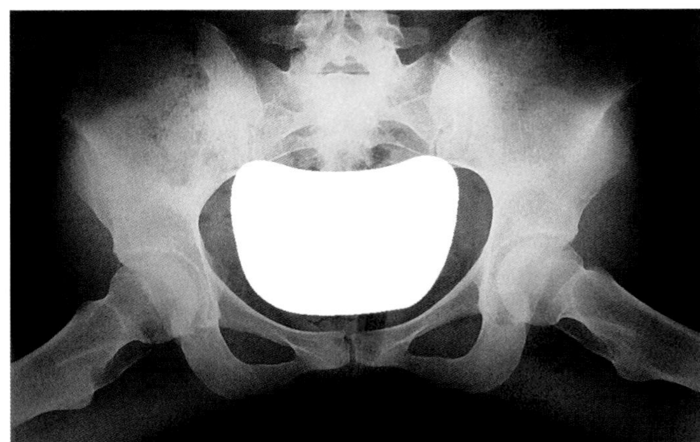

Fig. 8-41. Bilateral frog-leg. (Courtesy Kathy Martensen, RT.)

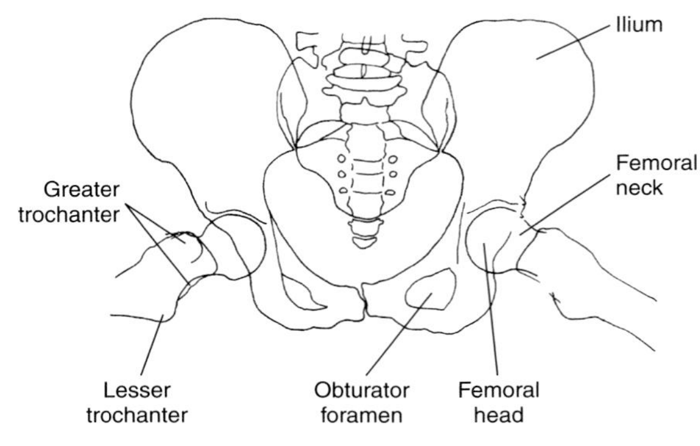

Fig. 8-42. Bilateral frog-leg.

Radiographic Criteria

Structures Shown: • Femoral heads and necks, acetabulum, and trochanteric areas are visible on one radiograph.

Position: • **No rotation** is evidenced by symmetric appearance of the pelvic bones, especially the ala of the ilium, two obturator foramina, and ischial spines, if visible. • The femoral heads and necks and greater and lesser trochanters should appear symmetric if both thighs were abducted equally. • The lesser trochanters should appear equal in size, as projected beyond the lower or medial margin of the femora. • The greater trochanters appear mostly superimposed over the femoral necks, which appear foreshortened (see Note 2).

Collimation and CR: • The pelvic girdle should be centered to the collimation field from right to left, with the midpoint being at about 2.5 cm (1 inch) superior to the symphysis pubis.

Exposure Criteria: • Optimal exposure visualizes the margins of the femoral head and the acetabulum through overlying pelvic structures, without overexposing the proximal femora. • Trabecular markings appear sharp, indicating no motion.

AP AXIAL "OUTLET" PROJECTION* (FOR ANTERIOR/INFERIOR PELVIC BONES): PELVIS

Taylor Method

Pelvis
SPECIAL
- AP axial outlet projection

Pathology Demonstrated

This projection presents an excellent view of the bilateral pubes and ischia to assess pelvic trauma for fractures and displacement.

Technical Factors

- IR size—24 × 30 cm (10 × 12 inches), crosswise, or 30 × 35 cm (11 × 14 inches)
- Moving or stationary grid
- 80 ± 5 kV range
- Technique and exposure:

cm	kV	mAs	Sk.	ML.	Gon.
17	85	10	124	33	M 124 F 31
					mrad

30 (35)
24 (30)
R

Shielding Gonadal shielding may be done if great care is taken not to obscure essential pelvic anatomy.

Patient Position With patient supine, provide pillow for head. With patient's legs extended, place support under knees for comfort.

Part Position

- Align midsagittal plane to CR and to midline of table and/or IR.
- Ensure **no rotation** of pelvis (ASIS-to-tabletop distance equal on both sides).
- Center IR to projected CR.

Central Ray

- Angle CR **cephalad 20° to 35° for males** and **30° to 45° for females.** (These different angles are due to differences in shapes between male and female pelves.)
- Direct CR to a midline point **1 to 2 inches (3 to 5 cm) distal to** the superior border of the **symphysis pubis** or **greater trochanters.**
- Minimum SID is 40 inches (100 cm).

Collimation Collimate closely on four sides to area of interest.

Respiration Suspend respiration during exposure.

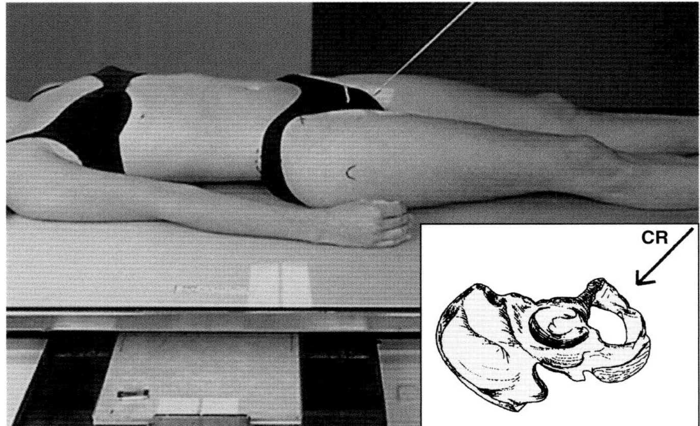

Fig. 8-43. AP axial outlet projection—CR 40° cephalad.

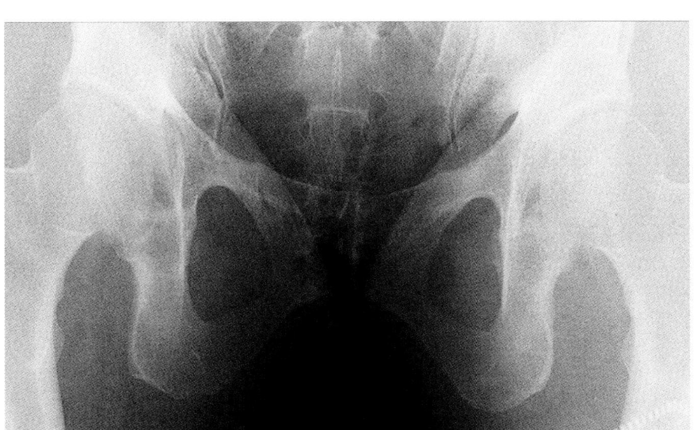
Fig. 8-44. AP axial outlet projection.

Radiographic Criteria

Structures Shown: • Superior and inferior rami of pubes and body and ramus of ischium are demonstrated well, with minimal foreshortening or superimposition.

Position: • **No rotation:** Obturator foramina and bilateral ischia are equal in size and shape.

Collimation and CR: • Correct CR angle evidenced by demonstration of the anterior/inferior pelvic bones, with minimal foreshortening. • Midpoint of symphysis joint should be in center of collimated field. • Lateral margins of collimation field should extend equally on both sides to just lateral to the femoral heads and acetabula. • Superior and inferior margins of field should include the body and superior pubic rami and the ischial tuberosities, respectively.

Exposure Criteria: • Body and superior rami of pubes are well demonstrated without overexposure of ischial rami. • Bony margins and trabecular markings of pubic and ischial bones appear sharp, indicating no motion.

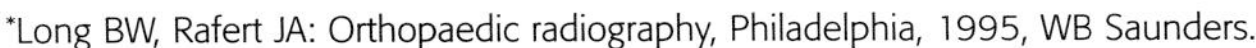

*Long BW, Rafert JA: Orthopaedic radiography, Philadelphia, 1995, WB Saunders.

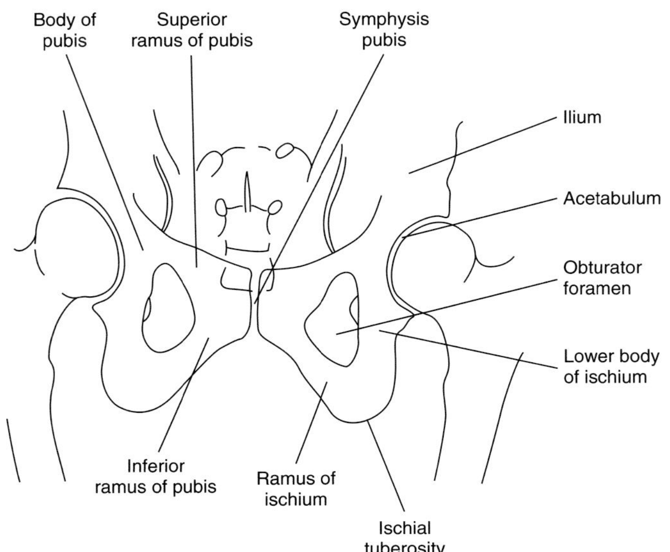

Fig. 8-45. AP axial outlet projection.

8

AP AXIAL "INLET" PROJECTION*: PELVIS

Pathology Demonstrated
This axial projection of the pelvic ring provides for an assessment of pelvic trauma for posterior displacement or inward or outward rotation of the anterior pelvis.

Pelvis
SPECIAL
• **AP axial outlet projection**
• AP axial inlet projection

Technical Factors

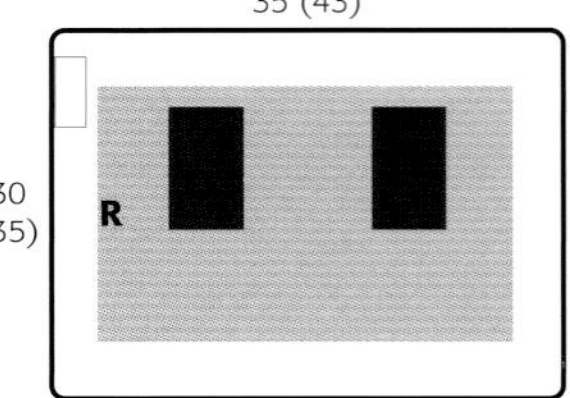

- IR size—30 × 35 cm (11 × 14 inches), crosswise, or 35 × 43 cm (14 × 17 inches)
- Moving or stationary grid
- 80 ± 5 kV range
- Technique and exposure:

cm	kV	mAs	Sk.	ML.	Gon.
17	85	12	149	40	M 149 F 37

mrad

Shielding Gonadal shielding is possible for males if care is taken not to obscure essential pelvic anatomy.

Patient Position With patient supine, provide pillow for head. With patient's legs extended, place support under knees for comfort.

Part Position
- Align midsagittal plane to CR and to midline of table and/or cassette.
- Ensure **no rotation** of pelvis (ASIS-to-tabletop distance equal on both sides).
- Center cassette to projected CR.

Central Ray
- Angle CR **caudad 40°** (near perpendicular to plane of inlet).
- Direct CR to a **midline point at level of ASISs.**
- Minimum SID is 40 inches (100 cm).

Collimation Collimate closely on four sides to area of interest.

Respiration Suspend respiration during exposure.

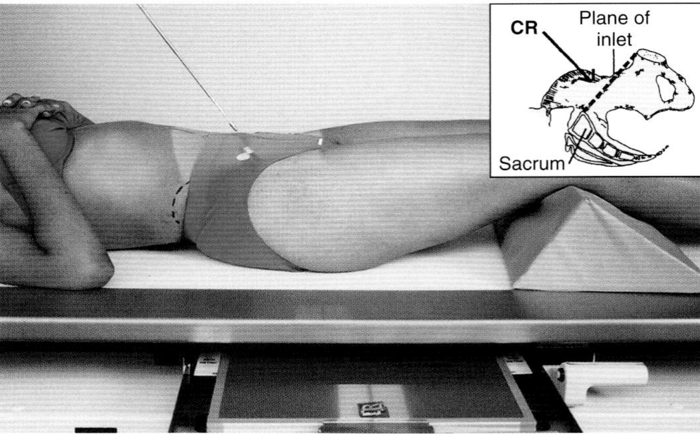

Fig. 8-46. AP axial inlet projection—CR 40° caudad (CR perpendicular to pelvic inlet).

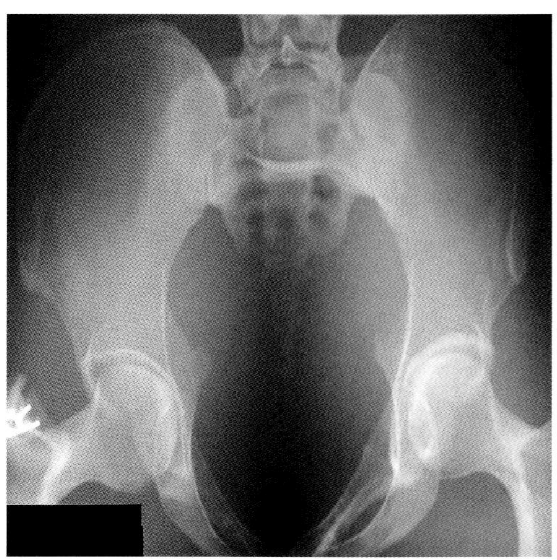

Fig. 8-47. AP axial inlet projection.

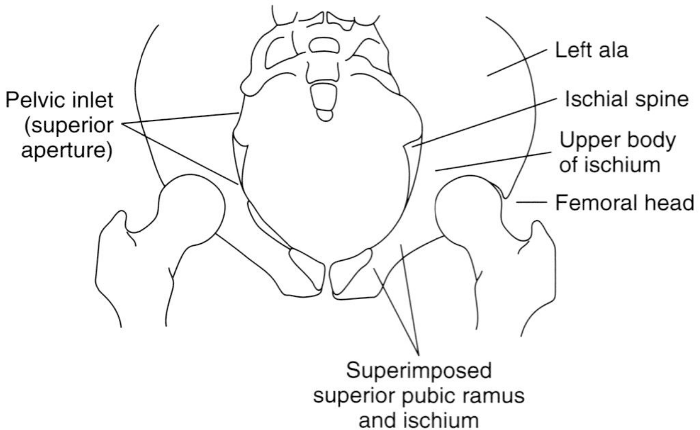

Fig. 8-48. AP axial inlet projection.

Radiographic Criteria

Structures Shown: • This is an axial projection that demonstrates pelvic ring or inlet (superior aperture) in its entirety.

Position: • **No rotation:** Ischial spines are fully demonstrated and equal in size and shape.

Collimation and CR: • Proper centering and angulation are evidenced by the demonstration of the superimposed anterior and posterior portions of the pelvic ring. • Center of pelvic inlet should be in center of collimated field. • Lateral margins of collimation field should extend equally on both sides to just lateral to the femoral heads and acetabula. • Superior and inferior margins of field should include the ala and the symphysis pubis, respectively.

Exposure Criteria: • Optimal exposure demonstrates the superimposed anterior and posterior portions of the pelvic ring. Lateral aspects of ala generally are overexposed. • Bony margins and trabecular markings of pubic and ischial bones appear sharp, indicating no motion.

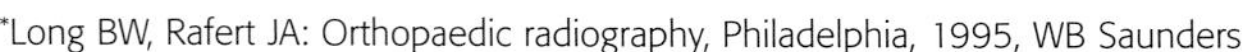

*Long BW, Rafert JA: Orthopaedic radiography, Philadelphia, 1995, WB Saunders.

POSTERIOR OBLIQUE PELVIS—ACETABULUM

Judet Method

Pathology Demonstrated

Position is useful to evaluate acetabular fracture or hip dislocation.

Both **right** and **left obliques** are generally taken for comparison, with both centered for upside or both for downside acetabulum, depending on anatomy to be visualized.

Pelvis
SPECIAL
- AP axial outlet
- AP axial inlet
- Posterior oblique acetabulum (Judet method)

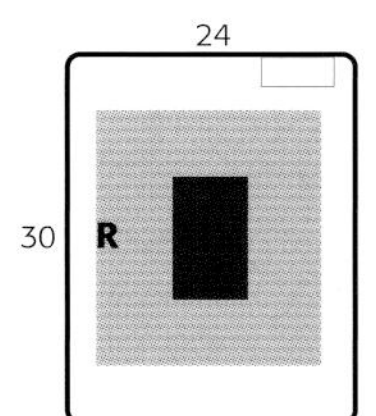

Technical Factors

- IR size—24 × 30 cm (10 × 12 inches), lengthwise
- Moving or stationary grid
- 80 ± 5 kV range
- Technique and exposure:

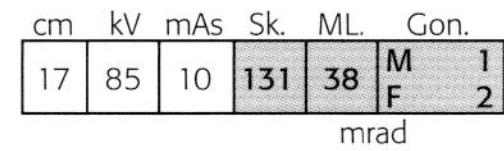

cm	kV	mAs	Sk.	ML.	Gon.
17	85	10	131	38	M 1 F 2
				mrad	

Shielding Shield gonads carefully without obscuring essential anatomy.

Patient Position—Posterior Oblique Positions

- With patient semisupine, provide pillow for head and position for **affected side up or down,** depending on anatomy to be demonstrated.

Part Position

- Place patient in **45° posterior oblique,** both pelvis and thorax 45° from tabletop. Support with wedge sponge.
- Align femoral head and acetabulum of interest to midline of tabletop and/or cassette.
- Center cassette longitudinally to CR at level of femoral head.

Central Ray

- When anatomy of interest is **downside,** direct CR perpendicular and centered to **2 inches** (5 cm) **distal and 2 inches** (5 cm) **medial to downside ASIS.**
- When anatomy of interest is upside, direct perpendicular and centered to **2 inches** (5 cm) **directly distal to upside ASIS.**
- Minimum SID is 40 inches (100 cm).

Collimation Collimate on four sides to anatomy of interest.

Respiration Suspend respiration for the exposure.

Radiographic Criteria

Structures Shown*: • When centered to the **downside** acetabulum, the **anterior rim** of the acetabulum and the **posterior ilioischial column** are demonstrated. The **iliac wing** is also well visualized (Fig. 8-51). • When centered to the **upside** acetabulum, the **posterior rim** of the acetabulum and the **anterior ilioischial column** are demonstrated. The **obturator foramen** is also visualized (Fig. 8-52).

Position: • Proper degree of obliquity is evidenced by an open and uniform hip joint space at the rim of acetabulum and femoral head. • The obturator foraman should be open, if obliqued correctly for the upside oblique, and appear closed on downside oblique.

Collimation and CR: • Acetabulum should be centered to IR and to collimation field. • The four-sided collimation should close to the anatomy of interest to reduce patient dose and scatter and obtain optimal contrast.

Exposure Criteria: • Optimal exposure should clearly demonstrate bony margins and trabecular markings of the acetabulum and femoral head regions; such markings should appear sharp, indicating no motion.

*Long BW, Rafert JA: Orthopaedic radiography, Philadelphia, 1995, WB Saunders.

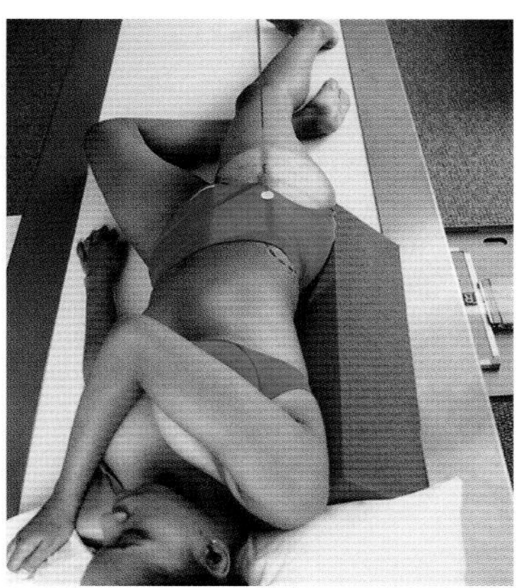

Fig. 8-49. RPO—centered for right (downside) acetabulum.

Fig. 8-50. LPO—centered for right (upside) acetabulum.

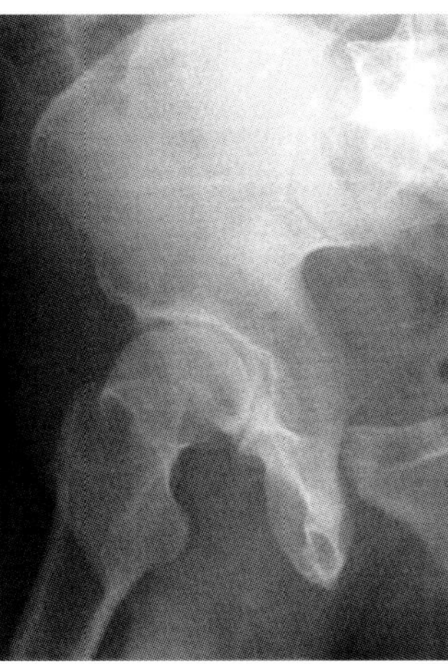

Fig. 8-51. RPO—downside (anterior rim and posterior ilioischial column).

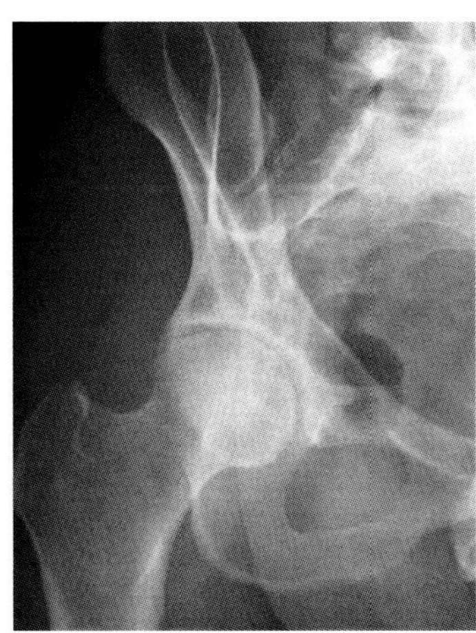

Fig. 8-52. LPO—upside (posterior rim and anterior ilioischial column).

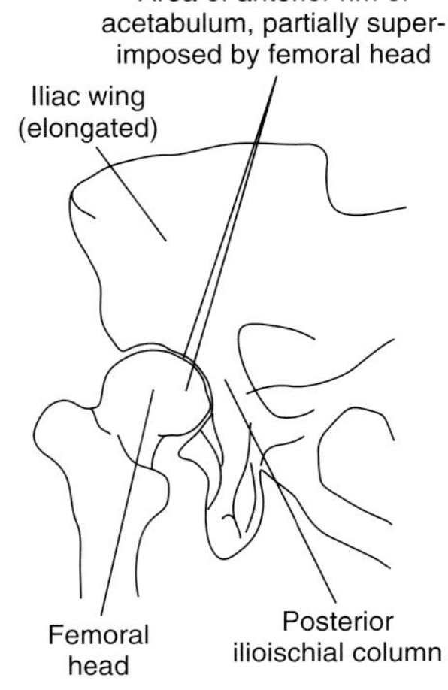

Fig. 8-53. RPO—downside acetabulum.

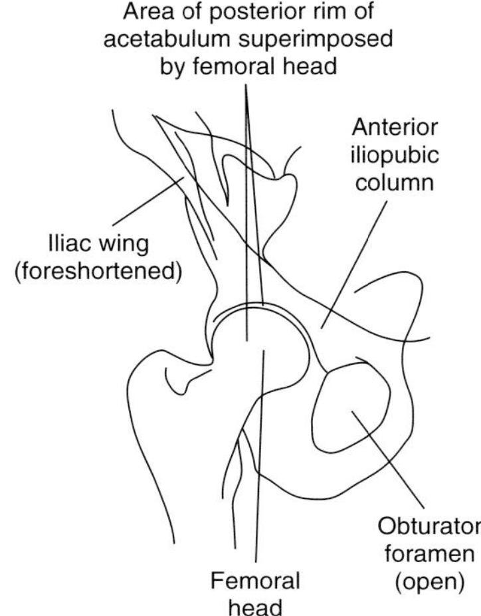

Fig. 8-54. LPO—upside acetabulum.

AP UNILATERAL HIP PROJECTION: HIP AND PROXIMAL FEMUR

Warning: Do **not** attempt to rotate legs if fracture is suspected. A basic AP pelvis to include both hips for comparison should be completed before an AP unilateral hip is performed for possible hip or pelvis trauma.

Hip and Proximal Femur
BASIC
- AP unilateral hip
- Axiolateral (trauma hip) (inferosuperior)

Pathology Demonstrated

This is a **postoperative** or **follow-up** exam to demonstrate the acetabulum, femoral head, neck and greater trochanter, and the condition and placement of any existing orthopedic appliance.

24
R
30

Technical Factors

- IR size—24 × 30 cm (10 × 12 inches), lengthwise
- Moving or stationary grid
- 80 ± 5 kV range
- Technique and exposure:

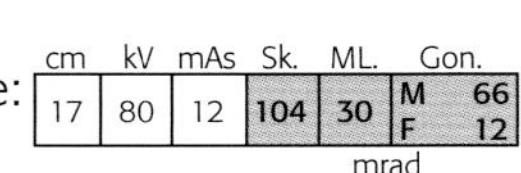

cm	kV	mAs	Sk.	ML.	Gon.
17	80	12	104	30	M 66 F 12
				mrad	

Shielding Place shield over gonads and pelvic area, **ensuring that affected hip is not obscured.**

Patient Position With patient supine, place arms at sides or across upper chest.

Part Position

- Locate **femoral neck** and align to CR and to midline of table and/or IR.
- Ensure **no rotation** of pelvis (equal distance from ASISs to table).
- Rotate affected leg **internally 15° to 20°** (see Warning above).

Central Ray

- CR is **perpendicular** to IR, directed to **1 or 2 inches (2.5 to 5 cm) distal to midfemoral neck** (to include all of orthopedic appliance of hip if present). Femoral neck can be located about **1 to 2 inches (3 to 5 cm) medial and 3 to 4 inches (8 to 10 cm) distal to ASIS** (see p. 269).
- Minimum SID is 40 inches (100 cm).

Collimation Collimate on four sides to area of interest.

Respiration Suspend respiration during exposure.

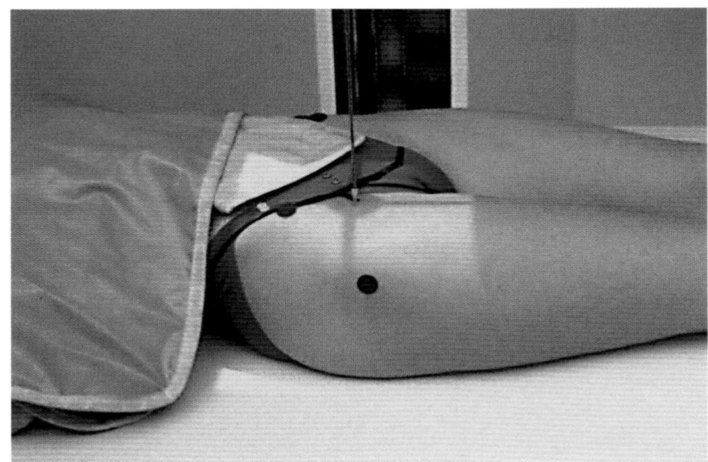

Fig. 8-55. AP right hip.

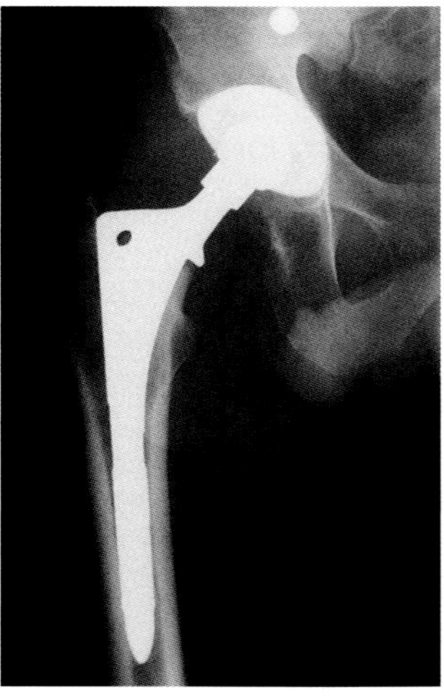

Fig. 8-56. AP hip. (Courtesy Bryan Mooneyham, RT [R].)

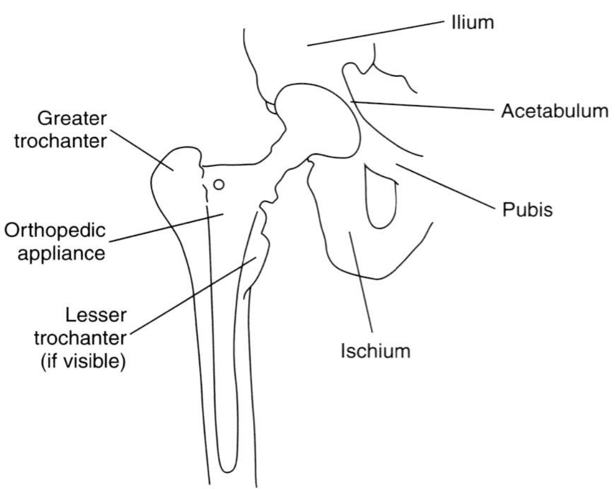

Fig. 8-57. AP hip.

Radiographic Criteria

Structures Shown: • The proximal one third of the femur should be visualized, along with the acetabulum and adjacent parts of the pubis, ischium, and ilium. • Any existing orthopedic appliance should be visible in its entirety.

Position: • The greater trochanter and femoral head and neck should be in full profile without foreshortening. • The lesser trochanter should not project beyond the medial border of the femur or on some patients only its very tip is seen with sufficient internal rotation of leg.

Collimation and CR: • Collimated field should demonstrate the entire hip joint and any orthopedic appliance in its entirety. • The femoral neck in the center of the collimation field is evidence of proper CR centering.

Exposure Criteria: • Optimal exposure visualizes the margins of the femoral head and the acetabulum through overlying pelvic structures without overexposing other parts of the proximal femur or pelvic structures. • Trabecular markings of greater trochanter and neck area appear sharp, indicating no motion.

8

AXIOLATERAL INFEROSUPERIOR PROJECTION: HIP AND PROXIMAL FEMUR–TRAUMA

Danelius-Miller Method

Warning: Do **not** attempt to internally rotate leg on initial trauma exam.

Note: This is a common projection for **trauma, surgery, and postsurgery patients,** as well as other patients who cannot move or rotate the affected leg for frog-leg lateral.

Hip and Proximal Femur
BASIC
• **AP unilateral hip**
• Axiolateral (trauma) (inferosuperior)

Pathology Demonstrated
Projection provides lateral view for fractures or dislocation assessment in trauma hip situations when affected leg cannot be moved.

Technical Factors

- IR size—24 × 30 cm (10 × 12 inches), lengthwise
- Stationary grid cassette (lead strips vertical to be able to center the CR to center line of grid to prevent grid cutoff)
- 80 ± 5 kV range
- Digital IR—requiring close collimation
- Technique and dose:

cm	kV	mAs	Sk.	ML.	Gon.
22	75	40	336	56	M 336 F 16

mrad

Shielding Gonadal shielding is not possible without obscuring essential anatomy; **close collimation is important.**

Patient Position May be done on stretcher or bedside if patient cannot be moved (see Chapter 19). Patient is supine, with pillow provided for head; elevate pelvis 1 to 2 inches (3 to 5 cm) if possible by placing supports under pelvis (more important for thin patients and for patients on a soft pad or in a bed).

Part Position

- Flex and elevate unaffected leg so that thigh is near-vertical position and outside collimation field. Support in this position. If foot is rested on collimator, as shown, provide folded sheets or padding to prevent burning of foot from **hot collimator.**
- Check to ensure **no rotation** of pelvis (equal ASIS-table distance).
- Place cassette in crease above iliac crest and adjust so that it is **parallel to femoral neck** and **perpendicular to CR.** Use cassette holder if available, or use sandbags to hold cassette in place.
- Internally rotate affected leg 15° to 20° **unless contraindicated** by possible fracture or other pathologic process (see Warning above).

Central Ray

- CR is **perpendicular** to femoral neck and to IR.
- Minimum SID is 40 inches (100 cm).

Collimation Collimate tightly on four sides to femoral head and neck region.

Respiration Suspend respiration during exposure.

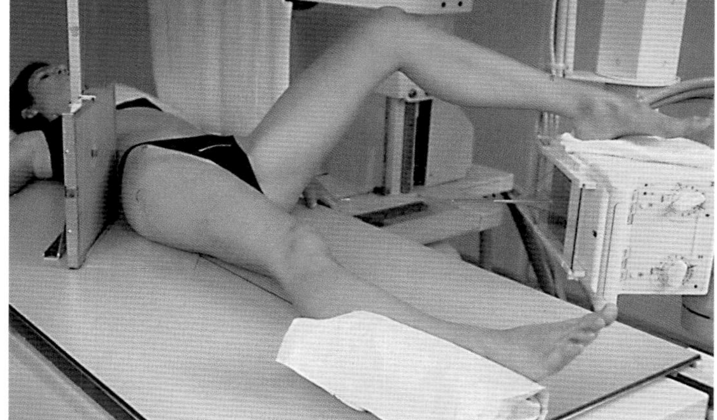

Fig. 8-58. Axiolateral hip.

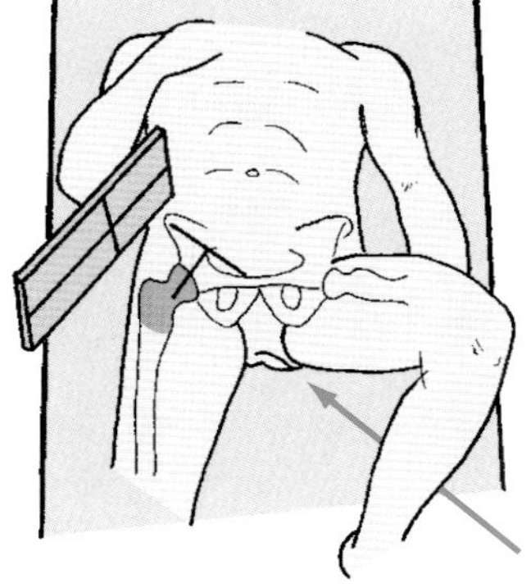

Fig. 8-59. Axiolateral hip.

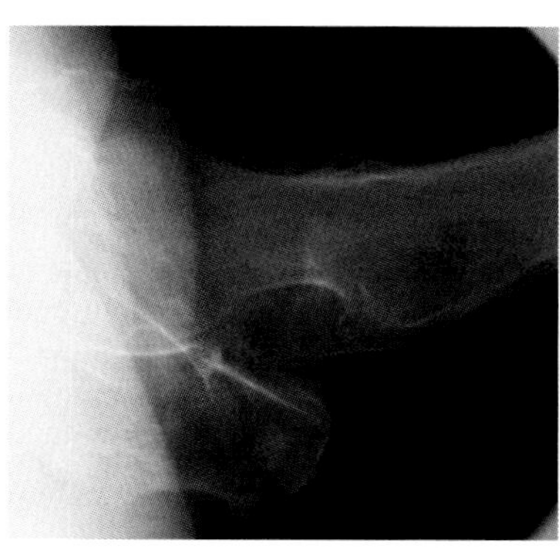

Fig. 8-60. Axiolateral hip.

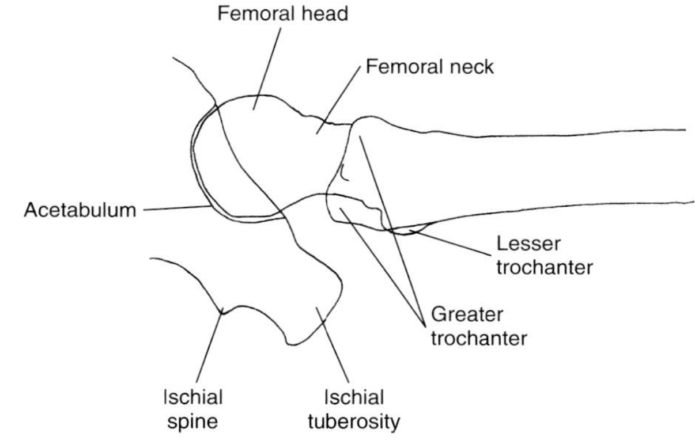

Fig. 8-61. Axiolateral hip.

Radiographic Criteria

Structures Shown: • Entire femoral head and neck, trochanter, and acetabulum should be visualized.

Position: • Only a small part if any of lesser trochanter is visualized with inversion of affected leg. • Only the most distal part of femoral neck should be superimposed by greater trochanter. • Soft tissue from raised unaffected leg is not superimposed over affected hip if leg is raised sufficiently and CR placed correctly.

Collimation and CR: • No grid lines are visible (grid lines indicate incorrect tube IR alignment).

Exposure Criteria: • Optimal exposure visualizes outline of entire femoral head and acetabulum without overexposing neck and proximal femoral shaft.

Note: Demonstrating the most proximal portion of femoral head and acetabulum on patient with thick thighs may be impossible.

UNILATERAL "FROG-LEG" PROJECTION—MEDIOLATERAL: HIP AND PROXIMAL FEMUR

Modified Cleaves Method

Warning: Do **not** attempt this position on patient with destructive hip disease or potential hip fracture or dislocation. This could result in significant displacement of fracture fragments (see lateral trauma projections).

Hip and Proximal Femur
SPECIAL—NONTRAUMA
• Unilateral frog-leg

Pathology Demonstrated
Projection provides lateral view to assess hip joint and proximal femur for **nontrauma hip** situations.

Technical Factors
- IR size—24 × 30 cm (10 × 12 inches), crosswise
- Moving or stationary grid
- 80 ± 5 kV range
- Technique and dose:

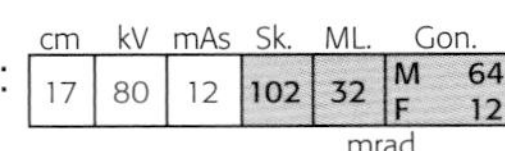

cm	kV	mAs	Sk.	ML.	Gon.
17	80	12	102	32	M 64 F 12
					mrad

Shielding Shield patient's gonads, ensuring affected hip is not obscured.

Patient Position With patient supine, position affected hip area to be aligned to CR and midline of table and/or IR.

Part Position
- Flex knee and hip on affected side, as shown, with sole of foot against inside of opposite leg, near knee if possible.
- Abduct femur **45° from vertical** for general proximal femur region (see Note 1).
- Center affected femoral neck to CR and midline of IR and tabletop. (Femoral neck is 3 to 4 inches or 7.5 to 10 cm distal to ASIS.)

Central Ray
- CR is **perpendicular** to IR (see Note 2), directed to **midfemoral neck** (center of IR).
- Minimum SID is 40 inches (100 cm).

Collimation Collimate closely on four sides to area of interest.

Respiration Suspend respiration during exposure.

Note 1: The optimum femur abduction for demonstration of the femoral neck without any foreshortening is 20° to 30° from vertical on most patients. This does result in significant foreshortening of the proximal femur region, which may be objectionable.

Note 2: A modification of this position is the Lauenstein/Hickey method, with the patient starting in a similar position, then rotating onto affected side until the femur is in contact with the tabletop and parallel to the IR. This position foreshortens the neck region but may demonstrate the head and acetabulum well if affected leg can be abducted sufficiently, as shown in Fig. 8-62, *inset.*

Radiographic Criteria

Structures Shown: • Lateral views of acetabulum and femoral head and neck, trochanteric area, and proximal one-third of femur are visible.

Position: • Proper abduction of femur is demonstrated by femoral neck seen in profile, superimposed by greater trochanter.

Collimation and CR: • Proper centering is evidenced by femoral neck in center of collimated field.

Exposure Criteria: • Optimal exposure visualizes the margins of the femoral head and the acetabulum through overlying pelvic structures without overexposing other parts of the proximal femur. • Trabecular markings and bony margins of proximal femur and pelvis should appear sharp, indicating no motion.

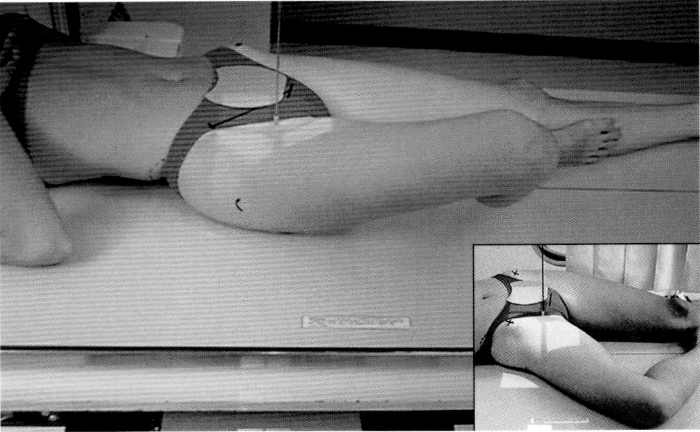

Fig. 8-62. Unilateral frog-leg position (femoral neck parallel to IR). *Inset,* demonstrates head and acetabulum well, but neck is foreshortened.

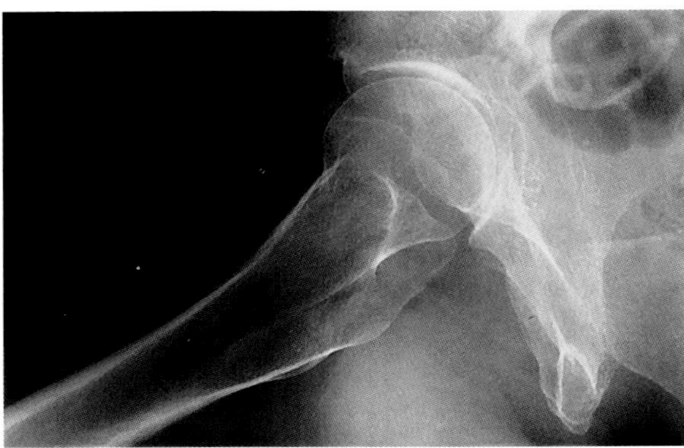

Fig. 8-63. For femoral neck—45° abduction.

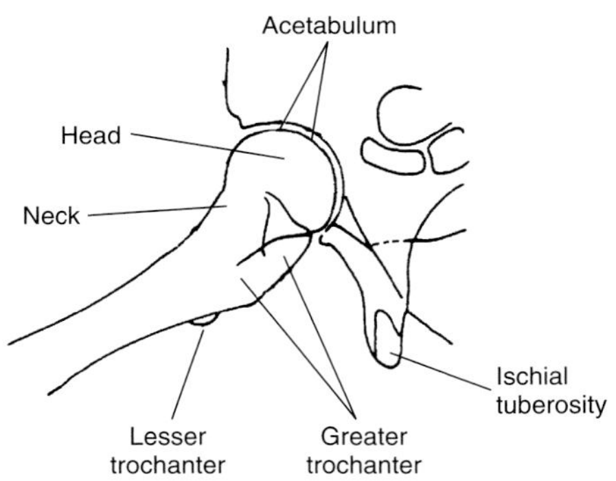

Fig. 8-64. Unilateral frog-leg.

MODIFIED AXIOLATERAL—POSSIBLE TRAUMA PROJECTION: HIP AND PROXIMAL FEMUR

Clements-Nakayama Method*

Hip and Proximal Femur
SPECIAL—NONTRAUMA
• Unilateral frog-leg
SPECIAL—TRAUMA
• Modified axiolateral (Clements-Nakayama method)

Pathology Demonstrated
This lateral oblique view is useful for assessment of possible **hip fractures** or with **arthroplasty** (surgery for hip prosthesis) when the patient has limited movement in both lower limbs and the inferosuperior projection cannot be obtained.

Technical Factors

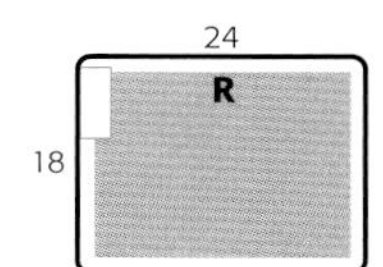

- IR size—18 × 24 cm (8 × 10 inches), crosswise
- Stationary grid cassette (cassette on edge with 15° tilt; grid lines lengthwise)
- 80 ± 5 kV range

Shielding Shield gonads as much as possible without obscuring essential anatomy.

Patient Position With patient supine, position affected side near edge of table with both legs fully extended. Provide pillow for head, and place arms across upper chest.

Part Position

- Maintain leg in neutral (anatomic) position. (15° posterior CR angle compensates for internal leg rotation.)
- Rest cassette on extended Bucky tray, which places the bottom edge of cassette about 2 inches (5 cm) below the level of the tabletop.
- Tilt cassette about 15° from vertical and adjust alignment of cassette to ensure that face of cassette is **perpendicular** to CR to prevent grid cutoff.
- Center centerline of cassette to projected CR.

Central Ray

- Angle CR **mediolaterally** as needed so that it is **perpendicular to** and **centered to femoral neck.** It should be angled posteriorly **15° to 20°** from horizontal.
- Minimum SID is 40 inches (100 cm).

Collimation Collimate closely on four sides to area of interest.

Respiration Suspend respiration during exposure.

Radiographic Criteria

Structures Shown: • Lateral oblique view of acetabulum, femoral head and neck, and trochanteric area are visible.

Position: • Femoral head and neck should be seen in profile, with only minimal superimposition by greater trochanter. • Lesser trochanter is seen projecting posterior to femoral shaft. (With leg in neutral or anatomic position, the amount of lesser trochanter seen is minimal, and with increased external rotation of leg, this amount decreases.)

Collimation and CR: • Femoral neck and trochanters should be centered to midimage area. • Collimation field should include from acetabulum to proximal femur, including both trochanters.

Exposure Criteria: • Optimal exposure visualizes femoral head and neck without overexposing proximal femoral shaft. • No excessive grid lines are visible on radiograph. • Bony margins and trabecular markings should be visible and sharp, indicating no motion.

*Clements RS, Nakayama HK: Radiographic methods in total hip arthroplasty, Radiol Technol 51:589-600, 1980.

Fig. 8-65. Modified axiolateral—CR **15° tilt** from horizontal perpendicular to femoral neck.

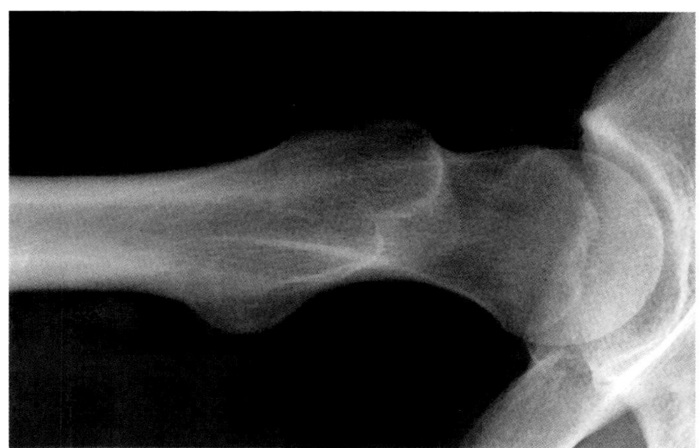

Fig. 8-66. Modified axiolateral.

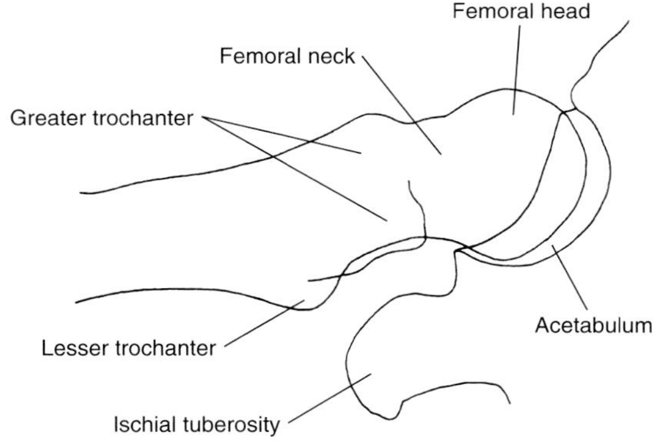

Fig. 8-67. Modified axiolateral.

AP AXIAL PROJECTION: SACROILIAC JOINTS

Sacroiliac Joints
BASIC
- AP axial
- **Posterior obliques**

Pathology Demonstrated
Projection is useful for assessment of fracture and joint dislocations or subluxation of the SI joints.

Technical Factors
- IR size—24 × 30 cm (10 × 12 inches), lengthwise
- Moving or stationary grid
- 85 ± 5 kV range
- Technique and dose:

cm	kV	mAs	Sk.	ML.	Gon.
17	85	9	106	30	M 9 F 26

mrad

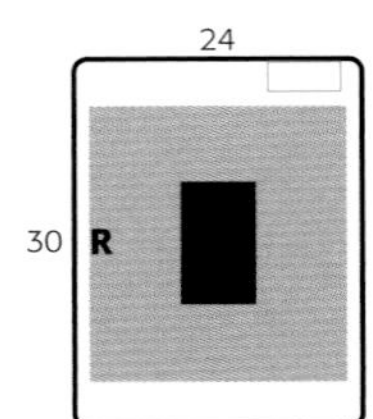

Shielding Carefully place gonadal shielding for males. Ovarian shielding on females is not possible because such shielding directly obscures area of interest.

Patient Position With patient supine, provide pillow for head; with patient's legs fully extended, provide support under knees for comfort.

Part Position
- Align midsagittal plane to CR and to midline of table and/or IR.
- Ensure **no rotation** of pelvis (ASIS-table distance equal on both sides).
- Angle center of IR to projected CR.

Central Ray
- Angle CR **30° to 35° cephalad** (generally males requiring about 30° and females 35°, with an increase in the lumbosacral curve).
- Direct CR to a midline point **about 2 inches (5 cm) below level of ASIS.**
- Minimum SID is 40 inches (100 cm).

Collimation Collimate to area of interest but ensure that side margins do not cut off sacroiliac joints.

Respiration Suspend respiration during exposure.

Alternative PA axial projection: If patient cannot assume the supine position, this image can be obtained as a PA projection with patient prone, using a 30° to 35° **caudad** angle. The CR would be centered to the level of L4 or slightly above the iliac crest.

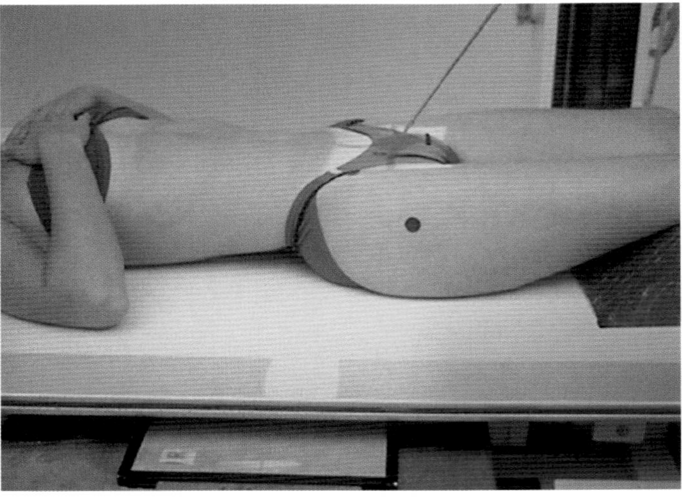

Fig. 8-68. AP axial of SI joints—CR 30° to 35° cephalad.

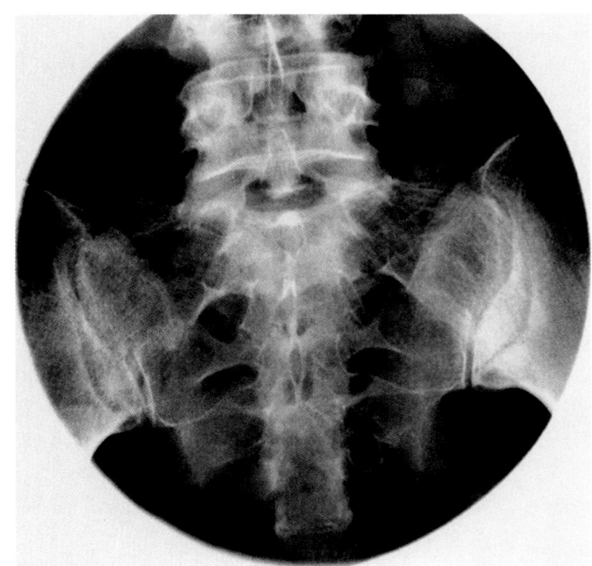

Fig. 8-69. AP axial.

Radiographic Criteria
Structures Shown: • Sacroiliac joints, L5-S1 junction, and entire sacrum are visible.

Position: • **No rotation** is evidenced by spinous process of L5 in center of vertebral body and symmetric appearance of bilateral wings (ala) of sacrum (SI joints being equally distant from midline of vertebrae).

Collimation and CR: • The sacroiliac joints spaces and the L5-S1 junction and sacral foramina should appear open, indicating correct CR angulation. • The SI joints and the first two segments of the sacrum should be centered to the collimation field and/or IR.

Exposure Criteria: • Optimal exposure should visualize all of the sacrum and the margins of the SI joint spaces. Bony margins and trabecular markings should be visible and sharp, indicating no motion.

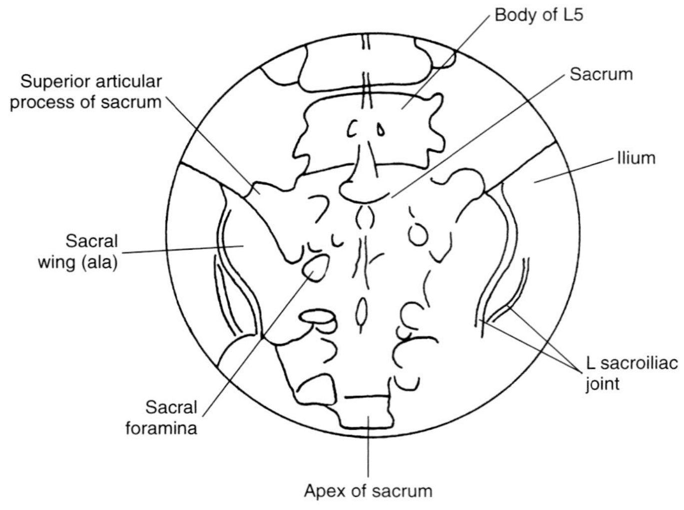

Fig. 8-70. AP axial.

POSTERIOR OBLIQUE POSITIONS (LPO AND RPO): SACROILIAC JOINTS

Sacroiliac Joints
BASIC
- **AP axial**
- Posterior obliques

Pathology Demonstrated

Position demonstrates sacroiliac joints **farthest from IR** to evaluate dislocation or subluxation of SI joint pathologic process.

Both sides are examined for comparison.

Technical Factors

- IR size—24 × 30 cm (10 × 12 inches), lengthwise
- Moving or stationary grid
- 80 ± 5 kV range
- Technique and dose:

cm	kV	mAs	Sk.	ML.	Gon.
17	80	12	125	26	M 9 F 29

mrad (per position)

24 30 R

Shielding Carefully shield gonads without obscuring sacroiliac joint area (can readily be done on males but requires more care with females). Ensure close collimation.

Patient Position With patient supine, provide pillow for head.

Part Position

- Turn into **25° to 30°** posterior oblique, **side of interest being elevated.**
- Visualize **right joint** with **LPO** and **left joint** with **RPO.**
- Use an angle-measuring device to ensure correct and consistent angles on **both** obliques.
- Place support under elevated hip and flex elevated knee.
- Align joint of interest to CR and to midline of table or IR.

Central Ray

- CR is **perpendicular,** directed to a point **1 inch (2.5 cm) medial** to upside ASIS (see Note for optional cephalad angle).
- Minimum SID is 40 inches (100 cm).

Collimation Collimate closely on four sides to area of interest.

Respiration Suspend respiration during exposure.

Note: To demonstrate the inferior or distal part of the joint more clearly, the CR may be angled 15° to 20° **cephalad.**

Radiographic Criteria

Structures Shown: • Sacroiliac joints farthest from IR are visible, with joint space appearing open.

Position: • The ala of the ilium and the sacrum should have no overlap, indicating the correct obliquity.

Collimation and CR: • Open SI joint should be in the center of collimation field.

Exposure Criteria: • Optimal exposure clearly visualizes the margins of the joint space along its entirety without overdensity or underdensity. • Bony margins and trabecular markings appear sharp, indicating no motion.

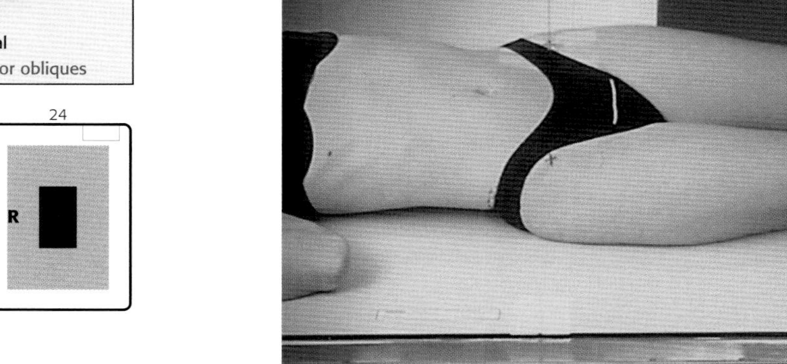

Fig. 8-71. RPO for left side (upside) SI joints.

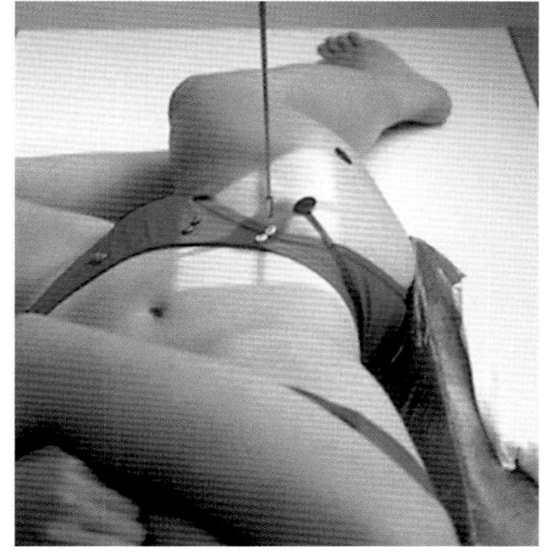

Fig. 8-72. LPO for right side (upside).

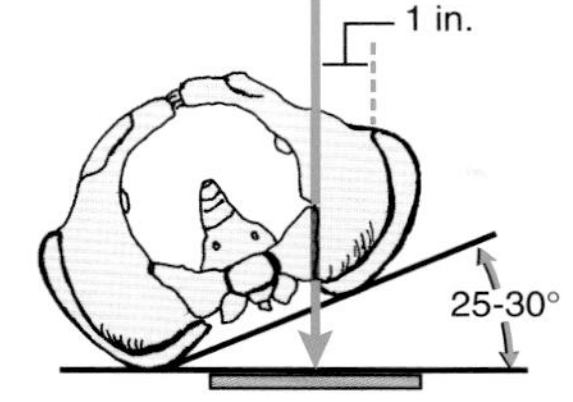

Fig. 8-73. LPO.

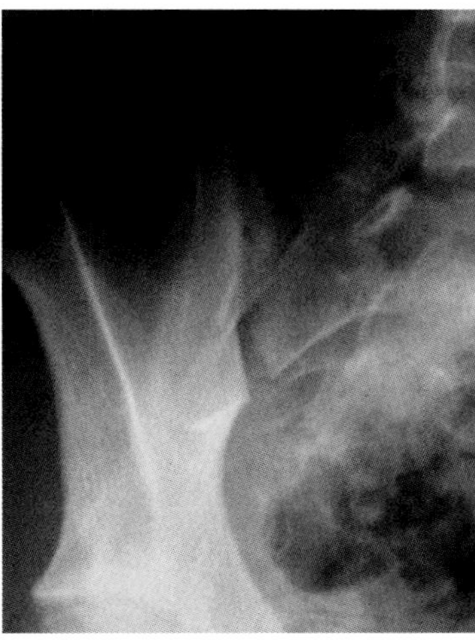

Fig. 8-74. LPO projection (upside). (Courtesy Kathy Martensen, RT)

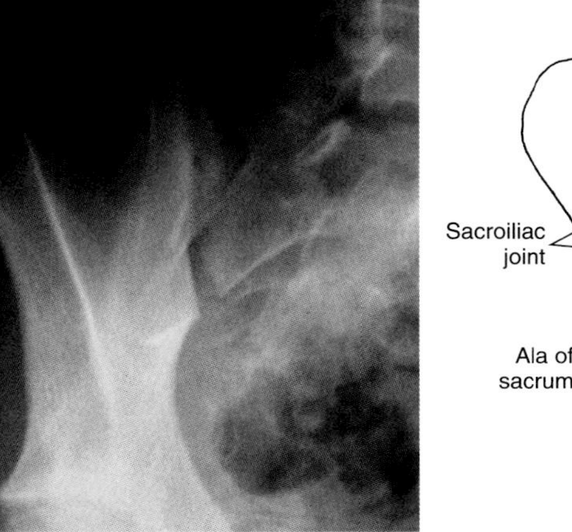

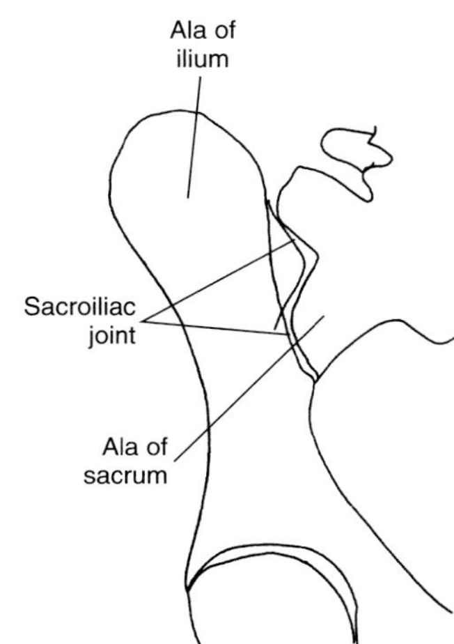

Fig. 8-75. LPO projection (upside). (Courtesy Kathy Martensen, RT)

8

RADIOGRAPHS FOR CRITIQUE

Students should determine whether they can critique each of these four radiographs based on the categories described in the textbook and outlined on the right. As a starting critique exercise, place a check in each category that demonstrates a **repeatable error** for that radiograph.

Student workbooks provide more space for writing critique comments and also provide complete critique answers for each of these radiographs. Answers are also provided in Appendix B, at the end of this textbook.

	RADIOGRAPHS A	B	C	D
1. Structures shown	____	____	____	____
2. Positioning	____	____	____	____
3. Collimation and CR	____	____	____	____
4. Exposure criteria	____	____	____	____
5. Markers	____	____	____	____

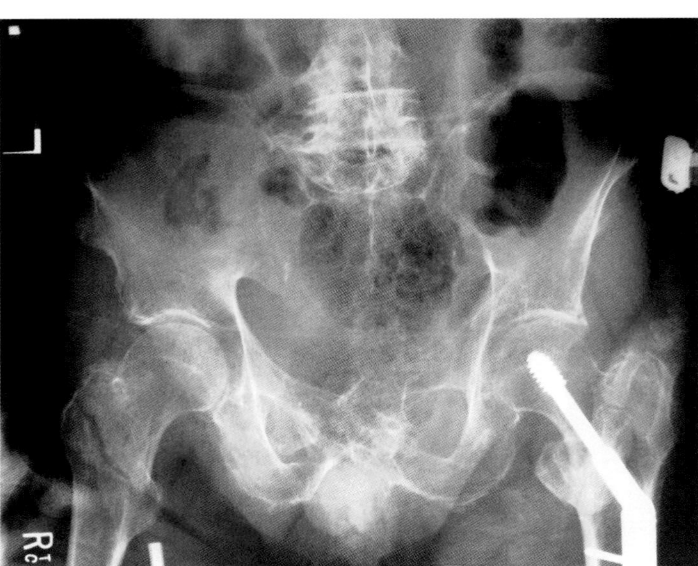

Fig. C8-76. AP pelvis (83-year-old). A

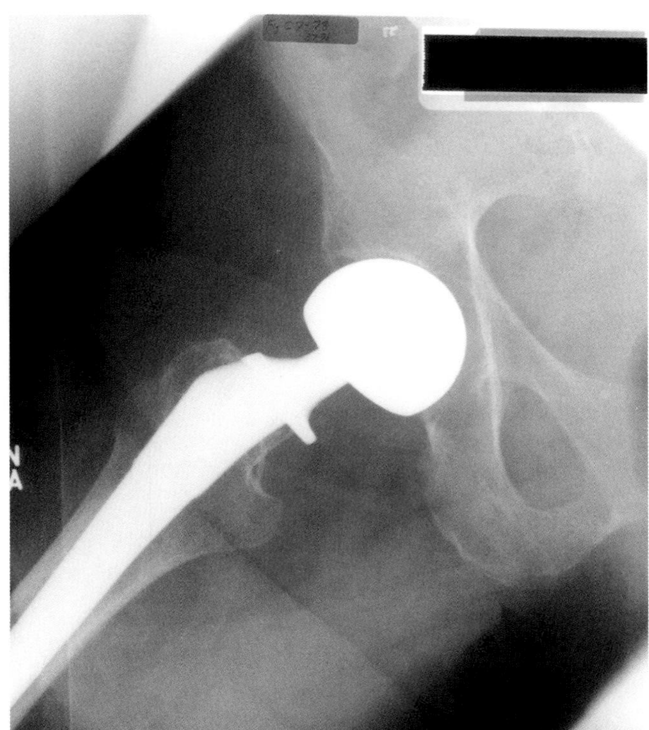

Fig. C8-77. Unilateral frog-leg (84-year-old). B

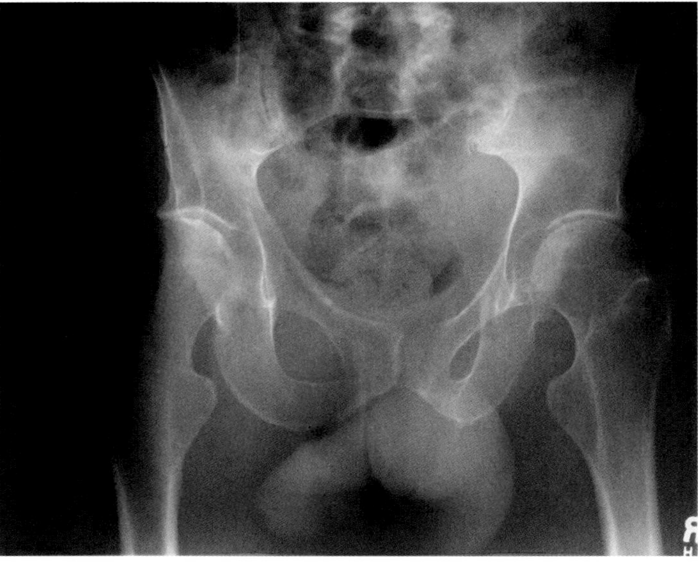

Fig. C8-78. AP pelvis (57-year-old). C

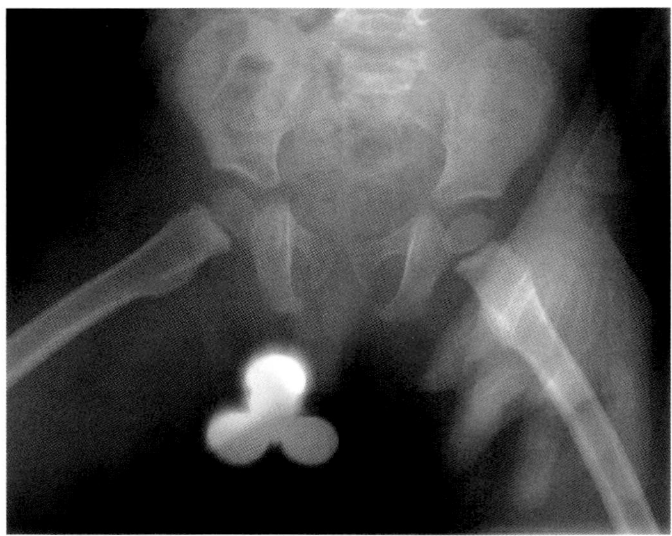

Fig. C8-79. Bilateral frog-leg (2-year-old). D

CHAPTER 9

Cervical and Thoracic Spine

CONTRIBUTIONS BY **Patti Ward,** MEd, RT(R)
CONTRIBUTORS TO PAST EDITIONS Alex Backus, MS, RT(R), April Apple, RT(R), Donna L. Wright, EdD, RT(R)

CONTENTS

RADIOGRAPHIC ANATOMY

Vertebral Column

The vertebral *(ver'te-bral)* column, commonly called the *spine* or *spinal column,* is a complex succession of many bones called **vertebrae** *(ver'te-bre)* (singular is **vertebra** *[ver'te-brah]*). It provides a flexible supporting column for the trunk and head and also transmits the weight of the trunk and upper body to the lower limbs. This column is located in the midsagittal plane, forming the posterior or dorsal aspect of the bony trunk of the body. As adjacent vertebrae are stacked vertically, openings in each vertebra line up to create a tubelike vertical spinal canal.

Spinal canal The spinal canal, which follows the various curves of the spinal column, begins at the base of the skull and extends distally into the sacrum. This canal contains the spinal cord and is filled with cerebrospinal fluid.

Spinal cord The spinal cord, which is enclosed and protected by the spinal canal, begins with the **medulla oblongata** *(me-dul'ah ob"long-ga'tah)* of the brain. It passes through the foramen magnum of the skull and continues through the **first cervical vertebra** all the way down to the **lower border of the first lumbar vertebra,** where it tapers off to a point called the **conus medullaris** *(ko'nus med'u"lar-is).*

Note: In some persons the conus medullaris may extend to as low as the body of L2. Therefore to avoid striking the spinal cord, the most common site for a lumbar puncture into the spinal canal is at the level of L3-L4. (See myelogram procedure description on p. 302.)

Intervertebral disks Tough fibrocartilaginous disks separate typical adult vertebrae. These cushion-like disks are tightly bound to the vertebrae for spinal stability but also allow for flexibility and movement of the vertebral column.

SECTIONS OF VERTEBRAL COLUMN

The vertebral column is divided into **five sections.** Within each of these five sections the vertebrae have distinctive characteristics.

Detailed anatomy and positioning of the first two sections, the cervical and thoracic vertebrae, are covered in this chapter. The last three sections, the lumbar vertebrae, sacrum, and coccyx, are covered in Chapter 10.

Cervical vertebrae The first seven vertebrae are known as **cervical vertebrae.** Although there may be a slight variation in the height of each vertebra among individuals, the average human has **seven** cervical vertebrae.

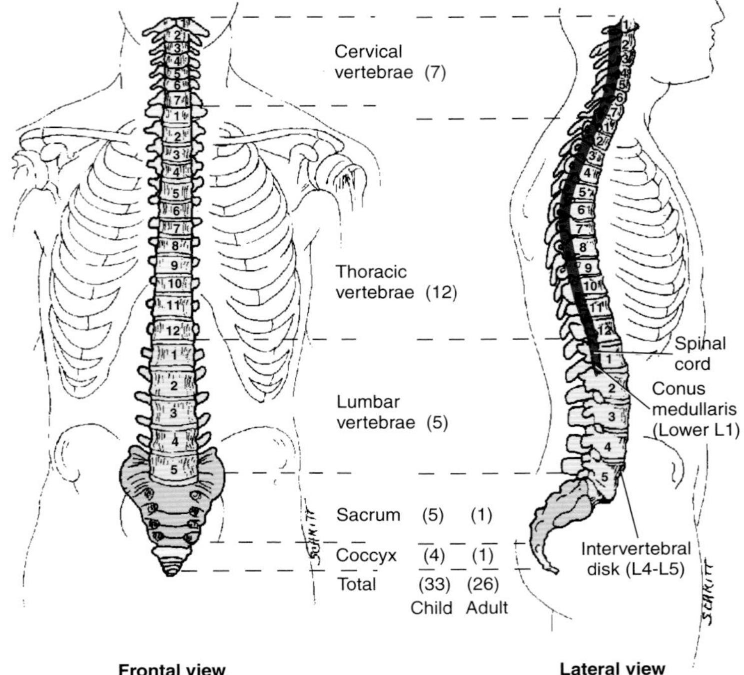

Fig. 9-1. Vertebral column.

Thoracic vertebrae The next **twelve** vertebrae are **thoracic vertebrae,** each connects to a pair of ribs. Because all vertebrae are posterior or dorsal in the body, the term *thoracic* is more correct when referring to this region rather than the older term, *dorsal spine.*

Lumbar vertebrae The largest individual vertebrae are the **five lumbar vertebrae.** These vertebrae are the strongest in the vertebral column because the load of body weight increases toward the inferior end of the column. For this reason the cartilaginous disks between the inferior lumbar vertebrae are common sites for injury and pathology.

Sacrum and coccyx The **sacrum** *(sa'krum)* and **coccyx** *(kok'siks)* develop as multiple separate bones and then fuse into two distinct bones. A newborn has **five** sacral *(sa'kral)* segments and from **three** to **five** (average of four) coccygeal *(kok-sij'e-al)* segments, for an average of **33** separate bones in the vertebral column of a young child. After fusion into a single sacrum and a single coccyx, the adult vertebral column is composed of an average of **26 separate bones.**

9

Vertebral Column Curvatures

The vertebral column is composed of a series of anteroposterior curves (Fig. 9-2). The terms **concave** (a rounded inward or depressed surface like a "cave") and **convex** (a rounded outward or elevated surface) are used to describe these curves. However, the curves are described as the opposite depending on whether you are describing them from an anterior perspective or a posterior perspective. For the purposes of this textbook, the curves will be described as if the patient is being evaluated from the posterior perspective. The cervical and lumbar regions have concave curvatures and are described as **lordotic.** The thoracic and sacral regions have **convex** curvatures.

Soon after birth the **thoracic** and **sacral** (pelvic) curves begin to develop. These two convex curves are called **primary curves.** As children begin to raise their head and sit up, the first **compensatory** concave curve forms in the cervical region. The second compensatory concave curve is the lumbar curvature, which develops when children learn to walk. Both of the inferior curves, the lumbar and sacral (pelvic), are usually more pronounced in women than in men.

These primary and compensatory curvatures are normal and serve an important function by increasing the strength of the vertebral column and helping maintain balance along a center line of gravity in the upright position.

Certain terms are commonly used to describe these curvatures when they become exaggerated or abnormal. These terms, **lordosis, kyphosis,** and **scoliosis,** are described as follows:

LORDOSIS*

The term **lordosis** *(lor-do'sis),* meaning *bent backward,* describes the **normal** anterior concavity of the lumbar and cervical spine as described above but also describes **abnormally increased "swayback" curvature** involving the lumbar spine.

KYPHOSIS*

Kyphosis *(ki-fo'sis),* meaning a *hump,* describes an **abnormal or exaggerated thoracic "humpback" curvature** with increased convexity.

SCOLIOSIS*

If the spine is viewed from the posterior or anterior perspective (Fig. 9-4), the vertebral column is usually nearly straight with little lateral curvature. Occasionally, a slight lateral curvature occurs in the upper thoracic region of a healthy adult. This curvature is usually associated with the dominant extremity, so this curvature may be convex to the right in a right-handed person and convex to the left in a left-handed person.

An abnormal or **exaggerated lateral curvature** is called **scoliosis** *(sko"le-o'sis).* This is a more serious type of problem that occurs when a pronounced S-shaped lateral curvature exists. This may cause severe deformity of the entire thorax. The effect of scoliosis is more obvious if it occurs in the lower vertebral column, where it may create a tilting of the pelvis with a resulting effect on the lower limbs, creating a limp or uneven walk.

*Dorland's illustrated medical dictionary, ed 28, Philadelphia, 1994, WB Saunders.

SUMMARY OF SPINAL CURVATURE TERMS

TERM	DESCRIPTION
Lordosis	Normal compensatory concave curvature of cervical and lumbar spine *or* Abnormal exaggerated lumbar curvature with increased concavity ("swayback")
Kyphosis	Abnormal exaggerated thoracic curvature with increased convexity
Scoliosis	Abnormal lateral curvature

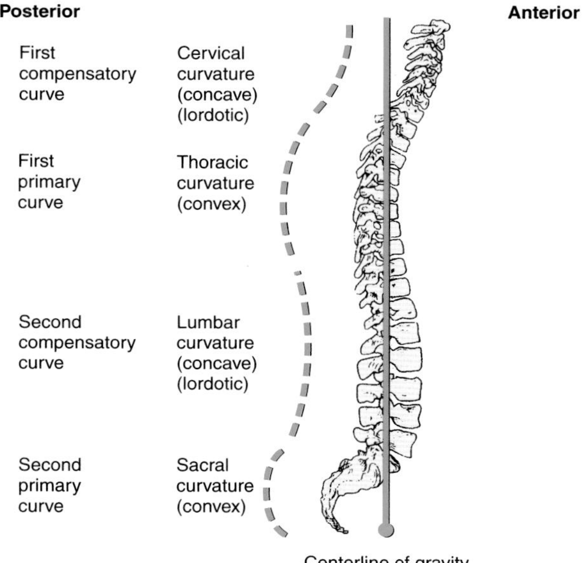

Fig. 9-2. Normal adult curvature (side view).

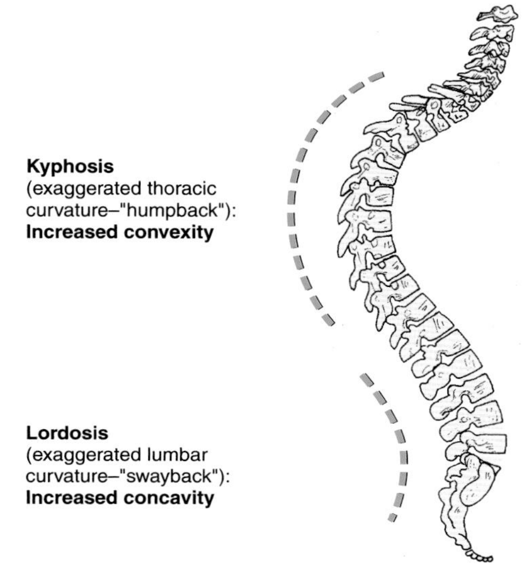

Fig. 9-3. Lordosis-kyphosis.

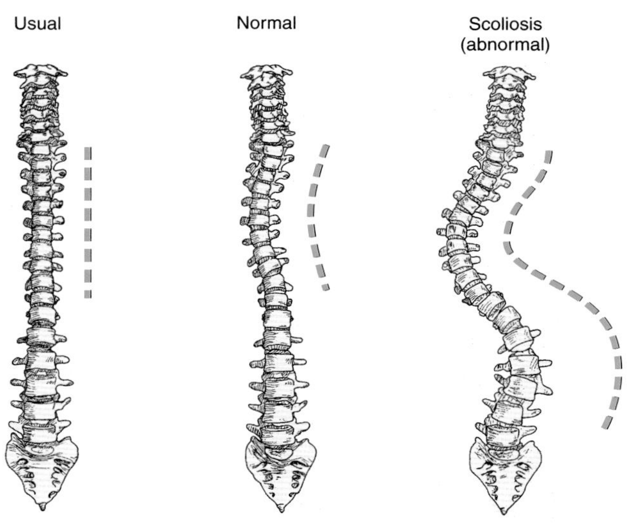

Fig. 9-4. Scoliosis—lateral curvatures (anterior view).

Typical Vertebral Anatomy

Although the vertebrae in the different regions vary in size and shape, all are similar in basic structure. A typical vertebra consists of two main parts, the **body** and the **vertebral arch.**

(1) BODY

The body is the thick, weight-bearing anterior part of the vertebra. Its superior and inferior surfaces are flat and rough for attachment of the intervertebral disks.

(2) VERTEBRAL ARCH

The second part of a typical vertebra consists of a ring or arch of bone extending posteriorly from the vertebral body. The posterior surface of the body and the arch form a circular opening, the **vertebral foramen,** that contains the spinal cord. When a number of vertebrae are stacked, as they are in the normal articulated vertebral column, the succession of vertebral foramina forms a tubelike opening, called the **vertebral** (spinal) **canal,** that encloses and protects the spinal cord (Fig. 9-5).

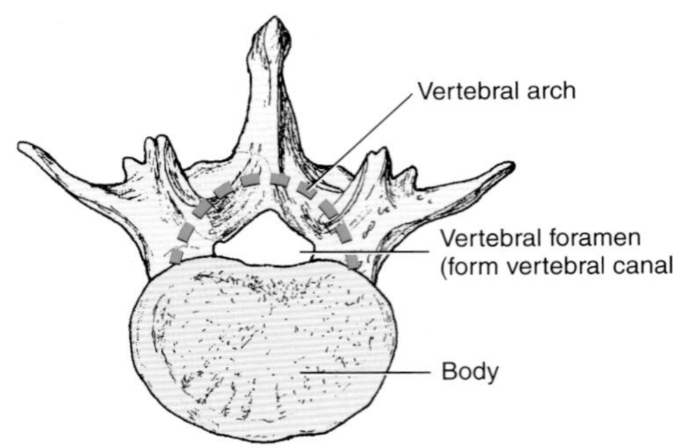

Fig. 9-5. Typical vertebra (demonstrates two main parts).

Superior perspective: Fig. 9-6 illustrates the various parts of the vertebral arch. **Pedicles** *(ped'i-kuls)* extend posteriorly from either side of the vertebral body. The pedicles form most of the sides of the vertebral arch.

The posterior part of the vertebral arch is formed by two somewhat flat layers of bone termed **laminae** *(lam'i-ne).* Each lamina extends posteriorly from each pedicle to unite in the midline.

Extending laterally from approximately the junction of each pedicle and lamina is a projection termed the **transverse process.**

The **spinous process** extends posteriorly at the midline junction of the two laminae. The spinous processes are the most posterior extensions of the vertebrae and can often be palpated along the posterior surface of the neck and back.

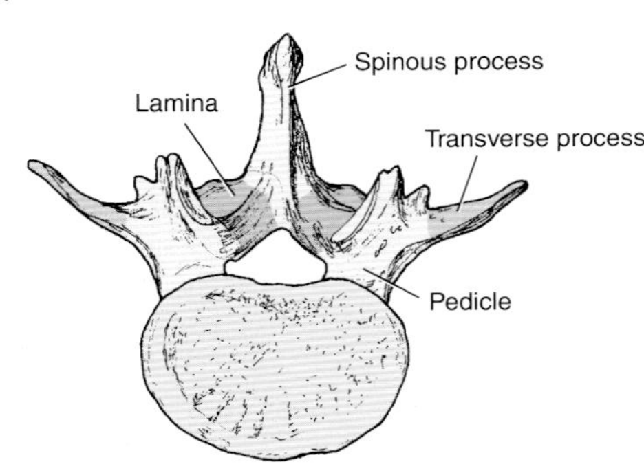

Fig. 9-6. Typical vertebra—superior view.

Lateral perspective: Fig. 9-7 illustrates a lateral orientation to the typical vertebra. The anterior vertebral body and the posterior spinous process are readily identified. Extending posteriorly directly from the vertebral body on each side are the **pedicles,** which terminate in the area of the **transverse process.** Continuing posteriorly from the origin of the transverse process on each side are the two **lamina,** which end at the spinous process.

Additional obvious parts seen on this lateral view are the right and left superimposed **superior articular processes** and the lower pair of right and left **inferior articular processes.** These processes provide for certain important joints that are unique and need to be visualized radiographically for each section of the vertebral column as described on the following pages.

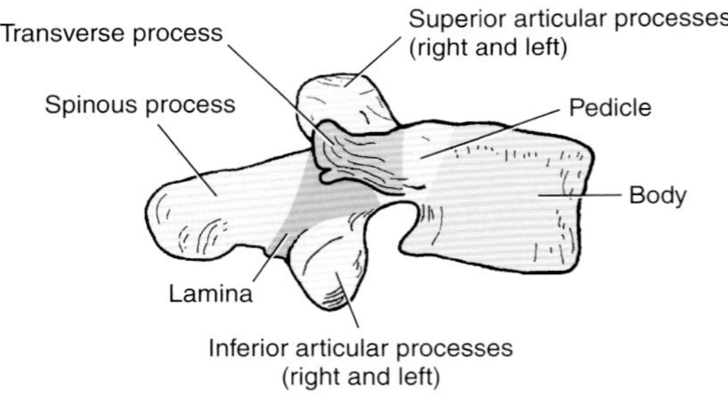

Fig. 9-7. Typical vertebra—lateral view.

9

Summary: The typical vertebra has **two pedicles** and **two laminae** that form the vertebral arch and the vertebral foramen containing the spinal cord, **two transverse processes** extending laterally, **one spinous process** extending posteriorly, and the large anterior **body.** Each typical vertebra also has **four articular processes,** two superior and two inferior, which formulate the important joints of the vertebral column.

(3) JOINTS IN THE VERTEBRAL COLUMN

In addition to the **body** and **vertebral arch,** the **joints** are a third important aspect of the vertebral column. The vertebral column would be rigidly immovable without the intervertebral disks and zygapophyseal joints. Respiration could not occur without the spine serving as a pivot point for arclike movement of the ribs.

Intervertebral Joints

The **intervertebral joints** are slightly movable joints between the vertebral bodies. The **intervertebral disks** located in these joints are tightly bound to the adjacent vertebral bodies for spinal stability but also allow for flexibility and movement of the vertebral column.

Zygapophyseal Joints (older term is apophyseal joints)

The **four articular processes** described on the preceding page are seen projecting from the area of the junction of the pedicles and laminae (Fig. 9-8). The term *facet (fas'et)* is sometimes used interchangeably with the term *zygapophyseal joints,* but the facet is actually only the articulating surface instead of the entire superior or inferior articular process.

Costal Joints

Although not directly involved in the stability of the spinal column itself, a third type of joint is also located along a portion of the vertebral column. In the thoracic region the twelve ribs articulate with the transverse processes and the vertebral bodies. These articulations of the ribs to the thoracic vertebra are **costal joints** and will be illustrated on later drawings of the thoracic vertebra.

(4) INTERVERTEBRAL FORAMINA

The fourth aspect of the vertebral column, which is important radiographically, involves the intervertebral foramina. Along the upper surface of each pedicle is a half moon–shaped area termed the ***superior vertebral notch,*** and along the lower surface of each pedicle is another half moon–shaped area termed the **inferior vertebral notch** (Fig. 9-8). When vertebrae are stacked, the superior and inferior vertebral notches line up. These two half-moon–shaped areas form a single opening, the **intervertebral foramen** (Fig. 9-9). Therefore between every two vertebrae are **two** intervertebral foramina, **one on each side,** through which important spinal nerves and blood vessels pass.

The zygapophyseal joints and the intervertebral foramina must be demonstrated radiographically by the appropriate projection in each of the three major portions of the vertebral column, as described and illustrated in later sections.

(5) INTERVERTEBRAL DISK

The fifth and final aspect of the vertebral column important radiographically is the intervertebral disks. The typical adult vertebrae are separated by tough fibrocartilaginous disks between the bodies of every two vertebrae except between the first and second cervical vertebrae. (The first cervical vertebra has no body.) These fibrocartilage disks provide a resilient cushion between the vertebrae, helping to absorb shock during movement of the spine.

As labeled in Fig. 9-10, each disk consists of an outer fibrous portion termed the **annulus fibrosus** *(an'u-lus fi-bro'sis)* and a soft, semigelatinous inner part called the **nucleus pulposus** *(nu'kle-us pul'po-sus).* When this soft inner part protrudes through the outer fibrous layer, it presses on the spinal cord and causes severe pain and numbness that radiates into the lower limbs. This condition, also known as a "slipped disk," is termed **herniated nucleus pulposus (HNP).** (See Pathologic Indications, p. 303.)

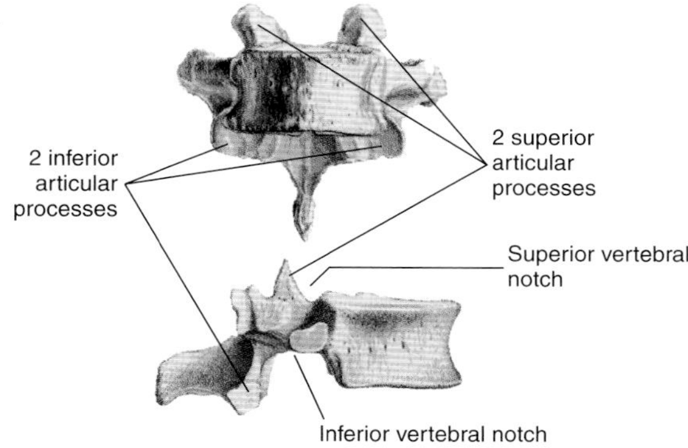

Fig. 9-8. Typical vertebra—articular processes (anterior and lateral views).

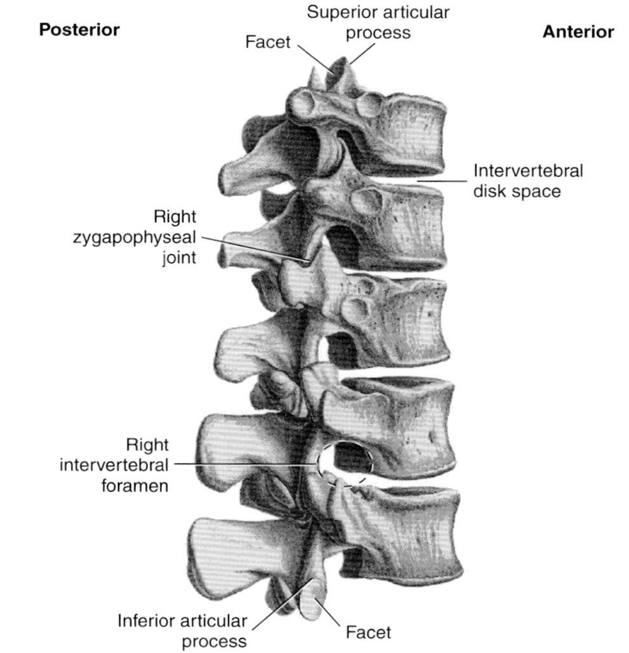

Fig. 9-9. Zygapophyseal joints and intervertebral foramina (lateral oblique view).

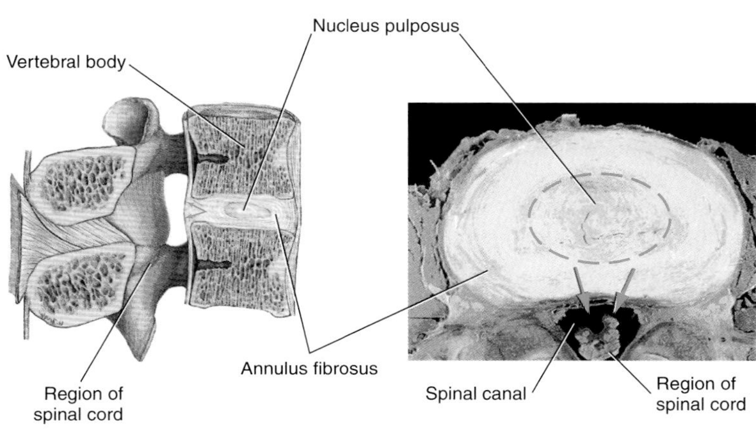

Fig. 9-10. Intervertebral disk.

Cervical Vertebrae Characteristics

The cervical vertebrae show little resemblance to either the lumbar or the thoracic vertebrae, which are more typical in appearance. Although most of the parts forming the typical vertebrae are present, various cervical vertebrae have unique characteristics such as **transverse foramina, bifid spinous process tips,** and **overlapping vertebral bodies.** Each cervical vertebra and vertebral body continues to get larger, progressing down to the seventh cervical.

C1 (the atlas) and C2 (the axis) are quite unusual and will be described separately. The third through sixth cervical vertebrae are typical cervical vertebrae. The last, or seventh, cervical vertebra, the **vertebra prominens,** has many features of the thoracic vertebrae, including an extra long and more horizontal spinous process that can be palpated at the base of the neck. This palpable bony landmark is useful for radiographic positioning (Fig. 9-11).

Superior perspective: Fig. 9-12 shows a typical cervical vertebra (C3 to C6) as viewed from above. The transverse processes are quite small and arise from both the pedicle and the body, rather than from the pedicle-lamina junction. The hole in each transverse process is called a **transverse foramen.** The vertebral artery, veins, and certain nerves pass through these successive transverse foramina. Therefore one unique characteristic of all cervical vertebrae is that they each have **three foramina** that run vertically: the right and left transverse foramina and the single large vertebral foramen.

The **spinous processes** of C2 through C6 are fairly short and end in double-pointed or **bifid tips,** a second unique characteristic typical of cervical vertebrae.

Lateral perspective (Fig. 9-13): When viewed from the lateral perspective, typical (C3 to C6) cervical vertebral bodies are small and oblong in shape, with the anterior edge slightly more inferior, which causes slight overlapping of vertebral bodies.

Located behind the transverse process at the junction of the pedicle and the lamina are the cervical articular processes. Between the superior and inferior articular processes is a short column ("pillar") of bone that is more supportive than the similar area in the rest of the spinal column. This column of bone is called the **articular pillar** (sometimes called the **lateral mass** when referring to C1).

CERVICAL ZYGAPOPHYSEAL JOINTS

The superior and inferior articular processes, as located over and under the articular pillars, are directly lateral to the large vertebral foramen. Therefore the zygapophyseal joints of the second through seventh cervical vertebrae are located at **right angles, or 90°,** to the midsagittal plane and thus are visualized only in a true lateral position (Fig. 9-14). However, unlike the other cervical zygapophyseal joints, those between C1 and C2 are visualized only on a **true AP projection** (see Fig. 9-18).

CERVICAL INTERVERTEBRAL FORAMINA

The intervertebral foramina can be identified by the pedicles, which form the superior and inferior boundaries of these foramina as shown in Figs. 9-12 and 9-14. The intervertebral foramina are situated at a **45° angle** to the midsagittal plane, open anteriorly, as shown on the drawings. They are also directed at a **15° inferior angle** because of the shape and the overlapping of the cervical vertebrae. Therefore to "open up" and radiographically demonstrate the cervical intervertebral foramina, a 45° oblique position combined with a 15° cephalad angle of the x-ray beam would be required (Figs. 9-31 and 9-33).

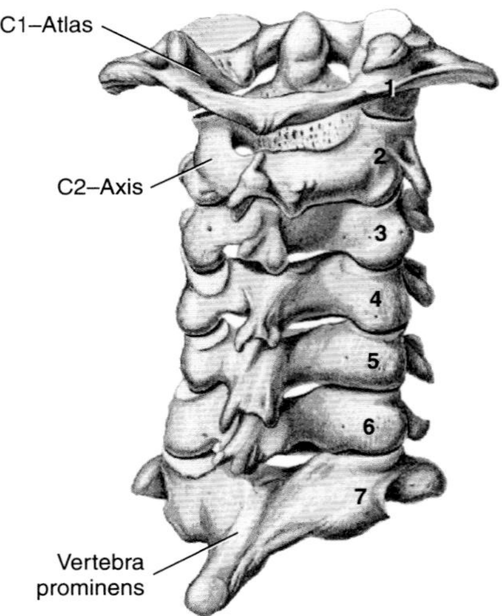

Fig. 9-11. Seven cervical vertebrae—oblique posterior view.

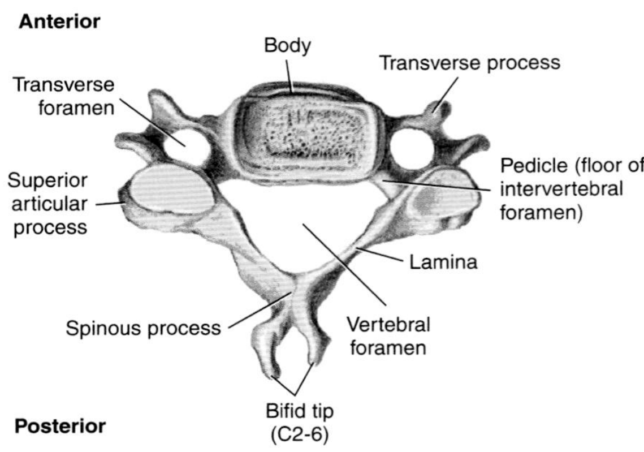

Fig. 9-12. Typical (C2-C6) cervical vertebra—superior view.

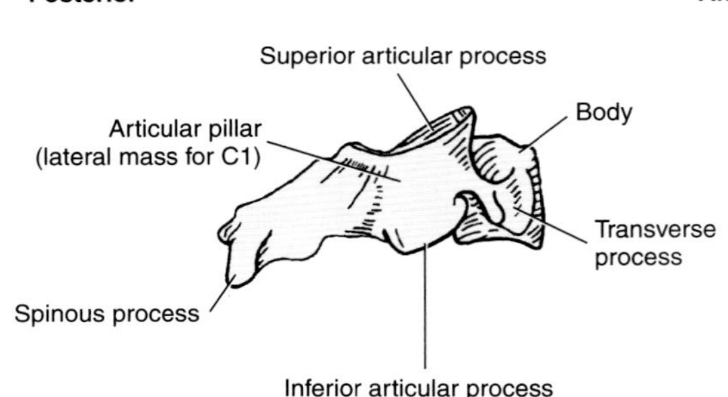

Fig. 9-13. Typical cervical vertebra—lateral view.

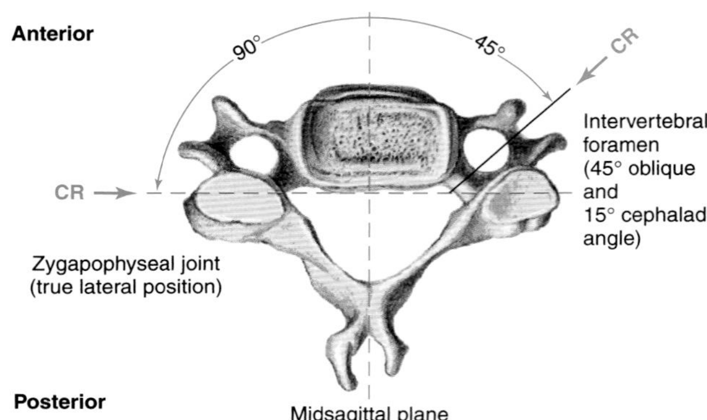

Fig. 9-14. Typical cervical vertebra (superior view).
—Zygapophyseal joints, 90° (true lateral).
—Intervertebral foramina, 45° oblique.

9

ATLAS (C1) (Fig. 9-15)

The first cervical vertebra, the **atlas,** a name derived from the Greek god who bore the world upon his shoulders, least resembles a typical vertebra. Anteriorly, there is no body but simply a thick arch of bone called the **anterior arch.** The anterior arch includes a small **anterior tubercle.**

The **dens** or **odontoid process** is part of the second cervical vertebra (Fig. 9-16) but is demonstrated in a superior perspective of C1 (Fig. 9-15) to show its location and how it is held in place by the **transverse atlantal ligament.** The positional relationship of C1 and C2 is also illustrated in Fig. 9-17 and radiographically in Fig. 9-18.

Rather than two laminae and a spinous process found in typical vertebrae, C1 has a **posterior arch** that generally bears a small **posterior tubercle** at the midline (Fig. 9-15).

Each of the left and right C1 **superior articular processes** presents a large depressed surface called a **superior facet** for articulation with the respective left and right occipital condyles of the skull. These articulations between C1 and the occipital condyles of the skull are called **atlantooccipital articulations.**

The **transverse processes** of C1 are smaller but still contain the **transverse foramina** distinctive of all cervical vertebrae.

The **articular pillars,** the segments of bone between the superior and inferior articular processes, are called **lateral masses** for C1. Because the lateral masses of C1 support the weight of the head and assist in rotation of the head, these portions are the most bulky and solid part of C1.

AXIS (C2)

The most distinctive feature of the second cervical vertebra, the **axis,** is the clinically important **dens** or **odontoid process,** the conical process projecting up from the upper surface of the **body.** Embryologically, the dens is actually the body of C1, but it fuses to C2 during development. Therefore it is considered part of C2 in mature skeletons.

Rotation of the head primarily occurs between C1 and C2, with the dens acting as a pivot. The superior facets of the superior articular processes articulating with the skull also assist in rotation of the head.

Severe stress as the possible result of a forced flexion-hyperextension, "whiplash" type of injury may cause a fracture of the dens. Any fracture of the vertebral column at this level could result in serious damage to the spinal cord as well.

As seen in Fig. 9-16, the **inferior articular process** for articulation with C3 lies inferior to the **lamina.** Below and lateral to the superior articular process is the transverse process with its **transverse foramen.** The blunt **spinous process** with its bifid tip extends posteriorly.

RELATIONSHIP OF C1 AND C2

Radiographically demonstrating the relationship of C1 to C2 and the relationship of C1 to the base of the skull is clinically important because injury this high in the spinal canal can result in serious paralysis and death. Fig. 9-18 is the radiographic image of an AP projection taken through an open mouth to demonstrate C1 and C2. The anterior arch of C1, which lies in front of the dens, is not clearly visible on this image because it is a fairly thin piece of bone compared with the larger, more dense dens.

Normally, articulations between C2 and C1, the **zygapophyseal joints,** are **perfectly symmetric.** Accordingly, the **relationship of the dens to C1 must also be perfectly symmetric.** Both injury and improper positioning can render these areas asymmetric. For example, **rotation of the skull** can alter the symmetry of these spaces and joints, thus imitating an injury. Therefore accurate positioning for this region is essential. The parts are labeled on the drawing of Fig. 9-17 and the radiographic image of Fig. 9-18 as follows:

A. Centrally located dens
B. Left transverse process of C1
C. Left lateral mass of C1
D. Inferior articular surface of C1
E. Left zygapophyseal joint
F. Body of C2
G. Right superior articular surface of C2

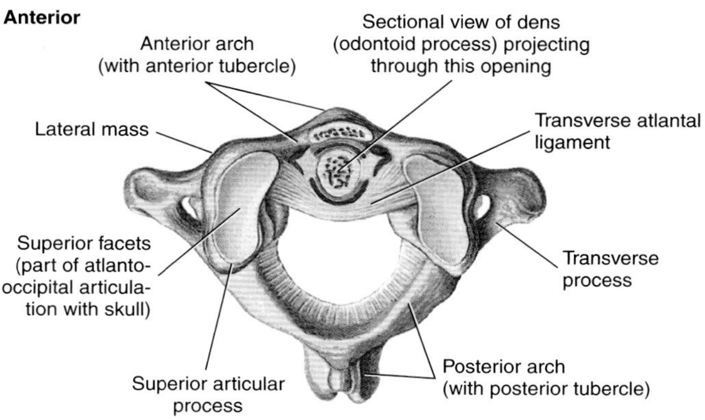

Fig. 9-15. Atlas (C1)—superior view.

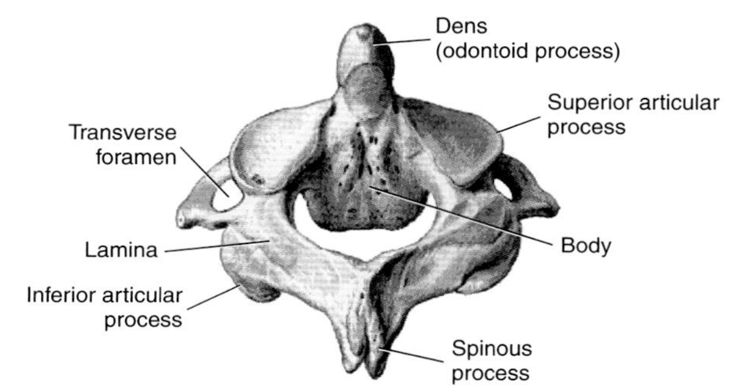

Fig. 9-16. Axis (C2)—posterior superior view.

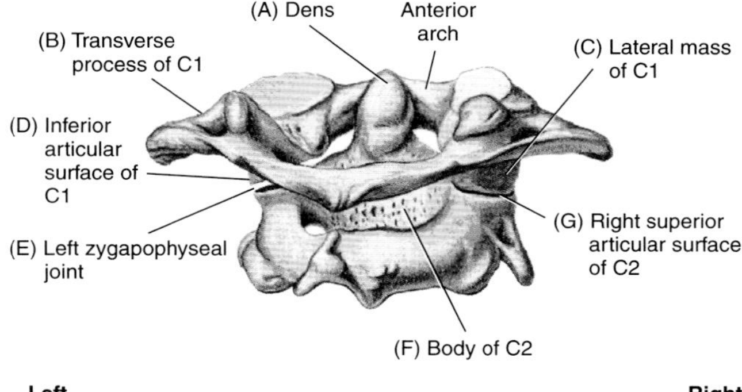

Fig. 9-17. C1 and C2—posterior oblique view.

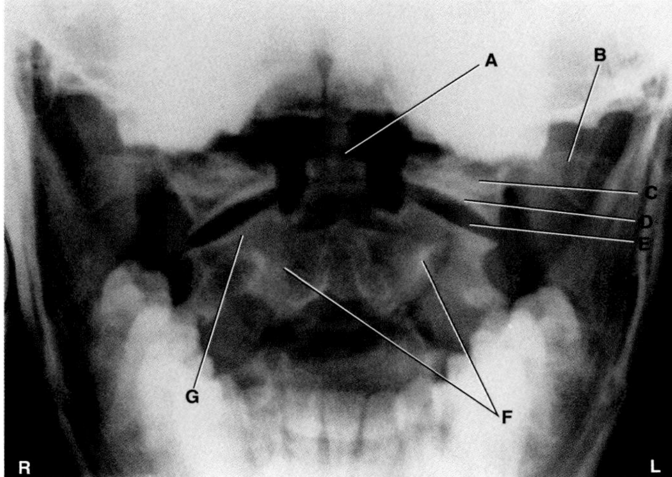

Fig. 9-18. AP open-mouth radiograph.

9

Thoracic Vertebrae Characteristics

An overview of the twelve thoracic vertebrae reveals marked progressive differences in size and appearance of upper vertebrae compared with lower ones, as demonstrated in Fig. 9-19.

T5, T6, T7, and T8 are considered typical thoracic vertebrae. The upper four thoracic vertebrae are smaller and share features of the cervical vertebrae. The lower four thoracic vertebrae are larger and share characteristics of the lumbar vertebrae.

RIB ARTICULATIONS

An important distinguishing feature of all thoracic vertebrae is their **facets for articulation with ribs.** Each of the 12 thoracic vertebrae is closely associated with one pair of ribs. Note in Fig. 9-20 that the two lumbar vertebrae, L1 and L2, do not show facets for rib articulations.

Costovertebral joints: Each thoracic vertebra has either **a full facet** *(fas'et)* or **two partial facets,** called **demifacets** *(dem"e-fas'ets),* on each side of the body. Each facet or combination of two demifacets accepts the head of a rib to form a **costovertebral joint** (Figs. 9-19, 9-20, and 9-21).

Vertebrae with two demifacets share articulations with the heads of ribs. For example, the head of the fourth rib "straddles" or articulates with demifacets on the vertebral bodies of both T3 and T4. The superior portion of the rib head articulates with the demifacet on the inferior margin of T3, and the inferior portion of the rib head articulates with the demifacet on the superior margin of T4.

Identifying ribs and the thoracic vertebrae is an important radiographic skill. T1 has a full facet and a demifacet on its inferior margin. T2 through T8 have demifacets on their upper and lower margins. T9 has only one demifacet on its upper margin. T10 through T12 have full facets. Knowing the facet arrangement makes it easy to predict the rib distribution. Rib 1 articulates with T1 only. Rib 2 articulates with T1 and T2, and so on. Ribs 11 and 12 articulate only with T11 and T12.

Costotransverse joints: In addition to costovertebral joints, all of the **first ten thoracic vertebrae** also have facets (one on each transverse process) that articulate with the tubercles of ribs 1 through 10. These articulations are termed **costotransverse joints.** Note in Figs. 9-19 and 9-20 that T11 and T12 do not show facets at the ends of the transverse process for rib articulations. Thus as the first ten pairs of ribs arch posteriorly from the upper ten vertebral bodies, the tubercle of each rib articulates with one transverse process to form a costotransverse joint. **Ribs 11 and 12, however, only articulate at the costovertebral joints.**

The superior cross-sectional perspective of typical rib articulations (Fig. 9-21) demonstrates that the articulations are closely spaced and enclosed in synovial capsules. These **synovial joints** are **diarthrodial** and allow slight **gliding movements.** This anatomy is further demonstrated and described in Chapter 11 on the bony thorax.

Superior and lateral perspectives *(Fig. 9-22):* Note the normal anatomic structures of a typical vertebra (vertebral body, pedicles, intervertebral foramina, superior and inferior articular processes, laminae, transverse processes, spinous processes). A unique characteristic of the thoracic region is that the long spinous process is projected so far inferiorly, as best seen on a lateral view. For example, when an AP radiographic projection of the thoracic spine is viewed, the spinous process of T4 will be superimposed on the body of T5.

Lateral oblique perspective *(Fig. 9-23):* The **superior articular processes** (facing primarily posteriorly) and the **inferior articular processes** (facing more anteriorly) are shown to connect the successive thoracic vertebrae to form the **zygapophyseal** (apophyseal) joints.

On each side, between any thoracic vertebrae, are **intervertebral foramina** defined on the superior and inferior margins by the pedicles (Fig. 9-23).

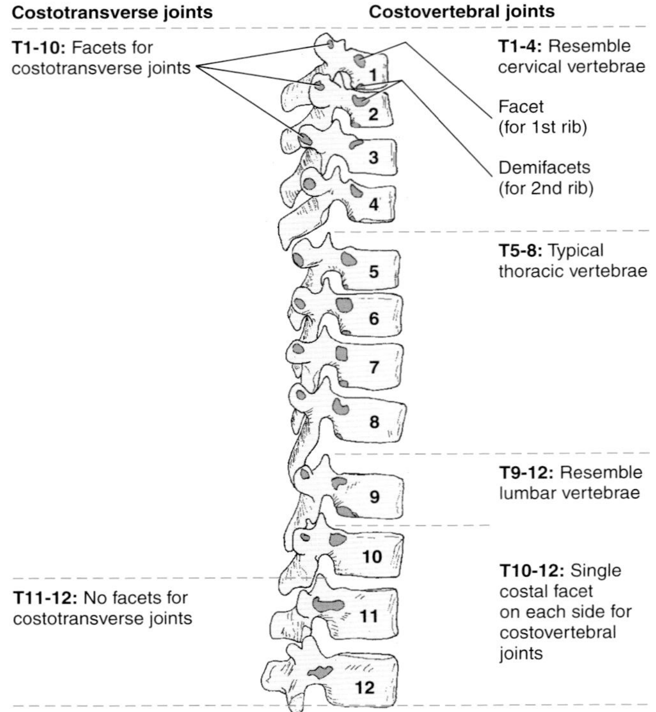

Fig. 9-19. Thoracic vertebrae (rib articulations).

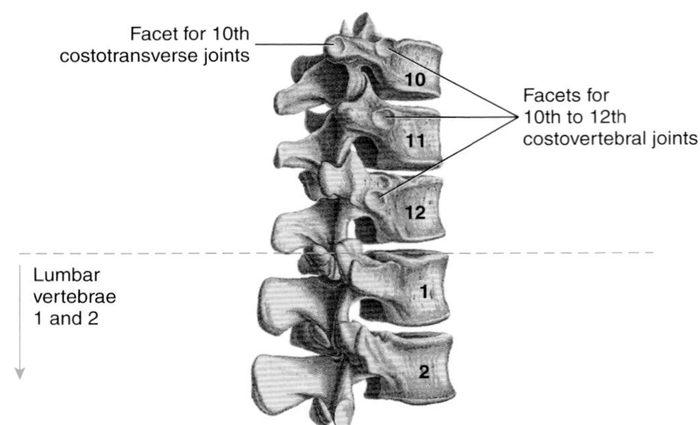

Fig. 9-20. T10-L2 (rib articulations on T10-12 only).

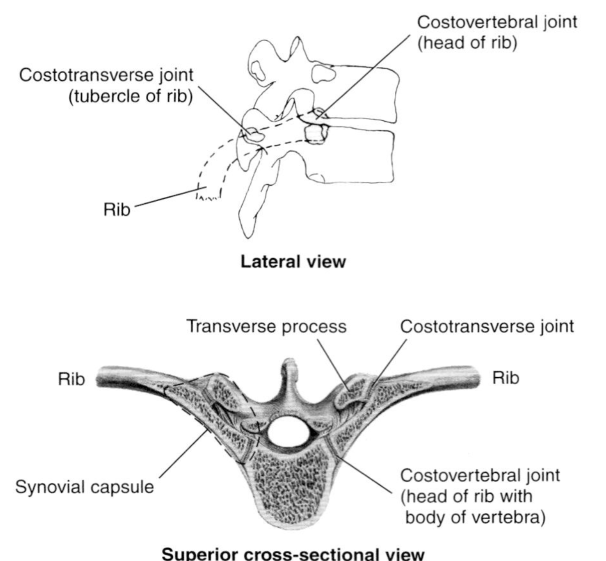

Fig. 9-21. Costovertebral and costotransverse joints—ribs 1 to 10.

9

THORACIC ZYGAPOPHYSEAL JOINTS

The structure and angles of the facets of the inferior and superior articular processes making up the zygapophyseal joints differ markedly from those of the cervical and lumbar vertebrae. In the thoracic vertebrae the zygapophyseal joints form an angle of **70° to 75° from the midsagittal plane** (MSP). Therefore, for example, to "open up" and radiographically demonstrate the thoracic zygapophyseal joints, a **70° to 75° oblique position** with a perpendicular central ray is required.

Fig. 9-35 on p. 299 is a photograph of the thoracic portion of a skeleton in an LPO position. Fig. 9-37 is a radiographic image of the same LPO position. On both one can easily see the right zygapophyseal joints.

THORACIC INTERVERTEBRAL FORAMINA

As demonstrated in Fig. 9-24, the openings of the intervertebral foramina on the thoracic vertebra are located at right angles, or **90°, to the midsagittal plane.** This is best demonstrated again on p. 299 with Fig. 9-34, a photograph of the thoracic portion of a skeleton in a lateral position. Fig. 9-36 is a radiographic image of the same lateral position. Both figures clearly show the left and right thoracic intervertebral foramina superimposed on each other.

UNIQUE C1-C2 JOINT CLASSIFICATIONS

The summary table below demonstrates that **three** joints or articulations with two different movement types are involved between C1 and C2 vertebrae. The first two joints are the **right and left lateral atlantoaxial joints** between the inferior articular surface of C1 (atlas) and the superior articular surface of C2 (axis). These are classified as **synovial** joints of **diarthrodial,** or freely movable, with **plane** (or **gliding**) movements. (Refer to Fig. 9-17 on p. 293.)

The third joint between C1 and C2 is the **medial atlantoaxial joint.** This articulation is between the dens of C2 and the anterior arch of C1 and is held in place by the transverse atlantal ligament, allowing a pivotal rotational movement between these two vertebrae. Therefore this joint or articulation is also classified as a **synovial** joint that is freely movable, or **diarthrodial,** with a **trochoid,** or **pivot,** type of movement. (See Figs. 9-15 and 9-17 on p. 293.)

SUMMARY OF VERTEBRAL JOINTS OF C AND T SPINE

JOINTS	CLASSIFICATION	MOBILITY TYPE	MOVEMENT TYPE
Skull-C1			
Atlantooccipital	Synovial	Diarthrodial	Ellipsoid (condyloid)
C1-C2			
R and L lateral atlantoaxial (2)*	Synovial	Diarthrodial	Plane (gliding)
Medial atlantoaxial (1)†	Synovial	Diarthrodial	Trochoid (pivot)
C2-T12			
Intervertebral	Cartilaginous (symphysis)	Amphiarthrodial (slightly movable)	N/A
Zygapophyseal	Synovial	Diarthrodial	Plane (gliding)
T1-T12			
Costovertebral	Synovial	Diarthrodial	Plane (gliding)
T1-T10			
Costotransverse	Synovial	Diarthrodial	Plane (gliding)

*Joint between dens of C2 and anterior arch of C1.

†Joints between lateral masses of C1 and superior facets of C2.

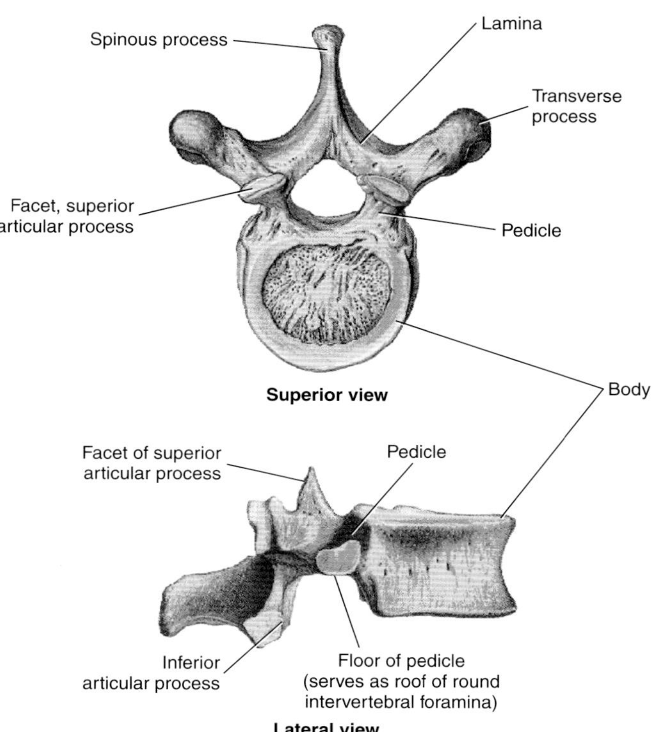

Fig. 9-22. Typical thoracic vertebrae.

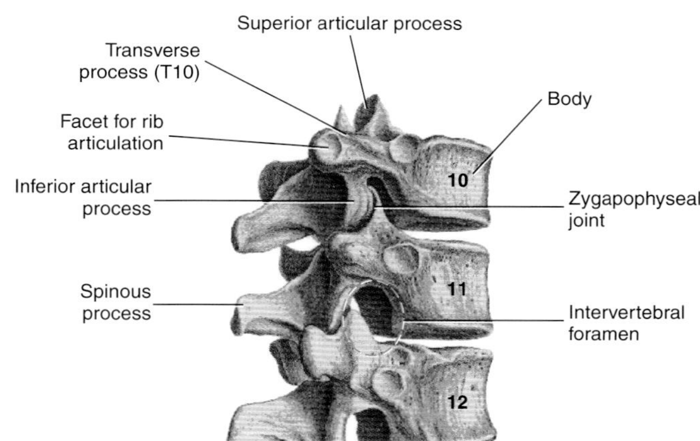

Fig. 9-23. Typical thoracic vertebrae (lateral oblique view).

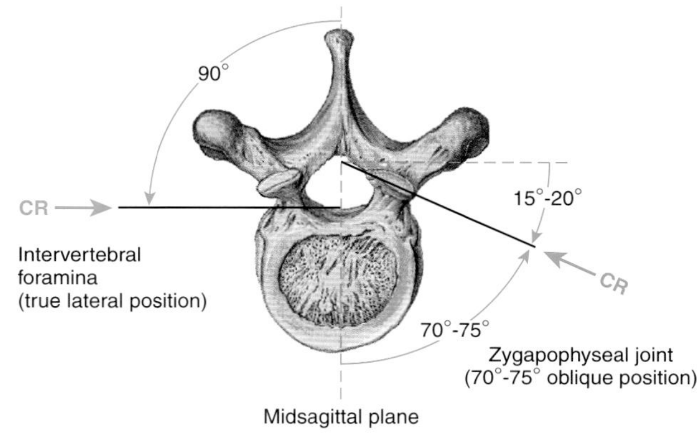

Fig. 9-24. Typical thoracic vertebrae.
—Intervertebral foramina, 90° (true lateral).
—Zygapophyseal joints, 70° to 75° (oblique).

Anatomy Review with Radiographic Images

AP CERVICAL SPINE IMAGE

Fig. 9-25 shows a conventional AP radiographic image of the cervical spine. Usually, the first two or three thoracic vertebrae, as well as C7 up to C3, are seen well on this projection. Identifying specific cervical vertebrae is possible by starting with T1, which can be identified by the attachment of the first pair of ribs. Therefore, to localize T1, locate the most superior ribs and find the vertebra to which they appear to connect. After T1 is located, visible cervical vertebrae can be identified by starting at C7 and counting upward.

A on this image is the first thoracic vertebra, determined by discovering that **B** is the first rib on the patient's right side.

C is the fourth cervical vertebra (count up from T1 and C7).

D is the articular pillar or lateral mass region of C3.

E is the spinous process of C3 seen on end.

Note: The white area at the top of the radiograph is created by the combined shadows of the base of the skull and the mandible. These structures effectively cover up the first two cervical vertebrae on this type of radiograph.

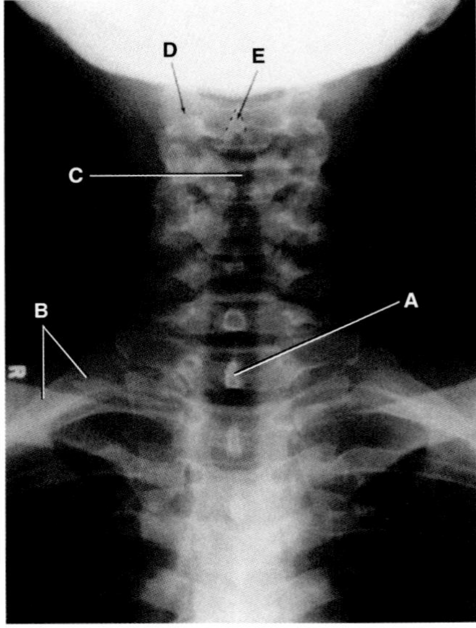

Fig. 9-25. AP C spine.

LATERAL CERVICAL SPINE IMAGE

The single most important radiograph clinically for a cervical spine series is a well-positioned lateral such as the one illustrated in Fig. 9-26. All seven cervical vertebrae and the alignment with T1 should be demonstrated on any lateral cervical spine radiograph. This is difficult on patients with thick, muscular, or wide shoulders and short necks. Additional projections may be necessary to supplement the routine lateral image. C1 and C7 have distinctive posterior structures that make it easier to identify them on radiographic images. The tubercle on the posterior arch of C1 resembles a spinous process and is easily identified. The spinous process of C7 is long and prominent, making it also easy to identify.

Fig. 9-26 also shows that the lower anterior margins of the last four or five cervical vertebral bodies have a slight lipped appearance. This characteristic, along with the general shape of the cervical vertebral bodies, requires that the central ray (CR) be angled approximately **20° cephalad** (toward the head) to "open up" these lower **intervertebral spaces** during an AP cervical spine projection.

A. Dens (odontoid process) enhanced with dotted lines on this radiographic image, seen extending up through the anterior ring of C1
B. Posterior arch and tubercle of the atlas, C1 (also see *A* in Fig. 9-27)
C. Body of C3
D. Zygapophyseal joint between C4 and C5 (best shown on a lateral projection for the cervical spine)
E. Body of C7
F. Spinous process of C7, vertebra prominens (a positioning landmark)

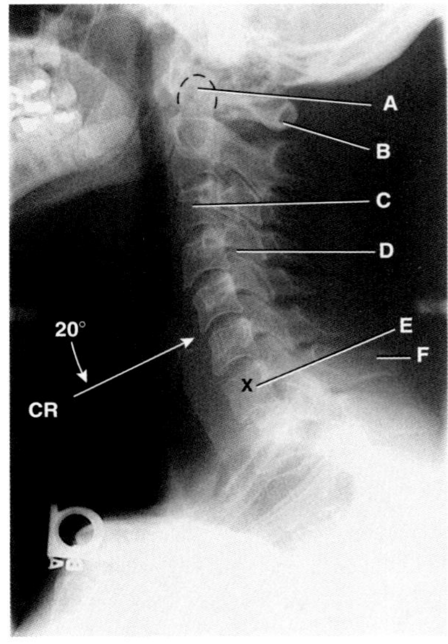

Fig. 9-26. Lateral C spine.

9

OBLIQUE CERVICAL SPINE IMAGE

Fig. 9-27 illustrates how well the oblique position demonstrates the cervical **intervertebral foramina.** Spinal nerves to and from the cord are transmitted through these intervertebral foramina.

A. Posterior arch and tubercle of C1
B. Intervertebral foramen between C4 and C5 (count down from C1)
C. Pedicle of C6
D. Body of C7

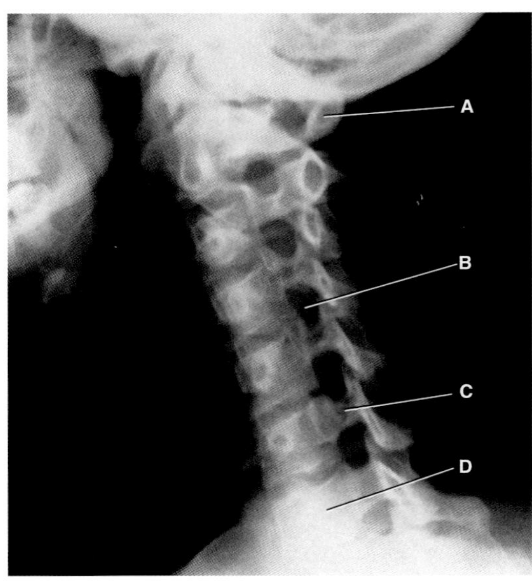

Fig. 9-27. Oblique C spine.

AP AND LATERAL THORACIC SPINE IMAGE

Individual thoracic vertebrae can best be identified on the AP projection because of visual cues provided by the posterior rib articulations. The first rib has a distinctive sharp curvature and attaches to T1. The twelfth rib is very short and attaches to T12. After identifying T1 or T12, one can count superiorly or inferiorly to identify the other thoracic vertebrae.

AP T spine image (Fig. 9-28)

A. First posterior rib
B. Tenth posterior rib
C. Spinous process of T11, faintly seen on edge through body
D. Body of T12
E. Intervertebral disk space between T8 and T9
F. Body of T7 (center of T spine and of average chest)
G. Body of T1 (Remember, heads of first ribs articulate with upper portion of T1.)

Lateral T spine (Fig. 9-29)

A. Body of T3. (Count up from T12, assuming the top edge of T12 is at the level of costophrenic angle [posterior tip] of diaphragm. An exception to this method of identifying thoracic vertebrae is necessary for patients who have lumbar ribs. These anomalous short ribs may be attached to the most superior lumbar vertebra.)
B. Body of T7
C. Intervertebral foramina between T11 and T12 (This is best demonstrated on a lateral image of the T spine.)

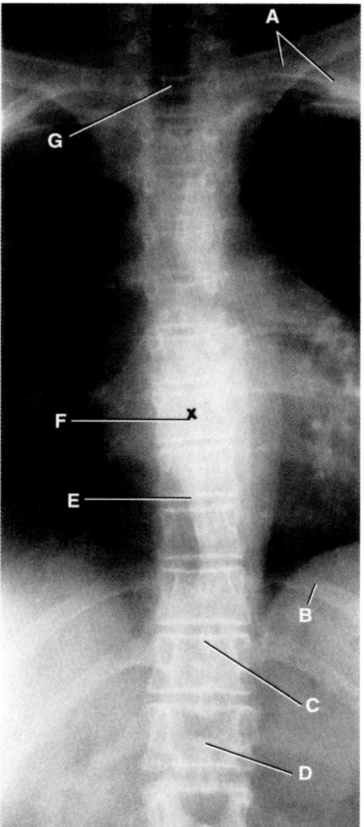

Fig. 9-28. AP T spine.

SUMMARY OF DISTINGUISHING FEATURES—C AND T SPINE

VERTEBRA	DISTINGUISHING FEATURE
Cervical Vertebrae	
All cervical vertebrae	Three foramina each
	More dominant articular pillars
C1, atlas	No body but anterior arch
	No spinous process but posterior tubercle with bifid tip
	Lateral masses (articular pillars)
	Superior facets for atlantooccipital articulations
C2, axis	Contains dens
C2-6	Short spinous processes with bifid tips
C7	Called *vertebra prominens* because of its long spinous process
Thoracic Vertebrae	
All thoracic vertebrae	Contain facets for rib articulations (facets or demifacets)
T1-10	Contain facets on transverse processes for rib articulations
T1-9	Contain demifacets for rib articulation
T10-12	Contain single facet for rib articulation

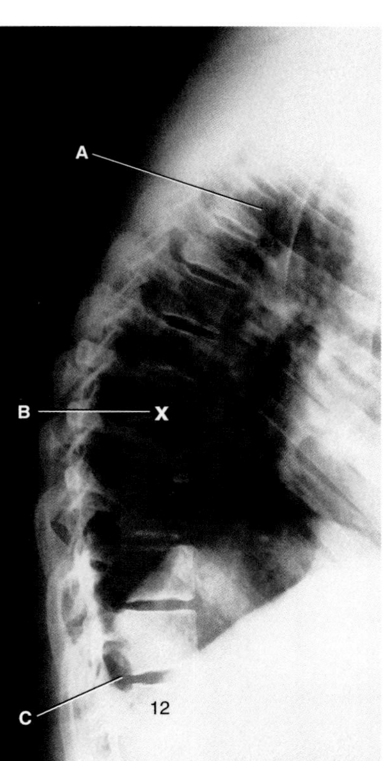

Fig. 9-29. Lateral T spine.

Intervertebral Foramina Versus Zygapophyseal Joints

Two anatomic areas of the spine that generally need to be demonstrated by the proper radiographs are the **intervertebral foramina** and the **zygapophyseal joints.** This is especially important for the cervical spine. The physician gains important information concerning the relationship of consecutive vertebrae by studying these two areas on the appropriate radiograph. To complicate matters, however, depending on the part of the spine to be radiographed (cervical, thoracic, or lumbar), a different body position is required to best show each anatomic area.

CERVICAL SPINE SKELETON

Two photographs of the cervical vertebrae (Figs. 9-30 and 9-31) are shown in position to visualize these areas on the cervical vertebrae. Fig. 9-30 is a cervical section of the vertebral column in a left lateral position, and Fig. 9-31 is a 45° left posterior oblique position (LPO). The **zygapophyseal joints** visualize well on the **lateral position** (see *arrow*).

On the right, the posterior oblique with a 45° rotation shows that the intervertebral foramina are clearly opened (see *arrow*). It is important to know that the **left posterior oblique** position opens up the foramina on the **right side,** and a **15° CR cephalad angle** is needed. Therefore on a **posterior oblique** cervical spine radiograph, the upside is the side on which the intervertebral foramina are opened well.

If this were taken in an **anterior** oblique position, with the foramina **closest** to the IR, the downside would be open and a 15° **caudad angle** would be required.

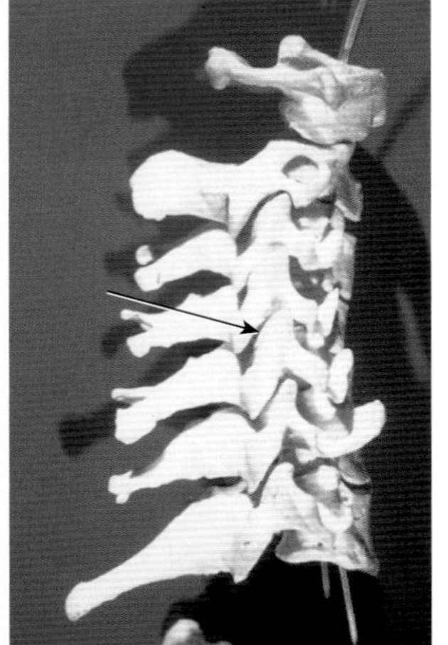

Fig. 9-30. Left lateral—zygapophyseal joints.

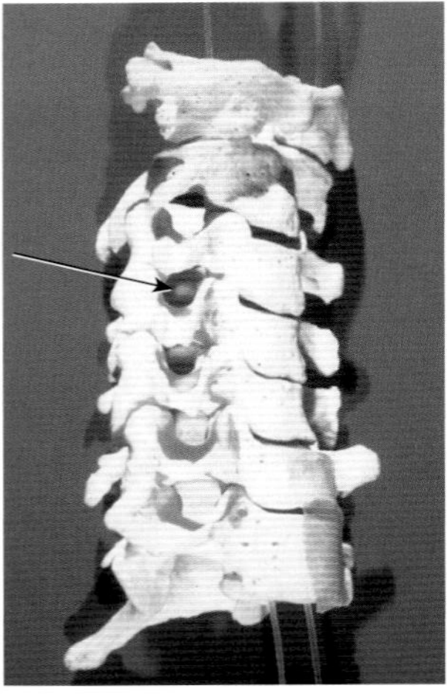

Fig. 9-31. Oblique (LPO)—right intervertebral foramina (upside).

CERVICAL SPINE RADIOGRAPHS

The two radiographs of the cervical spine (Figs. 9-32 and 9-33) illustrate the same anatomy in the same two positions as shown on the skeleton above. The lateral position on the right best shows the **zygapophyseal joints.** The joint on each side is superimposed upon the joint on the opposite side. It is important to remember that the zygapophyseal joints are located between the articular pillars of each vertebra.

The oblique cervical spine radiograph on the right shows the circular **intervertebral foramina** opened. In each oblique radiograph only one set of foramina are opened, whereas the ones on the opposite side are closed. Since this position is a **left posterior** oblique, the **right intervertebral foramina** or those on the **upside** are being shown.

Remember that the LPO will show the same anatomy as the RAO. Therefore, if the patient were placed in an **anterior** oblique position, the **downside** foramina to the film would be shown. Thus in either case, LPO or RAO, the right intervertebral foramina will be visualized.

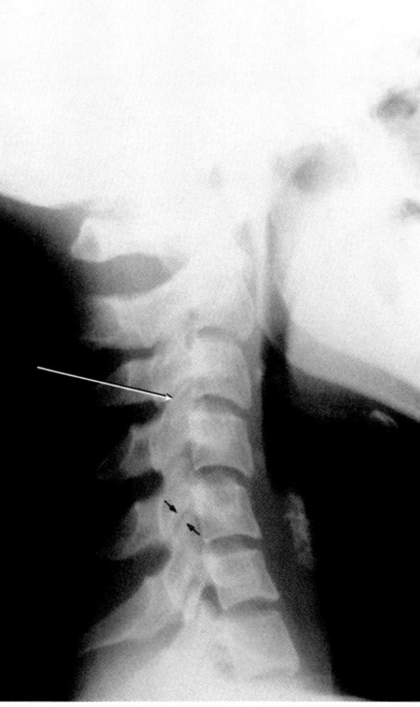

Fig. 9-32. Lateral (left)—zygapophyseal joints demonstrated.

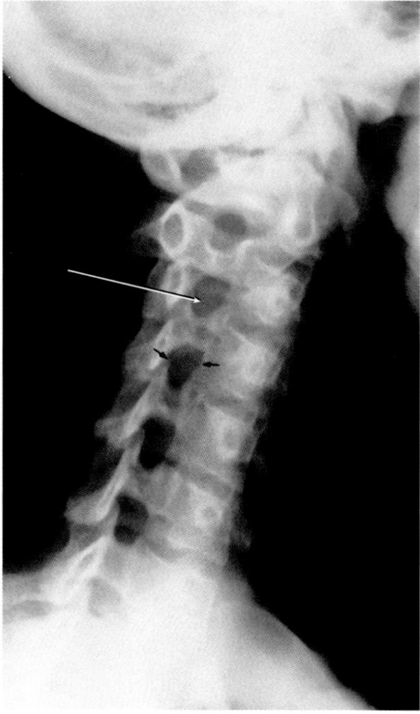

Fig. 9-33. Oblique (LPO)—right intervertebral foramina (upside).

9

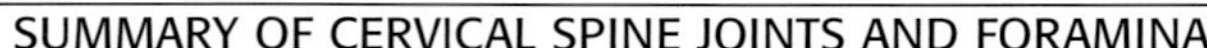

SUMMARY OF CERVICAL SPINE JOINTS AND FORAMINA	
Zygapophyseal Joints—	**Intervertebral Foramina—**
90° Lateral	**45° Oblique**
R or L lateral	**CR 15° cephalad—upside visualized**
	LPO—right foramina
	RPO—left foramina
	CR 15° caudad—downside visualized
	LAO—left foramina
	RAO—right foramina

THORACIC SPINE SKELETON

Two photographs of the thoracic vertebrae are shown (Figs. 9-34 and 9-35). The thoracic vertebrae on the left are in a lateral position; those on the right are in an oblique position. The **lateral position** of the thoracic spine best shows the **intervertebral foramina.** A **70° oblique** is necessary to open up the **zygapophyseal joints** on the thoracic spine.

The **posterior** oblique position on the right shows the zygapophyseal joint on the **upside. Anterior** obliques would demonstrate the **downside** joints.

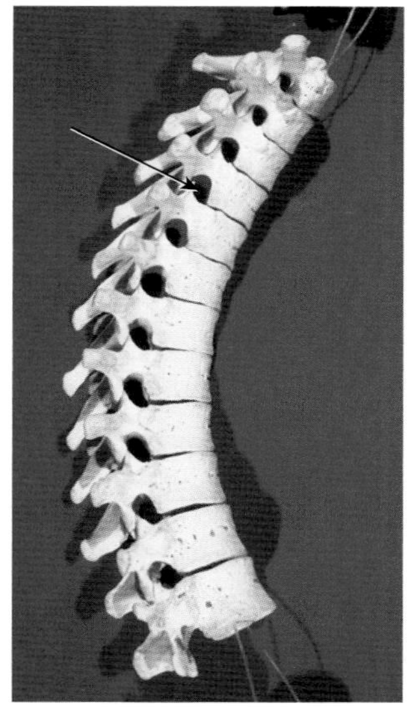

Fig. 9-34. Thoracic spine. Left lateral—intervertebral foramina.

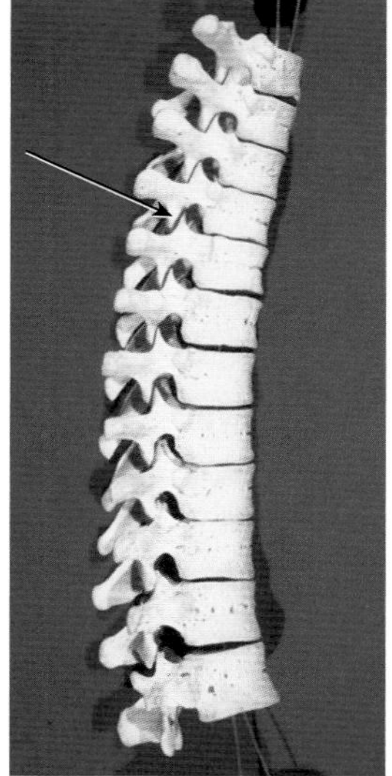

Fig. 9-35. Thoracic spine. Oblique (LPO)—upside zygapophyseal joints.

THORACIC SPINE RADIOGRAPHS

Radiographs of the thoracic spine in the lateral position and in the 70° oblique position (Figs. 9-36 and 9-37) correspond to the position of the thoracic skeleton directly above. Observe that the round openings of the superimposed **intervertebral foramina** are best visualized on the **lateral** radiograph on the left (see *arrow*).

The **zygapophyseal joints** are best visualized on the **oblique** radiograph on the right. The oblique radiograph is in a 70° LPO position, which should best visualize the zygapophyseal joints on the **upside,** or those farthest away from the IR. The LPO position best shows the **right zygapophyseal** joints.

If the obliques were taken as **anterior** obliques, the opposite would be true and the **downside** joints would be demonstrated. An **LAO** would demonstrate the **left** zygapophyseal joints. Therefore an LAO would demonstrate the same zygapophyseal joints as an RPO, as seen in the chart below.

SUMMARY OF THORACIC SPINE JOINTS AND FORAMINA

Intervertebral foramina—90° lateral	**Zygapophyseal joints—70° oblique**
R or L lateral	**Posterior obliques—upside**
	LPO—right zygapophyseal
	RPO—left zygapophyseal
	Anterior oblique—downside
	LAO—left zygapophyseal
	RAO—right zygapophyseal

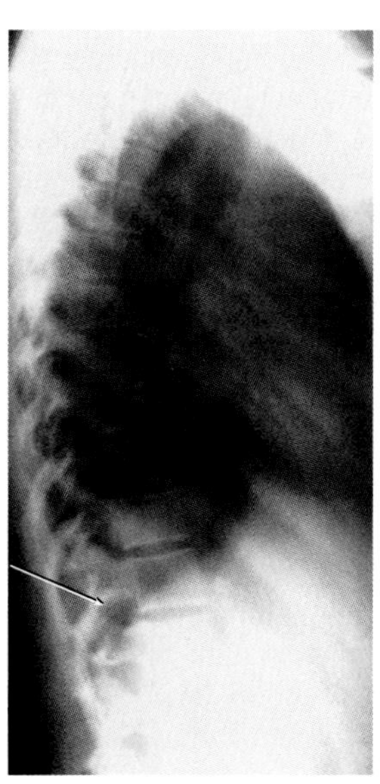

Fig. 9-36. Thoracic spine. Left lateral—intervertebral foramina.

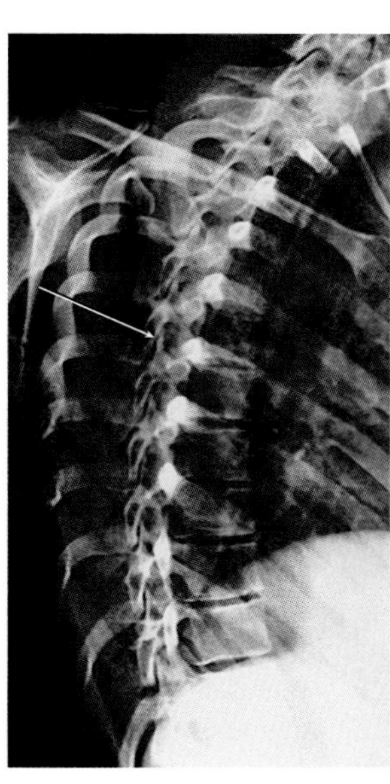

Fig. 9-37. Thoracic spine. Oblique (LPO)—right (upside) zygapophyseal joints.

RADIOGRAPHIC POSITIONING

Topographic Landmarks

Topographic landmarks provide useful, palpable guidepoints for radiographic positioning. Landmarks may be helpful when well-collimated radiographic images are required of specific vertebrae. There are variations between patients for different body habitus, but these landmarks represent anatomic relationships of an average patient.

CERVICAL LANDMARKS

Various anatomy correlates with levels of the cervical spine as illustrated in Figs. 9-38 and 9-39. The **mastoid tip** corresponds to the level of **C1.** Another way to localize the level of C1 is to go about 1 inch (2.5 cm) below the level of the **EAM** (external acoustic meatus).

With the head in a neutral position, the angle of the jaw, or **gonion,** is at the same level as **C3.** The most prominent part of the **thyroid cartilage,** or "Adam's apple," is at the approximate level of C5. This thyroid cartilage landmark varies between the levels of **C4 and C6.**

The spinous process of the last cervical vertebra, **C7 vertebra prominens,** is at about the same level as the **body of T1.** It is more obvious with the patient's head tipped forward and should be used to help locate C7 and T1 rather than the top of the shoulders. (Too much variability exists in the position of shoulders because of relative fitness and posture.) This is a useful landmark because of the importance of including all of C7 on a lateral cervical radiograph.

The shoulders should be depressed as much as possible for a lateral C spine radiograph; however, depending on the patient's body habitus, the shoulders may still occasionally superimpose the last cervical vertebra. Additional images may be necessary to demonstrate the alignment of C7 to T1 when the shoulders are too dense for adequate penetration on a routine lateral. In this case the jugular notch or the vertebra prominens can be used as a landmark for centering.

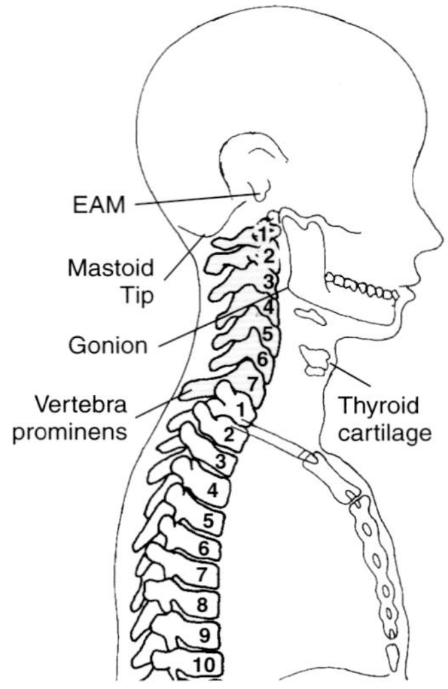

Fig. 9-38. Cervical spine landmarks.

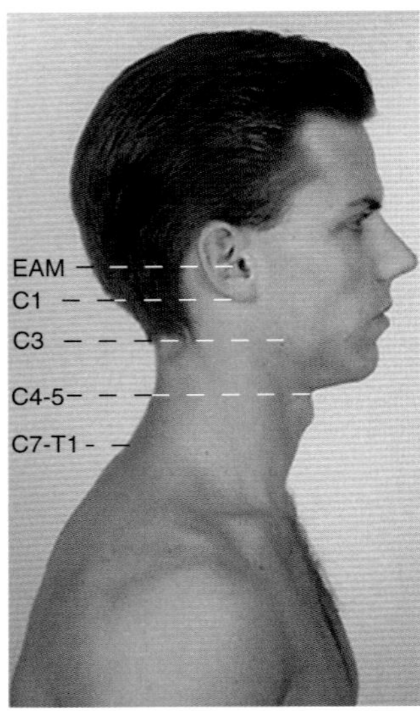

Fig. 9-39. Cervical spine landmarks.

STERNUM AND THORACIC SPINE LANDMARKS

Sternum anatomy correlates with levels of the thoracic spine as illustrated in Figs. 9-40 and 9-41. The sternum is divided into three basic sections. The upper section is the **manubrium.** The easily palpated **U-shaped** dip in the superior margin is the **jugular** (suprasternal) **notch** *(A).* The jugular notch is at the level of T2 and T3. T1 is about 1.5 inches (4 cm) superior to the level of the jugular notch.

9

The first thoracic vertebra can also be located by palpating posteriorly at the base of the neck for the prominent spinous process of C7, the **vertebra prominens.** Note that the long sloping vertebra prominens extends downward with its tip at the level of the body of T1.

The central portion of the sternum is called the **body.** The manubrium and body connect at a slight, easily located angle termed the **sternal angle** *(B),* about 2 inches (5 cm) inferior to the manubrial notch. Posteriorly, this is the level of junction of T4 and T5. Anteriorly, this is the level of the articulation of the second rib onto the sternum.

A frequently used landmark is the level of T7. Anteriorly, it is located about 3 to 4 inches (8 to 10 cm) inferior to the jugular notch or at the midpoint of the jugular notch and the xiphoid tip. Posteriorly, this is about 7 to 8 inches (18 to 20 cm) below the vertebra prominens *(C).* This landmark indicates the approximate center of the twelve thoracic vertebrae because the inferior vertebrae are larger than the superior ones.

The most inferior end of the sternum is called the **xiphoid process,** or **xiphoid tip.** Locating the xiphoid process on a patient requires some pressure *(D).* The xiphoid tip is at the level of T10.

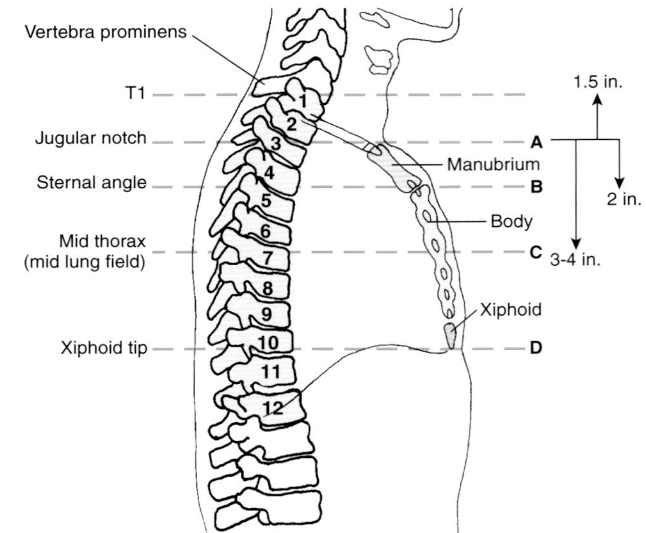

Fig. 9-40. Sternum and thoracic spine landmarks.

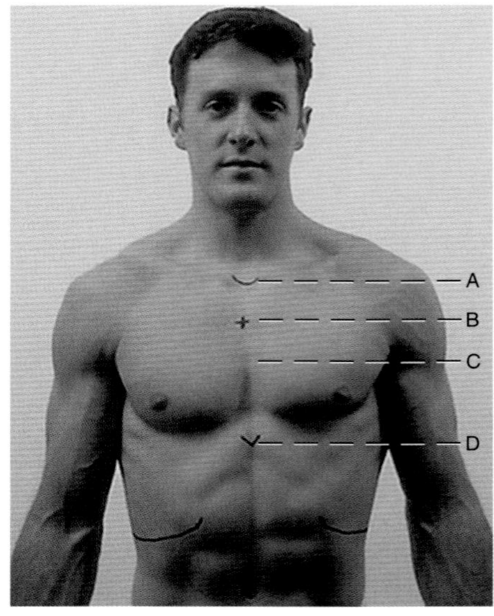

Fig. 9-41. Sternum and thoracic spine landmarks.

Positioning and Technical Considerations

ERECT VERSUS RECUMBENT

Radiographic examinations of the cervical spine are generally made with the patient erect to demonstrate alignment and ligament stability. An erect position also allows the natural curvature of the spine to be demonstrated, the shoulders to be depressed, and a 72-inch (180-cm) SID to be used to improve image quality and reduce magnification.

The patient may be either seated or standing in front of a vertical cassette holder, an upright Bucky, or a radiographic table. Some conditions, such as trauma, may require radiographing the cervical spine with the patient in a recumbent position.

Thoracic spines are most frequently radiographed with the patient recumbent, except for scoliosis exams, which need to be taken erect (described in Chapter 10).

PATIENT RADIATION PROTECTION

Exposure to radiosensitive tissues such as the thyroid, parathyroid, breasts, testes, and ovaries can be minimized during radiography of the cervical and thoracic spine by **close collimation,** the use of **proper exposure factors,** and **minimizing repeats.** Theoretically one can shield to protect radiosensitive organs (breast, thyroid, etc) from radiation, but because of the practicalities of maintaining such shields (erect positions, flexion/extension views, etc.) it is not a common practice, especially for the cervical spine projections. Also the source of secondary/scatter radiation for such regions is primarily from within the patient and surface shielding has little effect if correct collimation is utilized. However, to reassure the patient, lead contact shielding over the gonads and other radiosensitive areas is a good practice when it is clinically practical. Also, the thyroid dose can be reduced significantly during cervical oblique radiography by positioning the patient **in an anterior oblique rather than a posterior oblique** (see comparative patient dose icon boxes on p. 308).

TECHNICAL AND IMAGE QUALITY FACTORS (FILM-SCREEN IMAGING)

For the purposes of this discussion, technical and image quality factors include (1) exposure factors, (2) focal spot size, (3) compensating strategies, (4) SID, (5) scatter reduction, and (6) part/IR alignment.

During lateral and oblique spine radiography, the spinal column is unavoidably situated some distance from the IR (increased OID). The image geometry, therefore, results in reduction in sharpness because of magnification of the spine anatomy.

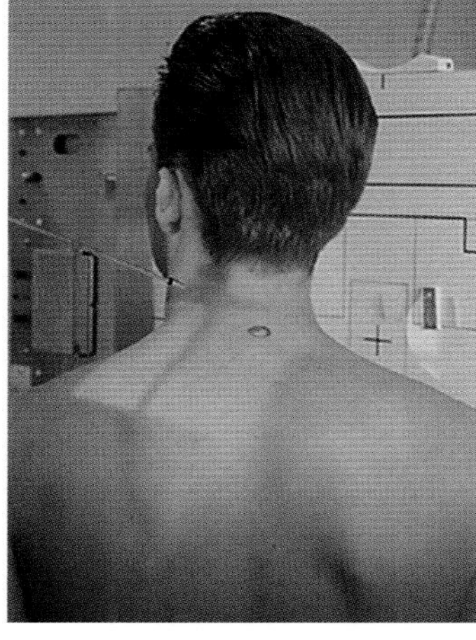

Fig. 9-42. Anterior cervical oblique.
—60-inch SID
—Small focal spot
—Anterior obliques reduce thyroid doses

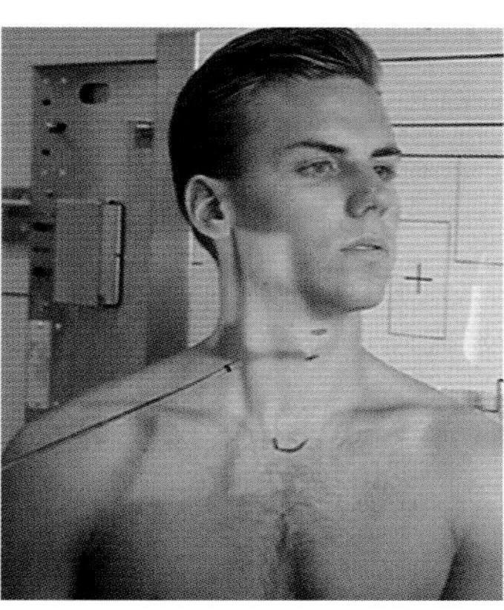

Fig. 9-43. Posterior cervical oblique—60-inch SID—small focal spot

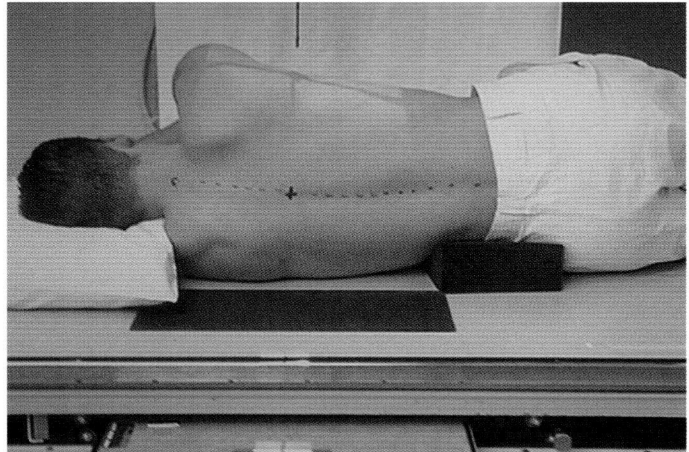

Fig. 9-44. Lateral T spine—with lead blocker behind patient—vertebral column near parallel to tabletop.

Exposure Factors

The kV range for a C spine is 70 to 80, and the range for a T spine is 80 to 90. The use of higher kV with high-latitude film-screen combinations can provide a wider range of densities on the image. Using higher kV can also reduce patient dose because lower mAs values can be used.

The lateral thoracic spine is most commonly obtained using a breathing technique to blur structures overlying the thoracic vertebrae. The breathing technique requires a minimum of 3 or 4 seconds exposure time with a low mA setting.

Focal Spot Size

Using a small focal spot can improve the recorded detail by reducing the effects of penumbra (image unsharpness). Breathing techniques involve a long exposure time at low mA settings that have smaller focal spot sizes.

Compensating Strategies

The range of vertebral sizes and the differing types of surrounding tissues in the thoracic region, in particular, present a radiographic challenge. For example, on an AP image, the exposure factors could overexpose the superior end (smaller vertebral bodies surrounded by air-filled lungs) and underexpose the inferior end (larger vertebral bodies surrounded by dense abdominal tissues below the diaphragm). This may result in a radiograph that is too dark (overexposed) at the superior end and too light (underexposed) at the inferior end.

"Wedge" filters provide more uniform density in the AP projection of the thoracic spine.

The anode-heel effect may be applied for AP thoracic spine projections by positioning the anode end of the tube (less intense portion of the field) over the thinner anatomic part (superior thoracic spine). However, the use of a wedge filter is generally a more effective method of equalizing density along an AP thoracic spine.

SID

Cervical spine radiographs should be taken with an increased SID of 60 to 72 inches (150 to 180 cm) to compensate for the increased OID, resulting in less magnification unsharpness.

Thoracic spine images are usually obtained at a minimum SID of 40 inches (100 cm).

9

Positioning and Technical Considerations—cont'd

Scatter Radiation

Use of higher kV and thick or dense tissue results in increased production of scatter radiation, which degrades the radiographic image. The effects of scatter radiation can be minimized in three ways: (1) with close collimation, (2) with a lead blocker placed on the tabletop next to the patient during lateral radiography (Fig. 9-44), and (3) with grids. Collimation reduces the amount of scatter produced while lead blockers and grids prevent the scatter radiation from reaching the IR.

Spine radiography requires a grid except for certain cervical spine radiographs, such as on small patients with necks measuring less than 10 cm. Another example is when considering the "air gap" phenomenon during lateral cervical radiography. The placement of the cassette far from the spine during lateral cervical radiography creates an air gap that reduces the amount of scatter radiation reaching the IR. This increased OID also contributes to more magnification of the image, which accounts for an increase in image receptor distance (SID) to compensate.

Part/IR Alignment

Correct part/IR alignment is important during spine radiography because the beam must pass through specific anatomic structures. For example, this may require placing a radiolucent sponge under the patient's waist to keep the spine near parallel to the cassette during lateral thoracic positioning (Fig. 9-44).

Optimal object/IR alignment is a challenge for lateral thoracic and lumbar spines because of the wide range of body builds among male and female patients. This is illustrated in the positioning pages for those projections.

Pediatric Applications

Two primary concerns in pediatric radiography are **patient motion** and **patient x-radiation dose.** A clear explanation of the procedure is required to obtain maximal trust and cooperation from the patient and guardian.

Careful immobilization is important to achieve proper positioning and to reduce patient motion. A **short exposure time** with optimal mA and kV helps reduce the chance of motion. To reduce dose to the pediatric patient, use as high a kV as possible while maintaining an acceptable level of radiographic contrast.

To ensure their safety from falls or other physical injury, continuously watch and care for pediatric patients. Refer to Chapter 20 for detailed communication strategies, immobilization techniques, and explanations.

Geriatric Applications

9

The physical effects associated with aging may result in the geriatric patient requiring additional assistance time and patience to obtain the required positions for spinal radiography. Patient care for the geriatric patient should include special attention in the areas of **communication, patient safety,** and **patient handling.** These patients may require extra time and assistance in achieving the required position.

Communication Varying degrees of vision and hearing loss can reduce patient understanding and cooperation. To improve communication: (1) avoid background noise; (2) face the patient; (3) gain the patient's attention; and (4) use clear, simple instructions. Allow the patient to retain hearing aids and eyeglasses if possible, or wait until the last moment if it is necessary to remove them. Use touch to emphasize positioning instructions. For the patient with significant hearing loss, a lowered voice with increased volume improves the likelihood the patient will hear. To verify understanding, ask the patient to repeat instructions. Always treat the geriatric patient with dignity and respect.

Safety The aging process can affect changes in balance and coordination that can bring about dizziness, vertigo, and an increased incidence of falling. Geriatric patients often fear falling. To ensure good patient safety, always assist the patient: (1) to get onto and off the radiographic table; (2) to change position; (3) to sit down. Reassurance and additional care from the technologist enables the patient to feel more secure and comfortable.

Patient handling and comfort The geriatric patient experiences skin changes and a diminished ability to regulate temperature. As the skin ages, it becomes thinner, is more easily broken, and is more prone to bleeding and bruising. Special care must be given when holding or moving the patient. Avoid using adhesive tape and use special care when removing tape from skin. Use a radiolucent pad on the exam table to minimize skin damage and to provide comfort and added warmth. Extra blankets may be required to keep the patient warm. The patient with exaggerated kyphosis needs extra pillows under the head or may be more comfortable if positioned in the erect position for some procedures.

Technical factors Because of the high incidence of osteoporosis in geriatric patients, the kV and/or mAs may require a decrease if manual exposure factors are being used. Older patients may have tremors or difficulty holding steady. Use of short exposure times (associated with the use of high mA) is recommended to reduce the risk of motion.

Digital Imaging Considerations

The following guidelines are important for digital imaging (CR and DR) of the cervical and thoracic spine:

1. **Correct centering** (to allow accurate postprocessing by the image reader)
2. **Close collimation, tabletop lead masking,** and **use of grids** (to reduce scatter exposure to the highly sensitive image receptors)
3. **Following the ALARA principle** in determining exposure factors, including the highest kV and the lowest mAs that result in desirable image quality (may require higher kV compared with film-screen imaging)
4. **Post-processing evaluation of exposure index values** (to ensure optimum image quality with the least radiation to the patient)

Alternative Modalities or Procedures

MYELOGRAM

A myelogram is an alternative radiographic procedure involving fluoroscopic and radiographic examination of the spinal canal to evaluate lesions in the spinal canal, intervertebral disks, or nerve roots. Water-soluble iodinated contrast is injected into the subarachnoid space of the spinal canal at the level of L3-L4. If no obstruction exists, the contrast will flow freely with the cerebrospinal fluid throughout the spinal canal and around nerve roots. Lesions will appear as filling defects.

Magnetic resonance imaging (MRI) and computed tomography (CT) are replacing myelography as the modality of choice for spinal canal–related symptoms, but myelograms are still being performed in some institutions and are described in more detail in Chapter 23.

COMPUTED TOMOGRAPHY

CT scans are useful for evaluating spinal trauma such as fractures, subluxations, herniated disks, tumors, and arthropathies such as rheumatoid arthritis and osteoarthritis.

MAGNETIC RESONANCE IMAGING

MRI of the cervical and thoracic spine is especially useful for demonstrating soft-tissue (noncalcified) structures associated with the spine, such as the intervertebral disks and the spinal cord itself.

The MRI sagittal section image of a cervical spine in Fig. 9-45 clearly demonstrates not only bony structure but soft tissue as well. The vertebral canal containing the spinal cord *(B)* is seen as a tube-like column directly posterior to the cervical vertebrae. The spinal cord is seen to be a continuation of the medulla oblongata of the brain *(A)*. A herniation of the disk between C5 and C6 is demonstrated by a slight posterior displacement, causing mild spinal cord displacement.

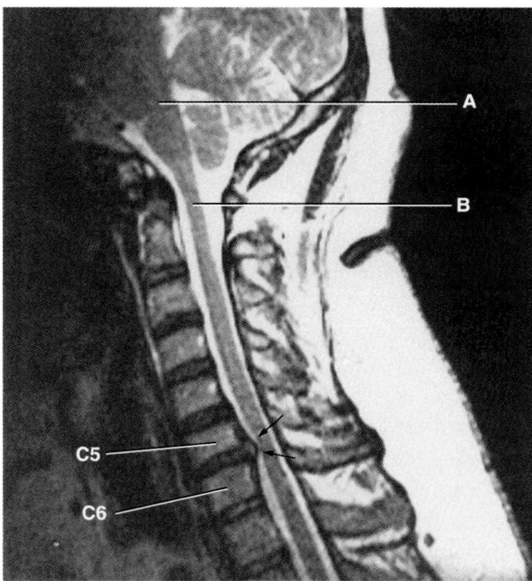

Fig. 9-45. MRI cervical spine (demonstrates herniated disk between C5 and C6).

NUCLEAR MEDICINE

Nuclear medicine studies involve injection of pharmaceuticals tagged with tracer elements to demonstrate specific physiologic processes including those that affect bone. For example, a technetium phosphate compound is injected and circulates with the blood. It will concentrate in areas of bone activity, creating a "hot spot" on the nuclear medicine scan image. Nuclear medicine scans can demonstrate several conditions related to the spine such as bone tumors, healing fractures, metastases of cancer to the spine, osteomyelitis (bone infections), or Paget's disease.

Pathologic Indications

Pathologic indications involving the cervical and thoracic spine that all technologists should be familiar with include the following (not necessarily an inclusive list):

Clay shoveler's fracture: This fracture results from hyperflexion of the neck and results in avulsion fractures on the spinous processes of C6 through T1. The fracture is best demonstrated on a lateral cervical spine radiograph.

Compression fracture: Frequently associated with osteoporosis, a compression fracture often involves collapse of a vertebral body resulting from flexion or axial loading, most often in thoracic or lumbar regions. It can also result from severe kyphosis caused by other diseases. The anterior edge collapses, changing the shape of the vertebral body into a wedge instead of a block. This results in an increase in kyphosis and may compromise respiratory and cardiac function; it also frequently results in injury to the spinal cord. Compression fractures are best demonstrated on a lateral projection of the affected region of the spine.

Hangman's fracture: This fracture extends through the pedicles of C2 with or without subluxation of C2 upon C3. This cervical fracture occurs when the neck is subjected to extreme hyperextension. The patient, if alive, is not stable because the intact dens is pressed posteriorly against the brain stem. A lateral projection of the cervical spine will demonstrate the anterior displacement of C2 characteristic of a hangman's fracture.

Jefferson fracture: This comminuted fracture (splintered or crushed at site of impact) occurs as a result of axial loading, such as landing on one's head or abruptly on one's feet. The anterior and posterior arches of C1 are fractured as the skull slams onto the ring. The AP open mouth projection and lateral cervical spine projections will demonstrate a Jefferson fracture.

Odontoid fracture: The odontoid fracture involves the dens, which can also extend into the lateral masses or arches of C1. An AP open mouth projection will demonstrate any disruption of the arches of C1.

Teardrop burst fracture: The mechanism of injury is compression with hyperflexion in the cervical region. The vertebral body is comminuted with triangular fragments avulsed from the anterointerior border and fragments from the posterior vertebral body displaced into the spinal canal. Neurologic damage (usually quadriplegia) is a high probability. Based on the extent of the fracture and possible spinal cord involvement, a CT scan is usually indicated once a baseline lateral and AP projection of the cervical spine has been taken.

Facets—unilateral subluxations and bilateral locks: Zygapophyseal joints in the cervical region can be disrupted during trauma. If the patient's injury involves flexion, distraction, and rotation, only one zygapophyseal joint may be out of alignment, with a unilateral subluxation. Radiographically the vertebral body will be rotated on its axis, creating a "bow tie" artifact on the lateral cervical spine image. If the patient's injury involves extreme flexion and distraction, both right and left zygapophyseal joints on the same level can be disrupted, creating bilateral locked facets. Radiographically, the vertebral body will appear to have "jumped" over the vertebral body immediate inferior to it. In either case the spine is not stable because the spinal cord is distressed by this manipulation. Following the AP and lateral projection of the cervical spine, a CT scan of the spine is generally indicated.

Herniated nucleus pulposus (HNP): If the soft inner part (nucleus pulposus) of an intervertebral disk protrudes through the fibrous cartilage outer layer (annulus) into the spinal canal, it may press on the spinal cord or spinal nerves and cause severe pain and possible numbness radiating into the extremities. This condition is sometimes called a "slipped disk." This is well demonstrated on an MR image of the cervical spine region in Fig. 9-45. Although it can affect cervical vertebrae, HNP more frequently involves levels L4 through L5. Although myelography has been traditionally performed for HNP, MRI now provides a noninvasive alternative for diagnosing this condition.

Kyphosis: Kyphosis is an abnormal or exaggerated convex curvature of the thoracic spine that results in stooped posture and reduction in height. Kyphosis may be caused by compression fractures of the anterior edges of the vertebral bodies in osteoporotic patients, particularly postmenopausal women. It may also be caused by poor posture, rickets, or other diseases involving the spine (see Scheuermann's disease). A lateral projection of the spine will best demonstrate the extent of kyphosis.

Lordosis: Lordosis describes the normal concave curvature of the lumbar spine and also describes an abnormal or exaggerated concave lumbar curvature. This condition may result from pregnancy, obesity, poor posture, rickets, or tuberculosis of the spine. A lateral projection of the spine will best demonstrate the extent of lordosis.

Scoliosis: Although many individuals normally have some slight lateral curvature of the thoracic spine, an **abnormal or exaggerated lateral curvature of the spine is called scoliosis.** Scoliosis is most common in children age 10 to 14 and more common in girls. It may require the use of a back brace for a period of time until the condition of vertebral stability improves. This deformity, if severe enough, may complicate cardiac and respiratory function. The effect of scoliosis is more obvious if it occurs in the lower vertebral column, where it may create a tilting of the pelvis with a resulting effect on the lower limbs, creating a "limp," or uneven walk. Procedures for diagnosing and determining the degree of scoliosis will be described later in the positioning section of this chapter.

Osteoarthritis: This is a type of arthritis characterized by degeneration of one or many joints. In the spine, changes may include bony sclerosis, degeneration of cartilage, and formation of osteophytes (bony outgrowths).

Osteoporosis: This is a condition characterized by loss of bone mass. Bone loss increases with age, immobilization, long-term steroid therapy, and menopause. The condition predisposes individuals to vertebral and hip fractures. Bone densitometry has become the gold standard for measuring the degree of osteoporosis as described in Chapter 23.

Scheuermann's disease: A relatively common disease of unknown origin that generally begins during adolescence, Scheuermann's disease results in the abnormal spinal curvature of kyphosis and scoliosis. It is more common in boys than girls. Most are mild cases that continue for several years, after which symptoms disappear but some spinal curvature remains.

Spondylitis: Spondylitis is the inflammation of the vertebrae.

Ankylosing spondylitis: This systemic illness of unknown etiology involves the spine and larger joints. It predominantly affects males ages 20 to 40 and results in pain and stiffness as a result of inflammation of the sacroiliac, intervertebral, and costovertebral joints, as well as paraspinal calcification, with ossification and ankylosis (union of bones) of the spinal joints. It may cause complete rigidity of the spine and thorax, usually first seen in sacroiliac joints.

SUMMARY OF PATHOLOGIC INDICATIONS

CONDITION OR DISEASE	MOST COMMON RADIOGRAPHIC EXAM	POSSIBLE RADIOGRAPHIC APPEARANCE	EXPOSURE FACTOR ADJUSTMENT*
Fractures			
Clay shoveler's fracture	Lateral and AP cervical, CT	Avulsion fracture of the spinous process of any vertebra C6-T1; may see "double spinous process sign" on AP radiograph because of displacement of avulsed fractured segment	None
Compression fracture	Lateral and AP of affected spine, CT	Wedge-shaped vertebral body from lateral perspective; irregular spacing from AP perspective	None
Hangman's fracture	Lateral cervical, CT	Fracture of the anterior C2 arch, usually also with anterior subluxation of C2 on C3	None
Jefferson fracture	AP open mouth C1-C2 image, CT	Bilateral offset or spreading of the lateral masses of C1 relative to the dens	None
Odontoid fracture	AP open mouth of C1-C2 and lateral cross-table, CT	Fracture line through base of dens, possibly extending into lateral masses or arches of C1	None
Teardrop burst fracture	Lateral cervical, CT	Comminuted vertebral body fragments avulsed from the anteroinferior border and fragments from the posterior vertebral body displaced into the spinal canal	None
Facets—unilateral subluxations and bilateral locks	Lateral cervical spine	Unilateral—"bow tie" deformity because the vertebra is rotated on its axis; bilateral—"jumped" deformity because the entire vertebra is located more anterior than it should be	None
Herniated nucleus pulposus (HNP)	AP and lateral of affected spine, CT, MRI	Possible narrowing in disk spacing between vertebrae and protrusion of disk into the spinal canal on CT or MRI	None
Kyphosis	Lateral thoracic spine, scoliosis series including erect PA/AP and lateral	Abnormal or exaggerated convex thoracic curvature	None
Lordosis	Lateral lumbar spine, scoliosis series including erect PA/AP and lateral	Normal concave lumbar curvature or abnormal or exaggerated lumbar curvature	None
Scoliosis	Erect AP/PA spine, scoliosis series including lateral bending	Abnormal or exaggerated lateral curvature of spine	None
Osteoarthritis	AP and lateral C and/or T spine	Degeneration of cartilage and formation of osteophytes (bony outgrowths)	None
Osteoporosis	DXA bone density exam of AP L spine and lateral hip	BMD (bone mineral density) loss	None or decrease (−) if severe
Scheuermann's disease	Scoliosis series	Mild kyphosis and/or scoliosis, most common involvement of thoracic spine	None
Spondylitis			
Ankylosing spondylitis	Sacroiliac joints, spinal series, nuclear medicine bone scan	Calcification with ossification (formation of bony ridges between vertebrae), creating stiffness and lack of joint mobility	None

*Depends on stage or severity of disease or condition.

9

Survey Information

Following are summaries of results of surveys conducted in years 1989, 1995, and 2000 to determine the most common standard or basic and special or optional projections/positions as performed in the United States and Canada

SUMMARY OF SURVEY RESULTS

Cervical spine: The three most common basic or routine cervical projections are the **AP, 15° to 20° cephalic angle** (99% U.S. and Canada), **AP open mouth** (98% U.S., 94% Canada), and **lateral** (98% U.S., 97% Canada).

The **anterior obliques** (68% U.S., 64% Canada) are slightly more common than the **posterior obliques** (62% U.S., 42% Canada). There is a significant difference in regions of the U.S. for the posterior versus anterior oblique. In the Eastern U.S., 75% do anterior obliques and 56% posterior obliques. In other U.S. regions the percentages were about the same for both obliques. This text recommends the anterior oblique because of its significantly lower thyroid dose (see p. 308). The **swimmer's lateral position** for C7 to T1 is becoming more common as part of the cervical routine in the U.S. (73% in 2000, 50% in 1995, and 59% in 1989).

The **AP** "wagging jaw" (Ottonello) continues as a special projection in the U.S. (36% in 2000, 31% in 1995, 10% in 1989). It is less common in Canada (only 15%).

Both the **AP dens** (Fuchs) and the **PA dens** (Judd) continue to be more common as specials in the U.S. (with 46% and 40%, respectively, in 2000, compared with only 33% and 25% in 1995). In Canada in 2000, they were much lower at 19% and 10%, respectively.

The **AP axial (pillar) vertebral arch** projection was added to the last two editions of this textbook because in the 2000 survey 39% in the U.S. and 24% in Canada indicated it as a special projection. This was very consistent in all regions of the U.S., varying only from 38% to 40%.

Thoracic spine: The lateral breathing technique is the most common lateral routine as indicated by 92% in U.S. and 88% in Canada. (It was 83% in the U.S. in 1995.)

The **posterior obliques** are slightly more common than anterior obliques in the U.S. (by 31% and 19%, respectively). The obliques are performed as special in Canada by only 8%. The text again recommends the anterior obliques because of significantly lower breast doses (see p. 318).

Standard and Special Operating Procedures

Protocols and operating procedures vary among facilities, depending on administrative structures, liabilities, and other factors. Radiographers should become familiar with the current standards of practice, protocols, and routine or basic and special projections for any facility in which they are working.

Certain basic and special projections for the cervical and thoracic spine are demonstrated and described on the following pages as suggested standard basic and special departmental routines or procedures.

BASIC PROJECTIONS

Standard or basic projections, also sometimes referred to as *routine projections* or *departmental routines,* are those projections commonly taken on average patients who are helpful and can cooperate in performing the procedure.

SPECIAL PROJECTIONS

Special projections are more common projections taken as extra or additional projections to better demonstrate certain pathologic conditions or specific body parts.

BASIC AND SPECIAL PROJECTIONS

Cervical Spine
BASIC
- AP open mouth (C1 and C2) 306
- AP axial 307
- Obliques 308
- Lateral 309
- Lateral, horizontal beam 310
- Swimmer's lateral (cervicothoracic) 311

Cervical Spine
SPECIAL
- Lateral hyperflexion and hyperextension 312
- AP (Fuchs method) 313 and PA (Judd method) 313
- AP "wagging jaw" (Ottonello method) 314
- AP axial (pillar) 315

Thoracic Spine
BASIC
- AP 316
- Lateral 317

SPECIAL
- Obliques 318

9

AP "OPEN MOUTH" PROJECTION—C1 AND C2: CERVICAL SPINE

Warning: Do **not** attempt any head or neck movement if cervical trauma is possible without first consulting with a physician who has reviewed a horizontal beam lateral radiograph.

Cervical Spine
BASIC
- **AP open mouth (C1 & C2)**
- **AP axial**
- **Obliques**
- **Lateral**
- **Swimmer's lateral**

Pathology Demonstrated

Pathology (particularly fractures) involving C1 and C2 and adjacent soft-tissue structures. Demonstrates odontoid and Jefferson fractures.

Technical Factors

- IR size—18 × 24 cm (8 × 10 inches), lengthwise
- Moving or stationary grid
- 75 ± 5 kV range
- Technique and dose:

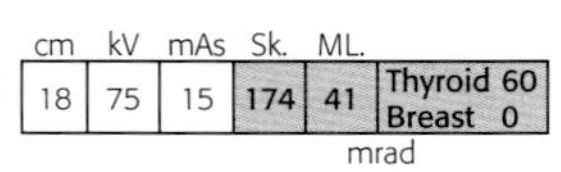

cm	kV	mAs	Sk.	ML.	
18	75	15	174	41	Thyroid 60 Breast 0

mrad

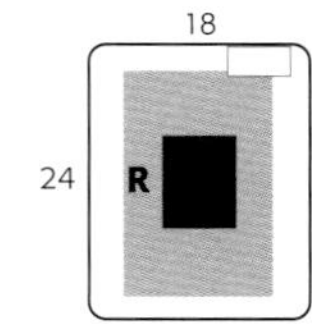

Patient Position Position patient in the supine or erect position with arms by sides. Place head on table surface, providing immobilization if needed.

Part Position

- Align midsagittal plane to CR and midline of table.
- Adjust head so that, with mouth open, a line from **lower margin of upper incisors to the base of the skull** (mastoid tips) **is perpendicular** to table and/or IR, or angle the CR accordingly.
- Ensure that **no rotation** of the head or thorax exists.
- Ensure that **mouth is wide open** during exposure. (Do this as the last step, and work quickly because it is difficult to maintain this position.)

Central Ray

- CR **perpendicular to IR,** directed through **center of open mouth**
- Cassette centered to CR
- Minimum SID of 40 inches (100 cm)

Collimation Close four-sided collimation to area of interest, approximately 4 × 4 inches or 10 × 10 cm

Respiration Suspend respiration.

Note: Make sure that when patient is instructed to open mouth that only the lower jaw moves. Instruct the patient to keep the tongue in the lower jaw to prevent its shadow from superimposing the atlas and axis.

If the upper dens cannot be demonstrated, see Fuchs or Judd method (p. 313).

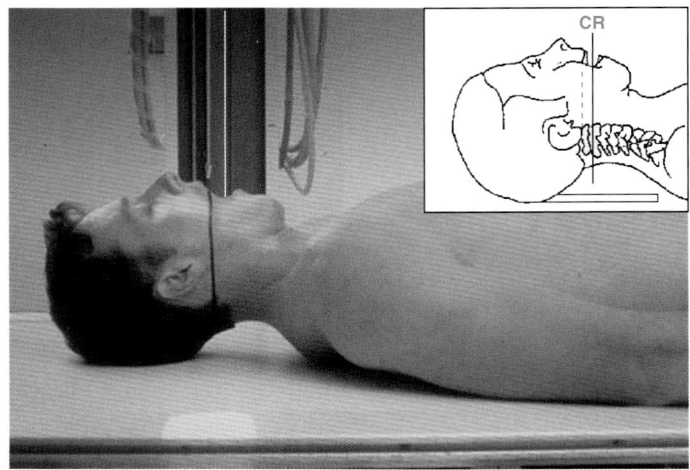

Fig. 9-46. AP open mouth—C1 to C2.

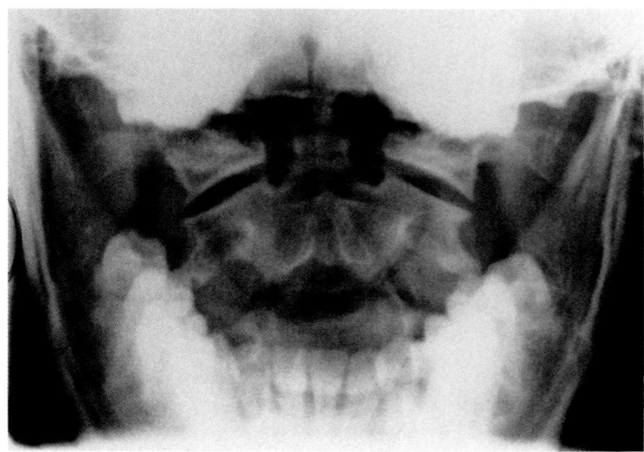

Fig. 9-47. AP open mouth—C1 to C2.

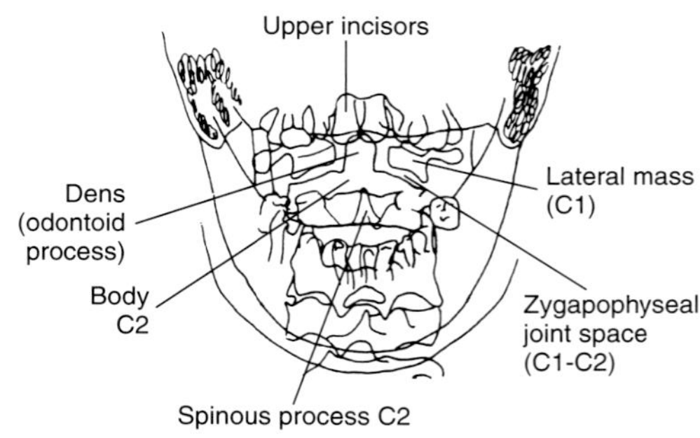

Fig. 9-48. AP open mouth—C1 to C2.

Radiographic Criteria

Structures Shown: • Dens (odontoid process) and vertebral body of C2, lateral masses of C1, and zygapophyseal joints between C1 and C2 should be clearly demonstrated through the open mouth.

Position: • Optimal flexion/extension of the neck, indicated by superimposition of the lower margin of the **upper incisors** on the **base of the skull.** Neither the teeth nor the skull base should superimpose the dens. • If the teeth are superimposed on the upper dens, reposition by slight hyperextension of the neck or angle the CR slightly cephalic • If the base of the skull is superimposed on the upper dens, reposition by slight hyperflexion of the neck or angle the CR slightly caudal (the base of the skull and/or the upper incisors will be projected about 1inch (2.5 cm) for every 5 degrees of caudal angulation). • **No rotation** is evidenced by equal distances from lateral masses and/or transverse processes of C1 to condyles of mandible, and by center alignment of spinous process of C2. Rotation can imitate pathology by causing unequal spaces between lateral masses and dens.

Collimation and CR: • Approximately 4 × 4 inches (10 × 10 cm) field with dens at the center of the collimation field.

Exposure Criteria: • Optimal exposure should demonstrate both bone and soft-tissue density. • Bony margins and trabecular marking should appear sharp, indicating no motion.

AP AXIAL PROJECTION: CERVICAL SPINE

Cervical Spine
BASIC
- AP open mouth (C1 & C2)
- AP axial
- Obliques
- Lateral
- Swimmer's lateral

Pathology Demonstrated

Pathology involving the mid- and lower cervical spine (C3 to C7). Demonstrates the clay shoveler's fracture, compression fractures, and herniated nucleus pulposus (HNP).

Technical Factors

- IR size—18 × 24 cm (8 × 10 inches), lengthwise
- Moving or stationary grid
- 75 ± 5 kV range
- Technique and dose:

cm	kV	mAs	Sk.	ML.	mrad
11	75	10	96	42	Thyroid 53 Breast 1

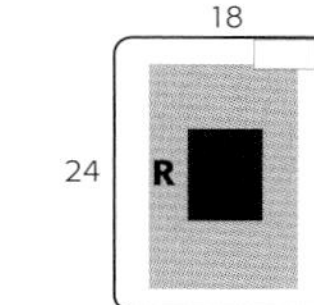

Patient Position Position patient in the supine or erect position, with arms by sides.

Part Position

- Align midsagittal plane to CR and midline of table and/or IR.
- Adjust head so that a line from the occlusal plane (chewing surface of teeth) to the base of the skull (mastoid tips) is perpendicular to table and/or IR. Line from tip of mandible to base of skull should be **parallel to angled CR.**
- Ensure that **no rotation** of the head or thorax exists.

Central Ray

- CR angled **15° to 20° cephalad,** to enter at the level of the **lower margin of thyroid cartilage** to pass through **C4** (see Note)
- Cassette centered to CR
- Minimum SID of 40 inches (100 cm)

Collimation Apply close lateral collimation to soft-tissue edges of the neck. Include as much of the spine lengthwise as possible to the edge of the IR.

Respiration Suspend respiration. Patient should not swallow during exposure.

Note: Cephalad angulation directs the beam between the overlapping cervical vertebral bodies to better demonstrate the intervertebral disk spaces. Angle the CR 15° when the patient is supine or if there is less lordotic curvature. Angle the CR 20° when the patient is erect or there is more lordotic curvature evident.

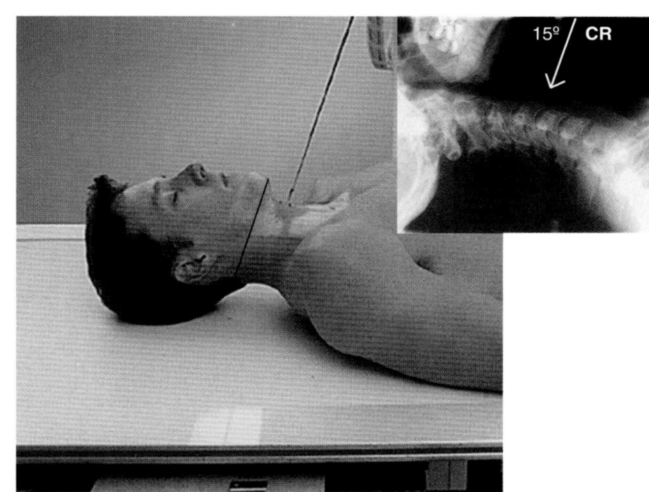

Fig. 9-49. AP supine, 15° cephalad angle. (Inset demonstrates 15° CR, parallel to plane of intervertebral disk spaces, centered to C4.)

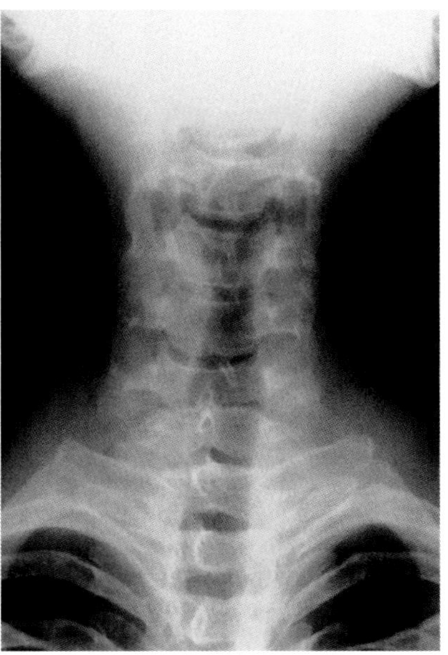

Fig. 9-50. AP, 15° cephalad angle.

Radiographic Criteria

Structures Shown: • C3 to T2 or T3 vertebral bodies, space between pedicles and intervertebral disk spaces clearly seen.

Position: • **No rotation:** Spinous processes and sternoclavicular joints (if visible) should be equidistant from the spinal column lateral borders. • The mandible and base of the skull will be superimposed over the first two cervical vertebrae.

Collimation and CR: • Close lateral collimation to soft-tissue margins of the neck, upper and lower collimation borders to IR margins. • Center of collimation field (CR) at C4 • Correct CR angle indicated by **open intervertebral disk spaces.**

Exposure Criteria: • Optimal exposure should demonstrate both bone and soft-tissue density. • Bony margins and trabecular marking should appear sharp, indicating no motion.

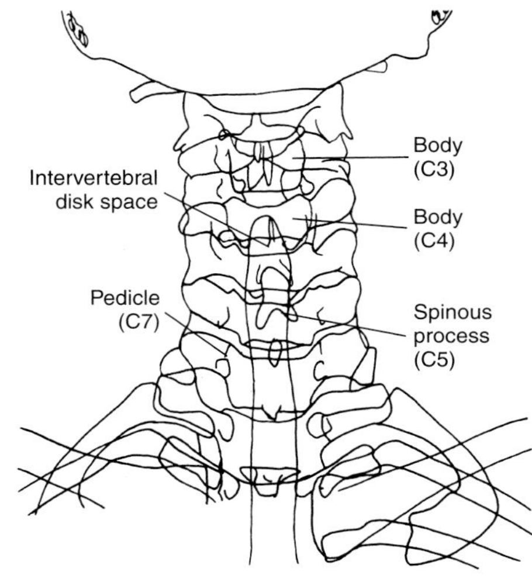

Fig. 9-51. AP, 15° cephalad angle.

9

ANTERIOR AND POSTERIOR OBLIQUE POSITIONS: CERVICAL SPINE

Warning: Do **not** attempt any head or neck movement if cervical trauma is possible without first consulting a physician who has reviewed a horizontal beam lateral radiograph (see p. 310).

Pathology Demonstrated

Pathology involving the cervical spine and adjacent soft-tissue structures. Stenosis involving the intervertebral foramen is demonstrated.

Both right and left obliques should be taken for comparison purposes. **Anterior obliques** are preferred because of reduced thyroid doses.

Cervical Spine
BASIC
- AP open mouth (C1 & C2)
- AP axial
- Obliques
- Lateral
- Swimmer's lateral

Technical Factors

- IR size—18 × 24 cm (8 × 10 inches), lengthwise
- Moving or stationary grid (optional because of air-gap)
- 75 ± 5 kV range
- Technique and dose per exposure: –Ant. obl. –Post. obl.

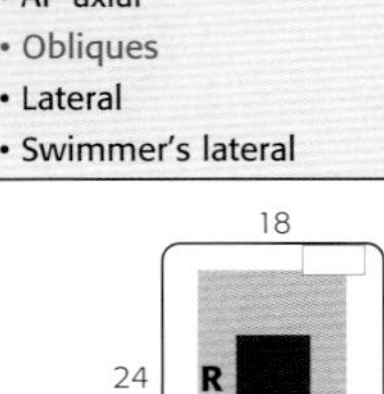

	cm	kV	mAs	Sk.	ML.	Dose (mrad)
Ant. obl.	11	75	10	129	50	Thyroid 5, Breast 0
Post. obl.	11	75	10	129	50	Thyroid 69, Breast 4

Patient Position The erect position is preferred (sitting or standing), but recumbent is possible if patient's condition requires this.

Part Position

- Center spine to **CR** and **midline** of table and/or IR.
- Place patient's arms at side; if patient is recumbent, place arms as needed to help maintain position.
- Rotate body and head 45°. (Use protractor or other angle gauge as needed to ensure 45° angle.) See Note about head rotation.
- Extend chin to prevent mandible from superimposing vertebrae. Elevating chin too much will superimpose base of skull over C1.

Central Ray

Anterior obliques:

- **15° caudad** to **C4** (level of upper margin of thyroid cartilage)

Posterior obliques:

- **15° cephalad** to **C4** (to lower thyroid cartilage)
- Cassette centered to projected CR
  SID of 60 to 72 inches (150 to 180 cm)

Collimation Collimate lateral borders to soft-tissue borders of neck and upper and lower margins to IR borders.

Respiration Patient should suspend respiration.

Note: Departmental option: The head may be turned toward IR to a near lateral position. This, however, results in some rotation of upper vertebrae but may help in preventing superimposition of vertebrae by mandible.

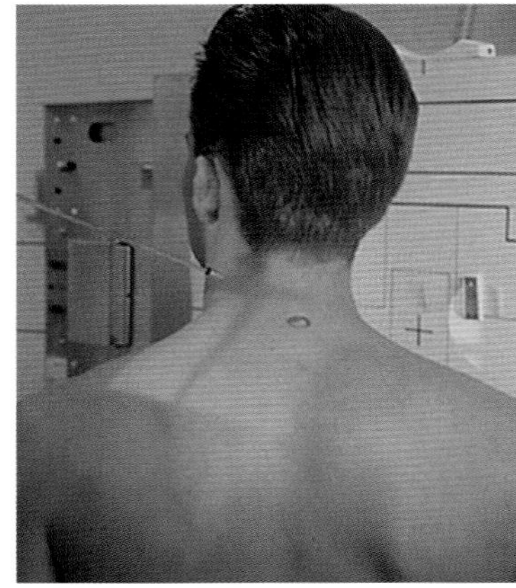

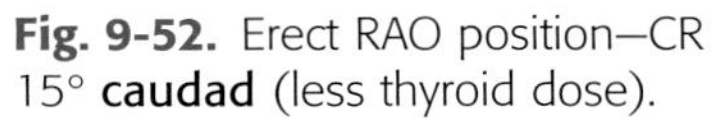

Fig. 9-52. Erect RAO position—CR 15° **caudad** (less thyroid dose).

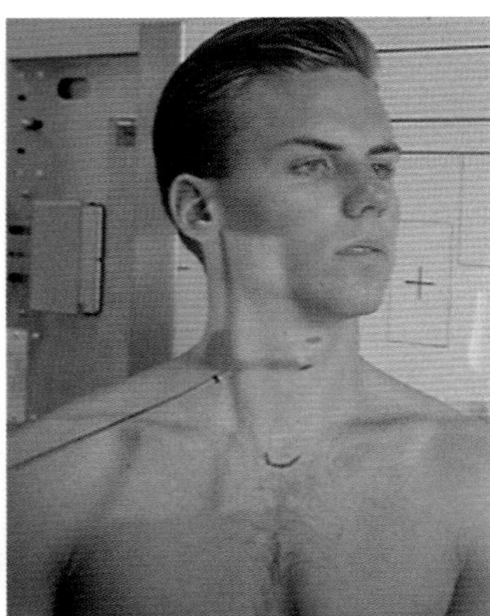

Fig. 9-53. Optional AP obliques, LPO—CR 15° **cephalad.**

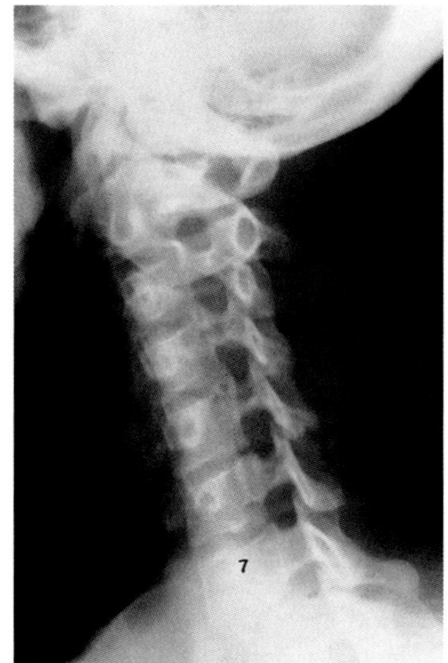

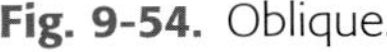

Fig. 9-54. Oblique.

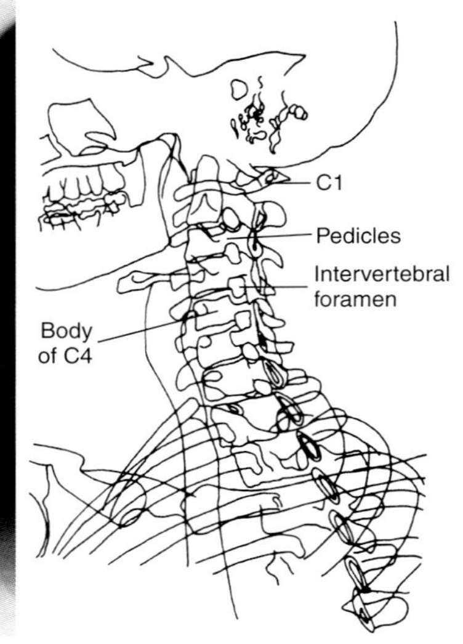

Fig. 9-55. Oblique.

Radiographic Criteria

Structures Shown: • **Anterior** obliques: intervertebral foramina and pedicles on the side of the patient **closest to IR.** • **Posterior** obliques: intervertebral foramina and pedicles on the side of the patient **farthest from the IR.**

Position: • To indicate correct rotation and CR angulation, intervertebral disk spaces and intervertebral foramina of interest (C2 through C7) should be open, and the pedicles of interest should be demonstrated in full profile. (Over or under rotation will narrow and partially obscure the intervertebral foramina.) • On-end pedicles aligned at the midline of the cervical body and visualization of zygapophyseal joints indicate over rotation. • Obscured intervertebral foramina and pedicles indicate under rotation • With correct elevation of the chin, the rami of the mandible should not superimpose the upper cervical vertebrae and the base of the skull should not superimpose C1.

Collimation and CR: • Apply close lateral collimation to soft-tissue edges of the neck. Include as much of the spine lengthwise as possible to the edge of the IR. • Correct CR angle will demonstrate open intervertebral foramina.

Exposure Criteria: • Optimal exposure should demonstrate soft tissue, as well as proper bone density of the entire cervical vertebrae. • Bony margins and trabecular marking should appear sharp, indicating no motion.

LATERAL POSITION: CERVICAL SPINE

Trauma patients: See lateral horizontal beam on next page.

Cervical Spine
BASIC
• AP open mouth (C1 & C2)
• AP axial
• Obliques
• Lateral
• Swimmer's lateral

Pathology Demonstrated
Pathology involving the cervical spine and adjacent soft-tissue structures. Spondylosis and osteoarthritis are demonstrated.

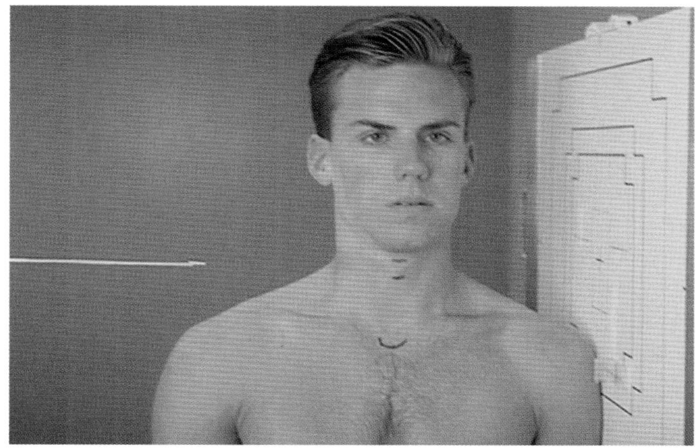

Fig. 9-56. Erect left lateral.

Technical Factors

- IR size—18 × 24 cm (8 × 10 inches), lengthwise
- Moving or stationary grid (optional because of air-gap)
- 75 ± 5 kV range
- Technique and dose at (72 inches):

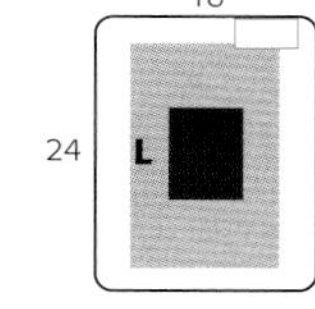

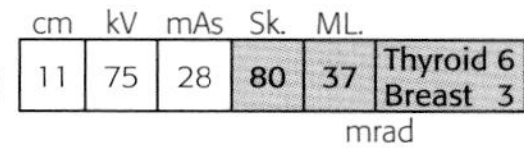

cm	kV	mAs	Sk.	ML.	
11	75	28	80	37	Thyroid 6 Breast 3
				mrad	

Patient Position Position patient in the erect lateral position, either sitting or standing with shoulder against vertical cassette holder.

Part Position

- Align midcoronal plane to CR and midline of table and/or IR.
- Centering IR to CR should place top of IR about 1 inch (2.5 cm) above EAM.
- Depress shoulders (for equal weights to both arms, see Note 1).
- Ask patient to **relax** and **drop shoulders down and forward as far as possible.** (Do this as the last step before exposure because this position is difficult to maintain.)
- Extend chin forward slightly (to prevent superimposition of the mandible on upper vertebrae).

Central Ray

- CR **perpendicular** to IR, directed horizontally to **C4** (level of upper margin of thyroid cartilage)
- Cassette centered to CR.
- SID of 60 to 72 inches (150 to 180 cm) (see Note 2)

Respiration Suspend respiration on **full expiration** (for maximum shoulder depression).

Collimation Perform four-sided collimation to area of interest. Collimate to near upper and lower IR borders.

Note 1: Adding 5- to 10-lb weights to each arm may help in pulling down shoulders.

Note 2: Long (72 inches or 180 cm) SID compensates for increased OID and provides for less magnification.

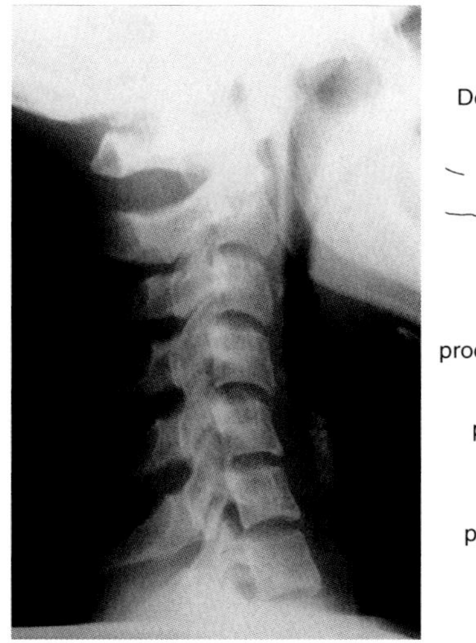

Fig. 9-57. Lateral.

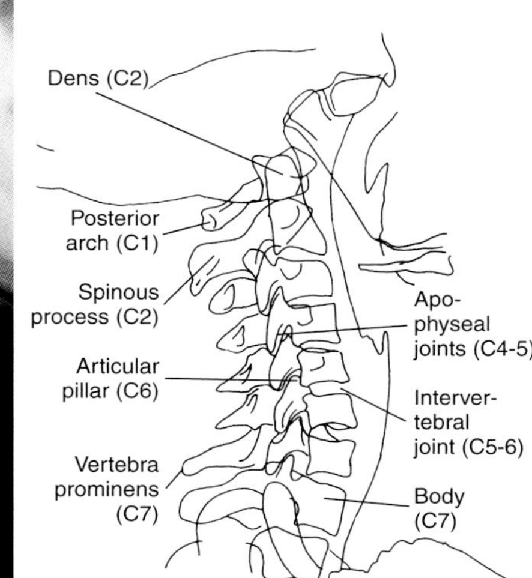

Fig. 9-58. Lateral.

Radiographic Criteria

Structures Shown: • Cervical vertebral bodies, intervertebral joint spaces, articular pillars, spinous processes, and zygapophyseal joints.

Position: • Depress shoulders or use weights so that C1 through C7 are clearly seen. If the junction of C7 to T1 is not demonstrated on the routine lateral projection, additional images such as the swimmer's lateral method radiograph should be obtained. • The chin is elevated sufficiently so the rami of the mandible do not superimpose C1 to C2. • **No rotation** of head is indicated by superimposition of both rami of the mandible. • Lower cervical rotation is evidenced by lack of superimposition of R and L side apophyseal joints, and posterior borders of bodies are not superimposed.

Collimation and CR: • Apply close lateral collimation to soft-tissue edges of the neck. • Adjust upper and lower collimation to IR borders. • Center of collimation field (CR) should be to C4 region.

Exposure Criteria: • Optimal exposure should demonstrate soft tissue, including margins of the air column, as well as proper bone density of the entire cervical vertebrae. • Bone margins and trabecular marking should appear sharp, indicating no motion.

LATERAL POSITION, HORIZONTAL BEAM: CERVICAL SPINE (TRAUMA PATIENT)

Warning: When radiographing trauma patients, do **not** remove cervical collar and do not move head or neck until a physician has evaluated this radiograph for fractures, subluxations, or evidence of cervical instability.

Cervical Spine (Trauma Patient)
BASIC
- Lateral (horizontal beam)

Pathology Demonstrated

Pathology involving the cervical spine is demonstrated, including clay shoveler's fracture, compression fracture, hangman's fracture, odontoid fracture, teardrop burst fracture, and subluxation.

Technical Factors

- IR size—18 × 24 cm (8 × 10 inches) or —24 × 30 cm (10 × 12 inches) lengthwise
- Nongrid cassette or grid (see Note 1)
- 75 ± 5 kV range with grid
- Technique and dose:

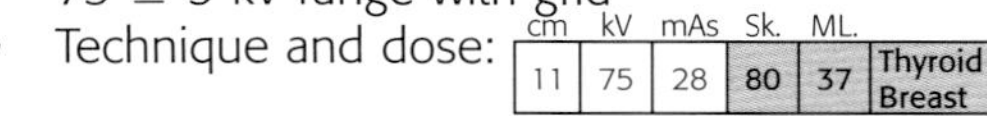

cm	kV	mAs	Sk.	ML.	
11	75	28	80	37	Thyroid 6 Breast 3

mrad

Patient Position Position patient in the supine position on stretcher or radiographic table.

Part Position

- Do **not** manipulate or move head or neck.
- Support cassette vertically against shoulder, or place stretcher next to vertical grid device.
- Center cassette to CR, which should place top of cassette about 1 to 2 inches (3 to 5 cm) above EAM.
- Depress shoulders (see Note 2).

Central Ray

- CR **perpendicular** to IR, directed horizontally to **C4** (level of upper margin of thyroid cartilage)
- SID of 60 to 72 inches (150 to 180 cm) (see Note 3)

Collimation Four-sided collimation to neck tissue borders and to include maximum proximal and distal spine regions

Respiration Suspend respiration on full **expiration** (this will help depress shoulders).

Note 1: Generally, a nongrid cassette can be used for smaller or average patients because of the increased OID and the resultant air-gap effect.

Note 2: Traction on arms will help depress shoulders but should only be done by a qualified assistant and/or with the consent or assistance of a physician.

Note 3: Longer SID results in less magnification with increased image sharpness.

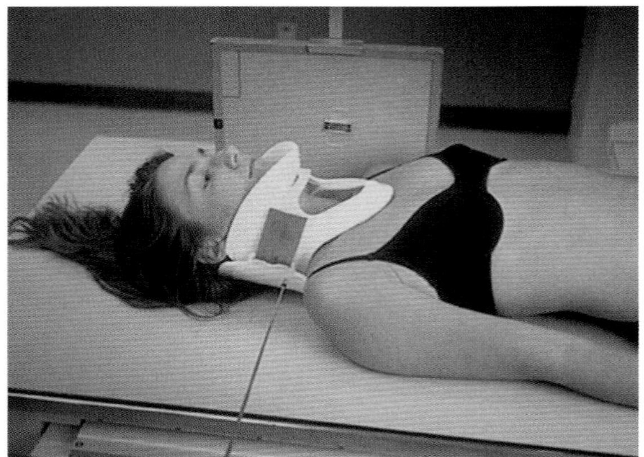

Fig. 9-59. Left lateral—horizontal beam.

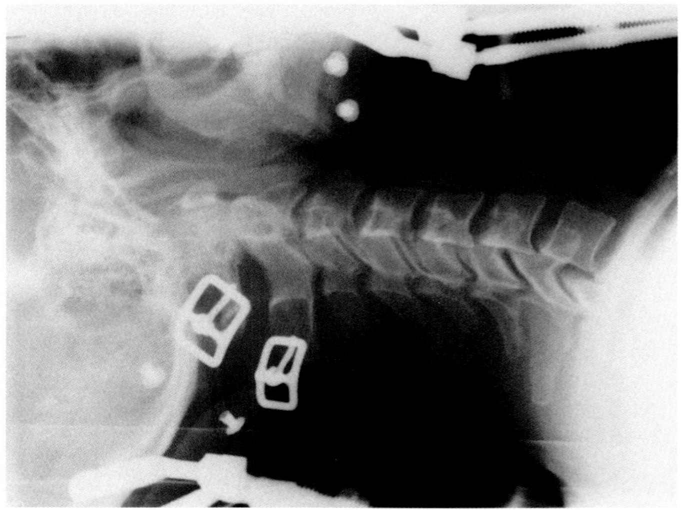

Fig. 9-60. Lateral—horizontal beam.

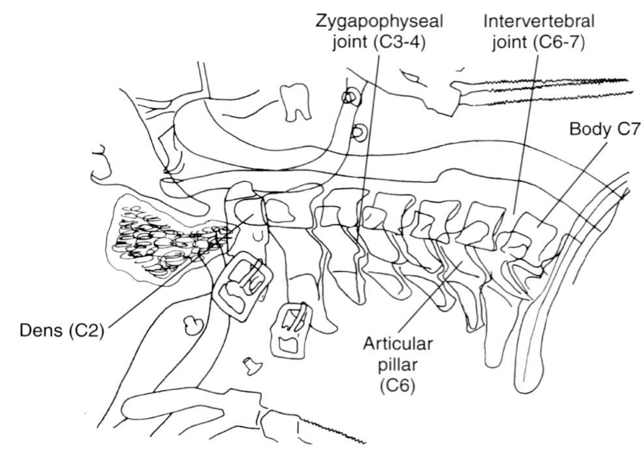

Fig. 9-61. Lateral—horizontal beam.

9

Radiographic Criteria

Structures Shown: • Cervical vertebral bodies, intervertebral joint spaces, articular pillars, spinous processes, and zygapophyseal joints.

Position: • C1 through C7 should be demonstrated. • If the junction of C7 to T1 is not demonstrated, additional images, such as the swimmer's lateral method radiograph, should be obtained. • The right and left articular pillars and zygapophyseal joints should be superimposed for each vertebra. • The bodies will be free of superimposition of the articular pillars and the spinous process will be seen in profile.

Collimation and CR: • Apply close lateral collimation to soft-tissue edges of the neck. • Include as much of the spine lengthwise as possible to the edge of the IR.

Exposure Criteria: • Optimal exposure should demonstrate soft tissue, as well as proper bone density of all aspects of the cervical vertebrae. • Bony margins and trabecular marking should appear sharp, indicating no motion.

CERVICOTHORACIC (SWIMMER'S) LATERAL POSITION: CERVICAL SPINE

Twining Method for C4-T3 Region

Cervical Spine
BASIC
- AP open mouth (C1 & C2)
- AP axial
- Obliques
- Lateral
- Swimmer's lateral

Pathology Demonstrated

Pathology involving the inferior cervical spine, superior thoracic spine, and adjacent soft-tissue structures. Various fractures (including compression fractures) and subluxation are demonstrated.

This is a good projection when C7 to T1 is not visualized on the lateral cervical spine or when the upper thoracic vertebrae are of special interest on a lateral thoracic spine.

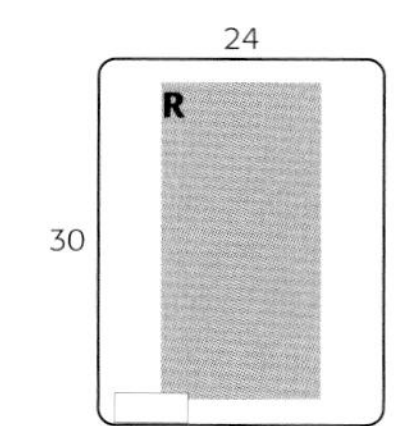

Technical Factors

- IR size—24 × 30 cm (10 × 12 inches), lengthwise
- Moving or stationary grid
- 80 ± 5 kV range (increase of 5 to 10 kV from lateral cervical)
- Technique and dose at 72 inches:

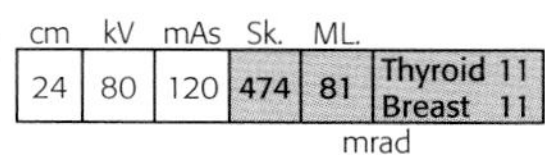

cm	kV	mAs	Sk.	ML.	mrad
24	80	120	474	81	Thyroid 11 Breast 11

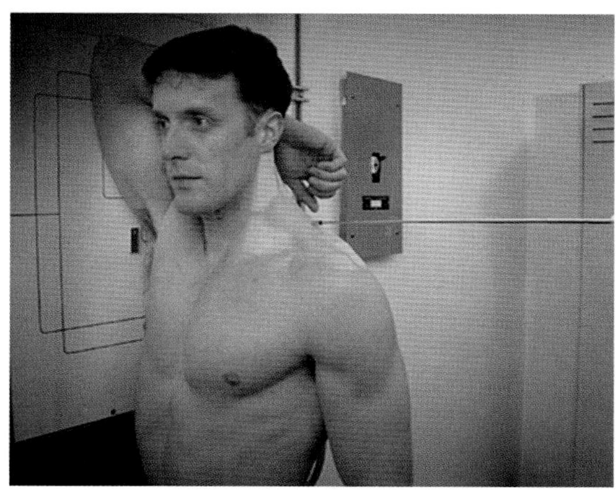

Fig. 9-62. Swimmer's lateral.

Patient Position Erect position is preferred (sitting or standing), but the radiograph may be done in the recumbent position if patient's condition requires this.

Part Position

- Align midcoronal plane to CR and midline of table or cassette holder.
- Place patient's arm and shoulder nearest IR up, flexing elbow and resting forearm on head for support.
- Position arm and shoulder away from IR, down and slightly anterior, to place humeral head anterior to vertebrae.
- Maintain thorax and head in as true a lateral position as possible.

Central Ray

- CR **perpendicular** to IR (see Note)
- CR centered to **T1,** which is approximately 1 inch (2.5 cm) above level of jugular notch anteriorly and at level of vertebra prominens posteriorly
- Cassette centered to CR
- SID of 60 to 72 inches (150 to 180 cm)

Collimation Close four-sided collimation to area of interest (field about 4 × 6 inches, or 10 × 15 cm)

Respiration Suspend breathing on full **expiration.**

Note: A slight caudad angulation of 3° to 5° may be necessary to help separate the two shoulders, especially on a patient with limited flexibility who cannot sufficiently depress the shoulder away from the IR.

Optional breathing technique: If patient can cooperate and remain immobilized, a low mA and 3- or 4-second exposure time can be used, with patient breathing short, even breaths during the exposure to blur out overlying lung structures.

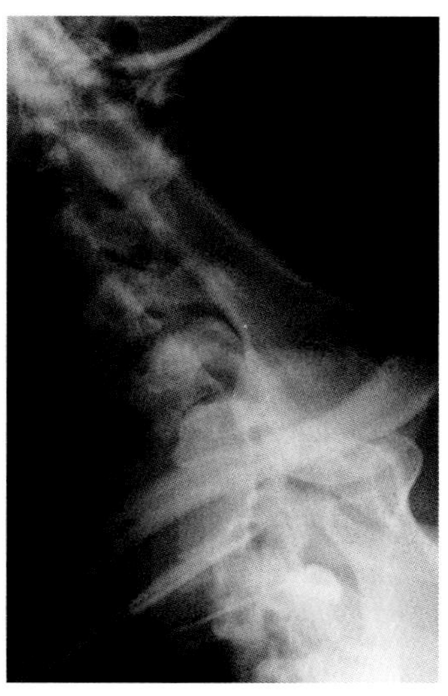

Fig. 9-63. Swimmer's lateral.

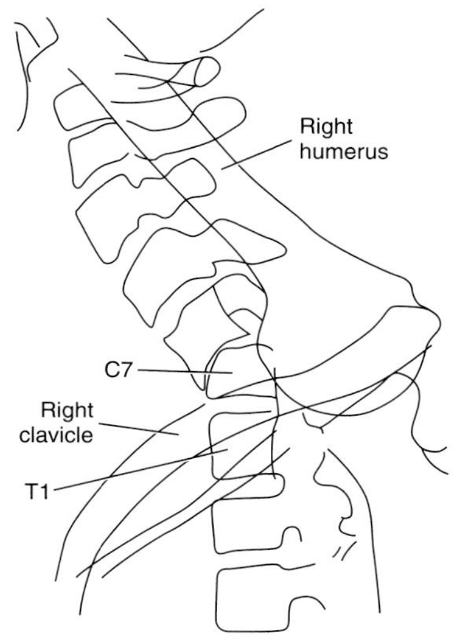

Fig. 9-64. Swimmer's lateral.

9

Radiographic Criteria

Structures Shown: • Vertebral bodies and intervertebral disk spaces of C4 to T3 are shown. • The humeral head and arm farthest from the IR are magnified and should appear distal to T4 or T5 (if visible).

Position: • Vertebral rotation should appear to be minimal. • The humeral heads should be separated vertically. The humeral head and arm closest to the IR are placed superiorly and thus superimpose the lower cervical to provide a more uniform density of the lower cervical and upper thoracic vertebrae.

Collimation and CR: • Apply close four-sided collimation to area of interest. • The center of collimation field (CR) should be to T1 region.

Exposure Criteria: • Optimal exposure should clearly visualize outlines of vertebrae, including intervertebral spaces of C4 to T3 through shoulder structures without overpenetrating upper vertebrae. • Bony margins and trabecular marking should appear sharp, indicating no motion.

LATERAL POSITIONS—HYPERFLEXION AND HYPEREXTENSION: CERVICAL SPINE

Warning: **Never** attempt these positions on trauma patient before cervical fractures have been ruled out.

Cervical Spine
SPECIAL
• Lateral–hyperflexion and hyperextension

Pathology Demonstrated

Functional study to demonstrate anteroposterior vertebral mobility. Frequently performed to rule out "whiplash" type of injuries or to follow up after spinal fusion surgery.

Technical Factors

- IR size—24 × 30 cm (10 ×12 inches), lengthwise
- Moving or stationary grid (optional)
- 75 ± 5 kV range (with grid)
- Technique and dose (per projection) at 72 inches:

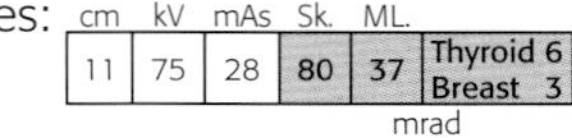

cm	kV	mAs	Sk.	ML.	mrad
11	75	28	80	37	Thyroid 6 Breast 3

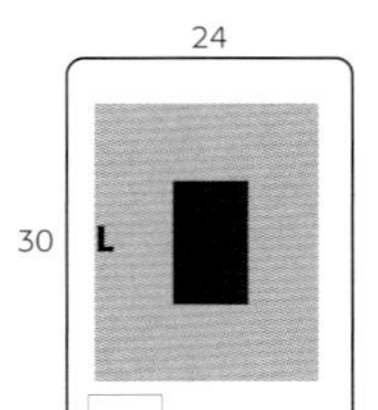

Patient Position Erect lateral, either sitting or standing, arms at sides.

Part Position

- Align midcoronal plane of vertebrae to CR and midline of IR.
- Ensure a **true lateral position,** no rotation of pelvis, shoulders, or head.
- **Relax** and **depress shoulders** as far as possible (weights on each arm may be used).
- For **hyperflexion:** Chin should be depressed until it touches the chest or as much as patient can tolerate (do not allow patient to move forward to ensure that entire cervical is included on IR).
- For **hyperextension:** Chin should be raised and head leaned back as much as possible (do not allow patient to move backward to ensure that entire cervical is included on IR).

Central Ray

- CR **perpendicular** to IR, directed horizontally to area of **C4** (level of upper margin of thyroid cartilage with head in neutral position)
- SID of 60 to 72 inches (150 to 180 cm)
- Height of cassette centered to level of CR (top of cassette about 2 inches or 5 cm above level of EAM)

Collimation Perform four-sided collimation to area of interest. Ensure that both upper and lower cervical vertebrae are included, especially on hyperflexion projection.

Respiration Suspend respiration on full expiration.

Note: These are uncomfortable for patient; do not keep in these positions longer than necessary.

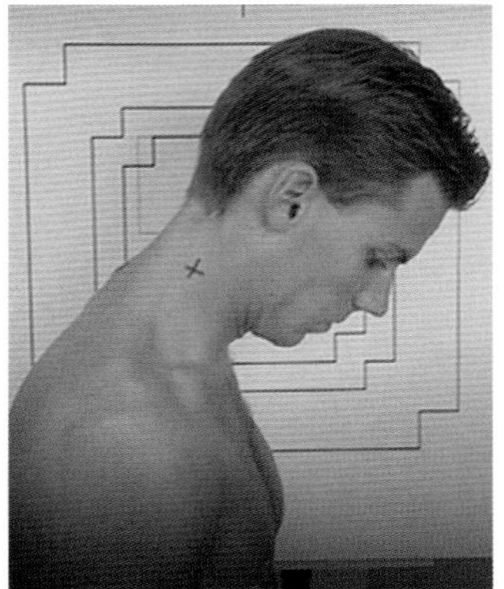

Fig. 9-65. Hyperflexion.

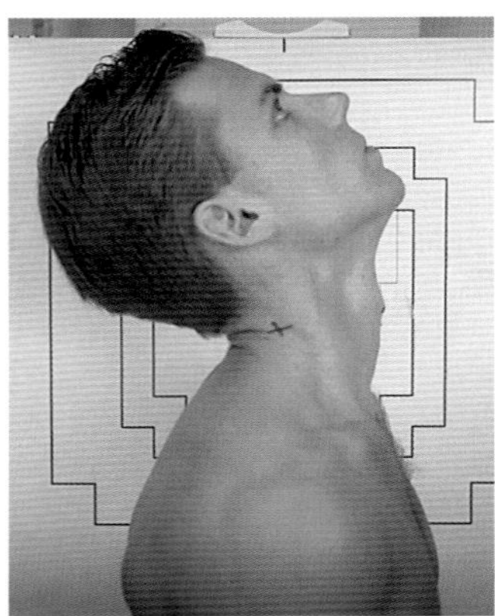

Fig. 9-66. Hyperextension.

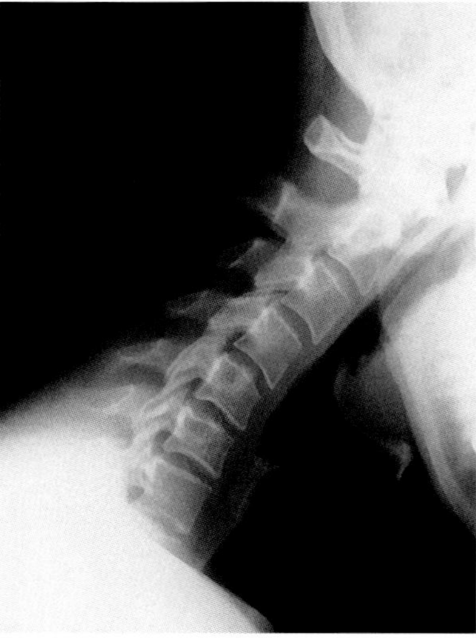

Fig. 9-67. Hyperflexion.

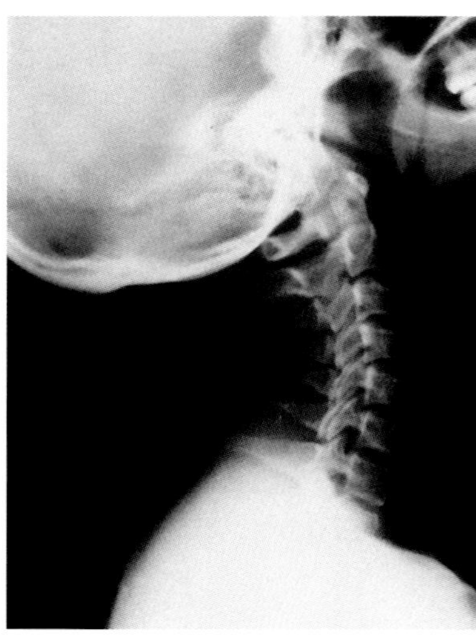

Fig. 9-68. Hyperextension.

Radiographic Criteria

Structures Shown: • Flexion and extension images demonstrate natural spinal curvature, range of spinal motion, and ligament stability. • C1 through C7 should be included on IR. C7, however, may not be completely visualized on some patients.

Position: • No rotation of head is indicated by superimposition of rami of mandible. • For **hyperflexion:** Spinous processes should be well separated. • For **hyperextension:** Spinous processes should be in close proximity.

Collimation and CR: • Apply close lateral collimation to soft-tissue edges of the neck. Include as much of the spine lengthwise as possible to the upper and lower IR margins. • Center of collimation field (CR) should be to region of C4.

Exposure Criteria: • Optimal exposure should demonstrate soft tissue, as well as proper bone density of entire cervical vertebrae. • Bony margins and trabecular markings should appear sharp, indicating no motion.

AP OR PA PROJECTION FOR C1-2 (DENS): CERVICAL SPINE

Fuchs Method (AP) or Judd Method (PA)

Warning: Do **not** attempt this head or neck movement if cervical trauma is possible without first consulting a physician who has reviewed a lateral cervical radiograph.

One of these projections is useful for demonstrating the superior portion of the dens when this area is not well visualized on the AP open mouth cervical spine projection.

Cervical Spine
SPECIAL
• Lateral–hyperflexion and hyperextension
• AP (Fuchs method)
• PA (Judd method)

Pathology Demonstrated

Pathology involving the dens and surrounding bony structures of the C1 ring is demonstrated.

Technical Factors

- IR size—18 × 24 cm (8 × 10 inches), crosswise
- Moving or stationary grid
- 75 ± 5 kV range
- Technique and dose—AP:
- Technique and dose—PA:

24 × 18, R; No AEC because of small field

	cm	kV	mAs	Sk.	ML.	Thyroid	Breast
AP	11	75	15	237	51	6	0
PA	11	75	15	173	40	3	0

mrad

Patient and Part Position

- Supine (AP) or prone (PA) with midsagittal plane aligned to CR and midline of table

AP (Fuchs method):

- Elevate chin as needed to bring **MML** (mentomeatal line) **near perpendicular to tabletop** (adjust CR angle as needed to be parallel to MML).
- Ensure that **no rotation** of head exists (angles of mandible equi-distant to tabletop).
- Center IR to projected CR.
- CR is **parallel to MML,** directed to **inferior tip of mandible.**

PA (Judd method):

- This is a reverse position to the AP. Chin is resting on tabletop and is extended to bring MML near perpendicular to table (may adjust CR as needed to be parallel to MML).
- Ensure that **no rotation of head** exists and that IR is centered to projected CR.
- Ensure that CR is **parallel to MML,** through midoccipital bone, about 1 inch (2.5 cm) inferoposterior to mastoid tips and angles of mandible.

Collimation Close four-sided collimation to C1 to C2 region

Respiration Suspend respiration on full expiration.

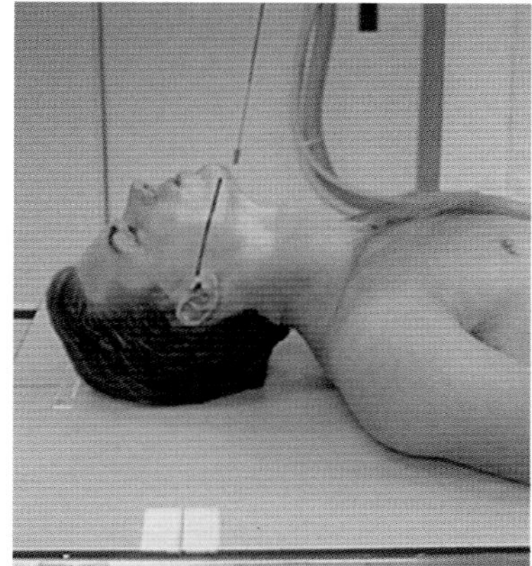

Fig. 9-69. AP—Fuchs method.

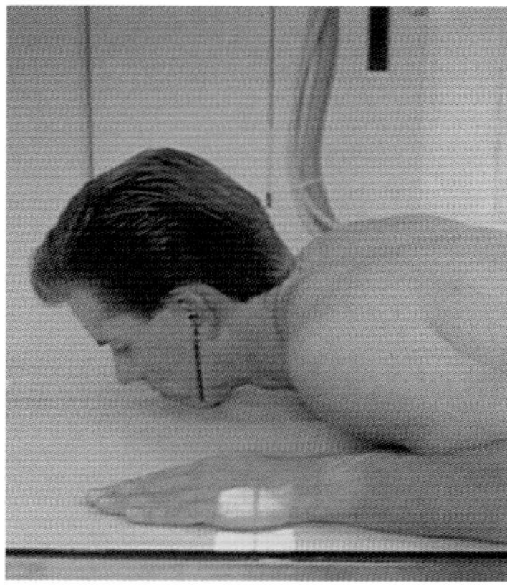

Fig. 9-70. PA—Judd method (less thyroid dose).

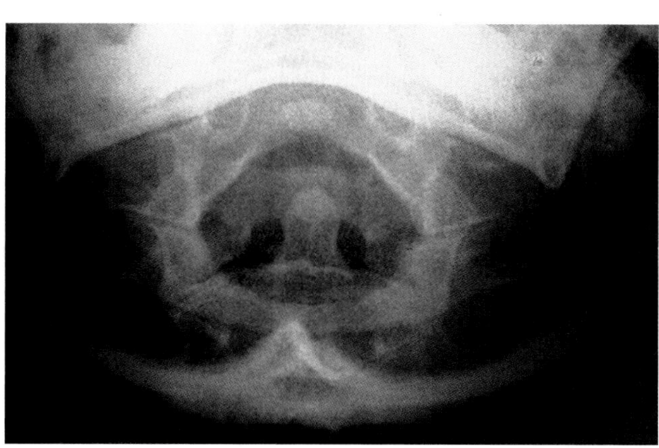

Fig. 9-71. AP or PA dens.

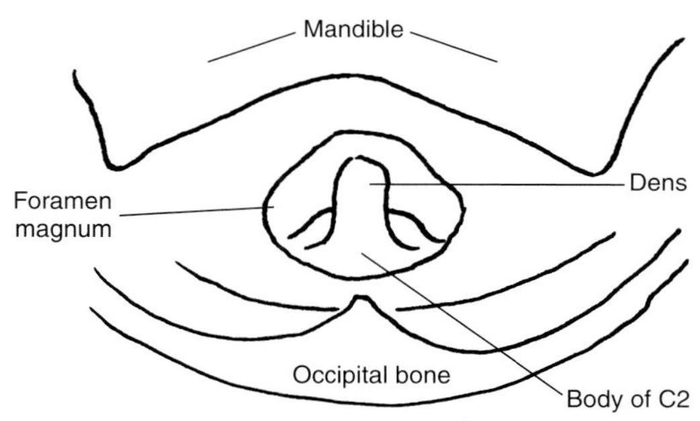

Fig. 9-72. AP or PA for C1 to C2, dens.

Radiographic Criteria

Structures Shown: • Demonstrates the dens (odontoid process) and other structures of C1 to C2 within the foramen magnum.

Position: • Dens process should be centered within the foramen magnum. • **No rotation:** This can be evaluated by the symmetric appearance of the mandible arched over the foramen magnum. • **Correct extension** of head and neck can be evaluated by checking that the tip of the mandible clears the superior portion of the dens and the foramen magnum.

Collimation and CR: • Close four-sided collimation to C1 to C2 region; center of collimation field (CR) to mid-dens region

Exposure Criteria: • Optimal exposure with no motion will demonstrate clear and sharp outline of dens and other structures of C1 and C2 within foramen magnum.

9

AP "WAGGING JAW" PROJECTION: CERVICAL SPINE

Ottonello Method

Warning: Do **not** attempt this head or neck movement if cervical trauma is possible without first consulting a physician who has reviewed a lateral cervical radiograph.

Cervical Spine
SPECIAL
- **Lateral–hyperflexion and hyperextension**
- **AP (Fuchs method), PA (Judd method)**
- AP moving or "wagging jaw" (Ottonello method)

Pathology Demonstrated

Pathology involving the dens and surrounding bony structures of the C1 ring, as well as the entire cervical column, is demonstrated.

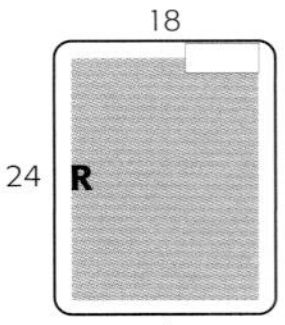

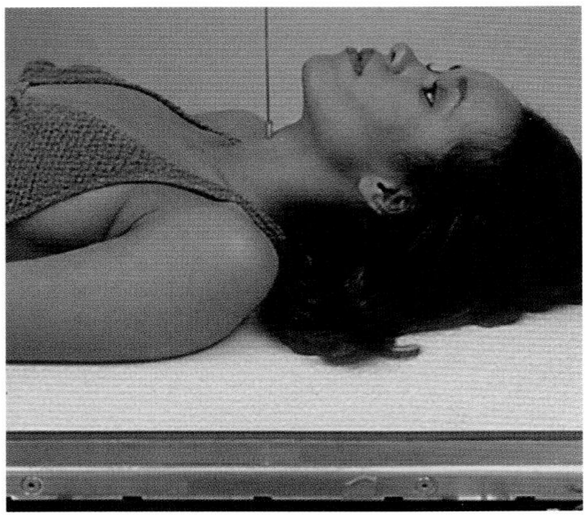

Fig. 9-73. Position for AP "wagging jaw."

Technical Factors

- IR size—18 × 24 cm (8 × 10 inches), lengthwise.
- Moving or stationary grid
- Low mA and long (>2 sec) exposure time
- 75 ± 5 kV range
- Technique and dose:

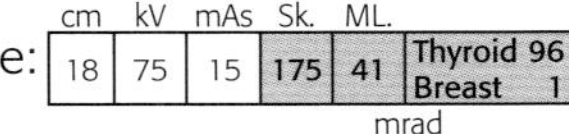

cm	kV	mAs	Sk.	ML.	
18	75	15	175	41	Thyroid 96 Breast 1

mrad

18 × 24 R

No AEC because of long exposure

Patient Position Position patient in the supine position with arms at side and head on table surface, providing immobilization if needed.

Part Position

- Align midsagittal plane to CR and midline of table.
- Adjust head so that a line drawn from **lower margin of upper incisors to the base of the skull is perpendicular** to table.
- Ensure that **no rotation** of the head or thorax exists.
- Mandible must be in **continuous motion** during exposure.
- Ensure that **only the mandible moves.** The head must not move, and the **teeth must not make contact.**

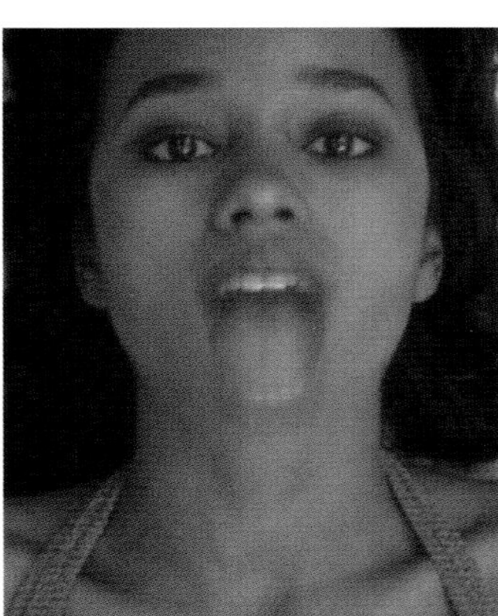

Fig. 9-74. AP "wagging jaw."

Central Ray

- CR **perpendicular** to IR, centered to **C4** (upper margin of thyroid cartilage)
- Cassette centered to CR
- Minimum SID of 40 inches (100 cm)

Collimation Four-sided collimation to area of entire cervical spine

Respiration Suspend respiration.

Note: Practice with patient before exposure to ensure that only the mandible is moving continuously, and that teeth do not make contact.

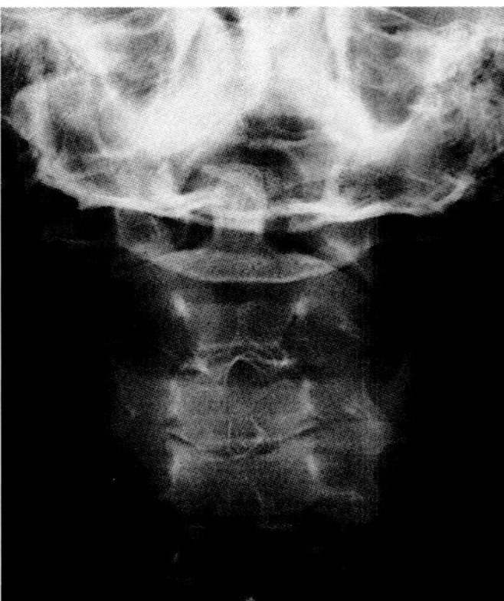

Fig. 9-75. AP radiograph of "wagging jaw" during exposure.

Radiographic Criteria

Structures Shown: • Entire cervical spine with mandible blurred.

Position: • Careful positioning is required to ensure C1 and C2 are well demonstrated. Immobilization of the head will reduce the likelihood of motion.

Collimation and CR: • Close lateral collimation to soft-tissue edges of the neck with lengthwise collimation to margins of IR • Center of collimation field (CR) to C4 region

Exposure Criteria: • Optimal exposure should demonstrate both the upper and lower cervical regions. • The C1 to C2 area should be lighter, yet still be well visualized. The lower vertebrae should appear somewhat darker, but not overexposed. • Bony margins should appear sharp, indicating no motion of vertebrae.

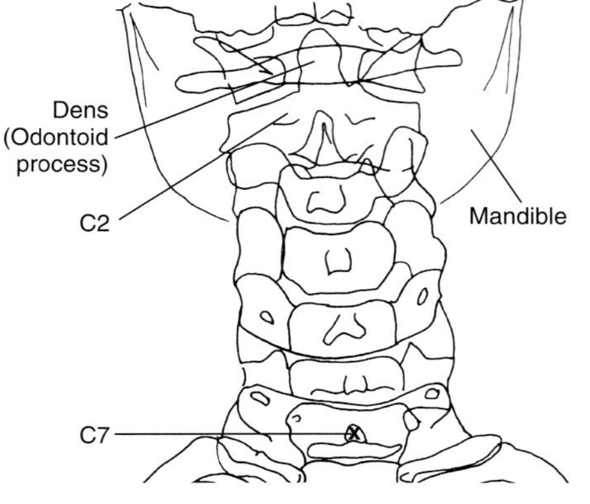

Fig. 9-76. AP "wagging jaw."

AP AXIAL PROJECTION—VERTEBRAL ARCH (PILLARS): CERVICAL SPINE

Warning: Do **not** attempt any head or neck movement if cervical trauma is possible without first consulting a physician who has reviewed a lateral cervical radiograph.

Cervical Spine
SPECIAL
• Lateral–hyperflexion and hyperextension
• AP (Fuchs method) PA (Judd method)
• AP "wagging jaw" (Ottonello method)
• AP axial (pillars)

Pathology Demonstrated

Pathology involving the posterior vertebral arch (particularly the pillars) of C4 to C7. Also used to demonstrate spinous processes of cervicothoracic vertebrae with whiplash-type injuries (see Warning above.)

24

R

36

Technical Factors

- IR size–24 × 36 cm (10 ×12 inches), lengthwise
- Moving or stationary grid
- 75 ± 5 kV range
- Technique and dose:

cm	kV	mAs	Sk.	ML.	
11	75	12	115	50	Thyroid 63 Breast 5
			mrad		

Patient Position Position patient in the supine position with arms at side.

Part Position

- Align midsagittal plane to CR and midline of table and/or IR.
- Hyperextend the neck if patient is able (see Warning above).
- Ensure **no rotation** of the head or thorax exists.

Central Ray

- CR angled **20° to 30° caudal,** to enter at the level of the **lower margin of the thyroid cartilage** and pass through **C5** (see Note)
- Cassette centered to CR
- Minimum SID of 40 inches (100 cm)

Collimation Close lateral collimation to soft-tissue edges of the neck and lengthwise collimation to margins of IR

Respiration Suspend respiration during exposure. Patient should not swallow during exposure.

Note: Sufficient hyperextension of neck and caudal CR angle is essential for demonstrating the posterior aspects of the mid- and lower cervical vertebra. The amount of CR angle (20° or 30°) is determined by the amount of natural cervical lordotic curvature. Some support may need to be placed under the shoulder for sufficient hyperextension.

Radiographic Criteria

Structures Shown: • Posterior elements of mid- and distal cervical and proximal thoracic vertebrae. In particular, the articulations (zygapophyseal joints) between the lateral masses (or pillars) are open and well demonstrated along with the laminae and spinous processes.

Position: • **No rotation:** Spinous processes should be equidistant from the spinal column lateral borders. • The mandible and base of the skull will be superimposed over the first two or three cervical vertebra.

Collimation and CR: • Lateral collimation to soft-tissue edges of the neck, and proximal and distal borders to margins of IR. • Center of collimation field (CR) at or near C5 vertebrae. • Zygapophyseal joints open, indicating correct CR angle.

Exposure Criteria: • Optimal exposure should demonstrate both bone and soft-tissue density. • Bony margins and trabecular marking should appear sharp, indicating no motion.

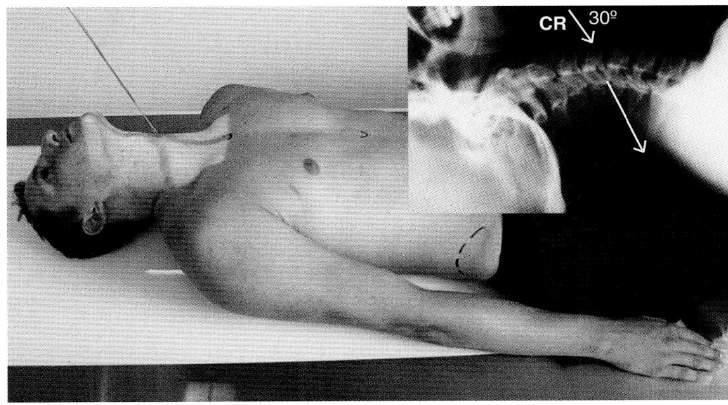

Fig. 9-77. AP axial (pillars), 20° to 30° caudal angle. *Inset,* Demonstrates caudal CR angle parallel with zygapophyseal joint spaces.

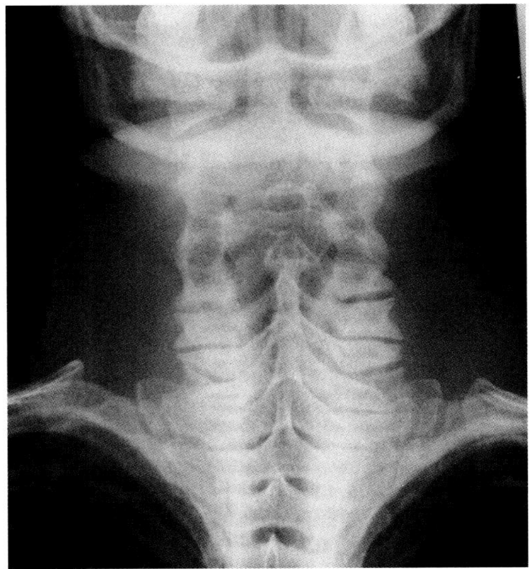

Fig. 9-78. AP axial (pillars). (Courtesy Teresa Easton-Porter.)

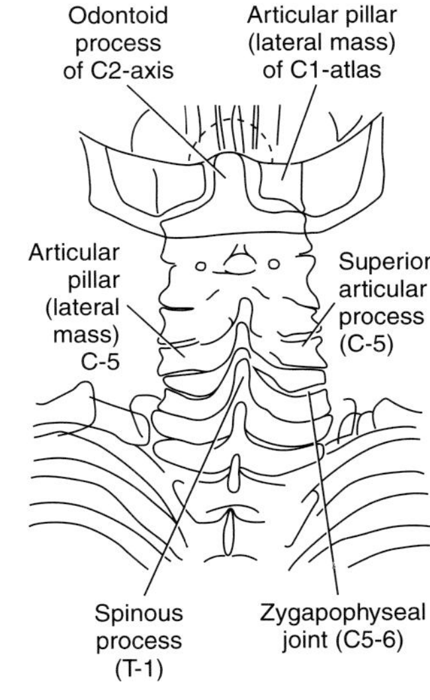

Fig. 9-79. AP axial (pillars).

AP PROJECTION: THORACIC SPINE

Thoracic Spine
BASIC
• AP
• Lateral

Pathology Demonstrated

Pathology involving the thoracic spine. Fractures (including compression fractures) and scoliosis are demonstrated.

Technical Factors

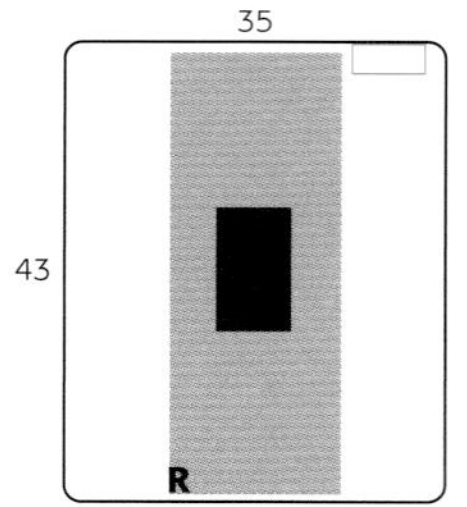

- IR size—35 × 43 cm (14 × 17 inches), lengthwise
- Moving or stationary grid
- 80 ± 5 or 90 ± 5 kV range
- May use wedge compensation filter with thicker part of filter at head end for more uniform density (especially for patients with thick or heavily muscled chests with greater difference in thickness between superior and mid-T spine region)
- Technique and dose—80 kV: / —90 kV:

	cm	kV	mAs	Sk.	ML.	mrad
80 kV	23	80	12	165	27	Thyroid 5, Breast 61
90 kV	23	90	7	125	23	Thyroid 4, Breast 49

Shielding Shield gonadal area without obscuring vertebral column.

The **anode-heel effect** will create more uniform density throughout the thoracic spine. Place patient so the more intense side of beam (cathode side) is over the abdominal end of patient.

Patient Position Position patient with arms at side and head on table or on a thin pillow.

Part Position

- Align midsagittal plane to CR and midline of table.
- **Flex knees and hips** to reduce thoracic curvature.
- Ensure that **no rotation** of the pelvis or thorax exists.

Central Ray

- CR **perpendicular** to IR
- CR centered to **T7,** which is 3 to 4 inches (8 to 10 cm) below jugular notch, or 1 to 2 inches (3 to 5 cm) below sternal angle (centering similar to that used with AP chest)
- Cassette centered to CR (top of cassette about 1 to 1½ inches, or 3 to 5 cm, above level of shoulder) on an average adult patient
- Minimum SID of 40 inches (100 cm)

Collimation Collimate on lateral margins to expose a field 4 or 5 inches (10 or 12 cm) wide, with upper and lower borders to IR margins.

Respiration Suspend respiration on **expiration.** (Expiration reduces air volume in thorax for more uniform density.)

Note: Higher kV with lower mAs decreases patient dose and also decreases overall contrast, which some radiologists may not prefer.

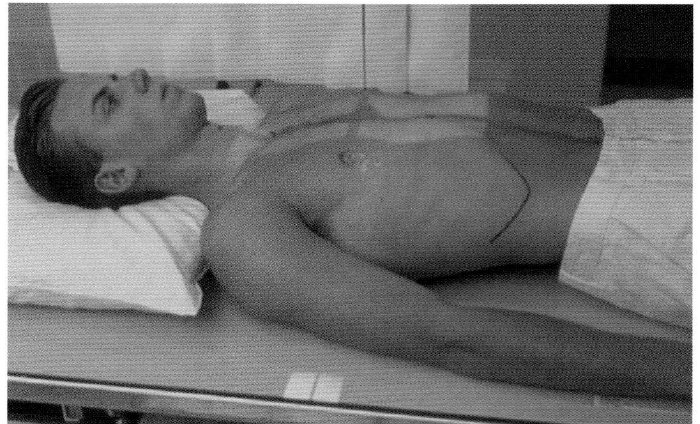

Fig. 9-80. AP T spine.

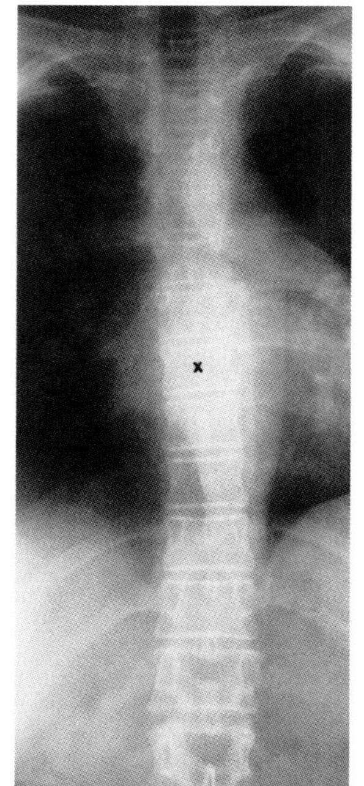

Fig. 9-81. AP.

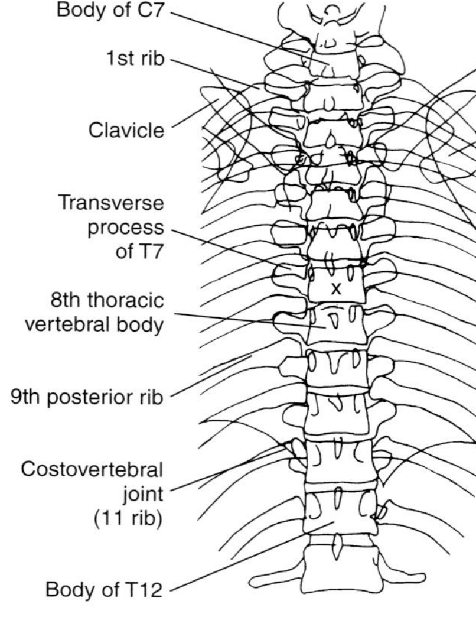

Fig. 9-82. AP.

Radiographic Criteria

Structures Shown: • Thoracic vertebral bodies, intervertebral joint spaces, spinous and transverse processes, posterior ribs, and costovertebral articulations.

Position: • The spinal column from C7 to L1 should be seen centered to the midline of the IR. • Sternoclavicular joints should be seen equidistant from the spine, indicating **no rotation.**

Collimation and CR: • Lateral collimation of 4 or 5 inches (10 to 12 cm) wide, with lengthwise collimation to IR margins.

Exposure Criteria: • Optimal exposure and use of wedge filter in addition to correct use of anode-heel effect should clearly demonstrate lower thoracic vertebral body margins and intervertebral joint spaces without overexposing upper thoracic vertebrae. • Bony margins and trabecular marking should appear sharp, indicating no motion.

LATERAL POSITION: THORACIC SPINE

Thoracic Spine
BASIC
• AP
• **Lateral**

Pathology Demonstrated
Pathology involving the thoracic spine, such as compression fractures, subluxation, or kyphosis is demonstrated.

Technical Factors
- IR size—35 × 43 cm (14 ×17 inches), lengthwise
- Moving or stationary grid
- 85 ± 5 kV range
- With breathing technique, low mA and 3 to 4 seconds of exposure
- Lead blocker placed on table behind patient to reduce scatter to IR (see Note 1)
- Technique and dose:

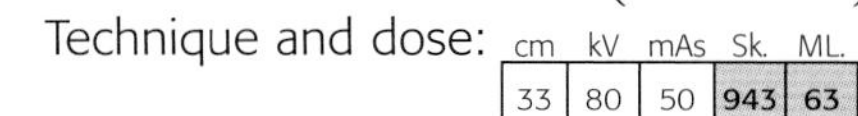

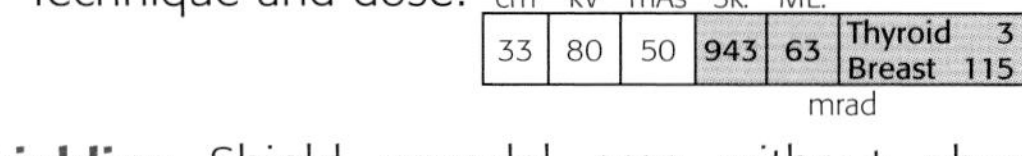

cm	kV	mAs	Sk.	ML.	
33	80	50	943	63	Thyroid 3 Breast 115

mrad

35 · 43 · L

No AEC with breathing technique.

Shielding Shield gonadal area without obscuring essential anatomy.

Patient Position Position patient in the lateral recumbent position, with head on pillow and knees flexed. The radiograph may be taken with the patient in the erect position with arms outstretched and weight evenly distributed on both feet.

Part Position
- Align midcoronal plane to CR and midline of table.
- Raise patient's arms to right angles to body with elbows flexed.
- Support patient's waist so entire spine is near parallel to table. (Palpate spinous processes to determine this.) (See Note 2.)
- Flex patient's hips and knees, with support between knees.
- Ensure that **no rotation** of shoulders or pelvis exists.

Central Ray
- CR **perpendicular to long axis** of thoracic spine (see Note 2)
- CR centered to **T7,** which is 3 to 4 inches (8 to 10 cm) below jugular notch or 7 to 8 inches (18 to 21 cm) below the vertebra prominens
- Cassette centered to CR (top of cassette about 2 inches or 5 cm above level of shoulders on average adult patient)
- Minimum SID of 40 inches (100 cm)

Collimation Collimate on lateral margins to expose a field 5 or 6 inches (13 to 15 cm) wide, with upper and lower borders to IR margins. (Greater kyphotic curvature requires wider collimation.)

Respiration Use breathing technique or suspend respiration after full expiration. Breathing technique blurs out unwanted rib and lung markings overlying thoracic vertebrae.

Note 1: Significant amounts of secondary/scatter radiation are generated. Close collimation and placement of a lead mat posterior to the part are essential to maintaining image quality. This is particularly important with digital imaging.

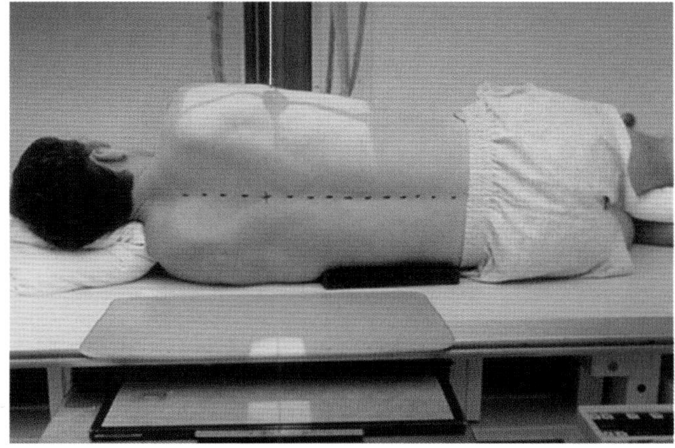

Fig. 9-83. Left lateral T spine, with proper waist support.

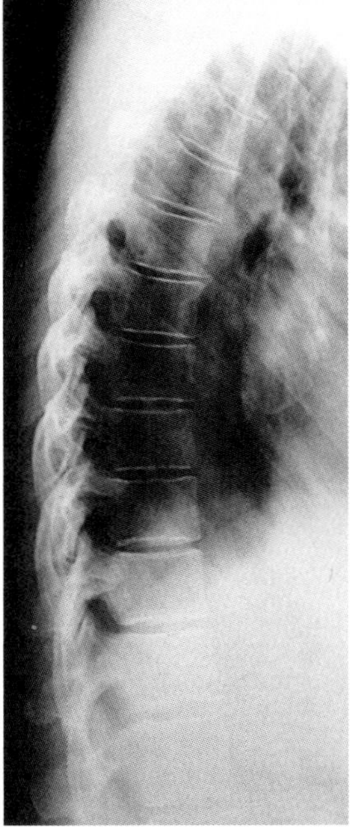

Fig. 9-84. Lateral with breathing.

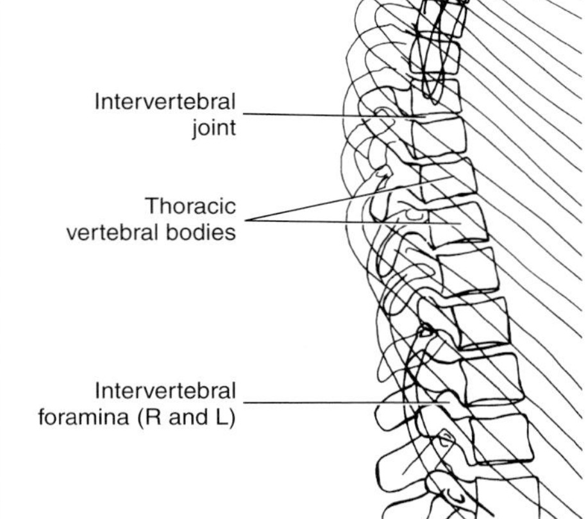

Fig. 9-85. Lateral.

Note 2: The optimal amount of support under the waist will cause the lower vertebrae to be the same distance from the tabletop as the upper vertebrae. A patient with wide hips will require substantially more support under waist to prevent "sag." A patient with broad shoulders may require a slight (3° to 5°) cephalic CR angle.

9

Radiographic Criteria

Structures Shown: • Thoracic vertebral bodies, intervertebral joint spaces, and intervertebral foramina are shown. • The most superior thoracic vertebrae (T1 to T3) will not be well visualized. • Obtain a lateral image using a swimmer's method if the upper thoracic vertebrae are of special interest.

Position: • Intervertebral disk spaces should be open. • Vertebral bodies should be in lateral profile without rotation as evidenced by superimposed posterior aspects of the vertebrae. • The posterior ribs will not be directly superimposed, especially if a patient has a wide thorax, because of the divergence of the x-ray beam.

Collimation and CR: • Apply close lateral collimation to the edges of the spine, without cutting off any pertinent anatomy. • Include as much of the spine lengthwise as possible to the IR margins.

Exposure Criteria: • Optimal exposure should demonstrate the thoracic vertebrae with blurring of the ribs and lung markings if breathing technique is used. • For most patients, T1 to T2 will be underexposed because of superimposition of shoulders. • Bony margins should appear sharp, indicating no motion of vertebrae.

OBLIQUE POSITION—ANTERIOR OR POSTERIOR OBLIQUES: THORACIC SPINE

Thoracic Spine
SPECIAL
• Obliques

Pathology Demonstrated
Pathology involving the zygapophyseal joints of the thoracic spine is demonstrated. Both right and left obliques are taken for comparison.

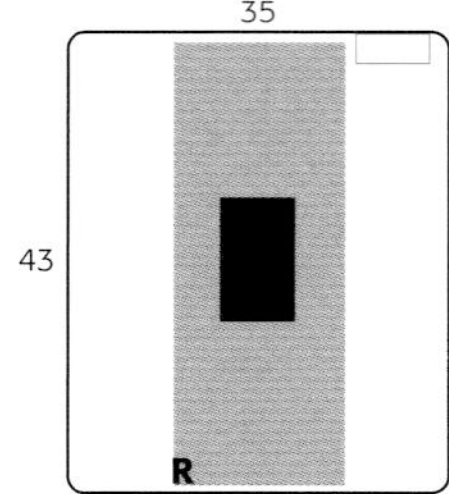

Technical Factors
- IR size—35 × 43 cm (14 × 17 inches), lengthwise
- Moving or stationary grid
- 80 ± 5 kV range
- Technique and dose:

	cm	kV	mAs	Sk.	ML.	mrad
Post. obl.	32	80	26	475	35	Thyroid 1 Breast 94
Ant. obl.	32	80	26	475	35	Thyroid 1 Breast 22

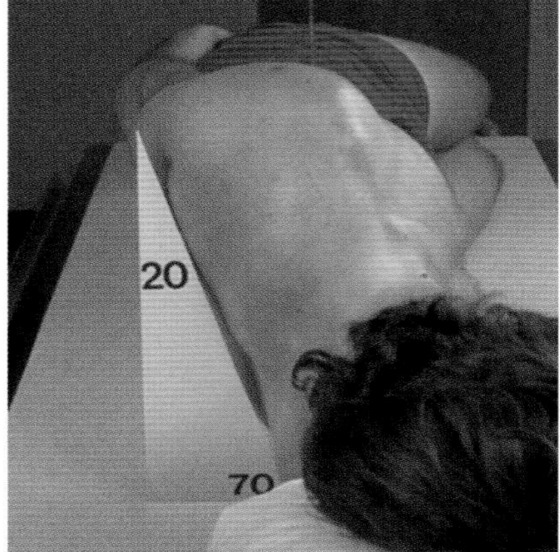

Fig. 9-86. Posterior oblique (RPO).

Shielding Shield gonadal area without obscuring essential spine anatomy.

Patient Position Position patient in the lateral erect or recumbent position, with head on pillow if recumbent.

Part Position
- Align **midaxillary plane to CR and midline of table** or IR.
- Rotate the body 20° from true lateral to create a **70° oblique** from plane of table. Ensure equal rotation of shoulders and pelvis.
- Flex hips, knees, and arms for stability as needed:

Posterior oblique (recumbent):
- LPO or RPO: Arm nearest table should be up and forward; arm nearest tube should be down and posterior.

Anterior oblique (recumbent):
- LAO or RAO: Arm nearest table should be down and posterior; arm nearest tube should be up and forward.

Erect anterior oblique:
- Distribute patient's weight equally on both feet.
- Rotate total body, shoulders, and pelvis 20° from lateral.
- Flex elbow, and place arm closest to IR on hip.
- Raise opposite arm and rest on cassette holder or on top of head.

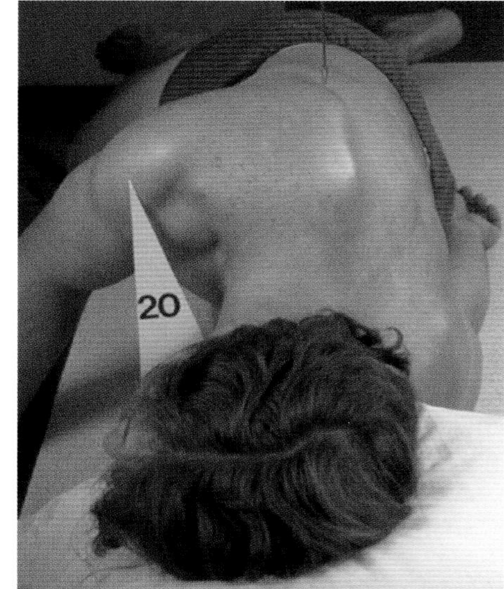

Fig. 9-87. Anterior oblique (LAO).

9

Central Ray
- CR **perpendicular** to IR
- CR centered to **T7**, which is 3 to 4 inches (8 to 10 cm) below jugular notch or 2 inches (5 cm) below sternal angle
- Cassette centered to CR (top of cassette about 1½ inches, or 3 cm, above level of shoulders)
- Minimum SID of 40 inches (100 cm)

Collimation Adjust for close four-sided collimation to area of interest. Greater kyphotic curvature requires wider collimation.

Respiration Suspend breathing on full expiration.

Note: Patient's thorax is 20° from lateral; some type of angle guide may be used to determine correct rotation (Figs. 9-86 and 9-87).

Radiographs may be taken as posterior or anterior obliques. **Anterior obliques** are recommended because of significantly lower breast dose.

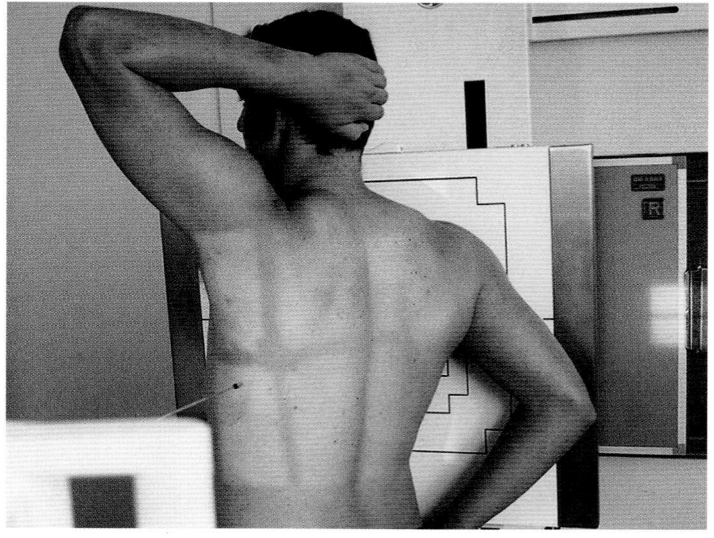

Fig. 9-88. Erect anterior oblique (LAO).

OBLIQUE POSITION—ANTERIOR OR POSTERIOR OBLIQUES

Radiographic Criteria

Structures Shown: • Zygapophyseal joints: **Anterior oblique** positions demonstrate the zygapophyseal joints closest to the IR, and **posterior oblique** positions demonstrate the joints farther from the IR.

Position: • All 12 thoracic vertebra should be seen and centered to the midline of the IR. • The zygapophyseal joints should be open and well demonstrated, but the amount of kyphosis will determine how many apophyseal joints will be clearly seen.

Collimation and CR: • Apply close lateral collimation to the edges of the spine without cutting off any pertinent vertebral anatomy. • Include as much of the spine lengthwise as possible to the margins of the IR.

Exposure Criteria: • Optimal exposure should demonstrate wide exposure latitude to visualize all parts of the 12 thoracic vertebrae. • Bony margins should appear sharp, indicating no motion.

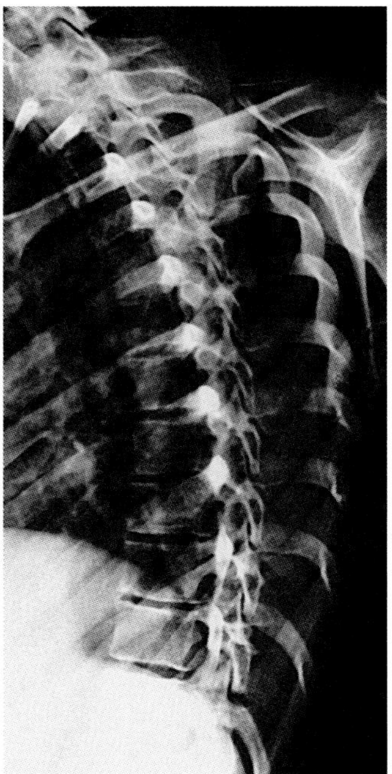

Fig. 9-89. Oblique T spine.

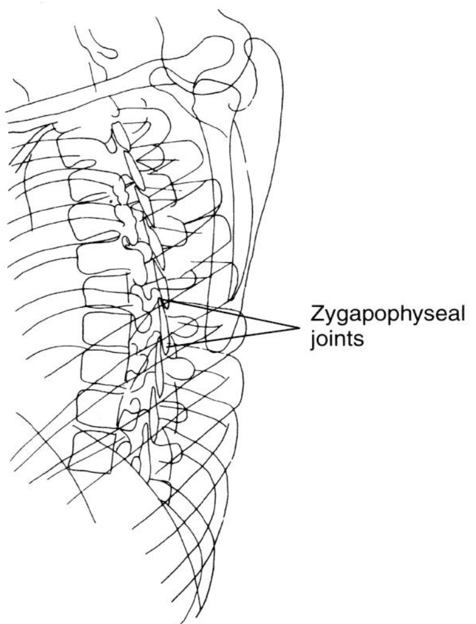

Fig. 9-90. Oblique T spine.

RADIOGRAPHS FOR CRITIQUE

Students should determine whether they can critique each of these six radiographs based on the categories as described in the textbook and as outlined on the right. As a starting critique exercise, place a check in each category that demonstrates a **repeatable error** for that radiograph.

Student workbooks provide more space for writing comments and complete critique answers for each of these radiographs. Answers are also provided in Appendix B, at the end of this textbook.

	RADIOGRAPHS					
	A	B	C	D	E	F
1. Structures shown	____	____	____	____	____	____
2. Positioning	____	____	____	____	____	____
3. Collimation and CR	____	____	____	____	____	____
4. Exposure criteria	____	____	____	____	____	____
5. Markers	____	____	____	____	____	____

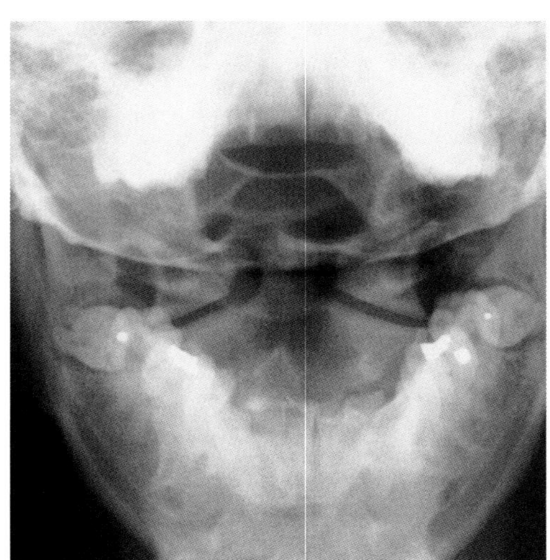

Fig. C9-91. AP open mouth (C1-C2). **A**

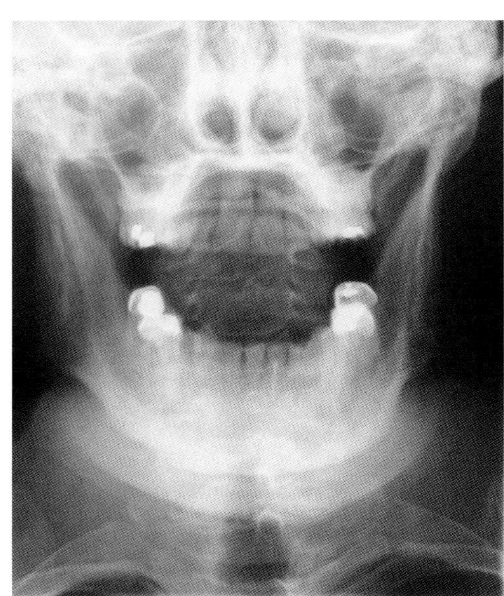

Fig. C9-92. AP open mouth (C1-C2). **B**

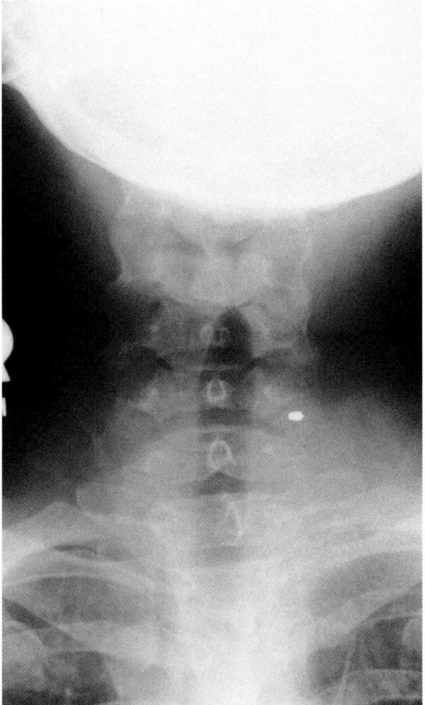

Fig. C9-93. AP C spine. **C**

9

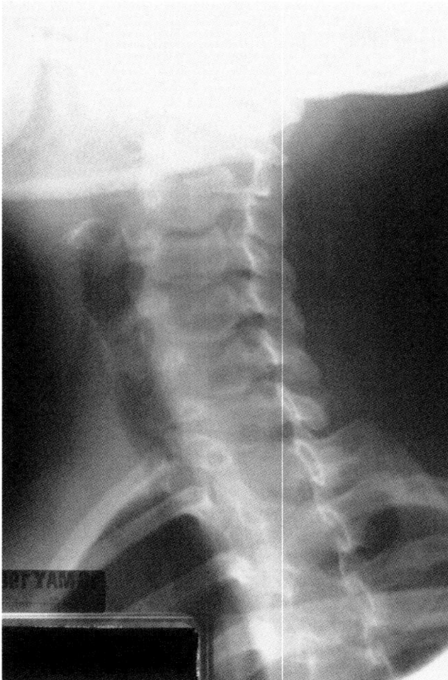

Fig. C9-94. Oblique C spine. **D**

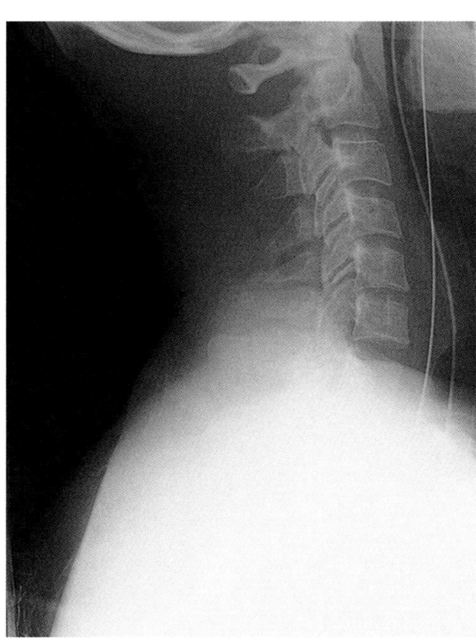

Fig. C9-95. Horizontal beam lateral C spine (with cervical collar). **E**

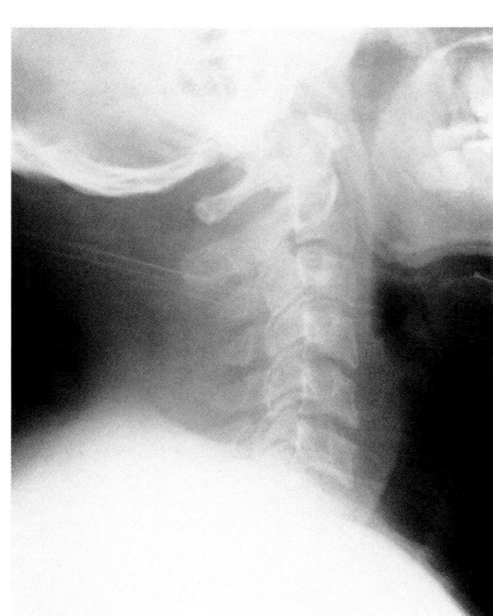

Fig. C9-96. Lateral C spine. **F**

CHAPTER 10

Lumbar Spine, Sacrum, and Coccyx

CONTRIBUTIONS BY **Patti Ward,** MEd, RT(R)
CONTRIBUTORS TO PAST EDITIONS Alex Backus, MS, RT(R), Cindy Murphy, RT R, ACR, BHSc

CONTENTS

RADIOGRAPHIC ANATOMY

This chapter describes anatomy and positioning of the **lumbar, sacrum,** and **coccyx** sections of the vertebral column. Refer to Chapter 9 for more detailed information about vertebral anatomy.

Lumbar Vertebrae

The largest individual vertebrae are the **five lumbar vertebrae.** These vertebrae are the strongest in the vertebral column because the load of body weight increases toward the inferior end of the column. For this reason the cartilaginous disks between the inferior lumbar vertebrae are common sites for injury and pathologic processes.

LATERAL AND SUPERIOR PERSPECTIVES

Patients typically have five lumbar vertebrae located just inferior to the 12 thoracic vertebrae. Fig. 10-1 illustrates the lateral perspective of a typical lumbar vertebra. Lumbar vertebral bodies are larger in comparison with thoracic and cervical vertebral bodies. The most inferior body, L5, is the largest. The **transverse processes** are fairly small, whereas the posteriorly projecting **spinous process** is bulky and blunt. The palpable lower tip of each lumbar spinous process lies at the level of the intervertebral disk space inferior to each vertebral body.

Intervertebral Foramina Fig. 10-2 shows the **intervertebral foramen** situated 90° relative to the midsagittal plane. Intervertebral foramina are spaces or openings between **pedicles** when two vertebrae are stacked on each other. Along the upper surface of each pedicle is a half-moon–shaped area termed the ***superior vertebral notch,*** and along the lower surface of each pedicle is another half-moon–shaped area termed the ***inferior vertebral notch.*** When vertebrae are stacked, the superior and inferior vertebral notches line up and the two half-moon–shaped areas form a single opening, the **intervertebral foramina** (see Chapter 9, Figs. 9-8 and 9-9). Therefore between every two vertebrae are two intervertebral foramina, one on each side, through which important spinal nerves and blood vessels pass. The intervertebral foramina in the lumbar region are demonstrated best on a lateral radiographic image.

Zygapophyseal Joints Each typical vertebra has four articular processes projecting from the area of the junction of the pedicles and laminae. The processes projecting upward are called the ***superior articular processes,*** and the processes projecting downward are the ***inferior articular processes.*** The term ***facet*** (*fas'et*) sometimes is used interchangeably with the term ***zygapophyseal joint;*** the facet is actually only the articulating surface instead of the entire superior or inferior articular process. Fig. 10-1 shows the relative positions of the superior and inferior lumbar articular processes from the lateral perspective.

The zygapophyseal joints form an angle open from **30° to 50°** to the midsagittal plane, as shown in Fig. 10-2. The upper lumbar are nearer the 50° angle, and the lower or distal lumbar are nearer 30°. Radiographic demonstration of the zygapophyseal joints is achieved by rotating the patient's body an average of 45°.

The **laminae** form a bridge between the transverse processes, lateral masses, and spinous process (Fig. 10-2). The portion of each lamina between the superior and inferior articular processes is the ***pars interarticularis.*** The pars interarticularis is demonstrated radiographically on the oblique lumbar image.

POSTERIOR AND ANTERIOR PERSPECTIVES

Fig. 10-3 demonstrates the general appearance of a lumbar vertebra as seen from the anterior and posterior perspectives. AP or PA radiographic projections of the lumbar spine demonstrate the **spinous processes** superimposed on the vertebral bodies. The **transverse processes** are demonstrated protruding laterally beyond the edges of the vertebral body.

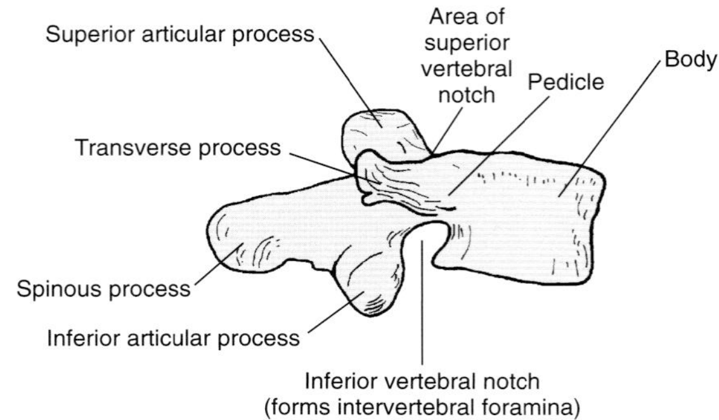

Fig. 10-1. Lumbar vertebra—lateral view.

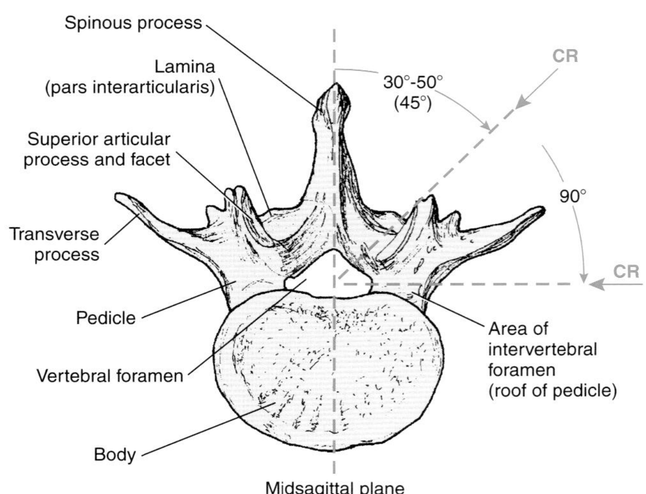

Fig. 10-2. Lumbar vertebra—superior view.

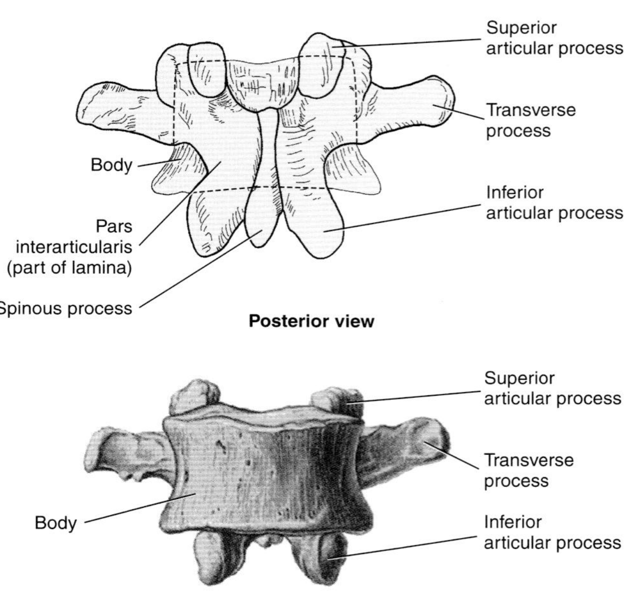

Fig. 10-3. Lumbar vertebra—posterior and anterior views.

Sacrum

The **sacrum** is inferior to the lumbar vertebrae.

ANTERIOR PERSPECTIVE

Fig. 10-4 illustrates the concave anterior surface of a sacrum. The bodies of the original five segments are fused into a single bone in the adult. The sacrum is shovel-shaped, with the apex pointed inferiorly and anteriorly. Four sets of **pelvic** (anterior) **sacral foramina** (similar to intervertebral foramen in more superior sections of the spine) transmit nerves and blood vessels.

The **alae,** or wings, of the sacrum are large masses of bone lateral to the first sacral segment. The two **superior articular processes** of the sacrum form zygapophyseal joints with the inferior articular processes of the fifth lumbar vertebrae.

LATERAL PERSPECTIVE

Fig. 10-5 clearly illustrates the dominant concave curve of the sacrum and the forward projection of the coccyx. These curves determine how the central ray must be angled differently for AP radiographic projections of the sacrum or coccyx.

The anterior ridge of the body of the first sacral segment helps form the posterior wall of the inlet of the true pelvis, and is termed the ***promontory*** of the sacrum, best demonstrated from a lateral perspective (see Fig. 10-5).

Posterior to the body of the first sacral segment is the opening to the **sacral canal,** which is a continuation of the vertebral canal and contains certain sacral nerves. The **median sacral crest** is formed by the fused spinous processes of the sacral vertebrae.

Figs. 10-5 and 10-6 illustrate the relative roughness and irregularity of the posterior surface of the sacrum, compared with the anterior or pelvic surface.

The sacrum articulates with the ilium of the pelvis at the **auricular surface** (marked *A* in Figs. 10-5 and 10-6). The auricular surface is named because of its resemblance in shape to the auricle of the ear.

The **sacral horns** (cornua) (marked *D* in Figs. 10-5 and 10-6) are small tubercles representing the inferior articular processes projecting inferiorly from each side of the fifth sacral segment. They project inferiorly and posteriorly to articulate with the corresponding **horns** (cornua) of the **coccyx.**

POSTERIOR SACRUM

Fig. 10-6 is a photograph of an actual sacrum, as seen from the posterior aspect. Clearly seen is the large, wedge-shaped *(A)* **auricular surface,** which articulates with a similar surface on the ilium to form the **sacroiliac joint.** Each sacroiliac joint opens **obliquely posteriorly at an angle of 30°.**

The **articulating facets of the superior articular processes** *(B)* also open to the rear and are shown on this photograph. There are eight—four on each side—**posterior sacral foramina** *(C),* corresponding to the same number of anterior sacral foramina.

The **sacral horns** (cornua; *D*) are seen as small bony projections at the very inferoposterior aspect of the sacrum. Remnants of the enclosed sacral canal *(E)* also can be seen. (Deteriorating bone leaves the canal partially open on this bone specimen.)

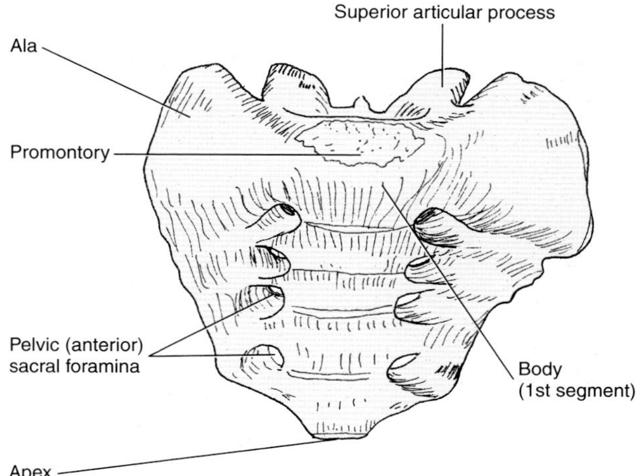

Fig. 10-4. Sacrum—anterior view.

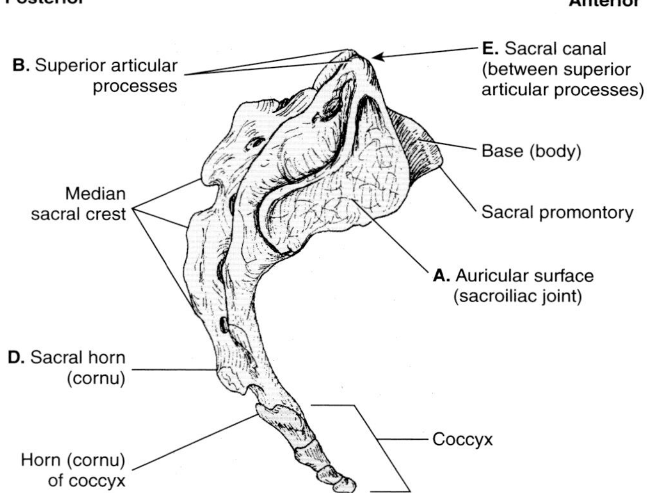

Fig. 10-5. Sacrum and coccyx—lateral view.

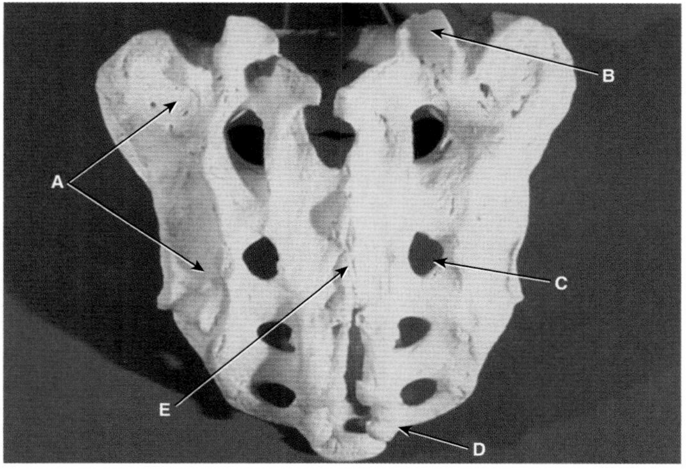

Fig. 10-6. Sacrum—posterior view.

Coccyx

ANTERIOR COCCYX

The most distal portion of the vertebral column is the **coccyx.** The anterior surface of the "tailbone," or coccyx, is illustrated in Fig. 10-7. This portion of the vertebral column has greatly regressed in the human, so there remains little resemblance to vertebrae. Three to five coccygeal segments (an average of four) have fused in the adult to form the single coccyx. The drawing in Fig. 10-7 demonstrates four formerly separate segments present in a youth, now fused into a single bone as an adult. The photograph of a coccyx in Fig. 10-8 demonstrates five segments now mostly fused in the adult coccyx.

The most superior segment is the largest and broadest of the four sections and even has two lateral projections that are small **transverse processes.** The distal pointed tip of the coccyx is termed the **apex,** whereas the broader, superior portion is termed the ***base.***

Occasionally the second segment does not fuse solidly with the larger first segment (see Fig. 10-8); however, the coccyx usually is one small, fairly insignificant end of the vertebral column.

POSTERIOR COCCYX

The posterior aspect of an actual coccyx is pictured in Fig. 10-8, along with a common U.S. postage stamp to allow comparison of the two sizes. (Note that a portion of the transverse process is missing on the upper right aspect of this specimen.)

LATERAL SACRUM AND COCCYX RADIOGRAPH

The lateral sacrum on this radiograph (Fig. 10-9) is seen as a large solid bone, as compared with the much smaller coccyx. The long axis of the sacrum is shown to be angled posteriorly, requiring a cephalad angle of the CR on an AP projection. This angle is greater on an average female, as compared with the average male.

Ordinarily the coccyx curves anteriorly, as seen and identified on this lateral radiograph so that the apex points toward the symphysis pubis of the anterior pelvis. This forward curvature is frequently more pronounced in males and less pronounced, with less curvature, in females. The coccyx projects into the birth canal in the female and, if angled excessively forward, can impede the birth process.

The most common injury associated with the coccyx results from a direct blow to the lower vertebral column when a person is in a sitting position. A wild ride on a toboggan might provide the type of force required to angulate the coccyx more forward than normal and make sitting down an action to be avoided for a period of time.

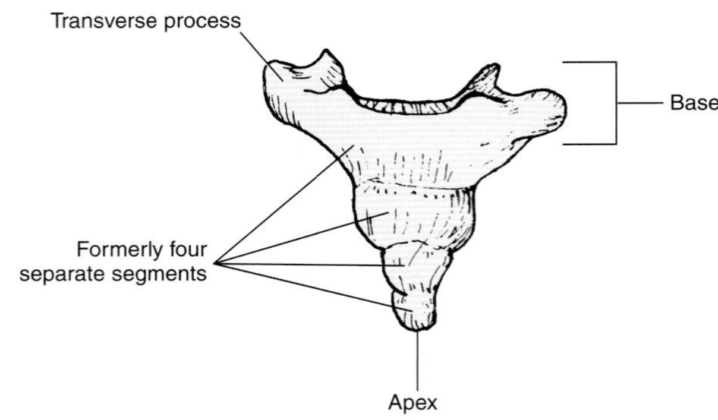

Fig. 10-7. Coccyx–anterior view.

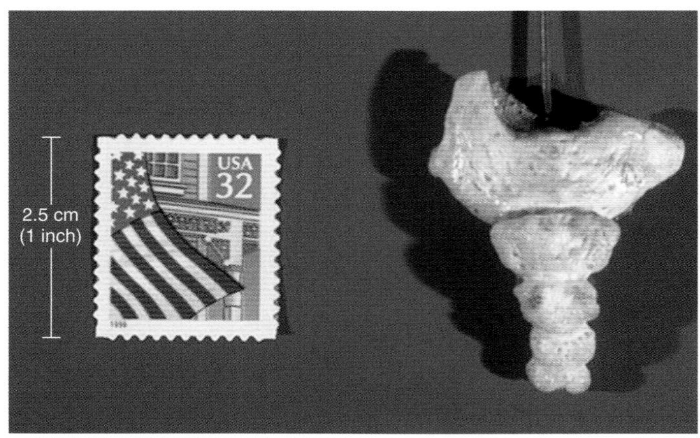

Fig. 10-8. Coccyx–posterior view (actual size).

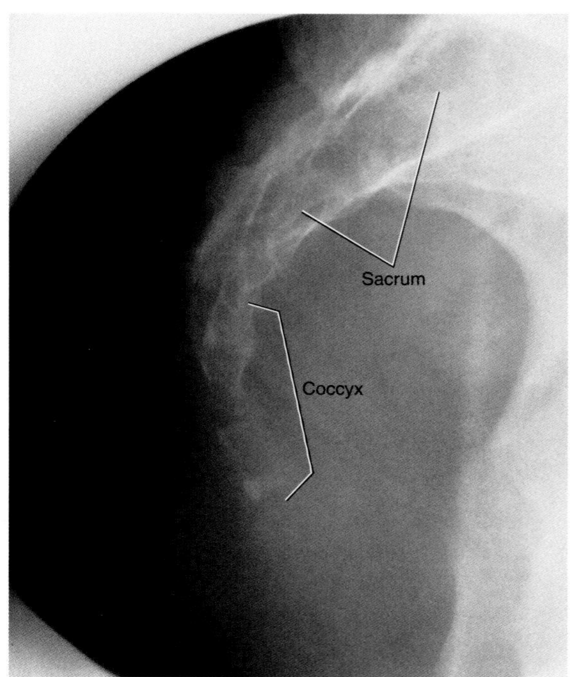

Fig. 10-9. Lateral sacrum and coccyx.

10

Anatomy Review

SUPEROINFERIOR PROJECTION (Fig. 10-10)

Certain parts on this radiograph of an individual lumbar vertebra taken from a disarticulated skeleton are labeled, as follows:

A. Spinous process
B. Lamina
C. Pedicle
D. Vertebral foramen
E. Body
F. Transverse process

LATERAL POSITION

Parts labeled *A* through *F* on the lateral view (Fig. 10-11) of a disarticulated lumbar vertebra are as follows:

A. Body
B. Inferior vertebral notch, or the floor of the pedicle making up the upper portion of the rounded intervertebral foramen
C. Area of the articulating facet of the inferior articular process (actual articular facet not shown on this lateral view); makes up the zygapophyseal joints when vertebrae are stacked
D. Spinous process
E. Superior articular process
F. Pedicle

Note that this lateral view would "open up" and demonstrate the intervertebral foramina well (the larger round opening directly under *B,* the inferior vertebral notch). However, it would not demonstrate the zygapophyseal joints, which would require a 45° oblique view.

AP PROJECTION

Individual structures are more difficult to identify when the vertebrae are superimposed by the soft tissues of the abdomen, as demonstrated on this AP lumbar spine radiograph (Fig. 10-12). Those structures labeled *A* through *F* are as follows:

A. Transverse process of L5
B. Lower lateral portion of the body of L4
C. Lower part of the spinous process of L4, as visualized on end
D. One inferior articular process of L3
E. Superior articular process of L4
F. L1-2 intervertebral disk space

The facets of the inferior and superior articular processes (*D* and *E*) make up one zygapophyseal joint not visualized on this AP projection. The joint is, however, demonstrated on a 45° oblique projection of lumbar vertebrae (see Fig. 10-16 on p. 326).

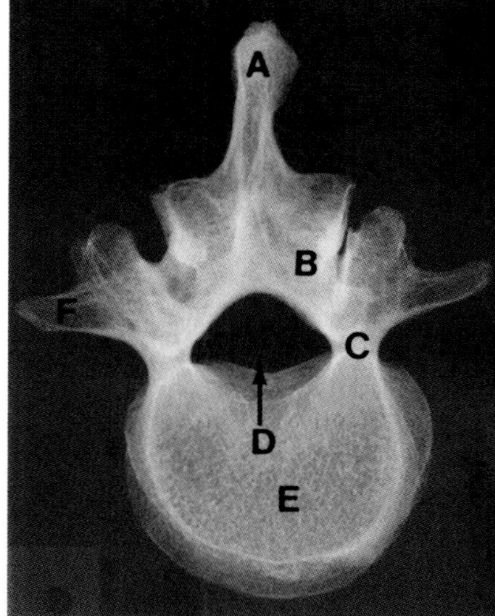

Fig. 10-10. Lumbar vertebra (superoinferior projection).

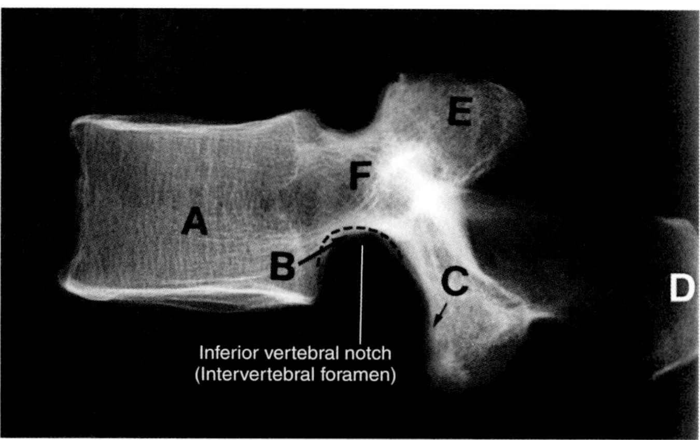

Fig. 10-11. Lumbar vertebra (lateral position).

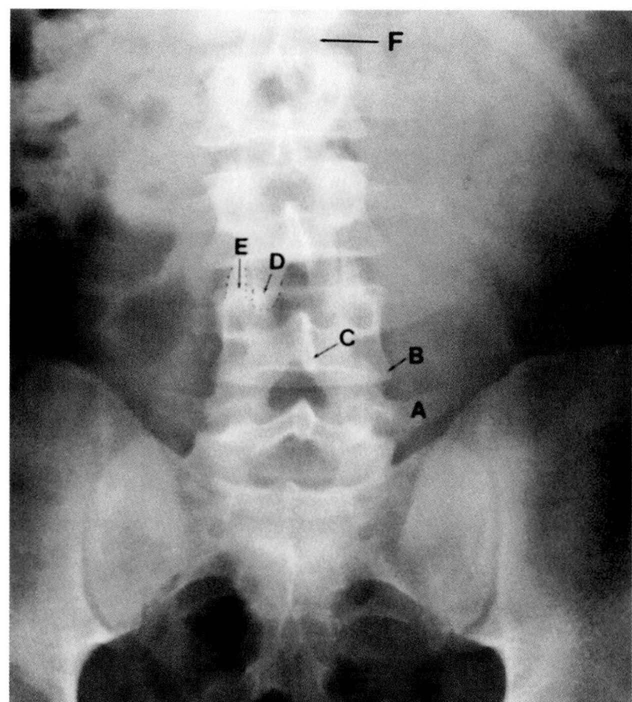

Fig. 10-12. Lumbar spine (AP projection).

10

LATERAL LUMBOSACRAL SPINE

Radiograph of entire lumbosacral spine in lateral position (Fig. 10-13) shows the following:

A. Body of L1
B. Body of L3
C. Intervertebral disk space between L4 and L5
D. Body of L5
E. Superimposed intervertebral foramina between L1 and L2

AP LUMBOSACRAL SPINE

AP projection of entire lumbosacral spine (Fig. 10-14) is labeled as follows:

A. Last thoracic vertebra (T12)
B. First lumbar vertebra
C. Third lumbar vertebra
D. Fifth lumbar vertebra

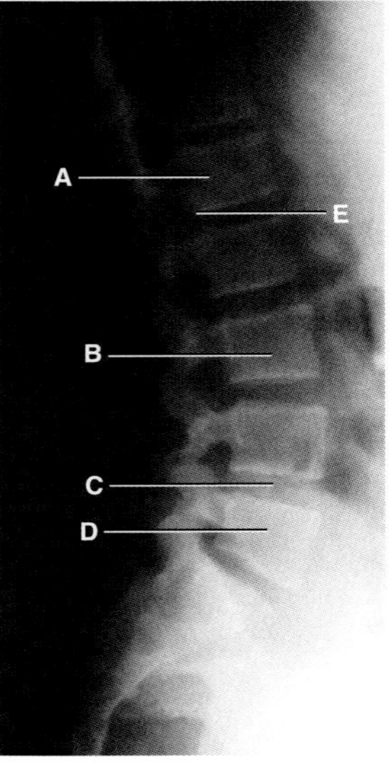

Fig. 10-13. Lumbosacral spine—lateral.

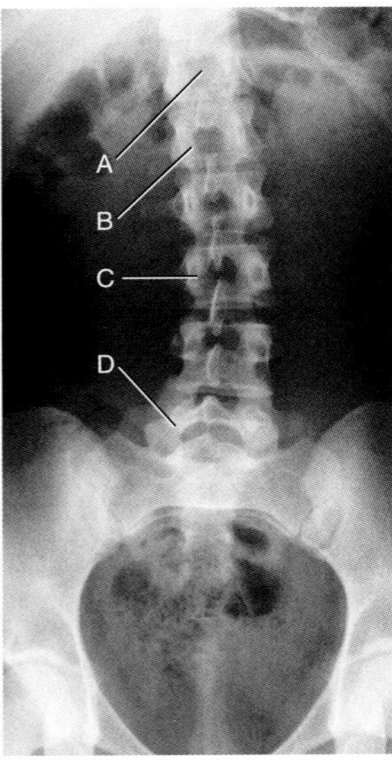

Fig. 10-14. Lumbosacral spine—AP.

Oblique Lumbar Vertebrae

APPEARANCE OF "SCOTTY DOG"

Any bone and its parts, when seen in an oblique position, are more difficult to recognize than the same bone seen in the conventional frontal or lateral view. A vertebra is no exception; however, imagination can help us in the case of the lumbar vertebrae. A good 45° oblique projects the various structures in such a way that a "Scotty dog" seems to appear. Fig. 10-15 shows the various components of the Scotty dog. The head and neck of the dog are probably the easiest features to recognize. The neck is one **pars interarticularis** (part of the lamina that primarily makes up the shoulder region of the dog). The **ear** of the dog is one **superior articular process,** whereas the **eye** is formed by one **pedicle.** One **transverse process** forms the **nose.** The **front legs** are formed by one **inferior articular process.**

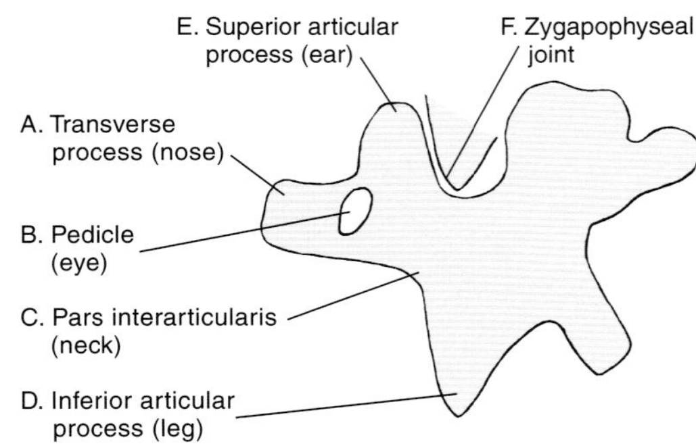

Fig. 10-15. The "Scotty dog."

OBLIQUE LUMBAR RADIOGRAPH

Fig. 10-16 shows the Scotty dog appearance that should be visible on a good oblique radiograph of the lumbar spine. The radiograph is labeled as follows:

A. Nose of the Scotty dog, formed by one transverse process
B. Eye, one pedicle seen on end
C. Neck of the dog, which is the pars interarticularis
D. Front leg of the dog, formed by one inferior articular process
E. Pointed ear, one of the superior articular processes
F. Zygapophyseal joint, formed by front leg of the Scotty above and ear of the Scotty below

Each of the five lumbar vertebrae should assume a similar Scotty dog appearance, with zygapophyseal joint spaces open on a correctly obliqued lumbar radiograph.

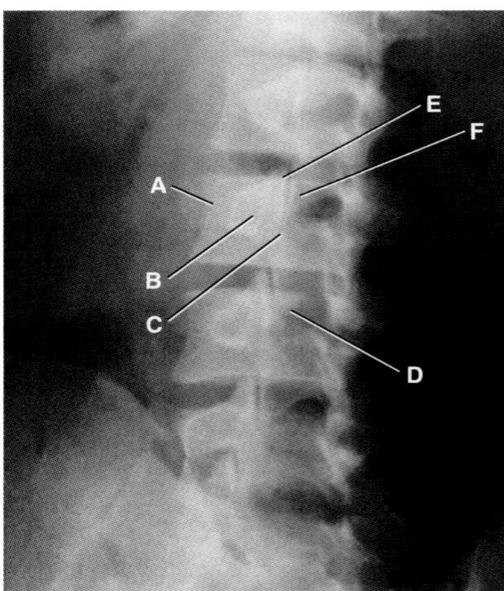

Fig. 10-16. Oblique lumbar spine (the "Scotty dog").

Classification of Joints

Two types of classifications of joints, or articulations, involve the vertebral column.

ZYGAPOPHYSEAL (APOPHYSEAL) JOINTS

The zygapophyseal joints between the superior and inferior articular processes are classified as **synovial** joints. These joints are lined with synovial membrane. They are **diarthrodial,** or freely movable, with a **plane (gliding) type** of movement.

INTERVERTEBRAL JOINTS

The intervertebral joints between the bodies of any two vertebrae contain intervertebral disks made up of fibrocartilage and are only slightly movable. These joints, which are tightly bound by cartilage, thus are classified as **cartilaginous joints.** They are **amphiarthrodial** (slightly movable) of the **symphysis subclass,** similar to the intervertebral joints of the cervical and thoracic spine as described in the preceding chapter.

There is not a great deal of motion between any two vertebrae, but the combined effect of all the vertebrae in the column does allow a considerable range of motion. The possible movements are flexion, extension, lateral flexion (bending), and rotation. Certain radiographic exams of the spinal column involving hyperflexion and hyperextension and/or right- and left-bending routines can measure this range of motion.

Intervertebral Foramina Versus Zygapophyseal Joints

INTERVERTEBRAL FORAMINA–LATERAL LUMBAR SPINE

The intervertebral foramina for the lumbar spine are visualized on a true lateral projection, as demonstrated in the Fig. 10-13 radiograph on the preceding page.

ZYGAPOPHYSEAL JOINTS–OBLIQUE LUMBAR SPINE

Positioning for oblique projections of the lumbar spine requires a good understanding of the anatomy of the vertebrae and the zygapophyseal joints. This is important to know how much to oblique the patient and which joint is being demonstrated.

Posterior Oblique As the drawing and photographs of the skeleton demonstrate, the **downside** joints are visualized on **posterior** obliques. The downside zygapophyseal joints are not visible on the skeleton because they are "under" the bodies of the vertebrae (Fig. 10-17), but as seen on the inferosuperior sectional drawing, the downside joints would be demonstrated on a posterior oblique. This is seen on the RPO radiograph in Fig. 10-19, which clearly shows the ears and legs of the Scotty dogs, or the right zygapophyseal joints (see *arrow*).

Anterior Oblique The anterior oblique position may be more comfortable for the patient and allow the natural lumbar curvature of the spine to coincide with the divergence of the x-ray beam.

As demonstrated, an **anterior** oblique visualizes the **upside** joints. Therefore a right anterior oblique (RAO) visualizes the upside, or left, zygapophyseal joints (Figs. 10-20 and 10-22).

The degree of obliquity depends on which area of the lumbar spine is of specific interest. A 45° oblique is for the general lumbar region, but if interest is specifically in **L1 or L2,** the degree of obliquity should be increased to **at least 50°**. If interest is in the **L5-S1** area, the obliquity would be **only about 30°** from an AP or PA projection. There is some variance among patients, but in general the upper lumbar region requires more degrees of obliquity than the lower regions. The reason is that the upper lumbar vertebrae take on some shape characteristics of the thoracic vertebrae, which require 70° of obliquity to demonstrate the zygapophyseal joints, as described in Chapter 9.

SUMMARY OF L SPINE JOINT AND FORAMINA POSITIONING

INTERVERTEBRAL FORAMINA–90° LATERAL	ZYGAPOPHYSEAL JOINTS–45° OBLIQUES
R or L Lateral	**Posterior obliques–downside**
	RPO–Right joints
	LPO–Left joints
	Anterior obliques–upside
	RAO–Left joints
	LAO–Right joints

SUMMARY OF JOINT CLASSIFICATIONS OF L SPINE

JOINTS	CLASSIFICATION	MOBILITY TYPE	MOVEMENT TYPE
Zygapophyseal joints	Synovial	Diarthrodial	Plane (gliding)
Intervertebral joints	Cartilaginous (symphysis)	Ampiarthrodial (slightly movable)	N/A

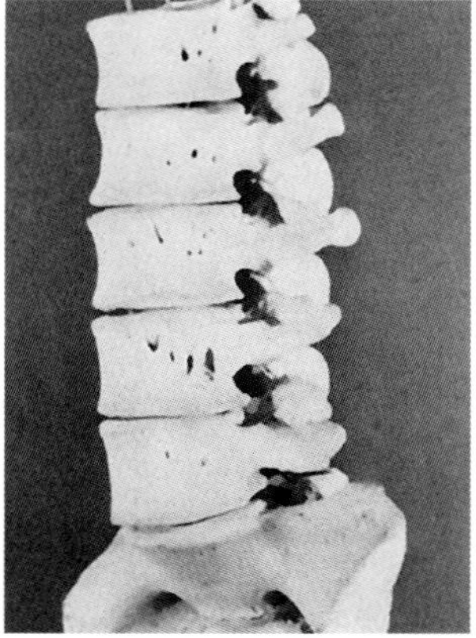

Fig. 10-17. Posterior oblique–downside joints.

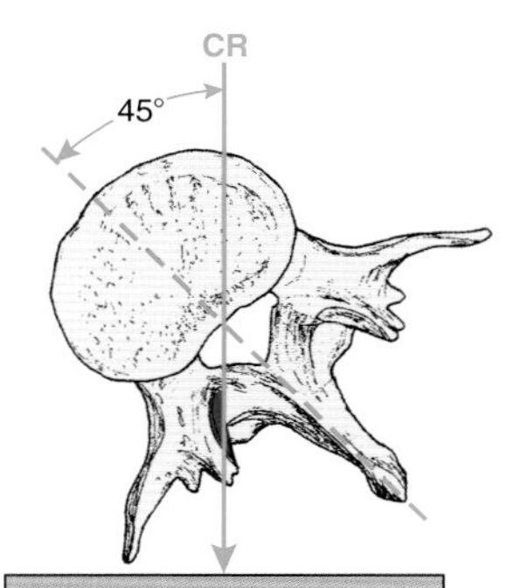

Fig. 10-18. Posterior oblique–downside joints.

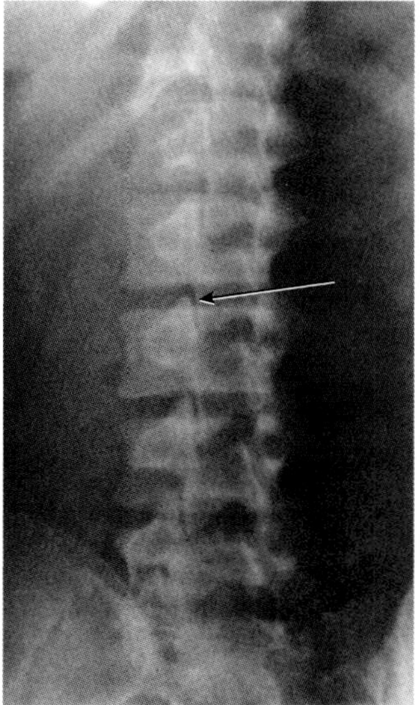

Fig. 10-19. Posterior oblique lumbar spine. **RPO**–downside, or **right,** joints.

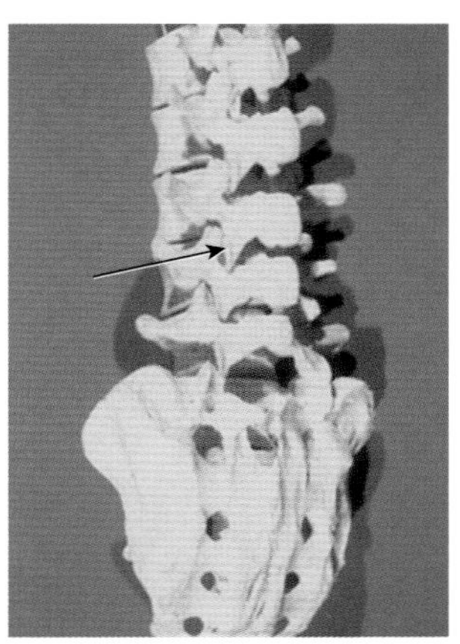

Fig. 10-20. Anterior oblique lumbar spine. **RAO**–upside, or **left,** joints.

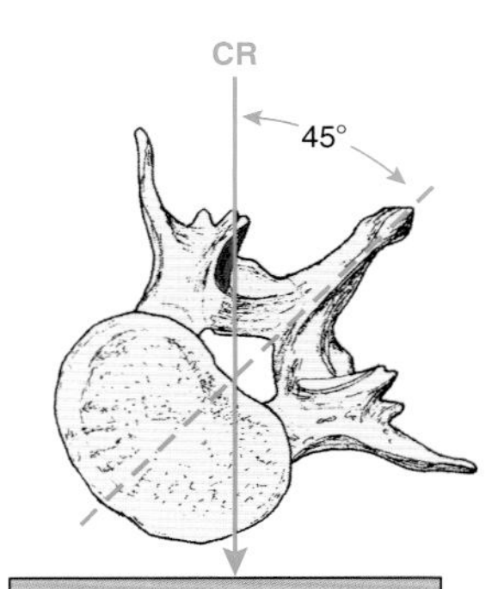

Fig. 10-21. Anterior oblique–upside joints.

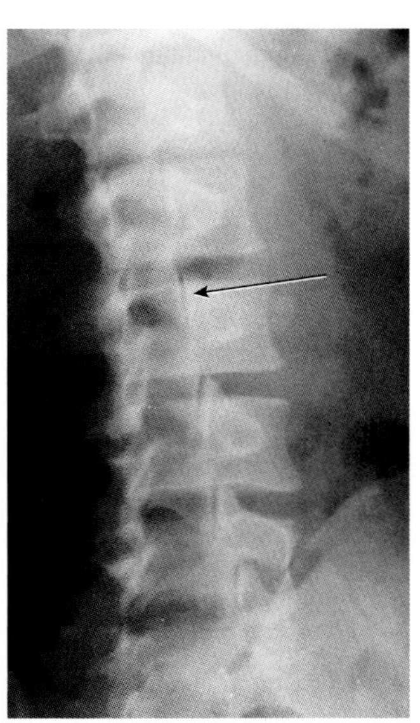

Fig. 10-22. Anterior oblique lumbar spine. **RAO**–upside, or **left,** joints.

10

RADIOGRAPHIC POSITIONING

Topographic Landmarks

Correct positioning for the coccyx, sacrum, and lumbar spine requires a thorough understanding of specific topographic landmarks that can be easily palpated.

The most reliable landmarks for the spine are various palpable bony prominences that are fairly consistent from one person to another. However, the landmarks presented refer to an average-sized, healthy, erect, normally developed adult male or female. These landmarks vary in subjects with anatomic and, especially, skeletal anomalies. The very young and the very old also have slightly different features than the average adult.

LOWER SPINE LANDMARKS

The drawings on the right illustrate various landmarks relative to the lower vertebral column.

A. **Level A** corresponds to the superior margin of the **symphysis pubis.** The size and shape of the **coccyx** vary greatly, but the midcoccyx is approximately at the level of the **symphysis pubis** or the **greater trochanter,** which is about 2.5 cm (1 inch) superior to the level of the symphysis pubis.
B. The **anterior superior iliac supine** (ASIS) is at about the same **level** *(B)* as the **first or second sacral segment.**
C. **Level C** is the most superior portion of the **iliac crest** and is at approximately the same level as the junction of the **fourth and fifth lumbar vertebrae.**
D. The lowest margin of the ribs or **lower costal margin** *(D)* is at the approximate level of **L2 or L3.**
E. The **xiphoid tip** is approximately at the level of **T9 or T10.**

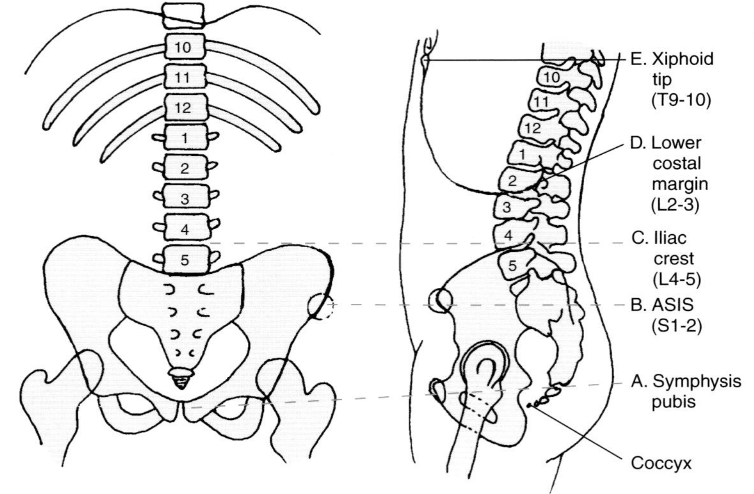

Fig. 10-23. Lower-spine landmarks.

10

Positioning Considerations

PATIENT RADIATION PROTECTION

Use of gonadal shielding and close collimation is especially important in dose reduction because of the proximity of the lumbar spine, sacrum, and coccyx to the gonads. Gonadal shielding can and should **always be used on males** of reproductive age on coccyx, sacrum, or lumbar-spine radiographs. The gonadal shield should be placed with the top edge of the shield at the lower margin of the symphysis pubis.

If the area of interest includes the sacrum and/or coccyx, gonadal shielding for females may not be possible without obscuring essential anatomy.

Females of childbearing age always must be questioned regarding the possibility of pregnancy before any radiographic exam of the lower vertebral column begins.

PATIENT POSITION

AP projections of the lumbar spine are obtained with the **knees flexed.** Flexing the knees (Fig. 10-26) reduces the lumbar curvature (lordosis), bringing the back closer to the radiographic exam table and the lumbar vertebral column more parallel to the IR. The incorrect position is shown in Fig. 10-25, where the pelvis is tipped forward slightly when the lower limbs are extended, exaggerating the lumbar curvature.

PA Versus AP Projections Even though the AP projection (with knees flexed) is a common part of the routine for the lumbar spine, there is an advantage to the PA projection. The prone position places the lumbar spine with its natural lumbar curvature in such a way that the intervertebral disk spaces are nearer parallel to the divergent x-ray beam. This position opens up and provides better visualization of the margins of the intervertebral disk spaces. Another advantage to the PA projection is a lower female ovarian dose of 25% to 30% less for a PA projection compared with an AP. (See icon boxes of patient dose comparisons for the AP [or PA] lumbar projection on p. 333 of this chapter.) However, a disadvantage of the PA projection is the increased OID of the lumbar vertebrae, which results in magnification unsharpness, especially for a patient with a large abdomen.

EXPOSURE FACTORS

The kV required for radiography of the lower vertebral column is dependent on the patient position. For example, the lateral position requires a higher kV than a supine position because of increased part thickness. Some department protocols require use of high-kV techniques. Increasing the kV and decreasing the mAs accordingly reduces patient doses but produces a lower-contrast image. Higher kV also increases scatter radiation, which tends to degrade the radiographic image. Close collimation is vital with high-kV technique to limit the amount of scatter radiation reaching the image and, as always, to reduce the patient dose. Recommended kV and comparative patient doses are listed on positioning pages.

Lead Mat on Tabletop See the following page, which details the importance of this practice along with close collimation, especially with digital imaging.

SID

The minimum SID is typically 40 inches (100 cm), but an increased SID of 42, 44, or even 46 inches (107, 112, or 117 cm) may be used in some departments to reduce magnification. This use depends on equipment specifications, as well as department protocol.

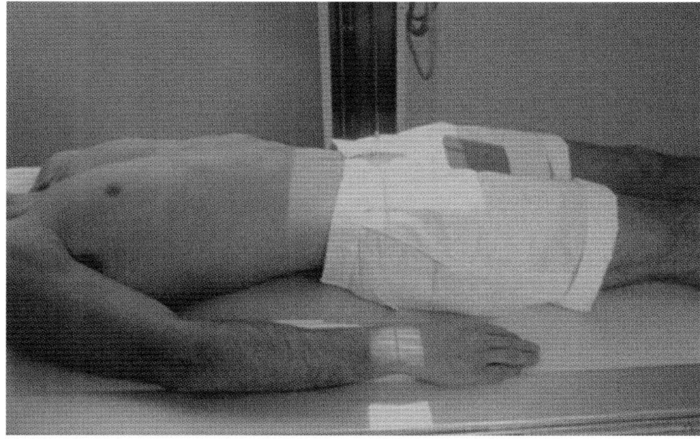

Fig. 10-24. Male gonadal shielding—lumbar spine.

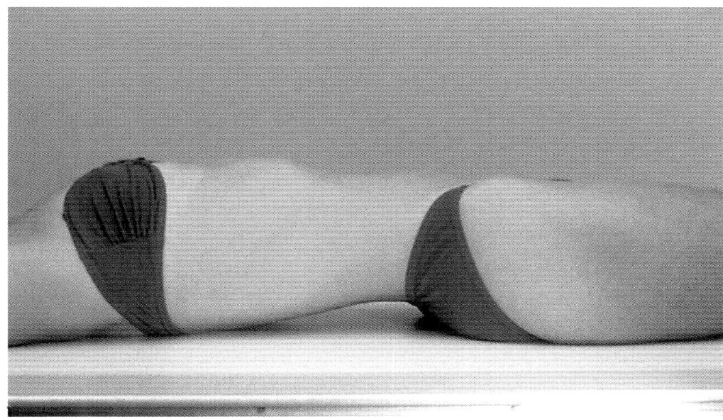

Fig. 10-25. Incorrect—lower limbs extended (AP lumbar spine).

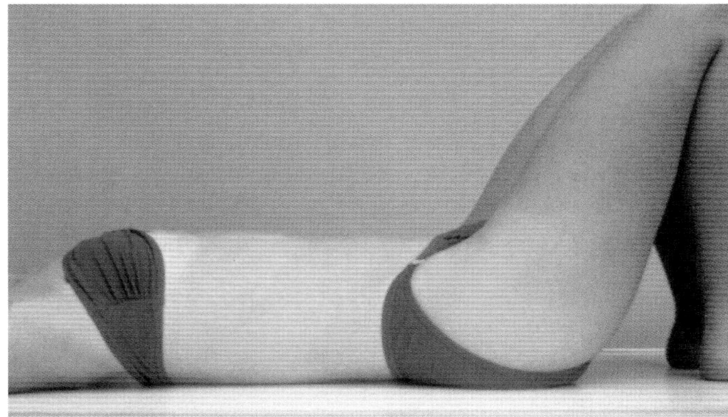

Fig. 10-26. Correct—knees and hips flexed (AP lumbar spine).

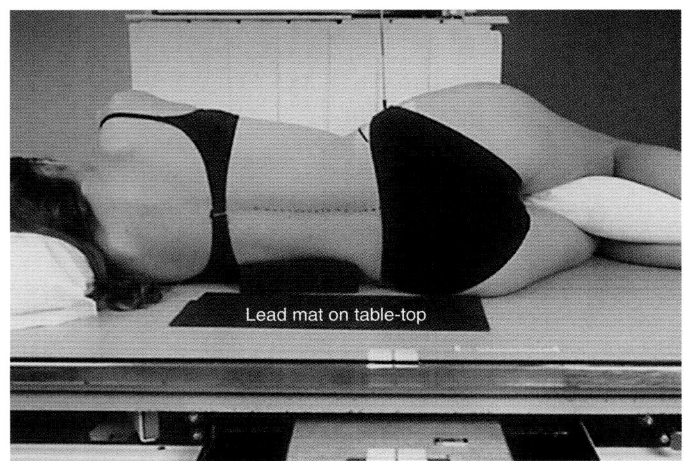

Fig. 10-27. Lateral lumbar spine with lead mat on tabletop.

10

PART/IR ALIGNMENT

Correct part/IR alignment is important during radiography of the lower vertebral column to ensure that the beam passes through the intervertebral disk spaces. This alignment may require a radiolucent sponge to be placed under the patient's waist to ensure that the spine is parallel with the IR. If a sponge is required, the size required is determined by the patient's body habitus.

DIGITAL IMAGING

As with other general skeletal radiographic examinations, CR and DR may be used to obtain images of the lumbar spine, sacrum, and coccyx. Because of the high sensitivity of these image-capture devices, **close collimation** and use of a **lead mat** posterior to the patient for a lateral lumbar spine position are important to reduce the amount of scatter reaching the IR (see Fig. 10-29), ensuring high-quality images.

PEDIATRIC APPLICATIONS

Patient Motion and Safety Two primary concerns in pediatric radiography are **patient motion** and **safety.** A clear explanation of the procedure is required to obtain maximal trust and cooperation from the patient and guardian.

Careful immobilization is important to achieve proper positioning and to reduce patient motion. A short exposure time helps reduce patient motion.

To secure their safety, pediatric patients should be continuously watched and cared for. Refer to Chapter 20 for detailed communication strategies, immobilization techniques, and explanations.

Communication Clear, simple instructions and communication are important, and distraction techniques that use toys, stuffed animals, etc., are effective in maintenance of patient cooperation.

Immobilization Pediatric patients (depending on age and condition) are often unable to maintain the required positions. Use of immobilization devices to support the patient is recommended to reduce the need for the patient to be held, thus reducing radiation exposure. (Chapter 20 provides an in-depth description of such devices.) If the patient must be held by the guardian, the technologist must provide a lead apron and/or gloves, and if the guardian is female, ensure that there is no possibility of pregnancy.

Technical Factors Technical factors vary with patient size. Use of **short exposures times** (associated with the use of high mA) is recommended to reduce the risk of patient motion.

GERIATRIC APPLICATIONS

Communication and Comfort Sensory loss (eyesight, hearing, etc.) associated with aging may result in the geriatric patient requiring additional assistance, time, and patience in achieving the required positions for spinal radiography. Decreased position awareness may cause these patients to fear falling off the radiography table when they are imaged in the recumbent position. Reassurance and additional care from the technologist help the patient to feel secure and comfortable.

If the examination is performed with the patient in the recumbent position, a radiolucent mattress or pad placed on the exam table provides comfort. Extra blankets may also be required to keep the patient warm. Patients with exaggerated kyphosis may be more comfortable if positioned for the images in the erect position.

Technical Factors Because of the high incidence of osteoporosis in geriatric patients, the kV or mAs may require a decrease if manual exposure factors are being used with film-screen imaging.

Older patients may have tremors or difficulty holding steady. Use of short exposure times (associated with the use of higher mA) is recommended to reduce the risk of motion.

Digital Imaging Considerations

The following guidelines are important for digital imaging (CR and DR) of the lumbar spine, sacrum, and coccyx:

1. **Correct central ray angle and centering:** This allows accurate post-processing by the image reader. This is especially important for projections such as the L5-S1 joint, the sacrum, and/or coccyx.
2. **Close collimation and tabletop lead masking:** This improves image quality by reducing scatter and secondary exposure to the highly sensitive digital image receptors.
3. **Adherence to the ALARA principle** in determining exposure factors: This may include increasing the kV for digital imaging over film-screen imaging, both for reducing patient exposure and for improving image quality.
4. **Post-processing evaluation of exposure index values:** This becomes an important consideration with lumbar spine, sacrum, and coccyx projections to ensure **optimum image quality with the least radiation** to the patient. (Remember, some of these projections may include primary exposure, as well as secondary and scatter radiation to the reproductive organs.)

Alternative Modalities and Procedures

COMPUTED TOMOGRAPHY

Computed tomography (CT) is useful in evaluation of the vertebral column. A wide range of pathologic conditions is demonstrated on the sectional images, including presence/extent of fractures, disk disease, and neoplastic disease.

MAGNETIC RESONANCE IMAGING

Magnetic resonance imaging (MRI) is superior for evaluation of the soft-tissue structures of the lumbar spine (that is, the spinal cord and intervertebral disk spaces).

NUCLEAR MEDICINE TECHNOLOGY

Nuclear medicine technology provides a sensitive diagnostic procedure (the radionuclide bone scan) for detection of skeletal pathologic processes. A radiopharmaceutical-tagged tracer element is injected that concentrates in areas of increased bone activity, demonstrating a "hot spot" on the nuclear medicine image. Any abnormal area is then further investigated with radiography.

Commonly, patients who are at risk or symptomatic for skeletal metastases undergo a bone scan (patients with multiple myeloma are an exception to this). The vertebral column is a common site of skeletal metastases. Inflammatory conditions, Paget's disease, neoplastic processes, and osteomyelitis may also be demonstrated on the bone scan.

BONE DENSITOMETRY

Bone densitometry is the noninvasive measurement of bone mass (see Chapter 23). The lumbar spine is one area often assessed in a bone-density study. Causes for loss of bone mass (osteoporosis) include long-term steroid use, hyperparathyroidism, estrogen deficiency, advancing age, and lifestyle factors (smoking, sedentary lifestyle, alcoholism). Bone densitometry is accurate to within 1%, and the radiation skin dose is very low. Conventional radiography does not detect loss of bone until the bone mass has been reduced by at least 30%.

MYELOGRAPHY

Myelography requires an injection of contrast media into the subarachnoid space via a lumbar or cervical puncture to visualize the soft-tissue structures of the spinal canal. Lesions of the spinal canal, nerve roots, and intervertebral disks are demonstrated.

The increase in availability of CT and MRI has greatly reduced the number of myelograms performed. In addition to the superior diagnostic quality of these modalities, the avoidance of the invasive puncture and contrast injection are benefits to the patient.

Pathologic Indications

Ankylosing spondylitis is an inflammatory condition that usually begins in the sacroiliac joints and progresses up the vertebral column. The spine may become completely rigid as the intervertebral and costovertebral joints fuse. It is most common in males in their 30s, and no cause is known.

Fractures are a lack in continuity of a structure:

- **Compression fractures** may be due to trauma, osteoporosis, or metastatic disease. The superior and inferior surfaces of the vertebral body are driven together, producing a wedge-shaped vertebra. For patients with osteoporosis or other vertebral pathologic processes, the force needed to cause this fracture type may be quite minor (for example, lifting light objects). This type of fracture rarely causes a neurologic deficit.
- **Chance fractures** result from a hyperflexion force, causing fracture through the vertebral body and posterior elements (spinous process, pedicles, facets, transverse processes). Patients wearing lap-type seat belts are at risk because these belts act as a fulcrum during sudden deceleration.

Herniated nucleus pulposus (HNP), also commonly known as a ***herniated lumbar disc*** (slipped disk) is usually due to trauma or improper lifting. The soft inner part of the intervertebral disk (nucleus pulposus) protrudes through the fibrous outer layer, pressing on the spinal cord or nerves. It occurs most frequently at L4 to L5 levels, causing **sciatica** (an irritation of the sciatic nerve that passes down the posterior leg). Plain radiographs do not demonstrate this condition but can be used to rule out other pathologic processes, such as neoplasia, spondylolisthesis, etc. Myelography once was indicated to visualize this pathologic process. CT and MRI are now the modalities of choice.

Metastases are primary malignant neoplasms that spread to distant sites via blood and lymphatics. The vertebrae are common sites of metastatic lesions, which may be characterized and visualized on the image as follows:

- **Osteolytic**—destructive lesions with irregular margins
- **Osteoblastic**—proliferative bony lesions of increased density
- **Combination osteolytic and osteoblastic**—"moth-eaten" appearance of bone resulting from the mix of destructive and blastic lesions

Scoliosis is a lateral curvature of the vertebral column, usually with some rotation of the vertebra. It involves the thoracic and lumbar regions.

Spina bifida is a congenital condition in which the posterior aspects of the vertebrae fail to develop, exposing part of the spinal cord. This condition varies greatly in severity and occurs most often at L5 (see Pathologic Indications in Chapter 20).

Spondylolisthesis involves forward movement of one vertebra in relation to another. It is commonly due to a developmental defect in the pars interarticularis or may result from spondylolysis or severe osteoarthritis. It is most common at L5-S1 but also occurs at L4-L5. Severe cases require a spinal fusion.

Spondylolysis is the dissolution of a vertebra, such as from aplasia (lack of development) of the vertebral arch and **separation of the pars interarticularis** of the vertebra. On the oblique projection the neck of the Scotty dog appears broken. It is most common at L4 or L5.

SUMMARY OF PATHOLOGIC INDICATIONS

CONDITION OR DISEASE	MOST COMMON IMAGING PROCEDURE	POSSIBLE RADIOGRAPHIC APPEARANCE	MANUAL EXPOSURE FACTOR ADJUSTMENT*
Ankylosing spondylitis	AP, lateral lumbar spine, sacroiliac joints Nuclear medicine bone scan	Vertebral column becoming fused, appearance of piece of bamboo; anterior longitudinal ligaments calcifying	None
Fractures:			
Compression	AP, lateral lumbar spine, CT	Anterior wedging of vertebrae; loss of body height	None or slight decrease depending on severity
Chance	AP, lateral lumbar spine, CT	Fracture through vertebral body and posterior elements	None
Herniated nucleus pulposus (HNP) (Herniated lumbar disc)	AP, lateral lumbar spine, CT, MRI	Possible narrowing of intervertebral disk spaces	None
Metastases	Bone scan, AP, lateral of spine	Dependent on lesion type: —Destructive—irregular margins and decreased density —Osteoblastic lesions—increased density —Combination—a moth-eaten appearance	None or increase or decrease, depending on type of lesion and stage of pathologic process
Scoliosis	Erect AP/PA and lateral spine	Lateral curvature of vertebral column	None
Spina bifida	Prenatal ultrasound, PA and lateral spine, CT or MRI	"Open" posterior vertebra, exposure of part of spinal cord	None
Spondylolisthesis	AP, lateral lumbar spine, CT	Forward slipping of one vertebra in relation to another	None
Spondylolysis	AP, lateral, oblique views of spine, CT	Defect in the pars interarticularis ("Scotty dog" appearing to wear a collar)	None

*Depends on stage or severity of disease or condition.

Survey Information

Following are summaries of results of surveys conducted in years 1989, 1995, and 2000 to determine the most common basic and special projections/positions as performed in the United States and Canada.

SUMMARY OF SURVEY RESULTS

Lumbar Spine The four most common **basic or routine projections** for the lumbar spine continue to be the **AP, lateral, lateral L5-S1,** and **oblique.** The **posterior obliques** are considered basic by **78%** of radiographic facilities in the U.S., but only **39%** in Canada. **Anterior obliques** are less common and are considered basic or routine by **20%** in the U.S. and **28%** in Canada.

The use of the **PA** rather than the AP projection increased to 11% in the total U.S. in 2000, from only 5% in 1995. The use of the PA in 2000 was much higher in the Western states (27%) than in the Midwest (10%) and the East (7%). In Canada the use of PA was only 9%.

The most common **special projections** for the lumbar spine listed in order of usage are as follows: **lateral flexion and extension** (64% in U.S., 46% in Canada); **AP fusion, R and L bending** (49% in U.S., 34% in Canada); **AP or PA scoliosis projection** (45% in U.S., 51% in Canada); and **AP L5-S1 axial** (26% in U.S., 13% in Canada).

Sacrum and Coccyx The three most common projections are the **AP axial sacrum** (98%-99%), **AP axial coccyx** (94%-96%), and **lateral sacrum and coccyx combined** (82% in U.S., 91% in Canada). The combined lateral of the sacrum and coccyx is much more common (82% in U.S., 91% in Canada) than separate laterals of the sacrum and coccyx (36% U.S., 22% in Canada).

Separate laterals are also **not recommended** by this textbook (unless they are specifically indicated) because of the relatively high gonadal doses from these projections.

Standard and Special Operating Procedures

Protocols and operating procedures vary among facilities, depending on administrative structures, liabilities, etc. Technologists should become familiar with the current standards of practice, protocols, and routine, or basic, and special projections for any facility in which they work.

Certain basic and special projections for the lumbar spine, sacrum, and coccyx are demonstrated and described on the following pages as suggested standard basic and special departmental routines or procedures.

BASIC PROJECTIONS

Standard, or basic, projections, also sometimes referred to as *routine projections* or *departmental routines,* are those projections commonly taken on average patients who are helpful and can cooperate in performing the procedure.

SPECIAL PROJECTIONS

Special projections are those more common projections taken as extra or additional projections to better demonstrate certain pathologic conditions or specific anatomic structures.

BASIC AND SPECIAL PROJECTIONS

10

AP (OR PA) PROJECTION: LUMBAR SPINE

Pathology Demonstrated
Pathology of the lumbar vertebrae, including fractures, scoliosis, and neoplastic processes, is demonstrated.

Lumbar Spine
BASIC
• AP (or PA)
• **Obliques–Anterior or posterior**
• **Lateral**
• **Lateral L5-S1**

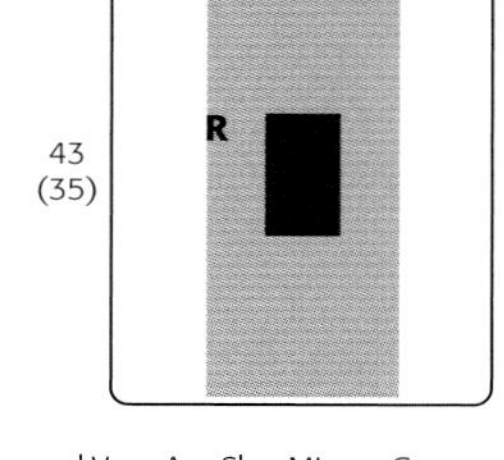

Technical Factors
- IR size—35 × 43 cm (14 × 17 inches), lengthwise, or 30 × 35 cm (11 × 14 inches)
- Moving or stationary grid
- 75-80 kV range (or 85-92 kV and reduction of mAs and dose)
- Technique and dose

	cm	kV	mAs	Sk.	ML.	Gon.
—AP at 80 kV:	17	80	15	175	45	M 1 F 19
—AP at 92 kV:	17	92	8	127	36	M 1 F 15
—PA at 92 kV:	17	92	8	127	36	M 0 F 11
						mrad

Shielding Place contact shield over gonads without obscuring area of interest. Female ovarian shielding obscures portions of sacrum and coccyx.

Patient Position Patient should be supine, with knees flexed and head on pillow (may also be done in prone or erect position; see Notes below).

Part Position
- Align midsagittal plane to CR and midline of table/grid.
- Place arms at side or up on chest.
- Ensure **no rotation** of torso or pelvis exists.

Central Ray
- Direct CR perpendicular to IR centered to following:

Larger IR (35 × 43): Center to **level of iliac crest** (L4-5 interspace). This larger IR will include lumbar vertebrae, sacrum, and possibly coccyx. Center IR to CR.

Smaller IR (30 × 35): Center to the **level of L3,** which may be localized by palpation of the lower costal margin (1½ inches, or 4 cm, above iliac crest). This smaller IR will include primarily the five lumbar vertebrae. Center IR to CR.

- Minimum SID is 40 inches (100 cm).

Collimation Four-sided collimation with superior and inferior borders to near IR margins

Respiration Suspend breathing on **expiration.**

Notes: Partial flexion of knees as shown straightens the spine, which helps open intervertebral disk spaces.

Radiograph may be done prone as a PA projection, which places intervertebral spaces more closely parallel to the diverging rays.

The erect position may be useful to demonstrate the natural weight-bearing stance of the spine.

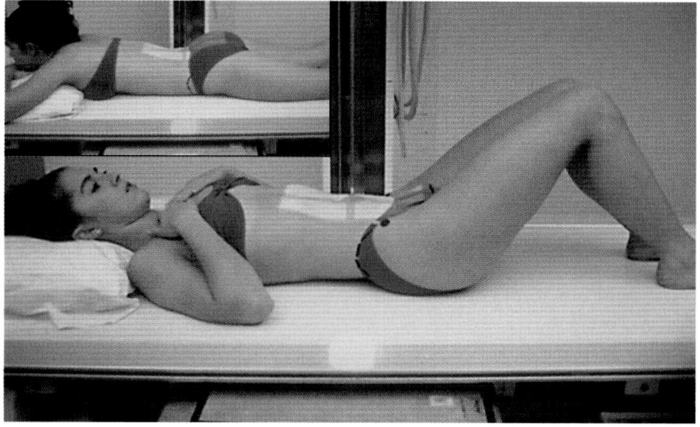

Fig. 10-28. AP projection (centered for 35 × 43 IR). *Inset,* Alternative PA projection.

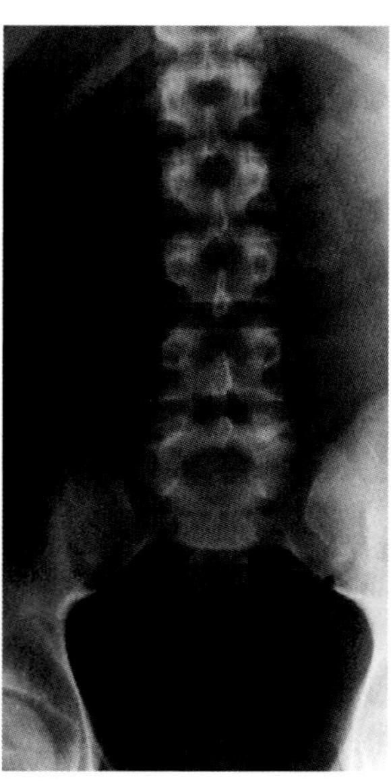

Fig. 10-29. AP projection (centered for 35 × 43 IR).

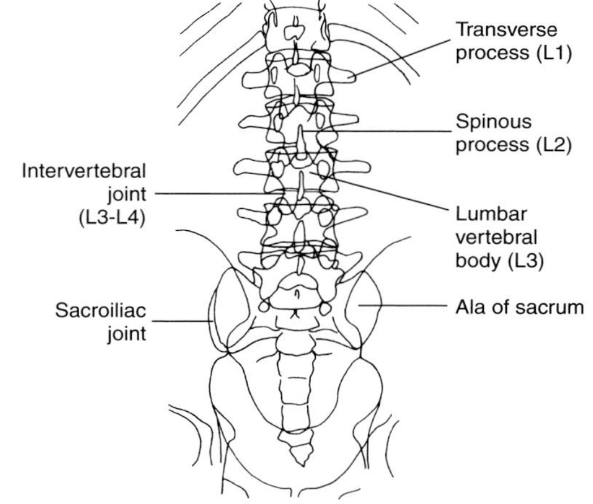

Fig. 10-30. AP projection.

Radiographic Criteria

Structures Shown: • Lumbar vertebral bodies, intervertebral joints, spinous and transverse processes, SI joints, and sacrum are shown. • 35 × 43 (14 × 17 inches) IR: Approximately T11 to the distal sacrum should be included. • 30 × 35 (11 × 14 inches) IR: T12 to S1 should be included.

Position: • **No patient rotation** is indicated by the following: SI joints equidistant from spinous processes; spinous processes in midline of vertebral column; R and L transverse processes equal in length.

Collimation and CR: • The vertebral column should be centered to the IR/collimated field, at the approximate level of L3-L4. • Lateral margins of collimated field should include the SI joints and psoas muscles.

Exposure Criteria: • Optimal density and contrast should demonstrate the lumbar vertebral bodies, intervertebral disk spaces, transverse processes, and psoas muscle shadows. • Sharp bony margins indicate no motion.

OBLIQUES—POSTERIOR (OR ANTERIOR) OBLIQUE POSITIONS: LUMBAR SPINE

Lumbar Spine
BASIC
- **AP (or PA)**
- Obliques–posterior or anterior
- **Lateral**
- **Lateral L5-S1**

30 (24)

35 (30)

R

Pathology Demonstrated

Defects of the pars interarticularis (for example, spondylolysis) are demonstrated.

Both right and left obliques obtained.

Technical Factors

- IR size—2 each 30 × 35 cm (11 × 14 inches), lengthwise, or 24 × 30 cm (10 × 12 inches)
- Moving or stationary grid
- 75-80 kV range (or 85-90 kV and reduction of mAs and dose)
- Technique and dose:

	cm	kV	mAs	Sk.	ML.	Gon.
Posterior oblique	21	85	15	222	45	M 0, F 22
Anterior oblique	21	85	15	222	45	M 0, F 15

mrad

Shielding Place contact shield over gonads without obscuring area of interest.

Patient Position Patient should be semisupine (RPO and LPO) or semiprone (RAO and LAO).

Part Position

- **Rotate body 45°** to place spinal column directly over midline of table/grid, aligned to CR.
- Flex knee for stability and comfort.
- Support lower back and pelvis with radiolucent sponges to maintain position. (This support is strongly recommended to prevent patients from grasping the edge of the table, which may result in their fingers being pinched.)

Central Ray

- Direct CR perpendicular to IR.
- Center to **L3 at the level of the lower costal margin (4 cm, or 1½ inches) above iliac crest.**
- Center 2 inches (5 cm) medial to upside ASIS.
- Center IR to CR.
- Minimum SID is 40 inches (100 cm).

Collimation Four-sided collimation to area of interest

Respiration Suspend breathing on expiration.

Note: A **50°** oblique from plane of tabletop best visualizes the zygapophyseal joints at **L1** to **L2,** and **30°** for **L5** to **S1.**

Fig. 10-31. 45° **RPO,** visualizing **right** (downside) zygapophyseal joints. Alternative anterior oblique, **LAO-right joints.**

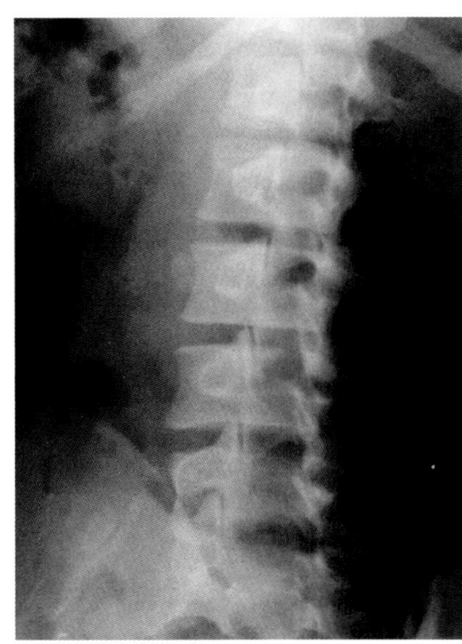

Fig. 10-32. 45° oblique.

Radiographic Criteria

Structures Shown: • Zygapophyseal joints are visible. (RPO and LPO show downside; RAO and LAO show upside.) • "Scotty dogs" should be visualized, and zygapophyseal joint should appear open.

Position: • Correct 45° patient rotation results in the pedicle ("eye") of the Scotty dog near the center of the vertebral body on the image. • The pedicle demonstrated posteriorly on the vertebral body indicates overrotation, and the pedicle demonstrated anteriorly on the vertebral body indicates underrotation.

Collimation and CR: • The vertebral column should be in the midline of the collimated field/IR, which is centered to L3.

Exposure Criteria: • Optimal density and contrast clearly demonstrate zygapophyseal joints from L1 to L5. • Sharp bony margins indicate no motion.

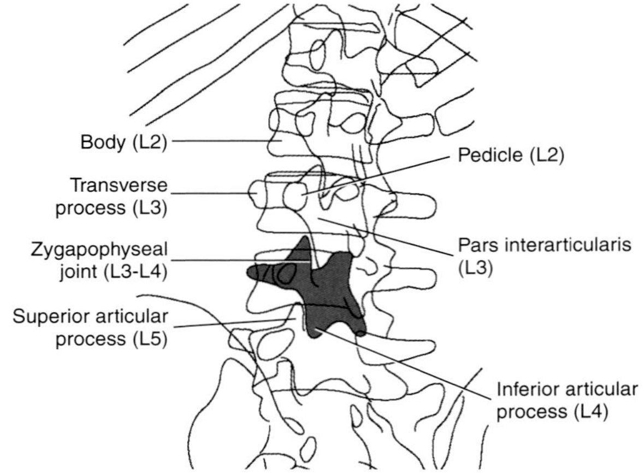

Fig. 10-33. 45° oblique.

LATERAL POSITION: LUMBAR SPINE

Lumbar Spine
BASIC
- AP (or PA)
- Obliques–posterior or anterior
- Lateral
- Lateral L5-S1

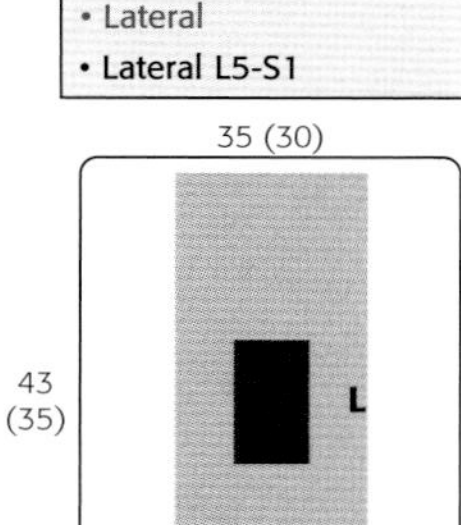

Pathology Demonstrated

Fractures, spondylolisthesis, neoplastic processes, and osteoporosis of lumbar vertebrae are demonstrated.

Technical Factors

- IR size–35 × 43 cm (14 × 17 inches), lengthwise, or 30 × 35 cm (11 × 14 inches)
- Moving or stationary grid
- 85-95 kV range
- Lead mat on tabletop behind patient
- Technique and dose:

	cm	kV	mAs	Sk.	ML.	Gon.
(Female)	27	90	50	1008	134	M 0 F 29
(Male)	30	90	65	1310	174	M 0 F 38

mrad

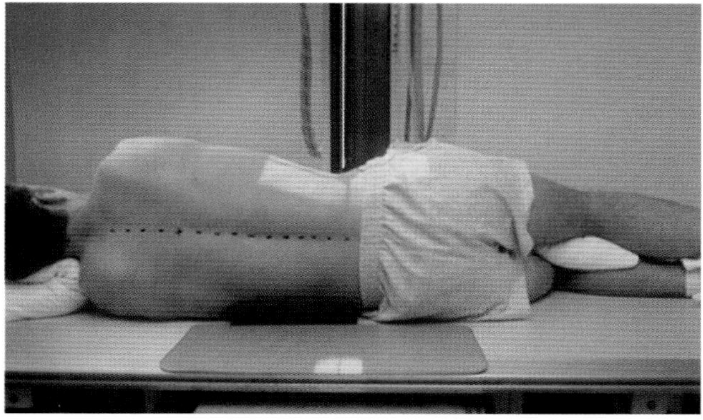

Fig. 10-34. L lateral (CR perpendicular to IR).

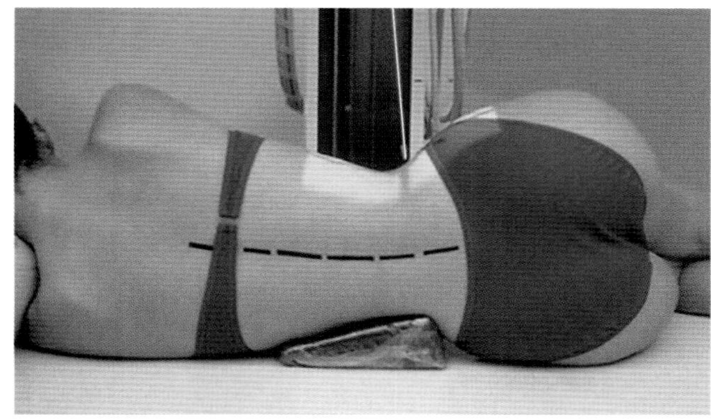

Fig. 10-35. L lateral (CR 5° caudad).

Shielding Shield gonads without obscuring area of interest.

Patient Position Position patient lateral recumbent, pillow for head, knees flexed, with support between knees and ankles to better maintain a true lateral position and ensure patient comfort.

Part Position

- Align midcoronal plane to CR and midline of table/grid.
- Place radiolucent support under waist, as needed to place the long axis of the spine near parallel to the table (palpating spinous processes to determine; see Notes).
- Ensure pelvis and torso are in **true lateral position.**

Central Ray

- Direct CR **perpendicular to long axis of spine.**

Larger IR (35 × 43): Center to **level of iliac crest** (L4-5). This position includes lumbar vertebrae, sacrum, and possibly coccyx. Center IR to CR.

Smaller IR (30 × 35): Center to L3 at the level of the lower costal margin (1½ inches, or 4 cm, above iliac crest). This position includes the five lumbar vertebrae. Center IR to CR.

- Minimum SID is 40 inches (100 cm).

Collimation Closely collimate on lateral borders. (Light field appears small because of the proximity of the patient to the x-ray tube and the divergence of the x-ray beam.)

Respiration Suspend breathing on expiration.

Notes: Although the average male patient (and some female patients) requires no CR angle, a patient with a wider pelvis and narrow thorax may require a 5° to 8° caudad angle even with support, as shown in Fig. 10-35.

If patient has a lateral curvature (scoliosis) of the spine (as determined by viewing of the spine from the back with the patient in the erect position and with hospital gown open) the patient should be placed in whichever lateral position **places the "sag," or convexity of the spine, down** to better open the intervertebral spaces.

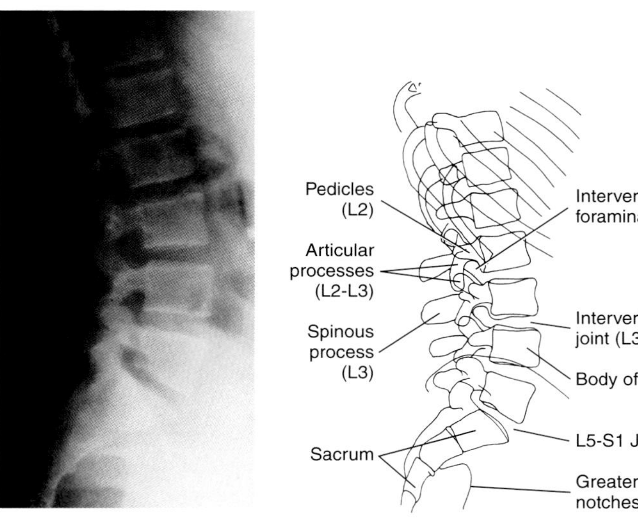

Fig. 10-36. Lateral. **Fig. 10-37.** Lateral.

Radiographic Criteria

Structures Shown: • Intervertebral foramina L1 to L4, vertebral bodies, intervertebral joints, spinous processes, and L5 to S1 junction are visible. • Depending on the IR size used, the entire sacrum may be included also.

Position: • Vertebral column is aligned parallel to the IR, as indicated by the following: intervertebral foramina appearing open; intervertebral joint spaces appearing open • No rotation is indicated by superimposed greater sciatic notches and posterior vertebral bodies.

Collimation and CR: • The vertebral column should be centered to the collimated field/IR, at the level of L3.

Exposure Criteria: • Optimal density and contrast should clearly demonstrate the vertebral bodies and joint spaces. • Sharp bony margins indicate no motion.

LATERAL L5 TO S1 POSITION: LUMBAR SPINE

Lumbar Spine
BASIC
- AP (or PA)
- Obliques–posterior or anterior
- Lateral
- Lateral L5-S1

Pathology Demonstrated
Spondylolisthesis involving L4 to L5 or L5 to S1 and other L5 to S1 pathologies is demonstrated.

Technical Factors
- IR size—18 × 24 cm (8 × 10 inches), lengthwise
- Moving or stationary grid
- 95-100 kV range
- Lead mat on tabletop behind patient
- Technique and dose:

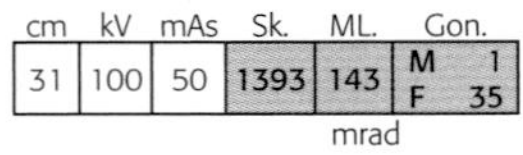

cm	kV	mAs	Sk.	ML.	Gon.
31	100	50	1393	143	M 1 F 35

mrad

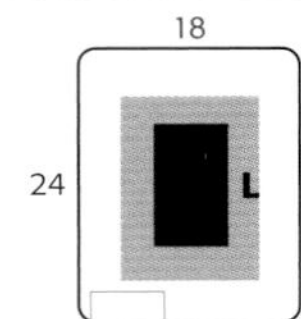

Shielding Shield gonads without obscuring area of interest.

Patient Position Patient should be in the lateral recumbent position, with a pillow for head and knees flexed. Provide support between knees and ankles to better maintain a true lateral position and ensure patient comfort.

Part Position
- Align midcoronal plane to CR and midline of table/grid.
- Flex knees.
- Place radiolucent support under waist (see Notes).
- Ensure pelvis and torso are in **true lateral** position.

Central Ray
- Direct CR **perpendicular** to IR with sufficient waist support, or angle **5° to 8° caudad** with less support (see Notes below).
- Center CR **1½ inches (4 cm) inferior to iliac crest** and **2 inches (5 cm) posterior to ASIS.** Center IR to CR.
- Minimum SID is 40 inches (100 cm).

Collimation Close four-sided collimation to area of interest

Respiration Suspend breathing.

Notes: If waist is not supported sufficiently, resulting in a sagging of the vertebral column, the CR must be angled 5° to 8° caudad to be parallel to interiliac plane (imaginary line between iliac crests, see Fig. 10-39)*

High amounts of secondary/scatter radiation are generated due to the part thickness. Close collimation is essential, along with placement of lead mat on tabletop behind patient. (This is especially important with digital imaging.)

*Francis C: Method improves consistency in L5-S1 joint space films. Radiol Technol 63:302, 1992.

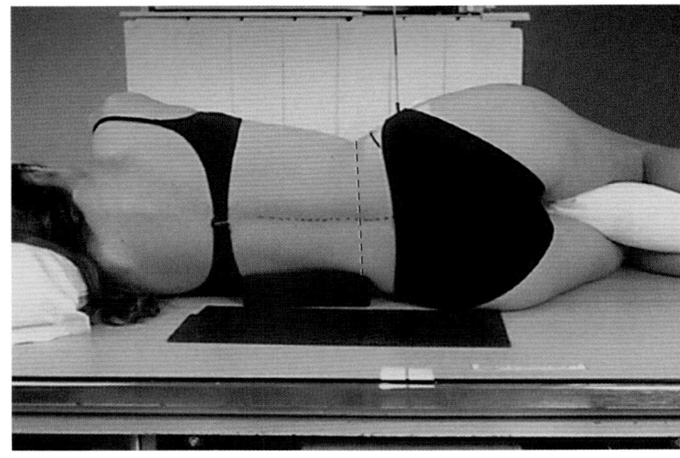

Fig. 10-38. L lateral L5-S1 with near-sufficient support—0° to 3° angle.

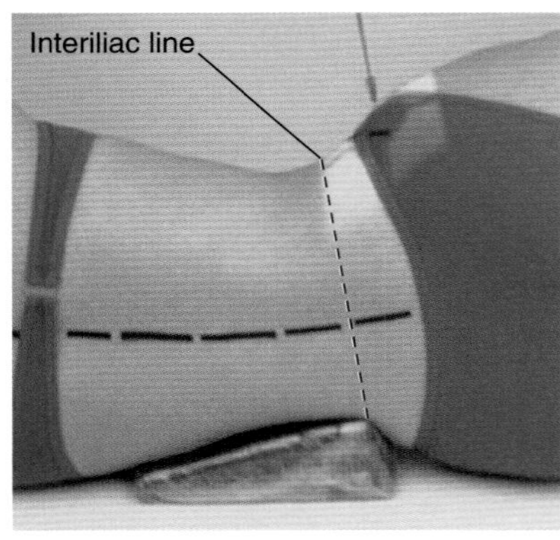

Fig. 10-39. L Lateral L5-S1 with less support—CR 5° to 8° caudad. (CR parallel to interiliac line.)

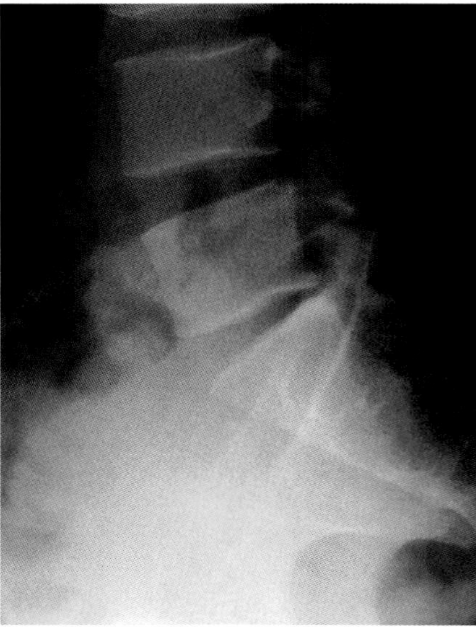

Fig. 10-40. Lateral L5-S1.

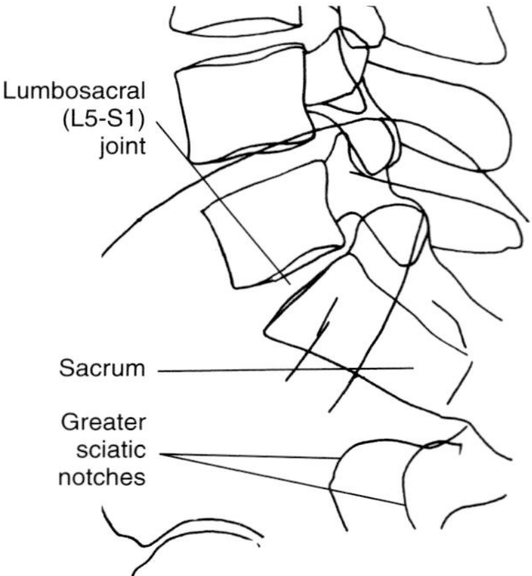

Fig. 10-41. Lateral L5-S1.

Radiographic Criteria

Structures Shown: • Open L4 to L5 and L5 to S1 joint space.

Position: • No rotation of the patient is evidenced by superimposed AP dimensions of greater sciatic notches of posterior pelvis and superimposed posterior borders of the vertebral bodies. • Correct alignment of the vertebral column and the IR/CR is indicated by open L4 to L5 and L5 to S1 joint spaces.

Collimation and CR: • L5 to S1 joint space in center of closely collimated field/IR.

Exposure Criteria: • Optimal contrast and density should clearly demonstrate the L5 to S1 joint space through the superimposed ilia of the pelvis. • Sharp bony margins indicate no motion.

AP AXIAL L5-S1 PROJECTION: LUMBAR SPINE

Lumbar Spine
SPECIAL
• AP axial L5-S1

Pathology Demonstrated
Pathology of L5 to S1 and the sacroiliac joints is demonstrated.

Technical Factors

- IR size—18 × 24 cm (8 × 10 inches), crosswise.
- Moving or stationary grid
- 80-85 kV range
- Technique and dose:

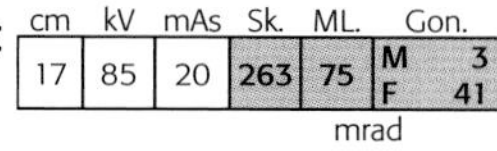

cm	kV	mAs	Sk.	ML.	Gon.
17	85	20	263	75	M 3 F 41

mrad

24
18 R

Shielding Shield gonads without obscuring area of interest. Female ovarian shielding obscures a portion of sacroiliac joints.

Patient Position Patient should be supine, with pillow for head and legs extended, with support under knees for comfort.

Part Position

- Place arms at side or on chest.
- Align midsagittal plane to CR and midline of table/grid.
- Ensure **no rotation** of torso or pelvis exists.

Central Ray

- Angle CR **cephalad, 30° (males)** to **35° (females).**
- CR should enter at the **level of the ASIS** centered to the **midline** of the body.
- Center IR to projected CR.
- Minimum SID is 40 inches (100 cm).

Collimation Close four-sided collimation to area of interest

Respiration Suspend breathing during exposure.

Notes: Angled AP projection "opens" L5 to S1 joint.

Lateral view of L5-S1 generally provides more information than the AP projection.

Radiograph also may be done **prone** with **caudal** angle of CR (increases OID).

Radiographic Criteria

Structures Shown: • L5 to S1 joint space and sacroiliac joints in AP projection

Position: • Sacroiliac joints demonstrate equal distance from spine, indicating no pelvic rotation. • Correct alignment of CR and L5-S1 is evidenced by an open joint space.

Collimation and CR: • L5 to S1 joint demonstrated in the center of a well-collimated field/IR.

Exposure Criteria: • Optimal density and contrast demonstrate the L5-S1 region and sacroiliac joints. • Sharp bony margins indicate no motion.

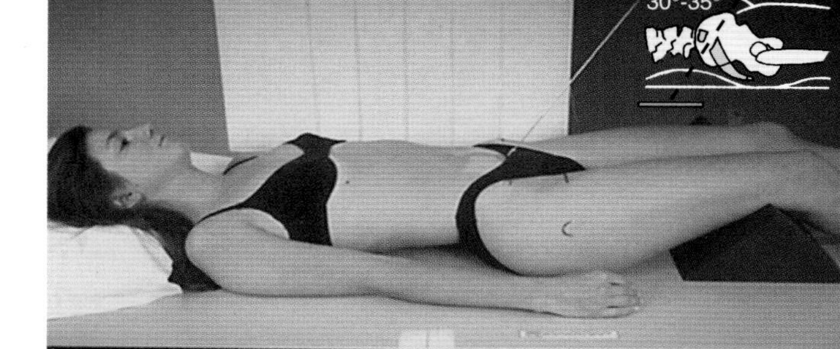

Fig. 10-42. AP axial L5-S1—30° to 35° cephalad.

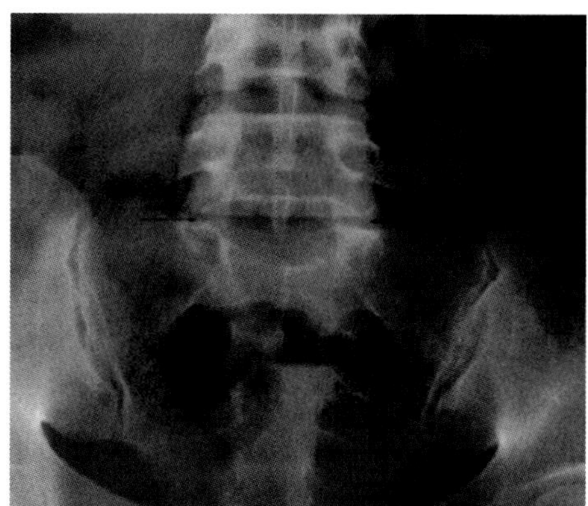

Fig. 10-43. AP axial L5-S1—30° cephalad.

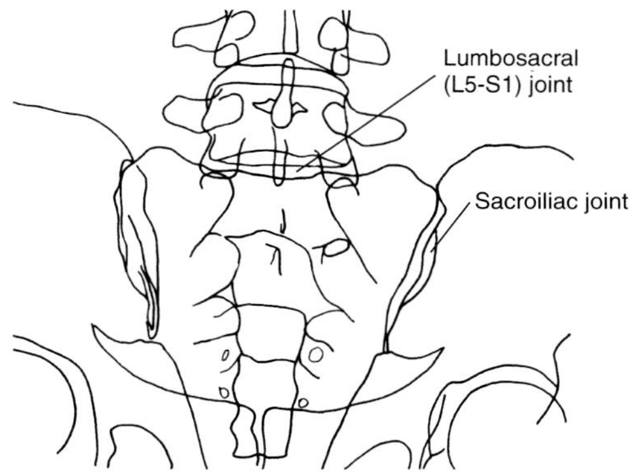

Fig. 10-44. AP axial L5-S1.

10

PA (AP) PROJECTION: SCOLIOSIS SERIES

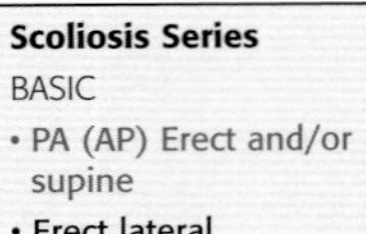
Scoliosis Series
BASIC
- PA (AP) Erect and/or supine
- Erect lateral

Pathology Demonstrated
Degree and severity of scoliosis are shown. A scoliosis series frequently includes **two AP (or PA) images** taken for comparison—one erect and one recumbent.

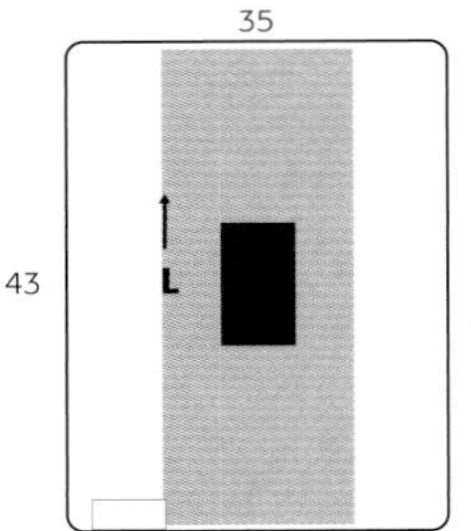

Technical Factors
- IR size—35 × 43 cm (14 × 17 inches), lengthwise; taller patients—35 × 90 cm (14 × 36 inches), if available
- Moving or stationary grid
- Compensating filters to obtain a more uniform density along the vertebral column
- kV as appropriate for patient size/age, to provide an image of optimal contrast and low patient dose
- Erect marker for erect position
- Technique and dose at 60 inches (152 cm) SID:

	cm	kV	mAs	Sk.	ML.	Breasts	Gon.
PA	23	90	25	447	81	16	M 1 F 43
AP	23	90	25	447	81	164	M 2 F 43

mrad

Shielding Shield gonadal region without obscuring area of interest. Use breast shields for young females. Shadow shields placed on collimator may be used as shown in Fig. 10-46 and as evident in Fig. 10-48.

Patient Position Position patient in the erect and recumbent position, with weight evenly distributed on both feet for the erect position.

Part Position
- Align midsagittal plane to CR and midline of IR, with arms at side.
- Ensure **no rotation** of torso or pelvis if possible. (Scoliosis may result in twisting and rotation of vertebrae, making some rotation unavoidable.)
- Place **lower margin of IR** a **minimum** of **1 to 2 inches (3 to 5 cm) below iliac crest** (centering height determined by IR size and/or area of scoliosis).

Central Ray
- CR perpendicular, directed to **midpoint of IR**
- SID of 40 to 60 inches (100 to 150 cm); longer SID required with larger IR to obtain required collimation

Collimation Collimate on four sides to area of interest. Too narrow a collimation is not recommended on **initial image** because deformities of adjacent areas of ribs and pelvis also must be evaluated.

Respiration Suspend breathing on **expiration.**

Notes: A PA rather than an AP projection is recommended because of the significantly reduced dose to radiation-sensitive areas, such as female breasts and the thyroid gland. Studies have shown this projection results in approximately 90% reduction in dosage to the breasts.* (Also see dose icon boxes above.)

Scoliosis generally requires repeat examinations over several years for pediatric patients, with emphasis on the need for careful shielding.

*Frank ED, Stears JG, Gray JE, and others: Use of the posteroanterior projection: a method of reducing x-ray exposures to radiosensitive organs, Radiol Technol 54:343-347, 1983.

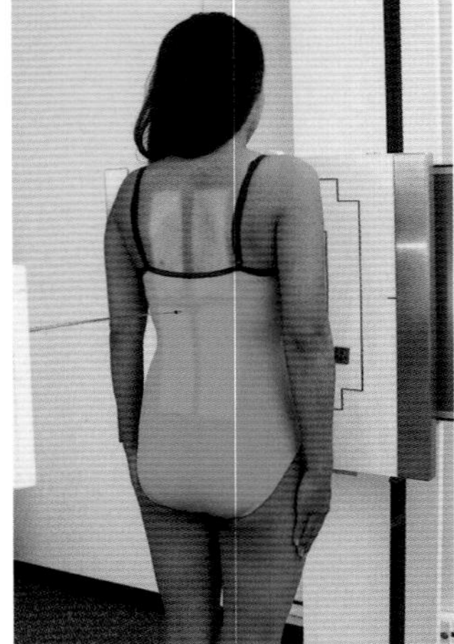
Fig. 10-45. PA erect.

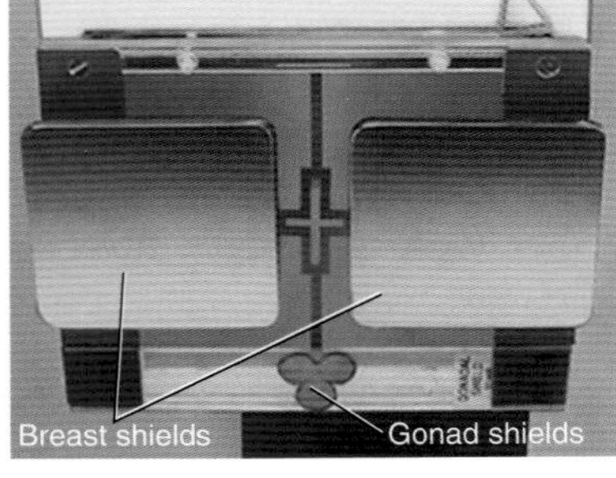

Fig. 10-46. Clear Pb compensating filters with breast and gonadal shields attached to bottom of collimator with magnets. (Courtesy Nuclear Associates, Carle, NY.)

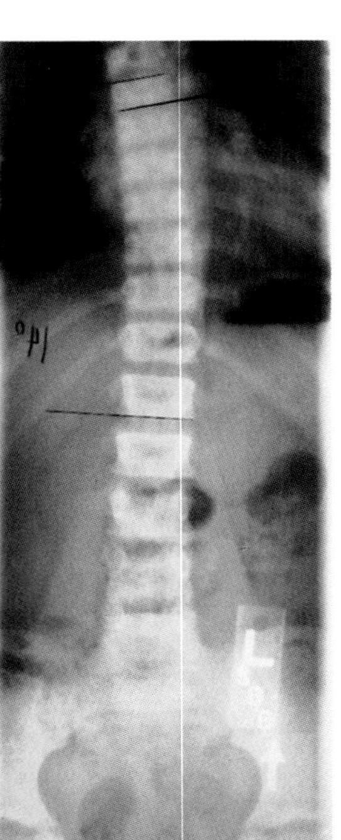
Fig. 10-47. PA erect—35 × 43 cm (14 × 17 inches) IR.

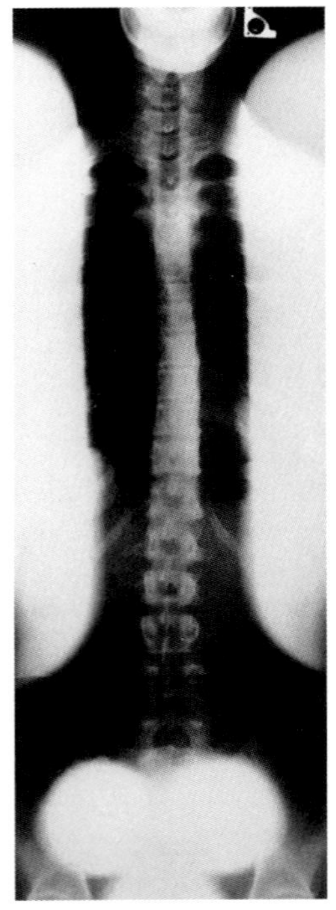
Fig. 10-48. PA erect—36 inches (90 cm) IR, shadow shields in place. (Courtesy Nuclear Associates, Carle, NY.)

Radiographic Criteria

Structures Shown: • The lumbar and thoracic vertebrae, as well as approximately 2 inches (5 cm) of the iliac crests.

Position: • Thoracic and lumbar vertebrae are demonstrated in as true an AP projection as possible. • Some rotation of pelvis and/or thorax may be apparent because scoliosis generally is accompanied by a twisting or rotation of involved vertebrae.

Collimation and CR: • Vertebral column should be in center of collimation field/IR.

Exposure Criteria: • Sufficient density and contrast should demonstrate the thoracic and lumbar vertebrae in their entirety. • A compensating filter assists in obtaining an even density throughout the length, if a 14 × 36 inch (35 × 90 cm) IR is used. • Sharp bony margins indicate no motion.

ERECT LATERAL POSITION: SCOLIOSIS SERIES

Scoliosis Series
BASIC
- **PA (AP) Erect and/or supine**
- Erect lateral

Structures Best Shown
Spondylolisthesis, degree of kyphosis, or lordosis.

Technical Factors
- IR size—35 × 43 cm (14 × 17 inches), lengthwise, or 35 × 90 cm (14 × 36 inches) on taller patients, if available
- Stationary or moving grid
- Erect marker
- Use of compensating filters to help obtain a more uniform density along the vertebral column
- 90-100 kV range
- Technique and dose at 60 inches (152 cm) SID:

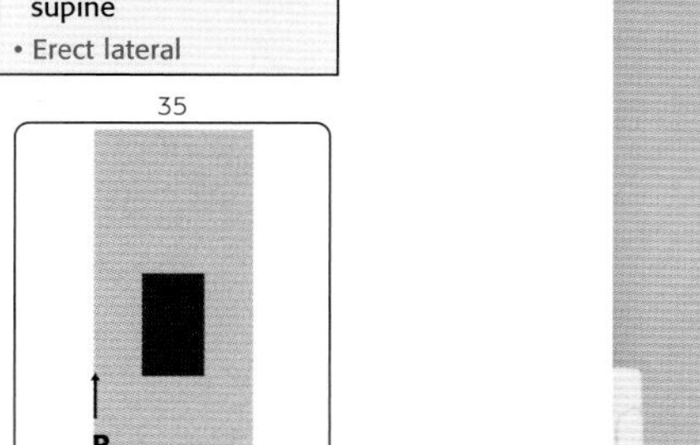

cm	kV	mAs	Sk.	ML.	Breasts	Gon.
27	90	50	1008	134	139	M 0 F 9

mrad

Shielding Place contact shield or shadow shield over gonads without obscuring area of interest. Use breast shields for young females.

Patient Position Position patient in erect lateral position with arms elevated, or if unsteady, grasping a support in front. The convex side of the curve is positioned against the IR.

Part Position
- Place pelvis and torso in as **true a lateral position** as possible.
- Align midcoronal plane of body to CR and midline of IR.
- Lower margin of IR should be a **minimum of 1 to 2 inches (3 to 5 cm) below level of iliac crests** (centering determined by IR size and patient size).

Central Ray
- CR **perpendicular,** directed to **midpoint of IR**
- SID of 40 to 60 inches (100 to 150 cm); longer SID required with larger IR to obtain required collimation

Collimation Perform four-sided collimation to area of interest. Use lateral collimation cautiously to prevent vertebral column cutoff.

Respiration Suspend breathing on **expiration.**

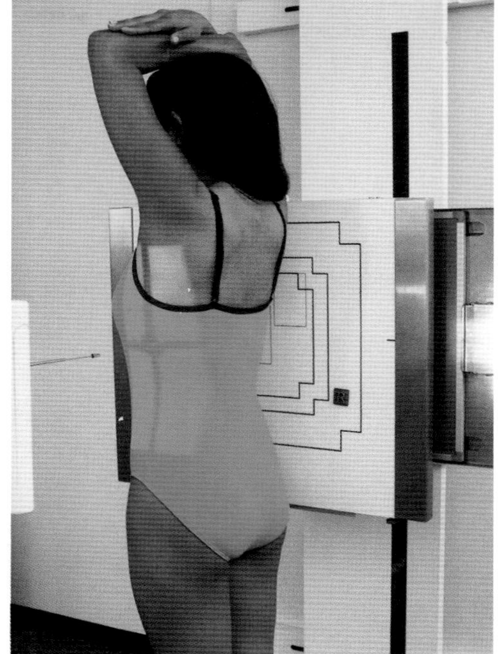

Fig. 10-49. Erect R lateral.

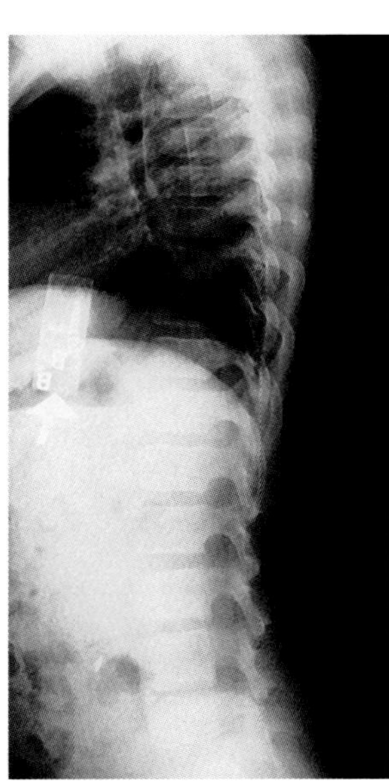

Fig. 10-50. Erect lateral.

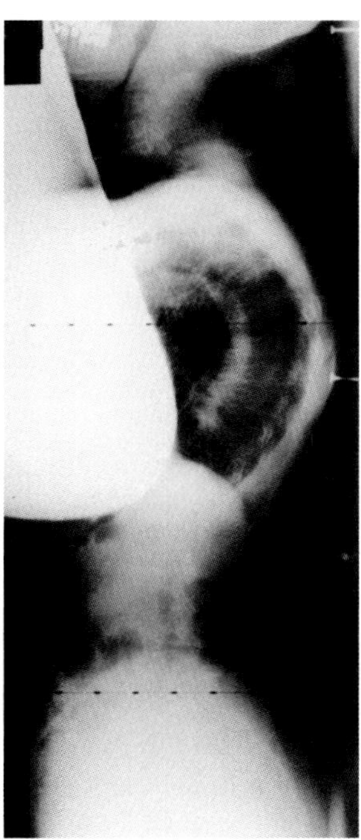

Fig. 10-51. Erect lateral. Clear Pb lateral thoracic compensating filter and breast shadow shield in place. (Courtesy Nuclear Associates, Carle, NY.)

Radiographic Criteria

Structures Shown: • Thoracic and lumbar vertebrae are demonstrated in a lateral position.

Position: • Thoracic and lumbar vertebrae are in as true a lateral position as possible. • Some rotation of pelvis and/or thorax may be apparent because scoliosis generally is accompanied by a twisting or rotation of involved vertebrae.

Collimation and CR: • Vertebral column should be in center of collimation field/IR. • A minimum of 1 inch (2.5 cm) of the iliac crests should be included.

Exposure Criteria: • Optimal density and contrast demonstrate lumbar vertebrae and thoracic vertebrae. • A compensation filter is useful to ensure an even density if a 35 × 90 cm (14 × 36 inch) IR is used. • Sharp bony margins indicate no motion.

PA (AP) PROJECTION—FERGUSON METHOD: SCOLIOSIS SERIES

Scoliosis Series
SPECIAL
- PA (AP) (Ferguson method)
- **AP (PA)—R and L bending**

Pathology Demonstrated

This method assists in differentiating deforming (primary) curve from compensatory curve.

Two images are obtained—one standard erect AP or PA and one with the foot or hip on the **convex side** of the curve elevated.

Technical Factors

- IR size—35 × 43 cm (14 × 17 inches), lengthwise, or 35 × 92 cm (14 × 36 inches)
- Moving or stationary grid
- Erect marker
- Use of compensating filters to help obtain a more uniform density along the vertebral column
- Technique and dose, per exposure at 60 inches (152 cm) in SID:

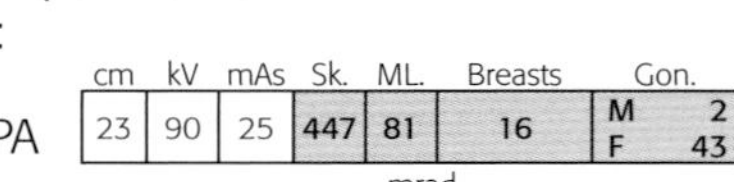

	cm	kV	mAs	Sk.	ML.	Breasts	Gon.
PA	23	90	25	447	81	16	M 2 F 43

mrad

Shielding Place contact shield or shadow shield over gonads without obscuring area of interest. Use breast shields for young females.

Patient Position

- Position patient, either seated or standing, with arms at side.
- For second image, place a block under foot (or hip if seated) on **convex side** of curve so that the patient can barely maintain position **without assistance.** A 3- to 4-inch (8- to 10-cm) block of some type may be used under the buttock if sitting or under the foot if standing (Fig. 10-53).

Part Position

- Align **midsagittal plane to CR and midline of table/grid,** with arms at side.
- Ensure **no rotation** of torso or pelvis, if possible.
- IR includes a minimum 1 to 2 inches (3 to 5 cm) below the iliac crest.

Central Ray

- Direct CR **perpendicular,** centered to **midpoint of IR.**
- SID is 40 to 60 inches (100 to 150 cm); longer SID is required to obtain adequate collimation if a 14 × 36 inch (35 × 90 cm) IR is used.

Collimation Four-sided collimation to area of interest

Respiration Suspend breathing on **expiration.**

Notes: No form of support (for example, compression band) is to be used in this exam. For second image, patient should stand or sit with block under one side, unassisted.

Radiographs should be done as PA projections, which reduce dosage to radiation-sensitive areas of thyroid and breast.

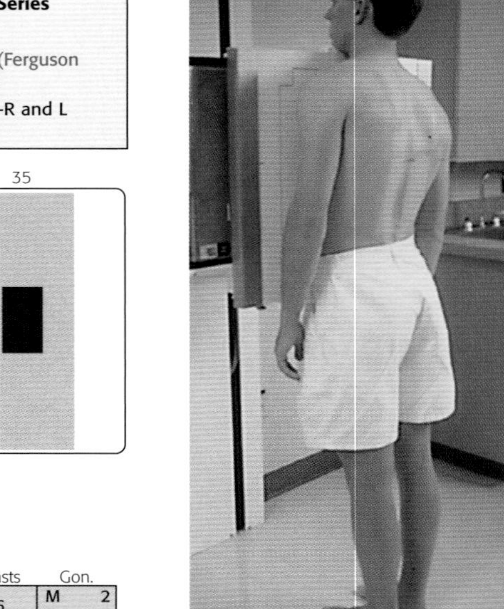

Fig. 10-52. PA erect.

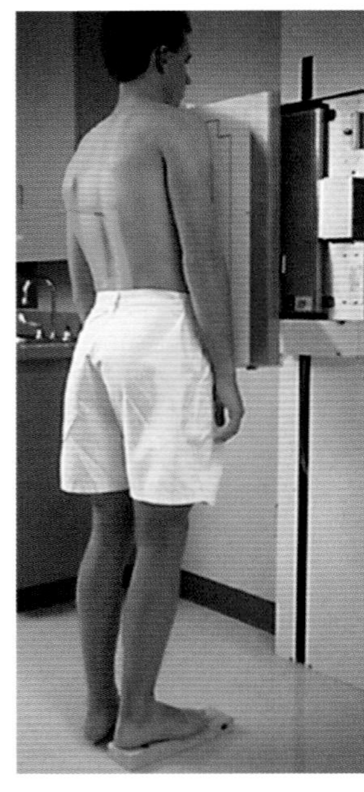

Fig. 10-53. PA with block under foot on **convex side** of curve.

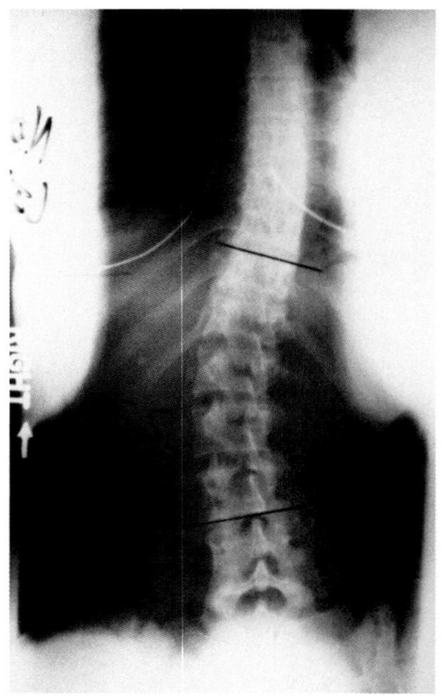

Fig. 10-54. Erect, with no lift.

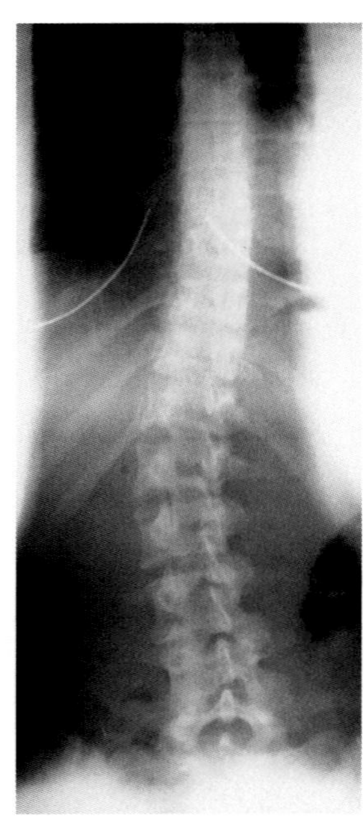

Fig. 10-55. Erect, with lift on right.

Radiographic Criteria

Structures Shown: • All thoracic and lumbar vertebrae should be demonstrated. • A minimum of 1 inch (2.5 cm) of iliac crest should be included on the image.

Position: • Thoracic and lumbar vertebrae should be demonstrated in as true a PA or AP projection as possible.

Collimation and CR: • Vertebral column should be in center of collimated field/IR.

Exposure Criteria: • Optimal density and contrast help clearly visualize the lumbar and thoracic vertebrae. • Use of a compensating filter may be useful to obtain a uniform density along the vertebral column. Sharp bony margins indicate no motion.

AP (PA) PROJECTION—RIGHT AND LEFT BENDING: SCOLIOSIS SERIES

Scoliosis Series
SPECIAL
- PA (AP) (Ferguson method)
- AP (PA)—R and L bending

Pathology Demonstrated

The range of motion of the vertebral column is assessed.

Technical Factors

- IR size—35 × 43 cm (14 × 17 inches), lengthwise, or 35 × 92 cm (14 × 36 inches)
- Moving or stationary grid
- Erect marker for erect position
- Use of compensating filters to help obtain a more uniform density along the vertebral column
- Technique and dose:

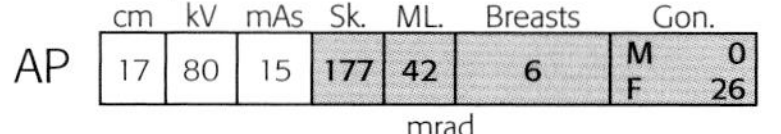

	cm	kV	mAs	Sk.	ML.	Breasts	Gon.
AP	17	80	15	177	42	6	M 0 / F 26
				mrad			

Shielding Place contact shield over gonads without obscuring area of interest.

Patient Position Take image with patient positioned erect or recumbent and as an AP or PA, with patient's arms at side.

Part Position

- Align midsagittal plane to CR and midline of table/grid.
- Ensure **no rotation** of torso or pelvis if possible
- Place bottom edge of IR **1 to 2 inches (3 to 5 cm) below iliac crest.**
- With the pelvis acting as a fulcrum, ask patient to bend laterally (lateral flexion) **as far as possible** to either side.
- If recumbent, move both the upper torso and the legs to achieve maximum lateral flexion.
- Repeat above steps when doing opposite side.

Central Ray

- CR **perpendicular,** directed to **midpoint of IR**
- SID of 40 to 60 inches (100 to 150 cm); longer SID required to obtain adequate collimation if using a 35 × 90 cm (14 × 36 inch) IR

Collimation Four-sided collimation to near borders of IR to not cut off any portion of vertebral column

Respiration Suspend breathing on **expiration.**

Notes: The pelvis must remain as stationary as possible during positioning. Pelvis acts as a fulcrum (pivot point) during changes of position.

Radiographs may be done as PA projections if taken erect, to significantly reduce exposure to radiation-sensitive organs.

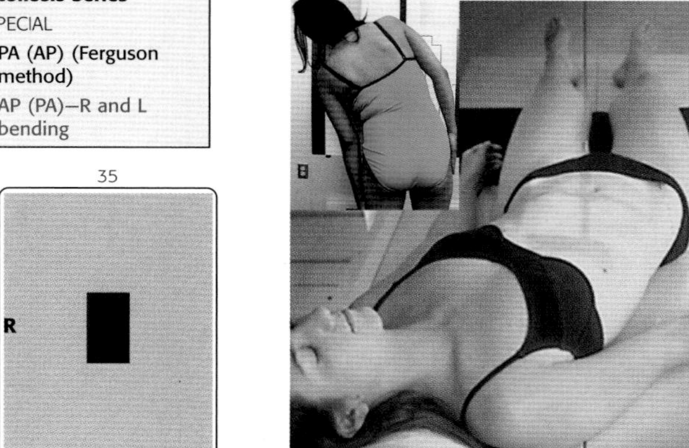

Fig. 10-56. AP supine—L bending. *Inset,* PA erect—L bending.

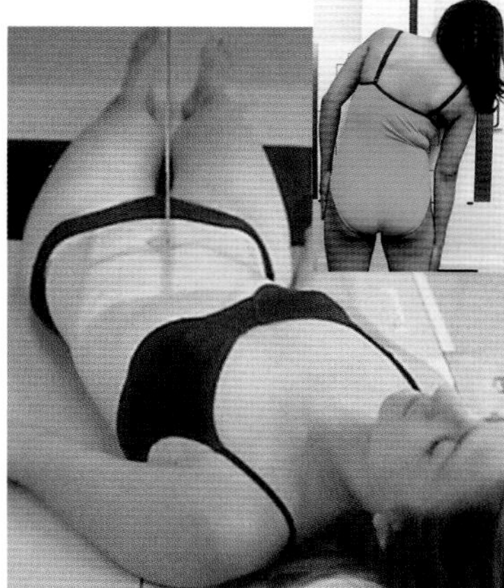

Fig. 10-57. AP supine—R bending. *Inset,* PA erect—R bending.

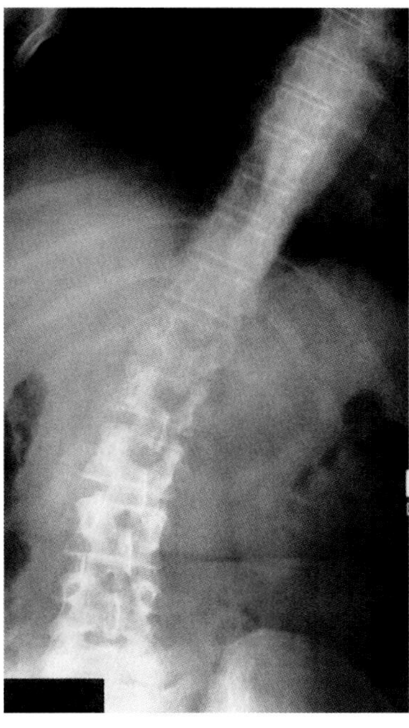

Fig. 10-58. AP—L bending.

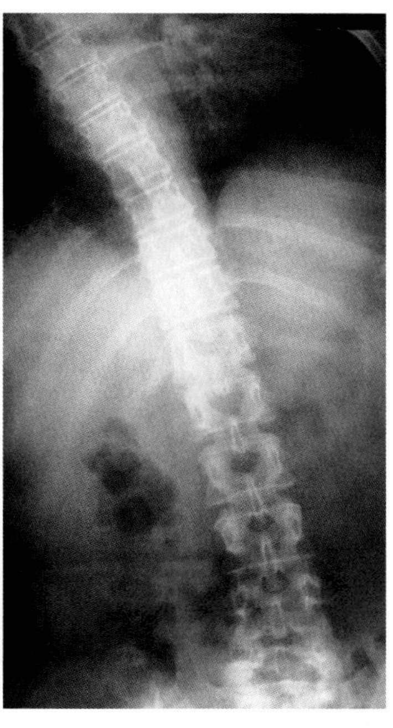

Fig. 10-59. AP—R bending.

Radiographic Criteria

Structures Shown: • An AP/PA projection of the thoracic and lumbar spine, with the patient in lateral flexion positions; minimum of 1 inch (2.5 cm) of the iliac crests visible on the image.

Position: • Thoracic and lumbar vertebrae should be demonstrated in lateral flexion (bending to the left and right). • Rotation of pelvis and/or thorax may be visible on the image because scoliosis often is accompanied by rotation of involved vertebrae.

Collimation and CR: • Vertebral column should be in center of collimated field/IR.

Exposure Criteria: • Optimal density and contrast help clearly demonstrate the lumbar and thoracic vertebrae. • A compensating filter may be useful to obtain a uniform density along the vertebral column. • Sharp bony margins indicate no motion.

LATERAL POSITIONS—HYPEREXTENSION AND HYPERFLEXION: SPINAL FUSION SERIES

Pathology Demonstrated
Projection is used to assess mobility at a spinal fusion site.

Two images are obtained with the patient in the lateral position (one in hyperflexion and one in hyperextension).

Right- and left-bending positions also are generally part of a spinal fusion series and are the same as for the scoliosis series on p. 341.

Spinal Fusion Series
BASIC
- AP (PA)—R and L bending (p. 341)
- Lateral— hyperextension and hyperflexion

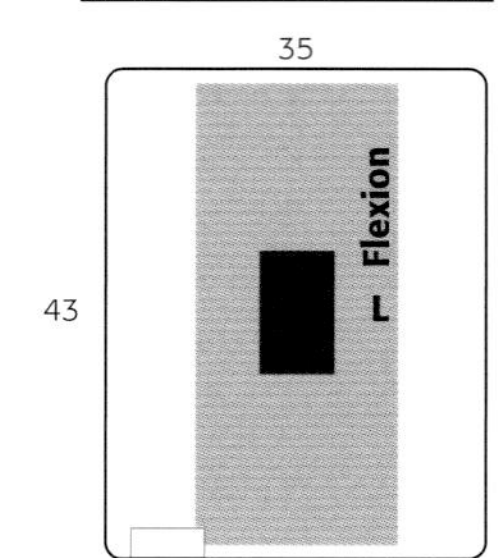

Technical Factors
- IR size—35 × 43 cm (14 × 17 inches)
- Stationary or moving grid
- 85-95 kV range; lead mat behind patient if recumbent
- Extension and flexion markers
- Technique and dose, per projection:

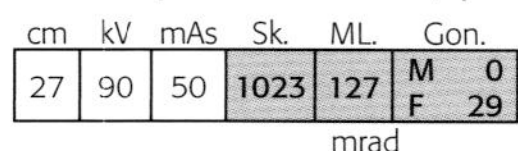

cm	kV	mAs	Sk.	ML.	Gon.
27	90	50	1023	127	M 0 F 29

mrad

Shielding Place contact shield over gonads without obscuring area of interest.

Patient Position Position patient in lateral recumbent position, with pillow for head and support between knees (see Notes for possible erect position).
- Place lower edge of IR 1 to 2 inches (3 to 5 cm) below iliac crest.

Part Position
- Align midcoronal plane to midline of grid.

Hyperflexion:
- Using pelvis as fulcrum, ask patient to assume fetal position (bend forward) and draw legs up **as far as possible.**

Hyperextension:
- Using pelvis as fulcrum, ask patient to move torso and legs posteriorly **as far as possible** to hyperextend long axis of body.
- Ensure no rotation of thorax or pelvis exists.

Central Ray
- Direct CR perpendicular to IR.
- Center CR to **site of fusion** if known or to center of IR.
- Minimum SID is 40 inches (100 cm).

Collimation Four-sided collimation to area of interest

Respiration Suspend breathing on expiration.

Notes: Projection also may be done with patient standing erect or sitting on a stool, first leaning forward as far as possible, gripping the stool legs, then leaning backward as far as possible, gripping the back of the stool to maintain this position.

The pelvis must remain as stationary as possible during positioning. The pelvis acts as a fulcrum (pivot point) during changes of position.

Radiographic Criteria

Structures Shown: • A lateral view of the lumbar vertebrae in hyperflexion and hyperextension.

Position: • True lateral position of patient is indicated by superimposed posterior vertebral bodies.

Collimation and CR: • Vertebral column should be in center of collimated field/IR.

Exposure Criteria: • Optimal density and contrast clearly demonstrate lumbar vertebrae and intervertebral joint spaces. • Sharp bony margins indicate no motion.

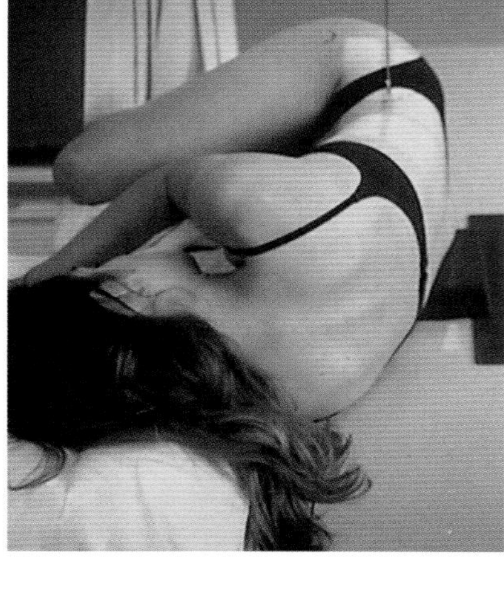

Fig. 10-60. Lateral—hyperflexion.

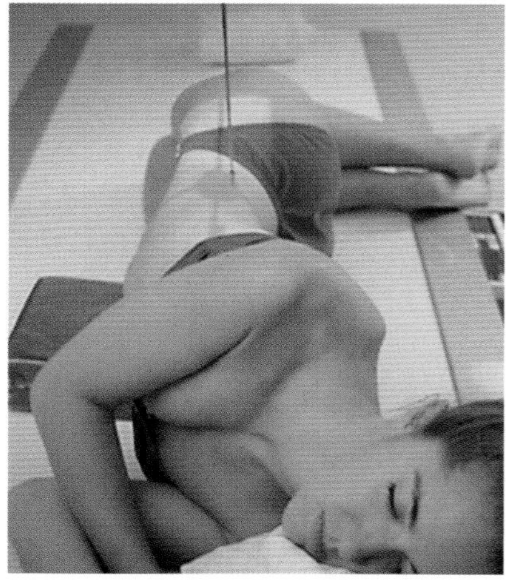

Fig. 10-61. Lateral—hyperextension.

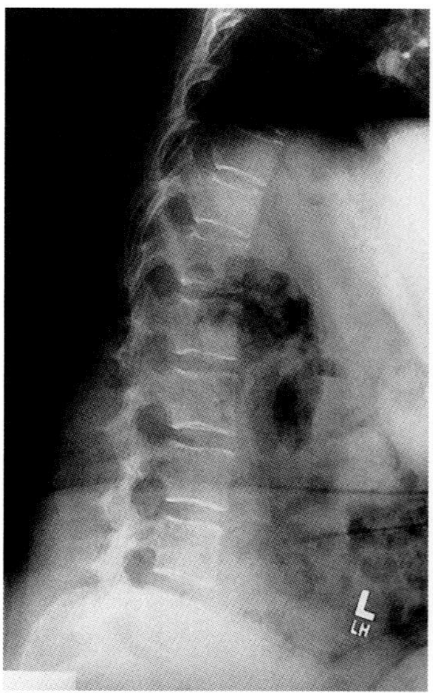

Fig. 10-62. Hyperflexion.

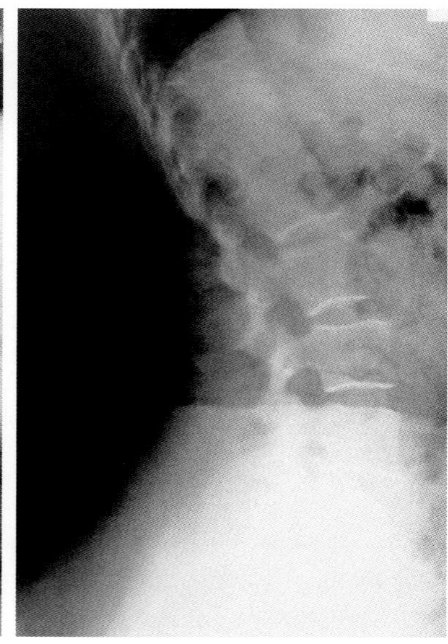

Fig. 10-63. Hyperextension.

10

AP AXIAL SACRUM PROJECTION: SACRUM

Sacrum and Coccyx
BASIC
- AP axial sacrum
- AP axial coccyx
- Lateral

24
R
30

Pathology Demonstrated
Pathology of the sacrum is demonstrated.

Note: The urinary bladder should be emptied before this procedure begins. Also desirable is to have the lower colon free of gas and fecal material, which may require a cleaning enema, as ordered by a physician.

Technical Factors
- IR size—24 × 30 cm (10 × 12 inches), lengthwise
- Moving or stationary grid
- 75-80 kV range (or 85-90 kV and reduction of mAs)
- Technique and dose at 80 kV:

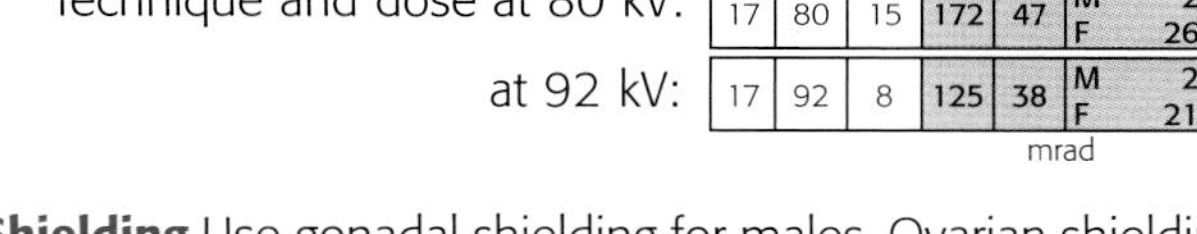

	cm	kV	mAs	Sk.	ML.	Gon. (mrad)
at 80 kV:	17	80	15	172	47	M 2, F 26
at 92 kV:	17	92	8	125	38	M 2, F 21

Shielding Use gonadal shielding for males. Ovarian shielding on females is not possible without obscuring area of interest.

Patient Position Position patient supine, with pillow for head and legs extended, with support under knees for comfort.

Part Position
- Align **midsagittal plane to CR and midline of table/grid.**
- Ensure **no rotation** of pelvis exists.

Central Ray
- CR angled **15° cephalad,** to enter at **midsagittal plane midway between level of symphysis pubis and ASIS**
- IR centered to projected CR
- Minimum SID of 40 inches (100 cm)

Collimation Close four-sided collimation to area of interest

Respiration Suspend breathing on expiration.

Notes: Technologist may need to increase CR angle to 20° cephalad for patients with an apparent greater posterior curvature or tilt of the sacrum and pelvis.

Female sacrum is generally shorter and wider than male sacrum (a consideration in close four-sided collimation).

Projection may be done **prone** (angle **15° caudad**) if necessary for patient's condition.

Radiographic Criteria

Structures Shown: • A nonforeshortened AP projection of the sacrum, the SI joints, and the L5-S1 junction.

Position: • Inferior portion of sacrum should be centered in the pelvic opening, indicating no rotation of pelvis. • Correct alignment of the sacrum and CR demonstrates the sacrum free of foreshortening, and the pubis and sacral foramina are not superimposed.

Collimation and CR: • The sacrum should be centered to IR and the field closely collimated.

Exposure Criteria: • Optimal density and contrast should demonstrate the sacrum and SI joints. • Sharp bony margins indicate no motion.

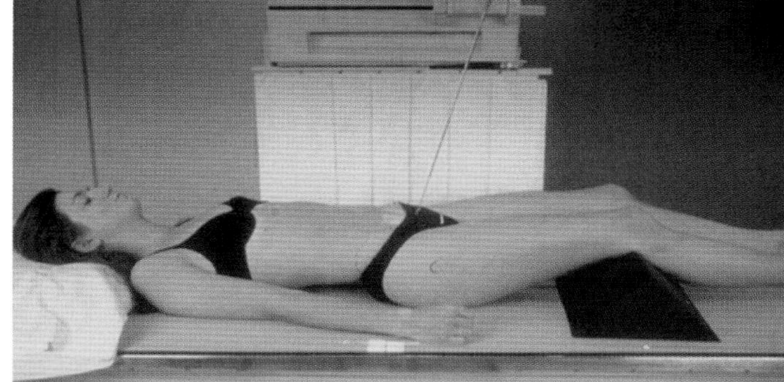

Fig. 10-64. AP—15° cephalad.

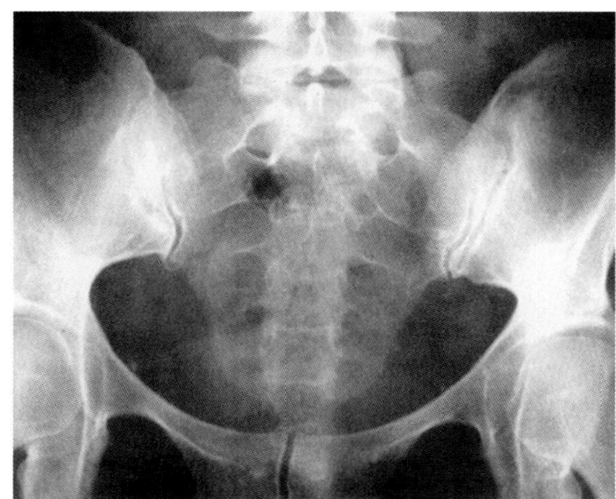

Fig. 10-65. AP—15° cephalad.

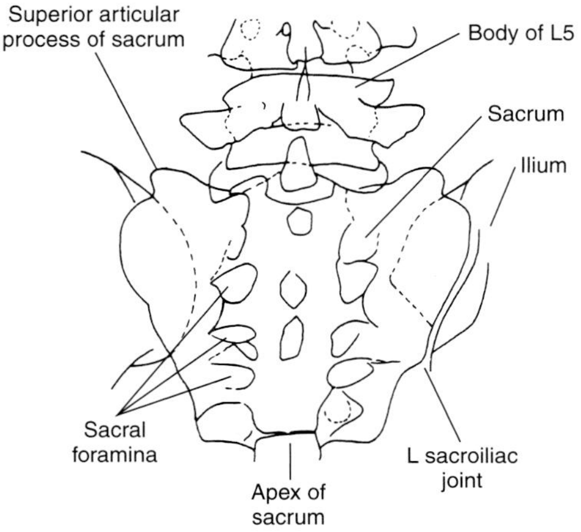

Fig. 10-66. AP sacrum—15° cephalad.

10

AP AXIAL COCCYX PROJECTION: COCCYX

Sacrum and Coccyx
BASIC
- **AP axial sacrum**
- AP axial coccyx
- LATERAL

24
30 R

Pathology Demonstrated

Pathology of the coccyx is demonstrated.

Note: The urinary bladder should be emptied before this procedure begins. Also desirable is to have the lower colon free of gas and fecal material, which may require a cleaning enema, as ordered by a physician.

Technical Factors

- IR size—24 × 30 cm (10 × 12 inches), lengthwise
- Moving or stationary grid
- 75-80 kV range (or 85-90 kV and reduction of mAs)
- Technique and dose at 80 kV / at 92 kV:

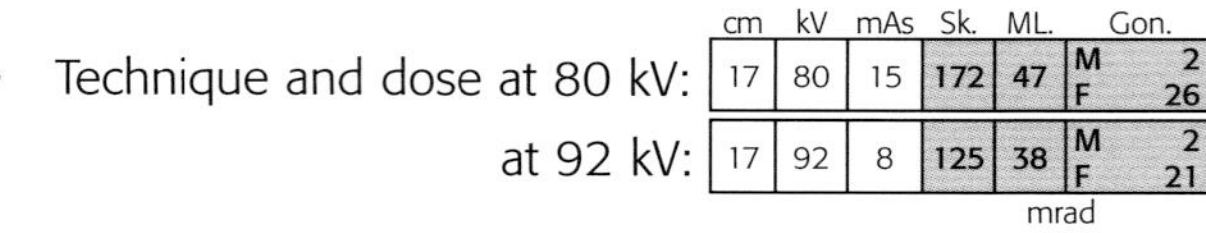

	cm	kV	mAs	Sk.	ML.	Gon.
at 80 kV:	17	80	15	172	47	M 2 F 26
at 92 kV:	17	92	8	125	38	M 2 F 21
					mrad	

Shielding Use gonadal shielding for males. Ovarian shielding on females is not possible without obscuring area of interest.

Patient Position Position patient supine, with a pillow for head and legs extended, with support under knees for comfort.

Part Position
- Align midsagittal plane to midline of table/grid.
- Ensure **no rotation** of pelvis.

Central Ray
- Angle CR **10° caudad,** to enter **2 inches** (5 cm) **superior to symphysis pubis.**
- Center IR to projected CR.
- Minimum SID is 40 inches (100 cm).

Collimation Close four-sided collimation to area of interest

Respiration Suspend breathing on expiration.

Notes: Technologist may need to increase CR angle to 15° caudad with a greater anterior curvature of the coccyx if apparent by palpation or as evidenced on the lateral.

Projection may be done **prone** (angle **10° cephalad**) if necessary for patient's condition, with CR centered to the coccyx, which can be localized using the greater trochanter.

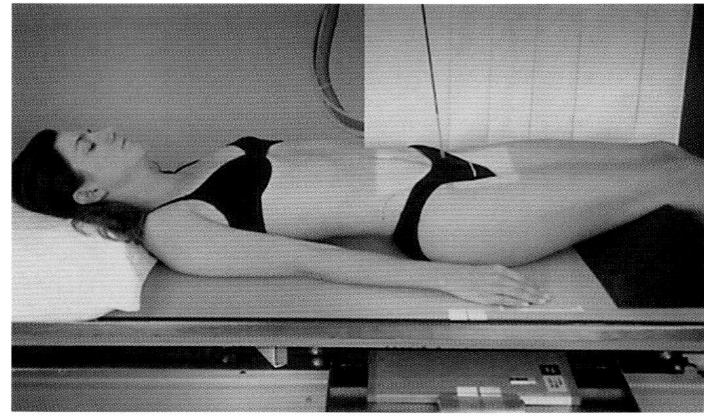

Fig. 10-67. AP coccyx—10° caudad.

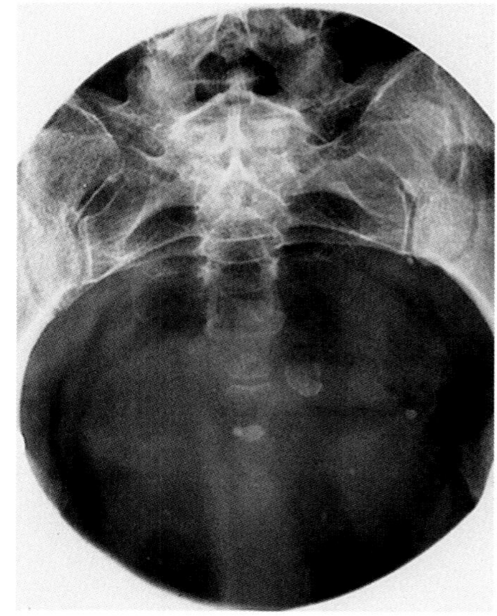

Fig. 10-68. AP coccyx—10° caudad. (Courtesy Jim Sanderson, RT.)

Radiographic Criteria

Structures Shown: • Coccyx free of self-superimposition and superimposition of symphysis pubis.

Position: • Correct coccyx and CR alignment demonstrates coccyx free of superimposition and projected superior to pubis. • Coccygeal segments should appear open. If not, they may be fused, or CR angle may need to be increased. (The greater the curvature of the coccyx, the greater the angulation needed.) • Coccyx should appear equidistant from the lateral walls of the pelvic opening, indicating no patient rotation.

Collimation and CR: • The coccyx should be centered to the closely collimated field.

Exposure Criteria: • Optimal density and contrast demonstrate the coccyx. • Sharp bony margins indicate no motion.

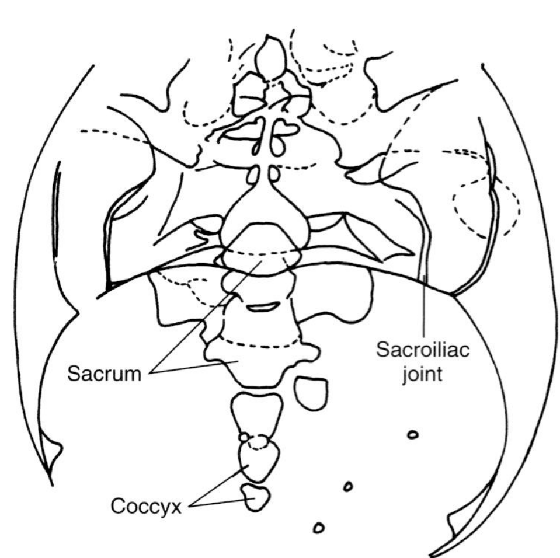

Fig. 10-69. AP coccyx—10° caudad.

10

LATERAL SACRUM AND COCCYX POSITION: SACRUM AND COCCYX

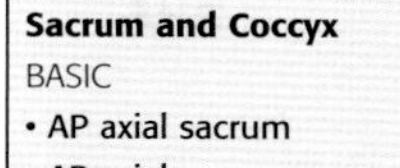

Sacrum and Coccyx
BASIC
- AP axial sacrum
- AP axial coccyx
- Lateral

Pathology Demonstrated
Pathology of the sacrum and coccyx is demonstrated.

Note: The sacrum and coccyx are commonly imaged together. Separate AP projections are required due to different CR angles, **but the laterals can be obtained with one exposure** centering to include both the sacrum and the coccyx. This projection is recommended to decrease gonadal doses.

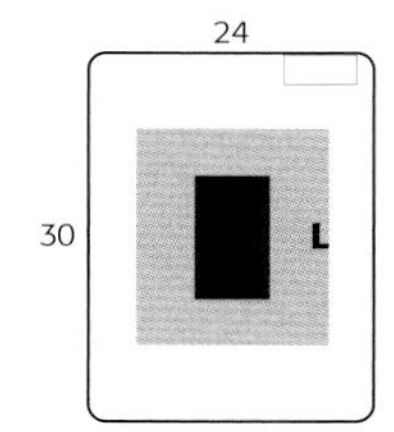

Technical Factors
- IR size—24 × 30 cm (10 × 12 inches), lengthwise
- Moving or stationary grid
- 90 ± 5 kV range
- Lead mat on table behind patient to reduce scatter to IR
- If coccyx is to be included, a boomerang-type filter is useful to ensure optimal density
- Technique and dose:

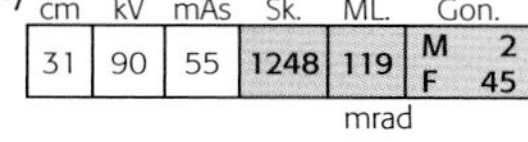

cm	kV	mAs	Sk.	ML.	Gon.
31	90	55	1248	119	M 2 F 45

mrad

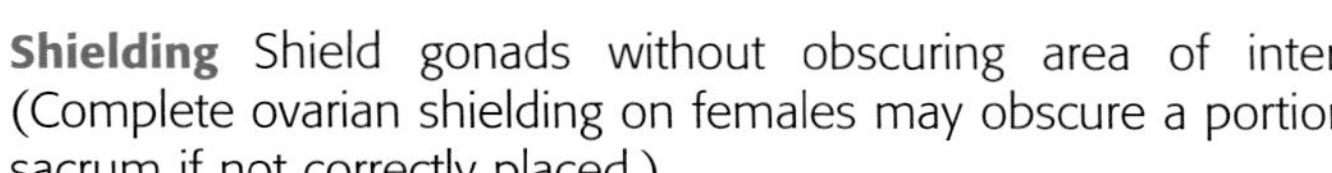

Shielding Shield gonads without obscuring area of interest. (Complete ovarian shielding on females may obscure a portion of sacrum if not correctly placed.)

Patient Position Position patient lateral recumbent, with a pillow for head.

Part Position
- Flex knees.
- Place support under waist and between knees and ankles to maintain patient position and ensure comfort.
- Align **long axis of sacrum and coccyx to CR and to midline** of table/grid.
- Ensure pelvis and body in **true lateral position.**

Central Ray
- Direct CR perpendicular to IR.
- Center CR 3 to 4 inches (8-10 cm) **posterior to ASIS** (centering for sacrum).
- Center IR to CR.
- Minimum SID is 40 inches (100 cm).

Collimation Close four-sided collimation to area of interest

Respiration Suspend breathing on expiration.

Note: High amounts of secondary and scatter radiation are generated. Close collimation is essential to reduce patient dose and obtain a high-quality image.

Radiographic Criteria

Structures Shown: • Lateral view of sacrum, L5-S1 joint, and coccyx.

Position: • Posterior margins of pelvis (greater sciatic notches and femoral heads) are superimposed, indicating no rotation of patient.

Collimation and CR: • Sacrum and coccyx appear in center of IR, with a closely collimated field.

Exposure Criteria: • Optimal contrast and density should clearly demonstrate the sacrum. • The coccyx may appear slightly overexposed, depending on patient size and filter use. • Sharp bony margins indicate no motion.

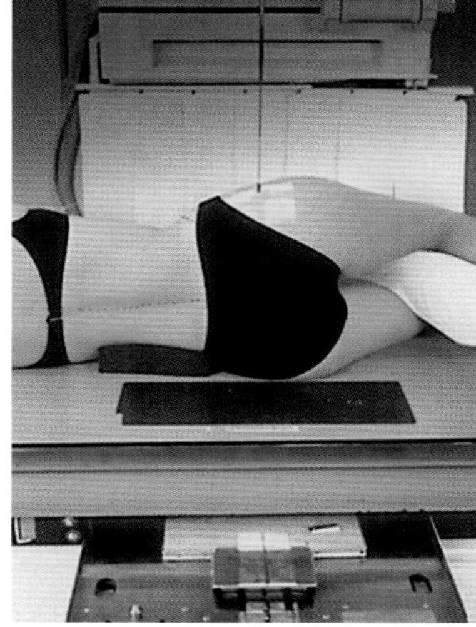

Fig. 10-70. Lateral sacrum and coccyx.

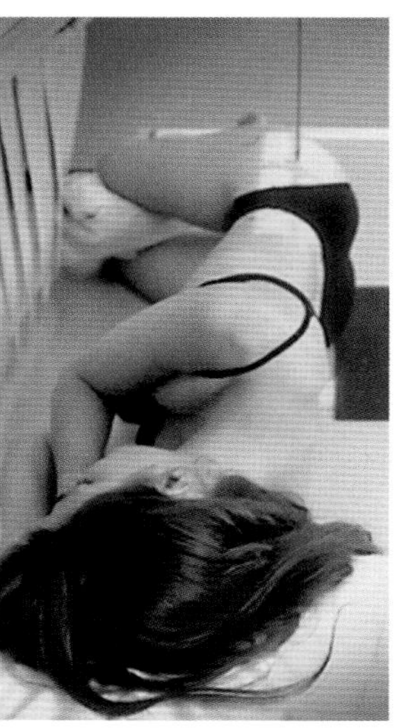

Fig. 10-71. Lateral sacrum.

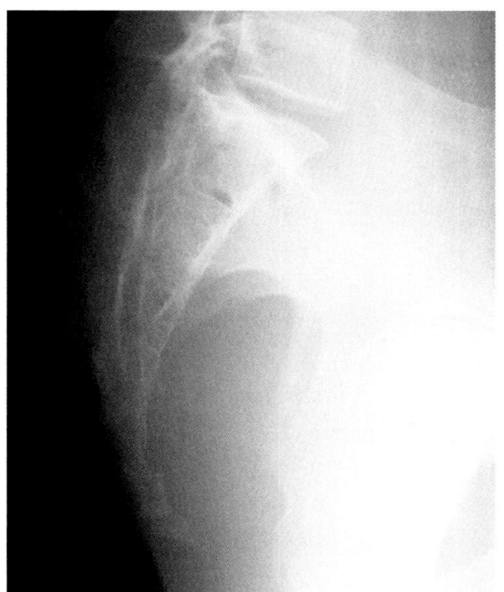

Fig. 10-72. Lateral sacrum and coccyx.

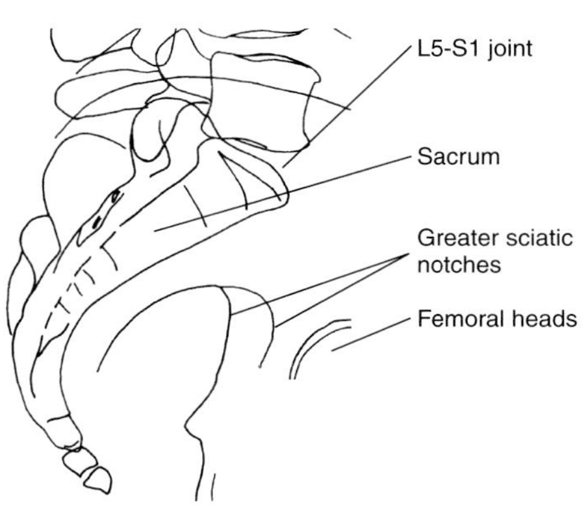

Fig. 10-73. Lateral sacrum and coccyx.

10

LATERAL COCCYX POSITION: COCCYX

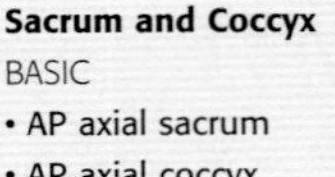

Sacrum and Coccyx

BASIC
- AP axial sacrum
- AP axial coccyx
- Lateral

Pathology Demonstrated
Pathology of the coccyx is demonstrated.

Note: The sacrum and coccyx are commonly ordered together, and a single lateral centered to **include both the sacrum and coccyx** can be obtained. This single lateral projection is recommended to decrease gonadal doses.

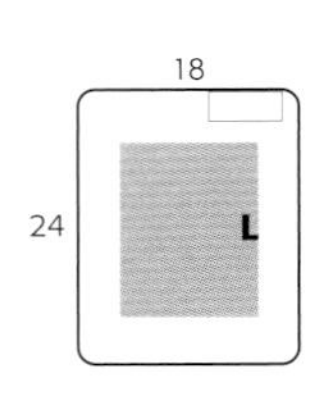

Technical Factors
- IR size—18 × 24 cm (8 × 10 inches), lengthwise
- Moving or stationary grid
- 80 ± 5 kV range
- Lead mat on table behind patient to reduce scatter to the IR
- Cautious use of AEC, if at all, due to location of body part
- Technique and dose:

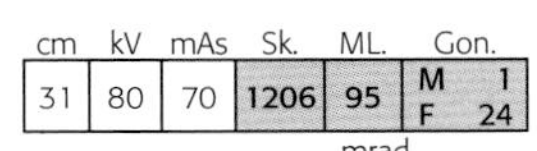

cm	kV	mAs	Sk.	ML.	Gon.
31	80	70	1206	95	M 1 F 24

mrad

Shielding Shield gonads without obscuring area of interest. Complete ovarian shielding on females may obscure a portion of sacrum and/or coccyx.

Patient Position Position patient lateral recumbent, with a pillow for head.

Part Position
- Flex knees.
- Place support under waist and between knees and ankles.
- Align **long axis of coccyx with CR table/grid.** (Remember superficial location of coccyx.)
- Ensure pelvis and body are in **true lateral** position.

Central Ray
- Direct CR perpendicular to table/grid.
- Center CR **3 to 4 inches (8 to 10 cm) posterior** and **2 inches (5 cm) distal to ASIS** (centering for coccyx).
- Center IR to CR.
- Minimum SID is 40 inches (100 cm).

Collimation Close four-sided collimation to area of interest

Respiration Suspend breathing on expiration.

Note: When the two are radiographed separately, the coccyx requires a lower kV and less mAs than the lateral sacrum.

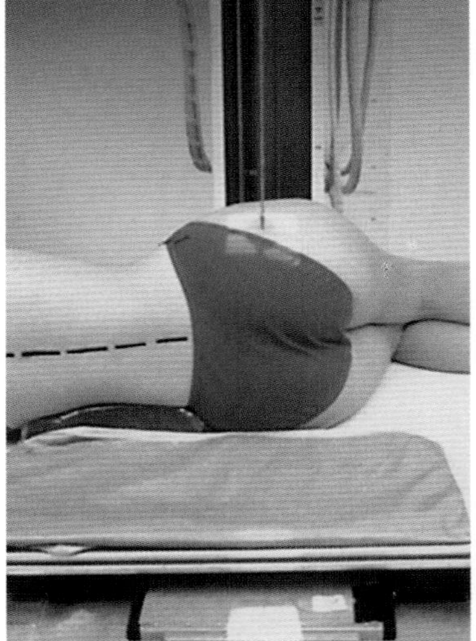

Fig. 10-74. Lateral coccyx.

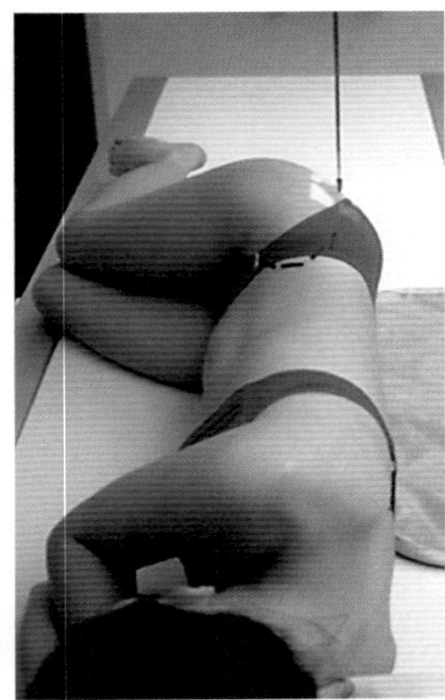

Fig. 10-75. Lateral coccyx.

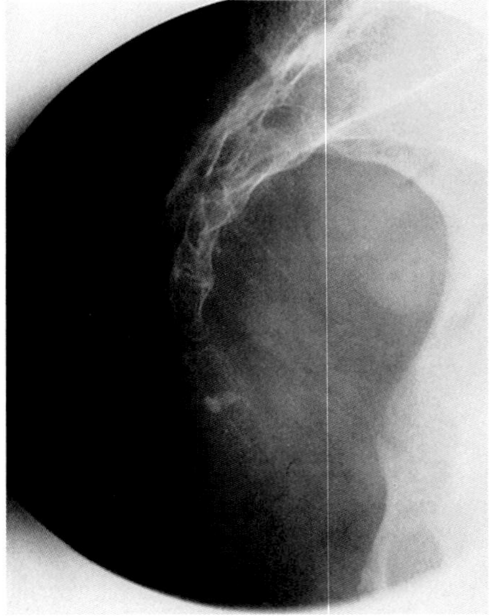

Fig. 10-76. Lateral coccyx. (Courtesy Jim Sanderson, RT.)

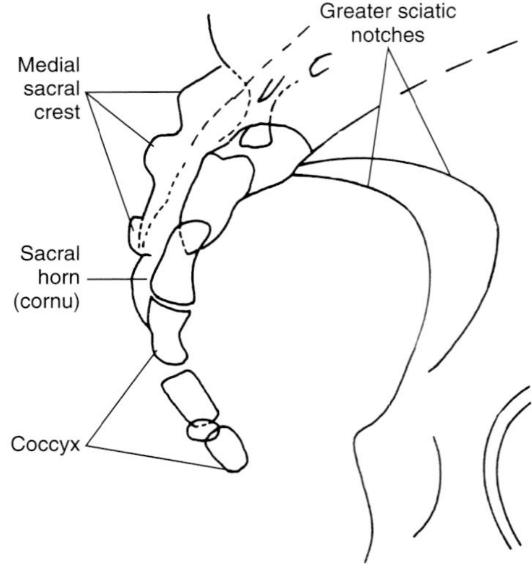

Fig. 10-77. Lateral coccyx.

Radiographic Criteria

Structures Shown: • Lateral view of the coccyx is visible (anterior concavity being demonstrated in this position). • Segment interspaces should appear open, if not fused.

Position: • No rotation of patient is indicated by superimposition of greater sciatic notches.

Collimation and CR: • Coccyx should appear in center of closely collimated field/IR.

Exposure Criteria: • Optimal density and contrast clearly demonstrate all coccyx segments. • Sharp bony margins indicate no motion.

10

RADIOGRAPHS FOR CRITIQUE

Students should determine whether they can critique each of these six radiographs based on the categories as described in the textbook and as outlined on the right. As a starting critique exercise, place a check in each category that demonstrates a **repeatable error** for that radiograph.

Student workbooks provide more space for writing critique comments and complete critique answers for each of these radiographs. Answers are also provided in Appendix B, at the end of this textbook.

	RADIOGRAPHS				
	A	B	C	D	E
1. Structures shown	____	____	____	____	____
2. Positioning	____	____	____	____	____
3. Collimation and CR	____	____	____	____	____
4. Exposure criteria	____	____	____	____	____
5. Markers	____	____	____	____	____

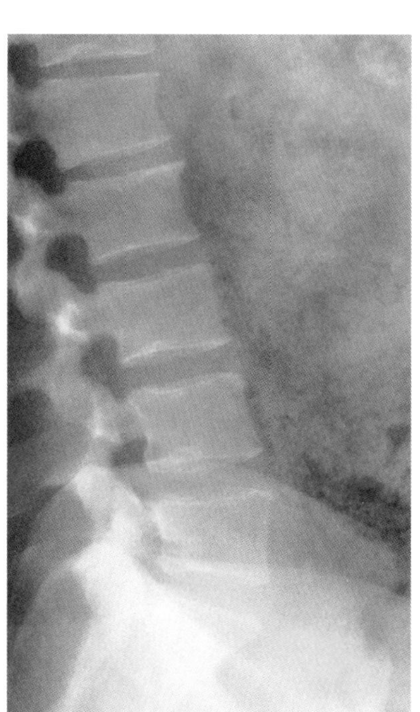

Fig. C10-78. Lateral L spine. A

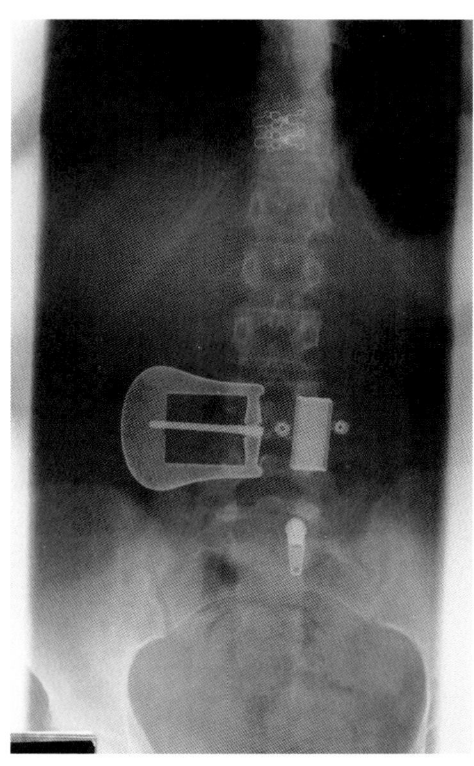

Fig. C10-79. AP lumbar spine. B

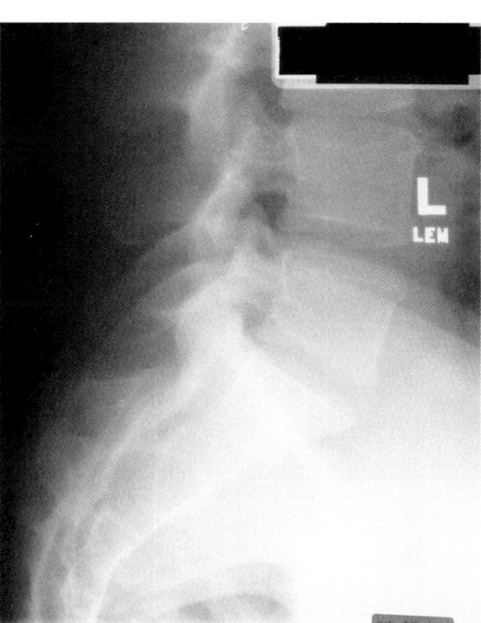

Fig. C10-80. Lateral L5-S1. C

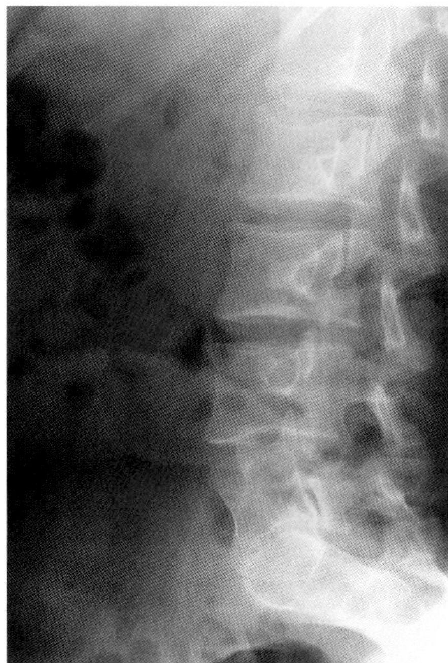

Fig. C10-81. Oblique L spine. D

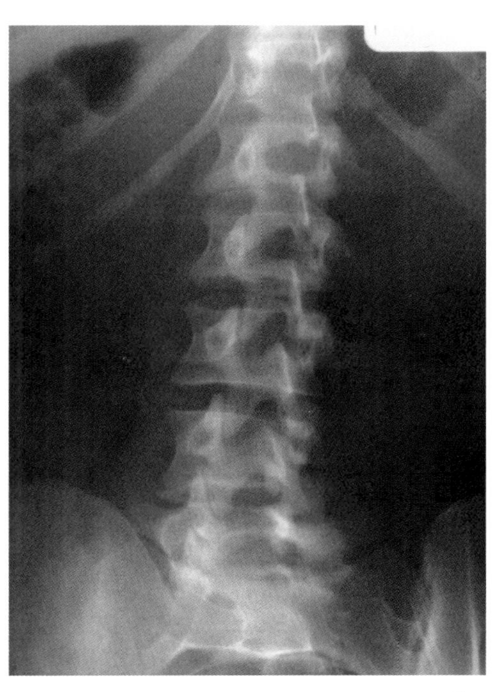

Fig. C10-82. Oblique L spine. E

CHAPTER 11

Bony Thorax—Sternum and Ribs

CONTRIBUTIONS BY **Patti Ward,** MEd, RT(R)
CONTRIBUTOR TO PAST EDITIONS Cindy Murphy, RT R, ACR, BHSc

CONTENTS

RADIOGRAPHIC ANATOMY

Bony Thorax

The main function of the bony thorax is to serve as an expandable, bellowslike chamber, wherein the interior capacity expands and contracts during inspiration and expiration, respectively. This is caused by alternate action of muscles attached to the rib cage and atmospheric pressure causing the air to move in and out of the lungs during respiration.

The bony thorax consists of the **sternum** anteriorly, the **thoracic vertebrae** posteriorly, and the **12 pairs of ribs** connecting the sternum to the vertebral column. The bony thorax protects important organs of the respiratory system and vital structures within the mediastinum, such as the heart and great vessels.

The sternum is also a common site for marrow biopsy, in which, under a local anesthetic, a needle is inserted into the marrow cavity of the sternum to withdraw a sample of red bone marrow.

The drawing in Fig. 11-3 shows the relationship of the sternum to the 12 pairs of ribs and 12 thoracic vertebrae. As demonstrated in the drawings on this page, the thin sternum superimposes the structures within the mediastinum and the dense thoracic spine in a direct frontal position. Therefore an AP or PA projection radiograph would demonstrate the thoracic spine but would show the sternum minimally, if at all.

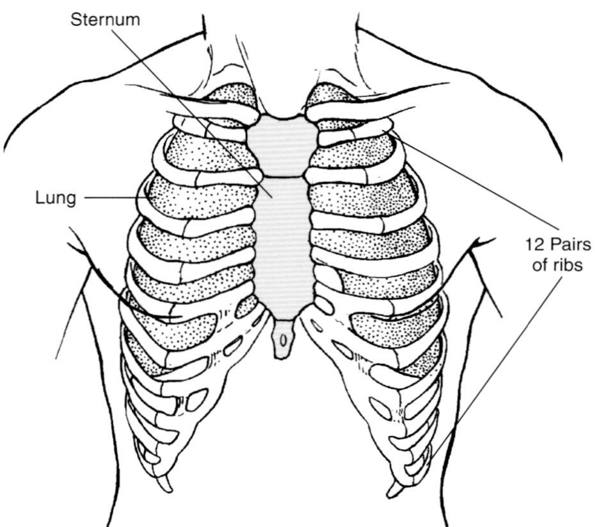

Fig. 11-1. Bony thorax, expandable enclosure for lungs.

STERNUM

The adult sternum is a thin, narrow, flat bone with three divisions. The upper portion is the **manubrium** *(mah-nu'bre-um).* The adult manubrium averages 2 inches, or 5 cm, in length.

The longest part of the sternum is the **body,** which is about 4 inches, or 10 cm, long. The union of the four segments of the body begins during puberty and is not completed until about the age of 25.

The most inferior portion of the sternum is the **xiphoid** *(zi'foid)* **process,** which is composed of cartilage during infancy and youth and usually does not become totally ossified until about age 40. The xiphoid process is generally rather small; however, it can vary in size, shape, and degree of ossification.

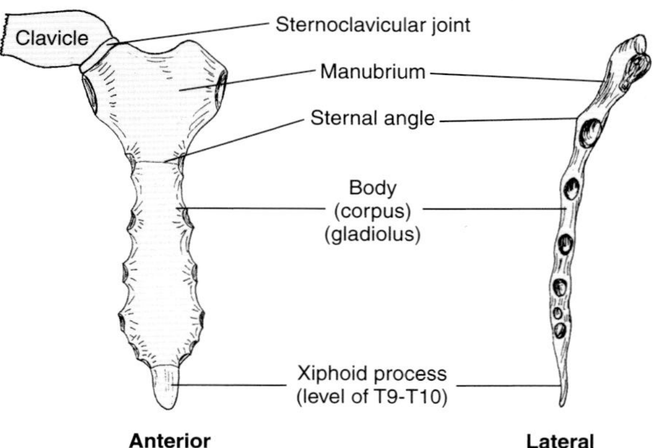

Fig. 11-2. Sternum.

Palpable Landmarks

The uppermost border of the manubrium is easy to palpate and is called the **jugular notch** (Fig. 11-3). Other secondary names for this area are **suprasternal** or **manubrial notch,** which describe the slightly notched area between the two clavicles along the upper border of the sternum. The jugular notch is at the level of T2-T3.

The lower end of the manubrium joins the body of the sternum to form a palpable prominence, the **sternal angle.** This is also an easily palpated landmark used for location of other structures of the bony thorax. The sternal angle is at the level of the disk space between **T4 and T5** for an average adult.

The **xiphoid tip** corresponds to the level of **T9-T10.** The **inferior rib angle** (lowest costal margin) corresponds to the level of **L2 or L3.**

Sternoclavicular articulation Each **clavicle** joins the manubrium lateral to the jugular notch on each side and is called the **sternoclavicular joint,** which is the only bony connection between each shoulder girdle and the bony thorax.

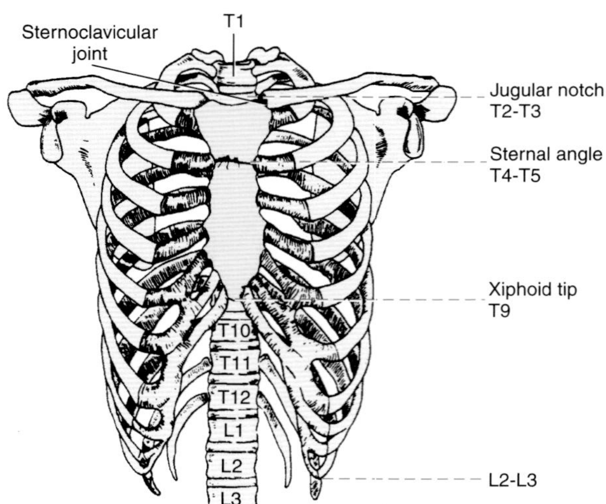

Fig. 11-3. Bony thorax—sternum, ribs, thoracic vertebrae (landmarks and associated vertebrae).

Sternal rib articulations The **clavicles** and the **cartilages** of the **first seven pairs of ribs** connect directly to the sternum. Below each clavicular notch and sternoclavicular joint is a depression or **facet** for articulation with the cartilage of the first rib.

The anterior ribs do not unite directly with the sternum but do so with a short piece of cartilage termed **costocartilage** (Fig. 11-4). The costocartilages and ribs have been added to one side of this drawing to show this relationship.

The second costocartilage connects to the sternum at the level of the sternal angle. An easy way to locate the anterior end of the second rib is to locate the sternal angle first, then feel laterally along the cartilage and the bone of the rib.

The third through the seventh costocartilages connect directly to the body of the sternum.

Ribs 8, 9, and 10 also possess costocartilage, but these connect to the number 7 costocartilage, which then connects to the sternum.

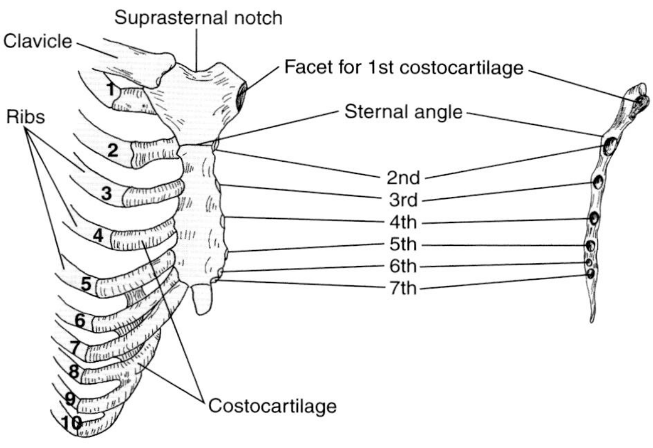

Fig. 11-4. Sternal rib articulations.

RIBS

Each rib is numbered according to the thoracic vertebra to which it attaches; therefore the ribs are numbered from the top down. The first seven pairs of ribs are considered **true ribs.** Each true rib attaches directly to the sternum by its own costocartilage. The term **false ribs** applies to the last five pairs of ribs, numbered 8, 9, 10, 11, and 12.

The drawing in Fig. 11-5 again clearly shows that, although ribs 8 through 10 have costocartilages, they connect to the costocartilage of the seventh rib.

The last two pairs of false ribs are unique in that they do not possess costocartilage. The term **floating ribs** can be used to designate these two pairs of ribs.

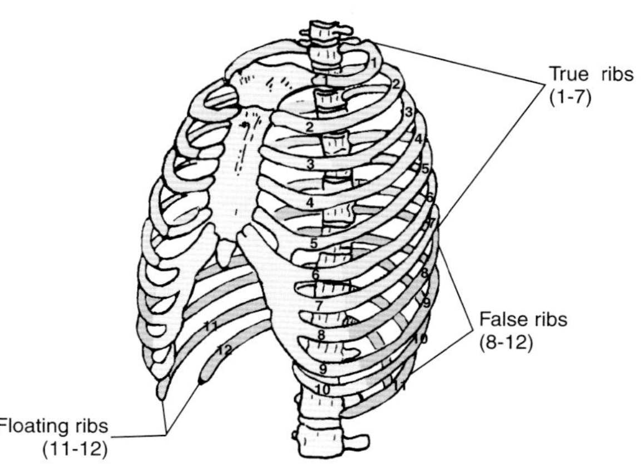

Fig. 11-5. Ribs.

Summary Ribs **1 to 7** are termed **true ribs** and connect directly to the sternum. The last five pair of ribs, **8 to 12,** are termed **false ribs.** The last two pair of ribs, **11 and 12,** which are also false ribs, are termed **floating ribs** because they are not connected anteriorly.

Typical Rib

Inferior view A typical rib viewed from its inferior surface is illustrated in Fig. 11-6. A central rib is used to show the common characteristics of a typical rib. Each rib has two ends: a posterior, or **vertebral, end** and an anterior, or **sternal, end.** Between the two ends is the **shaft,** or body, of the rib.

The vertebral end consists of a **head,** which articulates with one or two thoracic vertebral bodies, and a flattened **neck.** Lateral to the neck is an elevated **tubercle** that articulates with the transverse process of a vertebra and allows for attachment of a ligament. The body extends laterally from the tubercle, then angles forward and downward. The area of forward angulation is termed the **angle** of the rib.

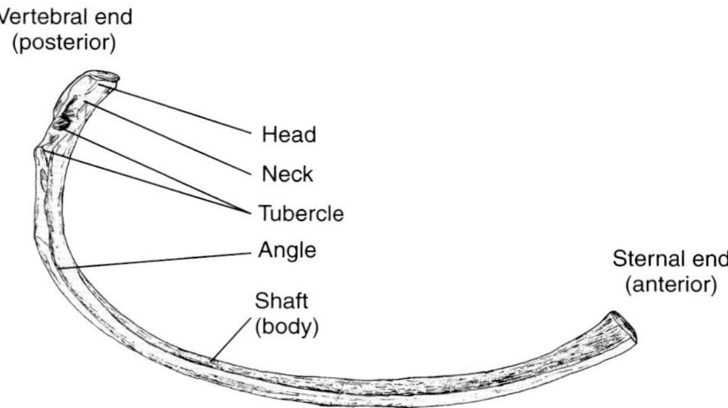

Fig. 11-6. Typical rib—inferior view.

Posterior view Seen on this posterior view are the **head, neck,** and **tubercles** at the vertebral end of the rib. Progressing laterally, the angle of the rib is that part where the shaft curves forward and downward toward the sternal end.

As seen in Fig. 11-7, the posterior or vertebral end of a typical rib is 3 to 5 inches (7.5 to 12.5 cm) **higher** than the anterior or sternal end. Therefore when viewing a radiograph of a chest or ribs, remember that the part of a rib most superior is the posterior end, or the end nearest the vertebrae. The anterior end is more inferior.

The lower inside margin of each rib protects an **artery,** a **vein,** and a **nerve;** therefore rib injuries are very painful and may be associated with substantial hemorrhage. This inside margin, containing the blood vessels and nerves, is termed the **costal groove.**

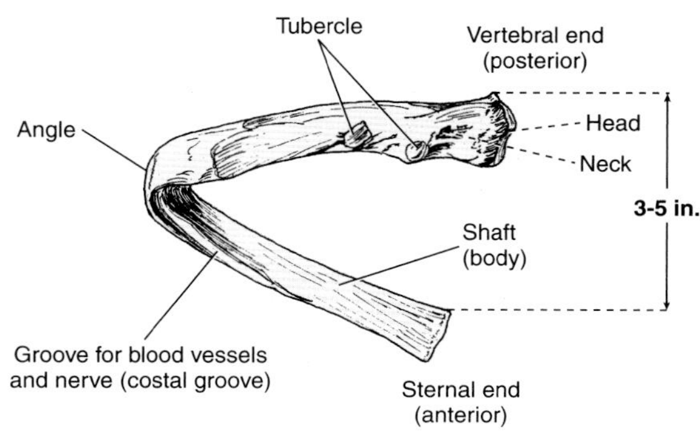

Fig. 11-7. Typical rib—posterior view.

RIB CAGE

Fig. 11-8 illustrates the bony thorax with the sternum and costocartilages removed. The fifth ribs have been shaded to better illustrate the downward angulation of the ribs.

Not all ribs have the same appearance. The first ribs are short and broad and are the most vertical of all the ribs. Counting downward from the short first pair, the ribs get longer and longer down to the seventh ribs. From the seventh ribs down, they get shorter and shorter through the fairly short twelfth, or last, pair of ribs. The first ribs are the most sharply curved. The bony thorax is **widest** at the lateral margins of the **eighth or ninth ribs.**

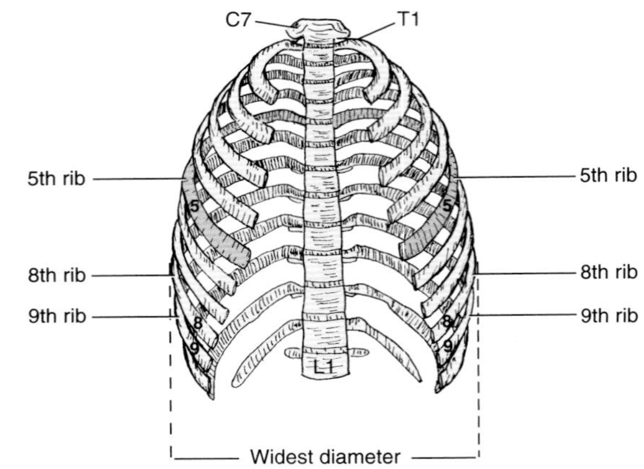

Fig. 11-8. Rib cage.

Articulations of Bony Thorax

ANTERIOR ARTICULATIONS

A frontal view of an articulated thorax is illustrated in Fig. 11-9. The joints or articulations of the anterior bony thorax are identified on this photograph. The joints along with the classification and the types of motion allowed are described as follows *(also see the summary chart at the bottom of the page):*

Part A (shown on left side at fourth rib) is the joint between costocartilage and the sternal end of the fourth rib and is called a **costochondral union** or **junction.** These ribs (1-10) form a unique type of union, wherein the cartilage and bone are bound together by the periosteum of the bone itself. This permits **no motion;** therefore they are termed **synarthrodial.**

Part B is one **sternoclavicular joint.** The sternoclavicular joints are **synovial** joints, containing articular capsules that permit a plane motion, or **gliding motion,** and are therefore **diarthrodial** joints.

Part C is the **sternocostal joint** of the first rib. The cartilage of the first rib attaches directly to the manubrium with no synovial capsule and allows **no motion (synarthrodial).** Therefore this is a **cartilaginous** class joint of the **synchondrosis** type.

Part D is the fourth sternocostal joint, typical of the second through the seventh joints between costocartilage and sternum. These are **synovial** joints, which allow a slight **plane (gliding) motion,** making them **diarthrodial** joints.

Part E represents the continuous borders of the **interchondral joints** between the costal cartilages of the anterior sixth through tenth ribs. These are all interconnected by a **synovial** type joint with a long thin articular capsule lined by synovial membrane. These allow a slight **plane (gliding) type of movement (diarthrodial),** facilitating movement of the bony thorax during the breathing process.

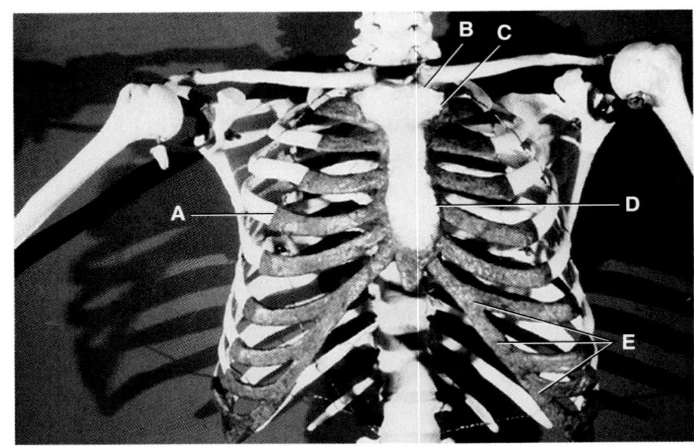

Fig. 11-9. Articulated thorax.

POSTERIOR ARTICULATIONS

The remaining posterior types of joints in the bony thorax, **parts F and G,** are illustrated in Fig. 11-10. The joints between the ribs and the vertebral column, the **costotransverse joints (F)** and the **costovertebral joints (G),** are **synovial** joints with articular capsules lined by synovial membrane, which allow a plane motion, or **gliding motion,** and are therefore **diarthrodial.**

Synovial joints

(F) Costotransverse joint
– Plane (gliding) motion
– Diarthrodial

(G) Costovertebral joint
– Plane (gliding) motion
– Diarthrodial

Fig. 11-10. Posterior articulations.

SUMMARY OF JOINT CLASSIFICATIONS OF THORAX

JOINTS	CLASSIFICATION	MOBILITY TYPE	MOVEMENT TYPE
(A) First–tenth costochondral unions (between costocartilage and ribs)	Unique type of union	Synarthrodial (immovable)	N/A
(B) Sternoclavicular joints (between clavicles and sternum)	Synovial	Diarthrodial	Plane (gliding)
(C) First sternocostal joint (between first rib and sternum)	Cartilaginous (synchondrosis)	Synarthrodial (immovable)	NA
(D) Second–seventh sternocostal joints (between second-seventh ribs and sternum)	Synovial	Diarthrodial	Plane (gliding)
(E) Sixth–tenth interchondral joints (between anterior sixth-tenth costal cartilages)	Synovial	Diarthrodial	Plane (gliding)
(F) First–tenth costotransverse joints (between ribs and transverse processes of T vertebrae)	Synovial	Diarthrodial	Plane (gliding)
(G) First–twelfth costovertebral joints (between heads of ribs and T vertebrae)	Synovial	Diarthrodial	Plane (gliding)

RADIOGRAPHIC POSITIONING

Positioning Considerations for the Sternum

The sternum is difficult to radiograph because of its bony composition and position within the thorax. It is an anterior midline structure that is in the same plane as the thoracic spine. Because the thoracic spine is much more dense, it is virtually impossible to see the sternum in a true AP or PA projection. Therefore the patient is rotated in a 15° to 20° RAO position to shift the sternum just to the left of the thoracic vertebrae and into the homogenous heart shadow (Fig. 11-11).

The degree of obliquity required is dependent on the size of the thoracic cavity. A patient with a shallow or thin chest requires more rotation than a patient with a deep one to cast the sternum away from the thoracic spine. For example, a patient with a large, barrel-chested thorax with a greater anteroposterior measurement requires less rotation (15°), whereas a thin-chested patient requires more rotation (20°). This principle is illustrated by the drawings in Figs. 11-11 and 11-12.

EXPOSURE FACTORS

It is difficult to obtain an optimal radiographic density and contrast on sternum images. The sternum is made up primarily of spongy bone with a thin layer of hard, compact bone surrounding it. This feature, combined with the close proximity of the easy-to-penetrate lungs and the harder-to-penetrate mediastinum/heart, makes exposure factor selection a challenge. Approximately 70 kV is recommended for sthenic patients to achieve acceptable contrast on the image.

Breathing technique may be used for radiographic examinations of the sternum. A breathing technique involves the patient taking shallow breaths during the exposure. If this is performed properly, the lung markings overlying the sternum will become obscured, whereas the image of the sternum remains sharp and well defined (Fig. 11-13.) This requires a low kV (65 ± 5) range, low mA, and a long exposure time of 3 or 4 seconds. The technologist must be sure the thorax in general is not moving during the exposure other than from the gentle breathing motion.

SID

A minimum SID for sternum radiography is 40 inches (100 cm). In the past, a common practice was to lower the SID to create magnification of overlying posterior ribs with resultant unsharpness (blurring). Although this produced quality images of the sternum, it also resulted in an increase in the radiation exposure to the patient. Therefore this practice is not recommended.

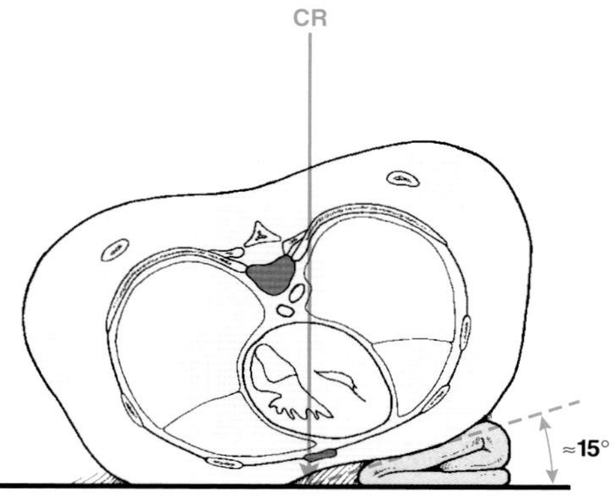

Fig. 11-11. Large, barrel-chested thorax, ≈ 15°.

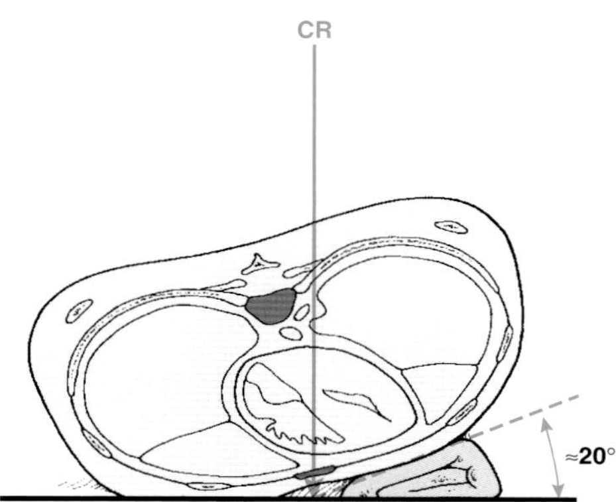

Fig. 11-12. Thin-chested thorax, ≈ 20°.

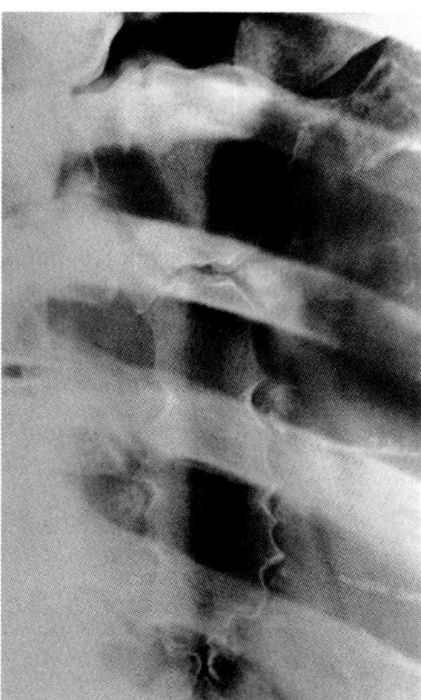

Fig. 11-13. RAO sternum, breathing technique.

11

Positioning Considerations for Ribs

Specific projections performed in a radiographic examination of the ribs are determined by the patient's clinical history and the department protocol.

If the patient's history is not provided by the referring physician, the technologist must obtain a complete clinical history that includes the following:

1. The nature of the trauma or patient complaint
2. The location of the rib pain or injury
3. Whether the patient has been coughing up blood

The technologist must also determine whether the patient is able to stand before beginning the procedure.

The following positioning guidelines will enable the technologist to produce a diagnostic radiologic examination of the ribs.

ABOVE OR BELOW DIAPHRAGM

The location of the trauma and/or patient complaint determines which region of the ribs is radiographed. Ribs above the diaphragm require different exposure factors, different breathing instructions, and generally different body positions than ribs located below the diaphragm.

The **upper 10 posterior ribs** are generally the minimum number of ribs above the dome or central portion of the diaphragm on a full inspiration, as described in Chapter 3. However, with painful rib injuries the patient may not be able to take as deep an inspiration; thus only nine or even eight posterior ribs may be seen above the diaphragm on inspiration.

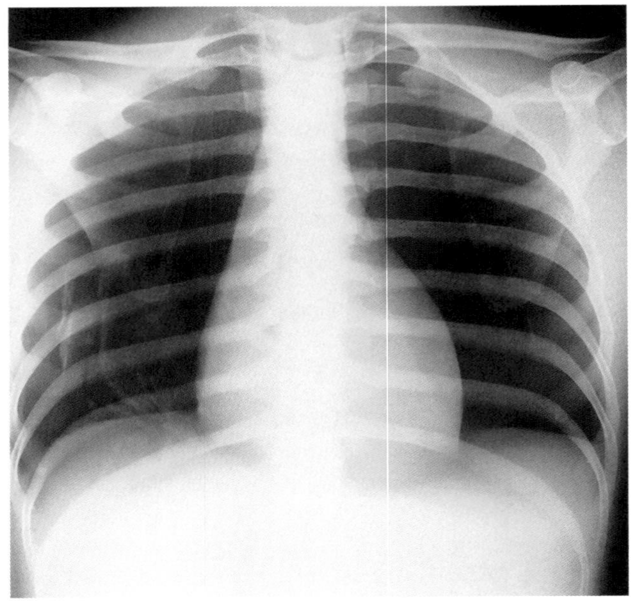

Fig. 11-14. Ribs above diaphragm
—Erect if possible;
—Inspiration;
—Low kV (65-75).

Above Diaphragm To best demonstrate the above-diaphragm ribs, the technologist should:

1. Take the radiographs **erect,** if patient is able to stand or sit. Gravity assists in lowering the diaphragm when the patient is in the erect position. This position also allows a deeper inspiration, which depresses the diaphragm to its lowest position. Also, rib injuries are very painful, and body movement creating pressure against the rib cage, such as from movements on the x-ray table, can cause severe pain and discomfort.
2. Suspend respiration and expose on **inspiration.** This should project the diaphragm below the ninth or tenth ribs on full inspiration.
3. Select a relatively **low kV** (65-75). Because the upper ribs are surrounded by lung tissue, a lower kV will preserve radiographic contrast and allow visualization of the ribs through the air-filled lungs. However, if the site of injury is over the heart area, a higher kV may be used to obtain a longer-scale contrast to visualize ribs both through the heart shadow and through the lung fields.

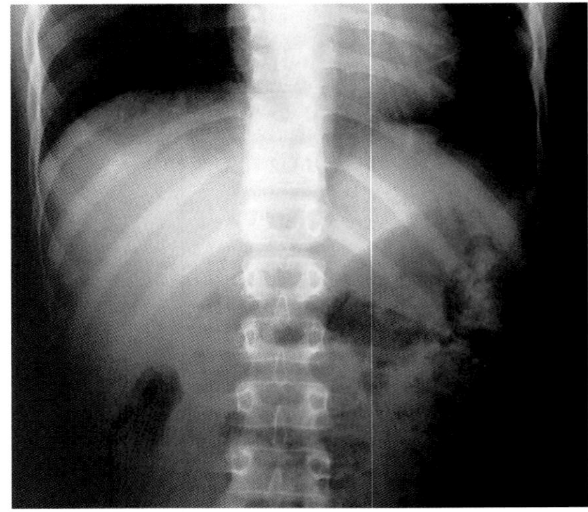

Fig. 11-15. Ribs below diaphragm;
—Recumbent;
—Expiration;
—Medium kV (75-85).

Below Diaphragm To best demonstrate these ribs below the diaphragm, the technologist should:

1. Take the radiographs with patient **recumbent** (supine). This allows the diaphragm to rise to the highest position and results in a "less thick" abdomen (especially on hypersthenic patients, because the abdomen flattens when recumbent). This provides better visualization of the lower ribs through abdominal structures.
2. Suspend respiration and expose on **expiration.** This should allow the diaphragm to rise to the level of the seventh or eighth posterior ribs, again providing a uniform density for below-diaphragm ribs.
3. Select a **medium kV** (75-85). Because the lower ribs are surrounded by the muscular diaphragm and dense abdominal structures, a medium kV will ensure proper penetration of these tissues.

RECOMMENDED PROJECTIONS

Departmental routines for ribs may vary depending on the preference of radiologists. One recommended routine is as follows:

Select the projections that will place the **area of interest closest to the image receptor,** and **rotate the spine away from the area of interest** (prevents the spine from superimposing region of interest).

For example, if a patient has a history of trauma to the **left posterior ribs,** the two preferred projections with this routine are a straight **AP** and a **left posterior oblique.** (Above- or below-diaphragm technique would be determined by the level of injured ribs.) The LPO will move the spinous processes **away from** the left side. The left posterior ribs are closest to the IR and more parallel to the IR to reduce foreshortening of these ribs.

A second example is a patient who has trauma to the **right anterior ribs.** Two preferred projections are a straight **PA** and a **left anterior oblique.** The **PA** will place the site of injury closest to the IR, and the **LAO** will rotate the spinous process **away from** the site of trauma.

MARKING THE SITE OF INJURY

Some department protocols request that the technologist tape a small, metallic "BB" or some other **small** type of radiopaque marker over the site of injury before obtaining the images. This ensures that the radiologist is aware of the location of the trauma or pathology as indicated by the patient.

Note: Each technologist should determine department protocol on this practice before using this method of identifying the potential site of injury.

CHEST RADIOGRAPHS

Departmental protocols also differ concerning the inclusion of chest x-rays as part of a rib exam. Injury to the bony thorax may result in an injury to the respiratory system, and patients with a history of rib injuries may require **erect PA and lateral** projections of the chest to rule out a possible pneumothorax, hemothorax, pulmonary contusion, or other chest pathology. If the patient cannot assume an erect position and the presence of air-fluid levels needs to be ruled out, an image obtained with the patient in a **decubitus position** using a horizontal beam should be included. This is described in Chapter 3.

PEDIATRIC APPLICATIONS

Two primary concerns in pediatric radiography are **patient motion** and **safety.** A clear explanation of the procedure is required to obtain maximal trust and cooperation from the patient and guardian.

Careful immobilization is important to achieve proper positioning and to reduce patient motion. A short exposure time with optimal mA and kV helps reduce patient motion.

To secure their safety, ensure that pediatric patients are continuously watched and cared for.

Communication A clear explanation of the procedure is required to obtain maximum trust and cooperation from the patient and guardian. Distraction techniques that use toys, stuffed animals, etc., are also effective in maintaining patient cooperation.

Immobilization Pediatric patients (depending on age and condition) are often unable to maintain the required positions. Use of immobilization devices to support the patient is recommended to reduce the need for the patient to be held, thus reducing radiation exposure. (Chapter 20 provides an in-depth description of such devices.) If the patient must be held by the guardian, the technologist must provide a lead apron and/or gloves and if the guardian is female, ensure no possibility of pregnancy.

Technical Factors Technical factors will vary as a result of various patient sizes. Use of short exposure times (associated with the use of high mA) is recommended to reduce the risk for patient motion. Breathing technique is not indicated for the young pediatric patient.

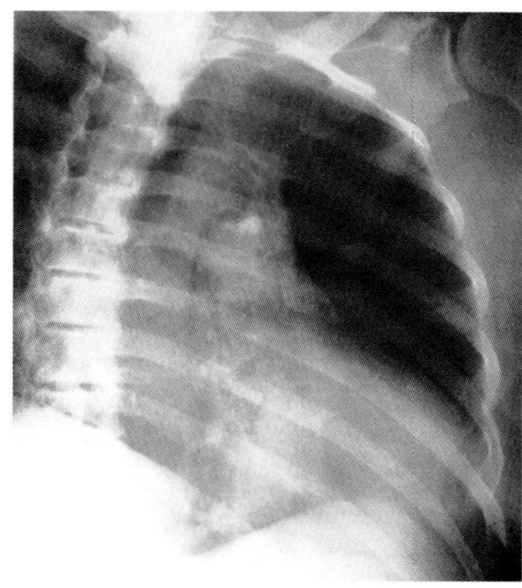

Fig. 11-16. LPO ribs—injury to left posterior ribs.

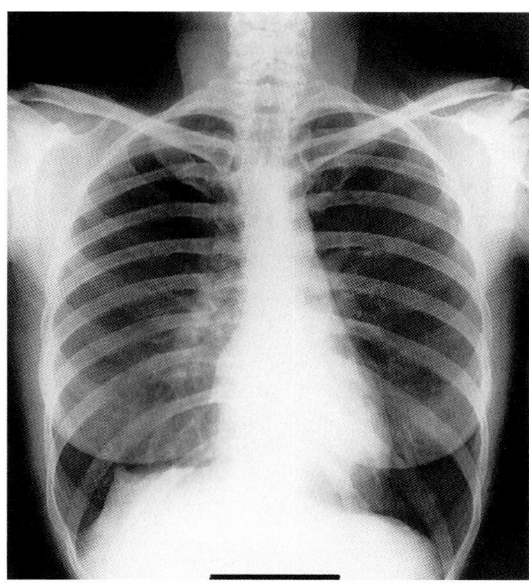

Fig. 11-17. PA erect chest, to rule out a possible pneumothorax and/or hemothorax.

GERIATRIC APPLICATIONS

Communication and Comfort Sensory loss (eyesight, hearing, etc.) associated with aging may result in the geriatric patient requiring additional assistance, time, and patience in achieving the required positions for the sternum and ribs. Decreased position awareness may cause these patients to fear falling off the radiography table when they are imaged in the recumbent position. Reassurance and additional care from the technologist will enable the patient to feel secure and comfortable.

If the examination is performed with the patient in the recumbent position, a radiolucent mattress or pad placed on the exam table will provide comfort. Extra blankets may also be required to keep the patient warm.

Technical Factors Because of the high incidence of osteoporosis in geriatric patients, the kV or mAs may require a decrease if manual exposure factors are being used with film-screen imaging. Older patients may have tremors or difficulty holding steady. Use of short exposure times (associated with the use of high mA) is recommended to reduce the risk for motion.

11

Digital Imaging Considerations

Guidelines for digital imaging (CR and DR) of the bony thorax, sternum, and ribs are similar to those described in previous chapters. These are:

1. **Correct centering and close collimation** (especially for sternum projections)
2. **Following ALARA principles** in determining **exposure factors** (may be desirable to increase kV over film-screen imaging both for reducing patient exposure and improving image quality)
3. **Post-processing evaluation of exposure index values** (for optimum quality image with least possible radiation to patient)

Alternative Modalities and Procedures

COMPUTED TOMOGRAPHY

Computed tomography provides sectional images of the bony thorax. Skeletal detail and associated soft tissues may be evaluated with CT when clinically indicated. CT is useful in visualizing pathology involving the sternum and/or sternoclavicular joints without obstruction by overlying dense structures.

NUCLEAR MEDICINE

Nuclear medicine technology provides a sensitive diagnostic procedure (the radionuclide bone scan) for detection of skeletal pathologies of the thoracic cage (e.g., metastases, occult fractures). A radiopharmaceutical-tagged tracer element is injected, which will concentrate in areas of increased bone activity, demonstrating a "hot spot" on the nuclear medicine image. Any abnormal area is then further investigated with radiography.

It is common practice for patients who are at risk or symptomatic for skeletal metastases to undergo a bone scan (patients with multiple myeloma are exceptions to this).

Pathologic Indications

Fractures The word *fracture* refers to a break in the structure of a bone. Fractures of the bony thorax can be particularly dangerous because of the proximity of the lungs, heart, and great vessels. Areas of common fracture include the following:

- **Ribs:** Rib fractures are most commonly caused by trauma or underlying pathology. Fractures to the first rib are often associated with injury to the underlying arteries/veins, whereas fractures to the lower ribs (8-12) may be associated with injuries to the adjacent organs: spleen, liver, or kidney. Any rib fracture runs the risk for causing injury to the lung or cardiovascular structures (e.g., pneumothorax, pulmonary, or cardiac contusion).
- **Flail chest:** This fracture of adjacent ribs, in two or more places, is caused by blunt trauma and is associated with underlying pulmonary injury.
- **Sternum:** Typically caused by blunt trauma, fractures of the sternum are associated with underlying cardiac injury.

Congenital anomalies

- **Pectus carinatum (pigeon chest):** This is a congenital defect characterized by anterior protrusion of the lower sternum.
- **Pectus excavatum:** Also referred to as **funnel chest,** this deformity is characterized by a depressed sternum.

Metastases These primary malignant neoplasms spread to distant sites via blood and lymphatics. The ribs are common sites of metastatic lesions, which may be characterized and visualized on the image as follows:

- **Osteolytic**—destructive lesions with irregular margins
- **Osteoblastic**—proliferative bony lesions of increased density
- **Combination osteolytic and osteoblastic**—"moth-eaten" appearance of bone resulting from the mix of destructive and blastic lesions

Osteomyelitis This localized infection of bone and marrow can be associated with postoperative complications of open heart surgery, which requires the sternum to be split.

SUMMARY OF PATHOLOGIC INDICATIONS

CONDITION OR DISEASE	MOST COMMON IMAGING PROCEDURE	POSSIBLE RADIOGRAPHIC APPEARANCE	MANUAL EXPOSURE FACTOR ADJUSTMENT*
Fractures:			
• Ribs/flail chest	Routine radiographic views of the ribs and chest	Disruption of bony cortex of the rib; linear lucency through the rib	None
• Sternum	Routine radiographic sternum views, CT	Disruption of bony cortex of the sternum; linear lucency or a displaced sternal segment	None
Congenital anomalies:			
• Pectus carinatum (pigeon chest)	Routine chest and possible lateral sternum	Anterior protrusion of lower sternum	None
• Pectus excavatum (funnel chest)	Routine chest and possible lateral sternum	Depressed sternum	None
Metastases	Routine radiographic views, nuclear medicine bone scan	Depends on lesion type: • Destructive—irregular margins and decreased density • Osteoblastic lesions—increased density • Combination—a "moth-eaten" appearance	None or increase or decrease, depending on type of lesion and stage of the pathology
Osteomyelitis	Routine sternum views, nuclear medicine bone scan	Erosion of bony margins	None

*Dependent on stage or severity of disease or condition.

Survey Information

Following are summaries of results of surveys conducted in years 1989, 1995, and 2000 to determine the most common basic and special or optional projections/positions as performed in the United States and Canada.

SUMMARY OF SURVEY RESULTS

Sternum The **lateral** continues to be the most common position (96%) in both the U.S. and Canada. The second most common position for the sternum is the **RAO,** with 83% indicating **breathing technique** in the U.S. and 28% RAO inspiration. In Canada 55% indicated breathing technique and 21% inspiration.

Tomograms were indicated to be special projections for the sternum and SC joints by 23% in the U.S. and 16% in Canada. Some significant regional differences occurred, with 20% in the Western United States indicating tomograms were routine or basic for the sternum and SC joints, but only **4%** in the Midwest and 6% in the Eastern states and 4% in Canada.

Sternoclavicular Joints The **PA** and the **right** and **left 10° to 15° anterior obliques** continue to be common basic projections in all regions of the U.S. and Canada.

Ribs The **AP or PA** (above or below diaphragm) continues to be the most common basic projection in all regions of the U.S. and Canada.

In the 1995 U.S. survey, **two obliques** (right and left) were more common (55%) than single obliques (45%). This changed in the 1999 survey to **65%, single oblique** in the U.S. **and 49%, two obliques.** This difference in rib routines was more dramatic in Canada in 1999, with 86% indicating the single oblique to be basic or routine and 18%, two obliques.

Including the erect **PA chest** as part of the rib routine increased in the U.S. to 67% in 2000 from 59% in 1995. In Canada 79% indicated the chest to be part of the rib series routine.

The practice of attaching a small metallic "BB" to the site of injury before imaging was indicated to be routine or basic by 20% and special by 23% in the U.S. In Canada this is less common, with only 3% indicating this to be routine and 9% to be special.

Standard and Special Operating Procedures

Protocols and operating procedures vary among facilities, depending on administrative structures, liabilities, and other factors. All technologists should become familiar with the current standards of practice, protocols, and routine or basic and special projections for any facility in which they are working.

Certain basic and special projections for the sternum, sternoclavicular joints, and ribs are demonstrated and described on the following pages as suggested standard basic and special departmental routines or procedures.

BASIC PROJECTIONS

Standard or basic projections, also sometimes referred to as routine projections or departmental routines, are those projections commonly taken on average patients who are helpful and can cooperate in performing the procedure.

SPECIAL PROJECTIONS

Special projections are those more common projections taken as extra or additional projections to better demonstrate certain pathologic conditions or specific body parts.

BASIC AND SPECIAL PROJECTIONS

Sternum
BASIC
- **RAO** 358
- **Lateral** 359

Sternoclavicular Joints
BASIC
- **PA** 360
- **Oblique** 361

Ribs
- **Posterior ribs (AP)** 362
  or
- **Anterior ribs (PA)** 363
- **Axillary ribs (anterior or posterior obliques)** 364
- **PA chest (Chapter 3)**

RAO POSITION: STERNUM

Sternum
BASIC
- RAO
- Lateral

Pathology Demonstrated

Pathology of the sternum, including fractures and inflammatory processes, is demonstrated.

Technical Factors

- IR size—24 × 30 cm (10 × 12 inches), lengthwise
- Moving or stationary grid
- Minimum 3-sec exposure if using breathing technique
- 65 ± 5 kV range
- Technique and dose:

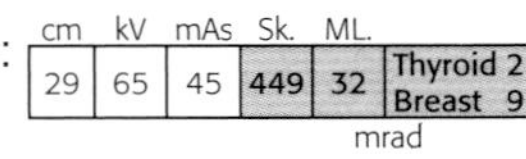

cm	kV	mAs	Sk.	ML.	mrad
29	65	45	449	32	Thyroid 2 Breast 9

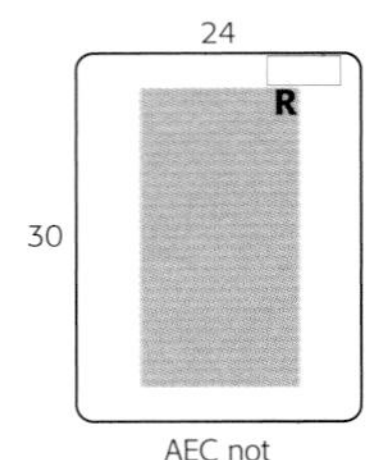

Shielding Shield gonadal region.

Patient Position Erect (preferred) with arms at side or semiprone position with slight rotation, right arm down by side, left arm up

Part Position

- Position patient oblique, **15° to 20°** to the right side, RAO (see Note 1).
- Align long axis of sternum to CR and to midline of table/upright Bucky.
- Place top of IR about 1 ½ inches (4 cm) above the jugular notch.

Central Ray

- CR perpendicular to IR
- CR directed to **center of sternum** (to left of midline and midway between the jugular notch and xiphoid process)
- Minimum SID of 40 inches (100 cm)

Collimation Collimate to sternum (about a 5-inch, or 13-cm, wide collimation field).

Respiration Breathing technique preferred if patient can cooperate. If breathing technique is not possible, suspend respiration on expiration.

Note 1—Rotation: A large deep-chested thorax requires less rotation than a thin-chested thorax to shift the sternum just to the left of vertebral column superimposed over the homogenous heart shadow. The amount of required rotation can also be determined by placing one hand on the sternum and the other on the spinous processes and determining that these two points are not superimposed as viewed from the position of the x-ray tube.

Note 2—Adaptation: This can be obtained in an **LPO position** if the patient's condition does not permit an RAO position. If the patient cannot be rotated, an oblique image may be obtained by angling the **CR 15°-20°** across the right side of the patient to project the sternum lateral to the vertebral column, onto the heart shadow (Fig. 11-18, *inset*). A portable grid would be required and should be **placed crosswise** on the stretcher or tabletop to prevent grid cutoff.

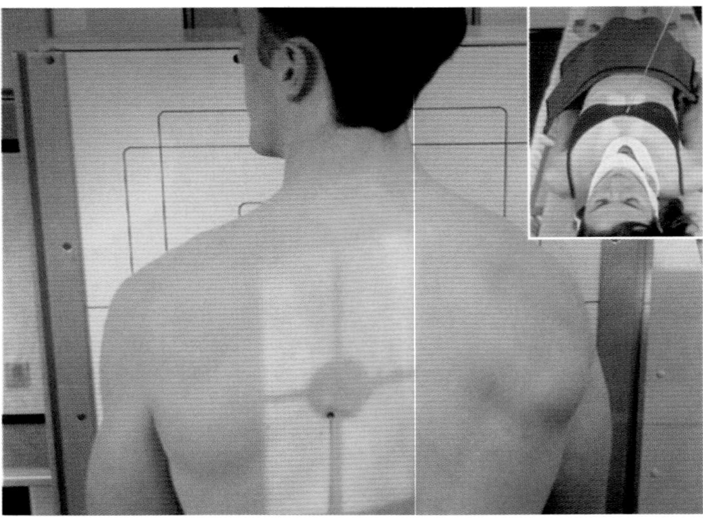

Fig. 11-18. Erect—RAO sternum. *Inset,* 15° to 20° cross angle, grid crosswise.

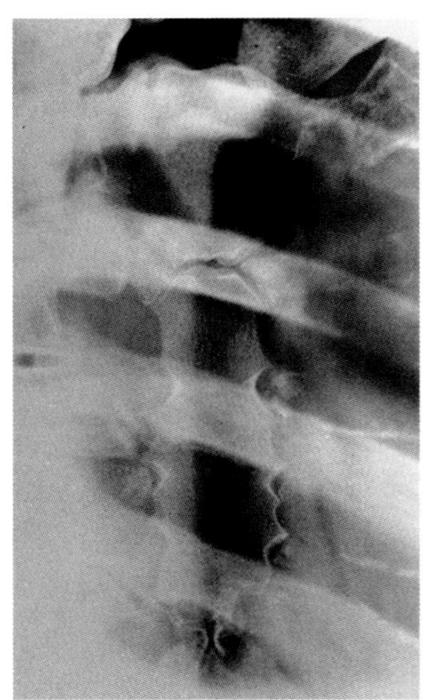

Fig. 11-19. RAO.

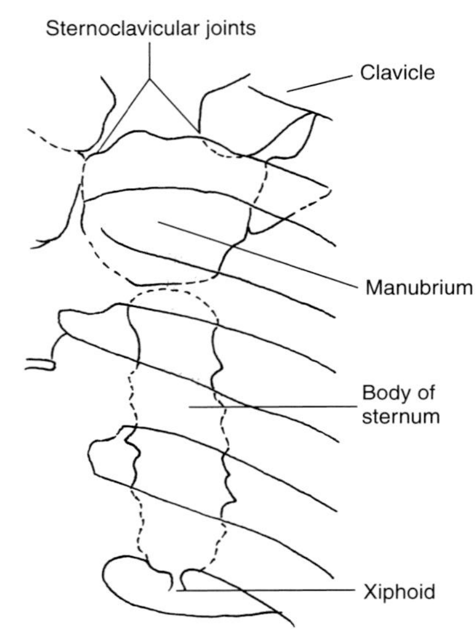

Fig. 11-20. RAO.

Radiographic Criteria

Structures Shown: • Sternum is visualized, superimposed on heart shadow.

Position: • Correct patient rotation is demonstrated by visualizing sternum alongside vertebral column with no superimposition by vertebrae.

Collimation and CR: • The sternum is centered to a closely collimated field.

Exposure Criteria: • Optimal contrast and density demonstrate outline of sternum through overlying ribs, lung, and heart. Bony margins appear sharp, but lung markings are blurred if breathing technique was used.

LATERAL POSITION—R OR L LATERAL: STERNUM

Sternum
BASIC
- RAO
- Lateral

Pathology Demonstrated
Pathology of the sternum, including fractures and inflammatory processes, is demonstrated.

Technical Factors
- IR size—24 × 30 cm (10 × 12 inches), lengthwise
  —30 × 35 cm (11 × 14 inches)
- Moving or stationary grid
- 70 to 75 kV
- Technique and dose:

cm	kV	mAs	Sk.	ML.	mrad
29	70	80	208	64	Thyroid 2 Breast 45

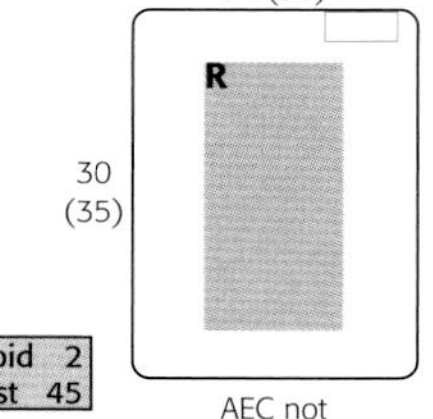

Shielding Shield gonadal region.

Patient Position Erect (preferred) or lateral recumbent

Part Position
Erect:
- Position patient standing or seated with shoulders and arms **drawn back.**

Lateral recumbent:
- Position patient lying on side with arms up above head, keep shoulders back.
- Place top of IR 1½ inches (4 cm) above the jugular notch.
- Align long axis of sternum to CR and midline of grid or table/upright Bucky.
- Ensure a true lateral, with **no rotation.**

Central Ray
- CR is perpendicular to IR.
- CR is directed to **center or sternum** (midway between the jugular notch and xiphoid process).
- SID of 60 to 72 inches (150 to 180 cm) is recommended to reduce magnification of sternum caused by increased OID. (If unable to obtain this SID and a minimum of 40 inches [100 cm] is used, a larger IR of 30 × 35 cm [11 × 14 inches] is recommended to compensate for the magnification.)
- Center IR to CR.

Collimation Close four-sided collimation to area of sternum

Respiration Suspend respiration on **inspiration.**

Note: Large, pendulous breasts of female patients may be drawn to the sides and held in position with a wide bandage if necessary.

Adaptation (Fig. 11-22): The lateral image can be obtained using a horizontal beam with patients in the supine position if their condition warrants this.

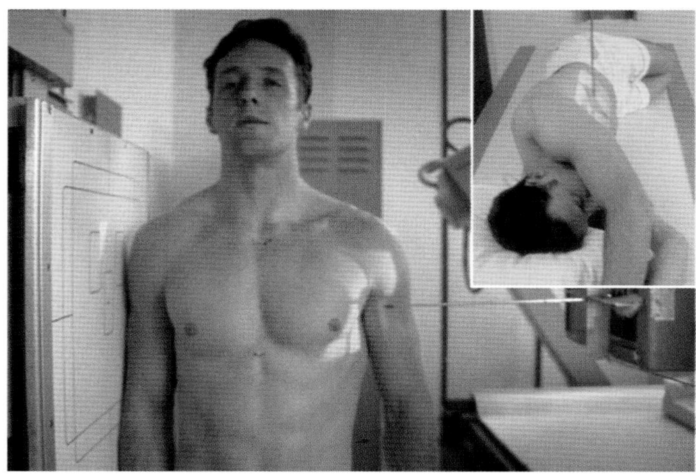

Fig. 11-21. Lateral—erect. *Inset,* Lateral recumbent.

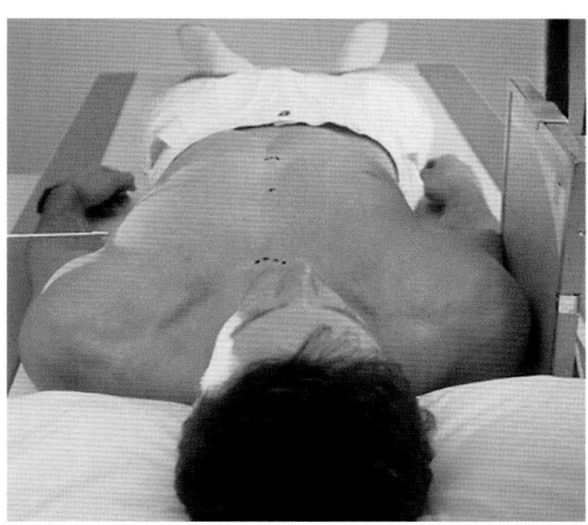

Fig. 11-22. Horizontal beam lateral.

Radiographic Criteria

Structures Shown: • Entire sternum with minimal overlap of soft tissues.

Position: • Correct patient position with no rotation demonstrates the following: • No superimposition of humeri, shoulders, or soft tissue on sternum • Entire sternum with no superimposition of the ribs.

Collimation and CR: • Sternum centered to closely collimated beam.

Exposure Criteria: • Optimal contrast and density to visualize the entire sternum • No motion, as indicated by sharp bony margins.

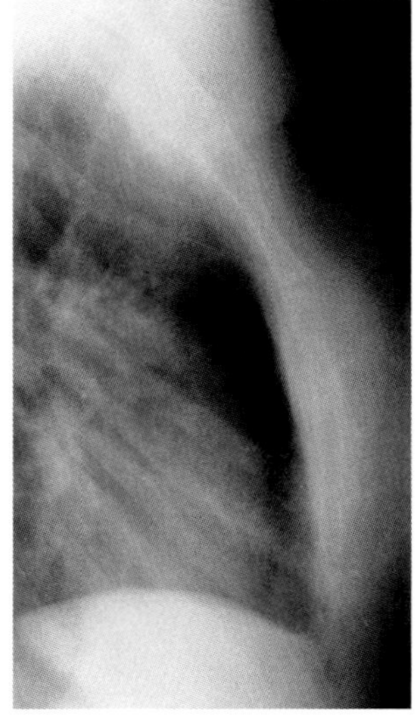

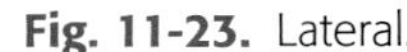

Fig. 11-23. Lateral.

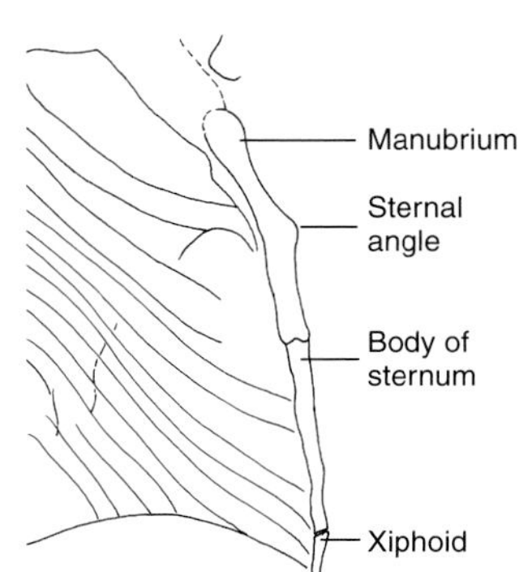

Fig. 11-24. Lateral.

PA PROJECTION: STERNOCLAVICULAR JOINTS

11

Sternoclavicular Joints
BASIC
- PA
- **Anterior obliques**

Pathology Demonstrated

Joint separation or other pathology of the sternoclavicular joints is demonstrated.

Technical Factors

- IR size—18 × 24 cm (8 × 10 inches), crosswise
- Moving or stationary grid
- 65 ± 5 kV
- Technique and dose:

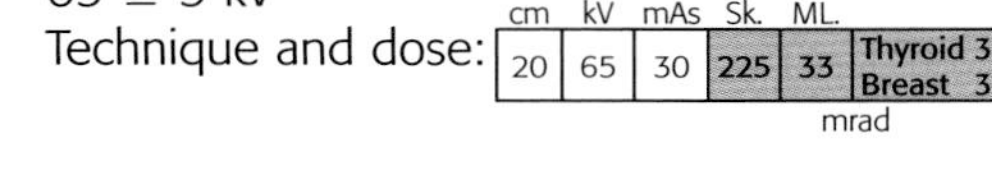
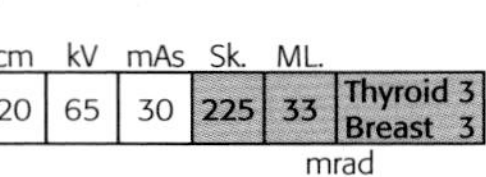

cm	kV	mAs	Sk.	ML.	mrad
20	65	30	225	33	Thyroid 3 Breast 3

24
L
18

Shielding Shield gonadal region.

Patient Position Patient prone, pillow for head turned to one side, arms up beside head, or down by side (may also be taken PA erect)

Part Position

- Align midsagittal plane to CR and to midline of grid or table/upright Bucky.
- Allow no rotation of shoulders.
- Center IR to CR (3 inches, or 7 cm, distal to vertebra prominens at level of T2 to T3).

Central Ray

- CR **perpendicular**, centered to **level of T2 to T3**, or 3 inches (7 cm) distal to vertebra prominens
- Minimum SID of 40 inches (100 cm)

Collimation Close collimation to area of interest

Respiration Suspend on **expiration** for a more uniform density.

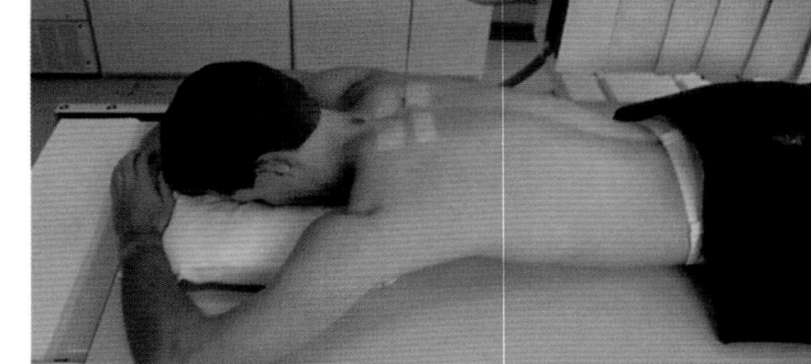

Fig. 11-25. PA bilateral, SC joints.

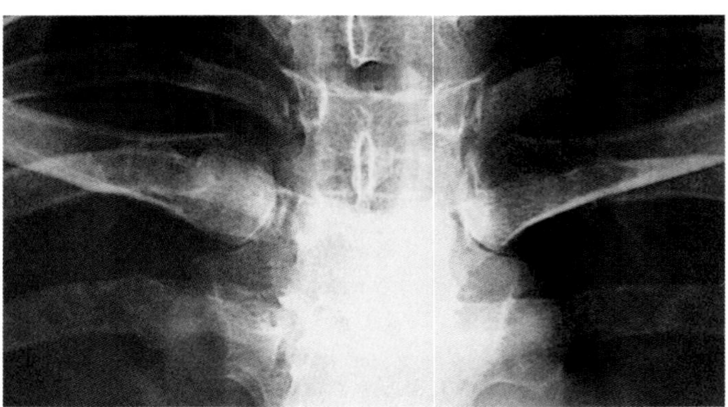

Fig. 11-26. PA bilateral, SC joints.

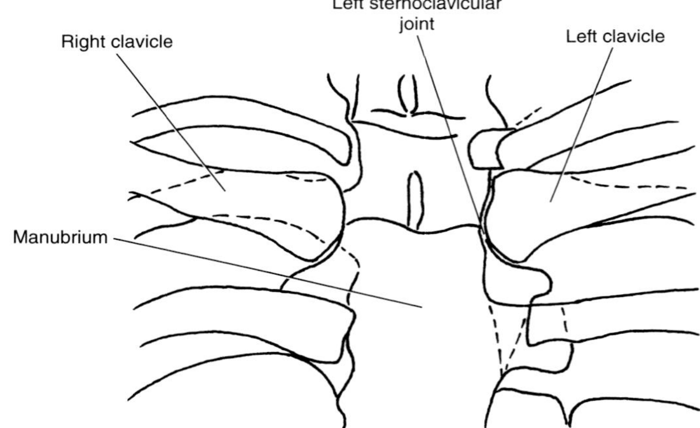

Fig. 11-27. PA bilateral, SC joints.

Radiographic Criteria

Structures Shown: • Lateral aspect of the manubrium and the medial portion of the clavicles are visualized lateral to the vertebral column, through superimposing ribs and lungs.

Position: • **No rotation** of patient, as demonstrated by equal distance of sternoclavicular joints from vertebral column on both sides.

Collimation and CR: • Closely collimated beam centered to the sternoclavicular joints.

Exposure Criteria: • Optimal contrast and density to visualize the manubrium and the medial portion of the clavicles through superimposing ribs and lungs • No motion, as indicated by sharp bony margins.

ANTERIOR OBLIQUE POSITIONS—RAO AND LAO: STERNOCLAVICULAR JOINTS

Images of the Right and Left Joints Are Obtained

Sternoclavicular Joints
BASIC
- PA
- Anterior obliques

Pathology Demonstrated

Joint separation or other pathology of the sternoclavicular joints; best visualizes the sternoclavicular joint on **downside**, which is also demonstrated closest to the spine on the radiograph (see Note 1) (see Note 2 for less obliquity to visualize upside joint).

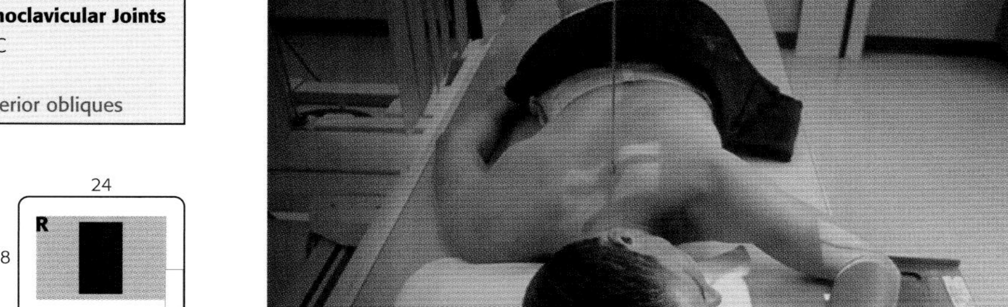

Fig. 11-28. 15° RAO, for right SC joints.

Technical Factors

- IR size—18 × 24 cm (8 × 10 inches), crosswise
- Moving or stationary grid
- 65 ± 5 kV
- Technique and dose:

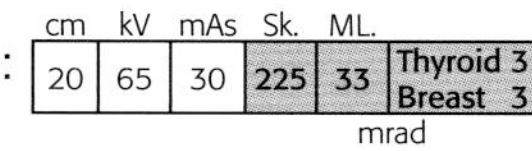

cm	kV	mAs	Sk.	ML.	
20	65	30	225	33	Thyroid 3 Breast 3

mrad

Shielding Shield gonadal region.

Patient Position Prone, with slight rotation (15°) of thorax with upside arm in front of patient and opposite arm behind the patient

Part Position

- With patient rotated 15°, align and center spinous process 1 to 2 inches (3 to 5 cm) lateral (toward upside) to CR and midline of grid or table/upright Bucky.
- Center IR to CR.

Central Ray

- CR perpendicular, to **level of T2 to T3,** or 3 inches (7.5 cm) distal to vertebra prominens, and 1 to 2 inches (3 to 5 cm) lateral (toward upside) to midsagittal plane
- Minimum SID of 40 inches (100 cm)

Collimation Close collimation to area of interest

Respiration Suspend on expiration for a more uniform density.

Adaptation: (1) If the patient's condition requires this, the oblique images may be obtained using posterior obliques with 15° rotation. (2) Oblique images may also be obtained by angling the CR 15° across the patient to project the SC joint lateral to the vertebrae. A portable grid would be required and should be placed crosswise on the stretcher or tabletop to prevent grid cutoff.

Note 1: A 15° rotation in an anterior oblique position will rotate the SC joint across the spine to the opposite side; thus an RAO will best demonstrate the right or downside SC joint.

Note 2: With less obliquity (5° to 10°) the opposite SC joint (the upside joint) would be visualized next to the vertebral column.

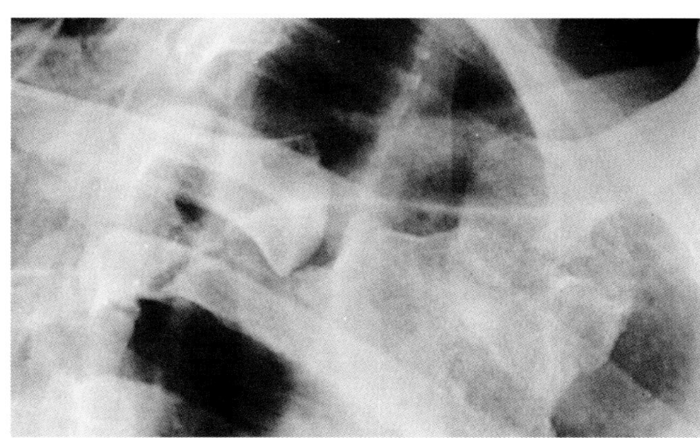

Fig. 11-29. 15° RAO, best demonstrates right (downside) SC joint.

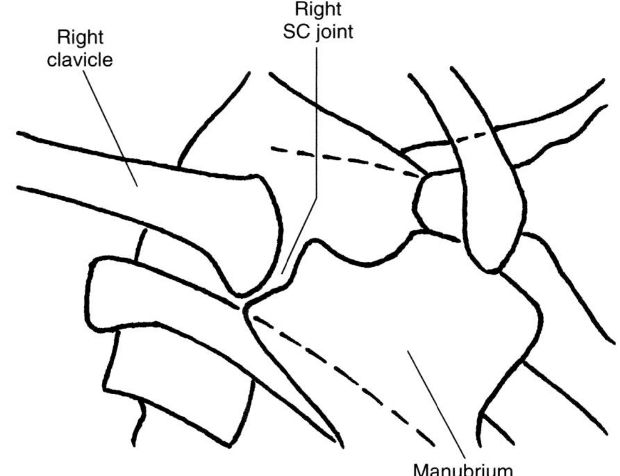

Fig. 11-30. 15° RAO.

Radiographic Criteria

Structures Shown: • The manubrium, medial portion of clavicles, and sternoclavicular joint are shown on the downside. The SC joint on the upside will be foreshortened.

Position: • Correct patient rotation demonstrates the downside sternoclavicular joint visualized with no superimposition of the vertebral column.

Collimation and CR: • Closely collimated beam centered to the SC joints.

Exposure Criteria: • Optimal contrast and density to visualize the sternoclavicular joints through overlying ribs and lungs • No motion, as indicated by sharp bony margins.

AP PROJECTION: POSTERIOR RIBS

Above or Below Diaphragm

Pathology Demonstrated
Pathology of the ribs, including fracture and neoplastic processes, is demonstrated.

Ribs
BASIC
• **Posterior ribs (AP) or anterior ribs (PA)**
• Axillary ribs (anterior or posterior obliques)
• PA chest (p. 96)

Technical Factors

- IR size—35 × 43 cm (14 × 17 inches) lengthwise or crosswise (see Note)
- Moving or stationary grid
- Above diaphragm: 65 to 75 kV
- Below diaphragm: 75 to 85 kV
- Technique and dose: at 72 inches (above diaphragm)

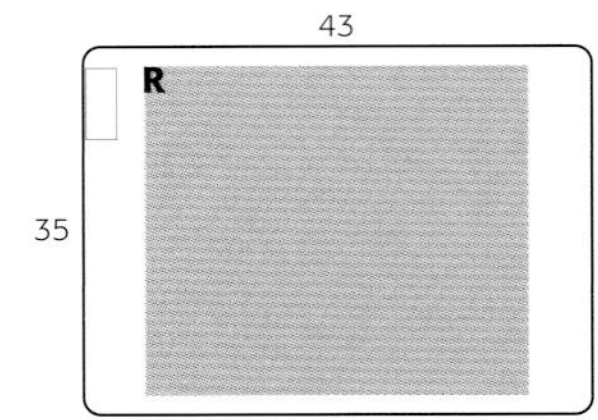

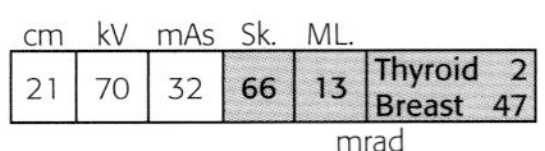

cm	kV	mAs	Sk.	ML.	mrad
21	70	32	66	13	Thyroid 2 Breast 47

Shielding Place lead shield over gonadal region.

Patient Position Erect preferred for above diaphragm if patient's condition allows and supine for below diaphragm

Part Position

- Align midsagittal plane to CR and to midline of grid or table/upright Bucky.
- Rotate shoulders anteriorly to remove scapulae from lung fields.
- **Raise chin** to prevent it superimposing upper ribs, look straight ahead.
- Allow **no rotation** of thorax or pelvis.

Central Ray

Above diaphragm:

- CR **perpendicular** to IR, centered to **3 or 4 inches** (8 to 10 cm) **below jugular notch** (level of T7)
- IR centered to level of CR (top of IR should be about 1½ inches, or 4 cm, above shoulders)

Below diaphragm:

- CR **perpendicular, centered to midway between xiphoid and lower rib cage**
- IR centered to level of CR (bottom of IR should be at iliac crest)
- Minimum SID of 40 inches (100 cm)

Collimation Collimate to outer margins of thorax.

Respiration Suspend respiration on **inspiration** for ribs **above** the diaphragm and **expiration** for ribs **below** the diaphragm.

Note: If doing a bilateral rib examination, place IR crosswise for large patients for both above and below diaphragm ribs to ensure that lateral rib margins are not cut off. This compensates for magnification caused by 40 inches (100 cm) of SID.

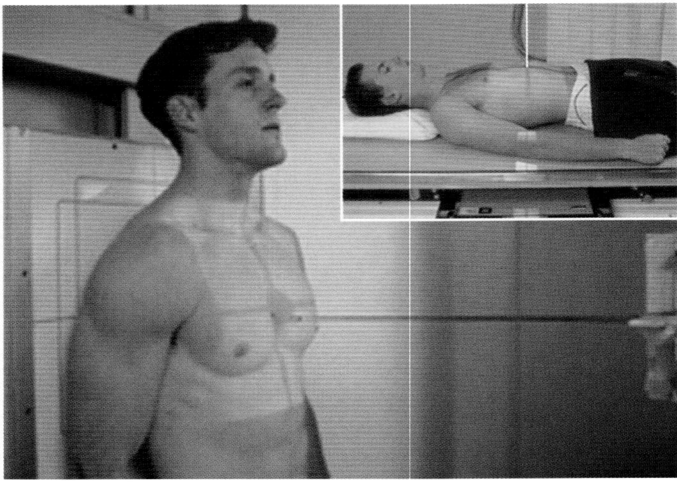

Fig. 11-31. AP erect—above diaphragm. *Inset,* AP supine—below diaphragm.

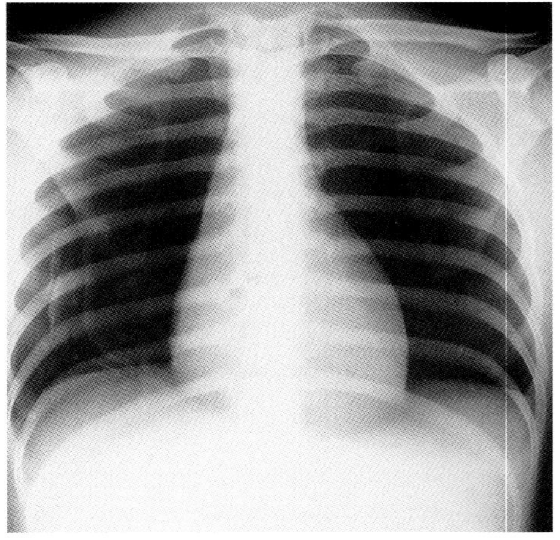

Fig. 11-32. AP—above diaphragm.

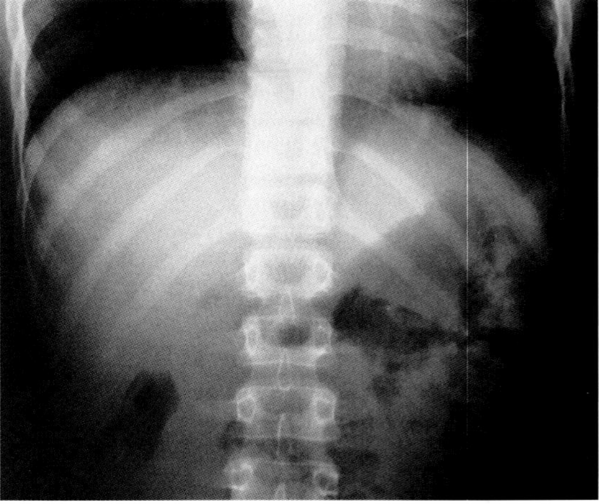

Fig. 11-33. AP—below diaphragm.

Radiographic Criteria

Structures Shown: • *Above diaphragm:* Ribs 1 through 9 or 1 through 10 should be visualized. • *Below diaphragm:* Ribs 8 through 12 should be visualized.

Position: • Rotation of the thorax should not be evident.

Collimation and CR: • Center collimation field appropriately, including ribs 1 through 9, or 1 through 10, or 8 through 12, depending on area of interest.

Exposure Criteria: • Optimal contrast and density to visualize ribs through the lungs and heart shadow or through the dense abdominal organs if below the diaphragm. • No motion, as demonstrated by sharp bony markings.

PA PROJECTION: ANTERIOR RIBS

Above Diaphragm

Ribs
BASIC
- Posterior ribs (AP) or anterior ribs (PA)
- Axillary ribs (anterior or posterior obliques)
- PA chest (p. 96)

Pathology Demonstrated

Pathology of the ribs includes fracture or neoplastic processes. (Injuries to ribs below the diaphragm are generally to posterior ribs; therefore AP projections are indicated.)

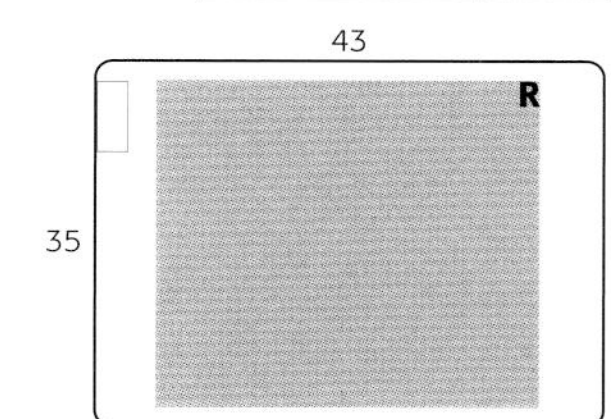

Technical Factors

- IR size—35 × 43 cm (14 × 17 inches), crosswise or lengthwise
- Moving or stationary grid
- 65 ± 75 kV range (above diaphragm)
- Technique and dose:

cm	kV	mAs	Sk.	ML.	
21	70	32	66	13	Thyroid 0 Breast 2
			mrad		

Shielding Place lead shield over gonadal region.

Patient Position Erect preferred or prone if necessary, with arms down to the side

Part Position

- Align midsagittal plane to CR and to midline of grid or table/ upright Bucky.
- Rotate shoulders anteriorly to remove scapulae from lung fields.
- Allow **no rotation** of thorax or pelvis.

Central Ray

- CR **perpendicular** to IR, centered to **T7** (7 to 8 inches, or 18 to 20 cm, below vertebra prominens as for PA chest)
- IR centered to level of CR (top of IR about 1½ inches, or 4 cm, above shoulders)
- Minimum SID of 40 inches (100 cm)

Collimation Collimate to outer margins of thorax.

Respiration Suspend respiration on **inspiration.**

PA erect chest: A common rib routine series (see Survey Results) includes an erect PA chest projection with lung exposure techniques to rule out respiratory trauma or dysfunctions such as a pneumothorax *(white arrows)* or hemothorax *(black arrows),* which may accompany rib injuries (Fig. 11-36.)

Radiographic Criteria

Structures Shown: • Ribs 1 through 9 or 10 visualized above the diaphragm.

Position: • No rotation of the thorax.

Collimation and CR: • Collimation field centered to T7, including ribs 1 through 9 or 1 through 10.

Exposure Criteria: • Optimal contrast and density to visualize ribs through the lungs and heart. • No motion, as demonstrated by sharp bony markings.

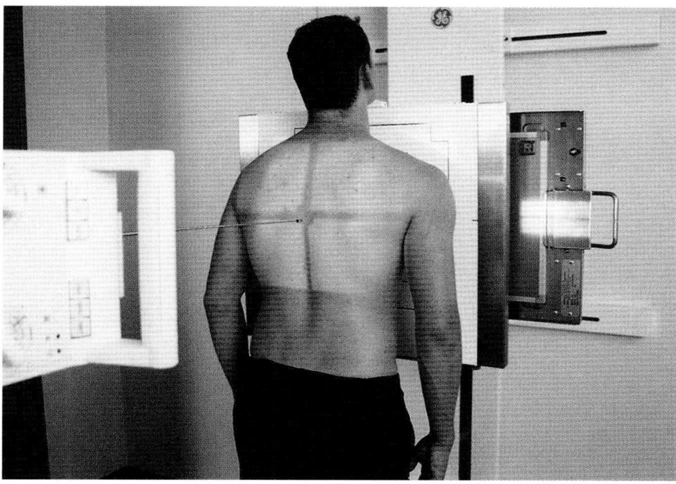

Fig. 11-34. PA ribs—above diaphragm.

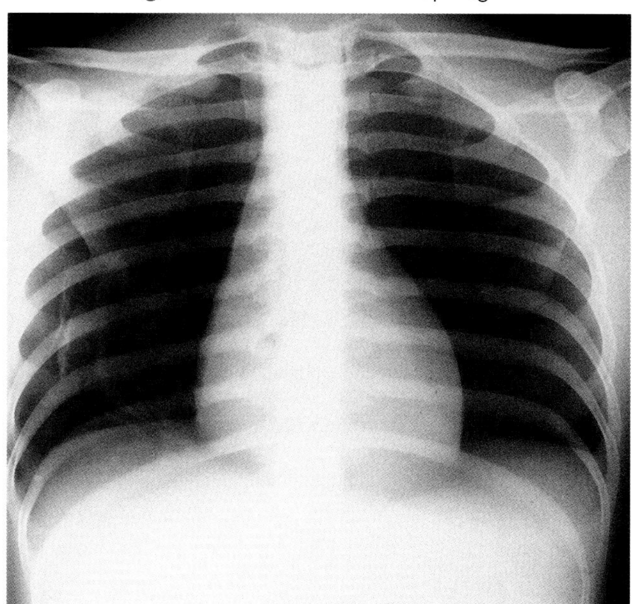

Fig. 11-35. PA ribs (rib technique).

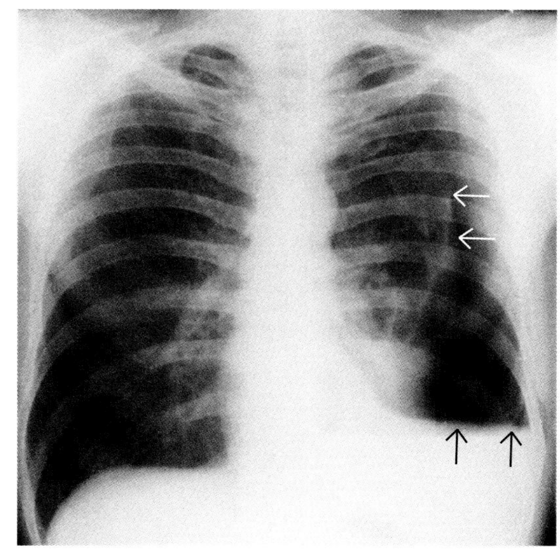

Fig. 11-36. PA erect chest (chest technique). Demonstrates a combination hemothorax and pneumothorax on left side.

POSTERIOR OR ANTERIOR OBLIQUE POSITIONS: RIBS

Above or Below Diaphragm

Ribs

BASIC

- **Posterior ribs (AP) or anterior ribs (PA)**
- Axillary ribs (anterior or posterior obliques)
- PA chest (p. 96)

Pathology Demonstrated

Pathology of the ribs, including fracture and neoplastic processes, is demonstrated.

Posterior/lateral injury: Posterior obliques, affected side toward IR

Anterior/lateral injury: Anterior obliques, affected side away from IR (see Note)

Technical Factors

- Film size—35 × 43 cm (14 × 17 inches), lengthwise
- Moving or stationary grid
- 70 to 75 kV above diaphragm, or 80 to 85 kV below diaphragm
- Technique and dose:

	cm	kV	mAs	Sk.	ML.	mrad
Post. Oblique	23	70	32	91	15	Thyroid 3 Breast 66
Ant. Oblique	23	70	32	91	15	Thyroid 1 Breast 3

35

43

R

Shielding Place lead shield over gonadal region.

Patient Position Erect preferred for above diaphragm if patient's condition allows or supine for below diaphragm

Part Position

- Rotate patient into 45° posterior or anterior oblique, **affected side closest to IR** on **posterior** oblique and **affected side away from IR** on **anterior** oblique. (Rotate spine **away** from site of injury.)
- Raise elevated side arm above head; extend opposite arm down and behind patient away from thorax.
- If recumbent, flex knee of elevated side to help maintain this position.
- Support body with positioning blocks if needed.
- Align a plane of the thorax midway between the spine and the lateral margin of thorax on side of interest to CR and to midline of the grid or table/Bucky. (Ensure that side of interest is **not** cut off.)

Central Ray

- CR **perpendicular** to IR, centered midway between lateral margin of ribs and spine

Above diaphragm:

- CR to level 3 or 4 inches (8 to 10 cm) below jugular notch **(T7)** (top of cassette about 1½ inches or 4 cm above shoulders)

Below diaphragm:

- CR to level midway between xiphoid and lower rib cage (bottom of cassette at about level of iliac crest)
- Minimum SID of 40 inches (100 cm)

Collimation Collimate to near IR borders on all four sides to not cut off rib cage for possible primary and secondary sites of rib injuries.

Respiration Suspend respiration on **inspiration** for above diaphragm ribs and on **expiration** for below diaphragm ribs.

Note: Following this routine, an injury (or other pathology) to the **right** side would require an **RPO** or an **LAO;** to the **left** side would require an **LPO** or an **RAO** to move the spine away from the area of interest. (Not all departments follow this routine. See pages 355 and 357.)

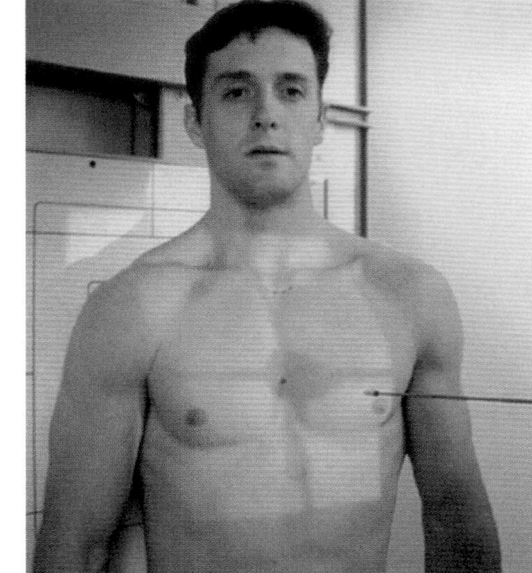

Fig. 11-37. RPO (injury to the **right posterior** ribs, above diaphragm).

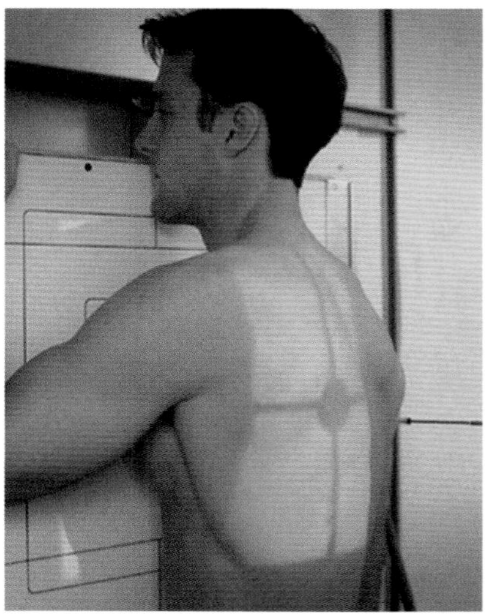

Fig. 11-38. RAO (injury to **left anterior** ribs, above diaphragm).

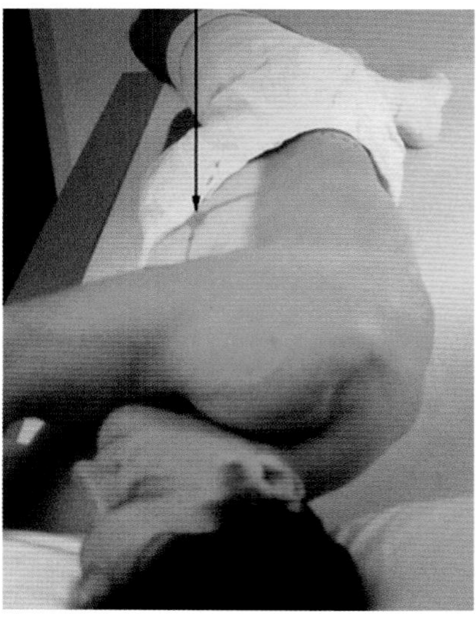

Fig. 11-39. LPO (injury to **left posterior** ribs, below diaphragm). Erect preferred if possible.

Additional collimated projection: Some departmental routines include one well-collimated projection of the region of injury taken on a smaller IR (Fig. 11-41).

Radiographic Criteria

Structures Shown: • *Above diaphragm ribs:* Ribs 1 through 9 or 10 should be included and seen above the diaphragm. • *Below diaphragm ribs:* Ribs 8 through 12 should be included and seen below the diaphragm; the axillary portion of the ribs under examination is projected without self-superimposition.

Position: • An accurate 45° oblique position should demonstrate the axillary ribs in profile with the spine shifted away from the area of interest.

Collimation and CR: • Collimation field centered appropriately, including ribs 1 through 9 or 10, or 8 through 12, depending on area of interest.

Exposure Criteria: • Optimal contrast and density to visualize ribs through the lungs and heart shadow or through the dense abdominal organs if below the diaphragm. • No motion, as demonstrated by sharp bony markings.

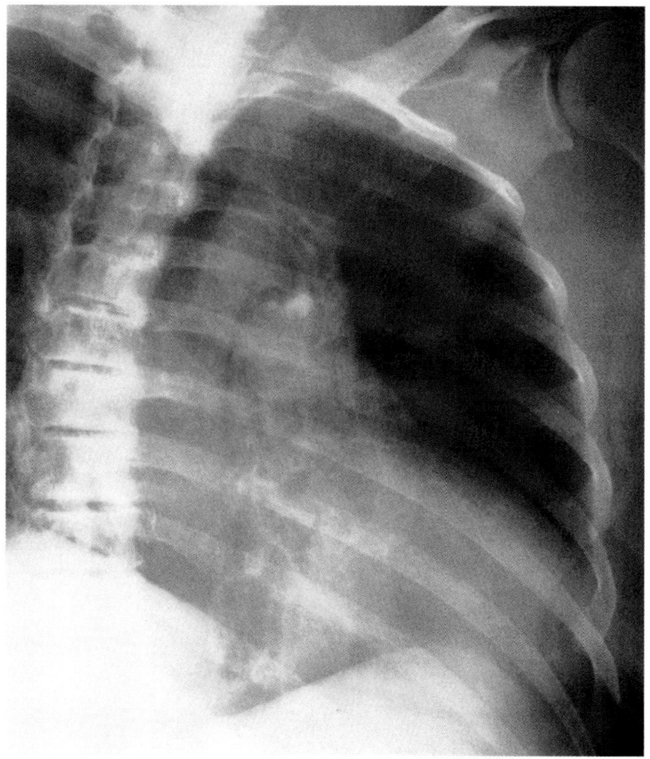

Fig. 11-40. LPO—above diaphragm.

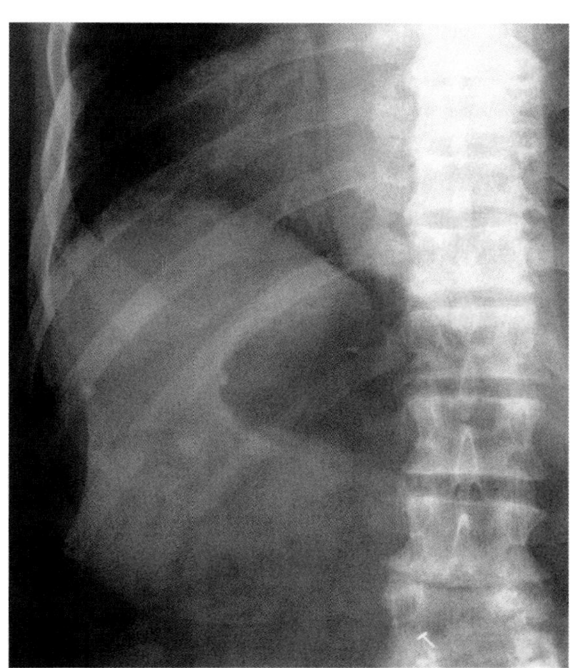

Fig. 11-41. AP below diaphragm centered for right ribs.

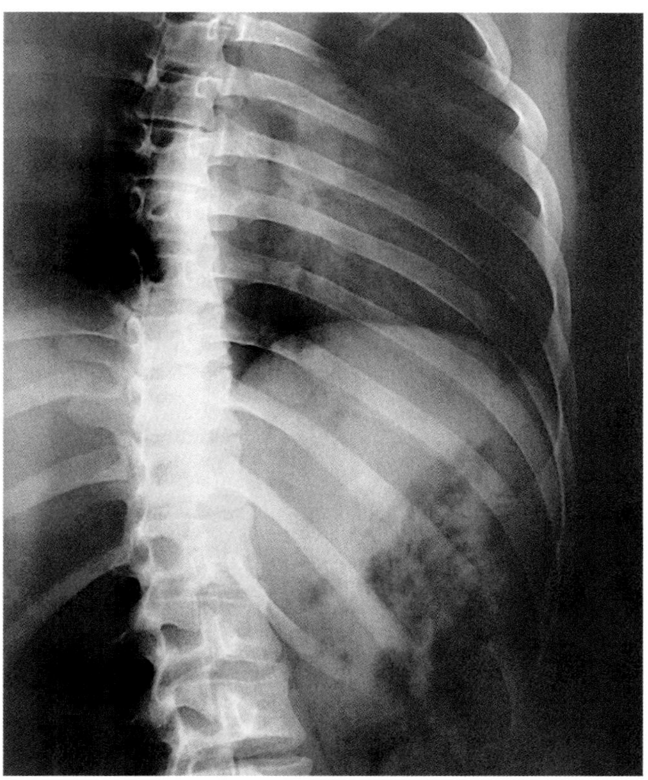

Fig. 11-42. LPO—below diaphragm, left ribs.

RADIOGRAPHS FOR CRITIQUE

Students should determine whether they can critique each of these four radiographs based on the categories as described in the textbook and as outlined on the right. As a starting critique exercise, place a check in each category that demonstrates a **repeatable error** for that radiograph.

Student workbooks provide more space for writing comments and complete critique answers for each of these radiographs. Answers are also provided in Appendix B, at the end of this textbook.

	RADIOGRAPHS A	B	C	D
1. Structures shown	____	____	____	____
2. Positioning	____	____	____	____
3. Collimation and CR	____	____	____	____
4. Exposure criteria	____	____	____	____
5. Markers	____	____	____	____

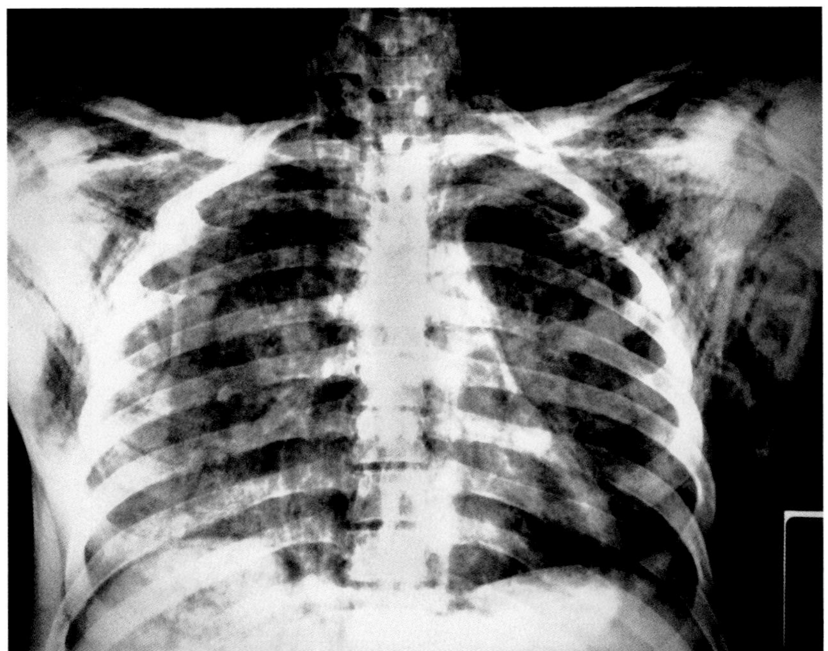

Fig. C11-43. Ribs—above diaphragm. (Mystery radiograph, Courtesy Bill Collins, RT.) **A**

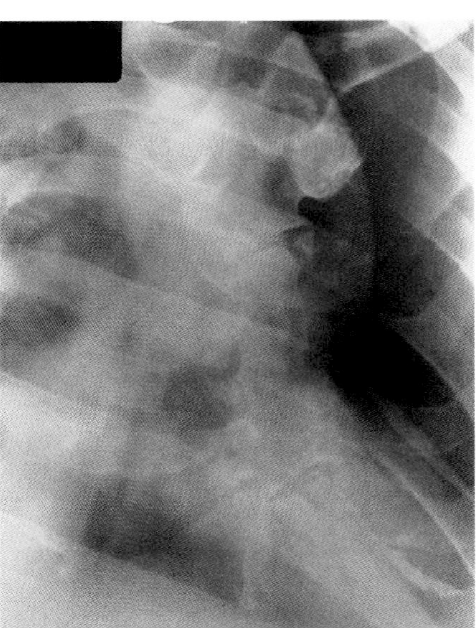

Fig. C11-44. Oblique sternum. **B**

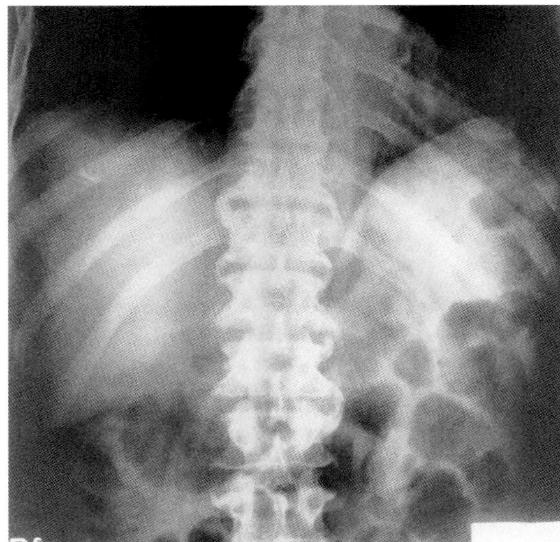

Fig. C11-45. Ribs—below diaphragm. **C**

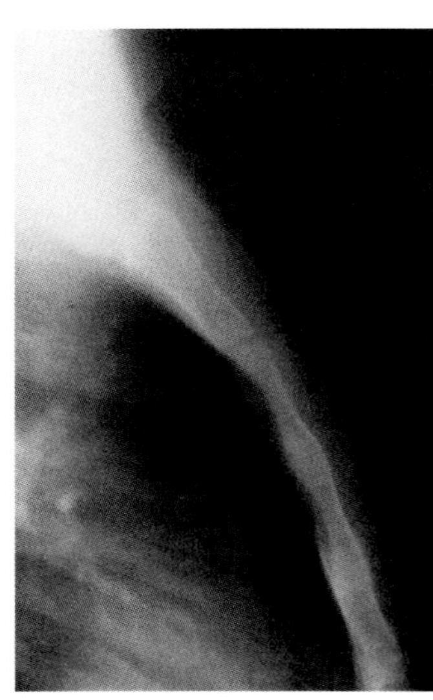

Fig. C11-46. Lateral sternum. **D**

CHAPTER 12

Skull and Cranial Bones

CONTRIBUTIONS BY **Renee F. Tossell,** PhD, RT(R)(M)(CV)
CONTRIBUTORS TO PAST EDITIONS Kathy M. Martensen, BS, RT(R), Barry T. Anthony, RT(R), Cindy Murphy, RT R, ACR, BHSc

CONTENTS

RADIOGRAPHIC ANATOMY

Skull

As with other body parts, radiography of the skull requires a good understanding of all related anatomy. The anatomy of the skull is very complex and requires specific attention to details.

The **skull,** or bony skeleton of the head, rests on the superior end of the vertebral column and is divided into two main sets of bones, the **8 cranial bones** and **14 facial bones.** Anatomy and positioning for the cranial bones are covered in this chapter; the facial bones will be covered in Chapter 13.

CRANIAL BONES (8)

The eight bones of the cranium are divided into the calvaria (skull cap) and floor. Each of these two areas primarily consists of four bones:

12

Calvaria (skull cap)

1. Frontal
2. Right parietal *(pah-ri'e-tal)*
3. Left parietal
4. Occipital *(ok-sip'i-tal)*

Floor

5. Right temporal
6. Left temporal
7. Sphenoid *(sfe'noid)*
8. Ethmoid *(eth'moid)*

The eight bones making up the calvaria (skull cap) and the floor or base of the cranium are demonstrated on these frontal, lateral, and superior cutaway view drawings. These cranial bones are fused in an adult to form a protective enclosure for the brain. Each of these cranial bones will be demonstrated and described individually in the pages that follow.

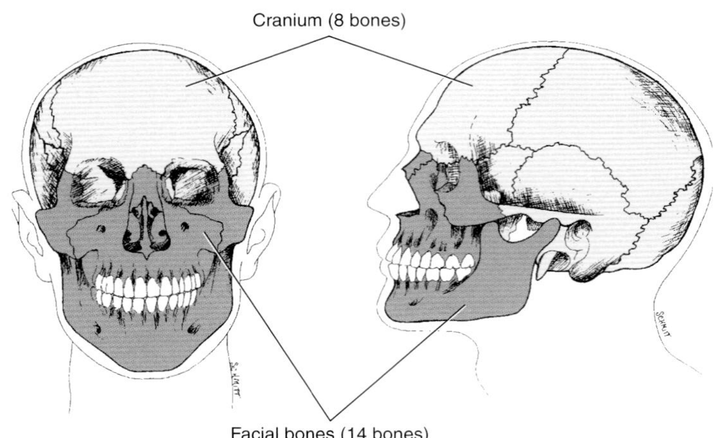

Fig. 12-1. Skull—bony skeleton of head (cranial and facial bones).

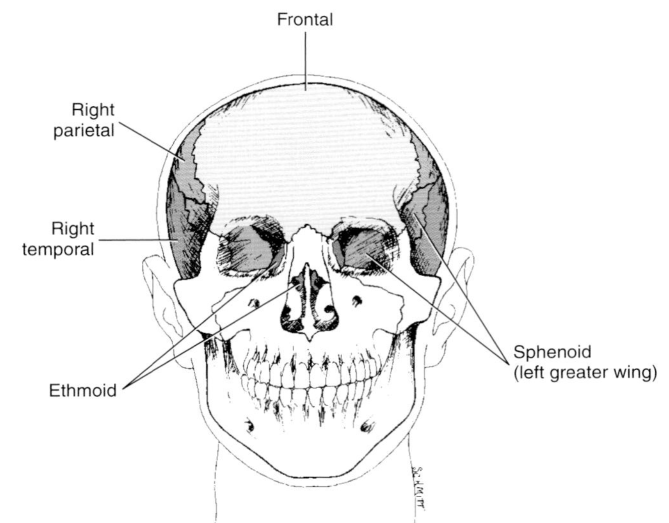

Fig. 12-2. Cranium—frontal view.

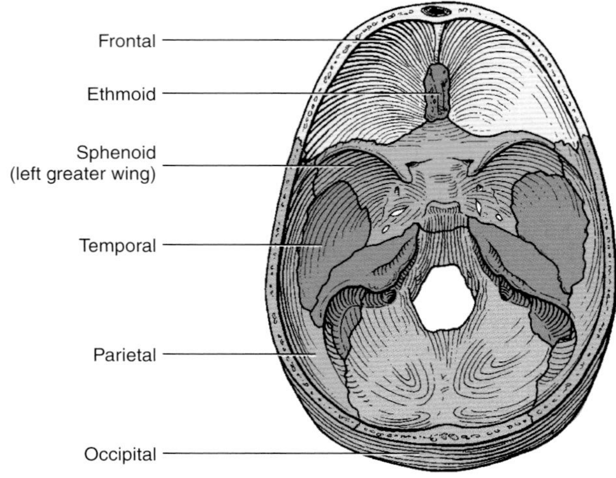

Fig. 12-3. Cranium—superior cutaway view.

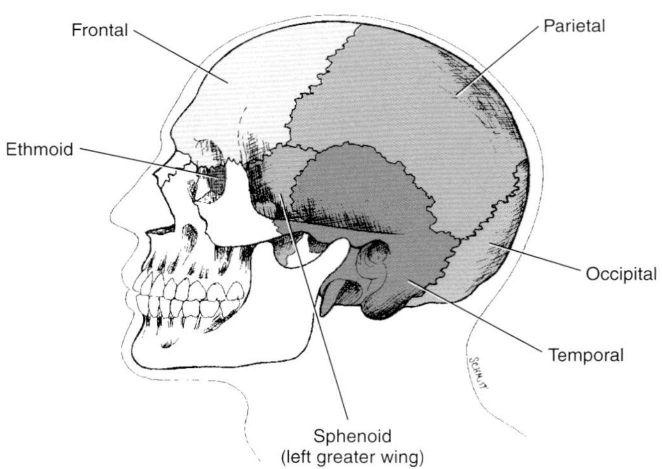

Fig. 12-4. Cranium—lateral view.

CRANIAL BONES

After the description of each of these eight bones appears a listing of specific adjoining bones. Some of the bones with which the cranial bones articulate are facial bones, which are described in Chapter 13. Knowledge of these articulations can help you learn the specific locations and relationships of each of these bones beginning with the frontal bone.

Frontal Bone

As viewed from the front, the bone of the calvaria most readily visible is the **frontal bone.** This bone contributes to the formation of the forehead and the superior part of each orbit. It consists of two main parts: the **squamous** or **vertical portion** (which forms the forehead) and the **orbital** or **horizontal portion** (which forms the superior part of the orbit).

Squamous or vertical portion (Figs. 12-5 and 12-6) The **glabella** is the smooth, raised prominence between the eyebrows just above the bridge of the nose.

The **supraorbital groove (SOG)** is the slight depression above each eyebrow. This becomes an important landmark because it corresponds to the floor of the anterior fossa of the cranial vault, which is also at the level of the orbital plate or the highest level of the facial bone mass (Fig. 12-7).

Note: You can locate this SOG on yourself by placing your finger against the length of your eyebrow and feeling the raised arch of bone, then allowing your finger to slide upward and drop slightly into the SOG.

The superior rim of each orbit is the **supraorbital margin,** or **SOM.** The **supraorbital notch** (foramen) is a small hole or opening within the supraorbital margin slightly medial to its midpoint. A nerve and an artery pass through this small opening.

That ridge of bone beneath each eyebrow is termed the **superciliary ridge** (arch). Between the superciliary arches is the **glabella.**

On each side of the squamous portion of the frontal bones above the supraorbital grooves is a larger rounded prominence termed the **frontal tuberosity** (eminence).

Orbital or horizontal portion (Fig. 12-7) As seen from the inferior aspect, the frontal bone shows primarily the horizontal or orbital portion, which consists of the **supraorbital margins, superciliary ridges, glabella,** and **frontal tuberosities.**

The **orbital plate** on each side forms the superior part of each orbit. Below the orbital plates lie facial bones, and above the orbital plates is the anterior part of the floor of the brain case.

Each orbital plate is separated from the other by the **ethmoidal notch.** The ethmoid bone, one of the bones of the floor of the cranium, fits into this notch. The **nasal** (frontal) **spine** is found at the anterior end of the ethmoidal notch.

Articulations The frontal bone articulates with **four** cranial bones: right and left parietals, the sphenoid, and the ethmoid. These can be identified on frontal, lateral, and superior cutaway drawings on p. 368. (The frontal bone also articulates with eight facial bones.)

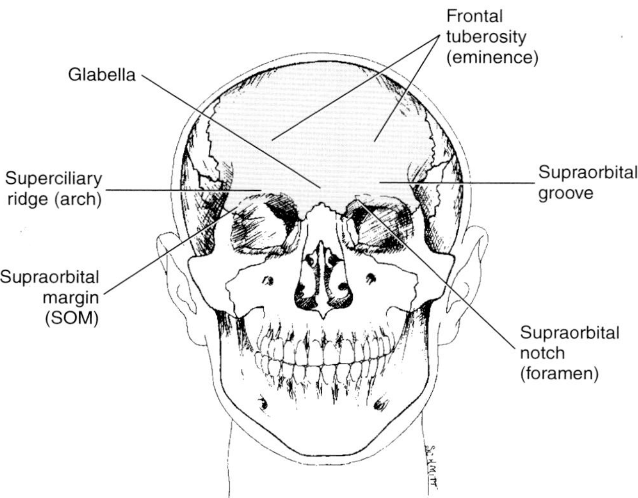

Fig. 12-5. Frontal bone—frontal view.

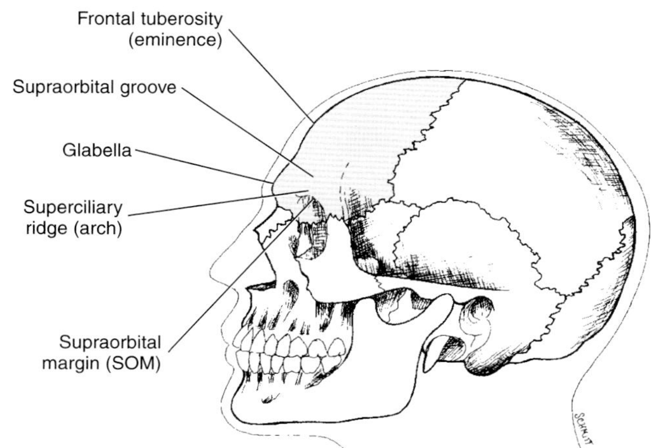

Fig. 12-6. Frontal bone—lateral view.

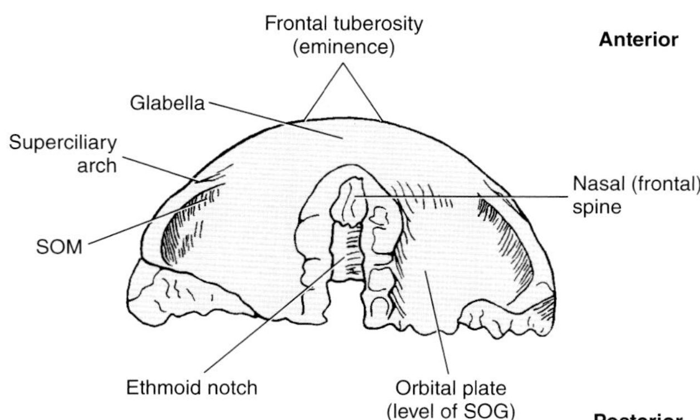

Fig. 12-7. Orbital portion of frontal bone—inferior view.

12

Parietal Bones

The paired **right** and **left parietal bones** are well demonstrated on the lateral and superior view drawings of Figs. 12-8 and 12-9. The lateral walls of the cranium and part of the roof are formed by the two parietal bones. The parietal bones are roughly square and have a concave internal surface.

The widest portion of the entire skull is located between the **parietal tubercles (eminences)** of the two parietal bones. The frontal bone is primarily anterior to the parietals; the occipital is posterior; the temporals are inferior; and the greater wings of the sphenoid are inferior and anterior.

Articulations Each parietal bone articulates with **five** cranial bones: the frontal, the occipital, a temporal, the sphenoid, and the opposite parietal.

Occipital Bone

The inferoposterior portion of the calvaria, or skull cap, is formed by the single occipital bone. The external surface of the occipital bone presents a rounded part termed the **squamous portion.** The squamous portion forms most of the back of the head and is that part of the occipital bone superior to the **external occipital protuberance,** or **inion,** which is the prominent bump or protuberance at the inferoposterior portion of the skull.

The large opening at the base of the occipital bone through which the spinal cord passes as it leaves the brain is termed the **foramen magnum,** literally meaning "great hole."

The two lateral **condylar portions (occipital condyles)** are oval processes with convex surfaces, with one on each side of the foramen magnum. These articulate with depressions on the first cervical vertebra, called the *atlas.* This two-part articulation between the skull and the cervical spine is called the **atlanto-occipital joint.**

Articulations The occipital articulates with **six** bones: the two parietals, the two temporals, the sphenoid, and the atlas (first cervical vertebra).

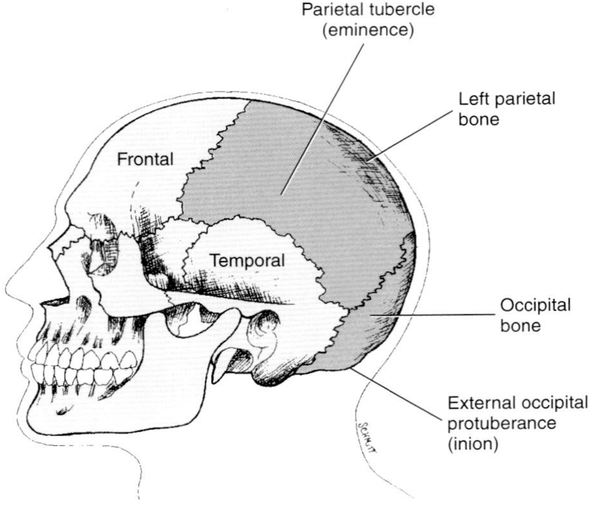

Fig. 12-8. Parietal and occipital bones—lateral view.

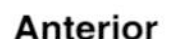

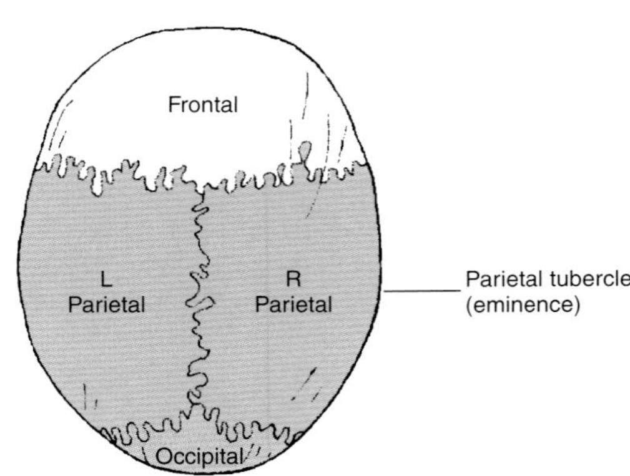

Fig. 12-9. Parietal and occipital bones—superior view.

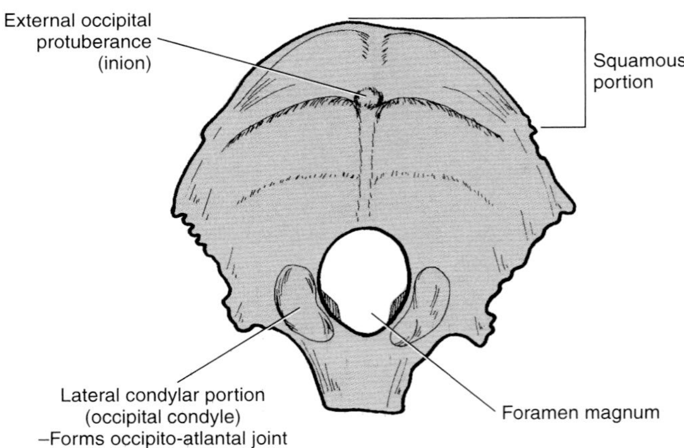

Fig. 12-10. Occipital bone—inferior view

Temporal Bones

Lateral view (Fig. 12-11) The paired **right** and **left temporal bones** are complex structures housing the delicate organs of hearing and balance. As seen from this lateral view drawing, the left temporal bone is situated between the greater wing of the sphenoid bone anteriorly and the occipital bone posteriorly.

Extending anteriorly from the squamous portion of the temporal bone is an arch of bone termed the **zygomatic** *(zi'go-mat'ik)* **process.** This process meets the temporal process of the zygomatic bone (one of the facial bones) to form the easily palpated **zygomatic arch.**

Inferior to the zygomatic process and just anterior to the **EAM,** external acoustic (auditory) meatus, is the **temporomandibular fossa,** into which the mandible fits to form the **TMJ,** or **temporomandibular joint.**

Projecting inferior to the mandible and anterior to the EAM is a slender bony projection called the **styloid process.**

Frontal cutaway view (Fig. 12-12) Each temporal bone is divided into **three primary parts.** First is the thin upper portion forming part of the wall of the skull, the **squamous portion.** This part of the skull is quite thin and is therefore the most vulnerable portion of the entire skull to fracture.

The second portion is the area posterior to the EAM, the **mastoid portion,** with a prominent **mastoid process,** or **tip.** Many air cells are located within the mastoid process.

The third main portion is the dense **petrous** *(pet'rus)* **portion,** also called the **petrous pyramid,** or **pars petrosa,** which house the organs of hearing and equilibrium including the mastoid air cells as described later in this chapter. Sometimes this is also called the **petromastoid portion** of the temporal bone because internally this includes the mastoid portion. The upper border or ridge of the petrous pyramids is commonly called the **petrous ridge,** or petrous apex.

Superior view (Fig. 12-13) The floor of the cranium is well visualized in this drawing. The single occipital bone resides between the paired temporal bones. The third main portion of each temporal bone, the **petrous portion,** is again shown in this superior view. This pyramid-shaped portion of the temporal bone is the thickest and most dense bone in the cranium. The **petrous pyramids** project anteriorly and toward the midline from the area of the **EAM.**

The **petrous ridge** of these pyramids **corresponds to the level of an important external landmark,** the **TEA** (top of the ear attachment). Near the center of the petrous pyramid on the posterior surface just superior to the **jugular foramen** is an opening or orifice termed the **internal acoustic meatus,** which serves to transmit the nerves of hearing and equilibrium.

Note: The openings of the external and internal acoustic meatus cannot be visualized on this superior view drawing because they are located on the posteroinferior aspect of the pyramid.

Articulations Each temporal bone articulates with **three** cranial bones: a parietal, the occipital, and the sphenoid. (Each temporal bone also articulates with two facial bones.)

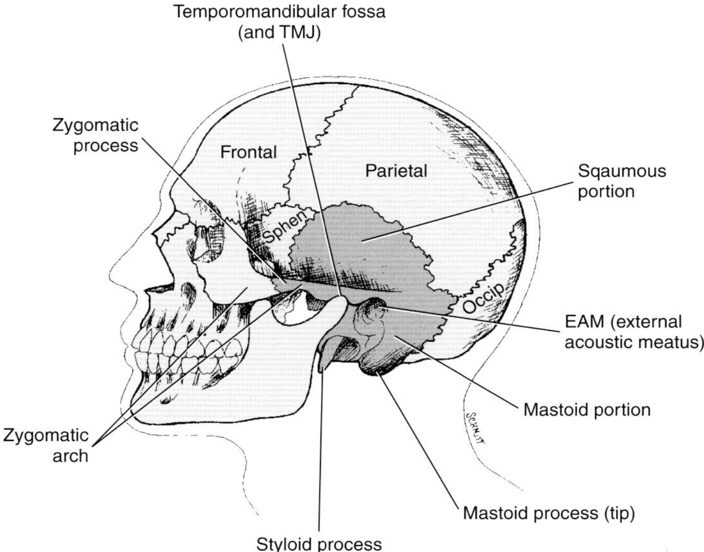

Fig. 12-11. Temporal bone—lateral view.

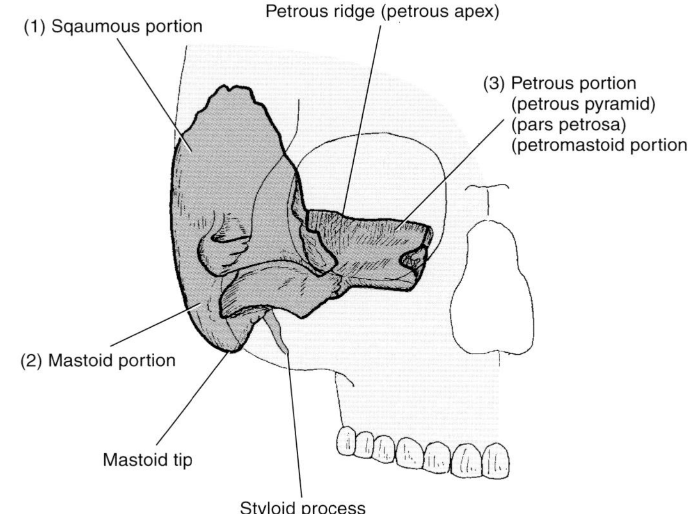

Fig. 12-12. Temporal bone, three primary parts—frontal cutaway view.

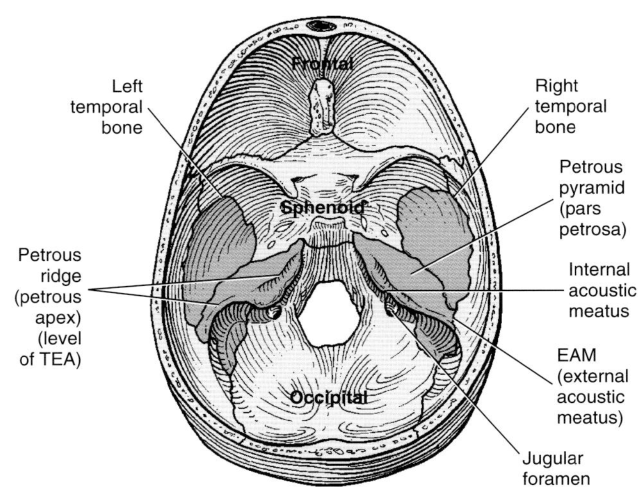

Fig. 12-13. Temporal bones—superior view.

12

12

Sphenoid Bone

Superior view The single centrally located **sphenoid bone** forms the anchor for all eight cranial bones. The central portion of the sphenoid is the body, which lies in the midline of the floor of the cranium and contains the sphenoid sinus, as best shown on the sagittal sectional drawing of Fig. 12-18 on p. 373.

The central depression on the body is termed the **sella turcica** *(sel'a-tur'si-ka).* This depression looks like a saddle from the side, as shown in Fig. 12-16 on p. 373, and derives its name from words meaning *Turkish saddle.* The sella turcica partially surrounds and protects a major gland of the body, the **hypophysis cerebri** or **pituitary gland.** Posterior to the sella turcica is the back of the saddle, the **dorsum sellae** *(dor'sum sel'e),* also best seen on the lateral drawing of Fig. 12-16.

The **clivus** *(kli'vus)* is a shallow depression that begins on the posterior aspect of the dorsum sellae of the sphenoid bone and extends posteriorly to the foramen magnum at the base of the occipital bone (Figs. 12-14 and 12-16). This slightly depressed area forms a base of support for the pons (a portion of the brain stem) and for the basilar artery.

Extending laterally from the body to either side are two pairs of wings. The smaller pair, termed the **lesser wings,** are triangular and nearly horizontal, ending medially in the two **anterior clinoid processes.** They project laterally from the upper, anterior portion of the body and extend to about the middle of each orbit. The **greater wings** extend laterally from the sides of the body and form a portion of the floor of the cranium and a portion of the sides of the cranium.

Three pairs of small openings or foramina exist in the greater wings for passage of certain nerves and blood vessels (Fig. 12-14). Lesions that can cause erosion of these foramina can be detected radiographically. The **foramen rotundum** *(ro-tun'dum)* and the **foramen ovale** *(o-va'le)* are seen as small openings on both the superior and oblique view drawings (Figs. 12-14 and 12-15). The locations of the pair of small rounded **foramen spinosum** *(spi-no'-sum)* are also seen on the superior view drawing (Fig. 12-14).

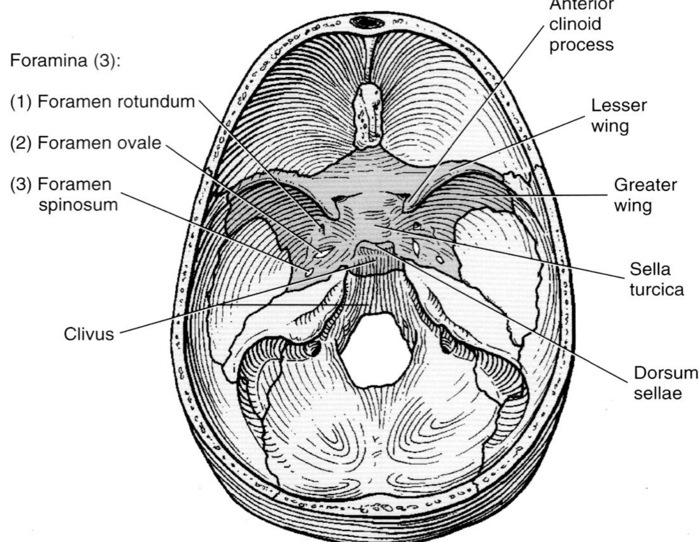

Fig. 12-14. Sphenoid bone—superior view.

Oblique view An oblique drawing of the sphenoid bone demonstrates the complexity of this bone. The shape of the sphenoid has been compared to a bat with its wings and legs extended as in flight. The centrally located depression, the **sella turcica,** is again seen on this view (Fig. 12-15).

Arising from the most posterior aspect of the **lesser wings** are two bony projections termed **anterior clinoid processes.** The anterior clinoids are somewhat larger and are spread farther apart than are the **posterior clinoid processes,** which extend superiorly from the **dorsum sellae,** best seen on the lateral drawing in Fig. 12-16.

Between the anterior body and the lesser wings on each side are groovelike canals through which the optic nerve and certain arteries pass into the orbital cavity. This begins in the center as the **chiasmatic** *(ki-az-mat'ik)* or **optic groove,** which leads on each side to an **optic canal,** which ends at the **optic foramen** or opening into the orbit. The optic foramina can be demonstrated radiographically with PA oblique projections of the orbits.

Slightly lateral and posterior to the optic foramina on each side are irregular-shaped openings, seen best on this oblique view, called **superior orbital fissures.** These openings provide additional communication with the orbits for numerous nerves and blood vessels. The foramen rotundum and the foramen ovale are seen again on this oblique view.

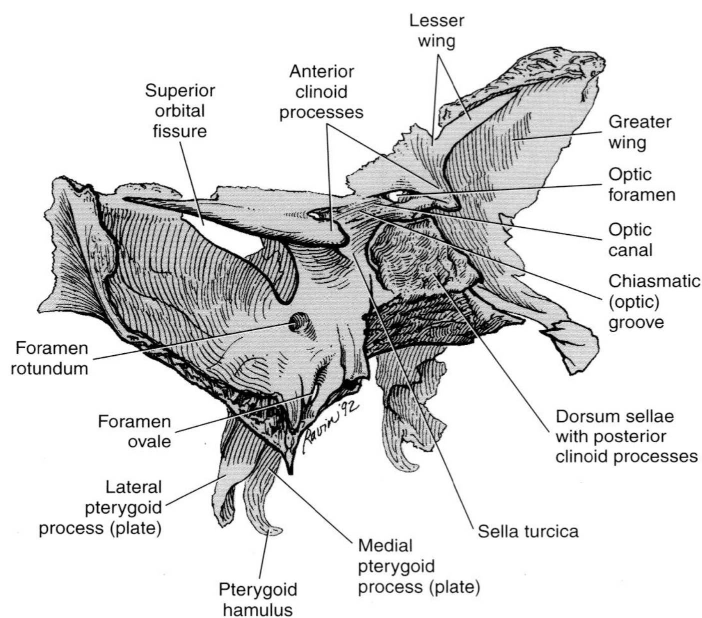

Fig. 12-15. Sphenoid bone—oblique view.

Projecting downward from the inferior surface of the body are four processes that correspond to the legs of the imaginary bat. The more lateral, somewhat flat extensions are termed the **lateral pterygoid** *(ter'i-goyd)* **processes,** sometimes called *plates.* Directly medial to these are two **medial pterygoid processes** or plates that end inferiorly in small hook-like processes, the **pterygoid hamuli.** The pterygoid processes or plates form part of the lateral walls of the nasal cavities.

Sella turcica—lateral view A true lateral view of the sella turcica would look similar to Fig. 12-16. Deformity of the sella turcica is often the only clue that a lesion exists intracranially; therefore radiography of the **sella turcica** may be very important. The depression of the **sella turcica** and the **dorsum sellae** are best seen on this view. The **anterior clinoid processes** are anterior and superior to the sella turcica, and the **posterior clinoid processes** are seen as small extensions located superior to the dorsum sellae. A portion of the **clivus** is also shown on the posterior aspect of the dorsum sellae.

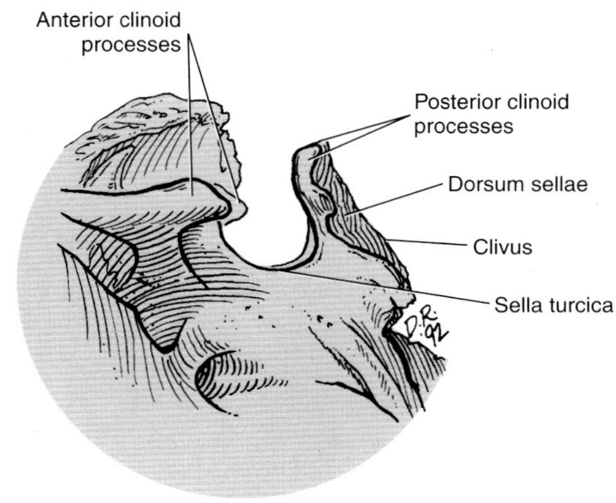

Fig. 12-16. Sella turcica of sphenoid bone—lateral view.

Articulations Because of its central location, the sphenoid articulates with **all seven** of the other cranial bones. (The sphenoid also articulates with five facial bones.)

Ethmoid Bone

The eighth and last cranial bone to be studied is the **ethmoid bone.** The single ethmoid bone lies primarily below the floor of the cranium. Only the top of the ethmoid is shown on a superior view situated in the ethmoidal notch of the frontal bone (Fig. 12-17).

A magnified coronal view of the entire ethmoid is shown on the right in Fig. 12-17. The small upper horizontal portion of the bone is termed the **cribriform plate** and contains many small openings or foramina through which the olfactory nerves, or the nerves of smell, pass. Projecting superiorly from the cribriform plate, similar to a rooster's comb, is the **crista galli** *(kris'ta gal'le).*

Note that the major portion of the ethmoid bone lies beneath the floor of the cranium. Projecting downward in the midline is the **perpendicular plate,** which helps to form the bony nasal septum. The two **lateral labyrinths** (masses) are suspended from the undersurface of the cribriform plate on each side of the perpendicular plate. The lateral masses contain the ethmoid air cells or sinuses and help form the medial walls of the orbits and the lateral walls of the nasal cavity. Extending medially and downward from the medial wall of each labyrinth are thin scroll-shaped projections of bone. These projections are termed the **superior** and **middle nasal conchae** *(kong'ha)* or **turbinates,** best shown on facial bone drawings in Chapter 13.

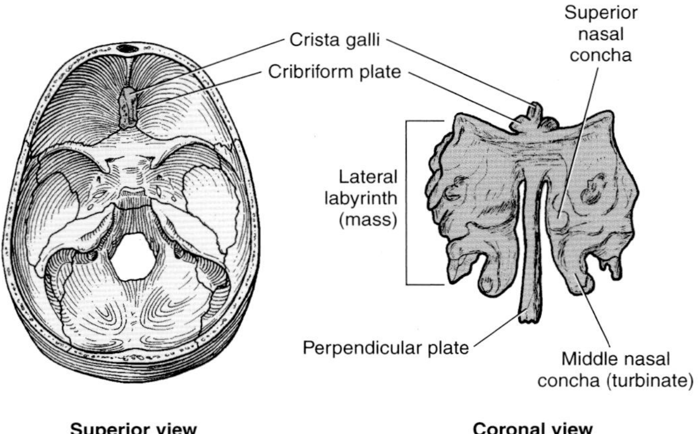

Fig. 12-17. Ethmoid bone.

Articulations The ethmoid articulates with **two** cranial bones: the frontal and the sphenoid. (It also articulates with 11 facial bones.)

Cranium—Sagittal View

Fig. 12-18 represents the right half of the skull, sectioned near the midsagittal plane. The centrally located **sphenoid** and **ethmoid** bones are well demonstrated, showing their relationship to each other and to the other cranial bones.

The **ethmoid bone** is located anterior to the sphenoid bone. The smaller **crista galli** and **cribriform plate** project superiorly, and the larger **perpendicular plate** extends inferiorly. The perpendicular plate forms the upper portion of the bony nasal septum.

The **sphenoid bone,** containing the saddle-shaped sella turcica, is located directly posterior to the ethmoid bone. Shown again is one of the two long slender-shaped **pterygoid processes** or plates extending down and forward, ending with the small pointed process called the **pterygoid hamulus.** Inferior and slightly anterior to the sella turcica of the sphenoid bone in this sagittal view is seen a hollow-like body area of the sphenoid, which houses the **sphenoid sinus.**

The larger **frontal bone** also demonstrates a cavity directly posterior to the glabella containing the **frontal sinus.** The vomer (a facial bone) is shown as a midline structure between parts of the sphenoid and ethmoid, as seen in Fig. 12-18.

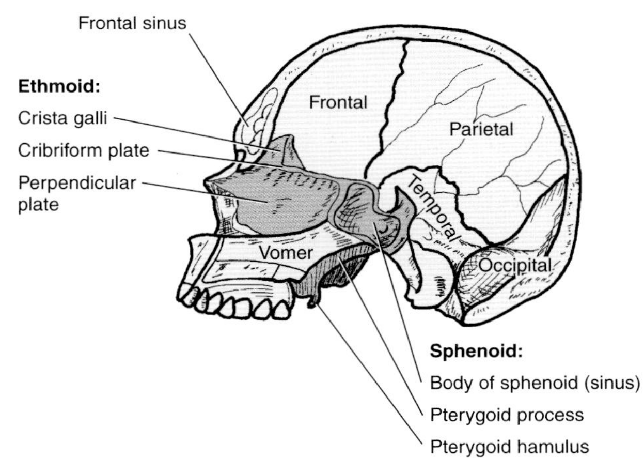

Fig. 12-18. Cranium—midsagittal view of sphenoid and ethmoid bones.

12

JOINTS OF THE CRANIUM—SUTURES

Adult Cranium

The articulations or joints of the cranium are called **sutures** and are classified as **fibrous joints.** In an adult they are immovable and therefore are **synarthrodial type joints.** These are demonstrated in Fig. 12-19 in lateral, superior oblique, and posterior views.

The **coronal** *(ko-ro'nal)* **suture** separates the frontal bone from the two parietals. Separating the two parietal bones in the midline is the **sagittal suture.**

Posteriorly the **lambdoidal** *(lam'doy-dal)* **suture** separates the two parietals from the occipital bone.

The **squamosal** *(skwa-mo'sal)* **sutures** are formed by the inferior junctions of the two parietal bones with their respective temporal bones.

Each end of the sagittal suture is identified as a point or area with a specific name as labeled. The anterior end of the sagittal suture is termed the **bregma** *(breg'mah),* and the posterior end is called the **lambda** *(lam'dah).* The right and left **pterions** *(ter're-ons)* are points at the junction of the parietals, temporals, and the greater wings of the sphenoid. (Note that the pterions are at the **posterior** end of sphenoparietal suture per *Gray's Anatomy.*)

12

The right and left **asterions** *(as-te're-ons)* are points posterior to the ear where the squamosal and lambdoidal sutures meet. These six recognizable bony points are used in surgery or other cases in which specific reference points for cranial measurements are necessary.

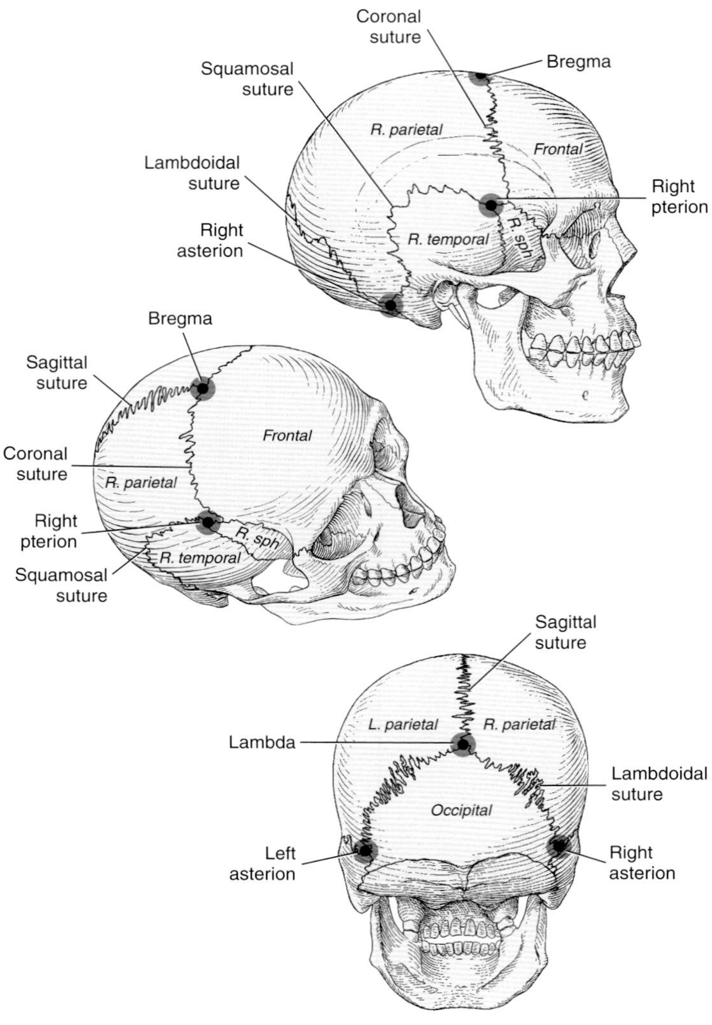

Fig. 12-19. Adult cranial sutures—**fibrous joints, synarthrodial** (immovable).

Infant Cranium

The calvaria, or skull cap, on an infant is very large in proportion to the rest of the body, but the facial bones are quite small, as seen on these drawings (Fig. 12-20). Ossification of the individual cranial bones is incomplete at birth and the sutures are membranous-covered spaces that fill in soon after birth. However, certain regions where sutures join are slower in their ossification and these are called **fontanels** *(fon"tah-nels').* The cranial sutures themselves generally do not completely close until about year 12 or 13, and some may not completely close until adulthood.

Fontanels Early in life, the bregma and lambda are not bony but are membrane-covered openings or "soft spots." These soft spots are termed the **anterior** and **posterior fontanels** in an infant. The anterior fontanel is the largest and at birth is about 2.5 cm wide and 4 cm long. It does not completely close until about 18 months of age.

Two smaller lateral fontanels that close soon after birth are the **sphenoid** (pterion in an adult) and **mastoid** (asterion in an adult) **fontanels,** located respectively at the sphenoid and mastoid angles of the parietal bones on each side of the head. Thus a total of **six fontanels** appear in an infant as follows:

INFANT	ADULT
1. Anterior fontanel	Bregma
2. Posterior fontanel	Lambda
3. Right sphenoid fontanel	Right pterion
4. Left sphenoid fontanel	Left pterion
5. Right mastoid fontanel	Right asterion
6. Left mastoid fontanel	Left asterion

Sutural, or Wormian, Bones

Certain small, irregular bones called *sutural,* or *Wormian, bones* sometimes develop in the adult skull sutures. These isolated bones are most often found in the lambdoidal suture but occasionally are also found in the region of the fontanels, especially the posterior fontanel. In the adult skull, these are completely ossified and are only visible by the sutural lines around their borders.

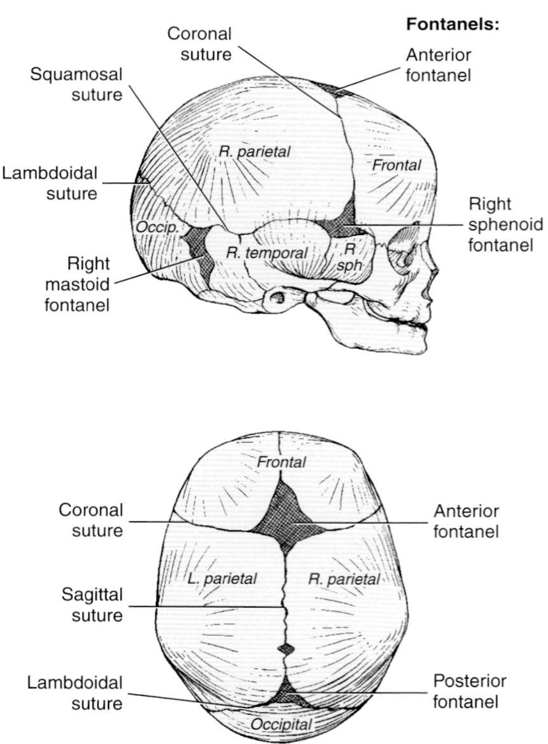

Fig. 12-20. Infant cranial sutures and **fontanels.**

ANATOMY REVIEW WITH RADIOGRAPHS

The following review exercises focus on the anatomy of the eight cranial bones as labeled on the radiographs on the right.

A recommended method of review and reinforcement is to cover the answers below and first attempt to identify each of the labeled parts from memory. Specific anatomic parts may be more difficult to recognize on radiographs as compared with drawings, but knowing locations and relationships to surrounding structures and bones should aid in identifying these parts.

Cranial Bones—PA Caldwell Projection

A. Supraorbital margin of right orbit
B. Crista galli of ethmoid
C. Sagittal suture (posterior skull)
D. Lambdoidal suture (posterior skull)
E. Petrous ridge

Cranial Bones—AP Axial Projection

A. Dorsum sella of sphenoid
B. Posterior clinoid processes
C. Petrous ridge or petrous pyramid
D. Parietal bone
E. Occipital bone
F. Foramen magnum

Cranial Bones—Lateral Projection

A. External acoustic meatus (EAM)
B. Mastoid portion of temporal bone
C. Occipital bone
D. Lambdoidal suture
E. Clivus
F. Dorsum sellae
G. Posterior clinoid processes
H. Anterior clinoid processes
I. Vertex of cranium
J. Coronal suture
K. Frontal bone
L. Orbital plates
M. Cribriform plate
N. Sella turcica
O. Body of sphenoid (sphenoid sinus)

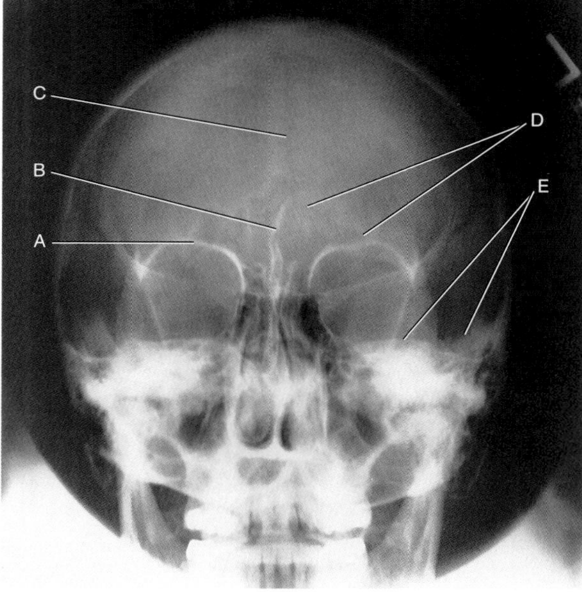

Fig. 12-21. PA Caldwell projection.

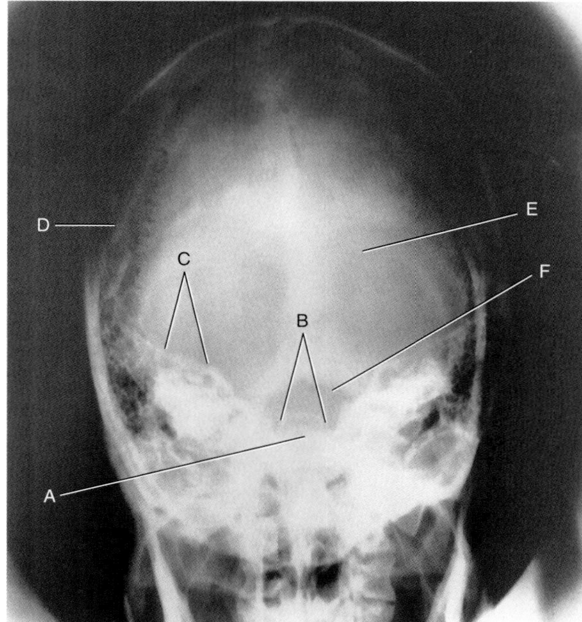

Fig. 12-22. AP axial projection.

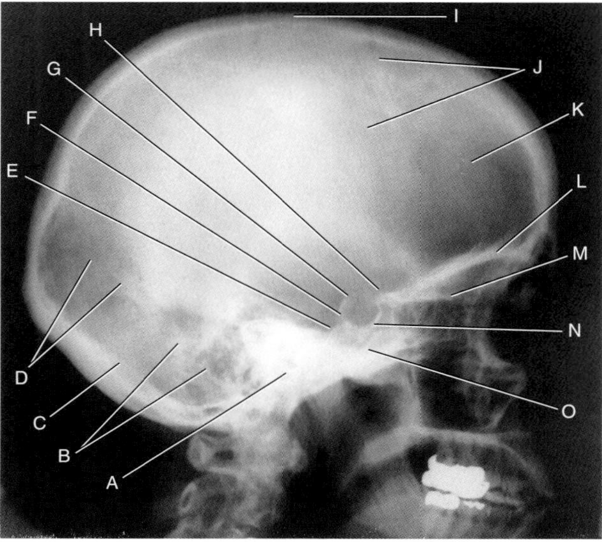

Fig. 12-23. Lateral projection.

12

Anatomy of Organs of Hearing and Equilibrium in Petrous Portion of Temporal Bones

Because of the density and relative location of the temporal bones, the mastoids and petrous portions are difficult to visualize with conventional radiography. Therefore, CT and MRI have largely replaced conventional radiography for imaging of these regions. However, much detailed and interrelated anatomy is present in these parts of the temporal bones that need to be understood to be recognizable either with conventional radiography or with CT or MRI sectional imaging.

The organs of hearing and equilibrium are the main structures found within the petrous portion of the temporal bones. The three divisions of the ear, the **external, middle,** and **internal portions,** are illustrated in Fig. 12-24.

External Ear

The **external ear** begins with the **auricle** or **pinna** on each side of the head. The **tragus** is part of this external structure. It is the small liplike structure located anterior to the EAM. This acts as a partial shield to the ear opening.

The opening and canal of the external ear is termed the **external acoustic meatus (EAM).** The external acoustic canal or meatus is about 2.5 cm long, half of which is bony in structure and half of which is cartilaginous.

The **mastoid process** and **mastoid tip** of the temporal bone are posterior and inferior to the EAM, whereas the **styloid process** is inferior and slightly anterior. The meatus narrows somewhat as it meets the **tympanic membrane** or **eardrum.** The eardrum is situated at an oblique angle, forming a depression, or well, at the lower medial end of the meatus.

Middle Ear

The **middle ear** is an irregularly shaped, air-containing cavity located between the external and the internal ear portions. The three main parts of the middle ear are the **tympanic membrane,** the three small bones called **auditory ossicles,** and the **tympanic cavity.** The tympanic membrane is considered part of the middle ear even though it serves as a partition between the external and middle ears.

The tympanic cavity is further divided into two parts. The larger cavity opposite the eardrum is called the **tympanic cavity proper.** The area above the level of the external auditory meatus and the eardrum is called the **attic,** or **epitympanic recess.** A structure important radiographically is the **drum crest,** or **spur.** The tympanic membrane is attached to this sharp, bony projection. The drum crest or spur separates the external acoustic meatus from the epitympanic recess.

The tympanic cavity communicates anteriorly with the nasopharynx by way of the **eustachian tube,** or **auditory tube.**

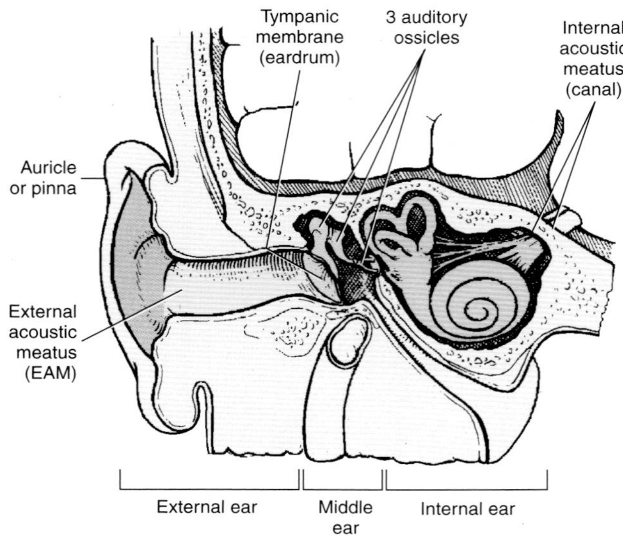

Fig. 12-24. Ear.

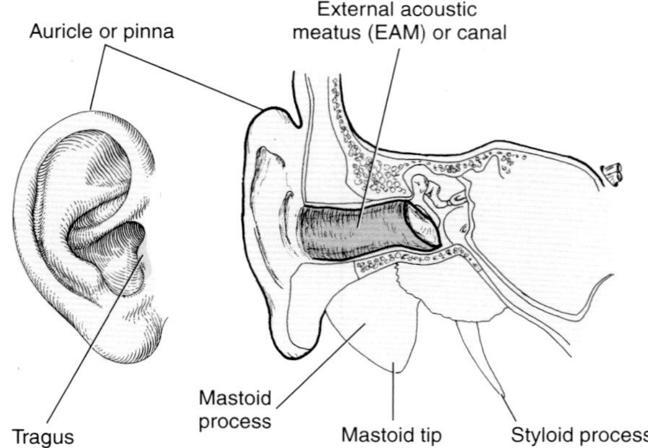

Fig. 12-25. External ear.

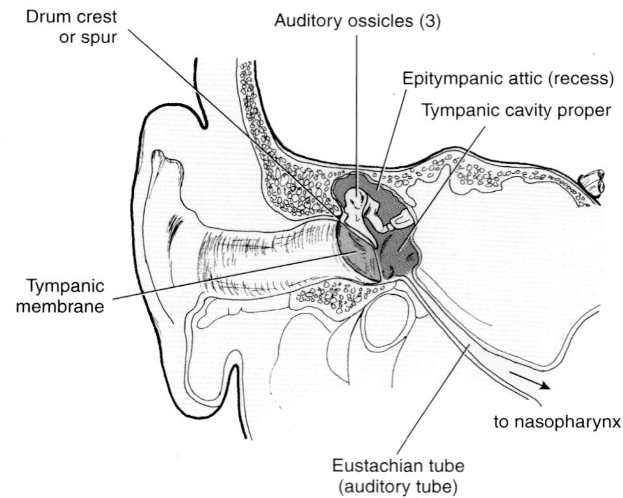

Fig. 12-26. Middle ear.

Eustachian tube The **eustachian tube** is the passageway between the middle ear and the nasopharynx. This tube is about 4 cm long and serves to equalize the pressure within the middle ear to the outside atmospheric air pressure through the nasopharynx. The sensation of one's ears popping is caused by the pressure being adjusted internally in the middle ear to prevent damage to the eardrum.

A problem associated with this direct communication between the middle ear and the nasopharynx is that disease organisms have a direct passageway from the throat to the middle ear. Therefore ear infections often accompany sore throats, especially in children whose immune system is still in development.

Internal acoustic meatus Fig. 12-28 illustrates the ear structures as they would appear in a **modified PA (Caldwell) projection.** A 5° to 10° CR caudad angle to the orbitomeatal line will project the petrous ridges to the **midorbital level** as shown in this drawing. This results in a special transorbital view, which may be taken to demonstrate the **internal acoustic meatus.** The opening to the internal acoustic meatus is an oblique aperture, smaller in diameter than the opening to the external acoustic meatus, and is very difficult to demonstrate clearly on any conventional radiographic projection. It is an important structure to visualize, however, because certain auditory and facial nerves and blood vessels pass through the internal acoustic meatus.

Note that in this drawing of a PA projection (Fig. 12-28) the internal acoustic meatus is projected into the orbital shadow slightly below the petrous ridge, allowing it to be visualized on radiographs taken in this position. Remember that the lateral portions of the petrous ridges are at approximately the level of the **TEA** (top of ear attachment).

The tubelike internal acoustic canal may be best demonstrated on plain radiographic images with an **axiolateral oblique projection,** or Stenvers method. Therefore both the modified PA Caldwell (with 5° to 10° caudal CR angle) and the axioanterior oblique (Stenvers) demonstrate the internal acoustic meatus or canal. However, as noted earlier in this chapter, CT and MRI have largely replaced conventional radiography in visualizing these hard-to-see temporal bone structures, and these two projections are less commonly performed today.

Mastoids A second direct communication into the middle ear occurs posteriorly to the **mastoid air cells.** The schematic drawing in Fig. 12-29 is a sagittal section showing the relationships of the mastoid air cells to the **attic,** or **epitympanic recess,** and the **tympanic cavity proper.** The **aditus** is the opening between the epitympanic recess and the mastoid portion of the temporal bone.

The aditus connects directly to a large chamber within the mastoid portion termed the **antrum.** The antrum then connects to the various **mastoid air cells.** This communication allows infection in the middle ear, which may have originated in the throat, to pass into the mastoid area. Once within the mastoid area, infection is separated from brain tissue only by thin bone. Before the common use of effective antibiotics, this was often a pathway for a serious infection of the brain, termed **encephalitis.** The thin plate of bone forming the roof of the antrum, aditus, and attic area of the tympanic cavity is called the **tegmen tympani.**

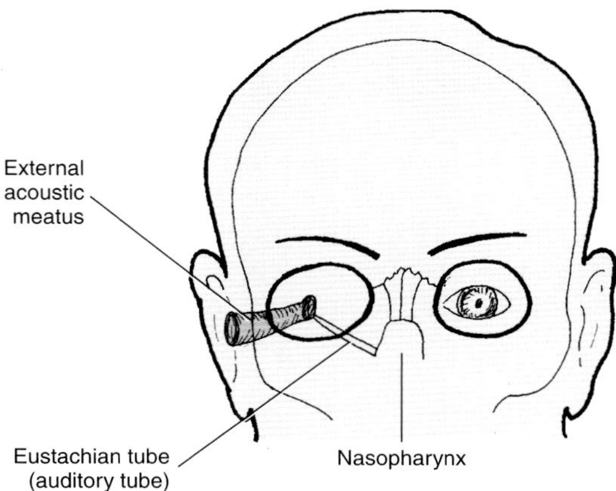

Fig. 12-27. Middle ear.

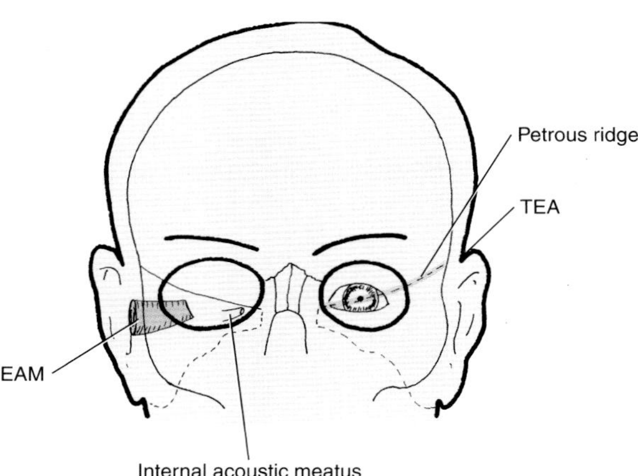

Fig. 12-28. Modified PA Caldwell projection (CR 5° to 10° caudad).

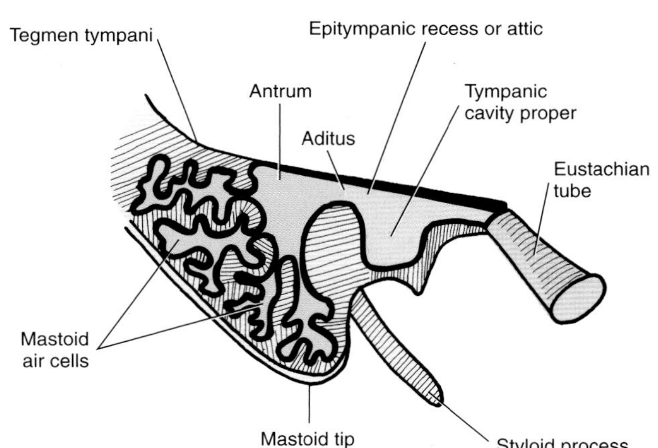

Fig. 12-29. Mastoid connection.

12

Auditory ossicles The **auditory ossicles** are three small bones that are prominent structures within the middle ear. Figs. 12-30 and 12-31 demonstrate that these three small bones are articulated to permit vibratory motion. The three auditory ossicles are located partly in the attic, or epitympanic recess, and partly in the tympanic cavity proper. These delicate bones bridge the middle ear cavity to transmit sound vibrations from the tympanic membrane to the oval window of the internal ear.

Vibrations are first picked up by the **malleus,** meaning "hammer," which is attached directly to the inside surface of the tympanic membrane. The head of the malleus articulates with the central ossicle, the **incus.** The incus receives its name from a supposed resemblance to an anvil, but it actually looks more like a premolar tooth with a body and two roots. The incus then connects to the stirrup-shaped **stapes,** which is the smallest of the three auditory ossicles. The foot plate of the stapes is then attached to another membrane called the **oval window** leading into the inner ear.

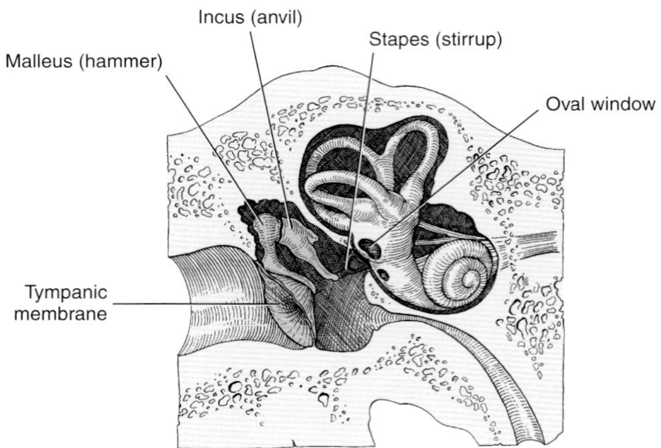

Fig. 12-30. Auditory ossicles—malleus, incus, and stapes.

12

Auditory ossicles—frontal and lateral view Fig. 12-31 illustrates the relationship of the auditory ossicles to one another in both a close-up frontal view and a lateral view. As seen from the front, the most lateral of the three bones is the **malleus,** whereas the most medial of the three bones is the **stapes.** The lateral-view drawing demonstrates how the ossicles would appear if one looked through the **external acoustic meatus** to see the bony ossicles of the middle ear. Note that the malleus, with its attachment to the eardrum, is located slightly anterior to the other two bones.

The resemblance of the **incus** to a premolar tooth with a body and two roots is well visualized in the lateral drawing. The longer root of the incus connects to the stapes, which in turn connects to the oval window of the cochlea, resulting in the sense of hearing.

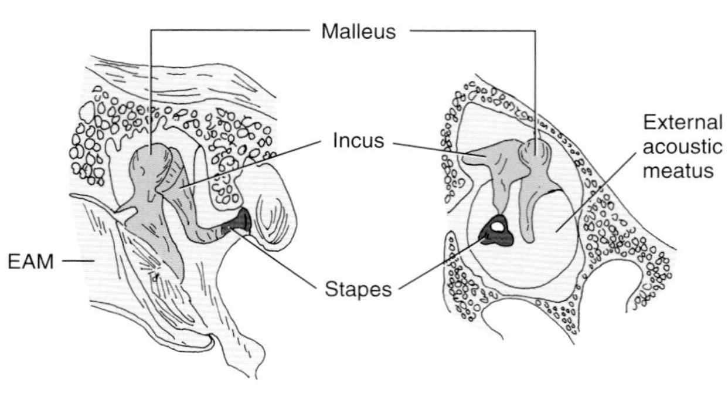

Fig. 12-31. Auditory ossicles.

Internal Ear

The complex **internal ear** contains the essential sensory apparatus of both **hearing** and **equilibrium.** Lying within the densest portion of the petrous pyramid, it can be divided into two main parts, the **osseous,** or **bony, labyrinth,** important radiographically, and the **membranous labyrinth.** The osseous labyrinth is a bony chamber housing the membranous labyrinth, a series of intercommunicating ducts and sacs. One such duct is the **endolymphatic duct,** a blind pouch or closed duct contained in a small canal-like, bony structure. The canal of the endolymphatic duct arises from the medial wall of the vestibule and extends to the posterior wall of the petrous pyramid, located both posterior and lateral to the **internal acoustic meatus.**

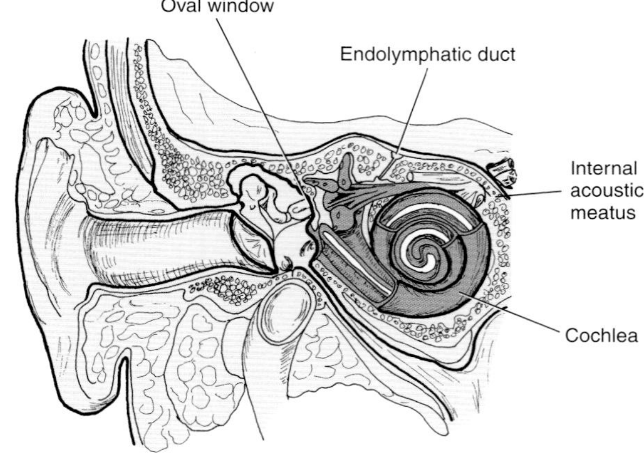

Fig. 12-32. Internal ear, osseous labyrinth—frontal view.

Osseous (bony) labyrinth The osseous, or bony, labyrinth is divided into **three** distinctly shaped parts: the **cochlea** (meaning "snail shell"), the **vestibule,** and the **semicircular canals.** The osseous labyrinth completely surrounds and encloses the ducts and sacs of the membranous labyrinth. As illustrated on the frontal cutaway view in Fig. 12-32, the snail-shaped, bony cochlea houses a long, coiled, tube-like duct of the membranous labyrinth.

The **cochlea** is the most anterior of the three parts of the osseous labyrinth. This is best shown on the lateral view of the osseous labyrinth in Fig. 12-33. The **round window,** sometimes called the **cochlear window,** is shown to be at the base of the cochlea.

The **vestibule** is the central portion of the bony labyrinth and contains the **oval window,** sometimes called the **vestibular window.**

Semicircular canals The **three semicircular canals** are located posterior to the other inner ear structures and are named according to their position; thus they are called the **superior, posterior,** and **lateral semicircular canals.** Each is located at a right angle to the other two, allowing for a sense of equilibrium as well as a sense of direction. Remember the **semicircular canals relate to the sense of direction or equilibrium,** and the **cochlea relates to the sense of hearing** because of its connection to the stapes through the oval window.

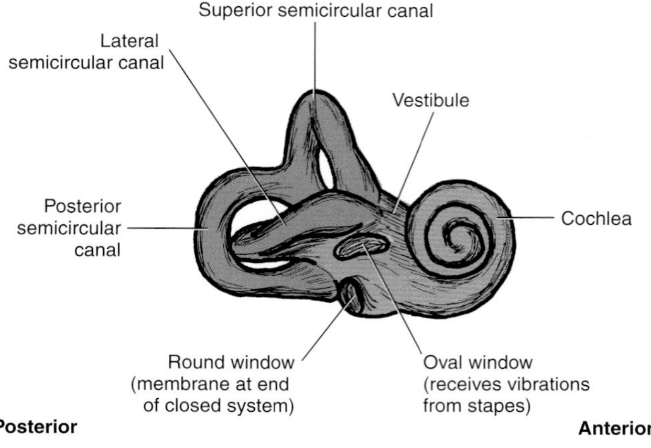

Fig. 12-33. Osseous (bony) labyrinth—lateral view.

"Windows" of internal ear (Fig. 12-33) The two openings into the internal ear are covered by membranes. The **oval,** or **vestibular, window** receives vibrations from the external ear through the distal aspect of the stapes of the middle ear and transmits these vibrations into the **vestibule** of the internal ear. The **round,** or **cochlear, window** is located at the base of the first coil of the cochlea. The round window is a membrane that allows movement of fluid within the closed duct system of the membranous labyrinth. As the oval window moves slightly inward with a vibration, the round window moves outward because this is a closed system and fluid does not compress. Vibrations and associated slight fluid movements within the cochlea produce impulses that are transmitted to the auditory nerve within the internal acoustic meatus, creating the sense of hearing.

ANATOMY REVIEW WITH RADIOGRAPHS

Specific anatomy of the temporal bone is difficult to recognize on conventional radiographs. However, knowing general shapes and relationships to recognizable structures allows for recognition of certain structures as follows:

Axiolateral Projection (Fig. 12-34)

A. EAM (external auditory meatus)
B. Mastoid antrum
C. Mastoid air cells
D. Downside mandibular condyle (just anterior to EAM)
E. Upside (magnified) mandibular condyle

Posterior Profile Position (Fig. 12-35)

A. Petrous ridge
B. Bony (osseous) labyrinth (semicircular canals)
C. EAM
D. Region of internal acoustic canal

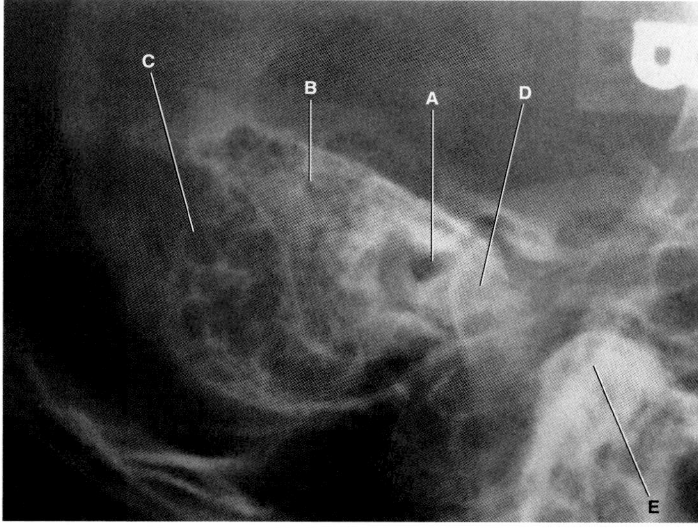

Fig. 12-34. Axiolateral projection for mastoids (modified Law method).

12

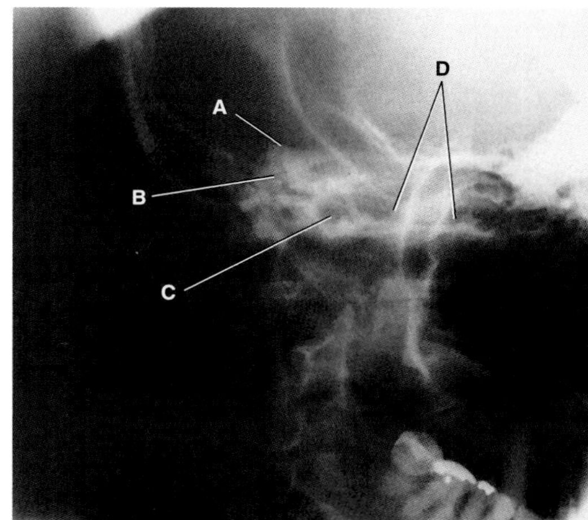

Fig. 12-35. Posterior profile projection for mastoids (Stenvers method).

RADIOGRAPHIC POSITIONING

Skull Radiography

Traditionally, the skull has been one of the most difficult and challenging parts of the body to radiograph. A good understanding of the anatomy and relationships of bones and structures of the skull as described in this chapter is essential before beginning a study of radiographic positioning of the cranium. Conventional radiography of certain parts of the skull, such as the more obscure internal structures, is less common today because of advances in other imaging modalities such as computed tomography (CT) and magnetic resonance imaging (MRI). However, in certain more remote areas of the country these imaging modalities may not be available and every technologist should be able to perform conventional skull radiography as described in this chapter.

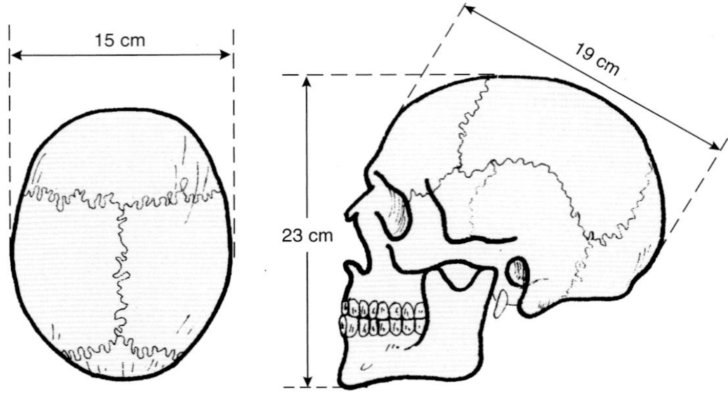

Fig. 12-36. Average skull (mesocephalic).

SKULL MORPHOLOGY (CLASSIFICATIONS BY SHAPE AND SIZE)

Mesocephalic Skull

The shape of the average head is termed **mesocephalic** *(mes'o-se-fal'ik)*. The average caliper measurements of the adult skull are 15 cm between the parietal eminences (lateral), 19 cm from frontal eminence to external occipital protuberance (AP or PA), and 23 cm from vertex to beneath the chin (SMV projection). Although most adults have a skull of the average size and shape, exceptions to the rule exist.

A general basis for describing skull types is by comparing the width of the skull at the parietal eminence with the length measured from the frontal eminence to the external occipital protuberance. For an average mesocephalic skull the **width is between 75% and 80% of the length.***

Brachycephalic and Dolichocephalic Skulls

Variations of the average-shaped or mesocephalic skull include the **brachycephalic** *(brak'e-se-fal'ik)* and the **dolichocephalic** *(dol'i-ko-se-fal'ik)* designations. The short, broad head is termed *brachycephalic,* and the long, narrow head is called *dolichocephalic.*

The width of the brachycephalic type **is 80% or greater** than the length. The width on the long, narrow dolichocephalic is **less than 75%** of the length.*

A second variation to remember is the **angle difference** between the petrous pyramids and the midsagittal plane. In the average-shaped, mesocephalic head, the petrous pyramids form an angle of **47°**. In the brachycephalic skull the angle is **greater than 47°** (approximately 54°), and in the dolichocephalic skull the angle is **less than 47°** (approximately 40°).

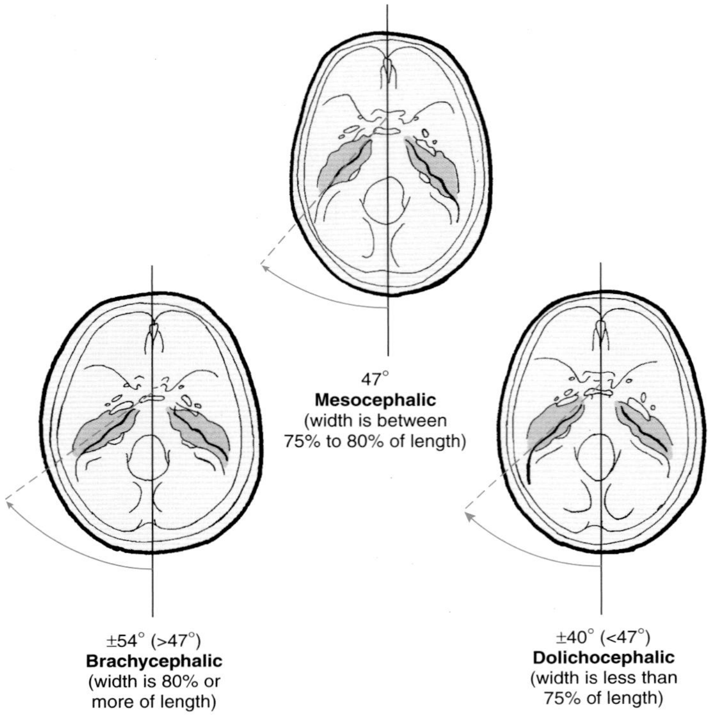

Fig. 12-37. Variable shapes.

Positioning Considerations Related to Skull Morphology

The positioning descriptions including CR angles and head rotations as described in this text are based on the average-shaped mesocephalic skull. For example, the axiolateral oblique projection (Law method) for the mastoids or the TMJs requires 15° of head rotation. A long, narrow, dolichocephalic head would require slightly more than 15° of rotation, and a short, broad, brachycephalic type would require less than 15°. The 45° oblique Stenvers method projection for the mastoids would also require a slight adjustment for these variations in skull shapes.

*Gray H: Gray's anatomy, ed 30, Philadelphia, 1985, Lea and Febiger.

CRANIAL TOPOGRAPHY (SURFACE LANDMARKS)

Certain surface landmarks and localizing lines must be used for accurate positioning of the cranium. Each of the following topographic structures can either be seen or palpated.

Body Planes

The **midsagittal,** or **median, plane (MSP)** divides the body into left and right halves. This plane is important in accurate positioning of the cranium because for every AP and PA or lateral projection, the midsagittal plane is either perpendicular to or parallel to the plane of the IR.

The **interpupillary (IPL),** or **interorbital, line** is a line connecting either the pupils or the outer canthi of the patient's eyes. When the head is placed in a **true lateral** position, the interpupillary line must be exactly perpendicular to the plane of the IR.

Anterior and Lateral View Landmarks

The **superciliary ridge (arch)** is that ridge or arch of bone extending across the forehead directly above each eye.

Slightly above this ridge is a slight groove or depression, termed the **supraorbital groove, or SOG.**

Note: The SOG is important because it corresponds to the highest level of the facial bone mass, which is also the level of the **floor of the anterior fossa** of the cranial vault.

The **glabella** *(glah-bel'ah)* is the smooth, slightly raised triangular area between and slightly superior to the eyebrows and above the bridge of the nose.

The **nasion** *(na'ze-on)* is the depression at the bridge of the nose. Anatomically, the nasion is the junction of the two nasal bones and the frontal bone.

The **acanthion** (*ah-kan'the-on,* little thorn) is the midline point at the junction of the upper lip and the nasal septum. This is the point where the nose and upper lip meet.

The **angle,** or **gonion** *(go'ne-on),* refers to the lower posterior angle on each side of the jaw or mandible.

A flat triangular area projects forward as the **chin,** or **mentum,** in the human. The midpoint of this triangular area of the chin as it appears from the front is termed the **mental point.**

Ear Parts of the ear that may be used as positioning landmarks are the **auricle,** or **pinna** (external portion of ear), the large flap of ear made of cartilage, and the **tragus,** the small cartilaginous flap covering the opening of the ear. The **TEA** (top of ear attachment) refers to the superior attachment of the auricle, or that part where the side frames of eyeglasses rest. This is an important landmark because it corresponds to the **level of the petrous ridge** on each side.

Eye The junctions of the upper and lower eyelids are termed **canthi** *(kan'thi).* Thus the **inner canthus** *(kan'thus)* is where the eyelids meet near the nose; the more lateral junction of the eyelids is termed the **outer canthus.**

The superior rim of the bony orbit of the eye is termed the **supraorbital margin,** or **SOM,** and the inferior rim is termed the **infraorbital margin,** or **IOM.** Another landmark is the **midlateral orbital margin,** that portion of the lateral rim near the outer canthus of the eye.

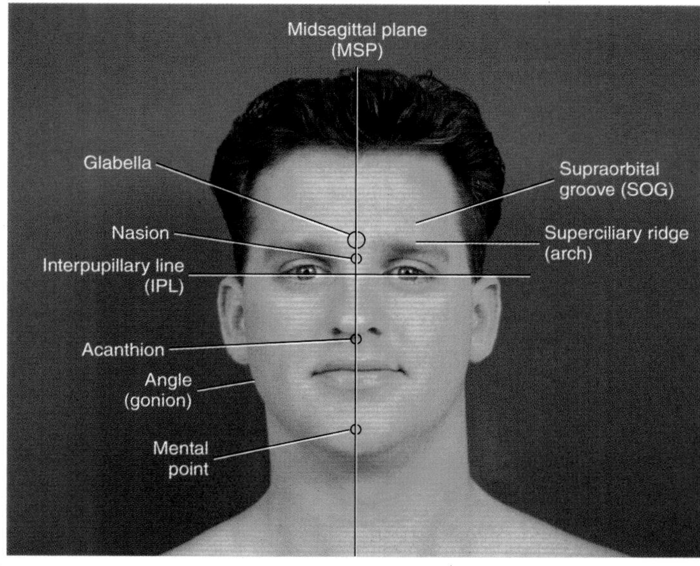

Fig. 12-38. Body planes and landmarks.

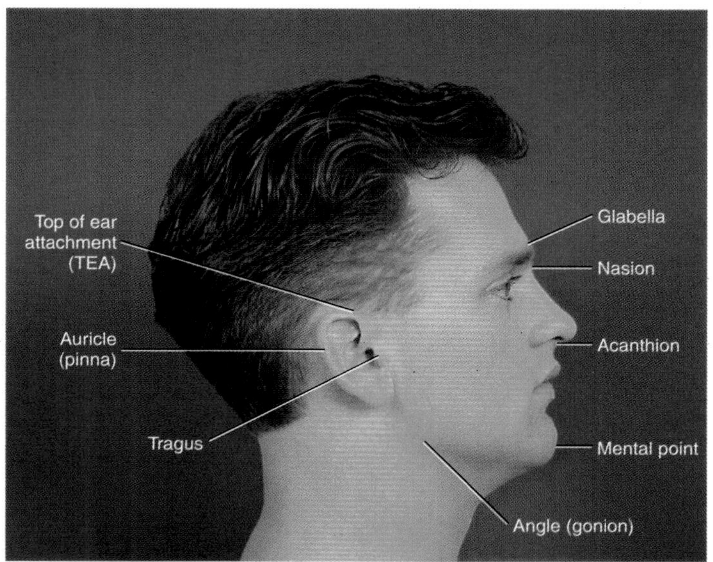

Fig. 12-39. Surface landmarks.

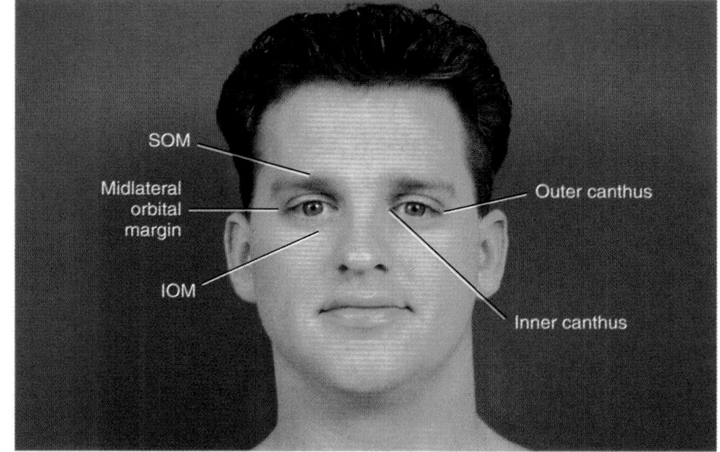

Fig. 12-40. Orbit landmarks.

12

Skull Positioning Lines

Certain positioning lines are important in skull radiography. These lines are formed by connecting certain facial landmarks to the midpoint of the **external acoustic (auditory) meatus (EAM).** The EAM is the opening of the external ear canal. The center point of this opening is called the **auricular point.**

The most superior of these positioning lines is the **glabellomeatal line (GML),** which is not as precise as the other lines because the glabella is an area and not a specific point. The GML refers to a line between the glabella and the EAM.

The **orbitomeatal line (OML)** is a frequently used positioning line located between the outer canthus (midlateral orbital margin) and the EAM.

The **infraorbitomeatal line (IOML)** is formed by connecting the infraorbital margin to the EAM. Two older terms identify this same line as **Reid's base line,** or **anthropologic base line.** Sometimes this is also referred to as simply the **base line** of the cranium, although these terms are not used in this text.

An average difference of **7° to 8°** exists between the angles of the orbitomeatal and the infraorbitomeatal lines. There is also an approximate 7° to 8° average angle difference between the orbitomeatal and glabellomeatal lines. Knowing the angle differences between these three lines is helpful in making positioning adjustments for specific projections of the cranium and facial bones.

The **acanthiomeatal line (AML)** and the **mentomeatal line (MML)** are important in radiography of the facial bones. Connecting the acanthion and the mental point respectively to the EAM forms these lines.

A line from the junction of the lips to the EAM, called the **lips-meatal line (LML)**, is a positioning line used in this textbook to position for a specific projection of the facial bones called a *modified acanthioparietal (Waters) projection* (see p. 422).

The **glabelloalveolar line (GAL)** connects the glabella to a point at the anterior aspect of the alveolar process of the maxilla. This line is used for positioning a tangential projection for the nasal bones.

The **inion** *(in'e-on)* is the most prominent point of the external occipital protuberance, a rise or bump along the midline of the lower back of the head near the junction of the head and neck where posterior muscles attach. An extension of the IOML posteriorly approximates the location of the inion.

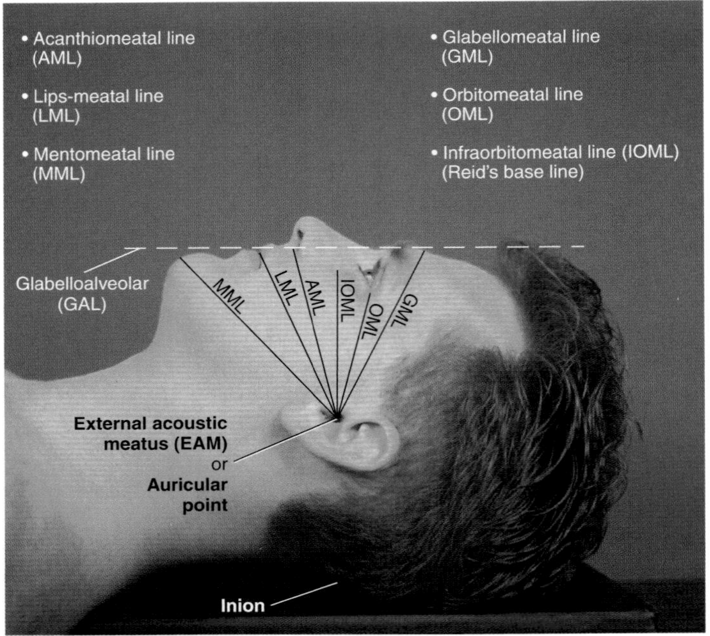

Fig. 12-41. Positioning lines.

Skull Positioning Aids

Various types of positioning aids can be used for determining precise angles required for accurate cranial or facial bones positioning. One common example of such a positioning aid is **a cardboard straightedge** cut at a specific angle to accurately position the cranium. In Fig. 12-42, a 90° straightedge is shown to determine that the orbitomeatal line has been placed perpendicular to the IR plane by depressing the chin as needed, or by placing a support under the back of the head if the chin cannot be depressed far enough. The chin can be raised or lowered to change the perpendicular reference line to be used in relationship to the central ray.

Other types of adjustable devices can be used for determining various degrees of angle in skull positioning. One example is the **angle finder** that indicates the number of degrees from horizontal; or in this example, the degrees between the IOML and the tabletop and/or image receptor (IR).

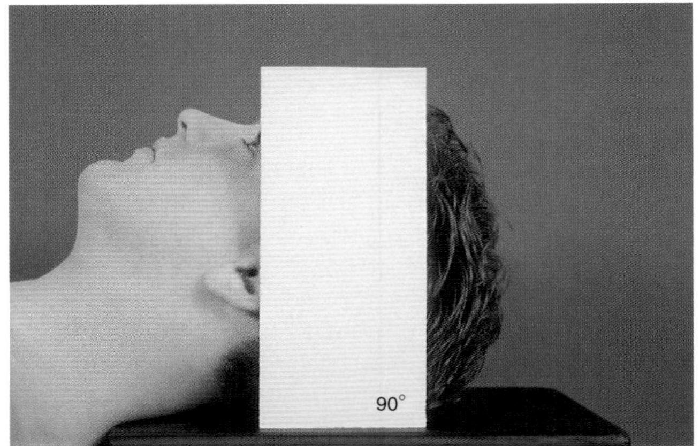

Fig. 12-42. Positioning aid—90° straightedge.

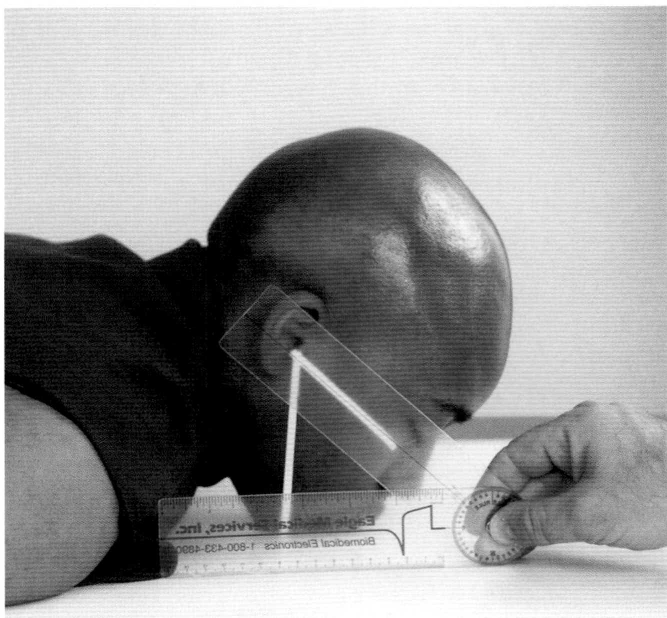

Fig. 12-43. Positioning aid—angle finder demonstrating degrees of IOML to IR.

POSITIONING CONSIDERATIONS

Erect versus Recumbent

Projections of the skull may be taken with the patient in the recumbent or erect position, depending on the patient's condition. Images in the erect position can be obtained by using a standard x-ray table in the vertical position or using an upright Bucky. The erect position allows the patient to be quickly and easily positioned and permits a horizontal beam to be used. A horizontal beam is necessary to visualize any existing air-fluid levels within the cranial or sinus cavities.

Patient Comfort

Patient motion almost always results in an unsatisfactory image. During skull radiography, the patient's head must be placed in precise positions and held motionless long enough to obtain an exposure. Always remember that a patient is attached to the skull being manipulated. Every effort should be made to make the patient's body as comfortable as possible, and positioning aids such as sponges, sandbags, and pillows should be used if needed.

Except in severe trauma cases, respiration should be suspended during the exposure to help prevent blurring of the image from breathing movements of the thorax. This is especially important when the patient is in a prone position. It is generally is not necessary for erect skull positions, however.

Hygiene Cranial and facial radiography may require the patient's face to be in direct contact with the table/upright Bucky surface. Therefore it is important that these surfaces be cleaned with disinfectant before use and on completion of the examination.

Exposure Factors

The principal exposure factors for radiographs of the skull include the following:

- Medium kV, 75-85
- Small focal spot (if equipment allows)
- Short exposure time with the highest mA possible

SID

The minimum SID with the image receptor in the table or upright Bucky is 40 inches (100 cm).

Radiation Protection

The best techniques for minimizing radiation exposure to the patient in skull radiography are to (1) use **good collimation practices** and (2) **minimize repeats.** Collimation should be adjusted closely to the area of interest.

The exposure factors and patient doses provided in the icon boxes on positioning pages are calculated for a SID of 40 inches, or 100 cm.

Gonadal shielding Generally, gonadal shielding does not need to be used in skull radiography. According to publication HEW 76-8031, *Handbook of Selected Organ Doses for Projections Common in Diagnostic Radiology,* with accurate collimation no detectable contribution to gonadal exposure occurs during radiography of the skull. However, lead shields may be used to reassure the patient.

Thyroid and breast shielding AP projections of the skull and facial bones can result in additional exposure to the radiosensitive thyroid (and breast on females). A contact shield placed over the neck and chest can be used for these projections. When there is a choice, PA rather than AP projections should be selected.

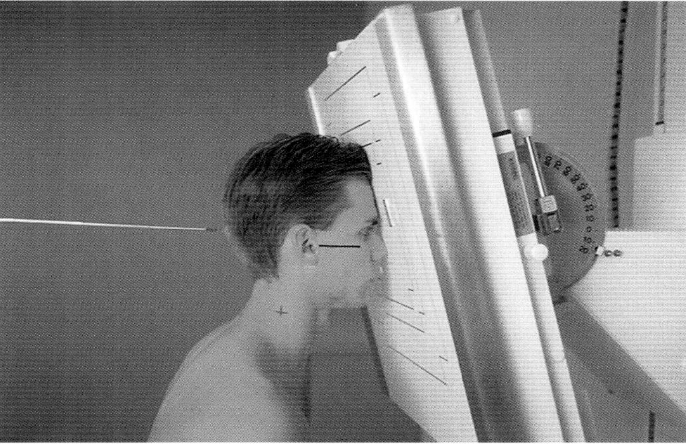

Fig. 12-44. Erect—upright Bucky.

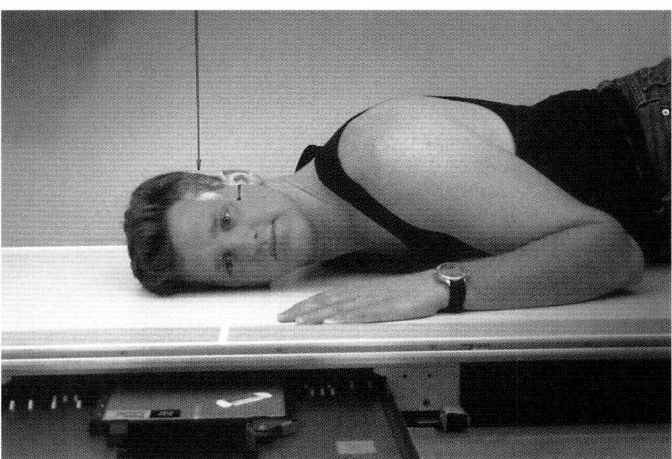

Fig. 12-45. Recumbent—table/Bucky.

12

Causes of Positioning Errors

When positioning a patient's head, look at various facial features and palpate anatomic landmarks to place the appropriate body plane precisely in relation to the plane of the IR. Although the human body is expected to be symmetric bilaterally (that is, the right half is identical to the left half), this is not always true. The ears, nose, and jaw are often asymmetric. The nose frequently deviates to one side of the midsagittal plane, and the ears are not necessarily in the same place or of the same size on each side.

The lower jaw or mandible is also often asymmetric. Bony parts, such as the mastoid tips and the orbital margins, are safer landmarks to use. Although you often use the patient's eyes as landmarks during positioning, do not use the nose, which may not be straight.

Five Common Positioning Errors

Five potential positioning errors related to skull positions are as follows:

1. Rotation
2. Tilt
3. Excessive flexion
4. Excessive extension
5. Incorrect CR angle

Rotation and **tilt** are two very common positioning errors, as demonstrated by the drawings on the right. Rotation of the skull almost always results in a retake; therefore the body planes should be correctly aligned (e.g., midsagittal plane is parallel to the tabletop and/or IR in a lateral position).

Tilt is a tipping or slanting of the midsagittal plane laterally, even though rotation may not be present (Fig. 12-47).

Excessive flexion or **extension** of the cervical spine (chin lowered or elevated too much, respectively), along with an **incorrect CR angle,** must be avoided.

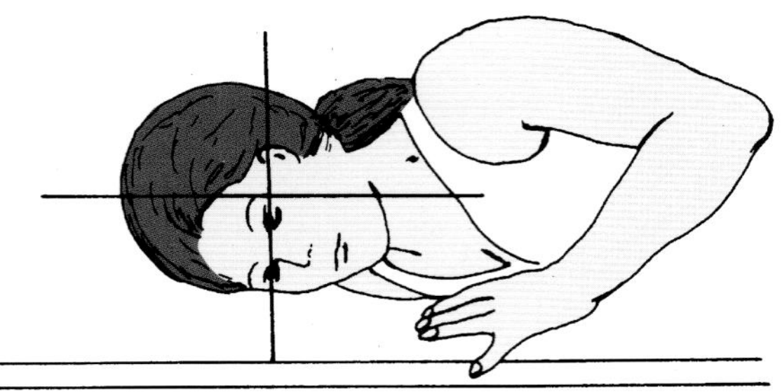

Fig. 12-46. Rotation—midsagittal plane is rotated, not parallel to tabletop and IR.

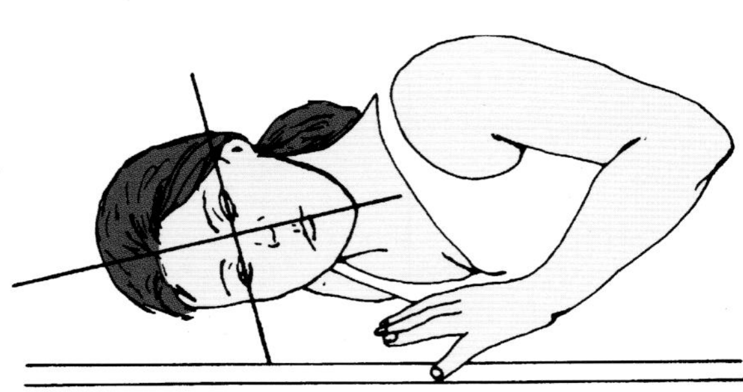

Fig. 12-47. Tilt—midsagittal plane is tipped or slanted, not parallel to tabletop or IR.

Pediatric Applications

Communication A clear explanation of the procedure is required to obtain the trust and cooperation of the patient and guardian. Distraction techniques using toys, stuffed animals, and other items are also effective in maintaining patient cooperation.

Immobilization Pediatric patients (depending on age and condition) are often unable to maintain the required positions. Use of immobilization devices to support the patient is recommended to reduce the need for the patient to be held, thus reducing radiation exposure. (Chapter 20 provides an in-depth description of such devices.) If it is necessary for the guardian to hold the patient, the technologist must provide a lead apron and/or gloves. If the guardian is female, the technologist must ensure that no possibility of pregnancy exists.

Technical factors Technical factors vary because of various patient sizes and pathologies. Use of short exposure times (associated with the use of high mA) is recommended to reduce the risk of patient motion.

Geriatric Applications

Communication and comfort Sensory loss (e.g., poor eyesight, hearing) associated with aging may result in the geriatric patient requiring additional assistance, time, and patience in obtaining the required positions for cranial radiography.

If the examination is performed with the patient in the recumbent position, decreased position awareness may cause the patient to fear falling off the radiography table. A radiolucent mattress or pad placed on the exam table will provide comfort, and extra blankets may be required for warmth. Reassurance and attention from the technologist help the patient feel secure and comfortable.

If the patient is able, attaining the required positions in the erect position (sitting) at an upright Bucky may be more comfortable, especially if they have an increased kyphosis. Lateral images obtained with a horizontal ray are often indicated for elderly patients who have limited movement.

Technical factors Because of the high incidence of osteoporosis in geriatric patients, the mAs may require a decrease if manual exposure factors are being used (a minimum adjustment of 25% to 30% is required to have a visible effect on the image).

Older patients may have tremors or signs of unsteadiness; use of short exposure times (associated with the use of high mA) is recommended to reduce the risk for motion.

Digital Imaging Considerations

Guidelines for digital imaging (CR and DR) of the skull are similar to those described in previous chapters. These are:

1. **Correct central ray angle and centering to body part and image receptor.** This provides for accurate post-processing of the image by the image reader.
2. **Close collimation.** Improves image quality by reducing scatter and secondary radiation to the highly sensitive digital image receptors (especially important for certain views of the sella turcica and mastoids).
3. **Following ALARA principles** in determining exposure factors (highest kV and lowest mAs that will result in desirable image quality). An increase in kV over film-screen imaging may be desirable, both for reducing patient exposure and improving image quality. (Sufficient mAs is required to produce a high-resolution image.)
4. **Post-processing evaluation of exposure index values** (for assurance that optimum quality image was achieved with least possible radiation to patient).

Alternative Modalities

COMPUTED TOMOGRAPHY

Computed tomography (CT) is the most common neuroimaging procedure performed. CT provides sectional images of the brain and bones of the skull in axial, sagittal, or coronal planes, whereas plain radiographic images provide a two-dimensional image of the bony skull only.

Because injury and pathology to the head often involve the brain and associated soft tissues, CT is a vital tool in full evaluation of the patient. It can differentiate between blood clots, white and gray matter, cerebrospinal fluid, cerebral edema, and neoplasms.

MAGNETIC RESONANCE IMAGING

Magnetic resonance imaging (MRI) also provides images of the brain and skull in axial, sagittal, and coronal planes. MRI provides increased sensitivity in detecting differences between normal and abnormal tissues in the brain and associated soft tissues.

The magnetic fields used in MRI are thought to be harmless, which means the patient is spared exposure to potentially harmful ionizing radiation.

ULTRASOUND (SONOGRAPHY)

Ultrasound of the brain of the neonate (through the fontanels) is an integral part of their management in the intensive care unit. It allows for rapid evaluation and screening of premature infants for intracranial hemorrhage. It is preferred over CT and MRI for this purpose because it is highly portable and less expensive, requires no sedation of the patient, and provides no ionizing radiation.

Ultrasound can also be valuable in the investigation and follow-up of hydrocephalus. Cranial sutures may also be evaluated, thus assisting in the diagnosis of premature suture closure (craniosynostosis).

NUCLEAR MEDICINE TECHNOLOGY

Nuclear medicine technology provides a sensitive screening procedure (the radionuclide bone scan) for detection of skeletal metastases, of which the skull is a common site. A bone scan is frequently ordered for patients who are at risk or symptomatic for metastases. Any focal abnormality on the bone scan is then investigated radiographically to further investigate the pathology. Patients with a history of multiple myeloma are often exceptions to this protocol.

Brain tissue may also be studied using nuclear medicine technology. New radiopharmaceuticals have allowed perfusion studies of the brain to be performed, typically on patients with Alzheimer's disease, seizure disorders, and dementia. Tumor response to treatment may also be assessed with this modality.

Pathologic Indications

SKULL AND CRANIAL PATHOLOGY

Indications for skull and cranial radiographic procedures have markedly decreased because CT and/or MRI is increasingly available. Smaller hospitals, clinics, and rural centers may still perform these procedures, however.

Skull fractures Skull fractures are disruptions in the continuity of bones of the skull.

Note: Although plain radiographic images of the skull do provide excellent spatial resolution of bone, the presence or absence of a fracture is in no way an indication of underlying brain injury. Additional imaging procedures must be performed (i.e., CT or MRI) to fully assess the brain tissue.

- **Linear fractures** are fractures of the skull that may appear as jagged or irregular lucent lines.
- **Depressed fractures** are sometimes called *ping-pong fractures.* A fragment of bone that is separated and depressed into the cranial cavity can occur. A tangential view may be used to determine the degree of depression if CT is unavailable.
- **Basal skull fractures** are fractures through the dense inner structures of the temporal bone. These fractures are very difficult to visualize because of the complexity of the anatomy through this area. If bleeding occurs, plain radiographic images may reveal an air-fluid level in the sphenoid sinus if a horizontal ray is used for the lateral view.

Gunshot wounds Gunshot wounds can be visualized by plain images that are typically performed to localize bullets in gunshot victims by an antemortem and/or postmortem examination. The bullet is easily recognizable because of lead content.

Neoplasms Neoplasms are new and abnormal growths:

- **Metastases** are primary malignant neoplasms that spread to distant sites via blood and the lymphatic system. The skull is a common site of metastatic lesions, which may be characterized and visualized on the image as follows:
  - **Osteolytic** are destructive lesions with irregular margins.
  - **Osteoblastic** are proliferative bony lesions of increased density.
  - **Combination osteolytic and osteoblastic lesions** have a "moth-eaten" appearance of bone because of the mix of destructive and blastic lesions.

Multiple myeloma This consists of one or more bone tumors that originate in the bone marrow. The skull is a commonly affected site.

Pituitary adenomas These are tumors of the pituitary gland that are investigated primarily by CT or MRI. Plain radiographic images may demonstrate enlargement of the sella turcica and erosion of the dorsum sella, often as an incidental finding.

Paget's disease (osteitis deformans) This is a disease of unknown origin that begins as a stage of bony destruction followed by bony repair. It involves many bony sites, including the skull. Radiographically, areas of lucency demonstrate the destructive stage, and a "cotton-wool" appearance with irregular areas of increased density (sclerosis) demonstrates the reparative stage.

TEMPORAL BONE PATHOLOGY

The more common pathologic indications for temporal bone radiographic procedures include the following:

Mastoiditis *(mas"toid-i'tis)* Acute mastoiditis is a bacteria infection of the mastoid process that can destroy the inner part of the mastoid process. Mastoid air cells are replaced with a fluid-filled abscess, which can lead to a progressive hearing loss. CT scans demonstrate fluid-filled abscess replacing air-filled mastoid air cells.

Neoplasms These are new and abnormal growths (tumors):

- **Acoustic neuroma:** This benign tumor of the auditory nerve sheath originates in the internal auditory canal. Patient complaints include hearing loss, dizziness, and loss of balance. It is typically diagnosed using CT or MRI, but it may be visualized on plain images in advanced cases with expansion and asymmetry of the affected IAC (internal acoustic canal).
- **Cholesteatoma** *(ko"le-ste"a-to'ma):* This benign cystlike mass or tumor, most common in the middle ear or mastoid region secondary to trauma to this region,* destroys bone, which can lead to serious complications, including hearing loss.
- **Polyp:** This growth arising from a mucous membrane and projecting into a cavity (sinus) may cause chronic sinusitis.

Otosclerosis *(o"to-skle-ro'sis)* This hereditary disease involving excessive spongy bone formation of the middle and inner ear is the most common cause of hearing loss in adults without eardrum damage. Symptoms first become evident in late adolescence or young adulthood.† It is best demonstrated on CT scans.

*Dorland's illustrated medical dictionary, ed 28, Philadelphia, 1994, WB Saunders.
†The Merck manual of medical information, 1997, Whitehouse Station, NJ, Merck.

12

CRANIUM—SUMMARY OF PATHOLOGIC INDICATIONS

CONDITION OR DISEASE	MOST COMMON RADIOGRAPHIC EXAM	POSSIBLE RADIOGRAPHIC APPEARANCE	MANUAL EXPOSURE FACTOR ADJUSTMENT*
Fractures	CT, routine skull series		None
• **Linear**	Routine skull series, CT	A jagged or irregular lucent line with sharp borders	None
• **Depressed**	Tangential projection sometimes helpful	Bone fragment depressed into the cranial cavity	None
• **Basal**	Horizontal ray lateral for potential air-fluid level in sphenoid sinuses and SMV projection if patient's condition allows	A fracture visualized in dense inner structures of temporal bone	None
Gunshot wound	Routine skull series, CT	High-density object in cranial cavity if bullet has not exited; skull fracture also present because of entrance of projectile	None
Metastases	Routine skull series, bone scan	Depends on lesion type: destructive lesions with decreased density or osteoblastic lesions with increased density or a combination with a moth-eaten appearance	(+) or (−) depending on type of lesion and stage of pathology
Multiple myeloma	Routine skull series	Osteolytic (radiolucent) areas	(−) or none depending on severity
Pituitary adenoma	CT, MRI, coned AP axial (Towne), and lateral	Enlarged sella turcica	(+) (because of decreased field size)
Paget's disease (osteitis deformans)	Routine skull series	Dependent on stage of disease; mixed areas of sclerotic (radiodense) and lytic (radiolucent); cotton-wool appearance	(+) if in advanced sclerotic stage
Mastoiditis	Radiographic mastoid views, CT, MRI	Increased densities (fluid-filled), replace mastoid air cells	None
Neoplasia			
• **Acoustic neuroma**	MRI, CT	Widened internal auditory canal	None
• **Cholesteatoma**	CT, MRI	Bone destruction involving middle ear	None
• **Polyp**	Routine radiographic sinus views, CT, MRI	Increased density in affected sinus, typically with rounded borders	None
Otosclerosis	CT, MRI	Excessive bone formation involving middle and inner ear	None

For the purpose of this table, a routine skull series is considered to be PA axial (Caldwell), AP axial (Towne), and lateral.
*Dependent on stage or severity of disease or condition.

Survey Information

Departmental standards (basic) and optional (special) routines for examinations of the cranium, sella turcica, and mastoids were somewhat consistent throughout the United States but demonstrate some difference in routines between U.S. and Canada (see lateral skull and PA 0° below). The results of this survey determined national norms for basic and special routines as presented in the positioning pages that follow.

Skull Series—Routine or Basic The most common basic projections for the routine skull series are as follows:

- **AP Towne** (98% in U.S., 96% in Canada)
- **Laterals, *both* R and L** (74% in U.S., 32% in Canada)
  or
  Single lateral, R *or* L (31% in U.S., 70% in Canada)
- **PA Caldwell** (79% in U.S., 70% in Canada)
- **PA 0°** (52% in U.S., 40% in Canada)

Both laterals routine was the consistent standard in all regions of the U.S., but the **single lateral** was more than twice as common in Canada.

The **PA 0°** was more common as a basic projection in the U.S. than in Canada and also indicated a significant regional difference in the U.S., with routine indicated by 73% in the West and only 51% in the East and 49% in the Midwest.

Special Skull Projections The **PA axial 25° cephalad (Haas method)** was indicated to be a special skull projection by 40% of survey responders in the U.S. and 26% in Canada. This was a higher frequency in the U.S. than in 1995, which was 30%.

The **SMV** continues to be a special skull projection as indicated by 38% in the U.S. and 33% in Canada. This has not changed significantly in the U.S. from previous surveys.

Sella Turcica The **lateral,** as expected, was still the most common basic position for the sella turcica, but less common in 1999 than in 1995, which was 80%, and 96% in 1989. (This reflects the trend of increased routine use of other modalities rather than conventional skull imaging for intracranial-type pathology.)

Mastoid and Temporal Bone Projections For those hospitals and/or clinics still performing these exams, the three *basic* projections most commonly performed throughout all regions of the U.S. and Canada are the **axiolateral (Law), axiolateral oblique (Stenvers),** and **AP axial (Towne).**

The two most common *special* projections are the **submentovertex (SMV)** and **axiolateral (Arcelin–reverse Stenvers).** The responses for all of these projections were similar throughout the U.S. and Canada.

Standard and Special Operating Procedures

Certain basic and special projections or positions for the cranium (skull series), mastoids, and sella turcica are demonstrated and described on the following pages as suggested standard basic and special departmental procedures.

BASIC PROJECTIONS

Standard or basic projections, also referred to as *routine projections* or *departmental routines,* are those projections commonly taken on patients who are able to cooperate in the performance of the procedure.

SPECIAL PROJECTIONS

Special projections are those projections obtained to better demonstrate certain pathologic conditions or specific body parts not well demonstrated in basic projections.

12

BASIC AND SPECIAL PROJECTIONS

(For trauma skull series, see Chapter 19—"Trauma, Mobile, and Surgical Radiography.")

Skull Series
BASIC
- AP axial (Towne method) 388
- Lateral 389
- PA axial 15° (Caldwell method) 390 or PA axial 25° to 30° 390
- PA 0° 391

SPECIAL
- Submentovertex (SMV) 392
- PA axial (Haas method) 393

Sella Turcica
BASIC
- Lateral 394
- AP axial (Towne method) 395

Mastoids
BASIC
- Axiolateral oblique (modified Law) 396
- Axiolateral oblique (posterior profile), Stenvers) 397
- AP axial (Towne) 388

SPECIAL
- Axiolateral oblique (Arcelin–reverse Stenvers) 398
- Submentovertex (SMV) 392

AP AXIAL PROJECTION; SKULL SERIES

Towne Method

Pathology Demonstrated

Skull fractures (medial and lateral displacement), neoplastic processes, and Paget's disease are demonstrated.

Skull Series
BASIC
- AP axial (Towne method)
- **Lateral**
- **PA 15° (Caldwell method) or PA 25° to 30°**
- **PA 0°**

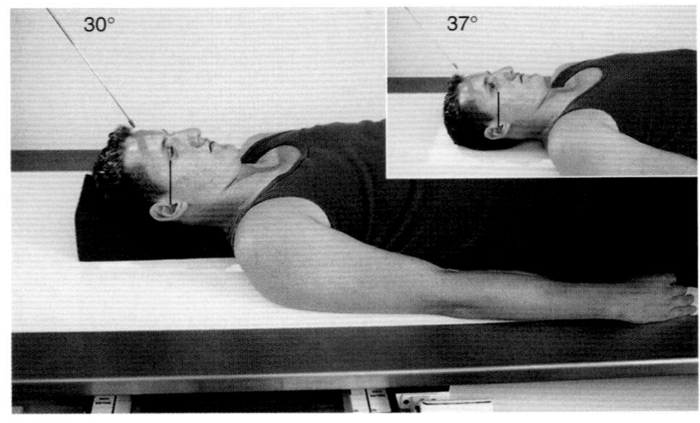

Fig. 12-48. Supine—AP axial. CR 30° to OML or 37° to IOML.

Technical Factors

24
30
R

- IR size—24 × 30 cm (10 × 12 inches), lengthwise
- Moving or stationary grid
- 70-80 kV range
- Small focal spot
- Technique and dose:

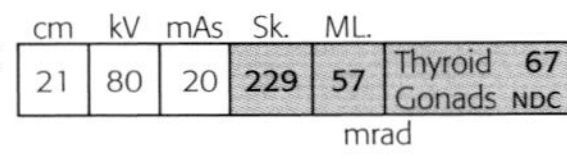

cm	kV	mAs	Sk.	ML.	
21	80	20	229	57	Thyroid 67 Gonads NDC
			mrad		

12

Patient Position Remove all metal, plastic, or other removable objects from patient's head. Take radiograph with the patient in the erect or supine position.

Part Position

- Depress chin, bringing **OML perpendicular** to IR. For patients unable to flex their neck to this extent, align the **IOML** perpendicular to the IR. Add radiolucent support under head if needed (see Note below).
- Align midsagittal plane to CR and to midline of the grid or the table/Bucky surface.
- Ensure that **no head rotation and/or no tilt** exists.
- Ensure that vertex of skull is in x-ray field.

Central Ray

- Angle CR **30° caudad to OML**, or **37° caudad to IOML** (see Note below).
- Center at midsagittal plane, **2½ inches** (6 cm) **above glabella,** or to pass through approximately ¾ inch (2 cm) superior to the level of EAMs (will exit the foramen magnum).
- Center IR to projected CR.
- Minimum SID is 40 inches (100 cm).

Collimation Collimate to outer margins of skull.

Respiration Suspend respiration.

Note: If patient is unable to depress the chin sufficiently to bring the **OML** perpendicular to the IR even with a small sponge under the head, the infraorbitomeatal line **(IOML)** can be placed perpendicular instead and the CR angle increased to **37°** caudad. This maintains the **30° angle between the OML and CR** and demonstrates the same anatomic relationships. (A 7° difference exists between the OML and IOML.)

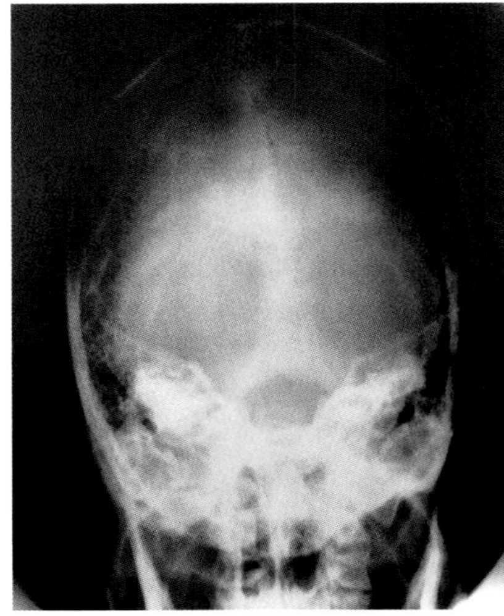

Fig. 12-49. AP axial.

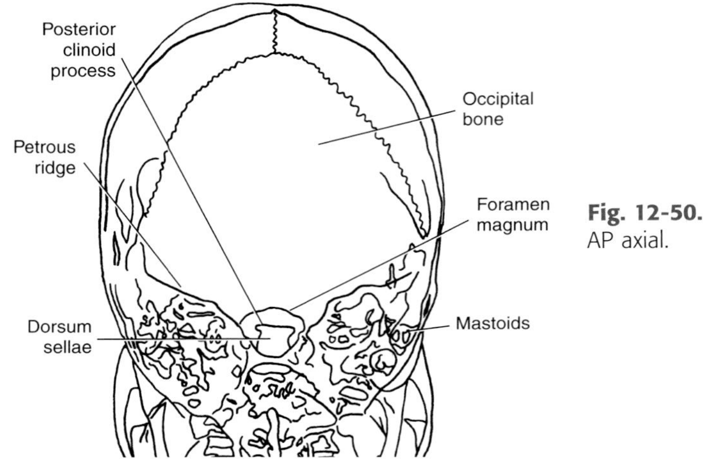

Fig. 12-50. AP axial.

Radiographic Criteria

Structures Shown: • Occipital bone, petrous pyramids, and foramen magnum are shown with the dorsum sellae and posterior clinoids visualized in the shadow of the foramen magnum.

Position: • Equal distance from foramen magnum to lateral margin of skull on both sides indicates **no rotation.** • Dorsum sella and posterior clinoids visualized in the foramen magnum indicate **correct CR angle and proper neck flexion/extension.** • **Underangulation** of the CR will project the dorsum sella **above the foramen magnum,** and **overangulation** will project the **anterior arch of C1** into the foramen magnum rather than the dorsum sella. • Petrous ridges should be symmetric and visualized superior to the mastoid processes.

Collimation and CR: • Entire skull is visualized on the image with the vertex near the top, and the foramen magnum is in the approximate center. • Collimation borders are to the outer margin of skull.

Exposure Criteria: • Density and contrast are sufficient to visualize occipital bone and sellar structures within foramen magnum. • Sharp bony margins indicate no motion.

LATERAL POSITION—RIGHT AND/OR LEFT LATERAL: SKULL SERIES

Skull Series
BASIC
- AP axial (Towne method)
- Lateral
- PA 15° (Caldwell method) or PA 25° to 30°
- PA 0°

Pathology Demonstrated

Skull fractures, neoplastic processes, and Paget's disease are demonstrated. A common general skull routine includes both right and left laterals.

Trauma routine: A horizontal beam is required to obtain a lateral view for trauma patients. This may demonstrate air-fluid levels in the sphenoid sinus, a sign of a basal skull fracture if intracranial bleeding occurs. See Chapter 19 for complete details on trauma skull.

Technical Factors

- IR size—24 × 30 cm (10 × 12 inches), crosswise
- Moving or stationary grid
- 70-80 kV range
- Small focal spot
- Technique and dose:

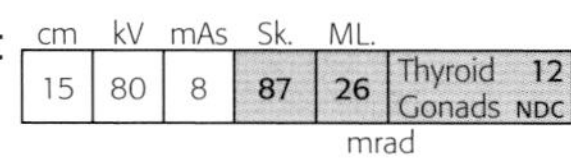

cm	kV	mAs	Sk.	ML.	
15	80	8	87	26	Thyroid 12 Gonads NDC

mrad

Patient Position Remove all metal, plastic, or other removable objects from patient's head. Take radiograph with patient in the erect or recumbent semiprone position.

Part Position

- Place the head in a **true lateral position,** with the side of interest closest to IR, with the patient's body as obliqued as needed for comfort. (A way to check for possible head rotation from a true lateral is to palpate the external occipital protuberance posteriorly and the nasion or glabella anteriorly and ensure that these two points are the same distance from the IR or tabletop.)
- Align **midsagittal plane parallel** to IR, ensuring **no rotation or tilt.**
- Align **interpupillary line perpendicular** to IR, ensuring no tilt of head (see Note below).
- Adjust neck flexion to align **IOML perpendicular** to front edge of IR. (GAL will be parallel to front edge of IR.)

Central Ray

- Align CR **perpendicular** to IR.
- Center to a point about **2 inches** (5 cm) **superior to EAM.**
- Center IR to CR.
- Minimum SID is 40 inches (100 cm).

Collimation Collimate to outer margins of skull.

Respiration Suspend respiration during exposure.

Note: For patients in the recumbent position, a radiolucent support placed under the chin will help in maintaining a true lateral position. A large-chested patient may require a radiolucent sponge under the entire head to prevent tilt, and a thin patient may require support under the upper thorax.

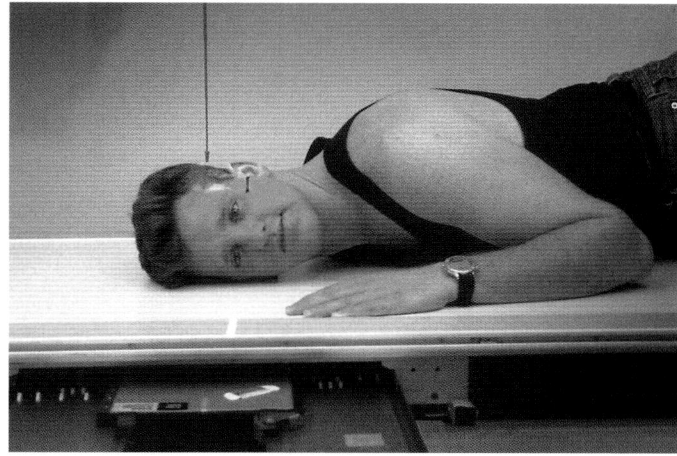

Fig. 12-51. Right lateral—recumbent.

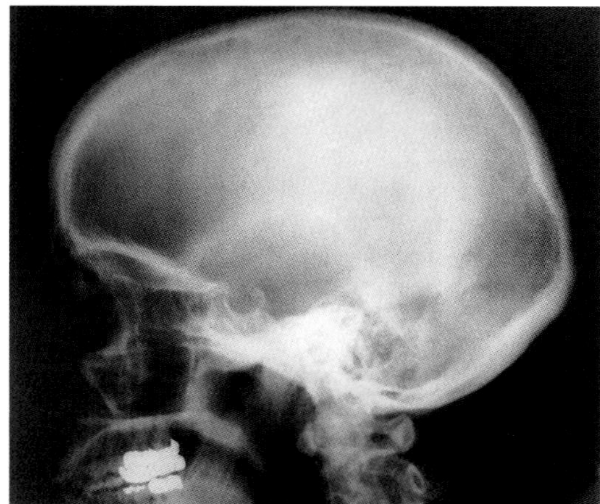

Fig. 12-52. Lateral.

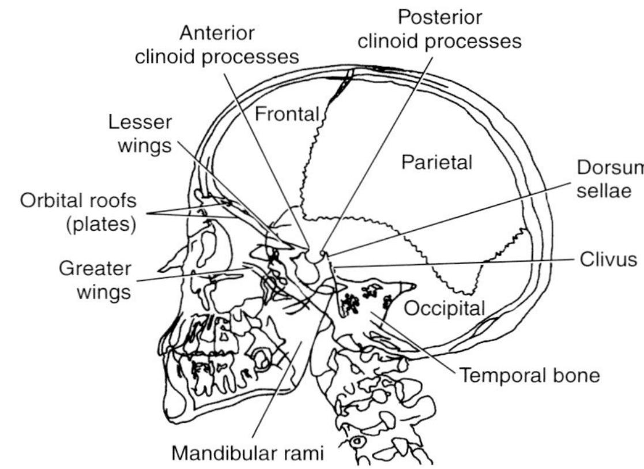

Fig. 12-53. Lateral.

Radiographic Criteria

Structures Shown: • Superimposed cranial halves with superior detail of the lateral cranium closest to the IR are demonstrated. The entire sella turcica, including anterior and posterior clinoids and dorsum sellae, is also shown. The sella turcica and clivus are demonstrated in profile.

Position: • See Fig. 12-67 for better visualization of central skull anatomy for determining tilt or rotation. • **No rotation or tilt** of the cranium is evident. • **Rotation** is evident by an **anterior and posterior separation** of symmetric bilateral structures such as the EAMs, mandibular rami, and greater wings of sphenoid. • **Tilt** is evident by **superior and inferior separation** of the orbital roofs (plates), EAMs, and lesser wings of sphenoid.

Collimation and CR: • Entire skull visualized on the image, with the region 2 inches (5 cm) superior to the EAM in the approximate center • Collimation borders to outer margin of skull.

Exposure Criteria: • Density and contrast are sufficient to visualize bony detail of sellar structures and surrounding skull. • Sharp bony margins indicate no motion.

12

PA AXIAL PROJECTION: SKULL SERIES

15° CR (Caldwell Method) or 25° to 30° CR

Pathology Demonstrated

Skull fractures (medial and lateral displacement), neoplastic processes, and Paget's disease are demonstrated.

Skull Series
BASIC
- AP axial (Towne method)
- Lateral
- PA 15° (Caldwell method) or PA 25° to 30°
- PA 0°

Technical Factors

- IR size—24 × 30 cm (10 × 12 inches), lengthwise
- Moving or stationary grid
- 70-80 kV range
- Small focal spot
- Technique and dose:

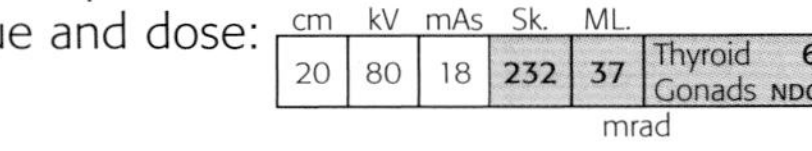

cm	kV	mAs	Sk.	ML.	
20	80	18	232	37	Thyroid 6 / Gonads NDC
			mrad		

24
30
R

Patient Position Remove all metal, plastic, or other removable objects from patient's head. Take radiograph with patient in the erect or prone position.

Part Position

- Rest patient's nose and forehead against table/Bucky surface.
- Flex neck as needed to align **OML perpendicular** to IR.
- Align **midsagittal plane perpendicular** to midline of the grid or table/Bucky surface to prevent head rotation and/or tilt.
- Center IR to CR.

Central Ray

- Angle CR **15° caudad** and **center to exit at nasion.**
- Alternate with **CR 25° to 30° caudad** and also center to **exit at nasion.**
- Minimum SID is 40 inches (100 cm).

Collimation Collimate to the outer margins of skull.

Respiration Suspend respiration.

Alternate 25° to 30°: An alternate projection is a **25° to 30° caudad** tube angle to better visualize the superior orbital fissures *(black arrows),* the foramen rotundum *(small white arrows),* and the inferior orbital rim region.

Note: A decreased caudal angulation of the CR and/or increased neck flexion (chin down) will result in the petrous pyramids being projected to the superior portion of the orbits.

Alternate AP axial projection: For patients who are unable to be positioned for a PA projection (e.g., trauma patients), an AP axial projection may be obtained using a 15° cephalic angle, positioning the OML perpendicular to the IR.

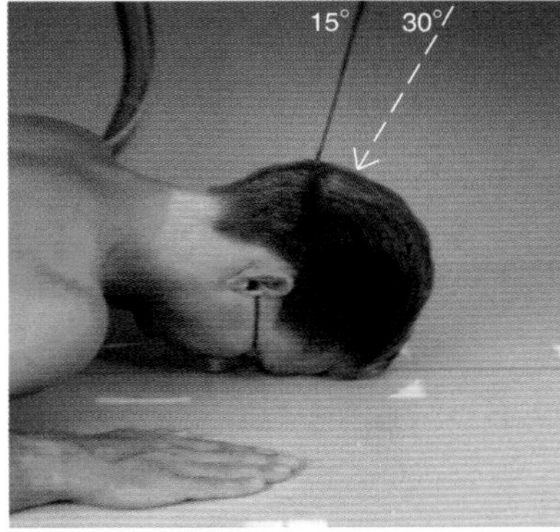

Fig. 12-54. PA—CR 15° caudad, OML perpendicular (and alternative CR 30° caudad—*dotted arrow*).

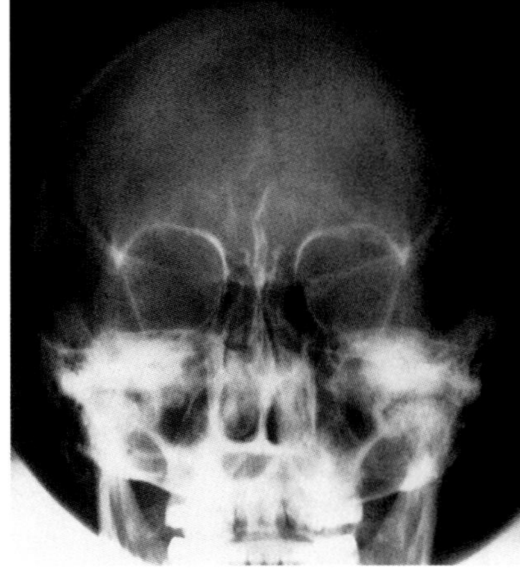

Fig. 12-55. PA—15° caudad (Caldwell).

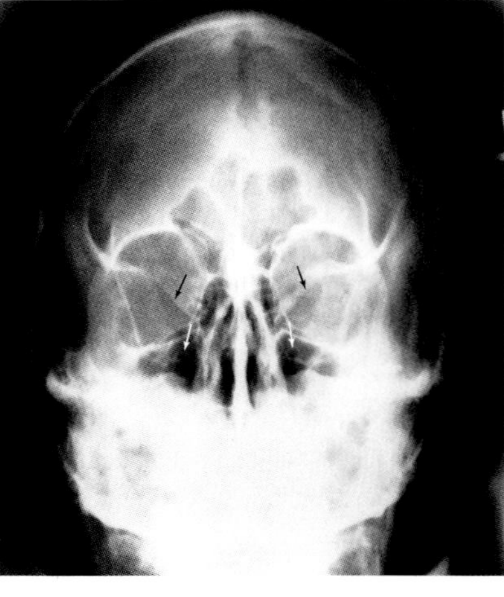

Fig. 12-56. Alternate PA—30° caudad.

Radiographic Criteria

Structures Shown: • Greater and lesser sphenoid wings, frontal bone, superior orbital fissures, frontal and anterior ethmoid sinuses, superior orbital margins, and crista galli are shown.

PA with 25° to 30° caudad angle: • In addition to the structures mentioned previously, the foramen rotundum adjacent to each inferior orbital rim is visualized (see *white arrows,* Fig. 12-56) and the entire superior orbital fissures (see *black arrows,* Fig. 12-56) are visualized within the orbits.

Position: • **No rotation** as assessed by equal distance from oblique orbital line to lateral margin of skull on each side, superior orbital fissures symmetric within the orbits, and correct extension of neck (OML alignment).

PA with 15° caudad angle: • Petrous pyramids are projected into the lower one-third of the orbits. • Superior orbital margin is visualized without superimposition.

PA with 25° to 30° caudad angle: • Petrous pyramids are projected at or just below the inferior orbital rim to allow visualization of the entire orbital margin.

Collimation and CR: • Entire skull is visualized on the image, with the nasion in the center. • Collimation borders are to outer margins of skull.

Exposure Criteria: • Density and contrast are sufficient to visualize the frontal bone and sellar structures without overexposure to perimeter regions of skull. • Sharp bony margins indicate no motion.

PA PROJECTION: SKULL SERIES

0° CR

Pathology Demonstrated

Skull fractures (medial and lateral displacement), neoplastic processes, and Paget's disease are demonstrated.

Skull Series
BASIC
• AP axial (Towne method)
• Lateral
• PA 15° (Caldwell method) or PA 25° to 30°
• PA 0°

Technical Factors

- IR size—24 × 30 cm (10 × 12 inches), lengthwise
- Moving or stationary grid
- 70-80 kV range
- Small focal spot
- Technique and dose:

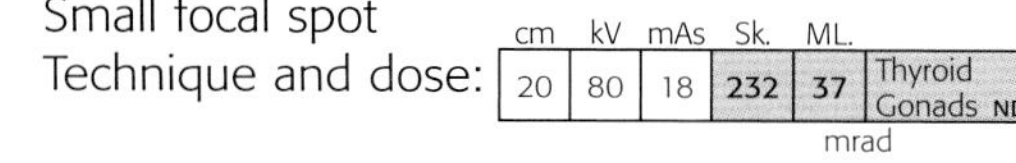

cm	kV	mAs	Sk.	ML.	
20	80	18	232	37	Thyroid 6 Gonads NDC
			mrad		

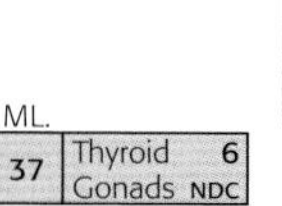

Patient Position Remove all metal, plastic, or other removable objects from patient's head.

Take radiograph with patient in the erect or prone position.

Part Position

- Rest patient's nose and forehead against table/Bucky surface.
- Flex neck aligning **OML perpendicular** to IR.
- Align **midsagittal plane perpendicular** to midline of table/Bucky to prevent head rotation and/or tilt (EAMs same distance from table/Bucky surface).
- Center IR to CR.

Central Ray

- CR is **perpendicular** to IR (parallel to OML) and **centered to exit at glabella.**
- Minimum SID is 40 inches (100 cm).

Collimation Collimate to outer margins of skull.

Respiration Suspend respiration during exposure.

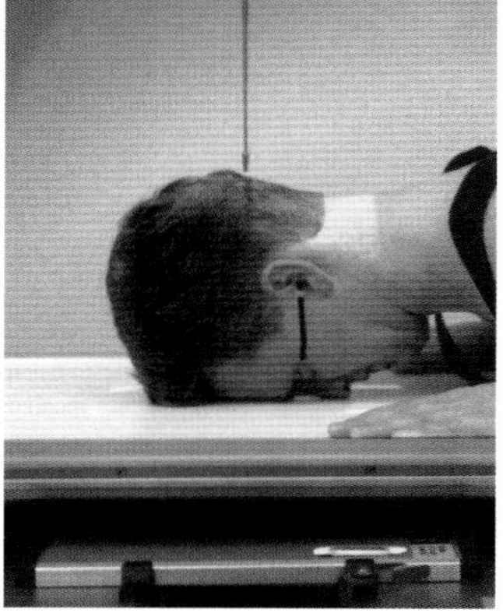

Fig. 12-57. PA—0° CR, OML perpendicular.

12

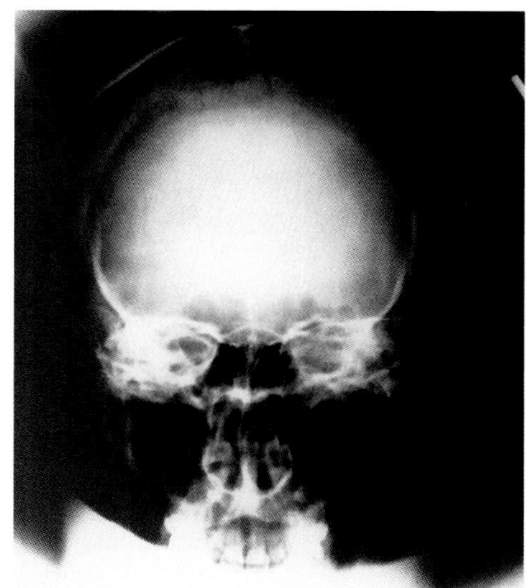

Fig. 12-58. PA—0° CR.

Radiographic Criteria

Structures Shown: • Frontal bone, crista galli, internal auditory canals, frontal and anterior ethmoid sinuses, petrous ridges, greater and lesser wings of sphenoid, and dorsum sellae are shown.

Position: • **No rotation** is evident, as indicated by equal distance bilaterally from oblique orbital line to lateral margin of skull. • Petrous ridges fill the orbits and superimpose the superior orbital region. • Posterior and anterior clinoids are visualized just superior to ethmoid sinuses.

Collimation and CR: • Entire skull is visualized on the image with the nasion in the center. • Collimation borders to outer borders of skull are visible.

Exposure Criteria: • Density and contrast are sufficient to visualize frontal bone and surrounding bony structures. • Sharp bony margins indicate no motion.

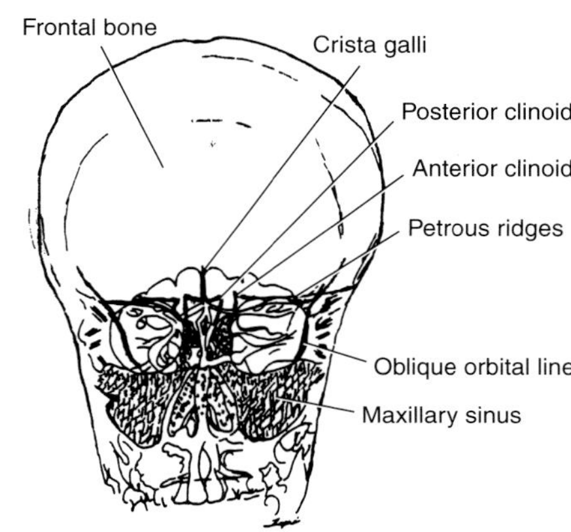

Fig. 12-59. PA—0° CR.

SUBMENTOVERTEX (SMV) PROJECTION: SKULL SERIES

Warning: Rule out cervical fracture or subluxation on trauma patient before attempting this projection.

Skull Series
SPECIAL
• Submentovertex (SMV)

Pathology Demonstrated

Advanced bony pathology of the inner temporal bone structures (skull base) and basal skull fracture are demonstrated.

Technical Factors

- IR size—24 × 30 cm (10 × 12 inches), lengthwise
- Moving or stationary grid
- 70-80 kV range
- Small focal spot
- Technique and dose:

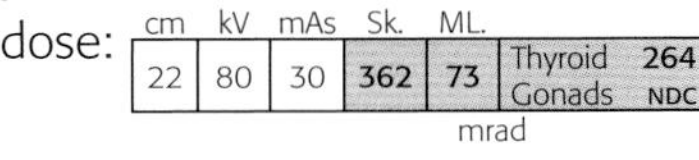

cm	kV	mAs	Sk.	ML.		
22	80	30	362	73	Thyroid	264
					Gonads	NDC

mrad

24 30 R

12

Shielding Shield patient's upper thorax region (shielding neck and thyroid will obscure area of interest).

Patient Position Remove all metal, plastic, and other removable objects from patient's head. Take radiograph with patient in an erect or supine position.

The erect position, which is easier for the patient, may be done with an erect table or an upright Bucky (see Fig. 12-60, inset).

Part Position

- Raise patient's chin and hyperextend the neck if possible until **infraorbitomeatal line (IOML) is parallel to IR** (see Notes below).
- Rest patient's head on vertex.
- Align **midsagittal plane perpendicular** to the midline of grid or table/Bucky surface, thus **avoiding tilt and/or rotation.**

Supine: With patient in the supine position, extend patient's head over end of table, and support grid cassette and head as shown, keeping **IOML parallel to IR** and **perpendicular to CR.** If table will not tilt as shown in Fig. 12-60, use a pillow under patient's back to allow sufficient neck extension.

Erect: If patient is unable to sufficiently extend the neck, compensate by angling the CR to remain **perpendicular to IOML.** Depending on the equipment being used, the IR may also be angled to maintain the perpendicular relationship with the CR (such as with an adjustable upright Bucky).

This position is very uncomfortable for patients in either the erect or the supine position; perform it as quickly as possible.

Central Ray

- CR is **perpendicular to infraorbitomeatal line.**
- Center **¾ inch (2 cm) anterior to level of EAMs** (midway between angles of mandible).
- Center image receptor to CR.
- Minimum SID is 40 inches (100 cm).

Collimation Collimate to outer margins of skull.

Respiration Suspend respiration.

Fig. 12-60. Submentovertex (SMV) tabletop with grid cassette. (*Inset,* Demonstrates use of upright Bucky.) CR perpendicular to IOML.

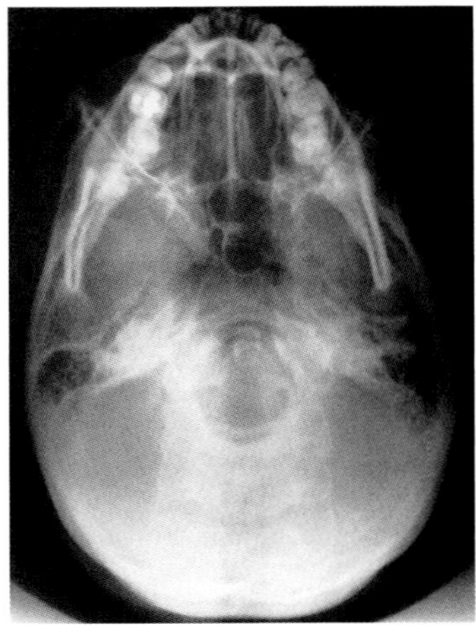

Fig. 12-61. Submentovertex.

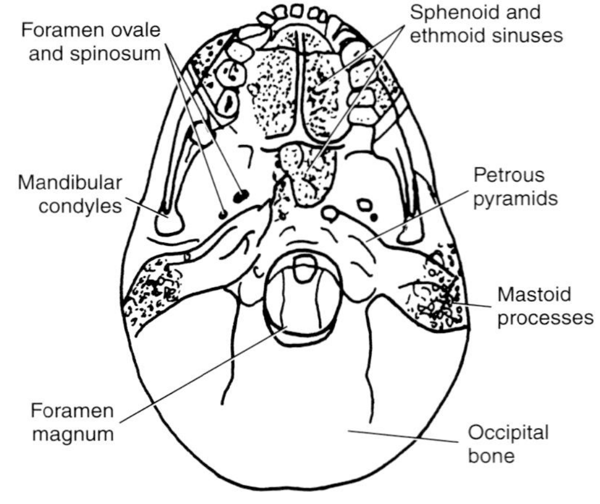

Fig. 12-62. Submentovertex.

Radiographic Criteria

Structures Shown: • Foramen ovale and spinosum, mandible, sphenoid and posterior ethmoid sinuses, mastoid processes, petrous ridges, hard palate, foramen magnum, and occipital bone are shown.

Position: • Correct extension of neck and relationship between IOML and CR as indicated by mandibular condyles projected anterior to petrous pyramids and frontal bone and mandibular symphysis superimposed. • **No rotation or tilt** as indicated by equal distance bilaterally from mandibular condyles to lateral border of skull.

Collimation and CR: • Entire skull should be visualized on the image, with the foramen magnum in the approximate center. • Collimation borders should be visible on outer margins of skull.

Exposure Criteria: • Density and contrast are sufficient to clearly visualize outline of foramen magnum. • Sharp bony margins indicate no motion.

PA AXIAL PROJECTION: SKULL SERIES

Haas Method

Skull Series
SPECIAL
- Submentovertex (SMV)
- PA axial (Haas method)

Pathology Demonstrated

Occipital bone, petrous pyramids, and foramen magnum, with dorsum sellae and posterior clinoids in its shadow, are shown.

This is an **alternative projection** for patients who cannot flex their necks sufficiently for AP axial (Towne). It results in magnification of the occipital area but results in lower doses to facial structures and thyroid gland.

This is not recommended when the occipital bone is the area of interest because of excessive magnification.

Technical Factors

- IR size—24 × 30 cm (10 × 12 inches), lengthwise
- Moving or stationary grid
- 70-80 kV range
- Small focal spot
- Technique and dose:

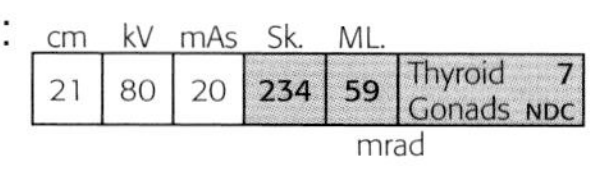

cm	kV	mAs	Sk.	ML.	
21	80	20	234	59	Thyroid 7 Gonads NDC

mrad

Patient Position Remove all metal, plastic, or other removable objects from patient's head. Take radiograph with patient in the erect or prone position.

Part Position

- Rest patient's nose and forehead against the table/Bucky surface.
- Flex neck, bringing **OML perpendicular** to IR.
- Align midsagittal plane to CR and to the midline of the grid or table/Bucky surface.
- Ensure that **no rotation or tilt** exists (midsagittal plane perpendicular to IR).

Central Ray

- Angle CR **25° cephalad to OML.**
- Center CR to midsagittal plane **through level of EAMs.**
- Center image receptor to projected CR.
- Minimum SID is 40 inches (100 cm).

Collimation Collimate to the outer margins of skull on all sides.

Respiration Suspend respiration.

Radiographic Criteria

Structures Shown: • Occipital bone, petrous pyramids, and foramen magnum are shown, with the dorsum sellae and posterior clinoids visualized in the shadow of the foramen magnum.

Position: • **No rotation** is evident, as indicated by equal distance from foramen magnum to the lateral margin of the skull on both sides. • Dorsum sellae and posterior clinoids are visualized in the foramen magnum, which indicates correct CR angle and proper neck flexion and extension. • Petrous ridges should be symmetric and visualized superior to the mastoid processes.

Collimation and CR: • Entire skull is visualized on the image with the vertex near the top and the foramen magnum and mastoid portions near the bottom. • Collimation borders are visible to outer margins of skull.

Exposure Criteria: • Density and contrast are sufficient to visualize occipital bone and sellar structures within foramen magnum. • Sharp bony margins indicate no motion.

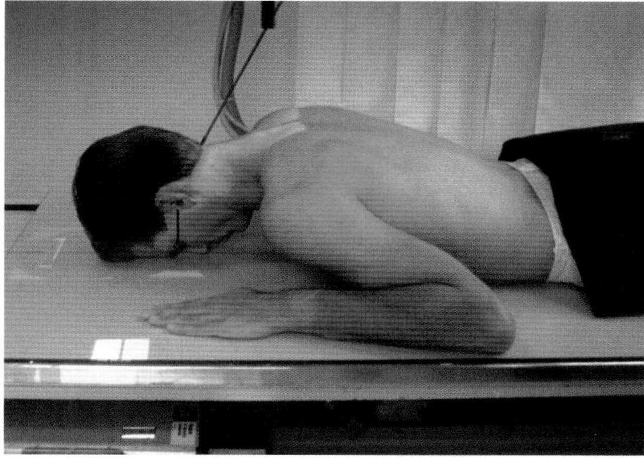

Fig. 12-63. PA axial—CR 25° cephalad to OML.

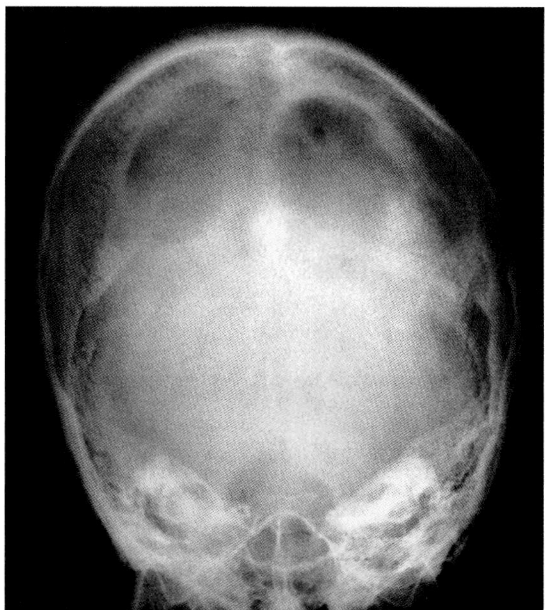

Fig. 12-64. PA axial.

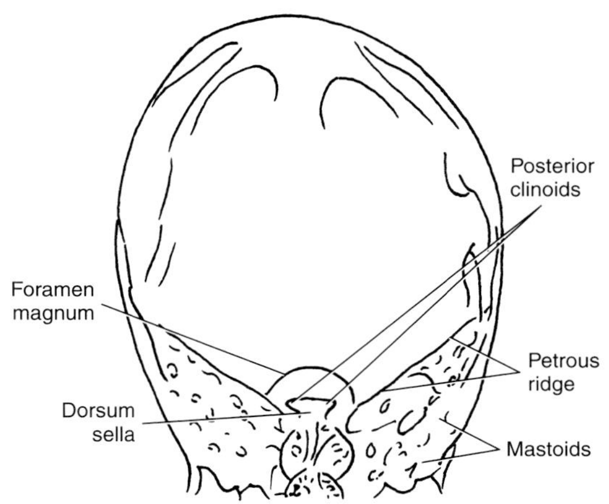

Fig. 12-65. PA axial.

LATERAL POSITION—RIGHT OR LEFT LATERAL: SELLA TURCICA

Sella Turcica
BASIC
- Lateral
- AP axial (Towne method)

Pathology Demonstrated

Pituitary adenomas may be demonstrated if involvement of the sella turcica occurs.

Technical Factors

- IR size—18 × 24 cm (8 × 10 inches), crosswise
- Moving or stationary grid
- 70-80 kV range
- Small focal spot
- Technique and dose:

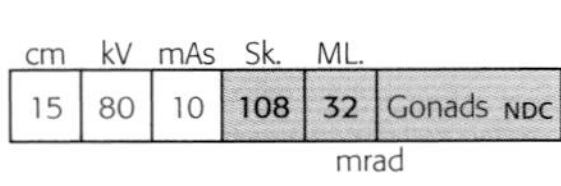

cm	kV	mAs	Sk.	ML.	
15	80	10	108	32	Gonads NDC
			mrad		

24 × 18 R

Patient Position Remove all metal, plastic, or other removable objects from patient's head. Take radiograph with patient in an erect or recumbent semiprone position.

Part Position

- Place patient's head in a **true lateral** position; position patient's body oblique as needed for comfort.
- Align **interpupillary line perpendicular** to table/Bucky surface.
- Align **midsagittal plane parallel** to table/Bucky surface.
- Place **IOML perpendicular** to front edge of IR.

Central Ray

- Align CR **perpendicular** to IR.
- Center to a **point ¾ inch** (2 cm) **anterior** and **¾ inch** (2 cm) **superior** to the external auditory meatus (EAM).
- Center image receptor to CR.
- Minimum SID is 40 inches (100 cm).

Collimation Collimate to a field size of approximately 4 inches (10 cm) square.

Respiration Suspend respiration during exposure.

Note: To obtain a sharply detailed image of the sella turcica, the use of a small focal spot and close collimation is essential.

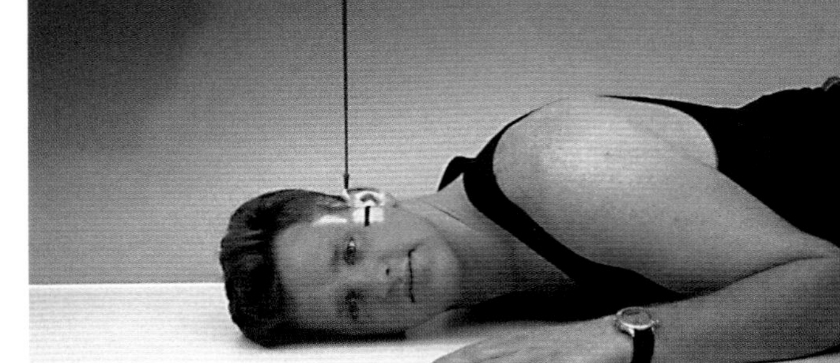

Fig. 12-66. Right lateral sella turcica—recumbent.

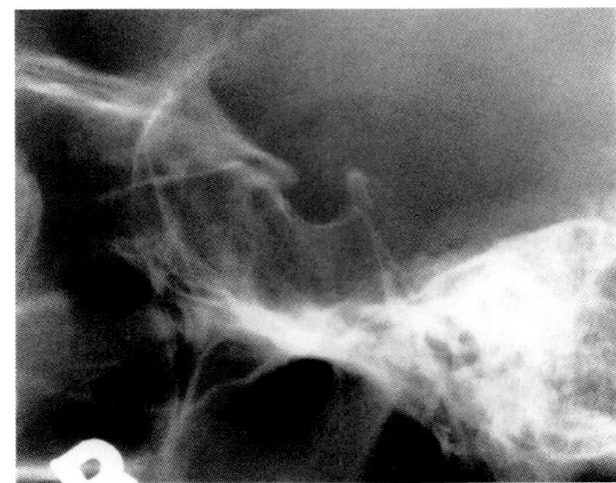

Fig. 12-67. Lateral sella turcica.

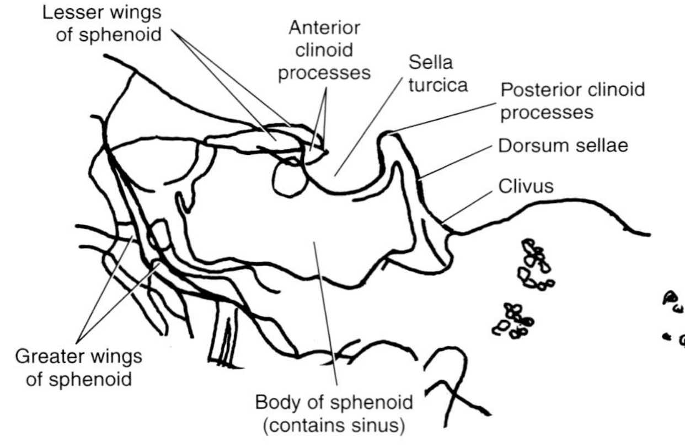

Fig. 12-68. Lateral sella turcica.

Radiographic Criteria

Structures Shown: • Sella turcica, anterior and posterior clinoid processes, dorsum sellae, and clivus are shown.

Position: • The sella turcica is visualized **without rotation or tilt** as indicated by the following: • The sella turcica and clivus are demonstrated in profile. • The anterior and the posterior clinoids are superimposed, and the greater wings and the lesser wings of the sphenoid are superimposed. • Rotation can be differentiated from tilt by the following: • **Rotation** is evident by an **anterior and posterior separation** of symmetric bilateral structures such as the EAMs, mandibular rami, and greater wings of sphenoid. • **Tilt** is evident by **superior and inferior separation** of the orbital roofs (plates), EAMs, and lesser wings of sphenoid.

Collimation and CR: • Closely collimated image, with the sella turcica in the center.

Exposure Criteria: • Density and contrast are sufficient to clearly visualize sella turcica and pituitary fossa. • Sharp bony margins indicate no motion.

AP AXIAL PROJECTION: SELLA TURCICA

Towne Method

Sella Turcica
BASIC
- **Lateral**
- AP axial (Towne method)

Pathology Demonstrated

Pituitary adenomas may be demonstrated if involvement of the sella turcica occurs.

Technical Factors

- IR size—18 × 24 cm (8 × 10 inches), lengthwise
- Moving or stationary grid
- 80 ± 5 kV range
- Small focal spot
- Technique and dose:

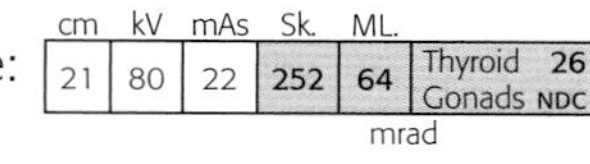

cm	kV	mAs	Sk.	ML.	
21	80	22	252	64	Thyroid 26 Gonads NDC
			mrad		

Shielding Shield patient's upper thorax region.

Patient Position Remove all metal, plastic, or other removable objects from patient's head. Take radiograph with patient in an erect or a supine position.

Part Position

- Rest patient's posterior skull against table/Bucky surface.
- Flex neck to bring **IOML perpendicular** to IR.
- Align **midsagittal plane perpendicular** to the midline of the grid or table/Bucky surface.

Central Ray

- Angle **CR 37° caudad** if **dorsum sellae** and **posterior clinoid processes** are of primary interest.
- Angle **CR 30° caudad** if the **anterior clinoids** are of primary interest.
- Center at midsagittal plane **1½ inches** (4 cm) above **superciliary arch.** (CR will exit the foramen magnum.)
- Center IR to projected CR.
- Minimum SID is 40 inches (100 cm).

Collimation Collimate to a field size of approximately 4 inches (10 cm) square.

Respiration Suspend respiration during exposure.

Note: To obtain a sharply detailed image of the dorsum sellae, a small focal spot and close collimation are essential.

Radiographic Criteria

Structures Shown: • Dorsum sella, anterior and posterior clinoid processes (depending on CR angulation), foramen magnum, petrous ridges, and occipital bone are shown.

Position: • **No rotation** is evident, as indicated by symmetric petrous ridges and by equal distances from the midsagittal plane (which can be identified by the perpendicular plate) to each anterior clinoid process. • A correctly positioned image will have the following features (CR angulation required depends on the structures of interest):

37° caudad angle: Dorsum sella and posterior clinoid processes are projected into the foramen magnum.

30° caudad angle: Anterior clinoids are clearly visualized, adjacent to each petrous ridge, directly above the foramen magnum; dorsum sella is projected above the foramen magnum, superimposing the occipital bone.

Collimation and CR: • A closely collimated image, with the dorsum sella located in the center.

Exposure Criteria: • Density and contrast are sufficient to visualize the dorsum sella through the adjacent skull structures. • Sharp bony margins indicate no motion.

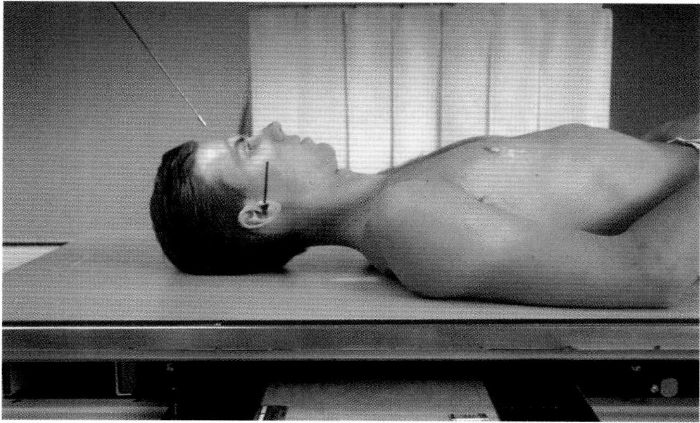

Fig. 12-69. AP axial—CR 30° to 37° caudad. IOML perpendicular.

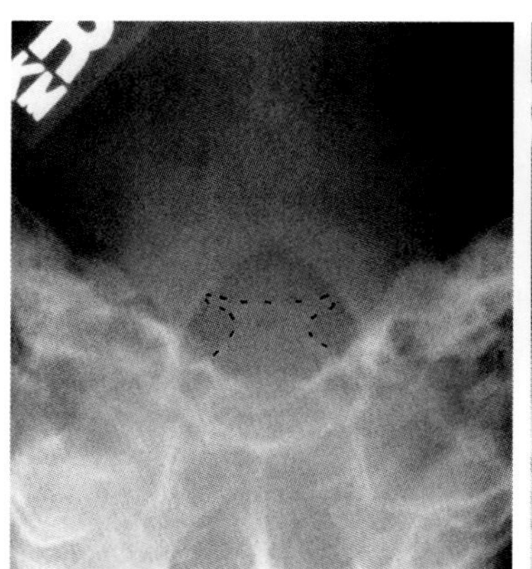

Fig. 12-70. 37° caudad.

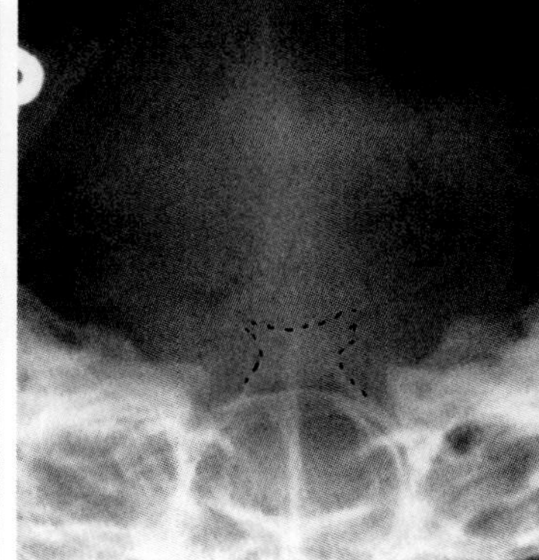

Fig. 12-71. 30° caudad.

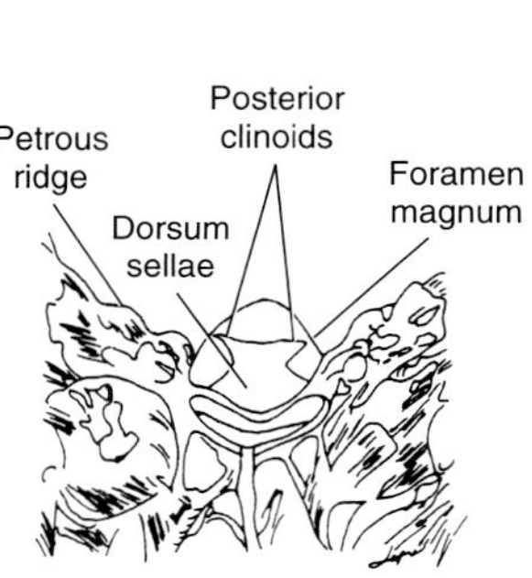

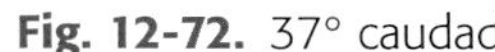

Fig. 12-72. 37° caudad.

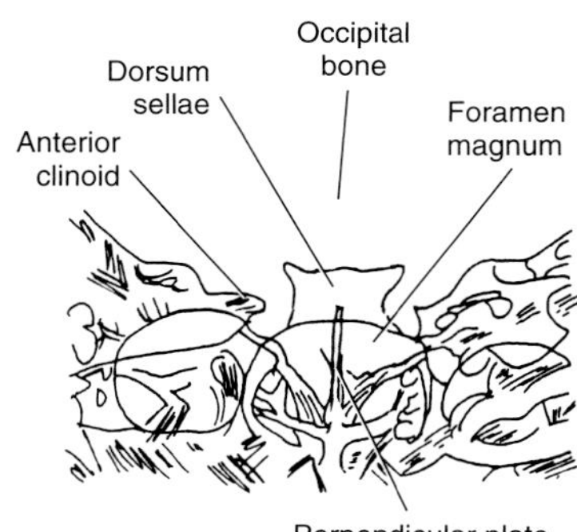

Fig. 12-73. 30° caudad.

AXIOLATERAL OBLIQUE PROJECTION: MASTOIDS

Modified Law Method

Mastoids
BASIC
- **Axiolateral oblique (modified Law)**
- **Axiolateral oblique (Stenvers)**
- **AP axial (Towne)** **(p. 388)**

Pathology Demonstrated

This projection demonstrates advanced bony pathology of the mastoid processes.

Both sides are generally examined for comparison.

Technical Factors

- IR size—18 × 24 cm (8 × 10 inches), lengthwise
- Moving or stationary grid
- 70-80 kV range
- Small focal spot
- Technique and dose:

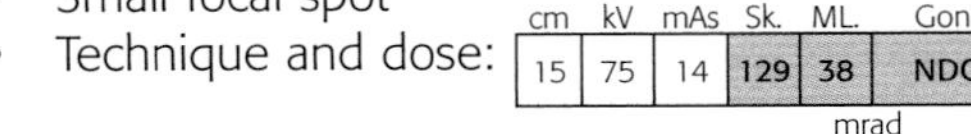

cm	kV	mAs	Sk.	ML.	Gon.
15	75	14	129	38	NDC
				mrad	

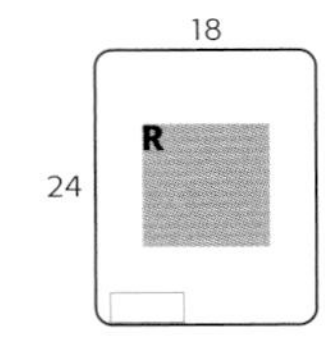

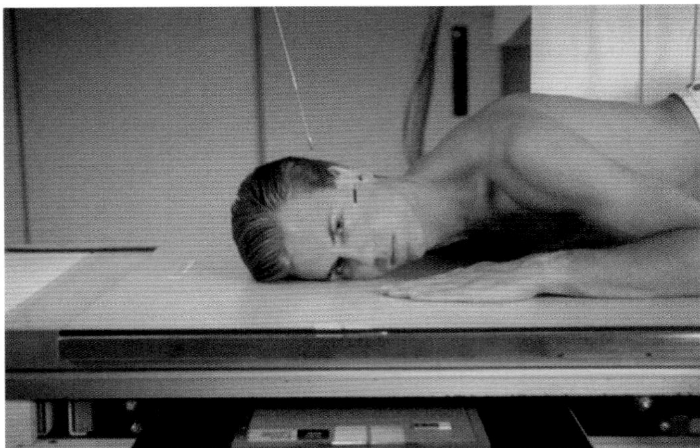

Fig. 12-74. Axiolateral oblique—15° oblique (head rotation), 15° caudad angle.

Patient Position Remove all metal, plastic, and other removable objects from head. Position the patient erect or prone. **Tape each auricle forward** to prevent superimposing mastoid.

Part Position

- Place lateral aspect of head against table/upright Bucky surface, with side of interest closest to IR; oblique body as needed for patient comfort.
- Align midsagittal plane parallel with table/upright Bucky surface. From the lateral position, **rotate face 15° toward IR.** Prevent tilt by maintaining the **interpupillary line perpendicular** to table/upright Bucky surface.
- Adjust chin to bring **IOML perpendicular** to front edge of IR.

Central Ray

- Angle CR **15° caudad.**
- Center CR to **exit at downside mastoid tip,** to enter **1 inch (2.5 cm) posterior and superior to upside EAM.**
- Center IR to projected CR.
- Minimum SID is 40 inches (100 cm).

Collimation Collimate to yield a field size of approximately 4 inches (10 cm) square.

Respiration Suspend respiration during exposure.

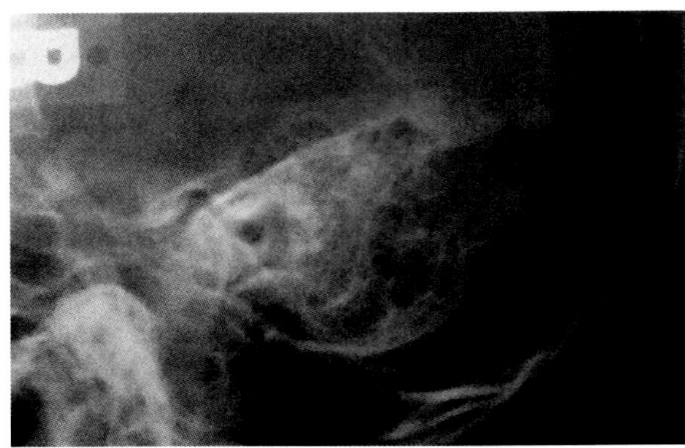

Fig. 12-75. Axiolateral oblique.

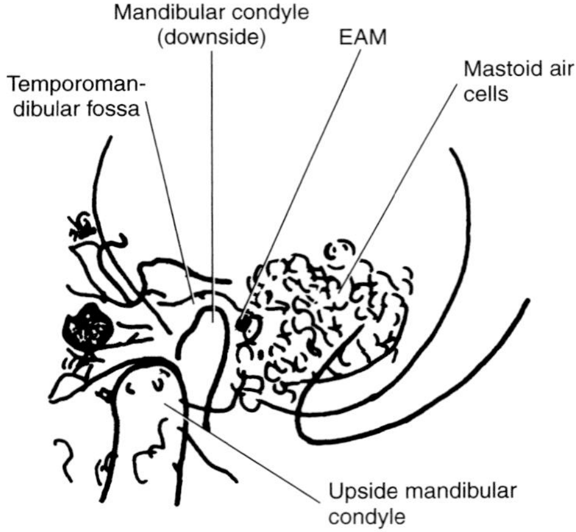

Fig. 12-76. Axiolateral oblique.

Radiographic Criteria

Structures Shown: • Lateral perspective of the mastoid air cells and bony labyrinths nearest the IR are shown.

Position: • Accurate positioning as indicated by the following: • Mastoid of interest (side down) visualized with no superimposition from opposite mastoid (side up) • Temporomandibular joint visualized anterior to mastoid of interest • Auricle of ear not superimposed on mastoid

Collimation and CR: • The mastoid air cells of interest are located in the center of the collimated field, centered just posterior to the EAM.

Exposure Criteria: • Density and contrast are sufficient to visualize mastoid air cells. • Sharp bony margins indicate no motion.

AXIOLATERAL OBLIQUE PROJECTION—POSTERIOR PROFILE: MASTOIDS

Stenvers Method

Pathology Demonstrated

This projection demonstrates advanced pathology of the temporal bone (e.g., advanced acoustic neuroma), which may cause the IACs (internal acoustic canals) to appear asymmetric.

Both sides are generally examined for comparison.

Mastoids
BASIC
- **Axiolateral oblique (modified Law)**
- Axiolateral oblique (Stenvers)
- **AP axial (Towne) (p. 388)**

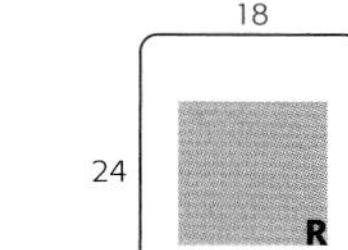

Technical Factors

- IR size—18 × 24 cm (8 × 10 inches), lengthwise
- Moving or stationary grid
- 70-80 kV range
- Small focal spot
- Technique and dose:

cm	kV	mAs	Sk.	ML.	Gon.
16	75	20	184	55	NDC
				mrad	

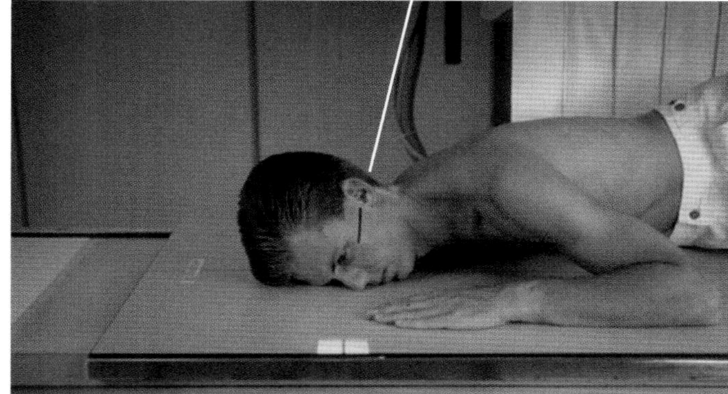

Fig. 12-77. Axiolateral oblique—posterior profile: 45° anterior oblique, 12° cephalad angle.

Patient Position Determine skull morphology for degree of rotation. Remove all metal, plastic, and other removable objects from head. Position the patient prone or erect.

Part Position

- Adjust chin to bring **IOML perpendicular** to IR.
- Rotate head **45° (mesocephalic) with the side of interest downside.** (Assess skull morphology to determine degree of rotation required.)
- Align downside mastoid region to CR and to center line of IR.

Central Ray

- Angle CR **12° cephalad,** centered to enter at about **3 to 4 inches (7 to 10 cm) posterior,** and **½ inch (1.25 cm) inferior to upside EAM,** to exit through downside mastoid process.
- Center IR to projected CR.
- Minimum SID is 40 inches (100 cm).

Collimation Collimate to yield a field size of approximately 4 inches (10 cm) square.

Respiration Suspend respiration during exposure.

Note: To obtain a sharply detailed image of the temporal bone structures, use of a small focal spot and close collimation is essential.

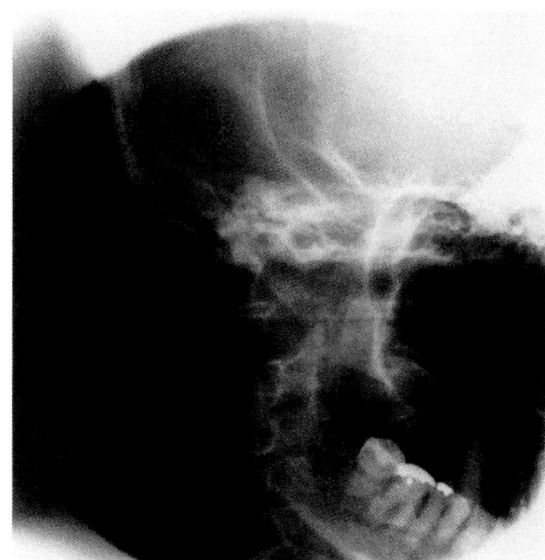

Fig. 12-78. Axiolateral oblique—posterior profile.

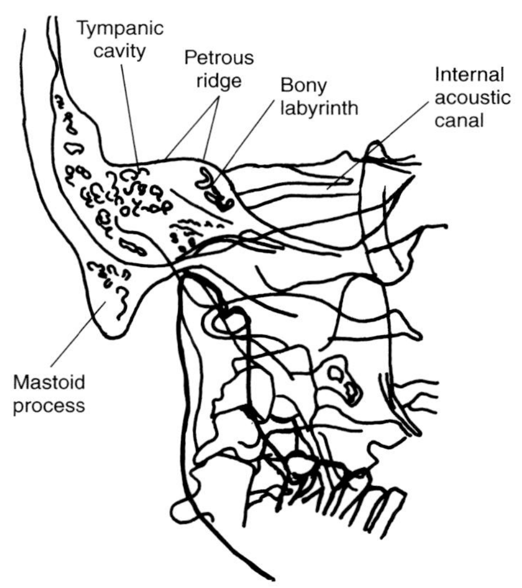

Fig. 12-79. Axiolateral oblique—posterior profile.

Radiographic Criteria

Structures Shown: • Petrous pyramid in profile, the bony labyrinth, the tympanic cavity, the internal auditory canal, and the mastoid air cells (with mastoid tip) projected clear of occipital bone on the side being examined are shown.

Position: • An accurately positioned image will demonstrate the following: • Mandibular condyle superimposing cervical spine • The internal acoustic canal, cochlea, and semicircular canals (bony labyrinths) below petrous ridge • Mastoid process in profile below the cranial margin • Posterior margin of mandibular ramus superimposing the posterior margin of the cervical spine

Collimation and CR: • Collimated field includes and is centered to the petrous ridge and mastoid process on the side being examined.

Exposure Criteria: • Density and contrast are sufficient to visualize the structures within bony labyrinth and petrous portions without overexposing mastoid process. • Sharp bony margins indicate no motion.

12

AXIOLATERAL OBLIQUE PROJECTION—ANTERIOR PROFILE: MASTOIDS

Arcelin Method (Reverse Stenvers Method)

Mastoids
SPECIAL
• Axiolateral oblique (Arcelin–reverse Stenvers)

Pathology Demonstrated

Advanced pathology of the temporal bone (e.g., advanced acoustic neuroma) is demonstrated.

This projection is primarily for patients who cannot be placed in a prone position for the PA oblique (Stenvers) projection.

The exam is performed bilaterally for comparison.

18
24
R

Technical Factors

- IR size—18 × 24 cm (8 × 10 inches), lengthwise
- Moving or stationary grid
- 70-80 kV range
- Small focal spot
- Technique and dose:

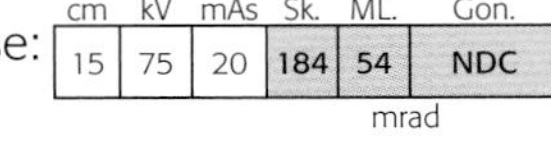

cm	kV	mAs	Sk.	ML.	Gon.
15	75	20	184	54	NDC

mrad

Patient Position Remove all metal, plastic, and other removable objects from head. Position the patient erect or supine.

Part Position

- Rotate head 45° away from side of interest (side elevated will be the side demonstrated).
- Adjust chin, bringing IOML perpendicular to table/upright Bucky surface.
- Align elevated mastoid region to CR and to center line of table/upright Bucky surface.

Central Ray

- Angle **CR 10° caudad,** centered to enter at **1 inch (2.5 cm) anterior and ¾ inch (2 cm) superior to elevated EAM.**
- Center IR to projected CR.
- Minimum SID is 40 inches (100 cm).

Collimation Collimate to a rectangle area of the petrous pyramid on the elevated side.

Respiration Suspend respiration during exposure.

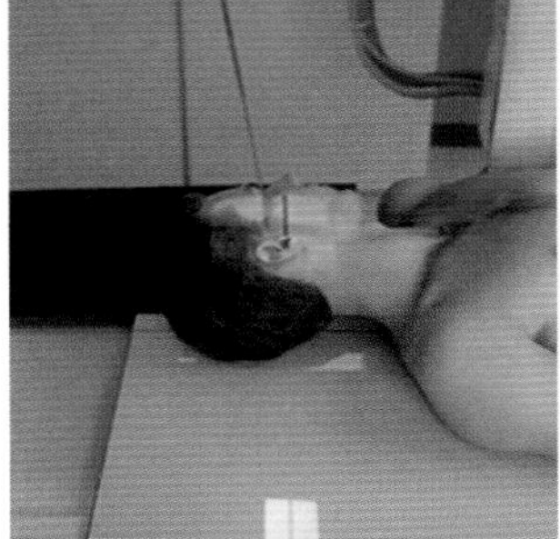

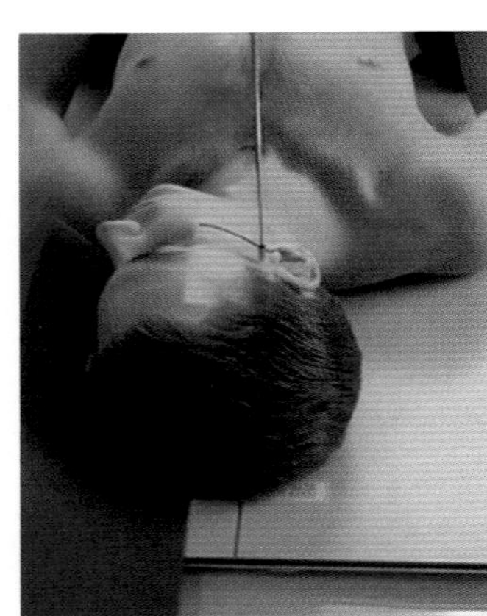

Fig. 12-80. Axiolateral oblique—right side up (upside): 45° oblique, CR 10° caudad.

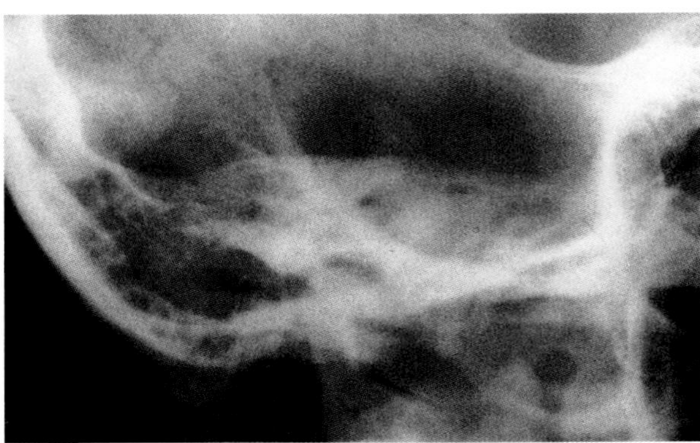

Fig. 12-81. Axiolateral oblique (anterior profile).

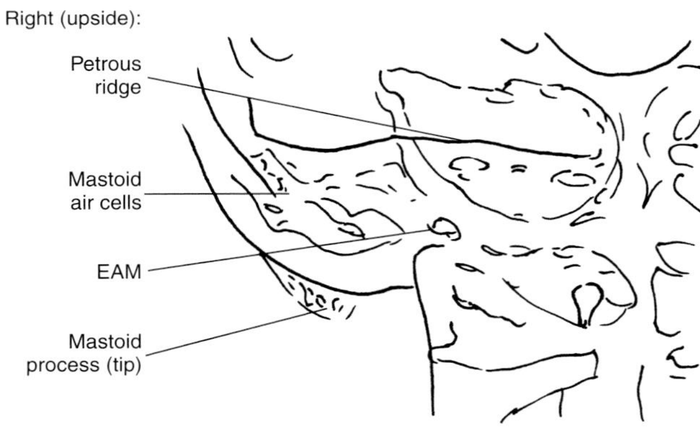

Fig. 12-82. Axiolateral oblique (anterior profile).

Radiographic Criteria

Structures Shown: • Elevated side petrous ridge is visualized because this position places it parallel to the IR. • The elevated side TMJ is visualized anterior to mastoid cell of interest.

Position: • An accurately positioned image will demonstrate the following: • Mandibular condyle superimposing the cervical spine • The internal acoustic canal, cochlea, and semicircular canals (bony labyrinths) below the petrous ridge • Mastoid process in profile below the cranial margin • Posterior margin of mandibular ramus superimposing the posterior margin of the cervical spine.

Collimation and CR: • The petrous ridge and mastoid process of the side being examined are centered to the well-collimated field.

Exposure Criteria: • Density and contrast are sufficient to visualize the temporal bone structures. • Sharp bony margins indicate no motion.

RADIOGRAPHS FOR CRITIQUE

Each of these skull radiographs demonstrates at least **one repeatable error.**

See whether you can critique each of these radiographs based on the categories as described in the textbook and as outlined on the right. As a starting critique exercise, place a check mark in each category that demonstrates a **repeatable error** for that radiograph.

Student workbooks provide more space for writing comments and complete critique answers for each of these radiographs. Answers are provided in Appendix B, at the end of this textbook.

	RADIOGRAPHS				
	A	B	C	D	E
1. Structures shown	____	____	____	____	____
2. Positioning	____	____	____	____	____
3. Collimation and CR	____	____	____	____	____
4. Exposure criteria	____	____	____	____	____
5. Markers	____	____	____	____	____

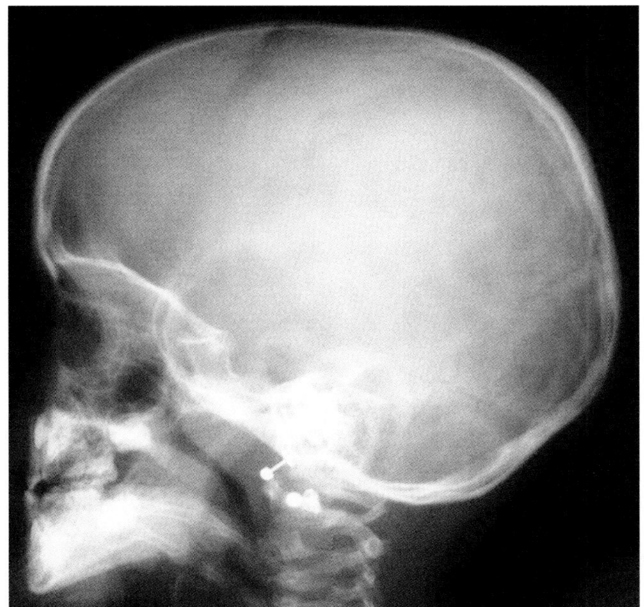

Fig. C12-83. Lateral skull—4-year-old patient. A

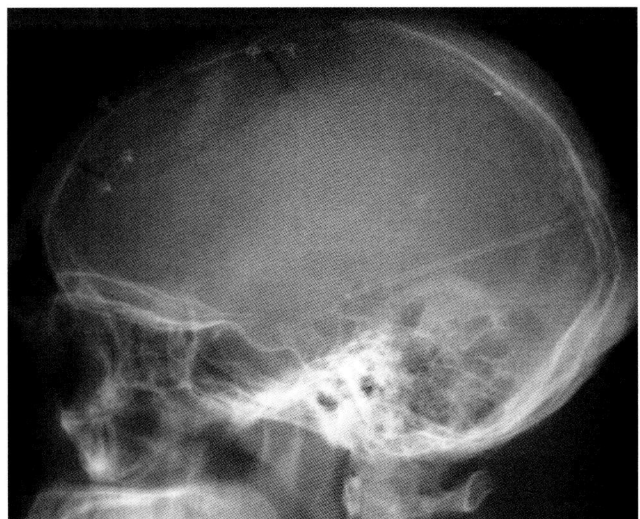

Fig. C12-84. Lateral skull—54-year-old posttrauma patient. B

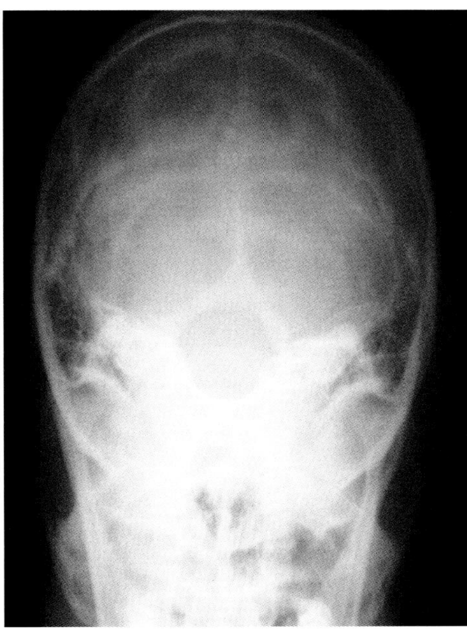

Fig. C12-85. AP Towne. C

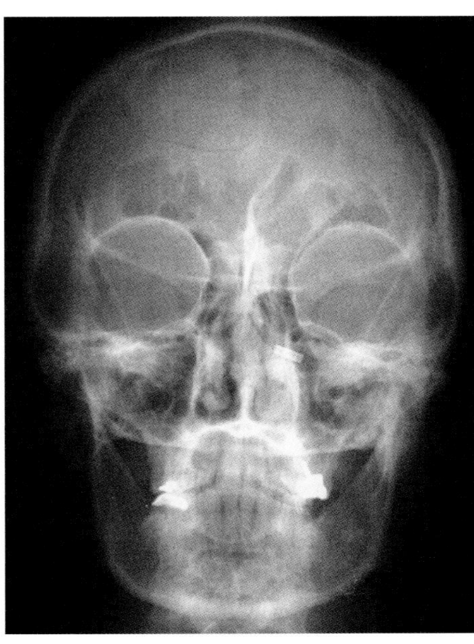

Fig. C12-86. Caldwell, PA or AP? D

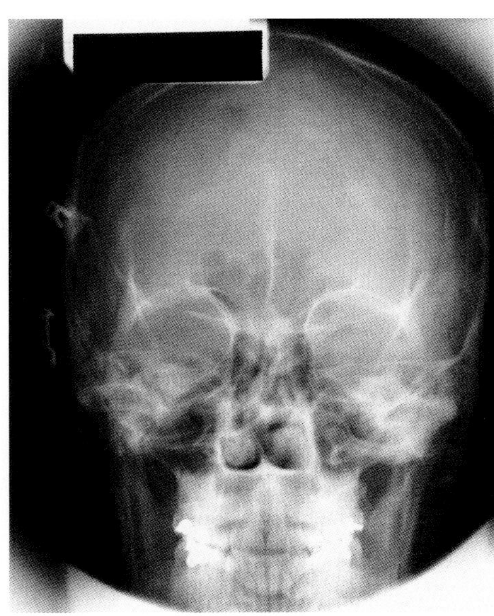

Fig. C12-87. Caldwell, PA or AP? E

CHAPTER 13

Facial Bones and Paranasal Sinuses

CONTRIBUTIONS BY **Renee F. Tossell,** PhD, RT(R)
CONTRIBUTORS TO PAST EDITIONS Kathy M. Martensen, BS, RT(R), Barry T. Anthony, RT(R), Cindy Murphy, RT R, ACR, BHSc

CONTENTS

RADIOGRAPHIC ANATOMY

Skull

In addition to the **eight cranial bones** described in Chapter 12, there are **14 facial bones** making up the skull, or bony skeleton of the head. Remember that the skull includes the total bony structure of the head, which includes both cranial and facial bones. The cranial bones are again identified on these drawings to demonstrate anatomic relationships of the total skull structure.

FACIAL BONES (14)

Each of the facial bones is identified on the frontal and lateral drawings of Figs. 13-1 and 13-2, except for the two palatine bones and the vomer, both of which are located internally and not visible on a dry skeleton from the exterior. These bones are identified on sectional drawings later in this chapter.

The 14 facial bones contribute to the shape and form of a person's face. In addition, the cavities of the orbits, nose, and mouth are largely constructed from the bones of the face. Of the 14 bones making up the facial skeleton, only 2 are single bones. The remaining 12 consist of six pairs of bones, with similar bones on each side of the face.

Facial Bones

2 Maxillae *(mak-sil-'e)* (upper jaw), or maxillary bones
2 Zygomatic bones *(zi'go-mat' ik)*
2 Lacrimal bones *(lak'-ri-mal)*
2 Nasal bones
2 Inferior nasal conchae *(kong'ke)*
2 Palatine bones *(pal'ah-tin)*
1 Vomer *(vo'mer)*
1 Mandible (lower jaw)
14 Total

Each of the facial bones is studied individually or in pairs. After the description of each is a listing of those specific adjoining bones with which they articulate. Knowing these anatomic relationships helps to understand the structure of the bony skeleton of the head.

13

Right and Left Maxillary Bones

The two **maxillae, or maxillary bones,** are the **largest immovable bones of the face.** The only facial bone larger than the maxilla is the movable lower jaw, or mandible. All the other bones of the upper facial area are closely associated with the two maxillae; thus they are structurally the most important bones of the upper face. The right and left maxillary bones are solidly united at the midline below the nasal septum. Each maxilla assists in the formation of three cavities of the face: (1) the mouth, (2) the nasal cavity, and (3) one orbit.

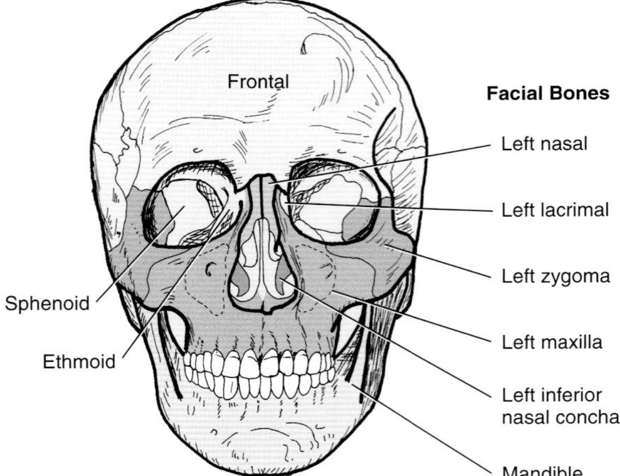

Fig. 13-1. Facial bones—frontal view.

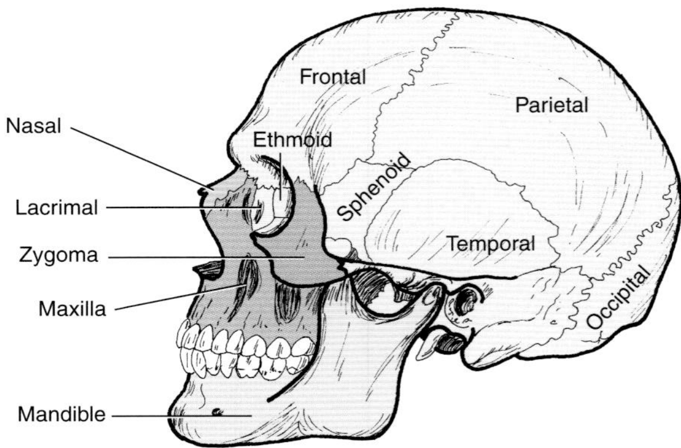

Fig. 13-2. Facial bones—lateral view.

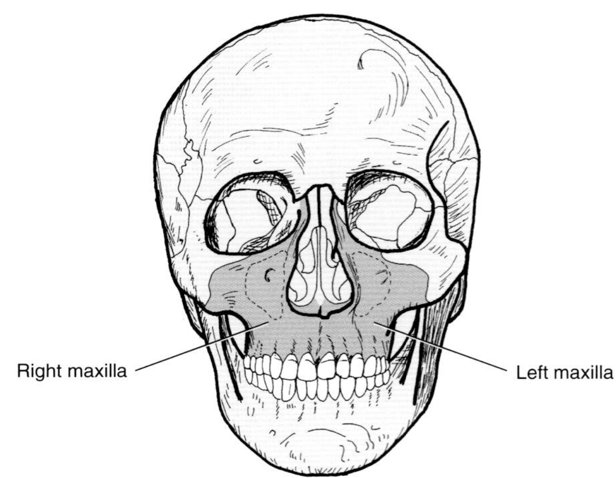

Fig. 13-3. Right and left maxillae.

Lateral view of left maxilla Each maxilla consists of a centrally located **body** and **four processes** projecting from that body. Three processes are more obvious and are visible on the lateral and frontal drawings. The fourth process, described below, is the palatine process, part of the hard palate.

The **body** of each maxilla is the centrally located portion that lies laterally to the nose. One of the three processes is the **frontal process,** which projects upward along the lateral border of the nose toward the frontal bone. The **zygomatic process** projects laterally to unite with the zygoma. The third process, the **alveolar process,** is the inferior aspect of the body of each maxilla. Along the inferior margin of each alveolar process are eight upper teeth.

The two maxillae are solidly united in the midline anteriorly. At the upper part of this midline union is the **anterior nasal spine.** A blow to the nose sometimes results in the nasal spine separating from the maxillae.

A point at the base of the anterior nasal spine is the **acanthion,** described later in this chapter as a surface landmark at the midline point where the nose and upper lip meet.

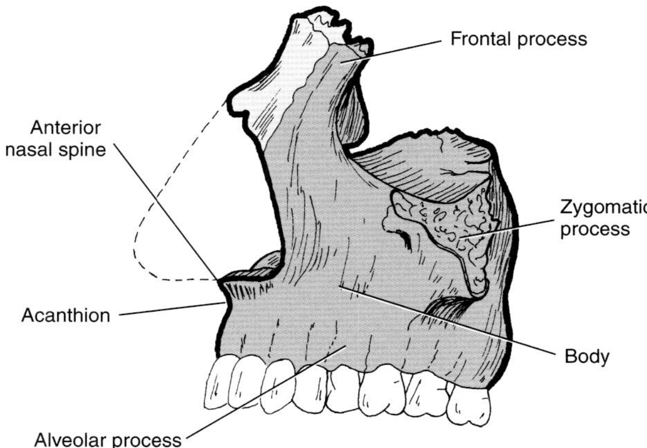

Fig. 13-4. Left maxilla—lateral view.

Frontal view The relationship of the two maxillary bones to the remainder of the bones of the skull is well demonstrated in the frontal view (Fig. 13-5). Note again **three processes,** as seen in the frontal view of the skull. Extending upward toward the frontal bone is the **frontal process.** Extending laterally toward the zygoma is the **zygomatic process,** and supporting the upper teeth is the **alveolar process.**

The body of each maxillary bone contains a large, air-filled cavity known as a **maxillary sinus.** There are several of these air-filled cavities in certain bones of the skull. These sinuses communicate with the nasal cavity and are collectively termed *paranasal sinuses;* they will be described further in this chapter.

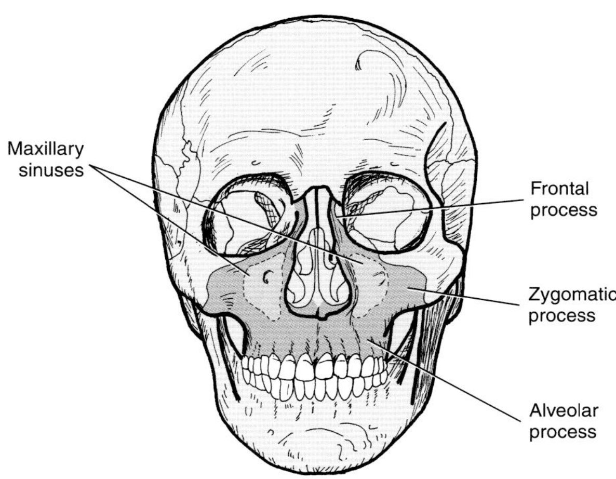

Fig. 13-5. Maxillae—frontal view.

Hard palate (inferior surface) The **fourth process** of each maxillary bone is the palatine process, which can only be demonstrated on an inferior view of the two maxillae (Fig. 13-6). The two palatine processes form the anterior portion of the roof of the mouth, called the *hard,* or *bony palate.* The two palatine processes are solidly united in the midline to form a synarthrodial (immovable) joint. A common congenital defect called a *cleft palate* is an opening between the palatine processes, caused by an incomplete joining of the two bones.

The horizontal portion of two other facial bones, the **palatine bones,** forms the posterior part of the hard palate. Only the horizontal portions of the L-shaped palatine bones are visible on this view. The vertical portions are demonstrated later on a cutaway drawing in Fig. 13-11.

Note the difference between the **palatine process** of the **maxillary bone** and the **separate palatine facial bones.**

The two small inferior portions of the sphenoid bone of the cranium are also shown on this inferior view of the hard palate. These two processes, the **pterygoid hamuli,** are similar to the feet of the outstretched legs of a bat, as described in an earlier drawing in Chapter 12 (see Fig. 12-15).

Articulations Each maxilla articulates with **two cranial bones** (frontal and ethmoid) and with **seven facial bones** (zygoma, lacrimal, nasal, palatine, inferior nasal concha, vomer, and the adjacent maxilla).

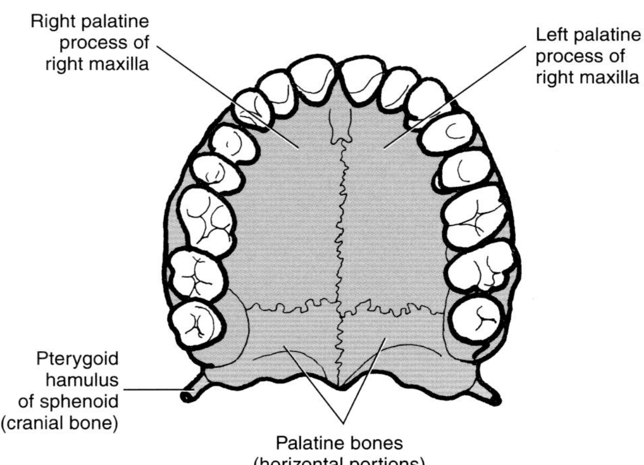

Fig. 13-6. Maxillae and palatine bones—hard palate (inferior surface).

13

Right and Left Zygomatic Bones

One **zygoma** is located lateral to the zygomatic process of each maxilla. These bones (sometimes termed *malar bones*) form the prominence of the cheeks and make up the lower outer portion of the orbits.

Projecting posteriorly from the zygoma is a slender process connecting with the zygomatic process of the temporal bone to form the **zygomatic arch.** The zygomatic arch is a fairly delicate structure and is sometimes fractured or "caved in" by a blow to the cheek. Note that the anterior portion of the arch is formed by the zygoma and the posterior portion by the zygomatic process of the temporal bone. The **zygomatic prominence** is a positioning landmark and refers to this prominent portion of the zygoma.

Articulations Each zygoma articulates with **three cranial bones** (frontal, sphenoid, and temporal) and with **one facial bone** (maxilla).

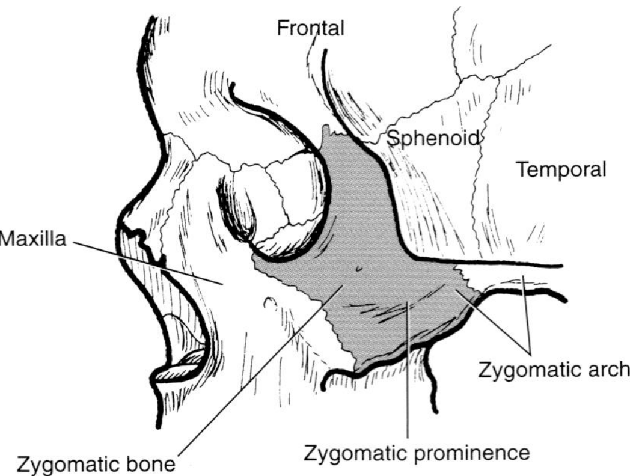

Fig. 13-7. Zygomatic bone—lateral view.

Right and Left Nasal and Lacrimal Bones

The lacrimal and nasal bones are the thinnest and most fragile bones in the entire body.

Lacrimal bones The two small and delicate lacrimal bones (about the size and shape of a fingernail) lie anteriorly on the medial side of each orbit just posterior to the frontal process of the maxilla. *Lacrimal,* derived from a word meaning "tear," is appropriate because the lacrimal bones are closely associated with the tear ducts.

Nasal bones The two fused nasal bones form the bridge of the nose and are somewhat variable in size. Some persons have very prominent nasal bones, whereas others' are quite small. Much of the nose is made up of cartilage, and only the two nasal bones form the upper part of the bridge of the nose. The nasal bones lie anterior and superomedial to the frontal process of the maxillae and inferior to the frontal bone. The point of junction of the two nasal bones with the frontal bone is a surface landmark termed the *nasion.*

Articulations

Lacrimal Each lacrimal bone articulates with **two cranial bones** (frontal and ethmoid) and with **two facial bones** (maxilla and inferior nasal concha).

Nasal Each nasal bone also articulates with **two cranial bones** (frontal and ethmoid) and **with two facial bones** (maxilla and adjacent nasal bone).

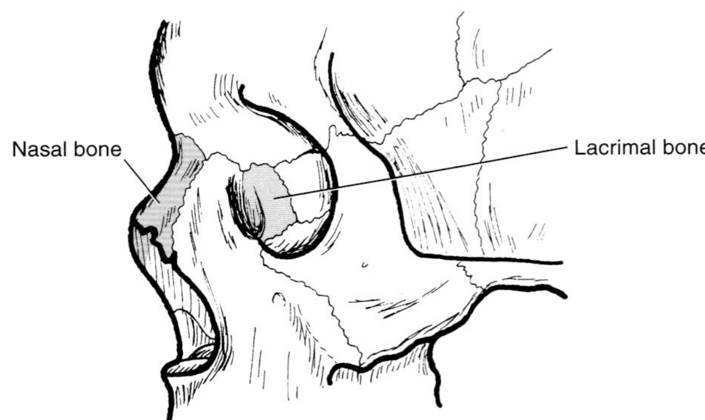

Fig. 13-8. Nasal and lacrimal bones—lateral view.

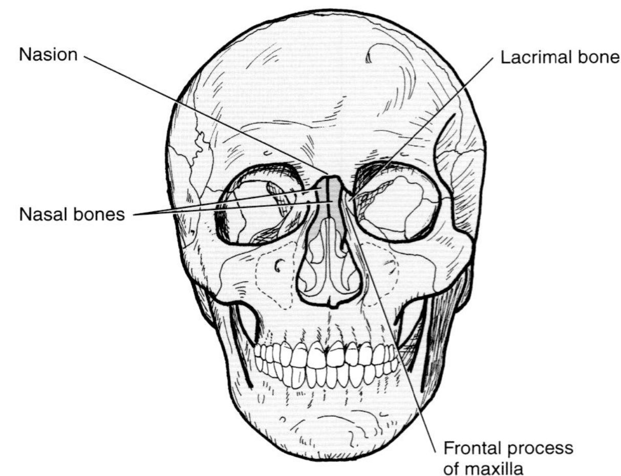

Fig. 13-9. Nasal and lacrimal bones—frontal view.

Right and Left Inferior Nasal Conchae

Within the nasal cavity are two thin, curved (or scroll-shaped) facial bones termed the **inferior nasal conchae** *(turbinates).* These two bones project from the lateral walls of the nasal cavity on each side and extend medially.

The **superior and middle nasal conchae** (turbinates) are similar scroll-like projections that extend from the **ethmoid bone** into the nasal cavities. (These two pairs are not shown separately on the frontal drawing but are shown in Fig. 13-11.)

In summary, there are three pairs of nasal conchae. The **superior and middle pairs are parts of the ethmoid bone,** whereas the **inferior pair are separate facial bones.**

The effect of the three pairs of nasal conchae is to divide the nasal cavities into various compartments. These irregular compartments tend to break up or mix the flow of air coming into the nasal cavities before it reaches the lungs. In this way the incoming air is somewhat warmed and cleaned as it comes in contact with the mucous membrane covering the conchae.

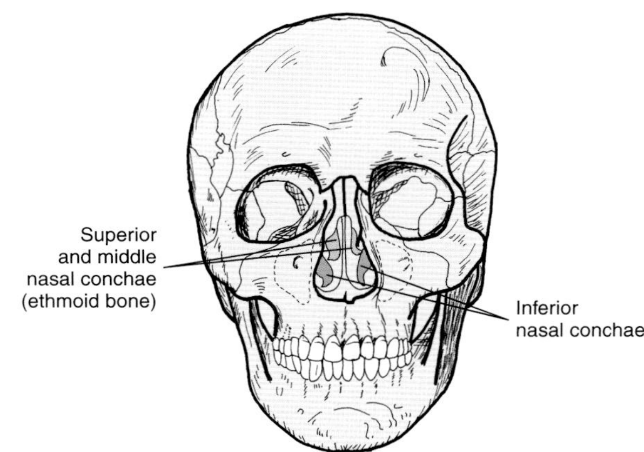

Fig. 13-10. Inferior nasal conchae.

Sectional drawing

Inferior nasal conchae The relationship between the various nasal conchae and the lateral wall of one nasal cavity is illustrated in this sectional drawing (Fig. 13-11). The midline structures making up the nasal septum have been removed so that the lateral portion of the right nasal cavity can be seen. Note that the **superior and middle conchae** are part of the ethmoid bone, and the **inferior nasal conchae** are separate facial bones. The **cribriform plate** and the **crista galli** of the ethmoid bone help to separate the cranium from the facial bone mass. The **palatine process** of the maxilla is again shown.

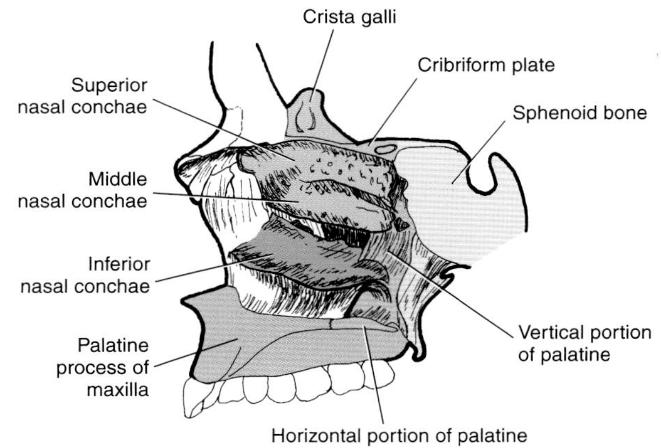

Fig. 13-11. Sectional view drawing—inferior nasal conchae and palatine bones.

Right and Left Palatine Bones

The two **palatine bones** are difficult to visualize in the study of a dry skeleton because they are located internally and are not visible from the outside. Each palatine bone is roughly L-shaped (Fig. 13-11). The vertical portion of the L extends upward between one maxilla and one pterygoid plate of the sphenoid bone. The horizontal portion of each L helps to make up the posterior portion of the hard palate, as shown in an earlier drawing (see Fig. 13-6).

Articulations

Inferior nasal conchae Each inferior nasal conchae articulates with **one cranial bone** (ethmoid) and with **three facial bones** (maxilla, lacrimal, and palatine).

Palatine Each palatine articulates with **two cranial bones** (sphenoid and ethmoid) and **four facial bones** (maxilla, inferior nasal conchae, vomer, and adjacent palatine).

Bony Nasal Septum

The midline structures of the nasal cavity, including the **bony nasal septum,** are shown on this sagittal-view drawing (Fig. 13-12). Two bones—the **ethmoid** and the **vomer**—form the bony nasal septum. This septum is formed superiorly by the **perpendicular plate** of the ethmoid bone and inferiorly by the single vomer bone. Anteriorly the nasal septum is cartilaginous and is termed the **septal cartilage.**

The perpendicular plate of the ethmoid bone and the vomer form the **bony nasal septum,** which can be demonstrated radiographically.

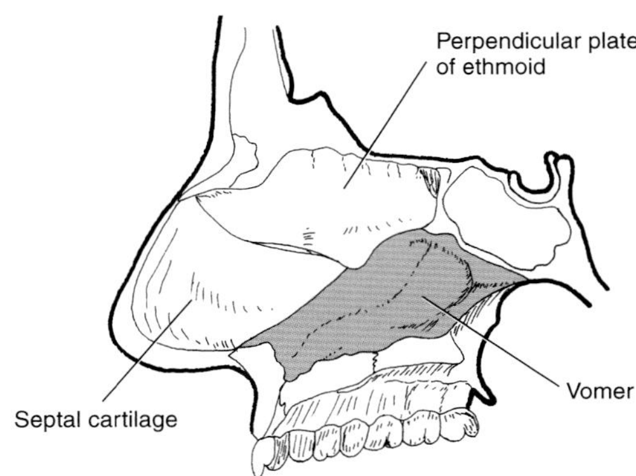

Fig. 13-12. Bony nasal septum and vomer.

Vomer

The single **vomer bone** (meaning "plowshare") is a thin, triangular-shaped bone that forms the inferoposterior part of the nasal septum. The surfaces of the vomer are marked by small furrow-like depressions for blood vessels, a source of nosebleed with trauma to the nasal area. A deviated nasal septum describes the clinical condition wherein the nasal septum is deflected or displaced laterally from the midline of the nose. This deviation usually occurs at the site of junction between the septal cartilage and the vomer. A severe deviation can entirely block the nasal passageway, making breathing through the nose impossible.

Articulations The vomer articulates with **two cranial bones** (sphenoid and ethmoid) and with **four facial bones** (right and left palatine bones and right and left maxillae). The vomer also articulates with the septal cartilage.

13

Mandible

The last and largest of the facial bones is the lower jaw, or **mandible.** It is the only movable bone in the adult skull. This large facial bone, which is a single bone in the adult, actually originates from two separate bones. The two bones in the infant join to become one at approximately 1 year of age.

Lateral view The **angle** (gonion) of the mandible divides each half of the mandible into two main parts. That area anterior to the angle is termed the **body** of the mandible, whereas the area superior to each angle is termed the **ramus.** Because the mandible is a single bone, the body actually extends from the left angle around to the right angle.

The lower teeth are rooted in the mandible; therefore an **alveolar process,** or ridge, extends along the entire superior portion of the body of the mandible.

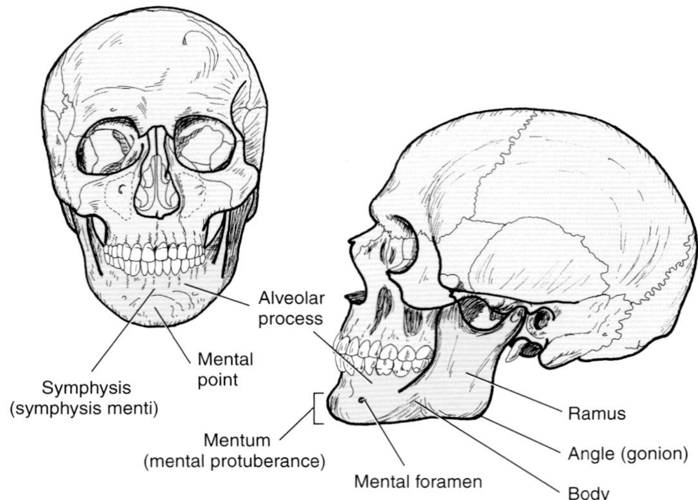

Fig. 13-13. Mandible—lateral and frontal views.

Frontal view The anterior aspect of the adult mandible is best seen on a frontal view. The single body forms from each lateral half and unites at the anterior midline. This union is called the **symphysis** of the mandible, or **symphysis menti.** The flat triangular area below the symphysis, projecting forward, is called the **mentum,** or **mental protuberance.** The center of the mental protuberance is described as the **mental point.** *Mentum* and *mental* are Latin words referring to the general area known as the chin. The mental point is a specific point of the chin, whereas the mentum is the entire area.

Located on each half of the body of the mandible are the **mental foramina.** These foramina serve as passageways for nerves and blood vessels.

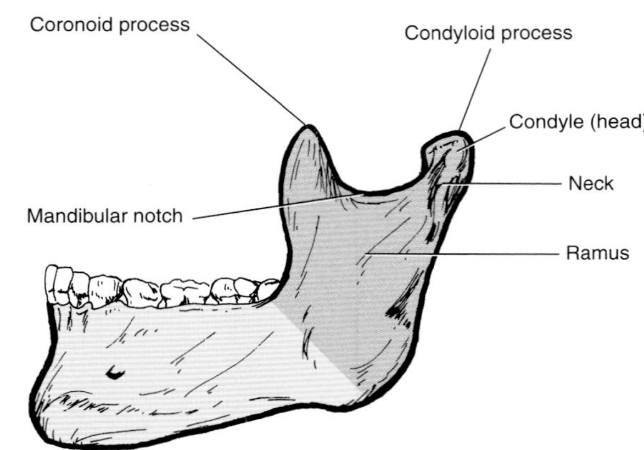

Fig. 13-14. Ramus of mandible—lateral view.

13

Ramus The upper portion of each **ramus** terminates in a U-shaped notch termed the **mandibular notch.** At each end of the mandibular notch is a process. The process at the anterior end of the mandibular notch is termed the **coronoid process.** This process does not articulate with another bone and cannot be easily palpated, because it lies just inferior to the zygomatic arch and serves as a site for muscle attachment.

Memory aid The **coronoid process** of the mandible must not be confused with the **coronoid process** of the proximal ulna of the forearm or the **coracoid process** of the scapula. One way to remember these terms is to associate *n* in coronoid with the *n* in each of the words *ulna* and *mandible.*

The posterior process of the upper ramus is termed the **condyloid process** and consists of two parts. The rounded end of the condyloid process is the **condyle** or **head,** whereas the constricted area directly below the condyle is the **neck.** The condyle of the condyloid process fits into the temporomandibular fossa of the temporal bone to form the **temporomandibular joint (TMJ)** (see following page).

Submentovertex projection The horseshoe shape of the mandible is well visualized on a **submentovertex** (SMV) projection (Fig. 13-15). Note that the mandible is a fairly thin structure, which explains why it is susceptible to fractures. The area of the **mentum** is well demonstrated, as are the **body** and **rami** of the mandible. The relative position of the upper ramus and its associated **coronoid process** and **condyle** are also demonstrated with this projection. Note that the condyle projects medial and the coronoid process slightly lateral on this view.

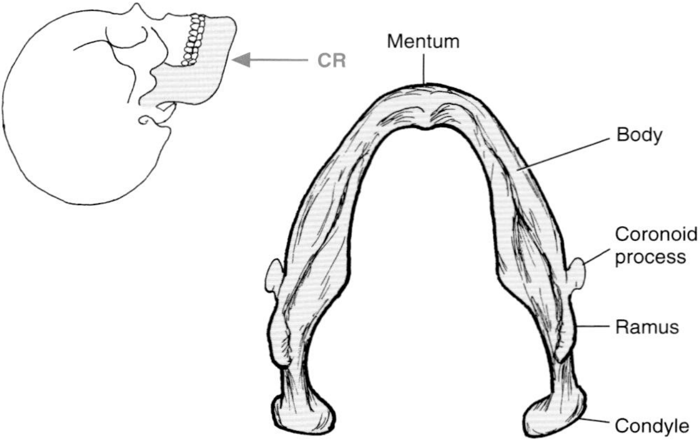

Fig. 13-15. Submentovertex (SMV) projection of mandible.

Temporomandibular Joint

The temporomandibular joint (TMJ), the only movable joint in the skull, is shown on this lateral drawing and on the lateral-view photograph of a dry skull (Figs. 13-16 and 13-17). The relationship of the mandible to the temporal bone of the cranium is well demonstrated.

The TMJ is formed by the **condyle,** (head) of the condyloid process of the mandible fitting into the **temporomandibular fossa** of the temporal bone. The TMJ is located just anterior and slightly superior to the **external acoustic meatus (EAM).**

JOINT CLASSIFICATIONS (MANDIBLE AND SKULL)

Synovial Joints (Diarthrodial)

The TMJ is classified as a **synovial type** of joint, which is **diarthrodial,** or freely movable. This synovial joint is divided into upper and lower synovial cavities by a single articular fibrous disk. A series of strong ligaments join the condylar neck of the mandible to the lower borders of the zygomatic process of the temporal bone.

The two-part articular capsule is lined by synovial membrane and divided by the articular disk. This complete two-part synovial joint, along with its fibrous articular disk, allows for not only a **hinge-type motion** but also a **gliding movement,** wherein the mandibular condyle glides forward as the mouth is opened. This movement is facilitated further by the shallow temporomandibular fossa with which the condyle of the mandible articulates.

Fibrous Joints (Synarthrodial)

There are two types of *fibrous* joints involving the skull, both of which are **synarthrodial,** or immovable. First are the **sutures** between cranial bones, as described in the preceding chapter. Second is a unique type of fibrous joint involving the teeth with the mandible and maxillae. This is a **gomphosis** *(gom-fo'sis)* subclass type of fibrous joint between the roots of the teeth and the alveolar processes of both the maxillae and the mandible.

TMJ motion The drawings and radiographs below illustrate the TMJ in both **open-** and **closed-mouth** positions. When the mouth is opened widely, the condyle moves forward to the front edge of the fossa. If the condyle slips too far anteriorly, the joint may dislocate. If the TMJ dislocates, either by force or by jaw motion, it may be difficult or even impossible to close the mouth, which returns the condyle to its normal position.

Radiographs (open and closed mouth) Two axiolateral projections (Schuller method) of the TMJ are shown below in closed- and open-mouth positions. The range of anterior movement of the condyle in relationship to the temporomandibular fossa is clearly demonstrated.

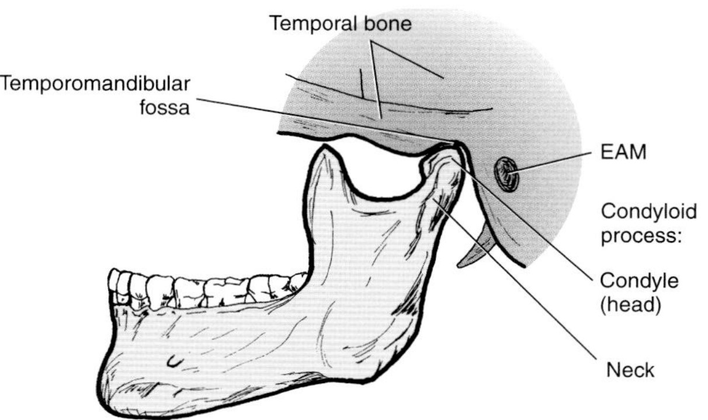

Fig. 13-16. Temporomandibular joint (TMJ).

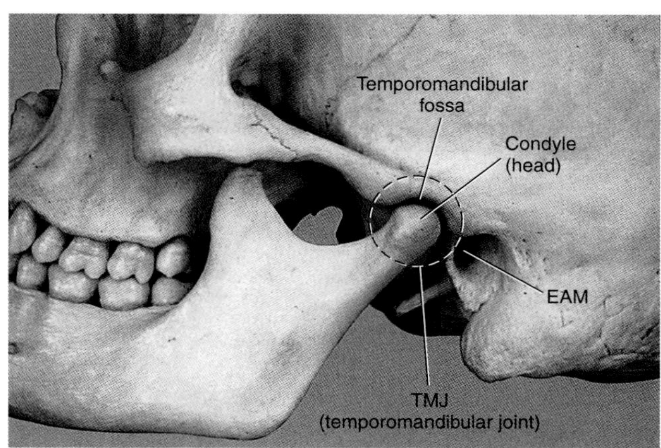

Fig. 13-17. Joints of mandible.

JOINTS OF MANDIBLE	
Temporomandibular Joint	**Alveoli and Roots of Teeth**
Classification:	Classification:
Synovial *(diarthrodial)*	***Fibrous*** *(synarthrodial)*
Movement types:	Subclass:
Ginglymus *(hinge)*	***Gomphosis***
Plane *(gliding)*	

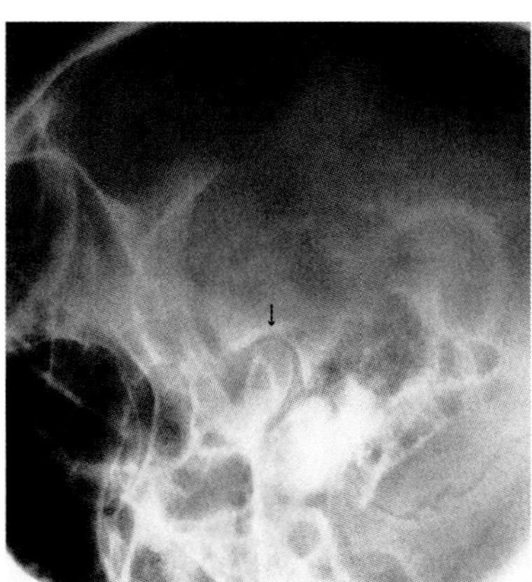

Fig. 13-18. Closed mouth.

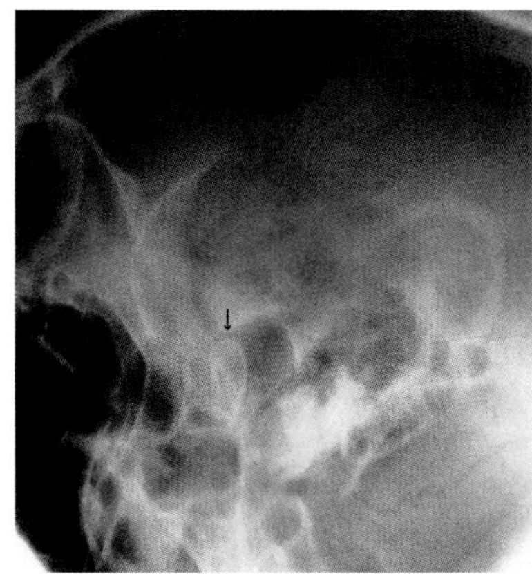

Fig. 13-19. Open mouth.

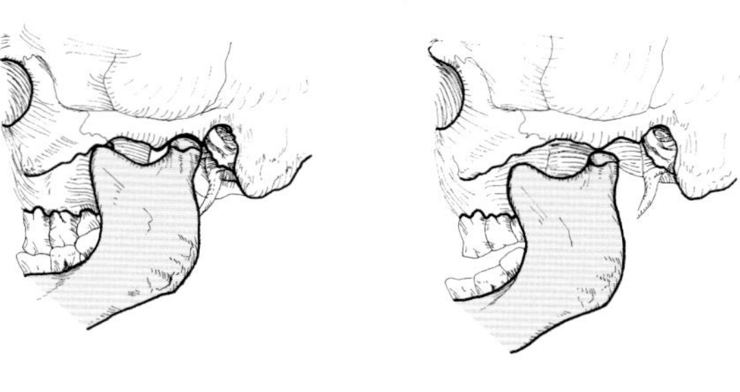

Fig. 13-20. TMJ motion.

13

PARANASAL SINUSES

The large, air-filled cavities of the **paranasal sinuses** are sometimes called the accessory nasal sinuses because they are lined with mucous membrane, which is continuous with the nasal cavity. These sinuses are divided into four groups, according to the bones that contain them:

1. **Maxillary** (2) — Maxillary (facial) bones
2. **Frontal** (usually 2) — Frontal (cranial) bones
3. **Ethmoid** (many) — Ethmoid (cranial) bones
4. **Sphenoid** (1 or 2) — Sphenoid (cranial) bone

Only the **maxillary sinuses** are part of the **facial bone** structure. The **frontal, ethmoid,** and **sphenoid** sinuses are contained within their respective **cranial bones.**

The paranasal sinuses begin developing in the fetus, but only the maxillary sinuses exhibit a definite cavity at birth. The frontal and sphenoid sinuses begin to be visible on radiographs at age 6 or 7. The ethmoid sinuses develop last. All the paranasal sinuses are generally fully developed by the late teenage years.

Each of these groups of sinuses will be studied, beginning with the largest, the maxillary sinuses.

Maxillary Sinuses

The large **maxillary sinuses** are paired structures, one being located within the body of each maxillary bone. An older term for maxillary sinus is **antrum,** an abbreviation of **"Antrum of Highmore."**

Each maxillary sinus is shaped somewhat like a pyramid on a frontal view. Laterally, they appear more cubic. The average total vertical dimension is between 3 and 4 cm, and the other dimensions are between 2.5 and 3 cm.

The bony walls of the maxillary sinuses are thin. The floor of each maxillary sinus is slightly below the level of the floor of each nasal fossa. The two maxillary sinuses vary in size from one person to another and from one side to the other.

Projecting into the floor of each maxillary sinus are several conic elevations relating to roots of the first and second upper molar teeth (Fig. 13-22). Occasionally, one or more of these roots can allow infections originating in the teeth, particularly in the molars and premolars, to travel upward into the maxillary sinus.

All the paranasal sinus cavities communicate with one another and with the **nasal cavity,** which is divided into two equal chambers, or **fossae.** In the case of the maxillary sinuses, this site of communication is the opening into the middle nasal meatus passageway located at the superior medial aspect of the sinus cavity itself, as demonstrated in Fig. 13-23. This is illustrated in more detail in Fig. 13-27 on the following page. When a person is erect, any mucus or fluid trapped within the sinus will tend to remain there and layer out, forming an air-fluid level. Therefore radiographic positioning of the paranasal sinuses should be accomplished with the patient in the **erect position,** if possible, to demonstrate any possible air-fluid levels.

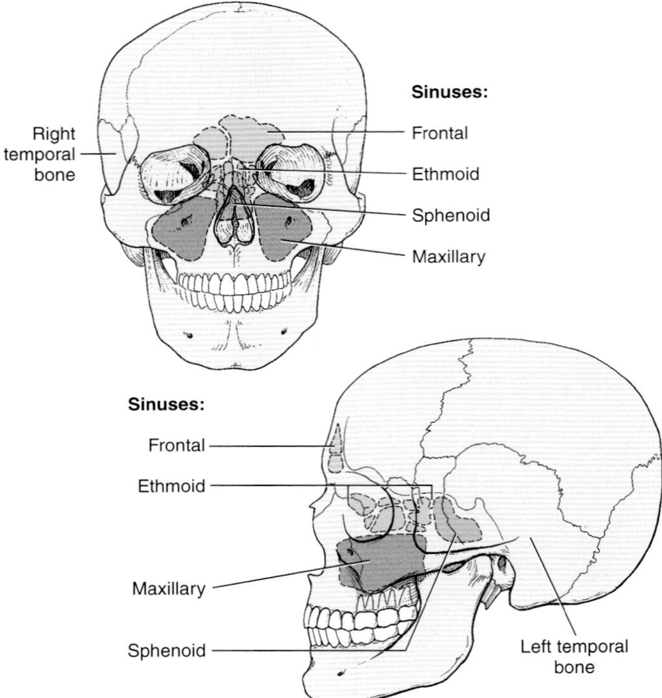

Fig. 13-21. Skull—paranasal sinuses and temporal bone.

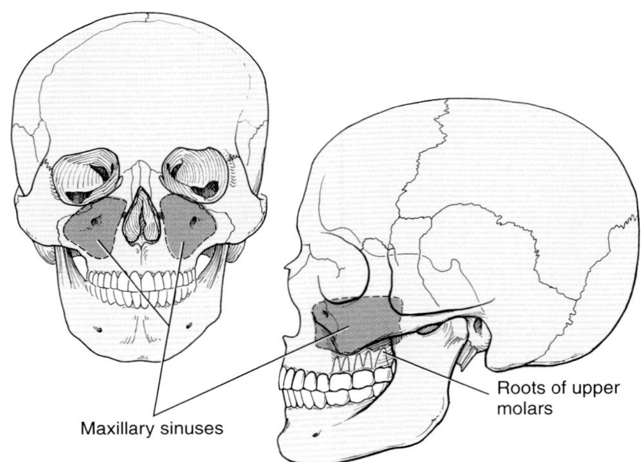

Fig. 13-22. Maxillary sinuses (2).

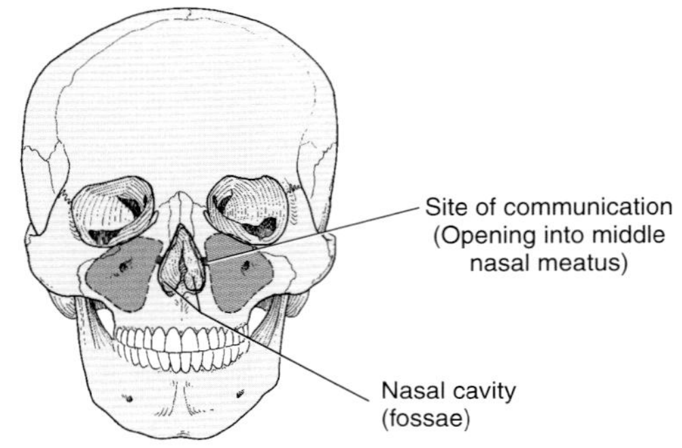

Fig. 13-23. Maxillary sinuses.

Frontal Sinuses

The **frontal sinuses** are located between the inner and outer tables of the skull, posterior to the glabella; they **rarely become aerated before age 6.** The maxillary sinuses are always paired and are usually fairly symmetric in size and shape; the frontal sinuses are rarely symmetric. The frontal sinuses are usually separated by a septum, which deviates from one side to the other or may be absent entirely, resulting in one single cavity. Generally, however, two cavities exist, varying in their sizes and shapes. They are generally larger in men than in women. They may be singular on either the right or left side, they may be paired as shown, or they may be absent.

Ethmoid Sinuses

The **ethmoid sinuses** are contained within the lateral masses or labyrinths of the ethmoid bone. These air cells are grouped into **anterior, middle,** and **posterior collections,** but they all intercommunicate.

When viewed from the side, the anterior ethmoid sinuses appear to fill the orbits. This is because portions of the ethmoid sinuses are contained in the lateral masses of the ethmoid bone, which helps to form the medial wall of each orbit.

Sphenoid Sinuses

The **sphenoid sinuses** lie in the body of the sphenoid bone directly below the sella turcica. The body of the sphenoid containing these sinuses is cubic and is frequently divided by a thin septum to form two cavities. This septum may be incomplete or absent entirely, however, resulting in only one cavity.

Since the sphenoid sinuses are so close to the base or floor of the cranium, sometimes pathologic processes make their presence known by the effect on these sinuses. An example is the demonstration of an air-fluid level within the sphenoid sinuses following skull trauma. This may be evidence that the patient has a basal skull fracture and that either blood or cerebrospinal fluid is leaking through the fracture into the sphenoid sinuses, a condition referred to as **sphenoid effusion.**

Osteomeatal complex The pathways of communication between the frontal, maxillary, and ethmoid sinuses provide drainage between these sinus cavities. These drainage pathways make up the **osteomeatal complex,** which can become obstructed and lead to infection of these sinuses, a condition termed **sinusitis.**

Fig. 13-27 illustrates **two key passageways** (infundibulum and middle nasal meatus) and their associated structures identified on coronal computed tomography (CT) sections.

As seen from this drawing, the **large maxillary sinus** drains through the **infundibulum** passageway down through the **middle nasal meatus** into the **inferior nasal meatus.** The **uncinate process** of the ethmoid bone makes up the medial wall of the infundibulum passageway. The **ethmoid bulla** receives drainage from the frontal and ethmoid sinus cells, which then drains down through the middle nasal meatus into the inferior nasal meatus, where it exits the body through the exterior nasal orifice.

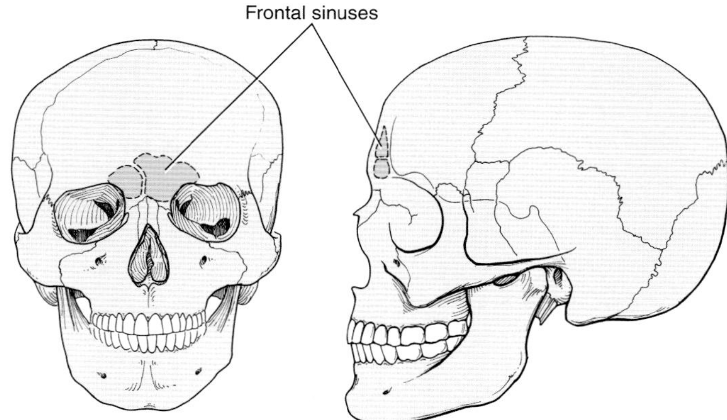

Fig. 13-24. Frontal sinuses.

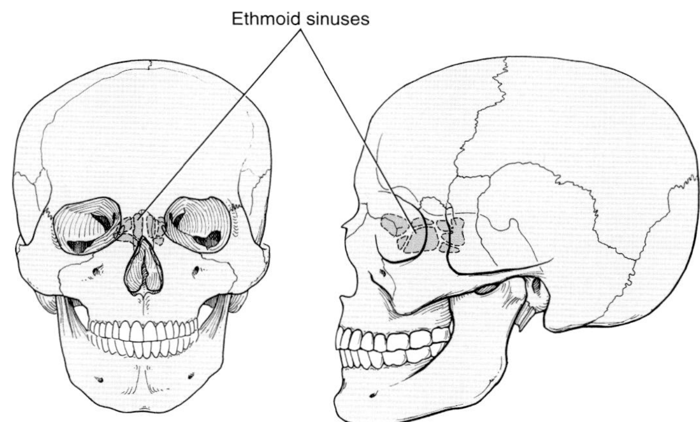

Fig. 13-25. Ethmoid sinuses.

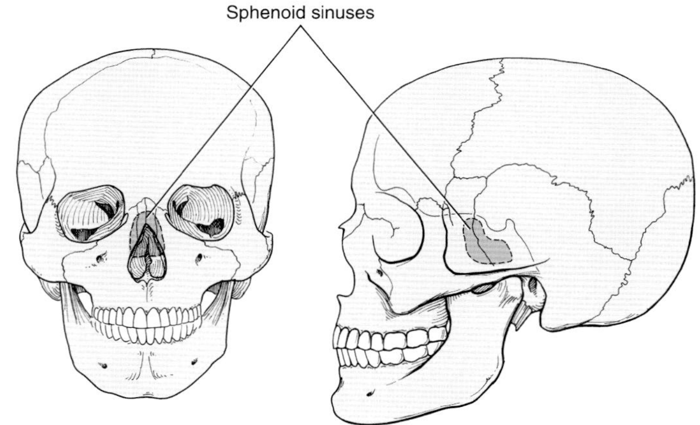

Fig. 13-26. Sphenoid sinuses.

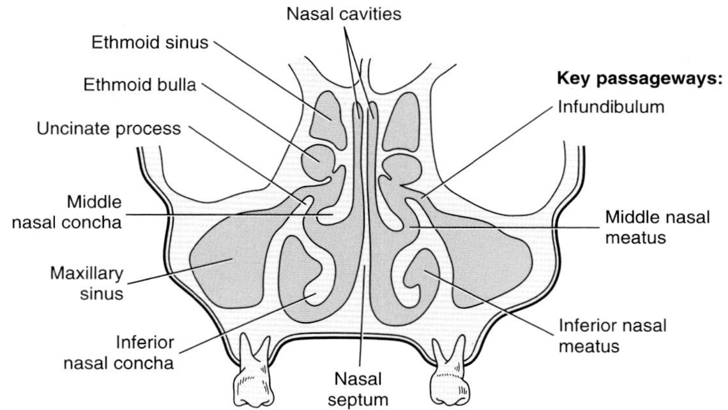

Fig. 13-27. Osteomeatal complex–coronal sectional view.

13

RADIOGRAPHS—PARANASAL SINUSES

Drawings of the sinuses on preceding pages included definite sizes and shapes of the sinuses with clear-cut borders. In actual radiographs these borders are not nearly as definite, because the various sinuses overlap and superimpose each other as seen on these radiographs of four common sinus projections. The labeled radiographs clearly demonstrate the relative locations and relationships of each of these sinuses. Note the following abbreviations: **F**—Frontal sinuses, **E**—Ethmoid sinuses, **M**—Maxillary sinuses, **S**—Sphenoid sinuses.

Lateral Position (Fig. 13-28)

The frontal sinuses are clearly visualized between the inner and outer tables of the skull.

The sphenoid sinuses appear to be continuous with the ethmoid sinuses anteriorly.

The large maxillary sinuses are clearly visualized. Note that the roots of the molars and premolars of the upper teeth appear to extend up through the floor of the maxillary sinuses.

PA (Caldwell) Projection (Fig. 13-29)

The frontal, ethmoid, and maxillary sinuses are clearly illustrated in this PA axial projection radiograph. The sphenoid sinuses are not demonstrated specifically, because they are located directly posterior to the ethmoid sinuses. This relationship is demonstrated on the lateral view (Fig. 13-28) and the SMV projection (Fig. 13-31).

PA Axial Transoral Projection (Open-Mouth Waters) (Fig. 13-30)

All four groups of sinuses are clearly demonstrated on this projection taken with mouth open and the head tipped back to separate and project the sphenoid sinuses inferior to the ethmoid sinuses. The open mouth also removes the upper teeth from direct superimposition of the sphenoid sinuses. The pyramid-shaped maxillary sinuses are clearly seen.

13

The mastoid air cells also visualize on each side, posterolateral to the mandible *(arrows).* They appear as small air-filled clusters within the mastoid portions of the temporal bone as described in Chapter 12, but they are not part of the paranasal sinuses.

Submentovertex (SMV) Projection (Fig. 13-31)

This projection is obtained with head tipped back so that the top of the head (vertex) is touching the table/upright Bucky surface and the CR is directed inferior to the chin (mentum).

The centrally located sphenoid sinuses are anterior to the large opening, the foramen magnum. The multiple clusters of ethmoid air cells extend to each side of the nasal septum. The mandible and teeth superimpose the maxillary sinuses. Portions of the maxillary sinuses visualize laterally.

The mastoid portions containing air cells are visualized in Fig. 13-30 (labeled *A*). Fig. 13-31 also demonstrates these air-filled mastoids and the dense petrous portions of the temporal bones (labeled *B*), as described in Chapter 12.

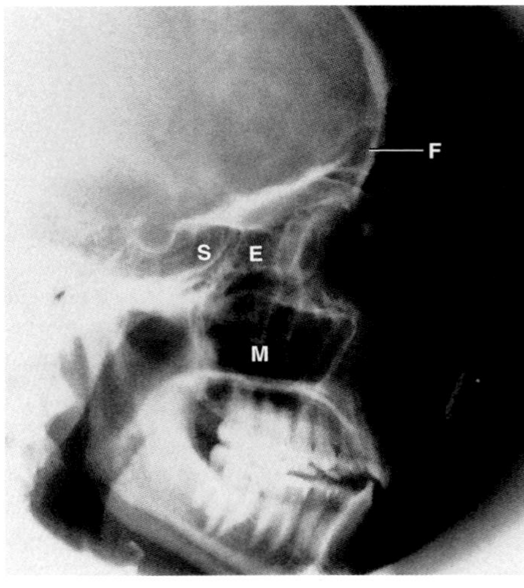

Fig. 13-28. Lateral sinuses position.

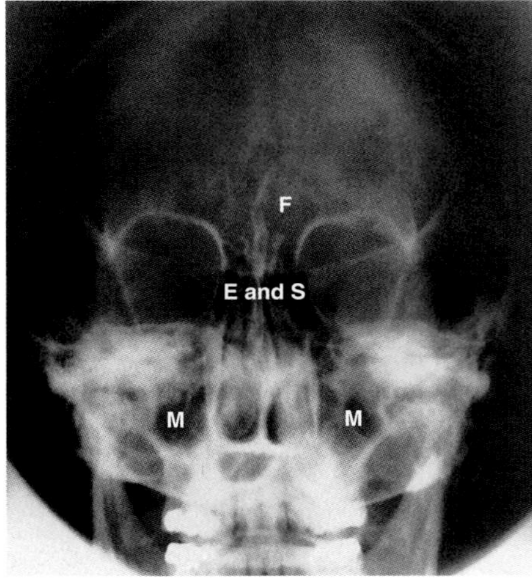

Fig. 13-29. PA Caldwell projection.

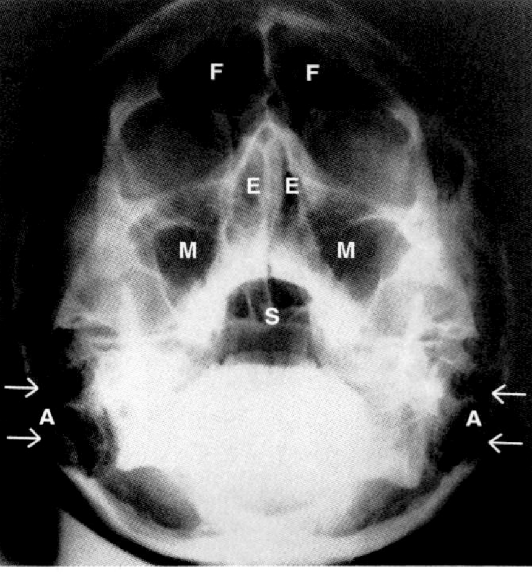

Fig. 13-30. PA axial transoral projection (open-mouth Waters).

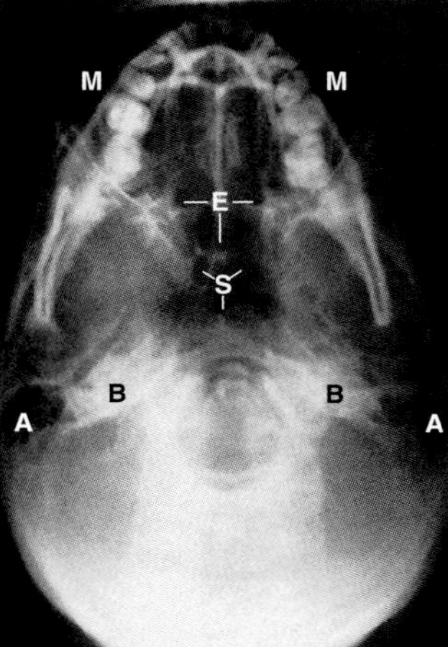

Fig. 13-31. SMV projection.

ORBITS

The complex anatomy of the 14 facial bones helps to form several facial cavities. Those cavities formed in total or in part by the facial bones are the mouth (oral cavity), the nasal cavities, and the orbits. The mouth and nasal cavities are primarily passageways and, as such, are rarely radiographed. The orbits, however, containing the vital organs of sight and associated nerves and blood vessels, are frequently imaged. The structure and shape of the orbits are illustrated in this simplified drawing (Fig. 13-32). Each orbit is a **cone-shaped,** bony-walled structure as shown on this drawing.

The rim of the orbit, corresponding to the outer circular portion of the cone, is called the **base.** The base of the orbit is seldom a true circle, however, and may even look like a figure with four definite sides. The posterior portion of the cone, the **apex,** corresponds to the **optic foramen,** through which the optic nerve passes.

The long axes of the orbits project both upward and toward the midline. With the head placed in an upright frontal or lateral position with the orbitomeatal line adjusted parallel to the floor, each orbit would project superiorly at an angle of **30°** and toward the midsagittal plane at an angle of **37°.** These two angles are important for radiographic positioning of the optic foramina. Remember that each optic foramen is located at the apex of its respective orbit. To radiograph either optic foramen, it is necessary to both extend the patient's chin by 30° and rotate the head 37°. The central ray then projects through the base of the orbit along the long axis of the cone-shaped orbit.

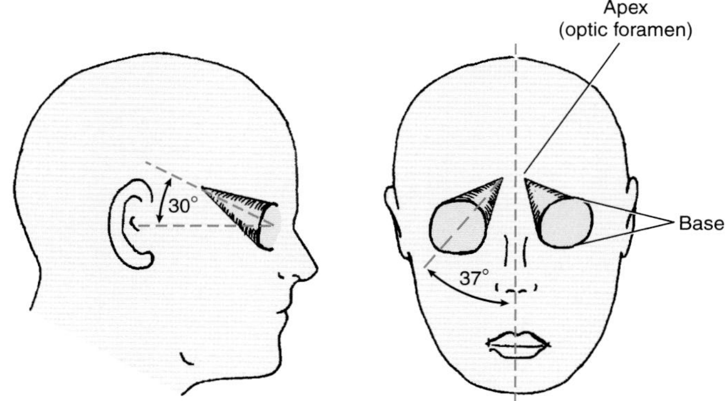

Fig. 13-32. Orbits (cone-shaped).

Bony Composition of Orbits

Each orbit is composed of parts of **seven bones.** The circumference or circular base of each orbit is composed of parts of **three** bones—the **frontal bone (orbital plate)** from the cranium and two from the facial bones—the **maxilla** and the **zygoma** (Fig. 13-33). Inside each orbital cavity are a roof, a floor, and two walls, parts of which are also formed by these three bones. The orbital plate of the frontal bone forms most of the roof of the orbit. The zygoma forms much of the lateral wall and some of the floor of the orbit, whereas a portion of the maxilla helps to form the floor.

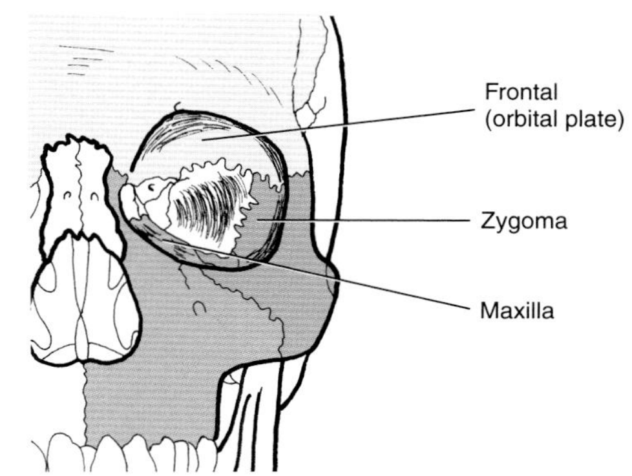

Fig. 13-33. Base of orbit—**three bones** (direct frontal view).

The slightly oblique frontal view in Fig. 13-34 demonstrates all seven bones that form each orbit. The **frontal, zygoma,** and **maxilla** bones, which form the base of the orbit, are again shown. A portion of the medial wall of the orbit is formed by the thin **lacrimal bone.** The **sphenoid** and **ethmoid** bones make up most of the posterior orbit, whereas only a small bit of the **palatine** bone contributes to the innermost posterior portion of the floor of each orbit.

In summary, the **seven** bones making up each orbit include **three cranial bones** and **four facial bones** as shown in the chart below.

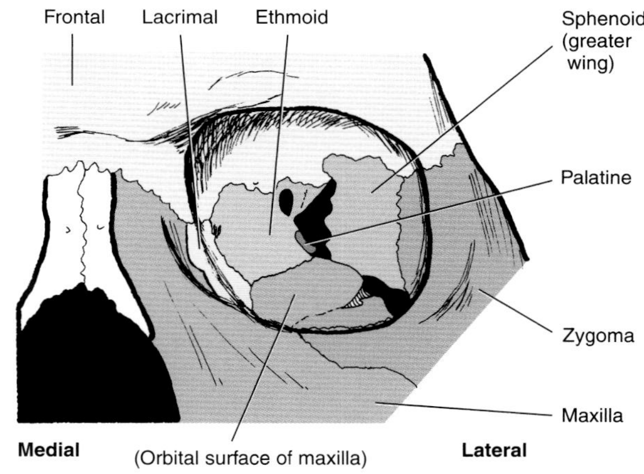

Fig. 13-34. Orbit—seven bones (slightly oblique frontal view).

SUMMARY CHART—BONES OF ORBITS

Cranial Bones	Facial Bones
1. Frontal	1. Maxilla
2. Sphenoid	2. Zygoma
3. Ethmoid	3. Lacrimal
	4. Palatine

Openings in Posterior Orbit

Each orbit also contains three holes or openings in the posterior portion, as demonstrated (Fig. 13-35). These openings provide for passage of specific cranial nerves. (The 12 pairs of cranial nerves are listed and described in the anatomy section of Chapter 22, Computed Tomography.)

The **optic foramen** is a small hole in the sphenoid bone, located posteriorly at the apex of the cone-shaped orbit. The optic foramen allows for passage of the optic nerve (CN II), which is a continuation of the retina.

The **superior orbital fissure** is a cleft or opening between the greater and lesser wings of the sphenoid bone, located lateral to the optic foramen. It allows for transmission of four primary cranial nerves (CN III–VI), which control movement of the eye and eyelid.

A third opening is the **inferior orbital fissure,** located between the maxilla, zygomatic bone, and greater wing of the sphenoid. It allows for transmission of the maxillary branch of CN V, which permits sensory innervation for the cheek, nose, upper lip, and teeth.

The small root of bone separating the superior orbital fissure and the optic canal is known as the **sphenoid strut.** The optic canal is a small canal into which the optic foramen opens. Therefore any abnormal enlargement of the optic nerve could cause erosion of the sphenoid strut, which is actually a portion of the lateral wall of the optic canal.

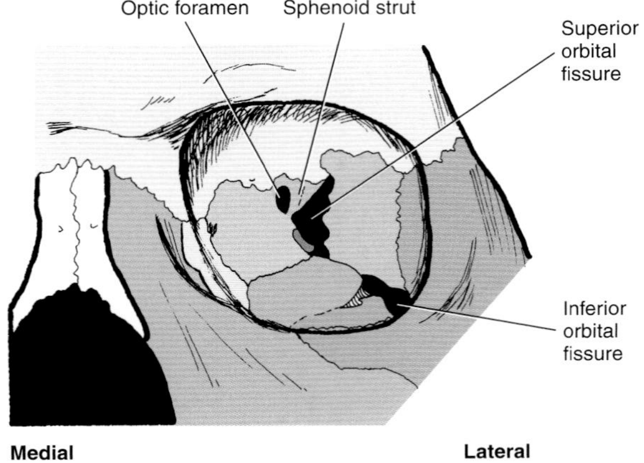

Fig. 13-35. Orbits—posterior openings (slightly oblique frontal view).

ANATOMY REVIEW

Review exercises for anatomy of the cranial and facial bones follow, as demonstrated on both a dry skull and on radiographs. Some anatomic parts identified on the dry skull are not visualized on these radiographs. Those parts that are identifiable are labeled as such. A good learning and/or review exercise is to carefully study both the dry skull illustrations and the radiographs and identify each part before looking at the answers below.

13

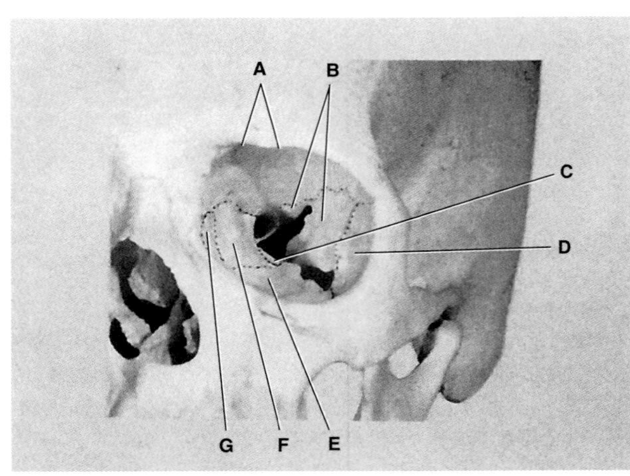

Fig. 13-36. Seven bones of left orbit.

Seven Bones of Left Orbit (Fig. 13-36)

A. Frontal bone (orbital plate)
B. Sphenoid bone
C. Small portion of palatine bone
D. Zygomatic bone
E. Maxillary bone
F. Ethmoid bone
G. Lacrimal bone

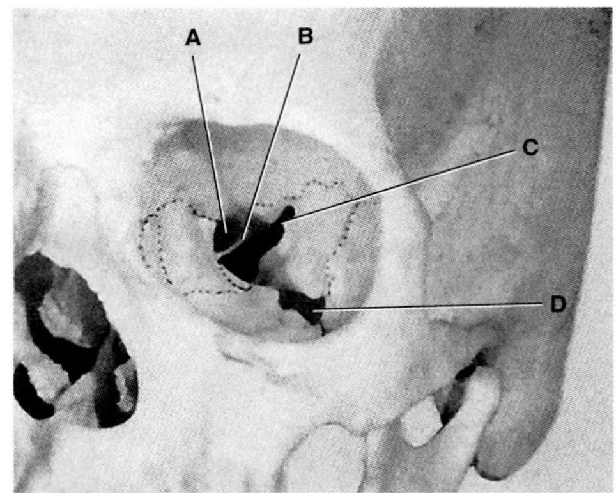

Fig. 13-37. Openings of left orbit.

Openings and Structures of Left Orbit (Fig. 13-37)

A. Optic foramen
B. Sphenoid strut
C. Superior orbital fissure
D. Inferior orbital fissure

Parietoorbital Oblique Projection of Orbits (Fig. 13-38)

A. Orbital plate of frontal bone
B. Sphenoid bone
C. Optic foramen and canal
D. Superior orbital fissure
E. Inferior orbital margin
F. Sphenoid strut (part of inferior and lateral wall of optic canal)
G. Lateral orbital margin
H. Superior orbital margin

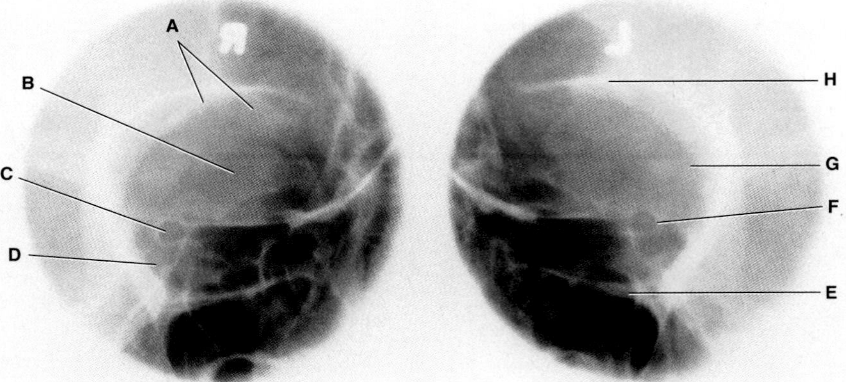

Fig. 13-38. Parietoorbital oblique projection of orbits.

Facial Bones—Lateral (Figs. 13-39 and 13-40)

*A. Zygomatic arch
*B. Right zygomatic bone
*C. Right nasal bone
*D. Frontal process of right maxilla
E. Anterior nasal spine
F. Alveolar process of maxilla
G. Alveolar process of mandible
H. Mentum or mental protuberance
*I. Mental foramen
J. Body of mandible
K. Angle (gonion)
L. Ramus of mandible
M. Coronoid process
*N. Mandibular notch
O. Neck of mandibular condyle
P. Condyle or head of mandible
Q. External acoustic meatus (EAM)
R. Temporomandibular fossa of temporal bone
†S. Greater wings of sphenoid
†T. Lesser wings of sphenoid with anterior clinoid processes
†U. Ethmoid sinuses between orbits
†V. Body of maxilla containing maxillary sinuses

Facial Bones—Parietoacanthial (Waters) (Figs. 13-41 and 13-42)

The photograph (Fig. 13-41) and radiograph (Fig. 13-42) represent the skull in a parietoacanthial projection (Waters position), with the head tilted back. This is one of the more common projections to visualize the facial bones, as follows:

A. Zygomatic prominence
B. Body of maxilla (contains maxillary sinuses)
C. Bony nasal septum (perpendicular plate of ethmoid and vomer bone)
D. Anterior nasal spine
E. Zygomatic arch
F. Coronoid process (Fig. 13-42 only)
G. Condyle (head)
H. Mastoid process of temporal bone
I. Angle of mandible
J. Foramen magnum (Fig. 13-42, which demonstrates the dens or odontoid process within foramen magnum)

*Skeleton only (Fig. 13-39).
†Radiograph only (Fig. 13-40)

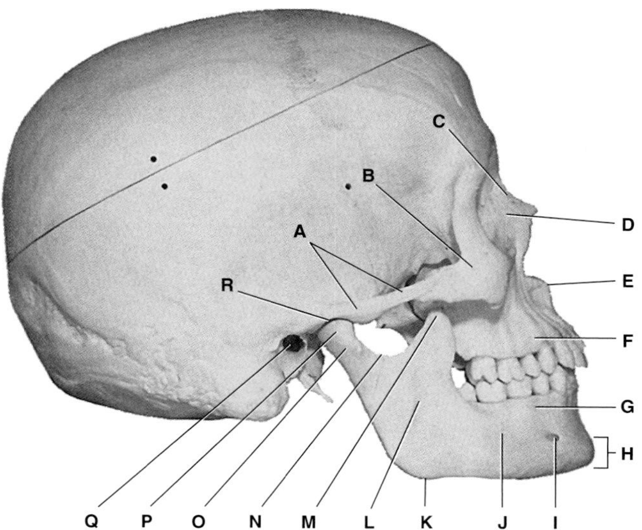

Fig. 13-39. Facial bones—lateral.

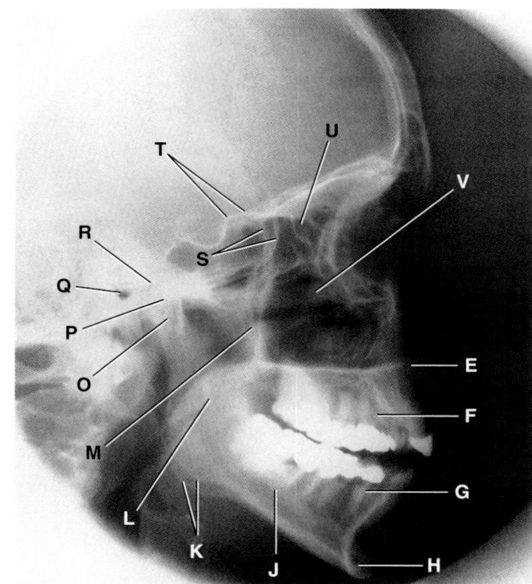

Fig. 13-40. Facial bones—lateral.

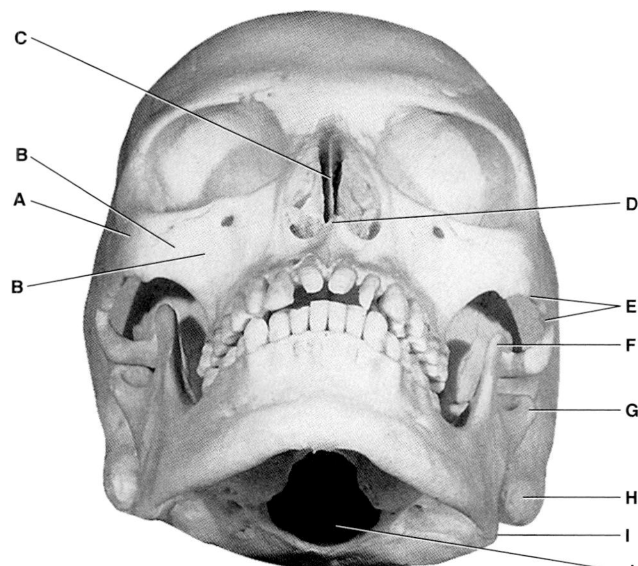

Fig. 13-41. Facial bones—parietoacanthial projection (Waters).

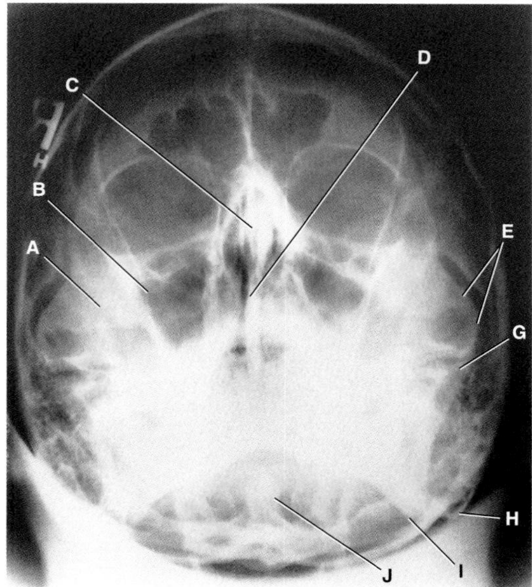

Fig. 13-42. Facial bones—parietoacanthial projection (Waters).

13

Facial Bones—SMV (Inferior View)

Fig. 13-43 illustrates an inferior view of the dry skull with the mandible removed. The SMV projection radiograph in Fig. 13-44 demonstrates positioning where the top of the head (vertex) is placed against the IR and the central ray enters under the chin (mentum).

Skull only (Fig. 13-43):

A. Zygomatic arch
B. Palatine process of maxilla
C. Horizontal process of palatine bone
D. Pterygoid hamulus of sphenoid

Radiograph only (Fig. 13-44):

E. Foramen ovale of sphenoid
F. Foramen spinosum of sphenoid
G. Foramen magnum
H. Petrous pyramid of temporal bone
I. Mastoid portion of temporal bone
J. Sphenoid sinus in body of sphenoid
K. Condyle (head) of mandible
L. Posterior border (vertical portion) of palatine bone
M. Vomer or bony nasal septum
N. Right maxillary sinuses
O. Ethmoid sinuses

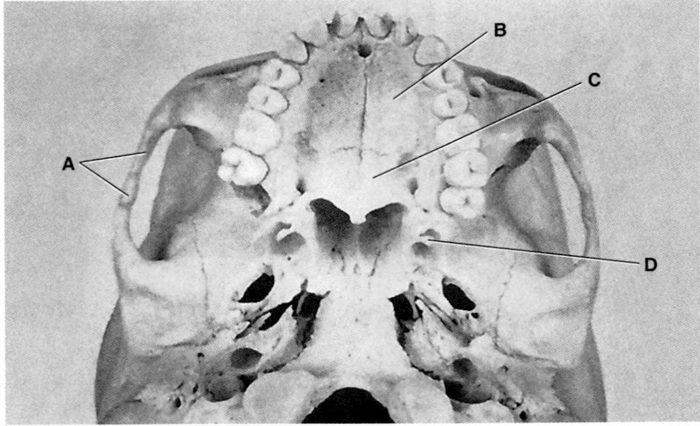

Fig. 13-43. Facial bones—inferior view.

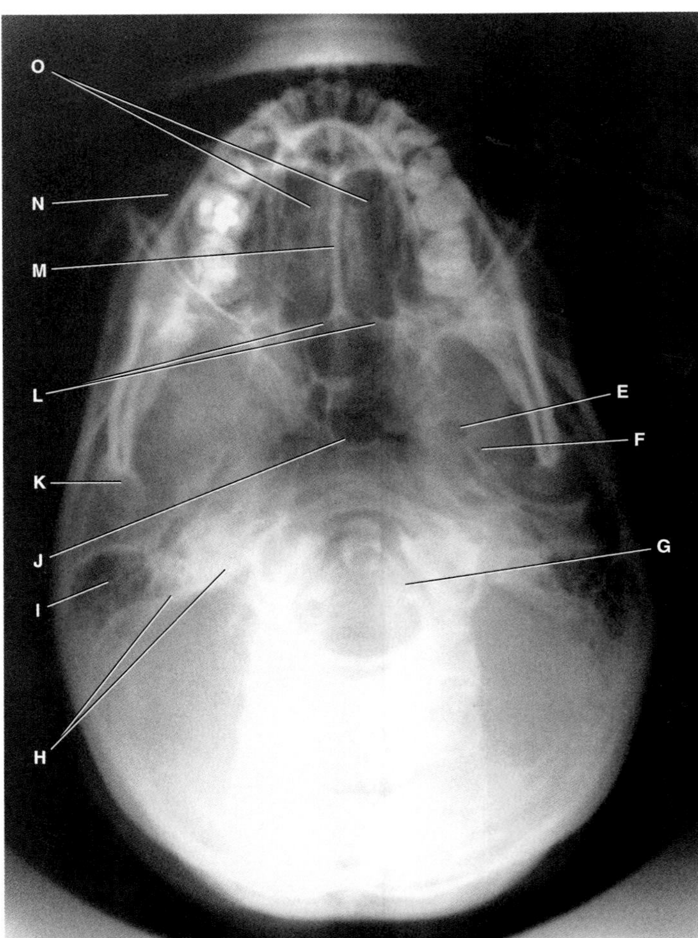

Fig. 13-44. Submentovertex (SMV) projection.

Facial Bones—Frontal View (Fig. 13-45)

A. Left nasal bone
B. Frontal process of left maxilla
C. Optic foramen
D. Superior orbital fissure
E. Inferior orbital fissure
F. Superior and middle nasal conchae of ethmoid bone
G. Vomer bone (lower portion of bony nasal septum)
H. Left inferior nasal conchae
I. Anterior nasal spine
J. Alveolar process of left maxilla
K. Alveolar process of left mandible
L. Mental foramen
M. Mentum or mental protuberance
N. Body of right mandible
O. Angle (gonion) of right mandible
P. Ramus of right mandible
Q. Body of right maxilla (contains maxillary sinuses)
R. Zygomatic prominence of right zygomatic bone
S. Outer orbit portion of right zygomatic bone
T. Sphenoid bone (cranial bone)

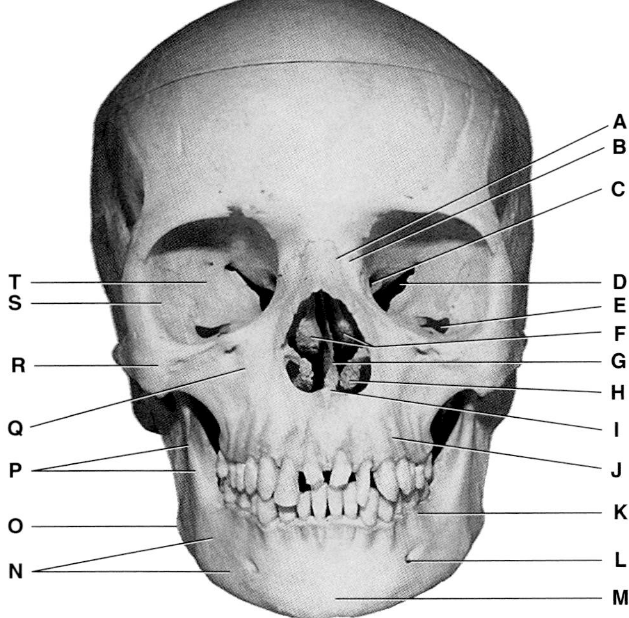

Fig. 13-45. Facial bones—frontal view.

13

RADIOGRAPHIC POSITIONING

Positioning Considerations

FACIAL BONES

Positioning considerations for the facial bones are similar to those of the skull, as described in the previous chapter.

Special Projections and Anatomic Relationships

Unobstructed radiographic images of various aspects of the cranium and facial bones are difficult to obtain because of the overall shape and structures of the skull. For example, dense internal bony structures of the skull will superimpose the delicate facial bones on a routine AP or PA projection. Therefore very specific CR angles and head positions are required, as described and illustrated below.

PA SKULL PROJECTION

The PA skull projection on the right (Fig. 13-47) was obtained with no tube angulation and with the OML (*dotted line* in Fig. 13-46) perpendicular to the plane of the image receptor. The central ray is therefore parallel to the OML. This position results in the **petrous pyramids being projected directly into the orbits.** Drawn on both images (see Figs. 13-46 and 13-47) is a line through the roof of the orbits and through the petrous ridges. With the orbits superimposed by the petrous pyramids, very little facial bone detail can be demonstrated radiographically. Therefore, with the head in this position, the PA projection with a perpendicular central ray has limited value for visualizing the facial bones.

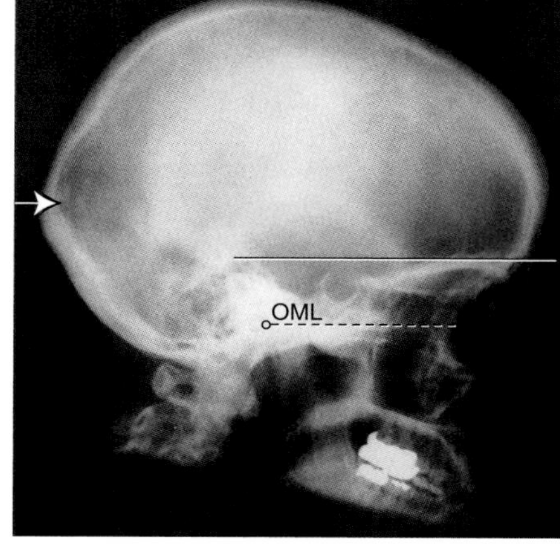

Fig. 13-46. Lateral skull for comparison of bony relationships—CR parallel to OML.

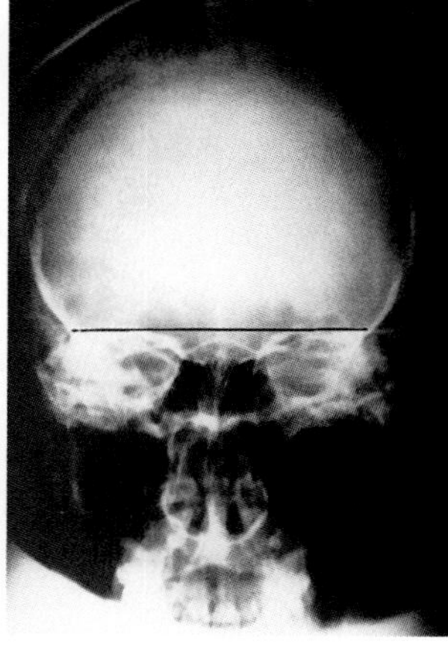

Fig. 13-47. Skull—PA projection.

PARIETOACANTHIAL (WATERS) PROJECTION

To visualize the facial bone mass with conventional radiography, the petrous pyramids must be removed from the facial bone area of interest. This can be done either by tube angulation or by extension of the neck. The radiographs to the right (Figs. 13-48 and 13-49) demonstrate the result. The neck is extended by raising the chin so that the **petrous pyramids are projected just below the maxillary sinuses.** The central ray is parallel to the mentomeatal line (MML). The radiograph on the right (Waters method, Fig. 13-49), if done correctly as described later in this chapter, demonstrates the petrous ridges (see *arrows*) projected below the maxillae and maxillary sinuses. Except for the mandible, the **facial bones are now projected superior to** the dense petrous pyramids and are **not superimposed by** them.

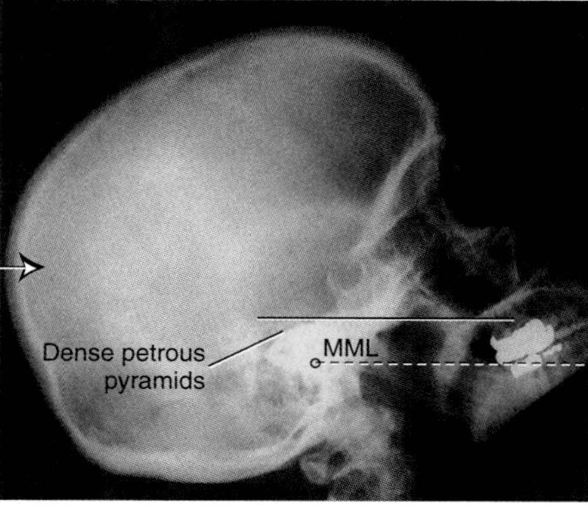

Fig. 13-48. Lateral skull for comparison of bony relationships—CR parallel to MML.

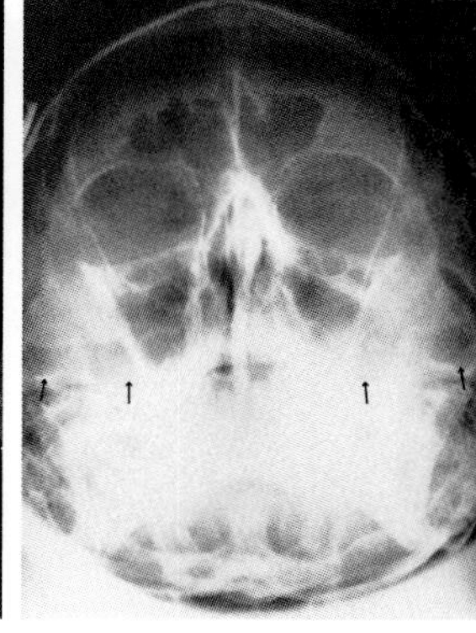

Fig. 13-49. Facial bones—parietoacanthial (Waters) projection.

Erect Versus Recumbent When positioning for facial bone projections, an **erect position is preferred** if the condition of the patient allows. This positioning can be done with an erect table or an upright Bucky. Often, moving the patient's entire body in the erect position (to adjust the various planes and positioning lines) is easier for accurate skull positioning. This is especially true with obese or hypersthenic patients. In addition, fluid levels in the sinuses or other cranial cavities that may indicate cranial pathologic conditions are visible in the erect position with a horizontal beam.

Trauma patients generally are radiographed in a recumbent (supine) position. Most facial bone projections can be obtained without moving the patient by compensating CR angles and/or CR-part-image receptor alignments, as demonstrated in Chapter 19 (Trauma, Mobile, and Surgical Radiography).

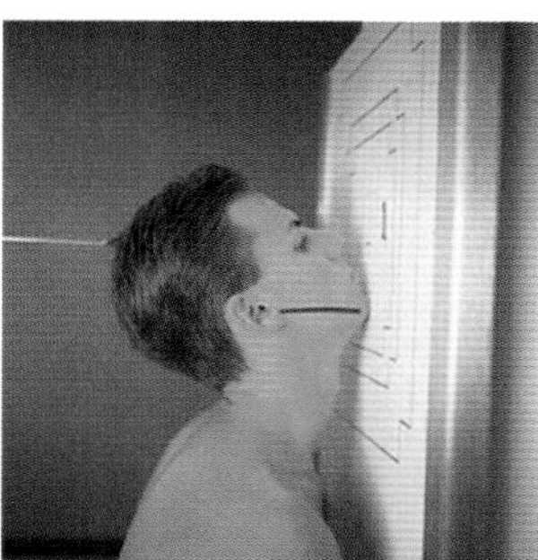

Fig. 13-50. PA, erect—upright Bucky.

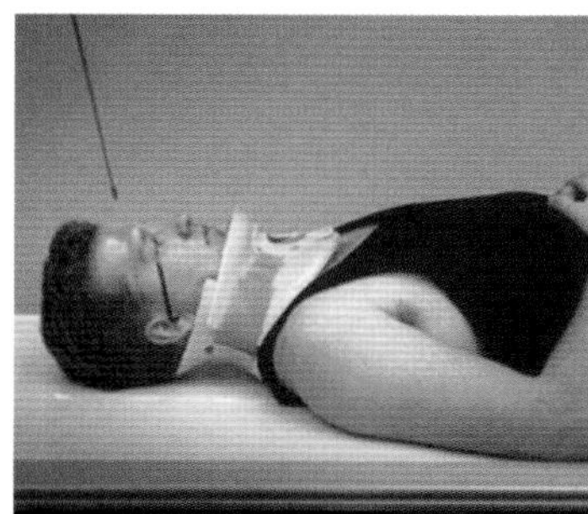

Fig. 13-51. AP, supine—trauma patient.

PARANASAL SINUSES

Technical Factors A medium kV range of 70 to 80 is commonly used to provide sufficient contrast of the air-filled paranasal sinuses. Optimum density as controlled by the mAs is especially important for sinus radiography to visualize pathology within the sinus cavities. A small focal spot should be used for maximum detail.

As with cranial and facial bone imaging, gonadal shielding is not useful in reducing gonadal exposure, but shields over the pelvic area may be used for patient reassurance. The gonadal doses in the dose icon boxes are listed as *NDC* (no detectable contribution). Close collimation and elimination of unnecessary repeats are the best measures for reducing radiation dose in sinus and temporal bone radiography.

Erect Position Images of the paranasal sinuses should be obtained with the patient in the **erect position** whenever possible to demonstrate air-fluid levels (if present) within the sinuses. This also requires the use of a **horizontal beam.** If the x-ray beam is not horizontal, air-fluid levels will not be visualized as clearly defined straight lines but will be seen as gradual density changes. Therefore rather than angling the central ray (CR) for a specific projection (such as for a PA Caldwell, which generally requires a 15° CR caudad angle), the CR remains horizontal and the head is tilted back as needed (Fig. 13-52).

If the patient's condition does not allow an upright position, then a horizontal beam lateral of the sinuses can be obtained to demonstrate air-fluid levels.

PEDIATRIC APPLICATIONS

Communication A clear explanation of the procedure is required to obtain cooperation from the patient and guardian. Distraction techniques using toys, stuffed animals, etc. are effective to maintain trust and cooperation (see Chapter 20, Pediatric Radiography).

13

Immobilization Pediatric patients (depending on the age and condition) are often unable to maintain the required positions. Use of immobilization devices to support the patient is recommended, reducing the need for the patient to be held. Chapter 20 provides an in-depth description of such devices. If the guardian is required to hold the patient, the technologist must provide lead aprons and/or gloves and ensure that there is no possibility of pregnancy if the guardian is female.

Technical Factors Technical factors vary because of various patient sizes. Use of short exposure times (associated with use of high mA) is recommended to reduce the risk of patient motion.

GERIATRIC APPLICATIONS

Communication and Comfort Sensory loss (poor eyesight, hearing, etc.) associated with aging may result in the geriatric patient requiring additional assistance, time, and patience to obtain the required positions for cranial radiography. Geriatric patients also frequently feel nervous and are afraid of falling off the exam table. Reassurance and additional care from the technologist enable the patient to feel secure and comfortable.

If the patient is able, it may be more comfortable to obtain the required positions in the erect position (sitting) at an upright Bucky, especially if the patient has an increased kyphosis. If the examination is performed with the patient in the recumbent position, a radiolucent mattress or pad placed on the exam table provides comfort. Extra blankets also may be required to keep the patient warm. Horizontal beam lateral views may be indicated for the elderly patient because of limitation in movement.

Technical Factors Because of the high incidence of osteoporosis in geriatric patients, the mAs may require a decrease if manual exposure factors are used. (A minimum adjustment of 25% to 30% is required to have a visible effect on the image.)

Older patients may have tremors or difficulty holding steady; use of short exposure times (associated with use of high mA) is recommended to reduce the risk of motion.

Digital Imaging Considerations

Guidelines for digital imaging (CR and DR) of the facial bones and sinuses are similar to those described in previous chapters. These are:

1. **Correct central ray angle and centering to body part and image receptor** provides for accurate post-processing of the image by the image reader.
2. **Close collimation is important** (especially for certain views of the nasal bones, optic foramina, orbits, and TMJs). This improves image quality by reducing scatter and secondary radiation to the highly sensitive digital image receptors.
3. **Follow ALARA principles** in determining exposure factors (highest kV and lowest mAs that will result in desirable image quality).
4. **Post-processing evaluation of exposure index values** ensures that optimum quality image was achieved with least possible radiation to patient.

Alternative Modalities and Procedures

COMPUTED TOMOGRAPHY

Computed tomography (CT) provides sectional images of the facial bones, orbits, mandible, and TMJs in axial, sagittal, or coronal planes. CT assists in full evaluation of these structures because skeletal detail, as well as associated soft tissues, may be visualized with CT.

Three-dimensional (3D) reconstruction of the slices is often useful when facial reconstructive surgery is required.

CT also allows visualization of the soft tissue planes of the sinuses and evaluation of the related bony structures. Coronal slices are most commonly indicated for CT of the sinuses.

MAGNETIC RESONANCE IMAGING

Magnetic resonance imaging (MRI) has limited usefulness in evaluation of bone; however, it is superior in evaluation of soft tissues.

MRI is useful for evaluation of TMJ syndrome to diagnose possible damage to the articular disk in the TMJ fossa (see indications on following page).

NUCLEAR MEDICINE

Nuclear medicine provides a sensitive diagnostic procedure (the radionuclide bone scan) for detection of osteomyelitis and occult fractures that may not be demonstrated on radiographic images.

ULTRASOUND

Research is ongoing concerning the use of ultrasound as a screening tool for maxillary sinusitis. Because it does not involve ionizing radiation exposure, it would be advantageous for pediatric and pregnant patients.

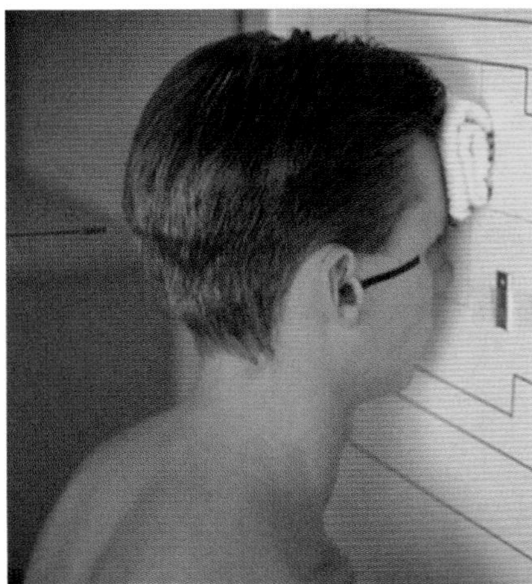

Fig. 13-52. Modified PA Caldwell—**horizontal CR,** OML tilted 15° from perpendicular. (A basic projection for sinuses.)

Pathologic Indications

In addition to CT and/or MRI procedures, conventional radiographic exams for the facial bones and paranasal sinuses are still commonly performed in smaller hospitals and clinics. For paranasal sinuses they are performed to demonstrate pathologies such as mucosal thickening, air-fluid levels, or erosion of bony margins of the sinuses.

Some of the more common pathologic indications for the various types of radiographic examinations for the facial bones and sinuses include the following:

Fracture is a break in the structure of a bone caused by a direct or indirect force. Examples of specific fractures involving the facial bones include the following:

- **Blowout** is a fracture of the floor of the orbit caused by an object striking the eyes straight on (Fig. 13-53). As the floor of the orbit ruptures, the inferior rectus muscle is forced through the fracture into the maxillary sinus, causing entrapment and diplopia (perception of two images).
- **Tripod** is a fracture caused by a blow to the cheek, resulting in a fracture of the zygoma in three places—the orbital process, the maxillary process, and the arch. The result is a "free-floating" zygomatic bone, or a tripod fracture (Fig. 13-54).
- **Le Fort** describes severe bilateral horizontal fractures of the maxillae resulting in an unstable detached fragment.
- **Contrecoup** is an injury/fracture to one side of a structure, caused by an impact to the opposite side. For example, a blow to one side of the mandible results in a fracture to the opposite side.

Foreign body of the eye refers to metal or other types of fragments in the eye, a relatively common industrial mishap. Plain images are useful to detect the presence of a metallic foreign object but are limited in their ability to demonstrate damage to tissues caused by these objects.

The patient interview before an MRI procedure includes questions regarding a history of a foreign object in the eye. Because the magnetic field causes the metal fragment to move, injury occurs to the soft tissues (even blindness may occur if the optic nerve is severed). Radiographic images may be obtained pre-MRI to confirm their presence.

Neoplasm describes a new and abnormal growth (tumor) that may occur in the skeletal structures of the face.

Osteomyelitis is a localized infection of bone/bone marrow. This infection may be caused by bacteria from a penetrating trauma or postoperative or fracture complications. It also may be spread by blood from a distant site.

Sinusitis *(si-nu-si-tis)* is an infection of the sinus mucosa and may be acute or chronic. The patient complains of headache, pain, swelling over the affected sinus(es), and possibly a low-grade fever.

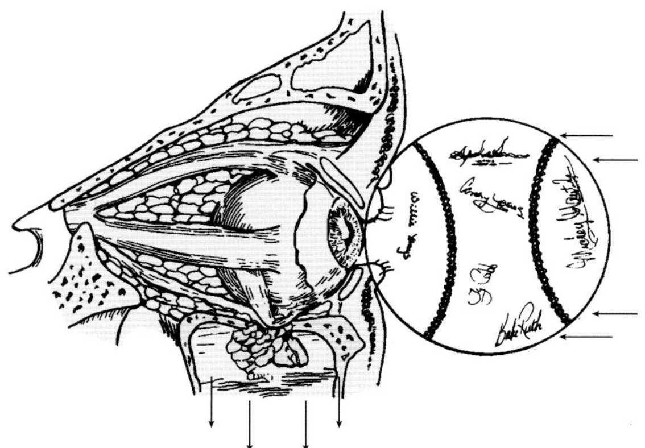

Fig. 13-53. "Blowout" fracture.

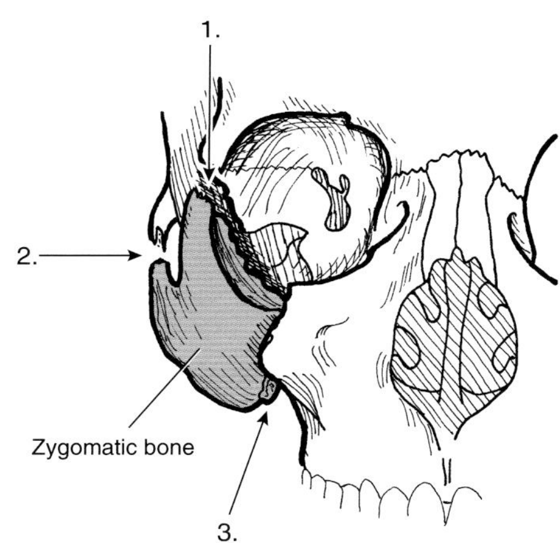

Fig. 13-54. Tripod fracture.

Secondary osteomyelitis, an infection of the bone and marrow secondary to sinusitis, results in erosion of the bony margins of the sinus.

TMJ syndrome is a term used to describe a set of symptoms, which may include pain and clicking, that indicates dysfunction of the TMJ. The condition may be caused by malocclusion, stress, muscle spasm, or inflammation.

FACIAL BONES—SUMMARY OF PATHOLOGIC INDICATIONS

CONDITION OR DISEASE	MOST COMMON RADIOGRAPHIC EXAM	POSSIBLE RADIOGRAPHIC APPEARANCE	MANUAL EXPOSURE FACTOR ADJUSTMENT
Fractures	Routine radiographic projections of affected area; CT	Disruption of bony cortex	None
Foreign body of the eye	Routine facial bone (orbits) projections, including modified parietoacanthial	Increased density if foreign body is metallic	None
Neoplasms	Routine radiographic projections of affected area, CT/MRI	Possible increase or decrease in density, depending on lesion type	None
Osteomyelitis	Nuclear medicine bone scan; routine radiographic projections of affected area	Soft-tissue swelling; loss of cortical margins	None
Sinusitis	Routine radiographic sinus views, CT, MRI	Sinus mucosal thickening, air-fluid levels, opacified sinus	None
Secondary osteomyelitis	Routine radiographic sinus views, CT	Erosion of bony margins of the sinus	None
TMJ syndrome	Axiolateral projection of TMJ (open and closed mouth position), CT/MRI	Abnormal relationship/range of motion between condyle and TM fossa	None

Survey Information

Departmental routines (basic and special) for exams involving the **facial bones** and **paranasal sinuses** are shown in the basic and special projection boxes shown below. These were quite consistent throughout all regions of the United States but did show some significant differences in certain projection routines between the U.S. and Canada, as shown on the right.

PARANASAL SINUSES

The three most common basic projections according to the 1999 survey were the **lateral, PA,** and **Waters,** with the **SMV** also basic by 62% in the U.S. and 20% in Canada. The **transoral Waters** was also basic by 39% in the U.S. and 42% in Canada.

Standard and Optional Operating Procedures

Certain basic and special projections or positions for exams involving the facial bones and paranasal sinuses are demonstrated and described on the following pages as suggested standard and special departmental procedures.

FACIAL BONES

PROJECTION	U.S. ROUTINE	CANADA ROUTINE
• Parietoorbital (Rhese oblique) for optic foramina	79%	34%
• Basilar (SMV) for zygomatic arches	74%	34%
• Basilar (SMV) for mandible	21%	8%
• Panorex for mandible (or TMJ)	41%	21%
• PA axial for mandible	37%	17%

BASIC PROJECTIONS

Standard, or basic, projections, also sometimes referred to as *routine projections* or *departmental routines,* are those projections commonly taken on average patients who are able to cooperate during the examination.

SPECIAL PROJECTIONS

Special projections are those more common projections taken as extra or additional projections to better demonstrate certain pathologic conditions or specific body parts.

BASIC AND SPECIAL PROJECTIONS

Trauma facial bone projections are included in Chapter 19 (Trauma, Mobile, and Surgical Radiography).

13

Facial Bones (Orbits)
BASIC
- Lateral 419
- Parietoacanthial (Waters method) 420
- PA (Caldwell method) 421

SPECIAL
- Modified parietoacanthial (modified Waters method) 422

Nasal Bones
BASIC
- Lateral 423
- Parietoacanthial (Waters method) 420

SPECIAL
- Superoinferior (axial) 424

Zygomatic Arches
BASIC
- Submentovertex (SMV) 425
- Oblique inferosuperior (tangential) 426
- AP axial (modified Towne method) 427
- Parietoacanthial (Waters method) 420

Optic Foramina
BASIC
- Parietoorbital (Rhese method) 428
- Parietoacanthial (Waters method) 420

SPECIAL
- Modified parietoacanthial (modified Waters method) 422

Mandible
BASIC
- Axiolateral 429
- PA 0° and 20°-25° cephalad 430
- AP axial (Towne method) 431

SPECIAL
- Submentovertex (SMV) 432
- Panorex 433

TMJs
BASIC
- AP axial (modified Towne method) 435

SPECIAL
- Axiolateral 15° oblique (modified Law method) 436
- Axiolateral (Schuller method) 437

Paranasal Sinuses
BASIC
- Lateral 438
- PA (Caldwell) 439
- Parietoacanthial (Waters) 440

SPECIAL
- Submentovertex (SMV) 441
- Parietoacanthial transoral (open-mouth Waters) 442

LATERAL POSITION—RIGHT OR LEFT LATERAL: FACIAL BONES

Facial Bones
BASIC
- Lateral
- Parietoacanthial (Waters method)
- PA axial (Caldwell method)

Pathology Demonstrated

Fractures and neoplastic/inflammatory processes of the facial bones, orbits, and mandible are shown.

The facial bone routine commonly includes only a single lateral, whereas the skull routine may include bilateral positions.

Technical Factors

- IR size—18 × 24 cm (8 × 10 inches), lengthwise
- Moving or stationary grid
- 70-80 kV range
- Small focal spot
- Technique and dose:

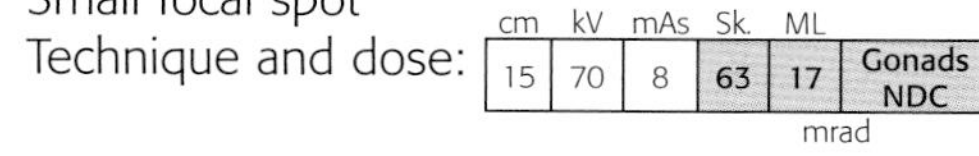

cm	kV	mAs	Sk.	ML	
15	70	8	63	17	Gonads NDC
			mrad		

18
24
R

Patient Position Remove all metal, plastic, and other removable objects from head. Patient position is erect or prone.

Part Position

- Rest lateral aspect of head against table or upright Bucky surface, **with side of interest closest to IR.**
- Adjust head into a **true lateral position** and oblique body as needed for patient's comfort. (Palpate the external occipital protuberance posteriorly and the nasion or glabella anteriorly to ensure that these two points are equidistant from the tabletop.) Place support sponge under chin if needed.
- Align **midsagittal plane parallel** to IR.
- Align **interpupillary line perpendicular** to IR.
- Adjust chin to bring the **IOML perpendicular** to front edge of IR.

Central Ray

- Align CR **perpendicular** to IR.
- Center CR to **zygoma,** midway between outer canthus and EAM.
- Center image receptor to CR.
- Minimum SID is 40 inches (100 cm).

Collimation Collimate on all sides to within 1 inch (2.5 cm) of facial bones.

Respiration Suspend respiration.

Note: Use radiolucent support under head if needed to bring IPL perpendicular to tabletop on large-chested patients.

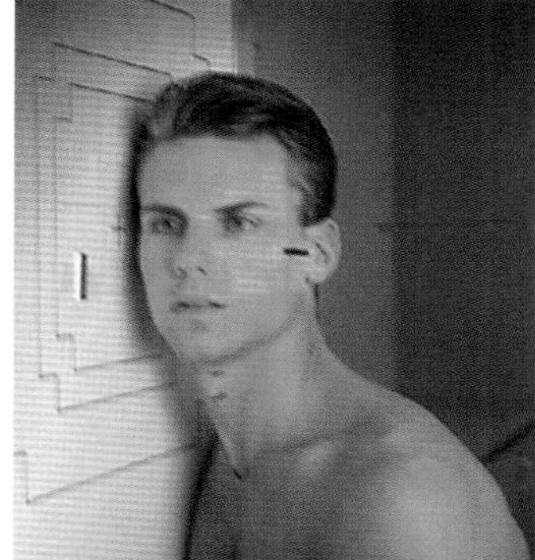

Fig. 13-55. Right lateral—erect.

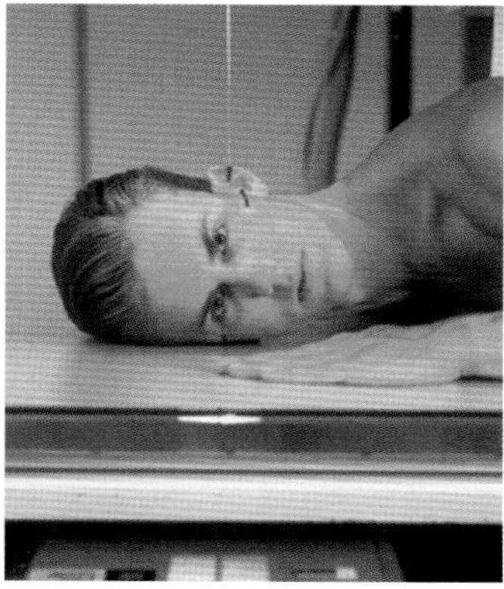

Fig. 13-56. Right lateral—recumbent.

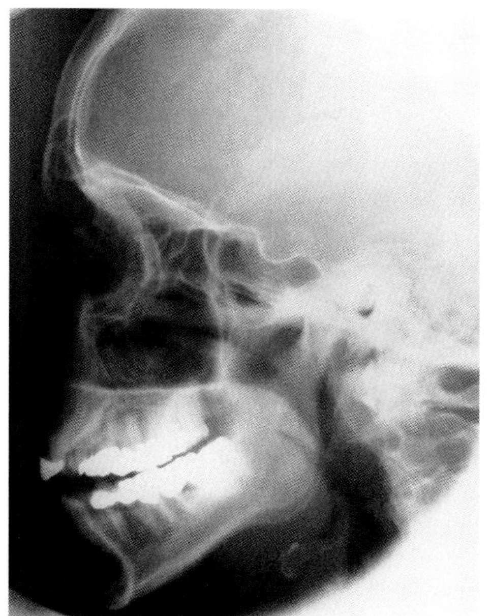

Fig. 13-57. Lateral facial bones.

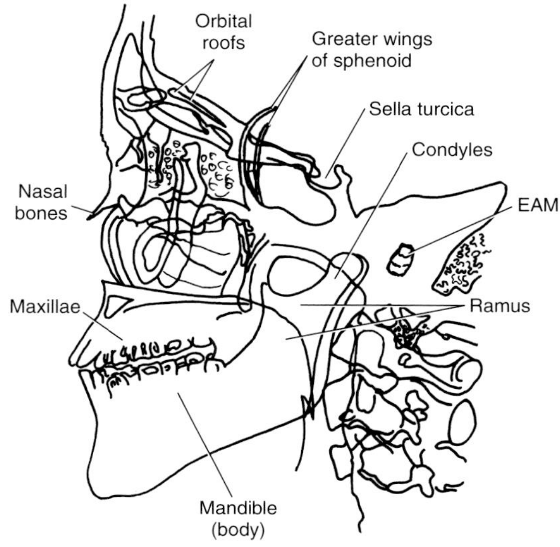

Fig. 13-58. Lateral facial bones.

Radiographic Criteria

Structures Shown: • Superimposed facial bones, greater wings of the sphenoid, orbital roofs, sella turcica, zygoma, and mandible.

Position: • An accurately positioned lateral image of the facial bones demonstrates no rotation (mandibular rami are superimposed) and no tilt (orbital roofs and greater wings of sphenoid are superimposed).

Collimation and CR: • Superimposed zygomatic bones should be in the center of the image, with the EAMs and orbital roofs included within the collimated field.

Exposure Criteria: • Contrast and density are sufficient to visualize the maxillary region. • Sharp bony margins indicate no motion.

13

PARIETOACANTHIAL PROJECTION: FACIAL BONES

Waters Method

Facial Bones
BASIC
- **Lateral**
- Parietoacanthial (Waters method)
- **PA axial (Caldwell method)**

Pathology Demonstrated

Fractures (particularly blowout, tripod, and Le Fort fractures) and neoplastic/inflammatory processes are shown. Foreign bodies in the eye may also be demonstrated on this image.

Technical Factors

- IR size—24 × 30 cm (10 × 12 inches), lengthwise,
  or
  —18 × 24 cm (8 × 10 inches)
- Moving or stationary grid
- 70-80 kV range
- Small focal spot
- Technique and dose:

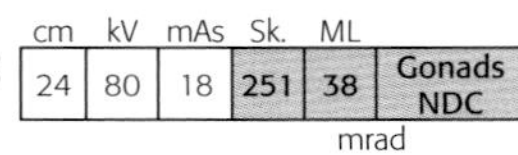

cm	kV	mAs	Sk.	ML	
24	80	18	251	38	Gonads NDC

mrad

24 (18)
30 (24)
R

Fig. 13-59. Parietoacanthial (Waters)—**MML perpendicular** (OML 37°).

Patient Position Remove all metal, plastic, and other removable objects from head. Patient position is erect or prone (erect is preferred if patient's condition allows).

Part Position

- Extend neck, resting chin against table/upright Bucky surface.
- Adjust head until **mentomeatal line (MML) is perpendicular to the plane of the image receptor.** OML will form a **37°** angle with the table/Bucky surface.
- Position the **midsagittal plane perpendicular** to the midline of the grid or the table/Bucky surface, preventing rotation and/or tilting of head. (One way to check for rotation is to palpate the mastoid processes on each side and the lateral orbital margins with the thumb and fingertips to ensure that these lines are equidistant from the tabletop.)

Central Ray

- Align CR **perpendicular** to IR, to **exit at acanthion.**
- Center image receptor to CR.
- Minimum SID is 40 inches (100 cm).

Collimation Collimate to outer margins of skull on all sides.

Respiration Suspend respiration.

Fig. 13-60. Parietoacanthial (Waters) projection.

Radiographic Criteria

Structures Shown: • Inferior orbital rim, maxillae, nasal septum, zygomatic bones, zygomatic arches, and anterior nasal spine.

Position: • Correct neck extension demonstrates petrous ridges just inferior to the maxillary sinuses. • No patient rotation exists, as indicated by equal distance from midsagittal plane (identified by the bony nasal septum) to the outer skull margin on each side.

Collimation and CR: • Entire skull included on the image, with the acanthion in the center • Collimation borders to the outer margins of the skull.

Exposure Criteria: • Contrast and density are sufficient to visualize maxillary region. • Sharp bony margins indicate no motion.

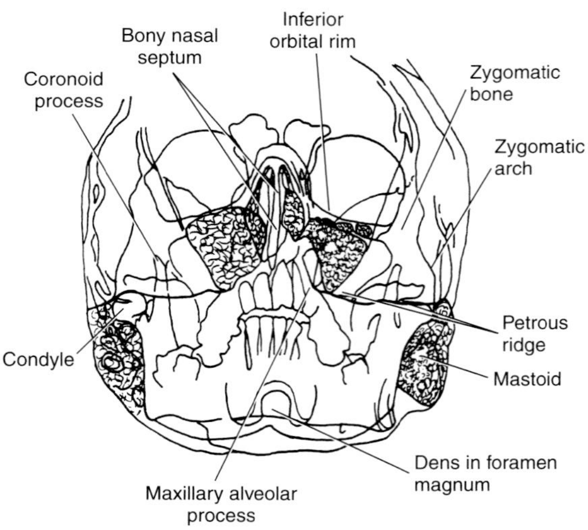

Fig. 13-61. Parietoacanthial (Waters) projection.

PA AXIAL PROJECTION: FACIAL BONES

Caldwell Method

Facial Bones
BASIC
- Lateral
- Parietoacanthial (Waters method)
- PA axial (Caldwell method)

Pathology Demonstrated

Fractures and neoplastic/inflammatory processes of the facial bones are shown.

Technical Factors

- IR size—24 × 30 cm (10 × 12 inches), lengthwise,
  or
  —18 × 24 cm (8 × 10 inches)
- Moving or stationary grid
- 70-80 kV range
- Small focal spot
- Technique and dose:

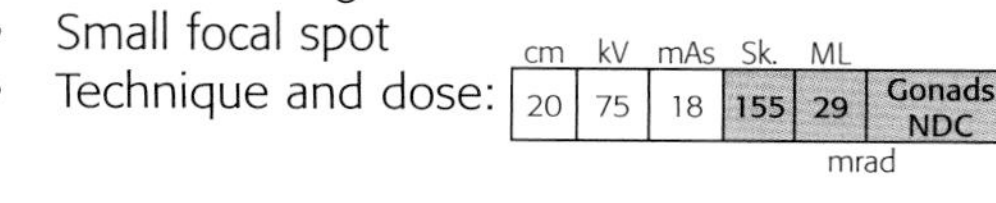

Patient Position Remove all metal, plastic, and other removable objects from head. Patient position is erect or prone (erect is preferred if patient's condition allows).

Part Position

- Rest patient's nose and forehead against tabletop.
- Tuck chin, bringing **OML perpendicular** to image receptor.
- Align **midsagittal plane perpendicular** to midline of grid or table/Bucky surface. Ensure **no rotation** or **tilt** of head.

Central Ray

- Angle **CR 15° caudad,** to **exit at nasion** (see Note below).
- Center CR to image receptor.
- Ensure minimum SID of 40 inches (100 cm).

Collimation Collimate on all sides to facial bones.

Respiration Suspend respiration.

Note: If area of interest is the orbital floors, use a 30° caudad angle to project the petrous ridges below the inferior orbital margin.

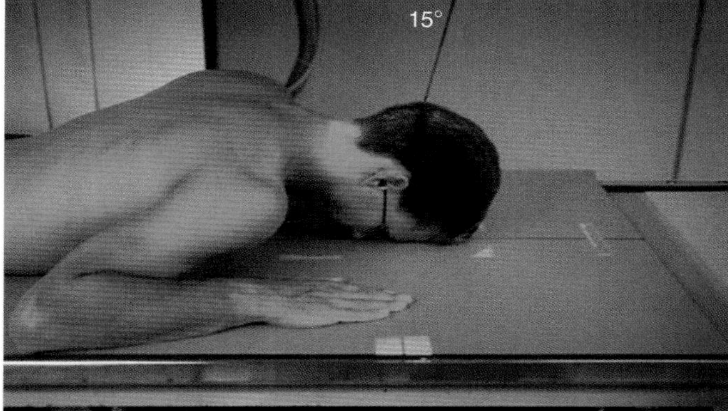

Fig. 13-62. PA axial Caldwell—**OML perpendicular, CR 15° caudad.**

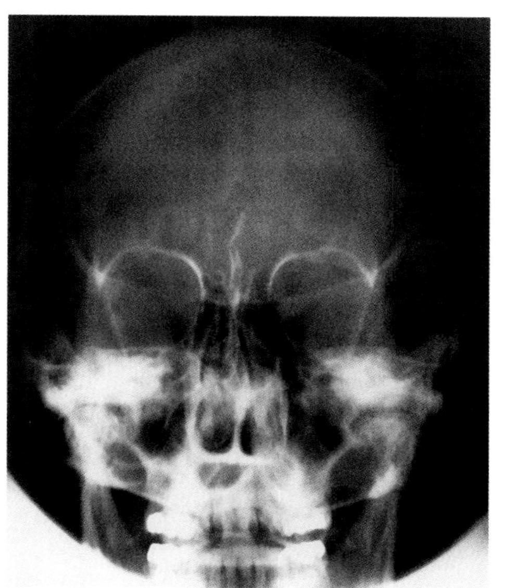

Fig. 13-63. PA axial Caldwell—CR 15°.

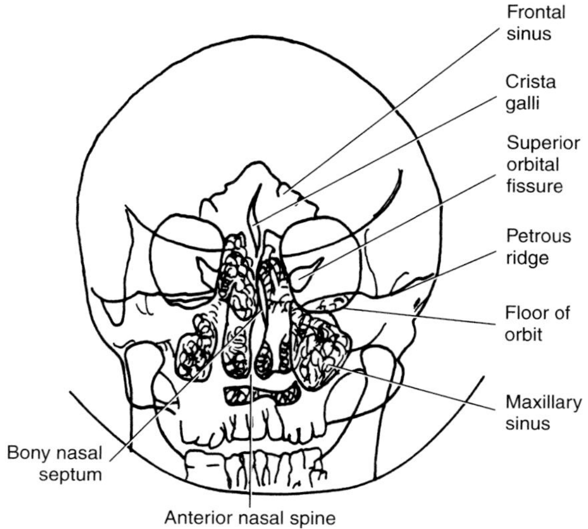

Fig. 13-64. PA axial Caldwell—CR 15°.

Radiographic Criteria

Structures Shown: • Orbital rim, maxillae, nasal septum, zygomatic bones, and anterior nasal spine.

Position: • Correct patient position/CR angulation is indicated by petrous ridges being projected into the **lower one third of orbits** with 15° caudad CR. If the orbital floors are the area of interest, the 30° caudad angle projects the petrous ridges below the inferior margins of the orbits. • No rotation of cranium is indicated by equal distance from midsagittal plane (identified by the crista galli) to the outer orbital margin on each side; superior orbital fissures are symmetric.

Collimation and CR: • The inferior orbital rim is located in the center of the image. • The collimated field includes the entire orbital margin and maxillae.

Exposure Criteria: • Contrast and density are sufficient to visualize maxillary region and orbital floor. • Sharp bony margins indicate no motion.

MODIFIED PARIETOACANTHIAL PROJECTION: FACIAL BONES

Modified Waters Method

Pathology Demonstrated
Orbital fractures (for example, blowout) and neoplastic/inflammatory processes are shown. Foreign bodies in the eye may also be demonstrated in this position.

Facial Bones
SPECIAL
• Modified parietoacanthial (modified Waters method)

Technical Factors
- IR size—18 × 24 cm (8 × 10 inches), lengthwise
- Moving or stationary grid
- 70-80 kV range
- Small focal spot
- Technique and dose:

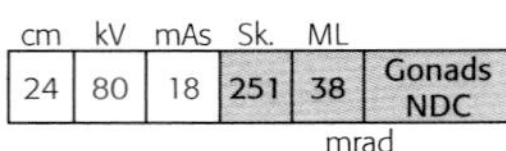

cm	kV	mAs	Sk.	ML	
24	80	18	251	38	Gonads NDC
			mrad		

Patient Position Remove all metal, plastic, and other removable objects from head. Patient position is erect or prone (erect is preferred if patient's condition allows).

Part Position
- Extend neck, resting chin and nose against table/upright Bucky surface.
- Adjust head until **lips-meatal line (LML) is perpendicular;** OML forms a **55°** angle with the image receptor.
- Position **midsagittal plane perpendicular** to the midline of the grid or the table/upright Bucky surface. Ensure **no rotation** or **tilt** of head.

Central Ray
- Align CR **perpendicular,** centered to **exit at acanthion.**
- Center image receptor to CR.
- Minimum SID is 40 inches (100 cm).

Collimation Collimate to within 1 inch (2.5 cm) of facial bones.

Respiration Suspend respiration during exposure.

Fig. 13-65. Modified parietoacanthial (Waters)—**LML perpendicular (OML 55°).**

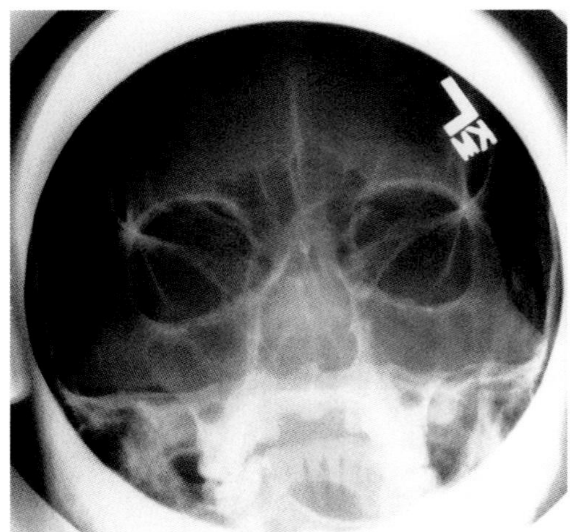

Fig. 13-66. Modified parietoacanthial (Waters).

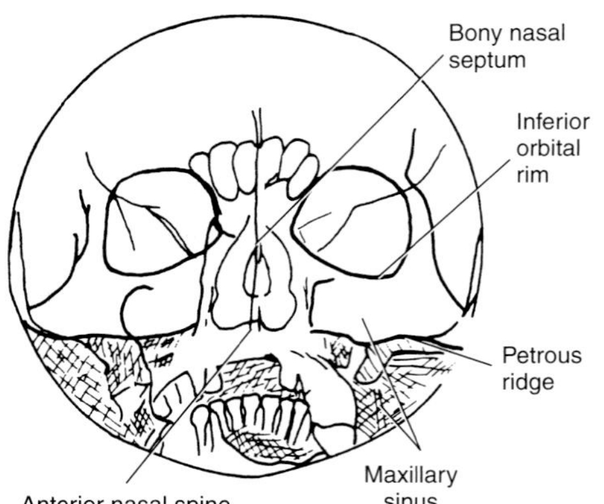

Fig. 13-67. Modified parietoacanthial (Waters).

Radiographic Criteria

Structures Shown: • Orbital floors are visible with this projection, which also provides a less distorted view of the entire orbital rims than a parietoacanthial (Waters) projection.

Position: • Correct position/CR angulation is indicated by petrous ridges projected into the lower half of the maxillary sinuses, below the inferior orbital rim. • No rotation of the cranium is indicated by equal distance from the midsagittal plane (identified by the bony nasal septum) to the outer orbital margin on each side.

Collimation and CR: • The inferior orbital rims should be located in the center of the image. • The entire orbital rim and maxillary bones should be included in the collimated field.

Exposure Criteria: • Contrast and density are sufficient to visualize the orbital floors. • Sharp bony margins indicate no motion.

LATERAL POSITION: NASAL BONES

Nasal Bones
BASIC
- Lateral
- Parietoacanthial (Waters method; see p. 420)

Pathology Demonstrated

Nasal bone fractures are shown.

Both sides should be examined for comparison, with the side closest to IR demonstrated.

Technical Factors

- IR size—18 × 24 cm (8 × 10 inches)
- **Detail screen** if conventional film-screen, tabletop being used
- 50-60 kV range
- Small focal spot
- AEC not recommended because of small exposure field
- Technique and dose:

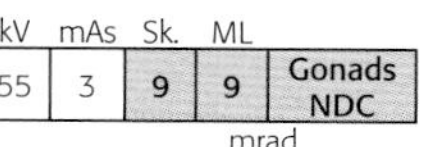

cm	kV	mAs	Sk.	ML	
2	55	3	9	9	Gonads NDC
			mrad		

24
18
L R
No AEC

Patient Position Remove all metal, plastic, and other removable objects from head. Patient position is prone or erect.

Part Position

- Rest lateral aspect of head against the table/upright Bucky surface, with side of interest closest to IR.
- Position nasal bones to center of image receptor.
- Adjust head into a **true lateral position** and oblique body as needed for patient's comfort (placing sponge block under chin if needed).
- Align **midsagittal plane parallel** with a table/upright Bucky surface.
- Align **interpupillary line perpendicular** to table/upright Bucky surface.
- Position **IOML perpendicular** to front edge of image receptor.

Central Ray

- Align CR **perpendicular** to IR.
- Center CR to ½ **inch (1.25 cm) inferior to nasion.**
- Minimum SID is 40 inches (100 cm).

Collimation Collimate on all sides to within 2 inches (5 cm) of nasal bone.

Respiration Suspend respiration during exposure.

Note: To obtain a sharply detailed image of the nasal bones, use a small focal spot, close collimation, and detail screens with film-screen imaging.

In addition, with **CR and DR digital imaging,** accurate central ray centering, tabletop masking, and close collimation are essential because of the image reader function and the sensitivity of the image receptor to scatter exposure.

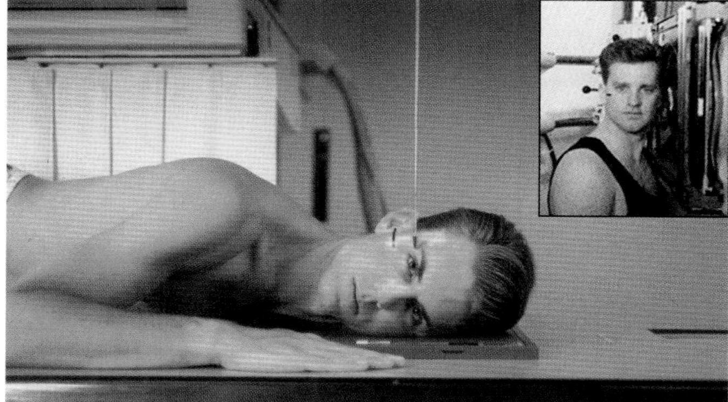

Fig. 13-68. Left lateral—prone or erect.

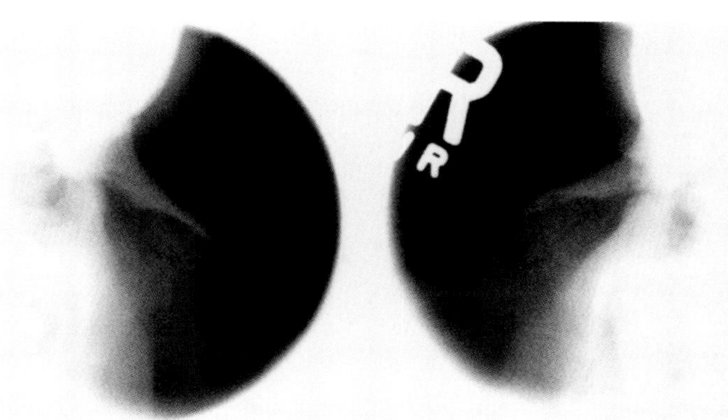

Fig. 13-69. Lateral (R and L).

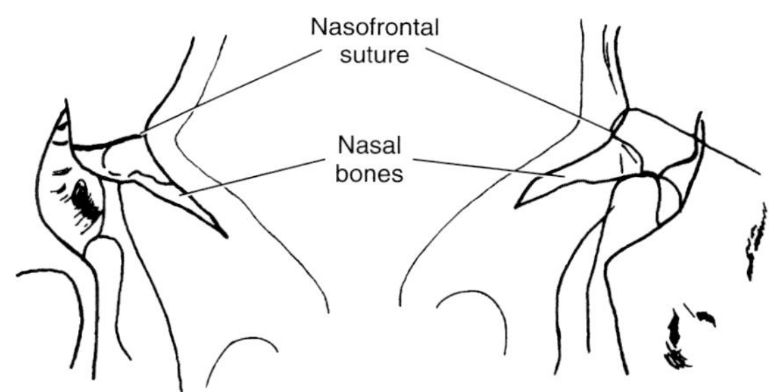

Fig. 13-70. Lateral (R and L).

Radiographic Criteria

Structures Shown: • Nasal bones with soft tissue nasal structures, the frontonasal suture, and the anterior nasal spine.

Position: • Nasal bones are demonstrated without rotation.

Collimation and CR: • The nasal bones are included in the center of the image. • The nasal soft tissue, anterior nasal spine, and frontonasal suture are included within the collimated field.

Exposure Criteria: • Contrast and density are sufficient to visualize nasal bone and soft-tissue structures. • Sharp bony structures indicate no motion.

13

SUPEROINFERIOR TANGENTIAL (AXIAL) PROJECTION: NASAL BONES

Nasal Bones
SPECIAL
• Superoinferior (axial)

Pathology Demonstrated
Fractures of the nasal bones (medial-lateral displacement)

Technical Factors
- IR size—18 × 24 cm (8× 10 inches), crosswise
- Detail screen if conventional film-screen system, tabletop being used
- 50-60 kV range
- Small focal spot
- AEC not recommended
- Technique and dose:

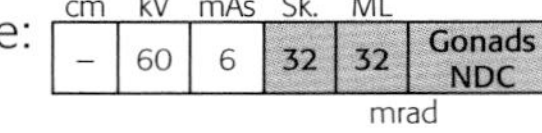

cm	kV	mAs	Sk.	ML	
–	60	6	32	32	Gonads NDC

mrad

24
18
L
No AEC

Shielding Place lead shield over lap or pelvic region to shield gonads.

Patient Position Patient is seated erect in a chair at end of table (Fig. 13-71, *inset*) or in the prone position on table.

Part Position
- Extend and rest chin on IR. Place angled support under IR, as demonstrated, to **place IR perpendicular to GAL** (glabelloalveolar line).
- Align midsagittal plane perpendicular to CR and to IR midline.

Central Ray
- Center CR to nasion and angle as needed to ensure it is **parallel to GAL.** (CR must just skim glabella and anterior upper front teeth.)
- Minimum SID is 40 inches (100 cm).

Collimation Collimate on all sides to nasal bones.

Respiration Suspend respiration during exposure.

Radiographic Criteria

Structures Shown: • Tangential projection of midnasal and distal nasal bones (with little superimposition of the glabella or alveolar ridge) and nasal soft tissue.

Position: • No patient rotation is evident, as indicated by equal distance from anterior nasal spine to outer soft-tissue borders on each side. • Incorrect neck position is indicated by visualization of alveolar ridge (excessive extension) or visualization of too much glabella (excessive flexion).

Collimation and CR: • Nasal bones should be centered to collimated field, which is limited to nasal bones and nasal soft tissue.

Exposure Criteria: • Contrast and density are sufficient to visualize nasal bones and nasal soft tissue. • Sharp bony margins indicate no motion.

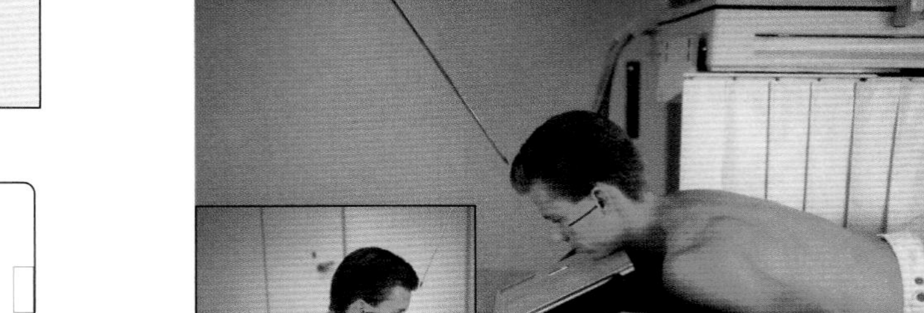

Fig. 13-71. Superoinferior projection—erect or prone.

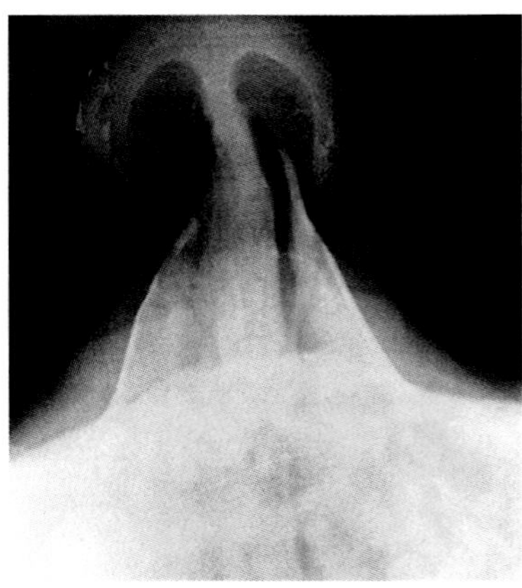

Fig. 13-72. Superoinferior projection.

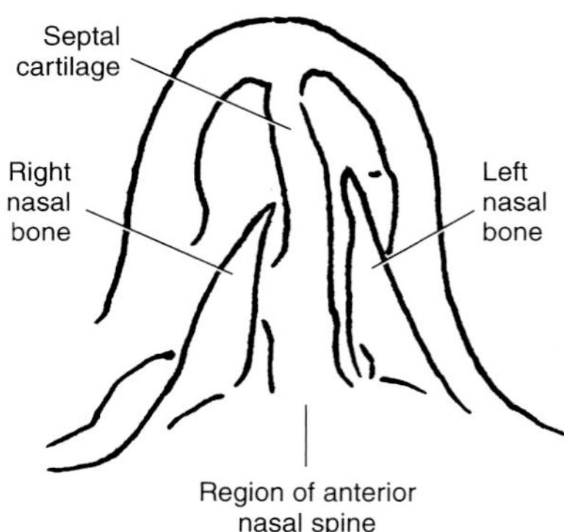

Fig. 13-73. Superoinferior projection.

13

SUBMENTOVERTEX (SMV) PROJECTION: ZYGOMATIC ARCHES

Zygomatic Arches
BASIC
- Submentovertex
- Oblique tangential
- AP axial (modified Towne)

Pathology Demonstrated

Fractures of the zygomatic arch and neoplastic/inflammatory processes are shown.

Technical Factors

- IR size—18 × 24 cm (8 × 10 inches), crosswise
- 60-70 kV range (soft-tissue technique)
- Small focal spot
- AEC not recommended
- Technique and dose:

24
R
18
No AEC

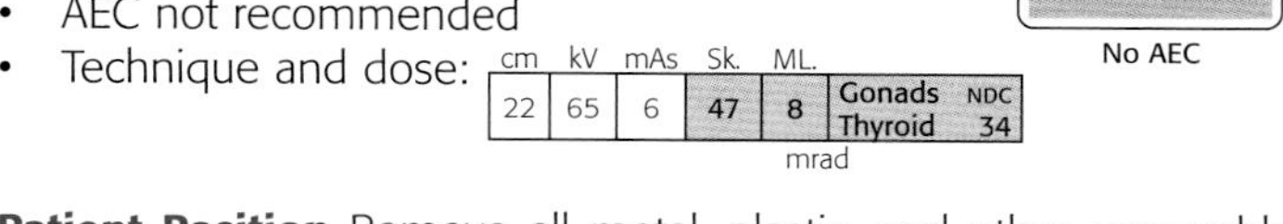

cm	kV	mAs	Sk.	ML.	Gonads NDC / Thyroid 34
22	65	6	47	8	Gonads NDC Thyroid 34

mrad

Patient Position Remove all metal, plastic, and other removable objects from head. This projection may be taken with the patient erect or supine. The erect position may be easier for the patient.

Part Position

- Raise chin, hyperextend neck until **IOML is parallel** to IR (see Notes).
- Rest head on vertex of skull.
- Align **midsagittal plane perpendicular** to midline of the grid or the table/upright Bucky surface, **avoiding all tilt and/or rotation.**

Central Ray

- Align CR **perpendicular** to IR (see Notes).
- Center CR **midway between zygomatic arches,** at a **level 1½ inches (4 cm) inferior to mandibular symphysis.**
- Center image receptor to CR, with plane of image receptor parallel to IOML.
- Minimum SID is 40 inches (100 cm).

Collimation Collimate to outer margins of zygoma.

Respiration Suspend respiration during exposure.

Notes: If patient is unable to extend neck adequately, angle CR **perpendicular to IOML.** If equipment allows, the image receptor should also be angled to maintain the CR/image receptor perpendicular relationship (see Fig. 13-74, *inset*).

This position is very uncomfortable for patients; complete the projection as quickly as possible.

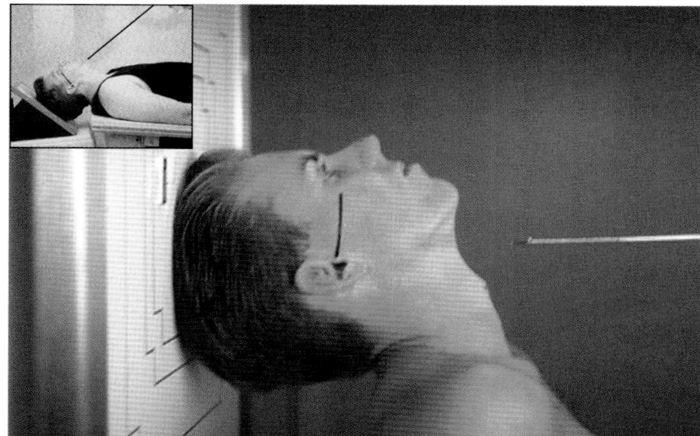

Fig. 13-74. SMV projection; supine or erect—**IOML parallel to IR; CR perpendicular to IOML.**

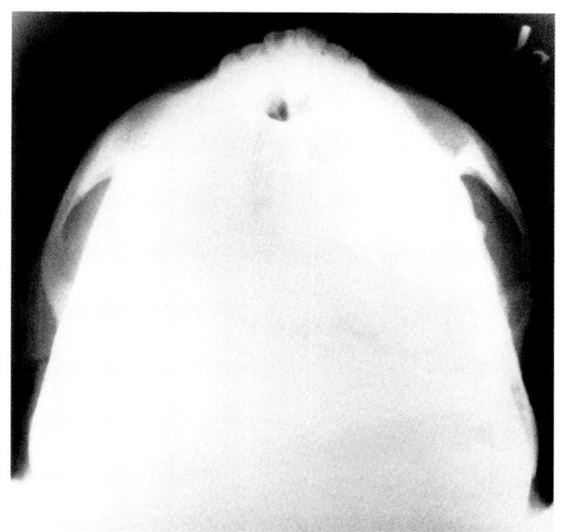

Fig. 13-75. SMV projection.

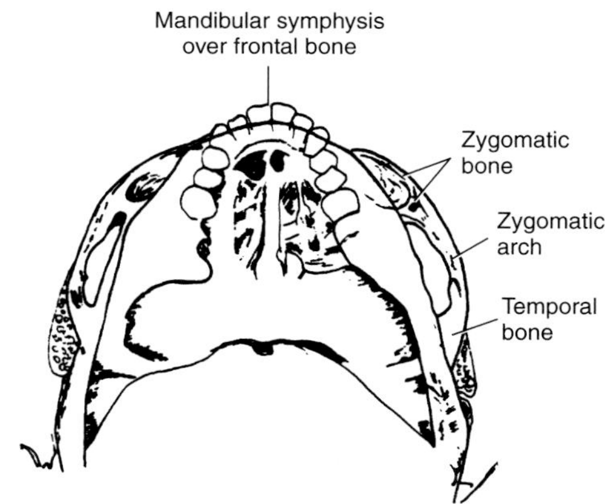

Fig. 13-76. SMV projection.

Radiographic Criteria

Structures Shown: • Zygomatic arches are demonstrated projecting laterally from each zygomatic and temporal bone (unless affected by trauma–for example, depressed fracture).

Position: • Correct IOML/CR relationship, as indicated by mandibular symphysis superimposing frontal bone. • No patient rotation, as indicated by zygomatic arches visualized symmetrically.

Collimation and CR: • Zygomatic arches should be centered to collimated field, which is limited to zygomatic arches.

Exposure Criteria: • Sufficient contrast and density to visualize zygomatic arches. • Sharp bony margins indicate no motion.

13

OBLIQUE INFEROSUPERIOR (TANGENTIAL) PROJECTION: ZYGOMATIC ARCHES

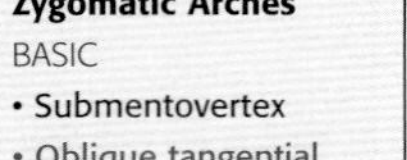
Zygomatic Arches
BASIC
- Submentovertex
- Oblique tangential
- AP axial (modified Towne)

Pathology Demonstrated

Fractures of the zygomatic arch are shown. This projection is especially useful for depressed zygomatic arches resulting from trauma or skull morphology.

Both sides are generally taken for comparison.

Technical Factors

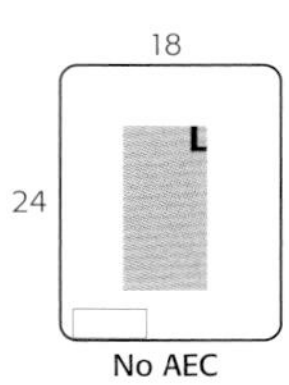

- IR size—18 × 24 cm (8 × 10 inches), lengthwise
- 60-70 kV range (soft-tissue technique)
- Small focal spot
- AEC not recommended
- Technique and dose:

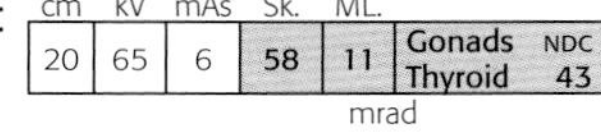

cm	kV	mAs	Sk.	ML.	
20	65	6	58	11	Gonads NDC Thyroid 43
			mrad		

Patient Position Remove all metal, plastic, and other removable objects from head. Patient position is erect or supine. Erect, which is easier for patient, may be done with an erect table or upright Bucky.

Part Position

- Raise chin, hyperextending neck until **IOML is parallel** to IR (see Notes).
- Rest head on vertex of skull.
- **Rotate head 15° toward side to be examined; then also tilt chin 15° toward side of interest.**

Central Ray

- Align **CR perpendicular** to **image receptor and IOML** (see Notes).
- Center CR to **zygomatic arch of interest** (CR skims parietal eminence and body of mandible).
- Adjust image receptor to be parallel to IOML and perpendicular to CR.
- Minimum SID is 40 inches (100 cm).

Collimation Collimate on all sides to within 1 inch (2.5 cm) of zygomatic bone and arch.

Respiration Suspend respiration.

Notes: If patient is unable to sufficiently extend neck, angle CR **perpendicular to IOML.** If equipment allows, the image receptor should also be angled to maintain the CR/image receptor perpendicular relationship.

This position is very uncomfortable for the patient; complete the projection as quickly as possible.

Radiographic Criteria

Structures Shown: • Single zygomatic arch, free of superimposition.

Position: • Correct patient position provides for demonstration of zygomatic arch without superimposition of parietal bone or mandible.

Collimation and CR: • Zygomatic arch should be visualized in the center of collimation field, which is limited to the zygomatic arch.

Exposure Criteria: • Contrast and density are sufficient to visualize zygomatic arch. • Sharp bony margins indicate no motion.

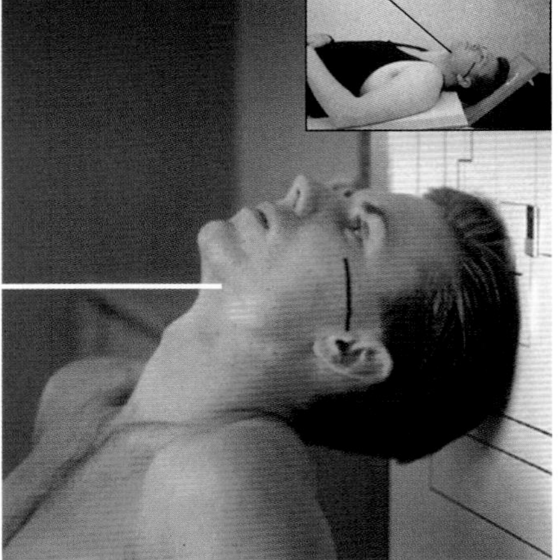

Fig. 13-77. Oblique tangential, upright Bucky.

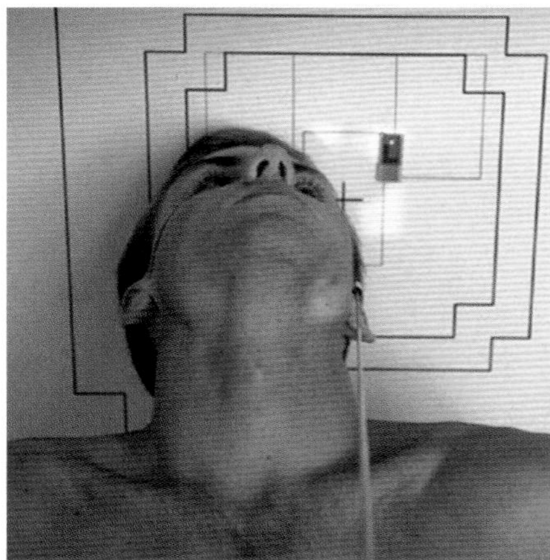

Fig. 13-78. Oblique tangential—15° tilt; 15° rotation; CR perpendicular to IOML.

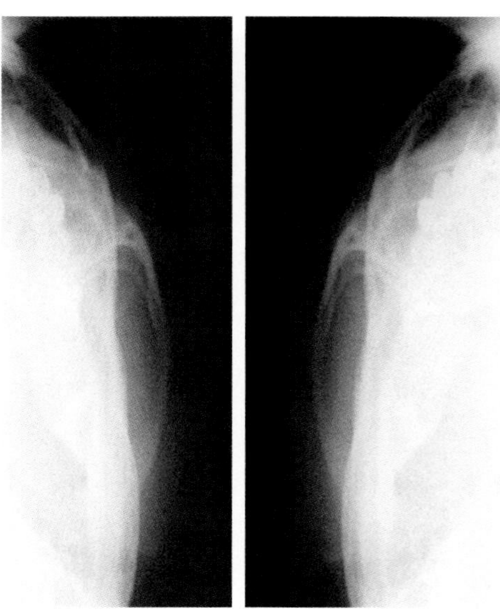

Fig. 13-79. Oblique tangential.

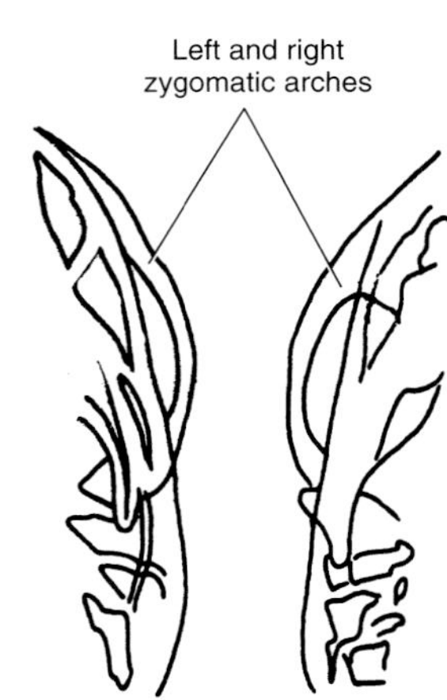

Fig. 13-80. Oblique tangential.

AP AXIAL PROJECTION: ZYGOMATIC ARCHES

Modified Towne Method

Zygomatic Arches
BASIC
- Submentovertex
- Oblique axial (tangential)
- AP axial (modified Towne)

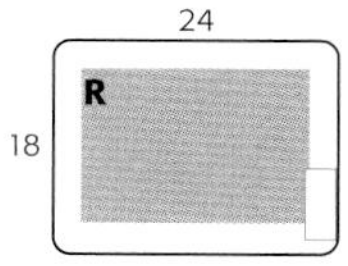

Pathology Demonstrated
Fractures and neoplastic/inflammatory processes of the zygomatic arch are shown.

Technical Factors
- IR size—18 × 24 cm (8 × 10 inches), crosswise
- Moving or stationary grid, near soft-tissue technique (if AEC is used, density should be decreased by approximately 50%)
- 60-70 kV range
- Small focal spot
- AEC not recommended
- Technique and dose:

cm	kV	mAs	Sk.	ML.	
17	70	30	255	65	Gonads NDC Thyroid 74

mrad

Patient Position Remove all metal, plastic, or other removable objects from head. Patient position is erect or supine.

Part Position
- Rest patient's posterior skull against table/upright Bucky surface.
- Tuck chin, bringing **OML (or IOML) perpendicular** to image receptor (see Note below).
- Align **midsagittal plane perpendicular** to midline of the grid or the table/upright Bucky surface to prevent head rotation or tilt.

Central Ray
- Angle CR **30° caudad to OML** or **37° to IOML** (see Note).
- Center **CR to 2.5 cm (1 inch) superior to glabella** (to pass through midarches).
- Center image receptor to projected CR.
- Minimum SID is 40 inches (100 cm).

Collimation Collimate to outer margins of zygomatic arches.

Respiration Suspend respiration during exposure.

Note: If patient is unable to depress the chin sufficiently to bring the OML perpendicular to the image receptor, the **IOML** can be placed perpendicular instead and the CR angle increased to 37° caudad. This positioning maintains the 30° angle between OML and CR and demonstrates the same anatomic relationships. (There is a 7° difference between the OML and IOML.)

Radiographic Criteria
Structures Shown: • Bilateral zygomatic arches.

Position: • Zygomatic arches are visualized without patient rotation as indicated by arches superimposing mandibular rami and symmetric appearance of arches.

Collimation and CR: • Zygomatic arches should be in center of the image. • Collimation field should be limited to the zygomatic arches.

Exposure Criteria: • Contrast and density are sufficient to visualize zygomatic arches. • Sharp bony margins indicate no motion.

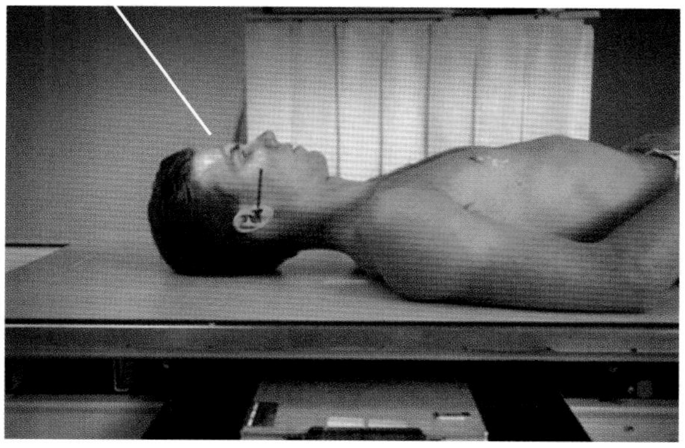

Fig. 13-81. AP axial—**CR 30° to OML** (37° to IOML).

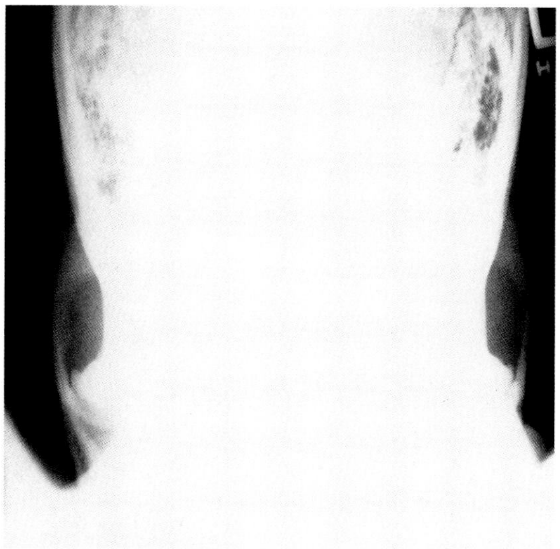

Fig. 13-82. AP axial.

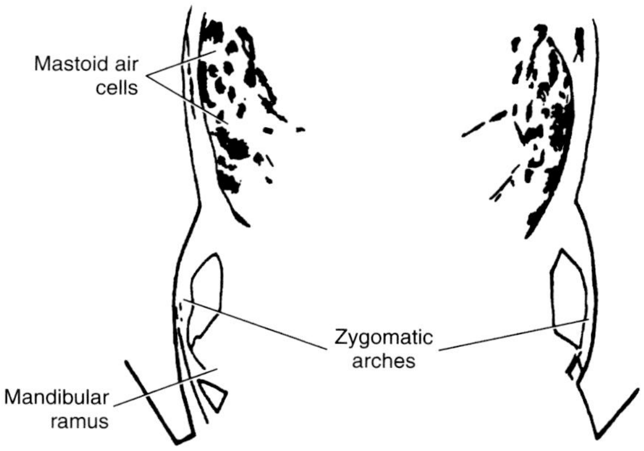

Fig. 13-83. AP axial.

PARIETOORBITAL OBLIQUE PROJECTION: OPTIC FORAMINA

Rhese Method

Pathology Demonstrated
Bony abnormalities of the optic foramen are shown.

Both sides are generally taken for comparison.

Optic Foramina
BASIC
- Parietoorbital (Rhese)
- Parietoacanthial (Waters method), p. 420

SPECIAL
- Modified parietoacanthial (modified Waters method), p. 422

Technical Factors
- IR size—18 × 24 cm (8 × 10 inches)
- Moving or stationary grid
- 70-80 kV range
- Small focal spot
- AEC not recommended due to small exposure field
- Technique and dose:

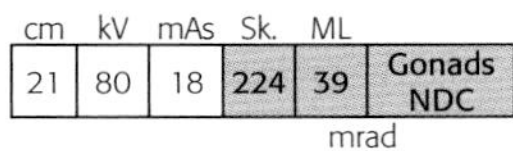

cm	kV	mAs	Sk.	ML	
21	80	18	224	39	Gonads NDC
			mrad		

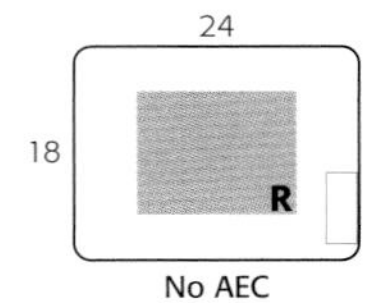

Patient Position Remove all metal, plastic, and other removable objects from head. Position patient erect or supine.

Part Position
- As a starting reference, position patient's chin, cheek, and nose against table/upright Bucky surface (see Notes).
- Adjust head as needed so that the midsagittal plane forms a **53° angle** with image receptor. (An angle indicator should be used to obtain an accurate angle of 53° from a lateral position.)
- Position **acanthiomeatal line perpendicular** to plane of image receptor.

Central Ray
- Align CR **perpendicular** to IR, centered to **downside orbit.**
- Minimum SID is 40 inches (100 cm).

Collimation Collimate on all sides to yield a field size of approximately 4 inches (10 cm) square.

Respiration Suspend respiration during exposure.

Notes: This projection is sometimes referred to as a "three-point landing" position (chin, cheek, and nose).

To obtain a sharply detailed image of the optic foramen, use of a **small focal spot** and **close collimation** is essential.

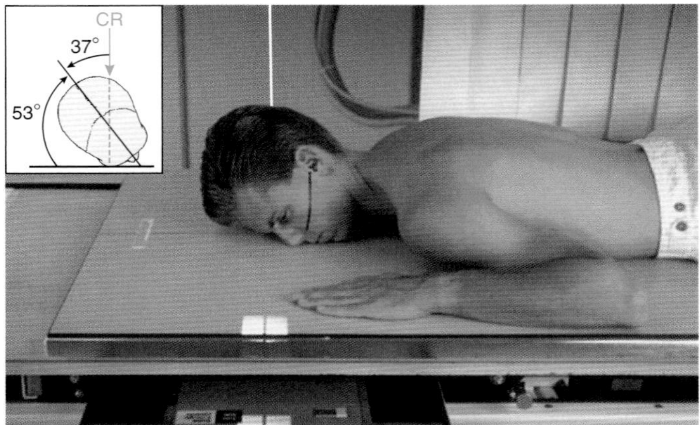

Fig. 13-84. Parietoorbital projection—53° rotation; acanthiomeatal line perpendicular; CR perpendicular.

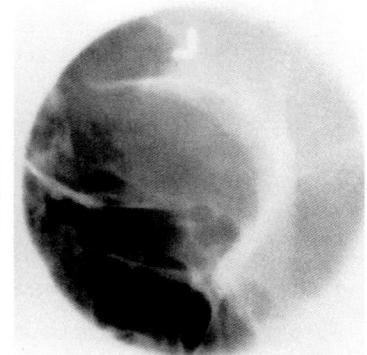

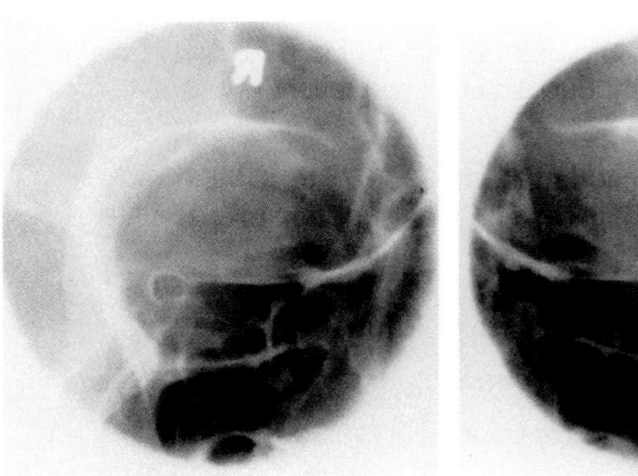

Fig. 13-85. Bilateral parietoorbital.

Radiographic Criteria

Structures Shown: • Cross section of each optic canal and a nondistorted view of the optic foramen.

Position: • Accurate positioning projects the optic foramen into the lower outer quadrant of orbit. (This projection results when acanthiomeatal line is correctly placed perpendicular to IR.)

Collimation and CR: • The optic foramen is located in the center of the image. • The orbital margins are included in the collimated field.

Exposure Criteria: • Contrast and density are sufficient to visualize the optic foramen. • Sharp bony margins indicate no motion.

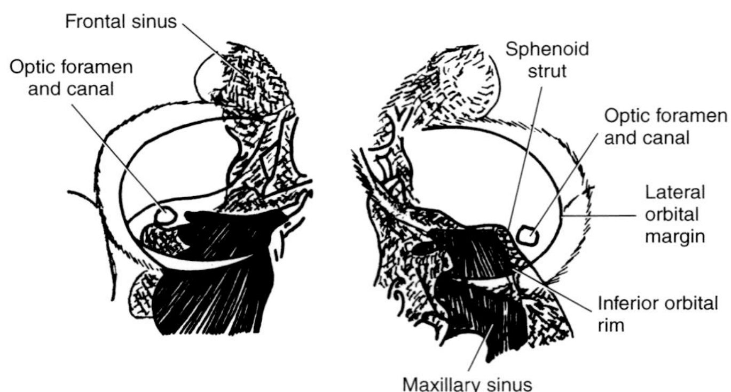

Fig. 13-86. Bilateral parietoorbital.

AXIOLATERAL PROJECTION: MANDIBLE

Mandible
BASIC
- Axiolateral
- PA (or PA axial)
- AP axial (Towne)

Pathology Demonstrated

Fractures and neoplastic/inflammatory processes of the mandible are shown.

Both sides are examined for comparison.

Technical Factors

- IR size—18 × 24 cm (8 × 10 inches), crosswise
- Moving or stationary grid
- 70-80 kV range
- Small focal spot
- AEC not used
- Technique and dose:

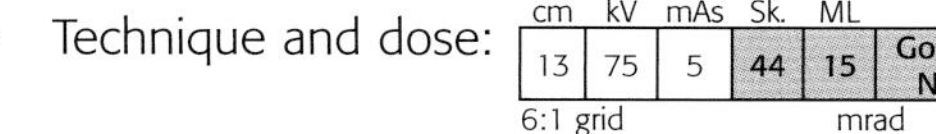

cm	kV	mAs	Sk.	ML	
13	75	5	44	15	Gonads NDC
6:1 grid			mrad		

24 / 18 / R / No AEC

Patient Position Remove all metal, plastic, and other removable objects from head. Patient position is erect or supine. (If supine, place image receptor on wedge sponge to minimize OID.) Use grid placed lengthwise for horizontal beam trauma position.

Part Position

- Place head in a lateral position, with side of interest against IR.
- If possible, have patient close mouth and bring teeth together.
- Extend neck to prevent cervical spine superimposition by chin.
- Rotate head in an oblique direction. The degree of obliquity depends on which section of the mandible is of interest. (Area of interest, if known, should be positioned parallel to IR.)
- Head in **true lateral** position best demonstrates **ramus.**
- **30°** rotation toward IR best demonstrates **body.**
- **45°** rotation best demonstrates **mentum.**
- **10° to 15°** rotation best provides a **general survey** of mandible.

Central Ray

- Angle CR **25° cephalad** from IPL; for the horizontal beam trauma position, angle the CR an additional **5° to 10° posteriorly.**
- Direct CR to exit mandibular region of interest.
- Center IR to projected CR.
- Minimum SID is 40 inches (100 cm).

Collimation Collimate on all sides to mandible.

Respiration Suspend respiration.

Note: For trauma patients who cannot assume erect or semisupine positions, see horizontal beam trauma projection (Fig. 13-89), as described in more detail in Chapter 19 (Trauma, Mobile, and Surgical Radiography).

Evaluation Criteria

Structures Shown: • Rami, condylar and coronoid processes, body, and mentum of mandible nearest the image receptor.

Position: • The appearance of the image/position of the patient depends on the structures under examination. For the ramus and body, the ramus of interest is demonstrated with no superimposition from opposite mandible (indicating correct CR angulation). • No superimposition of the cervical spine by the ramus should exist (indicating sufficient extension of neck). • The ramus and body should be demonstrated without foreshortening (indicating correct rotation of head). • The area of interest is demonstrated with minimal superimposition and minimal foreshortening.

Collimation and CR: • The entire mandible is located within the collimated field.

Exposure Criteria: • Contrast and density are sufficient to visualize the mandibular area of interest. • Sharp bony margins indicate no motion.

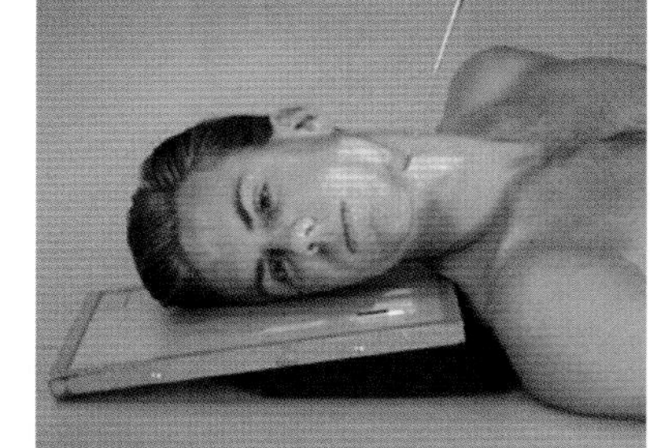

Fig. 13-87. Semisupine—15° **rotation** (general survey). Right lateral.

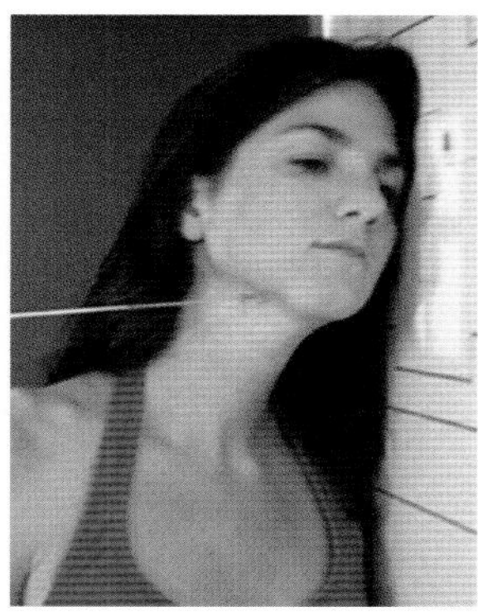

Fig. 13-88. Erect—**30° rotation** (for body). Left lateral.

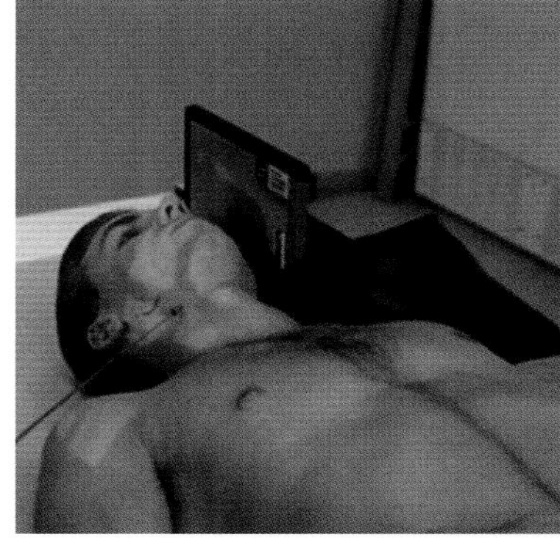

Fig. 13-89. Horizontal beam trauma projection—**25° cephalad; 5°-10° posteriorly.** Left lateral.

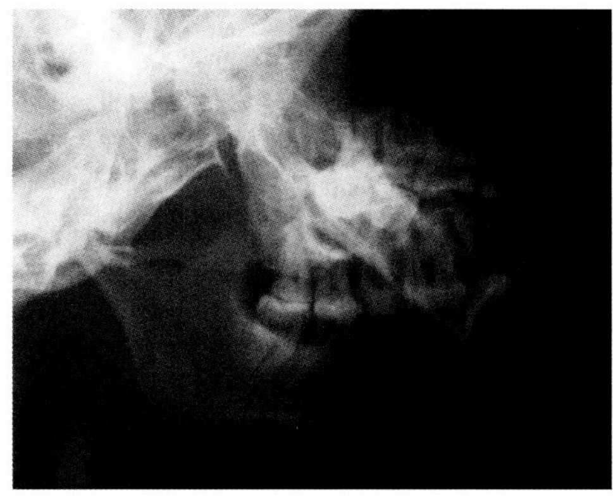

Fig. 13-90. Axiolateral (general survey).

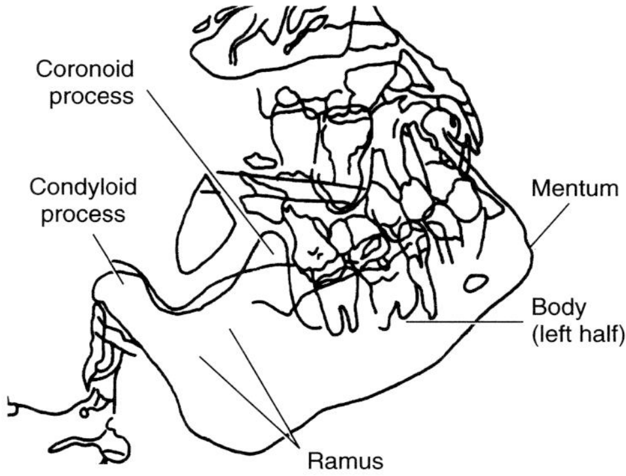

Fig. 13-91. Axiolateral (general survey).

PA OR PA AXIAL PROJECTION: MANDIBLE

Pathology Demonstrated

Fractures and neoplastic/inflammatory processes of the mandible are shown.

Optional PA axial best demonstrates proximal rami and elongated view of condyloid processes.

Mandible
BASIC
• **Axiolateral**
• PA (or PA axial)
• **AP axial (Towne)**

Technical Factors

- IR size—18 × 24 cm (8 × 10 inches), lengthwise
- Moving or stationary grid
- 70-80 kV range
- Small focal spot
- Technique and dose:

cm	kV	mAs	Sk.	ML	
17	75	12	120	32	Gonads NDC
			mrad		

18 × 24, R, No AEC

Patient Position Remove all metal, plastic, and other removable objects from head. Patient position is erect or prone.

Part Position

- Rest patient's forehead and nose against table/upright Bucky surface.
- Tuck chin, bringing **OML perpendicular** to IR (see Note).
- Align **midsagittal plane perpendicular** to midline of the grid or the table/Bucky surface (ensuring no rotation or tilt of head).
- Center image receptor to projected CR (to junction of lips).

Central Ray

- *PA:* Align CR **perpendicular** to IR, centered to **exit at junction of lips.**
- Minimum SID is 40 inches (100 cm).
- ***Optional PA axial:*** Angle CR 20° to 25° cephalad, centered to **exit at acanthion.**

Collimation Collimate to area of mandible.

Respiration Suspend respiration during exposure.

Note: For a true PA projection of the body (if this is area of interest), raise chin to bring acanthiomeatal line perpendicular to IR.

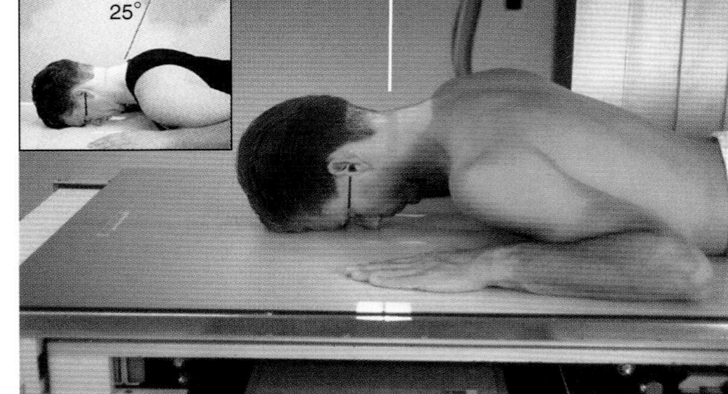

Fig. 13-92. PA—CR perpendicular, exit at junction of lips. *Inset,* Optional PA axial—CR 20° to 25° cephalad, exit at acanthion.

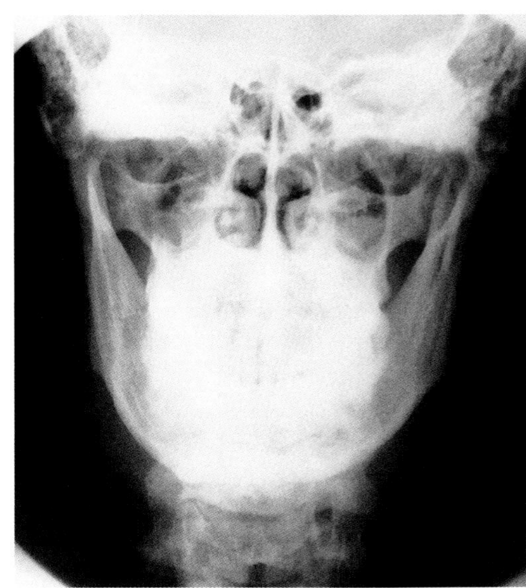

Fig. 13-93. PA—CR 0°.

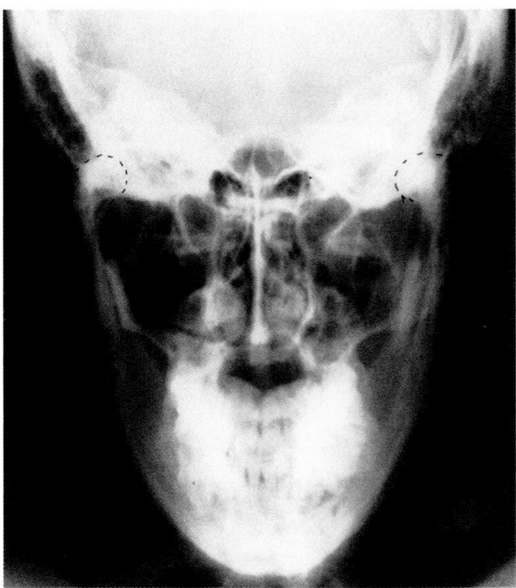

Fig. 13-94. Optional PA axial—CR 20° cephalad.

Radiographic Criteria

Structures Shown: • PA: Mandibular rami and lateral portion of body are visible. • Optional PA axial: TMJ region and heads of condyles are visible through mastoid processes; condyloid processes are well visualized (slightly elongated).

Position: • No patient rotation exists, as indicated by mandibular rami visualized symmetrically, lateral to the cervical spine. • Midbody and mentum are faintly visualized, superimposed on the cervical spine.

Collimation and CR: • The collimated image includes TMJs, mandibular rami, and mentum. • The mandibular rami are in the center of the collimated field.

Exposure Criteria: • Contrast and density are sufficient to visualize mandibular body and rami. • Sharp bony margins indicate no motion.

AP AXIAL PROJECTION: MANDIBLE

Towne Method

Mandible
BASIC
- **Axiolateral**
- **PA (or PA axial)**
- AP axial (Towne)

Pathology Demonstrated

Fractures and neoplastic/inflammatory processes of the condyloid processes of the mandible are shown.

Technical Factors

- IR size—18 × 24 cm (8 × 10 inches), lengthwise
- Moving or stationary grid
- 70-80 kV range (if AEC is used, reduce density 20% to 30%)
- Small focal spot
- Technique and dose:

cm	kV	mAs	Sk.	ML.	Gonads	Thyroid
21	80	16	232	42	NDC	57

mrad

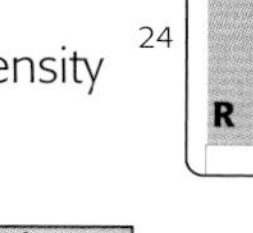

Patient Position Remove all metal, plastic, and other removable objects from head. Patient position is erect or supine.

Part Position

- Rest patient's posterior skull against table/upright Bucky surface.
- Tuck chin, bringing **OML perpendicular** to image receptor or place IOML perpendicular and add 7° to CR angle (see Note).
- Align **midsagittal plane perpendicular** to midline of the grid or the table/upright Bucky surface to prevent head rotation or tilt.

Central Ray

- Angle CR **35° to 40° caudad** (see Notes).
- Center CR to **glabella,** to pass through **midway between EAMs and angles of mandible.**
- Center image receptor to CR.
- Minimum SID is 40 inches (100 cm).

Collimation Collimate to mandible, including TMJs.

Respiration Suspend respiration during exposure.

Notes: If patient is unable to bring OML perpendicular to image receptor, align the IOML perpendicular and increase the CR angle 7°.

If the area of interest is the TM fossae, angle 40° to the OML to reduce superimposition of the TM fossae and mastoid portions of the temporal bone.

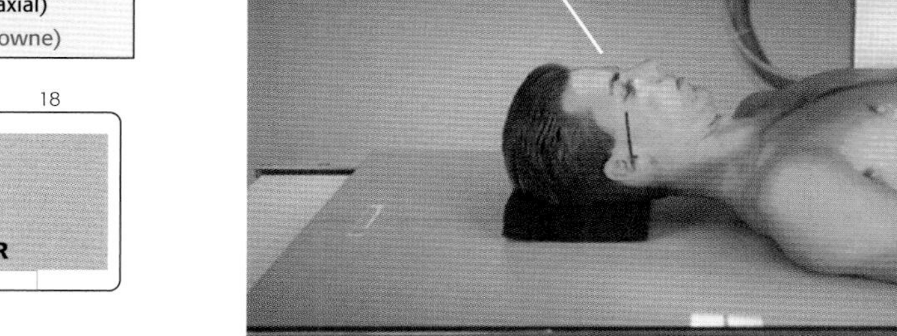

Fig. 13-95. AP axial—CR 35° to 40° to OML.

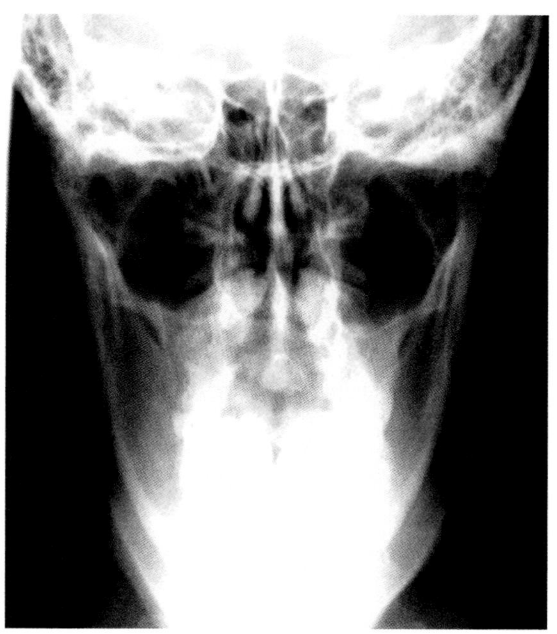

Fig. 13-96. AP axial.

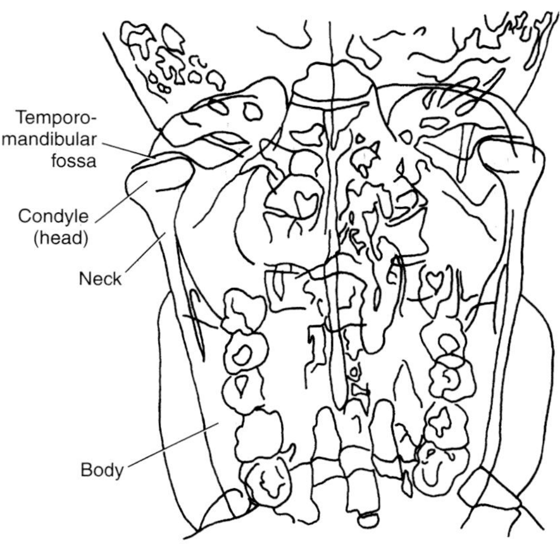

Fig. 13-97. AP axial.

Radiographic Criteria

Structures Shown: • Condyloid processes of mandible and temporomandibular fossae.

Position: • A correctly positioned image with no rotation demonstrates the following: condyloid processes visualized symmetrically, lateral to the cervical spine; clear visualization of condyle/temporomandibular fossae relationship, with minimal superimposition of the TM fossae and mastoid portions.

Collimation and CR: • Collimated field includes the condyloid processes of the mandible and the temporomandibular fossae.

Exposure Criteria: • Contrast and density are sufficient to visualize condyloid process and temporomandibular fossa. • No motion exists, as indicated by sharp bony margins.

13

SUBMENTOVERTEX (SMV) PROJECTION: MANDIBLE

Mandible
SPECIAL
- Submentovertex (SMV)
- Panorex (mandible and/or TMJs)

Pathology Demonstrated

Fractures and neoplastic/inflammatory process of the mandible are shown.

Technical Factors

- IR size—18 × 24 cm (8 × 10 inches), lengthwise
- Stationary or moving grid
- 70-80 kV range
- Small focal spot
- Technique and dose:

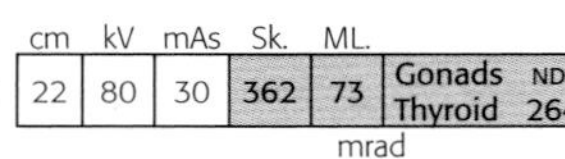

cm	kV	mAs	Sk.	ML.	
22	80	30	362	73	Gonads NDC Thyroid 264

mrad

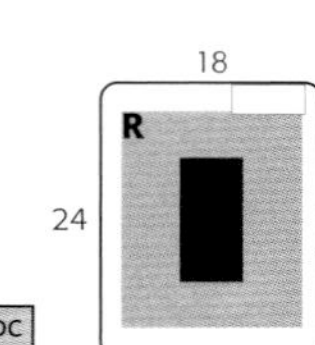

Patient Position Remove all metal, plastic, and other removable objects from head and neck. Patient position is erect or supine (erect preferred, if patient's condition allows). Erect may be done with an erect table or an upright Bucky (see photo *inset*).

Part Position

- Hyperextend neck until **IOML is parallel** to image receptor.
- Rest head on vertex of skull.
- Align **midsagittal plane perpendicular** to midline of the grid or the table/upright Bucky surface to prevent head rotation or tilt.

Central Ray

- Align CR **perpendicular to image receptor or IOML** (see Notes).
- Center CR to a point **midway between angles of mandible,** at a level **$1\frac{1}{2}$ inches (4 cm) inferior to mandibular symphysis.**
- Center image receptor to projected CR.
- Minimum SID is 40 inches (100 cm).

Collimation Collimate to area of mandible.

Respiration Suspend respiration.

Notes: If patient is unable to sufficiently extend the neck, angle tube to align CR **perpendicular to IOML.**

This position is very uncomfortable for the patient; complete the projection as quickly as possible.

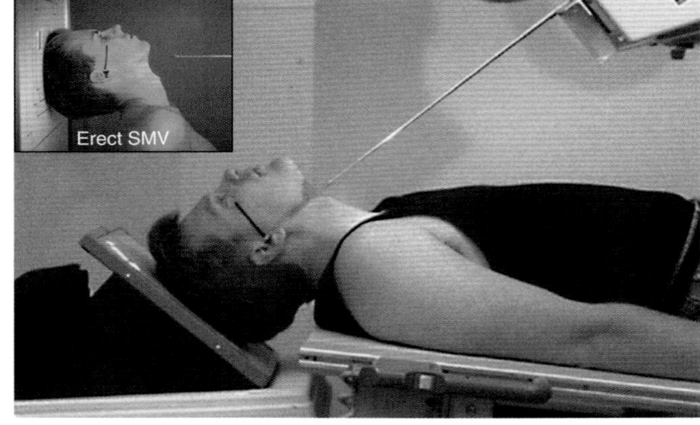

Fig. 13-98. Submentovertex (SMV).

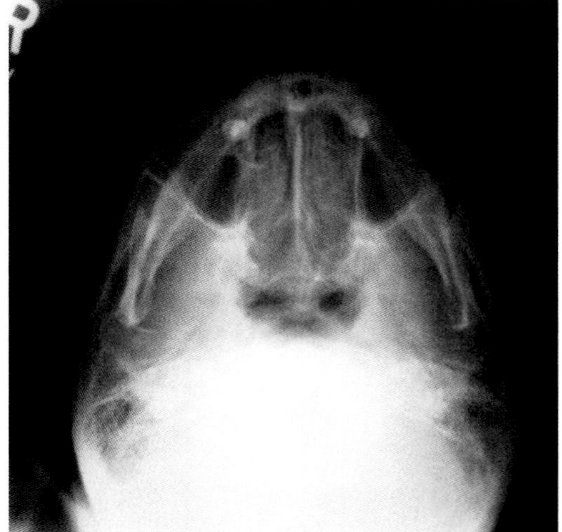

Fig. 13-99. Submentovertex (SMV).

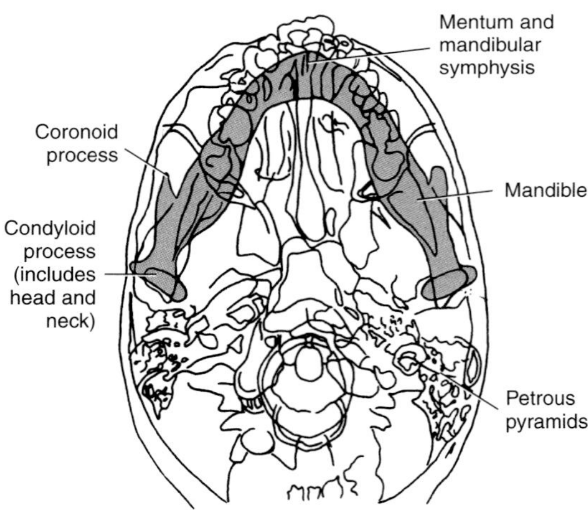

Fig. 13-100. Submentovertex (SMV).

Radiographic Criteria

Structures Shown: • Entire mandible and coronoid and condyloid processes.

Position: • Correct neck extension is indicated by the following: mandibular symphysis superimposing frontal bone; mandibular condyles projected anterior to petrous ridges • No patient rotation or tilt is indicated by the following: equal distance from mandible to lateral border of skull on both sides; mandibular coronoid processes visualized, projecting laterally from the rami area equally on each side of mandible.

Collimation and CR: • The collimated field includes, and is limited to, the mandible.

Exposure Criteria: • Contrast and density are sufficient to visualize the mandible superimposed on the skull. • Sharp bony margins indicate no motion.

PANOREX—PANORAMIC TOMOGRAPHY: MANDIBLE

Mandible
SPECIAL
- **Submentovertex (SMV)**
- Panorex (mandible and/or TMJs)

Pathology Demonstrated
Fractures of the mandible and TMJ pathology

Technical Factors
- IR size—23 × 30 cm (9 × 12 inches), crosswise
- Curved nongrid cassette
- 70-80 kV range

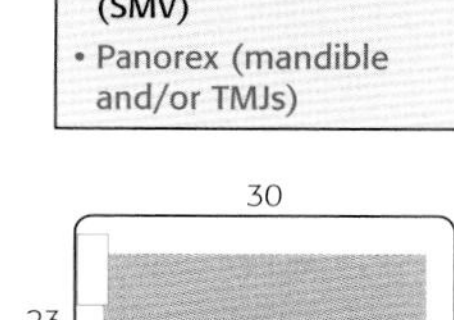

Unit Preparation
- Attach image receptor to panoramic unit.
- Position tube and image receptor at starting position.
- Raise chin rest to approximately same level as patient's chin.

Shielding Wrap vest-type lead apron around patient.

Patient Position
- Remove all metal, plastic, and other removable objects from head and neck.
- Explain to patient how tube and image receptor rotate and the time span needed for exposure.
- Guide patient into unit, resting patient's chin on bite block.
- Position patient's body, head, and neck as demonstrated below, in Fig. 13-103. Do not allow head and neck to stretch forward but have patient stand in close, with spine straight and hips forward.

Part Position
- Adjust height of chin rest until **IOML is aligned parallel with floor.** The occlusal plane (plane of biting surface of teeth) declines 10° from posterior to anterior.
- Align **midsagittal plane** with the vertical center line of the chin rest.
- Position bite block between patient's front teeth (see Note).
- Instruct patient to place lips together and position tongue on roof of mouth.

Central Ray
- X-ray beam direction is fixed and directed slightly cephalic to project anatomic structures, positioned at the same height, on top of one another.
- Fixed SID, per panoramic unit.

Collimation A narrow, vertical-slit diaphragm is attached to tube, providing collimation.

Note: When the TMJs are of interest, a second panoramic image is taken with the mouth open. This requires a larger bite block to be placed between the patient's teeth.

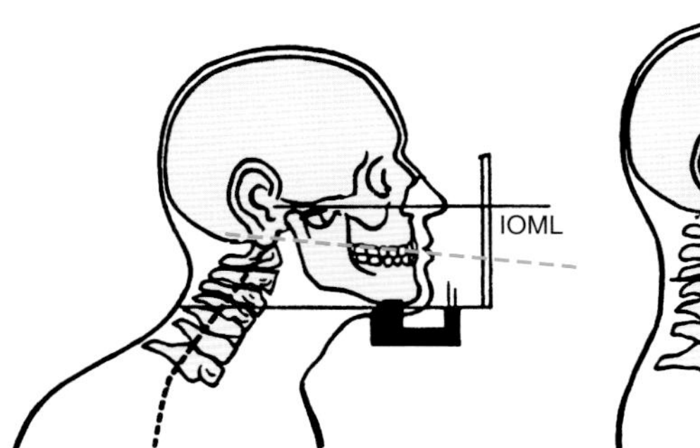

Fig. 13-102. Incorrect position.

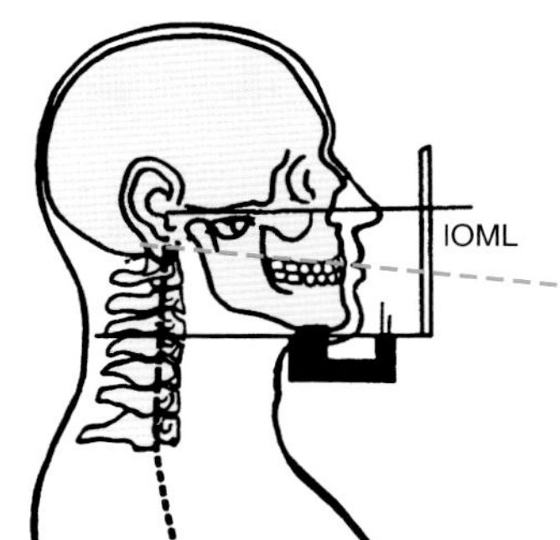

Fig. 13-103. Correct position.

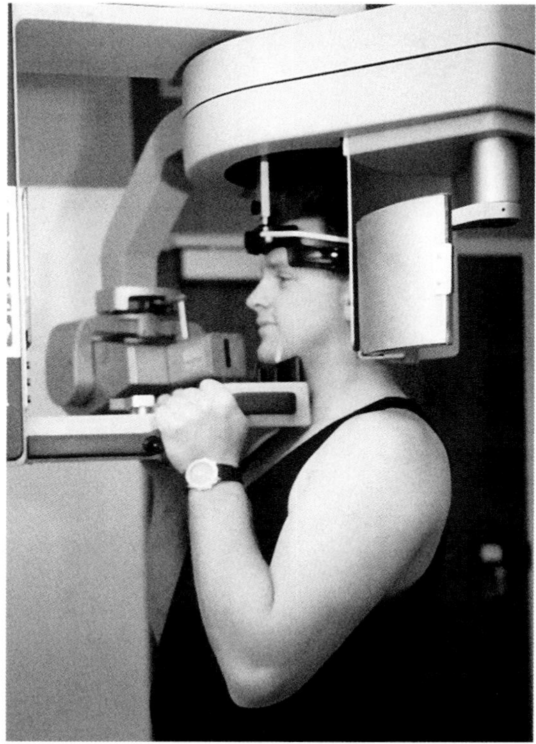

Fig. 13-101. Panorex—head correctly positioned.

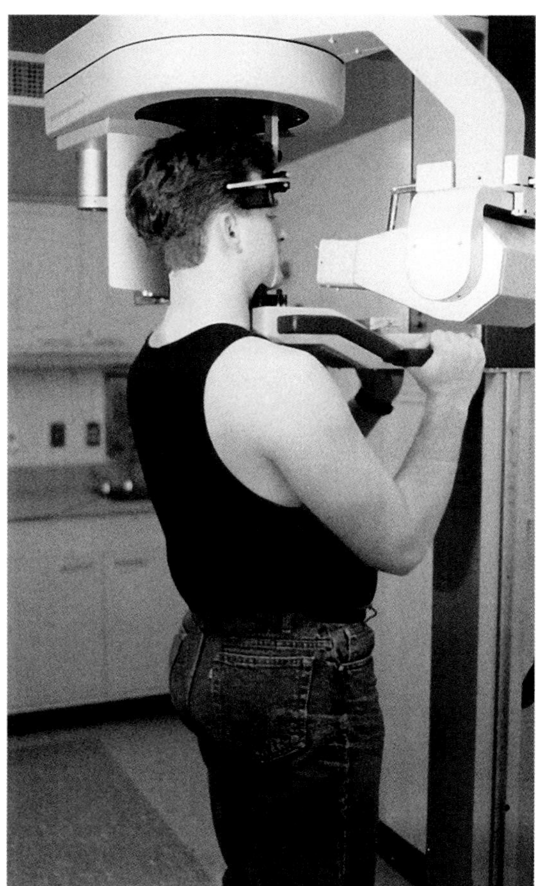

Fig. 13-104. Panorex—correct body position.

Radiographic Criteria

Structures Shown: • A single image of the teeth, mandible, TMJs, nasal fossae, maxillary sinus, zygomatic arches, and maxillae is shown. • A portion of the cervical spine is visualized.

Position: • The mandible visualized without rotation or tilting is indicated by the following: TMJs on the same horizontal plane in the image; rami and posterior teeth equally magnified on each side of the image; anterior and posterior teeth sharply visualized with uniform magnification. • Correct positioning of the patient is indicated by the following: mandibular symphysis projected slightly below the mandibular angles; mandible oval in shape; occlusal plane parallel with the long axis of the image; upper and lower teeth positioned slightly apart with no superimposition; cervical spine demonstrated with no superimposition of the TMJs.

Collimation and CR: • The mandible is located in the center of the image. • The entire mandible is included in the collimation field.

Exposure Criteria: • Density of mandible and teeth is uniform across entire image; no density loss is evident in the center. • No artifacts are superimposed on the image.

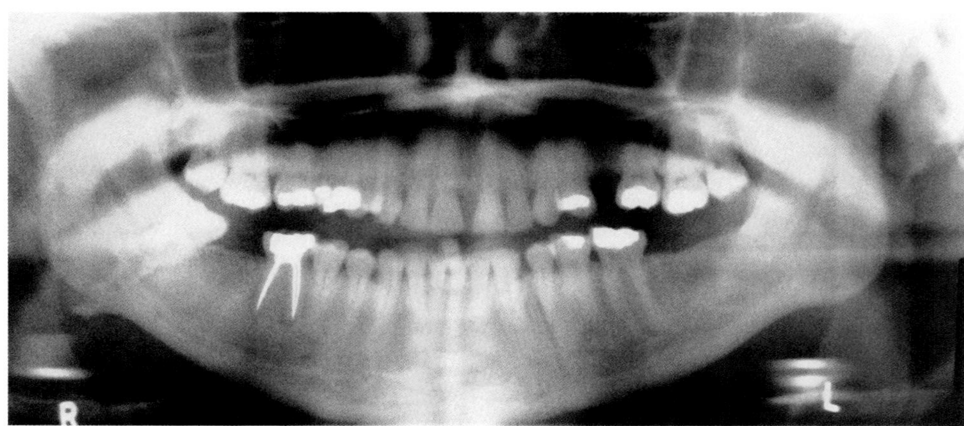

Fig. 13-105. Panorex.

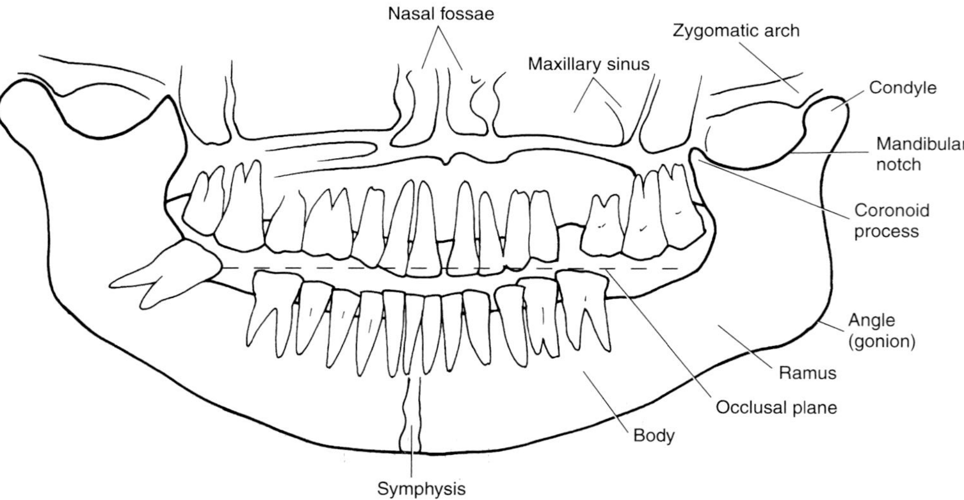

Fig. 13-106. Panorex.

AP AXIAL PROJECTION: TMJs

Modified Towne Method

Warning: Opening of the mouth should not be attempted with possible fracture.

TMJs
SPECIAL
- AP axial (modified Towne)
- Axiolateral oblique (modified Law)
- Axiolateral (Schuller)
- Panorex (p. 433)

Pathology Demonstrated

Fractures and abnormal relationship/range of motion between condyle and TM fossa

(See Note 1, concerning open- and closed-mouth comparisons.)

Technical Factors

- IR size—18 ×24 cm (8 × 10 inches), crosswise
- Moving or stationary grid
- 70-80 kV range (if AEC is used, reduce density by 20% to 30%)
- Small focal spot
- Technique and dose:

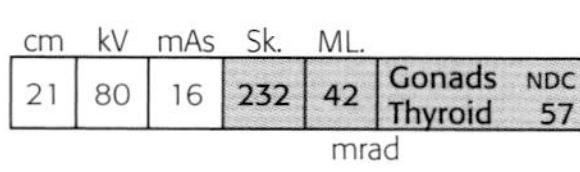

cm	kV	mAs	Sk.	ML.	Gonads NDC / Thyroid 57
21	80	16	232	42	Gonads NDC Thyroid 57

mrad

Patient Position Remove all metal, plastic, and other removable objects from head. Position patient erect or supine.

Part Position

- Rest patient's posterior skull against table/upright Bucky surface.
- Tuck chin, bringing **OML perpendicular** to table/ Bucky surface or bringing IOML perpendicular and increasing CR angle 7°.
- Align **midsagittal plane perpendicular** to midline of the grid or the table/upright Bucky surface to prevent head rotation or tilt.

Central Ray

- Angle CR **35° caudad from the OML** or **42° from IOML.**
- Direct CR to pass through 1 inch (2.5 cm) anterior to **level of TMJs** (2 inches [5 cm] anterior to EAMs).
- Center image receptor to projected CR.
- Minimum SID is 40 inches (100 cm).

Collimation Collimate on all sides to region of interest.

Respiration Suspend respiration during exposure.

Note 1: Some departmental protocols indicate, when patient's condition allows, that these projections be taken in both closed- and open-mouth positions for comparison purposes.

Note 2: An additional 5° increase of CR may best demonstrate the TM fossae and joint.

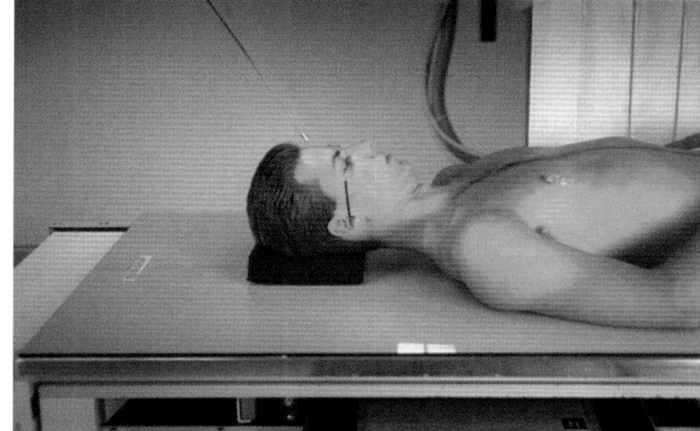

Fig. 13-107. AP axial—CR 35° to OML (closed-mouth position).

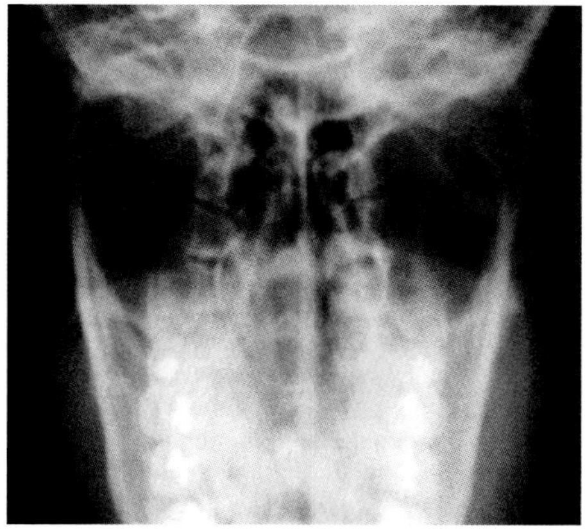

Fig. 13-108. AP axial (closed-mouth position).

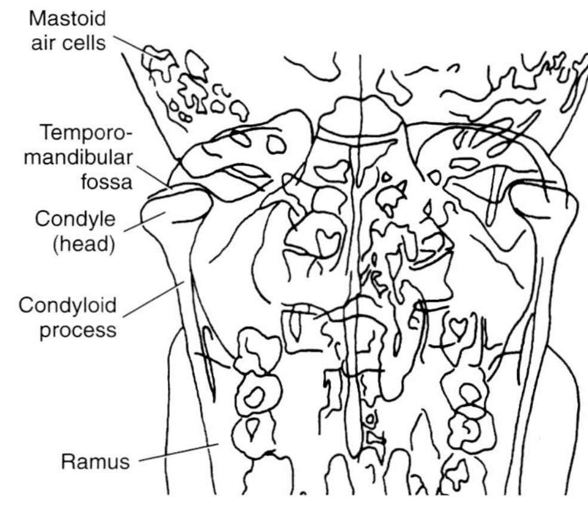

Fig. 13-109. AP axial.

Radiographic Criteria

Structures Shown: • Condyloid processes of mandible and temporomandibular fossae.

Position: • Correctly positioned patient, with no rotation, is indicated by the following: condyloid processes visualized symmetrically, lateral to the cervical spine; clear visualization of condyle and temporomandibular fossae relationship.

Collimation and CR: • Collimation field includes the condyloid process of the mandible and the temporomandibular fossa. • Center of the collimation field is the level of the TMJs.

Exposure Criteria: • Contrast and density are sufficient to visualize condyloid process and temporomandibular fossa. • Sharp bony margins indicate no motion.

AXIOLATERAL OBLIQUE PROJECTION: TMJs

Modified Law Method

Pathology Demonstrated

Abnormal relationship/range of motion between condyle and TM fossa is shown

Generally, images are obtained in the open- and closed-mouth positions.

TMJs

SPECIAL

- **AP axial (modified Towne)**
- Axiolateral 15° oblique (modified Law)
- **Axiolateral (Schuller)**
- **Panorex (p. 433)**

Technique Factors

- IR size—18 × 24 cm (8 × 10 inches), lengthwise
- Stationary or moving grid
- 70-80 kV range
- Small focal spot
- Technique and dose:

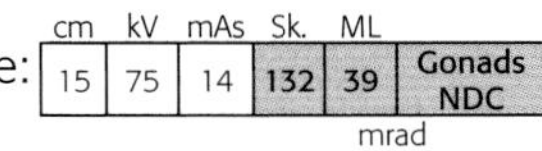

cm	kV	mAs	Sk.	ML	Gonads
15	75	14	132	39	NDC
			mrad		

Patient Position Patient position is erect or prone (erect is preferred if patient's condition allows). Rest lateral aspect of head against table/upright Bucky surface, with side of interest closest to image receptor.

Part Position

- Move patient's body in an oblique direction, as needed for patient's comfort.
- Prevent tilt by maintaining **interpupillary line perpendicular** to image receptor.
- Align **IOML perpendicular** to front edge of image receptor.
- From lateral position, **rotate face toward image receptor 15°** (midsagittal plane of head being rotated 15° from plane of IR).

Central Ray

- Angle CR **15° caudad,** centered to **1½ inches (4 cm) superior to upside EAM** (to pass through downside TMJ).
- Center image receptor to projected CR.
- Minimum SID is 40 inches (100 cm).

Collimation Collimate on all sides to yield a field size of approximately 4 inches (10 cm) square.

Respiration Suspend respiration during exposure.

Fig. 13-110. Right TMJ—closed and open mouth; **15° oblique; CR 15° caudad.**

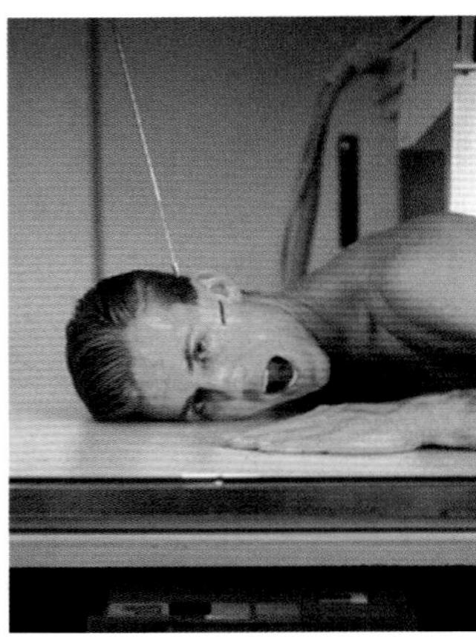

Fig. 13-111. Right TMJ—closed and open mouth; **15° oblique; CR 15° caudad.**

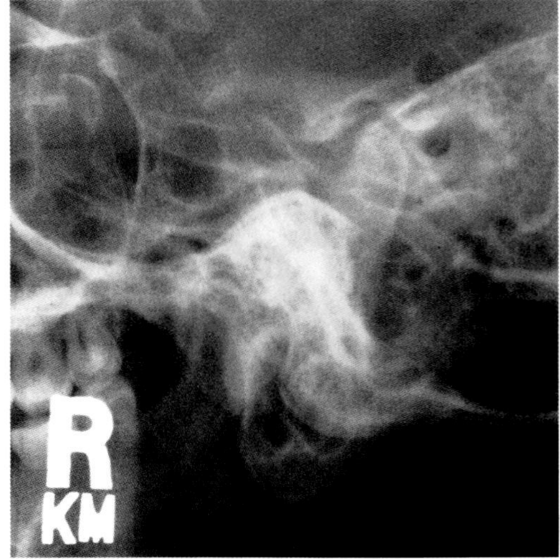

Fig. 13-112. TMJ—closed mouth.

Radiographic Criteria

Structures Shown: • TMJ nearest the image receptor is visible. • Closed-mouth image demonstrates condyle within mandibular fossa; the condyle moves to the anterior margin of the mandibular fossa in the open-mouth position.

Position: • Correctly positioned images demonstrate the TMJ closest to image receptor clearly, without superimposition of opposite TMJ (15° rotation preventing superimposition). • TMJ of interest is not superimposed by cervical spine.

Collimation and CR: • TMJ nearest to image receptor is located in the center of the tightly collimated field.

Exposure Criteria: • Contrast and density are sufficient to visualize TMJ. • Sharp bony margins indicate no motion.

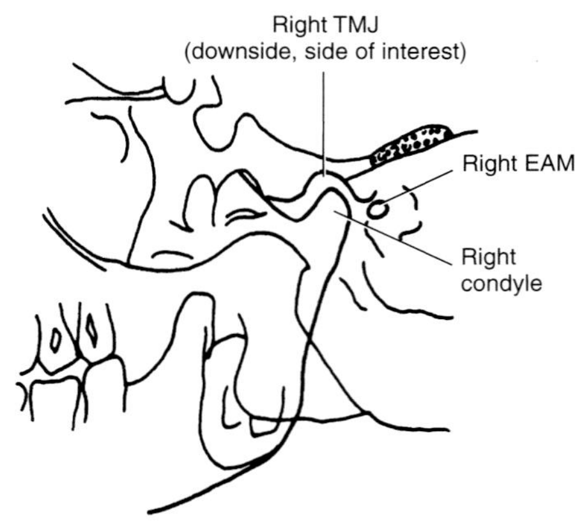

Fig. 13-113. TMJ—closed mouth.

AXIOLATERAL PROJECTION: TMJ

Schuller Method

TMJs
SPECIAL
- **AP axial (modified Towne)**
- **Axiolateral 15° oblique (modified Law)**
- Axiolateral (Schuller)
- **Panorex (p. 433)**

Pathology Demonstrated

Abnormal relationship/range of motion between condyle and TM fossa is shown.

Generally, images are obtained in the open- and closed-mouth positions.

Technical Factors

- IR size—18 × 24 cm (8 × 10 inches), lengthwise
- Stationary or moving grid
- 70-80 kV range
- Small focal spot
- Technique and dose:

cm	kV	mAs	Sk.	ML	
15	75	14	132	39	Gonads NDC
			mrad		

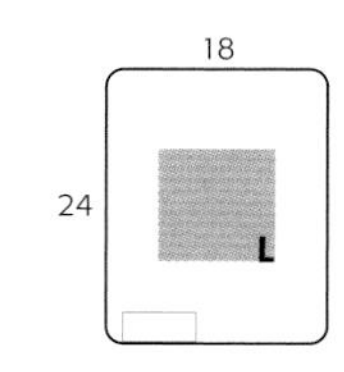

Patient Position Position patient erect or prone. Rest lateral aspect of head against table/Bucky surface, with side of interest nearest the image receptor.

Part Position

- Adjust head into a **true lateral position** and move patient's body in an oblique direction, as needed for patient's comfort.
- Align **interpupillary line perpendicular** to image receptor.
- Align **midsagittal plane parallel** with table/Bucky surface.
- Position **IOML perpendicular** to front edge of image receptor.

Central Ray

- Angle CR **25° to 30° caudad,** centered to ½ inch (1.3 cm) anterior and 2 inches (5 cm) superior to upside EAM.
- Center image receptor to projected TMJ.
- Minimum SID is 40 inches (100 cm).

Collimation Collimate on all sides to yield a field size of approximately 4 inches (10 cm) square.

Respiration Suspend respiration during exposure.

Note: This projection results in more elongation of the condyle, as compared with the modified Law method.

Radiographic Criteria

Structures Shown: • TMJ nearest the image receptor is visible. • The closed-mouth image demonstrates the condyle within the mandibular fossa; the condyle moves to anterior margin of fossa in the open-mouth position.

Position: • TMJs are demonstrated without rotation, as evidenced by superimposed lateral margins.

Collimation and CR: • TMJ nearest the image receptor is located in the center of the tightly collimated field.

Exposure Criteria: • Contrast and density are sufficient to visualize TMJ. • Sharp bony margins indicate no motion.

Fig. 13-114. Left TMJ—closed mouth; **true lateral, CR 25° to 30° caudad angle.**

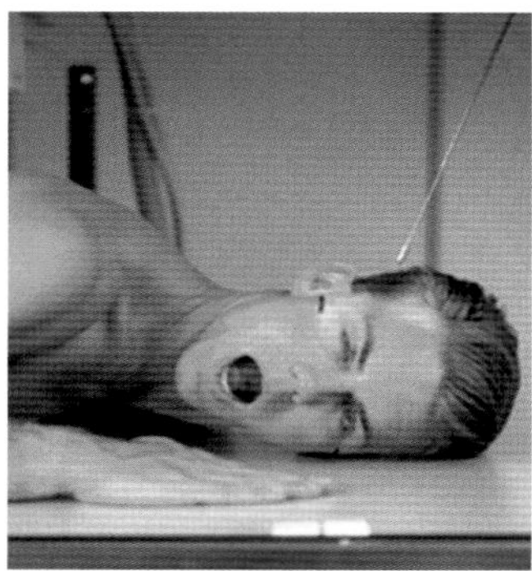

Fig. 13-115. Left TMJ—open mouth.

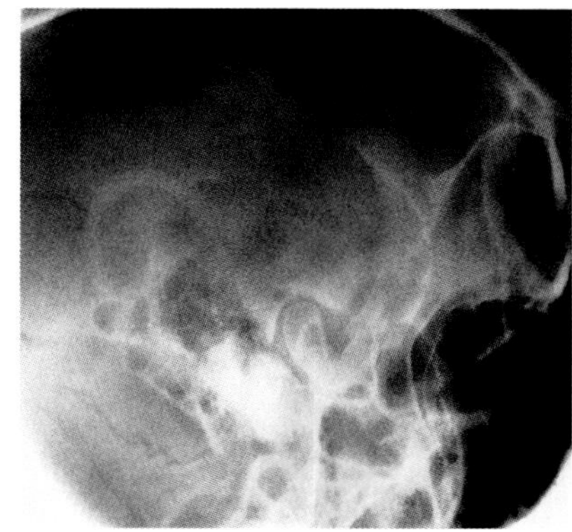

Fig. 13-116. Closed mouth.

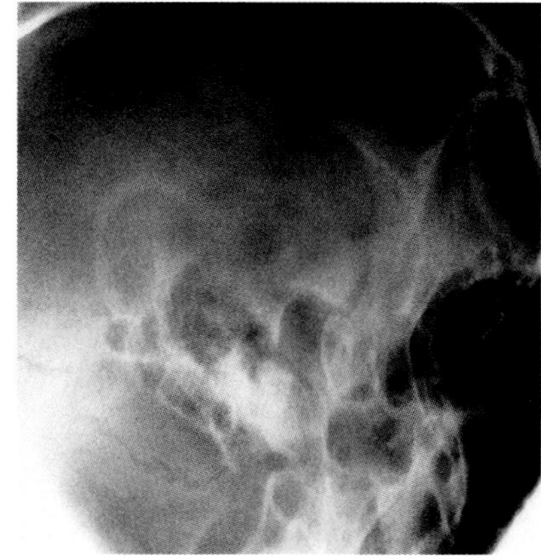

Fig. 13-117. Open mouth.

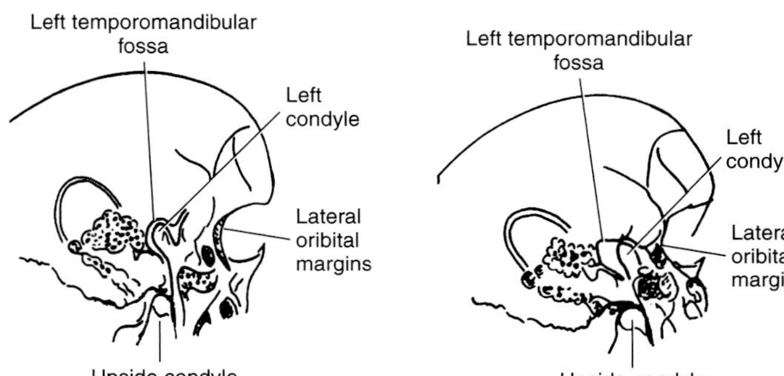

Fig. 13-118. Closed mouth. **Fig. 13-119.** Open mouth.

LATERAL POSITION—RIGHT OR LEFT LATERAL: SINUSES

Pathology Demonstrated
Inflammatory conditions (sinusitis, secondary osteomyelitis) and sinus polyps

Sinuses
BASIC
- Lateral
- PA (Caldwell)
- Parietoacanthial (Waters)

Technical Factors
- IR size—18 × 24 cm (8 × 10 inches), lengthwise
- Moving or stationary grid
- 70-80 kV range
- Small focal spot
- Technique and dose:

cm	kV	mAs	Sk.	ML	Gon.
15	70	5	39	10	NDC

mrad

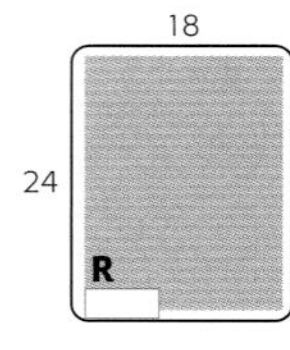

Patient Position Remove all metal, plastic, and other removable objects from head. Position patient **erect** (see Notes).

Part Position
- Place lateral aspect of head against table/upright Bucky surface, with side of interest closest to IR.
- Adjust head into a **true lateral** position, moving body in an oblique direction as needed for patient's comfort (midsagittal plane parallel to IR).
- Align **interpupillary line perpendicular to IR** (ensures no tilt).
- Adjust chin to align IOML perpendicular to front edge of IR.

Central Ray
- Align a **horizontal CR** perpendicular to the IR.
- Center CR to a point **midway between outer canthus and EAM.**
- Center IR to CR.
- Minimum SID is 40 inches (100 cm).

Collimation Collimate to area of sinus cavities.

Respiration Suspend respiration during exposure.

Notes: To visualize air-fluid levels, an erect position with a horizontal beam is required. Fluid within the paranasal sinus cavities is thick and gelatin-like, causing it to cling to the cavity walls. To visualize this fluid, allow a short time (at least 5 minutes) for the fluid to settle after a patient's position has been changed (i.e., from recumbent to erect).

If patient is unable to be placed in the upright position, the image may be obtained utilizing a horizontal beam, similar to trauma lateral facial bones, as described in Chapter 19 (Trauma, Mobile, and Surgical Radiography).

Radiographic Criteria

Structures Shown: • Sphenoid sinuses, superimposed frontal, ethmoid and maxillary sinuses, sella turcica, and orbital roofs.

Position: • An accurately positioned cranium without rotation or tilt is demonstrated by the following: superimposed mandibular rami, orbital roofs, and greater wings of the sphenoid; nonrotated sella turcica.

Collimation and CR: • Collimated field centered just posterior to the orbit and including the frontal, sphenoid, ethmoid, and maxillary sinuses.

Exposure Criteria: • Density and contrast are sufficient to visualize the sphenoid sinuses through the cranium without overexposing the maxillary and frontal sinuses. • Sharp bony margins indicate no motion.

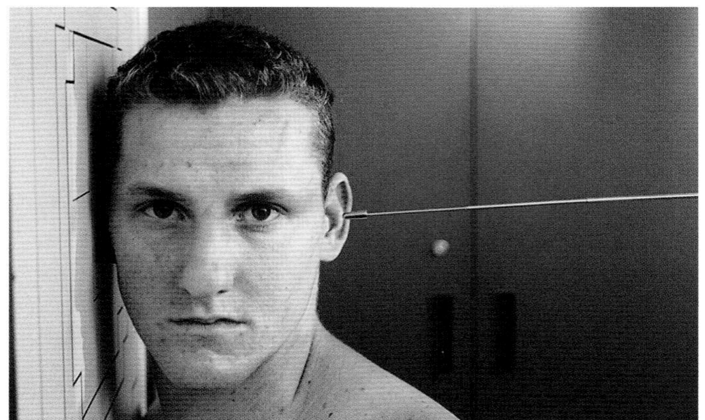

Fig. 13-120. Erect right lateral (upright Bucky).

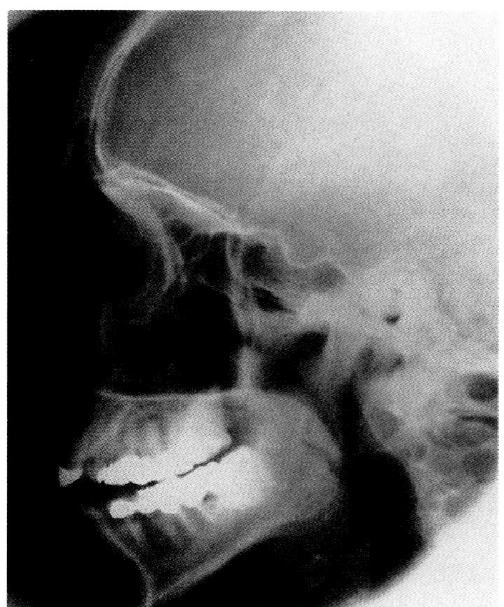

Fig. 13-121. Lateral sinuses.

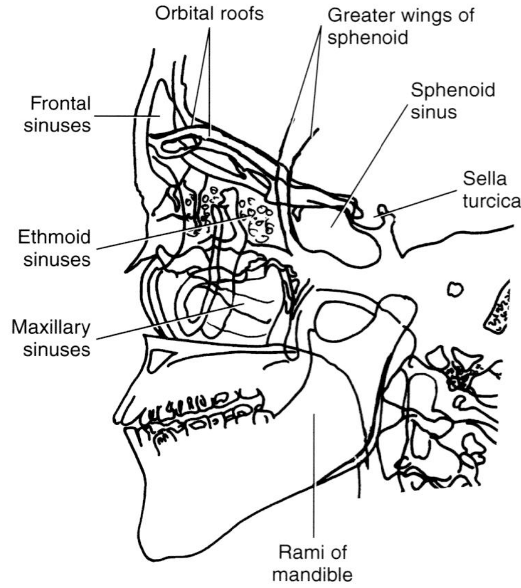

Fig. 13-122. Lateral sinuses.

13

PA PROJECTION: SINUSES

Caldwell Method

Sinuses
BASIC
- **Lateral**
- PA (Caldwell)
- **Parietoacanthial (Waters)**

Pathology Demonstrated
Inflammatory conditions (sinusitis, secondary osteomyelitis) and sinus polyps are shown.

Technical Factors
- IR size—18 × 24 cm (8 × 10 inches) lengthwise
- Moving or stationary grid
- 70-80 kV range
- Small focal spot
- Upright Bucky angled 15° if possible, CR horizontal (see Note)
- Technique and dose:

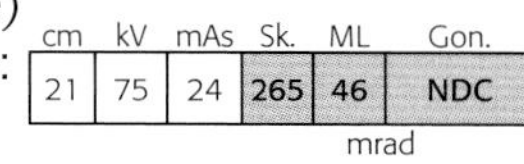

cm	kV	mAs	Sk.	ML	Gon.
21	75	24	265	46	NDC
				mrad	

Patient Position Remove all metal, plastic, and other removable objects from head. Position patient erect (see Note).

Part Position
- Place patient's nose and forehead against upright Bucky or table with neck extended to elevate the **OML 15° from horizontal.** A radiolucent support between forehead and upright Bucky or table may be used to maintain this position. **CR remains horizontal.** (See alternate method if Bucky can be tilted 15°.)
- Align **midsagittal plane perpendicular to midline** of grid or upright Bucky surface.
- Center IR to CR and to nasion, ensuring **no rotation.**

Central Ray
- Align **CR horizontal,** parallel with the floor (see Note).
- Center CR to **exit at nasion.**
- Minimum SID is 40 inches (100 cm).

Collimation Collimate to area of sinus cavities.

Respiration Suspend respiration.

Note: To accurately assess air-fluid levels, the **CR must be horizontal** and the **patient must be erect.**

Alternative method: An alternative method if the **Bucky can be tilted 15°** is shown in the inset photo (Fig. 13-123). The patient's forehead and nose can be supported directly against the Bucky with the **OML perpendicular to the Bucky surface** and **15° to the horizontal CR.**

Radiographic Criteria

Structures Shown: • Frontal sinuses projected above the frontonasal suture. • Anterior ethmoid air cells visualized lateral to each nasal bone, directly below the frontal sinuses.

Position: • Accurately positioned cranium with no rotation or tilt is indicated by the following: equal distance from the lateral margin of the orbit to the lateral border of the skull on both sides; equal distance from the midsagittal plane (identified by the crista galli) to the outer orbital margin on both sides; superior orbital fissures symmetrically visualized within the orbits. • Correct alignment of OML and CR projects petrous ridges into lower one third of orbits.

Collimation and CR: • Included and centered to the collimation field and IR are the frontal and anterior ethmoid sinuses.

Exposure Criteria: • Density and contrast are sufficient to visualize the frontal and ethmoid sinuses. • Sharp bony margins indicate no motion.

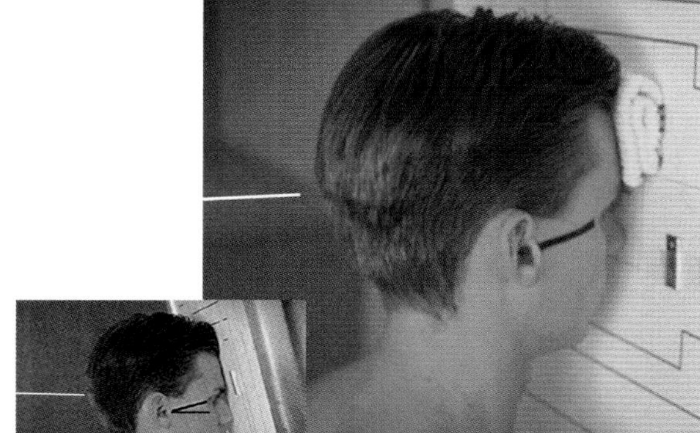

Fig. 13-123. CR horizontal, OML 15° to CR (if cannot be tilted). *Inset,* if upright, Bucky can be tilted 15°.

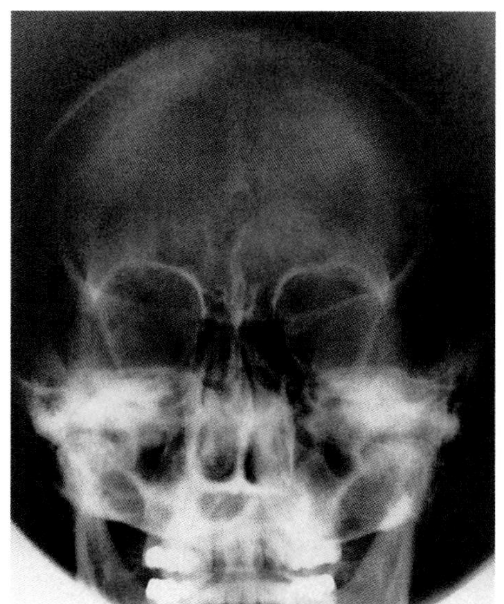

Fig. 13-124. PA projection.

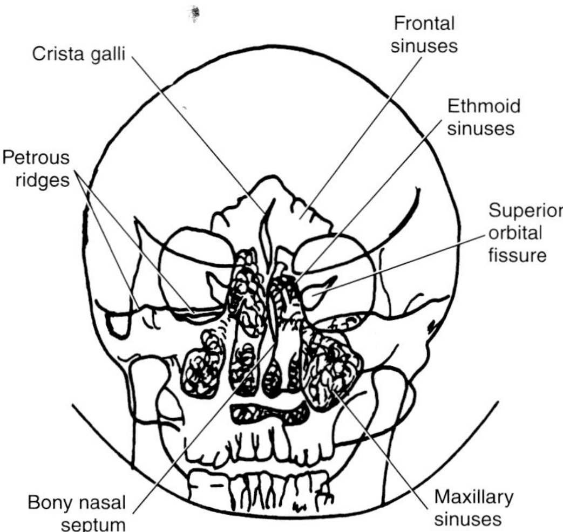

Fig. 13-125. PA projection.

PARIETOACANTHIAL PROJECTION: SINUSES

Waters Method

Sinuses
BASIC
- **Lateral**
- **PA (Caldwell)**
- Parietoacanthial (Waters)

Pathology Demonstrated

Inflammatory conditions (sinusitis, secondary osteomyelitis) and sinus polyps are shown.

Technical Factors

- IR size—18 × 24 cm (8 × 10 inches), lengthwise
- Moving or stationary grid
- 70-80 kV range
- Small focal spot
- Technique and dose:

cm	kV	mAs	Sk.	ML	Gon.
24	75	28	331	46	NDC
				mrad	

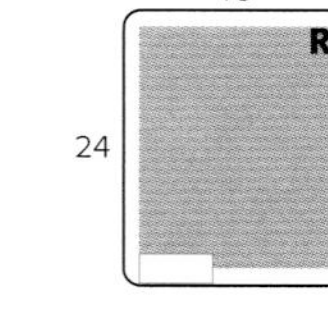

Patient Position Remove all metal, plastic, and other removable objects from head. Position patient erect (see Note).

Part Position

- Extend neck, placing chin and nose against table/upright Bucky surface.
- Adjust head until **mentomeatal line (MML) is perpendicular** to IR; OML will form a 37° angle with the plane of the IR.
- Position the **midsagittal plane perpendicular** to the midline of grid or table/upright Bucky surface.
- Ensure that **no rotation or tilt** exists.
- Center IR to CR and to acanthion.

Central Ray

- Align a **horizontal CR perpendicular** to the IR centered to **exit at acanthion.**
13
- Minimum SID is 40 inches (100 cm).

Collimation Collimate to area of sinus cavities.

Respiration Suspend respiration during exposure.

Note: CR must be horizontal and patient must be erect to demonstrate air-fluid levels within the paranasal sinus cavities.

Radiographic Criteria

Structures Shown: • Maxillary sinuses with the inferior aspect visualized free from superimposing alveolar processes and petrous ridges, the inferior orbital rim, and an oblique view of the frontal sinuses.

Position: • No rotation of the cranium is indicated by the following: equal distance from midsagittal plane (identified by the bony nasal septum) to the outer orbital margin on both sides; equal distance from the lateral orbital margin to the lateral border of the skull on both sides. • Adequate extension of neck demonstrates petrous ridges below the maxillary sinuses

Collimation and CR: • The collimated field, centered to the acanthion, includes the frontal and maxillary sinuses.

Exposure Criteria: • Density and contrast are sufficient to visualize maxillary sinuses. • Sharp bony margins indicate no motion.

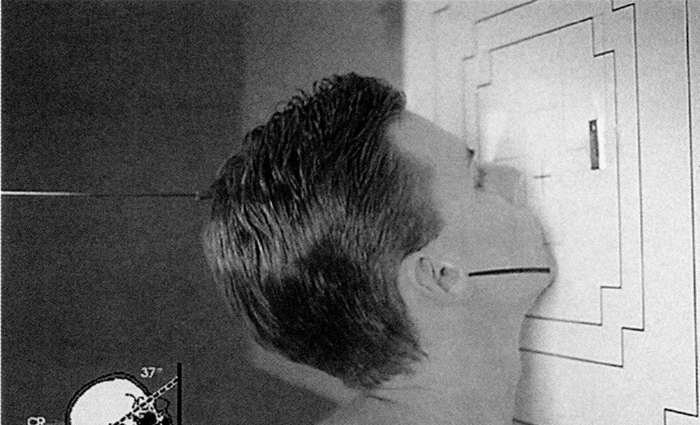

Fig. 13-126. Parietoacanthial projection (upright Bucky/table)—CR and MML perpendicular (OML 37° to IR).

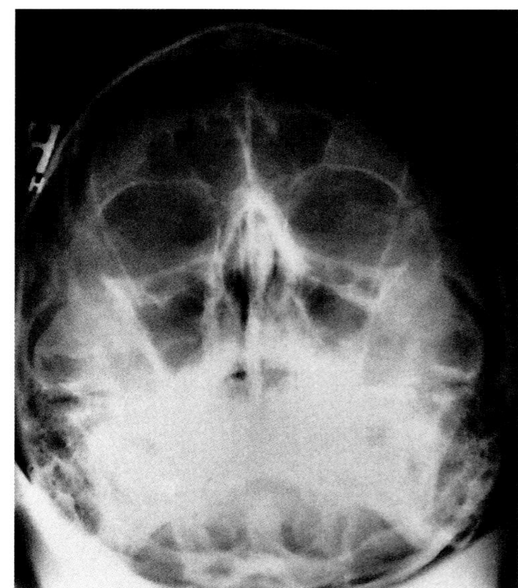

Fig. 13-127. Parietoacanthial projection.

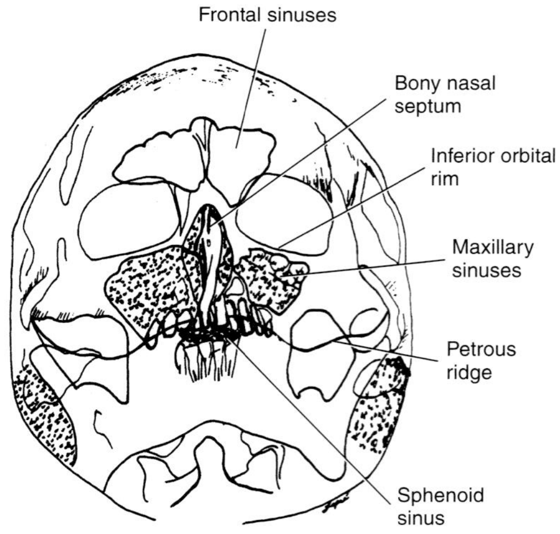

Fig. 13-128. Parietoacanthial projection.

SUBMENTOVERTEX (SMV) PROJECTION: SINUSES

Sinuses
SPECIAL
• Submentovertex (SMV)

Pathology Demonstrated
Inflammatory conditions (sinusitis, secondary osteomyelitis) and sinus polyps are shown.

Technical Factors
- IR size—18 × 24 cm (8 × 10 inches), lengthwise
- Moving or stationary grid
- 70-80 kV range
- Small focal spot
- Technique and dose:

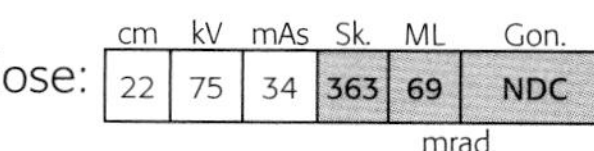

cm	kV	mAs	Sk.	ML	Gon.
22	75	34	363	69	NDC
			mrad		

18 × 24, R

Patient Position Remove all metal, plastic, and other removable objects from head and neck. Position patient erect, if possible, to show air-fluid levels.

Part Position
- Raise chin, hyperextend neck if possible until **IOML is parallel** to table/upright Bucky surface. (See Notes.)
- Head rests on vertex of skull.
- Align **midsagittal plane perpendicular** to midline of the grid or table/upright Bucky surface; ensure **no rotation or tilt.**

Central Ray
- CR directed **perpendicular to IOML** (see Notes)
- CR centered midway between angles of mandible, at a level 1½ to 2 inches (4 to 5 cm) inferior to mandibular symphysis
- CR centered to IR
- Minimum SID of 40 inches (100 cm)

Collimation Collimate on all sides to area of sinus cavities.

Respiration Suspend respiration during exposure.

Notes: If patient is unable to sufficiently extend neck, angle the tube from horizontal as needed to align the CR perpendicular to IOML.

This position is very uncomfortable for patient; have all factors set before positioning the patient and complete the projection as quickly as possible.

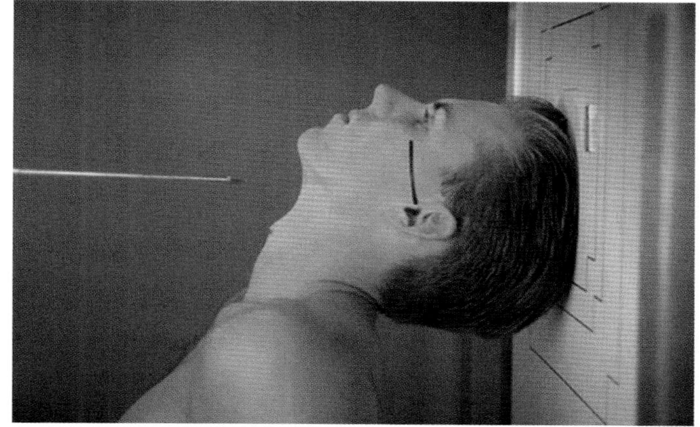

Fig. 13-129. SMV projection (upright Bucky/table).

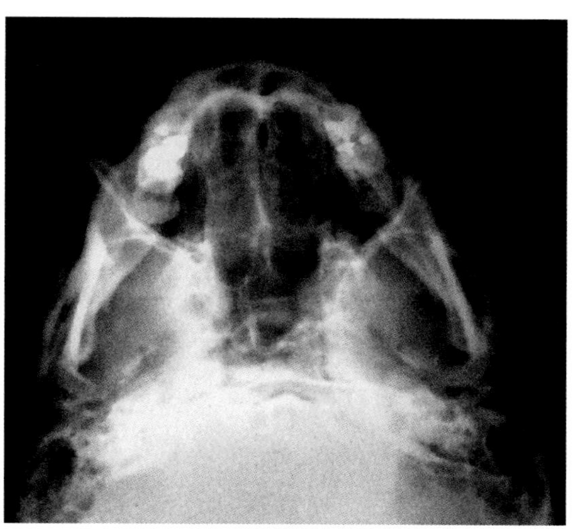

Fig. 13-130. SMV projection.

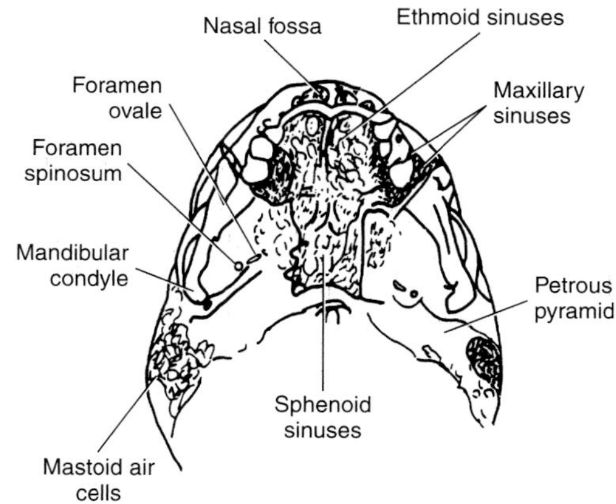

Fig. 13-131. SMV projection.

Radiographic Criteria

Structures Shown: • Sphenoid sinuses, ethmoid sinuses, nasal fossae, and maxillary sinuses.

Position: • Accurate IOML and CR relationship is demonstrated by the following: **mandibular condyles projected anterior to petrous ridges;** mandibular symphysis superimposing anterior frontal bone. • No rotation or tilt of the cranium is demonstrated by the following: petrous pyramids visualized symmetrically; distance from mandibular border to lateral border of skull equal on both sides.

Collimation and CR: • Collimated field includes sphenoid, maxillary, and ethmoid sinuses, with the sphenoid sinus in the approximate center.

Exposure Criteria: • Density and contrast are sufficient to visualize sphenoid and ethmoid sinuses. • Sharp bony margins indicate no motion.

PARIETOACANTHIAL TRANSORAL PROJECTION: SINUSES

Open-Mouth Waters Method

Sinuses
SPECIAL
- **Submentovertex (SMV)**
- Parietoacanthial transoral (open-mouth Waters)

Pathology Demonstrated

Inflammatory conditions (sinusitis, secondary osteomyelitis) and sinus polyps are shown.

Technical Factors

- IR size—18 × 24 cm (8 × 10 inches), lengthwise
- Moving or stationary grid
- 70-80 kV range
- Small focal spot
- Technique and dose:

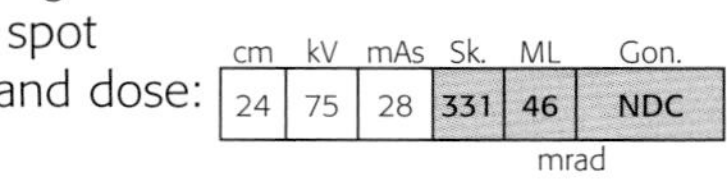

cm	kV	mAs	Sk.	ML	Gon.
24	75	28	331	46	NDC
				mrad	

18 × 24 (R)

Patient Position Remove all metal, plastic, and other removable objects from head. Position patient **erect** (see note).

Part Position

- Extend neck, placing chin and nose against table/upright Bucky surface.
- Adjust head until **OML forms a 37° angle** with IR (**MML will be perpendicular** with mouth closed).
- Position the **midsagittal plane perpendicular** to the midline of the grid or the table/upright Bucky surface; ensure **no rotation or tilt.**
- Instruct patient to open mouth by instructing to "drop jaw without moving head." (MML is no longer perpendicular.)
- Center IR to CR and to **acanthion.**

Central Ray

- Align a **horizontal CR perpendicular** to the IR.
- Center CR to **exit at acanthion.**
- Minimum SID is 40 inches (100 cm).

Collimation Collimate on all sides to area of sinus cavities.

Respiration Suspend respiration during exposure.

Fig. 13-132. Parietoacanthial transoral projection (upright Bucky/table).

Fig. 13-133. Parietoacanthial transoral projection.

Fig. 13-134. Parietoacanthial transoral projection.

Radiographic Criteria

Structures Shown: • Maxillary sinuses with the inferior aspect visualized, free from superimposing alveolar processes and petrous ridges, the inferior orbital rim, an oblique view of the frontal sinuses, and the sphenoid sinuses visualized through the open mouth.

Position: • No rotation of the cranium is indicated by the following: equal distance from the midsagittal plane (identified by the bony nasal septum) to the outer orbital margin on both sides; equal distance from the lateral orbital margin to the outer table of the skull on both sides; accurate extension of neck demonstrating petrous ridges below the maxillary sinuses.

Collimation and CR: • Collimated field includes the frontal, maxillary, and sphenoid sinuses, with the maxillary sinuses in the center.

Exposure Criteria: • Density and contrast are sufficient to visualize the maxillary and sphenoid sinuses. • Sharp bony margins indicate no motion.

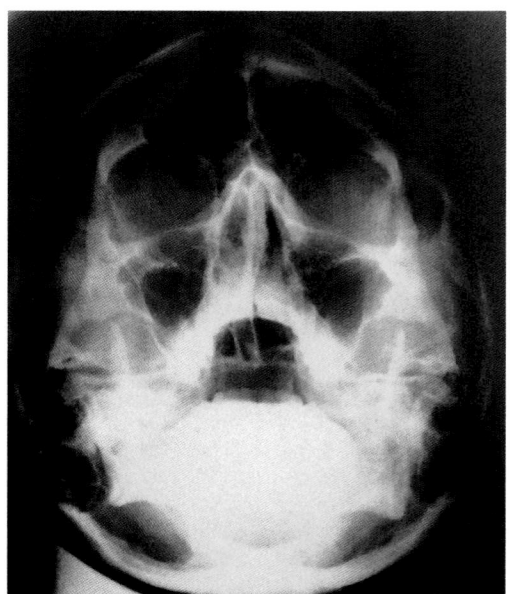

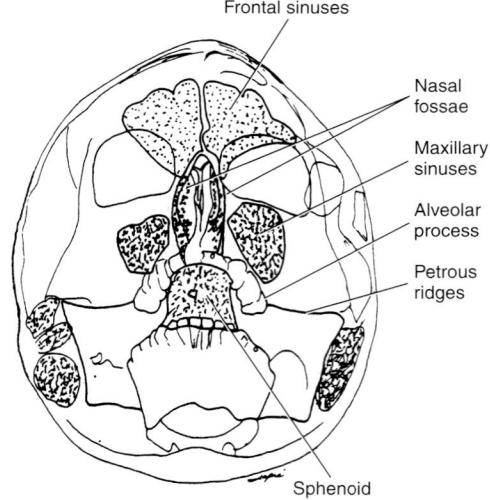

RADIOGRAPHS FOR CRITIQUE—FACIAL BONES

Note: Remember, CR must be horizontal and the patient erect to demonstrate air-fluid levels within the paranasal sinuses.

Students should determine whether they can critique each of these five radiographs based on the categories as described in the textbook and as outlined on the right. As a starting critique exercise, place a check in each category that demonstrates a **repeatable error** for that radiograph.

Student workbooks provide more space for writing comments and complete critique answers for each of these radiographs. Answers are provided in Appendix B, at the end of this textbook.

	RADIOGRAPHS				
	A	B	C	D	E
1. Structures shown	____	____	____	____	____
2. Positioning	____	____	____	____	____
3. Collimation and CR	____	____	____	____	____
4. Exposure criteria	____	____	____	____	____
5. Markers	____	____	____	____	____

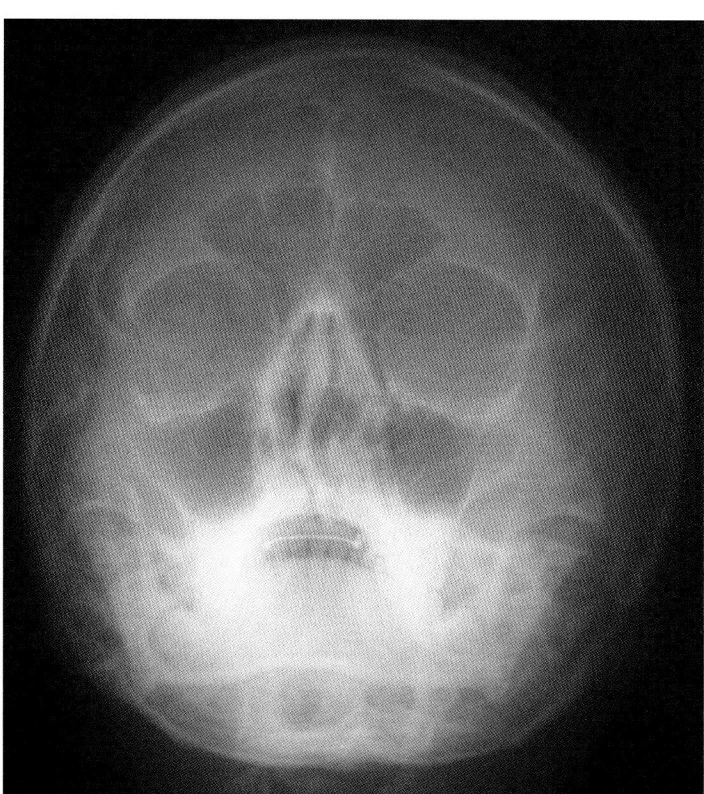

Fig. C13-135. Parietoacanthial (Waters)—facial bones. A

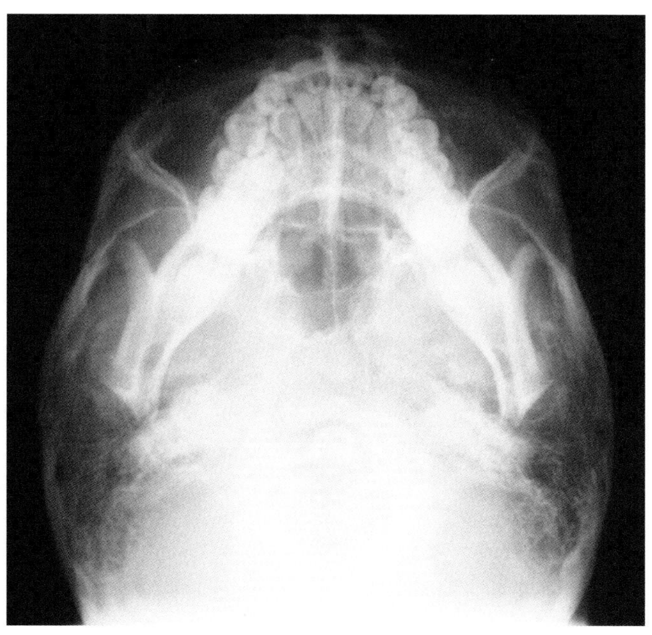

Fig. C13-136. SMV mandible. B

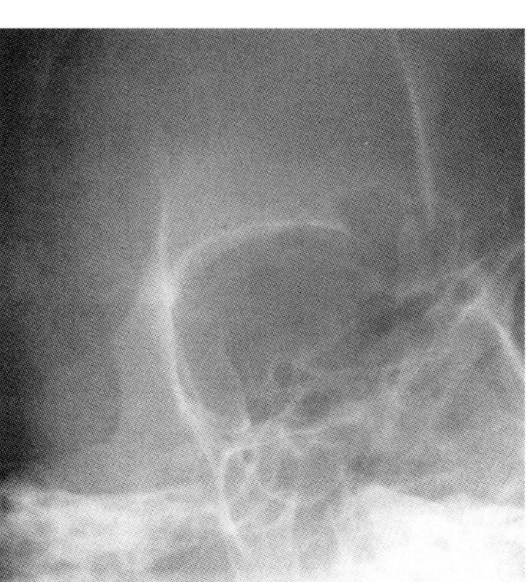

Fig. C13-137. Optic foramina—Rhese method. C

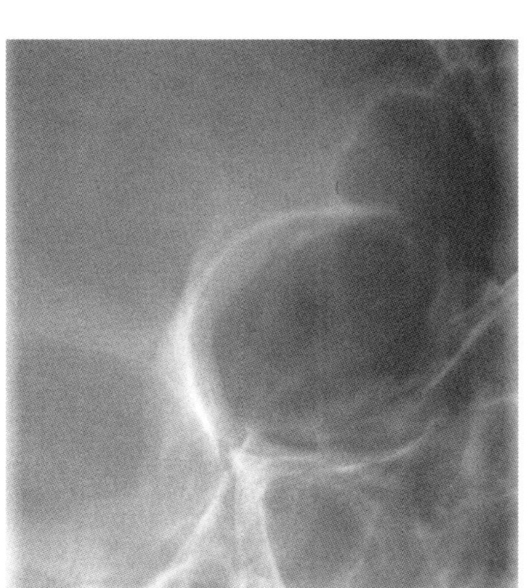

Fig. C13-138. Optic foramina—Rhese method. D

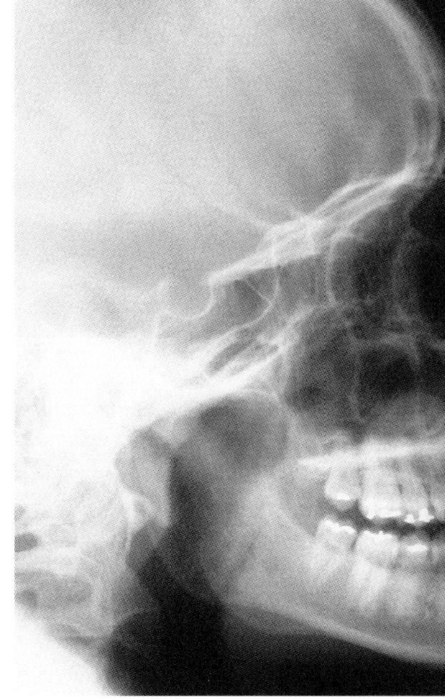

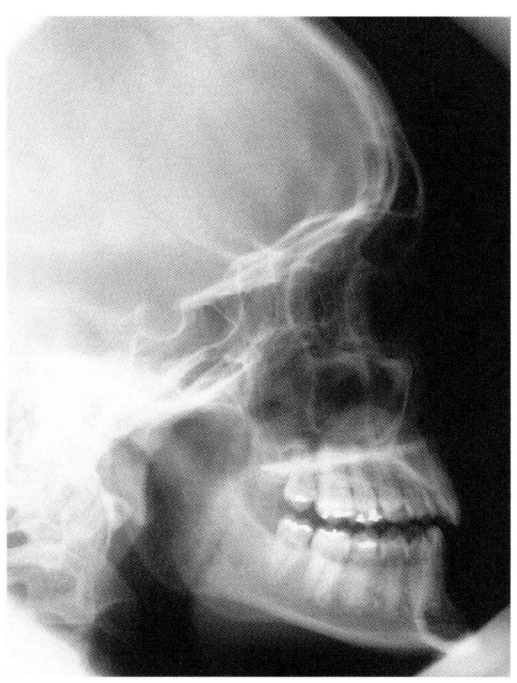

Fig. C13-139. Lateral facial bones. E

13

RADIOGRAPHS FOR CRITIQUE—SINUSES

Students should determine whether they can critique each of these four radiographs based on the categories as described in the textbook and as outlined on the right. As a starting critique exercise, place a check in each category that demonstrates a **repeatable error** for that radiograph.

Student workbooks provide more space for writing comments and complete critique answers for each of these radiographs. Answers are provided in Appendix B, at the end of this textbook.

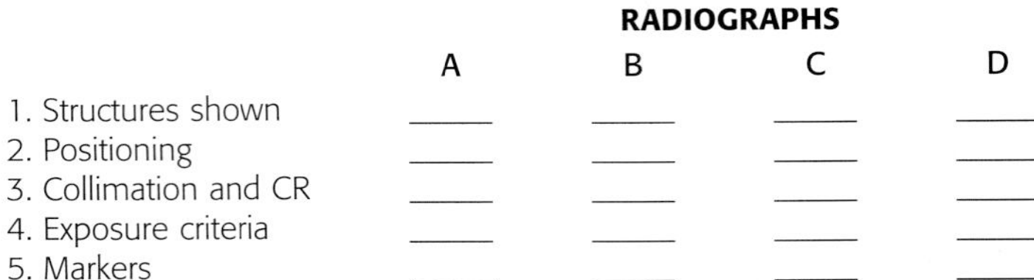

	RADIOGRAPHS			
	A	B	C	D
1. Structures shown	____	____	____	____
2. Positioning	____	____	____	____
3. Collimation and CR	____	____	____	____
4. Exposure criteria	____	____	____	____
5. Markers	____	____	____	____

Fig. C13-140. Sinuses—parietoacanthial transoral projection (open-mouth Waters). A

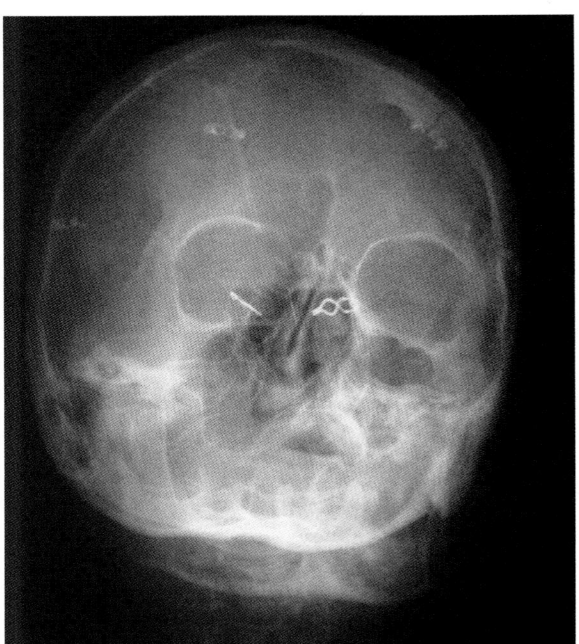

Fig. C13-141. Sinuses—parietoacanthial (Waters) projection. B

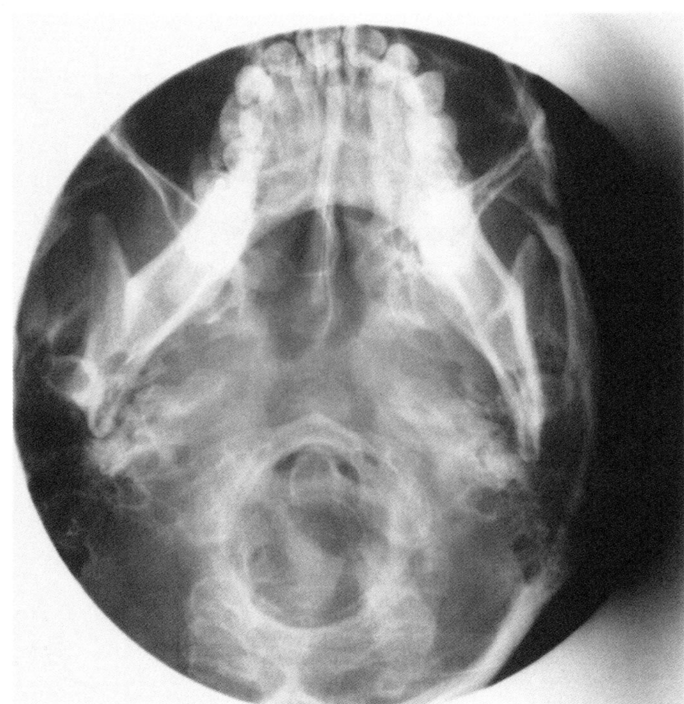

Fig. C13-142. Sinuses—SMV projection. C

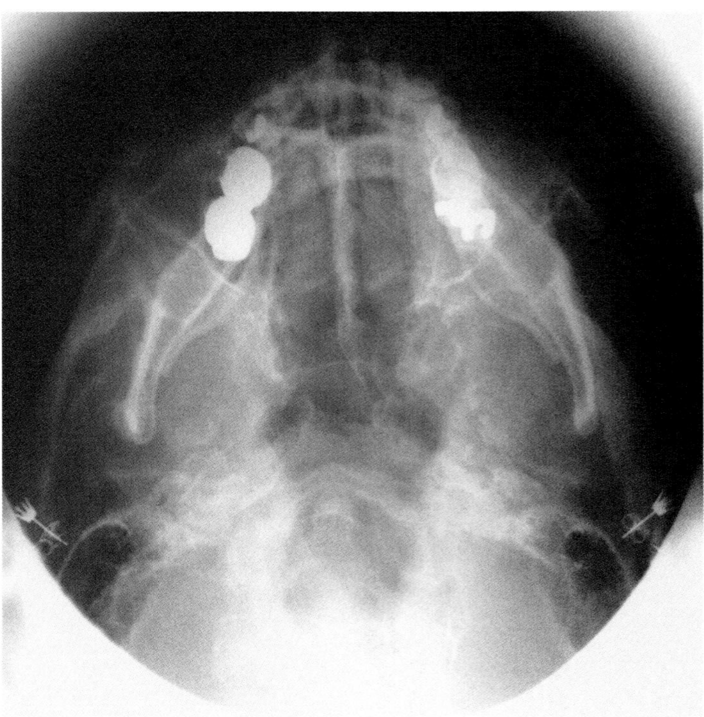

Fig. C13-143. Sinuses—SMV projection. D

CHAPTER 14

Upper Gastrointestinal System

CONTRIBUTOR TO PAST EDITIONS Barry T. Anthony, RT(R)

CONTENTS

Radiographic Anatomy

Radiographic Procedures

Radiographic Positioning

RADIOGRAPHIC ANATOMY

Digestive System

The digestive system includes the entire **alimentary canal** and several **accessory organs.**

ALIMENTARY CANAL

The alimentary canal begins at the (1) **oral cavity** (mouth); continues as the (2) **pharynx,** (3) **esophagus,** (4) **stomach,** and (5) **small intestine;** and ends as the (6) **large intestine,** which terminates as the (7) **anus.**

Anatomy and positioning of (1) the oral cavity through (5) the duodenum are covered in this chapter. The remainder of the small intestine, (6) the large intestine, and (7) the anus are covered in Chapter 15.

ACCESSORY ORGANS

Accessory organs of digestion include the **salivary glands, pancreas, liver,** and **gallbladder.**

FUNCTIONS

The digestive system performs the following **three primary functions:**

1. The **first** function is the **intake and/or digestion** of food, water, vitamins, and minerals. Food is ingested in the form of carbohydrates, lipids, and proteins. These complex food groups must be broken down, or digested, so that absorption can take place.
2. The **second** primary function of the digestive system is to **absorb** digested food particles, along with water, vitamins, and essential elements from the alimentary canal into the blood or lymphatic capillaries.
3. The **third** function is to **eliminate** any unused material in the form of semisolid waste products.

COMMON RADIOGRAPHIC PROCEDURES

Two common radiographic procedures involving the upper gastrointestinal system are presented in this chapter. These radiographic examinations involve the administration of a contrast medium.

Esophagram or Barium Swallow (a Study of the Pharynx and Esophagus)

A radiographic examination specifically of the pharynx and esophagus is termed an ***esophagram,*** or ***barium swallow.*** This procedure studies the form and function of the swallowing aspect of the pharynx and esophagus.

Upper Gastrointestinal Series (UGI) (Upper GI) (a Study of Distal Esophagus, Stomach, and Duodenum)

The procedure designed to study the distal esophagus, stomach, and duodenum in one examination is termed an ***upper gastrointestinal series.*** Alternative designations for upper gastrointestinal series include ***UGI, upper, GI,*** or, most commonly, ***upper GI.*** A PA radiograph from an upper GI series is shown in Fig. 14-2.

Barium sulfate mixed with water is the preferred contrast medium for the entire alimentary canal. The negative density area (appearing *white*) on the radiograph indicates the stomach and duodenum area filled with the barium-sulfate contrast media.

Alimentary Canal

Ch. 14
(1) Oral cavity (mouth)
(2) Pharynx
(3) Esophagus
(4) Stomach
(5) Duodenum and small intestine

Ch. 15
(6) Large intestine
(7) Anus

Accessory Organs
–Salivary glands
–Pancreas
–Liver
–Gallbladder

Functions
1. Intake and digestion
2. Absorption
3. Elimination

1 2 3 4 5 6 7

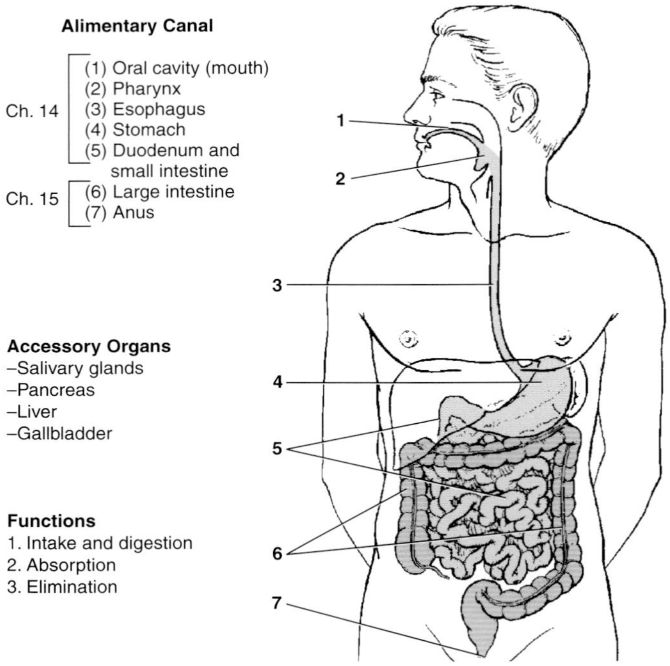

Fig. 14-1. Digestive system.

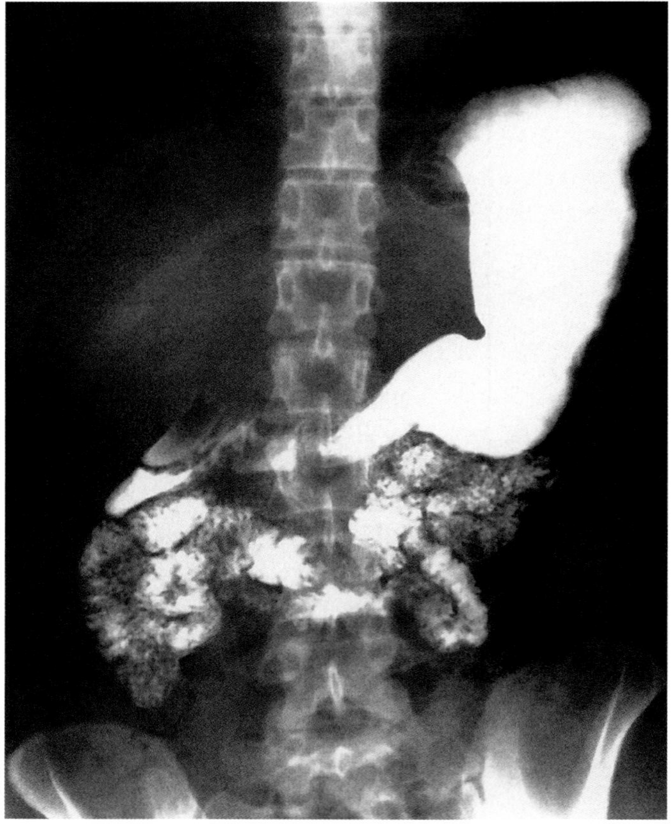

Fig. 14-2. PA–upper GI series (barium in stomach and duodenum).

14

Mouth (Oral Cavity)

The alimentary canal is a continuous hollow tube, beginning with the **oral cavity** (mouth). The oral cavity and surrounding structures are visualized in midsagittal section in Fig. 14-3.

The main cavity of the mouth is bounded in front and on the sides by the inner surfaces of the **upper** and **lower teeth.** The roof of the oral cavity is formed by the **hard** and **soft palates.** Hanging from the midposterior aspect of the soft palate is a small conical process termed the ***palatine uvula,*** commonly referred to as just the ***uvula*** *(u'-vu-lah).* The main part of the floor of the oral cavity is formed by the **tongue.** The oral cavity connects posteriorly with the **pharynx** *(far'inks),* as described below.

ACCESSORY ORGANS IN THE ORAL CAVITY (MOUTH)

The **salivary glands** are accessory organs of digestion associated with the mouth. The teeth and tongue cooperate in chewing movements to reduce the size of food particles and mix food with saliva. These chewing movements, termed ***mastication*** *(mas"ti-ka'shun),* initiate the mechanical part of digestion.

Three pairs of glands secrete most of the saliva in the oral cavity (Fig. 14-4). These glands are the (1) **parotid** *(pah-rot'id),* meaning *near the ear,* (2) **submandibular,** sometimes called *submaxillary* (below mandible or maxilla), and (3) **sublingual** *(sub-ling'gwal), below the tongue.*

Saliva is 99.5% water and 0.5% solutes or salts and certain digestive enzymes. Between 1000 and 1500 ml are secreted daily by the salivary glands. Saliva dissolves foods so that digestion can begin. It also contains an enzyme to begin digestion of starch.

Specific salivary glands secrete a thickened fluid containing mucus. This fluid lubricates food being chewed so that the food can form into a ball, or bolus, for swallowing. The act of swallowing is termed ***deglutition*** *(deg"loo-tish'un).*

Note: The salivary glands may be the site of infection, especially the parotid glands. **Mumps** is an inflammation and enlargement of the parotid glands caused by the mumps virus, which for about 30% of males past puberty also results in inflammation of the testes.

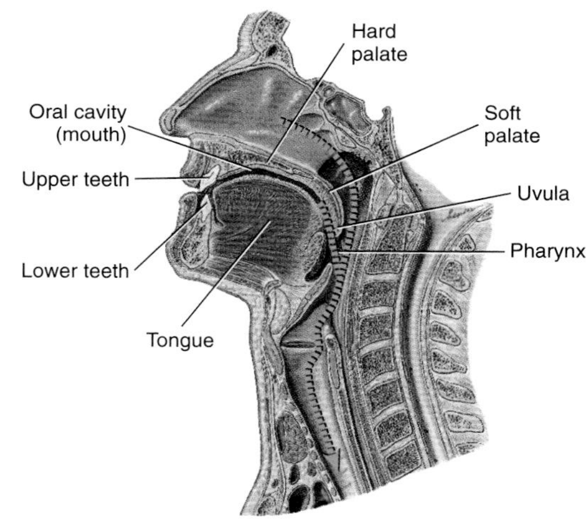

Fig. 14-3. Midsagittal section of mouth (oral or buccal cavity).

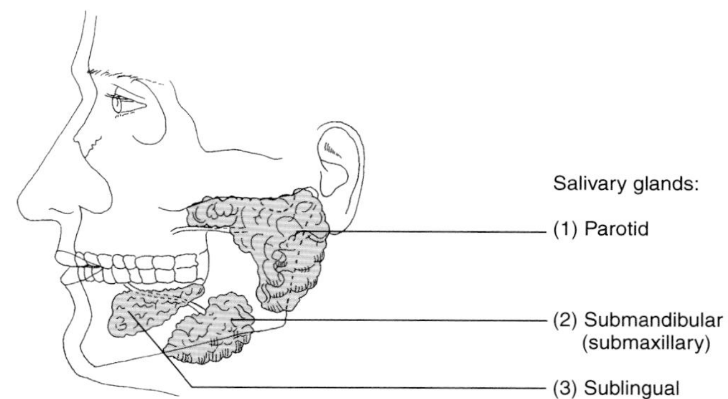

Fig. 14-4. Accessory organs in the mouth.

Pharynx

The alimentary canal continues as the pharynx posterior to the oral cavity. The **pharynx** is about 12.5 cm long and is that part of the digestive tube found posterior to the nasal cavity, mouth, and larynx. A midsagittal and a coronal section of the pharynx, as seen from the side and posterior, are shown in Fig. 14-5. The three parts of the pharynx are named according to their locations.

The **nasopharynx** is posterior to the bony nasal septum, nasal cavities, and soft palate. This portion of the pharynx is not part of the digestive system.

The **oropharynx** is directly posterior to the oral cavity proper. The oropharynx extends from the **soft palate** to the **epiglottis** *(ep"i-glot'is).* The epiglottis is a membrane-covered cartilage that moves down to cover the opening of the larynx during swallowing.

The third portion of the pharynx is termed the ***laryngopharynx,*** or *hypopharynx.* The laryngopharynx extends from the level of the epiglottis to the level of the lower border of the larynx (level of C6 as described in Chapter 3). From this point it continues as the **esophagus.** The **trachea** is seen anterior to the esophagus.

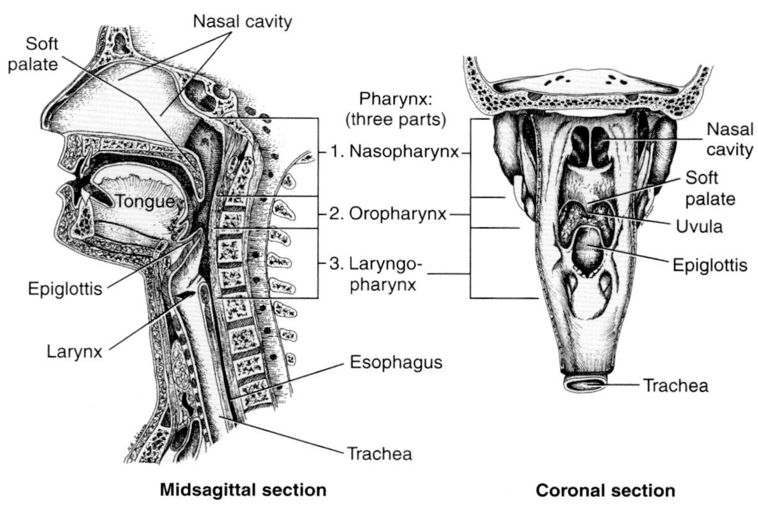

Fig. 14-5. Pharynx.

14

CAVITIES COMMUNICATING WITH THE PHARYNX

The drawing in Fig. 14-6 illustrates **seven cavities, or openings,** communicating with the three portions of the pharynx. The two **nasal cavities** and the two **tympanic cavities** connect to the **nasopharynx.** The tympanic cavities of the middle ears connect to the nasopharynx via the **auditory** or **eustachian tubes** (not shown on this drawing).

The **oral cavity** (mouth) connects posteriorly to the **oropharynx.** Inferiorly the **laryngopharynx** connects to the openings of both the **larynx** and the **esophagus.**

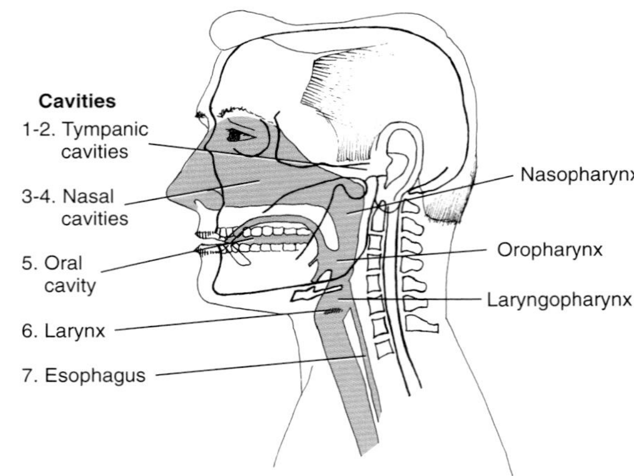

Fig. 14-6. Seven cavities, or openings, communicate with the pharynx.

DEGLUTITION (SWALLOWING)

Most important is that food and fluid travel from the oral cavity directly to the esophagus during the act of swallowing, or **deglutition.** During swallowing the **soft palate closes off the nasopharynx** to prevent swallowed substances from regurgitating into the nose. The tongue prevents the material from reentering the mouth.

During swallowing the **epiglottis is depressed to cover the laryngeal opening** like a lid. The vocal folds, or cords, also come together to close off the epiglottis. These actions combine to prevent food and fluid from being aspirated (entering the larynx, trachea, and bronchi).

Also, respiration is inhibited during deglutition to help prevent swallowed substances from entering the trachea and lungs. Occasionally, bits of material pass into the larynx and trachea during deglutition, causing a forceful episode of reflex coughing.

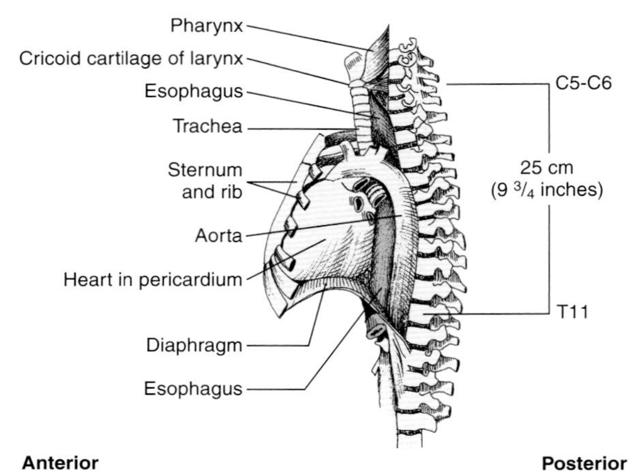

Fig. 14-7. Esophagus in mediastinum—lateral view.

Esophagus

The third part of the alimentary canal is the **esophagus.** The esophagus is a muscular canal, about 10 inches (25 cm) long and about ¾ inch (2 cm) in diameter, extending from the laryngopharynx to the stomach. The esophagus begins posterior to the level of the lower border of the **cricoid cartilage of the larynx** (C5 to C6), which is at the level of the upper margin of the thyroid cartilage. The esophagus terminates at its connection to the stomach, at the level of the **eleventh thoracic vertebra** (T11).

In Fig. 14-7, the esophagus is shown to be located **posterior to the larynx and trachea.** The spatial relationship of the esophagus to both the trachea and the thoracic vertebrae is an important relationship to remember. The esophagus is posterior to the trachea and just anterior to the cervical and thoracic vertebral bodies.

The descending **thoracic aorta** is between the distal esophagus and the lower thoracic spine. The **heart,** within its pericardial sac, is immediately posterior to the sternum, anterior to the esophagus, and superior to the diaphragm.

The esophagus is essentially vertical as it descends to the stomach. This swallowing tube is the narrowest part of the entire alimentary canal. The esophagus is most constricted first at its proximal end, where it enters the thorax, and second, where it passes through the diaphragm at the esophageal hiatus, or opening. The esophagus pierces the diaphragm at the **level of T10.** Just before passing through the diaphragm, the esophagus presents a distinct dilation, as shown in Fig. 14-8.

As the esophagus descends within the posterior aspect of the mediastinum, **two indentations** are present. One indentation occurs at the **aortic arch,** and the second is found where the esophagus crosses the **left primary bronchus.**

The lower portion of the esophagus lies close to the posterior aspects of the heart.

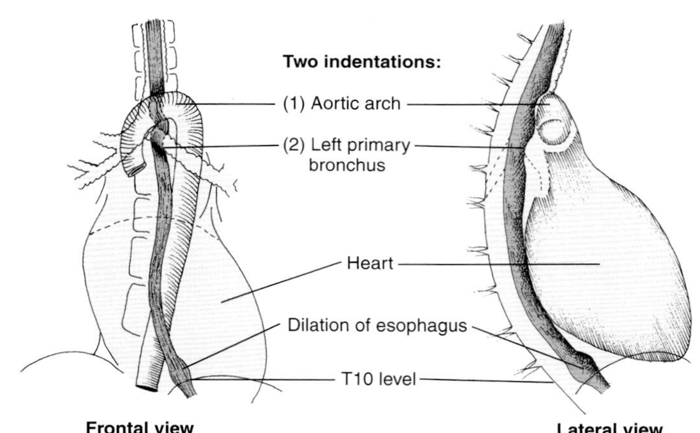

Fig. 14-8. Esophagus in mediastinum, demonstrating two indentations.

DIAPHRAGMATIC OPENINGS

The **esophagus** passes through the **diaphragm** slightly to the left and somewhat posterior to the midpoint of the diaphragm. The drawing on the left in Fig. 14-9 represents the inferior surface of the diaphragm and indicates the relative positions of the **esophagus, inferior vena cava,** and **aorta.**

The lateral-view drawing on the right shows the short abdominal portion of the esophagus below the diaphragm. The **abdominal segment of the esophagus,** termed the **cardiac antrum,** measures between 1 and 2 cm. The cardiac antrum curves sharply to the left after passing through the diaphragm to attach to the stomach.

The opening between the esophagus and the stomach is termed the **esophagogastric junction** *(cardiac orifice).* This opening is best shown in the drawing on the following page, Fig. 14-13. *Cardiac* is an adjective denoting a relationship to the heart; therefore the cardiac antrum and the cardiac orifice are located near the heart.

The junction of the stomach and the esophagus is normally securely attached to the diaphragm, so the upper stomach tends to follow the respiratory movements of the diaphragm.

SWALLOWING AND PERISTALSIS

The esophagus contains well-developed skeletal muscle layers (circular and longitudinal) in its upper third, skeletal and smooth muscle in its middle third, and smooth muscle in its lower third. Unlike the trachea, the esophagus is a collapsible tube that only opens when swallowing occurs. The process of deglutition continues in the esophagus after originating in the mouth and pharynx. Fluids tend to pass from the mouth and pharynx to the stomach primarily by gravity. A bolus of solid material tends to pass both by gravity and by peristalsis.

Peristalsis is a wavelike series of involuntary muscular contractions propelling solid and semisolid materials through the tubular alimentary canal. A solid bolus of barium sulfate filling the entire esophagus is seen in Fig. 14-10 descending to the stomach both by gravity and by peristalsis. Accumulation of barium in the stomach is seen on this PA radiograph.

Spot radiographs in an RAO position in Fig. 14-11 demonstrate the esophagus partially filled with barium, with normal peristaltic constrictions most evident in midportions and upper portions of the esophagus.

The relationship of the esophagus to the heart is seen on these radiographs. The esophagus is located immediately adjacent to the right and posterior heart borders.

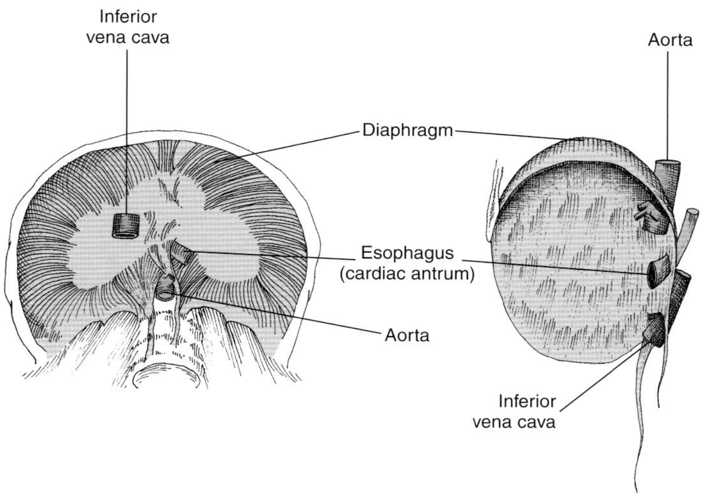

Fig. 14-9. Esophagus passing through diaphragm.

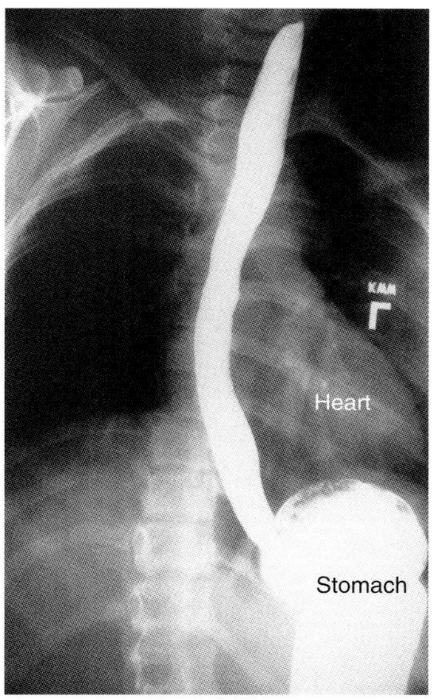

Fig. 14-10. PA esophagram (slightly obliqued).

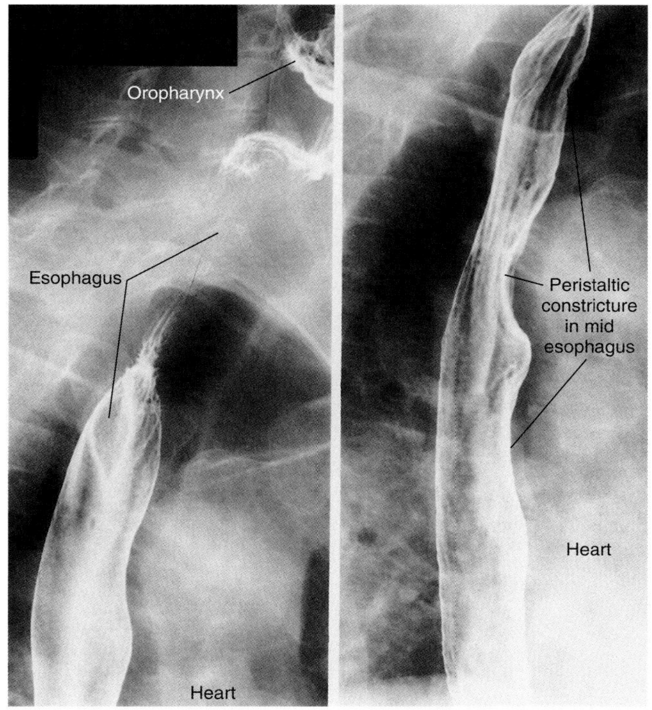

Fig. 14-11. RAO esophagram; upper esophagus. Midesophagus and lower esophagus just above diaphragm.

14

Stomach

The Greek word *gaster* means *stomach;* therefore *gastro* is a common term denoting stomach, thus the term ***gastrointestinal tract.***

The **stomach,** located between the **esophagus** and the **small intestine,** is the most dilated portion of the alimentary canal. When empty, the stomach tends to collapse. When the stomach must serve as a reservoir for swallowed food and fluid, it is remarkably expandable. After a very full meal the stomach stretches to what would appear to be almost the point of rupture.

Because the shape and position of the stomach are highly variable, the average shape and location are used in the following illustrations, with variations to follow later in this chapter.

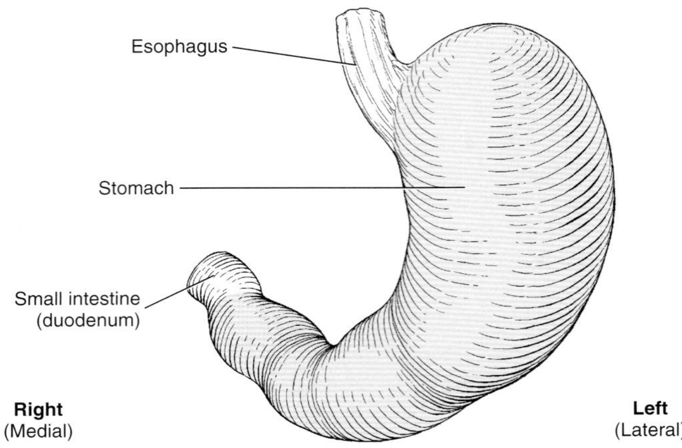

Fig. 14-12. Stomach—frontal view.

STOMACH OPENINGS AND CURVATURES

The **esophagogastric junction** (cardiac orifice) is the aperture, or opening, between the esophagus and the stomach (Fig. 14-13). A small, circular muscle, called the *cardiac sphincter,* allows food and fluid to pass through the cardiac orifice. This opening (esophagogastric junction) is commonly called the **cardiac orifice,** referring to the relationship of this orifice to that portion of the diaphragm near the heart, on which the heart rests.

Directly superior to this orifice is a notch called the **cardiac notch** *(incisura cardiaca).* This distal abdominal portion of the esophagus curves sharply into a slightly expanded portion of the terminal esophagus called the **cardiac antrum.**

The opening, or orifice, leaving the distal stomach is termed the **pyloric orifice,** sometimes just called **pylorus.** The pyloric sphincter at this orifice is a thickened muscular ring that relaxes periodically during digestion to allow stomach or gastric contents to move into the first part of the small intestine, the duodenum.

The **lesser curvature,** extending along the right, or medial, border of the stomach, forms a concave border as it extends between the cardiac and pyloric openings.

The **greater curvature** extends along the left, or lateral, border of the stomach. This greater curvature is four to five times longer than the lesser curvature.

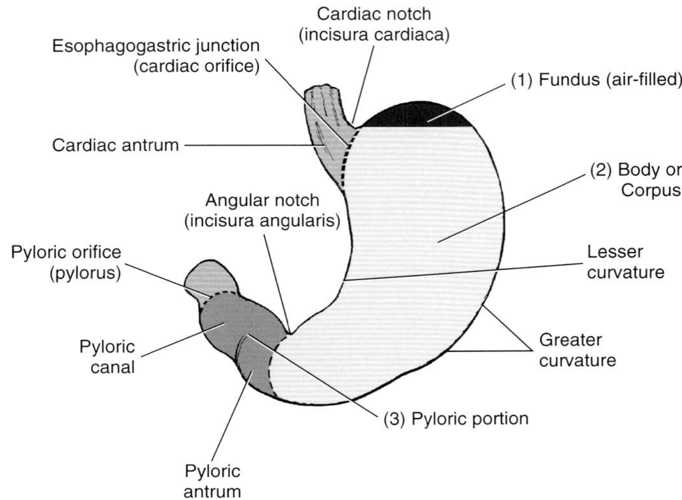

Fig. 14-13. Stomach—openings, greater and lesser curvatures, and subdivisions.

STOMACH SUBDIVISIONS

The stomach is composed of three main subdivisions: (1) the **fundus,** (2) the **body,** or **corpus,** and (3) the **pyloric portion** (Fig. 14-13). The fundus is that ballooned portion lying lateral and superior to the cardiac orifice. The upper portion of the stomach, including the cardiac antrum of the esophagus, is relatively fixed to the diaphragm and tends to move with motion of the diaphragm. In the upright, or erect, position, the fundus is usually filled by a bubble of swallowed air, referred to as a *gastric bubble.*

The lower end of the large body, or corpus, portion of the stomach has a partially constricted area separating the body from the pyloric portion of the stomach. This "notch," or constricted ringlike area, is called the **angular notch** *(incisura angularis).* The smaller terminal portion of the stomach to the right, or medial, of the angular notch is the pyloric portion of the stomach.

The pyloric portion of the stomach is frequently divided into two parts: (1) the **pyloric antrum,** shown as a slight dilation immediately distal to the angular notch, and (2) the narrowed **pyloric canal,** ending at the pyloric sphincter.

The barium-filled stomach in Fig. 14-14 demonstrates the actual appearance and shape of the stomach, as seen on a PA projection of the stomach and duodenum as part of an upper GI series. Review the labeled parts and compare them with the drawings in Figs. 14-12 and 14-13.

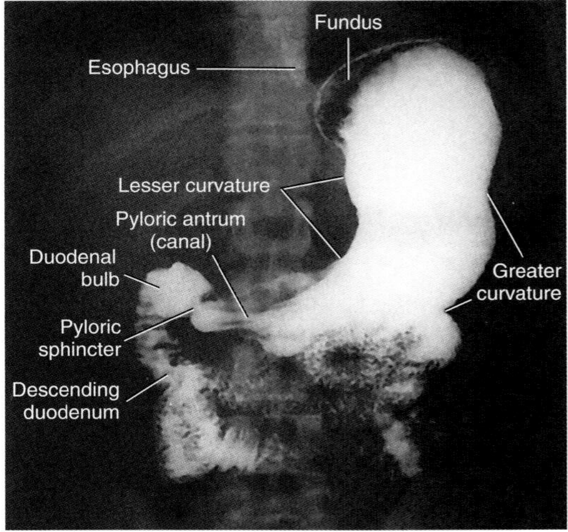

Fig. 14-14. Barium-filled stomach and duodenum.

GASTRIC FOLDS WITHIN STOMACH—RUGAE

When the stomach is empty, the internal lining is thrown into numerous longitudinal gastric folds termed **rugae,** pronounced *roo'je* (singular is ruga, *roo'gah*). These folds are shown in the drawing of Fig. 14-15 and are also demonstrated by the streaklike folds of the air-barium–filled stomach radiograph in Fig. 14-18 below. The rugae assist with mechanical digestion of food within the stomach.

A **gastric canal,** formed by rugae along the lesser curvature (Fig. 14-15), funnels fluids directly from the body of the stomach to the pylorus.

STOMACH POSITION

The illustration in Fig. 14-16 shows the typical orientation of an average, partially filled stomach in frontal and lateral views. The **fundus,** in addition to being the most superior portion of the stomach in general, is located posterior to the **body** of the stomach, as seen on the lateral view. The body can be seen to curve inferior and anterior from the fundus.

The **pyloric portion** is directed posteriorly. The pyloric valve (sphincter) and the first part of the small bowel are very near the posterior abdominal wall. The relationships of these components of the stomach are important in the distribution of air and barium in the stomach in specific body positions.

AIR-BARIUM DISTRIBUTION IN STOMACH

If an individual swallows a barium sulfate and water mixture, along with some air, as seen in Figs. 14-17 and 14-18, the position of the person's body determines the distribution of the barium and air within the stomach.

As already noted, from the lateral-view drawing one can see that in the **supine position** the fundus part of the stomach is the lowest part, where the heavy barium settles (Fig. 14-17).

In the **prone position** the fundus is in the highest position, causing the **air** to fill this part of the stomach, as seen in Fig. 14-18.

This appearance is also shown in the three position drawings in Fig. 14-19, where the air is shown as black and the barium as white, similar to the appearance of air and barium in a radiographic image.

The drawing on the lower left depicts the stomach of a person in a **supine** position.

The middle drawing shows the stomach of a person in a **prone** position.

The drawing on the lower right depicts the stomach of a person who is in an **erect** position. In the erect position, air rises to fill the fundus, whereas barium descends by gravity to fill the pyloric portion of the stomach. The air-barium line tends to be a straight line in the erect position, compared with the prone and supine positions.

When studying radiographic images of a stomach containing both air and barium, you can determine the patient's position by the relative locations of air versus barium within the stomach.

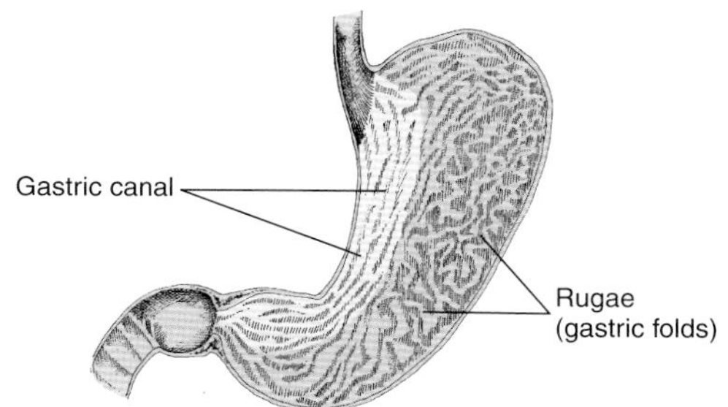

Fig. 14-15. Stomach—coronal section.

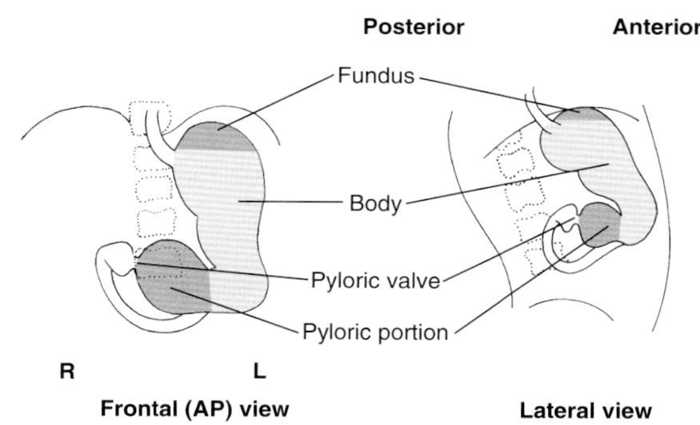

Fig. 14-16. Average empty stomach orientation.

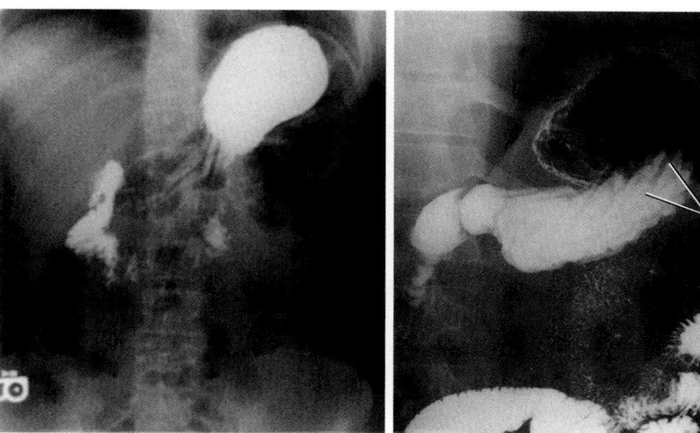

Fig. 14-17. AP—supine position (barium in fundus).

Fig. 14-18. RAO—prone position (air in fundus).

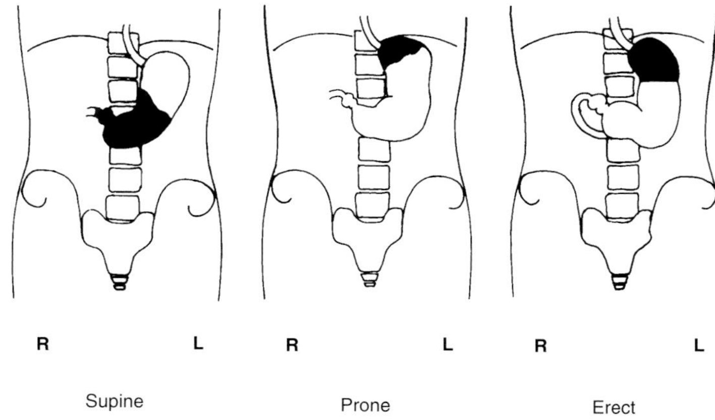

Fig. 14-19. Air-barium distribution in the stomach—frontal views in various body positions. Air = black; barium = white.

Duodenum

The fifth and final part of the upper GI system to be studied in this chapter is the **duodenum** *(du"o-de'num),* which is the first portion of the small intestine commonly called the *small bowel.* Because the duodenum is examined radiographically during the routine upper GI series, the duodenum is studied in this chapter, whereas the remainder of the small bowel is studied in Chapter 15 with the lower GI system.

The duodenum is about 8 to 10 inches (20 to 24 cm) long and is the shortest, widest, and most fixed portion of the small bowel.

The drawing in Fig. 14-20 demonstrates that the C-shaped duodenum is closely related to the **head of the pancreas.** The head of the pancreas, nestled in the C-loop of the duodenum, has been affectionately labeled the "romance of the abdomen" by certain authors.

The duodenum and the pancreas are *retroperitoneal* structures; that is, they are located *posterior to the parietal peritoneum,* as described in Chapter 4 (Abdomen).

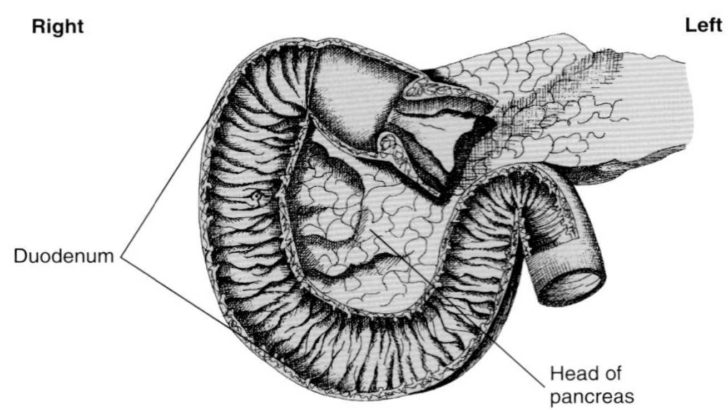

Fig. 14-20. Duodenum and pancreas.

FOUR PARTS OF THE DUODENUM

The duodenum is shaped like a letter C and consists of **four parts** (Fig. 14-21). The **first (superior) portion** begins at the pylorus of the stomach. The first part of the superior portion is termed the ***duodenal bulb,*** or ***cap.*** The duodenal bulb is easily located during barium studies of the upper GI tract and must be carefully studied because this area is a common site of ulcer disease.

The next part of the duodenum is the **second (descending) portion,** the longest segment. The descending portion of the duodenum receives the common bile and pancreatic ducts, as will be described in Chapter 16 (Gallbladder and Biliary Ducts).

The **third** part of the duodenum is the **horizontal portion.** This portion curves back to the left to join the final segment, the **fourth (ascending) portion** of the duodenum.

The junction of the duodenum with the second portion of small bowel, the **jejunum** *(jĕ-joo'-num),* is termed the **duodenojejunal flexure.** This portion is relatively fixed and held in place by a fibrous muscular band, the **suspensory ligament of the duodenum (ligament of Treitz).** This structure is a significant reference point in certain radiographic small-bowel studies.

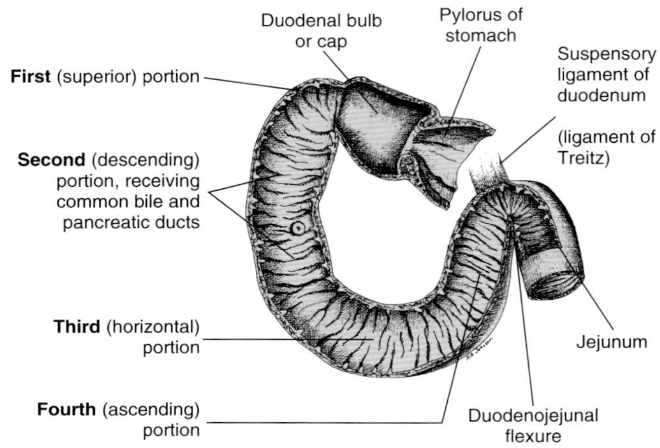

Fig. 14-21. Duodenum (four parts).

Anatomy Review

RADIOGRAPH OF STOMACH AND DUODENUM (Fig. 14-22)

This PA radiograph of the stomach and duodenum provides a good review of important radiographic anatomy. Identify the structures labeled on the radiograph and then compare your answers with those listed below:

A. Distal esophagus
B. Area of esophagogastric junction (cardiac orifice)
C. Lesser curvature of stomach
D. Angular notch (incisura angularis) of stomach
E. Pyloric portion of stomach
F. Pyloric valve or sphincter
G. Duodenal bulb of duodenum
H. Second (descending) portion of duodenum
I. Body of stomach
J. Greater curvature of stomach
K. Gastric folds, or rugae, of stomach
L. Fundus of stomach

14

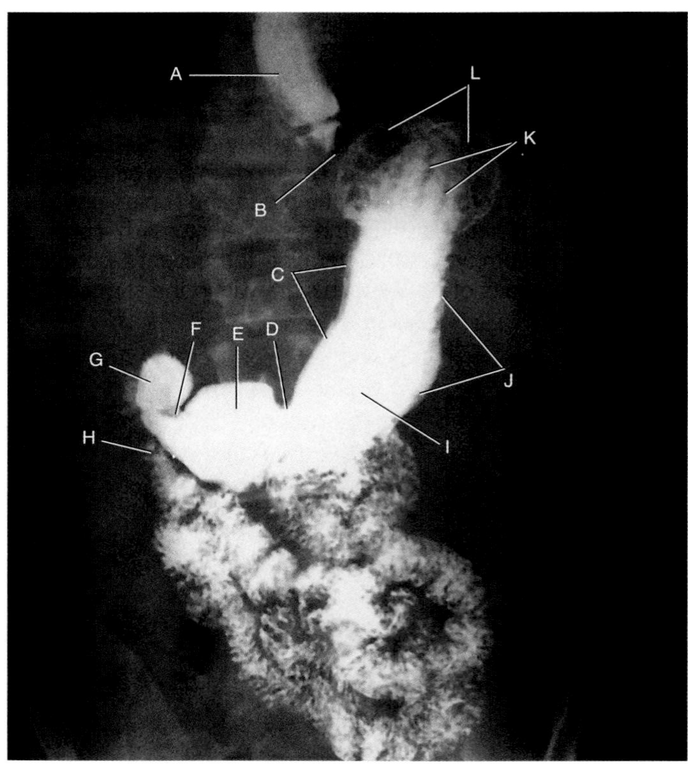

Fig. 14-22. PA projection.

Digestion

MECHANICAL DIGESTION

Digestion can be divided into a **mechanical process** and a **chemical component.** Mechanical digestion includes all movements of the GI tract, beginning in the oral cavity (mouth) with chewing, or **mastication** *(mas"ti-ka'shun),* and continuing in the pharynx and esophagus with swallowing, or **deglutition.**

Peristaltic activity can be detected in the lower esophagus and in the remainder of the alimentary canal. The passage of solid or semisolid food from the mouth to the stomach takes from 4 to 8 seconds, whereas liquids pass in about 1 second.

The stomach, acting as a reservoir for food and fluid, also acts as a large mixing bowl. Peristalsis tends to move the gastric contents toward the pyloric valve, but this valve opens selectively. If it is closed, the stomach contents are churned or mixed with stomach fluids into a semifluid mass termed ***chyme*** *(kim).* When the valve opens, small amounts of chyme are passed into the duodenum by **stomach peristalsis.** Gastric emptying is a fairly slow process, taking 2 to 6 hours to totally empty after an average meal. Food with high carbohydrate content leaves the stomach in several hours, whereas food with high protein or fat content moves through much more slowly.

The small intestine (small bowel) continues mechanical digestion with a churning motion within segments of the small bowel. This churning or mixing activity is termed ***rhythmic segmentation.*** Rhythmic segmentation tends to thoroughly mix food and digestive juices and bring the digested food into contact with the intestinal lining, or mucosa, to facilitate absorption. **Peristalsis** is again present to propel intestinal contents along the alimentary canal. Peristaltic contractions in the small intestine, however, are much weaker and slower than those in the esophagus and stomach, and the chyme moves through the small intestine at about 1 cm/minute. Therefore the chyme normally takes 3 to 5 hours to pass through the entire small intestine.

CHEMICAL DIGESTION

Chemical digestion includes all the chemical changes that food undergoes as it travels through the alimentary canal. Six different classes of substances are ingested: (1) **carbohydrates,** or complex sugars, (2) **proteins,** (3) **lipids** *(lip'id),* or **fats,** (4) **vitamins,** (5) **minerals,** and (6) **water.** Only the carbohydrates, proteins, and lipids need to be chemically digested to be absorbed. Vitamins, minerals, and water are used in the form in which the body ingests them.

Chemical digestion is speeded up by various **enzymes.** Enzymes are **biologic catalysts** found in the various digestive juices that are produced by salivary glands in the mouth and by the stomach, small bowel, and pancreas. The various enzymes are organic compounds, which are proteins. They accelerate chemical changes in other substances without actually appearing in the final products of the reaction.

Digested Substances and Resultant By-Products

1. **Carbohydrate** digestion of starches begins in the mouth and stomach and is completed in the small intestine. The end products of digestion of these complex sugars are **simple sugars.**
2. **Protein** digestion begins in the stomach and is completed in the small intestine. The end products of protein digestion are **amino acids.**
3. **Lipid,** or fat, digestion essentially takes place only in the small bowel, although small amounts of the enzyme necessary for fat digestion are found in the stomach.

SUMMARY OF MECHANICAL DIGESTION

Oral Cavity (Teeth and Tongue)	Mastication (chewing) Deglutition (swallowing)
Pharynx	Deglutition
Esophagus	Deglutition Peristalsis (waves of muscular contraction) (1 to 8 sec)
Stomach	Mixing (chyme) Peristalsis (2 to 6 hr)
Small Intestine (Small Bowel)	Rhythmic segmentation (churning) Peristalsis (3 to 5 hr)

SUMMARY OF CHEMICAL DIGESTION

Substances Ingested, Digested, and Absorbed

1. Carbohydrates (complex sugars) → simple sugars (mouth and stomach)
2. Proteins → amino acids (stomach and small bowel)
3. Lipids (fats) → fatty acids and glycerol (small bowel only)

Substances Ingested But NOT Digested

4. Vitamins
5. Minerals
6. Water

Enzymes (digestive juices)

- Biologic catalysts

Bile (from GB)

- Emulsification of fats

Bile, manufactured by the liver and stored in the gallbladder, is discharged into the duodenum to assist in the breakdown of lipids. Bile contains no enzymes, but it does emulsify fats. During emulsification, large fat droplets are broken down to small fat droplets, which have greater surface area (to volume) and give enzymes greater access for the breakdown of lipids. The end products of fat (or lipids), during digestion are **fatty acids** and **glycerol** *(glis'-er-ol).*

Most absorption of digestive end products takes place in the small intestine. Simple sugars, amino acids, fatty acids, glycerol, H_2O, and most salts and vitamins are absorbed into the bloodstream or the lymphatic system through the lining of the small intestine. Limited absorption takes place in the stomach and may include some water, alcohol, and certain drugs but no nutrients. Any residues of digestion or unabsorbed digestive products are eliminated from the large bowel as a component of feces.

SUMMARY

In general, **three primary functions** of the digestive system are accomplished within the alimentary canal.

First, ingestion and/or **digestion** takes place in the oral cavity, pharynx, esophagus, stomach, and small intestine.

Second, digestive end products, along with water, vitamins, and minerals, are **absorbed** primarily by the small intestine and to a very small degree by the stomach and are transported into the circulatory system.

Third, unused or unnecessary solid material is **eliminated** by the large intestine. (Digestive functions of the large intestine are described in Chapter 15.)

SUMMARY: PRIMARY FUNCTIONS OF DIGESTIVE SYSTEM

1. **Ingestion** and/or **digestion**
   - Oral cavity
   - Pharynx
   - Esophagus
   - Stomach
   - Small intestine
2. **Absorption**
   - Small intestine (and stomach)
3. **Elimination**
   - Large intestine

Body Habitus

The type of body habitus has a great effect on the location of the GI organs within the abdominal cavity. To accurately and consistently position for GI procedures, one must know and understand the characteristics of each of these classes of body habitus.

The four general classes of body habitus are shown in Fig. 14-23.

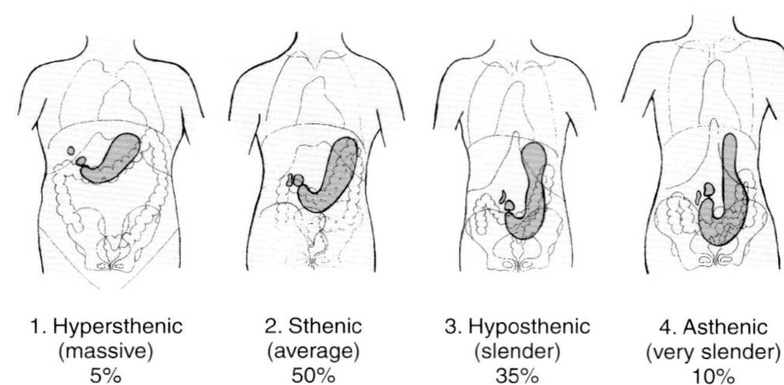

Fig. 14-23. Body habitus—four body types.

HYPERSTHENIC VERSUS HYPOSTHENIC/ASTHENIC (Fig. 14-24)

Hypersthenic The hypersthenic type designates the 5% of the population with the most **massive body build,** with the chest and abdomen being very broad and deep from front to back. The lungs are short, and the diaphragm is high. The transverse colon is quite high, and the entire **large intestine** extends to the periphery of the abdominal cavity. This type generally requires two radiographs placed crosswise to include the entire large intestine.

The **gallbladder** (GB) tends to associate in location with the duodenal bulb and pylorus region of the stomach. For the hypersthenic patient the GB is high and almost transverse and lies well to the right of the midline. The **stomach** is also very high and assumes a transverse position. The level of the stomach extends from approximately T9 to T13, with the center of the stomach about 1 inch (2.5 cm) distal to the xiphoid process. The duodenal bulb is at approximately the level of **T11 or T12,** to the right of the midline.

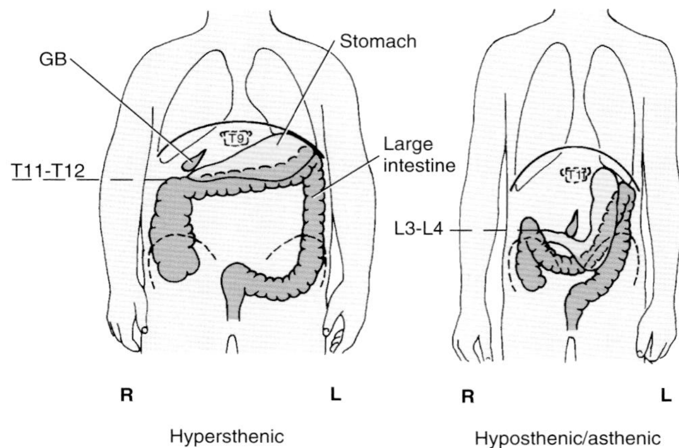

Fig. 14-24. Hypersthenic, compared with hyposthenic/asthenic.

Hyposthenic/Asthenic This body type is essentially the opposite of the hypersthenic type. Hyposthenic/asthenic individuals are more slender and have narrow and longer lungs, with a low diaphragm. This placement causes the **large intestine** to be very low in the abdomen, which has its greatest capacity in the pelvic region.

The **stomach** is J-shaped and low in the abdomen, extending from about T11 down below the level of the iliac crests to approximately L5 or even lower. The vertical portion of the stomach is to the left of midline, with the duodenal bulb near the midline at the level of **L3 or L4.**

The **gallbladder** is near the midline or slightly to the right and just above it, at the level of the iliac crest, or approximately at L3 to L4.

Sthenic (Fig. 14-25) The **average body build** is the sthenic type, which is a more slender version of the hypersthenic classification. The **stomach** is also somewhat J-shaped, is located lower than in the massive body type, and generally extends from the level of T10 or T11 down to about L2. The duodenal bulb is at the approximate level of **L1 to L2,** to the right of the midline. The **gallbladder** is less transverse and lies midway between the lateral abdominal wall and the midline. The **left colic (splenic) flexure** of the **large intestine** is often quite high, resting under the left diaphragm.

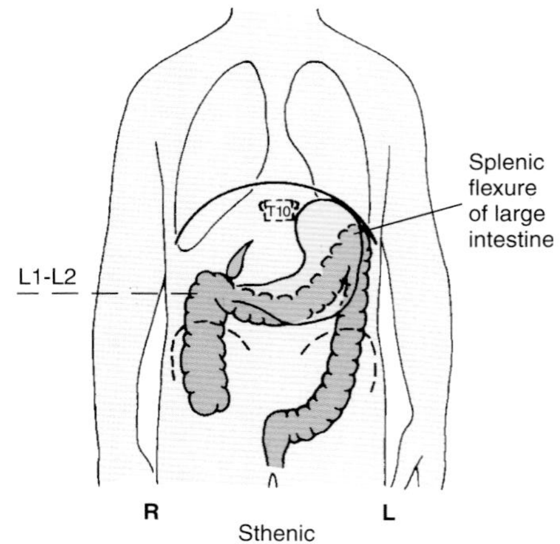

Fig. 14-25. Sthenic (average).

ADDITIONAL FACTORS

In addition to body habitus, other factors affecting the position of the stomach include **stomach contents, respiration, body position** (erect versus recumbent), and **age.** Because the upper stomach is attached to the diaphragm, whether one is in full inspiration or expiration affects the superior extent of the stomach. All abdominal organs tend to drop 1 to 2 inches (2.5 to 5 cm) in an erect position, or even more with age and loss of muscle tone. As a technologist, correct localization of the stomach and other organs for different body types in various positions comes with positioning practice.

14

Radiographs of Upper Gastrointestinal Tract Demonstrating Body Types

Most persons do not fall clearly into one of the distinct four body types but are a combination of these types, and the technologist needs to be able to evaluate each patient for probable stomach and/or gallbladder locations.

The three radiographic and photographic body type examples below demonstrate the position and location of the stomach on the three most common body types. The location of the stomach and duodenal bulb to specific vertebrae should be noted, in addition to the iliac crest and lower costal margin positioning landmarks.

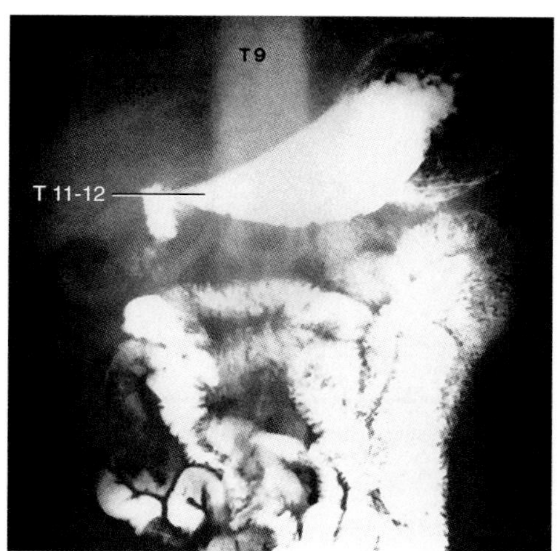

Fig. 14-26. Hypersthenic.
General stomach—high and transverse, level T9 to T12.
Pyloric portion—level of T11 to T12, at midline.
Duodenal bulb location—level of T11 to T12, to right of midline.

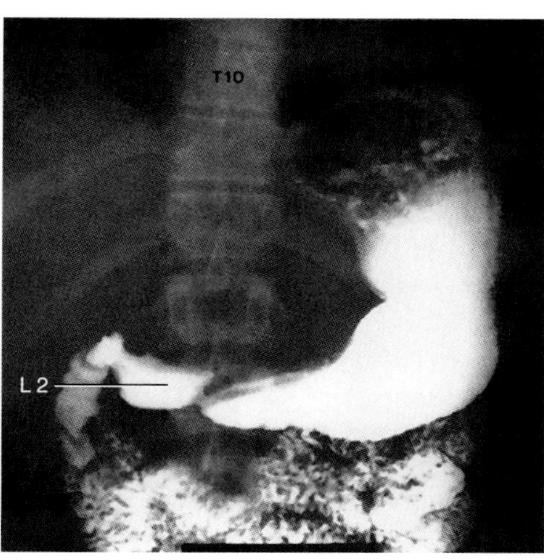

Fig. 14-27. Sthenic.
General stomach—level T10 to L2.
Pyloric portion—level of L2, near midline.
Duodenal bulb location—level of L2, near midline.

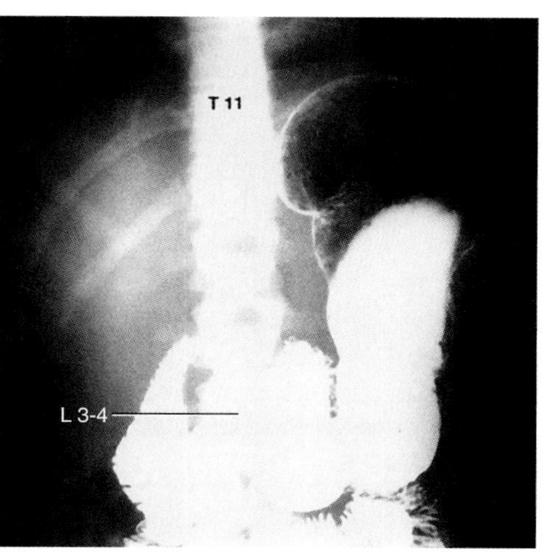

Fig. 14-28. Hyposthenic/asthenic.
General stomach—low and vertical, level T11 to L4.
Pyloric portion—level of L3 to L4, to left of midline.
Duodenal bulb location—level of L3, at midline.

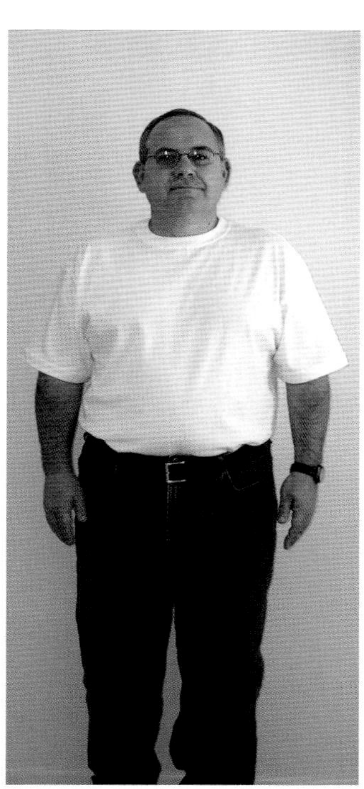

Fig. 14-29. Hypersthenic. Generally shorter in height, with broad shoulders and hips and short torso (less distance between lower rib cage and iliac crest). Abdominal cavity is widest at upper margin.

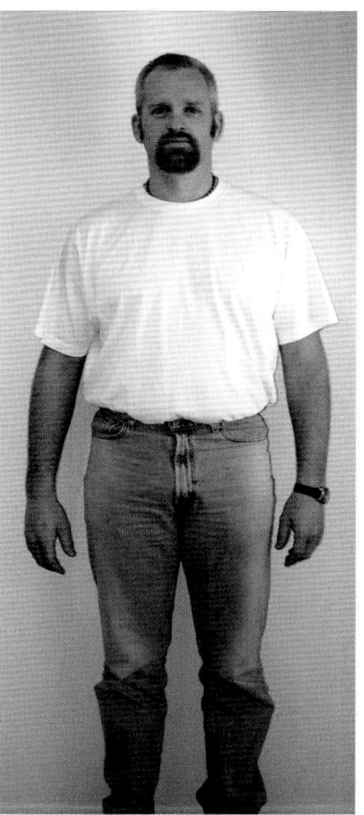

Fig. 14-30. Sthenic. Near average in height, weight, and length of torso (may be somewhat heavier than average, with some hypersthenic characteristics).

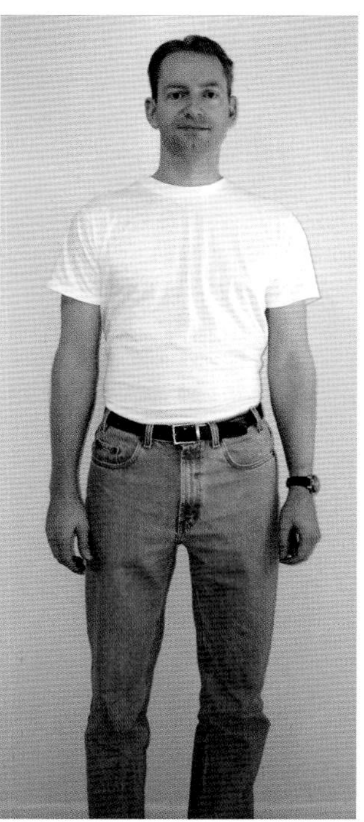

Fig. 14-31. Hyposthenic/asthenic. Generally tall and thin, with long torso. (This example is somewhere between a hyposthenic and an asthenic.) Abdominal cavity is widest at lower margin for a true asthenic.

RADIOGRAPHIC PROCEDURES

Similarities

Radiographic procedures or examinations of the entire alimentary canal are similar in three general aspects.

First, because most parts of the GI tract are comparable in density to those tissues surrounding them, some type of **contrast medium** must be added to visualize these structures. Ordinarily, the only parts of the alimentary canal that can be seen on plain radiographs are the fundus of the stomach (in the upright position), due to the gastric air bubble, and parts of the large intestine, due to pockets of gas and collections of fecal matter.

Most of the alimentary canal simply blends in with the surrounding structures and cannot be visualized without the use of contrast media. This fact is illustrated by comparison of a plain abdominal radiograph (Fig. 14-32) to an upper GI series radiograph with barium sulfate used as a contrast medium (Fig. 14-33).

A **second** similarity is that the initial stage of each radiographic examination of the alimentary canal is carried out with **fluoroscopy.** Fluoroscopy allows the radiologist to (1) observe the GI tract in motion, (2) produce radiographic images during the course of the examination, and (3) determine the most appropriate course of action for the complete radiographic examination. To view organs in motion and isolate anatomic structures is absolutely essential for radiographic examination of the upper GI tract. The structures in this area assume a wide variety of shapes and sizes, depending on body habitus, age, and other individual differences.

In addition, the functional activity of the alimentary canal exhibits a wide range of differences that are considered within normal limits. In addition to these variations, a large number of abnormal conditions exist, making it important that these organs be viewed directly by fluoroscopy.

A **third** similarity is that **radiographic images are recorded during, and frequently after, the fluoroscopic examination** to provide a permanent record of the normal or abnormal findings. A postfluoroscopy "overhead" radiograph is being readied for exposure by the technologist after performance of fluoroscopy for an upper GI series in Fig. 14-35. The positioning section of this chapter describes the most common postfluoroscopy routine projections for esophagram and upper GI procedures.

With the increased use of **digital fluoroscopy,** the number of postfluoroscopy radiographs has diminished greatly. Some departments rely strictly on the digital image produced during fluoroscopy rather than any additional postfluoroscopy radiographs. Digital fluoroscopy is described in more detail later in this chapter.

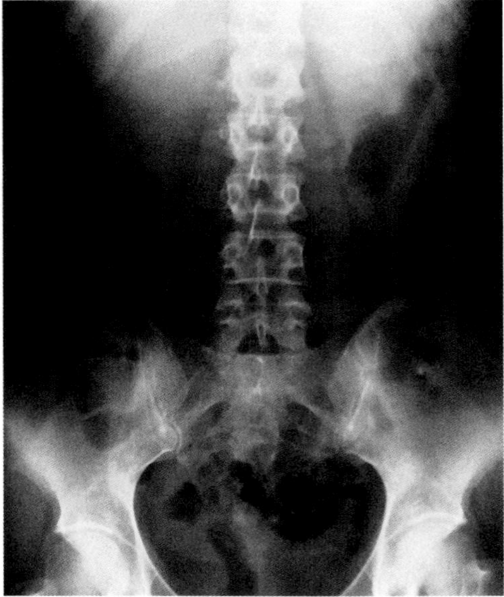

Fig. 14-32. Plain abdomen.

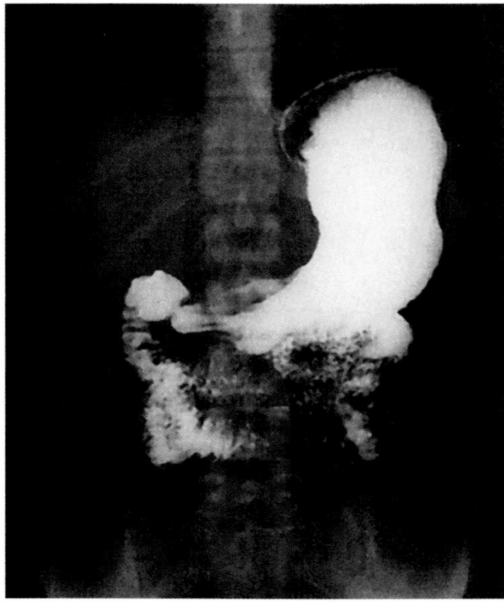

Fig. 14-33. Barium in stomach.

14

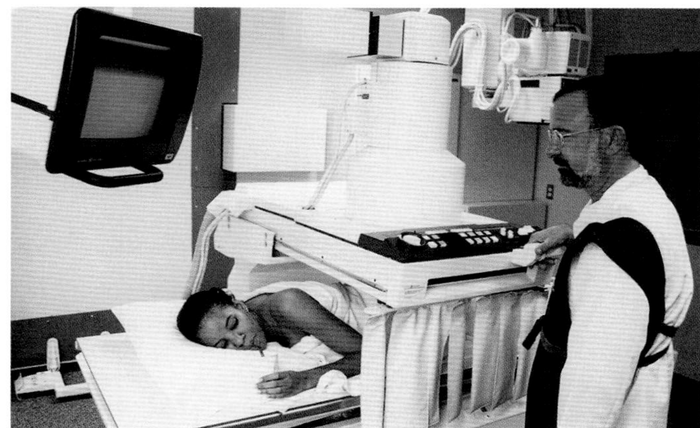

Fig. 14-34. Patient and radiologist ready to begin upper GI fluoroscopy procedure. (Combination digital/spot film system.)

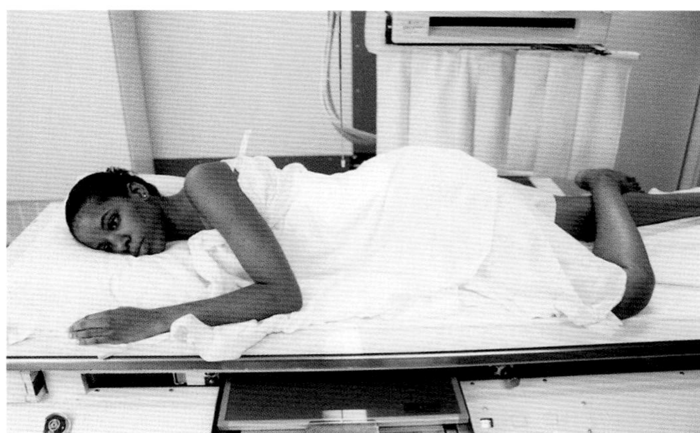

Fig. 14-35. Patient in position for postfluoroscopy "overhead" radiograph.

Contrast Media

Radiolucent and **radiopaque** contrast media are utilized to render the GI tract visible radiographically.

Radiolucent, or **negative, contrast** media include **swallowed air, CO_2 gas crystals,** and the normally present **gas bubble** in the stomach. Calcium and magnesium citrate carbonate crystals are most commonly used to produce CO_2 gas.

BARIUM SULFATE (BARIUM)

The most common **positive, or radiopaque, contrast medium** used to visualize the gastrointestinal system is **barium sulfate** ($BaSO_4$), commonly referred to as just *barium.* As illustrated in Fig. 14-36, barium sulfate is a powdered, chalklike substance. The powdered barium sulfate is mixed with water before ingestion by the patient.

This particular compound, which is a salt of barium, is relatively inert because of its extreme insolubility in water and other aqueous solutions, such as acids. All other salts of barium tend to be toxic or poisonous to the human system. Therefore the barium sulfate used in radiology departments must be chemically pure.

A mixture of barium sulfate and water forms a **colloidal suspension,** not a solution. For a solution, the molecules of the substance added to water must actually dissolve in the water. **Barium sulfate never dissolves in the water.** In a colloidal suspension, however (such as barium sulfate and water), the particles suspended in the water may tend to settle out when allowed to sit for a period of time.

The radiograph shown in Fig. 14-37 shows cups of four different brands of barium that were mixed with a ratio by volume of one part water to one part barium sulfate and then allowed to sit for 24 hours. Because different brands of barium sulfate were used, some cups exhibit more separation or settling than others. This settling demonstrates that when the barium sulfate and water are mixed before they are actually needed, each cup must be thoroughly stirred before actual use.

Many special barium sulfate preparations are available commercially. Most of these preparations contain finely divided barium sulfate in a special suspending agent, so they tend to resist settling out and therefore stay in suspension longer. Each suspension must be well mixed before use, however. Various brands have different smells and different flavors, such as chocolate, chocolate malt, vanilla, lemon, lime, or strawberry.

THIN BARIUM

Barium sulfate may be prepared or purchased in a relatively thin or thick mixture. The thin barium sulfate and water mixture contained in a cup, as illustrated in Fig. 14-38, contains **one part $BaSO_4$ to one part water.** Thin barium is the consistency of a thin milkshake and is used to study the entire GI tract.

The motility, or speed, with which barium sulfate passes through the GI tract depends on the suspending medium and additives, the temperature, and the consistency of the preparation, as well as on the general condition of the patient and the GI tract. Mixing the preparation exactly according to radiologist preferences and departmental protocol is most important. When the mixture is cold, the chalky taste is much less objectionable.

THICK BARIUM

Thick barium contains **three or four parts $BaSO_4$ to one part water** and should be the consistency of cooked cereal. Thick barium is more difficult to swallow but is well suited for use in the esophagus because it descends slowly and tends to coat the mucosal lining.

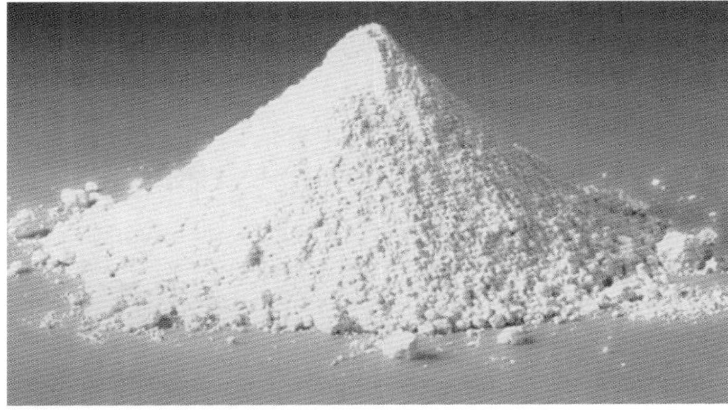

Fig. 14-36. Barium sulfate ($BaSO_4$).

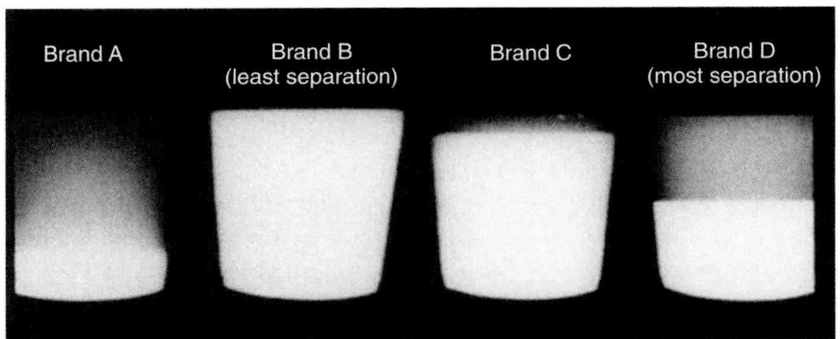

Fig. 14-37. Cups of barium.

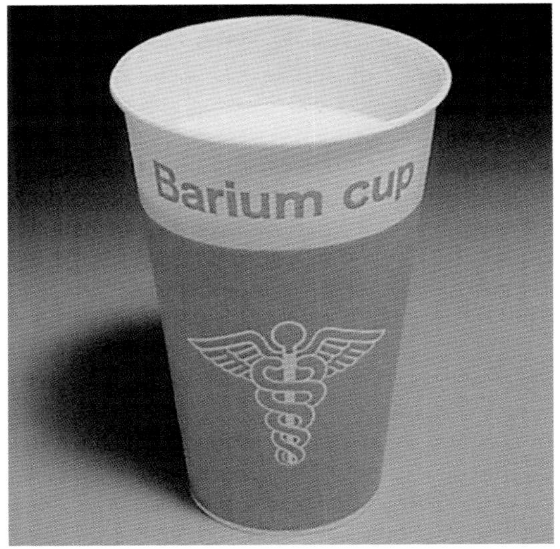

Fig. 14-38. Thin barium sulfate and water mixture (one part barium to one part water).

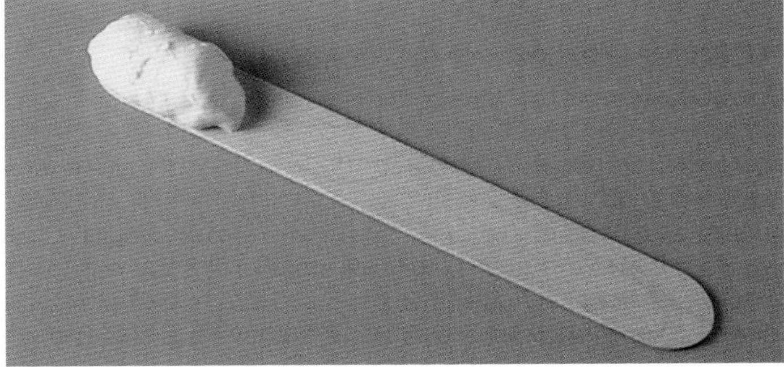

Fig. 14-39. Thick barium sulfate mixture (three or four parts barium to one part water).

CONTRAINDICATIONS TO BARIUM SULFATE

Barium sulfate mixtures are contraindicated if **any chance exists that the mixture might escape into the peritoneal cavity.** This escape may occur through a perforated viscus or during surgery that follows the radiographic procedure. In either of these two cases, **water-soluble, iodinated contrast media** should be used. Two examples of this type are Gastrografin and Gastroview, which is shown in Fig. 14-40. Both of these water-soluble contrast agents can be easily removed by aspiration before or during surgery. If any of this water-soluble material escapes into the peritoneal cavity, the body can readily absorb it. Barium sulfate, on the other hand, is not absorbed.

One drawback to the water-soluble materials is their bitter taste. Although these iodinated contrast media sometimes are mixed with carbonated soft drinks to mask the taste, they often are used "as is" or diluted with water. The patient should be forewarned that the taste may be slightly bitter.

The technologist should be aware that water-soluble contrast agents travel through the GI tract faster than barium sulfate. The shorter transit time of water-soluble contrast agents should be kept in mind if delayed images of the stomach of duodenum are ordered.

Warning Water-soluble iodinated contrast media **should not be used** if the patient is sensitive to iodine. It has also been reported that a small number of patients are hypersensitive to barium sulfate or the additives. Although this is a rare occurrence, the patient should be observed for any signs of allergic reaction.

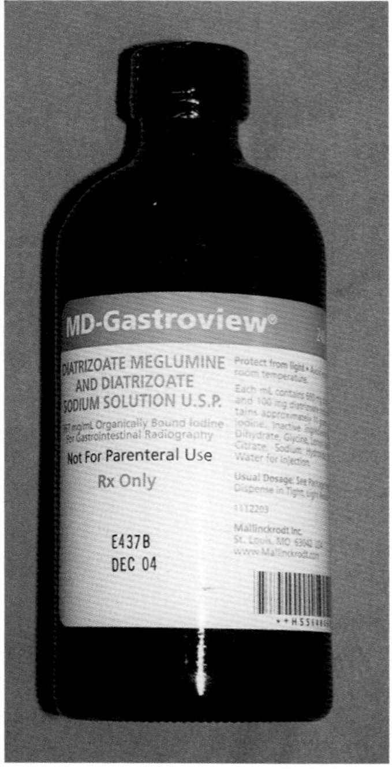

Fig. 14-40. Example of water-soluble iodinated contrast medium.

DOUBLE CONTRAST

The use of **double-contrast techniques** has been employed widely to enhance the diagnosis of certain diseases and conditions during upper GIs. Some departments are also performing double-contrast esophagrams. The use of double-contrast procedures employing both radiolucent and radiopaque contrast media was developed in Japan, where a high incidence of stomach carcinoma exists.

The **radiopaque** contrast medium is **barium sulfate.** High-density barium is used to provide good coating of the stomach mucosa. A pre-measured, commercially produced cup of barium sulfate is most often provided by the department, to which the technologist needs only to add water and mix thoroughly.

The **radiolucent** contrast medium is either **room air** or **carbon dioxide gas.** To introduce room air, small pin-prick holes are placed in the patient's straw. As the patient drinks the barium mixture, air is drawn into the body.

Carbon dioxide gas is created when the patient ingests gas-producing crystals. Two common forms of these crystals are **calcium and magnesium citrate.** On reaching the stomach, these crystals **form a large gas bubble.** The gas mixes with the barium and forces the barium sulfate against the stomach mucosa, providing better coating and visibility of the mucosa and its patterns (Fig. 14-41). Longitudinal mucosal folds (rugae) of the stomach are seen in Fig. 14-42 *(arrows).* Potential polyps, diverticula, and ulcers are demonstrated better with a double-contrast technique.

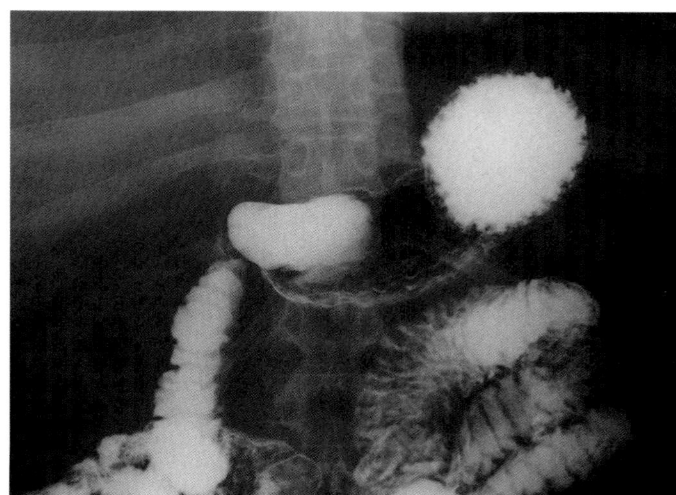

Fig. 14-41. UGI—double contrast; demonstrates air- and barium-filled stomach.

POSTEXAM ELIMINATION (DEFECATION)

One of the normal functions of the large intestine is the absorption of water. Any barium sulfate mixture remaining in the large intestine after either an upper GI series or a barium enema may become hardened and somewhat solidified in the large bowel and consequently be difficult to evacuate. Some patients may require a laxative after these examinations to help remove the barium sulfate. If laxatives are contraindicated, the patient should force fluids or use mineral oil until stools are free from all traces of the white barium.

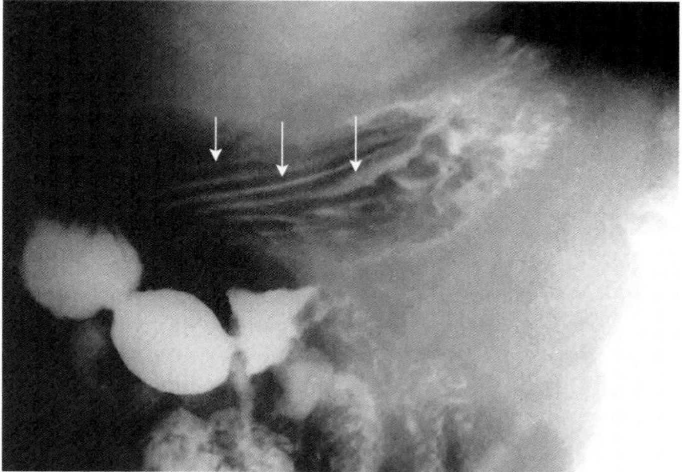

Fig. 14-42. UGI—double contrast; demonstrates air- and barium-filled stomach, with mucosal folds lined with barium.

Radiography–Fluoroscopy (R/F) Equipment

CONVENTIONAL/NONDIGITAL FLUOROSCOPY UNIT (WITH IMAGE INTENSIFICATION, TV, AND SPOT FILMS)

A conventional nondigital combination radiography-fluoroscopy (R/F) unit is illustrated in Fig. 14-43 in an upright position. The **x-ray fluoroscopy tube** is located under the table. This general-purpose fluoroscopy room is equipped with a variety of electronic devices. These include an **image intensifier, spot film devices, television,** and a **photospot camera** that moves as the table is tilted up or down. The electronically enhanced image can be viewed with a **television monitor.**

Spot Film-Screen Cassettes The conventional nondigital fluoroscopic unit is equipped with a **spot film device** to permanently record optimal images on film-screen cassettes. Cassettes of various sizes can be moved into position to permit a conventional, photo-timed radiographic exposure. When fluoroscopy is being performed, these cassettes are in a lead-protected park position within the fluoroscopic unit ready for use when the fluoroscopist wishes to record on film a specific fluoroscopic image.

Television Fluoroscopy A television monitor system is shown, with the video pickup tube (television camera) located in the fluoro tower unit in combination with the image intensifier. Because these television video systems are always closed-circuit, monitors can also be placed outside the fluoroscopy room for simultaneous live viewing during the examination.

Photospot Images Some nondigital fluoroscopic systems also use a **photospot camera** for photospot images (such as small stationary spot frames taken on 105 mm film). These photospot images are recorded by the photospot camera on the **output side** of the image intensifier, whereas conventional spot films taken on 18 × 24 cm (8 × 10 inches) or similar-sized film-screen cassettes are direct images taken on the **input side** of the image intensifier (Fig. 14-43). Therefore spot film-screen images don't utilize the image intensifier and lack the brightness of photospot images.

Cinefluoroscopy Cinefluoroscopy, or cine, cameras are similar to movie cameras. They provide rapid filming to capture fast physiologic processes or functions. Before the advent of digital fluoroscopy, this method of film imaging was ideal for cardiac catheterization procedures. Cine camera devices generally use 16 or 35 mm film, but today filmless digital cinefluoroscopy systems are available.

Image Intensification In the early 1950s the invention of the **image intensifier** revolutionized fluoroscopy. The image intensifier utilizes the radiation that passes through the patient and enhances the resultant image by electronically making this image 1000 to 6000 times brighter than the older fluoroscopy screen techniques. The image produced through image intensification is bright enough to be seen with photopic or day vision. The room lights are dimmed, and the fluoroscopic examination is carried out in a comfortably illuminated room.

The image intensifier is located in the fluoroscopy tower above the tabletop, whereas the x-ray tube is located beneath the tabletop (Figs. 14-43 and 14-44).

An important hanging leaded tower drape shield is shown in position in Fig. 14-44 to protect the operator.

Note: Newer digital fluoroscopy systems are in common use today wherein these spot film-screen cassettes or photospot camera images are not used. These digital imaging systems are shown and described on following pages.

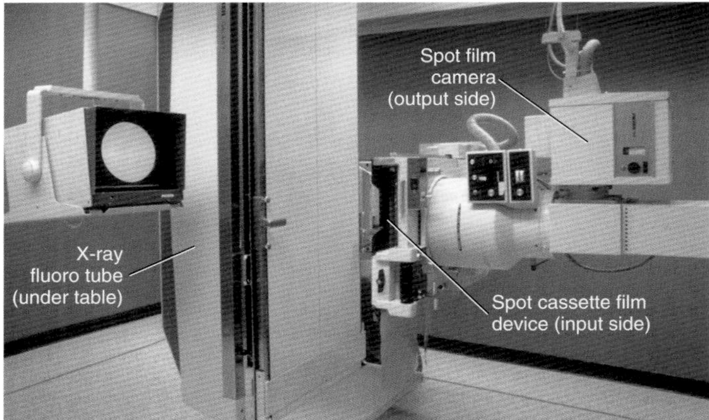

Fig. 14-43. Conventional nondigital fluoroscopy system.

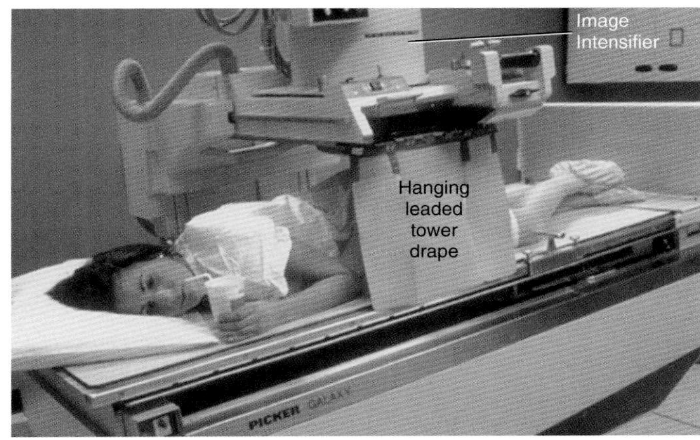

Fig. 14-44. Patient in horizontal position for GI fluoroscopy.

14

DIGITAL FLUOROSCOPY

With the increased use of computers and digital imaging, the use of digitized fluoroscopy equipment is becoming more common. A **C-arm digital fluoroscopy unit** is shown in Fig. 14-45. In this position the x-ray tube is on the lower portion of the C-arm and the image intensifier is on the upper portion. This type of digital fluoroscopy unit is very flexible in that it can be rotated around the patient in any position for various types of special procedures, including invasive angiography studies, as described in Chapter 21.

Digital Radiography-Fluoroscopy (R/F) A digital R/F system is shown in Fig. 14-46. This type of combination radiography-fluoroscopy system is commonly used for GI procedures. This system incorporates digital fluoroscopy capabilities with a conventional type of x-ray table and "under-the-table" fluoro x-tube. It also includes a separate **radiography tube** for conventional "overhead" radiography applications.

Digital fluoroscopy is similar to the television fluoroscopy system described in this chapter, with the addition of a **digital converter** and a **computer** for image manipulation and/or storage. An analog-to-digital converter is incorporated into the fluoroscopy tower on the **output side** of the image intensifier. From there the image information is transmitted into a computer for manipulation and/or storage. The computer's hard disk stores the images produced during the study. Because of limited disk space, the images are generally only kept on the hard disk for a limited period of time before they are transferred to either a magnetic or optical disk for longer-term storage.

A computer workstation provides a keyboard and usually a mouse or trackball for image manipulations. Images can then be displayed on high-resolution monitors located in the fluoroscopy room as well and on monitors located in other locations for remote viewing.

The use of digital fluoroscopy permits GI studies to remain in a digital format that can be sent to various locations inside and outside the hospital. Digital fluoroscopy has led to the expanded use of PACS (Patient Archiving and Communications Systems), which is a digital imaging network that provides the ability to store, retrieve, manipulate, and print specific examinations at various locations. As described in more detail in Chapter 2, PACS ties together all the digital imaging modalities, such as ultrasound, nuclear medicine, magnetic resonance, and computed radiography, into a digital community that allows radiologists, technologists, and referring physicians to view these images. The concept of the "film room" is becoming obsolete with PACS because with digital imaging, the handling and storage of hard-copy images are no longer required.

ADVANTAGES OF DIGITAL OVER CONVENTIONAL FILM-SCREEN FLUOROSCOPY

No Cassettes Are Required Radiographic images can be recorded during the fluoroscopy procedure similar to "spot films," except that no cassettes are required. Specific images are captured instead in digital form for display on high-resolution monitors and/or for storage and manipulation as needed, then printed on film if desired. Thus these digital still-frame images replace the conventional spot films taken on cassettes on the input side of the image intensifier. They also can replace the need for photo spots or cine films taken during an upper GI study. This feature saves time and radiation dose to the patient.

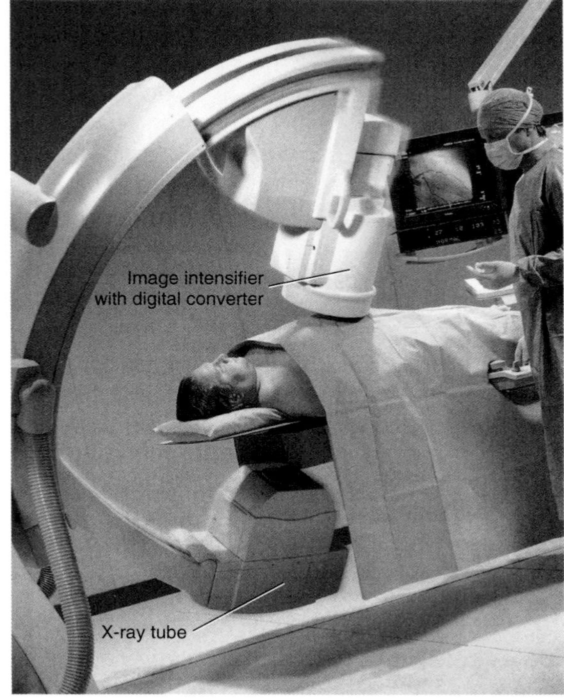

Fig. 14-45. C-arm digital fluoroscopy. (Courtesy Philips Medical Systems.)

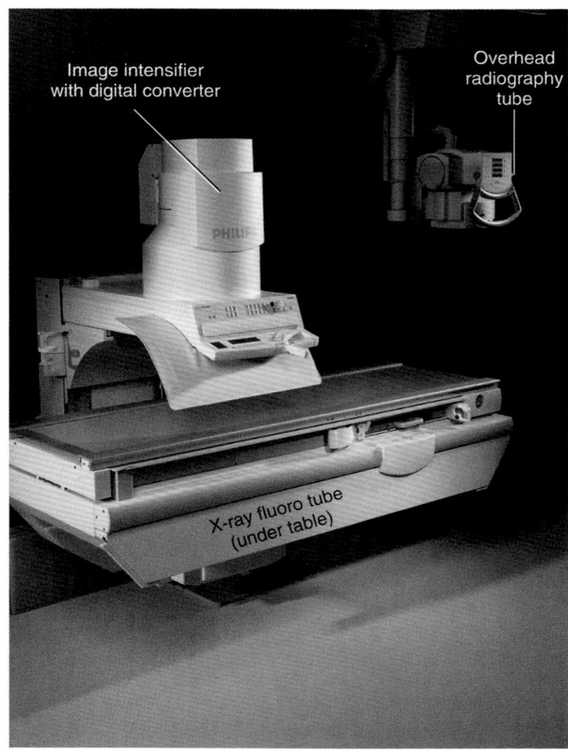

Fig. 14-46. Combination digital R/F system. (Courtesy Philips Medical Systems.)

Optional Postfluoroscopy "Overhead" Images The question of routinely taking these "overhead" images following fluoroscopy is determined by the radiologist or by departmental protocol. Frequently, sufficient digital images are recorded of the entire GI tract in various positions during fluoroscopy that no postfluoroscopy "overhead" larger format images are required. This elimination can result in significant film cost savings, as well as time savings for upper and lower GI series procedures.

Multiple Frame Formatting and Multiple "Original" Films Multiple images can be formatted and printed on one film. This format can be four on one (Fig. 14-47), six on one, nine on one, or even 12 on one. "Hard-copy" films can be printed at any time and as often as desired. Therefore if radiographs are lost or misplaced or if duplicates are needed, additional "original" films can be reprinted at any time.

Cine Loop Capability Individual images can also be recorded in rapid succession and then be displayed as moving or cine images. This feature is beneficial for certain studies, such as an esophagram for possible esophageal reflux or impaired swallowing mechanisms. This capability replaces the need for spot film cameras or video recording. Once the study has been completed, the technologist can play back the cine loop to demonstrate dynamic flow of barium through the esophagus or stomach. The radiologist can then also interpret the study from a monitor located in the reading room.

Image Enhancement and Manipulation Digital fluoroscopy images can be enhanced and/or manipulated by the use of equalization filters (Figs. 14-48 and 14-49). These image-enhancement and manipulation features include edge enhancement, overall brightness and contrast controls, masking, and digital subtraction study possibilities. Other options include shifting from a negative to a positive image, motion artifact control, and margin (edge) enhancement. With the study saved on the hard disk, the technologist or radiologist has the ability to alter these imaging parameters at will.

Reduced Patient Exposure Digital fluorographic imaging **can reduce patient exposure 30% to 50%,** compared with conventional fluoroscopy because of the increased sensitivity of image receptors resulting from a "pulsed progressive" scanning process.* This can be an important consideration in pediatric applications.

"Road mapping" is also possible with digital fluoroscopy, wherein a specific fluoroscopic image can be held on one monitor in combination with continuous imaging on a second monitor or on different portions of the same monitor. This feature is an advantage in certain interventional procedures requiring the placement of catheters and guidewires. This type of intermittent "road mapping" or "frame hold" capability also decreases patient exposure by reducing the need for continuous x-ray exposure of the patient.*

*Hendee WR, Ritenour R: Medical imaging physics, ed 3, St. Louis, 1992, Mosby-Year Book.

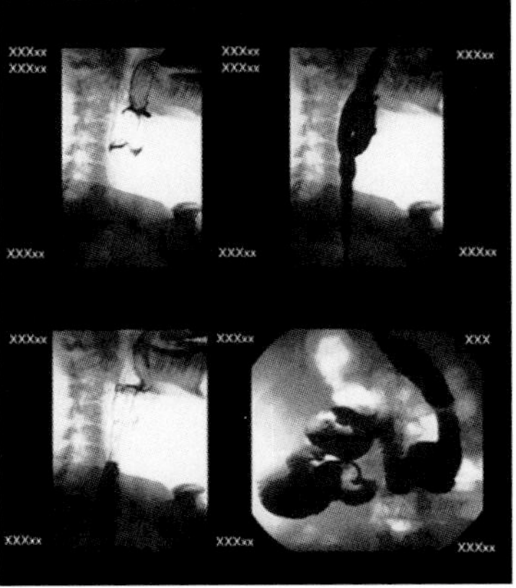

Fig. 14-47. Multiple-frame images—four images on one 35- × 43-cm (14- × 17-inch) film.

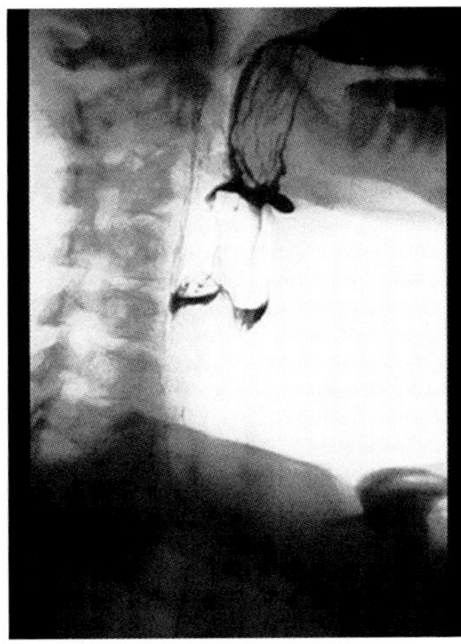

Fig. 14-48. Without equalization filter.

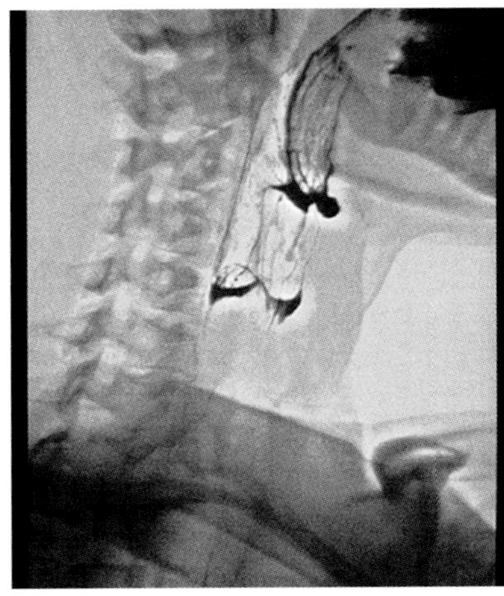

Fig. 14-49. With equalization filter.

14

WORKER PROTECTION DURING FLUOROSCOPY

Radiation protection practices during fluoroscopy are described in Chapter 2.

Exposure Patterns Exposure patterns and related doses within the fluoroscopy room are also provided in Chapter 2, indicating where one should stand or not stand in the room during fluoroscopy. Fig. 14-50 demonstrates these exposure patterns, which remind the assisting technologist **not** to stand close to the table on either side of the radiologist but rather to **stay back** from **the higher scatter fields** as much as possible throughout the fluoroscopy procedure.

Lead Drape Shield The flexible **lead tower drape shield** attached to the front of the fluoroscopic and spot-film device is very important and should be inspected regularly to ensure that it is not damaged or improperly placed (see Fig. 14-44 on p. 459).

Bucky Slot Shield The technologist should always ensure that the **Bucky is all the way to the end of the table** before the beginning of a fluoroscopic procedure, which then brings out the metal **Bucky slot shield** to cover the approximately 2 inch (5 cm) space directly under the tabletop (Fig. 14-51). This shield significantly reduces the scatter radiation resulting from the fluoroscopy x-ray tube located under the table. Leakage or scatter rays can escape through this waist-high Bucky space if the Bucky shield is not completely out on this type of system.

This Bucky-at-end-of-table requirement during fluoroscopy is not only important for worker protection but also necessary to keep the Bucky mechanism from the path of the fluoroscopy x-ray tube under the table.

Lead Aprons **Protective aprons** of 0.5-mm lead equivalency must always be worn during fluoroscopy. Some technologists and radiologists may also choose to wear **lead-equivalent glasses** and **thyroid shields.**

Before the radiologist or technologist places a hand into the fluoroscopy beam, a **leaded glove** must always be worn and the beam must be first attenuated by the patient's body. The use of a **compression paddle** (described on p. 467) is an even better alternative to placement of a gloved hand in the fluoroscopy primary beam when compression of parts of the patient's abdomen is required.

Cardinal Principles of Radiation Protection

One of the best ways to reduce worker dose during fluoroscopy is to apply the following three "Cardinal Principles of Radiation Protection." If these principles are applied correctly, dose to both the fluoroscopist and the technologist can be reduced greatly.

1. **Time:** Reduce the amount of time the fluoroscopy tube is energized. Although most procedures are performed by radiologists and the amount of fluoroscopy time is controlled by them, the technologist should also keep track of fluoroscopy time. If fluoroscopy time becomes excessive, the situation should be discussed with a supervisor.

   The use of "intermittent fluoroscopy" reduces dose to the patient and workers. With digital fluoroscopy, the "Image Freeze" function should be used, which allows the last energized image to remain visible on the monitor. Then the fluoroscopy tube is activated only when a new image is required.
2. **Shielding:** Follow all the shielding precautions described above, including correct use of the **lead drape shield,** the **Bucky slot shield,** and **lead gloves.**
3. **Distance:** The most effective method of reducing dose during fluoroscopy procedures is to increase the distance between the x-ray tube and the technologist. By applying the Inverse Square Law, technologists can significantly reduce dose to themselves. Doubling the distance between the x-ray tube and the worker can reduce dose by a factor of four. When not changing cassettes or managing the patient, technologists should maximize their distance from the x-ray tube.

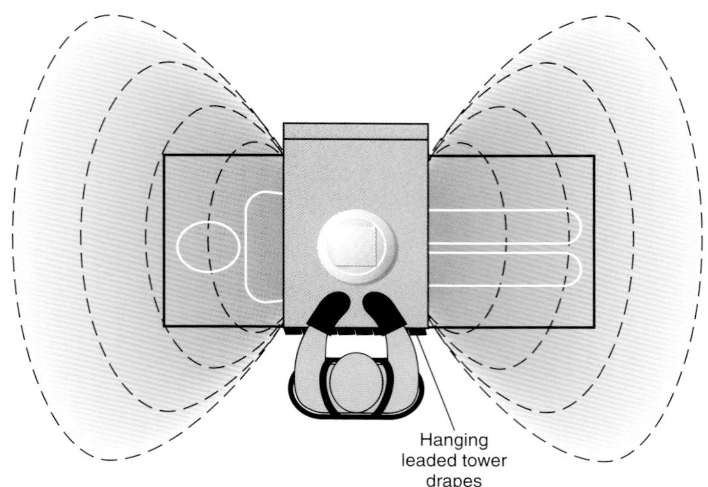

Fig. 14-50. Fluoroscopy exposure patterns.

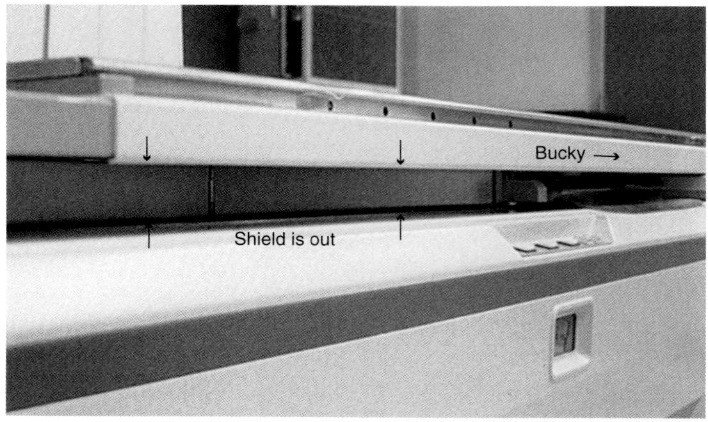

Fig. 14-51. Close-up view of Bucky slot shield completely out, with Bucky tray at far end of table.

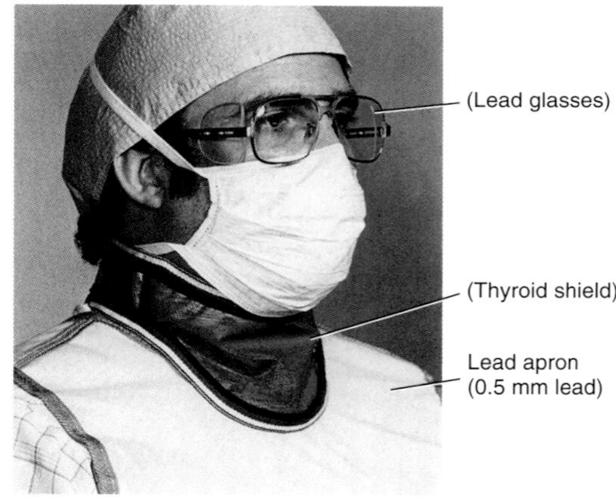

Fig. 14-52. Lead apron, with thyroid shield and lead glasses. (Courtesy Nuclear Associates, Carle, NY.)

WORKER PROTECTION SUMMARY CHART

PROTECTIVE DEVICE	BENEFIT
Fluoroscopy leaded tower drape	Greatly reduces exposure to the fluoroscopy personnel
Lead apron (0.5-mm Pb)	Reduces exposure to the torso
Lead gloves	Reduces exposure to the hands and wrists
Bucky slot shield	Reduces exposure to the gonadal region
Lead goggles	Reduces exposure to the lenses of the eye
Thyroid shield	Reduces exposure to the thyroid gland
Compression paddle	Reduces exposure to arm and hand of fluoroscopist

14

Esophagram Procedure

Two common radiographic procedures of the upper GI system involving the administration of contrast media are the **esophagram,** or *barium swallow,* as it is sometimes referred to, and the **upper GI series.** Each of these procedures is described in detail, beginning with the esophagram.

DEFINITION AND PURPOSE

An esophagram, or barium swallow, is the common radiographic procedure or examination of the **pharynx** and **esophagus,** utilizing a radiopaque contrast medium. Occasionally, a negative or radiolucent contrast medium may be used.

The purpose of an esophagram is to study radiographically the form and function of the swallowing aspects of the pharynx and esophagus.

CONTRAINDICATIONS

No major contraindications exist for esophagrams except possible sensitivity to the contrast media used. The technologist should determine whether the patient has a history of sensitivity to barium sulfate or water-soluble contrast media.

Pathologic Indications for Esophagram

The more common pathologic indications for an esophagram procedure include the following:

Achalasia *(ak"a-la'zha),* also termed *cardiospasm,* is a motor disorder of the esophagus in which peristalsis is reduced along the distal two thirds of the esophagus. Achalasis is evident at the esophagogastric sphincter because of its inability to relax during swallowing. The thoracic esophagus may also lose its normal peristaltic activity and become dilated (megaesophagus). Video and rapid digital fluoroscopy are most helpful in diagnosis of achalasia.

Anatomic anomalies may be congenital or caused by disease, such as cancer of the esophagus. Patients suffering from a stroke often develop impaired swallowing mechanisms. Certain foods and contrast agents are administered during the examination to evaluate swallowing patterns. A speech pathologist may witness the study to better understand the speech and swallowing patterns of the patient. Video and digital fluoroscopy are used during these studies.

Barrett's esophagus, or *Barrett's syndrome,* is the replacement of the normal squamous epithelium with columnar-lined epithelium ulcer tissue in the lower esophagus. This replacement may produce a stricture in the distal esophagus. In advanced cases, the development of a peptic ulcer in the distal esophagus may occur.

The esophagram may demonstrate subtle tissue changes in the esophagus, but **nuclear medicine** is the modality of choice for this condition. The patient is injected with technetium 99m pertechnetate to demonstrate the shift in tissue types in the esophagus.

Carcinoma of the esophagus includes one of the most common malignancies of the esophagus, **adenocarcinoma.** Advanced symptoms include dysphagia (difficulty in swallowing) and localized pain during meals and bleeding. Other tumors of the esophagus include **carcinosarcoma,** which often produces a large, irregular polyp, and **pseudocarcinoma.**

Esophagram and endoscopy are performed to detect these tumors. The esophagram may demonstrate atrophic changes in the mucosa due to the invasion of the tumor as well as stricture. CT may be performed in staging of the tumor and in determining whether it has extended beyond the inner layer of mucosa of the esophagus.

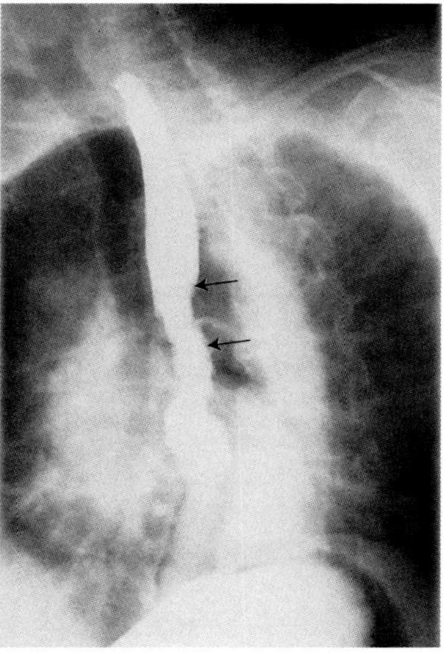

Fig. 14-53. Esophagram—LAO demonstrating a constricted area of the esophagus; probable carcinoma *(arrows).*

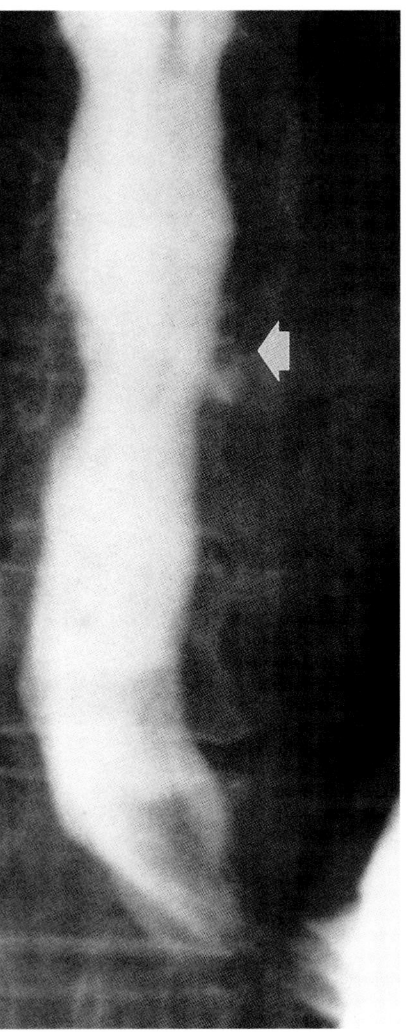

Fig. 14-54. Barrett's esophagus. Ulcerations *(arrow)* have developed at some distance from esophagogastric junction. (From Eisenberger RL, Johnson NM: Comprehensive radiographic pathology, ed 3, St. Louis, 2003, Mosby.)

14

Dysphagia *(dis-fa'je-a)* is difficulty in swallowing. This difficulty may be due to a congenital or acquired condition, a trapped bolus of food, paralysis of the pharyngeal or esophageal muscles, or inflammation. Narrowing or an enlarged, flaccid appearance of the esophagus may be seen during the esophagram, depending on the cause of the dysphagia. Video and digital fluoroscopy are the modalities of choice.

Esophageal varices are characterized by dilation of the veins in the distal esophagus. This condition is often seen with acute liver disease, such as cirrhosis due to increased portal hypertension. With restriction in the venous flow through the liver, the coronary veins in the distal esophagus become dilated, tortuous, and engorged with blood. In advanced cases the veins may begin to bleed. Esophageal varices present with narrowing of the distal third of the esophagus and a "wormlike" or "cobblestone" appearance due to the enlarged veins during an esophagram.

Foreign bodies, of which patients may ingest a variety, include a bolus of food, metallic objects, and other materials lodging in the esophagus. Their locations and dimensions may be determined during the esophagram. Radiolucent foreign bodies, such as fish bones, may require the use of additional materials and techniques to detect them. Cotton may be shredded and placed in a cup of barium and drunk by the patient. The intent of this technique is to allow a tuft of the cotton to be suspended by the radiolucent foreign body and visible during fluoroscopy. Although this technique has been used for decades, most gastroenterologists prefer the use of endoscopy to isolate and remove these foreign bodies.

Gastroesophageal reflux disease (GERD), or **esophageal reflux,** is the entry of gastric contents into the esophagus, irritating the lining of the esophagus. Esophageal reflux is reported as heartburn by most patients. This condition may lead to **esophagitis** demonstrated by an irregular and/or ulcerative appearance of the mucosa of the esophagus.

Although specific causes for GERD or esophageal reflux have not been confirmed, cigarette smoking and excessive intake of aspirin, alcohol, and caffeine increase the incidence of reflux.

Specific methods used to demonstrate esophageal reflux during fluoroscopy are discussed later in this chapter. With advanced cases, the distal esophagus demonstrates longitudinal streaks during an esophagram because of changes in the mucosa. Endoscopy is often performed to detect early signs of esophageal reflux or GERD.

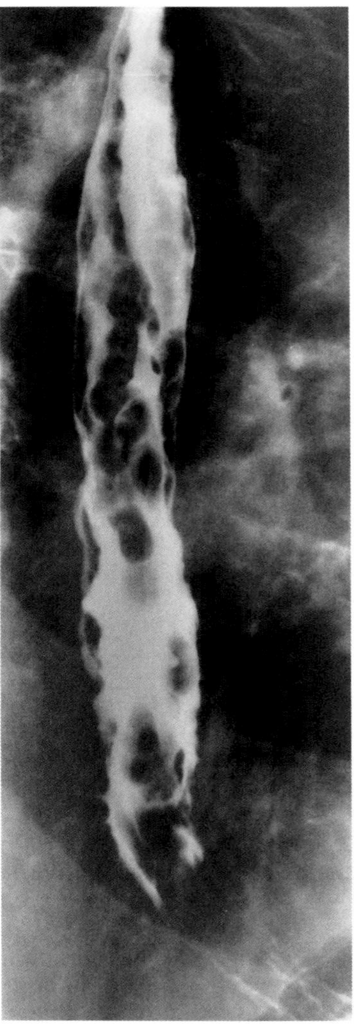

Fig. 14-55. Esophageal varices with diffuse round and oval filling defects. (From Eisenberger RL, Johnson NM: Comprehensive radiographic pathology, ed 3, St. Louis, 2003, Mosby.)

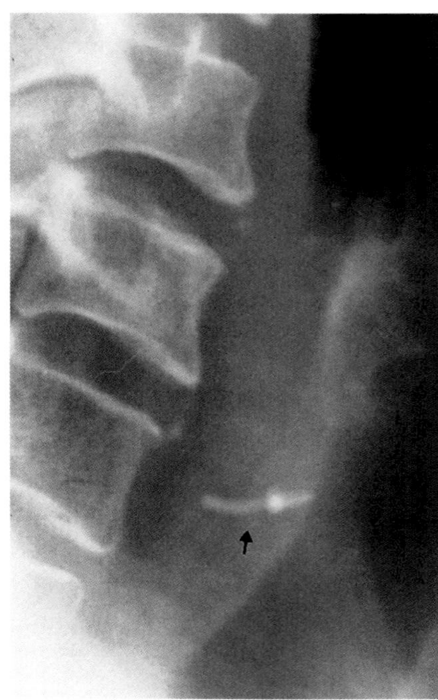

Fig. 14-56. Fish bone *(arrow)* in lower cervical portion of esophagus. (From Eisenberger RL, Johnson NM: Comprehensive radiographic pathology, ed 3, St. Louis, 2003, Mosby.)

14

Zenker's diverticulum is characterized by a large outpouching of the esophagus just above the upper esophageal sphincter. It is believed to be caused by a weakening of the muscle wall. Because of the size of the diverticulum, the patient may experience dysphagia, aspiration, and regurgitation of food eaten hours earlier. Although medication can reduce the symptoms of Zenker's diverticulum, surgery may be required.

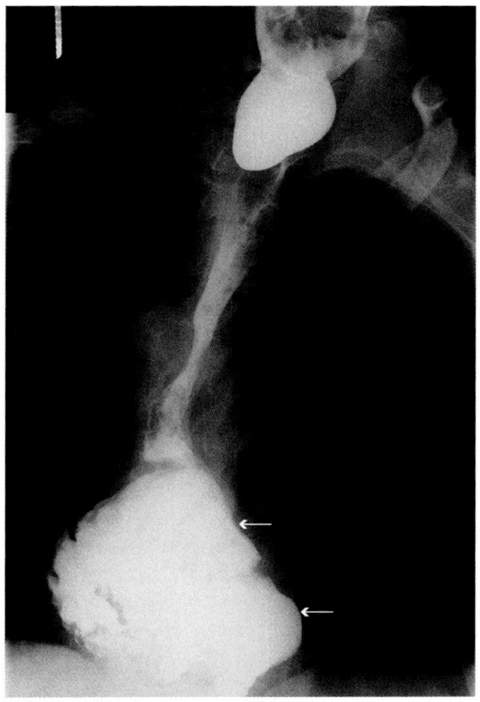

Fig. 14-57. Zenker's diverticulum.

ESOPHAGRAM—SUMMARY OF PATHOLOGIC INDICATIONS

CONDITION OR DISEASE	MOST COMMON RADIOGRAPHIC EXAM	POSSIBLE RADIOGRAPHIC APPEARANCE	MANUAL EXPOSURE FACTOR ADJUSTMENT*
Achalasia	Esophagram with video or digital fluoroscopy	Stricture or narrowing of the esophagus	None
Anatomic anomalies (including foreign bodies)	Esophagram with video or digital fluoroscopy (functional study) endoscopy employed for foreign bodies	Abnormal peristaltic patterns A variety of foreign bodies—both radiopaque and radiolucent	None None
Barrett's esophagus	Esophagram and/or nuclear medicine scan	Stricture or "streaked" appearance of distal esophagus	None
Carcinoma	Esophagram and CT scan	Point of stricture, narrowing, or atrophic changes of mucosa	None
Dysphagia	Esophagram with video or digital fluoroscopy (functional study)	Narrowing or enlargement of the esophagus, depending on etiology	None
Esophageal varices	Esophagram (and endoscopy)	Narrowing and "wormlike" appearance of esophagus	None
Zenker's diverticulum	Esophagram (and endoscopy)	Enlarged recess or cavity in proximal esophagus	None

*Dependent on stage or severity of disease or condition.

PATIENT AND ROOM PREPARATION FOR ESOPHAGRAM

Because the esophagus is empty most of the time, **patients need no preparation for an esophagram unless an upper GI series is to follow.** When combined with an upper GI, or if the primary interest is the lower esophagus, preparation for the UGI takes precedence.

For an esophagram only, all clothing and anything metallic between the mouth and the waist should be removed, and the patient should wear a hospital gown. Before the fluoroscopic procedure a pertinent history should be taken and the examination carefully explained to the patient.

The first part of an esophagram involves fluoroscopy with a positive-contrast medium. The examination room should be clean, tidy, and appropriately stocked before the patient is escorted to the room. The appropriate amount and type of contrast medium should be ready. Esophagrams generally use **both thin and thick barium.** Additional items useful in the detection of a radiolucent foreign body are (1) cotton balls soaked in thin barium, (2) barium pills or gelatin capsules filled with $BaSO_4$, and (3) marshmallows. After swallowing any one of these three substances, the patient is asked to swallow an additional thin barium mixture.

Because the esophagram begins with the table in the vertical position, the footboard should be in place and tested for security. Lead aprons, compression paddle, and lead gloves should be provided for the radiologist, as well as lead aprons for all other personnel in the room. Proper radiation protection methods must be observed at all times during fluoroscopy.

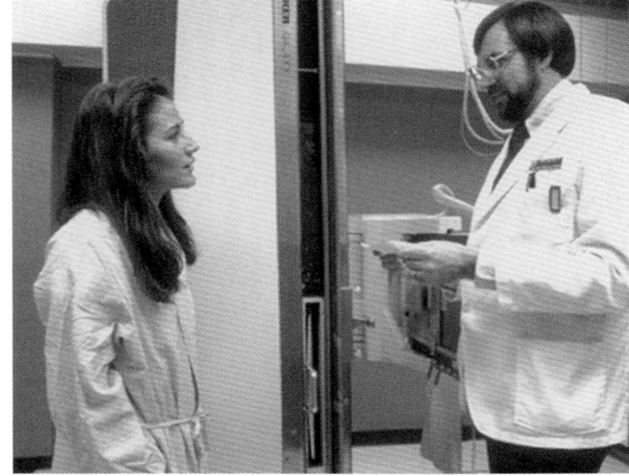

Fig. 14-58. Prepare patient; explain procedure to patient.

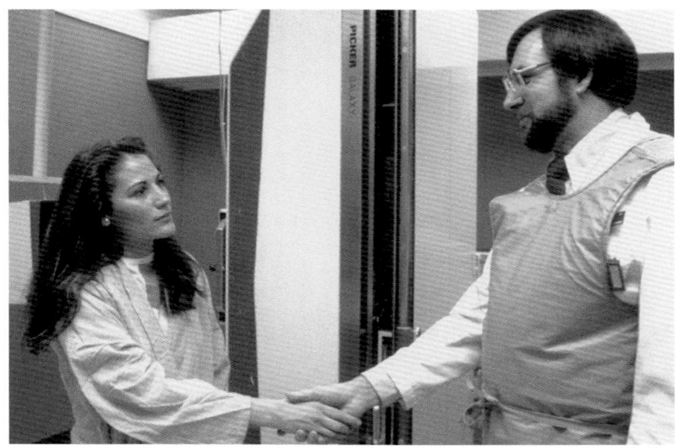

Fig. 14-59. Introduce and assist the radiologist.

GENERAL PROCEDURE

Fluoroscopy With the room prepared and the patient ready, the patient and radiologist are introduced and the patient's history and the reason for the exam discussed. The fluoroscopic examination usually begins with a general survey of the patient's chest, including heart, lungs, and diaphragm, and the abdomen.

During fluoroscopy, the technologist's duties, in general, are to follow the radiologist's instructions, assist the patient as needed, and expedite the procedure in any manner possible. Because the examination is begun in the upright or erect position, a cup of thin barium is placed in the patient's left hand close to the left shoulder. The patient then is instructed to follow the radiologist's instructions concerning how much to drink and when. The radiologist observes the flow of barium with the fluoroscope.

Swallowing (deglutition) of thin barium is observed with the patient in various positions. Similar positions may be used while the patient swallows thick barium. The use of thick barium allows better visualization of mucosal patterns and any lesion within the esophagus. The type of barium mixture to be used, however, is determined by the radiologist.

14

After the upright studies, horizontal and Trendelenburg positions with thick and thin barium may follow. A patient is shown in position for an **RAO projection** with a cup of thin barium (Fig. 14-60). The pharynx and cervical esophagus are usually studied fluoroscopically with spot films, whereas the main portion of the esophagus down to the stomach is studied both with fluoroscopy and with postfluoroscopy "overhead" radiographs.

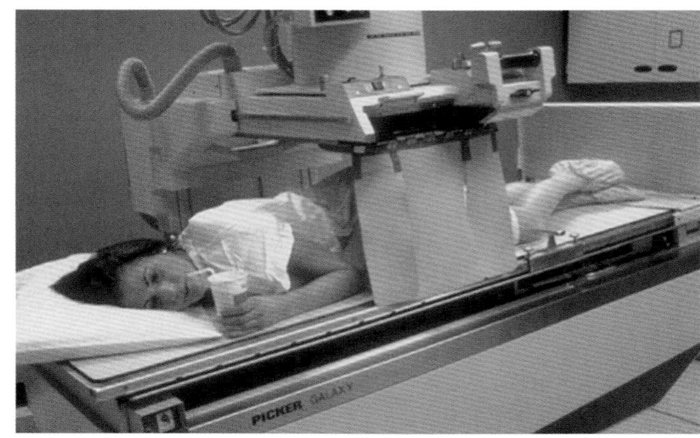

Fig. 14-60. RAO, with cup of thin barium.

DEMONSTRATION OF ESOPHAGEAL REFLUX

The diagnosis of possible esophageal reflux or regurgitation of gastric contents may occur during fluoroscopy or an esophagram. One or more of the following procedures may be performed to detect esophageal reflux:

1. Breathing exercises
2. The water test
3. Compression paddle technique
4. The toe-touch maneuver

Breathing Exercises

The various breathing exercises are all designed to increase both the intrathoracic and the intraabdominal pressures. The most common breathing exercise is the **Valsalva maneuver.** The patient is asked to take a deep breath and, while holding the breath in, to bear down as though trying to move the bowels. This maneuver forces air against the closed glottis. A modified Valsalva maneuver is accomplished as the patient pinches off the nose, closes the mouth, and tries to blow the nose. The cheeks should expand outward as though the patient were blowing up a balloon.

A **Mueller maneuver** can also be performed as the patient exhales and then tries to inhale against a closed glottis.

With both methods, the increase of intraabdominal pressure may produce the reflux of ingested barium that would confirm the presence of esophageal reflux. The radiologist carefully observes the esophagogastric junction during these maneuvers.

Water Test

The water test (Fig. 14-61) is done with the patient in the supine position and turned up slightly on the left side. This slight LPO position fills the fundus with barium. The patient is asked to swallow a mouthful of water through a straw. Under fluoroscopy the radiologist closely observes the esophagogastric junction. A positive water test occurs when significant amounts of barium regurgitate into the esophagus from the stomach.

Compression Technique

A compression paddle (Fig. 14-62) can be placed under the patient in the prone position and inflated as needed to provide pressure to the stomach region. The radiologist can demonstrate the obscure esophagogastric junction during this process to detect possible esophageal reflux.

Toe-Touch Maneuver

The toe-touch maneuver (Fig. 14-63) is also performed to study possible regurgitation into the esophagus from the stomach. Under fluoroscopy the cardiac orifice is observed as the patient bends over and touches the toes. Esophageal reflux and hiatal hernias are sometimes demonstrated with the toe-touch maneuver.

Postfluoroscopy Imaging

After the fluoroscopy portion of the esophagram, radiographs are obtained of the entire barium-filled esophagus. Positioning routines and descriptions for postfluoroscopy "overhead" imaging are described in detail in the positioning section of this chapter.

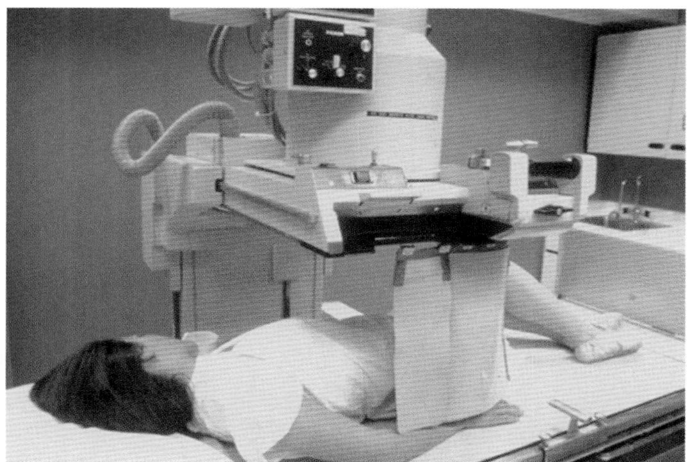

Fig. 14-61. Water test—LPO position.

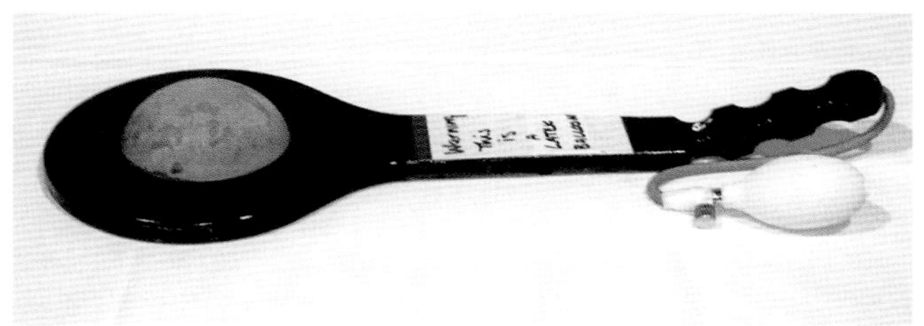

Fig. 14-62. Compression paddle.

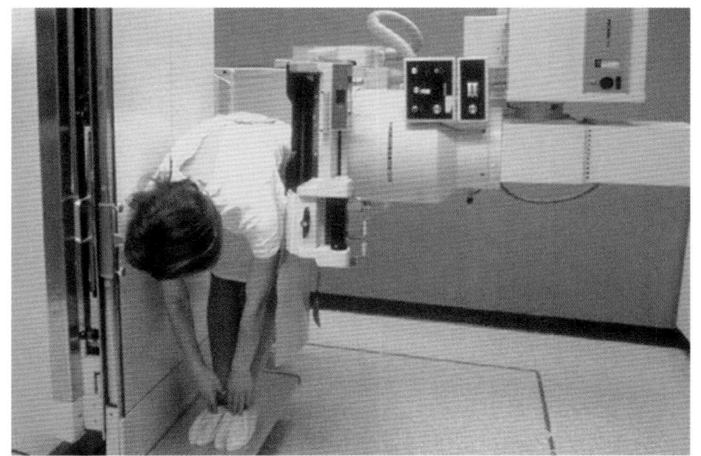

Fig. 14-63. Toe-touch maneuver.

Upper GI Series Procedure

In addition to the esophagram, the second and very common radiographic procedure or examination of the upper GI system involving contrast media is the **upper GI series** (UGI).

DEFINITION AND PURPOSE

Radiographic examination of the **distal esophagus, stomach,** and **duodenum** is called a UGI, or upper GI.

The purpose of the upper GI is to study radiographically the form and function of the distal esophagus, stomach, and duodenum, as well as to detect abnormal anatomic and functional conditions.

CONTRAINDICATIONS

Contraindications for upper GI examinations apply primarily to the type of contrast media used. If the patient has a history of bowel perforation, laceration, or viscus rupture, the use of barium sulfate may be contraindicated. An oral, water-soluble, iodinated contrast media may be used in place of barium sulfate.

Pathologic Indications for Upper GI Series

The more common pathologic indications for an upper GI series include the following:

Bezoar describes a mass of **undigested material** that becomes trapped in the stomach. This mass is usually made up of hair, certain vegetable fibers, or wood products. The material builds up over time and may form an obstruction in the stomach.

Specific terms for bezoars include the ***trichobezoar,*** made up of ingested hair, and the ***phytobezoar,*** which is ingested vegetable fiber or seeds.[*] Some patients are unable to break down or process certain vegetable fibers or seeds.

The upper GI demonstrates the bezoar. Radiographic appearances include a mass defined as a filling defect within the stomach. The bezoar retains a light coating of barium even after the stomach has emptied most of the barium (Fig. 14-64)

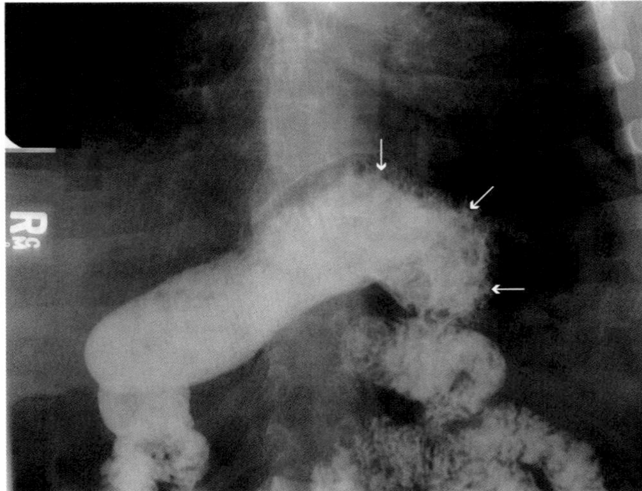

Fig. 14-64. AP axial projection—trichobezoar; very large.

Diverticula are weakenings and blind **outpouchings** of a portion of the mucosal wall. They can occur in the stomach or small intestine. Gastric diverticula generally range between 1 and 2 cm but may be as small as a few millimeters to 8 cm in diameter. Nearly 70% to 90% of gastric diverticula arise in the posterior aspect of the fundus. Consequently, the lateral position taken during an upper GI study may be the only projection to demonstrate gastric diverticula. Most gastric diverticula are asymptomatic and are discovered accidentally.

Although benign, diverticula can lead to perforation if untreated.[*] Other complications include inflammation and ulceration at the site of neoplasm formation. A double-contrast upper GI is recommended to diagnose any tumors or diverticula. An air-filled, barium-lined diverticulum of the duodenal bulb is shown in Fig. 14-65.

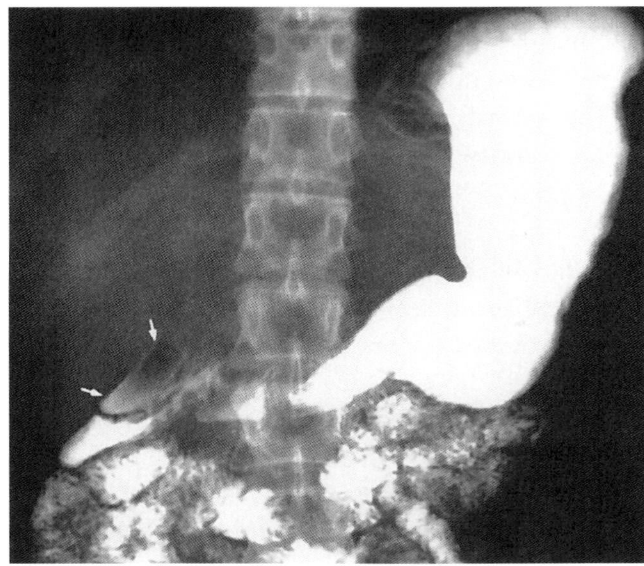

Fig. 14-65. PA projection—diverticulum in duodenum *(arrows).*

Emesis *(em'e-sis)* is the act of vomiting. Blood in vomit is called ***hematemesis,*** which may indicate other forms of pathologic processes present in the GI tract.

Gastric carcinomas comprise 70% of all stomach neoplasms. Radiographic signs include a large irregular filling defect within the stomach, marked or nodular edges of the stomach lining, rigidity of the stomach, and associated ulceration of the mucosa.

The double-contrast upper GI remains the gold standard for the detection of gastric carcinoma. CT and/or endoscopy may be performed to determine the degree of invasion of the tumor into tissues surrounding the stomach.

[*]Meschan I: Synopsis of analysis of roentgen signs in general radiology, Philadelphia, 1976, WB Saunders.

Gastritis is an inflammation of the lining or mucosa of the stomach. Gastritis may develop in response to various physiologic and environmental conditions. **Acute gastritis** presents severe symptoms of pain and discomfort. **Chronic gastritis** is an intermittent condition that may be brought on by changes in diet, stress, or other factors.

Gastritis is best demonstrated with a double-contrast upper GI. The fine coating of barium demonstrates subtle changes to the mucosal lining. Specific radiographic appearances may include, but are not restricted to, absence of rugae, thin gastric wall, and "speckled" appearance of the mucosa. Endoscopy may also be performed to visually inspect the mucosa for signs of gastritis.

Hiatal hernia is a condition in which a portion of the stomach herniates through the diaphragmatic opening. The herniation may be slight, but in severe cases a majority of the stomach is found within the thoracic cavity above the diaphragm.

Hiatal hernia may be due to a congenitally short esophagus or a weakening of the muscle that surrounds the diaphragmatic opening, allowing the passage of the esophagus.* This form of hiatal hernia may occur in the pediatric as well as the adult patient. An adult moderate-size hiatal hernia is shown in Fig. 14-67, in which a portion of the stomach containing air and barium is seen above the diaphragm.

Sliding hiatal hernia is a second type of hiatal hernia due to a weakening of a small muscle (esophageal sphincter) located between the terminal esophagus and the diaphragm. The purpose of the esophageal sphincter is to keep the cardiac portion of the stomach below the diaphragm and produce a high-pressure zone to prevent esophageal reflux. Because of aging or other factors, this sphincter may weaken and permit a portion of the stomach to herniate through the esophageal hiatus. Because the degree of herniation may vary from time to time, it is termed a ***sliding hiatal hernia.*** The condition is frequently present at birth, but symptoms of difficulty in swallowing usually don't begin until young adulthood.

Note: A sliding hiatal hernia may produce a radiographic sign termed ***Schatzki's ring,*** which is a ringlike constriction at the distal esophagus (Fig. 14-68).

*__Hypertrophic pyloric stenosis (HPS)__ is the most common type of gastric obstruction in infants. It is caused by hypertrophy of the antral muscle at the orifice of the pylorus. Hypertrophy of this muscle produces an obstruction at the pylorus. Symptoms of HPS include projectile vomiting following feedings, acute pain, and possible distention of the abdomen. HPS can be diagnosed during an upper GI. Often, HPS will present as distention of the stomach with a small channel (if any at all) of barium passing through the pylorus into the duodenum. Ultrasound has become the modality of choice in diagnosing HPS. Ultrasound can measure the diameter and length of the antral muscle to determine whether it is larger (hypertrophic) than normal. It is reported that a muscle thickness greater than 4 mm is a positive sign of HPS†. In addition, ultrasound does not require radiation exposure to the infant or use of contrast media.

*Meschan I: Synopsis of analysis of roentgen signs in general radiology, Philadelphia, 1976, WB Saunders.
†Ell R: Handbook of gastrointestinal and genitourinary radiology, St. Louis, 1992, Mosby.

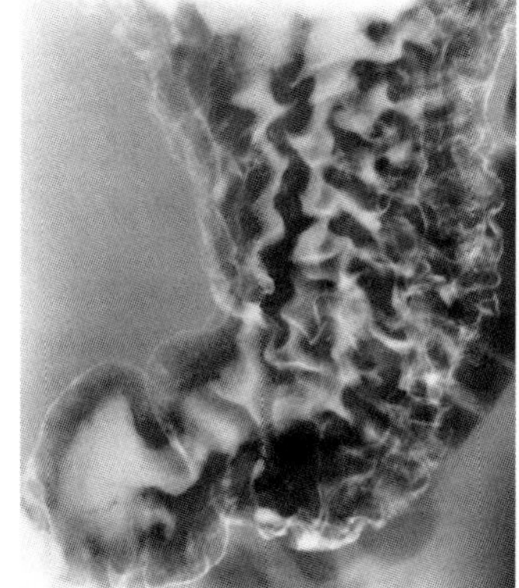

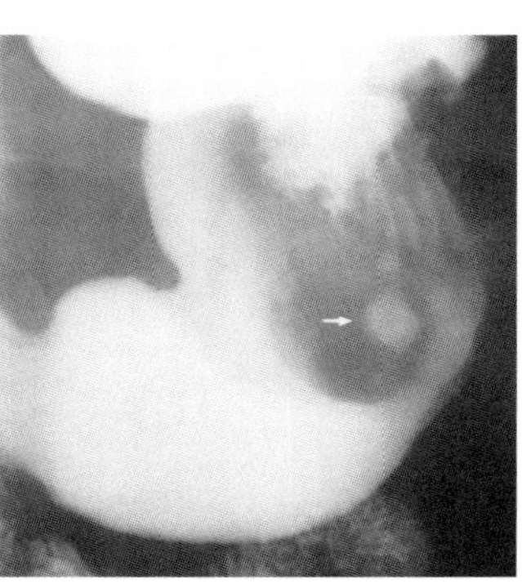

Fig. 14-66. Gastritis. **A,** In this example appearance includes thickening of rugal folds throughout stomach. **B,** Appearance includes some absence of rugal folds. (From Eisenberger RL, Johnson NM: Comprehensive radiographic pathology, ed 3, St. Louis, 2003, Mosby.)

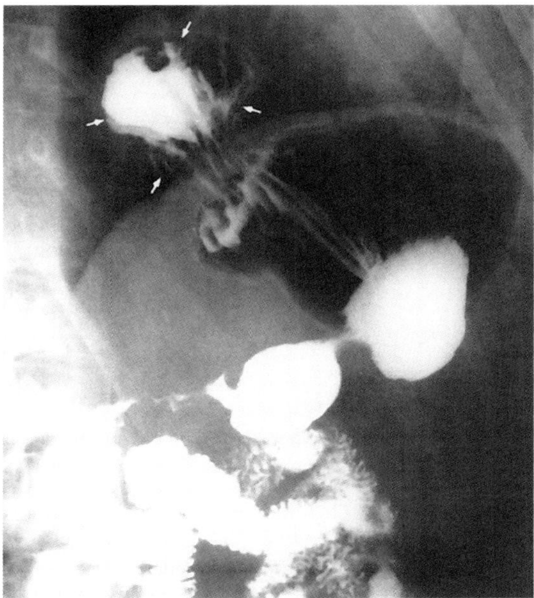

Fig. 14-67. Upper GI—demonstrating hiatal hernia *(arrows).*

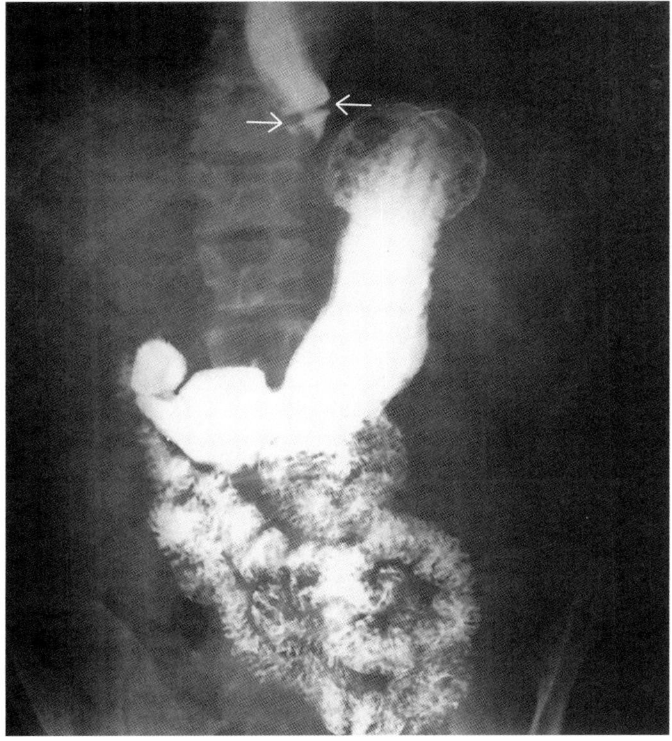

Fig. 14-68. Sliding hiatal hernia with Schatzki's ring *(arrows).*

14

Ulcers are erosions of the stomach or duodenal mucosa due to various physiologic or environmental conditions, such as excessive gastric secretions, stress, diet, and smoking. Some more recent studies suggest that ulcers may be caused by bacteria and thus can be treated with antibiotics. If untreated, the ulcer may lead to a perforation of the stomach or duodenum.

During an upper GI study, the ulcer appears as a punctate barium collection that may be surrounded by a "lucent-halo" appearance. A small peptic ulcer filled with barium is seen in Fig. 14-69. The double-contrast upper GI is recommended for most ulcer studies. It may be preceded or followed by endoscopy of the upper GI tract. Types of ulcers include the following:

- **Duodenal ulcer** is a peptic ulcer situated in the duodenum. These ulcers are frequently located in the second or third aspect of the duodenum. Duodenal ulcers are rarely malignant.*
- **Peptic ulcer** describes ulceration of the mucous membrane of the esophagus, stomach, or duodenum, caused by the action of the acid gastric juice. Therefore the term *peptic ulcer* can be synonymous with *gastric ulcer,* or *duodenal ulcer.* Peptic ulcer disease is often preceded by gastritis and is secondary to hyperacidity.
- **Gastric ulcer** is an ulcer of the gastric mucosa.
- **Perforating ulcer** is an ulcer that involves the entire thickness of the wall of the stomach or intestine, creating an opening on both surfaces. Only 5% of all ulcers lead to perforation.* If an ulcer does become perforated, it will create an opening between the intestine and the peritoneal cavity. Radiographic signs include the presence of free air under the diaphragm, as seen with an erect abdomen radiograph. If untreated, this ulcer may lead to peritonitis and eventual death.

*Ell R: Handbook of gastrointestinal and genitourinary radiology, St. Louis, 1992, Mosby.

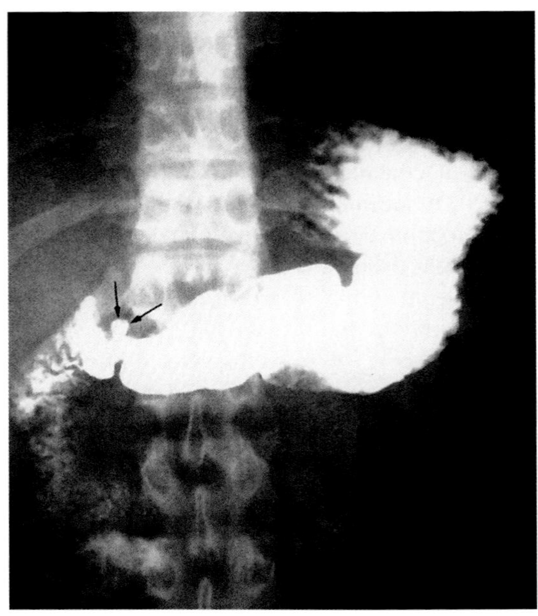

Fig. 14-69. PA projection—peptic ulcer *(arrows).*

UPPER GI SERIES—SUMMARY OF PATHOLOGIC INDICATIONS

CONDITION OR DISEASE	MOST COMMON RADIOGRAPHIC EXAM	POSSIBLE RADIOGRAPHIC APPEARANCE	MANUAL EXPOSURE FACTOR ADJUSTMENT*
Bezoar • Phytobezoar • Trichobezoar	Upper GI and/or endoscopy	Filling defect or ill-defined mass within stomach	None
Diverticula	Double-contrast upper GI	Outpouchings of the mucosal wall	None
Gastric carcinoma	Double-contrast upper GI	Irregular filling defect within stomach	None
Gastritis	Double-contrast upper GI	Absence of rugae, thin gastric wall, and "speckled" appearance of the mucosa	None
Hiatal hernia (sliding hiatal hernia)	Single- or double-contrast upper GI	Gastric bubble above diaphragm or Schatzki's ring	None
Hypertrophic pyloric stenosis (HPS)	Upper GI or ultrasound	Distention of stomach due to obstruction of pylorus	None
Ulcer	Double-contrast upper GI	Punctate collection of barium and "halo" sign	None

*Dependent on stage or severity of disease or condition.

PATIENT PREPARATION FOR UPPER GI SERIES

The goal of patient preparation for an upper GI series is for the patient to arrive in the radiology department with a completely empty stomach. For an examination scheduled in the morning hours, the patient should be **NPO** (*non per os,* meaning "nothing by mouth") from midnight until time of the examination. Food and fluids should be withheld for at least 8 hours prior to the exam. **The patient is also instructed not to smoke cigarettes or chew gum during the NPO period.** These activities tend to increase gastric secretions and salivation, which prevent proper coating of the barium to the gastric mucosa.

The upper GI series is often a time-consuming procedure, so the patient should be forewarned about the time the examination may take when the appointment is made. This time is especially true if the UGI is to be followed by a small bowel series. The importance of an empty stomach should also be stressed when the appointment is made so that the patient arrives properly prepared both physically and psychologically.

PREGNANCY PRECAUTIONS

If the patient is a female, then a menstrual history must be obtained. Irradiation of an early pregnancy is one of the most hazardous situations in diagnostic radiography.

X-ray examinations such as the upper GI series that include the pelvis and uterus in the primary beam and include fluoroscopy should only be done on pregnant females when absolutely necessary.

In general, abdominal radiographs of a known pregnancy should be delayed at least until the third trimester or, if patient's condition allows (as determined by the physician), until after the pregnancy. This waiting period is especially important if fluoroscopy, which greatly increases patient exposure, is involved.

ROOM PREPARATION AND FLUOROSCOPY PROCEDURE

Room setup for a UGI series is very similar to that for an esophagram. The thin barium sulfate mixture is the usual contrast medium necessary for an upper GI series. On occasion, thick barium may be used in addition to some type of gas-forming preparation. On rare occasions, water-soluble contrast media are used in preference to the barium sulfate mixture.

The fluoroscopy table is raised to the vertical position, although with some very ill patients the exam must be started with the table horizontal. Therefore the foot board should be placed at the end of the table. The room should be clean and tidy, and the control panel should be set up for fluoroscopy. If conventional fluoroscopy is being used, the spot-film mechanism and the photospot (105 mm) camera should be properly loaded and in working condition. All cassettes for the entire exam should be provided. Lead aprons, lead gloves, and the compression paddle should be provided for the radiologists, as well as lead aprons for all other personnel in the room.

Before introduction of the patient and the radiologist, the examination procedure should be carefully explained to the patient and the patient's history obtained.

General duties during fluoroscopy for an upper GI series are similar to those for an esophagram. The technologist should follow the radiologist's instructions, assist the patient as needed, and expedite the procedure in any manner possible.

The fluoroscopic routine followed by radiologists varies greatly but usually begins with the patient in the upright position. A wide variety of table and patient movements and special maneuvers follow until fluoroscopy is complete.

Patient Instructions

____ **I.V. CHOLANGIOGRAM AND/OR INTRAVENOUS PYELOGRAM**
1. Bowel Prep Kit III - 24 hour prep. All instructions are contained in kit.

____ **BARIUM ENEMA**
1. Bowel Prep Kit III - 24 hour prep. All instructions are contained in kit. May have a clear liquid breakfast.

____ **GALLBLADDER SERIES (ORAL CHOLECYSTOGRAM)**
1. Fat free supper evening before examination.
2. Take one iodinated contrast tablet every ½ hour starting at 2:00 p.m. day before exam.
3. Nothing by mouth after midnight.

____ **UPPER G.I. SERIES AND/OR SMALL BOWEL SERIES**
1. Do not eat, drink, smoke or chew gum after midnight. Any antispasmodic medication should be preferably discontinued at least 24 hours before exam. Bowel Prep Kit III may be purchased at most drug stores. Baptist Medical Center Pharmacy carries this kit along with Revco and Thrifty Drugs. Please call ahead to your pharmacy if you have any questions.

____ **ULTRASOUND PREPS:**
Ultrasound of the ABDOMEN: **Fat free clear** liquid diet from 6:00 p.m. the evening before examination.
Ultrasound of the PELVIS: **MUST** have a full bladder. Finish drinking 38 to 42 ounces of liquid one hour before exam. **DO NOT** empty bladder until after exam.

C.T. PREPS:
Abdomen - Clear liquids after midnight
Chest - Clear liquids only four hours prior to exam
Head - Clear liquids only four hours prior to exam
Pelvis - Clear liquids after midnight
Spine - no prep

Appointment date ____________ Appointment time ____________

Fig. 14-70. Sample patient instruction form. (Courtesy Phoenix Baptist Hospital and Medical Center, Phoenix, Ariz.)

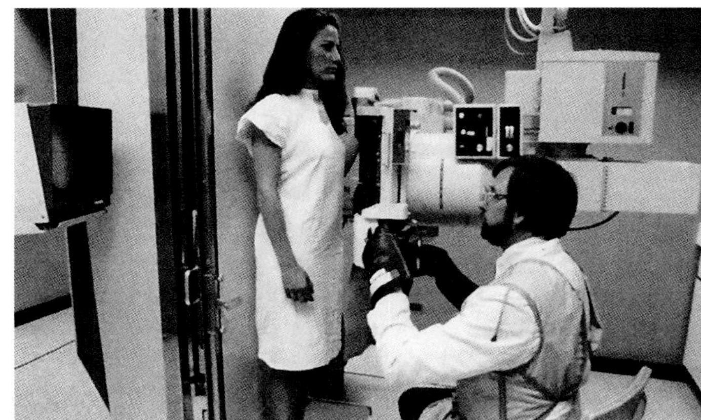

Fig. 14-71. Fluoroscopy of upper GI tract—digital fluoroscopy system. (Courtesy Philips Medical Systems.)

PATIENT AND TABLE MOVEMENTS

Various patient positions combined with table movements are made during the fluoroscopic procedure. The technologist must help the patient with the barium cup, provide a pillow when the patient is lying down, and keep the patient adequately covered at all times. The barium cup should be held by the patient in the left hand near the left shoulder whenever the patient is upright. The cup must be taken from the patient when the table is tilted up or down.

Part of the technologist's responsibility is to watch the patient's hands and fingers during table movements. Sometimes holding onto the edge of the table can result in pinched fingers. The radiologist is occupied watching the fluoroscopy screen or the monitor during these moves and doesn't see the patient's hands.

The right anterior oblique position, illustrated in Fig. 14-73, allows barium to migrate toward the pyloric portion or distal stomach, whereas any air in the stomach will shift toward the fundus.

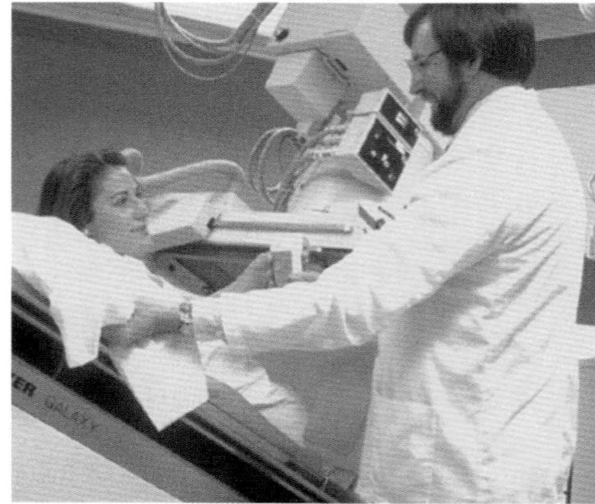

Fig. 14-72. Assisting patient with table movements.

POSTFLUOROSCOPY ROUTINES

After fluoroscopy, certain routine positions or projections may be obtained to further document any tentative diagnosis concluded fluoroscopically. These overhead radiographs, such as the RAO shown in Fig. 14-73, must be obtained immediately after fluoroscopy, before too much of the barium meal has passed into the jejunum.

With **digital fluoroscopy** the routine postfluoroscopy overhead radiographs may not be requested by the radiologist, as described earlier in this chapter.

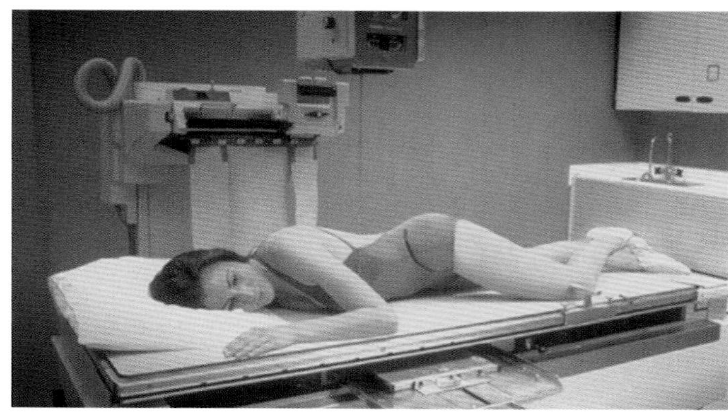

Fig. 14-73. Postfluoroscopy overhead RAO position.

PEDIATRIC APPLICATIONS

Refer to Chapter 20 for further details.

Pediatric Patient Preparation for Upper GI The following guidelines are suggested, but department protocol should be followed:

- Infant under 1 year: NPO for 4 hours
- Children older than 1 year: NPO for 6 hours

Barium Preparation Dilution of the barium may be required if the child will be fed through a bottle. A larger hole may be required in the nipple to ensure a smooth flow of barium. Following are some suggested barium volume guidelines, but specific department protocol should be followed:

- NB to 1 year: 2 to 4 oz.
- 1 to 3 years: 4 to 6 oz.
- 3 to 10 years: 6 to 12 oz.
- Older than 10 years: 12 to 16 oz.

Room Preparation Most upper GIs for pediatric patients are performed with the table in the horizontal position. Protective aprons must be provided for all persons in the fluoroscopy room. Individuals feeding or restraining the child during fluoroscopy should wear protective gloves and be instructed **not** to stand at the head or foot of the table, where the radiation exposure is the greatest.

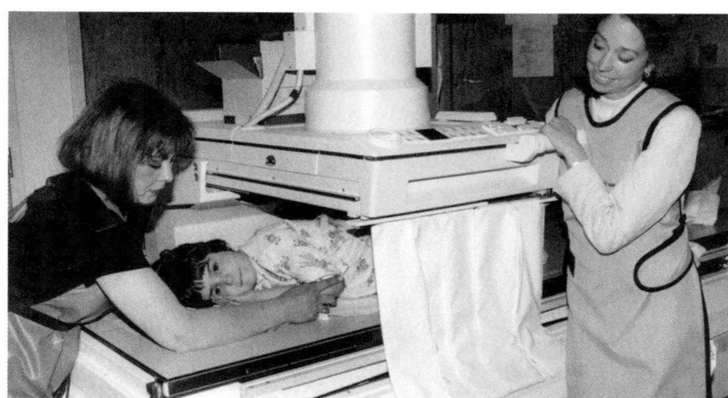

Fig. 14-74. Preparing a pediatric patient for GI fluoroscopy. Parent must step back before fluoroscopy begins.

GERIATRIC APPLICATIONS

The risk of dehydration during GI studies is a concern for geriatric patients, who may require additional attention and monitoring because of the normal patient preparation of withholding of fluids and ingestion of barium. The use of water-soluble contrast agents such as Gastrografin® may further increase the risk of dehydration. Geriatric patients should be scheduled for GI studies early in the morning to allow them to return to normal fluid intake and diet following the procedure.

Geriatric patients may require additional time and assistance in changing positions on the table because they frequently feel nervous and are afraid of falling off the exam table.

Some decrease in exposure factors also may be required for geriatric patients with lower tissue density or with asthenic-type body habitus.

SUMMARY OF POSITIONING TIPS FOR UPPER GI EXAMINATIONS

Clinical History

Obtain clinical history from the patient or chart to determine clinical indications for the study and any past or recent abdominal surgery of the GI tract. Surgery or resection of the bowel or stomach alters its normal position. Pay close attention to the fluoroscopy monitor to detect such differences, which may affect positioning and centering on the postfluoroscopy imaging.

Review the patient's chart to ensure that the correct procedure has been ordered. Also identify specific allergies and determine other pertinent information.

Body Habitus

Consider the body habitus of the patient. Remember that the stomach is high and transverse with the hypersthenic patient and low and vertical with the hyposthenic patient. The sthenic or average patient has the duodenum bulb near the L2 region. Usually, L2 is located 2.5 to 5 cm (1 to 2 inches) above the lower lateral rib cage margin. Centering points in this text are designed for the average sthenic patient.

Fluoroscopy

During fluoroscopy, identify the stomach on the fluoroscopy monitor. Pinpoint surrounding structures to gain clues about location of the stomach and duodenum. For example, if the body of the stomach is adjacent to the iliac wing, center lower than the average or sthenic patient.

High kV and Short Exposure Time

High kV of 100 to 125 is required to penetrate adequately and increase visibility of barium-filled structures. A kV below 100 will not provide visibility of the mucosa of the esophagus, stomach, or duodenum. Short exposure times are needed to control peristaltic motion. With double-contrast or water-soluble contrast GI studies, reduction of the kV to an 80 to 90 range is common with film-screen imaging to provide higher-contrast images without overpenetrating the anatomy (determine departmental kV preferences)

Digital Imaging Considerations

With the use of digital fluoroscopy, postfluoroscopy overhead projections are taken less frequently during the esophagram and upper GI procedures. If such projections are requested and computed radiography (CR) is used, the following technical considerations should be followed:

1. **Collimation:** To ensure that the image plate (IP) is read correctly by the image plate reader and a good diagnostic image is produced, **correct collimation is essential.** By eliminating extraneous tissue or signal from the IP, the laser reader is able to reproduce the analog image correctly without artifact. Because of the proximity of the spine, without accurate collimation the IR reader may use a bony rather than a soft-tissue algorithm to reconstruct the image. This may lead to certain soft-tissue structures and pathology being obscured during the image reconstruction process. Careful collimation to the organs being imaged will minimize this by improving the diagnostic quality of the final radiographic image.
2. **Accurate centering:** Most CR systems will scan the IP from the center outward. To reproduce the analog image correctly, **the anatomy must be properly centered.** Careful analysis of body habitus is crucial during an esophagram and upper GI procedure. Keep in mind how the position of the stomach will vary between a hypersthenic and asthenic patient. If the stomach is not centered to the IP, the laser reader will not reproduce it correctly. It is important to ensure the **central ray, body part,** and **IP are aligned** for correct centering of the anatomy of interest.
3. **Exposure factors:** With CR systems, a minimum kV and mAs must be used to create an acceptable image. Inadequate kV or mAs will produce a "mottled" image; however the technologist must not increase mAs needlessly, because this will increase patient dose. Departments should have established technical charts to ensure that adequate kV and mAs are used for these procedures. Once images have been produced, the exposure index values should be verified to determine whether they are within the acceptable range to ensure that sufficient exposure factors were used without overexposing the patient needlessly.

Alternative Modalities and Procedures

COMPUTED TOMOGRAPHY

Computed tomography (CT) is an excellent modality used to demonstrate tumors of the GI tract, as well as the liver, spleen, and pancreas. With the use of diluted oral contrast media, CT can demonstrate diverticula, hiatal hernia, and bowel perforation.

CT has become the modality of choice to demonstrate trauma and tumors of the GI tract and accessory organs.

MAGNETIC RESONANCE IMAGING

Tumor and vascular disease of the liver and esophageal varices are demonstrated with magnetic resonance imaging (MRI) by use of a flow-sensitive, short flip angle pulse sequence.

Hemochromatosis, or iron overload, which can occur with patients undergoing multiple blood transfusions or may be due to a genetic condition, is well visualized with MRI. This condition leads to an abnormal amount of iron being deposited within the liver parenchyma. Excessive iron deposited in tissue produces a strong signal in MR images.

SONOGRAPHY

Intraesophageal sonography for esophageal varices and carcinoma of the esophagus is becoming an alternative to the esophagram. By passing a small transducer into the esophagus, detailed images of the inner mucosa layer can be acquired. Small varices and polyps of the esophagus and upper stomach can be evaluated. As stated earlier, sonography has become an effective diagnostic tool for hypertrophic pyloric stenosis in infants.

Doppler ultrasound can be used to detect vascular flow to specific accessory organs in the GI tract.

NUCLEAR MEDICINE

The use of specific radionuclides demonstrates cirrhosis of the liver, splenic tumors, GI bleeding, and gastric emptying studies. Gastric emptying studies are performed to determine the rate of emptying of food from the stomach.

Also, esophageal reflux can be diagnosed by addition of a radionuclide to a drink, such as milk. With a compression band placed along the upper abdomen, the nuclear medicine camera can measure any return of gastric contents through the esophagogastric junction. Nuclear medicine is also very effective in demonstrating Barrett's esophagus.

RADIOGRAPHIC POSITIONING

Survey Information

A 2000 survey of the operating procedures (department routines) was conducted throughout the United States and Canada. The information on the right was compiled from the survey, indicating the norm for basic projections for esophagrams and upper GI exams. The survey results were very consistent throughout all regions of the United States but did show significant differences between the U.S. and Canada. The most obvious difference was the exclusion of postfluoroscopy overhead imaging when digital fluoroscopy was used in the U.S. (40%) compared with Canada (72%).

The **double-contrast technique** for the upper GI is a common procedure, as indicated on the U.S. survey conducted in 1989 (62%). This question was not included in the 1995 and 2000 surveys, but the results are presumed to be similar or even higher. Generally the double-contrast positioning routines are similar to the regular single-contrast upper GI, with the only difference being the lower kV exposure techniques, as described.

Basic and Special Postfluoroscopy Projections

Certain **basic** and **special** positions or projections of the esophagus, stomach, and duodenum are described and demonstrated on the following pages.

The three basic postfluoroscopy projections for the **esophagram** are described in the following positioning section, along with the one special oblique position.

The five projections for the **upper GI series** are listed in order of suggested clinical usefulness when postfluoroscopy overhead projections are requested. As the above survey indicates, with the increased use of digital fluoroscopy, these postfluoroscopy overhead projections are not as common as in the past, but technologists should be able to perform them when requested.

ESOPHAGRAM ROUTINE

	U.S. Average			Canada
	Basic			Basic
	2000	1995	1989	2000
Esophagus				
RAO	91%	87%	88%	39%
Left lateral	70%	65%	55%	42%
AP	58%	59%	48%	45%
PA	29%	32%	30%	12%
LAO	46%	44%	–	24%

UPPER GI ROUTINE

	U.S. Average			Canada
	Basic			Basic
	2000	1995	1989	2000
Stomach and Duodenum				
AP scout (supine)	66%	54%	–	11%
RAO (recumbent)	90%	89%	93%	28%
PA (recumbent)	81%	79%	85%	22%
Right lateral (recumbent)	82%	82%	80%	23%
LPO (recumbent)	52%	59%	55%	24%
AP (recumbent)	56%	63%	50%	26%
Double-contrast techniques	–	–	62%	–
Digital fluoroscopy; no overheads	40%	–	–	72%

RAO POSITION: ESOPHAGRAM

Pathology Demonstrated

Strictures, foreign bodies, anatomic anomalies, and neoplasms of the esophagus are shown.

Esophagram
BASIC
• RAO (35° to 40°)
• Lateral
• AP (PA)

Technical Factors

- IR size—35 × 43 cm (14 × 17 inches), lengthwise
- Moving or stationary grid
- 100-110 kV range
- Technique and dose:

cm	kV	mAs	Sk.	ML.	Gon.
22	110	3	79	18	M <0.01 F 0.1

mrad

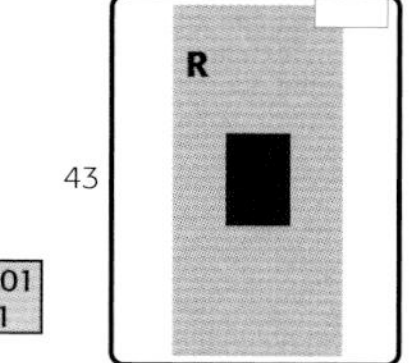

Shielding Place lead shield over patient's pelvic region to protect gonads.

Patient Position Position patient recumbent or erect. Recumbent is preferred because of more complete filling of the esophagus (due to the gravity factor with the erect position).

Part Position

- Rotate **35° to 40°** from a prone position, with the right anterior body against IR or table.
- Place right arm down and left arm flexed at elbow and up by the patient's head, holding cup of barium, with a straw in patient's mouth.
- Flex left knee for support.
- Align midline of thorax in the oblique position to midline of IR and/or table.
- Place top of IR about 2 inches (5 cm) above level of shoulders to place center of IR at CR.

Central Ray

- CR **perpendicular** to IR
- CR to center of cassette at **level of T5 or T6** (2 to 3 inches, or 5 to 7.5 cm, inferior to jugular notch)
- Minimum SID of 40 inches (100 cm) or 72 inches (180 cm) if patient is erect

Collimation Collimate the lateral borders to create two-sided collimation about 5 or 6 inches (12 to 15 cm) wide. Collimate end borders to IR margins, with L or R placed within collimation field.

Respiration Suspend respiration and expose on expiration (see Notes).

Note 1: Thick barium—Two or three spoonfuls of thick barium should be ingested and the exposure made immediately after last bolus is swallowed. (Patient generally does not breathe immediately after a swallow.)

Note 2: Thin barium—For complete filling of the esophagus with thin barium, the patient may need to drink through a straw, with continuous swallowing and exposure made after three or four swallows without suspending respiration (using as short an exposure time as possible).

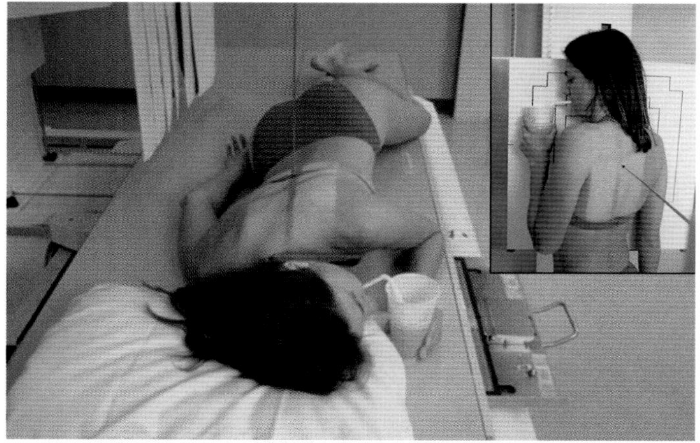

Fig. 14-75. 35° to 40° RAO—recumbent or erect.

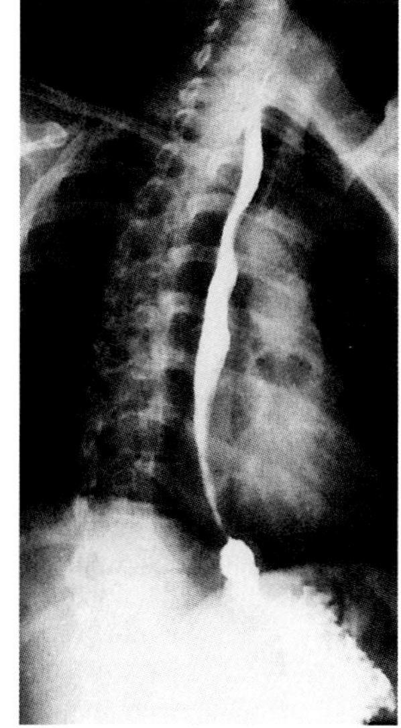

Fig. 14-76. RAO.

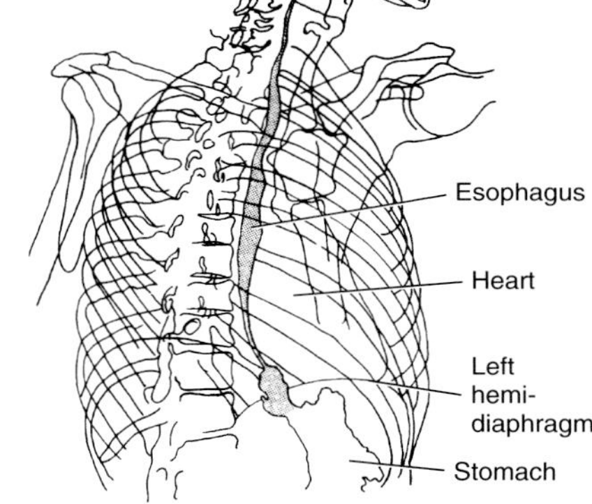

Fig. 14-77. RAO.

14

Radiographic Criteria

Structures Shown: • Esophagus should be visible between the vertebral column and heart. (RAO provides more visibility of pertinent anatomy between vertebrae and heart than does the LAO.)

Position: • Adequate rotation of body projects esophagus between vertebral column and heart. If esophagus is situated over the spine, more rotation of the body is required. • Entire esophagus is filled or lined with contrast media. • Upper limbs should not superimpose the esophagus.

Collimation and CR: • Collimation margins are seen laterally on radiograph. • CR is centered at level of T5 or T6 to include the entire esophagus.

Exposure Criteria: • Appropriate technique is used to clearly visualize borders of the contrast media–filled esophagus; sharp structural margins indicate no motion.

LATERAL POSITION: ESOPHAGRAM

Esophagram
BASIC
- RAO (35° to 40°)
- **Lateral**
- AP (PA)

Pathology Demonstrated

Strictures, foreign bodies, anatomic anomalies, and neoplasms of the esophagus are shown.

Technical Factors

- IR size—35 × 43 cm (14 × 17 inches), lengthwise
- Moving or stationary grid
- 100-110 kV range
- Technique and dose:

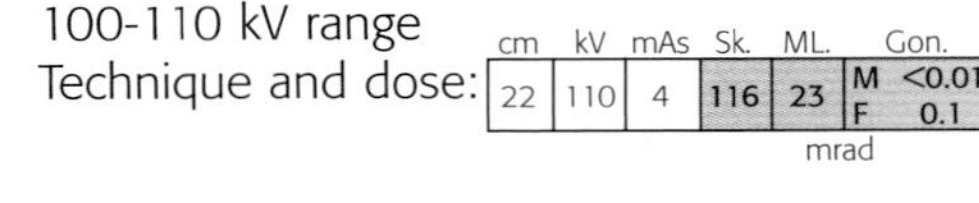

cm	kV	mAs	Sk.	ML.	Gon.
22	110	4	116	23	M <0.01 F 0.1

mrad

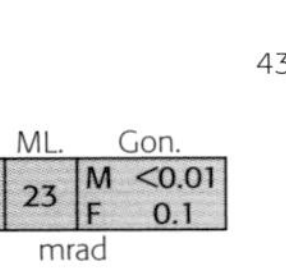

Shielding Position lead shield over gonadal area.

Patient Position Position patient recumbent or erect (recumbent preferred).

Part Position

- Place patient's arms over the head, with the elbows flexed and superimposed.
- Align **midcoronal plane to midline** of IR and/or table.
- Place shoulders and hips in a true lateral position.
- Place top of IR about 2 inches (5 cm) above level of shoulders, to place center of IR at CR.

Central Ray

- CR **perpendicular** to IR
- CR to **level of T5 or T6** (2 to 3 inches, or 5 to 7.5 cm, inferior to jugular notch)
- Minimum SID of 40 inches (100 cm) or 72 inches (180 cm) if erect

Collimation Collimate along the lateral borders to create two-sided collimation about 5 or 6 inches (12 to 15 cm) wide.

Respiration Suspend respiration and expose on expiration.

Note: See preceding page for barium swallow instructions.

Optional swimmer's lateral position (Fig. 14-79) allows for better demonstration of the upper esophagus without superimposition of arms and shoulders.

Position hips and shoulders in true lateral position; then separate shoulders from esophageal region by placing upside shoulder down and back, with arm behind back. Place downside shoulder and arm up and in front to hold cup of barium.

Radiographic Criteria

Structures Shown: • Entire esophagus is seen between thoracic spine and heart.

Position: • True lateral is indicated by direct superimposition of posterior ribs. • The patient's arms should not superimpose the esophagus. • Entire esophagus is filled or lined with contrast media.

Collimation and CR: • Collimation margins are seen laterally on radiograph. • CR is centered at level of T5 or T6 to include the entire esophagus.

Exposure Criteria: • Appropriate technique is used to clearly visualize borders of the contrast media–filled esophagus. • Sharp structural margins indicate no motion.

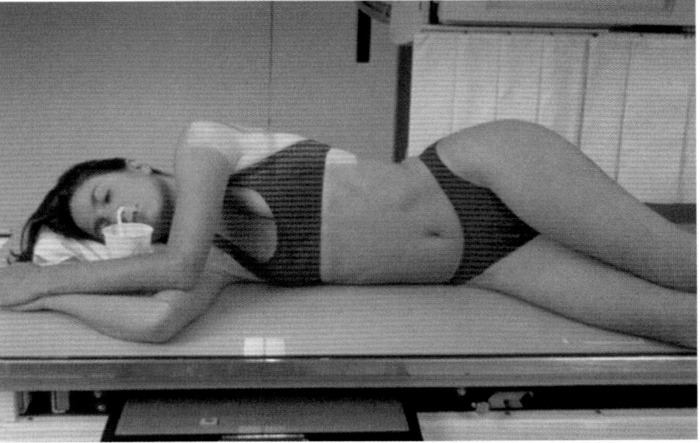

Fig. 14-78. Right lateral—arms up.

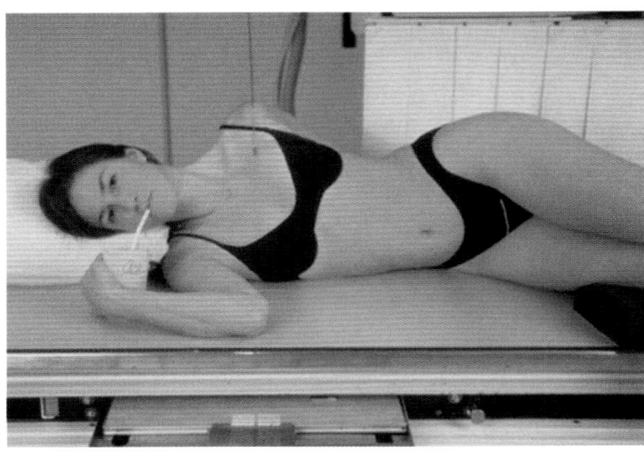

Fig. 14-79. Optional—swimmer's lateral for better visualization of upper esophagus.

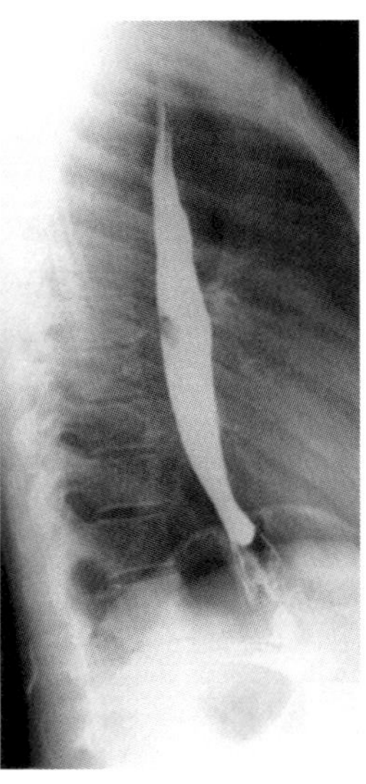

Fig. 14-80. Lateral—arms up.

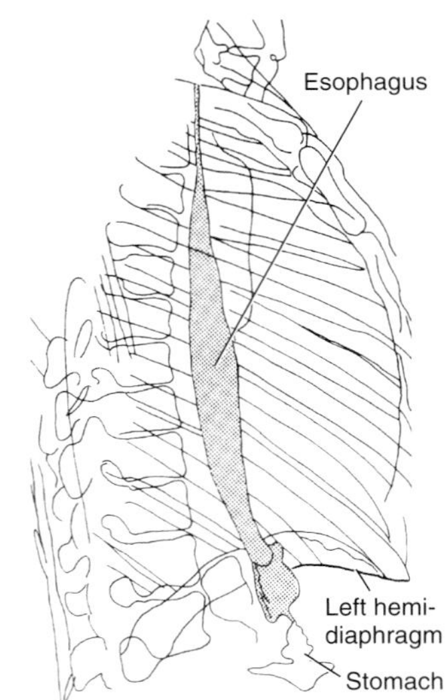

Fig. 14-81. Lateral.

14

AP (PA) PROJECTION: ESOPHAGRAM

Esophagram
BASIC
- RAO (35° to 40°)
- Lateral
- AP (PA)

Pathology Demonstrated

Strictures, foreign bodies, anatomic anomalies, and neoplasms of the esophagus are shown.

This projection may not be as diagnostic as the RAO or lateral positions.

Technical Factors

- IR size—35 × 43 cm (14 × 17 inches), lengthwise
- Moving or stationary grid
- 100-110 kV range
- Technique and dose:

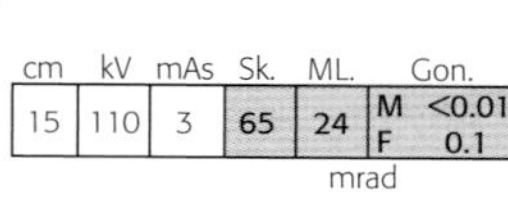

cm	kV	mAs	Sk.	ML.	Gon.
15	110	3	65	24	M <0.01 F 0.1

mrad

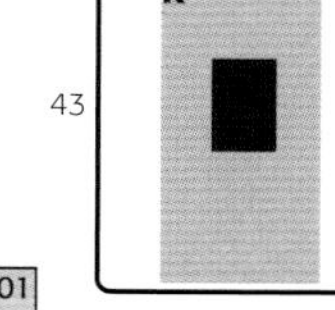

Shielding Place lead shield over patient's pelvic region to shield gonads.

Patient Position Position patient recumbent or erect (recumbent preferred).

Part Position

- Align **midsagittal plane to midline** of IR and/or table.
- Ensure that shoulders and hips are **not rotated.**
- Place right arm up to hold cup of barium.
- Place top of IR about 2 inches (5 cm) above top of shoulder, to place CR at center of IR.

Central Ray

- CR **perpendicular** to IR
- CR to midsagittal plane, **1 inch** (2.5 cm) **inferior to sternal angle** (T5-6) or approximately 3 inches (7.5 cm) inferior to jugular notch
- Minimum SID of 40 inches (100 cm) or 72 inches (183 cm) if erect

Collimation Use tight side collimation to result in a collimation field that is about 5 or 6 inches (12 to 15 cm) wide. Collimate end borders to IR margins.

Respiration Suspend respiration and expose on expiration.

Alternative PA: This image can also be taken as a PA projection with similar positioning, centering, and CR locations.

Notes: Two or three spoonfuls of thick barium should be ingested and the exposure made immediately after the last bolus is swallowed. (Patient generally does not breathe immediately after a swallow.)

For complete filling of the esophagus with thin barium, the patient may need to drink through a straw, with continuous swallowing and exposure made after three or four swallows without suspending respiration.

Radiographic Criteria

Structures Shown: • The entire esophagus is filled with barium.

Position: • No rotation of the patient's body is evidenced by the symmetry of the sternoclavicular (SC) joints.

Collimation and CR: • Collimation margins are seen laterally on radiograph. • CR is centered at level of T5 or T6 to include the entire esophagus.

Exposure Criteria: • Appropriate technique is used to visualize the esophagus through the superimposed thoracic vertebrae. • Sharp structural margins indicate no motion.

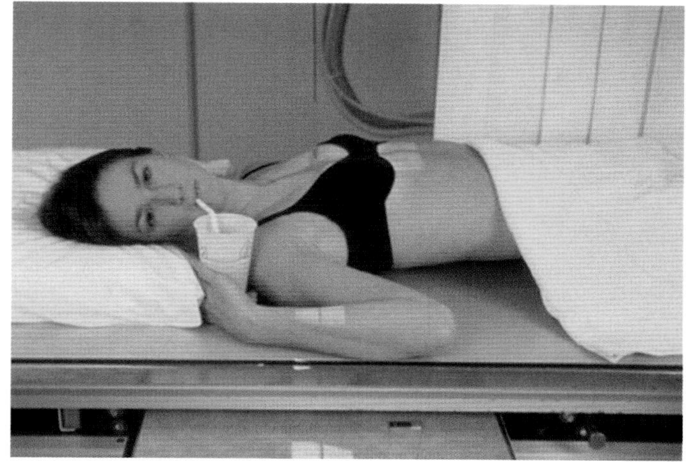

Fig. 14-82. Recumbent AP projection.

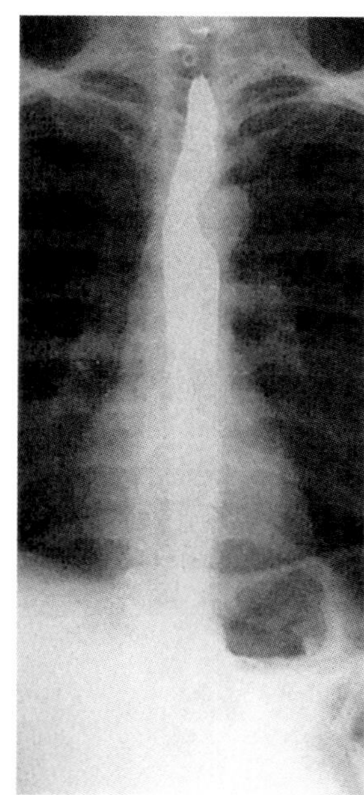

Fig. 14-83. AP projection.

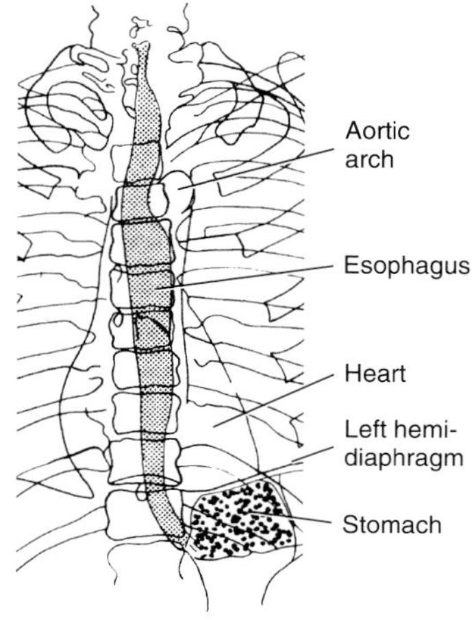

Fig. 14-84. AP projection.

14

LAO POSITION: ESOPHAGRAM

Esophagram
SPECIAL
• LAO

Pathology Demonstrated
Strictures, foreign bodies, anatomic anomalies, and neoplasms of the esophagus are shown.

Technical Factors
- IR size—35 × 43 cm (14 × 17 inches), lengthwise
- Moving or stationary grid
- 100-110 kV range
- Technique and dose:

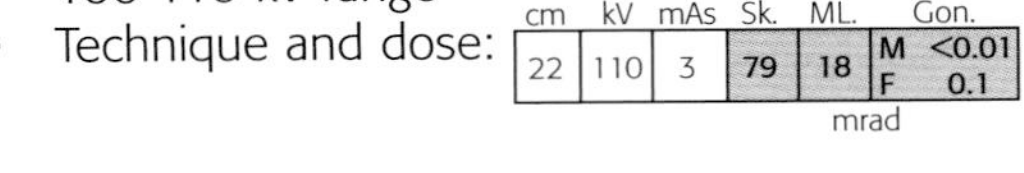

cm	kV	mAs	Sk.	ML.	Gon.
22	110	3	79	18	M <0.01 F 0.1

mrad

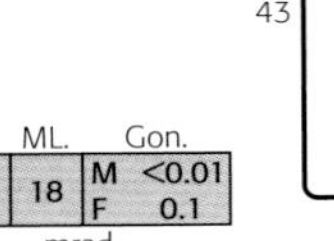

Shielding Place lead shield over gonadal area.

Patient Position Position patient recumbent or erect (recumbent preferred).

Part Position
- Rotate **35° to 40°** from a PA, with the left anterior body against IR or table.
- Place left arm down by the patient's side, right arm flexed at elbow and up by the patient's head.
- Flex right knee for support.
- Place top of cassette about 2 inches (5 cm) above level of shoulders, to place CR at center of IR.

Central Ray
- CR **perpendicular** to IR
- CR to level of **T5** or **T6** (2 to 3 inches, or 5 to 7.5 cm, inferior to jugular notch)
- Minimum SID of 40 inches (100 cm) or 72 inches (180 cm) if erect

Collimation Collimate lateral borders to create two-sided collimation about 5 or 6 inches (12 to 15 cm) wide. Collimate end borders to IR margins.

Respiration Suspend respiration and expose on expiration.

Note 1: Thick barium—Two or three spoonfuls of thick barium should be ingested and the exposure made immediately after last bolus is swallowed. (Patient generally does not breathe immediately after a swallow.)

Note 2: Thin barium—For complete filling of the esophagus with thin barium, the patient may need to drink through a straw, with continuous swallowing and exposure made after three or four swallows without suspending respiration (using as short an exposure time as possible).

14

Radiographic Criteria

Structures Shown: • Esophagus is seen between hilar region of lungs and thoracic spine. • The entire esophagus is filled with contrast medium.

Position: • The patient's upper limbs should not superimpose the esophagus.

Collimation and CR: • Collimation margins are seen laterally on radiograph. • CR is centered at level of T5 or T6 to include the entire esophagus.

Exposure Criteria: • Appropriate technique is used to clearly visualize borders of the contrast media–filled esophagus through the heart shadow. • Sharp structural margins indicate no motion.

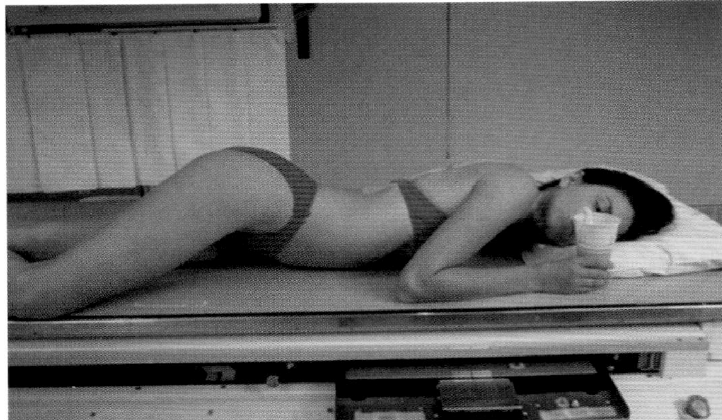

Fig. 14-85. Recumbent LAO position.

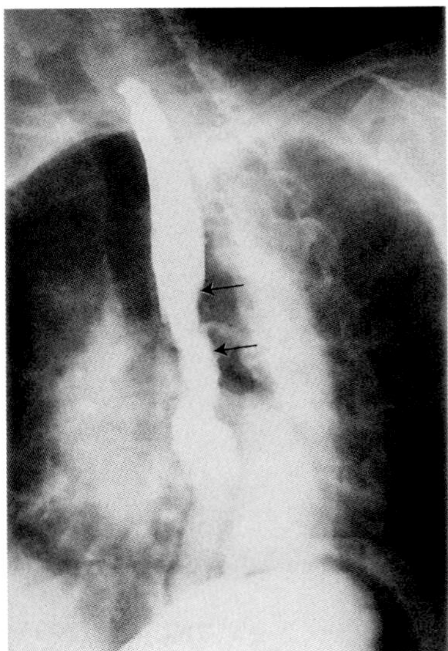

Fig. 14-86. LAO—demonstrating a constricted area of esophagus, probably carcinoma *(arrows)*.

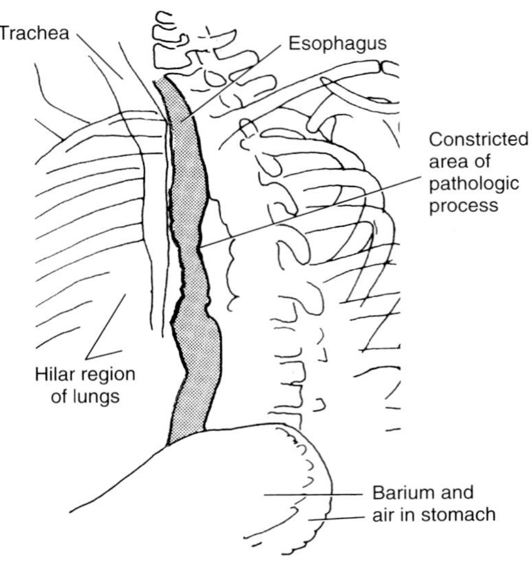

Fig. 14-87. LAO position.

RAO POSITION: UPPER GI SERIES

Upper GI Series
BASIC
- RAO
- PA
- Right lateral
- LPO
- AP

Pathology Demonstrated

This is the ideal position to demonstrate polyps and ulcers of the pylorus, duodenal bulb, and C-loop of the duodenum.

Technical Factors

- IR size—24 × 30 cm (10 × 12 inches), lengthwise or—30 × 35 cm (11 × 14 inches)
- Moving or stationary grid
- 100-110 kV range (80-90 kV for double-contrast study)
- Technique and dose:

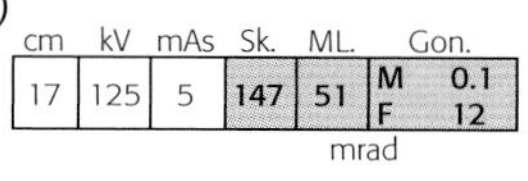
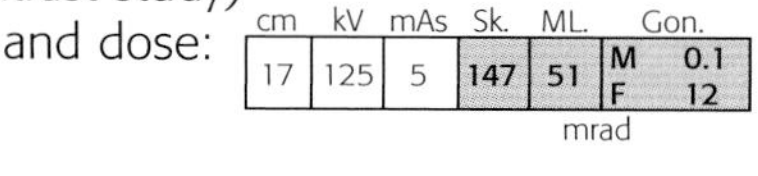

cm	kV	mAs	Sk.	ML.	Gon.
17	125	5	147	51	M 0.1 F 12

mrad

24 (30)

30 (35)

R

Shielding Place lead shield over patient's pelvic region to protect gonads **without covering pertinent anatomy.**

Patient Position Position patient recumbent, with the body partially rotated into an RAO position; provide pillow for head.

Part Position

- From a prone position, rotate **40° to 70°**, with right anterior body against IR or table (more rotation sometimes required for heavy hypersthenic-type patients and less for thin asthenic types).
- Place right arm down and left arm flexed at elbow and up by the patient's head.
- Flex left knee for support.

Central Ray

- Direct CR **perpendicular** to IR.
- *Sthenic type:* Center CR and IR to duodenal bulb at **level of L1** (1 to 2 inches, or 2.5 to 5 cm, above lower lateral rib margin), **midway between spine and upside lateral border of abdomen,** 45° to 55° oblique.
- *Asthenic:* Center about 2 inches (5 cm) below level of L1, 40° oblique.
- *Hypersthenic:* Center about 2 inches (5 cm) above level of L1 and nearer midline, 70° oblique.
- Center cassette to CR.
- Minimum SID is 40 inches (100 cm).

Collimation Collimate on four sides to outer margins of IR or to area of interest on larger IR.

Respiration Suspend respiration and expose on expiration.

Radiographic Criteria

Structures Shown: • Entire stomach and C-loop of duodenum are visible.

Position: • Duodenal bulb is in profile.

Collimation and CR: • Collimation is seen along the four margins of the radiograph. • CR is centered to level of L1, with body of stomach and C-loop centered on radiograph.

Exposure Criteria: • Appropriate technique is used to clearly visualize the gastric folds without overexposing other pertinent anatomy. • Sharp structural margins indicate no motion.

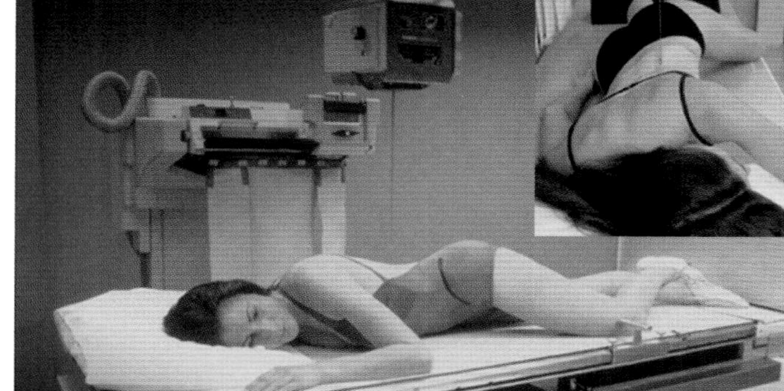

Fig. 14-88. RAO position.

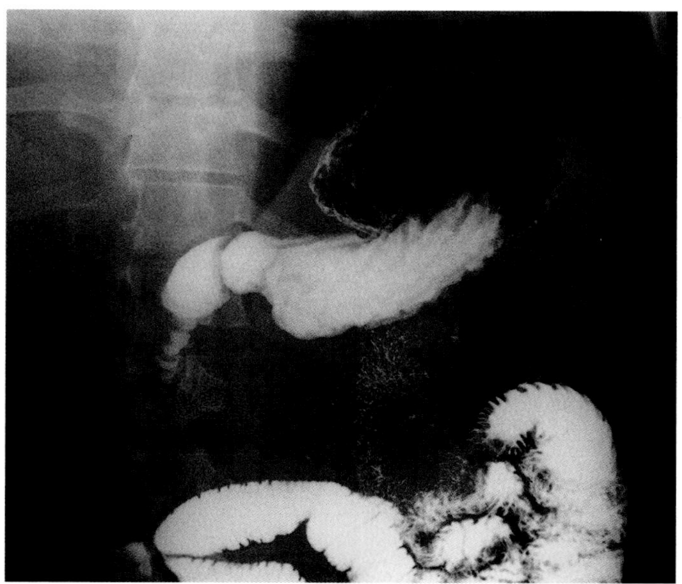

Fig. 14-89. RAO position.

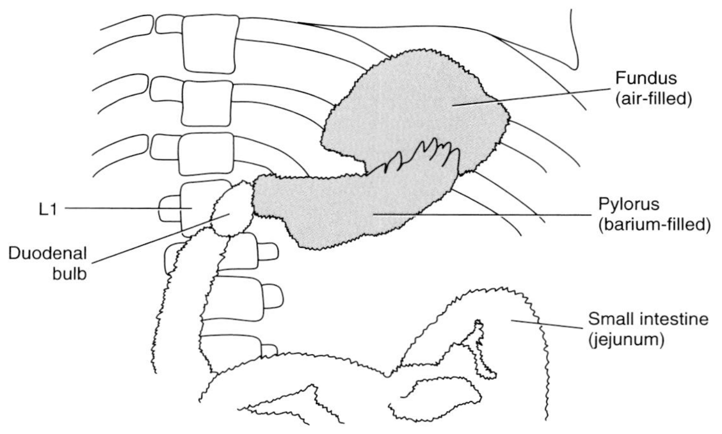

Fig. 14-90. RAO.

14

PA PROJECTION: UPPER GI SERIES

Upper GI Series
BASIC
- RAO
- PA
- Right lateral
- LPO
- AP

Pathology Demonstrated
Polyps, diverticula, bezoars, and signs of gastritis in the body and pylorus of the stomach are shown.

Technical Factors
- Film size—24 × 30 cm (10 × 12 inches), lengthwise
  or—30 × 35 cm (11 × 14 inches)
  or—35 × 43 cm (14 × 17 inches) if small bowel is to be included
- Moving or stationary grid
- 100 to 110 kV range (80-90 kV range for double-contrast study)
- Technique and dose:

cm	kV	mAs	Sk.	ML.	Gon.
18	125	4	113	38	M 0.1 F 9

mrad

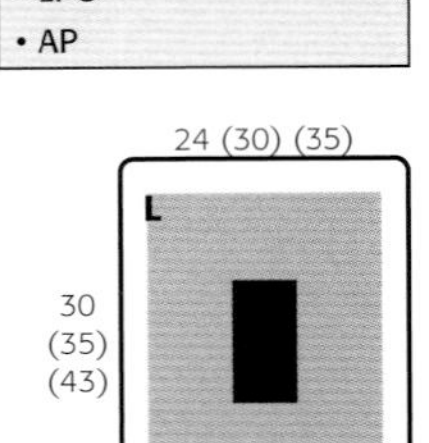

Shielding Place lead shield over patient's pelvic region to protect gonads **without covering pertinent anatomy.**

Patient Position Position patient prone, with arms up beside head; provide pillow.

Part Position
- Align midsagittal plane to CR and to table.
- Ensure that the **body is not rotated.**

Central Ray
- Direct CR **perpendicular** to IR.
- ***Sthenic type:*** Center CR and IR to level of pylorus and duodenal bulb at **level of L1** (1 to 2 inches, or 2.5 to 5 cm, above lower lateral rib margin) and about **1 inch (2.5 cm) left of the vertebral column.**
- *Asthenic:* Center about 5 cm or 2 inches below level of L1.
- *Hypersthenic:* Center about 5 cm or 2 inches above level of L1 and nearer midline.
- Center cassette to CR.
- Minimum SID is 40 inches (100 cm).

Collimation Collimate on four sides to outer margins of IR or to area of interest on a larger IR.

Respiration Suspend respiration and expose on expiration.

Alternate PA axial: The position of the high transverse stomach on a **hypersthenic**-type patient causes almost an end-on view, with much overlapping of the pyloric region of the stomach and the duodenal bulb with a 90∞ PA projection. Therefore a **35° to 45° cephalic angle** of the central ray separates these areas for better visualization. The greater and lesser curvatures of the stomach are also better visualized in profile.

For **infants** a **20° to 25° cephalic CR angle** is recommended to open the body and pylorus of stomach.

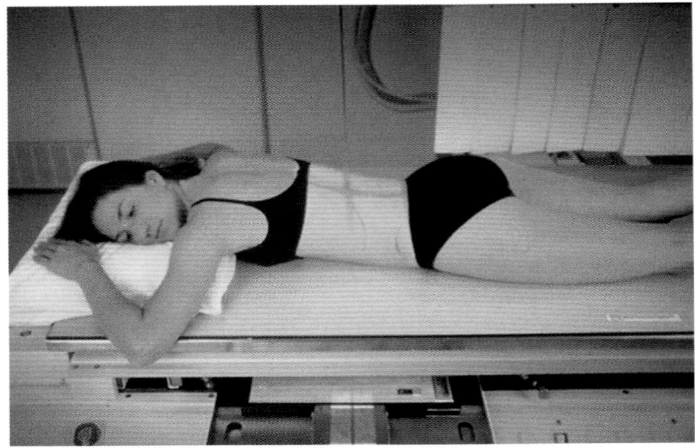

Fig. 14-91. PA projection.

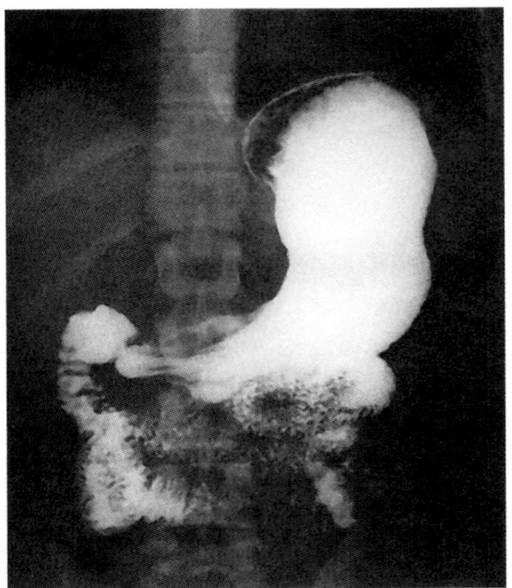

Fig. 14-92. PA projection.

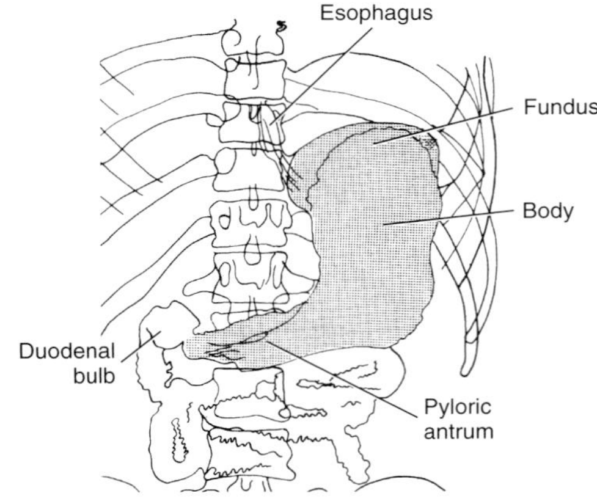

Fig. 14-93. PA projection.

Radiographic Criteria

Structures Shown: • Entire stomach and duodenum are visible.

Position: • Body and pylorus of the stomach are barium filled.

Collimation and CR: • Collimation is seen along the four margins of the radiograph. • CR is centered to level of L2, with body and pylorus of stomach and C-loop centered on radiograph.

Exposure Criteria: • Appropriate technique is used to visualize the gastric folds without overexposing other pertinent anatomy; sharp structural margins indicate no motion.

RIGHT LATERAL POSITION: UPPER GI SERIES

Upper GI Series
BASIC
- RAO
- PA
- Right lateral
- LPO
- AP

Pathology Demonstrated
Pathologic processes of the **retrogastric space** (space behind the stomach) are shown. Diverticula, tumors, gastric ulcers, and trauma to the stomach may be demonstrated along the posterior margin of the stomach.

Technical Factors
- IR size—24 × 30 cm (10 × 12 inches), lengthwise
  or—30 × 35 cm (11 × 14 inches)
- 110 to 125 kV range (85-95 kV range for double-contrast study)
- Technique and dose:

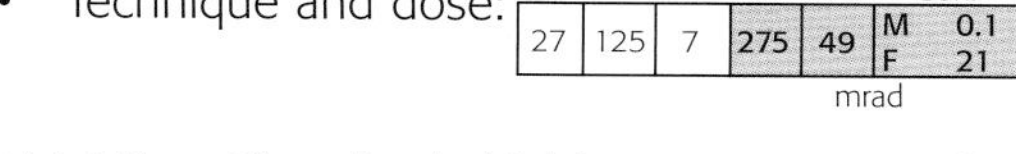

cm	kV	mAs	Sk.	ML.	Gon.
27	125	7	275	49	M 0.1 F 21

mrad

24 (30)
R
30 (35)

Shielding Place lead shield over patient's pelvic region to protect gonads **without covering pertinent anatomy.**

Patient Position Position patient recumbent in a right-lateral position. Provide pillow for head. Place arms up by the patient's head and flex knees.

Part Position
- Ensure that shoulders and hips are in a true lateral position.
- Center IR at CR (bottom of cassette about at level of iliac crest).

Central Ray
- Direct CR **perpendicular** to IR.
- *Sthenic type:* Center CR and IR to duodenal bulb at level of **L1** (level of lower lateral margin of the ribs) and **1 to 1½ inches (2.5 to 4 cm) anterior to midcoronal plane** (near midway between anterior border of vertebrae and the anterior abdomen).
- *Hypersthenic:* Center about 2 inches (5 cm) above L1.
- *Asthenic:* Center about 2 inches (5 cm) lower below L1.
- Minimum SID is 40 inches (100 cm).

Collimation Collimate on four sides to outer margins of IR or to area of interest on larger IR.

Respiration Suspend respiration and expose on expiration.

Note: Stomach generally is located about one vertebra higher in this position than in PA or oblique positions.

Radiographic Criteria
Structures Shown: • Entire stomach and duodenum are visible. • **Retrogastric space** is demonstrated. • Pylorus of stomach and C-loop of duodenum should be visualized well on hypersthenic-type patients.

Position: • **No rotation** should be present; vertebral bodies should be seen for reference purposes. The intervertebral foramen should be open, indicating a true lateral position.

Collimation and CR: • Collimation is seen along the four margins of the radiograph. • CR is centered at level to duodenal bulb at level of L1.

Exposure Criteria: • Appropriate technique is used to visualize the gastric folds without overexposing other pertinent anatomy; sharp structural margins indicate no motion.

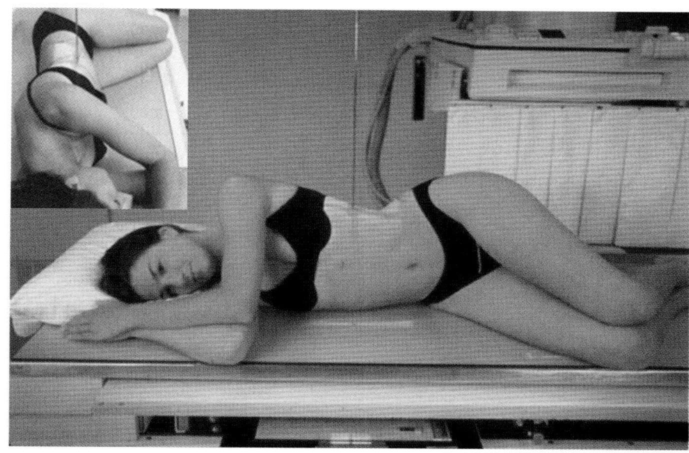

Fig. 14-94. Right lateral position.

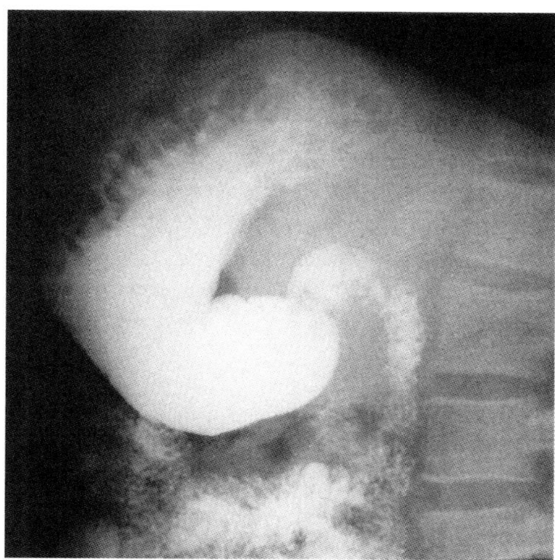

Fig. 14-95. Right lateral position.

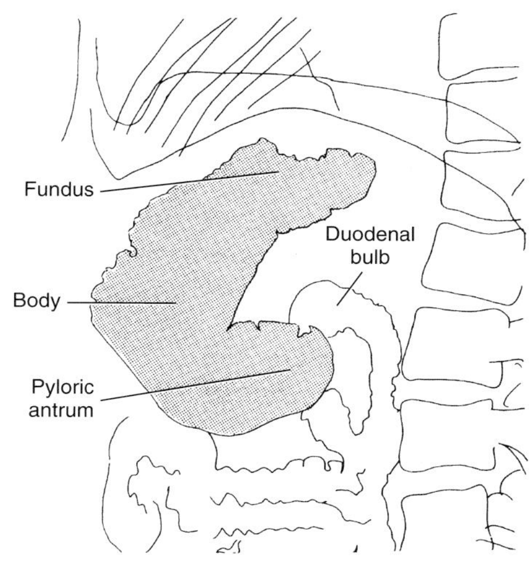

Fig. 14-96. Right lateral position.

14

LPO POSITION: UPPER GI SERIES

Upper GI Series
BASIC
- RAO
- PA
- Right lateral
- LPO
- AP

Pathology Demonstrated

When a double-contrast technique is used, the air-filled pylorus and duodenal bulb may better demonstrate signs of gastritis and ulcers.

Technical Factors

- IR size—24 × 30 cm (10 × 12 inches), lengthwise
  or—30 × 35 cm (11 × 14 inches)
- Moving or stationary grid
- 100-110 kV range (80-90 kV range for double-contrast study)
- Technique and dose:

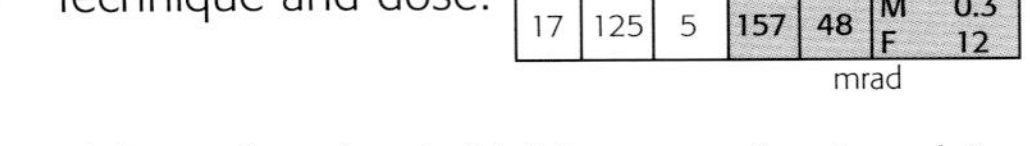

cm	kV	mAs	Sk.	ML.	Gon.
17	125	5	157	48	M 0.3 F 12
				mrad	

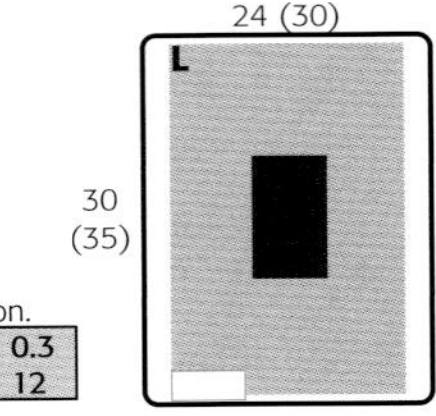

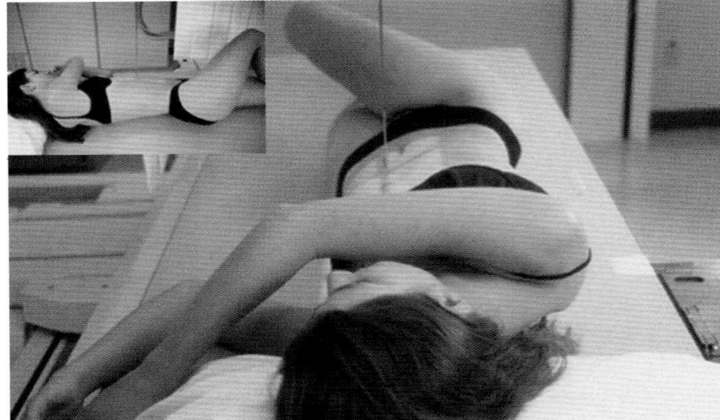

Fig. 14-97. LPO position.

Shielding Place lead shield over patient's pelvic region.

Patient Position Position patient recumbent, with the body partially rotated into an LPO position; provide pillow for head.

Part Position

- Rotate **30° to 60°** from supine position, with left posterior against IR or table (more rotation possibly required for heavy hypersthenic-type patients and less for thin asthenic types).
- Flex right knee for support.
- Extend left arm from body and raise right arm high across chest to grasp end of table for support. (Do not pinch fingers when moving Bucky.)
- Center IR at CR (bottom of cassette at level of iliac crest).

Central Ray

- Direct CR **perpendicular** to IR.
- ***Sthenic type:*** Center CR and IR to **level of L1** (about midway between xiphoid tip and lower lateral margin of ribs) and **midway between midline of body** and **left lateral margin** of abdomen, 45° oblique.
- ***Hypersthenic:*** Center about 2 inches (5 cm) above L1, 60° oblique.
- ***Asthenic:*** Center about 2 inches (5 cm) below L1 and nearer to midline, 30° oblique.
- Minimum SID is 40 inches (100 cm).

Collimation Collimate on four sides to outer margins of IR or to area of interest on larger IR.

Respiration Suspend respiration and expose on expiration.

Note: Stomach is generally located higher in this position than in the lateral; therefore center one vertebra higher than on PA or RAO positions.

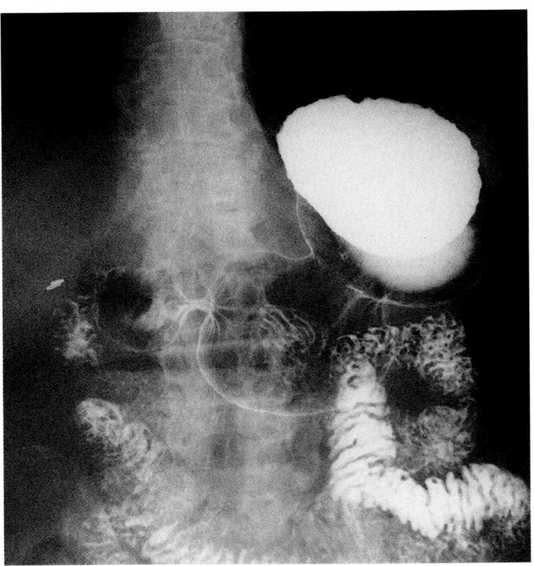

Fig. 14-98. LPO position.

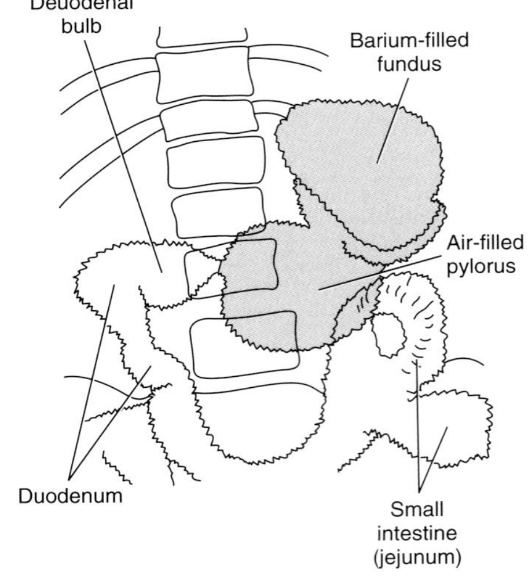

Fig. 14-99. LPO.

Radiographic Criteria

Structures Shown: • Entire stomach and duodenum are visible. • An unobstructed view of the duodenal bulb should be seen, without superimposition by the pylorus of the stomach.

Position: • The fundus should be filled with barium. • With a double-contrast procedure the body and pylorus and occasionally the duodenal bulb are air filled.

Collimation and CR: • Collimation is seen along the four margins of the radiograph. • CR is centered level to duodenal bulb.

Exposure Criteria: • Appropriate technique is used to visualize the gastric folds without overexposing other pertinent anatomy; sharp structural margins indicate no motion.

AP PROJECTION: UPPER GI SERIES

Pathology Demonstrated

Possible **hiatal hernia** may be demonstrated in **Trendelenburg position.**

Upper GI Series
BASIC
• RAO
• PA
• Right lateral
• LPO
• AP

Technical Factors

- IR size—30 × 35 cm (11 × 14 inches), lengthwise
  or—35 × 43 cm (14 × 17 inches)
- Moving or stationary grid
- 100-110 kV range
  (80-90 kV range for double-contrast study)
- Technique and dose:

cm	kV	mAs	Sk.	ML.	Gon.
18	125	4	114	39	M 0.1 F 10

mrad

30 (35)
35 (43)
R

Shielding Place lead shield over patient's pelvic region to protect gonads without covering pertinent anatomy.

Patient Position Position patient supine, arms at sides; provide pillow for head.

Part Position

- Align **midsagittal plane to midline** of table.
- Ensure that **body is not rotated.**
- Center cassette to CR. (Bottom of 11- × 14-inch [30- × 35-cm] cassette should be about at level of iliac crest.)

Central Ray

- Center CR **perpendicular** to IR.
- *Sthenic type:* Center CR and IR to **level of L1** (about midway between xiphoid tip and lower margin of ribs), **midway between midline and left-lateral margin** of abdomen.
- *Hypersthenic:* Center about 1 inch (2.5 cm) above L1.
- *Asthenic:* Position CR about 2 inches (5 cm) below and nearer to midline.
- Minimum SID is 40 inches (100 cm).

Collimation Collimate on four sides to outer margins of IR or to area of interest if larger IR is used.

Respiration Suspend respiration and expose on expiration.

Alternative AP Trendelenburg: A partial Trendelenburg (head down) position may be necessary to fill the fundus on a thin asthenic patient. A full Trendelenburg angulation facilitates the demonstration of hiatal hernia. (Install shoulder braces for patient safety.)

Radiographic Criteria

Structures Shown: • Entire stomach and duodenum are visible. • Diaphragm and lower lung fields are included for demonstration of possible hiatal hernia.

Position: • Fundus of the stomach is filled with barium and is near center of IR.

Collimation and CR: • Collimation is seen along the four margins of the radiograph. • CR is centered to duodenal bulb at level of L1.

Exposure Criteria: • Appropriate technique is used to visualize the gastric folds without overexposing other pertinent anatomy. • Sharp structural margins indicate no motion.

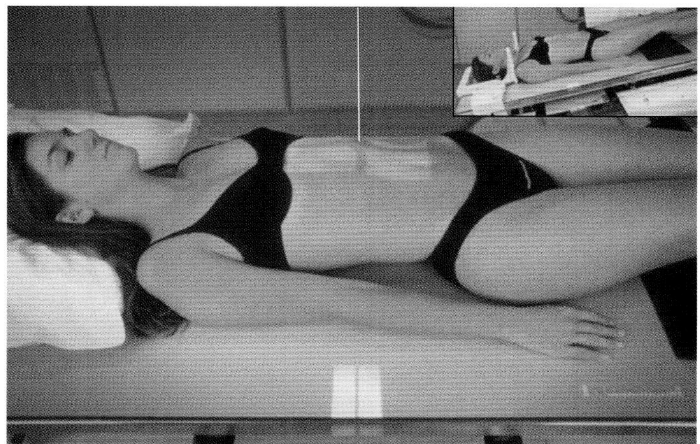

Fig. 14-100. AP supine. *Inset,* Trendelenburg option.

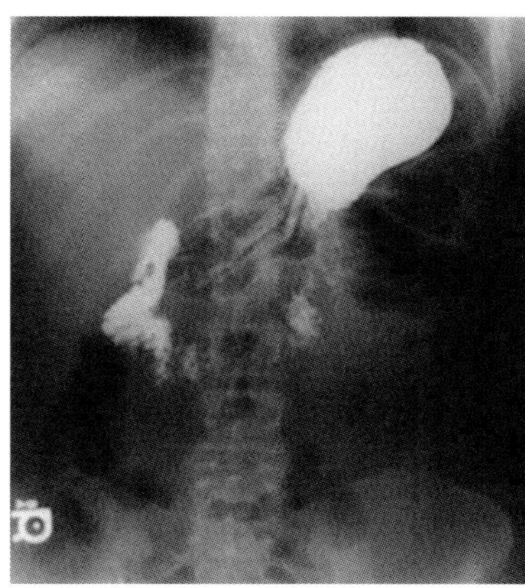

Fig. 14-101. AP, supine.

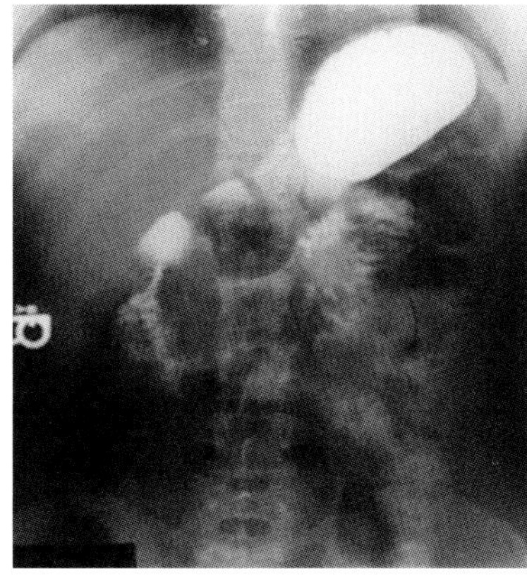

Fig. 14-102. AP, Trendelenburg.

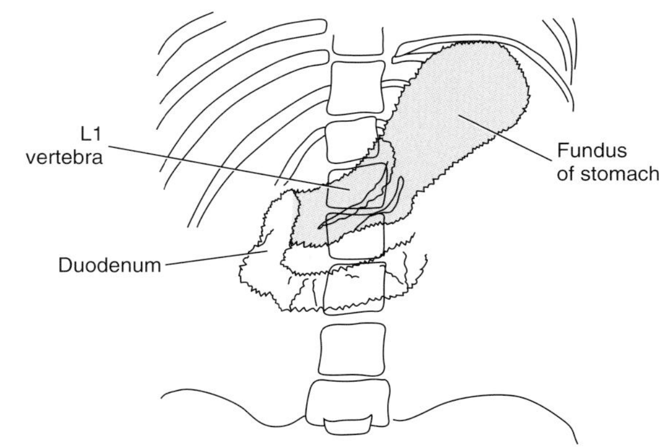

Fig. 14-103. AP, supine.

14

CHAPTER 15

Lower Gastrointestinal System

CONTRIBUTOR TO PAST EDITIONS Barry T. Anthony, RT(R)

CONTENTS

RADIOGRAPHIC ANATOMY

Digestive System

The first five parts of the alimentary canal (through the stomach and first part of the small intestine, the duodenum) were described in the preceding chapter.

This chapter continues with the alimentary canal of the digestive system beyond the stomach, beginning with the **small intestine** (small bowel). If the entire small intestine were removed from the body at autopsy, separated from its mesenteric attachment, uncoiled, and stretched out, it would average 7 meters, or 23 feet, in length. During life, with good muscle tone the actual length of the small intestine is shorter, measuring between 4.5 and 5.5 meters, or 15 to 18 feet. Tremendous individual variation does exist, however. In one series of 100 autopsies, the small bowel varied in length from 15 to 31 feet. Its diameter varies from 1.5 inches (3.8 cm) at the proximal aspect to about 1 inch (2.5 cm) at the distal end.

The **large intestine** (large bowel) begins in the lower right quadrant near its connection with the small intestine. The large intestine extends around the periphery of the abdominal cavity to end at the **anus.** The large intestine is about 1.5 meters (5 feet) long and about 6 cm (2.5 inches) in diameter.

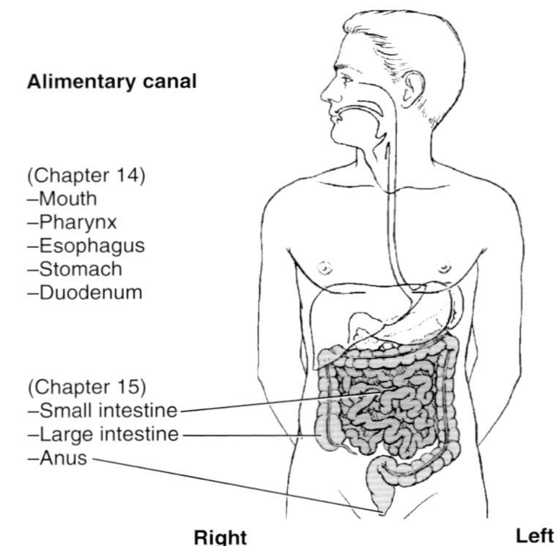

Fig. 15-1. Digestive system.

COMMON RADIOGRAPHIC PROCEDURES

Two common radiographic procedures involving the lower gastrointestinal (GI) system are presented in this chapter. Both procedures involve administration of a contrast medium.

Small Bowel Series (SBS)—Study of Small Intestine Radiographic examination specifically of the small intestine is termed a ***small bowel series,*** or ***SBS.*** This examination is often combined with an upper GI series and under these conditions may be termed a *small bowel follow-through.* A radiograph of the barium-filled small bowel is shown in Fig. 15-2.

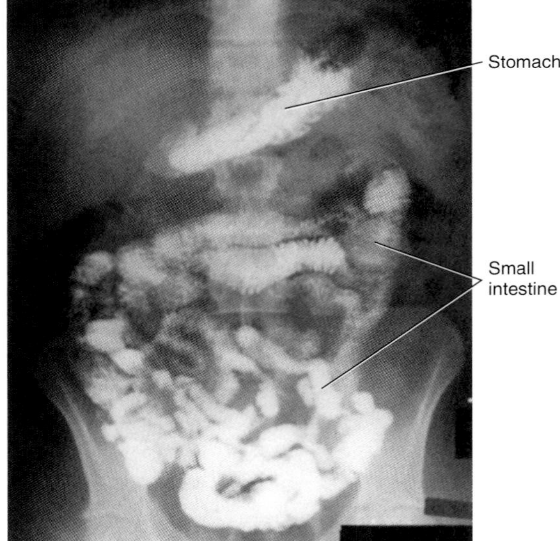

Fig. 15-2. Small bowel series—PA.

Barium Enema (BE, Lower GI Series, Colon)—Study of Large Intestine The radiographic procedure designed to study the large intestine is most commonly termed a ***barium enema.*** Alternate designations include *BE, BaE,* or *lower GI series.* Fig. 15-3 demonstrates a large bowel or colon filled with a combination of air and barium, referred to as a *double-contrast barium enema.*

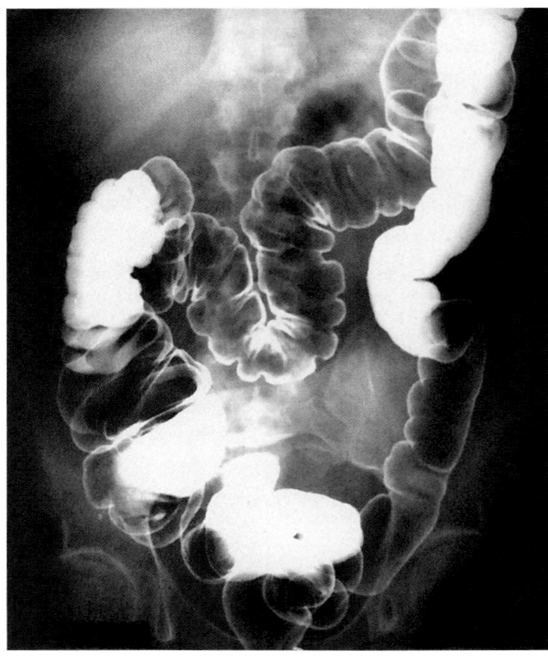

Fig. 15-3. Double-contrast barium enema—AP.

Small Intestine

Beginning at the pyloric valve of the stomach the three parts of the small intestine, in order, are the **duodenum, jejunum,** and **ileum.**

The relative location of the three parts of the small intestine in relationship to the four abdominal quadrants is demonstrated.

DUODENUM (RUQ AND LUQ)

The **duodenum** is the first part of the small intestine, as studied in detail in Chapter 14, and it is the shortest, widest, and most fixed portion of the small bowel. It is primarily located in the right upper quadrant (RUQ). It also extends into the left upper quadrant (LUQ), where it joins the jejunum at a point termed the *duodenojejunal flexure.*

JEJUNUM (LUQ AND LLQ)

The **jejunum** is located primarily to the left of midline in the left upper and left lower quadrants (LUQ and LLQ), making up about **two fifths** of the small bowel.

The jejunum begins at the site of the duodenojejunal junction slightly to the left of the midline in the left upper quadrant (under the transverse colon on the drawing in Fig. 15-4). This relatively fixed site of the small bowel becomes a radiographic reference point for certain small bowel studies.

ILEUM (RLQ AND LLQ)

The **ileum** is located primarily in the right upper and right and left lower quadrants (RUQ, RLQ, and LLQ). Approximately **three fifths** of the small bowel is ileum. Therefore the ileum is the longest portion of the small intestine. The terminal ileum joins the large intestine at the **ileocecal valve** in the right lower quadrant, as shown in Fig. 15-4.

SECTIONAL DIFFERENCES

The various sections of small intestine can be identified radiographically both by their **location** and by their **appearance.** The C-shaped duodenum is fairly fixed in position immediately distal to the stomach and is easily recognized on radiographs. The internal lining of the second and third (descending and horizontal) portions of the duodenum is gathered into tight circular folds formed by the mucosa of the small intestine containing numerous small fingerlike projections termed ***villi,*** resulting in a "feathery" appearance when filled with barium.

Jejunum The circular folds of the distal duodenum are found in the jejunum as well. Although there is no abrupt end to the circular feathery folds, the ileum tends not to have this appearance. This difference in appearance between the jejunum and ileum can be seen in the barium-filled small bowel radiograph in Fig. 15-5.

Ileum The internal lining of the ileum appears on a radiograph as smoother, with fewer indentations and therefore a less feathery appearance.

Another observable difference in the three sections of small intestine is that the internal diameter gets progressively smaller from duodenum to ileum.

CT Cross-Sectional Image A computed tomogram (CT) axial or cross-sectional image through the level of the second portion of the duodenum is seen in Fig. 15-6. This image demonstrates the relative positions of the stomach and duodenum in relationship to the head of the pancreas. A portion of cross-sections of loops of jejunum is also shown on the patient's left, along with a loop of colon.

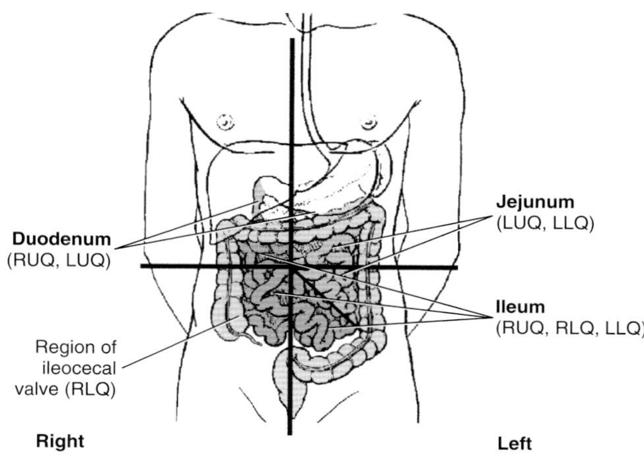

Fig. 15-4. Small intestines—four quadrants.

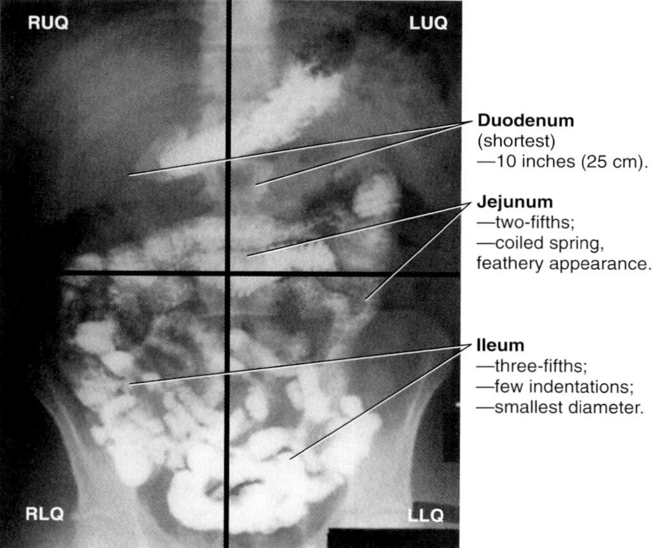

Fig. 15-5. Barium-filled stomach and small intestine (four quadrants).

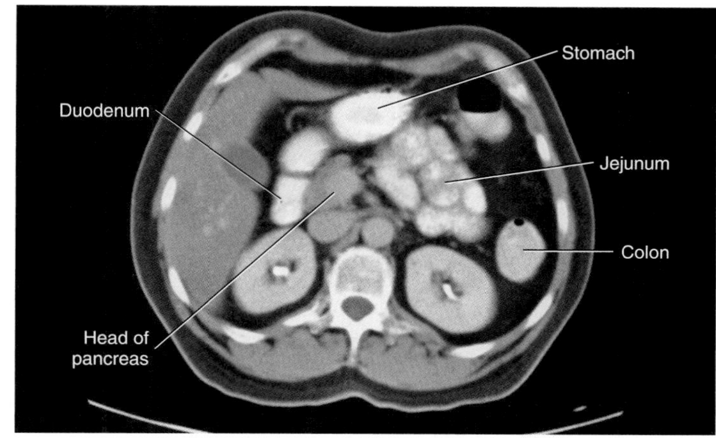

Fig. 15-6. CT axial section—level of second portion of duodenum.

Large Intestine

The large intestine begins in the right lower quadrant, just lateral to the ileocecal valve. The large intestine consists of four major parts: **cecum, colon, rectum,** and **anal canal** (see Fig. 15-7).

The final segment of the large intestine is the **rectum.** The distal rectum contains the **anal canal,** which ends at the **anus.**

COLON VERSUS LARGE INTESTINE

Large intestine and *colon* are NOT synonyms, although many technologists use these terms interchangeably. The **colon** consists of **four sections** and **two flexures** and does **not** include the cecum and rectum. The four sections of the colon are (1) the **ascending colon,** (2) the **transverse colon,** (3) the **descending colon,** and (4) the **sigmoid colon.** The **right** (hepatic) and **left** (splenic) **colic flexures** thus are also included as part of the colon.

The transverse colon has a wide range of motion and normally loops down more than shown on this drawing.

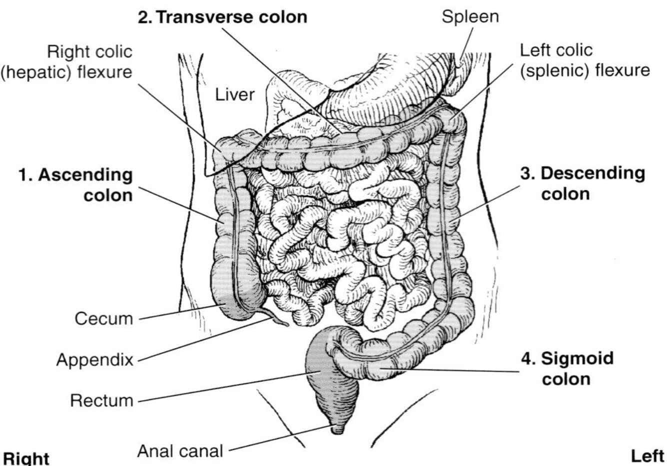

Fig. 15-7. Large intestine (includes colon).

CECUM

At the proximal end of the large intestine is the **cecum,** a large blind pouch located inferior to the level of the ileocecal valve. The vermiform **appendix** (commonly referred to as just the appendix) is attached to the cecum. The internal appearance of the cecum and **terminal ileum** is shown in Fig. 15-8. The most distal part of the small intestine, the ileum, joins the cecum at the **ileocecal valve.** The ileocecal valve consists of two lips that extend into the large bowel.

The ileocecal valve acts as a sphincter to prevent the contents of the ileum from passing too quickly into the cecum. A second function of the ileocecal valve is to prevent reflux, or a backward flow of large intestine contents, into the ileum. The ileocecal valve does only a fair job of preventing reflux because some barium can almost always be refluxed into the terminal ileum when a barium enema is performed. The **cecum** is the widest portion of the large intestine and is fairly free to move about in the right lower quadrant.

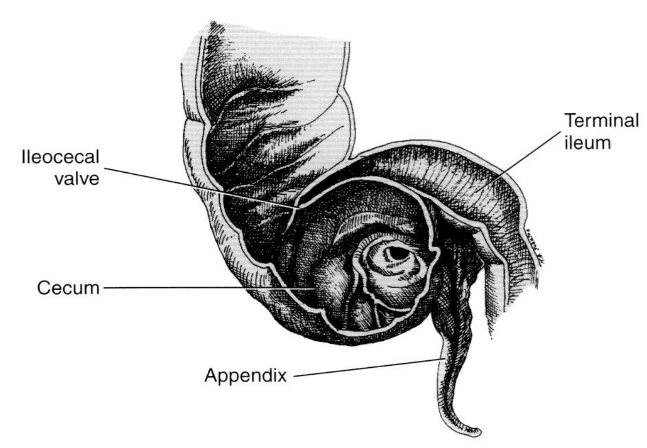

Fig. 15-8. Cecum, terminal ileum, and appendix.

Appendix The **vermiform appendix** (appendix) is a long (2 to 20 cm), narrow, worm-shaped tube extending from the cecum. The term, *vermiform,* in fact, means "wormlike." The appendix is usually attached to the posteromedial aspect of the cecum and commonly extends toward the pelvis. It may, however, pass posterior to the cecum. Because the appendix has a blind ending, infectious agents may enter the appendix, which cannot empty itself. The result is **appendicitis.** An inflamed appendix may require surgical removal, termed an ***appendectomy,*** before the diseased structure ruptures and causes peritonitis. Acute appendicitis accounts for about 50% of all emergency abdominal surgeries and is 1½ times more common in men than in women.

Occasionally, fecal matter or barium sulfate from a GI tract study may fill the appendix and remain there indefinitely.

LARGE INTESTINE—BARIUM-FILLED

A barium-enema radiograph is shown in Fig. 15-9, demonstrating the barium-filled **appendix;** the four parts of the colon—**ascending, transverse, descending,** and **sigmoid;** and the two flexures—the **right colic** (hepatic) **flexure** and the **left colic** (splenic) **flexure.** The remaining three parts of the large intestine are also shown—the **cecum, rectum,** and **anal canal.** As shown on this radiograph, these various parts are not neatly arranged around the periphery of the abdomen as shown on the drawings. Instead they demonstrate a wide range of specific structure locations and relative sizes of the various portions of the large intestine dependent on the body habitus and the contents of the intestine.

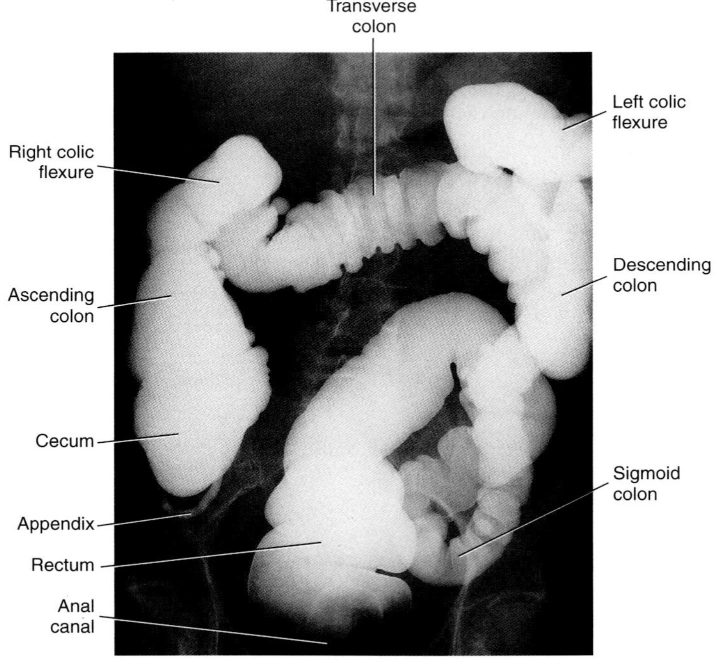

Fig. 15-9. Barium enema of large intestine.

15

RECTUM AND ANAL CANAL

The **rectum** extends from the sigmoid colon to the **anus.** The rectum begins at the level of S3 (third sacral segment) and is about 4½ inches (12 cm) long. The final 1 to 1½ inches (2.5 to 4 cm) of large intestine is constricted to form the **anal canal.** The anal canal terminates as an opening to the exterior, the **anus.** The rectum closely follows the sacrococcygeal curve, as demonstrated in the lateral view in Fig. 15-10.

The **rectal ampulla** is a dilated portion of the rectum located anterior to the coccyx. The initial direction of the rectum along the **sacrum** is down and back; however, in the region of the rectal ampulla, the direction changes to down and forward. A second abrupt change in direction occurs in the region of the anal canal, which is directed downward and backward. Therefore the rectum presents **two anteroposterior curves.** This fact must be remembered when a rectal tube or enema tip is inserted into the lower GI tract by the technologist for a barium-enema procedure. Serious injury can occur if the enema tip is forced into the anus and anal canal incorrectly at the wrong angle.

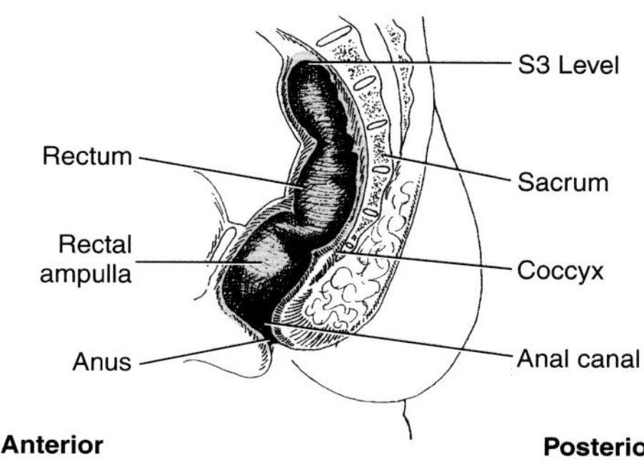

Fig. 15-10. Rectum—lateral view.

LARGE VERSUS SMALL INTESTINE

Three characteristics readily differentiate the large intestine from the small intestine.

First, the **internal diameter** of the large intestine is usually greater than the diameter of the small bowel.

Second, the muscular portion of the intestinal wall contains three external bands of longitudinal muscle fibers of the large bowel to form three bands of muscle called ***taeniae coli,*** which tend to pull the large intestine into pouches. Each of these pouches, or sacculations, is termed a ***haustrum.*** Therefore a second primary identifying characteristic of the large bowel is the presence of multiple haustra. This characteristic is demonstrated in the enlarged drawing of the proximal large intestine in Fig. 15-11.

The **third** differentiation is the **relative positions** of the two structures. The **large intestine** extends around the **periphery** of the abdominal cavity, whereas the **small intestine** is more **centrally** located.

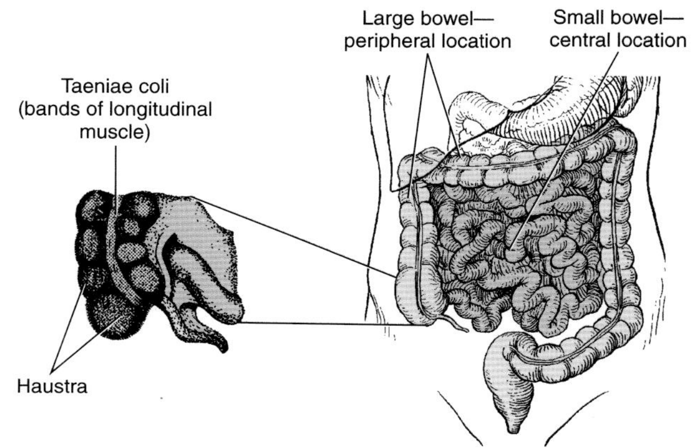

Fig. 15-11. Intestinal differences—large versus small intestine.

RELATIVE LOCATIONS OF AIR AND BARIUM IN LARGE INTESTINE

The simplified drawings in Fig. 15-12 represent the large intestine in **supine** and **prone** positions. If the large intestine contained both air and barium sulfate, the air would tend to rise and the barium would tend to sink because of gravity. The displacement and ultimate location of **air** is shown as **black** and the **barium** as **white.**

When a person is **supine,** air rises to fill those structures that are most anterior, which are the transverse and loops of sigmoid colon. The barium sinks to fill primarily the ascending, descending, and parts of the sigmoid colon.

When a patient is **prone,** barium and air reverse positions. The drawing on the right illustrates the prone position; hence air has risen to fill the rectum, ascending colon, and descending colon.

Recognizing these spatial relationships is important both during fluoroscopy and during radiography when barium-enema examinations are performed.

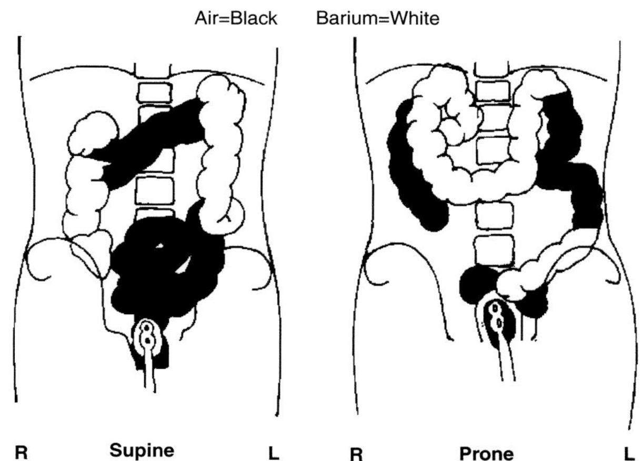

Fig. 15-12. Barium versus air in the large intestine.

15

Anatomy Review

SMALL BOWEL RADIOGRAPHS

Three parts of the small bowel are demonstrated in these 30-minute and 2-hour small bowel radiographs, taken 30 minutes and 2 hours after ingestion of barium (Figs. 15-13 to 15-15). Note the characteristic feathery-appearing sections of duodenum *(A)* and jejunum *(C)*. The smoother appearance of the ileum is also evident *(D)*.

The terminal portion of the ileum *(D)*, the ileocecal valve *(E)*, and the cecum of the large intestine are best shown on a spot film of this area (Fig. 15-15). A spot film such as this, using a compression cone, is frequently taken of the ileocecal valve area at the end of a small bowel series to best visualize this region. These figures illustrate the following labeled parts of the small intestine:

A. Duodenum
B. Area of suspensory muscle of the duodenum (ligament of Treitz; site of duodenojejunal flexure, superimposed by stomach on these radiographs)
C. Jejunum
D. Ileum
E. Area of ileocecal valve

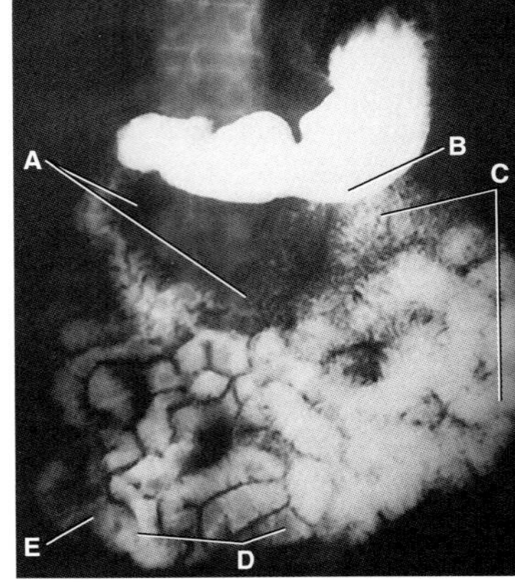

Fig. 15-13. PA, 30-minute small bowel.

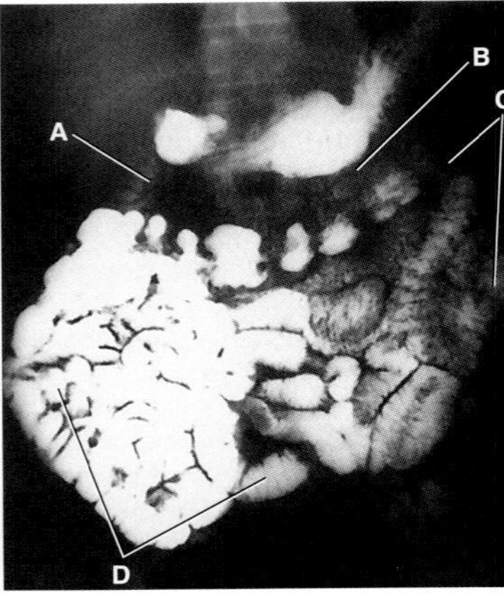

Fig. 15-14. PA, 2-hour small bowel.

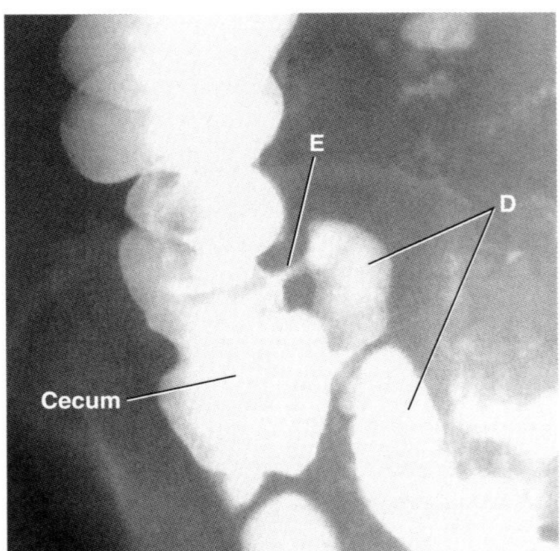

Fig. 15-15. Spot film of ileocecal valve. (Courtesy Jim Sanderson, RT.)

BARIUM ENEMA (Figs. 15-16, 15-17, and 15-18)

Anteroposterior (AP), lateral, and right anterior oblique (RAO) radiographs of a barium enema exam (Figs. 15-16 to 15-18) illustrate the key anatomy of the large intestine, labeled as follows:

a. Cecum
b. Ascending colon
c. Right colic (hepatic) flexure (usually located lower than left colic flexure due to presence of large space occupying liver)
d. Transverse colon
e. Left colic (splenic) flexure
f. Descending colon
g. Sigmoid colon
h. Rectum

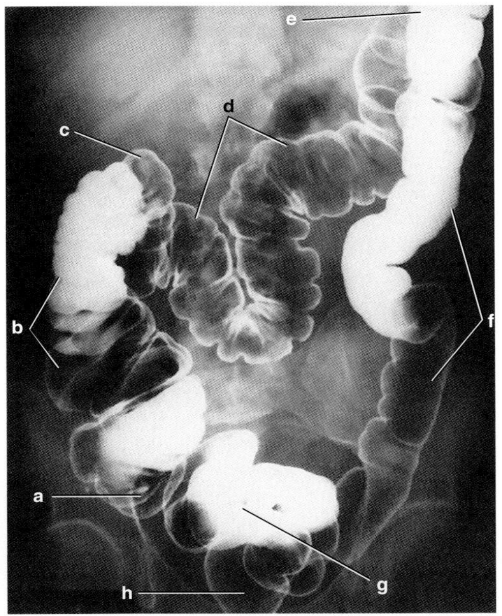

Fig. 15-16. AP, barium enema (double-contrast study).

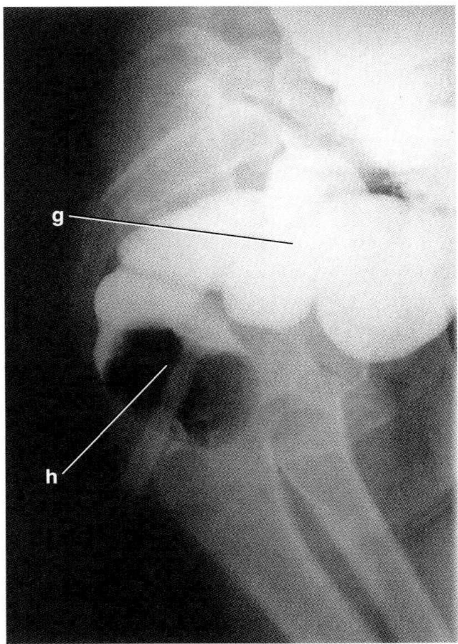

Fig. 15-17. Lateral rectum; barium enema.

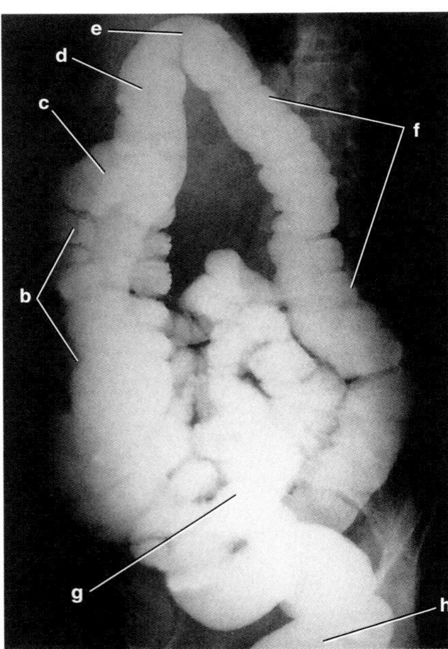

Fig. 15-18. LAO, barium enema (single-contrast study).

15

Digestive Functions

DIGESTIVE FUNCTIONS OF THE INTESTINES

Four primary digestive functions that are accomplished largely by the small and large intestines are as follows:

1. **Digestion** (chemical and mechanical)
2. **Absorption**
3. **Reabsorption** of water, inorganic salts, vitamin K, and amino acids
4. **Elimination** (defecation)

Most **digestion** and **absorption** take place within the **small intestine.** Also the majority of the **salts** and approximately **95% of H_2O are reabsorbed** in the small intestine. Some minimal reabsorption of H_2O and inorganic salts also occurs in the large intestine, along with the elimination of unused or unnecessary materials.

The primary function of the **large intestine,** however, is the **elimination of feces** (defecation). Feces consist normally of 65% water and 35% solid matter, such as food residues, digestive secretions, and bacteria. Other specific functions of the large intestine are some absorption of water, absorption of inorganic salt, and absorption of vitamin K in addition to certain amino acids. These vitamins and amino acids are produced by a large collection of naturally occurring microorganisms (bacteria) found in the large intestine.

Therefore the last stage of digestion occurs in the large intestine through **bacterial action,** which converts the remaining proteins into amino acids. Some vitamins, such as B and K, are also synthesized by bacteria and absorbed by the large intestine. A by-product of this bacterial action is the release of hydrogen, carbon dioxide, and methane gas. These gases are called ***flatus*** *(fla'tus)* and aid in breaking down the remaining proteins to amino acids.

MOVEMENTS OF DIGESTIVE TRACT

Of the various digestive functions of the intestine, digestive movements, sometimes referred to as *mechanical digestion,* are best demonstrated and evident on radiographic studies.

Small Intestine Digestive movements throughout the length of the small bowel consist of (1) **peristalsis** *(per"i-stal'sis)* and (2) **rhythmic segmentation.** Peristalsis describes wavelike contractions that propel food from the stomach through the small and large intestines and eventually expel it from the body. Barium sulfate entering the stomach reaches the ileocecal valve between 2 and 3 hours after inception.

Rhythmic segmentation describes localized contractions in areas or regions containing food. For example, food within a specific aspect of the small intestine is contracted to produce segments of a particular column of food. Through rhythmic segmentation, digestion and reabsorption of select nutrients are more effective.

Large Intestine In the large intestine, digestive movements continue with (1) **peristalsis,** (2) **haustral** *(haws'tral)* **churning,** (3) **mass peristalsis,** and (4) **defecation** *(def"e-ka'shun).* Haustral churning produces movement of material within the large intestine. During this process a particular group of haustra (bands of muscle) remains relaxed and distended while the bands are filling up with material. When the distention reaches a certain level, the intestinal walls contract or "churn" to squeeze the contents into the next group of haustra. Mass peristalsis tends to move the entire large bowel contents into the sigmoid colon and rectum, usually once every 24 hours. Defecation is a so-called bowel movement, or emptying of the rectum.

SUMMARY OF LOWER DIGESTIVE SYSTEM FUNCTIONS

RESPONSIBLE COMPONENT OF INTESTINE	FUNCTION
Small intestine:	**1. Digestion:** Chemical and mechanical
Duodenum	**2. Absorption:** Nutrients, H_2O, salts, proteins
and	
Jejunum (primarily)	**3. Reabsorption:** H_2O and salts
Large intestine:	Some reabsorption of H_2O and inorganic salts
	Vitamins B and K, Amino acids } Produced by bacterial action; release of gases (flatus)
	4. Elimination (defecation)

SUMMARY OF DIGESTIVE MOVEMENTS AND ELIMINATION

RESPONSIBLE COMPONENT OF INTESTINE	FUNCTION
Small intestine	**1. Peristalsis**
	2. Rhythmic segmentation
Large intestine	**1. Peristalsis**
	2. Haustral churning
	3. Mass peristalsis
	4. Defecation

RADIOGRAPHIC PROCEDURES

Small Bowel Series

The plain abdominal radiograph shown in Fig. 15-19 is of a healthy, ambulatory adult. The many meters of small intestine are generally not visible in the central portion of the abdomen. In the average ambulatory adult a large collection of gas in the small intestine is considered abnormal. Without any gas present the small bowel simply blends in with other soft tissue structures. Therefore radiographic examination of the alimentary canal requires the introduction of contrast media for visualization.

DEFINITION

A radiographic study specifically of the small intestine is termed a ***small bowel series,*** or ***SBS.*** The upper GI and small bowel series are most often combined. Under these circumstances the small bowel portion of the exam may be called a *small bowel follow-through,* or *SBFT.* A radiopaque contrast media is required for this study.

PURPOSE

The purpose of the small bowel series is **to study the form and function of the three components of the small bowel,** as well as **detect any abnormal conditions.**

Because this study also examines **function** of the small bowel, the procedure **must be timed.** The time should be noted when the patient has ingested a substantial amount (at least ¾ cup) of the contrast media.

CONTRAINDICATIONS

Two strict contraindications exist to contrast media studies of the intestinal tract.

First, presurgical patients and patients suspected of having a **perforated hollow viscus** (intestine or organ) should **not** receive barium sulfate. The water-soluble, iodinated media should be used instead. With young or dehydrated patients, care must be taken when a water-soluble contrast media is used. Because of these patients' hypertonic nature, they tend to draw water into the bowel, leading to increased dehydration.

Second, barium sulfate by mouth is contraindicated in patients with a possible **large bowel obstruction.** An obstructed large bowel should first be ruled out with an acute abdominal series and a barium enema.

PATHOLOGIC INDICATIONS

The more common pathologic indications for a small bowel series include the following:

Enteritis *(en"ter-i'tis)* is a term describing inflammation of the intestine, primarily the small intestine. Enteritis may be caused by bacterial or protozoan organisms or other environmental factors. When the stomach is also involved, the condition is described as ***gastroenteritis.*** Chronic irritation may cause the lumen of the intestine to become thickened, irregular, and narrowed.

Regional enteritis (**segmental enteritis,** or **Crohn's disease**) is a chronic inflammatory disease of unknown etiology, involving any part of the GI tract but commonly involving the terminal ileum, with scarring and thickening of the bowel wall. This scarring produces the "cobblestone" appearance visible during a small bowel series, or enteroclysis. Radiographically, these lesions resemble gastric erosions or ulcers seen in barium studies as minor variations in barium coating. In advanced cases, segments of the intestine become narrowed due to chronic spasm, producing the "string sign" evident during a small bowel series, or enteroclysis. Regional enteritis frequently leads to intestinal obstruction and fistula and abscess formation and has a high rate of recurrence after treatment.

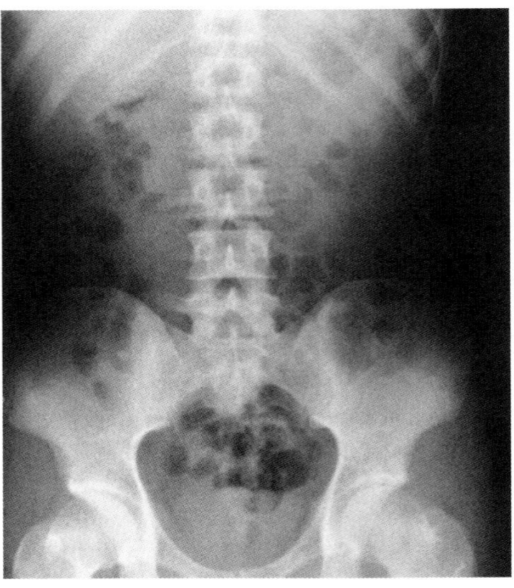

Fig. 15-19. Plain abdominal radiograph—normal (some gas seen in large intestine).

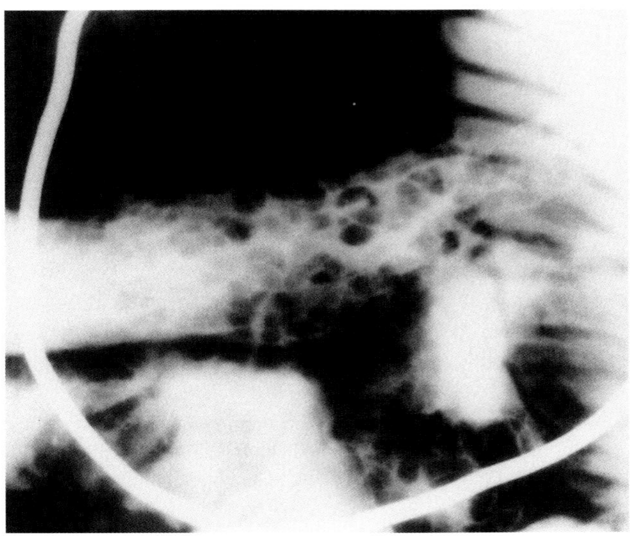

Fig. 15-20. Crohn's Disease involving ileum, Cobblestone appearance. (From Eisenberg RL, Johnson NM: Comprehensive radiographic pathology, ed 3, St. Louis, 2003, Mosby.)

Giardiasis *(je"ahr-di-a-sis)* is a common infection of the lumen of the small intestine due to the flagellate protozoan *(Giardia lamblia)*. It is often spread by contaminated food and water and/or person-to-person contact. Symptoms of giardiasis include nonspecific GI discomfort, mild to profuse diarrhea, nausea, anorexia, and weight loss. The organism usually involves the duodenum and jejunum and is associated with spasm, irritability, and increased secretions. On the small bowel series, giardiasis produces dilation of the intestine, with thickening of the circular folds. Often, lab analysis of a stool specimen is required to detect the presence of the *Giardia* organism.

Ileus *(il'e-us)* is an **obstruction of the small intestine,** as seen in Fig. 15-22, wherein the proximal jejunum is markedly expanded with air. There are two types of ileus: (1) **adynamic,** or **paralytic** and (2) **mechanical.**

Adynamic, or **paralytic,** ileus is due to the **cessation of peristalsis.** Without these involuntary, wavelike contractions, the bowel is flaccid and unable to propel its contents forward. Causes for adynamic ileus include infection, such as peritonitis or appendicitis, presence of certain drugs, or a postsurgical complication. Adynamic ileus usually involves the entire GI tract. With adynamic ileus, usually no fluid levels are demonstrated on the erect abdomen projection. However, the intestine is distended with a thin bowel wall.

A **mechanical obstruction** is a physical blockage of the bowel. It may be due to tumors, adhesions, or hernias. The loops of intestine proximal to the site of obstruction are markedly dilated with gas. This dilation produces the radiographic sign commonly called "circular staircase or herringbone" pattern evident on an erect or decubitus abdomen projection. Air-fluid levels are usually present as seen on these projections.

Meckel's diverticulum* is a fairly common birth defect found in the ileum of the small bowel. It may measure as large as 10 or 12 cm in diameter, usually 2 to 4 feet proximal to the ileocecal valve. It is found in about 2% of adults during surgery for other reasons. It is a persistence of the yolk sac (umbilical vesicle), resulting in a saclike outpouching of the intestinal wall. Usually the condition does not cause symptoms unless it becomes inflamed (diverticulitis) or causes bowel obstruction. It is rarely seen on barium studies of the small bowel because of the rapid emptying on a barium study. It is best diagnosed with a radionuclide (nuclear medicine) scan.

*Merck manual of medical information, 1997, White House Station, NJ, Merck and Co, p 1288.

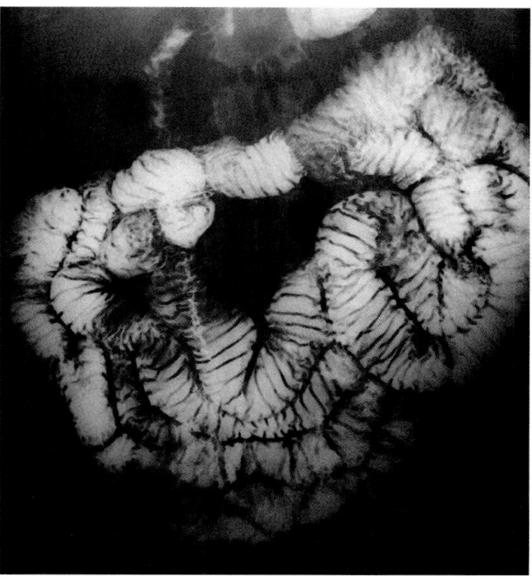

Fig. 15-21. Giardiasis of small intestine, jejunum, and ileum. (Dilation of intestine, with thick circular folds, is visible.)

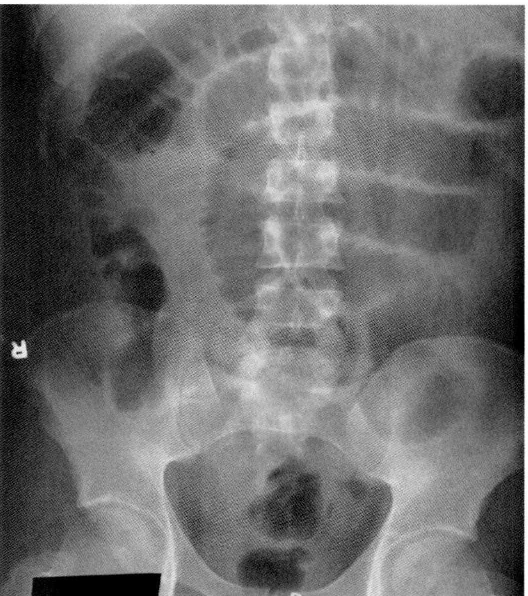

Fig. 15-22. Ileus (obstruction) of small bowel demonstrated by greatly extended air-filled loops of small bowel.

Neoplasm *(ne'o-plazm)* is a term meaning "new growth." This growth may be benign or malignant (cancerous). Common benign tumors of the small intestine include **adenomas** and **leiomyomas**. The majority of benign tumors are found in the jejunum and ileum.

Carcinoid tumors are the most common tumors of the small bowel. They have a benign appearance but have the potential to become malignant. They are small-size lesions that tend to grow submucosally and are frequently missed radiographically.

Lymphoma and **adenocarcinoma** are malignant tumors of the small intestine. Lymphomas are demonstrated during a small bowel series as producing the "stacked coin" sign, which is caused by thickening, coarsening, and possible hemorrhage of the mucosal wall. Other segments of intestine may become narrowed and ulcerative. Adenocarcinomas produce short and sharp "napkin-ring" defects within the lumen and may lead to complete obstruction. These radiographic signs of neoplasm are demonstrated during a barium enema procedure. The most frequent sites for adenocarcinoma are the duodenum and proximal jejunum.

The small bowel series, or **enteroclysis,** may demonstrate a stricture or blockage due to the neoplasm. CT of the abdomen may further isolate the location and size of the tumor.

Sprue *(spru)* and **malabsorption syndromes*** are conditions in which the patient's GI tract is unable to process and absorb certain nutrients. Sprue is a group of intestinal malabsorption diseases involving the inability to absorb certain proteins and dietary fat. The malabsorption may be due to an intraluminal (digestive) defect, a mucosal abnormality, or a lymphatic obstruction. Often malabsorption syndrome is experienced in patients with lactose and sucrose sensitivities. Deficiency syndromes may result from excessive loss of vitamins, electrolytes, iron, calcium, etc. During the small bowel series the mucosa may appear to be thickened as a result of the constant irritation.

*Ell SR: Handbook of gastrointestinal and genitourinary radiology, St. Louis, 1992, Mosby, pp 55, 63.

Celiac disease is a form of sprue or malabsorption disease affecting the proximal small bowel, especially the proximal duodenum. It commonly involves the insoluble protein (gluten) found in cereal grains.

Whipple's disease* is a disorder of the proximal small bowel. Its cause is unknown. Symptoms include dilation of the intestine, edema, malabsorption, deposits of fat in the bowel wall, and mesenteric nodules. Whipple's disease is best diagnosed with the small bowel series, which demonstrates the distorted loops of small intestine.

*Ell SR: Handbook of gastrointestinal and genitourinary radiology, St. Louis, 1992, Mosby, pp 55, 63.

SMALL INTESTINE—SUMMARY OF PATHOLOGIC INDICATIONS

CONDITION OR DISEASE	MOST COMMON RADIOGRAPHIC EXAM	POSSIBLE RADIOGRAPHIC APPEARANCE	MANUAL EXPOSURE FACTOR ADJUSTMENT*
Enteritis	Small bowel series, enteroclysis	Thickening of mucosal folds and poor definition of circular folds	None
Regional enteritis (Crohn's disease)	Small bowel series, enteroclysis	Segments of lumen narrowed and irregular; "cobblestone" appearance and "string sign" being common	None
Giardiasis	Small bowel series, enteroclysis	Dilation of the intestine, with thickening of the circular folds	None
Ileus (obstruction) **Adynamic** **Mechanical**	Acute abdomen series, small bowel series, enteroclysis	Abnormal gas patterns, dilated loops of bowel, "circular staircase" or "herringbone" pattern	(−) Decrease if large segments of intestine are gas-filled
Malabsorption syndromes (sprue)	Small bowel series, enteroclysis, or CT of the abdomen	Thickening of mucosal folds and poor definition of normal "feathery" appearance	None
Meckel's diverticulum	Nuclear medicine scan, small bowel series, enteroclysis	Large diverticulum of the ileum, proximal to ileocecal valve; rarely seen on barium studies	None
Neoplasm	Small bowel series, enteroclysis, or CT of the abdomen	Narrowed segments of intestine; "apple-core" or "napkin-ring sign"; partial or complete obstruction	None
Whipple's disease	Small bowel series	Dilation and distorted loops of small bowel	None

*Dependent on stage or severity of disease or condition.

Small Bowel Procedures

Four methods are used to study the small intestine radiographically. Methods 1 and 2 are the more common methods. Methods 3 and 4 are special small bowel studies done if Methods 1 and 2 are unsatisfactory or contraindicated.

1. UGI–small bowel combination
2. Small bowel only series
3. Enteroclysis
4. Intubation method

CONTRAST MEDIA

A thin mixture of barium sulfate is used for most small bowel series. In the case of suspected perforated bowel or if surgery is going to follow the SBS, a water-soluble, iodinated contrast media may be given. If the patient has hypomotility of the bowel, ice water or another stimulant may be provided to increase the transit of the barium. Also, water-soluble, iodinated contrast media can be added to the barium to increase peristalsis and the transit time of the contrast media through the small intestine.

1. UPPER GI–SMALL BOWEL COMBINATION

For an upper GI–small bowel combination procedure a routine upper GI series is done first. After the routine stomach study, progress of the barium is followed through the entire small bowel. During a routine upper GI series, the patient generally should have ingested 1 full cup or 8 ounces of barium sulfate mixture. For any small bowel examination the time that the patient ingested this barium should be noted because timing for sequential radiographs is frequently based on the ingestion of this first cup during the UGI procedure. Some departments, however, begin the timing on ingestion of the second cup.

After completion of fluoroscopy and routine radiography of the stomach, the patient is given 1 additional cup of barium to ingest. The time that this is done should also be noted. Then, 30 minutes after the initial barium ingestion, a PA radiograph of the proximal small bowel is obtained. This first radiograph of the small bowel series (marked "30 minutes") is usually obtained about 15 minutes after completion of the UGI series.

Radiographs are obtained at specific intervals throughout the small bowel series until the barium sulfate column passes through the ileocecal valve and progresses into the ascending colon. For the first 2 hours in the small bowel series, radiographs are usually obtained at 15- to 30-minute intervals. If continuing the examination beyond the 2-hour time frame becomes necessary, then radiographs are usually obtained every hour until barium passes through the ileocecal valve. (See procedure summary on upper right.)

Review of Images As soon as each radiograph in the small bowel series is processed, it should be reviewed by the radiologist. The physician may wish to examine any suspicious area under the fluoroscope or request additional radiographs.

Fluoroscopic Study The region of the terminal ileum and ileocecal valve is generally studied fluoroscopically. Spot filming of the terminal ileum usually indicates completion of the examination.

The patient shown in Fig. 15-23 is in position under the compression cone, which, when lowered against the abdomen, spreads out loops of ileum to better visualize the ileocecal valve.

Delayed Radiographs The radiologist may request delayed radiographs to follow the barium through the entire large bowel. A barium meal given by mouth usually reaches the rectum in 24 hours.

PROCEDURE SUMMARY

1. Upper GI—Small Bowel Combination

Basic:
- Routine UGI first
- Notation of time patient ingested first cup (8 oz) of barium
- Ingestion of second cup of barium
- 30-minute PA radiograph (centering high for proximal SB)
- Half-hour interval radiographs, centered to iliac crest, until barium reaches large bowel (usually 2 hours)
- 1-hour interval radiographs if more time is needed after 2 hours

Optional:
- Fluoroscopy and spot filming of ileocecal valve and terminal ileum (compression cone may be used)

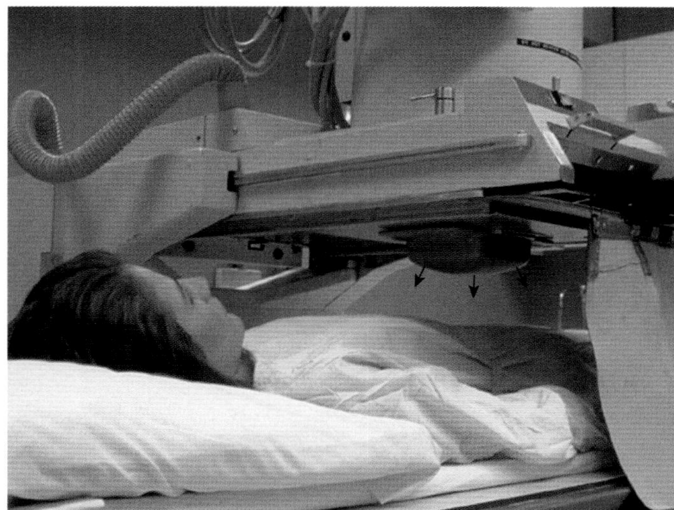

Fig. 15-23. Fluoroscopy of ileocecal region with compression cone.

15

2. SMALL BOWEL ONLY SERIES

The second possibility for study of the small intestine is the small bowel only series, as summarized on the right. For every contrast medium examination, including the small bowel series, a plain radiograph should be obtained before introduction of the contrast medium.

For the small bowel only series, 2 cups (16 ounces) of barium are generally ingested by the patient, and the time is noted. Depending on departmental protocol, the first radiograph is taken either 15 or 30 minutes after completion of barium ingestion. This first radiograph requires high centering to include the diaphragm. From this point on, the exam is exactly like the follow-up series of the UGI. Half-hour radiographs are generally taken for 2 hours, with 1-hour radiographs thereafter, until barium reaches the cecum and/or ascending colon.

Note: Some routines may include continuous half-hour imaging until the barium reaches the cecum.

In the routine small bowel series, regular barium sulfate ordinarily reaches the large intestine within 2 or 3 hours, but this time varies greatly among patients.

Fluoroscopy with spot filming and use of a compression cone may again be an option to better visualize the ileocecal valve.

3. ENTEROCLYSIS–DOUBLE-CONTRAST SMALL BOWEL PROCEDURE

A third method of a small bowel study is the **enteroclysis** *(en"ter-ok'li-sis)* procedure, which is a **double-contrast method** used to evaluate the small bowel.

Enteroclysis describes the injection of a nutrient or medicinal liquid into the bowel. In the context of a radiographic small bowel procedure, it refers to a study wherein the patient is intubated under fluoroscopic control with a special **enteroclysis catheter** that passes through the stomach into the duodenum to the region of the duodenojejunal junction (suspensory ligament). With fluoroscopy guidance, a Bilbao or Sellink tube is placed into the terminal duodenum.

First, a high-density suspension of **barium** is injected through this catheter at a rate of 100 ml/minute. Fluoroscopic and conventional radiographs may be taken at this time. Then, either **air** or **methylcellulose** is injected into the bowel to distend it and provide a double-contrast effect. Methylcellulose is preferred because it adheres to the bowel while distending it. This double-contrast effect dilates the loops of small bowel, while increasing visibility of the mucosa. This action leads to increased accuracy of the study.

The disadvantages of enteroclysis are increased patient discomfort and the possibility of bowel perforation during catheter placement.

Enteroclysis is indicated for patients with clinical histories of **small bowel ileus, regional enteritis,** or **malabsorption syndrome.**

On proper filling of the small bowel with the contrast media, the radiologist takes the appropriate fluoroscopy spot images. The technologist may be asked to produce various projections of the small bowel to include AP, PA, obliques, and possibly erect projections.

After the procedure is completed, the catheter is removed and the patient encouraged to increase water intake and possibly laxatives.

The radiograph seen in Fig. 15-24 is an example of an enteroclysis. The end of the catheter *(small arrows)* is seen in the distal duodenum, not yet reaching the duodenojejunal junction (ligament of Treitz; *large upper arrow*). The introduction of the methylcellulose dilates the lumen of the bowel, while the barium coats the mucosa.

PROCEDURE SUMMARY

2. Small Bowel Only Series

Basic:
- Plain abdomen radiograph (scout)
- 2 cups (16 oz) of barium ingested (noting time)
- 15- to 30-minute radiograph (centered high for proximal SB)
- Half-hour interval radiographs (centered to crest) until barium reaches large bowel (usually 2 hours)
- 1-hour interval radiographs, if more time is needed (some routines including continuous half-hour intervals)

Optional:
- Fluoroscopy with compression sometimes required

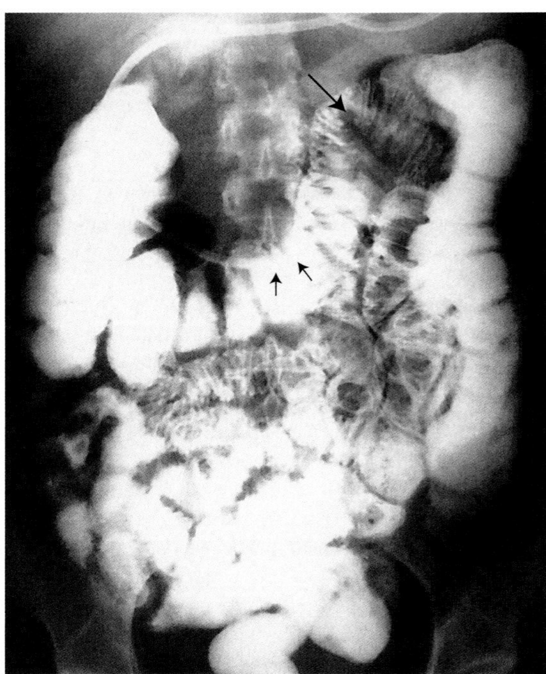

Fig. 15-24. PA radiograph–enteroclysis.

PROCEDURE SUMMARY

3. Enteroclysis (Double-Contrast Small Bowel Series)

Procedure:
- Special catheter advanced to duodenojejunal junction
- Thin mixture of barium sulfate instilled
- Air or methylcellulose instilled
- Fluoroscopic spot films and conventional radiographs taken
- On successful completion of exam, intubation tube removed

15

4. INTUBATION METHOD—SINGLE-CONTRAST MEDIA STUDY

The fourth and final method of small bowel study is GI **intubation** *(in"tu-ba'shun),* sometimes referred to as a *small bowel enema.* This is a technique whereby a **nasogastric tube** is passed through the patient's nose, through the esophagus, stomach, duodenum, and into the jejunum (Fig. 15-25). This radiograph demonstrates the end of the tube *(small arrows)* still looped in the lower part of the stomach, having not yet passed into the duodenum. The extended air-filled loops of small bowel demonstrating air-fluid levels indicate some type of small bowel obstruction.

This procedure is performed for both diagnostic and therapeutic purposes. The **diagnostic intubation** procedure may be referred to as a ***small bowel enema.*** A **single-lumen tube** is passed into the proximal jejunum. Placing the patient into an RAO position may aid in passing the tube from the stomach into the duodenum by gastric peristaltic action. Either a water-soluble iodinated agent or a thin-barium sulfate suspension is then injected through the tube. Radiographs are taken at timed intervals, similar to a standard small bowel series.

The **therapeutic intubation** procedure is often performed to relieve postoperative distention or decompress a small bowel obstruction. A **double-lumen** catheter, termed a ***Miller-Abbott (M-A) tube,*** is advanced into the stomach. Mercury may be instilled on the outer lumen to aid in the advancement of the catheter. Through peristalsis the catheter is advanced into the jejunum. The technologist may be asked to take radiographs at timed intervals to determine whether the catheter is advancing. Gas and excessive fluids can be withdrawn through the catheter.

An optional part of this study may include fluoroscopy, wherein the tube can be guided into the duodenum by the use of compression and manual manipulation.

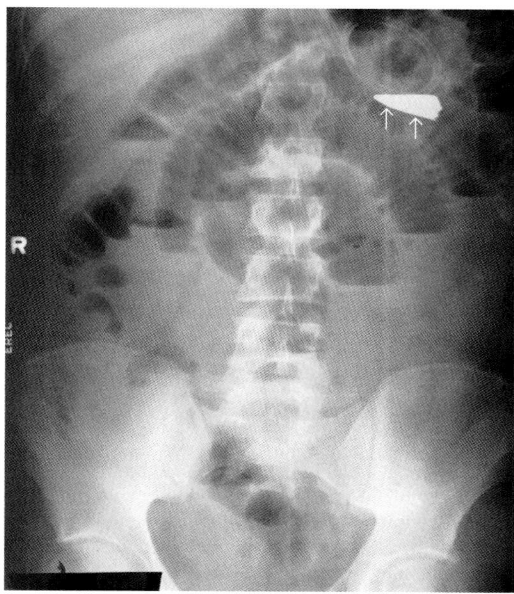

Fig. 15-25. AP erect abdomen—intubation method.

PROCEDURE SUMMARY

4. Intubation Method (Single-Contrast Small Bowel Series)

Procedure:
- Single lumen catheter advanced to proximal jejunum (double lumen catheter for therapeutic intubation)
- Water-soluble iodinated agent or thin mixture of barium sulfate instilled
- Time noted at which that contrast media instilled
- Conventional radiographs or optional fluoroscopic spot films taken at specific time intervals

PATIENT PREPARATION

Patient preparation for a small bowel series is identical to that for an upper GI series. In fact, the most common method of small bowel study is a combination of the two examinations into one long examination, with the small bowel series following the UGI series.

The goal of patient preparation for either the upper GI series or the small bowel series is an **empty stomach.** Food and fluid must be withheld for at least **8 hours** before these exams. Ideally, the patient should be on a low-residue diet 48 hours before the small bowel series. In addition, the patient should not smoke cigarettes or chew gum during the NPO period. Before the procedure the patient should be asked to void, so as not to cause displacement of the ileum due to a distended bladder.

PREGNANCY PRECAUTIONS

If the patient is a female, a menstrual history must be obtained. Irradiation of an early pregnancy is one of the most hazardous situations in diagnostic radiography. X-ray examinations such as the small bowel series or the barium enema that include the pelvis and uterus in the primary beam and also include fluoroscopy **should not be done on pregnant females unless absolutely necessary.** If the patient is unsure whether she may be pregnant, the technologist should bring this to the attention of the radiologist. A pregnancy test may be ordered before the procedure.

METHOD OF IMAGING

Imaging for any overhead radiograph during a small bowel series is done on 35- × 43-cm (14- × 17-inch) image receptors to visualize as much of the small intestine as possible. Spot imaging of selected portions of the small bowel is done on smaller-sized IRs.

The prone position is usually used during a small bowel series, unless the patient is unable to assume that position. The **prone position** allows abdominal compression **to separate the various loops of bowel and create a higher degree of visibility.** Asthenic patients may be placed in the Trendelenburg position to separate overlapping loops of ileum.

For the 30-minute radiograph, the IR is placed high enough to include the stomach on the finished radiograph. This placement requires longitudinal centering to the duodenal bulb and side-to-side centering to the midsagittal plane. Approximately three fourths of the IR should extend above the iliac crest. Because most of the barium is in the stomach and proximal small bowel, a high-kV technique should be utilized on this initial radiograph.

All radiographs after the initial 30-minute exposure should be centered to the iliac crest. For the 1-hour and later radiographs, medium-kilovoltage techniques may be used because barium is spread through more of the alimentary canal and not concentrated in the stomach. Spot imaging of the terminal ileum usually completes the examination.

Barium Enema (BE or Lower GI Series)

DEFINITION

The radiographic study of the large intestine is commonly termed a *barium enema.* It requires the use of a contrast media to demonstrate the large intestine and its components. Alternative names include *BE* (BaE) and *lower GI series*.

PURPOSE

The purpose of the barium enema is to **radiographically study the form and function of the large intestine to detect any abnormal conditions.** Both the single-contrast and the double-contrast barium enema include a study of the **entire large intestine.**

CONTRAINDICATIONS

The two strict contraindications for the barium enema are similar to those described for the small bowel series. These were described as a **possible perforated hollow viscus** and a **possible large bowel obstruction.** These patients should not be given barium as a contrast media agent. Although not as radiopaque as barium sulfate, water-soluble contrast media can be used for these conditions.

A careful review of the patient's chart and clinical history may help prevent problems during the procedure. The radiologist should be informed of any conditions or disease processes noted in the patient's chart. This information may dictate the type of study that will be performed.

Also important is to review the patient's chart to determine whether the patient had a **sigmoidoscopy** or **colonoscopy** before the barium enema. If a **biopsy of the colon** was performed during these procedures, the involved section of the colon wall may be weakened, which may lead to perforation during the barium enema. The **radiologist must be informed of this** situation before beginning the procedure.

Appendicitis The barium enema is generally not performed in cases of acute appendicitis because of the danger of perforation.

High-resolution **ultrasound** with graded compression and CT have become the modalities of choice for the diagnosis of acute appendicitis when clinical indications are unclear.

PATHOLOGIC INDICATIONS (BARIUM ENEMA)

Common pathologic indications for a barium enema include the following:

Colitis *(ko-li'tis)* is an **inflammatory condition of the large intestine** that may be caused by many factors, including bacterial infection, diet, stress, and other environmental conditions. The intestinal mucosa can appear rigid and thick, and haustral markings may be missing along the involved segment. Because of chronic inflammation and spasm, the intestinal wall has a "saw-tooth" or jagged appearance.

Ulcerative colitis describes a severe form of colitis that is most common in young adults. It is a chronic condition that often leads to coinlike ulcers developing within the mucosal wall. These ulcers may be seen during the barium enema as multiple ring-shaped filling defects, creating a "cobblestone" appearance along the mucosa. Patients with long-term bouts of ulcerative colitis may develop "stovepipe" colon, in which the haustral markings and flexures are mostly absent.

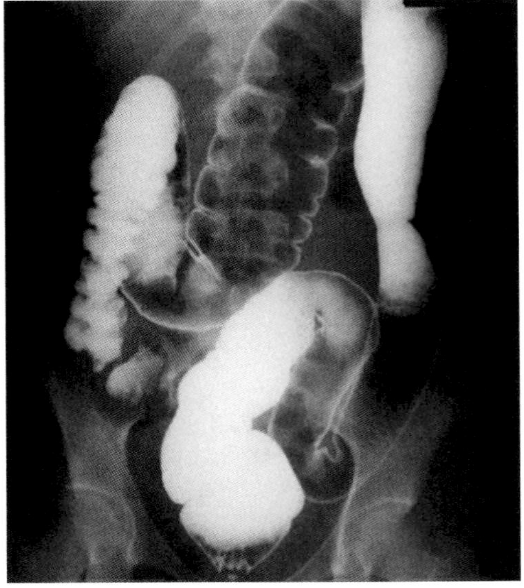

Fig. 15-26. BE, double-contrast study.

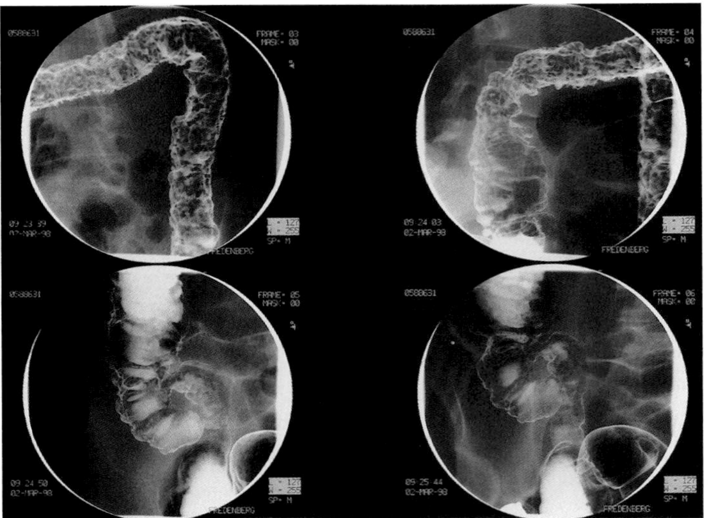

Fig. 15-27. Ulcerative colitis.

15

Diverticulum *(di"ver-tik'u-lum)* is an **outpouching of the mucosal wall** resulting from a herniation of the inner wall of the colon. Although a relatively benign condition, it may become widespread throughout the colon but is most prevalent in the sigmoid colon. It is most common in adults past the age of 40 years. The condition of having numerous diverticula is termed ***diverticulosis.*** If these diverticula become infected, the condition is then referred to as ***diverticulitis.*** Inflamed diverticula may become a source of bleeding, in which case surgical removal may be necessary. A patient may develop peritonitis if a diverticulum perforates through the mucosal wall.

Diverticula appear as small barium-filled circular defects projecting **outward** from the colon wall during a barium enema (see small *arrows* in Fig. 15-28). The double-contrast barium enema provides an excellent view of the intestinal mucosal and demonstrates small diverticula present. The double-contrast barium enema clearly demonstrates the presence of most diverticula.

Intussusception *(in"ta-sa-sep'shan)* is a telescoping or invagination of one part of the intestine into another. It is most common in infants under 2 years of age but can occur in adults. A barium enema or an air/gas enema may play a therapeutic role in reexpanding the involved bowel. Radiographically the barium column terminates into a "mushroom-shaped" dilation with very little barium/gas passing beyond it. This dilation marks the point of the obstruction. Intussusception must be resolved quickly so that it does not lead to obstruction and necrosis of the bowel (see Chapter 20). If the condition recurs, surgery may be needed.

Neoplasms are common in the large intestine. Although benign tumors do occur, carcinoma of the large intestine is a leading cause of death in both males and females. A majority of carcinomas of the large intestine occur in the rectum and sigmoid colon. These cancerous tumors often encircle the lumen of the colon, producing an irregular channel through it. The radiographic appearance of these tumors as demonstrated during a barium enema leads to descriptive terms such as "apple-core" or "napkin-ring" lesions. Both benign and malignant tumors may begin as **polyps.**

Annular carcinoma (adenocarcinoma) is one of the most typical forms of colon cancer that may form an "apple-core" or "napkin-ring" appearance as the tumor grows and infiltrates the bowel walls. It frequently results in large bowel obstruction.

Polyps are saclike projections similar to diverticula except that they project **inward** into the lumen rather than outward as do diverticula. Like diverticula, polyps can become inflamed and be a source of bleeding, in which case they may need to be surgically removed. Barium enema, endoscopy, and CT are the most effective modalities in demonstrating neoplasm in the large intestine.

Volvulus *(vol'vu-lus)* is a twisting of a portion of the intestine on its own mesentery, leading to a mechanical-type obstruction. Blood supply to the twisted portion is compromised, leading to obstruction and necrosis, or localized death of tissue. A volvulus may be found in portions of the jejunum or ileum or in the cecum and sigmoid colon. Volvulus is more likely to occur in males than females and is most common between the ages of 20 and 50 years. The classic sign is called a "beak" sign, a tapered narrowing at the volvulus site as demonstrated during a barium enema. A volvulus will produce an air-fluid level, as well demonstrated on an erect abdomen projection.

Cecal volvulus describes the ascending colon and the cecum having a long mesentery, making them more susceptible to a volvulus.

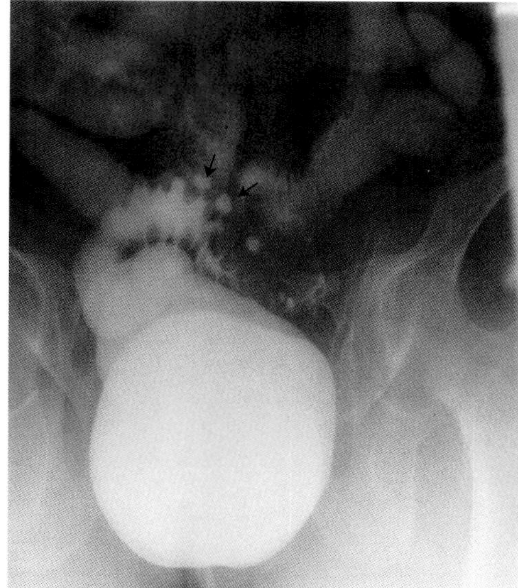

Fig. 15-28. Diverticulum of sigmoid colon.

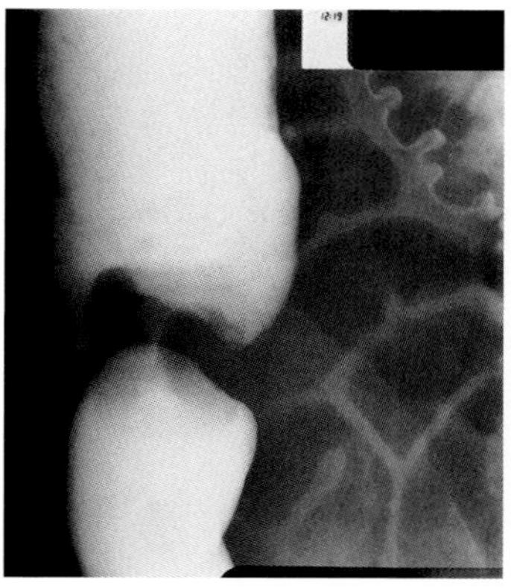

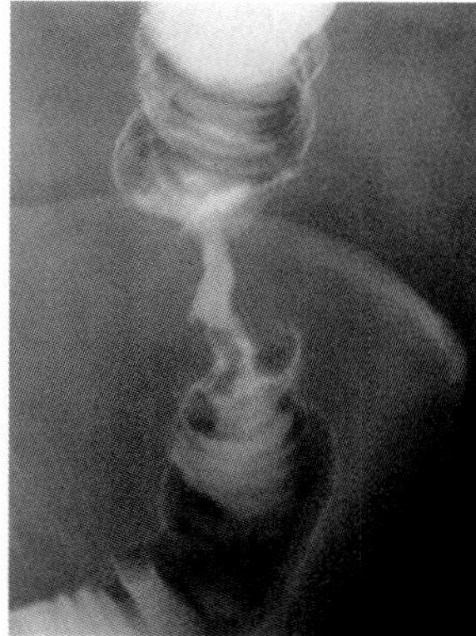

Fig. 15-29. Neoplasm—colon cancer with "apple-core" lesion *(left).* Advanced carcinoma of the colon *(right).*

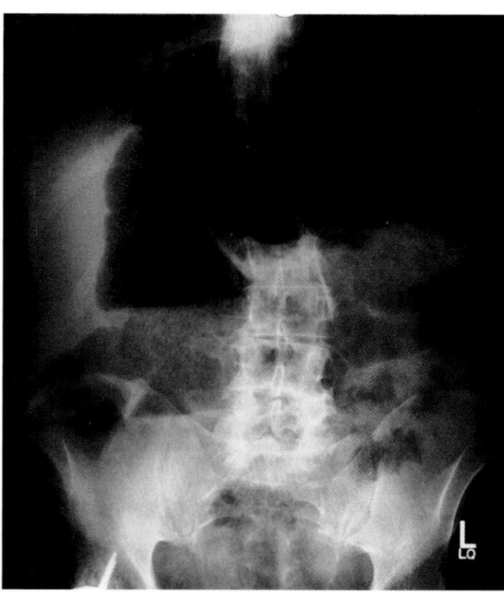

Fig. 15-30. Cecal volvulus.

15

LARGE INTESTINE—SUMMARY OF PATHOLOGIC INDICATIONS

CONDITION OR DISEASE	MOST COMMON RADIOGRAPHIC EXAM	POSSIBLE RADIOGRAPHIC APPEARANCE	MANUAL EXPOSURE FACTOR ADJUSTMENT*
Colitis	Single- and double-contrast (preferred) BE	Thickening of mucosal wall with loss of haustral markings	None
Ulcerative colitis	Single- and double-contrast (preferred) BE	"Cobblestone" and possible "stovepipe" appearance with severe forms	None
Diverticulum (diverticulosis/ diverticulitis)	Double-contrast BE recommended	Barium-filled circular defects projecting outward from colon wall; jagged or "sawtooth" appearance of the mucosa	None
Intussusception	Single or air/gas contrast enema recommended	"Mushroom-shaped" dilation at the distal aspect of the intussusception, with very little barium or gas passing beyond it	None
Neoplasm	Double-contrast BE recommended to detect small polyps	Filling defects; narrowness or tapering of lumen; "apple-core" or "napkin-ring" lesions	None
Polyps	Double-contrast BE recommended	Barium-filled, saclike projections projecting inward into the lumen of bowel	None
Volvulus	Single-contrast BE	Tapered or "corkscrew" appearance, with air-filled distended bowel	None

*Dependent on stage or severity of disease or condition.

Barium Enema Procedure

PATIENT PREPARATION

Preparation of the patient for a barium enema is more involved than is preparation for the stomach and small bowel. The final objective, however, is the same. The **section of alimentary canal to be examined must be empty.** Thorough cleansing of the entire large bowel is of paramount importance to the satisfactory contrast-medium study of the large intestine.

CONTRAINDICATIONS TO LAXATIVES (CATHARTICS)

Certain conditions contraindicate the use of very effective cathartics or purgatives needed to thoroughly cleanse the large bowel. These exceptions are (1) gross bleeding, (2) severe diarrhea, (3) obstruction, and (4) inflammatory conditions such as appendicitis.

A laxative is a substance that produces frequent soft or liquid bowel movements. These substances increase peristalsis in the large bowel and occasionally in the small bowel as well by irritating the sensory nerve endings in the intestinal mucosa. This increased peristalsis dramatically accelerates the passage of intestinal contents through the digestive system.

TWO CLASSES OF LAXATIVES

Two different classes of laxatives may be prescribed. First are the irritant laxatives, such as castor oil; second are the saline laxatives, such as magnesium citrate or magnesium sulfate. The use of irritant laxatives is rare today. For best results, bowel-cleansing procedures should be specified on patient instruction sheets for both inpatients and outpatients. A technologist should be completely familiar with the type of preparation used in each radiology department. The importance of a clean bowel for a barium enema, and especially for a double-contrast barium enema, cannot be overstated. Any retained fecal matter may obscure the normal anatomy or give false diagnostic information and lead to a rescheduling of the procedure after the colon has been properly cleaned.

RADIOGRAPHIC ROOM PREPARATION

The radiographic room should be prepared in advance of the patient's arrival. The fluoroscopic room and examination table should be clean and tidy for each patient. The control panel should be set for fluoroscopy, with the appropriate technical factors selected. The fluoroscopy timer may be set up to its maximum time, which is usually 5 minutes. If conventional fluoroscopy is used, the photospot mechanism should be in proper working order and a supply of spot-film cassettes handy. The appropriate number and size of conventional cassettes should be provided. Protective lead aprons and lead gloves should be provided for the radiologist, as well as lead aprons for all other personnel to be in the room. The fluoroscopic table should be placed in the horizontal position, with waterproof backing or disposable pads placed on the tabletop. Waterproof protection is essential in case of premature evacuation of the enema.

The Bucky tray must be positioned at the foot end of the table if the fluoroscopy tube is located beneath the tabletop. This will expand the Bucky slot shield, reducing gonadal dose to the fluoroscopist, as described in Chapter 14 (see Fig. 14-51). The radiation foot control switch should be placed appropriately for the radiologist or the remote control area prepared. Tissues, towels, replacement linen, bedpan, extra gowns, a room air freshener, and a waste receptacle should be readily available. The appropriate contrast medium or media, container, tubing, and enema tip should be prepared. A proper lubricant should be provided for the enema tip. The type of barium sulfate used and the concentration of the mixture vary considerably, depending on radiologist preferences and the type of examination to be performed.

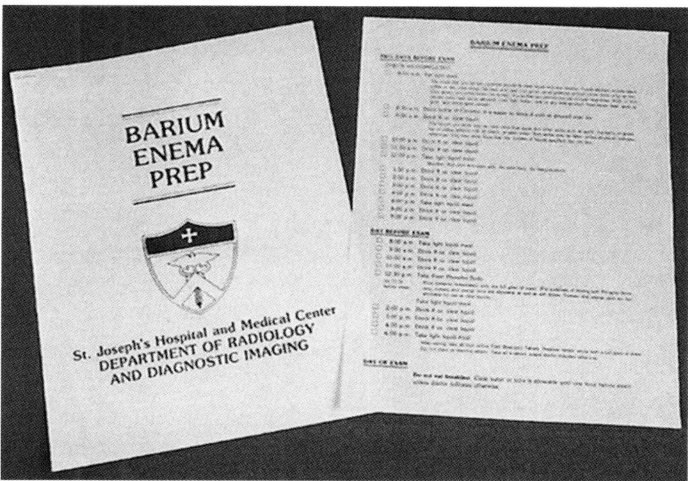

Fig. 15-31. Patient preparation instructions. (Courtesy St. Joseph's Hospital and Medical Center, Phoenix, Ariz.)

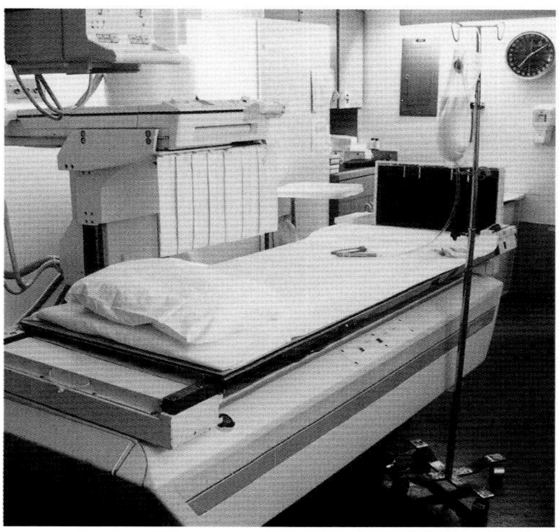

Fig. 15-32. Room preparation.

EQUIPMENT AND SUPPLIES

Barium Enema Containers A closed-system enema container is used to administer the barium sulfate or the air and barium sulfate combination during the barium enema (Fig. 15-33). This closed-type disposable barium enema bag system has replaced the older open-type system for convenience and to reduce the risk of cross-infection.

This system, shown in the photograph, demonstrates the disposable enema bag with a pre-measured amount of barium sulfate. Once mixed, the suspension travels down its own connective tubing, and flow is controlled by a plastic stopcock. An enema tip is placed on the end of the tubing and inserted in the patient's rectum.

After the examination, much of the barium can be drained back into the bag by lowering the system below tabletop level. The entire bag and tubing are disposed of after a single use.

Enema Tips Various types and sizes of enema tips are available (Fig. 15-34). The three most common enema tips are *(A)* plastic disposable, *(B)* rectal retention, and *(C)* air-contrast retention enema tips. All these are considered single-use, disposable enema tips.

Rectal disposable retention tips *(B and C),* sometimes called *retention catheters,* are used on those patients who have relaxed anal sphincters or those who cannot for any reason retain the enema. These rectal-retention catheters consist of a double-lumen tube with a thin rubber balloon at the distal end. After rectal insertion, this balloon is carefully inflated with air through a small tube to assist the patient in retaining the barium enema. These retention catheters should be **fully inflated only with fluoroscopic guidance by the radiologist** because of the potential dangers of intestinal rupture. Because of the discomfort to the patient, the balloon should not be fully inflated until the fluoroscopy procedure begins.

A special type of rectal tip *(C)* is needed to inject air through a separate tube into the colon, where it mixes with the barium for a **double-contrast BE exam.**

LATEX ALLERGIES

Today most products are primarily latex-free, but determination of whether the patient is sensitive to natural latex products is still important. Patients with sensitivity toward latex experience anaphylactoid-type reactions that include sneezing, redness, rashes, difficulty in breathing, and even death.

If the patient has a history of latex sensitivity, the technologist must ensure that the enema tip, tubing, and gloves are latex-free. Even the dust produced by removal of gloves may introduce latex protein into the air, which could be inhaled by the patient.

Technologists with latex sensitivity must be keenly aware of the type of gloves, catheters, and other latex devices found in the department. If a rash develops while wearing gloves or handling certain objects, they should consult their physician to determine whether they have latex sensitivity.

CONTRAST MEDIA

Barium sulfate is the most common type of positive-contrast media used for the barium enema. The concentration of the barium sulfate suspension varies according to the study performed. A standard mixture used for single-contrast media barium enemas ranges between 15% and 25% weight-to-volume (w/v). The thicker barium used for double-contrast barium enemas has a weight-to-volume concentration between 75% and 95% or higher. The evacuative proctogram (see p. 508) requires a contrast media with a minimum weight-to-volume of 100%.

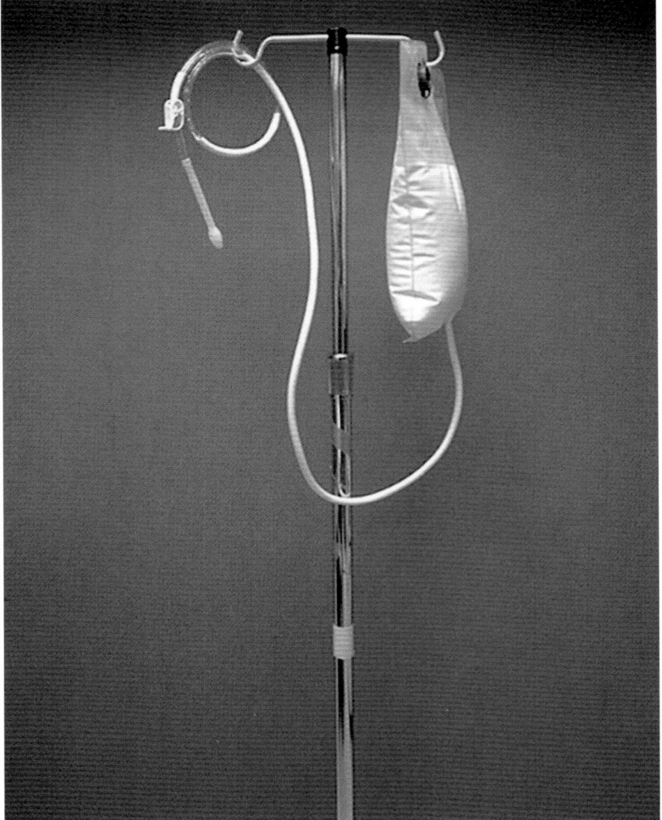

Fig. 15-33. Closed-system enema container.

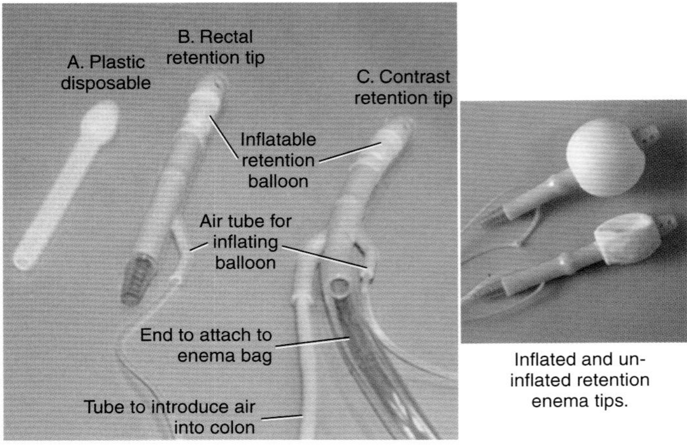

Fig. 15-34. Enema tips, three types.

Negative-Contrast Agent The double-contrast media also uses a number of negative-contrast agents in addition to the barium sulfate. Room air, nitrogen, and carbon dioxide are the most common forms of negative-contrast media used. Carbon dioxide is gaining wide use because it is well tolerated by the large intestine and is absorbed rapidly after the procedure. Carbon dioxide and nitrogen gas are stored in a small tank and can be introduced into the rectum through an air-contrast retention enema tip.

An iodinated, water-soluble contrast media may be used in the case of a perforated or lacerated intestinal wall or if the patient is scheduled for surgery after the barium enema. Remember that a lower kV (70 to 80) should be used with a water-soluble and negative-contrast agent.

Contrast Media Preparation The mixing instructions as supplied by the manufacturer should be followed precisely.

A debate has evolved over the temperature of the water used to prepare the barium sulfate suspension. Some experts recommend the use of cold water (40°-45° F) in the preparation of the contrast media. The cold water is reported to have an anesthetic effect on the colon and increase retention of the contrast media. Critics have stated that the cold water may lead to colonic spasm.

Room-temperature water (85°-90°) is recommended by most experts to produce a more successful examination with maximal patient comfort. The technologist should NEVER use hot water to prepare the contrast media. The hot water may scald the mucosal lining of the colon.

Because the barium sulfate produces a colloidal suspension, shaking the enema bag before tip insertion is important to prevent separation of the barium sulfate and water.

Spasm during the barium enema is a common side effect. Patient anxiety, overexpansion of the intestinal wall, discomfort, and related disease process all may lead to colonic spasm. To minimize the possibility of spasm, a topical anesthetic such as lidocaine may be added to the contrast media. If spasm does occur during the study, glucagon can be given intravenously and should be kept in the department for these situations.

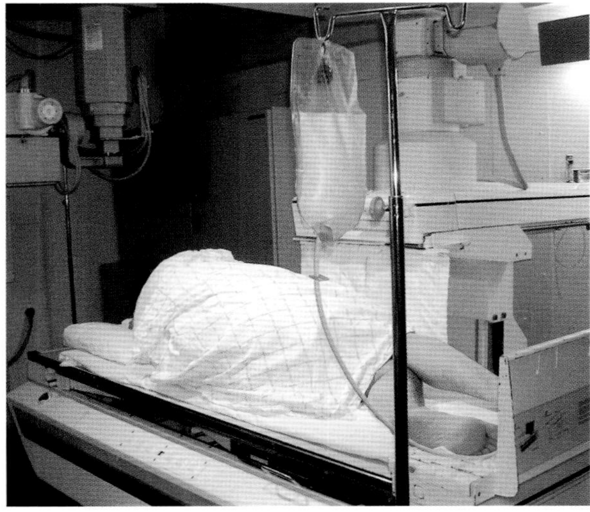

Fig. 15-35. Procedure preparation.

PROCEDURE PREPARATION

A barium enema patient is examined in an appropriate hospital gown. A cotton gown with the opening and ties in the back is preferable. The type of gown that must be pulled over the patient's head to remove should never be used. Sometimes the gown becomes soiled during the examination. The outpatient is instructed to remove all clothing, including shoes and socks or hose. Disposable slippers should be provided in case some barium is lost on the way to the rest room.

After the fluoroscopic room is completely prepared and the contrast medium ready, the patient is escorted to the examination room. Before insertion of the enema tip, a pertinent history should be taken and the examination carefully explained. Because complete cooperation is essential and this examination can be somewhat embarrassing, every effort should be made to reassure the patient at every stage of the exam.

Any previous radiographs should be available for the radiologist. The patient is placed in the **Sims position** before insertion of the enema tip.

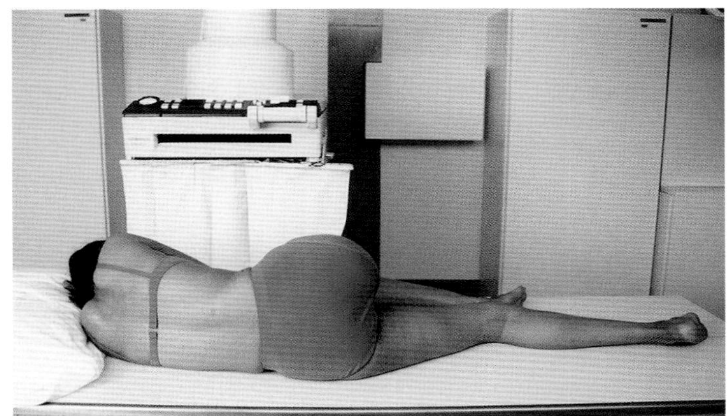

Fig. 15-36. Sims position (for rectal tip insertion).

Sims Position The Sims position is shown in Fig. 15-36. The patient is asked to roll onto the left side and lean forward. The right leg is flexed at the knee and hip and is placed in front of the left leg. The left knee is comfortably flexed. The Sims position relaxes the abdominal muscles and decreases pressure within the abdomen.

Each phase of the rectal-tube insertion must be explained to the patient. Before insertion, the barium sulfate solution should be well mixed and a little of the barium mixture run into a waste receptacle to ensure that no air remains in the tubing or enema tip.

Preparation for Rectal Tip Insertion The technologist wears a rectal glove and enfolds the enema tip in several sheets of paper toweling. The rectal tip is well lubricated with a water-soluble lubricant.

Before the examination the patient should be instructed to (1) keep the anal sphincter tightly contracted against the rectal tube to hold it in position and prevent leakage; (2) relax the abdominal muscles to prevent increased intraabdominal pressure, and (3) concentrate on breathing by mouth to reduce spasms and cramping. The patient must be assured that barium flow will be stopped if cramping should occur.

ENEMA TIP INSERTION

To insert the enema tip, the opening in the back of the patient's gown should be adjusted to expose only the anal region. The rest of the patient should be well covered when the rectal tube is inserted. The patient's modesty should be protected in any way possible during the barium enema examination. The right buttock should be raised to open the gluteal fold and expose the anus. The patient should take in a few deep breaths before actual insertion of the enema tip. If the tip will not enter with gentle pressure, the patient should be asked to relax and assist if possible. The tip should **NEVER** be forced in such a manner that could cause injury to the patient. Because the abdominal muscles relax on expiration, the tip should be inserted during the exhalation phase of respiration.

The rectum and anal canal present a double curvature; therefore the tube is first inserted in a forward direction approximately 1 to 1½ inches (2.5 to 4 cm). This initial insertion should be **aimed toward the umbilicus.** After the initial insertion the rectal tube is directed **superiorly and slightly anteriorly** to follow the normal curvature of the rectum. The total insertion of the tip should **not exceed 3 to 4 cm** to prevent possible injury to the wall of the rectum. The rectal tube may be taped in place or held to prevent it from slipping out while the patient turns back into a supine position for the start of fluoroscopy. This position is usually supine but may be prone, depending on the preference of the radiologist.

If the retention-type tip is necessary, most departments allow the technologist to instill one or two puffs of air into the balloon end to help hold it in place. However, the bulb should be **filled to its maximum only under fluoroscopic control** as the fluoroscopy procedure begins. As the procedure begins, the IV pole supporting the enema bag should be **no higher than 24 inches (60 cm)** above the radiographic table.

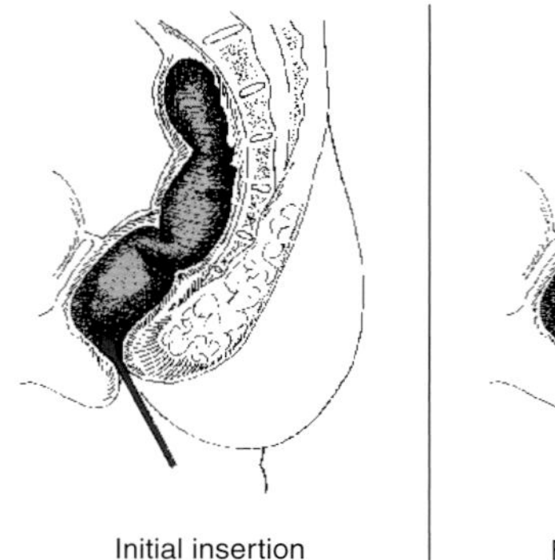

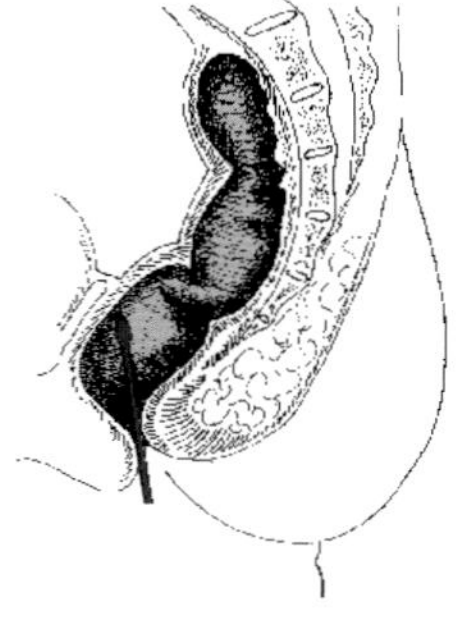

Fig. 15-37. Enema tip insertion.

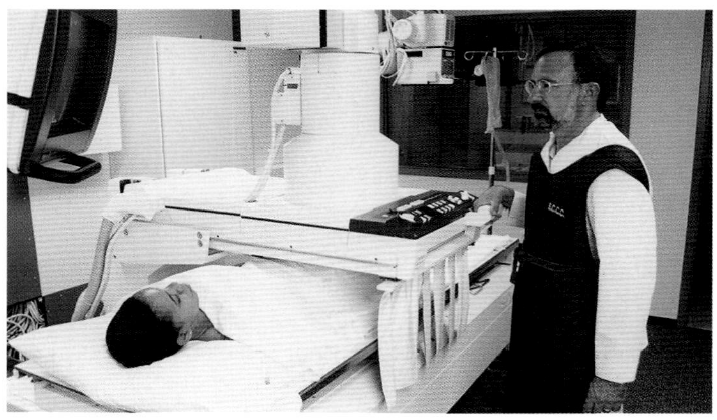

Fig. 15-38. Barium enema fluoroscopy.

SUMMARY OF ENEMA TIP INSERTION PROCEDURE

Step 1 Describe the tip insertion procedure to the patient. Answer any questions.

Step 2 Place patient in Sims position. Patient should lie on the left side, with the right leg flexed at the knee and hip.

Step 3 Shake enema bag once more to ensure proper mixing of barium sulfate suspension. Allow barium to flow through the tubing and from tip to remove any air in the system.

Step 4 Wearing gloves, coat enema tip well with water-soluble lubricant. Wrap proximal aspect of enema tip in paper towel.

Step 5 On expiration, direct enema tip toward the umbilicus approximately 1 to 1½ inches (2.5 to 4 cm).

Step 6 After initial insertion, advance up superiorly and slightly anteriorly. The total insertion should not exceed 3 to 4 cm. Do NOT force enema tip.

Step 7 Tape tubing in place to prevent slippage. Do NOT inflate retention tip unless directed by radiologist.

Step 8 Ensure IV pole/enema bag is no more than 24 inches (60 cm) above the table. Ensure tubing stopcock is in the closed position and no barium flows into the patient.

FLUOROSCOPY ROUTINE

Note: The following routine may differ for those countries or those facilities in which the expanded scope of technologists includes the barium enema fluoroscopy.

The radiologist is summoned to the radiographic room after all room and patient preparations are completed. Following introduction of the physician and patient, the patient's history and the reason for the examination are discussed.

During barium-enema fluoroscopy the general duties of the technologist are to follow the radiologist's instructions, assist the patient as needed, and expedite the procedure in any way possible. The technologist must also control the flow of barium and/or air and change fluoroscopy spot cassettes. The flow of barium is started and stopped several times during the BE. Each time the technologist asks that the flow be started, the technologist should say "barium on" after the clamp or hemostat is released. Each time the technologist requests that the flow be stopped, the technologist should say "barium off" after the tubing is clamped.

Many changes in patient position are made during fluoroscopy. These positional changes are made to better visualize superimposed sections of bowel and aid in advancement of the barium column. The technologist may need to assist the patient with positional moves and ensure that the tubing is not kinked or accidentally pulled out during the examination.

The fluoroscopic procedure begins with a general survey of the patient's abdomen and chest. For some departmental routines, if the retention-type enema tip is required, the air balloon may be inflated under fluoroscopic control at this point.

Various spot radiographs are obtained of selected portions of the large intestine as the barium column proceeds in retrograde fashion from rectum to cecum. At the end of the fluoroscopic procedure a little barium is refluxed through the ileocecal valve and fluoroscopy spots are obtained of that area. Moderate discomfort is usually experienced when the large bowel is totally filled, so the examination must be concluded as rapidly as possible.

Routine overhead radiographs are obtained with the bowel filled unless digital fluoroscopy is used, in which case overhead postfluoroscopy radiographs are generally not required.

TYPES OF LOWER GI EXAMINATIONS (PROCEDURES)

Three specific types of radiographic examinations or procedures of the lower GI described in this chapter are as follows:

1. Single-contrast barium enema
2. Double-contrast barium enema
3. Evacuative proctography (defecogram)

1. SINGLE-CONTRAST BARIUM ENEMA PROCEDURE

The **single-contrast barium enema** is a procedure using only a positive-contrast medium. In most cases the contrast material is barium sulfate in a thin mixture. Occasionally the contrast medium must be a water-soluble contrast material. For example if the patient is to be taken to surgery after the single-contrast enema procedure, then a water-soluble contrast medium must be used.

An example of a single-contrast barium enema using barium sulfate as the contrast medium is shown in Fig. 15-39.

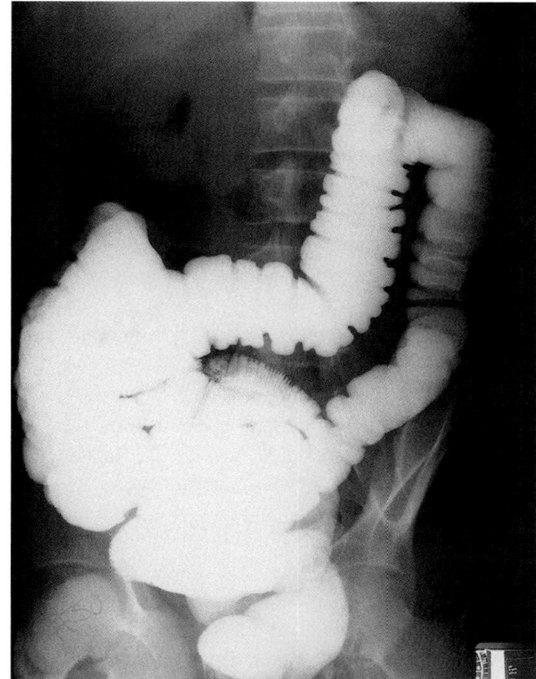

Fig. 15-39. Single-contrast barium enema.

2. DOUBLE-CONTRAST BARIUM ENEMA PROCEDURE

A second common type of barium enema procedure is the **double-contrast type.** Double-contrast studies are more effective in demonstrating polyps and diverticula than the single-contrast barium enema procedure. Radiographic and fluoroscopic procedures for a double-contrast barium enema are somewhat different in that both air and barium must be introduced into the large bowel. Fig. 15-40 is a double-contrast barium enema radiograph taken in the right lateral decubitus position. An absolutely **clean large bowel is essential** to the double-contrast study, and a **much thicker barium mixture is required.** Although exact ratios depend on the commercial preparations used, the ratio approaches a one-to-one mix so that the final product is like heavy cream.

Two-Stage Procedure One preferred method used to coat the bowel is a two-stage, double-contrast procedure. Initially the thick barium is allowed to fill the left side of the intestine, including the left colic flexure. (The purpose of the thick-barium mixture is to facilitate adherence to the mucosal lining.) Air is then instilled into the bowel, pushing the barium column through to the right side. At this time the radiologist may ask that the enema bag be lowered below the table to allow any excess barium to be drained from the large intestine to provide better visualization of the intestinal mucosa.

The second stage consists of inflation of the bowel with a large amount of air/gas that moves the main column of barium forward, leaving only the barium adhering to the mucosal wall. These steps are carried out under fluoroscopic control because the air column cannot be allowed in front of the barium column.

This procedure demonstrates neoplasms or polyps that may be forming on the inner wall of the bowel projecting into the lumen or opening of the bowel. These formations generally would not be visible during a single-contrast, full-column barium enema study.

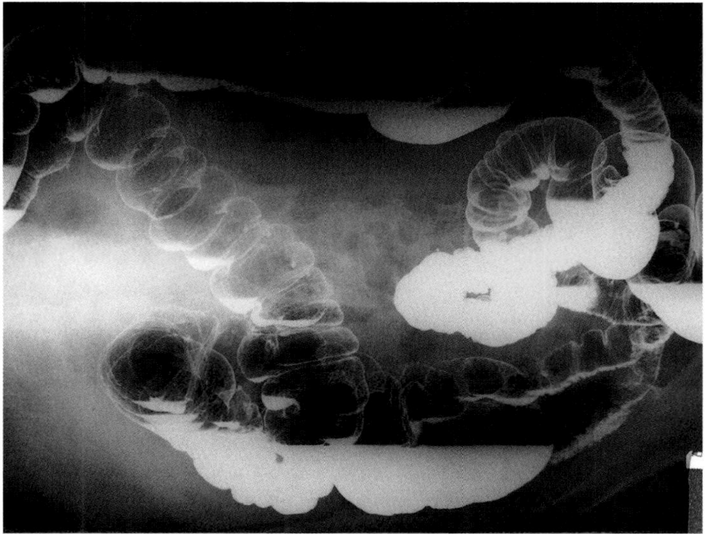

Fig. 15-40. Double-contrast barium enema (right lateral decubitus).

Single-Stage Procedure A single-stage, double-contrast procedure may also be used, wherein the barium and air are instilled in a single procedure that reduces time and radiation exposure to the patient. With this method, some high-density barium is first instilled into the rectum with the patient in a slight Trendelenburg position. The barium tube is then clamped, and with the table in a horizontal position, the patient is placed into the various oblique and lateral positions after the addition of various amounts of air with the double-contrast procedure.

Spot Films (During Fluoroscopy) With both the single-contrast and the double-contrast studies, spot radiographs are obtained to document any suspicious area. The patient may be asked to rotate several times to distribute the barium and air better with the double-contrast procedure.

Digital Fluoroscopy With **digital fluoroscopy** these "spot" images are obtained digitally rather than with separate spot-film cassettes and image intensification. Images taken during the study are then stored in the memory of the computer. Once the images have undergone quality assurance, they are transferred to the PACS system for interpretation. The radiologist can then review all the recorded images and print only images that have diagnostic importance. With PACS, images can be reviewed, read, and stored within the database system without having to produce hard-copy prints.

Postfluoroscopy Radiographs After fluoroscopy and before the patient is allowed to empty the large bowel, if digital fluoroscopy is not used, one or more additional radiographs of the filled bowel should be obtained for either single-contrast or double-contrast procedures. The standard enema tip can be removed before these radiographs because removal may make it easier to hold in the enema. However, some departmental routines keep the enema tip in during the overhead filming procedure. The retention-type tip, however, is generally not removed until the large bowel is ready to be emptied when the patient is placed on a bed pan or on the commode.

Fig. 15-41 demonstrates the most common position for a routine barium enema. This is the **PA projection** with a full-sized 35- × 43-cm (14- × 17-inch) IR centered to the iliac crest. The PA projection with the patient in a prone position is preferred over an AP in a supine position because compression of the abdomen in the prone position results in a more uniform radiographic density of the entire abdomen.

The cassette or IR should be centered to include the rectal ampulla on the bottom of the image. This positioning usually includes the entire large intestine, with the exception of the left colic flexure. Cutting off the left colic flexure on the radiographs may be acceptable if this area is well demonstrated on a previously obtained spot film. However, some departmental routines may include a second image centered higher to include this area on larger patients or two images, with IR placed crosswise.

Other projections are also obtained before evacuation of the barium. Double-contrast procedures generally require right and left lateral decubitus AP or PA projections, with a horizontal x-ray beam to better demonstrate the upside or air-filled portions of the large intestine.

Note: Because of the vast difference in density between the air-filled and the barium-filled aspects of the large intestine, there may be a tendency to overexpose the air-filled region. The recommendation is that the technologist consider using a compensating filter for the decubitus and ventral lateral projections taken during an air-contrast study. One version of a compensating filter that works well attaches to the face of the collimator by two small magnetic disks. The disks can be adjusted to place the filter over the air-filled portion of the large intestine.

All postfluoroscopy radiographs must be obtained as rapidly as possible because the patient may have difficulty retaining the barium.

Once the routine preevacuation radiographs and any supplemental radiographs have been obtained, the patient is allowed to expel the barium. For the patient who has had the enema tip removed, a quick trip to a nearby restroom is necessary. For the patient who cannot make such a trip, a bedpan should be provided. For the patient who is still connected to a closed system, simple lowering of the plastic bag to floor level to allow most of the barium to drain back into the bag is helpful. Department protocol determines how a retention tip should be removed. One way is to first clamp off the retention tip, and then disconnect it from the enema tubing and container. Once the patient is safely on a bedpan or commode, air is released from the bulb and the tip is removed.

Postevacuative Radiograph After most of the barium has been expelled, a postevacuation radiograph is obtained. The postevacuative radiograph is usually taken in the prone position, but may be taken supine if needed. Most of the barium should have been evacuated. If too much barium is retained, the patient is given more time for evacuation, and a second postevacuation image is obtained.

Postprocedure instructions to patients should include increased liquid intake and a high-fiber diet because of the possibility of constipation from the barium (most important for geriatric patients).

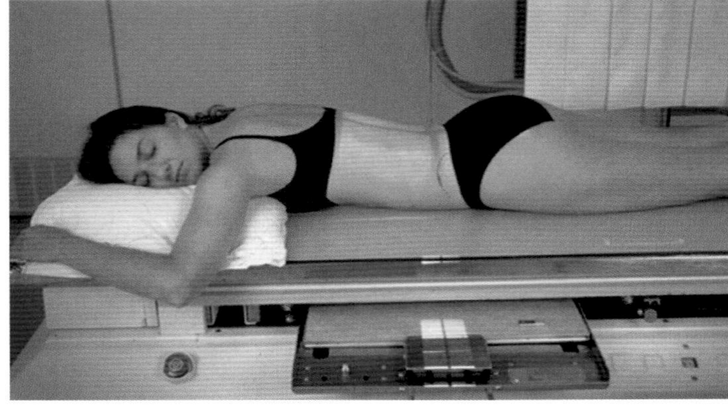

Fig. 15-41. Postfluoroscopy radiography—PA projection.

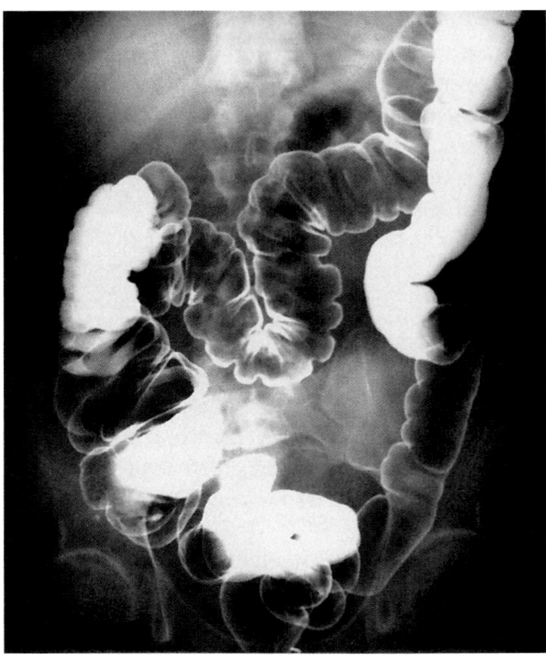

Fig. 15-42. AP, double-contrast barium enema.

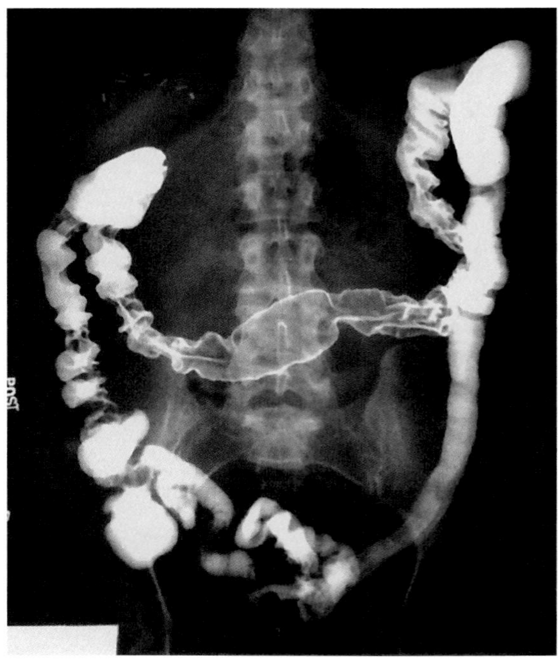

Fig. 15-43. AP supine, postevacuation.

3. EVACUATIVE PROCTOGRAPHY–DEFECOGRAPHY

A third, less common type of radiographic study involving the lower GI tract is **evacuative proctography,** sometimes called ***defecography.*** This study is a more specialized procedure performed in some departments, especially on children or younger adult patients.

Definition and Purpose The evacuative proctography is a **functional study of the anus and rectum during the evacuation and rest phases of defecation** (bowel movement).

Pathologic Indications Pathologic indications for evacuative proctography include **rectoceles, rectal intussusception,** and **prolapse** of the rectum. A rectocele, a common form of the pathologic process, is a blind pouch of the rectum caused by weakening of the anterior or posterior wall. Rectoceles may retain fecal material even after evacuation.

Special Equipment A special commode is required for this study (Fig. 15-44). It consists of a toilet seat built onto a frame that contains a waste receptacle or a disposable plastic bag *(A).* The commode demonstrated has wheels or casters *(B)* so that it can be rolled into position over the extended footboard and platform *(C)* attached to the tabletop *(D).* The entire commode with patient can then be raised or lowered by raising of the tabletop with the attached footboard and commode during the procedure *(arrows).* Clamps should be used (not shown in these photographs) to secure the commode to the footboard platform for stability during the procedure. The clamps allow the commode to be attached to the footboard and raised as needed to utilize the table Bucky and fluoroscopy unit. The seat is often cushioned *(E)* for patient comfort. The filters found beneath the seat (not shown) compensate for tissue differences and help maintain acceptable levels of density and contrast.

Contrast Media To study the process of evacuation, a very high-density barium sulfate mixture is required. Some departments produce their own contrast media by mixing barium sulfate with either potato starch or commercially produced additives. The potato starch thickens the barium sulfate to produce a mashed-potato consistency. The normal barium sulfate suspension evacuates too quickly to detect any pathologic processes.

A ready-to-use contrast media, **Anatrast,** is available (Fig. 15-46). This contrast media is premixed and packaged in a single-use tube. Some departments also introduce a thick liquid barium, such as **Polibar Plus** or **EZ-HD,** before the Anatrast to evaluate the sigmoid colon and the rectum.

Applicator The mechanical applicator (Fig. 15-46) resembles a caulking gun similar to that used in the building industry. The premixed and prepackaged tube of Anatrast is inserted in the applicator and a flexible tube with an enema tip is attached to the opened tip of the tube *(B-1).*

The thick liquid barium is drawn into a syringe and inserted through a rectal tube and tip. In this example an inner plastic tube *(C)* is being used, inserted in an outer rectal tube *(D),* to which the enema tip is attached. The syringe is then used to instill the thick liquid contrast media. The inner plastic tube is attached to the syringe filled with the liquid Polibar Plus or equivalent and inserted within the rectal tube, to which is attached a standard enema tip for insertion into the rectum.

Labeled parts (Fig. 15-46) are as follows:

A. Mechanical applicator
B. Tube of Anatrast (B-1 tip to be opened)
C. Inner plastic tube (for insertion of syringe or tube of Anatrast)
D. Rectal tube (to which enema tip is attached, D-1)
E. Syringe

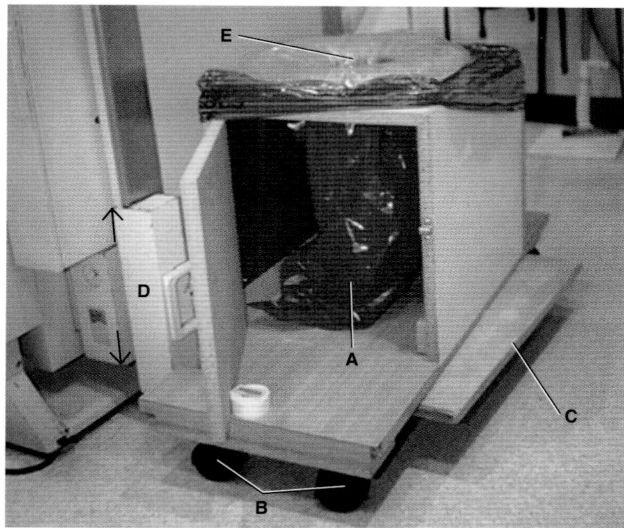

Fig. 15-44. Commode for defecogram.

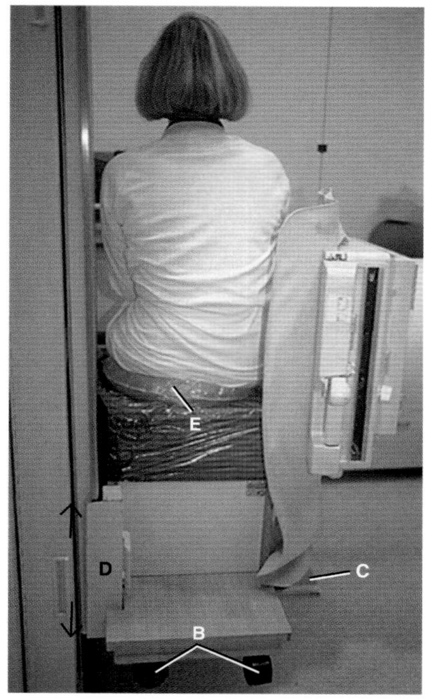

Fig. 15-45. Patient in position.

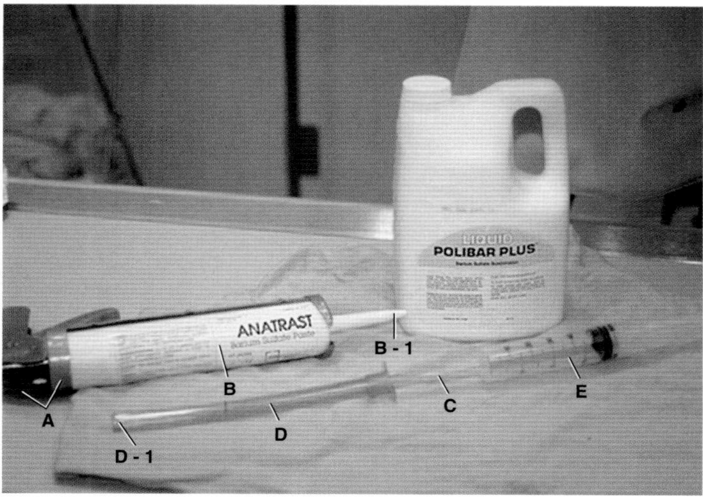

Fig. 15-46. Applicator.

EVACUATIVE PROCTOGRAM PROCEDURE

With the patient in a lateral recumbent position on a cart, the contrast media is instilled into the rectum with the applicator. A nipple marker (small BB) may be placed at the anal orifice.

The patient is quickly placed on the commode for filming during defecation. Lateral video fluoroscopy spot images and standard radiographic projections are taken during the study. The lateral rectum position is usually preferred by most radiologists (Fig. 15-47).

The anorectal angle or junction must be demonstrated during the procedure. This angle is the alignment between the anus and rectum that shifts between the rest and evacuation phases. The radiologist measures this angle during these phases to determine whether any abnormalities exist.

A lateral recumbent postevacuation radiograph is taken as the final part of this procedure (Fig. 15-48).

SUMMARY OF EVACUATIVE PROCTOGRAM PROCEDURE

1. Place radiographic table vertical and attach commode with clamps.
2. Prepare contrast medium according to department specifications.
3. Set up imaging equipment (fluoroscopy, 105-mm spot film camera, spot cassette, or video recorder), or use digital fluoroscopy.
4 Ask patient to remove all clothing and change into a hospital gown.
5. Take a scout image using conventional x-ray tube. (Scout image must include the region of the anorectal angle.)
6. Place patient in a lateral recumbent position on a cart and instill contrast medium.
7. Position patient on the commode and take radiographs in the rest and strain phases, with patient in a lateral position.
8. Using fluoroscopy imaging devices or video recorder, image patient during defecation.
9. Assist in taking of postevacuation radiograph.

Colostomy Barium Enema

Colostomy *(ka-los'ta-me)* is a surgical formation of an artificial or surgical connection between two portions of the large intestine.

In the case of disease, tumor, or inflammatory processes, a section of the large intestine may have been removed or altered. Often, because of a tumor in the sigmoid colon or rectum, this part of the lower intestine is removed. The terminal end of the intestine is then brought to the anterior surface of the abdomen, where an artificial opening is created. This artificial opening is termed a ***stoma.***

In some cases a temporary colostomy is performed to allow healing of the involved section of large intestine. The involved region is bypassed through the use of a the colostomy. Once healing is complete, the two sections of the large intestine are reconnected. Fecal matter is then discharged from the body via the stoma into a special appliance bag that is attached to the skin over the stoma. Once healing is complete, an anastomosis (reconnection) of the two sections of the large intestine is performed surgically. For select patients, the colostomy is permanent due to the amount of large intestine removed or other factors.

CLINICAL INDICATIONS AND PURPOSE

The clinical indications and purpose for the colostomy barium enema are **to assess for proper healing, obstruction, or leakage or to perform a presurgical evaluation.** Sometimes, in addition to the colostomy barium enema, another enema may be given rectally at the same time. This type of study evaluates the terminal large intestine before it is reconnected surgically.

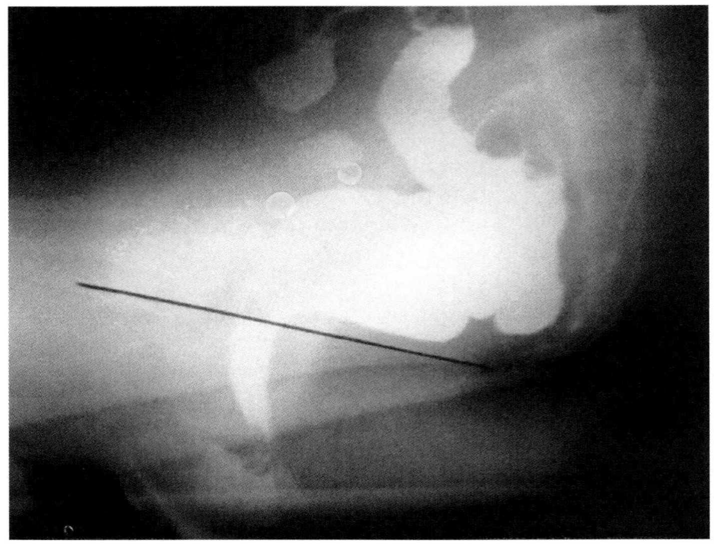

Fig. 15-47. Lateral defecogram (during strain or evacuation).

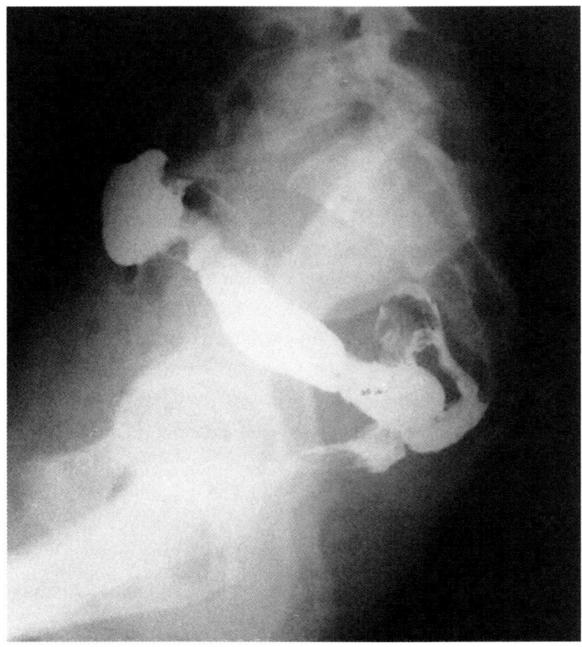

Fig. 15-48. Lateral defecogram (same patient as above—postevacuation).

SPECIAL SUPPLIES FOR COLOSTOMY BARIUM ENEMA

Ready-to-use colostomy barium enema kits (Fig. 15-49) are available that contain stoma tips, tubing, premeasured barium enema bag, adhesive disks, lubricant, and gauze. Because the stoma has no sphincter to retain the barium, a special tapered irrigation tip is inserted into the stoma. Once the irrigation tip has been inserted, a special adhesive pad holds it in place. The enema bag tubing is then attached directly to the irrigation tip.

Small balloon retention catheters (Fig. 15-50) can also be used instead of the tapered irrigation tip. Care must be taken during insertion and inflation of these catheters into the stoma. The stoma is delicate and can be perforated if too much pressure is applied. Most departments require that the radiologist perform this task.

PATIENT PREPARATION

If the barium enema is for nonacute reasons, the patient is asked to irrigate the ostomy before the procedure. The patient may be asked to bring an irrigation device and additional appliance bags. The patient should follow the same dietary restrictions as required for the standard barium enema.

PROCEDURE

Barium sulfate remains the contrast media of choice. A single- or double-contrast media procedure may be performed as with any routine barium enema. Iodinated, water-soluble contrast media may be used if indicated. The colostomy barium enema requires that the contrast media take a different route through the stoma. As a result of bowel resection, anatomic structures and landmarks are often altered. The technologist must observe the anatomy during fluoroscopy to plan for alterations in the positioning routine. Before reattaching the resected bowel (thus eliminating the need for the colostomy), barium may be delivered through both the stoma and the rectum during the procedure to ensure healing is complete. Finally, the technologist should have a clean appliance bag available for the postevacuation phase of the study. Some patients are unable to use the restroom.

SUMMARY OF COLOSTOMY BARIUM ENEMA PROCEDURE

1. Dress the patient in a hospital gown. Depending on the location of the stoma, leave gown open in front or back.
2. Prepare fluoroscopic room, open up tray, and lay out contents.
3. Mix contrast media according to department specifications.
4. Take preliminary scout image using conventional x-ray tube.
5. Wearing gloves, remove and discard dressings covering stoma.
6. Once radiologist has inserted irrigation tip into stoma, tape enema tubing in place.
7. Assist during fluoroscopic phase of study.
8. Take postfluoroscopic "overhead" images as requested.
9. After imaging, lower enema bag, allowing contrast media to flow back into enema bag.
10. Once the intestine is drained, assist in taking of a postevacuation image.
11. Assist patient with cleanup and in securing the appliance bag over the stoma.

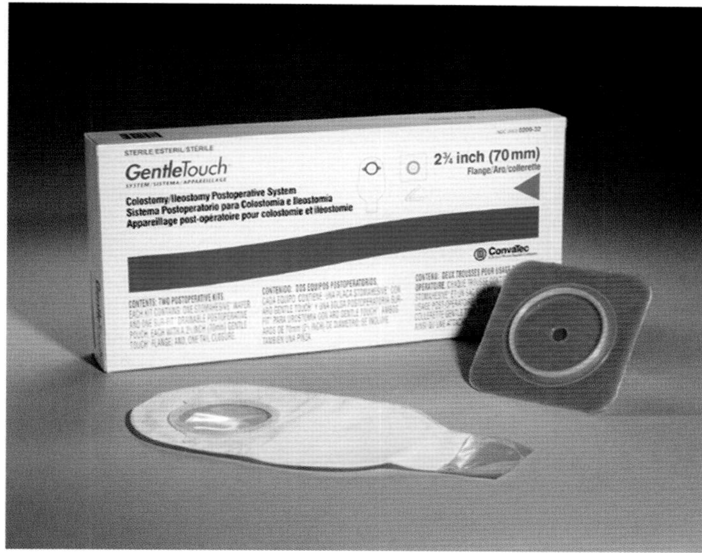

Fig. 15-49. Colostomy postoperative kit. (Courtesy Cona Tec.)

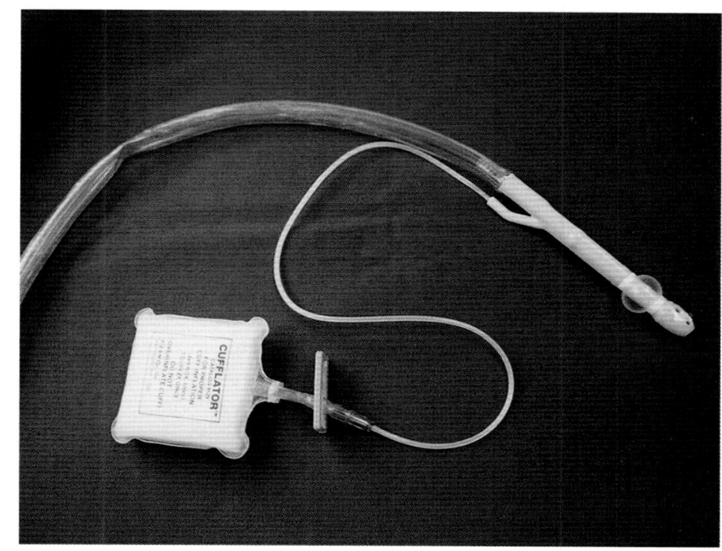

Fig. 15-50. Colostomy tip.

SUMMARY OF SAFETY CONCERNS DURING ALL BARIUM ENEMA PROCEDURES

Safety during any barium enema procedure is of utmost importance. Five of these important safety concerns are as follows:

1. **Review Patient's Chart** Note any pertinent clinical history on the exam requisition and inform the radiologist if the patient had a sigmoidoscopy or colonoscopy before the barium enema, especially if a biopsy was performed. Determine whether the patient has any known allergies to the contrast media or natural latex products.
2. **Never Force Enema Tip Into Rectum** This action may lead to a perforated rectum. The radiologist inserts the enema tip under fluoroscopy guidance, if needed.
3. **The Height of Enema Bag Does Not Exceed 24 Inches (60 cm) Above Table** This distance should be maintained before the beginning of the procedure. The radiologist may wish to raise bag height during the procedure based on the rate of flow of the contrast media.
4. **Verify Water Temperature of Contrast Media** Water that is too hot or cold may injure the patient or compromise the procedure.
5. **Escort Patient to the Restroom After Completion of Study** A barium enema can be stressful for some patients. Patients have been known to faint during or after evacuation.

PEDIATRIC APPLICATIONS

Small Bowel Series and Barium Enema The pediatric small bowel series and barium enema are similar in many ways to those for an adult. However, keep in mind that the transit time of barium from the stomach to the ileocecal region is faster for children as compared with adults. Therefore during the small bowel series images should be taken **every 20 to 30 minutes** to avoid missing critical anatomy and possible pathology during the study. Often, the barium will reach the ileocecal sphincter within 1 hour.

For the barium enema, care must be taken when inserting the enema tip into the rectum. For the infant, often a #10 French, flexible silicone catheter is used. For the older child, a flexible enema tip is recommended to minimize injury to the rectum during insertion.

For both the small bowel series and barium enema, these procedures should be scheduled early in the morning to permit the child to return to normal fluid intake and diet.

Review Chapter 20, Pediatric Radiography, for specific information on bowel and procedure preparation for the small bowl series and barium enema.

GERIATRIC APPLICATIONS

Lower GI procedures such as the barium enema and evacuative proctogram are especially stressful for the geriatric patient. The technologist must exhibit patience and explain the procedure completely. As with all patients, the technologist should provide every opportunity to maintain the modesty of the patient during the procedure. Extra care and patience are frequently required as geriatric patients are turned and moved around on the x-ray table. Because of space disorientation, these patients may experience a fear of falling off the table. Escort the patient to the restroom following the procedure.

Because many geriatric patients have limited sphincter control, the retention balloon enema tip is recommended.

Postprocedural instructions of increased intake of liquids and a high-fiber diet are important for geriatric patients to prevent or minimize possible impaction of the barium. These cautions apply to both upper and lower GI studies or small bowel series, whenever large amounts of barium are ingested by mouth or given retrograde, as with the barium enema.

DIGITAL IMAGING CONSIDERATIONS

With the use of digital fluoroscopy, postfluoroscopy projections taken during the small bowel series and barium enema procedures are less frequently required. However, if overhead projections are requested and computed radiography (CR) is used, the technical considerations concerning **collimation, accurate centering, exposure factors,** and postprocessing **verification of exposure index values** to ensure that the patient was not needlessly overexposed are all important, as described in preceding chapters.

1. **Collimation:** To ensure that the imaging plate (IP) is read correctly by the imaging plate reader and a good diagnostic image is produced, **correct collimation is essential.** By eliminating extraneous tissue or signal from the IP, the laser reader is able to reproduce the analog image correctly without artifact.
2. **Accurate centering:** Most CR systems will scan the IP from the center outward. To reproduce the analog image correctly, **the anatomy must be properly centered.** Careful analysis of body habitus is crucial during a small bowel series or a barium enema procedure. Keep in mind how the position of the small and large bowel will vary between hypersthenic and asthenic patients. If the specific regions of the small or large bowel are not centered to the IP, the laser reader will not reproduce it correctly. It is important to ensure the **central ray, body part,** and **IP are aligned** to permit correct centering of the anatomy of interest.
3. **Exposure factors:** With the CR system, adequate radiation must reach the IP to form a diagnostic image. With most CR systems, a minimum kV and mAs must be used to create an acceptable image. Inadequate kV or mAs will produce a "mottled" image. However, the technologist must not increase mAs needlessly, which will increase patient dose. Departments should have established technical charts to ensure that adequate kV and mAs are used for these procedures. Once images have been produced, the sensitivity numbers (S numbers) should be verified to determine whether they are within the acceptable range to ensure that sufficient exposure factors were used without overexposing the patient needlessly.

Alternative Modalities or Procedures

COMPUTED TOMOGRAPHY

Computed tomography (CT) provides a comprehensive evaluation of the lower GI tract for tumors, GI bleeds, and abscesses caused by infection. Although most CT studies of the abdomen utilize intravenous contrast media, the use of rectal contrast media continues to be debated. Some experts state that the use of rectal contrast media during a CT of the abdomen obscures subtle types of pathologic processes within the intestine. Others argue that a fully distended large intestine may pinpoint the location of tumors and abscesses adjacent to the large intestine.

The use of CT has become a common means of diagnosing acute appendicitis. Thin, consecutive slices taken in the region of the cecum may demonstrate a coprolith or abscess surrounding the vermiform appendix. To better delineate the vermiform appendix, rectal contrast media is often required.

NUCLEAR MEDICINE

A number of nuclear medicine procedures can be performed for various lower GI conditions and diseases. The use of radionuclides can assist in the diagnosis of Meckel's diverticulum, GI bleeding, and gastric emptying and bowel motility studies.

MAGNETIC RESONANCE IMAGING

Although magnetic resonance imaging (MRI) is not the gold standard for imaging of the GI tract, it has been used in limited applications. MRI cannot detect mucosal lesions, but it can demonstrate primary tumors of the bowel and adjacent structures. It can also assist with the planning for surgical excision of these tumors. Abscesses in the mesentery or retroperitoneum can be easily demonstrated on T2-weighted MRI.

SONOGRAPHY (ULTRASOUND)

Although the large intestine is too gaseous for ultrasound, the detection of tumors and collections of fluid and cysts is quite feasible. A filled urinary bladder provides an acoustic window to study structures and regions that surround the large intestine. Ultrasound with graded compression may be useful, along with clinical evaluation for diagnosis of appendicitis.

RADIOGRAPHIC POSITIONING

Survey Information

Surveys of the operating procedures (department routines) were conducted throughout the United States and Canada. The following information was compiled from these surveys, indicating the norm for basic and special projections for small bowel and barium enema series. The results were generally quite consistent throughout all regions of the U.S. and Canada.

SMALL BOWEL SERIES

	U.S. AVERAGE						CANADA	
	BASIC			SPECIAL			BASIC	SPECIAL
	2000	1995	1989	2000	1995	1989	2000	2000
Small bowel series								
• PA scout	80%	71%	—	—	—	—	5%	—
• PA (½ hr to 2 hr, hourly after 2 hr)	96%	93%	85%	—	—	—	91%	—
• Ileocecal spots	78%	69%	79%	—	—	—	68%	—
• Enteroclysis procedure, double contrast	—	—	—	48%	38%	25%	—	23%
• Intubation method	—	—	—	35%	21%	17%	—	13%

SUMMARY

Small Bowel Series **Enteroclysis** procedures are shown to be increasingly performed as special small bowel procedures in the U.S., as shown above. The **intubation method** also shows an increase in usage. Both of these procedures are performed less frequently in Canada, as shown.

Barium Enema Routine The survey indicated that both the **double-contrast** and the **single-contrast** barium enema are considered basic or routine in most departments in the U.S. and Canada, with the double-contrast continuing to receive a slightly higher indication of usage.

Digital Fluoroscopy Digital fluoroscopy without any conventional overhead radiographs is shown as basic or routine in 2000 by 26% in the U.S. and 27% in Canada. This percentage was much lower than for upper GI series (as described in Chapter 14), in which 40% in the U.S. and 72% in Canada indicated that digital fluoroscopy was routine or basic. These percentages also have most likely increased in more recent years as digital fluoroscopy systems are more commonly available for both upper and lower GI exams.

BARIUM ENEMA ROUTINE

	U.S. Average			Canada
	Basic			Basic
	2000	1995	1989	2000
Barium enema				
• Double contrast	96%	87%	76%	84%
• Single contrast	94%	81%	72%	62%
• PA	99%	93%	86%	84%
• Lateral rectum	88%	89%	77%	48%
• Right lateral decubitus	94%	76%	73%	88%
• Left lateral decubitus	94%	85%	73%	87%
• LPO and RPO	89%	78%	18%	45%
• RAO and LAO	59%	58%	58%	32%
• PA postevacuation	90%	85%	71%	61%
• AP axial (butterfly)	62%	45%	18%	31%
• PA Axial (butterfly)	55%	40%	15%	42%
• Ventral decubitus	51%	16%	—	32%
• Digital fluoroscopy, no overhead	26%	—	—	27%

Basic and Special Projections

Certain basic and special projections of the small and large intestine are demonstrated and described on the following pages. The radiologist and technologist must closely coordinate their efforts during both the small bowel series and the barium enema. A great deal of individual variation exists among radiologists. The routine or basic projections listed may vary from hospital to hospital. The radiographic routine for the barium enema, in particular, must be thoroughly understood by the technologist in advance of the examination, because any radiographs needed must be obtained as rapidly as possible.

Small Bowel Series
BASIC

Barium Enema
BASIC

PA PROJECTION: SMALL BOWEL SERIES

Small Bowel Series
BASIC
- PA (every 15 to 30 minutes) enteroclysis and intubation

Pathology Demonstrated
Inflammatory processes, neoplasms, and obstructions of the small intestine are shown.

Upper GI–small bowel combination: Commonly done in combination, wherein additional barium is ingested after completion of the upper GI (see p. 495)

Small bowel only series: Includes a scout abdomen radiograph followed by ingestion of barium and timed interval radiographs (see p. 496)

Enteroclysis and intubation procedures: See descriptions on pp. 496 and 497.

35 × 43, **30 min.**, **L**

Technical Factors
- IR size—35 × 43 cm (14× 17 inches), lengthwise
- Moving or stationary grid
- 100-125 kV range
- Time markers to be used
- Technique and dose:
  –PA, 30 minutes SB

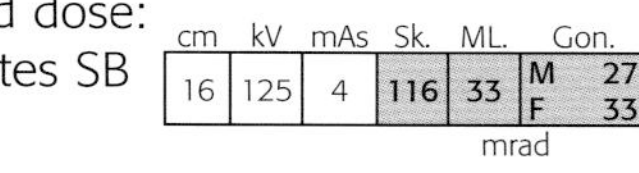

cm	kV	mAs	Sk.	ML.	Gon.
16	125	4	116	33	M 27 F 33

mrad

Shielding Shield gonads only if such shielding does not cover pertinent anatomy.

Patient Position Patient is prone (or supine if patient can't lie in prone position) with a pillow for the head.

Part Position
- Align midsagittal plane to midline of table/grid and/or CR.
- Place arms up beside head and legs extended, with support under ankles.
- Ensure that **no rotation** exists.

Central Ray
- CR is **perpendicular** to IR. (1) **15 or 30 min:** Center to about **2 inches** (5 cm) **above iliac crest** (see Note). (2) **Hourly:** Center CR and midpoint of IR to **iliac crest.**
- Center IR to CR.
- Minimum SID is 40 inches (100 cm).

Collimation Collimate on four sides to outer margins of IR.

Respiration Suspend respiration and expose on expiration.

Note: Timing begins with ingestion of barium. Timed intervals of radiographs depend on transit time of specific barium preparation used and on departmental protocol. **For the first 30-minute radiograph,** center high to include entire stomach.

Subsequent 30-minute interval radiographs are taken until barium reaches large bowel (usually 2 hours). The study is generally completed once the contrast media reaches the cecum and/or the ascending colon.

Fluoroscopy and spot imaging of the **ileocecal valve** and terminal ileum after barium reaches this area is a common part of small bowel series routine. This procedure, however, is determined by the radiologist's preference and departmental routines.

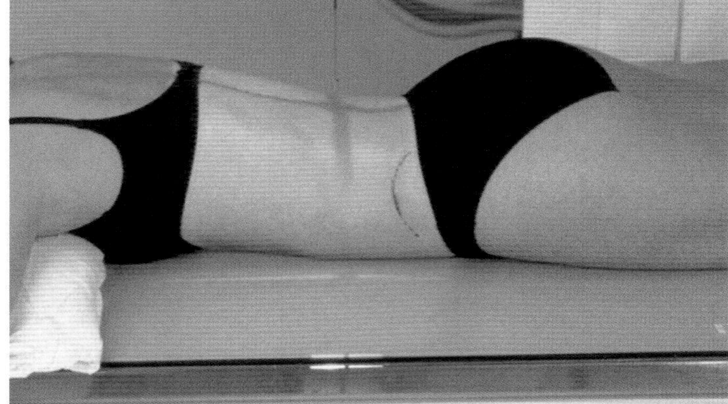

Fig. 15-51. PA, 15 or 30 minutes—centered approximately 2 inches (5 cm) above iliac crest.

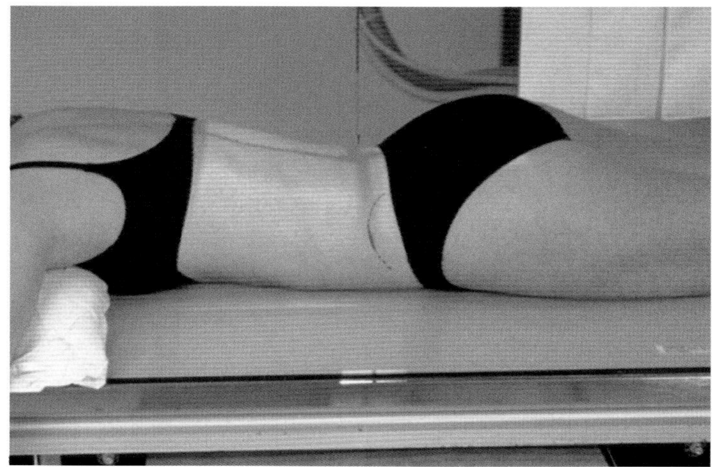

Fig. 15-52. PA, hourly—centered to iliac crest.

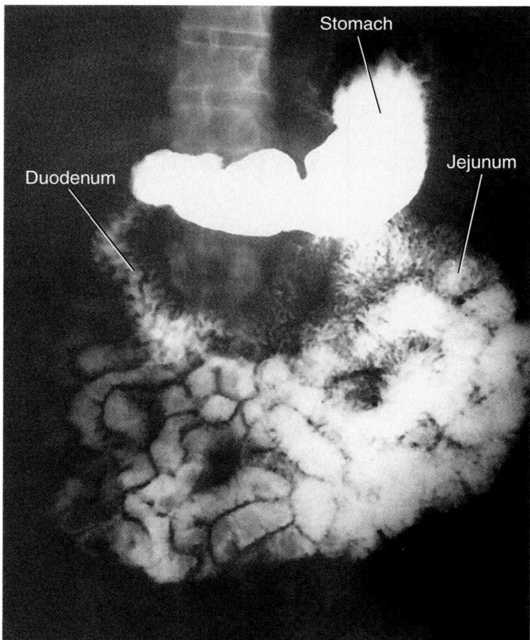

Fig. 15-53. PA SBS—30 minutes (most barium located in stomach, duodenum, and jejunum).

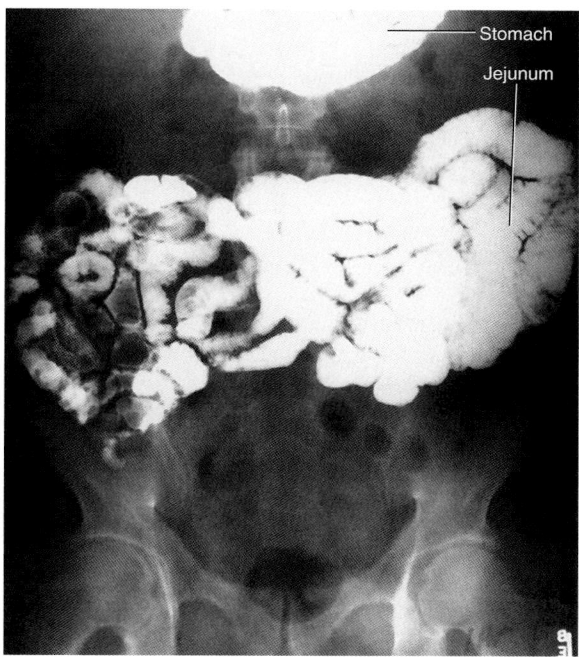

Fig. 15-54. PA SBS—1 hour (most barium located in jejunum).

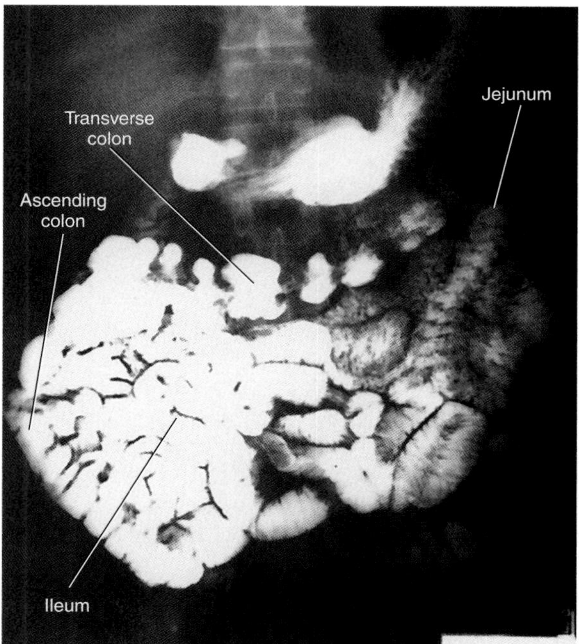

Fig. 15-55. PA, 2 hour (most barium located in ileum and proximal colon).

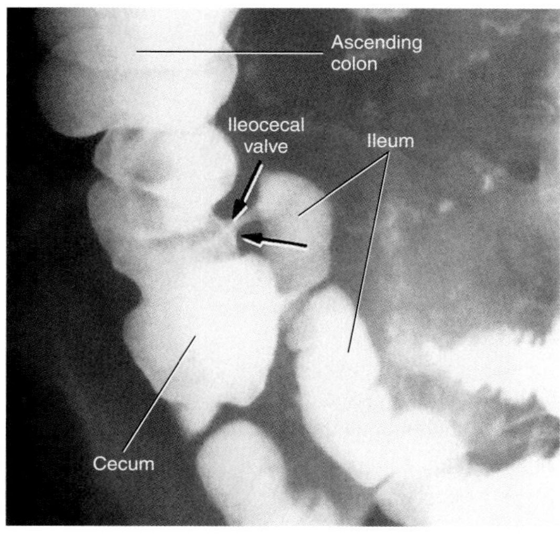

Fig. 15-56. PA (ileocecal spot). (Courtesy James Sanderson, RT.)

Radiographic Criteria

Structures Shown: • Entire small intestine is demonstrated on each radiograph, with the stomach included on the first 15- and/or 30-minute radiograph.

Position: • **No rotation** is present. The ala of the ilium and the lumbar vertebrae are symmetric.

Collimation and CR: • Only minimal collimation margins are seen on all four sides for adults. • CR is centered approximately 5 cm (2 inches) above the iliac crest for the initial radiographs. • CR is centered at iliac crest for remaining radiographs.

Exposure Criteria and Markers: • Appropriate technique is employed to visualize the contrast-filled small intestine without overexposing those parts that are only partially filled with barium. • Sharp structural margins indicate no motion. • Patient ID information **time interval markers,** and R or L marker are visible without superimposition of essential anatomy.

PA AND/OR AP PROJECTION: BARIUM ENEMA

Barium Enema
BASIC
• PA and/or AP

Pathology Demonstrated
Obstructions, including ileus, volvulus, and intussusception, are demonstrated. Double-contrast media barium enema is ideal for demonstrating diverticulosis, polyps, and mucosal changes.

35
43
L

Technical Factors
- IR size—35 × 43 cm (14 × 17 inches), lengthwise
- Moving or stationary grid
- 100-125 kV range (single contrast)
- 80-90 kV range (double contrast)
- Technique and dose:

cm	kV	mAs	Sk.	ML.	Gon.
16	125	4	116	33	M 27 F 33
					mrad

Shielding Place lead shields over gonads **only** if such shielding does not cover pertinent anatomy. (Female ovarian shielding is not possible for full-size BE radiographs.)

Patient Position Patient is prone or supine, with a pillow for head.

Part Position
- Align midsagittal plane to midline of table.
- Ensure that **no** body **rotation** exists.

Central Ray
- CR is **perpendicular** to IR.
- Center CR to level of **iliac crest.**
- Center IR to CR.
- Minimum SID is 40 inches (100 cm).

Collimation Collimate on four sides to margins of IR.

Respiration Suspend respiration and expose on expiration.

Notes: For most patients the enema tip can be removed before overhead filming unless a retention-type tip is being used. This type should generally not be removed until the patient is ready to evacuate.

Include rectal ampulla at lower margin of radiograph. Determine departmental policy regarding inclusion of the left colic flexure on all patients if this area is adequately included in spot images during fluoroscopy. (Most adult patients require 2 images if this area is to be included.)

For hypersthenic patients, use two 35 × 43 cm (14 × 17 inches) cassettes placed crosswise to include entire large intestine.

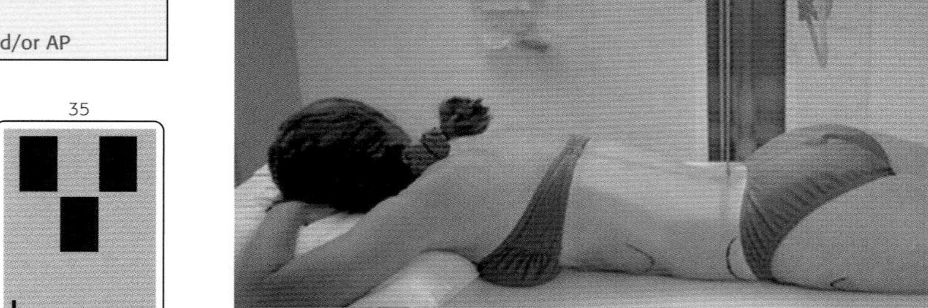

Fig. 15-57. PA or AP *(inset)* projections.

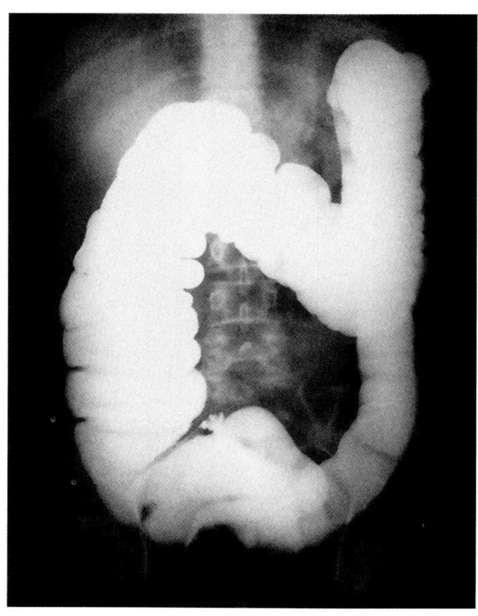

Fig. 15-58. PA projection—single-contrast BE.

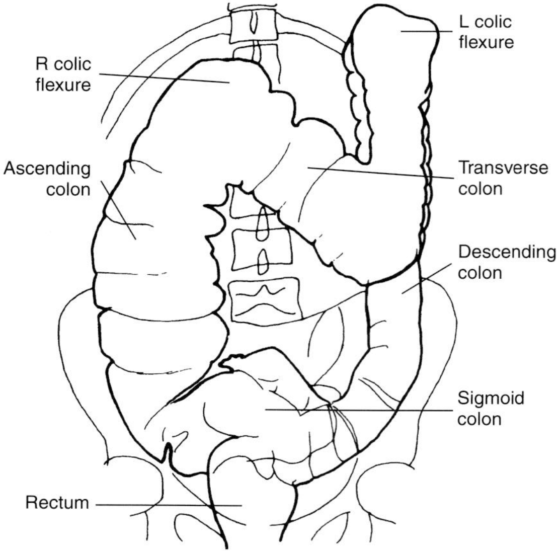

Fig. 15-59. PA projection.

Radiographic Criteria

Structures Shown: • The transverse colon should be primarily barium-filled on the PA and air-filled on the AP with a double-contrast study. • Entire large intestine should be demonstrated, including the left colic flexure (see Notes).

Position: • No rotation should exist. • The ala of the ilium and the lumbar vertebrae are symmetric.

Collimation and CR: • Only minimal collimation margins are seen on all four sides for adults. • CR is centered at level of iliac crest.

Exposure Criteria: • Appropriate technique should visualize the entire air- and barium-filled large intestine without overexposing the mucosal outlines of those sections of primarily air-filled bowel on a double-contrast study. • Sharp structural margins indicate no motion.

RAO POSITION: BARIUM ENEMA

Barium Enema
BASIC
- PA and/or AP
- RAO

Pathology Demonstrated

Obstructions, including ileus, volvulus, and intussusception, are often demonstrated. Double-contrast media barium enema is ideal for demonstrating diverticulosis, polyps, and mucosal changes.

Technical Factors

- IR size—35 × 43 cm (14 × 17 inches), lengthwise
- Moving or stationary grid
- 80-90 kV range (double-contrast study; 100-125 kV range for single-contrast study)
- Technique and dose:

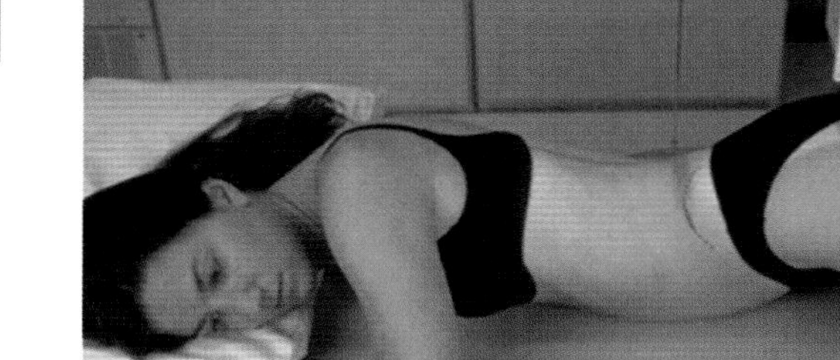

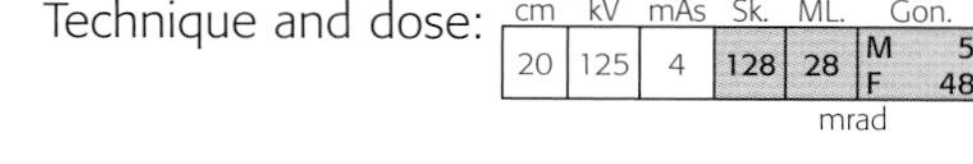
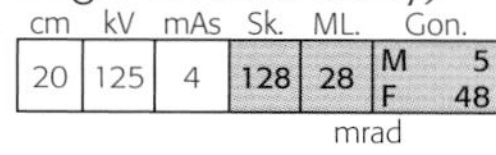

cm	kV	mAs	Sk.	ML.	Gon.
20	125	4	128	28	M 5 / F 48
				mrad	

Shielding Shield gonads only if this is possible without covering pertinent anatomy.

Patient Position Patient is semiprone, rotated into a 35° to 45° right anterior oblique, with a pillow for head.

Part Position

- Align midsagittal plane along long axis of table, with right and left abdominal margins equidistant from center line of table and/or CR.
- Place left arm up on pillow, right arm down behind patient, and left knee partially flexed.
- Check posterior pelvis and trunk for **35° to 45° rotation.**

Central Ray

- Direct CR **perpendicular** to IR to a point about **1 inch** (2.5 cm) **to the left** of midsagittal plane.
- Center CR and IR to **level of iliac crest** (see Note).
- Minimum SID is 40 inches (100 cm).

Collimation Collimate to outer margins of IR.

Respiration Suspend respiration and expose on expiration.

Note: Ensure that rectal ampulla is included on lower margin of IR. This action may require centering 1 or 2 inches (5 to 10 cm) below the iliac crest on larger patients and taking a second image centered 1 to 2 inches (5 to 10 cm) above the crest to include the right colic flexure (Figs. 15-61 and 15-62).

Fig. 15-60. 35° to 45° RAO.

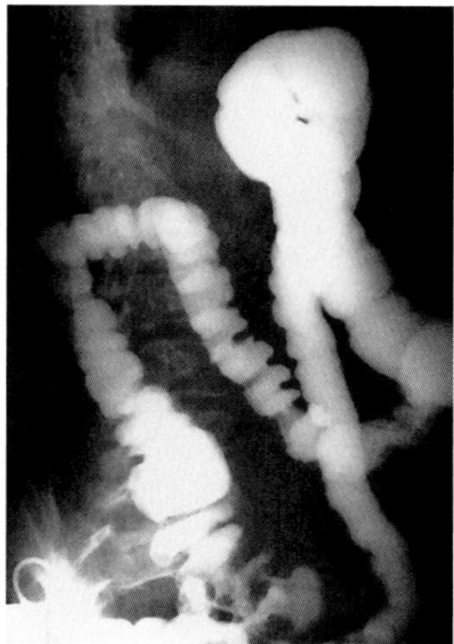

Fig. 15-61. RAO (centered high to include R and L colic flexures).

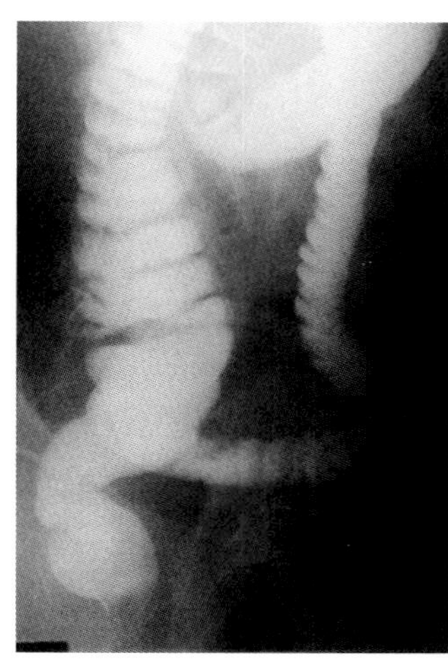

Fig. 15-62. RAO (centered low to include rectal ampulla).

Radiographic Criteria

Structures Shown: • The **right colic flexure** and the **ascending** and **sigmoid colon** are seen "open" without significant superimposition. • The entire large intestine is included, with the possible exception of the left colic flexure, which is best demonstrated in LAO position (or may require a second image centered higher). • The rectal ampulla should be included on lower margin of radiograph.

Position: • The spine is parallel to the edge of radiograph (unless scoliosis is present). • Ala of right ilium is elongated, while the left side is foreshortened; and right colic flexure is seen in profile if included.

Collimation and CR: • Only minimal collimation margins are seen on all four sides for adults. • CR is centered at level of iliac crest.

Exposure Criteria: • Appropriate technique should visualize the entire air- and barium-filled large intestine without overexposing the mucosal outlines of those sections of primarily air-filled bowel on a double-contrast study. • Sharp structural margins indicate no motion.

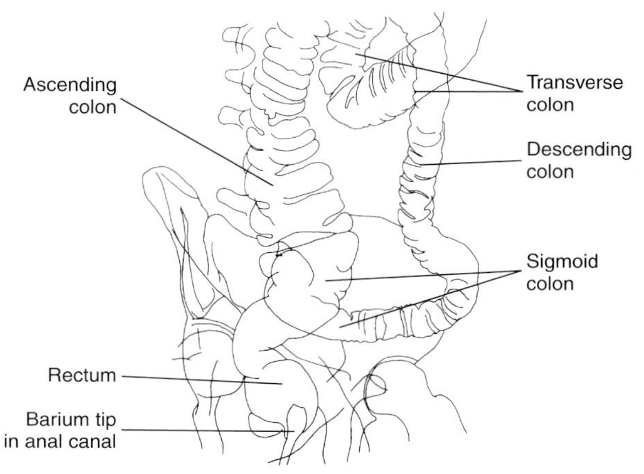

Fig. 15-63. RAO (to include rectal ampulla).

15

LAO POSITION: BARIUM ENEMA

Barium Enema
BASIC
- PA and/or AP
- RAO
- LAO

Pathology Demonstrated
Obstructions, including ileus, volvulus, and intussusception, are often demonstrated. Double-contrast media barium enema is ideal for demonstrating diverticulosis, polyps, and mucosal changes.

Technical Factors
- IR size—35 × 43 cm (14 × 17 inches), lengthwise
- Moving or stationary grid
- 100-125 kV range (single-contrast study)
  80-90 kV range (double-contrast study)
- Technique and dose:

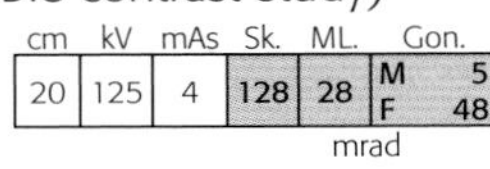
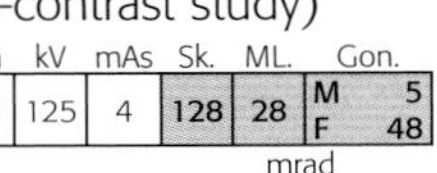

cm	kV	mAs	Sk.	ML.	Gon.
20	125	4	128	28	M 5 F 48

mrad

35
43
L

Shielding Place lead shield over gonads only if possible without covering pertinent anatomy.

Patient Position Patient is semiprone, rotated into a 35° to 45° left anterior oblique, with a pillow for head.

Part Position
- Align midsagittal plane along long axis of table, with right and left abdominal margins equidistant from center line of table and/or CR.
- Place right arm up on pillow, left arm down behind patient, and right knee partially flexed.
- Check posterior pelvis and trunk for **35° to 45° rotation.**

Central Ray
- CR is **perpendicular** to IR, directed to a point about 1 inch (2.5 cm) **to the right** of midsagittal plane.
- Center CR and IR to **1 to 2 inches** (2.5 to 5 cm) **above iliac crest** (see Note).
- Center cassette to CR.
- Minimum SID is 40 inches (100 cm).

Collimation Collimate on four sides to outer margins of IR.

Respiration Suspend respiration and expose on expiration.

Note: Most adult patients require about 2 inches (5 cm) higher centering to include the **left colic flexure,** which generally cuts off the lower large bowel; then a second image centered 2 or 3 inches (5 to 7.5 cm) lower is required to include the rectal area.

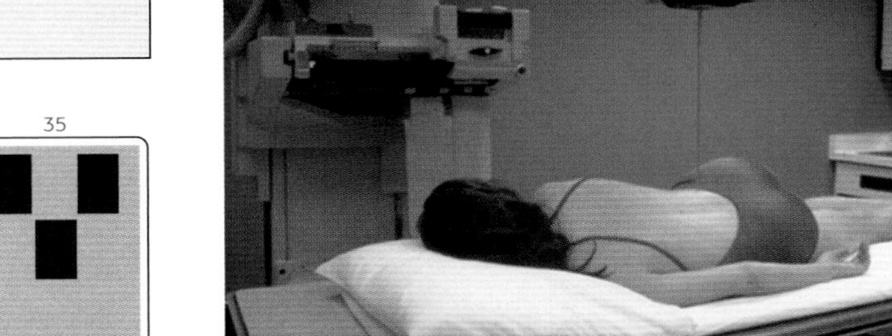

Fig. 15-64. LAO position.

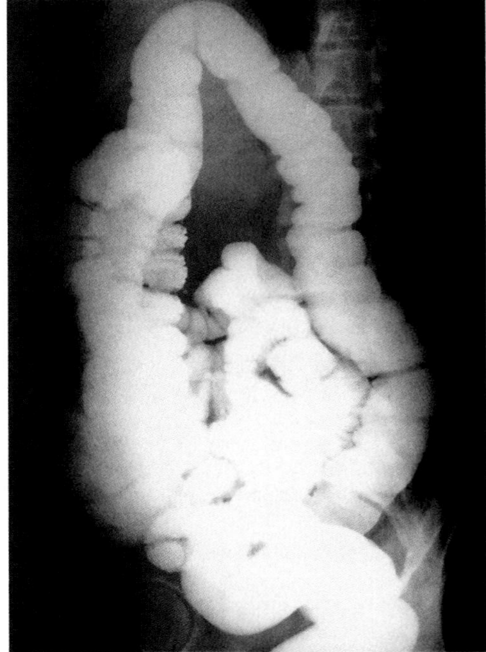

Fig. 15-65. LAO (centered high to include L colic flexure).

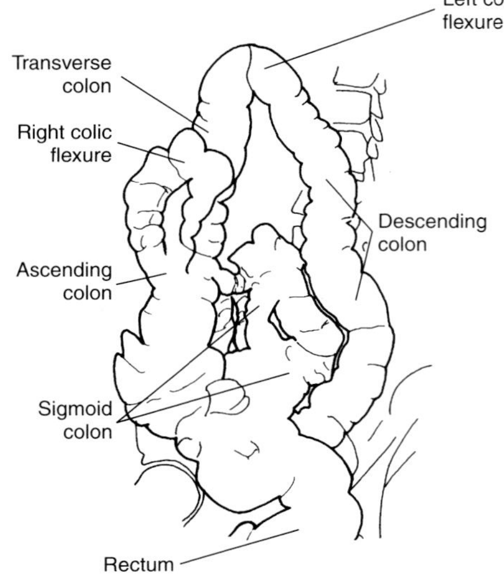

Fig. 15-66. LAO position.

Radiographic Criteria
Structures Shown: • The **left colic flexure** should be seen as open without significant superimposition. • The descending colon should be well demonstrated. • The entire large intestine should be included (see Notes).

Position: • Spine is parallel to the edge of radiograph (unless scoliosis is present). • Ala of left ilium is elongated, whereas the right side is foreshortened and left colic flexure is seen in profile.

Collimation and CR: • Only minimal collimation margins are seen on all four sides for adults. • CR is centered at level of iliac crest, or centered 2 inches (5 cm) above iliac crest to include entire left colic flexure.

Exposure Criteria: • Appropriate technique should visualize the contrast-filled large intestine without significant overexposure of any portion. • Sharp structural margins indicate no motion.

LPO AND RPO POSITIONS: BARIUM ENEMA

Barium Enema
BASIC
- PA and/or AP
- RAO
- LAO
- LPO and/or RPO

Pathology Demonstrated

Obstructions, including ileus, volvulus, and intussusception, are often demonstrated. Double-contrast barium enema is ideal for demonstrating diverticulosis, polyps, and mucosal changes.

Technical Factors

- IR size—35 × 43 cm (14 × 17 inches), lengthwise
- Moving or stationary grid
- 100-125 kV range (single-contrast study) 80-90 kV range (double-contrast study)
- Technique and dose:

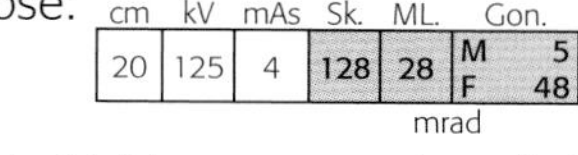
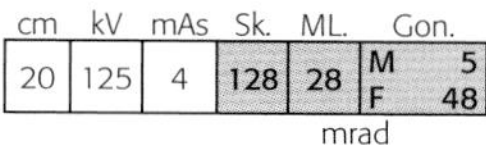

cm	kV	mAs	Sk.	ML.	Gon.
20	125	4	128	28	M 5 F 48

mrad

35 × 43, R

Shielding Place lead shield over gonads only if possible without covering pertinent anatomy.

Patient Position Patient is semisupine, rotated 35° to 45° into right and left posterior obliques, with a pillow for head.

Part Position
- Flex elevated side elbow and place in front of head; place opposite arm down by patient's side.
- Partially flex elevated side knee for support to maintain this position.
- Align **midsagittal plane along long axis of table,** with right and left abdominal margins equidistant from center line of table.

Central Ray
- Direct CR **perpendicular** to IR.
- Angle CR and center of IR to level of **iliac crests** and about **1 inch** (2.5 cm) **lateral to elevated side** of midsagittal plane (see Note).
- Minimum SID is 40 inches (100 cm).

Collimation Collimate on four sides to outer margins of IR.

Respiration Expose on expiration.

Note: Ensure that rectal ampulla is included. Most adult patients require a second IR centered 2 or 3 inches (5 to 7.5 cm) higher on the **RPO** if the left colic (splenic) flexure is to be included (Fig. 15-71).

Radiographic Criteria

Structures Shown: • *LPO*—The **right colic** (hepatic) **flexure** and ascending and rectosigmoid portions should appear "open" without significant superimposition. • *RPO*—The **left colic** (splenic) **flexure** and the descending portions should appear "open" without significant superimposition. (A second IR centered lower to include the rectal area is required on most adult patients if this area is to be included on these postfluoroscopy overheads.) • The rectal ampulla should be included on the lower margins of the radiograph. • Entire contrast-filled large intestine, including the rectal ampulla, should be included (see Notes).

Position: • LPO—No tilt is evident, and spine is parallel to the edge of radiograph. • Ala of left ilium is elongated and right side is foreshortened. • RPO—Tilt is present; spine is parallel to the edge of radiograph. • Rotation exists; ala of right ilium is elongated and left side is foreshortened.

Collimation and CR: • Only minimal collimation margins are seen on all four sides for adults. • CR is centered at level of iliac crest. • CR may be centered 2 inches (5 cm) above iliac crest to include entire left colic flexure for the RPO position.

Exposure Criteria: • Appropriate technique should visualize the contrast-filled large intestine without significant overexposure of any portion. • Sharp structural margins indicate no motion.

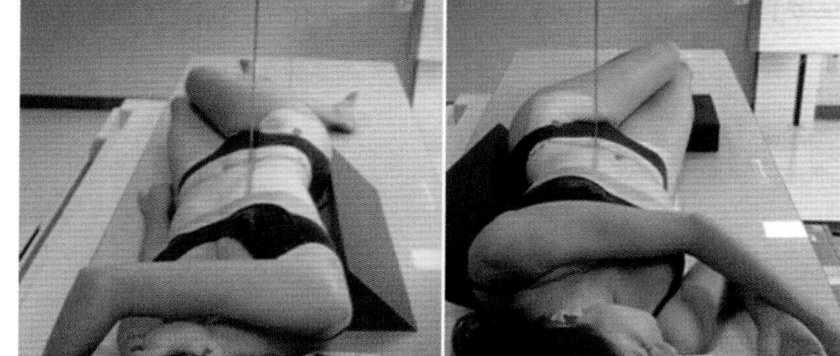

Fig. 15-67. Left, LPO. Right, RPO.

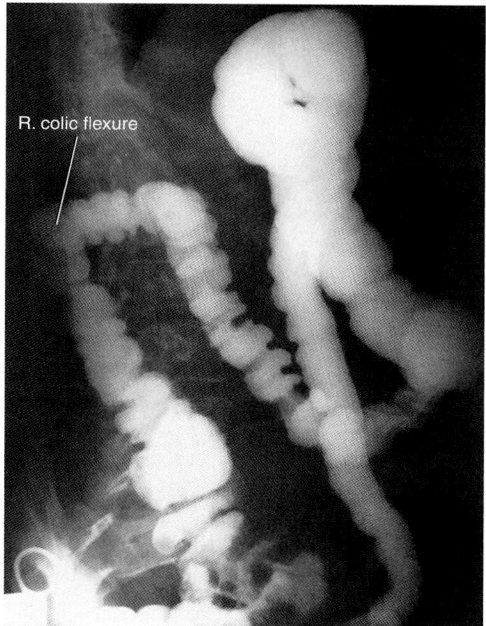

Fig. 15-68. LPO—for right colic flexure. (Image centered high to include both right and left colic flexures.)

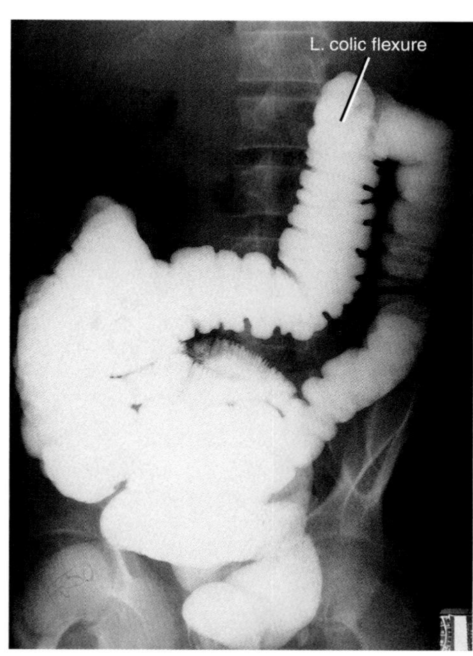

Fig. 15-69. RPO—for left colic flexure. (Image centered high to include both right and left colic flexures.)

15

LATERAL RECTUM POSITION OR VENTRAL DECUBITUS LATERAL: BARIUM ENEMA

Barium Enema
BASIC
- PA and/or AP
- RAO
- LAO
- LPO and/or RPO
- Lateral rectum

Pathology Demonstrated

Lateral position is ideal for demonstrating polyps, strictures, and fistulae between the rectum and the bladder/uterus. The ventral decubitus position is best for double-contrast study.

Technical Factors

- IR size—24 × 30 cm (10 × 12 inches), lengthwise
- Moving or stationary grid
- 100-125 kV range
- A compensating or wedge filter for more uniform density on ventral decubitus lateral
- Technique and dose:

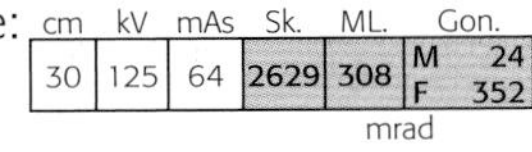
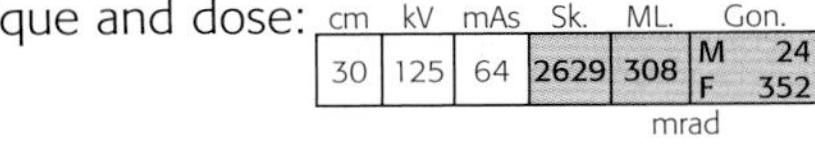

cm	kV	mAs	Sk.	ML.	Gon.
30	125	64	2629	308	M 24 F 352

mrad

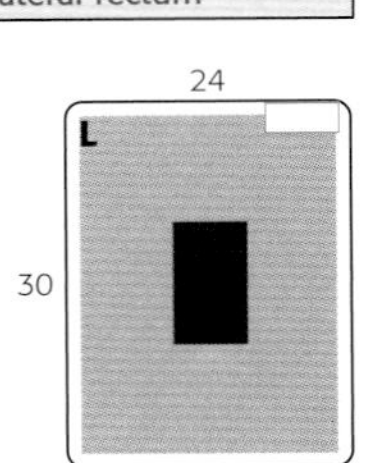

Shielding Lead shielding of gonads without covering pertinent anatomy may not be possible, especially for females. This inability makes close and accurate collimation especially important.

Patient Position Patient position is lateral recumbent, with a pillow for head.

Part Position (Lateral Position)

- Align midaxillary plane to midline of table and/or IR.
- Flex and superimpose knees; place arms up in front of head.
- Ensure **no rotation** exists; superimpose shoulders and hips.

Central Ray

- CR is **perpendicular** to IR (CR is **horizontal** for ventral decubitus).
- Center CR to level of **ASIS** and **midcoronal plane** (midway between ASIS and posterior sacrum).
- Center IR to CR.
- Minimum SID is 40 inches (100 cm).

Alternative ventral decubitus lateral horizontal beam positions are beneficial for double-contrast studies. Centering for the ventral decubitus is similar to the lateral rectum position.

Collimation Collimate on four sides to area of interest, generally near outer margins of IR.

Respiration Suspend respiration and expose on expiration.

Radiographic Criteria

Structures Shown: • Contrast-filled rectosigmoid region is demonstrated.

Position: • No rotation is evident; femoral heads are superimposed.

Collimation and CR: • Only minimal collimation margins are seen on all four sides for adults. • Rectosigmoid region is in center of image.

Exposure Criteria: • Appropriate technique is used to visualize both the contrast-filled rectum and sigmoid regions, with adequate penetration to demonstrate these areas through the superimposed pelvis and hips. • Sharp structural margins indicate no motion.

Fig. 15-70. Left lateral rectum. *Inset,* Ventral decubitus (double-contrast study).

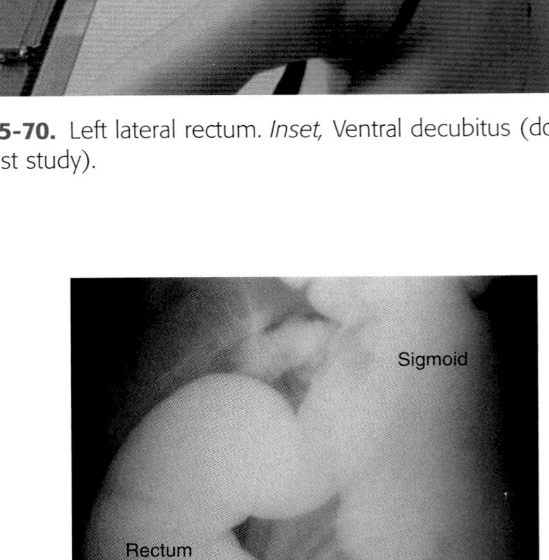

Fig. 15-71. Left lateral rectum.

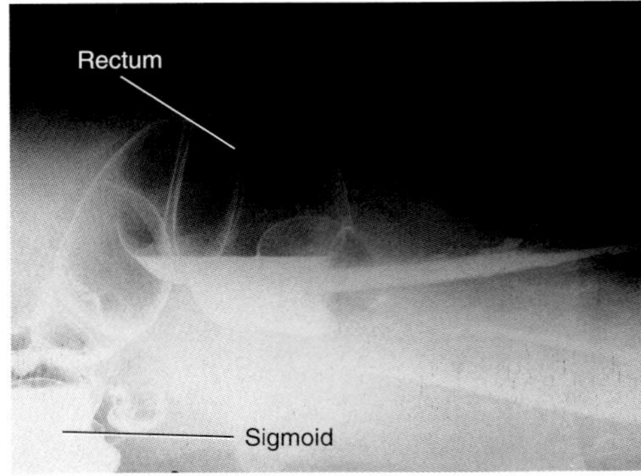

Fig. 15-72. Ventral decubitus lateral rectum.

15

RIGHT LATERAL DECUBITUS POSITION (AP OR PA): BARIUM ENEMA–DOUBLE CONTRAST

Barium Enema
BASIC
- PA and/or AP
- RAO
- LAO
- LPO and/or RPO
- Lateral rectum
- R and L lateral decubitus (double-contrast study)

Pathology Demonstrated

This position is especially helpful in demonstrating polyps of the left side or air-filled portions of the large intestine.

Both right and left decubitus positions are generally taken with the double-contrast study.

Technical Factors

- IR size—35 × 43 cm (14 × 17 inches), lengthwise with patient
- Bucky or grid cassette
- 80-90 kV (double-contrast study)
- Compensating filter placed on upside of abdomen (attached to collimator face with magnets)
- Technique and dose:

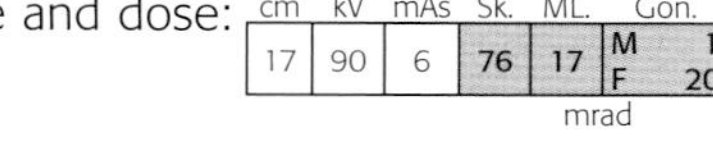
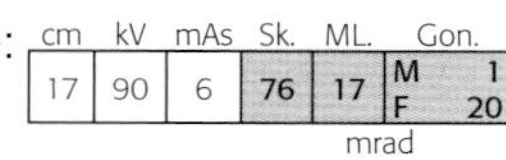

cm	kV	mAs	Sk.	ML.	Gon.
17	90	6	76	17	M 1 F 20
					mrad

Shielding Place lead shield over gonadal region only if possible without covering pertinent anatomy.

Patient Position Patient is in lateral recumbent position, with a pillow for head and lying on **right** side on a radiolucent pad, with portable grid placed behind patient's back for an AP projection. The patient also can be facing the portable grid or the vertical table for a PA projection. (If patient is on a cart, **lock wheels** or secure cart to prevent patient from falling.)

Part Position
- Position patient and/or IR so that iliac crest is to center of IR and to CR.
- Place arms up, with knees flexed.
- Ensure **no rotation** exists; superimpose shoulders and hips from above.

Central Ray
- Direct CR **horizontal,** perpendicular to IR.
- Center CR to **level of iliac crest** and **midsagittal plane.**
- Minimum SID is 40 inches (100 cm).

Collimation Collimate on four sides to outer margins of IR.

Respiration Suspend respiration and expose on expiration.

Note: Proceed as rapidly as possible.

For hypersthenic patients, use 2 each 34 × 43 cm (14 × 17 inches) IRs placed crosswise to include all of large intestine.

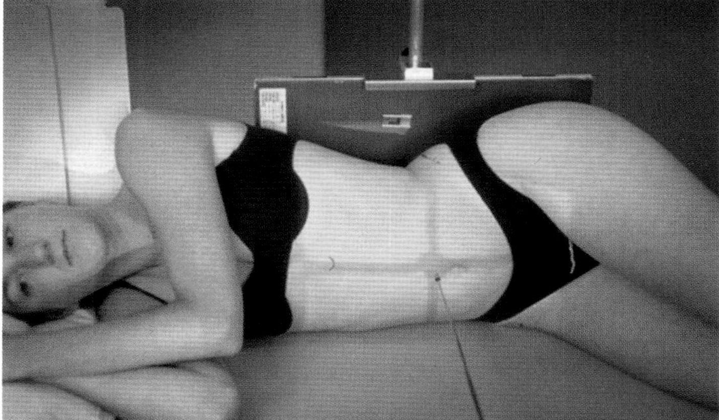

Fig. 15-73. Right lateral decubitus—AP (with portable grid).

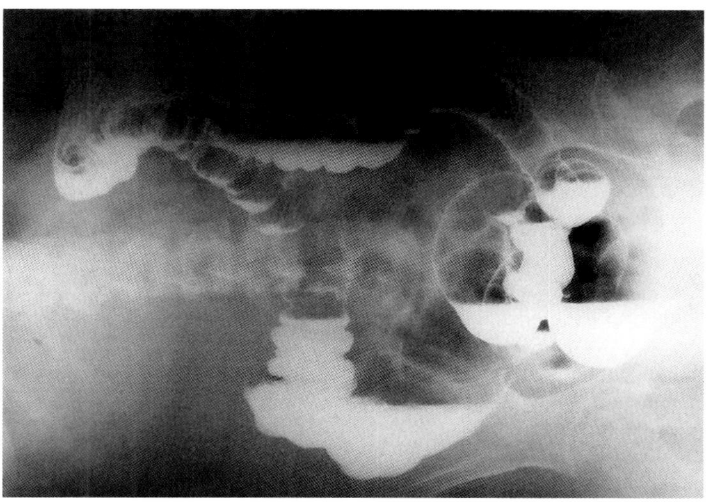

Fig. 15-74. Right lateral decubitus.

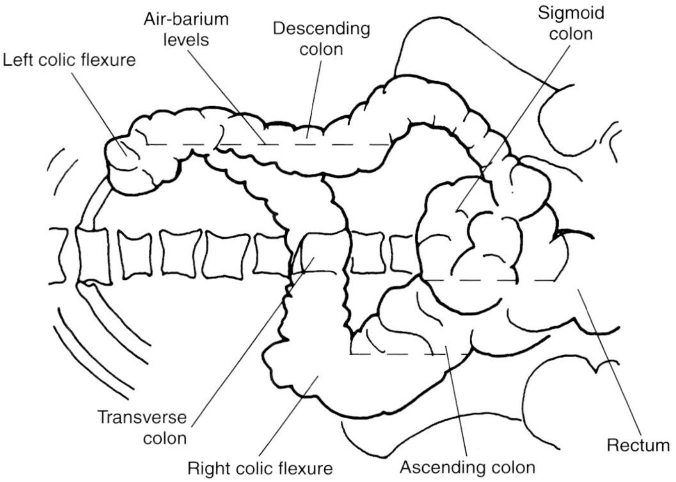

Fig. 15-75. Right lateral decubitus.

Radiographic Criteria

Structures Shown: • Entire large intestine is demonstrated to include air-filled left colic flexure and descending colon.

Position: • No rotation is evident by symmetric appearance of pelvis and ribcage.

Collimation and CR: • Only minimal collimation margins are seen on all four sides for adults. • Entire large intestine is centered on radiograph.

Exposure Criteria: • Appropriate technique is used to visualize borders of entire large intestine, including barium-filled portions, but to not overpenetrate the air-filled portion of the large intestine. • Mucosal patterns of air-filled colon should be clearly visible. • If air-filled portion of large intestine is overpenetrated consistently, a compensating filter should be considered. • Sharp structural margins indicate no motion.

15

LEFT LATERAL DECUBITUS POSITION (AP OR PA PROJECTION): BARIUM ENEMA

Barium Enema
BASIC
- PA and/or AP
- RAO
- LAO
- LPO and/or RPO
- Lateral rectum
- R and L lateral decubitus (double-contrast study)

Pathology Demonstrated

This position demonstrates the entire contrast-filled large intestine and is especially helpful in demonstrating polyps. It best demonstrates the **right side,** which includes air-filled portions of the large intestine.

Both right and left decubitus positions (AP or PA) are generally taken with the double-contrast study.

Technical Factors

- IR size—35 × 43 cm (14 × 17 inches), lengthwise with patient
- Bucky or grid cassette
- 80-90 kV range (double-contrast study)
- Technique and dose:

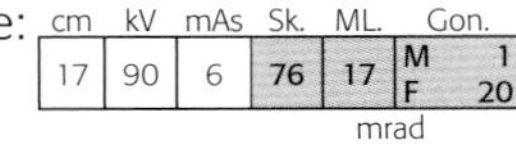

cm	kV	mAs	Sk.	ML.	Gon.
17	90	6	76	17	M 1 F 20

mrad

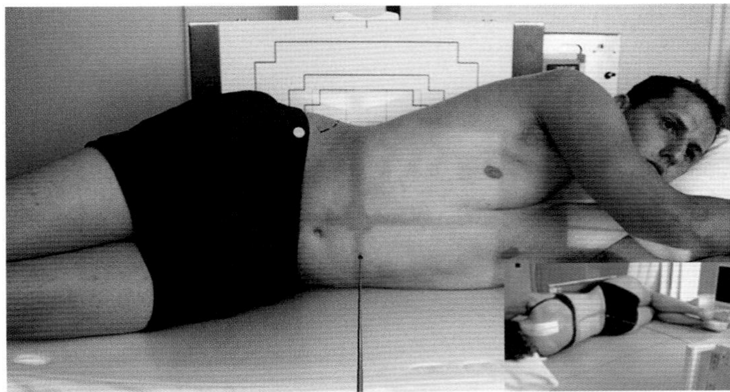

Fig. 15-76. Left lateral decubitus—AP projection. *Inset,* PA projection.

Shielding Place lead shield over gonadal region only if possible without covering pertinent anatomy.

Patient Position Position patient lateral recumbent, with a pillow for head, lying on **left** side on a radiolucent pad. (If on a cart, **lock wheels** or secure cart to prevent patient from falling.)

Part Position

- Position patient and/or IR so that iliac crest is to center of IR and to CR.
- Place arms up, with knees flexed.
- Ensure **no rotation** exists; superimpose shoulders and hips from above.

Central Ray

- Direct CR **horizontal,** perpendicular to IR.
- Center CR to **level of iliac crest** and **midsagittal plane.**
- Minimum SID is 40 inches (100 cm).

Collimation Collimate on four sides to outer margins of IR.

Respiration Suspend respiration and expose on expiration.

Note: Because most double-contrast barium enema studies include both right and left lateral decubitus positions, it is generally easier to take one projection with the back against the table or film holder and then have the patient roll over on the other side and move the cart around, with patient's head at the other end of the table. This task may be easier than sitting the patient up and turning the patient end-to-end on the cart or table.

For hypersthenic patients, use 2 IRs (each 35 × 43 cm; 14 × 17 inches) placed crosswise to include all of large intestine.

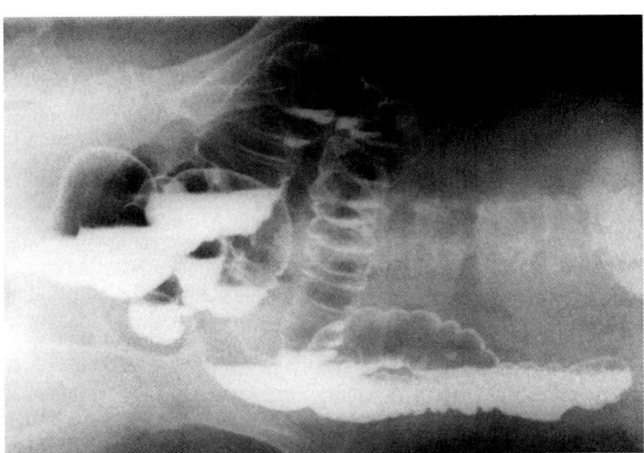

Fig. 15-77. Left lateral decubitus.

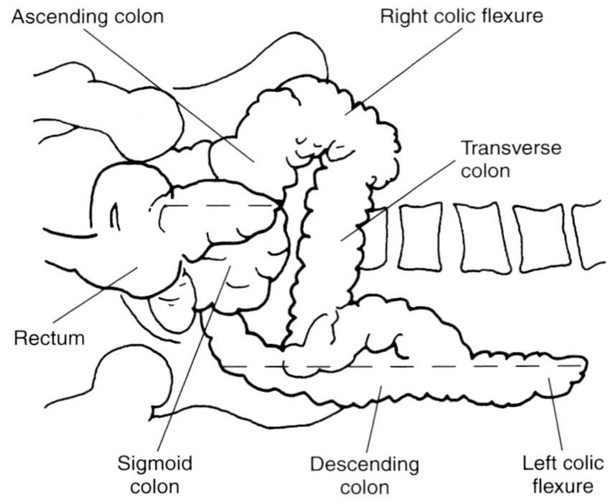

Fig. 15-78. Left lateral decubitus.

Radiographic Criteria

Structures Shown: • Entire large intestine is demonstrated, with air-filled right colic flexure, ascending colon, and cecum.

Position: • No rotation exists, evidenced by symmetric appearance of pelvis and ribcage.

Collimation and CR: • Only minimal collimation margins are seen on all four sides for adults. • Entire large intestine is centered on radiograph.

Exposure Criteria: • Appropriate technique is used to visualize borders of entire large intestine, including barium-filled portions, but to not overpenetrate the air-filled portion of the large intestine. • Mucosal patterns of air-filled colon should be clearly visible. • If air-filled portion of large intestine is overpenetrated, a compensating filter should be considered. • Sharp structural margins indicate no motion.

PA (AP) PROJECTION—POSTEVACUATION: BARIUM ENEMA

Barium Enema
BASIC
- PA and/or AP
- RAO
- LAO
- LPO and/or RPO
- Lateral rectum
- R and L lateral decubitus (double-contrast study)
- PA postevacuation

Pathology Demonstrated

This position demonstrates the mucosal pattern of large intestine with residual contrast media for demonstrating small polyps and defects.

It is most commonly taken prone as a PA, but may be taken with patient supine as an AP, if necessary.

Technical Factors

- IR size—35 × 43 cm (14 × 17 inches), lengthwise
- Moving or stationary grid
- 80-90 kV range
- Use postevacuation marker
- Technique and dose:

cm	kV	mAs	Sk.	ML.	Gon.
16	100	4	74	19	M 12 / F 18

mrad

35
43
L Post-evac

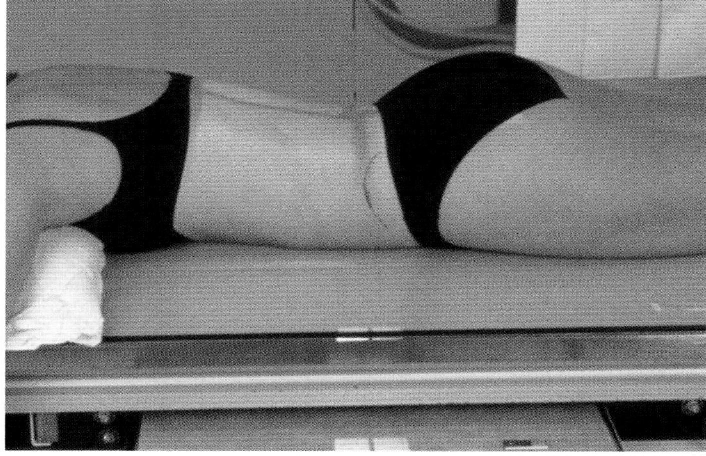

Fig. 15-79. PA postevacuation.

Shielding Place lead shield over gonads only if possible without covering pertinent anatomy.

Patient Position Patient is prone or supine, with a pillow for head.

Part Position

- Align midsagittal plane to midline of table and/or CR.
- Ensure **no** body **rotation exists.**

Central Ray

- CR is **perpendicular** to IR.
- Center CR and center of IR to **iliac crest.**
- Minimum SID is 40 inches (100 cm).

Collimation Collimate on four sides to outer margins of IR.

Respiration Suspend respiration and expose on expiration.

Note: Image should be taken after patient has had sufficient time for adequate evacuation. If radiograph shows insufficient evacuation to clearly visualize mucosal pattern, a second radiograph should be obtained after further evacuation. Sometimes coffee or tea can be given as a stimulant for this purpose. Include rectal ampulla on lower margin of radiograph.

Use lower kV to prevent overpenetration, with only the residual contrast media remaining in large bowel.

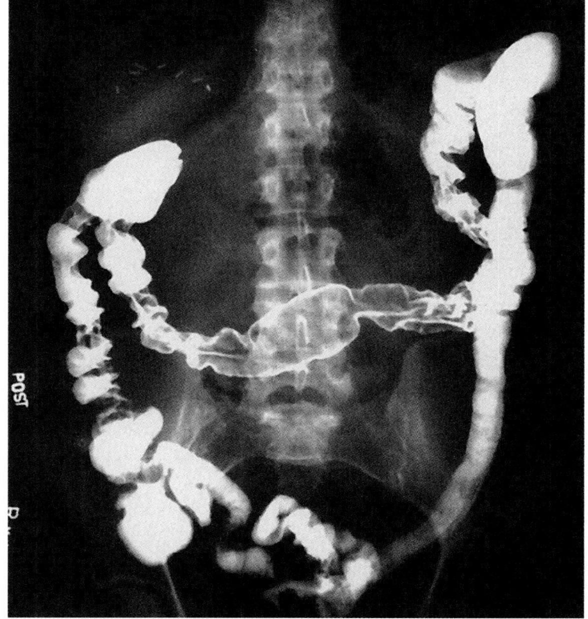

Fig. 15-80. PA postevacuation.

Radiographic Criteria

Structures Shown: • Entire large intestine should be visualized, with only a residual amount of contrast media.

Position: • Spine is parallel to the edge of radiograph (unless scoliosis is present). • No rotation exists; the ala of the ilium and the lumbar vertebrae are symmetric.

Collimation and CR: • Only minimal collimation margins are seen on all four sides for adults. • CR is centered at level of iliac crest.

Exposure Criteria and Markers: • Appropriate technique is used to visualize outline of entire mucosal pattern of the large intestine without overexposure of any parts. • Sharp structural margins indicate no motion. • Markers: Postevacuation and right or left markers should be visible.

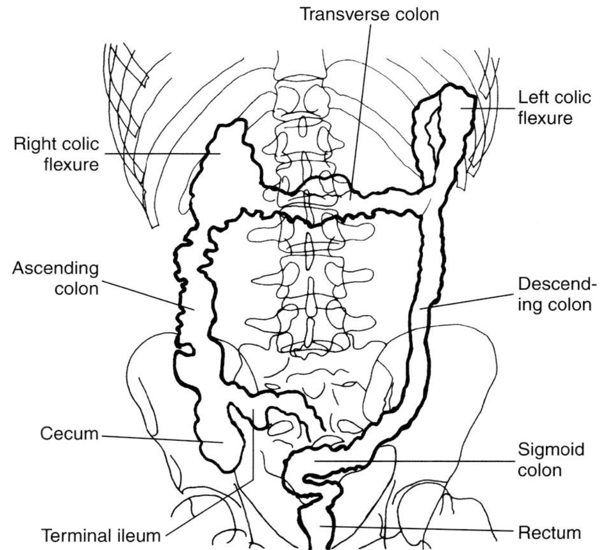

Fig. 15-81. PA postevacuation.

15

AP AXIAL OR AP AXIAL OBLIQUE (LPO) PROJECTIONS: BARIUM ENEMA

"Butterfly" Positions

Pathology Demonstrated
Polyps or other pathologic processes in the rectosigmoid aspect of the large intestine are often demonstrated with this position.

Barium Enema
SPECIAL
- AP or LPO axial

Technical Factors
- IR size—28 × 35 cm (11 × 14 inches), lengthwise
- Moving or stationary grid
- 100-125 kV range for single contrast (or 90-100 kV range, double contrast)
- Technique and dose:

cm	kV	mAs	Sk.	ML.	Gon.
16	125	6	172	52	M 6 F 65

mrad

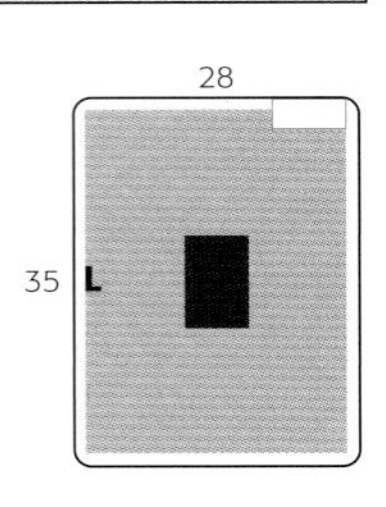

Shielding Place lead shield over gonads without covering pertinent anatomy (may not be possible).

Patient Position Position patient supine or partially rotated into an LPO position, with a pillow for head.

Part Position
AP axial:
- Position patient supine and align midsagittal plane to midline of table.
- Extend legs; place arms down by patient's side or up across chest; ensure **no rotation.**

LPO:
- Rotate patient **30°** to **40°** into LPO (left posterior side down).
- Raise right arm, with left arm extended, and right knee partially flexed.

Central Ray
Angle CR **30°** to **40° cephalad.**
AP:
- Direct CR **2 inches** (5 cm) **inferior** to **level of ASIS,** and to **midsagittal plane.**

LPO:
- Direct CR **2 inches** (5 cm) **inferior** and **2 inches** (5 cm) **medial to right ASIS.**
- Center IR to CR.
- Minimum SID is 40 inches (100 cm).

Collimation Collimate on four sides to outer margins of IR.

Respiration Suspend respiration and expose on expiration.

Note: Proceed as rapidly as possible. Similar views can also be obtained with a **PA axial** and an **RAO** with **30°** to **40° caudad** CR angle (see following page).

Radiographic Criteria
Structures Shown: • Elongated views of the rectosigmoid segments should be visible with less overlapping of sigmoid loops than with a 90° AP projection.
Position: • *AP axial*—Adequate CR angulation is evidenced by elongation of rectosigmoid segments of large intestine. • *LPO axial*—Adequate CR angulation and patient obliquity are evidenced by elongation and less superimposition of rectosigmoid segments of large intestine.
Collimation and CR: • Only minimal collimation margins are seen on all four sides for adults. • Rectosigmoid region is centered in near midaspect of radiograph; all of rectum is included on lower margin.
Exposure Criteria: • Appropriate technique is used to visualize outlines of all rectosigmoid segments of large intestine. • Sharp structural margins indicate no motion.

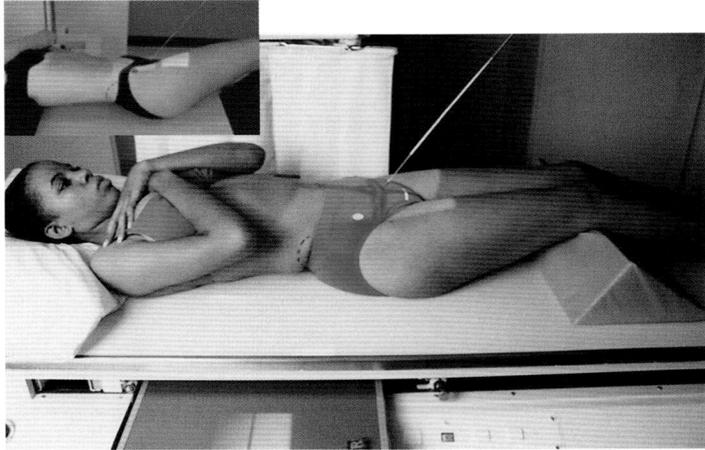

Fig. 15-82. AP axial—CR 30° to 40° cephalad. Inset—30° to 40° LPO.

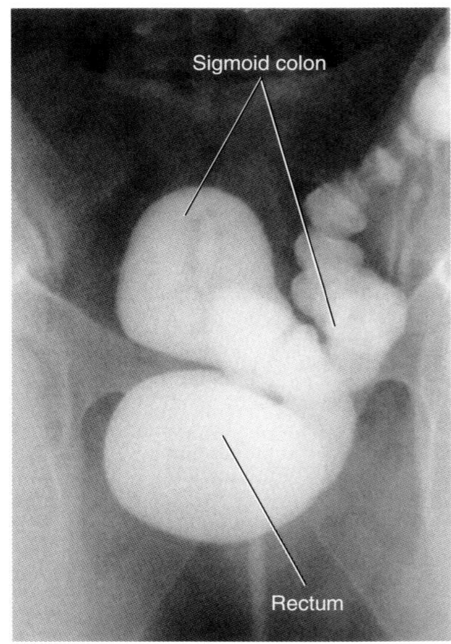

Fig. 15-83. AP axial.

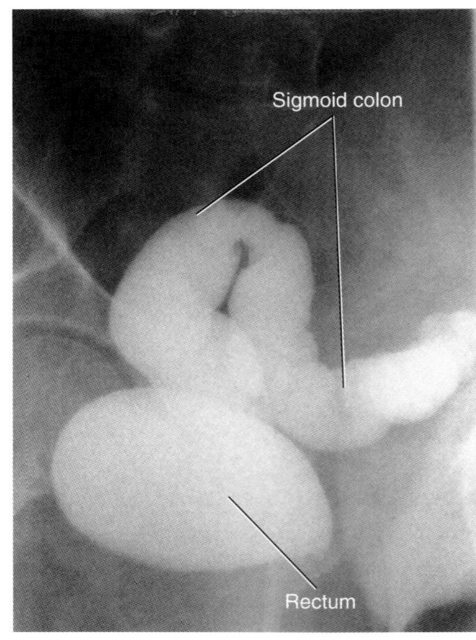

Fig. 15-84. AP axial oblique (LPO).

PA AXIAL OR PA AXIAL OBLIQUE (RAO) PROJECTIONS: BARIUM ENEMA

"Butterfly" Positions

Barium Enema
SPECIAL
- **AP or LPO axial**
- PA or RAO axial

Pathology Demonstrated

This projection demonstrates polyps or other pathologic processes in the rectosigmoid aspect of the large intestine; air contrast best visualizes for this pathologic process.

Technical Factors

- IR size—28 × 35 cm (11 × 14 inches), lengthwise
- Moving or stationary grid
- 100-125 kV range for single contrast (or 90-100 kV range for double contrast)
- Technique and dose:

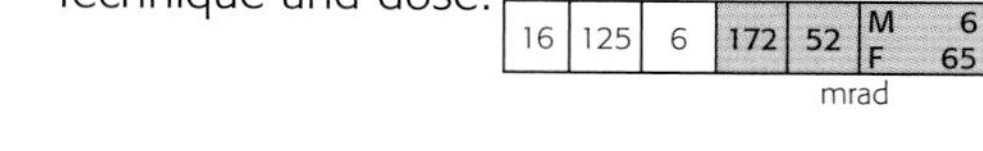
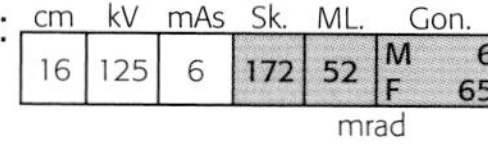

cm	kV	mAs	Sk.	ML.	Gon.
16	125	6	172	52	M 6 F 65

mrad

Shielding Placement of lead shield over gonads is generally not possible without covering pertinent anatomy.

Patient Position Position patient prone or partially rotated into an RAO position with a pillow for head.

Part Position

PA: • Position patient prone and align midsagittal plane to midline of table.
- Place arms up beside head or down by sides away from body.
- Ensure **no rotation** of pelvis or trunk.

RAO: • Rotate patient **35° to 45°** into **RAO** (right anterior side down).
- Place left arm up, right arm down by side, and left knee partially flexed.

Central Ray

Angle CR **30° to 40° caudad.**

PA: • Align CR to exit at **level of ASIS** and to **midsagittal plane.**

RAO: • Align CR to exit at **level of ASIS** and **2 inches** (5 cm) to **left of lumbar spinous processes.**
- Center film holder to CR.
- Minimum SID is 40 inches (100 cm).

Collimation Collimate on four sides to outer margins of IR.

Respiration Suspend respiration and expose on expiration.

Note: Proceed as rapidly as possible.

Similar views of rectosigmoid region, AP and LPO with 30° to 40° cephalad angle, are described on preceding page.

Radiographic Criteria

Structures Shown: • Elongated views of rectosigmoid segments of the large intestine are shown without excessive superimposition. • The double-contrast study best visualizes this region of overlapping loops of bowel.

Position: • Adequate CR angulation and patient obliquity on the oblique are evidenced by elongation and less superimposition of rectosigmoid segments of large intestine.

Collimation and CR: • Minimal collimation margins are seen on all four sides for adults. • Rectosigmoid region is centered in near midaspect of radiograph and all of rectum is included on lower margins of IR.

Exposure Criteria: • Appropriate technique is used to visualize outlines of all rectosigmoid segments of large intestine without overpenetrating the air-filled outlines of these segments of large intestine with air-contrast study. • Sharp structural margins indicate no motion.

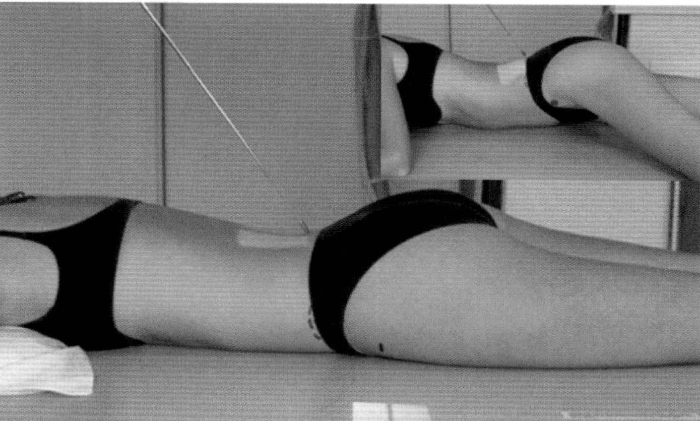

Fig. 15-85. PA axial—CR 30° to 40° caudad. Inset—RAO axial.

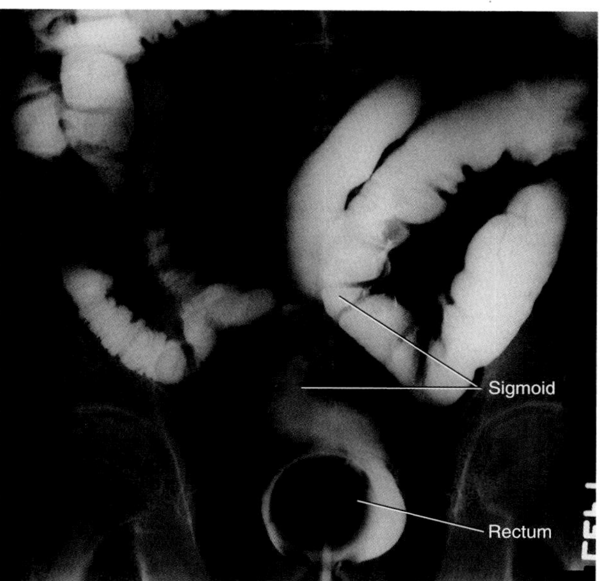

Fig. 15-86. PA axial (single-contrast study).

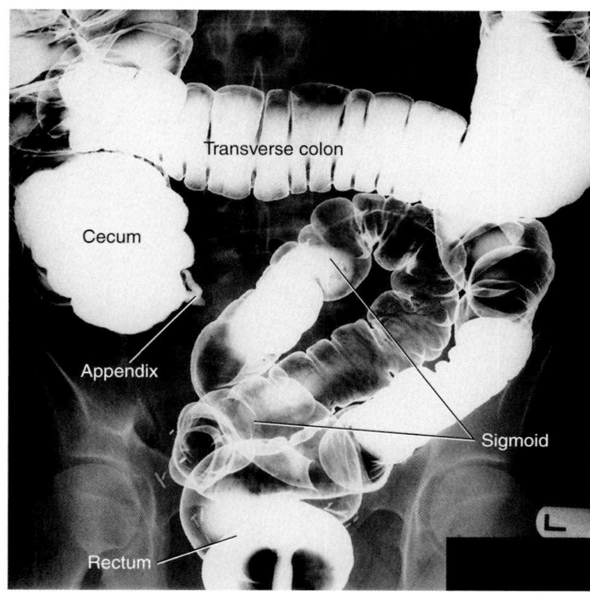

Fig. 15-87. PA axial (double-contrast study).

15

CHAPTER 16

Gallbladder and Biliary Ducts

CONTRIBUTOR TO PAST EDITIONS Barry T. Anthony, RT(R)

CONTENTS

RADIOGRAPHIC ANATOMY

16

Liver

Radiographic examination of the biliary system involves studying the manufacture, transport, and storage of bile. Bile is manufactured by the liver, transported by the various ducts, and stored in the gallbladder. Understanding radiographic examination of the biliary system requires knowledge of the basic anatomy and physiology of the liver, gallbladder, and connecting ducts.

The liver is the largest solid organ in the human body and weighs 3 or 4 pounds (1.5 kg), or $^1/_{36}$ of the total body weight in an average adult. It occupies most of the **right upper quadrant.** Of the nine abdominal regions, the liver occupies almost all of the right hypochondrium, a major part of the epigastrium, and a significant part of the left hypochondrium.

As viewed from the front in Fig. 16-1, the liver is triangular in shape. The upper border is the widest part of the liver (approximately 8 to 9 inches, or 20 to 23 cm) and is convex to conform to the inferior surface of the right hemidiaphragm.

The right border of the liver is its greatest vertical dimension, approximately 6 to 7 inches (15 to 17.5 cm). In the average person it extends to slightly below the lateral portion of the tenth rib just above the right kidney. The liver is fairly well protected by the lower right rib cage. Because the liver is highly vascular and easily lacerated, protection by the ribs is very necessary.

The distal end of the gallbladder extends slightly below the anterior, inferior margin of the liver. The rest of the gallbladder lies along the inferior and posterior surface of the liver (Fig. 16-3).

LOBES OF THE LIVER

The liver is partially divided into two major lobes and two minor lobes. As viewed from the front in Fig. 16-2, only the two major lobes can be seen. A much larger **right lobe** is separated from the smaller **left lobe** by the **falciform** *(fal'si-form)* **ligament.**

Associated with the large right lobe posteriorly are the two minor lobes, which can be seen only when viewing the visceral or inferior and posterior surface of the liver (Fig. 16-3). The first of these is the small **quadrate lobe** located on the inferior surface of the right lobe between the gallbladder and the falciform ligament. Just posterior to the quadrate lobe is the second minor lobe, the **caudate lobe,** which extends **superiorly** to the diaphragmatic surface. The large **inferior vena cava** contours over the surface of this caudate lobe. The midinferior surface includes the hepatic bile ducts, which are described and illustrated on the following page.

FUNCTION OF THE LIVER

The liver is a complex organ and is absolutely essential to life. The liver performs more than 100 different functions, but the one function most applicable to radiographic study is the **production of large amounts of bile.** It secretes from 800 to 1000 ml, or about 1 quart of bile per day.

The major function of bile is to aid in the digestion of fats by emulsifying or breaking down fat globules and the absorption of fat following its digestion. Bile also contains cholesterol, which is made soluble in the bile by the bile salts.

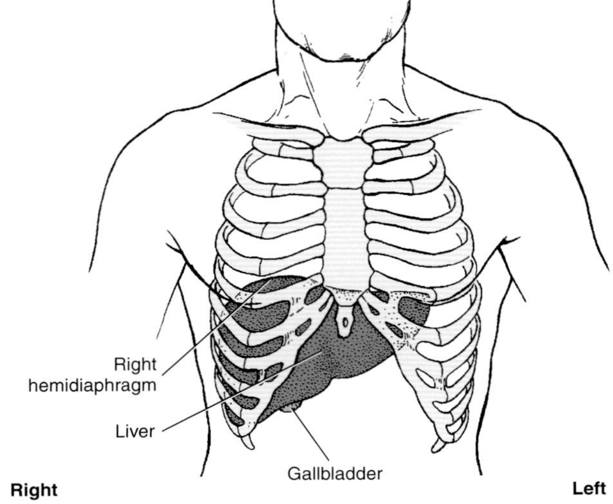

Fig. 16-1. Liver and gallbladder—anterior view.

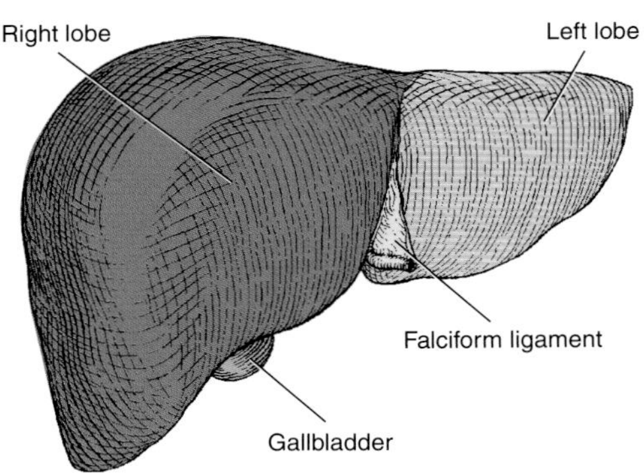

Fig. 16-2. Liver—anterior view.

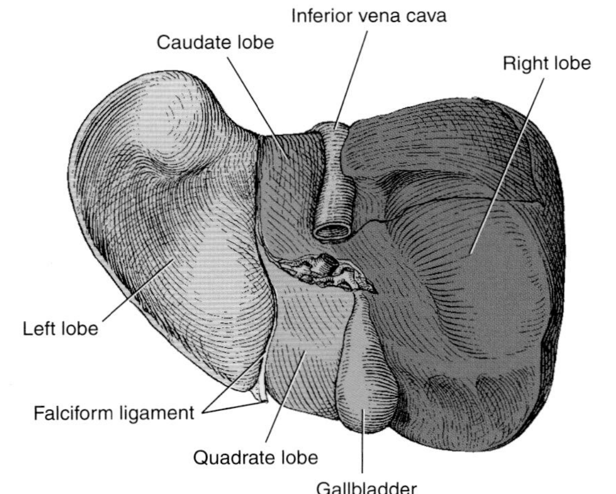

Fig. 16-3. Liver and gallbladder—inferior and posterior view.

Gallbladder and Biliary Ducts

The gallbladder and the extrahepatic biliary ducts (located outside of the liver) are shown in Fig. 16-4. Bile is formed in small lobules of the liver and travels by small ducts to either the **right** or **left hepatic duct.** The right and left hepatic ducts join to continue as the **common hepatic duct.** Bile is either carried to the **gallbladder** via the **cystic duct** for temporary storage or secreted directly into the **duodenum** by way of the **common bile duct,** which is joined by the main **pancreatic duct.**

The **gallbladder** (GB) is a pear-shaped sac composed of three parts: **fundus, body,** and **neck** (Fig. 16-5). The fundus is the distal end and the broadest part of the gallbladder. The main section of the gallbladder is termed the *body.* The narrow proximal end is termed the *neck,* which continues as the **cystic duct.** The cystic duct is 3 to 4 centimeters long, containing several membranous folds along its length. These folds are called the **spiral valve,** which functions to prevent distention or collapse of the cystic duct.

The normal gallbladder is from 7 to 10 centimeters long, about 3 centimeters wide and normally holds 30 to 40 ml of bile.

FUNCTIONS OF THE GALLBLADDER

The **three** primary functions of the gallbladder are to (1) **store** bile, and (2) to **concentrate** bile, and (3) to **contract when stimulated.**

First If bile is not needed for digestive purposes, it is stored for future use in the gallbladder.

Second Bile is concentrated within the gallbladder as a result of hydrolysis (removal of water). In the abnormal situation, if too much water is absorbed or if the cholesterol becomes too concentrated, gallstones (choleliths) may form in the gallbladder. (Cholesterol coming out of solution forms the most common type of gallstones.*)

Third The gallbladder normally contracts when foods such as fats or fatty acids are in the duodenum. These foods stimulate the duodenal mucosa to secrete the hormone cholecystokinin (CCK). Increased levels of CCK in the blood cause the gallbladder to contract and the terminal opening of the common bile duct to relax. In addition, CCK causes increased exocrine activity by the pancreas.

COMMON BILE DUCT

The **common bile duct** averages about 7.5 centimeters in length and has an internal diameter about the size of a drinking straw. The common bile duct descends behind the superior portion of the duodenum and the head of the pancreas to enter the second or **descending portion of the duodenum.**

The end of the common bile duct is closely associated with the end of the **pancreatic duct (duct of Wirsung)** *(Vér'soong),* as shown in Fig. 16-6.

In about 40% of individuals these two ducts remain separated as they pass into the duodenum as two separate ducts with separate openings. In the remaining 60% the common bile duct joins the pancreatic duct to form one common passageway through the single papilla into the duodenum.* In these individuals, this short, single channel becomes narrower as it passes into the duodenum, and is therefore a common site for impaction of gallstones.* Some references refer to this common passageway as an ampulla, the **hepatopancreatic ampulla,** or the older term **ampulla of Vater.**

Near the terminal opening of this passageway into the duodenum, the duct walls contain circular muscle fiber, termed the **hepatopancreatic sphincter** or **sphincter of Oddi** *(Od'e).* This sphincter relaxes when levels of CCK increase in the bloodstream. The presence of this ring of muscle causes a protrusion into the lumen of the duodenum termed the **duodenal papilla** or **papilla of Vater.**

*Clemente CD, editor: Gray's anatomy, ed 30, Philadelphia, 1985, Lea and Febiger, p. 1502.

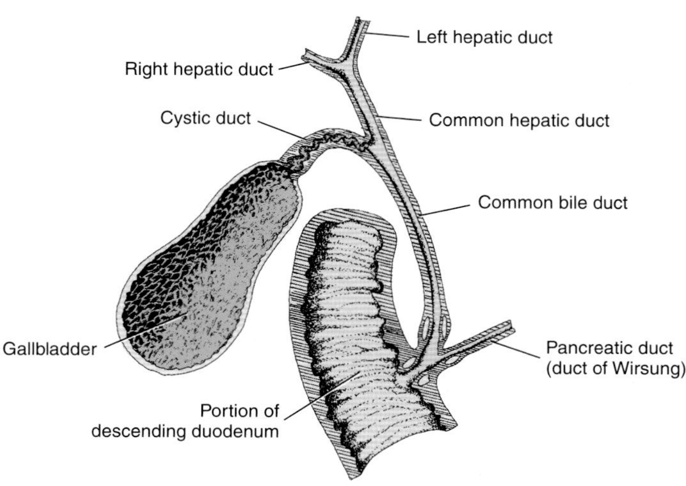

Fig. 16-4. Gallbladder and extrahepatic biliary ducts.

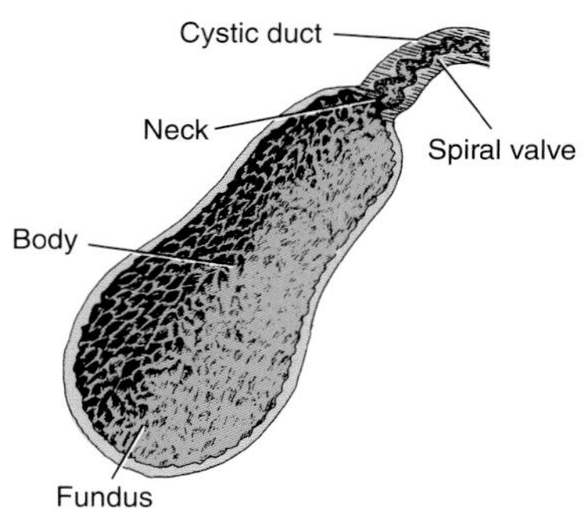

Fig. 16-5. Gallbladder and cystic duct.

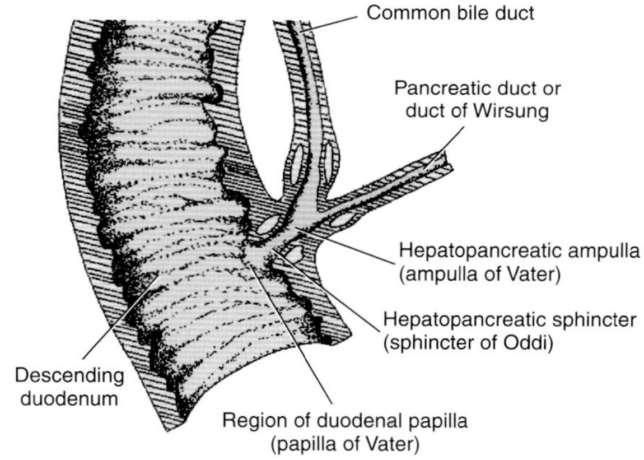

Fig. 16-6. Common bile duct.

16

GALLBLADDER AND BILIARY DUCTS (LATERAL VIEW)

The simplified lateral-view drawing in Fig. 16-7 illustrates the arrangement of the **liver, gallbladder,** and **biliary ducts** as seen from the right side. The gallbladder is **anterior** to the midcoronal plane, whereas the duct system is about midway between the front and the back. This spatial relationship influences optimal positioning of either the gallbladder or the biliary ducts. If necessary to place the gallbladder as close to the image receptor as possible, the prone position would be much better than the supine position. If the primary purpose is to **drain the gallbladder** into the duct system, the patient would be placed **supine** to assist this drainage.

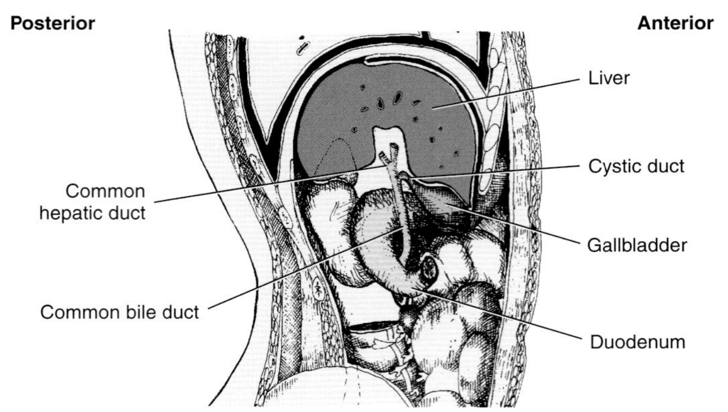

Fig. 16-7. Side view of gallbladder and biliary ducts.

BODY HABITUS AND GALLBLADDER LOCATION

The usual position of the gallbladder varies according to the body build of the patient (Fig. 16-8).

Hypersthenic In the **hypersthenic** body habitus, the gallbladder is usually located higher and more lateral than average. The most common basic position for the gallbladder is the LAO, and only a slight rotation of **15° to 20°** will shift the gallbladder away from the spine for the hypersthenic patient.

Sthenic/Hyposthenic In the average body builds, which includes the **sthenic** and **hyposthenic** types, the gallbladder is usually located about halfway between the xiphoid tip and the lower lateral rib margin. A **20° to 25°** LAO position is required to shift the gallbladder away from the spine.

Asthenic In the **asthenic** body habitus, the gallbladder is much lower, near the level of the iliac crest and near the midline. A **35° to 40°** rotation LAO is required to shift the gallbladder away from the spine.

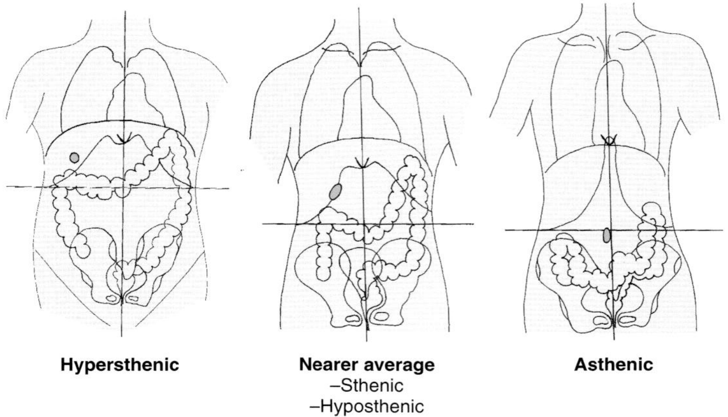

Fig. 16-8. Body habitus and gallbladder variation.

Anatomy Review

RADIOGRAPH OF THE GALLBLADDER

This LAO position of the gallbladder in Fig. 16-9 demonstrates the cystic duct and the three major divisions of the gallbladder as labeled:

A. Cystic duct
B. Neck
C. Body
D. Fundus

Note by the low position of the gallbladder near the level of the iliac crest, and by the 35° to 40° LAO position, that this patient represents a near asthenic body habitus type.

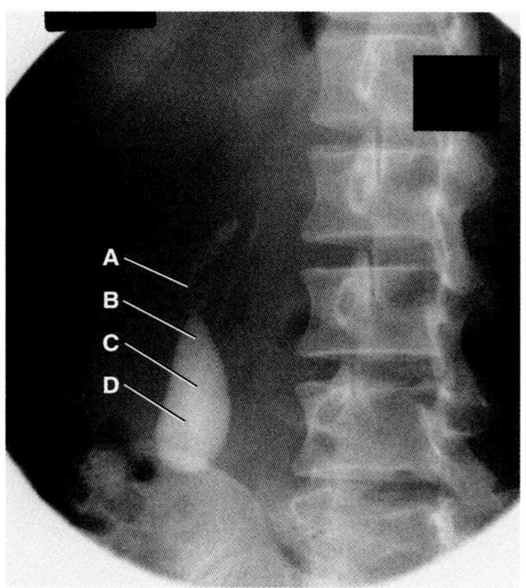

Fig. 16-9. Cholecystogram (gallbladder); 35°-40° LAO position.

RADIOGRAPH OF THE BILIARY DUCTS

Fig. 16-10 demonstrates two spot images of the various divisions and components of the biliary tract. This was taken during a surgical procedure, wherein contrast media was injected via a catheter directly into the biliary ducts. This does not represent normal duct positions but visualizes certain identifiable duct components and demonstrates the complexity of the biliary system as it may be seen on radiographs taken during an operative cholangiogram.

A. Right hepatic duct
B. Left hepatic duct
C. Common bile duct
D. Region of duodenal papilla (papilla of Vater)
E. Duodenum (descending loop)

Note: The common bile duct and the duodenal papilla cannot be definitely determined from this radiograph alone.

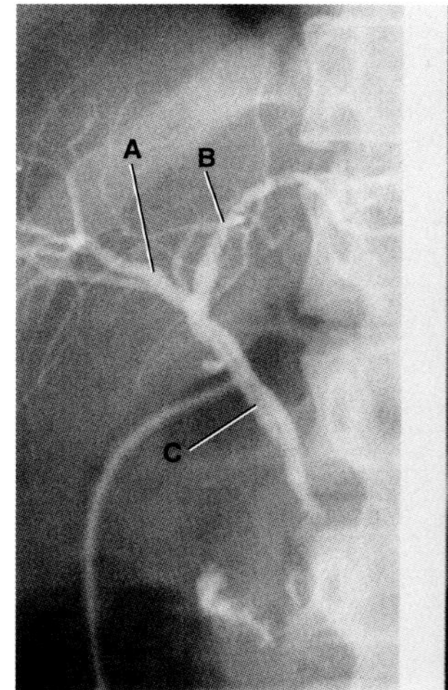

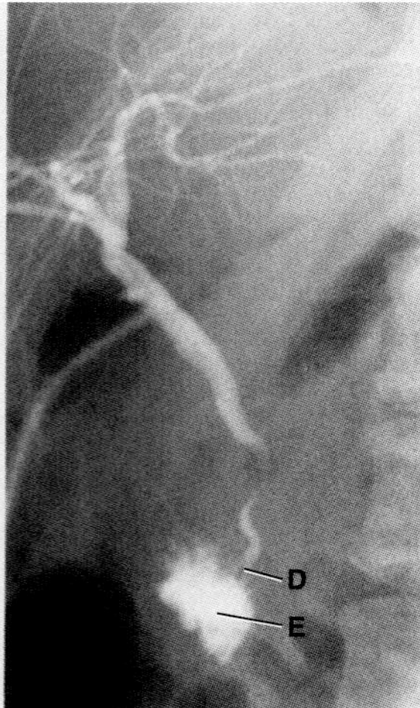

Fig. 16-10. Biliary ducts.

16

RADIOGRAPHIC PROCEDURES AND POSITIONING

Gallbladder and Biliary Duct Radiography

Because the liver is such a large, solid organ, it can be easily located in the upper right quadrant on abdominal radiographs. The gallbladder and biliary ducts, however, blend in with other abdominal soft tissues and in most cases cannot be visualized without the addition of contrast media. Only about 10% to 15% of all gallstones contain enough calcium to be visualized on a plain abdominal radiographic image (see description of cholelithiasis on following page). Fig. 16-11 demonstrates gallstones within the gallbladder on this oral cholecystogram scout radiograph.

TERMINOLOGY

Radiographic examination of the gallbladder and biliary ducts is referred to by different terms. It is important to identify a specific examination by the correct term. The following biliary terminology chart lists and defines commonly used terms:

BILIARY TERMINOLOGY

TERM	MEANING
Chole- *(ko'le)*	Prefix denoting relationship to bile
Cysto- *(sis'to)*	Prefix denoting sac or bladder
Cholecystogram *(ko"le-sis'to-gram)* (Oral cholecystogram —OCG)	Radiographic examination of the gallbladder
Cholangiogram *(ko-lan'je-o-gram")*	Radiographic examination of the biliary ducts
Cholecystocholangiogram *(ko"-le-sis"to-ko-lan'je-o-gram)*	Study of both the gallbladder and biliary ducts
Choleliths *(ko'le-liths)*	Gallstones
Cholelithiasis *(ko"le-li-thi'ah-sis)*	Condition of having gallstones
Cholecystitis *(ko"le-sis-ti'tis)*	Inflammation of the gallbladder
Cholecystectomy *(ko"le-sis-tek'ta-me)*	Surgical removal of the gallbladder

Oral Cholecystogram–Historical Review

Contrast media is ingested orally for a **cholecystogram;** thus this procedure is termed an oral cholecystogram, abbreviated **OCG** (Fig. 16-11).

A common way to get contrast media into the biliary system has been orally (by mouth). Cholecystography of this type is accomplished following ingestion of four to six tablets or capsules during the evening preceding the examination. These oral contrast media for visualization of the gallbladder are termed **cholecystopaques.**

Note: The number of oral cholecystograms being ordered has declined greatly because of the increased use of sonography. However, they may still be performed in certain institutions and technologists should be familiar with this procedure.

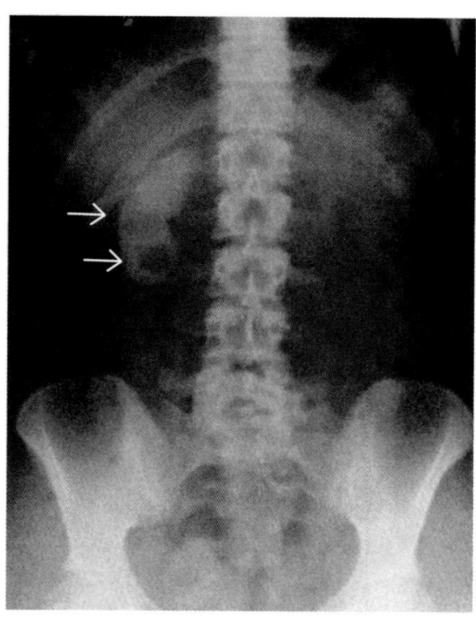

Fig. 16-11. Oral cholecystogram (OCG) (with gallstones—cholelithiasis, *arrows*).

PURPOSE

The purpose of the oral cholecystogram is to study radiographically the anatomy and function of the biliary system. The oral cholecystogram measures the following:

1. The **functional ability** of the liver to remove the orally administered contrast medium from the bloodstream and to excrete it along with the bile
2. The **patency and condition of the biliary ducts**
3. The **concentrating and contracting ability of the gallbladder**

CONTRAINDICATIONS

Contraindications to cholecystography are few, but do include the following:

1. Advanced hepatorenal disease, especially with renal impairment (e.g., severe jaundice, acute or chronic liver failure, renal failure, and hepatocellular disease)
2. Active gastrointestinal (GI) disease, such as vomiting, severe diarrhea, or malabsorption syndrome, which would prevent absorption of the oral contrast medium
3. Hypersensitivity to iodine-containing compounds
4. Pregnancy, which requires referral for ultrasound

Pathologic Indications

GALLBLADDER AND BILIARY DUCT RADIOGRAPHY

Clinical indications for oral cholecystogram include **nausea, heartburn,** and **vomiting.** A number of abnormal conditions may be demonstrated using various imaging modalities. They include the following:

Biliary Calculi (Gallstones)

Choledocholithiasis is the presence of stones in the **biliary ducts.** Biliary stones may form in the biliary ducts or migrate from the **gallbladder.** Often, these stones produce a blockage in the ducts. Symptoms include pain, tenderness in the right upper quadrant, jaundice, and sometimes pancreatitis.

Cholelithiasis is the condition of having abnormal calcifications or stones in the gallbladder. Cholelithiasis is the most common abnormality diagnosed during an OCG. Increased levels of bilirubin, calcium, or cholesterol may lead to the formation of gallstones. Female and obese patients are at a higher risk for developing gallstones. Ninety percent of all gallbladder and duct disorders are due to cholelithiasis. Symptoms of cholelithiasis include right upper quadrant pain usually after a meal, nausea, and possibly vomiting. Patients with complete blockage of the biliary ducts may develop jaundice.

Approximately 60% of gallstones are primarily made up of cholesterol, making them highly radiolucent; another 25% to 30% are primarily cholesterol and/or crystalline salts, which also are radiolucent. These radiolucent gallstones produce filling defects within the gallbladder during the OCG. This leaves a smaller percentage (approximately 10% to15%) of gallstones that are composed of crystalline calcium salts, which are often visible on an abdominal radiographic image without contrast media.

Milk calcium bile is the emulsion of biliary stones in the gallbladder. This emulsion buildup of calcium deposits within the gallbladder may be difficult to diagnose during an OCG. Milk calcium bile may be best demonstrated on the PA scout image. It will be seen as a diffuse collection of sand-like calcifications or sediment.

Although drugs have been developed that will dissolve these stones, most patients will have their gallbladder removed. A laparoscopic technique for removing the gallbladder (cholecystectomy) has greatly reduced the convalescence of the patient.

With **sonography,** any stones within the gallbladder or biliary ducts produce a "shadowing" effect. The shadowing effect is created by the partial blockage of the sound wave as it passes by.

Cholecystitis Cholecystitis, acute or chronic, is inflammation of the gallbladder. In **acute cholecystitis,** often a blockage of the cystic duct restricts the flow of bile from the gallbladder into the common bile duct. The blockage is frequently due to a stone lodged in the neck of the gallbladder. After a period of time, the bile begins to irritate the inner lining of the gallbladder and it becomes inflamed. Symptoms of acute cholecystitis include abdominal pain, tenderness in the right, upper quadrant, and fever. Bacterial infection and ischemia (obstruction of blood supply) of the gallbladder may also produce acute cholecystitis. Gas-producing bacteria may lead to a gangrenous gallbladder. The gallbladder with acute cholecystitis rarely becomes radiopaque during an OCG.

Chronic cholecystitis is almost always associated with gallstones but may also be an outcome of pancreatitis or carcinoma of the gallbladder. Symptoms of right upper quadrant pain, heartburn, and nausea may occur following a meal. Calcified plaques, thickening or calcification of the wall of the gallbladder may be related to chronic cholecystitis. Chronic cholecystitis may produce repetitive attacks following meals and typically subside in 1 to 4 hours.

Neoplasms Neoplasms are new growths, which may be benign or malignant. Malignant or cancerous tumors of the gallbladder can be aggressive and spread to the liver, pancreas, or GI tract. Fortunately, neoplasms of the gallbladder are relatively rare. Of the malignant tumors of the gallbladder, 9% are adenocarcinomas and 10% are squamous cell carcinomas. Common benign tumors of the gallbladder include adenomas and cholesterol polyps.

Approximately 80% of patients with carcinoma of the gallbladder have stones. As the tumor grows, it may obstruct the biliary system. Patients may experience pain, vomiting, and jaundice. Sonography and computed tomography are the best modalities to demonstrate neoplasms of the gallbladder. Sometimes, a stent or drain needs to be inserted within the common bile duct to provide a pathway for the buildup of bile resulting from obstruction.

Biliary Stenosis Biliary stenosis is a narrowing of one of the biliary ducts. The flow of bile may be restricted by this condition. In the case of gallstones, the stenosis may prevent the passage of the small gallstones into the duodenum, leading to obstruction of the ducts. Cholecystitis and jaundice may result from biliary stenosis. During cholangiography, the common bile duct may appear elongated, tapered, and narrow. A gallstone lodged at the distal common bile duct often presents a filling defect with a small channel of contrast media passing around it.

Congenital Anomalies Congenital anomalies of the gallbladder are conditions that the patient possesses at birth. Although most are benign, some may affect the production, storage, or release of bile.

SUMMARY OF PATHOLOGIC INDICATIONS—GALLBLADDER AND BILIARY DUCT RADIOGRAPHY

CONDITION OR DISEASE	MOST COMMON RADIOGRAPHIC EXAM	POSSIBLE RADIOGRAPHIC APPEARANCE	MANUAL EXPOSURE FACTOR ADJUSTMENT*
Choledocholithiasis (stones in **biliary ducts**)	Oral cholecystogram (OCG) Sonography	Nonvisualization of gallbladder on OCG	None
Cholelithiasis (stones in **gallbladder**)	Oral cholecystogram (OCG) Sonography Radionuclide studies	Both radiolucent and radiopaque densities seen in the region of the gallbladder; "shadowing" effect with sonography	None
Acute cholecystitis	Oral cholecystogram (OCG) Sonography Radionuclide studies	Nonvisualized gallbladder during OCG Thickened wall of gallbladder with sonography	None
Chronic cholecystitis	Oral cholecystogram (OCG) Sonography	Calcified plaques or calcification of the wall of the gallbladder	None
Neoplasms	Sonography Computed tomography	Mass seen within gallbladder, liver, and/or biliary ducts	N/A
Biliary stenosis	Operative cholangiogram	Elongated, tapered, and narrowing of common bile duct	None
Congenital anomalies	Oral cholecystogram (OCG) Sonography	Possible nonvisualization of gallbladder on OCG	None

*Dependent on stage or severity of condition.

Oral Cholecystogram Procedure

PATIENT PREPARATION

Patient preparations for the oral cholecystogram (OCG) correlate well with preparations for an upper GI series, so these exams are commonly scheduled on the same morning. Patients who have been on a fat-free diet should eat some fats for 1 or 2 days before the gallbladder examination. Ingestion of fats causes the gallbladder to contract. By making sure that the gallbladder has emptied before the administration of contrast medium, chances are increased that the newly formed bile, with contrast medium added, will be stored in the gallbladder.

Laxatives are to be avoided during the 24-hour period before the exam. The evening meal before the examination should be a light one and should not contain any fats or fried foods. When combined with an upper GI, **the patient must be NPO** (*nil per os,* meaning "nothing by mouth") for at least 8 hours and **must refrain from chewing gum or smoking** until after the exam.

Depending on the contrast medium used, either four or six tablets or capsules are taken after the evening meal but before 9 p.m. The usual cholecystopaques are most effective **taken 10 to 12 hours before the exam.** No breakfast is permitted, and the patient reports to radiology in the early morning. The exact patient prep and amount of contrast medium used will vary from hospital to hospital.

When the patient arrives in the radiology department for oral cholecystography, they should be instructed to remove all clothing from the chest and abdomen areas and put on a hospital gown.

PATIENT INTERVIEW

Before the scout radiograph, the patient must be questioned about taking the contrast medium. **First,** ask the patient how many pills were taken and at what time. It may be necessary to have the patient describe the capsules or tablets to confirm that they were the correct ones.

Second, question the patient regarding any reaction from the pills. Nausea followed by vomiting would prevent adequate absorption, as would active diarrhea. Any anaphylactoid or allergic reactions should be noted.

Third, determine that the patient has not had breakfast.

Fourth, make sure that the patient still has a gallbladder. A cholecystogram is not needed on those rare occasions when the patient has already had the gallbladder surgically removed.

Fifth, question the female patient of childbearing age regarding a possible pregnancy with precautions taken as for other abdominal radiographic exams.

IMAGING ROUTINE

Scout A scout image is generally taken first with the patient in a prone position on a 24 × 30 cm (10 × 12 inches) or 35 × 43 cm (14 × 17 inches) IR at 70 to 80 kV. The scout image must be checked to determine the presence or absence of an opacified gallbladder.

If the gallbladder shadow is present, the technologist should determine (1) its exact location, (2) presence of any overlap by intestine or bone, (3) sufficient concentration of contrast medium for additional imaging, and (4) quality of the exposure factors. If the gallbladder did not opacify adequately for imaging, question the patient again in detail about preparation and especially about diet for the past 24 hours.

Nonvisualization on the first day may result in a 2-day study with a second dose of contrast medium or, perhaps, a trip to the sonography department for cholecystosonography.

LAO and Right Lateral Decubitus (PA) or Erect PA A common imaging routine as described and illustrated later in this chapter includes the **left anterior oblique** position, in addition to **either a right lateral decubitus or an erect PA** projection. The lateral decubitus or erect position is important to stratify or "layer out" gallstones and also to allow the gallbladder to assume a different position within the abdomen in relationship to the spine or other abdominal structures.

Patient Instructions

____ **I.V. CHOLANGIOGRAM AND/OR INTRAVENOUS PYELOGRAM**
1. Bowel Prep Kit III - 24 hour prep. All instructions are contained in kit.

____ **BARIUM ENEMA**
1. Bowel Prep Kit III - 24 hour prep. All instructions are contained in kit. May have a clear liquid breakfast.

____ **GALLBLADDER SERIES (ORAL CHOLECYSTOGRAM)**
1. Fat free supper evening before examination.
2. Take one iodinated contrast media tablet every ½ hour starting at 2:00 p.m. day before exam
3. Nothing by mouth after midnight.

____ **UPPER G.I. SERIES AND/OR SMALL BOWEL SERIES**
1. Do not eat, drink, smoke or chew gum after midnight. Any anti-spasmodic medication should be preferably discontinued at least 24 hours before exam. Bowel Prep Kit III may be purchased at most drug stores. Baptist Medical Center Pharmacy carries this kit along with Revco and Thrifty Drugs. Please call ahead to your pharmacy if you have any questions.

____ **ULTRASOUND PREPS:**
Ultrasound of the ABDOMEN: **Fat free clear** liquid diet from 6:00 p.m. the evening before examination.
Ultrasound of the PELVIS: **MUST** have a full bladder. Finish drinking 38 to 42 ounces of liquid one hour before exam. **DO NOT** empty bladder until after exam.

C.T. PREPS:
Abdomen - Clear liquids after midnight
Chest - Clear liquids only four hours prior to exam
Head - Clear liquids only four hours prior to exam
Pelvis - Clear liquids after midnight
Spine - no prep

Appointment date ____________ Appointment time ____________

Fig. 16-12. Sample patient instruction form.

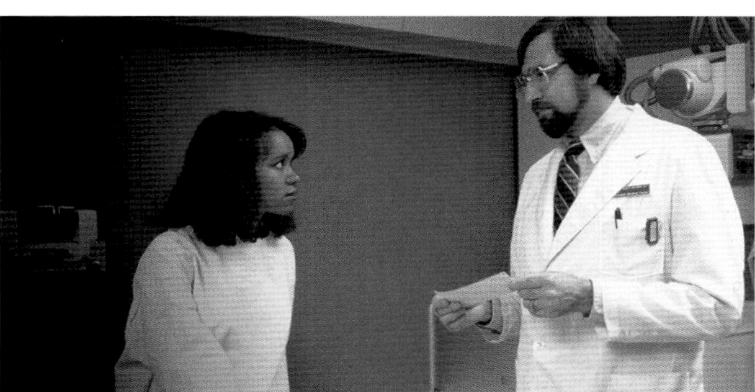

Fig. 16-13. Patient interview.

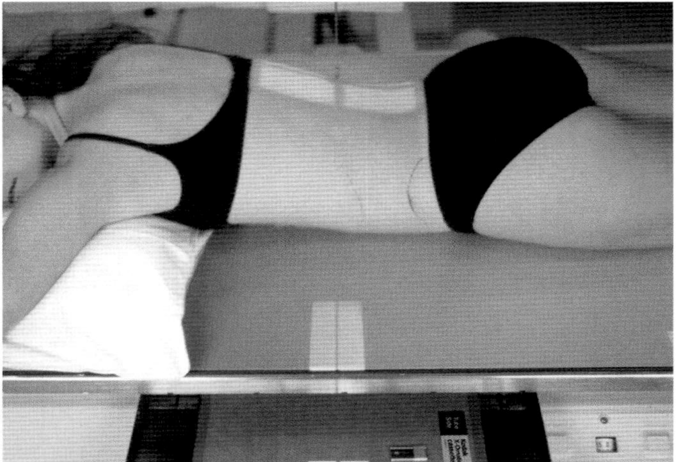

Fig. 16-14. Positioning for a cholecystogram scout.

Some radiologists also request **fluoroscopy and spot images** of the gallbladder in the upright position in addition to the conventional imaging routine. Fluoroscopy and spot imaging allows use of compression and small positional changes to optimally visualize the gallbladder.

16

Sonography (Ultrasound)

Sonography of the gallbladder provides a noninvasive means to study the gallbladder and the biliary ducts (Figs. 16-15).

Four advantages of sonography over conventional OCG imaging are as follows:

1. **No ionizing radiation:** Sonography is a nonionizing radiation imaging modality that eliminates radiation exposure to the patient, radiologist, and technologist (if fluoroscopy is performed with conventional OCG).
2. **Detection of small calculi:** Sonography can detect small calculi in the gallbladder and biliary ducts that generally are not visualized during an OCG.
3. **No contrast medium:** No contrast medium is required with sonography. Therefore this is an ideal alternative for patients who are sensitive to iodinated contrast agents.
4. **Less patient preparation:** Patient preparation with sonography is greatly reduced as compared with the OCG. For sonography, the patient should be NPO 4 hours before the exam, whereas the patient preparation and contrast media administration for an OCG can require 2 or more days to complete. Therefore sonography provides a quick diagnosis for gallbladder disease and the physician can make a surgical decision in hours rather than days.

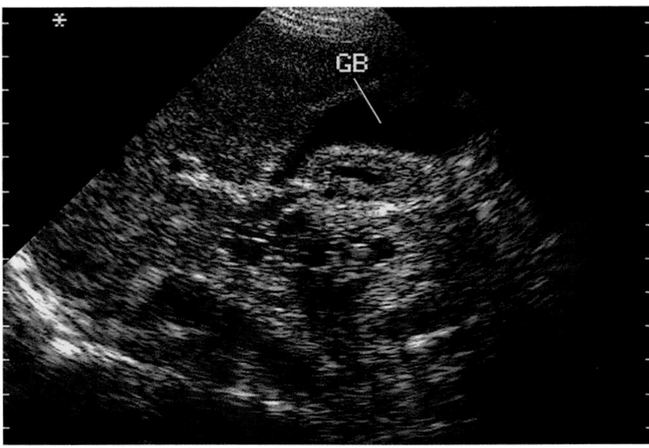

Fig. 16-15. Ultrasound of gallbladder.

Special Radiographic Biliary Duct Procedures

The following four special radiographic biliary duct procedures are being performed in such significant numbers that technologists should be able to perform them when requested. The first one listed in the box at right and on p. 533 is the **operative cholangiogram,** which is performed in surgery under the direction of the surgeon and will be described in more detail in the Surgical Radiographic Procedures section of Chapter 19.

The remaining three biliary duct special procedures are described in the box at right and on pp. 533-535 and are generally performed in the radiology department.

SPECIAL RADIOGRAPHIC BILIARY DUCT PROCEDURES AND PATHOLOGIC INDICATIONS

Operative Cholangiogram

Operative cholangiograms are performed to accomplish the following:

1. Reveal any choleliths not previously detected (primary purpose)
2. Investigate the patency of the biliary tract
3. Determine the functional status of the papilla of Vater
4. Demonstrate small lesions, strictures, or dilatations within the biliary ducts

Postoperative T-Tube Cholangiogram

T-tube cholangiograms are performed to accomplish the following:

1. Visualize any residual or previously undetected choleliths
2. Evaluate the status of the biliary duct system
3. Demonstrate small lesions, strictures, or dilatations within the biliary ducts
4. Extract small stone from biliary duct during the T-tube procedure using a special basket catheter

Percutaneous Transhepatic Cholangiography (PTC)

The PTC is performed in the following cases:

1. Obstructive jaundice: If the patient is jaundiced and the ducts are suspected to be dilated, an obstruction of the biliary ducts may be the cause. The obstruction may be due to calculi or biliary stenosis.
2. Stone extraction and biliary drainage: PTC allows the radiologist to diagnose the condition and, using specialized equipment, remove the stone or dilate the restricted portion of the biliary tract. Excess bile may be drained during a PTC to decompress the biliary ducts.

Endoscopic Retrograde Cholangiopancreatography (ERCP)

The diagnostic ERCP is performed to accomplish the following:

1. Investigate the patency of the biliary/pancreatic ducts
2. Reveal any choleliths not previously detected
3. Demonstrate small lesions, strictures, or dilatations within the biliary/pancreatic ducts

Operative (or Immediate) Cholangiogram

First performed in 1932, the **operative** or **immediate cholangiogram** is performed during surgery, usually during a cholecystectomy, wherein the surgeon removes the gallbladder. The surgeon may suspect that residual stones are located in one of the biliary ducts. After the gallbladder is removed, a small catheter is inserted into the remaining portion of the cystic duct. Iodinated contrast media is injected and radiographic images are obtained. This procedure is described in detail and illustrated in Chapter 19 under Surgical Radiographic Procedures.

Postoperative (T-Tube or Delayed) Cholangiography

Postoperative, also termed *T-tube,* or *delayed cholangiography,* is usually performed in the radiology department following a cholecystectomy. The surgeon may be concerned about residual stones in the biliary ducts that went undetected during the surgery. If these concerns exist, the surgeon will place a special T-tube catheter into the common bile duct during the cholecystectomy. The catheter extends to the outside of the body and is clamped off.

SUMMARY OF POSTOPERATIVE (T-TUBE) CHOLANGIOGRAPHY PROCEDURE

The following steps are taken in the performance of a postoperative cholangiogram:

1. Prepare the fluoroscopic suite.
2. Set up the examination tray.
3. Select and prepare the contrast media. Determine whether the patient is hypersensitive to iodinated contrast media.
4. Take the appropriate scout images to verify position and technique.
5. Provide lead aprons for those persons remaining in the room during the procedure.
6. Monitor the patient during the procedure.
7. Change fluoro spot film-screen cassettes as needed.
8. Produce conventional radiographs as requested.

Because the T-tube catheter has been clamped off, drainage of excess bile is performed at the beginning of the procedure. An emesis basin should be provided for this task. **Follow standard precautions when handling bile.**

After duct drainage and under fluoroscopic control, the iodinated contrast media is injected fractionally and fluoro spot films are taken. It is important not to introduce any air bubbles while injecting contrast media because these bubbles may be confused for radiolucent stones.

If residual stones are detected, the radiologist may elect to remove them. Similar to the percutaneous transhepatic cholangiography (PTC) procedure described on the following page, a basket catheter may be passed over a guide wire and the stones removed.

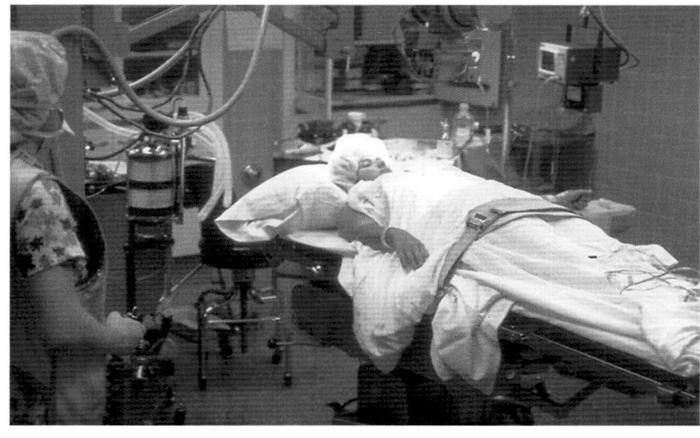

Fig. 16-16. Obtaining a scout image for an operative cholangiogram.

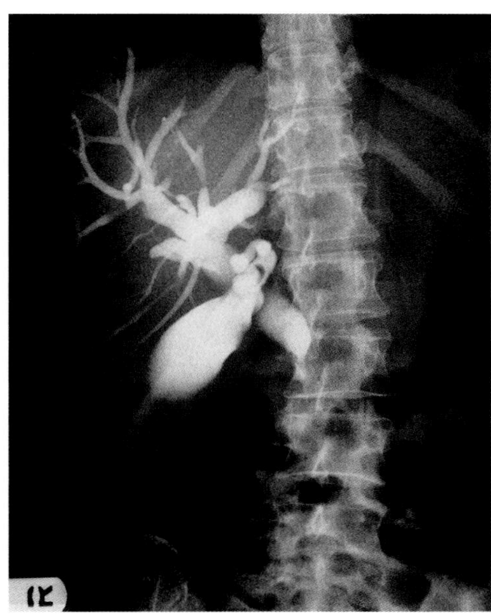

Fig. 16-17. T-tube cholangiogram.

16

Percutaneous Transhepatic Cholangiography

Percutaneous transhepatic cholangiography **(PTC)** is another type of cholangiography that demonstrates the biliary ducts. Also generally performed in the radiology department, PTC is more invasive than other forms of cholangiography and performed less frequently. However, it gives the radiologist more options in the diagnosis and treatment of biliary conditions.

The PTC involves a **direct puncture of biliary ducts** with a needle passing through the liver. Once the needle is within a duct, iodinated contrast media is injected under fluoroscopic control. Fluoroscopic spot images and conventional radiographic images are taken during the procedure.

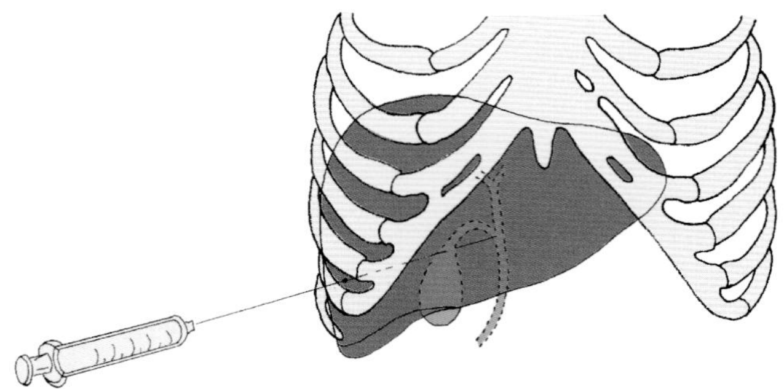

Fig. 16-18. PTC puncture through liver into biliary ducts.

PROCEDURE

A certain amount of risk is associated with the PTC because of the needle puncture into the liver tissue. The three major risks include the following:

1. **Liver hemorrhage:** The liver may hemorrhage internally, or bile may escape into the peritoneal cavity.
2. **Pneumothorax:** Because the liver is near the right hemidiaphragm, the needle puncture may result in a pneumothorax. Therefore, after the procedure, a chest radiograph may be ordered.
3. **Escape of bile:** Bile may escape into the peritoneal cavity, leading to inflammation of surrounding tissue. In addition to studying the biliary ducts, the PTC may serve as a therapeutic procedure to extract stones or decompress dilated ducts.

Both during and after the procedure, the patient's vital signs are closely monitored to detect deterioration.

The site of the puncture is surgically prepared. After the local anesthetic is given, the radiologist inserts the needle into the liver in the approximate location of the biliary ducts. More than one puncture may be necessary to locate the appropriate duct. Under fluoroscopic view, the radiologist adjusts the needle while slowly injecting the contrast media. Once the ducts are filled, fluoroscopic spot images and conventional radiographic images are taken.

A larger needle may be inserted into a duct containing a stone. A special basket or loop catheter is passed over a guide wire and is positioned near the stone. Under fluoroscopic control, the stone can be extracted from the duct.

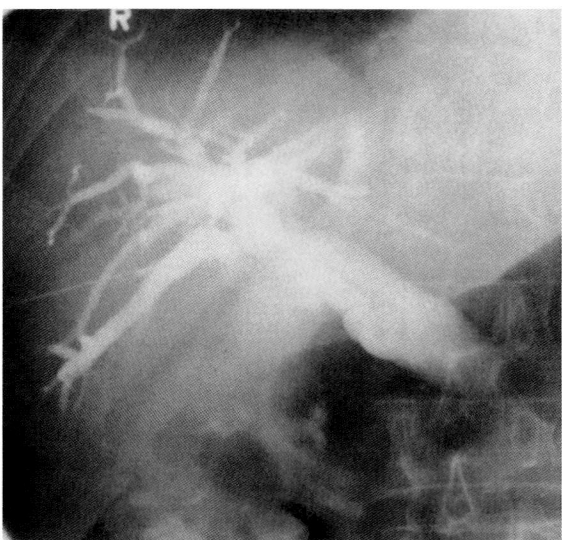

Fig. 16-19. Percutaneous transhepatic cholangiogram (PTC).

SUMMARY OF PTC PROCEDURE

Although the percutaneous transhepatic puncture is performed by the radiologist, the technologist has specific responsibilities. These responsibilities include the following:

1. Prepare the fluoroscopic suite.
2. Set up the sterile tray and include the long, thin-walled needle used for the puncture. (The needle is a Chiba, or "skinny" needle. It has a flexible shaft that allows for easy manipulation of the needle during the puncture.)
3. Select and prepare the contrast media. Determine whether the patient is hypersensitive to iodinated contrast media.
4. Provide lead aprons for those persons remaining in the room during the exposure.
5. Take the appropriate scout images to verify position and technique.
6. Monitor the patient during the procedure.
7. Change fluoroscopy films as needed, if spot film-screen cassettes are being used.
8. Take chest radiographic image following procedure if requested.

Endoscopic Retrograde Cholangiopancreatography

Another procedure for examination of the biliary and main pancreatic ducts that is performed more frequently is endoscopic retrograde cholangiopancreatography, or simply **ERCP.**

ENDOSCOPY

Endoscopy *(en-dos'ko-pe)* is inspection of any cavity of the body by means of an endoscope, an instrument that allows illumination of the internal lining of an organ. Various fiber-optic endoscopes are available to examine the interior lining of the stomach, duodenum, and colon. Older types of endoscopes allow for individual viewing only through an eyepiece, but newer **video endoscopes** project the image onto video monitors for multiple viewing. Also, a special type of fiber-optic endoscope, called a **duodenoscope,** is commonly used for an ERCP exam. This instrument, when inserted into the duodenum through the mouth, esophagus, and stomach, provides a wide-angle side view that is useful for locating and inserting a catheter or cannula into the small opening of the sphincter of Oddi, leading from the duodenum into the common bile duct and the main pancreatic ducts.

DIAGNOSTIC OR THERAPEUTIC

The ERCP can be either a diagnostic or a therapeutic procedure. Therapeutically, ERCP can be performed to relieve certain pathologic conditions. This can be either the removal of choleliths or small lesions, or for other purposes such as to repair a stenosis (narrowing or blockage of a duct or canal) of the hepatopancreatic sphincter or associated ducts.*

For diagnostic purposes, in general, the ERCP procedure includes the insertion endoscopically of the catheter or injection cannula into the common bile duct or main pancreatic duct under fluoroscopic control, followed by retrograde injection (backward or reverse direction) of contrast media into the biliary ducts. The procedure is usually performed by a gastroenterologist assisted by a team including the technologist, one or more nurses, and perhaps a radiologist.

SUMMARY OF ERCP PROCEDURE

The ERCP typically involves the following steps:

1. Prepare the fluoroscopic suite.
2. Set up the examination tray.
3. Select and prepare the contrast media. Determine whether the patient is hypersensitive to iodinated contrast media.
4. Take the appropriate scout images to verify position and technique.
5. Assist the gastroenterologist with fluoroscopy for the placement of the catheter or injection cannula.
6. Monitor the patient during the procedure.
7. Change fluoroscopy spot films as needed, if a film-screen system is being used.
8. Produce conventional radiographic images as requested.

PRECAUTIONS

1. Because the patient's throat is anesthetized during the procedure, the patient should remain NPO for at least 1 hour (or more) after the procedure. This will prevent aspiration of food or liquid into the lungs.
2. Review the clinical history of the patient to determine whether the patient has pancreatitis or, specifically, a pseudocyst of the pancreas. Injecting contrast media into a pseudocyst may lead to a rupture.
3. Ensure that all persons in the fluoroscopy room wear protective aprons.

*Tortorici MR, Apfel PJ: Advanced radiographic and angiographic procedures with an introduction to specialized imaging, Philadelphia, 1995, FA Davis.

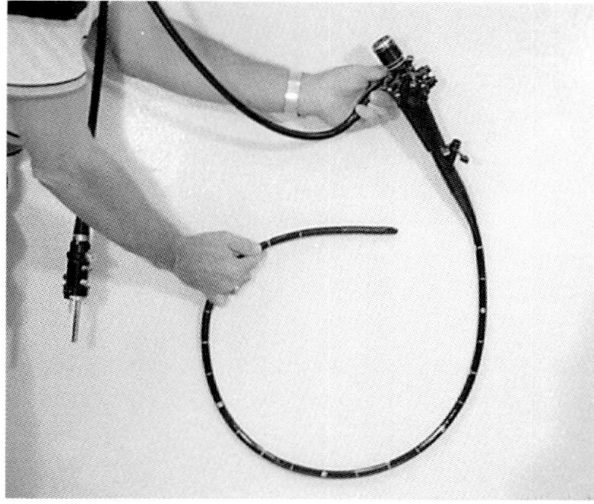

Fig. 16-20. Duodenoscope (can be connected to video monitor). (Modified from Tortorici MR, Apfel PJ: Advanced radiographic and angiographic procedures with an introduction to specialized imaging, Philadelphia, 1995, FA Davis, p. 49, with permission.)

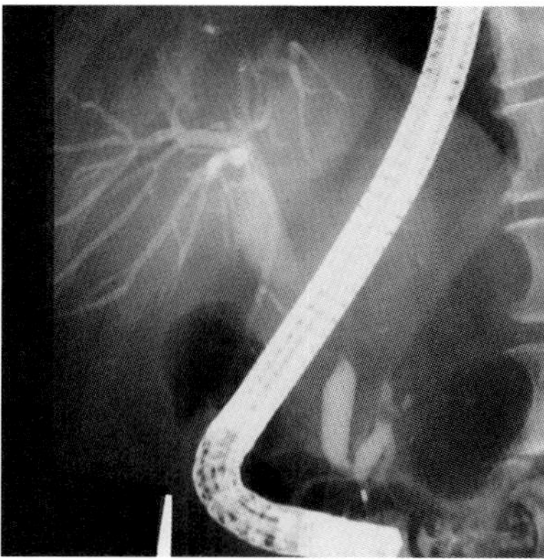

Fig. 16-21. ERCP radiograph demonstrating biliary tree.

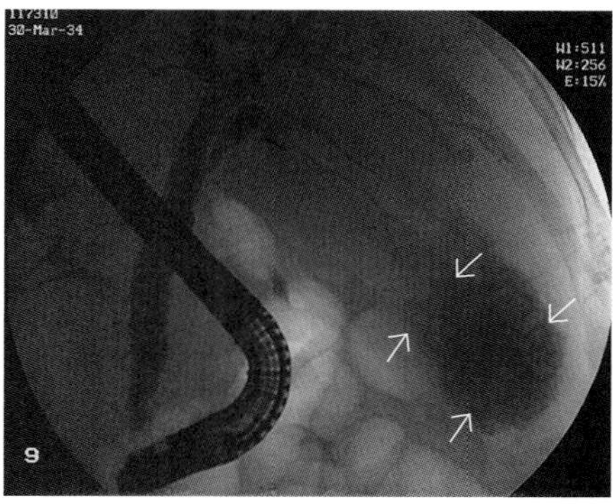

Fig. 16-22. ERCP digital positive image of biliary tree and gallbladder filled with gallstones *(arrows).*

Summary of Radiographic Procedures

GALLBLADDER AND BILIARY SYSTEM RADIOGRAPHY

In summary, **cholecystography and cholangiography** may be categorized by the method of contrast medium administration. Contrast medium is usually administered orally for cholecystography (gallbladder exam). For cholangiography, the biliary ducts are usually studied after intravenous infusion or various methods of direct injection of contrast medium.

PEDIATRIC APPLICATIONS

Although it rarely happens, children can develop gallstones. The presence of gallstones is often secondary to childhood diseases or conditions such as hemolytic anemia and sickle cell anemia. Oral cholecystograms (OCG) are seldom performed on children because of the increased use of sonography.

GERIATRIC APPLICATIONS

The contrast media ingested for an oral OCG may be irritating to the GI tract of certain patients, especially older individuals. The technologist should carefully interview the patient before the procedure. Note any history of severe vomiting and diarrhea after the ingestion of the oral contrast media.

SUMMARY TABLE OF GALLBLADDER AND BILIARY SYSTEM PROCEDURES

PROCEDURE	ANATOMY VISUALIZED	ADMINISTRATION OF CONTRAST MEDIA
Cholecystography—Gallbladder		
1. Oral cholecystogram (OCG)	Gallbladder	Oral ingestion
Cholangiography—Biliary Ducts		
1. Sonography procedure	Gallbladder and biliary ducts	None needed
2. Operative (immediate) cholangiogram or laparoscopic cholangiogram	Biliary ducts	Direct injection through catheter during surgery
3. T-tube cholangiogram	Biliary ducts	Direct injection through indwelling drainage tube
4. Percutaneous transhepatic cholangiogram (PTC)	Biliary ducts	Direct injection by a needle puncture through the liver into the biliary ducts
5. Endoscopic retrograde cholangiopancreatogram (ERCP)	Biliary/pancreatic ducts	Direct injection through catheter placed during endoscopic procedure

Alternative Modalities and Procedures

NUCLEAR MEDICINE

A **hepatobiliary** or **HIDA** scan is a scan of the gallbladder and biliary system. Patients with a history of abdominal pain, nausea, and vomiting, or chest pain resulting from gallbladder or biliary disease are candidates for this procedure. Patients are injected with a radioactive isotope and images are taken approximately 1 to 2 hours after injection. After the completion of the examination, another procedure may be performed to indicate the response of the gallbladder to hormonal stimulation. It requires a second injection.

Liver and spleen nuclear medicine scans evaluate functional liver disorders that include cirrhosis, hepatitis, and metabolic disorders.

COMPUTED TOMOGRAPHY

Computed tomography (CT) of the biliary system is an excellent modality for demonstrating a variety of conditions and diseases. CT is especially effective in demonstrating neoplasms of the liver, gallbladder, and pancreas. Stones can also be demonstrated with CT, but because of cost and radiation exposure, sonography is often preferred.

MAGNETIC RESONANCE IMAGING

Whereas CT and sonography are used to screen for neoplasms of the biliary system, magnetic resonance imaging (MRI) serves as an excellent modality in demonstrating select conditions. Specifically, MRI is effective in detecting hepatocellular carcinoma, cholangiocarcinoma, hepatic metastases, intrahepatic lymphoma, and adenocarcinoma of the gallbladder.

Gallstones can be demonstrated with MRI as a signal void with T2-weighted images. But because of cost and time factors, sonography should be considered over MRI for the patient with cholelithiasis.

RADIOGRAPHIC POSITIONING

Survey Information

A 2000 survey of the operating procedures (department routines) was conducted throughout the United States and Canada. The following information was compiled from the survey indicating the norm for basic routines for oral cholecystography and operative cholangiography. The results were somewhat consistent throughout all regions of the U.S. but demonstrated significant differences between the U.S. and Canada in two areas. This was in the use of ultrasound exclusively for gallbladder procedures and in the frequency of performing PTC and ERCP procedures.

REGIONAL DIFFERENCES IN U.S.

Some significant differences also existed in the exclusive use of ultrasound for gallbladder procedures in the Midwest (51%) compared with the East (46%) and the West (33%). See appendix at end of the textbook for more regional differences.

ORAL CHOLECYSTOGRAM (OCG OR GALLBLADDER) ROUTINE

	U.S. Average			Canada
	Basic			Basic
	2000	1995	1989	2000
Gallbladder (OCG)				
PA scout	54%	70%	78%	14%
LAO	39%	74%	63%	8%
R lat. decub.	32%	34%	31%	2%
PA erect	23%	30%	19%	7%
Fatty meal or CCK-PZ injection	29%	23%	20%	7%
Sonogram in combination with oral cholecystogram	25%	19%	—	6%
Sonogram exclusively	47%	—	—	59%

OPERATIVE CHOLANGIOGRAM ROUTINE

	U.S. Average			Canada
	Basic			Basic
	2000	1995	1989	2000
OR Cholangiogram				
AP	74%	81%	87%	55%
RPO	32%	27%	28%	13%

PERCUTANEOUS TRANSHEPATIC CHOLANGIOGRAM (PTC)

	U.S. Average			Canada
	Basic			Basic
	2000	1995	1989	2000
PTC				
Post-injection OP fluoro and spots	49%	65%	—	36%

T-TUBE POSTOPERATIVE CHOLANGIOGRAM

	U.S. Average			Canada
	Basic			Basic
	2000	1995	1989	2000
T-tube				
Fluoro and spot films	76%	86%	—	64%
AP	51%	67%	—	17%
RPO	39%	49%	—	12%

ENDOSCOPIC RETROGRADE CHOLANGIOPANCREATOGRAM (ERCP)

	U.S. Average			Canada
	Basic			Basic
	2000	1995	1989	2000
ERCP				
Post-injection AP fluoro and spots	74%	75%	—	2%
AP	37%	42%	—	4%
RPO	21%	19%	—	5%

Basic and Special Projections

Certain basic projections or positions of the gallbladder and biliary ducts are demonstrated and described on the following pages. The radiologist and technologist must closely coordinate their efforts during examinations of this part of the body. Individual variations exist among radiologists, and the routine or basic positions or projections listed may vary from hospital to hospital.

Gallbladder (Oral Cholecystogram—OCG)

BASIC

- **PA scout** 538
- **LAO** 539
- **Right lateral decubitus (PA)** 540
- **PA erect** 541

Special Biliary Duct Procedures

Percutaneous transhepatic cholangiography (PTC), endoscopic retrograde cholangiopancreatogram (ERCP), and T-tube cholangiography are described in the preceding pages of this chapter. These exams are performed primarily by the radiologist, with the radiographer assisting, therefore they are not described in the positioning pages of this chapter. Certain of these procedures that may be performed in the operating room with the use of mobile digital fluoroscopy (C-arm) are described in Chapter 19 in the section on surgical radiography.

PA PROJECTION: GALLBLADDER (ORAL CHOLECYSTOGRAM)

Scout

Gallbladder (Oral Cholecystogram)
BASIC
- PA scout
- LAO
- Right lateral decubitus (PA)
- PA erect

Pathology Demonstrated
A PA scout is taken to determine presence and location of gallbladder, presence of choleliths, adequate concentration of contrast media, and correctness of exposure factors.

Technical Factors
- IR size—24 × 30 cm (10 × 12 inches), lengthwise
  or—35 × 43 cm (14 × 17 inches), lengthwise
- Moving or stationary grid
- 70-80 kV range
- Technique and dose:

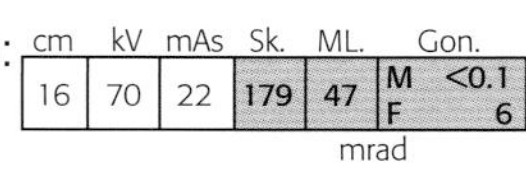

cm	kV	mAs	Sk.	ML.	Gon.
16	70	22	179	47	M <0.1 F 6
			mrad		

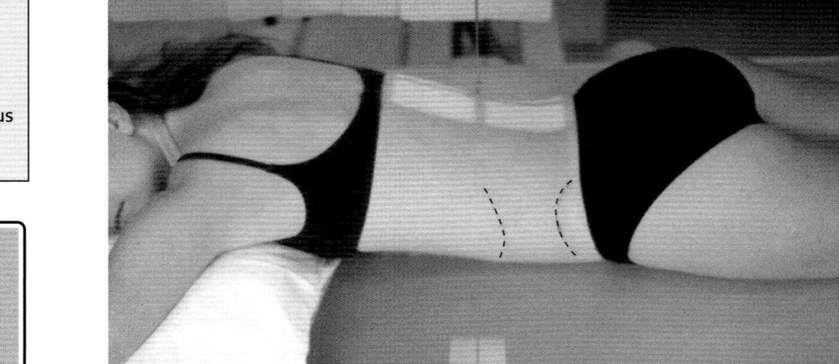

Fig. 16-23. PA scout (sthenic type)—centered to GB.

Exception: Some departmental routines include a full abdomen scout on a 35- × 43-cm (14- × 17-inch) IR, with positioning as for a PA abdomen centered to level of iliac crest or slightly above.

Shielding Place lead shield over gonadal area, not obscuring area of interest.

Patient Position Position patient prone (or erect), with a pillow for head, arms up beside head, and legs extended with support under ankles.

Part Position
- Align midsagittal plane to long axis of table with right half of abdomen centered to CR and to midline of table for sthenic type patient (see Note).
- Ensure that no rotation of pelvis or trunk exists.

Central Ray
- CR **perpendicular** to IR
- For average sthenic patient, CR to **level of L2** (which is about ½ to 1 inch, or 1.25 to 2.5 cm, above lowest margin of rib cage) **about 2 inches,** or 5 cm, **to right of midsagittal plane** (see Note on body habitus)
- Image receptor centered to CR
- Minimum SID of 40 inches (100 cm)

Collimation Collimate on four sides to cassette margins.

Respiration Suspend respiration upon expiration.

Note: Body habitus variation: **hypersthenic** (broad)—gallbladder more horizontal, 2 inches (5 cm) higher and more lateral; **asthenic** (thin)—gallbladder vertical, 2 inches (5 cm) lower, near the midline.

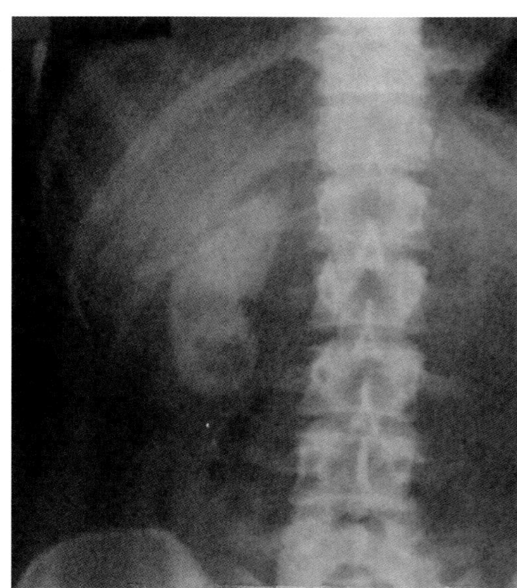

Fig. 16-24. PA scout.

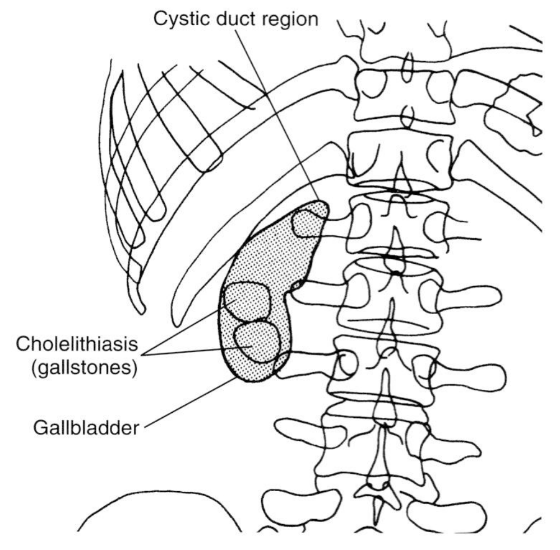

Fig. 16-25. PA scout.

Radiographic Criteria

Structures Shown: • Region of opacified gallbladder and area of cystic duct is demonstrated centered to IR.

Position: • Spine is parallel to the edge of radiograph. • **No rotation** is evident; the lumbar vertebrae, including the transverse processes, appear symmetric.

Collimation and CR: • Only minimal collimation margins are seen on all four sides of IR. • CR is centered at level of gallbladder.

Exposure Criteria: • No motion of gallbladder or abdominal contents is evident. • Appropriate technique is used with short-scale contrast to clearly visualize gallbladder, even through overlying rib if present. Choleliths (gallstones) may be visible, as seen in Fig. 16-24.

16

LAO POSITION: GALLBLADDER (ORAL CHOLECYSTOGRAM)

Gallbladder (Oral Cholecystogram)
BASIC
- PA scout
- LAO
- Right lateral decubitus (PA)
- PA erect

Pathology Demonstrated
Projects opacified gallbladder away from vertebral column; ideal projection to delineate between gas trapped in bowel and radiolucent stones in the gallbladder.

Technical Factors:
- IR size—24 × 30 cm (10 × 12 inches), lengthwise
- Moving or stationary grid
- 70-80 kV range
- Technique and dose:

cm	kV	mAs	Sk.	ML.	Gon.
19	70	30	262	54	M <1.0 F 9

mrad

Shielding Place lead shield over gonadal area, not obscuring area of interest.

Patient Position Patient semiprone, left anterior side down; pillow for head, right arm up, left arm down, right knee partially flexed to maintain this position

Part Position
- Rotate patient **15° to 40°** into LAO (less rotation on broad hypersthenic, more rotation on thin asthenic type).
- Align midsagittal plane to long axis of table, approximate right half of abdomen to CR and to midline of table (determine from scout and resultant marking on skin).

Central Ray
- CR **perpendicular** to IR
- CR to gallbladder as determined from scout
- IR centered to CR
- Minimum SID of 40 inches (100 cm)

Collimation Collimate on four sides to area of interest.

Respiration Suspend respiration upon expiration.

Note: Accurate centering and collimation should be possible with skin marking from preceding scout image.

An RPO may be performed if patient is not able to lie in a prone or semiprone position.

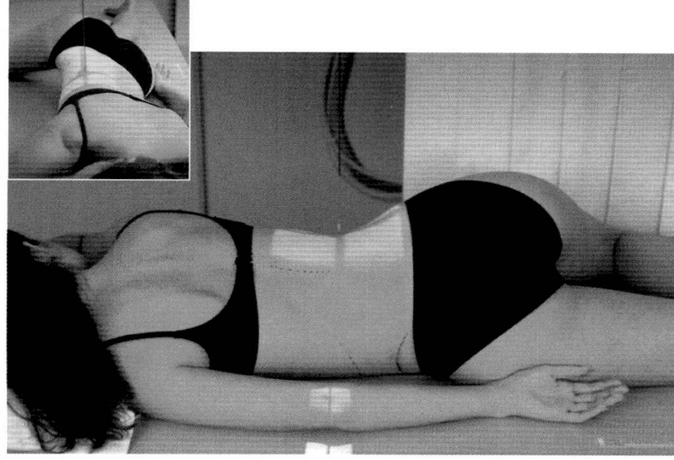

Fig. 16-26. LAO.

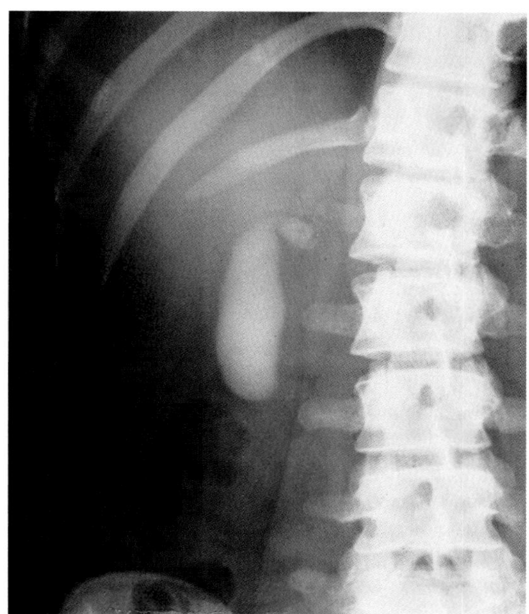

Fig. 16-27. LAO.

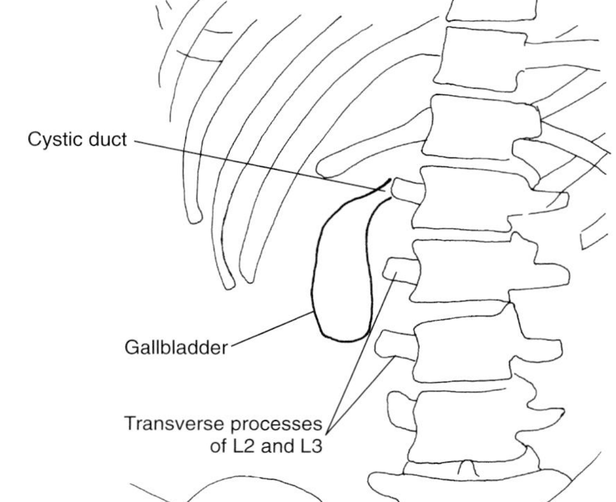

Fig. 16-28. LAO.

Radiographic Criteria

Structures Shown: • Entire opacified gallbladder and area of cystic duct are included centered to IR.

Position: • Spine is parallel to the edge of radiograph. • Gallbladder is adequately rotated away from spine. • If gallbladder is superimposed over any part of spine, the patient is underobliqued.

Collimation and CR: • Only minimal collimation margins are seen on all four sides for adults. • Gallbladder is centered within collimation field.

Exposure Criteria: • No evidence of motion. • Appropriate technique is used with short-scale contrast to clearly visualize gallbladder.

16

RIGHT LATERAL DECUBITUS POSITION (PA PROJECTION): GALLBLADDER (ORAL CHOLECYSTOGRAM)

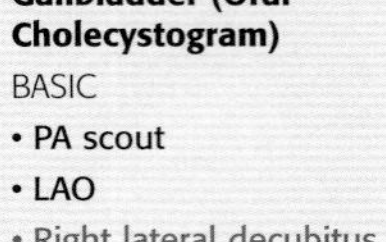
Gallbladder (Oral Cholecystogram)
BASIC
- PA scout
- LAO
- Right lateral decubitus (PA)
- PA erect

Pathology Demonstrated

Opacified gallbladder is projected away from the vertebral column. Right lateral decubitus position will stratify or layer any possible choleliths (gallstones) within the gallbladder.

This may be performed when the patient cannot stand erect.

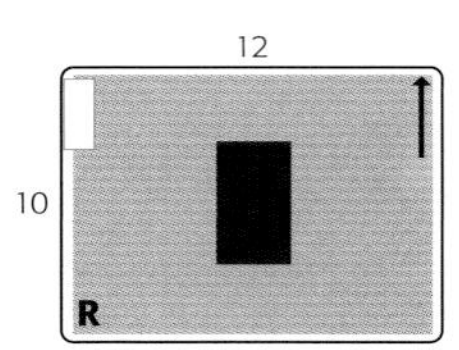

Technical Factors

- IR size—24 × 30 cm (10 × 12 inches), lengthwise
- Moving or stationary grid
- 70-80 kV range
- Decubitus marker used
- Technique and dose:

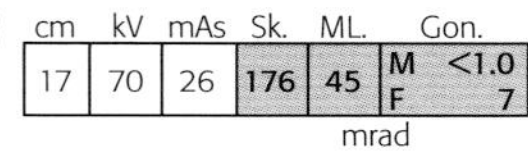

cm	kV	mAs	Sk.	ML.	Gon.
17	70	26	176	45	M <1.0 F 7
			mrad		

Shielding Place lead shield over gonadal area, not obscuring area of interest.

Patient Position Patient is placed on radiolucent pads, lying on right side facing the table and/or IR. (Separate pads for hips and shoulders allow gallbladder to drop more freely away from vertebrae.) Provide pillow for head, arms above head, knees flexed one on the other. Secure cart wheels so that patient will not fall.

Part Position

- Adjust cart and/or IR to center gallbladder to IR and to CR. (Gallbladder location is determined from scout radiograph.)
- **No rotation**—ensure that hips and shoulders are in a true lateral position.

Central Ray

- CR **horizontal,** directed to right half of abdomen to gallbladder, location determined from scout radiograph
- Image receptor centered to CR
- Minimum SID of 40 inches (100 cm)

Collimation Collimate on four sides to area of interest.

Respiration Suspend respiration upon expiration.

Note: This may be taken as an AP if necessary, but a PA projection is preferred because of the more anterior location of gallbladder.

Decubitus position provides for "dropping" of gallbladder away from spine, and for stratification of gallstones, wherein the stones heavier than bile layer out or separate from those lighter than bile (Fig. 16-30). These stones may not be visible on other projections.

Radiographic Criteria

Structures Shown: • Entire opacified gallbladder and area of cystic duct are included, centered to IR. • Gallbladder is seen located below vertebral column. • Stratification lines of choleliths should be visible if present.

Position: • Spine is parallel to the edge of radiograph. • No rotation occurs. • Bony lumbar spine structures are symmetric.

Collimation and CR: • Only minimal collimation margins are seen on all four sides for adults. • Gallbladder is centered within collimation field.

Exposure Criteria: • No evidence of motion. • Appropriate technique is used with short-scale contrast to clearly visualize gallbladder without overpenetrating and burning out possible choleliths.

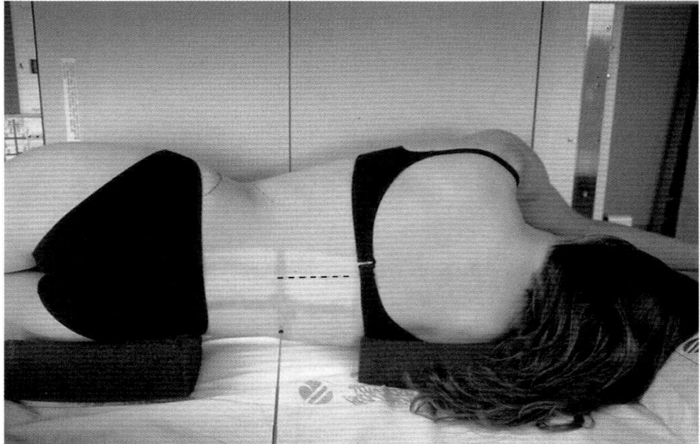

Fig. 16-29. Right lateral decubitus (PA).

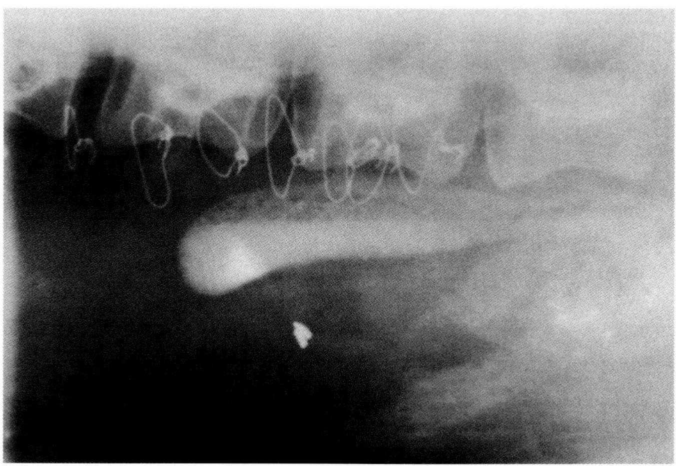

Fig. 16-30. Right lateral decubitus (PA).

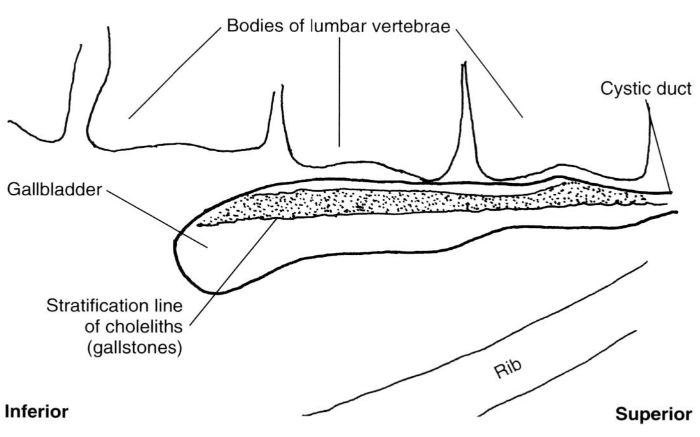

Fig. 16-31. Right lateral decubitus (PA).

PA PROJECTION—ERECT POSITION: GALLBLADDER (ORAL CHOLECYSTOGRAM)

Pathology Demonstrated
Opacified gallbladder and possible stratification or layering of any choleliths (gallstones) within the gallbladder are demonstrated.

Gallbladder (Oral Cholecystogram)
BASIC
- PA scout
- LAO
- Right lateral decubitus (PA)
- PA erect

Technical Factors
- IR size—24 × 30 cm (10 × 12 inches), lengthwise
- Moving or stationary grid
- 70-80 kV range
- Erect marker used
- Technique and dose:

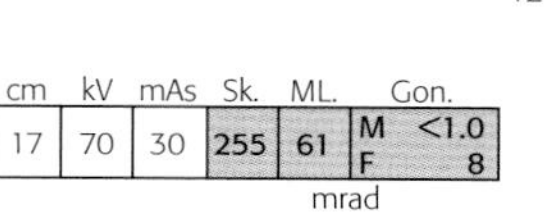

cm	kV	mAs	Sk.	ML.	Gon.
17	70	30	255	61	M <1.0 F 8

mrad

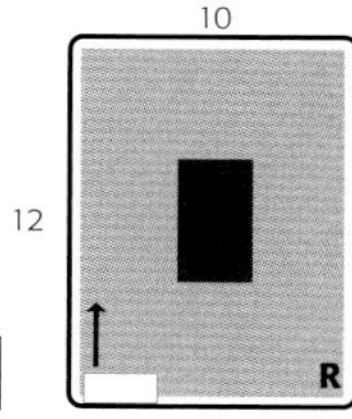

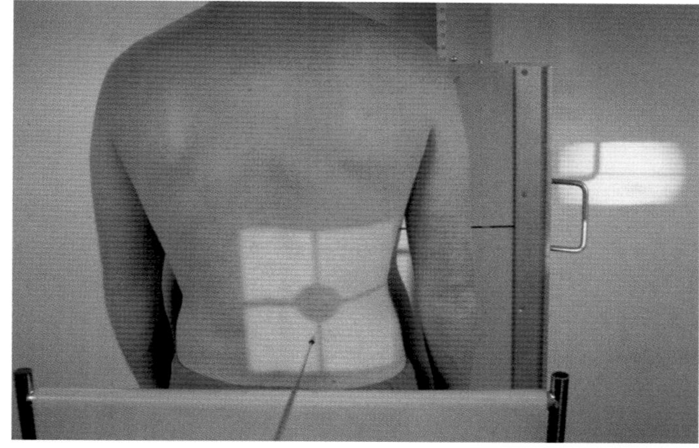

Fig. 16-32. PA erect.

Shielding Place lead shield over gonadal area, not obscuring area of interest (may use freestanding shield as shown in Fig. 16-32).

Patient Position Patient erect, facing the table and/or IR, arms at side

Part Position
- Align a point on abdomen about 2 inches (5 cm) **to right of midsagittal plane to CR and to midline of erect table.**
- Spread feet and distribute body weight evenly on both legs for stabilization.
- For asthenic type patient, rotate into 10° to 15° LAO to shift gallbladder away from spine.

Central Ray
- CR **horizontal,** directed to gallbladder, which will be 1 to 2 inches (2.5 to 5 cm) more inferior than on scout radiograph taken recumbent
- Image receptor centered to CR
- Minimum SID of 40 inches (100 cm)

Collimation Collimate on four sides to area of interest. (More collimation borders are visible on larger IR.)

Respiration Suspend respiration upon expiration.

Note: This may be taken as an AP if necessary, but the PA projection is preferred because of the more anterior location of the gallbladder.

Change centering as needed for extremes of body habitus.

Erect position with horizontal beam provides for stratification of possible gallstones similar to that of decubitus position. (Decubitus may be taken instead of erect if patient cannot stand.)

This may be taken as a spot image with fluoroscopy (Fig. 16-34).

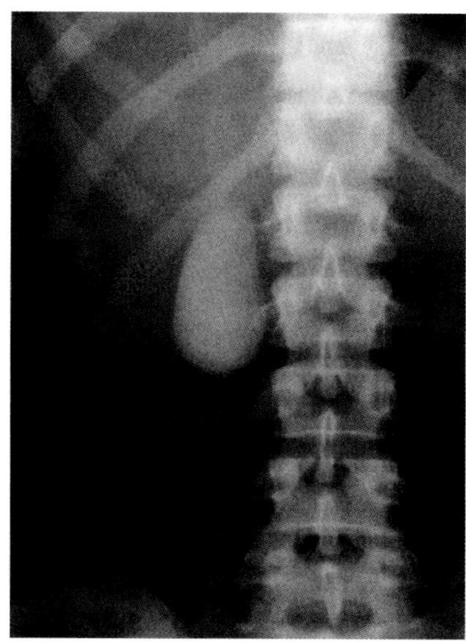

Fig. 16-33. PA erect.

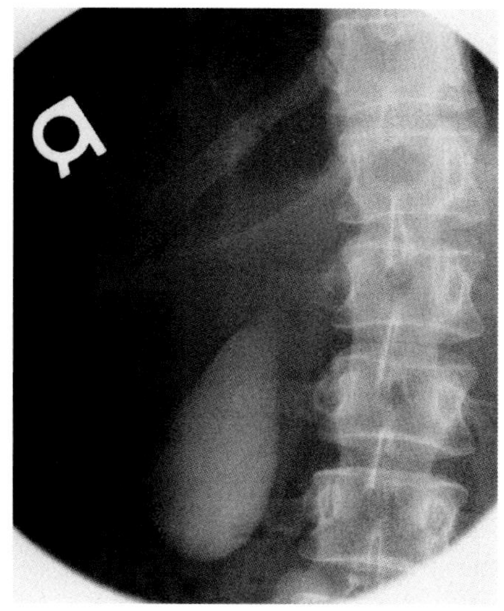

Fig. 16-34. AP erect fluoro spot.

Radiographic Criteria

Structures Shown: • Entire opacified gallbladder and area of cystic duct are included centered to IR. • Gallbladder is located 1 to 2 inches (2.5 to 5 cm) more inferior than in recumbent position. • Stratification lines of choleliths should be visible if present.

Position: • No tilt is evident. • Spine is parallel to the edge of radiograph

Collimation and CR: • Gallbladder should not be superimposed by vertebra. • Only minimal collimation margins are seen on all four sides for adults.

Exposure Criteria: • Appropriate technique is used with short-scale contrast to clearly visualize gallbladder without over penetrating and burning out possible choleliths. • No motion evident.

CHAPTER 17

Urinary System and Venipuncture

CONTRIBUTORS TO PAST EDITIONS Jenny A. Kellstrom, MEd, RT(R), Barry T. Anthony, RT(R)

CONTENTS

17

RADIOGRAPHIC ANATOMY

Urinary System

Radiographic examinations of the urinary system are among the most common contrast media procedures performed in radiology departments. The urinary system consists of **two kidneys, two ureters** *(u-re'ter* or yoo-ret'er†),* **one urinary bladder,** and **one urethra** *(u-re'thrah* or yoo-re'thra†).*

Note: Determine which of the possible pronunciations of these terms are most common in your region.

The two kidneys and the ureters are organs lying in the retroperitoneal space. These two bean-shaped organs lie on either side of the vertebral column in the most posterior part of the abdominal cavity. The right kidney is generally slightly lower or more inferior than the left due to the presence of the liver. Near the upper medial part of each kidney is a **suprarenal** (adrenal) **gland.** These important glands of the endocrine system are located in the fatty capsule surrounding each kidney.

Each kidney connects to the single urinary bladder by its own ureter. Waste material, in the form of urine, travels from the kidneys to the bladder via these two narrow tubes, termed *ureters.* The saclike urinary bladder serves as a reservoir to store urine until it can be eliminated from the body via the **urethra.**

The Latin designation for kidney is *ren,* and *renal* is a common adjective referring to kidney.

KIDNEYS

The various organs of the urinary system and their relationship to the bony skeleton are shown from the back in Fig. 17-2 and from the left side in Fig. 17-3. The posteriorly placed **kidneys** lie on either side of the vertebral column in the upper posterior abdomen. They lie posterior to the lower portion of the **liver** on the right and posterior to the lower **spleen** on the left (Fig. 17-2). The lower ribcage thus forms a protective enclosure for the kidneys.

URETERS

Most of each **ureter** lies anterior to its respective kidney. The ureters follow the natural curve of the vertebral column. Each ureter initially curves forward, following the lumbar lordotic curvature, and then curves backward on entering the pelvis. After passing into the pelvis, each ureter follows the sacrococcygeal curve before entering the posterolateral aspect of the bladder.

URETHRA

The **urethra** connects the bladder to the exterior. The urethra exits from the body inferior to the symphysis pubis.

The entire urinary system is either posterior to or below the peritoneum. The **kidneys and ureters are retroperitoneal structures,** whereas the **bladder and urethra are infraperitoneal structures.**

*Dorland's illustrated medical dictionary, ed 28, Philadelphia, 1994, WB Saunders.
†Webster's new world dictionary, ed 3 (college), New York, 1994, Macmillan.

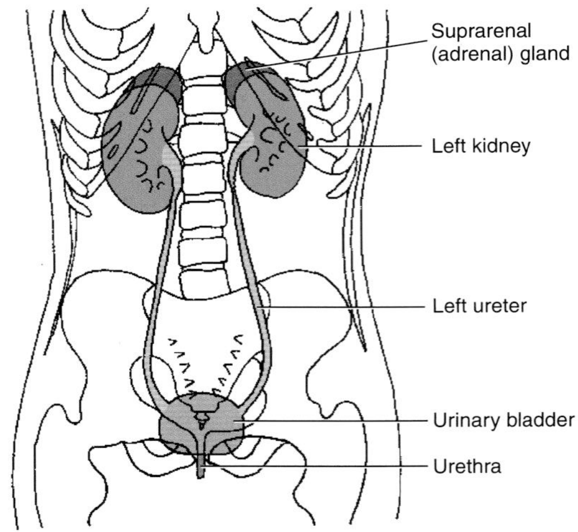

Fig. 17-1. Urinary system—anterior view.

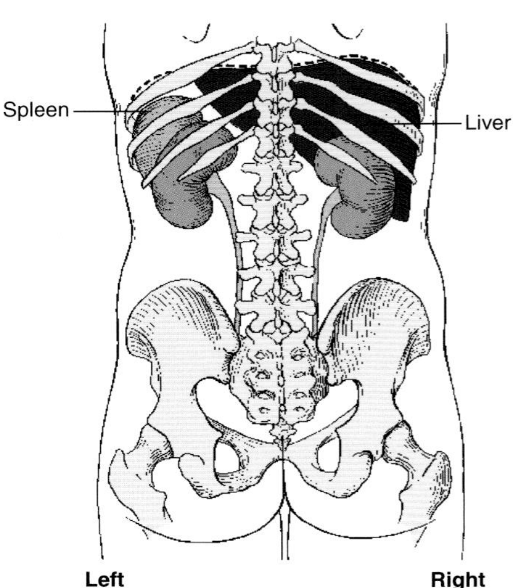

Fig. 17-2. Urinary system—posterior view.

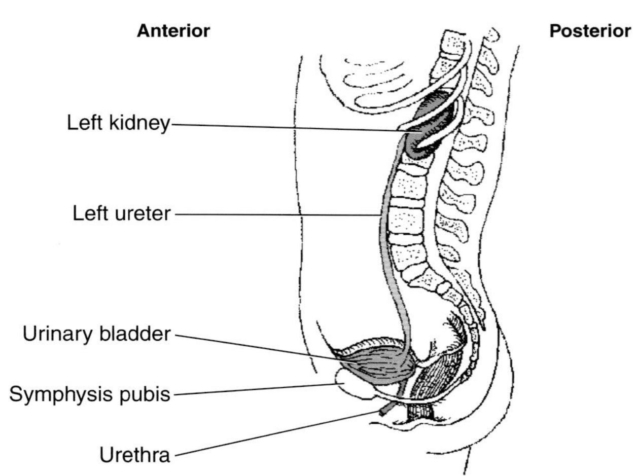

Fig. 17-3. Urinary system—lateral view.

Kidneys

The average adult kidney is fairly small, weighing about 150 grams. The measurements are 4 to 5 inches (10 to 12 cm) long, 2 to 3 inches (5 to 7.5 cm) wide, and 1 inch (2.5 cm) thick. The left kidney is a little longer but narrower than the right. Despite the small size, at least one functional kidney is absolutely essential for normal well-being. Failure of both kidneys, unless corrected, means inevitable death.

KIDNEY ORIENTATION

The usual orientation of the kidneys in the supine individual is shown in Fig. 17-4. The large muscles on either side of the vertebral column cause the longitudinal plane of the kidneys to form a vertical angle of about 20° with the midsagittal plane. These large muscles include the two **psoas** *(so'es)* **major muscles.** These muscle masses grow larger as they progress inferiorly from the upper lumbar vertebrae. This gradual enlargement causes the 20° angle, wherein the upper pole of each kidney is closer to the midline than its lower pole (Fig. 17-4).

These large posterior abdominal muscles also cause the kidneys to rotate backward within the retroperitoneal space. As a result, the medial border of each kidney is more anterior than the lateral border (Fig. 17-5).

The **aorta** and **inferior vena cava** are also indicated to show their relationship to the kidneys.

CROSS-SECTIONAL VIEW

Transverse cross-sectional views through the level of L2 illustrate the usual amount of backward rotation of the kidneys (Figs. 17-5 and 17-6). The normal kidney rotation of about **30°** is due to the midline location of the vertebral column and the large **psoas major muscles** on either side. The **quadratus lumborum muscles** are also shown on each side just posterior to the kidneys. The deep muscles of the back include the group of **erector spinae muscles** on each side of the spine.

When posterior oblique projections are used during radiographic studies of the urinary system, each kidney in turn is placed parallel to the plane of the image receptor. The body is rotated about **30° in each direction** to place one kidney, and then the other, parallel to the IR plane. A 30° LPO positions the right kidney parallel to the IR, and a 30° RPO positions the left kidney parallel.

Each kidney is surrounded by a mass of fatty tissue termed the **adipose capsule,** or **perirenal fat.** The presence of these fatty capsules around the kidneys permits radiographic visualization of the kidneys on plain abdominal radiographs. There is sufficient density difference between fat and muscle to visualize the outline of each kidney on most technically satisfactory abdominal radiographs.

CT Axial Section Fig. 17-6 represents a CT (computed tomogram) axial section through the level of the midkidneys at L2. This section demonstrates anatomic relationships of the kidneys to adjoining organs and structures. The anatomy that should be recognizable is as follows:

A. Pancreas
B. Gallbladder
C. Inferior portion of right lobe of the liver
D. Right kidney
E. Psoas major muscle
F. Erector spinae muscles
G. L2 vertebra
H. Quadratus lumborum muscle
I. Renal pelvis of left kidney
J. Descending colon
K. Abdominal aorta
L. Small intestine (jejunum)

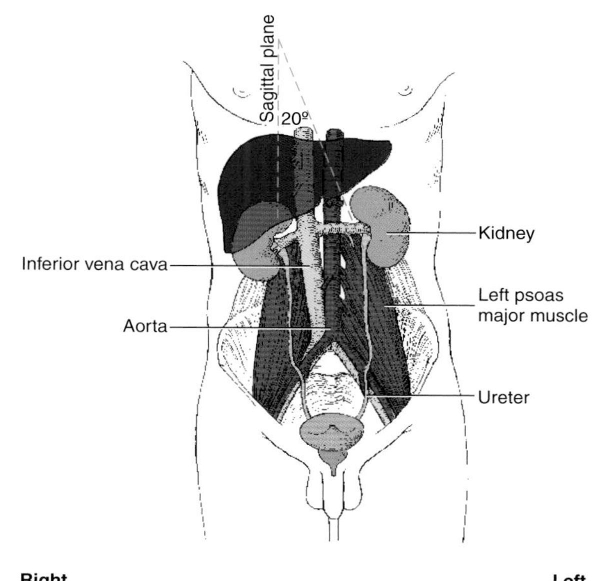

Fig. 17-4. Kidney orientation—frontal view.

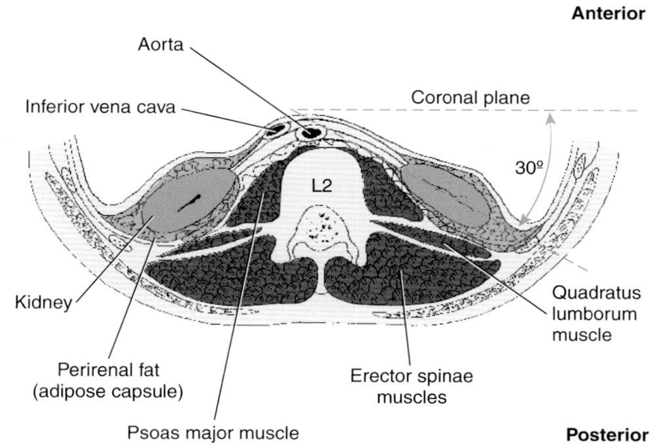

Fig. 17-5. Kidney orientation—cross-sectional view.

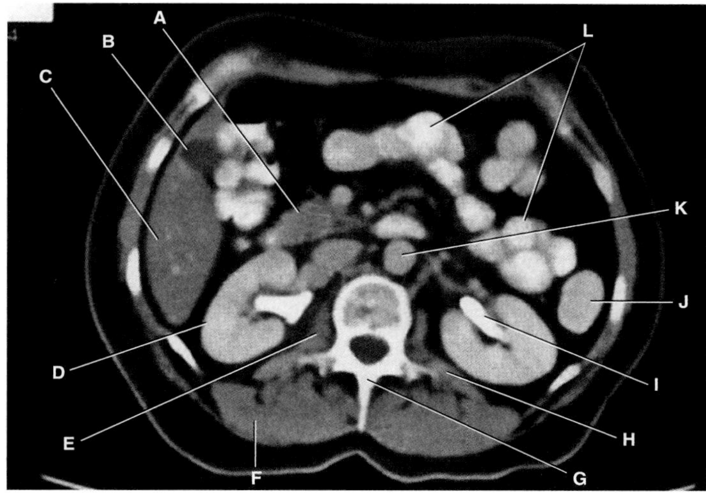

Fig. 17-6. CT axial section at level of L2.

NORMAL KIDNEY LOCATION

Most abdominal radiographs, including urograms, are performed on expiration with the patient supine. The combined effect of expiration and a supine position allow the kidneys to lie fairly high in the abdominal cavity. Under these conditions the kidneys normally lie about **halfway between the xiphoid process and the iliac crest.** The left kidney normally lies about 1 cm more superior than does the right one. The top of the left kidney is usually at the level of the **T11-T12 interspace.** The bottom of the right kidney is most often level with the upper part of **L3.**

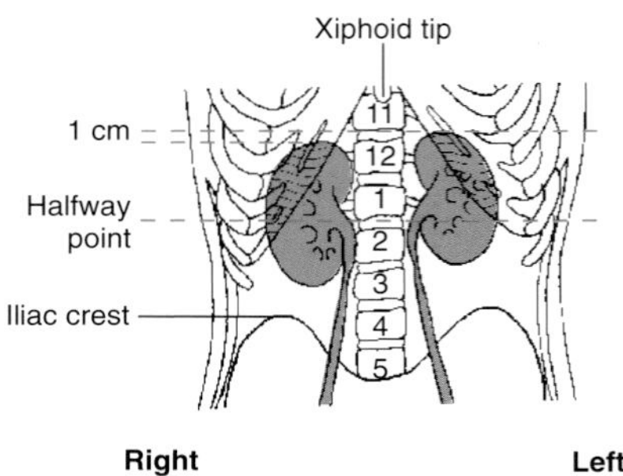

Fig. 17-7. Normal kidney location.

Kidney Movement Because the kidneys are only loosely attached within their fatty capsule, they tend to move up and down with movements of the diaphragm and position changes. When one inhales deeply or stands upright, the kidneys normally drop about one lumbar vertebrae, or 5 cm (2 inches). If the kidneys drop more than this, a condition termed ***nephroptosis*** *(nef″rop-to′sis)* is said to exist. With some very thin and older patients in particular, the kidneys may drop dramatically and end up within the pelvis, which may create problems from a "kinking" or twisting of the ureters.

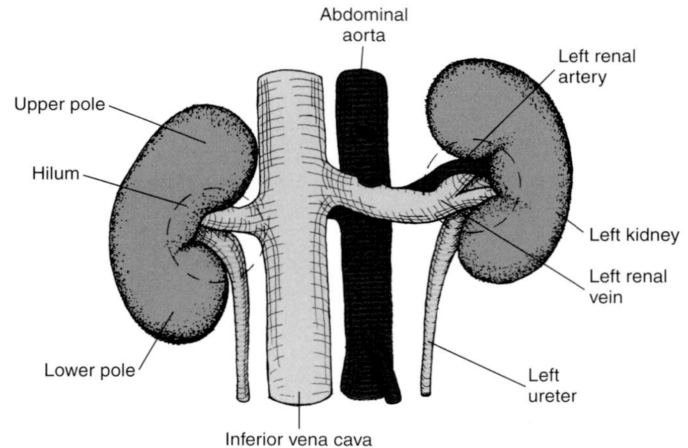

Fig. 17-8. Renal blood vessels.

FUNCTIONS OF URINARY SYSTEM

The primary function of the urinary system is the **production of urine and its elimination** from the body. During production of urine, the kidneys perform the following functions:

1. Remove nitrogenous wastes
2. Regulate water levels in the body
3. Regulate acid-base balance and electrolyte levels of the blood

Nitrogenous waste products such as urea and creatinine are formed during the normal metabolism of proteins. Buildup of these nitrogenous wastes in the blood results in the clinical condition termed **uremia.**

RENAL BLOOD VESSELS

Large blood vessels are needed to handle the vast quantities of blood flowing through the kidneys daily. At rest, about 25% of the blood pumped from the heart with each beat passes through the kidneys. Arterial blood is received by the kidneys directly from the **abdominal aorta** via the left and right renal arteries. Each **renal artery** branches and re-branches until a vast capillary network is formed in each kidney.

Because most of the blood volume entering the kidneys is returned to the circulatory system, the **renal veins** must also be large vessels. The renal veins connect directly to the large **inferior vena cava** to return the blood to the right side of the heart. The renal veins are anterior to the renal arteries.

Along the medial border of each kidney is a centrally located, longitudinal fissure termed the **hilum** *(hi′lum).* The hilum serves to transmit the renal artery and renal vein, lymphatics, nerves, and ureter.

Each kidney is arbitrarily divided into an upper part and a lower part, called the **upper pole** and the **lower pole,** respectively.

SUMMARY CHART OF URINE PRODUCTION

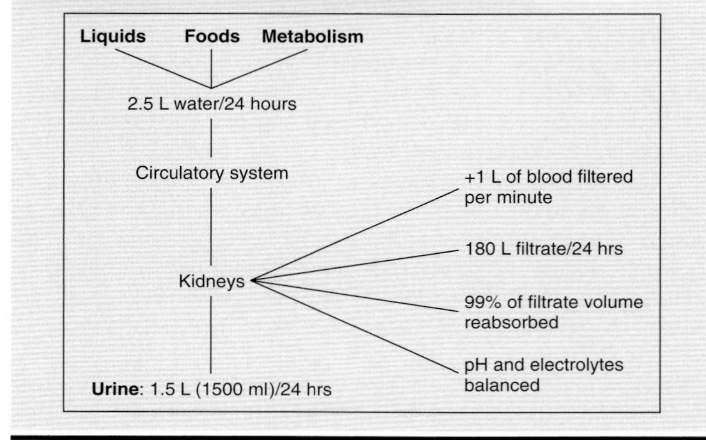

Urine Production

The average water intake for humans during each 24-hour period is about 2.5 L (2500 ml). This water comes from ingested liquids and foods and from the end products of metabolism. These 2.5 L of water eventually end up in the bloodstream. Vast quantities of blood are filtered every 24 hours. At rest, more than 1 L of blood flows through the kidneys every minute of the day, which results in about 180 L of filtrate being removed from the blood every 24 hours. More than 99% of this filtrate volume is reabsorbed by the kidneys and returned to the bloodstream. During the reabsorption process the blood pH and amounts of various electrolytes, such as sodium, potassium, and chloride, are regulated.

From the large amount of blood flowing through the kidneys daily, about **1.5 L, or 1500 ml,** of urine is formed. This amount is average and varies greatly depending on fluid intake, amount of perspiration, and other factors.

MACROSCOPIC STRUCTURE

The macroscopic internal structure of the kidney is shown in Fig. 17-9. Directly under the **fibrous capsule** surrounding each kidney is the **cortex,** forming the peripheral, or outer, portion of the kidney substance. Under the cortex is the internal structure termed the **medulla,** which is composed of from 8 to 18 conical masses termed **renal pyramids.** The cortex periodically dips between the pyramids to form the **renal columns,** which extend to the **renal sinus.**

The renal pyramids are primarily a collection of tubules that converge at an opening at the **renal papilla** (apex) and drain into the **minor calyx** (*kal'lis* or *ka'liks*[†]). Calyces appear as hollowed, flattened tubes. From 4 to 13 minor calyces unite to form two to three **major calyces.** The major calyces unite to form the **renal pelvis,** which appears in the shape of a larger flattened funnel. Each expanded renal pelvis narrows to continue as the **ureter.** Thus urine formed in the microscopic or nephron portion of the kidney finally reaches the ureter by passing through the various collecting tubules, to a minor calyx, to a major calyx, and then to the renal pelvis.

The term **renal parenchyma** *(par-eng'ki-mah)* is a general term used to describe the total functional portions of the kidneys, such as those visualized during an early phase of an intravenous urogram procedure.

MICROSCOPIC STRUCTURE

The structural and functional unit of the kidney is the microscopic **nephron.** One million nephrons exist in each kidney. One such nephron is shown in Fig. 17-10, a greatly magnified but very small cutaway section of the kidney. A more detailed view of a single nephron and its collecting ducts is shown in Fig. 17-11. Small arteries in the kidney **cortex** form tiny capillary tufts, termed **glomeruli** *(glo-mer'u-li).* Blood is initially filtered through the many glomeruli.

Afferent arterioles supply blood **to** the glomeruli, and **efferent** arterioles take blood away to a secondary capillary network in close relationship to the straight and convoluted tubules. Each glomerulus is surrounded by a **glomerular capsule** (Bowman's capsule), which is the proximal portion of each nephron collecting filtrate. (The glomerulus is also part of the **nephron,** which is made up of the glomerulus **and** the long tubules.) The glomerular filtrate travels from the **glomerular capsule** to a **proximal convoluted tubule,** to the **descending** and **ascending limbs** of the **loop of Henle*** *(Hen'le),* to a **distal convoluted tubule,** to a **collecting tubule,** and finally, into a **minor calyx.** The filtrate is termed *urine* by the time it reaches the minor calyx. Between Bowman's capsule and minor calyces, more than 99% of the filtrate is reabsorbed into the kidney's venous system.

Microscopically the glomeruli, glomerular capsules, and proximal and distal convoluted tubules of the many nephrons are located within the **cortex** of the kidney. The loop of Henle and the collecting tubules are located primarily within the **medulla.** The renal pyramids within the medulla are primarily a collection of tubules.

*Fredrich Gustav Jakob Henle was a German anatomist who lived between 1809 and 1885.
[†]Webster's new world dictionary, ed 3 (college), New York, 1994, Macmillan.

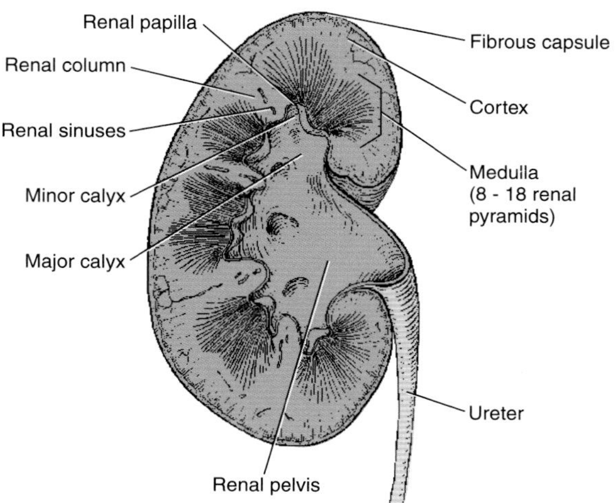

Fig. 17-9. Renal structure.

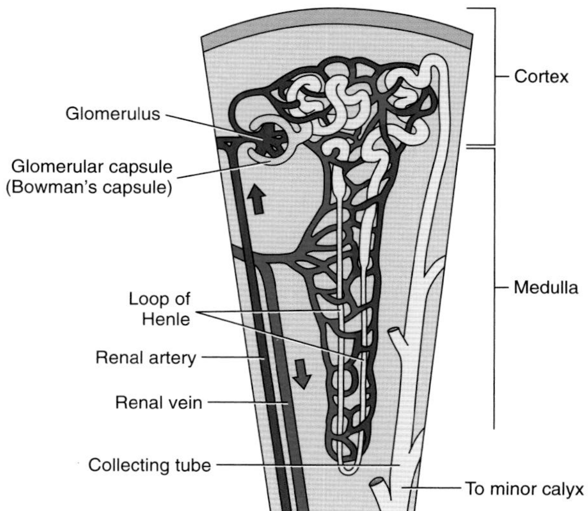

Fig. 17-10. Microscopic structure (nephron).

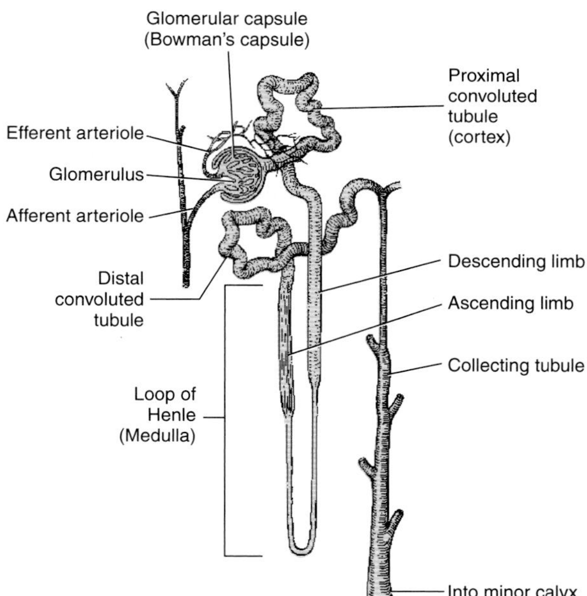

Fig. 17-11. Nephron and collecting duct.

17

17

Ureters

The **ureters** convey urine from the kidneys to the urinary bladder. Slow peristaltic waves and gravity force urine down the ureters into the bladder, as demonstrated in Fig. 17-12. This is an image taken 10 minutes after injection of contrast media into the bloodstream as part of an intravenous urogram procedure.

The **renal pelvis** leaves each kidney at the hilum to become the **ureter.** The ureters vary in length from 28 to 34 cm, with the right one being slightly shorter than the left.

As the ureters pass inferiorly, they **lie on the anterior surface of each psoas major muscle** (Fig. 17-13). Continuing to follow the curvature of the vertebral column, the ureters eventually enter the posterolateral portion of each side of the **urinary bladder.**

URETER SIZE AND POINTS OF CONSTRICTION

The ureters vary in diameter from 1 mm to almost 1 cm. Normally, **three constricted points** exist along the course of each ureter. If a kidney stone attempts to pass from kidney to bladder, it may have trouble passing through these three spots (see Fig. 17-13).

The **first** point is the **ureteropelvic** *(u-re'ter-o-pel-vic)* **(UP) junction,** where the renal pelvis funnels down into the small ureter. This section is best seen on the radiograph of Fig. 17-12.

The **second** is near the **brim of the pelvis,** where the iliac blood vessels cross over the ureters (see Fig. 17-13).

The **third** is where the ureter joins the bladder, termed the **ureterovesical** *(u-re"ter-o-ves'i-kal)* **junction,** or *UV junction.* Most kidney stones passing down the ureter tend to hang up at the third site, the UV junction, and once the stone passes this point into the bladder, it generally has little trouble passing from the bladder and through the urethra to the exterior.

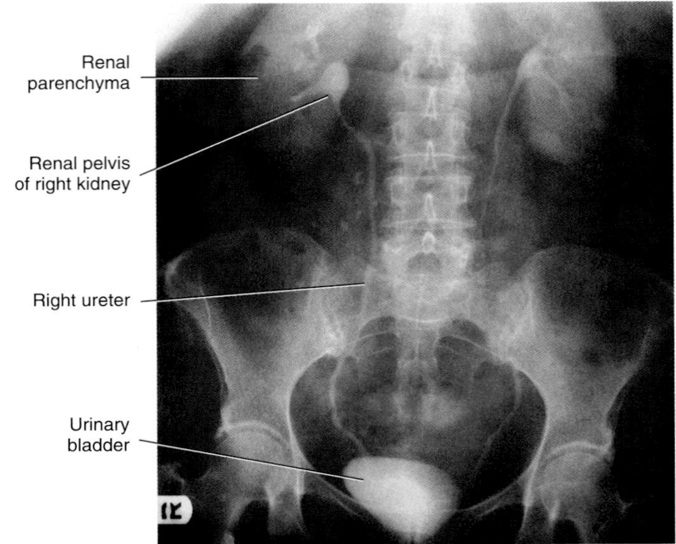

Fig. 17-12. IVU radiograph, demonstrating kidneys, ureters, and bladder.

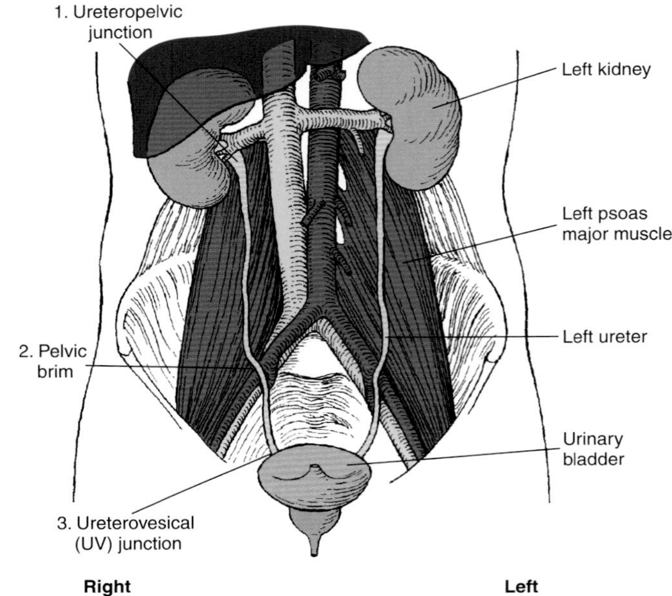

Fig. 17-13. Ureters; three possible points of constriction (possible sites for kidney stone lodging).

Urinary Bladder

The urinary bladder is a musculomembranous sac that serves as a reservoir for urine. The empty bladder is somewhat flattened and only assumes the more oval shape as in Figs. 17-13 and 17-14 when partially or fully distended.

The triangular portion of the bladder along the inner, posterior surface is termed the **trigone** *(tri'gon).* The trigone is the muscular area formed by the entrance of the two **ureters** from behind and the exit site of the **urethra** (Fig. 17-14). The trigone is firmly attached to the floor of the pelvis. The mucosa of the trigone is smooth, whereas the remaining aspect of the inner mucosa of the bladder has numerous folds termed *rugae.* As the bladder fills, the top of the bladder expands upward and forward toward the abdominal cavity.

The gland surrounding the proximal urethra is the **prostate gland.** It is situated inferior to the bladder measuring 1.5 inches (3.8 cm) in diameter and 1 inch (2.5 cm) in height. Only males possess a prostate gland, so this drawing represents a male bladder, although the internal structure of the bladder in both sexes is similar. The prostate produces a fluid that aids with the motility of sperm during reproduction.

BLADDER FUNCTIONS

The **bladder** functions as a reservoir for urine and, aided by the urethra, expels urine from the body. Normally some urine is in the bladder at all times, but as the amount reaches 250 ml, the desire to void arises. The act of voiding (urination) is normally under voluntary control, and the desire to void may pass if the bladder cannot be emptied right away. The total capacity of the bladder varies from **350** to **500 ml.** As the bladder becomes more and more full, the desire to void becomes more and more urgent. If the internal bladder pressure rises too high, involuntary urination occurs.

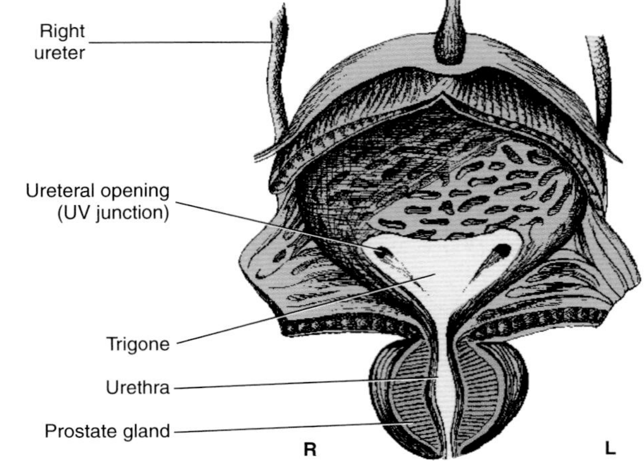

Fig. 17-14. Male urinary bladder—anterior cutaway view.

SIZE AND POSITION OF THE BLADDER

The size, position, and functional status of the bladder depend somewhat on surrounding organs and on how full the bladder is. When the rectum contains fecal matter, the bladder is pushed up and forward. A term pregnancy, as shown in Fig. 17-15, exerts tremendous downward pressure on the bladder.

Note: This drawing is only to show anatomy and the location of the urinary bladder in relationship to the symphysis pubis and the fetus. Remember that **no** radiographic urinary system exams or procedures are performed during pregnancy unless in special cases in which the benefits outweigh the risks, as determined by a physician.

FEMALE PELVIC ORGANS

The female pelvic organs are shown in the midsagittal section in Fig. 17-16. The **urinary bladder** lies posterior to and just above the upper margin of the **symphysis pubis,** depending on the amount of bladder distention. The female **urethra** is a narrow canal, about 4 cm long, extending from the internal urethral orifice to the external urethral orifice. The single function of the female urethra is the passage of urine to the exterior.

Female Reproductive Organs The female reproductive organs include the paired **ovaries** (female gonads), **uterine** (fallopian) **tubes,** and **vagina** (Fig. 17-16).

A close relationship exists between the urethra and bladder, and the uterus and vagina. The urethra is imbedded in the anterior wall of the vagina. The spatial relationship of the three external openings becomes important during certain radiographic procedures. The anal opening is most posterior, the urethral opening is most anterior, and the vaginal opening is in between.

Retroperitoneal and Infraperitoneal Organs The **kidneys** and **ureters** are shown to be **retroperitoneal organs** located posterior to the peritoneal cavity for both males and females. The **urinary bladder, urethra,** and **male reproductive organs** are **infraperitoneal** (inferior to the peritoneal cavity).

As described in Chapter 4, the female **uterus, uterine tubes,** and **ovaries** pass **into** the peritoneal cavity. The male reproductive organs, however, are located totally **below** the peritoneum, separating them completely from those organs within the peritoneal cavity. Thus the lower aspect of the peritoneum is a **closed sac in the male but not in the female.**

MALE PELVIC ORGANS

The male pelvic organs are shown in the midsagittal section in Fig. 17-17. When the **urinary bladder** is empty, most of the bladder lies directly posterior to the upper margin of the **symphysis pubis.** As the bladder distends, as it would during a cystogram or radiographic study of the bladder, more and more of the bladder lies above the level of the symphysis pubis.

Male Reproductive Organs The male reproductive organs include the **testes** (male gonads), **seminal vesicles and related ducts, ejaculatory ducts** and **ductus deferens** (vas deferens), **penis,** and **scrotum** (containing the testes). The relative location of these organs is shown in Fig. 17-17.

The male **urethra** extends from the internal urethral orifice to the external urethral orifice at the end of the penis. The urethra extends through the **prostate gland** and through the length of the penis. The male urethra averages 17.5 to 20 cm in length and serves two functions—to help eliminate urine stored in the bladder and to serve as a passageway for semen.

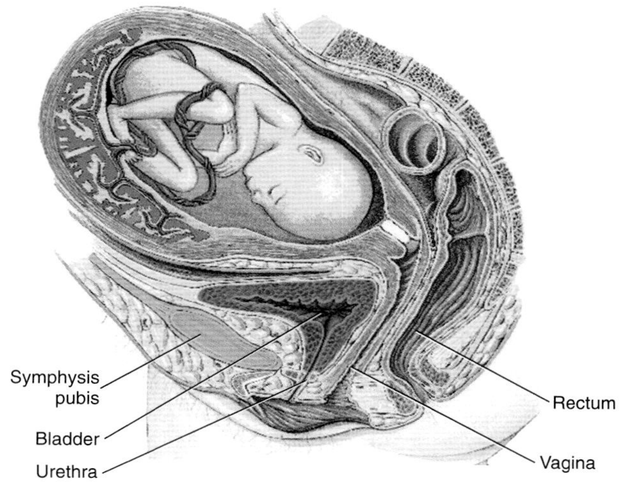

Fig. 17-15. Term pregnancy and relationship to bladder.

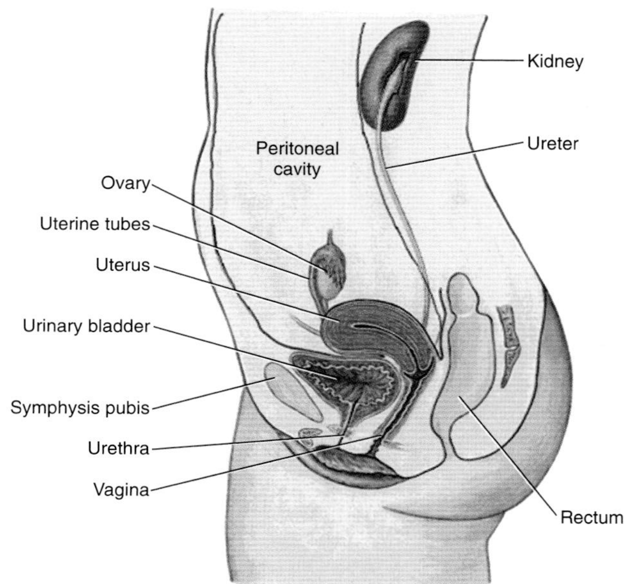

Fig. 17-16. Female pelvic organs.

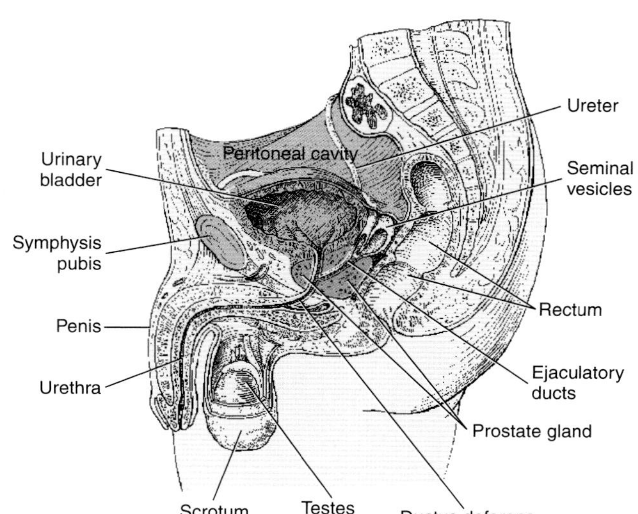

Fig. 17-17. Male pelvic organs.

17

Anatomy Review With Radiographs

RETROGRADE PYELOGRAM

Identify the following anatomic structures as labeled on this retrograde pyelogram (Fig. 17-18) in which contrast media is being injected through a catheter inserted (retrograde) through the urethra, bladder, and ureter to the level of the renal pelvis:

A. Minor calyces
B. Major calyces
C. Renal pelvis
D. Ureteropelvic junction (UPJ)
E. Proximal ureter
F. Distal ureter
G. Urinary bladder

VOIDING CYSTOURETHROGRAM

Identify the following anatomic structures labeled on this radiograph of the urinary bladder and urethra (Fig. 17-19), taken as the young male patient is voiding the contrast media:

A. Distal ureter
B. Urinary bladder
C. Trigone area of bladder
D. Area of prostate gland
E. Urethra

CT AXIAL SECTION

Anatomic structures of the abdomen are seen in a cross-sectional view of an axial CT image (Fig. 17-20). Identifying the following abdominal organs and structures provides a good review of all abdominal anatomic structures and their relative relationships to one another:

A. Liver (lower portion of right lobe)
B. Colon (ascending)
C. Small bowel
D. Colon (descending)
E. Left kidney (lower lobe)
F. Left ureter
G. Aorta
H. Major psoas muscle
I. Right ureter
J. Right kidney

17

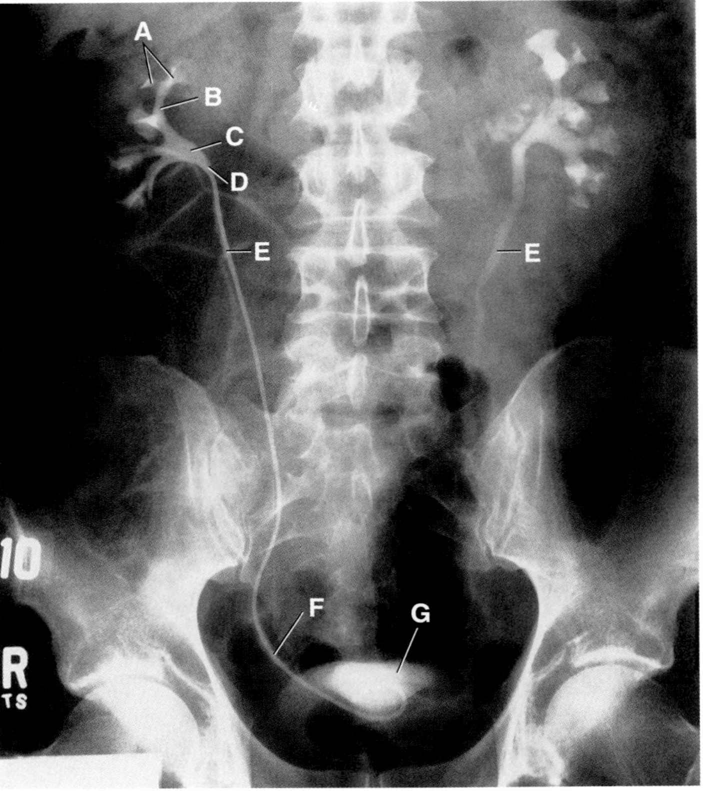

Fig. 17-18. Retrograde pyelogram (catheter in right ureter).

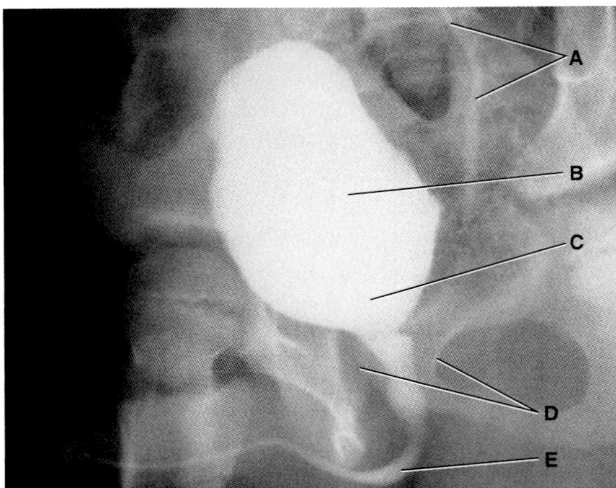

Fig. 17-19. Voiding cystourethrogram—RPO (male).

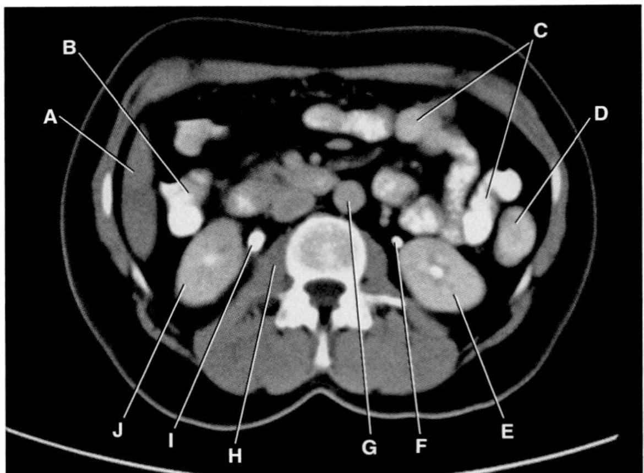

Fig. 17-20. CT axial section.

VENIPUNCTURE

INTRODUCTION

Venipuncture can be defined as **the puncture of a vein for withdrawal or injection of a substance** such as contrast media for urographic procedures, In the past, this venipuncture for urography was performed by physicians and laboratory or nursing personnel. However, in recent years, venipuncture has become part of the scope of practice for the diagnostic imaging professional. The American Society of Radiologic Technologists (ASRT) includes venipuncture in its curriculum guide for educational programs in radiography.

Canada: In Canada, technologists and radiologists are supportive of this additional responsibility. Because venipuncture and contrast media injection are considered delegated medical acts, technologists in the profession must be certified competent after attending an organized training program. Annual recertification is also required. Entry-level technologists are taught this skill during their training in an accredited radiologic technology training program.

PREPARATION FOR ADMINISTRATION OF CONTRAST AGENTS

Before withdrawing contents from any vial or bottle, **confirmation of the correct contents** and the **expiration date** is important. Also, all air must be removed from the syringe before drawing in the bottle or vial contents.

Iodinated contrast agents may be administered by either **bolus injection** or **drip infusion.**

Bolus Injection Bolus injections provide a rapid introduction of the contrast agent into the vascular system. This method requires drawing of the agent into a syringe for manual injection.

The **rate** of bolus injection is controlled by the following:

- Gauge of needle or connecting tubing
- Amount of contrast agent being injected
- Viscosity of contrast agent
- Stability of vein
- Force applied by the individual performing the injection

Drip Infusion Drip infusion permits a larger amount of contrast agent to be introduced over a longer period of time. It is used most commonly when the drip-infusion catheter is already in place for repeated or continuous infusions. This method delivers the contrast agent to the vascular system through a length of tubing connected to an over-the-needle insertion into a vein.

The contrast agent is contained in an intravenous (IV) solution bag or bottle that is inverted and connected to the tubing (Fig. 17-23). The rate of infusion, which may be gradual or rapid, depending on the needs of the study, is controlled by a clamp device located below the drip meter on the IV tubing.

EQUIPMENT AND SUPPLIES

Before the actual procedure, the technologist must have all necessary materials assembled and the room prepared, including an emergency cart in the immediate vicinity with necessary equipment and supplies. This cart should include an emesis basin and epinephrine or Benadryl for emergency injection in the event of patient reactions.

Venipuncture requires the following equipment and supplies:

- Tourniquets
- 70% isopropyl alcohol, 1% to 2% iodine, or Betadine wipes
- Various sizes of butterfly and over-the-needle catheters (Jelco, angiocath, or heparin lock)
- Disposable syringes
- IV infusion tubing
- Arm board
- Cotton balls or 2 × 2–inch gauze
- Hypoallergenic tape
- Gloves (latex-free recommended)
- Contrast agent

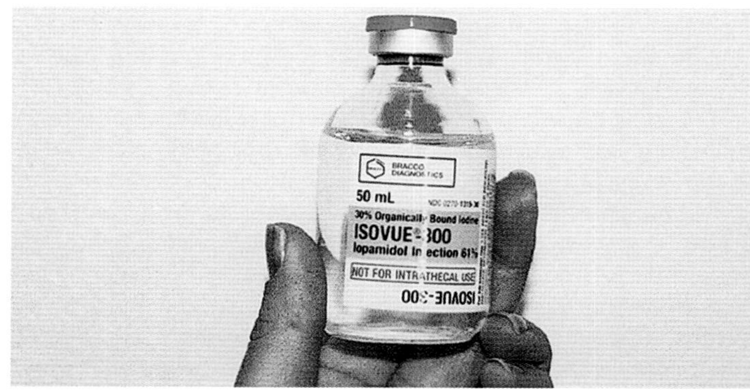

Fig. 17-21. Confirm contents and expiration date.

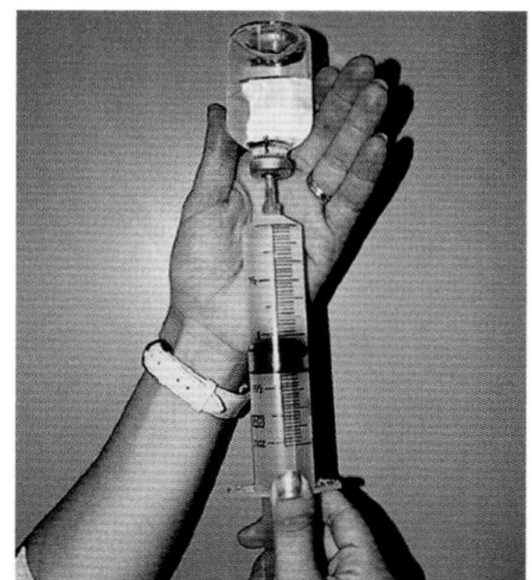
Fig. 17-22. Drawing into syringe for bolus injection.

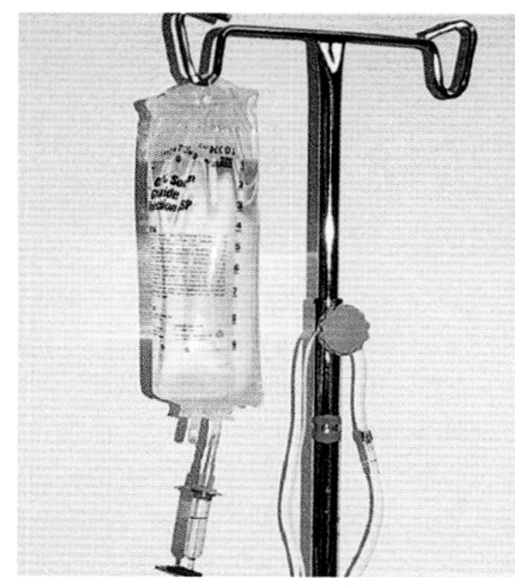
Fig. 17-23. Inverted solution bag or bottle for drip infusion.

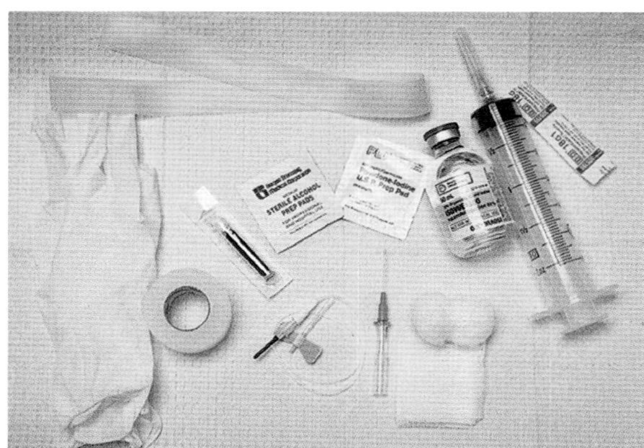
Fig. 17-24. Venipuncture supplies.

PATIENT PREPARATION

Many people are phobic of needles and experience some discomfort during venipuncture. After **introductions** and **proper identification of the patient** (as with all radiographic procedures), the mental and emotional status of the patient must be assessed. This assessment may confirm that the patient is more comfortable lying down, especially if fainting is a possibility.

For a child the technologist must determine the level of cooperation. If the technologist believes the child may become combative or move during needle insertion, the guardian or other personnel should be asked to help keep the child calm and help immobilize the limb. However, attempts to gain the cooperation of the child through proper and complete communication are always preferable. The technologist should not lie to a child about the procedure, because venipuncture may hurt. The technologist should be open and frank to questions and concerns.

SIGNING INFORMED CONSENT FORM

Venipuncture is an invasive procedure that carries the risk for complications when contrast agents are injected. The technologist must ensure that the patient is fully aware of these potential risks and has signed an **informed consent form** before the procedure. If a child is undergoing venipuncture, the procedure should be explained to both the child and the guardian, and the guardian should sign the informed consent form.

SELECTION OF VEIN

For most intravenous urograms, veins in the **antecubital fossa** are recommended. The veins in this region are generally large, easy to access, and durable enough to withstand a bolus injection of contrast agents without extravasation (a discharge of the injected agent from a blood vessel into the surrounding tissues).

Veins located in the antecubital fossa commonly used during venipuncture include the **median cubital, cephalic,** and **basilic veins.** The technologist should be prepared for problems with any type of venipuncture. As a result of flexion of the elbow, a needle may become dislodged if left in during the procedure. In other cases the veins in the antecubital fossa may have been overused for other laboratory tests and injections, and other veins must be selected, such as the **radial vein** of the anterior wrist. Veins on the posterior hand or lower forearm, such as the **cephalic** or **basilic veins,** may also provide a more reliable route for contrast agents.

The technologist should avoid veins that are sclerotic (hardened), tortuous (twisted), rolling, or overused. Areas of vein bifurcation or veins that lie directly over an artery should not be used. **Do not** inject directly into a shunt, central line, or vascular catheter unless directed to do so by a physician.

Ensure Vein and Not an Artery In selecting an injection site, ensure that the vessel is **not an artery,** as evident by the amount of pressure that can frequently be felt on careful palpation of a vessel. In addition, veins are typically closer to the skin surface in the elbow as compared with arteries.

TYPE AND SIZE OF NEEDLE

For bolus injections of 50 to 100 ml of contrast media on adults, an **18- to 20-gauge butterfly needle** is most often used. The butterfly needle provides the technologist a better sense of "feel" during the actual venipuncture because of the two side flaps provided with it. The size of the needle is determined by the size of the vein. For pediatric patients a smaller 23- to 25-gauge needle is often used. The technologist may also choose to use an **over-the-needle catheter** or **straight needle** instead of the butterfly.

Note: *A butterfly needle or over-the-needle catheter is recommended so that a line in the vein is established in case an allergic reaction occurs.*

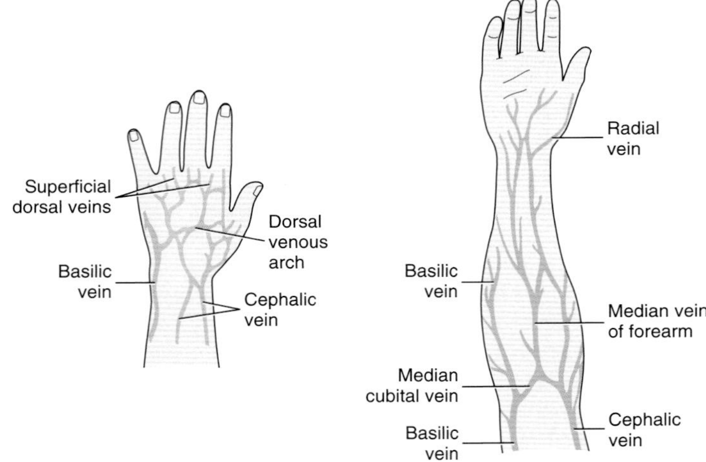

Fig. 17-25. Possible veins for venipuncture.

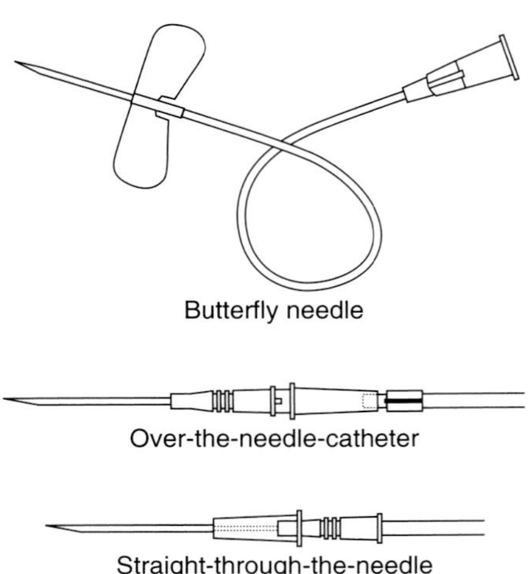

Fig. 17-26. Three types of needles.

VENIPUNCTURE PROCEDURE

Step 1: Wash Hands and Put on Gloves

After making introductions, checking patient ID, explaining the procedure, and obtaining a signature for the consent form, the technologist must do as follows:

A. Wash the hands thoroughly.
B. Put on gloves. (Avoid latex gloves if possible due to possible allergies by technologist or patient.)

Step 2: Select Site and Apply Tourniquet

A. Make patient comfortable, supporting the arm using an arm board. Select the injection site and place tourniquet **3 to 4 inches (8 to 10 cm)** above the site. Tighten the tourniquet sufficiently to dilate the veins.

Step 3: Confirm Puncture Site and Cleanse

A. Palpate the vein after the tourniquet is in place to confirm the site.
B. Cleanse the site with alcohol, iodine, or Betadine wipe, using a circular motion from the center outward.

Step 4: Initiate Puncture

A. Using the nondominant hand, anchor the vein by making the skin taut just below the puncture site.
B. With the **bevel** of the needle **facing upward,** approach the vein at an angle between 20° and 45°. Advance the needle until a slight "pop" or release of pressure is sensed. (Do not "jab" the needle too hard because it may puncture completely through the vein.)

Decrease the angle of the needle, advancing it slightly further into the vein.

Alternative site—cephalic or basilic veins of posterior hand: Locate vein by fingertip palpation and gently insert needle into vein (Figs. 17-34 and 17-35).

Note: If extravasation (infiltration) does occur or if for other reasons the venipuncture must be terminated, withdraw the needle or catheter and apply light pressure on the site with gauze or a cotton ball. Always use a new needle for any subsequent punctures.

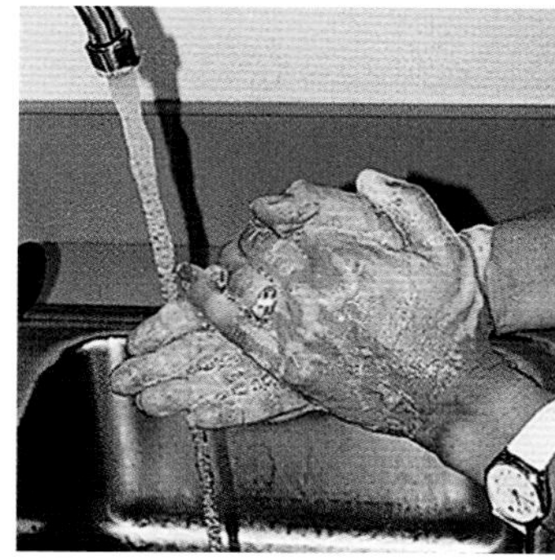

Fig. 17-27. Wash hands.

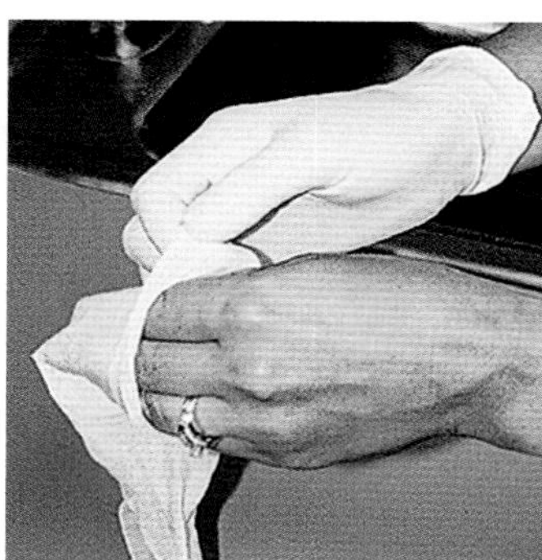

Fig. 17-28. Put on gloves.

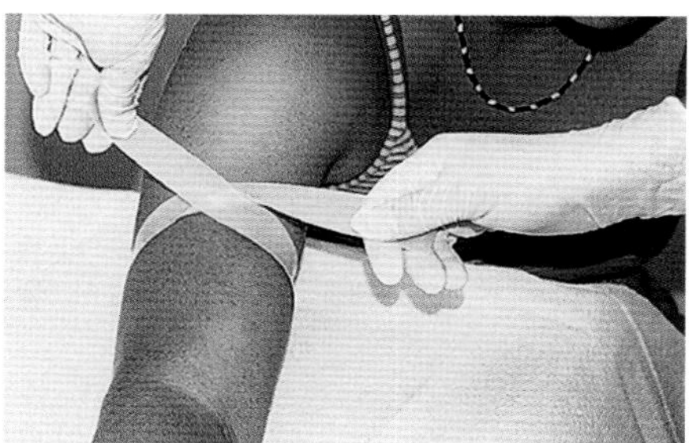

Fig. 17-29. Apply tourniquet.

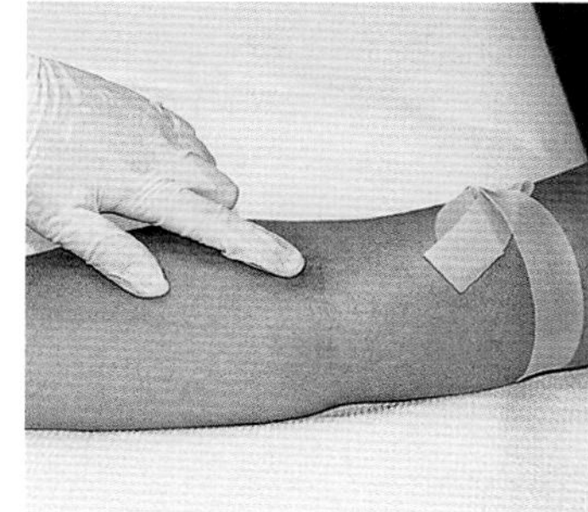

Fig. 17-30. Palpate vein to confirm site.

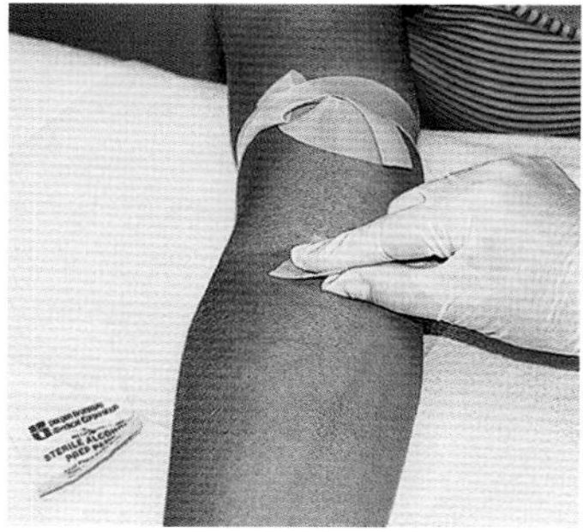

Fig. 17-31. Cleanse site.

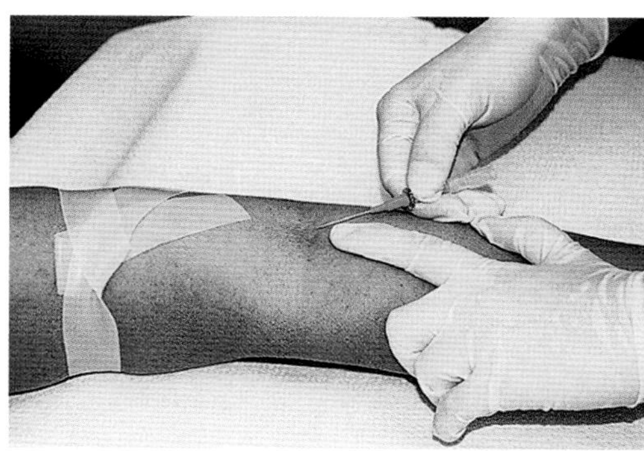

Fig. 17-32. Anchor vein with opposite hand.

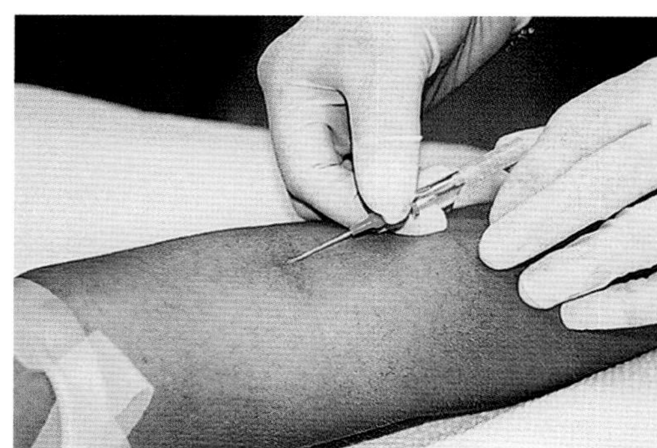

Fig. 17-33. Insert needle with **bevel up,** 20° to 25°, and advance slightly.

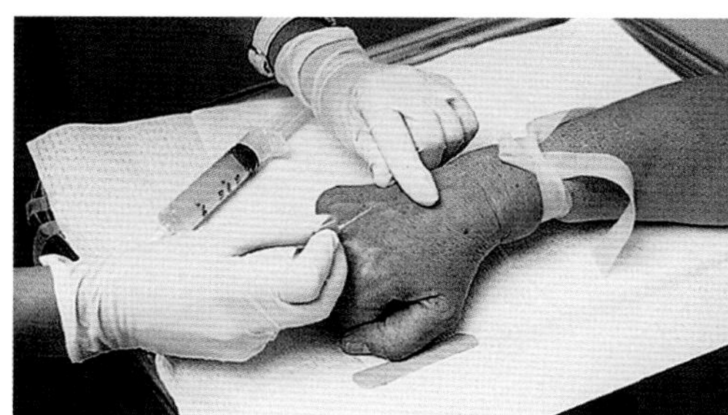

Fig. 17-34. With butterfly needle (posterior hand site)—anchor vein with opposite hand.

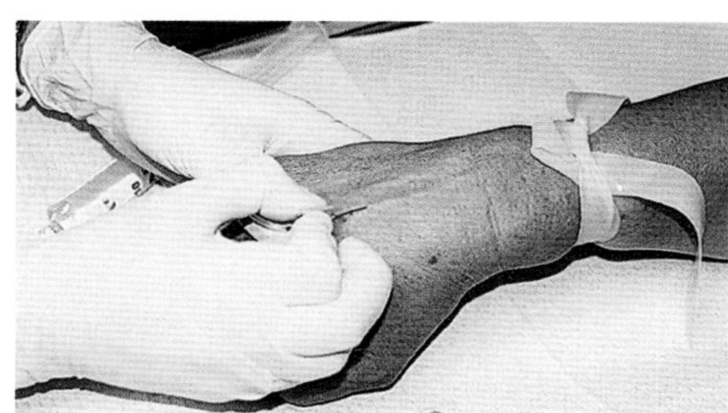

Fig. 17-35. With butterfly needle (posterior hand site)—insert needle with **bevel up,** 20° to 25°, and advance slightly.

17

Step 5: Confirm Entry and Secure Needle

A. **Butterfly needle** method (Fig. 17-36): Observe the tubing attached to the needle for retrograde flow of blood. If no blood is seen, make slight adjustment to the needle position until blood backflow is seen in the tubing. Tape needle in place.

B. **Over-the-needle catheter** (Fig. 17-37): Once the needle is in the vein, firmly grasp the catheter with the thumb and index finger. Withdraw the stylet or needle while advancing the catheter into the vein. Tape needle and catheter in place.

Step 6: Prepare for Injection

A. **Butterfly needle:** With needle in place, release the tourniquet, uncap the hub of the catheter, and connect the syringe, ready to proceed with the injection.

B. **Over-the-needle-catheter:** Observe the tubing attached to the needle or outer cannula for retrograde flow of blood. Release the tourniquet, tape the catheter in place, uncap the hub of the catheter, and connect the syringe or IV tubing.

Step 7: Proceed With Injection

Ensure that the contrast media is administered at the established rate, watching the injection site for possible signs of extravasation (see Note on preceding page).

The person performing the venipuncture must write in the patient's chart the **starting time of injection,** the **type and amount of contrast media injected,** the **site of injection,** and **sign the full name** (initials are not sufficient).

Step 8: Needle or Catheter Removal

For patient safety, leave the needle or catheter in place for the entire examination or until the physician directs its removal.

First, put on gloves to remove the needle or the catheter, and then gently remove the tape. Press slightly over the injection site using a 2 × 2 inch gauze or cotton ball and quickly but carefully withdraw needle from the vein. Place pressure immediately over the puncture site and hold until the bleeding stops. Tape the gauze or cotton ball securely in place.

Summary of Safety Considerations

1. Always wear gloves during all aspects of the procedure.
2. Follow Occupational Safety and Health Administration (OSHA) Standard Precautions and dispose of all materials containing blood or body fluids properly.
3. Do not attempt to remove needles from syringes. Place needle and syringe in sharps container. Do not let sharps container overflow. Replace container when half full.
4. If unsuccessful during initial puncture, use a new butterfly or over-the-needle catheter for the second attempt. (The needle or catheter may have been damaged during the insertion.) Also select another puncture site.
5. If extravasation of contrast agent occurs, provide a warm compress over injection site.
6. Document injection, including all complications and the injection site, time, and amount and type of contrast agent injected.

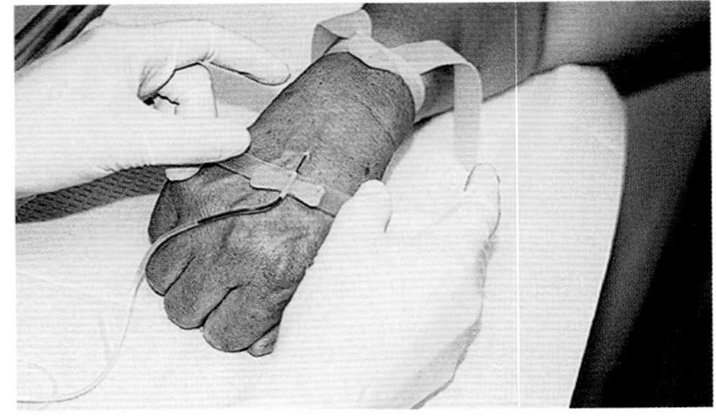

Fig. 17-36. With butterfly needle. Observe backflow of blood and tape needle in place.

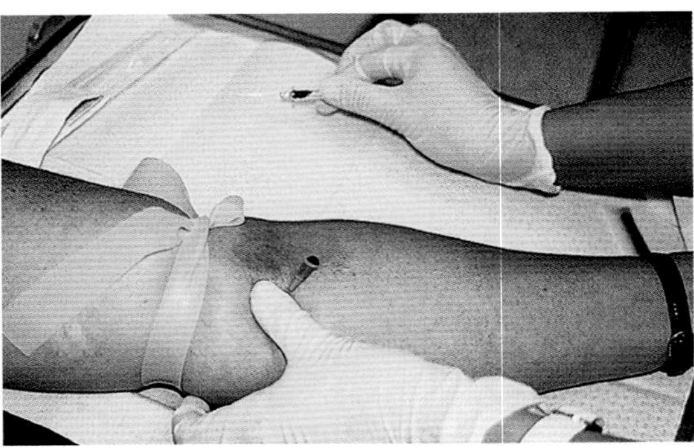

Fig. 17-37. With over-the-needle catheter. Withdraw stylet or needle.

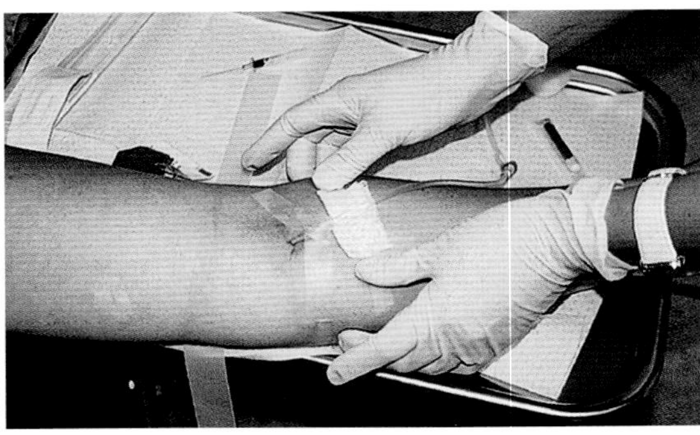

Fig. 17-38. Tape needle and catheter in place.

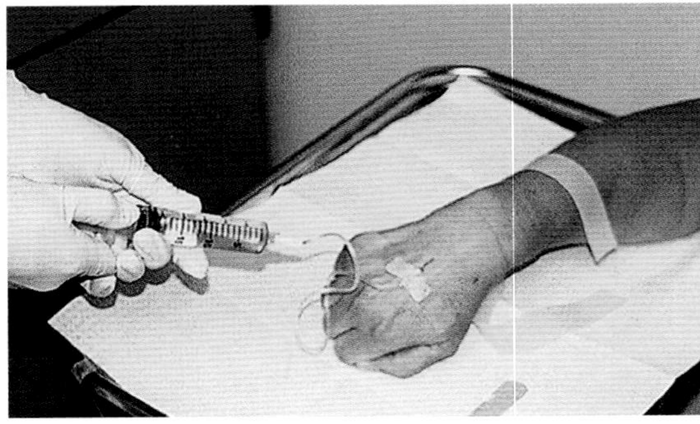

Fig. 17-39. Tape butterfly needle in place. Release tourniquet, ready to begin injection.

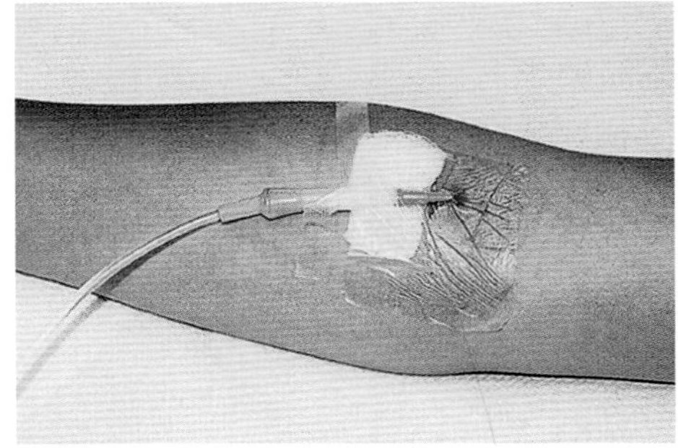

Fig. 17-40. Release tourniquet for over-the-needle catheter. Tape needle and catheter in place, ready to begin injection.

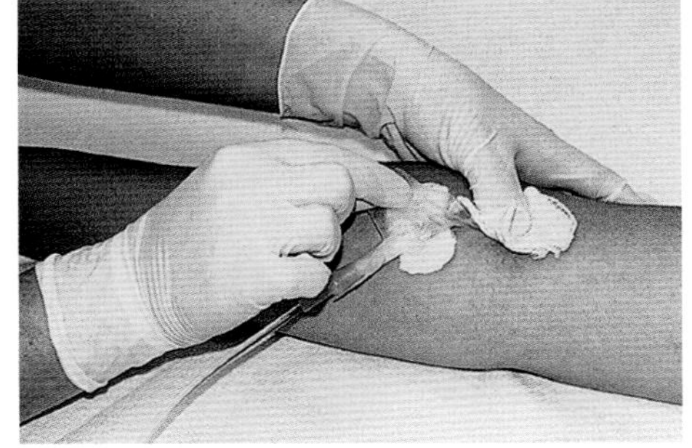

Fig. 17-41. Remove needle or catheter.

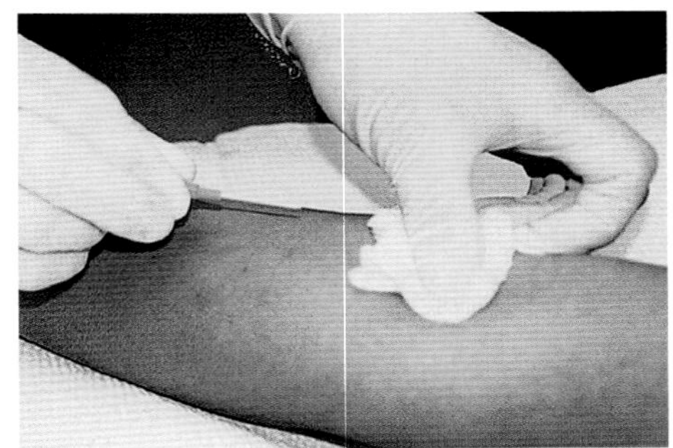

Fig. 17-42. Apply immediate pressure over injection site.

Contrast Media and Urography

INTRODUCTION TO THE INTRAVENOUS UROGRAM

The plain abdominal radiographic image demonstrates very little information of the urinary system. The gross outline of the kidneys may be faintly demonstrated due to the fatty capsule surrounding the kidneys. However, in general, the urinary system blends in with the other soft tissue structures of the abdominal cavity, thus requiring contrast media to visualize the internal, fluid-filled portion of the urinary system radiographically. This radiographic procedure using contrast media injected intravenously is termed an **intravenous urogram (IVU).** Radiographic examination of the urinary system in general is termed **urography** *(u'rog'rah-fe)*. *Uro-* is a prefix denoting a relationship to urine or to the urinary tract.

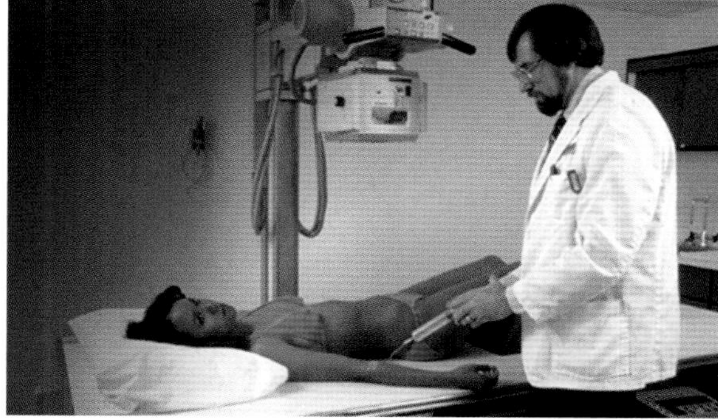

Fig. 17-43. Intravenous urogram (IVU); injection of contrast media.

TYPES OF CONTRAST MEDIA

The two major types of iodinated contrast media used in urology are **ionic** and **nonionic.** The chemical structures of the two types are somewhat different and behave differently in the body.

IONIC ORGANIC IODIDES

For many years, patients received a type of organic, iodinated contrast media referred to as **ionic.** This contrast agent contains **iodine** as the **opacifying element** and other chemical components to create a complex molecule. The parent compound of the molecule is a carboxyl group, in the form of benzoic acid, to which other chemical components (side chains) are attached. Ionic, iodinated contrast media contain a positively charged side chain element called the **cation.** The cation is a salt, usually sodium or meglumine, or a combination of both. These salts increase the solubility of the contrast media.

The cation is combined with a negatively charged component called the **anion.** Diatrizoate and iothalamate are common anions that help stabilize the contrast media compound. The cation and anion are side chains that attach to the parent, benzoic acid ring, along with **three iodine atoms,** the contrast media agents, thus the term *tri-iodinated contrast media* (Fig. 17-44).

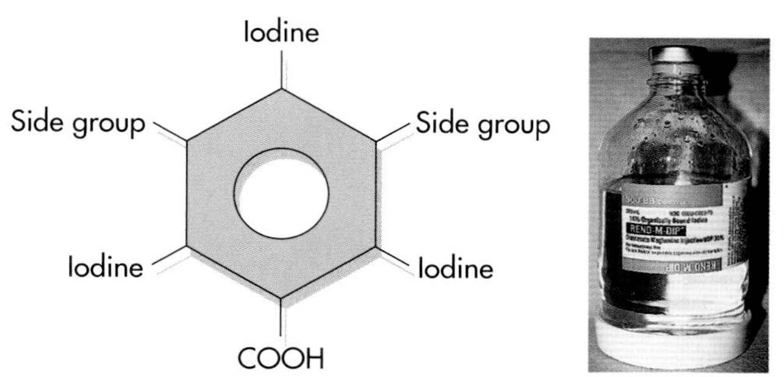

Fig. 17-44. Ionic tri-iodinated (ionic) contrast media. (Left modified from Jensen SC, Peppers MP: Pharmacology and drug administration for imaging technologists, St. Louis, 1998, Mosby.)

Higher Osmolality and Greater Chance of Reaction Once injected, the cation dissociates from the parent compound or anion, thus creating two separate ions in the blood. This action creates a hypertonic condition, or an increase in the blood plasma **osmolality.** This increase in osmolality can cause vein spasm, pain at the injection site, and fluid retention. More important, ionic contrast agents may increase the probability that a patient will experience a contrast media reaction. Any disruption to the delicate balance of the body's physiologic functions may result in a reaction. This concept is the basis of the chemotoxic theory, which states that any disruption to that physiologic balance, called **homeostasis,** may lead to reaction. Increasing the number of ions in the plasma can disrupt homeostasis and create a reaction.

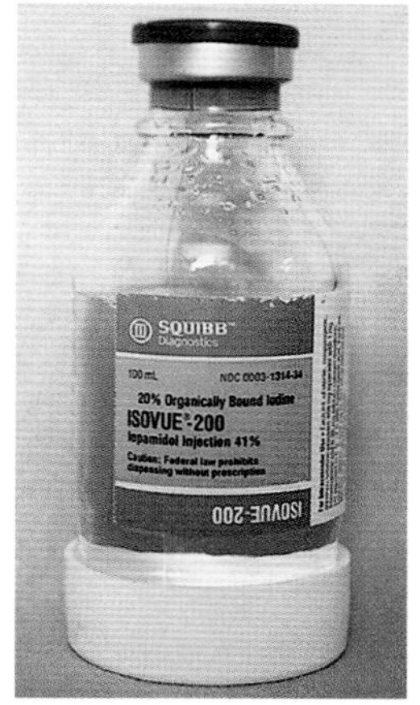

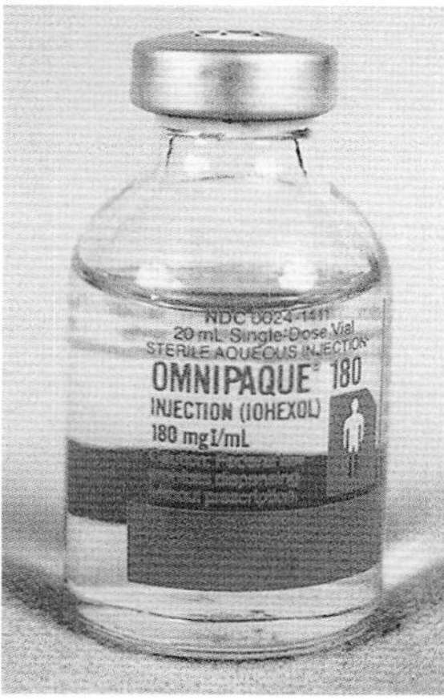

Fig. 17-45. Two examples of water-soluble nonionic contrast media.

NONIONIC ORGANIC IODIDE

In 1984 a new generation of contrast media was introduced in the United States that also contains iodine as needed for opacity but **contains no positive-charged cations.** The ionizing carboxyl group is replaced with a nondisassociated group, such as amide or glucose. When dissolved in water, a nonionic compound forms with each molecule, also containing **three iodine atoms.** Therefore when injected into the blood or other body cavities, the contrast media remains intact. The term **nonionic** was coined to describe this type of contrast media based on its nonionizing characteristic.

Low Osmolality and Less Chance of Reaction Because of their nonionizing nature, these contrast agents are of **low osmolality** and therefore do not increase the osmolality of the blood plasma. Nonionic contrast media are thus near isotonic and are better tolerated by the body. Research indicates that patients are less likely to have contrast media reactions or more likely to have less severe reactions or side effects when nonionic contrast agents are used. The cost for nonionic contrast media, however, is greater than for ionic agents. Therefore although many radiology departments use nonionic contrast media exclusively, others base their decisions to use nonionic contrast media on patient history and the potential for reactions.

COMMON SIDE EFFECTS

Side effects occur in many patients as an expected outcome to the injected iodinated contrast media. They are brief and self-limiting.

Two common side effects occurring after an intravenous injection of iodinated contrast media are a **temporary hot flash** and a **metallic taste in the mouth.** Both the hot flash, particularly in the face, and the metallic taste in the mouth usually pass quickly. Discussion of these possible effects and careful explanation of the examination help reduce patient anxiety and prepare the patient psychologically.

Patient History A careful patient history may serve to alert the medical team to a possible reaction. Patients with histories of allergy are more likely to experience adverse reactions to contrast media than those who have no allergies. Questions to ask the patient should include the following:

1. Are you allergic to anything?
2. Have you ever had hay fever, asthma, or hives?
3. Are you allergic to any drugs or medications?
4. Are you **allergic to iodine**?
5. Are you allergic to other foods?
6. Are you currently taking **Glucophage**?
7. Have you ever had an x-ray examination that required an injection into an artery or vein?

A positive response to any of these questions alerts the injection team to an increased probability of reaction.

BLOOD CHEMISTRY

The technologist must check the patient's chart to determine the **creatinine** and **BUN** (blood urea nitrogen) **levels.** These laboratory tests should have been drawn and reported in the patient's chart before the urinary study. Creatinine and BUN levels are diagnostic indicators of kidney function. Elevated creatinine or BUN levels may indicate acute or chronic renal failure, tumor, or other conditions of the urinary system. Patients with elevated blood levels have a greater chance of experiencing an adverse contrast media reaction. **Normal creatinine levels** for the adult are **0.6 to 1.5 mg/dl. BUN levels** should range between **8 and 25 mg/100 ml.**

GLUCOPHAGE*

Glucophage (metformin hydrochloride) is a drug given for the management of noninsulin-dependent diabetes mellitus. Patients currently taking Glucophage should **not** be given iodinated contrast media. The combination of iodinated contrast media and Glucophage may increase the risk for contrast media–induced acute renal failure. The American College of Radiology recommends that Glucophage be withheld for at least **48 hours** before a contrast media procedure. The taking of Glucophage may be reinstituted **48 hours after the procedure,** provided that kidney functions are judged to be normal.

The technologist must review the patient chart and ask the patient whether he or she is taking Glucophage. If the patient says "yes," this information should be brought to the immediate attention of the radiologist before injection.

SELECTION AND PREPARATION OF CONTRAST MEDIA

Selection and preparation of the correct contrast medium are important steps before injection. Because labels on various media containers are similar, one should **always read the label very carefully** several times. In addition, the **empty container should be shown to the radiologist or the person making the actual injection.**

Whenever contrast medium is drawn into a syringe, the sterility of the medium, the syringe, and the needle must be maintained.

*ACR Bulletin, American College of Radiology, August 1995; American College of Radiology Bulletin, 1995; and Prescribing information, Bristol-Myers Squibb Company, Princeton, NJ, revised, July, 2002.

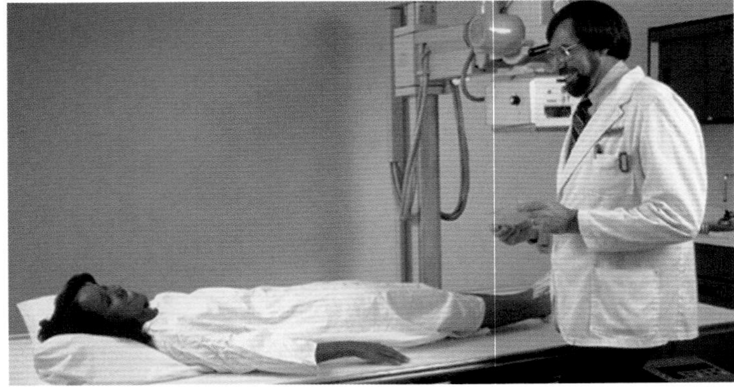

Fig. 17-46. Obtain patient history.

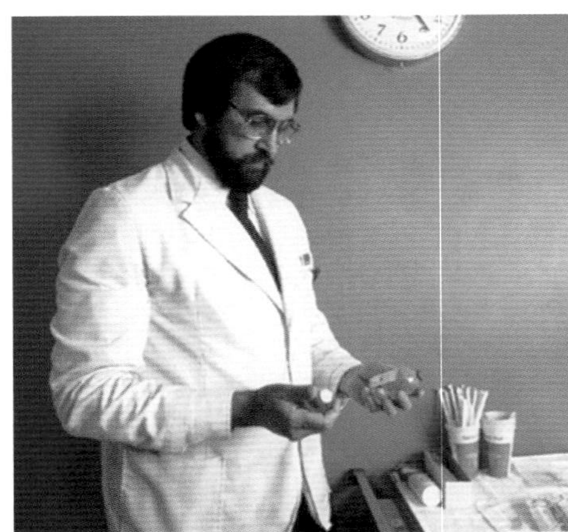

Fig. 17-47. Selection and preparation of contrast media; checking of label.

Reactions to Contrast Media

PREPARATION FOR POSSIBLE REACTION

Because contrast medium reaction is possible and unpredictable, a fully stocked **emergency response cart** must be readily available whenever an intravenous injection is made. In addition to emergency drugs, the cart should contain cardiopulmonary resuscitation equipment, portable oxygen, a suction and blood pressure apparatus, and possibly a defibrillator and monitor.

The technologist is responsible for ensuring that the emergency drug cart is complete and available in the room. Masks and cannula for oxygen support, suction tips, needles, and syringes must be readily available in the room. The status of this equipment and emergency drug cart should be verified before any contrast media procedure.

A common emergency drug is **epinephrine,** which should be available along with a syringe and needle ready for use.

Premedication Procedure To reduce the risk for contrast media reactions, some patients may be premedicated before an iodinated contrast media procedure. The patient is given a number of medications at different stages to reduce the risk of an allergic reaction to the contrast media. One of the common premedication protocols includes a combination of Benadryl and prednisone over a period of 12 hours before the procedure. Patients who have a history of hay fever, asthma, or food allergy may be candidates for the premedication procedure. The technologist should ask patients whether they have received any premedication prior to the procedure and note it in the patient's chart.

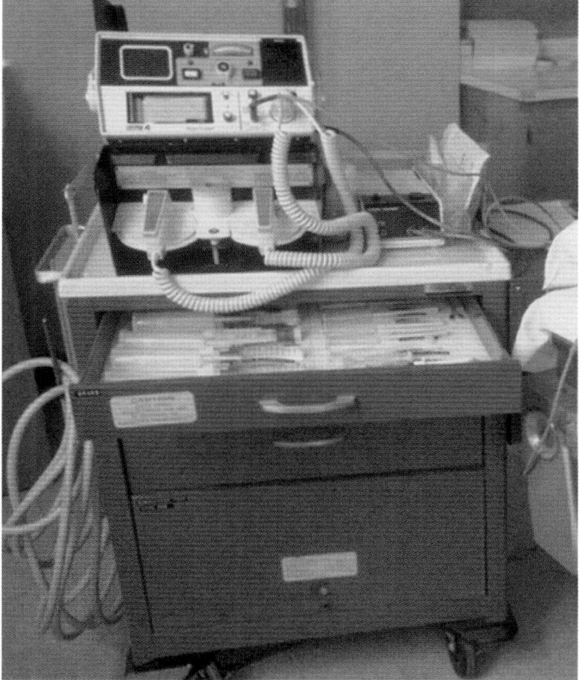

Fig. 17-48. Emergency response cart.

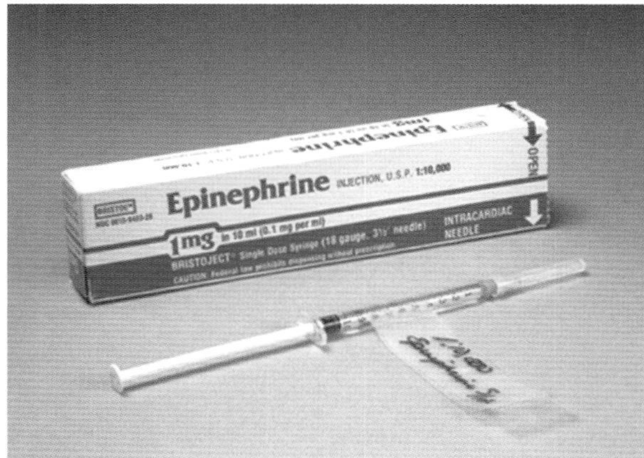

Fig. 17-49. Emergency drug.

Categories of Contrast Media Reactions* There are four general categories of contrast media reactions: (1) **vasomotor effect,** (2) **anaphylactic reaction,** (3) **vasovagal reaction,** and (4) **acute renal failure.** These four reaction types are classified according to the body system affected, the nature of the reaction (e.g., allergic versus nonallergic), and its severity.

The severity of each reaction is also defined as being **mild, moderate,** or **severe.** These levels of severity are explained later in this section with examples of related symptoms for each.

Regardless of the type of contrast media reaction that a patient may experience, it is important to report any symptoms in the patient's chart.

1. **Vasomotor effect:** This **nonallergic reaction** often does not require drug intervention or medical assistance. This type of reaction is based on anxiety and/or fear. Although this may not be a life-threatening situation, the technologist must be attentive to all needs of the patient. Symptoms of a vasomotor reaction include:
   - Anxiety
   - Lightheadedness
   - Nausea
   - Syncope
   - Mild, scattered hives

   Treatment for a vasomotor effect includes having the patient breathe slowly, providing a cool wash cloth, and reassuring the patient. Continue to observe the patient to ensure these symptoms do not advance into a more serious reaction.
2. **Anaphylactic reaction:** This second type of reaction is a **true allergic reaction** resulting from the introduction of iodinated contrast media. Symptoms of an anaphylactic reaction include:
   - Urticaria (moderate to severe hive)
   - Laryngospasm
   - Bronchospasm
   - Angioedema
   - Hypotension
   - Tachycardia (>100 beats per minute)

   Since anaphylactic reactions may lead to a life-threatening condition, medical assistance must be provided without delay. Treatment often involves drug intervention to counter the effects of the reaction.
3. **Vasovagal reaction:** This third type of reaction is a **life-threatening condition.** The introduction of iodinated contrast agents stimulates the vagus nerve, which may cause the heart rate to drop and the blood pressure to fall dangerously. Fast and prompt response from the medical team is required.

   Symptoms of a vasovagal reaction include:
   - Hypotension (systolic blood pressure <80 mm Hg)
   - Bradycardia (<50 beats/minute)
   - No detectable pulse

   A medical emergency must be declared immediately. Ensure that the emergency drug cart is nearby and that oxygen and suction equipment are available.
4. **Acute renal failure:** This is the fourth and final type of anaphylactic reaction, in which **the kidneys shut down.** The start of this reaction follows contrast media injection and may not be obvious for as long as 48 hours after the study has been completed.

   Treatment includes hydration, administration of Lasix (diuretic), and possible renal dialysis. Since this reaction occurs after the urographic procedure is completed, the patient should be told to alert the physician of any difficulty in producing urine or other unusual symptoms.

*Sharon H. Inman, RT (R) (GM), *Emergency Pharmacology,* lecture given at ACERT Annual Education Conference, January 30, 2003.

VASOMOTOR EFFECT SUMMARY

SYMPTOMS	TECHOLOGIST RESPONSIBILITIES
Anxiety	Have patient take slow breaths and reassure patient. Continue to monitor patient.
Lightheadedness	Comfort and reassure patient.
Nausea	Provide emesis basis and cool wash cloth.
Syncope (fainting)	Comfort and support patient and monitor vital signs.
Mild urticaria (scattered hives)	Inform nurse or physician. Continue to monitor patient.

ANAPHYLACTIC REACTION SUMMARY

SYMPTOMS	TECHNOLOGIST RESPONSIBILITIES
Moderate to severe urticaria (hives)	Call for medical assistance. Continue to monitor patient.
Laryngospasm (choking sensation from closure of larynx)	Call for medical assistance. Continue to monitor patient.
Angioedema (swelling of soft tissues)	Call for medical assistance. Continue to monitor patient.
Hypotension (low BP), moderate	Call for medical assistance. Continue to monitor patient.
Tachycardia (rapid heart beat), moderate	Call for medical assistance. Continue to monitor patient.

VASOVAGAL REACTION

SYMPTOMS	TECHNOLOGIST RESPONSIBILITIES
Hypotension (systolic BP <80)	Declare medical emergency **(code).** Continue to monitor vital signs.
Bradycardia (heart rate <50 bpm)	Declare medical emergency **(code).** Continue tomonitor vital signs.
No detectable pulse	Declare medical emergency **(code).** Continue to monitor vital signs.

ACUTE RENAL FAILURE

SYMPTOMS	TECHNOLOGIST RESPONSIBILITIES
Diminished urine output	Notify physician.
Anuria (no urine output)	Notify physician

SEVERITY LEVELS OF REACTIONS

In addition to the four categories of reactions to contrast media used in urography as described, there are also three levels of severity—**mild, moderate,** and **severe.** Any reaction, however, regardless of how minor it may seem, deserves careful observation. Mild reactions sometimes signal a more serious reaction to follow. Most reactions to contrast media occur rapidly if they happen at all, but on occasion a delayed reaction may occur.

The patient should **never be left alone** after an intravenous injection. As the necessary radiographs are obtained, the patient should be observed and questioned regarding any changes. The radiologist or other responsible physician should be within immediate reach for 1 hour after an injection. **The physician must be summoned immediately for any moderate or severe reaction.**

Mild Reactions (Vasomotor or Anaphylactic)

The majority of reactions to contrast media are mild vasomotor types usually requiring no treatment other than support and verbal reassurance. These mild reactions, such as **nausea and vomiting,** are fairly common. One should not forewarn the patient of their possible occurrence, however. Sometimes the power of suggestion is enough to bring on this type of reaction. An emesis basin should be handy in case of vomiting and a cold towel for the forehead in case of nausea. The patient should never vomit while supine; have the patient sit up or turn onto the side, as shown in Fig. 17-50.

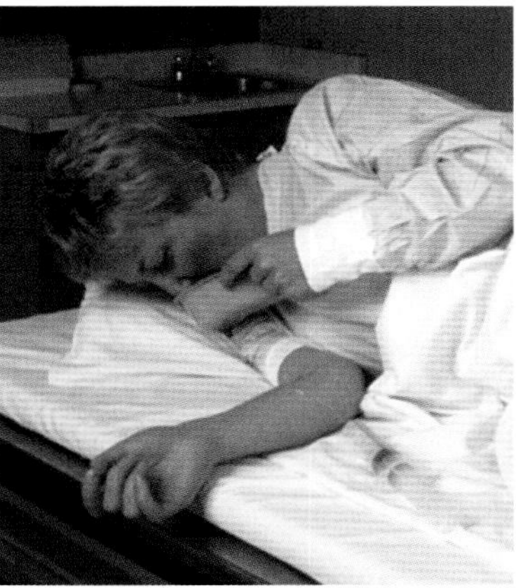

Fig. 17-50. Mild reaction—nausea.

Other mild vasomotor or anaphylactic type reactions include **hives** or **urticaria** *(ur"ti-ka're-ah),* **itching,** and **sneezing.** These reactions cause some concern because they may signal a more severe response.

Another form of mild reaction may also occur at the injection site, particularly if some of the contrast medium leaks from the vein into the surrounding tissue. Such leakage is termed **extravasation** *(eks-trav"ah-sa'shun).* Pain, burning, or numbness may result when extravasation occurs. A warm towel over the injection site may speed absorption of the contrast material.

Sometimes the sight of a needle or the sensation of a needle stick may trigger a mild form of **vasomotor** reaction. Symptoms include a sensation of weakness or dizziness, sweating, and the feeling that precedes fainting. Explanation of the procedure and a confident injection team often deter this type of reaction. The patient's blood pressure should be taken during even a mild form of vasomotor reaction because a marked drop in pressure indicates a more serious reaction.

Moderate Reactions (Anaphylactic)

A moderate reaction is one that requires treatment for both the symptoms and the comfort of the patient. Moderate anaphylactic-type reactions include **excessive urticaria** (hives); **tachycardia** *(tak"e-kar'de-ah),* or rapid heartbeat; **giant hives;** and **excessive vomiting.** Medical assistance should be summoned for any signs of these moderate reactions, which usually require administration of some type of **medication** while the patient is still in radiology. These symptoms usually respond rapidly and completely to the appropriate medication.

Someone should always remain with the patient to monitor and provide comfort, and the patient's reaction and all drugs administered during the treatment should be documented.

Severe Reactions (Vasovagal or Acute Renal Failure)

Severe reactions occur approximately in 1 of every 14,000 contrast procedures. Fatal reactions occur in approximately 1 in every 40,000 contrast procedures.* Severe reactions are all **life-threatening** and require **immediate, intensive treatment.** Any reaction that produces life-threatening symptoms requiring vigorous, active treatment is classified as a severe reaction. Very **low blood pressure, cardiac or respiratory arrest, loss of consciousness, convulsions, laryngeal edema, cyanosis, difficulty in breathing,** and **profound shock** are examples of severe reactions. Delayed or inappropriate treatment for any of these symptoms or conditions could result in the patient's death. If a severe reaction is suspected, the physician should be summoned immediately. If needed, the appropriate **emergency response code** as designated for that institution or department also should be called.

Note: Department protocol for response to all reactions to contrast media should be documented and understood by all students and technologists. In-service training must be provided to ensure this understanding.

*Tortorici M, Administration of imaging pharmaceuticals, Philadelphia, 1996, WB Saunders.

17

Excretory Urography—Intravenous Urogram

The **excretory** or **intravenous urogram (IVU)** is the most common radiographic examination of the urinary system. This examination has often been referred to as an *intravenous pyelogram, or IVP. Pyelo,* however, refers only to the renal pelves. Because the excretory urogram normally visualizes more anatomy than just the renal pelvis, the term IVP is not an accurate term for this procedure and should not be used.

The IVU visualizes the minor and major calyces, renal pelves, ureters, and urinary bladder after an intravenous injection of contrast medium. The IVU is a **true functional test** because the contrast medium molecules are rapidly removed from the bloodstream and excreted completely by the normal kidney.

PURPOSE

The three purposes of an IVU are as follows:

1. To visualize the collecting portion of the urinary system
2. To assess the functional ability of the kidneys
3. To evaluate the urinary system for pathology or anatomic anomalies

CONTRAINDICATIONS

Even though present-day contrast media are considered relatively safe, the technologist must take extra care in obtaining the patient history. Through the patient history, the technologist may become aware of certain conditions that prevent the patient from having an IVU. The major contraindications include the following:

1. Hypersensitivity to iodinated contrast media
2. Anuria, or absence of urine excretion
3. Multiple myeloma
4. Diabetes, especially diabetes mellitus
5. Severe hepatic or renal disease
6. Congestive heart failure
7. Pheochromocytoma *(fe-o-kro"mo-si-to'mah)*
8. Sickle cell anemia
9. Patients taking Glucophage (must be withheld 48 hours prior to the contrast media study)
10. Renal failure, acute or chronic (see Glossary of Urinary Pathologic Terms, following section)

Certain conditions on this list, such as (3) **multiple myeloma** and (7) **pheochromocytoma,** warrant additional consideration. Multiple myeloma is a malignant condition of the plasma cells of the bone marrow, and a pheochromocytoma is a tumor of the adrenal gland. Research indicates that these patients are at greater risk during the IVU. Because (8) **sickle cell anemia** can compromise the function of the kidney, these patients are also at a higher risk. A patient with one of the above contraindications may need to be examined with some other imaging modality. However, a patient with any of these high-risk conditions may still have an IVU if the physician believes the benefit of the procedure outweighs the risks.

A hydration therapy of a saline IV drip and diuretic before the procedure may reduce the risk for patients with multiple myeloma, diabetes mellitus, and other conditions. These patients may also be candidates for the premedication protocol prior to the contrast media study.

GLOSSARY OF URINARY PATHOLOGIC TERMS

Following are common pathologic terms related to the urinary system that may be used to describe possible reactions to contrast media. These terms may be encountered in the patient's chart, the examination requisition, or the exam results report:

Acute renal failure (ARF): See term below under *renal failure.*

Angioedema (*an'je-o-e-de-ma*): Regions or areas of subcutaneous swelling due to allergic reaction to foods or drugs. Swelling of the lips and other parts of the mouth, the eyelids, and the hand and feet may occur.

Anuria *(an-ur'e-a):* Complete cessation of urinary secretion by the kidneys; also called **anuresis.**

Bacteriuria *(bak-ter"e-u-re-a):* Presence of bacteria in the urine.

Bradycardia *(brak-e-kar'de-a):* Slowness of heartbeat, usually <50 beats per minute.

Bronchospasm *(brong'ko-spazm):* Contraction of the muscles within the walls of the bronchi and bronchioles, producing a restriction of air passing through them.

Diuretic *(di"u-ret'ik):* An agent that increases excretion of urine.

Fecaluria *(fe"kal-u're-a):* Presence of fecal matter in the urine.

Glucosuria *(gloo"ko-su're-a):* Presence of glucose in the urine.

Hematuria *(he"ma-tu're-a):* Blood in the urine.

Hypotension *(hi'po-ten'shun):* Below normal arterial blood pressure.

Laryngospasm *(la-ring-go-spazm):* Closure of the glottic aperture within the glottic opening within the larynx.

Lasix *(la'siks):* A brand name for a diuretic used in treatment of renal disease.

Lithotripsy *(lith'o-trip"se):* A technique using acoustic (sound) waves to shatter large kidney stones into small particles that can be passed.

Micturition *(mik"tu-ri'shan):* The act of voiding or urination.

Nephroptosis *(nef"rop-to'sis):* Excessive downward movement of kidney when erect.

Oliguria *(ol"i-gu're-a):* Excretion of a diminished amount of urine in relation to the fluid intake, usually defined as less than 400 ml per 24 hours; also called **hypouresis** and **oligouresis.**

Pneumouria *(noo"mo-u're-a):* Presence of gas in the urine, usually as a result of a fistula between the bladder and intestine.

Polyuria *(pol"e-u're-a):* Passage of a large volume of urine in a given period; a common symptom of diabetes.

Proteinuria *(pro"te-nu're-a):* The presence of an excess of serum proteins in the urine; also termed **albuminuria.**

Renal agenesis *(re'nal a-jen'a-sis):* The absence of a functioning kidney.

Renal failure (acute or chronic): The inability of a kidney to excrete metabolites at normal plasma levels, or the inability to retain electrolytes under conditions of normal intake.

- **Acute renal failure:** Marked by uremia and usually by oliguria or anuria, with hyperkalemia and pulmonary edema; the IVU demonstrating little or no contrast media reaching the kidney; possible further complication of the patient's condition with use of iodinated contrast media; ultrasound considered a safer alternative to look for signs of renal failure.
- **Chronic renal failure:** Results from a wide variety of conditions and may require hemodialysis or transplantation.

Retention: The inability to void, which may be due to obstruction in the urethra or the lack of sensation to urinate.

Syncope *(sin'ko-pe):* Loss of consciousness due to reduced cerebral blood flow; also called "fainting."

Tachycardia *(tak-i-kar'de-a):* Rapid heart beat, usually >100 beats per minute.

Uremia *(u-re'me-a):* An excess in the blood of urea, creatinine, and other nitrogenous end products of protein and amino acid metabolism; often present with chronic renal failure; **also may be called *azotemia.***

Urinary incontinence: Constant or frequent involuntary passage of urine; commonly caused by failure of voluntary control of the vesical and urethral sphincters.

Urinary reflux: A backward or return flow of urine from bladder into ureter and kidney; also termed **vesicoureteral reflux;** a common cause of pyelonephritis, in which the backflow of urine may carry bacteria that can produce infection in the kidney.

Urinary tract infection (UTI): Infections that frequently occur in both adults and children and are caused by bacteria, viruses, fungi, or certain parasites; commonly caused by vesicoureteral reflux.

Urticaria *(er'ti-kar'i-a):* An eruption of wheals (hives) often due to a hypersensitivity to food or drugs.

Pathologic Indications

The more common pathologic indications for radiographic urinary system procedures include the following:

Benign prostatic hyperplasia (BPH) is an age-associated enlargement of the prostate generally beginning in the fifth decade of life. Although it is a benign condition, it may cause urethral compression and obstruction. This obstruction often produces painful and frequent urination and possible vesicoureteral reflux.

The postvoid, erect projection taken during an IVU or cystogram produces a defect along the base of the bladder indicative of BPH. The floor of the bladder may appear elevated and indented.

Bladder calculi are stones that form in the urinary bladder. These stones are not as common as renal calculi, but they can grow quite large in the bladder (Fig. 17-51) and may be radiolucent or radiopaque. The radiolucent stones are most often uric acid stones. The presence of bladder stones can make urination difficult. These stones may be demonstrated during an IVU or retrograde cystogram. They are seen clearly during a CT scan of the pelvis as well.

Bladder carcinoma is a tumor that is three times more common in males than females.* The tumor is usually diagnosed after the age of 50 years. Symptoms of bladder carcinoma include hematuria and frequency in urination. The tumor is often a solid or papillary mass with mucosal involvement. Although the cystogram may be performed, CT and MR are used to stage the tumor and determine the amount of tissue involved.

Congenital anomalies are structural or chemical imperfections or alterations present at birth.

- **Duplication of ureter and renal pelvis** involves two ureters and/or the renal pelvis originating from the same kidney. It is the most common type of congenital anomaly of the urinary system.* Usually, this anomaly does not create a health concern for the patient. The IVU confirms this condition.
- **Ectopic kidney** describes a normal kidney that fails to ascend into the abdomen but rather remains in the pelvis. This type of kidney has a shorter than normal ureter. Although this condition does not pose a health concern for the patient, it may interfere with the birth process in females. Although an IVU will confirm the location of the ectopic kidney, sonography and CT of the pelvis will also demonstrate this anomaly.
- **Horseshoe kidney** is a fusion of the kidneys during the development of the fetus. Nearly 95% of the cases have the lower poles of the kidneys fused.* This fusion does not usually affect the function of the kidney. Because of the fusion of the lower poles, the kidneys do not ascend to their normal position in the abdomen and are typically situated in the lower abdomen/upper pelvis. CT and sonography of the abdomen will demonstrate this congenital condition in addition to the IVU.
- **Malrotation** is an abnormal rotation of the kidney evident with the renal pelvis turned from a medial into an anterior or posterior direction. The ureteropelvic junction (UPJ) may be seen lateral to the kidney. Usually malrotation does not produce any major problems for the patient.

Cystitis *(sis-ti'tis)* describes an inflammation of the urinary bladder due to a bacterial or fungal infection. It is seen most often in females because of the shorter urethra that permits the retrograde passage of bacteria into the bladder.

Laboratory tests confirm the presence of infection. The cystogram may demonstrate signs of chronic cystitis in the form of mucosal edema.

*Ell SR: Handbook of gastrointestinal and genitourinary radiology, St. Louis, 1992, Mosby.

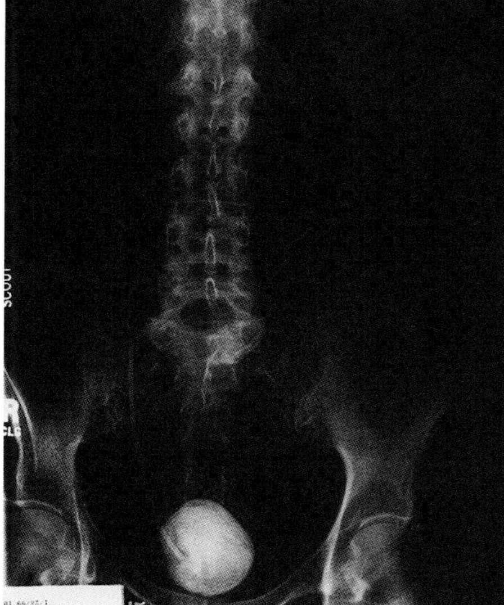

Fig. 17-51. Large stone in bladder.

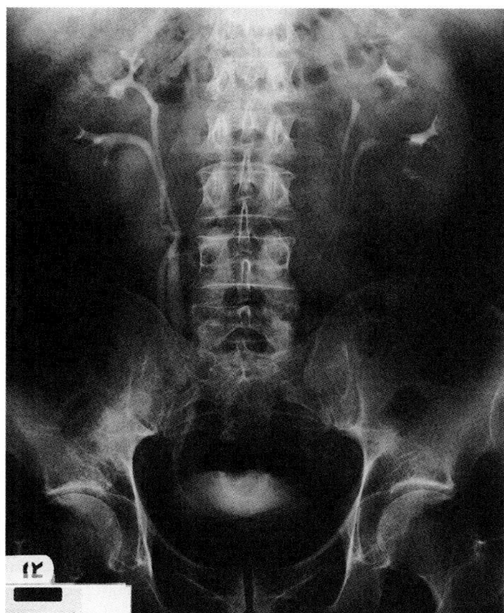

A

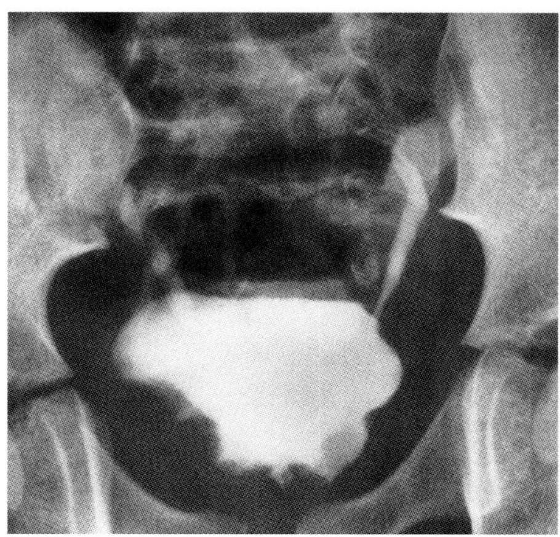

B

Fig. 17-52. A, Bilateral dual renal pelvis and ureters. **B,** Cystitis shows irregular lobulated filling defects at base of bladder. (**B** from Eisenberg RL, Johnson NM: Comprehensive radiographic pathology, ed 3, St. Louis, 2003, Mosby.)

17

Glomerulonephritis *(glo-mer"u-lo-na·fri'tis)* (also known as *Bright disease*) is an inflammation of the capillary loops of the glomeruli of the kidneys. (*Nephritis* indicates inflammation of the nephron.)

- It occurs in acute, subacute, and chronic forms. With **acute glomerulonephritis** the IVU may demonstrate an **enlarged kidney** with reduced concentration of contrast media in the collecting system. Ultrasound is the modality of choice and may show an enlarged, echolucent kidney with the acute conditions.
- With the **chronic condition,** ultrasound demonstrates **small kidney size** caused by fibrosis and cortex destruction from long-standing inflammation. Thus chronic forms of this disease result in **small kidneys with blunt, rounded calyces.** This condition is the most common cause of undeveloped kidneys in young adults.* This condition is characterized by hypertension with increased amounts of albumin, BUN, and creatinine levels in the urine.
- Nuclear medicine may be performed to demonstrate functional changes within the nephron due to infection or restriction of blood flow through the capillary beds.

Polycystic kidney disease is a disorder marked by cysts scattered throughout one or both kidneys. This disease is the **most common cause of enlarged kidneys.*** Its cause may be either genetic or congenital, depending on the type of polycystic disease. These cysts alter the appearance of the kidney and may alter renal function. In some cases the liver may have cysts as well.

The appearance of polycystic disease is described as a "bunch of grapes" scattered throughout the kidney.† Three major types of polycystic kidney disease include **infantile, childhood,** and **adult.** (See Chapter 20 for a description of infantile and childhood types.)

- **Adult:** This form of polycystic disease is inherent. Although the condition is present at birth, symptoms are not seen until later in life.

Symptoms include renal hypertension, proteinuria, and signs of chronic renal failure. If a cyst ruptures into a calyx, it may produce hematuria. The nephrogram or nephrotomogram taken during an IVU may provide an indirect sign of cysts. High-resolution CT does an excellent job in demonstrating radiolucent regions characteristic of cysts, as does ultrasound.

Renal calculi describe calcifications that occur in the luminal aspect of the urinary tract. These calcifications often lead to renal obstruction. Calcifications occur in the renal parenchyma as well.

The causes for stone formation remain uncertain. Research indicates that patients with very acidic urine (pH 5-6) and elevated levels of calcium in the urine have a greater incidence of renal stones. Conditions that may produce elevated levels of calcium in the urine include hyperparathyroidism, bone metastasis, and multiple myeloma. Abnormal ingestion of calcium may increase the risk for renal calculi.

Although the IVU demonstrates obstruction caused by renal calculi, CT of the urinary tract is becoming the gold standard to detect stones.

- **Staghorn calculus** is a large stone that grows and completely fills the renal pelvis, blocking the flow of urine.

*Linn-Watson TA: Radiographic pathology, Philadelphia, 1996, WB Saunders.
†Ell SR: Handbook of gastrointestinal and genitourinary radiology, St. Louis, 1992, Mosby.

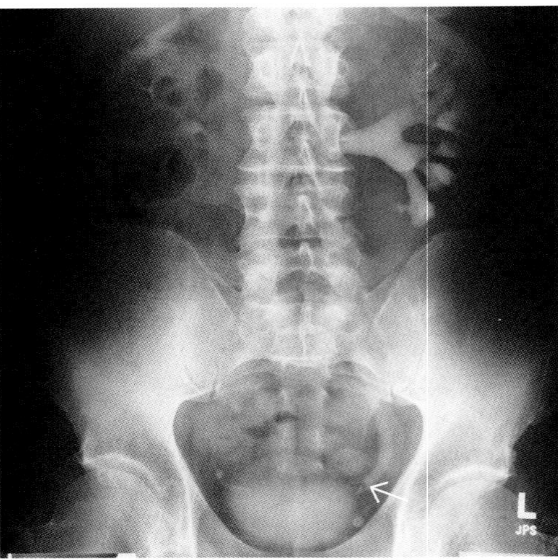

Fig. 17-53. Small triangular-shaped calculus in distal left ureter blocking flow of urine and contrast media *(arrow).*

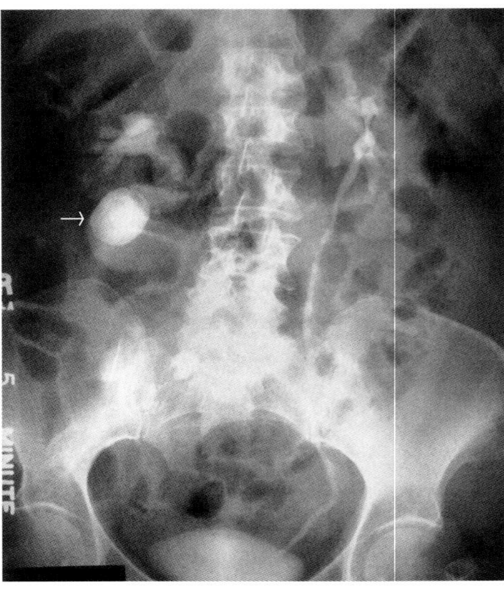

Fig. 17-54. Unusually large calculus in right ureter *(arrow).* (Courtesy Gateway Community College, Phoenix.)

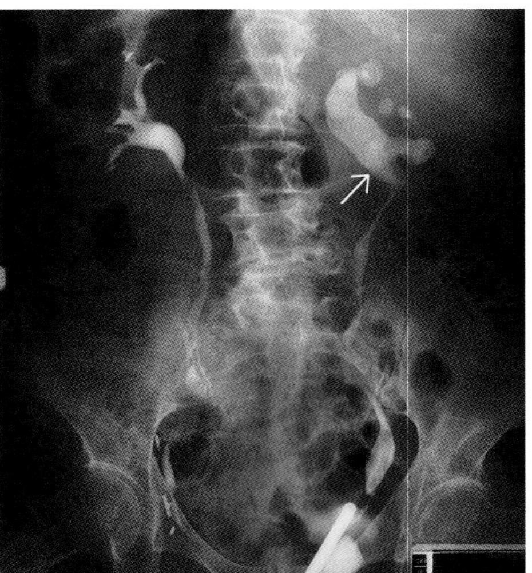

Fig. 17-55. Staghorn calculus in left kidney *(arrow).*

Renal cell carcinoma (hypernephroma) is the most frequent type of malignant tumor of the kidney.* It is three times more frequent in males than females. Symptoms include flank pain and hematuria. The tumor itself is typically a large, irregular mass with internal areas of necrosis and hemorrhage.

The IVU may demonstrate a reduced excretion of contrast media due to tumor involvement, but ultrasound and CT are the modalities of choice in demonstrating the extent of the tumor and its impact on surrounding tissues.

Hydronephrosis *(hi″dro-na-fro′sis)* is a distention of the renal pelvis and calyces of the kidneys as a result of some obstruction of the ureters or renal pelvis. It may be present in both kidneys in a female when the ureters are compressed by the fetus. Other more common causes are calculi (stones) in the renal pelvis or ureter, tumors, and structural or congenital abnormalities (Fig. 17-57).

Pyelonephritis *(pi″a-lo-na-fri′tis)* describes an inflammation of the kidney and renal pelvis caused by pyogenic (pus-forming) bacteria. The inflammation process primarily affects the interstitial tissue between the tubules, whereas glomerulonephritis, described on the preceding page, involves the glomeruli and tubules themselves.

With acute pyelonephritis the IVU is frequently normal, but with chronic pyelonephritis the hallmark urographic sign is patchy and blunting or rounding of the calyces with atrophy and thinning of renal parenchyma.

Renal hypertension is increased blood pressure to the kidney through the renal artery due to atherosclerosis. A form of hypertension results from an increased excretion of renin, which results in excessive vasoconstriction.

Severe hypertension can result in localized necrosis of the renal parenchyma and **small kidneys,** with **delayed excretion** and overconcentration of the contrast media. Diabetes in conjunction with renal hypertension can accentuate the damage to the kidney.

Renal hypertension often requires an alteration of the normal IVU routine. The filming sequence for the study allows for shorter spans of time between images. (The hypertensive IVU exam, which has largely been replaced by alternative modalities, will be described more completely in a later section of this chapter.)

Renal obstruction may be caused by necrotic debris, calculus, blood thrombus, or trauma. Renal obstruction from any source may lead to renal damage. The longer the obstruction persists, the greater the chance of functional injury.

- **Acute obstruction:** During an IVU the nephrogram demonstrates a reduced perfusion of contrast media throughout the kidney. Delayed opacification of the collecting system is another sign of acute obstruction. It may be hours after injection before the contrast media is visible in the collecting system. This delay may require the technologist to take delayed films several hours after injection.
- **Chronic or partial obstruction:** During the IVU the collecting system may be opacified, but the calyces may show signs of enlargement and hydronephrosis.

Vesicorectal (vesicocolonic) fistula is a fistula (artificial opening) between the urinary bladder and rectum or aspects of the colon. This condition may be due to trauma or tumor, or it may be a congenital defect.

Approximately 60% of fistulas result from diverticulosis (outpouching or herniation of an organ wall usually in the small or large intestine). Another 20% are a result of an invading carcinoma, colitis, and trauma.* Pneumaturia and fecaluria are symptoms of a fistula.

Although the barium enema and cystogram are performed to determine whether a fistula is present, they only visualize approximately 50% of the condition. CT is recommended to demonstrate signs of inflammation or air in the bladder, which indicate a fistula.

*Ell SR: Handbook of gastrointestinal and genitourinary radiology, St. Louis, 1992, Mosby.

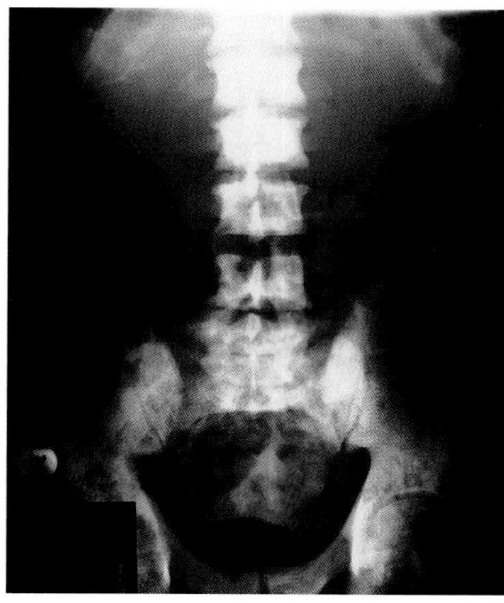

Fig. 17-56. Cancer of prostate with metastasis to pelvis and spine.

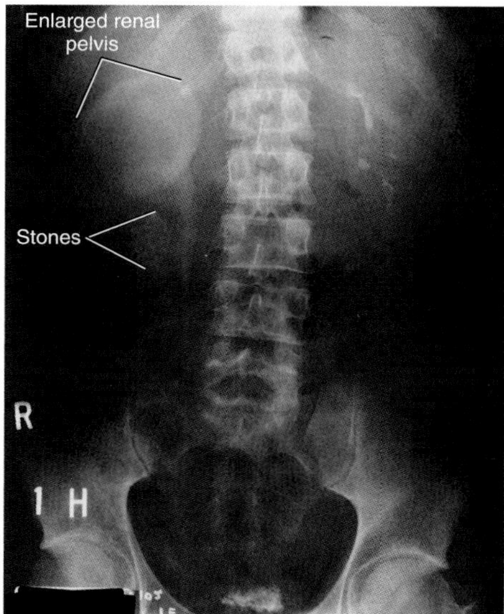

Fig. 17-57. 1-hour delayed IVU; large hydronephrosis, evidently, due to stones in right kidney.

17

17

URINARY SYSTEM—SUMMARY OF PATHOLOGIC INDICATIONS

CONDITION OR DISEASE	MOST COMMON RADIOGRAPHIC EXAM	POSSIBLE RADIOGRAPHIC APPEARANCE	MANUAL EXPOSURE FACTOR ADJUSTMENT
Benign prostatic hyperplasia (BPH)	IVU—erect postvoid or recumbent bladder, cystogram	Elevated or indented floor of the bladder	None
Bladder calculi	Cystogram, ultrasound/CT (preferred)	Calcifications within bladder	None
Bladder carcinoma	Cystogram, CT, and MRI (preferred)	Mucosal change within bladder	None
Congenital anomalies • **Duplication of ureter and renal pelvis** • **Ectopic kidney** • **Horseshoe kidney** • **Malrotation**	IVU, ultrasound/CT	Appearance dependent on the nature of the anomaly	None
Cystitis	Cystogram	Mucosal changes within bladder	None
Glomerulonephritis (Bright disease)	IVU, ultrasound/nuclear medicine	Acute—normal or enlarged kidneys with normal calyces; chronic—bilateral small kidneys, blunted calyces	None
Hydronephrosis	IVU (nephrogram), ultrasound, retrograde urogram	Enlarged renal pelvis and calyces and ureter proximal to obstruction; nephrogram becoming abnormally dense	None
Polycystic kidney disease (infantile, childhood, or adult)	IVU (nephrogram), CT	Enlarged kidneys, elongated renal pelvis, radiolucents (cysts) throughout cortex	None
Pyelonephritis	IVU (nephrogram), ultrasound	Chronic—patchy, blunting of calyces, with atrophy and thinning parenchyma	None
Renal calculi	IVU, CT (preferred), nuclear medicine	Signs of obstruction of the urinary system	None
Renal cell carcinoma	IVU, ultrasound/CT (preferred)	Irregular appearance of parenchyma or collecting system	None
Renal hypertension	Hypertensive IVU series, ultrasound (preferred)	Small kidneys, with delayed excretion and overconcentration of contrast media	None
Renal obstruction	IVU, CT (tumor, stones)	Signs of obstruction of the urinary system	None
Vesicorectal fistula (vesicocolonic)	Cystogram/barium enema, CT (preferred)	Signs of inflammation or fluid collections	None

PATIENT PREPARATION

Patient preparation for the IVU and the barium enema is similar. The intestinal tract should be free of gas and fecal material for both examinations. If both examinations are to be performed on the same patient, they can be done on the same day. The IVU is done first, with the barium enema to follow.

The general patient preparation for the IVU includes the following:

1. Light evening meal before the procedure
2. Bowel-cleansing laxative
3. NPO after midnight (a minimum of 8 hours)
4. Enema on the morning of the examination

Before the excretory urogram, all clothing except shoes and socks should be removed and replaced with a short-sleeved hospital gown. The opening and ties should be in the back.

The patient should void just before the examination for the following two reasons:

1. A bladder that is too full could rupture, especially if compression is applied early in the exam.
2. Urine already present in the bladder dilutes the contrast medium accumulating there.

PREGNANCY PRECAUTIONS

If the patient is a female, a menstrual history must be obtained. Irradiation of an early pregnancy is one of the most hazardous situations in diagnostic radiography.

X-ray examinations such as the IVU, which include the pelvis and uterus in the primary beam, should be done on pregnant females **only** when absolutely necessary and when the benefits exceed the risk. Abdominal radiographs of a known pregnancy should be delayed until the third trimester, if done at all.

In certain cases an IVU on a pregnant patient may be requested. Frequently, it is to rule out urinary obstruction. In these situations the technologist should communicate with the radiologist to determine whether the number of radiographs taken during the IVU can be reduced. A reduction in the number of projections taken may be the best way to reduce dose to the fetus. The use of higher kV, with lower mAs exposure factors, also reduces patient exposure.

PREPARATION OF RADIOGRAPHIC EQUIPMENT AND SUPPLIES

Equipment and supplies needed for urography, in addition to a suitable radiographic room, are the following:

1. Correct type and amount of contrast medium drawn up in an appropriate syringe
2. The empty container of contrast medium to show the physician or assistant doing the injection
3. A selection of sterile needles to include 18-, 21-, and 23-gauge butterfly needles and tubing
4. Alcohol sponges or wipes
5. Tourniquet
6. Towel or sponge to support the elbow
7. Male gonadal shield
8. Emesis basin
9. Lead numbers, minute marker, and R and L markers
10. Emergency cart handy
11. Epinephrine or Benadryl ready for emergency injection
12. Ureteric compression device (if used by department)
13. A cold towel for the forehead or a warm towel for the injection site, if necessary
14. Oxygen and suction devices operational and ready.

These items should be assembled and ready before the patient is escorted to the radiographic room.

URETERIC COMPRESSION

A method used to enhance filling of the pelvicalyceal system and proximal ureters is ureteric compression. Furthermore, ureteric compression allows the renal collecting system to retain the contrast medium longer for a more complete study. One such compression device is shown on the model in Fig. 17-59. It is a Velcro band that wraps around two inflatable pneumatic paddles. These paddles are held in place by a piece of Plexiglas and sponge.

Fig. 17-58. Excretory urography supplies.

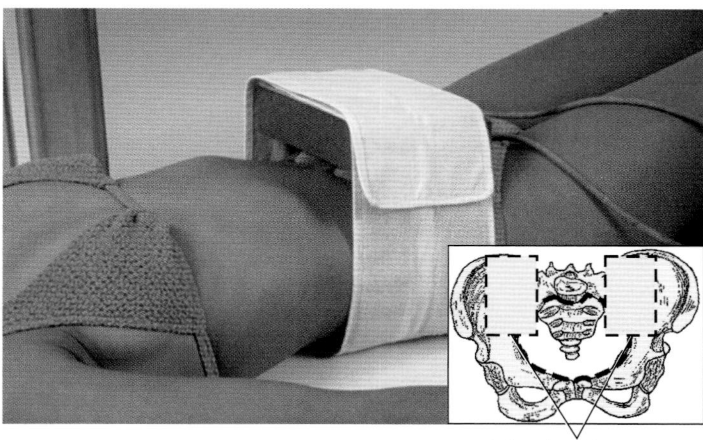

Fig. 17-59. Ureteric compression. *Inset,* Inflated paddles over outer pelvic brim.

Before injection of the contrast medium, the device is placed on the patient, with the paddles deflated. The two paddles must be **placed over the outer pelvic brim** on each side to allow for compression of the ureters. The inner edges of the paddles should nearly touch just lateral to the vertebral spine on each side. The greatest pressure is exerted in the center of the inflated paddles, which should be positioned over the point where the ureters cross the psoas muscles. Without proper placement of the paddles, the contrast medium is excreted at its normal rate (see Fig. 17-59, *inset*).

Once the contrast media is introduced, the paddles are inflated and remain in place until the postcompression images are ready to be obtained.

CONTRAINDICATIONS TO URETERIC COMPRESSION

Certain conditions exist that contraindicate the use of ureteric compression. These include the following:

1. **Possible ureteric stones** (difficult to distinguish between the effects of compression versus the appearance due to a stone)
2. **Abdominal mass** (may also present the same radiographic appearance as ureteric compression)
3. **Abdominal aortic aneurysm** (compression device possibly leading to leakage or rupture of the aneurysm)
4. **Recent abdominal surgery**
5. **Severe abdominal pain**
6. **Acute abdominal trauma**

Alternative Trendelenburg The Trendelenburg position (wherein the head end of the table is lowered about 15°) provides some of the same results as the compression procedure without as much risk to the patient whose symptoms contraindicate ureteric compression.

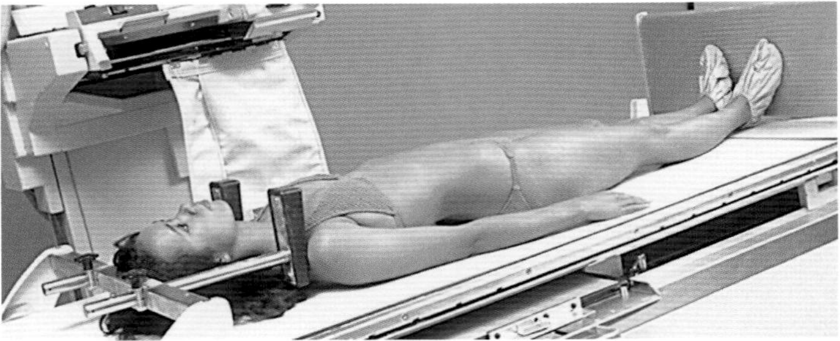

Fig. 17-60. IVU—Trendelenburg position.

General IVU Procedure

Department routines vary for the IVU. This section introduces a generic procedure for the IVU. The department supervisor should be consulted for specific differences from the following description.

SCOUT IMAGE AND INJECTION

17

The patient's clinical history and other pertinent information are discussed with the radiologist before injection. The scout radiograph is taken to (1) verify patient preparation, (2) determine whether exposure factors are acceptable, (3) verify positioning, and (4) detect any abnormal calcifications. These scout radiographs should be shown to the radiologist before injection. If the patient has a catheter in place, it should be clamped before injection.

When the injection is made, **the exact starting time and the length of injection** should be noted. Timing for the entire series is based on the start of the injection, not the end of it. The injection usually takes between 30 seconds and 1 minute to complete. As the examination proceeds, the patient should be observed carefully for any signs or symptoms indicating a reaction to the contrast medium. The chart should note the amount and type of contrast medium given to the patient.

After the full injection of contrast medium, radiographs are taken at specific time intervals. Each image must be marked with a lead number indicating the time interval when the radiograph was taken.

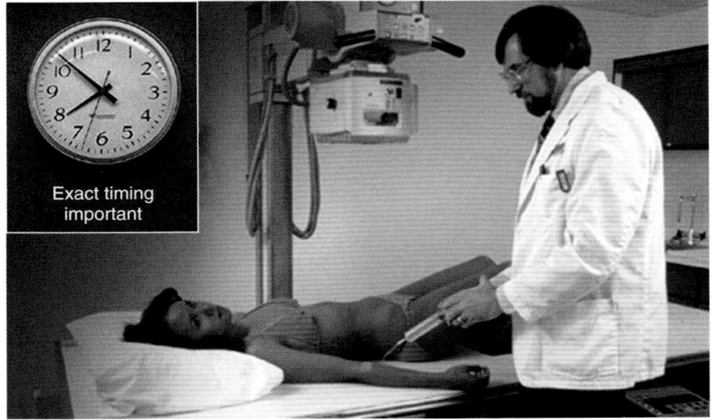

Fig. 17-61. IVU injection.

BASIC IMAGING ROUTINE (SAMPLE IVU PROTOCOL)

A common basic routine for an IVU is as follows:

1. **Nephrogram** or **nephrotomogram** is taken immediately after completion of injection (or 1 minute after start of injection) to capture the early stages of the contrast medium entering the collecting system. (Additional description on following page.)
2. **5-minute image** requires a full KUB to include the entire urinary system. The supine position (AP) is the preferred position.
3. **15-minute image** requires a full KUB to include the entire urinary system. Once again, the supine position (AP) is most commonly requested.
4. **20-minute obliques** should use the LPO and RPO positioning to provide a different perspective of the kidneys and project the ureters away from the spine.
5. **Postvoid** radiograph is taken after the patient has voided. The positions of choice may be a prone (PA) or erect AP. The bladder should be included on this final radiograph.

Note: Ensure that time markers are placed on IR prior to exposure to record the time of exposure.

SUMMARY OF SAMPLE IVU PROTOCOL

1. **Clinical History Taken**
2. **Scout Radiograph Taken**
3. **Injection of Contrast Media Performed**
   (Note starting time of injection and type and amount of contrast media injected.)
4. **Basic Imaging Routine Performed**
   1-minute nephrogram or nephrotomogram
   5-minute AP supine
   15-minute AP supine
   20-minute posterior obliques
   Postvoid (prone or erect)

ALTERNATIVES TO ROUTINE

Many variations or alternatives to the basic routine exist, and the radiologist may order specific positions at any time during the study. Three common variations include the following:

1. Postrelease or "Spill" Procedure With Ureteric Compression A full-size radiograph is taken after the release of compression. The procedure is explained to the patient, and the air pressure is released, as illustrated in Fig. 17-62. The spill radiograph or any other delayed imaging is usually done in the supine position.

To assess for asymmetric renal function, compression may be applied immediately after the 5-minute exposure (unless contraindicated), then removed immediately before the 15-minute image.

2. Erect Position for Bladder If the patient has a history of prolapse of the bladder or enlarged prostate gland, the erect bladder position taken **before voiding** may confirm these conditions.

3. Delayed Radiographs Often with urinary calculi, the filling of the involved ureter is slow. The patient may be brought back to the department on a 1- or 2-hour basis. The radiology staff should be aware of when the next radiograph is due before leaving the department for the day.

After the completion of the usual IVU series, a postvoid radiograph is often obtained in either the prone or upright position. By emptying of the bladder, small abnormalities of the bladder may be detected. The upright position also demonstrates any unusual movement of the kidneys.

The radiologist should confirm that no additional images are required before releasing the patient from the department.

NEPHROGRAM VERSUS NEPHROTOMOGRAM

Radiographs taken very early in the series are termed **nephrograms** *(nef'ro-grams).* The renal parenchyma or functional portion of the kidney consists of many thousands of nephrons. Because individual nephrons are microscopic, the nephron phase is a blush of the entire kidney substance. This blush results from contrast medium being dispersed throughout the many nephrons but not into the collecting tubules as yet. The usual nephrogram is obtained with a radiograph at 1 minute after the start of injection. Ureteric compression, if used, tends to prolong the nephron phase to as long as 5 minutes in the normal kidney.

The most common imaging during the nephron phase is a "tomographic" nephrogram, called a **nephrotomogram,** as opposed to a "nontomographic" nephrogram. With a nephrotomogram (Fig. 17-63), three separate focal levels are commonly taken during this phase of the study. (See Chapter 23 for principles of conventional tomography.)

Because the primary interest in nephrography is the kidneys, centering and IR size should be confined to the kidneys. Centering should be halfway between the iliac crest and the xiphoid process unless a better centering point is determined after the scout radiograph is viewed.

In determination of the initial fulcrum level, one method is to measure the thickness of the midabdomen using calipers. Once this number is obtained, it is divided by 3. Therefore an abdomen that is 24 cm thick would begin with the fulcrum setting at 8 cm. If the patient is lying on a thick pad or mattress, 1 cm is added to this calculation, which would then result in the initial fulcrum being set at 9 cm.

Timing is critical on this radiograph, so the exposure must be made exactly 60 seconds after the start of the injection. The table, IR, and control panel must be in readiness even before the injection is begun because the injection sometimes takes nearly 60 seconds to complete.

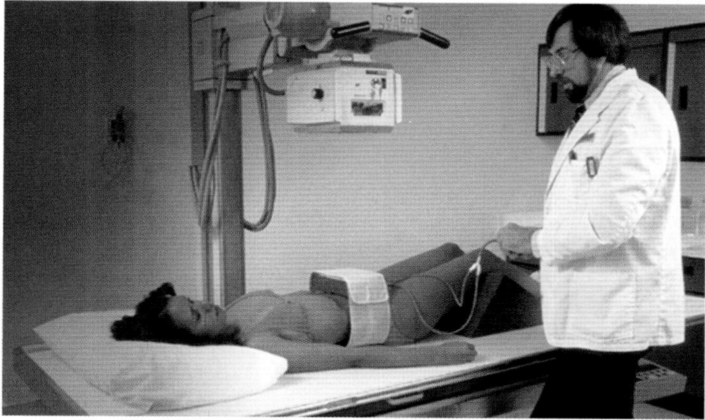

Fig. 17-62. Postrelease, or "spill," procedure.

17

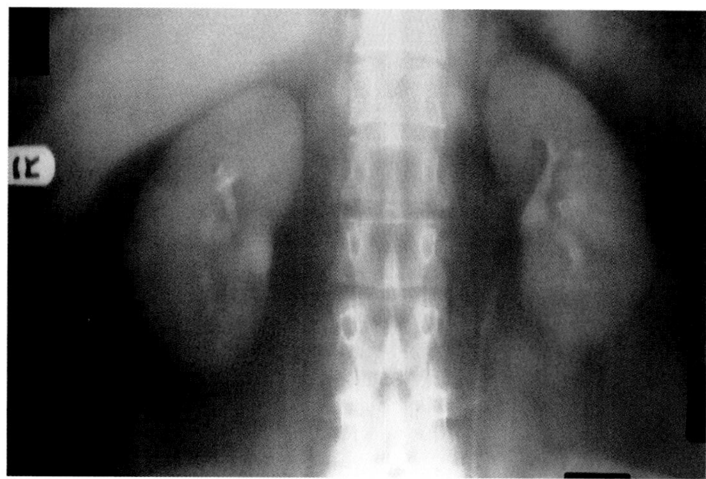

Fig. 17-63. Nephrotomogram—1 minute.

Hypertensive IVU

PURPOSE

One special type of IVU is the **hypertensive urogram.** This examination is performed on patients with high blood pressure (hypertension) to determine whether the kidneys are the cause of the hypertension. There is a much shorter time between projections for a hypertensive IVU, as compared with a standard IVU procedure.

PROCEDURE

During the hypertensive urogram, several early radiographs must be obtained. All cassettes must be available and marked with lead numbers to reflect the time sequence of each image. Once the procedure begins, radiographs must be taken at a set interval.

The hypertensive study includes at least **1-, 2-,** and **3-minute radiographs,** with the possibility of additional radiographs every 30 seconds. In most cases, timing begins at the start of injection.

After the very early radiographs, the imaging sequence may be similar to a standard IVU with imaging of the ureters and bladder.

Note: This procedure is not commonly performed today but may be done when other alternative modalities are unavailable.

Retrograde Urography

PURPOSE

Retrograde urography is a **nonfunctional examination of the urinary system** during which contrast medium is introduced directly retrograde (backward, against the flow) into the pelvicalyceal system **via catheterization** by a urologist during a minor surgical procedure. Retrograde urography is nonfunctional because the patient's normal physiologic processes are not involved in the procedure. This procedure is performed to determine the location of urinary calculi or other types of obstruction.

Note: This procedure is less frequently performed today because of the increased use of CT for locating urinary calculi or obstruction within the urinary system.

PROCEDURE

Surgery personnel place the patient on the combination cystoscopic radiographic table, usually located in the surgery department. The patient is placed in the modified lithotomy position, which requires that the legs be placed in stirrups, as illustrated in Fig. 17-64. The patient is usually either sedated or anesthetized for this examination. More details of this procedure are covered under surgical procedures discussed in Chapter 19.

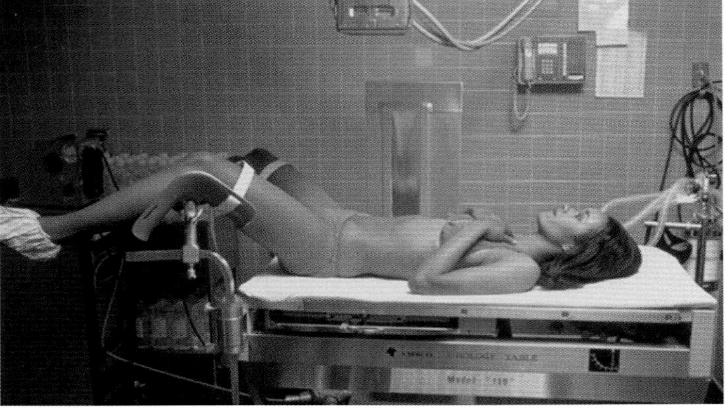

Fig. 17-64. Retrograde urogram (scout position).

Retrograde Cystography (Cystogram)

PURPOSE

A retrograde cystogram *(sis'to-gram)* is a **nonfunctional** radiographic examination of the **urinary bladder** after instillation of an iodinated contrast medium via a urethral catheter. The cystogram is a common procedure performed to rule out trauma, calculi, tumor, and inflammatory disease of the urinary bladder.

PROCEDURE

There is no patient preparation for this examination, although the patient should empty the bladder before catheterization. After routine bladder catheterization under aseptic conditions, the bladder is drained of any residual urine. The bladder is then filled with dilute contrast medium, as illustrated in Fig. 17-65. The contrast material is allowed to flow in **by gravity only.** One should never hurry or attempt to introduce the contrast medium under pressure, which could result in rupture of the bladder.

After the bladder is filled, which may require 150 to 500 ml, either fluorographic spot radiographs are taken by the radiologist or various overhead positions are exposed by the technologist.

Routine positioning for a cystogram includes an **AP, with a 15° caudad angle** and **bilateral posterior obliques.**

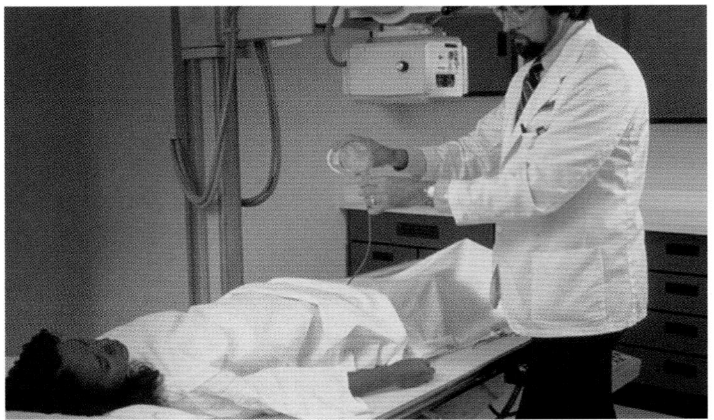

Fig. 17-65. Cystogram—technologist instilling contrast medium.

Voiding Cystourethrography (VCU)

PURPOSE

Voiding radiographs may be taken after the routine cystogram. When the images are combined in this manner, the examination is termed a **cystourethrogram** *(sist"o-u-re'thro-gram),* or **voiding cystourethrogram (VCU).** This exam provides a study of the urethra and evaluates the patient's ability to urinate; therefore it is a **functional study** of the bladder and urethra.

PATHOLOGIC INDICATIONS

Trauma and **incontinence** are common pathologic indications for a VCU exam.

PROCEDURE

The voiding phase of the examination is best done with fluoroscopy with image-acquisition capability. The procedure is sometimes performed with the patient supine, although the upright position makes voiding easier. Before removal of the catheter from the bladder and urethra, any liquid must first be removed from the balloon portion of the catheter, if this type of catheter is being used. Then the catheter is **very gently** removed. The urethra can be traumatized if care is not exercised.

The female is usually examined in the AP or slight oblique position, as shown on the radiograph in Fig. 17-66. The male is best examined in a 30° right posterior oblique position. An adequate receptacle or absorbent padding must be provided for the patient. Conventional or digital fluoroscopy may be used to capture specific phases of voiding.

After voiding is complete and adequate imaging is obtained, a postvoiding AP may be requested.

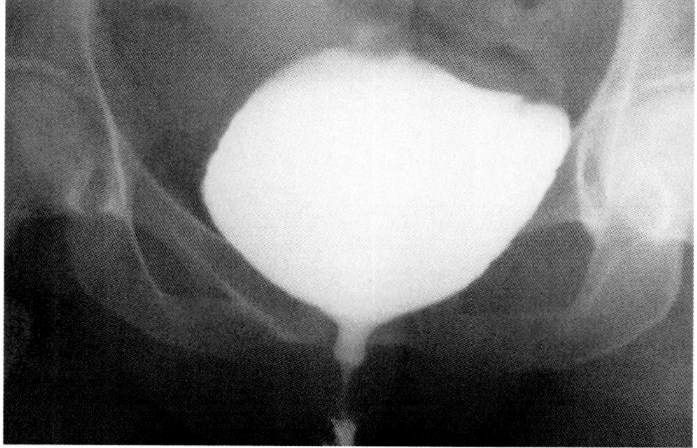

Fig. 17-66. Female voiding cystourethrogram.

Retrograde Urethrography

PURPOSE

A retrograde urethrogram is sometimes performed on the **male patient** to demonstrate the full length of the urethra. Contrast medium is injected retrograde into the distal urethra until the entire urethra is filled (Fig. 17-67).

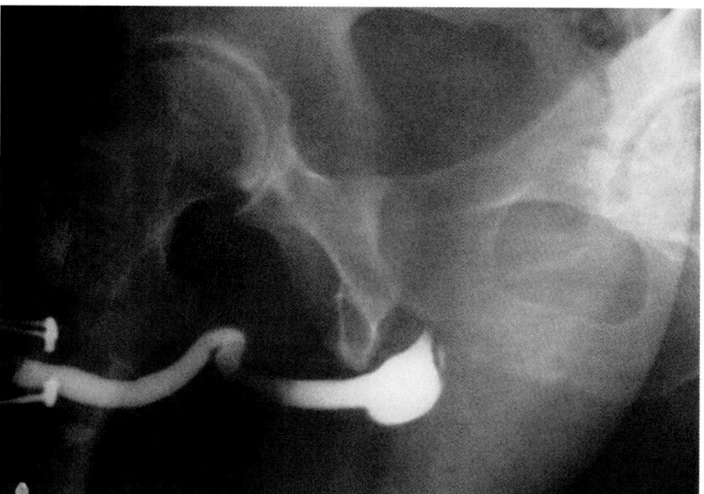

Fig. 17-67. Male retrograde urethrogram.

PATHOLOGIC INDICATIONS

Trauma and **obstruction of the urethra** are pathologic indications for this procedure.

PROCEDURE

Injection of contrast material is sometimes facilitated by a special device termed a **Brodney clamp** (Fig. 17-68), which is attached to the distal penis.

A **30° right posterior oblique** is the position of choice, and centering is to the symphysis pubis. The special catheter is inserted into the distal urethra, and the injection is made. Ample contrast medium is used to fill the entire urethra, and exposures are made. An RPO retrograde urethrogram on a male patient is shown in Fig. 17-67. Ideally, the urethra is superimposed over the soft tissues of the right thigh. This position prevents superimposition of any bony structures except for the lower pelvis and proximal femur.

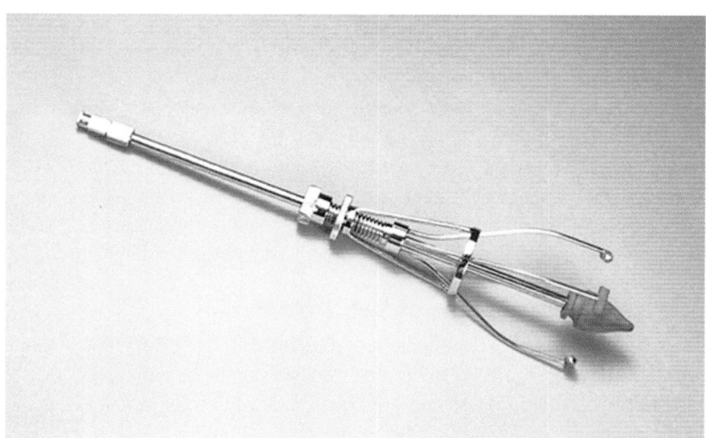

Fig. 17-68. Brodney clamp.

Summary of Urinary System Procedures

Urographic procedures may be categorized by the method of contrast medium administration. Contrast medium is introduced either (1) into the circulatory system or (2) directly into the structure to be studied.

SUMMARY OF UROGRAPHIC PROCEDURES

PROCEDURE	CONTRAST MEDIA DELIVERY
IVU	Intravenous injection: antegrade flow of contrast media through superficial vein in arm
Retrograde urography	Retrograde injection through ureteral catheter by a urologist as a surgical procedure
Retrograde cystography	Retrograde flow into bladder through urethral catheter driven by gravity
Voiding cystourethrography	Retrograde flow into bladder through urethral catheter, followed by withdrawal of catheter for imaging during voiding
Retrograde urethrography (male)	Retrograde injection through Brodney clamp or special catheter

PEDIATRIC APPLICATIONS

The physiology of the pediatric patient is sensitive to changes in diet, fluid intake, and the presence of iodinated contrast media. Therefore the patient preparation for an IVU for the infant and young child must be carefully monitored. Restricting fluids for a long period of time before the procedure may lead to severe dehydration, which can lead to an added risk for contrast media reaction. Pediatric patients need to be scheduled early in the day so that they can return to a normal diet after the procedure. Furthermore, the technologist needs to carefully monitor the patient throughout the procedure.

The increased use of ultrasound for a variety of urinary conditions has provided a safer method (without radiation) for the evaluation of the pediatric patient.

GERIATRIC APPLICATIONS

As with pediatric patients the older patient may be affected negatively by the change in diet and fluid intake before the IVU. The technologist must monitor the geriatric patient carefully during this procedure.

Because many geriatric patients have a clinical history of diabetes, the technologist must ask whether they are taking Glucophage. As stated earlier, the use of iodinated contrast media is contraindicated for the patient taking this drug.

Digital Imaging Considerations

Digital imaging considerations for all urographic procedures, including the more common IVU exam, are similar to those for other abdominal projections such as described in detail in Chapter 4 on the abdomen.

These include (1) **close collimation,** (2) **accurate centering** of central ray to body part of interest and to IR, (3) **optimal exposure factors** remembering the ALARA principle, which is confirmed by (4) **post-processing evaluation of exposure index values.**

Alternative Modalities and Procedures

COMPUTED TOMOGRAPHY

The use of CT for renal calculi studies is growing. It provides a means to rule out stones in the urinary system without the use of iodinated contrast media. High-speed, helical CT scanners are able to examine the complete urinary system quickly and efficiently. Contiguous, fine transverse slices from the kidneys to the urinary bladder provide a safe assessment for stones without the use of iodinated contrast media.

In many imaging departments, CT of the urinary system for renal calculi is replacing the IVU study. The patient does not require an extensive bowel prep, and the location of the stone can be pinpointed accurately.

CT also continues to be an ideal imaging modality for the evaluation of tumors and obstructions.

SONOGRAPHY (ULTRASOUND)

Ultrasound provides a means to evaluate the kidney and bladder in a noninvasive manner. The filled bladder provides an acoustic "window" to demonstrate bladder calculi or masses within the bladder or organs that surround the bladder, such as the uterus. Ultrasound can also evaluate the kidney to determine whether cysts or masses are present. Ultrasound is the modality of choice for evaluation of the transplanted kidney. Ultrasound, along with nuclear medicine, can also be used to measure parenchymal perfusion. Reduced blood flow or perfusion may be an indication of tissue rejection.

Endorectal ultrasound is highly effective for imaging of the prostate. It can distinguish among solid, cystic, and mixed tissue masses in the prostate gland.

MAGNETIC RESONANCE IMAGING

MRI is used to demonstrate subtle tissue changes of the urinary bladder and kidney and to evaluate tumors, renal transplants, and patency of the renal artery and veins. On T1 weighted images, the kidney is well defined in contrast to the fat-laden perirenal space. Coronal, sagittal, and transverse perspectives of the urinary system provide a means to determine the spread of select tumors of the kidney to adjacent structures.

NUCLEAR MEDICINE

Specific nuclear medicine procedures can measure renal function and excretion rates. Nuclear medicine studies provide a functional evaluation of the kidneys. This method provides a less hazardous method to evaluate the kidneys for signs of chronic and acute renal failure without the use of iodinated contrast media, especially true in the evaluation of transplanted kidney. Subtle signs of organ rejection can be measured by the degree of perfusion of radionuclides in the nephrons.

Radionuclides are also being used to determine whether a physical blockage exists in the ureter and evaluate for vesicoureteral reflux. In the case of vesicoureteral reflux, the patient's bladder is filled with saline, and a very small amount of radioactive material is instilled. During the act of voiding, any trace of reflux can be tracked and filmed.

In general, the role of nuclear medicine in evaluating renal anatomy is decreasing, but it is being used more to confirm and analyze renal function.

RADIOGRAPHIC POSITIONING

Survey Information

A 2000 survey of the operating procedures (department routines) was conducted throughout the United States and Canada. The survey results were very consistent throughout all regions of the United States but did show some significant differences in the **IVU oblique positions** between the U.S. and Canada. In the U.S., 82% indicated that these were routine. In Canada 18% indicated that they were routine, and 42% indicated that they were special positions.

The **nephrotomograms** also were indicated as routine or basic much less in Canada than in the U.S., both with and without ureteric compression. This indication was also true for the cystogram routine.

Venipuncture by technologists for IVU exams was more common in 2000 in all regions of the U.S. than it was in Canada. More than 75% in the U.S. indicated technologists performed more than 24 venipunctures annually in their departments.

Basic and Special Projections

Certain basic or special projections of the urinary system are demonstrated and described on the following pages. The radiologist and technologist must closely coordinate their efforts during examinations of this anatomy.

17

17

AP PROJECTION (SCOUT AND SERIES): INTRAVENOUS (EXCRETORY) UROGRAPHY

Pathology Demonstrated
Scout demonstrates abnormal calcifications that may be urinary calculi. After injection, the AP projection may demonstrate signs of obstruction, hydronephrosis, tumor, or infection.

See p. 566 for IVU routine.

Intravenous (Excretory) Urography—IVU
BASIC
- AP (scout and series)
- **Nephrotomogram**
- **RPO and LPO (30°)**
- **AP—postvoid**

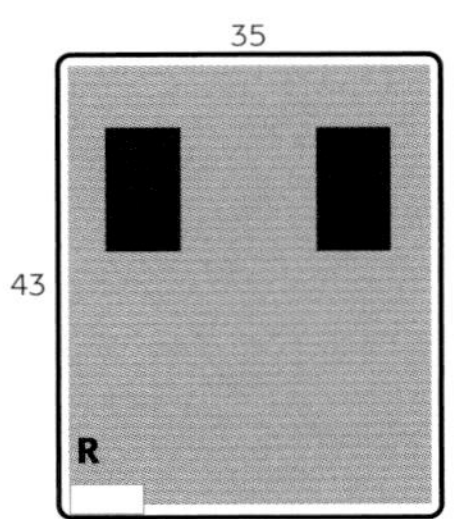

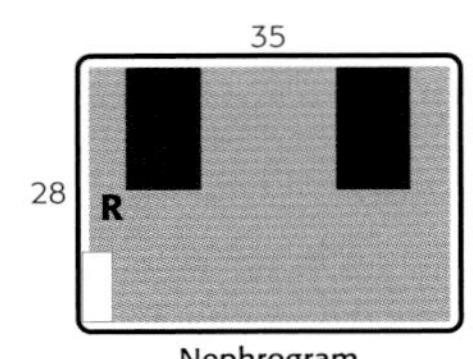

Nephrogram

Technical Factors
- IR size—35 × 43 cm (14 × 17 inches), lengthwise; for nephrogram—28 × 35 cm (11 × 14 inches), crosswise
- Moving or stationary grid
- 70-75 kV range
- Minute markers where applicable
- Technique and dose:

cm	kV	mAs	Sk.	ML.	Gon.
19	75	15	152	36	M 3 F 34

mrad

Shielding Shield gonads on males, keeping the shield below the superior margin of the symphysis pubis. Shield both males and females for nephrogram.

Patient Position Situate patient supine, with pillow for head, arms at sides away from body, support under knees to relieve back strain.

Part Position
- Align midsagittal plane to center line of table and to CR.
- Ensure **no rotation** of trunk or pelvis.
- Include symphysis pubis on bottom of cassette without cutting off upper kidneys. (A second smaller IR for bladder area may be necessary on hypersthenic patients.)

Central Ray
- CR is **perpendicular** to IR.
- Center CR and IR to **level of iliac crest** and to midsagittal plane.
- Minimum SID is 40 inches (100 cm).

Collimation Collimate to IR or smaller if possible.

Respiration Suspend respiration and expose on expiration.

Note: Have patient empty bladder immediately before beginning exam so that contrast medium in the bladder is not diluted. Explain procedure and obtain clinical history before injection of contrast medium. Be prepared for possible reaction to contrast medium.

Radiographic Criteria

Structures Shown: • Entire urinary system is visualized from upper renal shadows to distal urinary bladder. The symphysis pubis should be included on lower margin of the IR. • After injection, only a portion of the urinary system may be opacified on a specific radiograph in the series.

Position: • **No rotation** as evidenced by symmetry of iliac wings and ribcage.

Collimation and CR: • Collimation borders to IR margins on top and bottom to prevent cutoff of essential anatomy. • Complete arch of symphysis pubis visible on bottom margin of radiograph, with center of image at level of iliac crest.

Exposure Criteria and Markers: • No motion due to respiration or movement. • Appropriate technique with short-scale contrast demonstrating the urinary system. • Minute markers and R or L markers visible on all series radiographs.

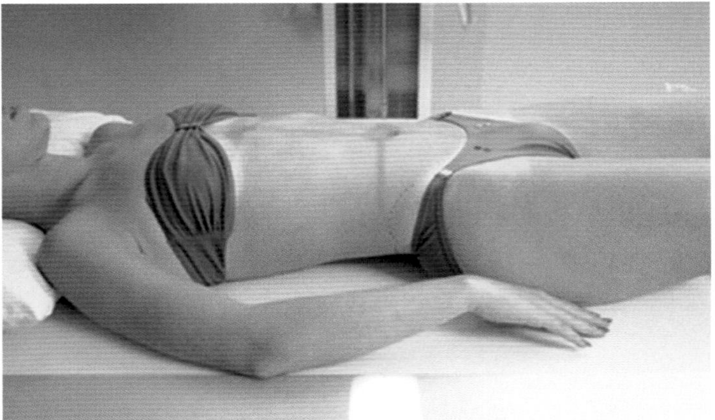

Fig. 17-69. IVU scout and series.

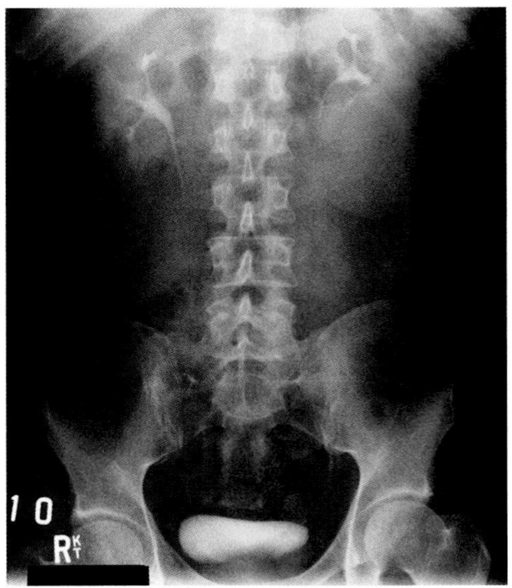

Fig. 17-70. IVU (10 minutes).

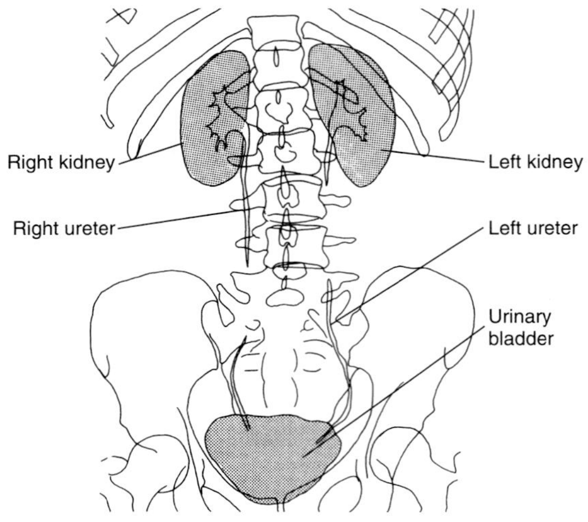

Fig. 17-71. IVU.

NEPHROTOMOGRAM AND NEPHROGRAM: INTRAVENOUS (EXCRETORY) UROGRAPHY

Intravenous (Excretory) Urography—IVU
BASIC
- AP (scout and series)
- Nephrotomogram
- RPO and LPO (30°)
- AP—postvoid

30 (35)
24 (28)
R

Pathology Demonstrated

Nephrogram or nephrotomogram demonstrate conditions and trauma to the renal parenchyma. Renal cysts and/or adrenal masses may be demonstrated during this phase of the IVU.

A **nephrogram** involves a single AP radiograph of the kidney region taken within 60 seconds after injection.

Technical Factors

- Linear tomography
- IR size—24 × 30 cm (10 × 12 inches), or 28 × 35 cm (11 × 14 inches), crosswise
- Moving or stationary grid
- 70-75 kV range
- Select correct exposure angle:
  —10° angle or less, producing larger section of tissue in relative focus
  —40° exposure angle, producing thinner sections of tissue in relative focus; therefore more tomographic exposures required to demonstrate the entire kidney
  —If only three tomograms to be taken, 10° exposure angle or less (known as **zonography**)

Shielding Shield gonadal area for both males and females.

Patient Position Position patient supine, with pillow for head, arms at side away from body, and support under knees to relieve back strain.

Part Position

- Align midsagittal plane to center line of table/grid.
- Ensure **no rotation** of trunk or pelvis.

Central Ray

- Center CR **midway between xiphoid tip and iliac crest.**
- Minimum SID is 40 inches (100 cm) (or distance as required by specific tomographic equipment).

Collimation Collimate to IR size or smaller if possible.

Respiration Suspend respiration and expose on expiration.

Note: Explain tomographic procedure to reduce anxiety for patient. Obtain clinical history before injection of contrast medium. Remind patient to remain immobile between exposures. Check scout image to verify focus level, optimal technique, and position of kidneys. Tomography procedures including equipment setup and procedure are described in Chapter 23.

Radiographic Criteria

Structures Shown: • Entire renal parenchyma is visualized, with some filling of collecting system with contrast medium.

Position: • **No motion** due to respiration or movement is evident.

Collimation and CR: • Collimation borders should be to IR margins on top and bottom to prevent cutoff of essential anatomy. • CR is centered midway between xiphoid tip and iliac crest, with both kidneys demonstrated.

Exposure Criteria and Markers: • Appropriate technique is used to demonstrate renal parenchyma. • The specific focus level markers should be visible on each radiograph, along with R or L and minute markers.

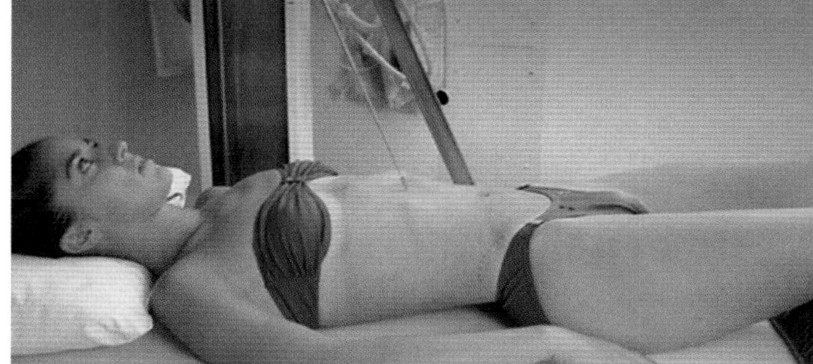

Fig. 17-72. Nephrotomogram (tube in starting position).

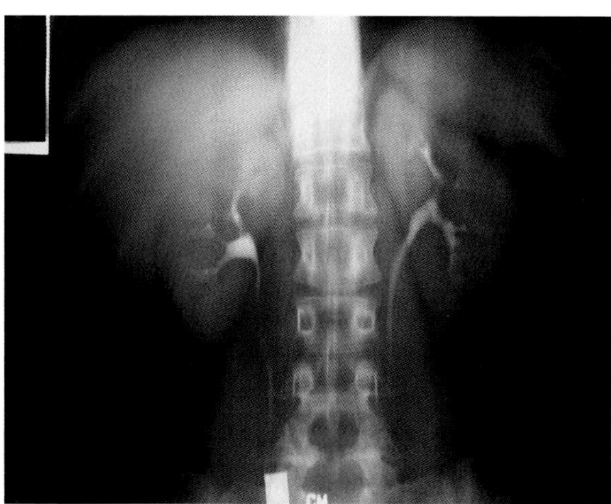

Fig. 17-73. Nephrotomogram (linear motion tomogram).

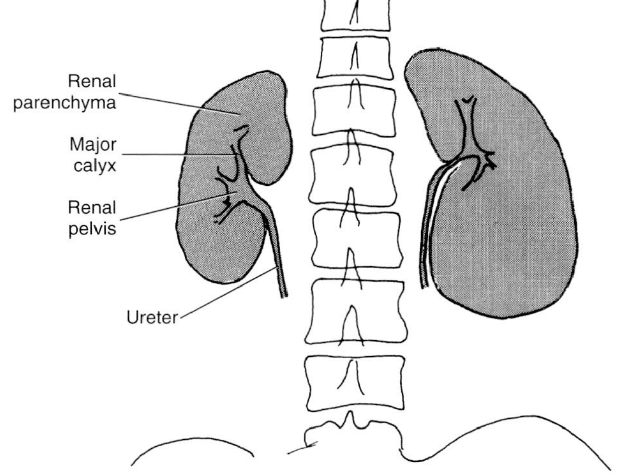

Fig. 17-74. Nephrotomogram.

17

RPO AND LPO POSITIONS: INTRAVENOUS (EXCRETORY) UROGRAPHY

Intravenous (Excretory) Urography—IVU
BASIC
- AP (scout and series)
- Nephrotomogram
- RPO and LPO (30°)
- AP—postvoid

Pathology Demonstrated

Signs of infection, trauma, and obstruction of the elevated kidney are shown. Also demonstrates trauma or obstruction of the downside ureter.

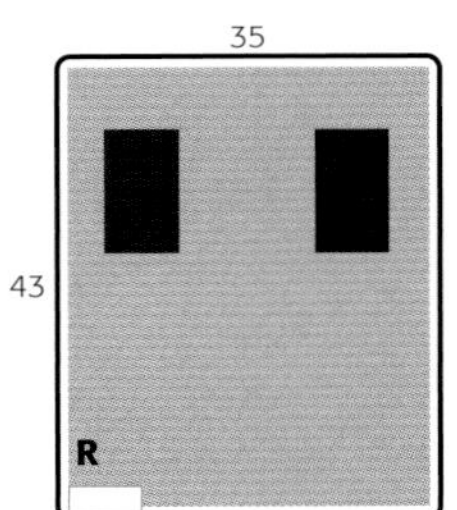

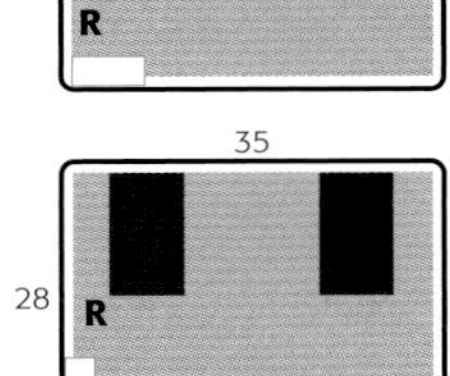

Technical Factors

- IR size—35 × 43 cm (14 × 17 inches), lengthwise, or 28 × 35 cm (11 × 14 inches), crosswise (see Note)
- Moving or stationary grid
- 70-75 kV range
- Minute marker
- Technique and dose (35- × 43-cm IR):

cm	kV	mAs	Sk.	ML.	Gon.
19	75	25	266	53	M 5 F 60
			mrad		

Shielding Shield gonads on males (see Note).

Patient Position Patient is supine and partially rotated toward the right or left side.

Part Position

- Rotate body 30° for both R and L posterior oblique positions.
- Flex elevated side knee for support of lower body.
- Raise arm on elevated side and place across upper chest.
- Center vertebral column to midline of table/grid and to CR.

Central Ray

- CR is **perpendicular** to IR.
- Center CR and cassette to **level of iliac crest** and vertebral column.
- Minimum SID is 40 inches (100 cm).

Collimation Collimate to IR or smaller if possible.

Respiration Suspend respiration and expose on expiration.

Note: Some departmental routines include a smaller IR placed crosswise to include the kidneys and proximal ureters, thus allowing gonadal shielding for both males and females. Centering would then be midway between xiphoid and iliac crests.

Radiographic Criteria

Structures Shown: • The kidney on elevated side is placed in profile or parallel to the IR and is best demonstrated with each oblique. • The downside ureter is projected away from the spine, providing an unobstructed view of this ureter.

Position: • No excessive obliquity is evident. • The elevated kidney is parallel to the plane of IR and not projected into the vertebral bodies of the lumbar spine. • Complete arch of symphysis pubis is visible on bottom margin of radiograph, and the kidneys are included at the upper margin.

Collimation and CR: • Collimation borders should be to IR margins on top and bottom to prevent cutoff of essential anatomy. • Center of image (CR) is at level of iliac crest.

Exposure Criteria: • No motion due to respiration or movement is evident. • Appropriate technique with short-scale contrast is used to visualize the urinary system. • Minute markers and R or L markers should be visible.

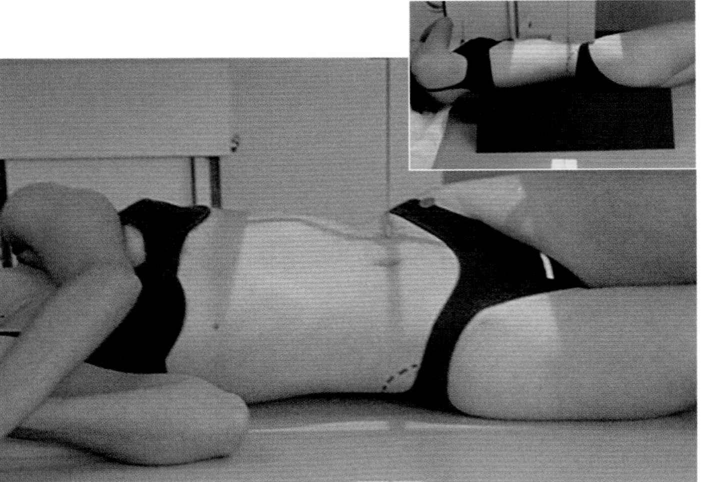

Fig. 17-75. RPO—30°. *Inset,* 30° LPO.

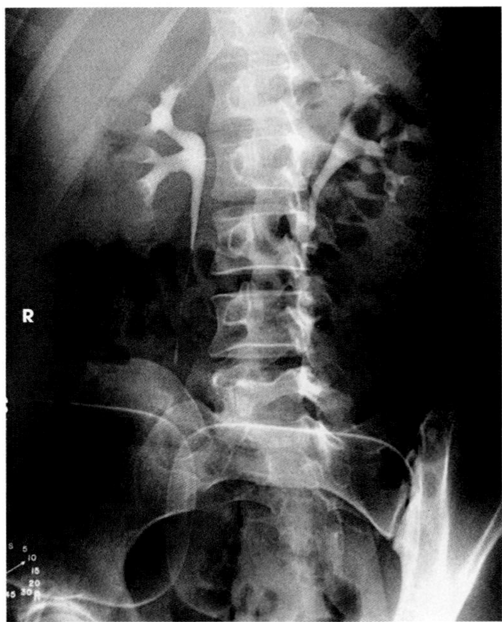

Fig. 17-76. RPO. (From Ballinger PW, Frank ED: Merrill's atlas of radiographic positions and radiologic procedures, ed 10, St. Louis, 2003, Mosby.)

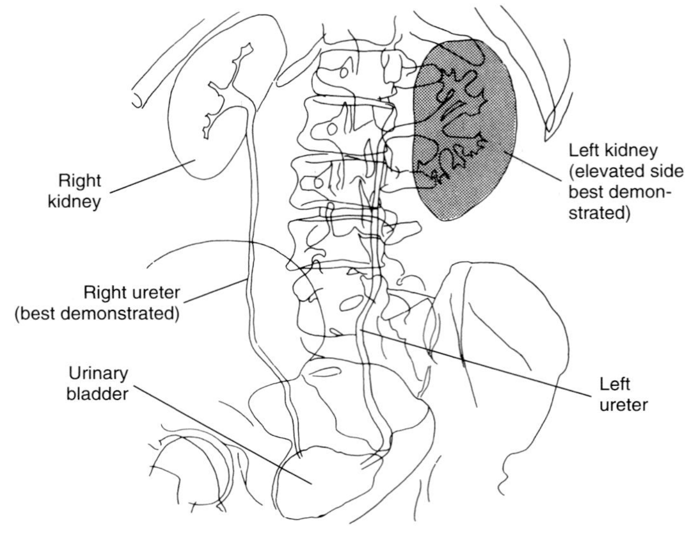

Fig. 17-77. RPO.

AP PROJECTION: INTRAVENOUS (EXCRETORY) UROGRAPHY

Postvoid

Intravenous (Excretory) Urography—IVU
BASIC
- AP (scout and series)
- Nephrotomogram
- RPO and LPO (30°)
- AP—postvoid

Pathology Demonstrated

Position may demonstrate enlarged prostate (possible BPH) or prolapse of the bladder.

The erect position demonstrates nephroptosis (positional change of kidneys).

Technical Factors

- IR size—35 × 43 cm (14 × 17 inches), lengthwise
- Moving or stationary grid
- 70-75 kV range
- Erect and/or postvoid markers
- Technique and dose:

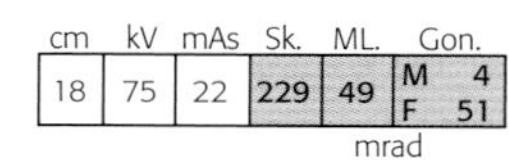

cm	kV	mAs	Sk.	ML.	Gon.
18	75	22	229	49	M 4 F 51

mrad

35

43

Post-void

R

Shielding Shield gonads on males if such shielding does not cover essential anatomy.

Patient Position Patient is erect, with back against table, or in prone position.

Part Position

- Align midsagittal plane to center of table/grid or IR, with no rotation.
- Position arms away from body.
- Ensure that symphysis pubis is included on bottom of IR.
- Center low enough to include prostate area, especially on older males.

Central Ray

- Direct CR **perpendicular** to IR.
- Center to level of **iliac crest** and midsagittal plane, or for larger patients, 1 inch (2.5 cm) lower to ensure that bladder area is included.
- Minimum SID is 40 inches (100 cm).

Collimation Collimate to IR size or smaller if possible.

Respiration Suspend respiration and expose on expiration.

Alternative PA or AP recumbent: This image may also be taken as a PA or AP projection in the recumbent position, with centering similar to that described above.

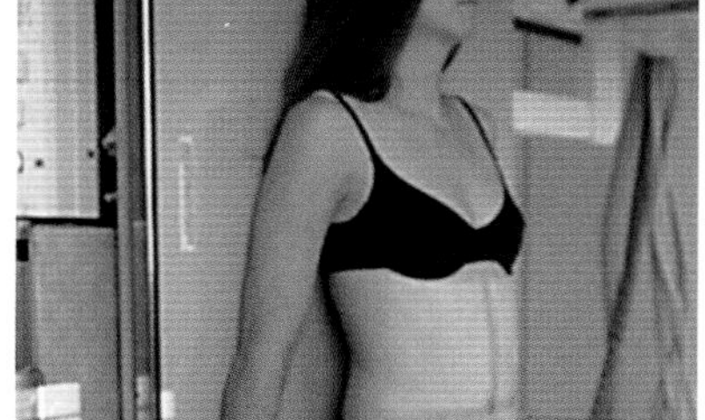

Fig. 17-78. AP erect (postvoid)—center at iliac crest to include symphysis pubis.

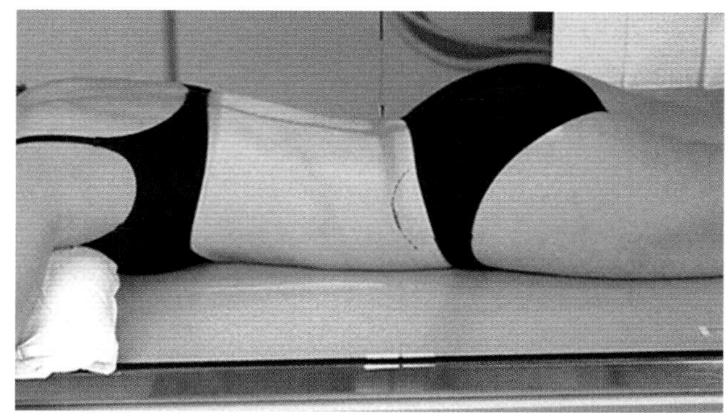

Fig. 17-79. Alternative: PA prone (postvoid).

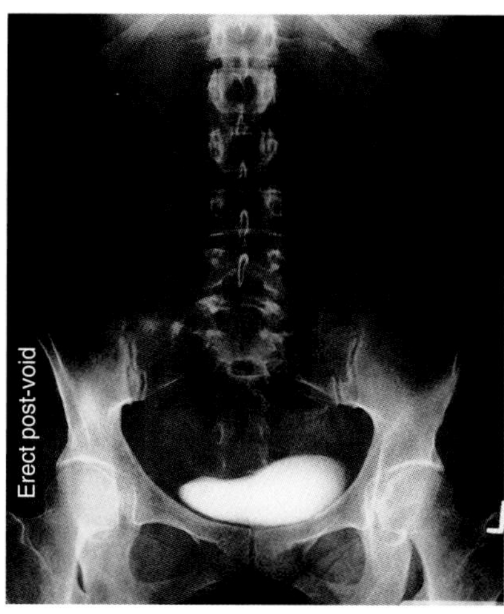

Fig. 17-80. AP erect (postvoid).

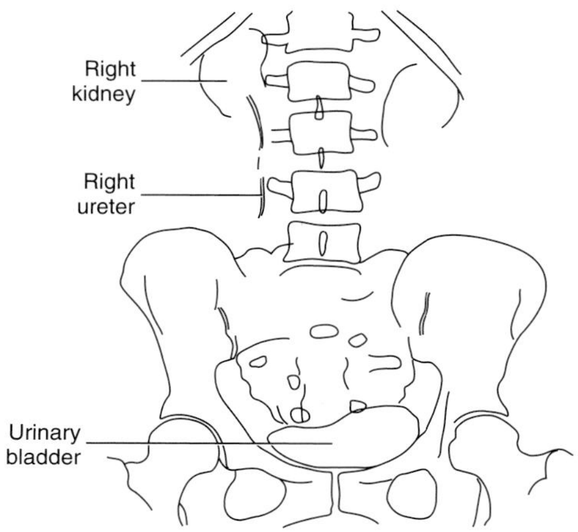

Fig. 17-81. AP erect (postvoid).

Radiographic Criteria

Structures Shown: • Entire urinary system is included, with only residual contrast media visible. • All of symphysis pubis (to include prostate area on males) is included on radiograph.

Position: • **No rotation** is evident by symmetry of iliac wings.

Collimation and CR: • Collimation borders should be to IR margins on top and bottom to prevent cutoff of essential anatomy. • Center of image (CR) is at level of iliac crest.

Exposure Criteria and Markers: • **No motion** due to respiration or motion is evident. • Appropriate technique is used to demonstrate residual contrast media in the urinary system. • Erect and/or postvoid markers and R or L markers are visible.

17

AP PROJECTION: INTRAVENOUS (EXCRETORY) UROGRAPHY

Ureteric Compression

Warning Compression should **not** be used for patients with a history of abdominal masses, obstructions (such as stones), abdominal aortic aneurysms, or recent surgery. (See Contraindications to Ureteric Compression, p. 565. A Trendelenburg position with 15° tilt, which approximates the same effect, can be used for such patients.)

Intravenous (Excretory) Urography—IVU
SPECIAL
- AP ureteric compression

Pathology Demonstrated

Pyelonephritis and other conditions involving the collecting system of the kidney are shown.

Technical Factors

- IR size—30 × 35 cm (11 × 14 inches), crosswise
- Moving or stationary grid
- 70-75 kV range
- Technique and dose (with 35- × 43-cm) IR:

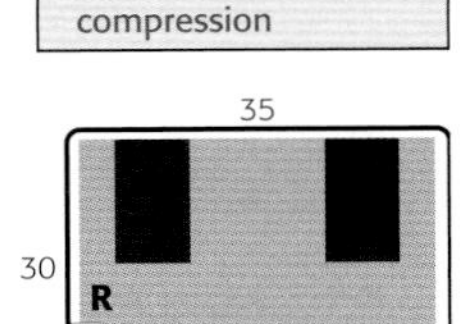

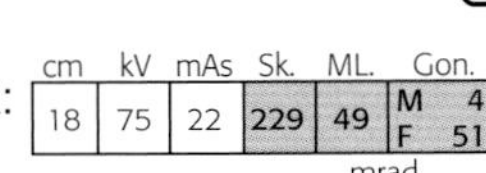

cm	kV	mAs	Sk.	ML.	Gon.
18	75	22	229	49	M 4 F 51
				mrad	

Shielding For males, place lead shield over gonadal area.

Patient Position Position patient supine, with compression device in place.

Part Position

- Align midsagittal plane to center line of table/grid and to CR.
- Flex and support knees.
- Position arms away from body.
- Place upper edge of compression paddles at level of iliac crests. Inner edges of paddles should nearly touch just lateral to the vertebral spine on each side. (This places maximum pressure over the area of the ureters, which are just lateral to the lumbar spine and medial to the SI joints.)

Central Ray

- CR is **perpendicular** to IR.
- Center to **midway between xiphoid and iliac crests.**
- Minimum SID is 40 inches (100 cm).

Collimation Collimate to IR size or smaller if possible.

Respiration Suspend respiration and expose on expiration.

Note: Immediately after injection of contrast media, the paddles are inflated and remain in place until the radiologist indicates they be released. Imaging sequence is to be determined by department protocol or as determined by radiologist.

Radiographic Criteria

Structures Shown: • Entire urinary system visualized, with enhanced pelvic calyceal filling.

Position: • **No rotation,** as evident by symmetry of iliac wings and/or lumbar spine.

Collimation and CR: • Collimation borders are to IR margins on top and bottom to prevent cutoff of essential anatomy. • CR is centered midway between xiphoid tip and iliac crest, with both kidneys demonstrated.

Exposure Criteria • No motion due to respiration or movement is evident. • Appropriate technique is employed, with short-scale contrast to visualize the urinary system.

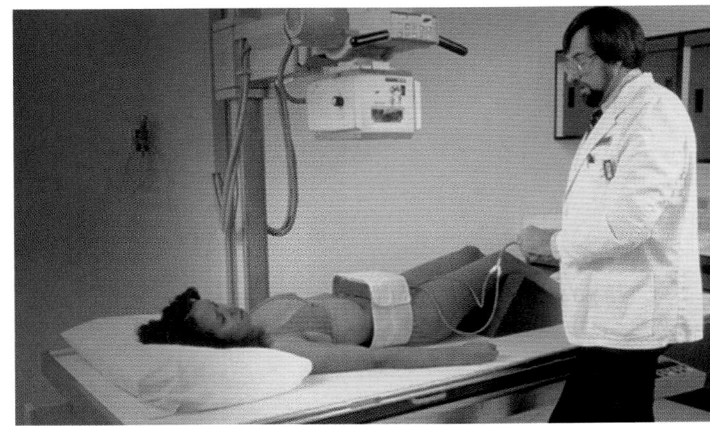

Fig. 17-82. AP—ureteric compression being applied.

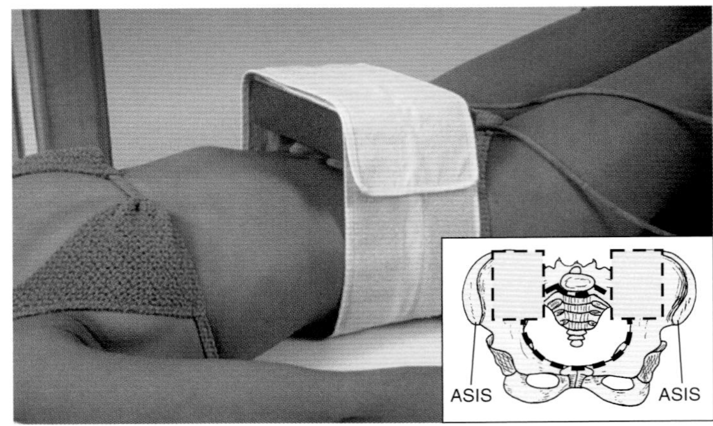

Fig. 17-83. Ureteric compression, with inflated paddles placed correctly.

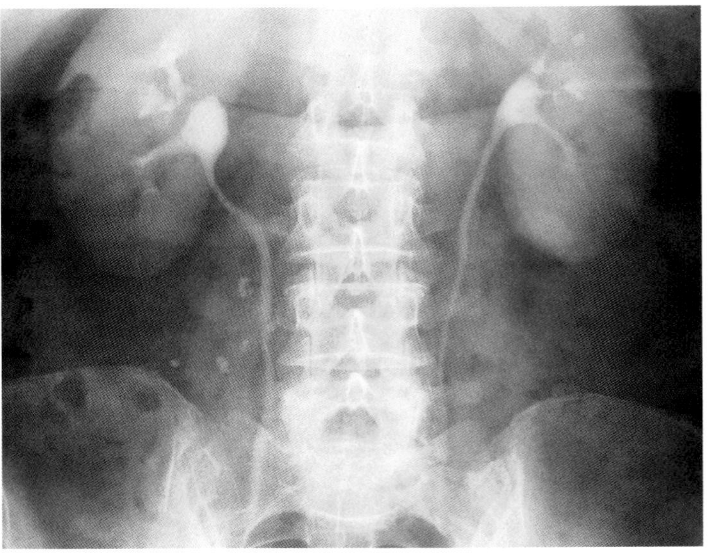

Fig. 17-84. AP—ureteric compression.

AP PROJECTION • LPO AND RPO POSITIONS • LATERAL POSITION (OPTIONAL): CYSTOGRAPHY

Cystography
BASIC
- AP (10°-15° caudad)
- Both obliques (45°-60°)

SPECIAL
- Lateral (optional)

Pathology Demonstrated

Signs of cystitis, obstruction, vesicoureteral reflux, and bladder calculi are visualized. Lateral demonstrates possible fistulae between bladder and either uterus or rectum.

See p. 568 for detailed procedure descriptions.

Technical Factors

- IR size—30 × 35 cm (11 × 14 inches) for a child, or 35 × 43 cm (14 × 17 inches) for an adult, lengthwise (to demonstrate urinary reflux)
- Moving or stationary grid
- 70-75 kV range (80-90 kV for lateral)
- Technique and dose:

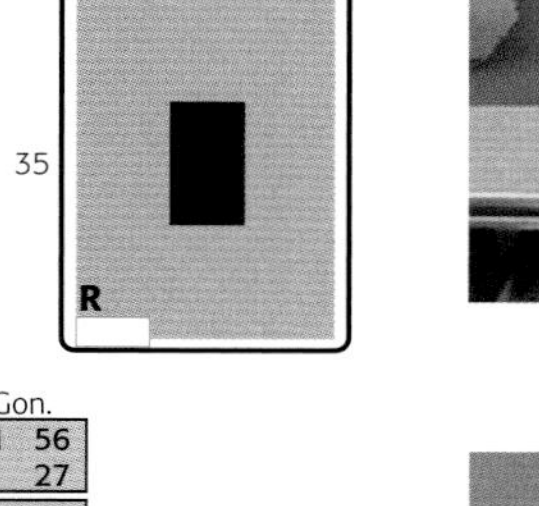

	cm	kV	mAs	Sk.	ML.	Gon.
AP:	16	75	15	143	41	M 56 F 27
Obliques:	20	75	20	215	42	M 83 F 41
Lateral:	31	90	48	1084	101	M 101 F 101
				mrad		

Patient and Part Position

AP:
- Patient is supine, with legs extended and midsagittal plane to center of table.

Posterior Obliques:
- 45° to 60° body rotation. (Steep obliques are used to visualize posterolateral aspect of bladder, especially UV junction.)
- Partially flex downside leg for stabilization.

Note: Do not flex elevated side leg more than necessary to prevent superimposition of leg over bladder.

Lateral (optional due to large gonadal radiation dose):
- Position patient in true lateral (no rotation).

Central Ray

AP:
- For bladder projections only, center **2 inches** (5 cm) **superior to symphysis pubis,** with **10° to 15° caudad** tube angle (to project symphysis pubis inferior to bladder).
- To demonstrate urinary reflux, center higher at level of iliac crest.

Posterior Obliques:
- For bladder projections only, **CR perpendicular**—center **2 inches** (5 cm) **superior to symphysis pubis** and 5 cm **(2 inches) medial to ASIS.**
- To demonstrate urinary reflux, center higher at level of iliac crest.

Lateral (optional):
- **CR perpendicular**—center **2 inches** (5 cm) **superior to and posterior to symphysis pubis.**

Collimation Collimate to IR size or smaller if possible.

Respiration Suspend respiration and expose on expiration.

Note: Unclamp and drain bladder before filling with contrast medium.

Contrast medium should **never** be injected under pressure but allowed to fill slowly by gravity in the presence of an attendant.

Include prostate area just distal to pubis on older males.

Radiographic Criteria Summary

• Distal ureters, urinary bladder, and proximal urethra on males should be included. • Appropriate technique is employed to visualize the urinary bladder.

AP: • Urinary bladder is **not** superimposed by pubic bones.

Posterior Obliques: • Urinary bladder is **not** superimposed by partially flexed elevated side leg.

Lateral (optional): • Hips and femurs are superimposed.

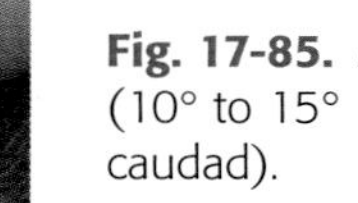

Fig. 17-85. AP (10° to 15° caudad).

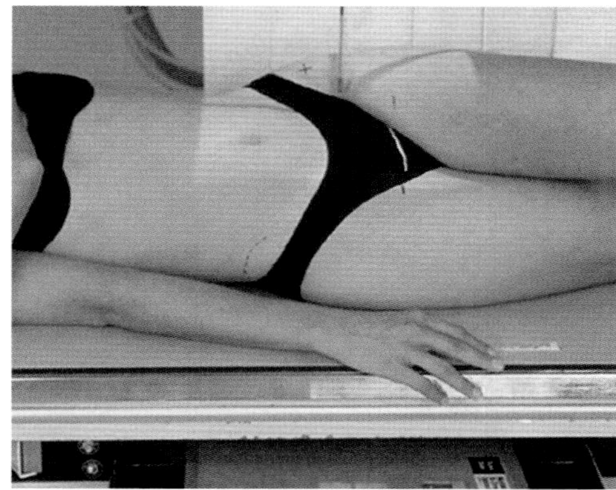

Fig. 17-86. RPO (45° to 60°).

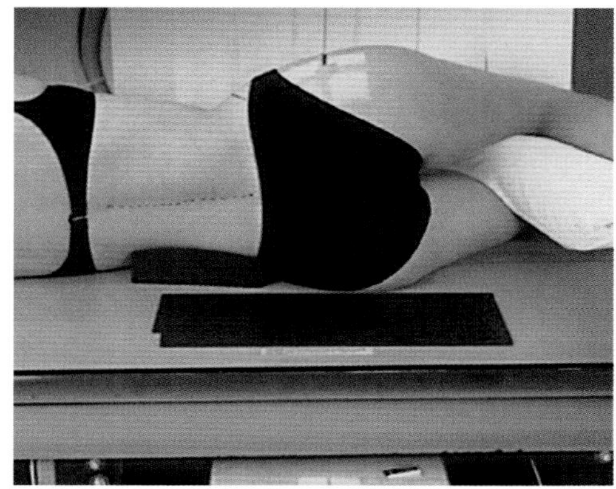

Fig. 17-87. Left lateral (optional).

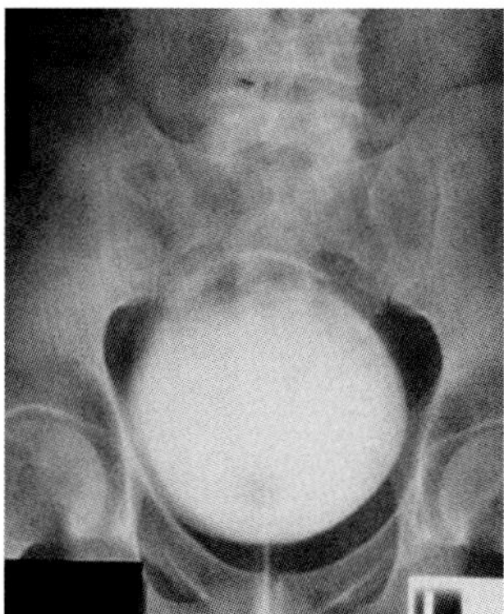

Fig. 17-88. AP (10° to 15° caudad).

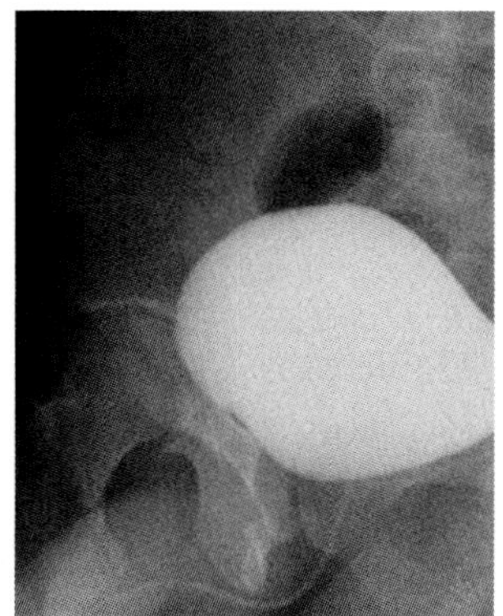

Fig. 17-89. 45° posterior oblique.

17

RPO (30°) POSITION–MALE • AP PROJECTION–FEMALE: VOIDING CYSTOURETHROGRAPHY

Pathology Demonstrated
Functional study of the urinary bladder and urethra determines cause of urinary retention and evaluates for possible vesicoureteral reflux.

See p. 569 for additional procedure descriptions.

Voiding Cystourethrography
BASIC
- Male–RPO (30°)
- Female–AP

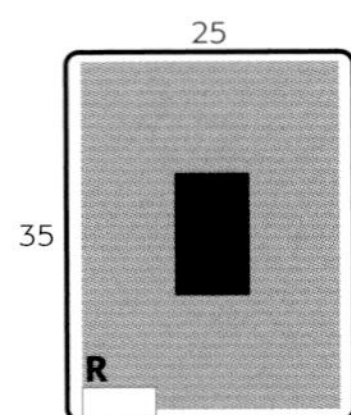

Technical Factors
- IR size–25 × 35 cm (10 × 12 inches), lengthwise
- Moving or stationary grid
- 70-75 kV range
- Technique and dose:

	cm	kV	mAs	Sk.	ML.	Gon. (mrad)
Oblique:	20	75	20	215	42	M 83 F 41
AP:	16	75	15	143	41	M 56 F 27

Shielding Because bladder and urethra are primary areas of interest, gonadal shielding isn't possible.

Patient Position Take image with patient **recumbent or erect.**

Part Position
Male:
- Oblique body **30° into the right** posterior oblique (RPO) position.
- Superimpose urethra over soft tissues of right thigh.

Female:
- Position patient supine or erect.
- Center midsagittal plane to table or film holder.
- Extend and slightly separate legs.

Central Ray
- CR is **perpendicular** to IR.
- Center CR and IR to **symphysis pubis.**
- Minimum SID is 40 inches (100 cm).

Collimation Collimate to IR size or smaller if possible.

Respiration Suspend respiration and expose on expiration.

Note: Fluoroscopy and spot imaging are best for this procedure. Catheter must be gently removed before voiding procedure. Radiolucent receptacle or absorbent padding should be provided for patient. After voiding is complete, a post voiding AP may be requested.

Radiographic Criteria

Structures Shown: • Contrast-filled urinary bladder and urethra are visualized.

Position: • *RPO:* Male urethra containing contrast medium is superimposed over soft tissues of right thigh. • *AP:* Female urethra containing contrast medium is demonstrated inferior to the symphysis pubis.

Collimation and CR: • Collimation borders are to lateral tissue margins of abdomen. • Center of collimation field (CR) is to midaspect of urinary bladder.

Exposure Criteria • Appropriate technique is employed to visualize the urinary bladder without overexposing the male prostate area and the contrast-filled urethra of either the male or female.

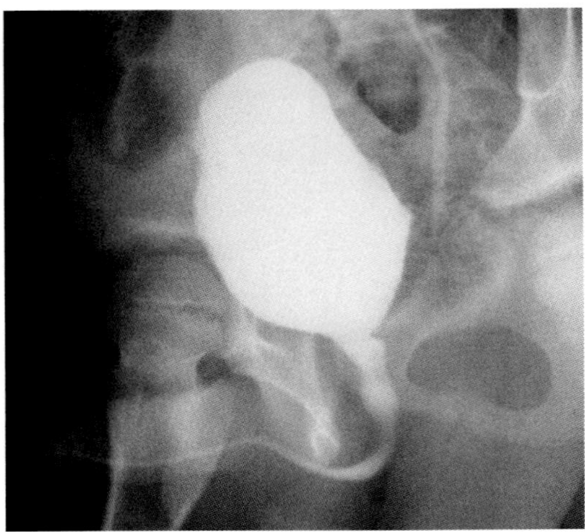

Fig. 17-90. RPO–male.

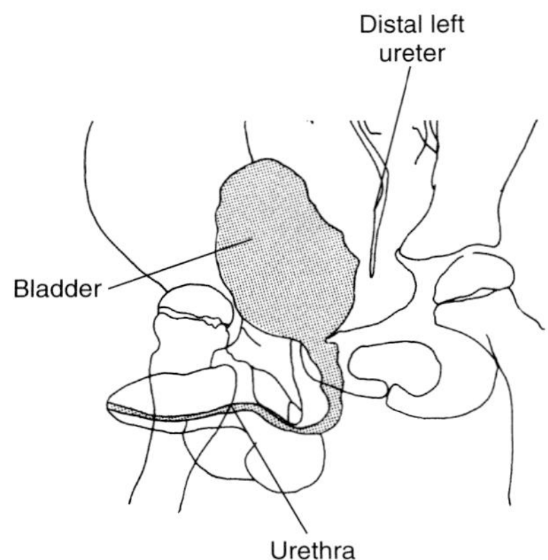

Fig. 17-91. RPO–male.

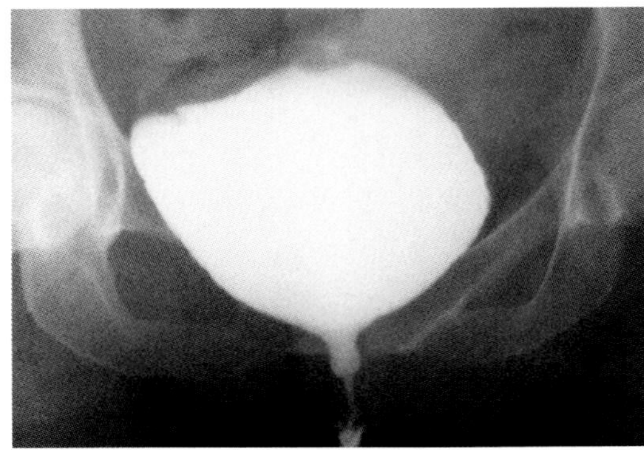

Fig. 17-92. AP–female.

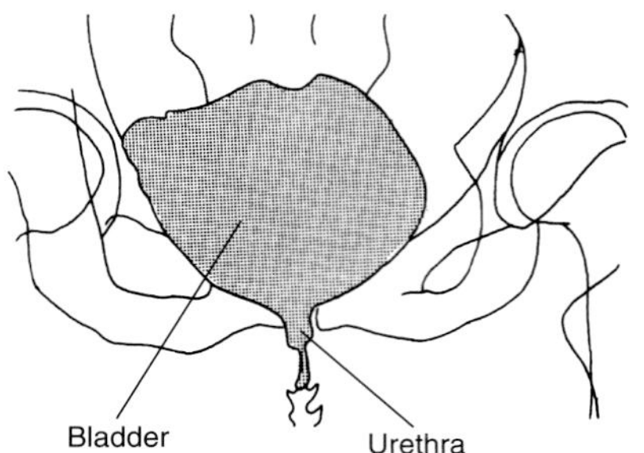

Fig. 17-93. AP–female.

CHAPTER 18

Mammography

CONTRIBUTIONS BY **Eugene D. Frank,** MA, RT(R), FASRT, FAERS, **Sandra J. Nauman,** RT(R)(M)
CONTRIBUTOR TO PAST EDITIONS Nancy L. Dickerson, RT(R)(M)

CONTENTS

RADIOGRAPHIC ANATOMY

Breast Cancer

Until recently, breast cancer was the leading cause of death from cancer among women. Lung cancer has now become the leader. Breast cancer accounts for 32% of all new cancers detected in women and 18% of all cancer deaths. The American Cancer Society (ACS) estimates that one in eight American women will develop breast cancer sometime in her life. Worldwide, there are over 1 million cases of breast cancer documented.*

The best defense against the disease is for women to have regular mammograms so that early detection is possible.

Men can also develop breast cancer but their chances are between 1% and 2% of a woman's chances. Because it is more uncommon, the symptoms are not recognized as early and often male breast cancer progresses to advanced stages before it is diagnosed.

Regular mammography is the key to survival with breast cancer because breast lesions may be detected before they become symptomatic or metastasize. Mammograms can detect a lesion as small as 2.0 mm, which may take 2 to 4 years to become palpable. It is reported that once a breast tumor has reached 2 cm in size, it often has metastasized. Unfortunately, the average survival time for a patient with metastatic breast cancer is only 2 years.* Therefore, it is critical for older women and at-risk males to have annual mammograms performed to detect breast lesions before they can metastasize.

Mammography has evolved into one of the most critical and demanding x-ray examinations performed. Mammographic procedures are highly dependent on the knowledge and skills of the mammographer. A mammographer is a radiologic technologist who has received additional training in mammography. Accurate and careful positioning of the breast during mammography is imperative in diagnosing breast cancer. The maximum amount of breast tissue must be clearly demonstrated on each projection. Mammography images must contain maximum contrast, exhibit superb resolution, and have no artifacts. Mammographers must be certified through professional training, experience, and continuing education in mammography.

Current recommendations from the ACS, the American College of Radiology (ACR), and other health organizations are that all women over the age of 40 undergo an annual screening mammogram. High-risk patients with a family history of breast cancer may be advised to have screening mammograms at an earlier age. The good news is that although the number of new breast cancer cases is increasing, the mortality rate has dropped over recent years, as reported by the National Cancer Institute (NCI). The conclusion is that screening mammography is one of the best diagnostic tools in detecting early breast cancers before they can spread.

Mammography Quality Standards Act

In 1992 the US federal government enacted the **Mammography Quality Standards Act (MQSA).** This came about as a result of both the ACS's high-visibility public relations campaign that all women over 40 undergo screening mammography and federal legislation that provided reimbursement for screening mammography in women eligible for Medicare. The Act was written because of lobbying from the ACR resulting from the great concern about the poor quality mammography being performed. The Act went into effect on **October 1, 1994,** and requires all sites (except VA facilities) that provide mammography service to meet quality standards and become certified for operation by the secretary of the Department of Health and Human Services (DHHS). Enactment of the MQSA marks the first time the use of an x-ray machine and a specific examination were regulated by the federal government.

*Andolina VF, Lille S, Willison KM: Mammographic imaging: a practical guide, ed 2, Philadelphia, 2001, Lippincott Williams & Wilkins.

The final rules of the Act went into effect on **April 28, 1999,** and are now known as Public Law 105-248.

In Canada, mammography guidelines are set by the Canadian Association of Radiologists (CAR).

The technical aspects of mammography are tightly controlled and mammography must be performed on a dedicated mammography unit. The mammography unit must be state-of-the-art and monitored regularly through an intensive quality assurance program. Although film-based systems are still the gold-standard in breast imaging, digital mammography is becoming more common. These digital units provide the ability to localize small lesions and guide the radiologist during biopsy. Information on digital mammography will be discussed later in this chapter.

Anatomy of the Breast

In the adult female, each of the mammary glands or breasts is a conic or hemispheric eminence located on the anterior and lateral chest walls. Breast size varies from one individual to another and even in the same woman, depending on her age and the influence of various hormones. However, the usual breast extends from the anterior portion of the **second rib** down to the **sixth** or **seventh rib** and from the lateral border of the sternum well into the axilla.

SURFACE ANATOMY

The surface anatomy includes the **nipple,** a small projection containing a collection of duct openings from the secretory glands within the breast tissue. The pigmented area surrounding the nipple is termed the **areola,** a circular area of different color surrounding a central point. The junction of the inferior part of the breast with the anterior chest wall is called the **inframammary fold** (IMF). The **axillary tail** is a band of tissue that wraps around the pectoral muscle laterally (Fig. 18-1).

The width of the breast, called the **mediolateral diameter,** on most patients is greater than the vertical measurement, from top to bottom. The vertical measurement, which may be described as the **craniocaudad diameter,** averages from 12 to 15 centimeters at the chest wall. The mammographer must realize that more breast tissue exists than the obvious tissue that extends from the chest. Mammary tissue is overlying the costocartilages near the sternum, and breast tissue is extending well up into the axilla. This breast tissue extending into the axilla is called the **tail of the breast** or the **axillary prolongation** of the breast. See Fig. 18-11 for a description of the base of the breast.

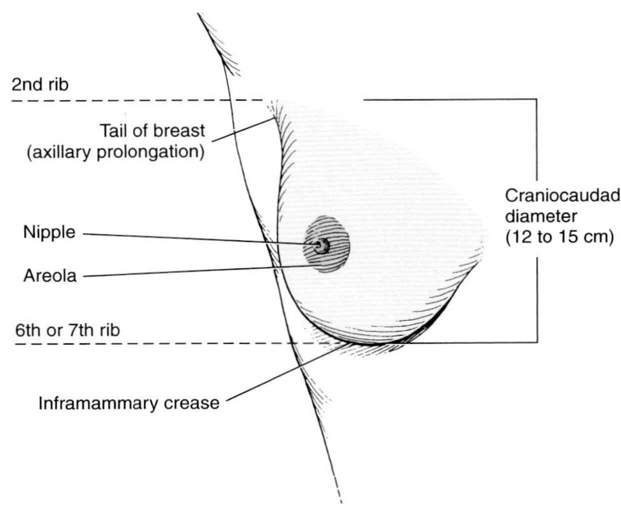

Fig. 18-1. Surface anatomy.

METHODS OF LOCALIZATION

Two methods are commonly used to subdivide the breast into smaller areas for localization purposes. The **quadrant system,** shown in Fig. 18-2, is easiest to use. Four quadrants can be described by using the nipple as the center. These quadrants are the **UOQ** (upper outer quadrant), the **UIQ** (upper inner quadrant), the **LOQ** (lower outer quadrant), and the **LIQ** (lower inner quadrant).

A second method, called the **clock system,** shown on the right in Fig. 18-2, compares the surface of the breast to the face of a clock. A problem with the clock method arises when a medial or lateral portion of either breast is described. What is described at 3 o'clock in the right breast has to be described at 9 o'clock in the left breast.

If either the referring physician or the patient has felt a mass of any suspicious area in either breast, one of these methods is used to describe the area of special interest to radiology personnel.

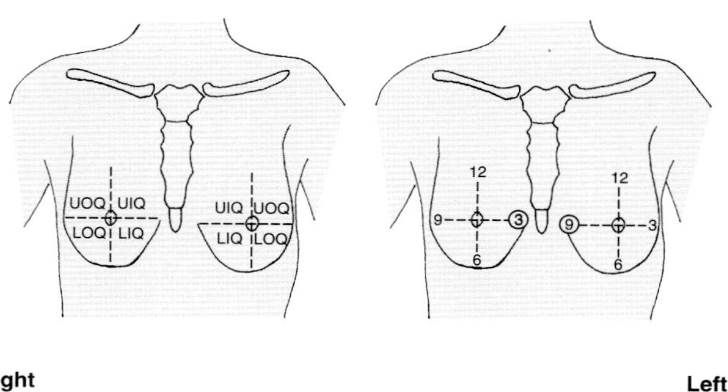

Fig. 18-2. Breast localization—quadrant and clock system methods.

SAGITTAL SECTION ANATOMY

A sagittal section through a mature breast is illustrated in Fig. 18-3, showing the relationship of the mammary gland to the underlying structures of the chest wall. On this drawing the **IMF** is at the level of the sixth rib, but a great deal of variation does exist among individuals.

The large **pectoralis major muscle** is seen overlying the bony thorax. A sheet of fibrous tissue surrounds the breast below the skin surface. A similar sheet of tissue covers the pectoralis major muscle. These two fibrous sheets connect in an area termed the **retromammary space.** This retromammary space must be demonstrated on at least one projection during the radiographic study of the mammary gland. Because the connections within the retromammary space are fairly loose, the normal breast exhibits considerable mobility on the chest wall.

The relative position of glandular tissue versus adipose (fatty) tissue is illustrated in Fig. 18-4. The central portion of the breast is primarily **glandular tissue.** Varying amounts of **adipose,** or **fatty, tissue** surround the glandular tissue. Size variation from individual to individual is due primarily to the amount of adipose tissue in the breast. The amount of glandular tissue is fairly constant from one female to another.

Because lactation or the secretion of milk is the primary function of the mammary gland, the amount of glandular and fatty tissue, or the size of the female breast, has no bearing on the functional ability of the gland.

The skin covering the breast is seen to be uniform in thickness, except in the area of the areola and nipple, where the skin is somewhat thicker.

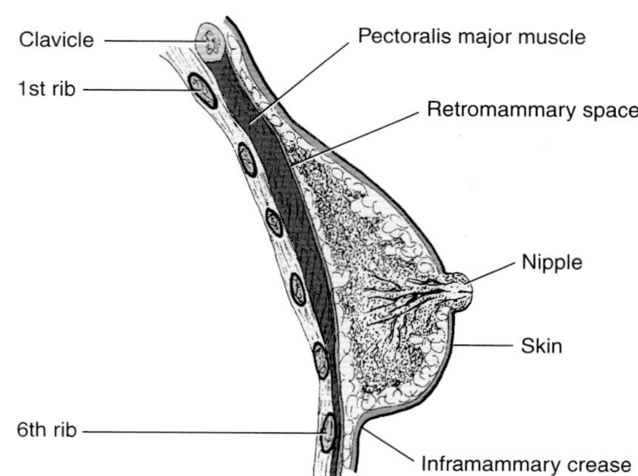

Fig. 18-3. Breast sagittal section.

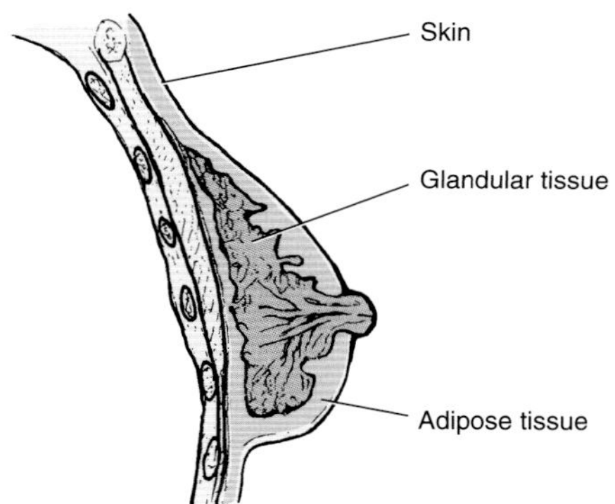

Fig. 18-4. Breast tissue sagittal section.

FRONTAL VIEW ANATOMY

The glandular tissue of the breast is divided into **15** or **20 lobes** arranged like the spokes of a wheel surrounding the nipple (Fig. 18-5).

The glandular lobes, made up of a number of individual **lobules,** are not clearly separated but are grouped in a radial arrangement as shown on this drawing. Distally, the smallest lobules consist of clusters of rounded **alveoli.** Upon glandular stimulation, peripheral cells of the alveoli form oil globules in their interior, which when ejected into the lumen of the alveoli constitute milk globules. The clusters of alveoli that make up the lobules are interconnected and drain by individual **ducts.** Each duct enlarges into a small **ampulla** that serves as a reservoir for milk just before terminating in a tiny opening on the surface of the **nipple.**

The various subdivisions of these ducts and associated ampullae are activated during pregnancy to prepare for lactation and, following birth, to produce milk for the newborn.

A layer of adipose tissue just under the skin surrounds and covers the glandular tissue. Lobular mammary fatty tissue, **subcutaneous fat,** is interspersed between the glandular elements. **Interlobular connective** or fibrous tissues surround and support the lobes and other glandular structures. Band-like extensions of this fibrous tissue are known as **Cooper's** (suspensory) **ligaments** of the breast and function to provide support for the mammary glands.

Each breast is abundantly supplied by blood vessels, nerves, and lymphatic vessels. The veins of the mammary gland are usually larger than the arteries and are located more peripherally. Some of the larger veins can usually be seen distinctly on a mammogram. The term **trabeculae** is used by radiologists to describe various small structures seen on the finished radiograph, such as small blood vessels, fibrous connective tissues, ducts, and other small structures that cannot be differentiated.

18

BREAST TISSUE TYPES

One of the major problems in radiography of the breast is that the various tissues have low inherent subject contrast. Breast tissue can be divided into three main types of tissues: (1) **glandular,** (2) **fibrous** or **connective,** and (3) **adipose** (Fig. 18-6). Because these tissues are all "soft tissues," no bone or air-filled tissue is present to provide contrast. The fibrous and glandular tissues are of similar density—that is, radiation is absorbed by these two tissues in a similar fashion.

The major difference in the breast tissues is the fact that adipose or fatty tissue is less dense than either the fibrous or glandular tissue. This difference in density between the fatty tissue and the remaining tissues provides for the photographic density differences apparent on the finished radiograph.

SUMMARY

Three types of breast tissue exist:

1. Glandular 2. Fibrous or connective	} Similar higher density (lighter)
3. Adipose	Less density (darker)

The film-screen mammogram image (Fig. 18-7) demonstrates differences in tissue densities. These differences provide the basis for the radiographic image of the breast. Note that the more dense glandular and fibrous or connective tissues appear as "light" structures or regions. The less dense adipose or fatty tissues appear light to dark gray, depending on the thickness of these tissues.

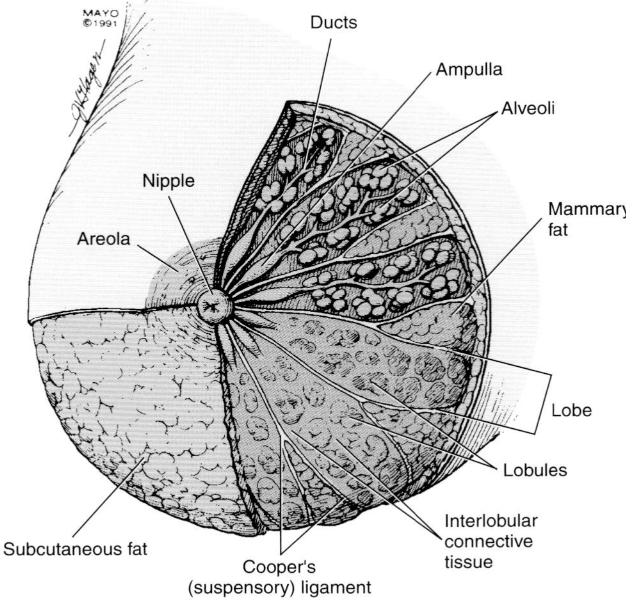

Fig. 18-5. Breast—anterior view (glandular tissue).

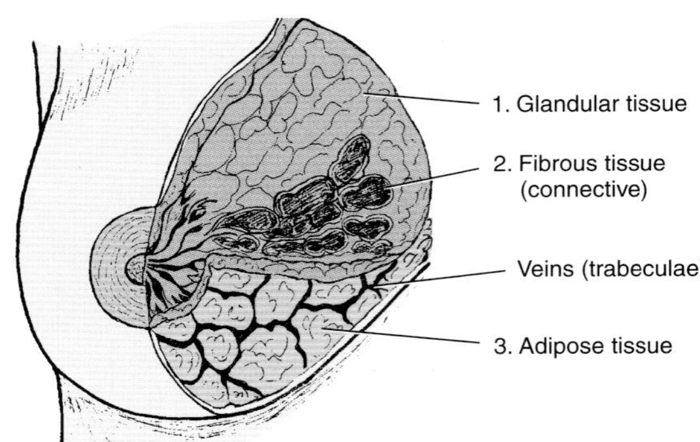

Fig. 18-6. Breast—anterior view (three tissue types).

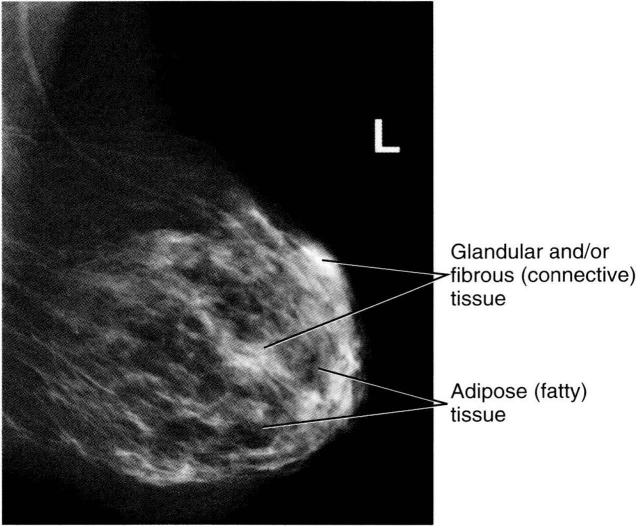

Fig. 18-7. Film-screen mammogram.

Breast Classifications

Technical radiographic factors for any one part of the body are determined mainly by the thickness of that particular part. A large elbow, for example, will require greater exposure factors than a small elbow. In mammography, however, **both** the **compressed breast thickness** and the **tissue density** contribute to technique selection. The breast size or thickness is easy to determine, but breast density is less obvious and requires additional information.

The relative density of the breast is primarily affected by the patient's inherent breast characteristics, hormone status, age, and pregnancies. The mammary gland undergoes cyclic changes associated with the rise and fall of hormonal secretions during the menstrual cycle, changes during pregnancy and lactation, and gradual changes that occur throughout a woman's lifetime.

Generally speaking, however, breasts can be classified into **three broad categories,** depending on the relative amounts of fibro-glandular tissue versus fatty tissue. These three categories are described as follows:

1. Fibro-Glandular Breast

The first category is the fibro-glandular breast. The younger breast is usually quite dense, because it contains relatively little fatty tissue. The common age grouping for the fibro-glandular category is post-puberty to about age 30. However, those females over the age of 30 who have never given birth to a live infant will probably also be in this general grouping. Pregnant or lactating females of any age are also placed in this grouping, because they possess a very dense type of breast (see Fig. 18-8).

2. Fibro-Fatty Breast

A second general category is the fibro-fatty breast. As the female ages and more changes occur in the breast tissues, the low amount of fatty tissue gradually shifts to a more equal distribution of fat and fibro-glandular tissue. Therefore, in the 30- to 50-year-old group, the breast is not quite as dense as in the younger group.

Radiographically, this breast is of average density and requires less exposure than the fibro-glandular type of breast.

Several pregnancies early in a woman's reproductive life will accelerate her breast development toward this fibro-fatty category (see Fig. 18-9).

3. Fatty Breast

A third and final grouping is the fatty breast that occurs following menopause, commonly age 50 and above. After a female's reproductive life, most of the glandular breast tissue atrophies and is converted to fatty tissue in a process called *involution.* Even less exposure is required on this type of breast than is required on the first two types of breasts (see Fig. 18-10).

The breasts of children and most males contain mostly fat in small proportions and therefore fall into this category also. Although most mammograms are performed on the female patient, it is important to recognize that between 1% and 2% of all breast cancer is found in the male; therefore, mammograms will occasionally be performed on a male.

SUMMARY

In addition to breast size or thickness upon compression, the average density of the tissues of the breast will determine exposure factors. The most dense breast is the **fibro-glandular** type. The least dense is the **fatty** type, and the breast with equal amounts of fatty and fibro-glandular tissue is termed **fibro-fatty.**

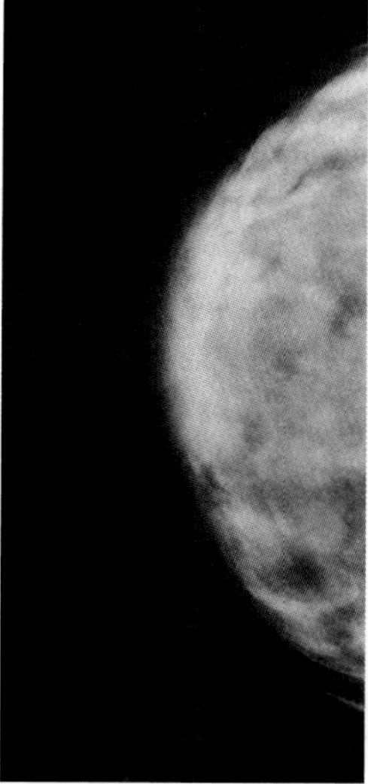

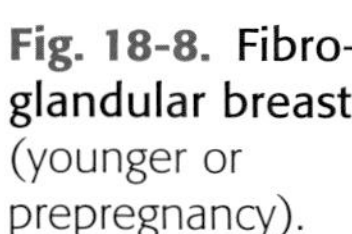

Fig. 18-8. **Fibro-glandular breast** (younger or prepregnancy).

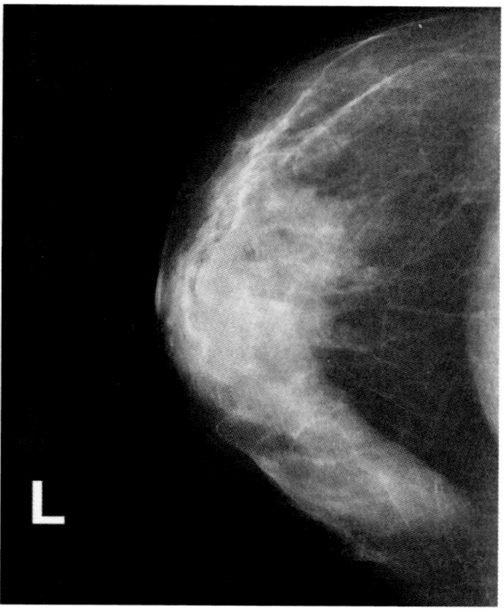

Fig. 18-9. **Fibro-fatty breast** (30-50 years old, post-pregnancy).

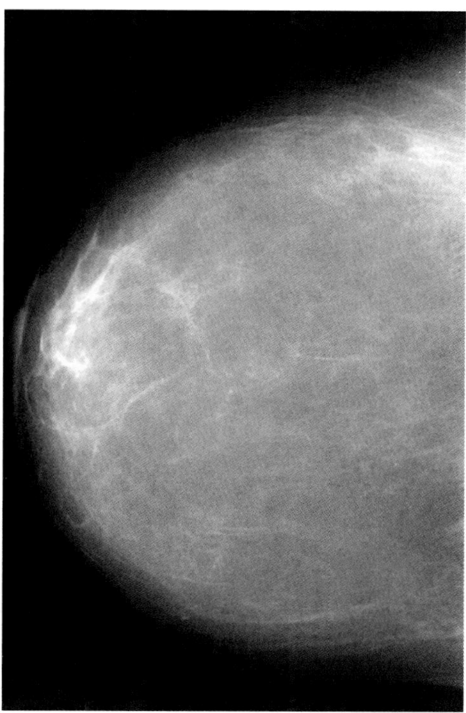

Fig. 18-10. **Fatty breast** (68 year old). (From Ballinger PW, Frank ED: Merrill's atlas of radiographic positions and radiographic procedures, ed 10, St. Louis, 2003, Mosby.)

SUMMARY OF BREAST CLASSIFICATIONS

1. Fibro-Glandular Breast

- Common age group—15 to 30 years (and childless females over age 30)
- Pregnant or lactating females
- Radiographically dense
- Very little fat

2. Fibro-Fatty Breast

- Common age group—30 to 50 years
- Young women with 3 or more pregnancies
- Average density, radiographically
- 50% fat and 50% fibro-glandular

3. Fatty Breast

- Common age group—50 years and over
- Postmenopausal
- Minimal density, radiographically
- Breasts of children and males

RADIOGRAPHIC POSITIONING

Positioning and Technical Considerations

PATIENT PREPARATION

Before the examination begins, the mammographer will explain the procedure and ask the patient to put on a gown, preferably one designed for mammography, which allows exposure of only the breast that is being examined. The patient will be instructed to remove any jewelry, talcum powder, or antiperspirant that may cause artifacts on the radiographic image.

The mammographer will document relevant patient history as per departmental protocol. Generally this patient history will include the following:

- Number of pregnancies
- Family history of cancer including breast cancer
- Medications (e.g., hormone therapy) currently taking
- Previous surgery
- Previous mammograms, when and where performed
- Description of problem, such as screening mammogram, lumps, pain, and discharge

The mammographer should also note location of scars, palpable masses, moles, warts, tattoos, etc.

BREAST POSITIONING

In mammography, the great variability of the breast, with respect to the proportion of fatty tissue to fibro-glandular tissue, presents certain technical difficulties. In producing a superior-quality mammogram, the shape and contour of the normal breast poses additional problems to the mammographer.

The **base** of the breast is that portion near the chest wall, whereas the area near the nipple is termed the **apex.** In either the craniocaudad or the mediolateral projection, the base of the breast is much thicker and contains much denser tissues than at the apex.

To overcome this anatomic difference, compression is used in combination with a specially designed tube so that the more intense central ray (CR) of the x-ray beam penetrates the thicker base of the breast.

X-RAY TUBE

The most distinctive aspect of the mammography machine is the unique design of the x-ray tube, which has a **molybdenum target** with small focal spots of **0.3** and **0.1 mm. Rhodium** has recently been introduced as an optional anode material. The focal spots must be this size because of the size of the cancer calcifications, which are typically less than 1.0 mm in size.

The anode configuration produces a **prominent heel effect** resulting from the short source-to-image receptor distance (SID) and the use of a narrow reference target angle. Because the x-ray tube is aligned with the cathode placed over the base of the breast (at the chest wall) and the anode outward toward the apex (nipple area), the heel effect fortunately can be used to maximum advantage (Fig. 18-11). Because the cathode side of the x-ray beam has significantly greater intensity of x-rays compared with the anode side, a more uniform-density breast image can be produced, because the more intense x-rays are at the base, where tissue thickness is greater.

Most mammograms utilize **grids, automatic exposure control** (AEC), and the important **breast compression device.**

AEC Chamber Selection The AEC chambers on most mammography systems are adjustable in up to 10 positions from the chest wall to the nipple region. To ensure adequate exposure of the more dense/thick tissues, generally the **chamber under the chest wall,** or to the **more dense tissue area** should be selected. Exceptions to this include special projections, such as magnification and spot compression views.

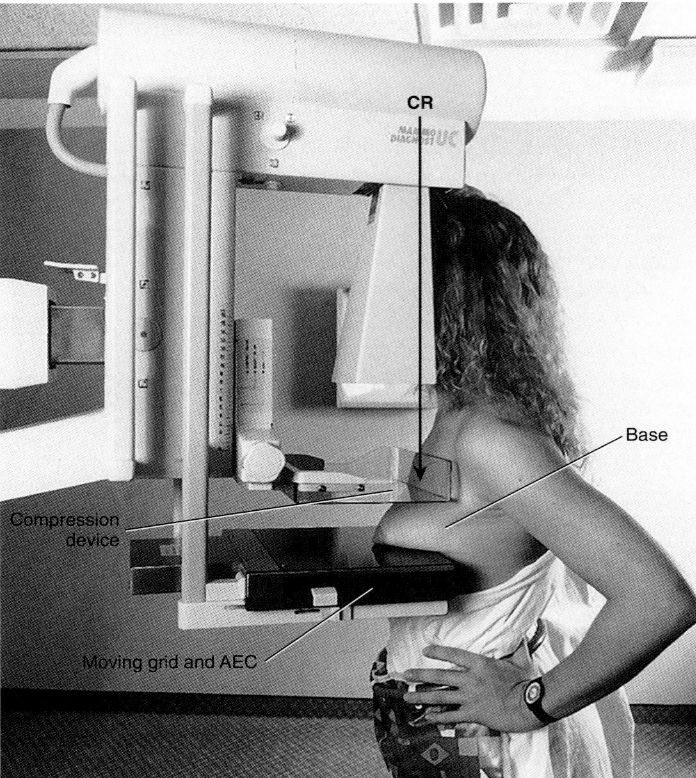

Fig. 18-11. Placement of patient on a dedicated mammography unit for a craniocaudal (CC) projection. (Compression is not firmly applied for this photo.)
Note: Vertical CR is placed directly over the chest wall structures, which allows the posterosuperior breast structures to be imaged.

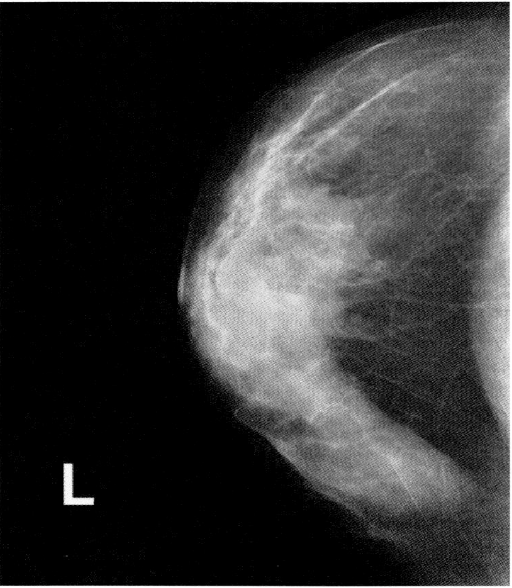

Fig. 18-12. Example of AEC nearer nipple (more dense tissue area).

For the most part, the AEC chamber selection is dependent on tissue density. For example, in Fig. 18-12 the breast tissue is more dense toward the nipple, and in this case the detector would be placed nearer the more dense tissue to ensure adequate exposure.

COMPRESSION*

All mammography machines contain a compression device that is used to compress the breast. Improvements in breast compression technology in recent years have greatly improved the visibility of detail in breast images. The compression device is made of a plastic that allows transmission of the low-energy x-rays. The device should have a straight chest wall edge to allow the compression to grasp the breast tissues close to the chest wall. Compression is controlled by the technologist and is typically applied at **25 to 45 pounds** of force.

In addition to the standard compression device, a smaller "spot" device may be used to compress localized areas. The compression device should be checked regularly to ensure that it is working properly and applying the correct amount of pressure.

Appropriately applied compression is one of the critical components in the production of a high-quality mammogram. Six benefits of using compression are to:

1. Decrease the thickness of the breast
2. Bring the breast structures as close to the IR as possible
3. Decrease dose and scattered radiation
4. Decrease motion and geometric unsharpness
5. Increase contrast
6. Separate breast structure

These six factors identify how image quality or resolution is improved by reducing scatter and also by reducing magnification of breast structures. This is illustrated by comparing the uncompressed and compressed drawings in Fig. 18-13. Note the location of the microcalcifications and lesion that are surrounded by dense breast tissue on the left drawing *(A),* and how compression has brought them closer to the IR in drawing *B.* Therefore the overall breast thickness has also been greatly reduced, which reduces the ratio of scatter to primary radiation by one half.

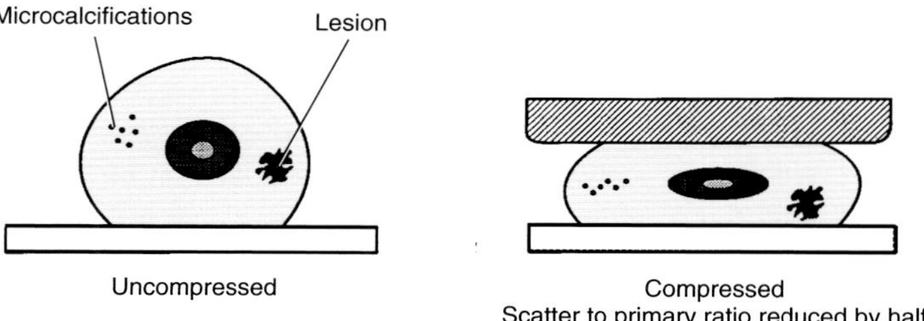

Fig. 18-13. The effect of breast compression:
1. Decreased tissue thickness (less scatter, better resolution)
2. Breast structures closer to IR

MAGNIFICATION (Fig. 18-14)

The magnification method is used to enlarge specific areas of interest such as small lesions or microcalcifications. This requires an x-ray tube with a **0.1-mm focal spot** to maintain image resolution. Magnification of 1½ to 2 times can be obtained by inserting a magnification platform between the image receptor and the breast, thereby magnifying the part resulting from **increased OID.** This magnification technique can be used with most mammogram projections.

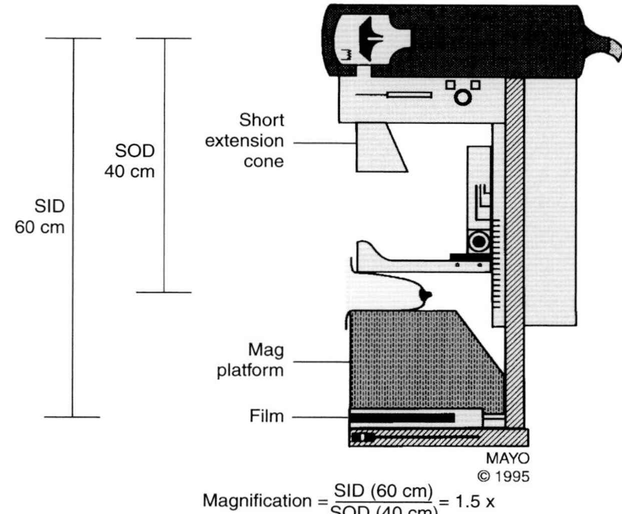

Fig. 18-14. Magnification—breast in position on a raised platform to produce a 1.5 × magnification image. (Courtesy Mayo Foundation.)

PATIENT DOSE

Patient dose is significant in mammography, as seen by the dose icon boxes included on each positioning page. A skin dose of 800 to 900 mrad and a mean glandular dose (MGD) of 130 to 150 mrad is common for a 4-cm thickness mammogram (p. 591), which is much higher than for most other body parts. For example, a much thicker 30-cm lateral lumbar spine at 90 kV, 50 mAs, has a skin dose of 1000 to 1300 and a midline dose of 130 to 180 mrad (p. 335). The reason for the relatively high dose for mammograms is the very low kV (25 to 28) and the high mAs (75 to 85) required.

The principal way patient dose is controlled in mammography is by careful and accurate positioning, which minimizes the need for repeats. The ACR recommends a repeat rate of **less than 5%** for mammography. The only shielding possible is a waist apron for shielding the gonadal region.

Note: Mean glandular dose is the average breast tissue dose, rather than a specific midline dose as for the lumbar spine and other body parts.

*Frank ED: Technical aspects of mammography. In Carlton RL, Adler AM, editors: Principles of radiographic imaging, ed 3, Albany, 2001, Delmar.

18

FILM-SCREEN MAMMOGRAPHY

Film-screen mammography continues to be the standard in current breast radiography. The greatest benefit of the film-screen system is an **excellent image with a low radiation dose,** allowing women to have this examination regularly. The ability to see **fine detail, edge sharpness,** and **soft tissue** is a hallmark of a good film-screen mammogram. However, digital mammography (computed radiography and/or digital radiography) is developing rapidly and has certain distinct advantages over film-screen mammography.

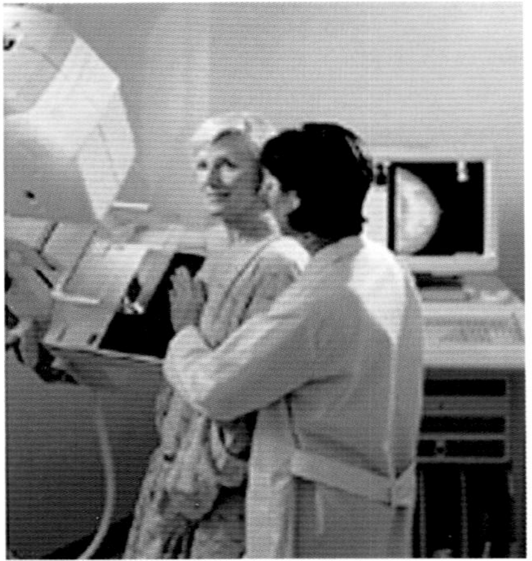

Fig. 18-15. Digital mammography unit. (Courtesy G.E. Medical Systems.)

Digital Mammography

COMPUTED RADIOGRAPHY MAMMOGRAPHY

Computed radiography (CR) can be used for mammography similar to the way it is used in general radiography with its imaging plate (IP) and image processor, as described in Chapter 2. CR cassettes containing imaging plates can be used in existing mammographic systems. CR mammography has certain advantages over film-screen systems, such as the following:

Operating Costs One advantage of CR over film-screen systems is that the imaging plates can be exposed many times before they need to be replaced. Therefore, considering the cost of film and associated expenses, the use of CR becomes more economical. In addition, the need for chemical processing is eliminated, which is more ecologically sound.

Teleradiology Options A second important advantage of CR mammography is its ability to retrieve and/or transfer images to remote locations for interpretation or consultation. This is referred to as **teleradiology,** or more specifically for transmitting mammogram images electronically, the term *telemammography* is sometimes used.

18

Archiving and PACS Options After the images have been interpreted, they can be stored electronically at any desired location through the PACS (also described in Chapter 2). This is a third advantage of digital imaging compared with film-screen systems, because the need for physical storage space for hardcopy films is eliminated as mammogram images are incorporated into existing PACS.

DIRECT DIGITAL RADIOGRAPHY

Direct digital radiography (DR) is a second form of digital imaging that continues to be refined and developed but is not yet in common use. These mammographic systems contain a flat detector that is permanently mounted on the x-ray unit. Comparison studies have shown that newer DR mammographic systems have improved contrast resolution with reductions in patient dose compared with film-screen imaging. There is no imaging plate as required with CR. The flat detector captures the remnant x-rays and produces a digital image. The digital image is then projected on a monitor at the mammographer's workstation for direct viewing and post-processing as needed.

CONCLUSION—DIGITAL VERSUS FILM-SCREEN MAMMOGRAPHY

Although contrast resolution is outstanding with a digital system, the overall spatial resolution of the digital image at this time still falls short of the film-screen system. As a result, confidence in detecting microcalcifications and tissue changes in the breast has been questioned by radiologists when examining the digital breast image. However, improvements in detector technology and monitor design may soon match film-screen resolution. Also certain post-processing features such as magnification (all or part of the image), edge enhancement, image reversal (reversing the dark and light pixel values of the image), and adjustment of image contrast and brightness, all can be used to enhance specific mammographic images and improve their diagnostic quality.

Digital mammography, as with digital imaging in general radiography, will in all likelihood eventually replace film-screen mammography.

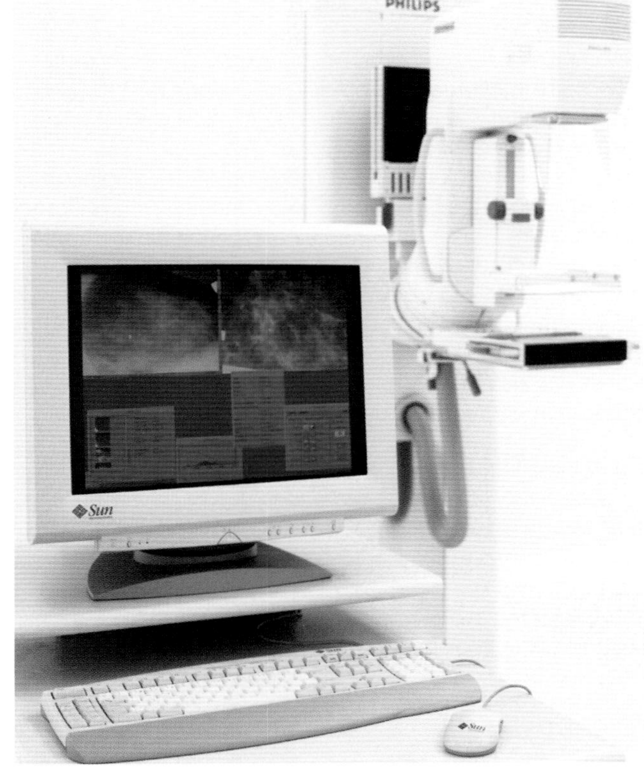

Fig. 18-16. Digital mammography unit workstation for direct viewing and post-processing options. (Courtesy Philips Medical Systems.)

COMPUTER-AIDED DETECTION SYSTEMS

Today, the computer is being used as the "second opinion" in mammographic interpretation. Computer-aided detection (CAD) is a technology that has the potential to impact dramatically the diagnosis of breast cancer. CAD systems use a computerized detection algorithm to analyze digital images for various suspicious lesions and provide the radiologist with an estimate of the probability of malignancy. Certain studies have shown that using a second reader to interpret screening mammograms improves the cancer detection rate by as much as 10%.*

Using computers is advantageous because they do not get fatigued or distracted, nor do they demonstrate intraobserver variation. Clusters of microcalcifications are a good example of objects appropriate for CAD viewing because they differ from normal anatomic structures in density, shape, and size. Detection and classification of microcalcifications and borders of lesions are possible with CAD. Some studies show improvement in microcalcification detection rates. The use of CAD systems is increasing, but they are not expected to replace the radiologist.

*Anderson EDC, Muir BB, Walsh JS, et al: The efficacy of double-reading mammograms in breast screening, *Clin Radiol* 49:248, 1994.

Alternative Modalities and Procedures

SONOGRAPHY (ULTRASOUND)

Sonography has been used to image the breast since the mid-1970s. It provides valuable adjunct information for the radiologist, along with the film-screen mammogram and physical examination. Today sonography is an integral part of the mammography department and the mammogram examination. Its major value is its ability to **distinguish between a cyst and a solid lesion.** It is also used extensively to determine fluid, abscess, hematoma, and silicone gel. Ultrasound has the ability to find cancers in women with dense breasts. Mammographers may also be trained to perform sonography of the breast in addition to film-screen mammography. Image quality is heavily dependent on sonographer expertise.

Conventional Scanner and Hand-Held Transducer When a high-resolution conventional scanner (Fig. 18-17) is used, the patient is positioned supine or rolled slightly onto one side. The hand-held transducer is placed on a palpable mass or an area noted on a mammogram. Fig. 18-18 shows an image from such a scanner.

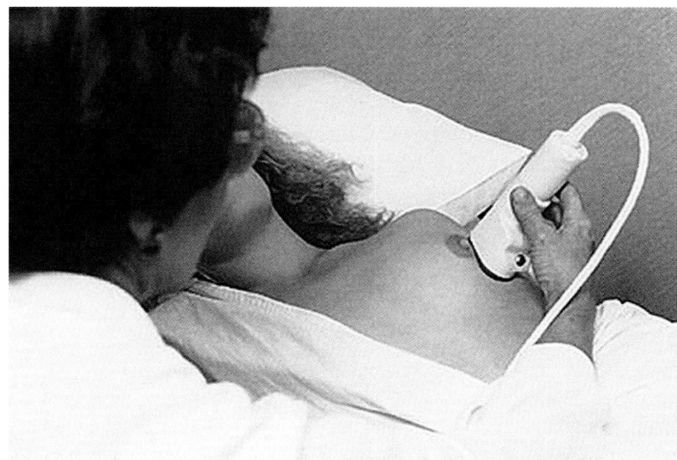

Fig. 18-17. Conventional ultrasound scanner with hand-held transducer.

NUCLEAR MEDICINE

Two nuclear medicine procedures are relevant to breast imaging, as follows:

Mammoscintigraphy may be helpful in confirming breast cancer diagnosis. Technetium-99m-sestamibi is injected as a tracer into the arm opposite the affected breast; breast images are obtained 10 minutes later. This procedure has fallen slightly out of favor because of the high number of false-positive results.

Sentinal node studies are useful for patients with melanoma, and they are also becoming increasingly useful for breast cancer. This procedure involves injecting sulfur colloid around the lesion subcutaneously. (Patients must have had a localization procedure previously.) The flow is then observed through the lymph vessels to assess which nodes are affected by the cancer.

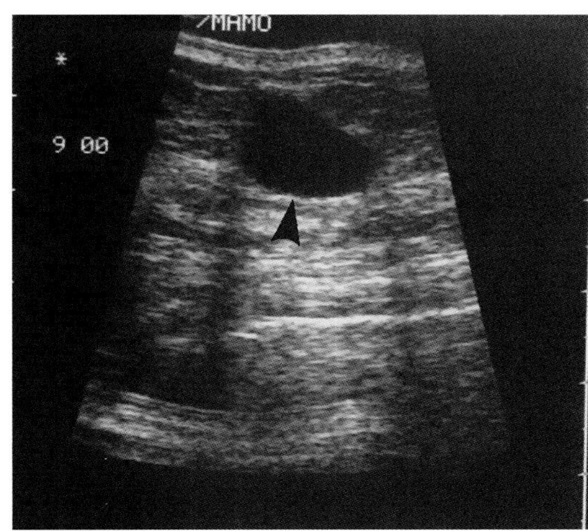

Fig. 18-18. Breast sonogram obtained with conventional scanner showing a cyst *(arrow).*

18

POSITRON EMISSION TOMOGRAPHY

Positron Emission Tomography (PET) is being used to detect early signs of cancerous growth within the breast. Using the tracer fluorodeoxyglucose (FDG), early cancerous cells can be detected by their increased metabolism. This increased metabolism uses sugar and the FDG tracer molecules at a greater rate as compared with normal breast tissue, making the cancer's location visible with PET. PET also is used following surgery or treatment for breast cancer to determine whether recurrent disease is present in the breast or other parts of the body.

Two disadvantages of using PET for breast imaging are **higher cost** and **radiation exposure.** Therefore even though PET has certain valuable applications for early detection of breast disease, the cost of the equipment required and use of short half-life radioactive tracers make the use of PET impractical as a screening tool. Radiation exposure from FDG tracer is approximately 6 times greater than that from a technetium-99m-sestamibi study as used in nuclear medicine.

MAGNETIC RESONANCE IMAGING

MRI has received approval from the FDA as an adjunct screening tool for breast imaging. The number of breast MRI scans performed in the U.S. is increasing annually. Although its cost makes it prohibitive for general clinical use, MRI has been clinically proven to be effective for certain special applications.

Advantages of MRI

One advantage of MRI is that it can **show the whole breast maximally** with greater comfort for the patient. Also, recent work with contrast indicates that MRI can show evidence of **vascularization of lesions.** Furthermore, it provides better sensitivity and specificity than ultrasound and x-ray mammography.

Additional advantages of MRI involve its superior ability to visualize pathology on patients with **dense breast tissue** (Fig. 18-19) and with **breast implants** (Fig. 18-20).

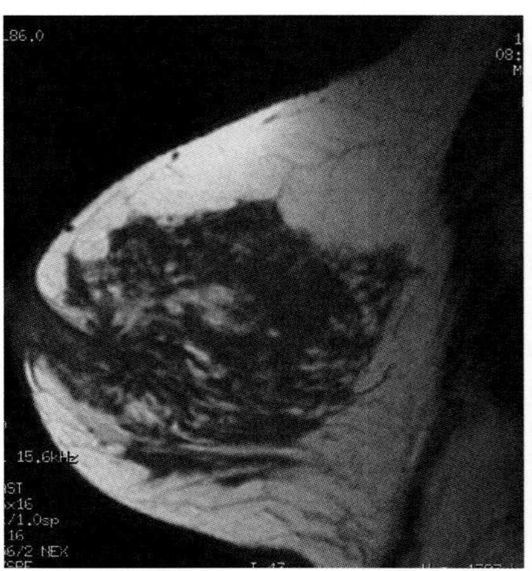
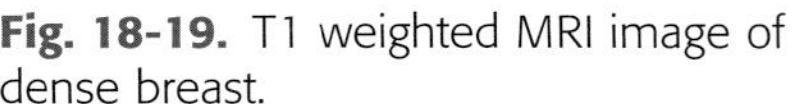

Fig. 18-19. T1 weighted MRI image of dense breast.

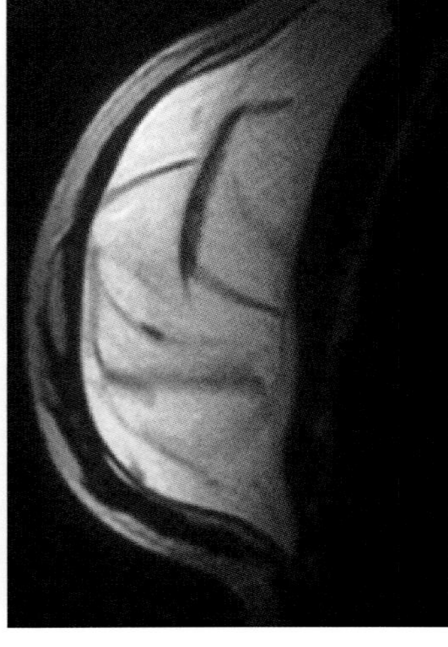

Fig. 18-20. MRI image—normal silicone implant.

Dense Breast Tissue As an adjunct to mammographic studies, MRI has shown to be useful for classifying suspicious lesions and microcalcifications that have been identified on mammograms. MRI is especially helpful in evaluating small breasts and very dense breast tissue.

Breast Implants More than 1 million women in the U.S. and Canada have undergone breast augmentation (surgical implants). Silicone and saline implants are radiopaque, requiring implant displaced (ID) views (Eklund method). Compression is more difficult with implants, and extra care must be taken by the mammographer not to rupture the implant. Automatic exposure control (AEC) also cannot be used with augmented breasts, all of which makes imaging of breast tissue with implants a challenge using conventional screening mammograms or ultrasound techniques.

MRI has been clinically proven to be most effective in diagnosing problems related to breast implant imaging. For example, with MRI it is possible to evaluate potential intracapsular and extracapsular rupture, including the area posterior to the implant, which is very problematic with either mammography or sonography studies. The MRI images in Figs. 18-21 and 18-22 clearly demonstrate intracapsular and extracapsular ruptures of silicone implants.

In addition to diagnosing implant rupture, it is also important to demonstrate the breast tissue surrounding and posterior to the implants for possible malignant growth. Physical examination is more difficult with implants, which also increases the risk for cancer growth without detection. MRI, unlike mammography or sonography, is not hindered by the presence of an implant.

Clinical testing is being done with a new kind of radiolucent implant that will allow more effective use of film-screen mammography, including the use of automatic exposure controls. However, the more than 1 million women with radiopaque implants, many of whom are nearing the life expectancy limits of the implants, will require more and more evaluations of breast implants for possible rupture or other related problems. This in turn increases the potential role of MRI in breast implant imaging.

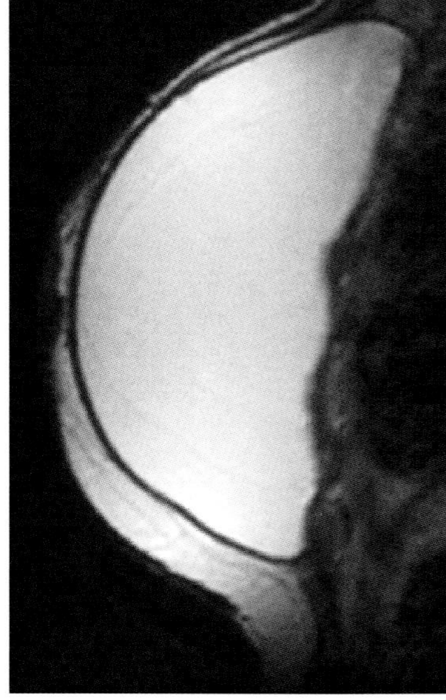

Fig. 18-21. MRI image—intracapsular rupture (silicone contained by fibrous capsule).

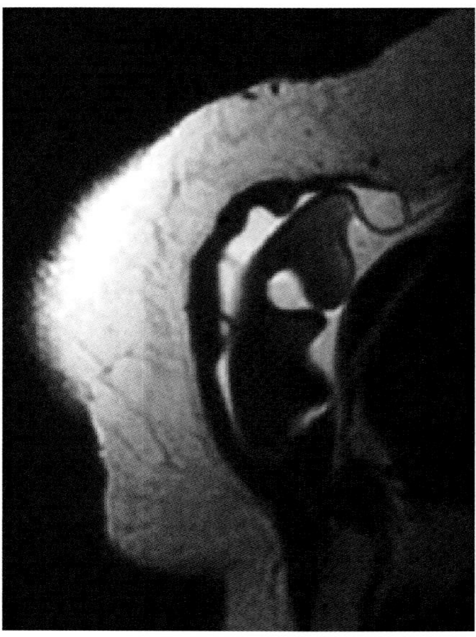

Fig. 18-22. MRI image—saline component inside, silicone outside.

Disadvantages of MRI

Two primary disadvantages of MRI are its **high false-positive rate** and the **high cost,** both of which limit its use as a breast screening procedure. However, research and clinical use continue as MRI evolves into playing a larger role in the diagnostic workup for breast lesions.

Pathologic Indications

Screening mammography is important for the early detection of pathologic changes in the breast. These changes can be either benign (noncancerous), or malignant (cancerous). The most common pathologic indications for mammography include the following:

Breast carcinoma (cancer): Carcinoma of the breast is divided into two categories, **noninvasive** and **invasive.** Noninvasive carcinoma is a distinct lesion of the breast that has the potential to become invasive cancer. These lesions are restricted to the glandular lumen and do not have access to the lymphatic system or blood vessels. Noninvasive cancer may also be termed ***in situ.*** **Ductal carcinoma in situ (DCIS)** is isolated within the breast duct and has not spread to other areas of the breast. **Lobular carcinoma in situ (LCIS)** is abnormal cells that have been detected in one or more of the breast lobes. Noninvasive cancers (DCIS and LCIS) comprise approximately 15% to 20% of all breast cancer diagnoses.

The most common form of breast cancer is invasive or infiltrating ductal carcinoma. This type comprises approximately 80% of all breast cancer diagnoses. Invasive cancer is believed to arise in the terminal duct lobular unit. The majority of these cancers cannot be specified without histologic evaluation. Invasive cancer of the breast carries the worst overall prognosis of the invasive cancers.

Cysts: Cysts are **fluid-filled sacs** that are benign and appear as well-circumscribed masses. Their density is usually that of the surrounding tissue; however, they may also appear denser. To positively diagnose a cyst, ultrasonography and needle biopsies are required.

Fibroadenoma: Fibroadenomas are the most common benign, solid lumps or tumors composed of fibrous and glandular tissue. They are well-circumscribed lesions with clearly defined edges that can be felt during palpation. They typically have the same density as the surrounding tissue. The mass is an overgrowth of the fibrous tissue of the breast lobule.

Fibrocystic changes: This common, benign condition is usually bilateral in premenopausal women. It includes a variety of conditions; the most obvious are fibrosis and cystic dilation of ducts. Multiple cysts with increased fibrous tissue are commonly distributed throughout the breasts.

Gynecomastia: Gynecomastia is from a Greek term meaning "woman-like breasts." This is a benign condition of the male breast in which there is a benign glandular enlargement of the breast. Gynecomastia may be unilateral or bilateral but seems to be more pronounced in one breast. It typically presents as a palpable mass by the nipple.

Intraductal papilloma: This is a small growth inside the duct of the breast near the nipple. The symptoms may include spontaneous, unilateral nipple discharge that may be bloody to clear in color. The mammographic appearance is typically normal. Sonography of the breast may be helpful. When performing a galactography or ductography, a contrast agent is injected into the duct in order to reveal a filling defect that would indicate the presence of an intraductal papilloma.

Paget's disease of the nipple: This condition first appears as a crust or scaly nipple sore or as a discharge from the nipple. Slightly more than half of the persons having this cancer also have a lump in the breast. Paget's disease may be invasive or noninvasive.

SUMMARY OF PATHOLOGIC INDICATIONS

CONDITION OR DISEASE	MOST COMMON RADIOGRAPHIC EXAM	POSSIBLE RADIOGRAPHIC APPEARANCE	MANUAL EXPOSURE FACTOR ADJUSTMENT*
Breast carcinoma	Bilateral mammogram	Mass with spiculated border, architectural distortion, or calcifiations.	None
Cysts	Bilateral mammogram and sonogram	Well-defined margins have only slightly higher density than surrounding tissues.	None
Fibroadenoma	Bilateral mammogram and sonogram to differentiate solid versus fluid-filled cysts	Breast tumor has smooth, well-defined margins.	None
Fibrocystic changes	Bilateral mammogram and sonogram	Multiple fibrous cysts are high-density areas throughout breasts.	None
Gynecomastia	Bilateral mammography and sonogram	Flame-shaped opacity extending and expanding posterior to the nipple.	None
Intraductal papilloma	Bilateral mammography and sonogram, galactography; mammogram typically normal	Galactography may have filling defect.	None
Paget's disease of the nipple	Bilateral mammogram	If masses are present, they will appear as breast carcinoma.	None

*Dependent on severity and stage of disease.

TERMINOLOGY AND ABBREVIATIONS

Certain positioning terminology, some of which is unique to mammography, needs to be understood and used correctly. These terms and their abbreviations are used to identify images and are standard nomenclature as approved by the ACR in October 1995. It is important to use these **terms** and **abbreviations** correctly when applying for ACR accreditation.

MAMMOGRAPHY TERMINOLOGY CHART

ACR NOMENCLATURE	DESCRIPTION
AT	**Axillary tail view:** A mediolateral 20°-30° oblique projection
AX	**Axillary view:** For lymph nodes and other axillary content
CC	**Craniocaudal:** A basic superior to inferior projection
CV	**Cleavage view:** A double breast compression view (demonstrates breast tissue anterior to the sternum and the medial aspects of both breasts)
FB	Caudocranial, **from below** (sometimes in practice also abbreviated as CCFB
ID	**Implant displaced:** The Eklund method views for augmented breast
LM	**Lateromedial** projection
LMO*	**Lateromedial oblique** (inferolateral-superomedial): With pacemaker
ML	**Mediolateral** projection
MLO	**Mediolateral oblique** (superomedial-inferolateral oblique): The basic oblique
RL†	**Rolled lateral** (superior breast tissue rolled laterally)
RM†	**Rolled medial** (superior breast tissue rolled medially)
SIO*	**Superolateral-inferomedial oblique:** Reverse oblique
TAN	**Tangential** (also mark image with view and degree of angulation)
XCCL	**Exaggerated craniocaudal (laterally):** A special CC projection with emphasis on the axillary tissue

*Image should be marked with any deviation from 0° with *LMO* or *SIO*.

†Used as a suffix after the projection.

Survey Information

Routine (basic projections): As expected, the **craniocaudal (CC)** and the **mediolateral oblique (MLO)** were the two most commonly performed routine projections throughout all regions of the U.S. and Canada.

The next most common projection was the **mediolateral (ML)**. This is listed as a special projection in this chapter.

Additional special projections: The second and third most common special projections were the **exaggerated craniocaudal (laterally)** (XCCL) and the **Eklund method CC** and **MLO.**

The remaining special projections not described in this chapter are the **axillary tail (AT), cleavage view (CV),** and **rolled lateral** and **rolled medial CC** projections.

BASIC PROJECTIONS

Standard or basic projections, also sometimes referred to as routine projections or departmental routines, are those projections or positions commonly performed in most mammography departments.

SPECIAL PROJECTIONS

Special projections are those more common projections or positions taken as extra or additional projections to better demonstrate certain pathologic conditions or specific body parts.

18

CRANIOCAUDAL (CC) PROJECTION: MAMMOGRAPHY

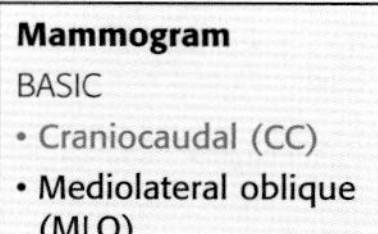
Mammogram
BASIC
- Craniocaudal (CC)
- **Mediolateral oblique (MLO)**

Pathology Demonstrated

This projection allows detection and/or evaluation of calcifications, cysts, carcinomas, or other abnormalities or changes in the breast tissue.

Both breasts are imaged separately for comparison.

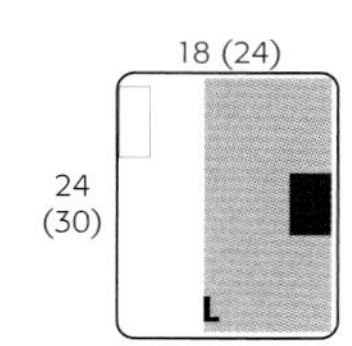

Technical Factors

- IR size—18 × 24 cm, crosswise
  or
  —24 × 30 cm, crosswise
- Grid
- 25 to 28 kV
- Technique and dose:

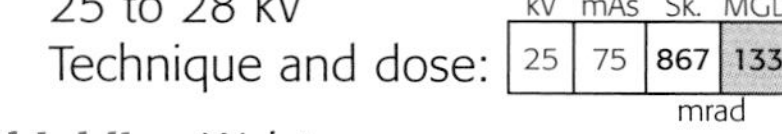

kV	mAs	Sk.	MGD
25	75	867	133
		mrad	

Shielding Waist apron

Patient Position Standing; if not possible, seated

Part Position

- IR height is determined by **lifting the breast** to achieve a 90° angle to the chest wall. The IR will be at the level of **the inframammary fold at its upper limits.**
- The breast is pulled forward onto the IR centrally with the **nipple in profile.**
- The arm on the side being imaged is relaxed at the side and the shoulder is back out of the way.
- The head is turned away from the side being imaged.
- Medial tissue of opposite breast to be draped on the corner of the image receptor.
- Wrinkles and folds on the breast should be smoothed out and compression applied until taut.
- The marker and patient ID information are always placed on the **axillary side.**

Central Ray

- Perpendicular, centered to the base of the breast, the chest wall edge of the IR; CR not movable
- SID: Fixed, varies with manufacturer, about 60 cm (24 inches)

Collimation Use appropriate cone/collimation.

Respiration Suspend breathing.

Note: Position AEC chamber to ensure adequate exposure of various tissue densities.

PNL (posterior nipple line): To evaluate the depth of breast tissue. This is determined by an imaginary line from the nipple to the pectoris muscle or edge of image, whichever is the shorter distance. The PNL on CC projection (Fig. 18-24) should be within 1 cm of that on MLO projection (Fig. 18-28).

Radiographic Criteria

Structures Shown: • Entire breast tissue should be visualized, including the central, subareolar, and medial breast • Pectoral muscle should be visualized on 20-30% of patients. The posterior nipple line (PNL) measurement must be within 1 cm of the MLO measurement.

Position and Compression: • Nipple is seen in profile. • Tissue thickness is distributed evenly on the IR, indicating optimum compression.

Collimation and CR: • CR and collimation chamber are fixed and will be centered correctly if breast tissue is properly centered and visualized on IR.

Exposure Criteria: • Dense areas are adequately penetrated, resulting in optimal contrast. Sharp tissue markings indicate no motion. • R or L marker and patient information are correctly placed at axillary side of IR; no artifacts are visible.

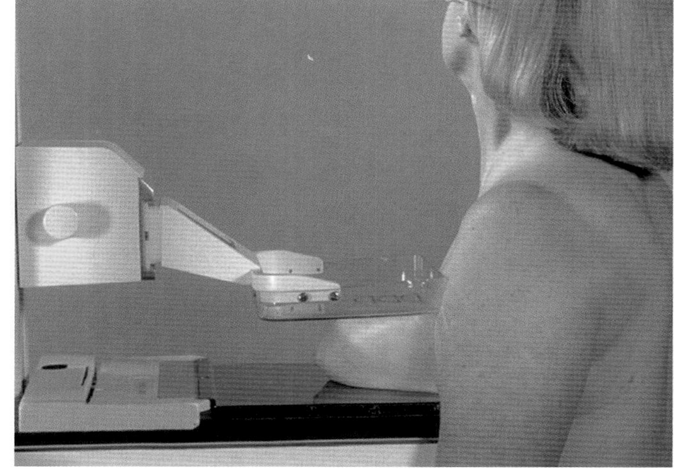

Fig. 18-23. CC projection.

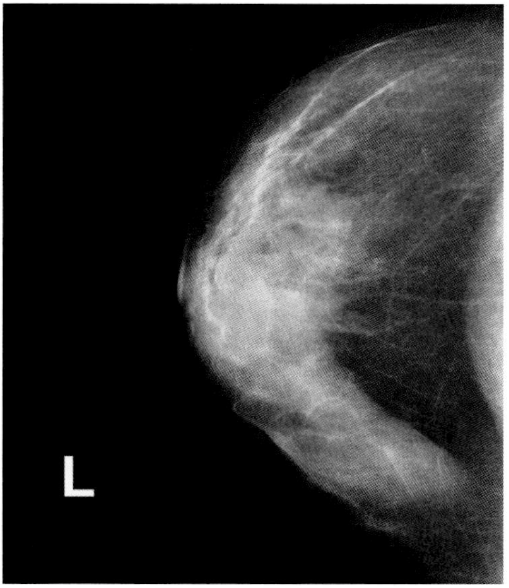

Fig. 18-24. CC projection.

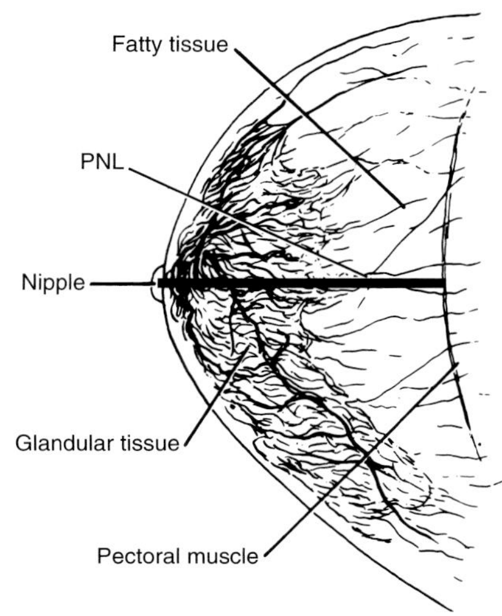

Fig. 18-25. CC projection.

MEDIOLATERAL OBLIQUE (MLO) PROJECTION: MAMMOGRAM

Superomedial–Inferolateral Oblique

Mammogram
BASIC
- Craniocaudal (CC)
- Mediolateral oblique (MLO)

Pathology Demonstrated

Projection allows detection and/or evaluation of calcifications, cysts, carcinomas, or other abnormalities or changes in the deep lateral aspect of breast tissue.

Both breasts are imaged separately for comparison.

Technical Factors

- IR size—18 × 24 cm, crosswise or
  —24 × 30 cm, crosswise
- Grid
- 25 to 28 kV
- Technique and dose:

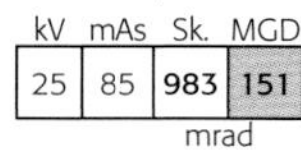

kV	mAs	Sk.	MGD
25	85	983	151
		mrad	

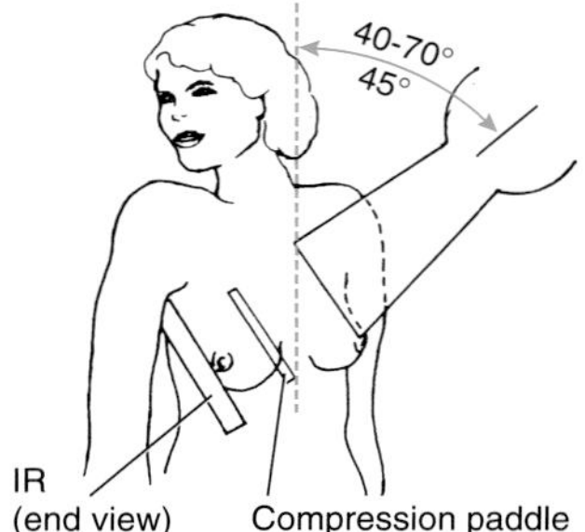

Fig. 18-26. MLO projection.

18 (24)
R
24
(30)

Shielding Waist apron

Patient Position Standing; if not possible, seated

Part Position

- Tube and IR remain at right angles to each other; **CR is angled about 45°.** CR enters the breast **medially,** perpendicular to the patient's pectoral muscle.
  –For heavy and large-breasted women, angle 40° to 60° from vertical.
  –For thin and small-breasted women, angle 60° to 70° from vertical.
- Adjust IR height so that top of IR will be at the level of the axilla.
- With the patient facing the unit and feet forward exactly like CC view, place the arm of the side being imaged forward and hand on the bar toward the front.
- Pull breast tissue and pectoral muscle **anteriorly** and **medially away from chest wall.** Push the patient slightly toward the angled IR until the inferolateral aspect of the breast is touching the IR. The nipple should be in profile.
- Apply compression slowly with the **breast held away from the chest wall and up** to prevent sagging.
- The upper edge of the compression device will rest under the clavicle and the lower edge will include the inframammary fold.
- Wrinkles and folds on the breast should be smoothed out and compression applied until taut.
- If necessary, have patient gently retract opposite breast with other hand to prevent superimposition.
- The marker should be placed high and at the axilla.

Central Ray

- Perpendicular, centered to the base of the breast, the chest wall edge of the IR; CR not movable
- **SID:** Fixed, varies with manufacturer, about 60 cm (24 inches)

Collimation Use appropriate cone/collimation.

Respiration Suspend breathing.

Note: To show **all** of the breast tissue on this projection with a large breast, two IRs may be needed, one positioned higher to get all of the axillary region and a second IR positioned lower to include the main part of the breast. Position AEC chamber to appropriate position to ensure adequate exposure of various tissue densities.

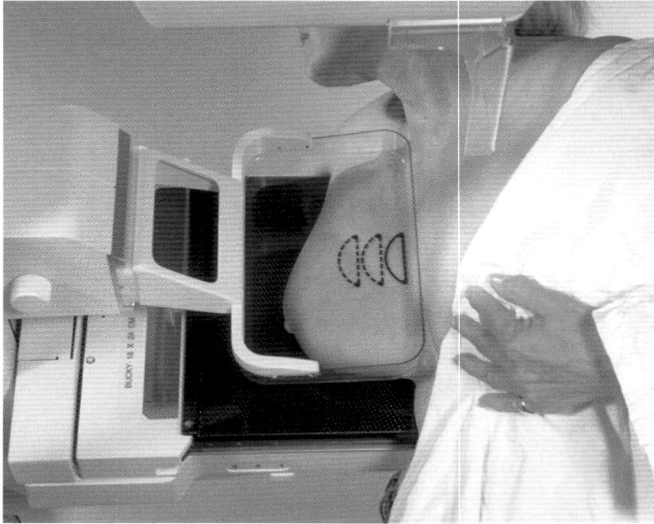

Fig. 18-27. MLO projection. (Note x-ray tube/film unit angled about 45°; see Fig. 18-26.)

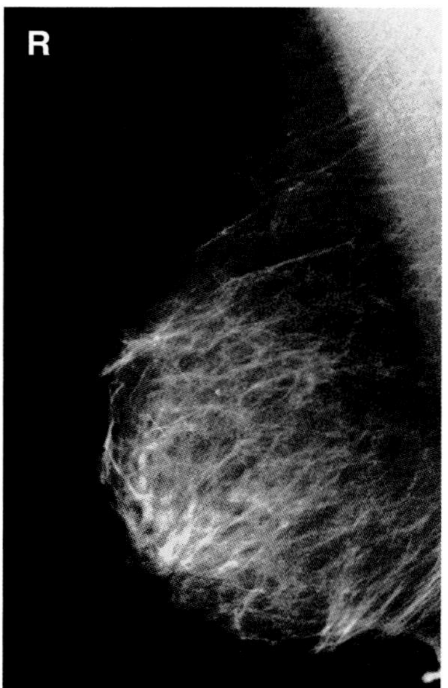

Fig. 18-28. MLO projection. (Modified from Ballinger PW, Frank ED: Merrill's atlas of radiographic positions and radiographic procedures, ed 10, St. Louis, 2003, Mosby.)

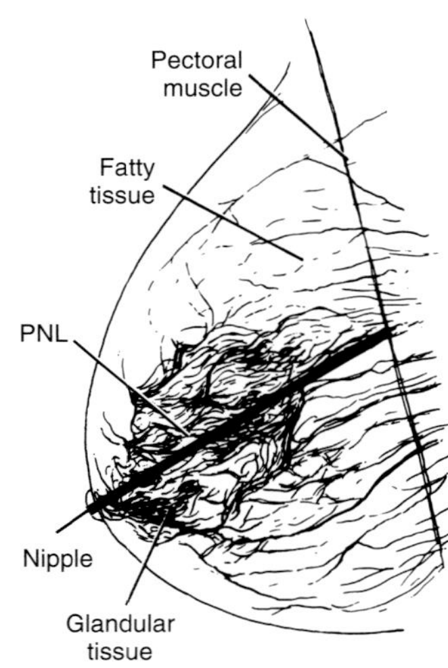

Fig. 18-29. MLO projection. PNL should be within 1 cm of the PNL of CC projection (Fig. 18-25).

Radiographic Criteria

Structures Shown: • Entire breast tissue is visible, from the pectoral muscle to level of nipple. • The inframammary fold (IMF) must be seen and the breast must not be drooping.

Position and Compression: • Nipple is seen in profile. • Breast is seen to be pulled out and away from chest with even thickness indicating optimum compression.

Collimation and CR: • CR and collimation are fixed and will be centered correctly if breast tissue is correctly centered and visualized on IR.

Exposure Criteria: • Dense areas are adequately penetrated, resulting in optimal contrast. • Sharp tissue markings indicate no motion. • R or L marker and patient information are correctly placed at axillary side; no artifacts are visible.

MEDIOLATERAL (ML) PROJECTION—TRUE LATERAL BREAST POSITION

Mammogram
SPECIAL
• Mediolateral (ML)

Pathology Demonstrated
Breast pathology is demonstrated, especially inflammation or other pathology in the lateral aspect of breast.

This projection may be requested by the radiologist as an optional projection to confirm an abnormality seen only on the MLO. This is also useful for evaluating air-fluid levels in structures, such as milk of calcium.

Technical Factors

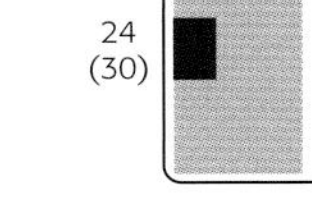

- IR size—18 × 24 cm, crosswise, or 24 × 30 cm, crosswise
- Grid
- 25 to 28 kV
- Technique and dose:

kV	mAs	Sk.	MGD
25	85	983	151

mrad

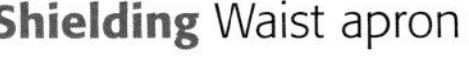

Shielding Waist apron

Patient Position Standing; if not possible, seated

Part Position
- Tube and IR remain at right angles to each other as **CR is angled 90°** from vertical.
- Adjust IR height to be centered to midbreast.
- With patient facing the unit feet forward, place arm of the side being imaged forward and the hand on the bar toward the front.
- Pull breast tissue and pectoral muscle anteriorly and medially away from the chest wall. Push the patient slightly toward IR until the inferolateral aspect of the breast is touching the IR. The nipple should be in profile.
- Apply compression slowly with the breast held away from the chest wall and up to prevent sagging. After paddle has passed the sternum, rotate patient until breast is in a true lateral position.
- Wrinkles and folds on the breast should be smoothed out and compression applied until taut.
- Open inframammary fold by pulling abdominal tissue down.
- If necessary, have patient gently retract opposite breast with other hand to prevent superimposition.
- The marker should be placed high and at the axilla.

Central Ray
- Perpendicular, centered to the base of the breast, the chest wall edge of the IR; CR not movable
- SID: Fixed, varies with manufacturer, about 60 cm (24 inches)

Collimation Use appropriate cone/collimation.

Respiration Suspend breathing.

Note: Position AEC chamber to ensure adequate exposure of various tissue densities.

Radiographic Criteria

Structures Shown: • Lateral view of entire breast tissue includes axillary region, pectoral muscle, and open IMF.

Position and Compression: • Nipple is seen in profile; tissue thickness is evenly distributed on the IR indicating optimum compression. • Axillary breast tissue (generally including pectoral muscle) is included, indicating correct centering and IR vertical placement.

Collimation and CR: • CR and collimation chamber are fixed and will be centered correctly if breast tissue is correctly centered and visualized on IR.

Exposure Criteria: • Dense areas are adequately penetrated, resulting in optimal contrast. • Sharp tissue markings indicate no motion. • R and L markers and patient information are correctly placed at axillary side of IR. No artifacts are visible.

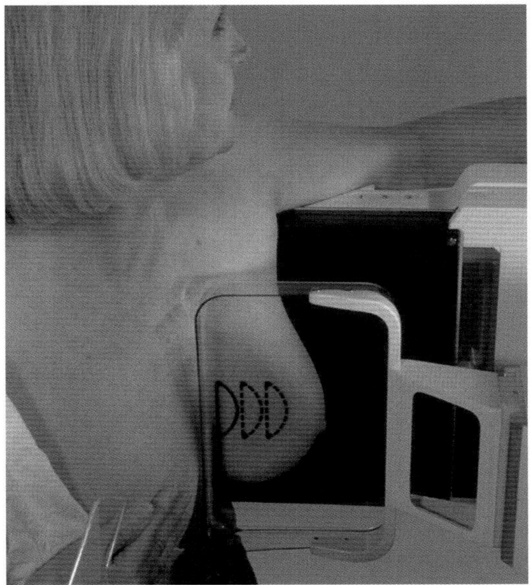

Fig. 18-30. ML projection.

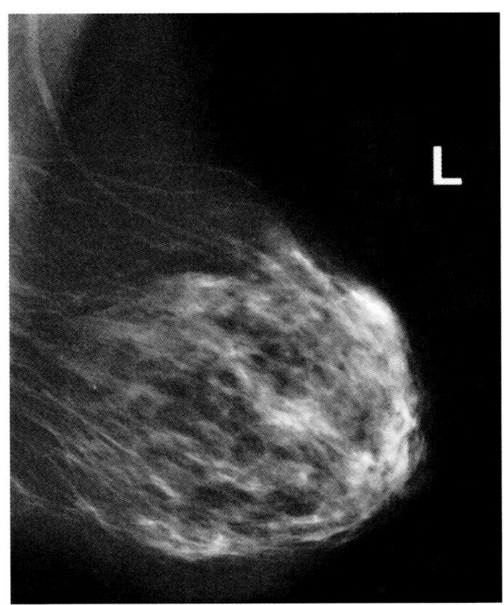

Fig. 18-31. ML projection.

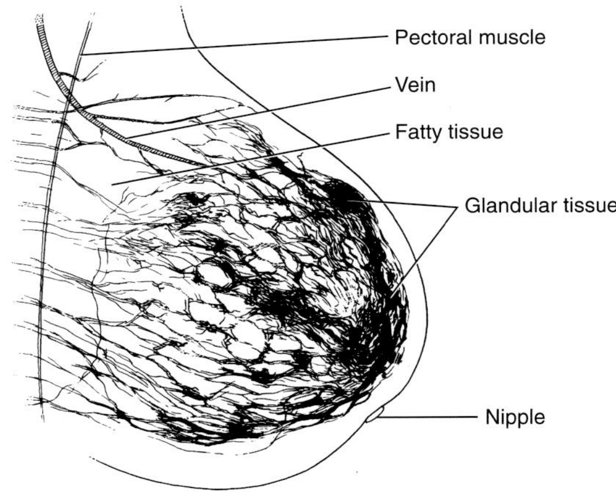

Fig. 18-32. ML projection.

18

EXAGGERATED CRANIOCAUDAL (LATERALLY) (XCCL) PROJECTION: MAMMOGRAM

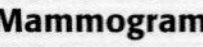

Mammogram
SPECIAL
• **Mediolateral (ML)**
• Exaggerated craniocaudal (laterally) (XCCL)

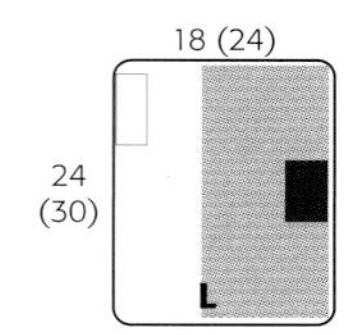

Pathology Demonstrated
Projection demonstrates potential breast pathology or change in breast tissue. It also emphasizes axillary tissue.

This is the most frequently requested optional projection when the CC projection does not show all the axillary tissue or when a lesion is seen on the MLO but not on the CC.

Technical Factors
- IR size—18 × 24 cm, crosswise or 24 ×30 cm, crosswise
- Grid
- 25 to 28 kV
- Technique and dose:

kV	mAs	Sk.	MGD
25	75	867	133

mrad

Shielding Waist apron

Patient Position Standing; if not possible, seated

Part Position
- Begin as if to do a CC projection, then **rotate the body** slightly as needed to include more of the **axillary** aspect of breast (Fig. 18-33).
- Put the patient's hand on the bar toward the front and relax the shoulder. (Some recommend angling the tube 5° mediolaterally.)
- The head is turned away from the side being imaged.
- The breast is pulled forward onto the IR, wrinkles and folds should be smoothed out, and compression is applied until taut. The nipple should be in profile.
- The marker is always placed on the axillary side.

18

Central Ray
- Perpendicular, centered to the base of the breast, the chest wall edge of the cassette; CR not movable
- SID: Fixed, varies with manufacturer, about 60 cm (24 inches)

Collimation Use appropriate cone/collimation.

Respiration Suspend breathing.

Note: If a lesion is deeper, do an **AT (axillary tail)** view.

If a lesion is not found on lateral aspect of breast, do **medially exaggerated craniocaudad** view.

Position AEC chamber to appropriate position to ensure adequate exposure of various tissue densities.

Radiographic Criteria

Structures Shown: • Axillary breast tissue, pectoral muscle, and central and subareolar tissues are included.

Position and Compression: • Nipple is seen in profile. • Tissue thickness is evenly distributed, indicating optimum compression. • Axillary tissues, including pectoral muscle, are visualized, indicating correct positioning with sufficient body rotation.

Collimation and CR: • CR and collimation are fixed and will be centered correctly if breast tissue is correctly centered and visualized on IR.

Exposure Criteria: • Dense areas are adequately penetrated, resulting in optimal contrast. • Sharp tissue markings indicate no motion. • R and L markers and patient information are correctly placed at axillary side of IR. • No artifacts are visible.

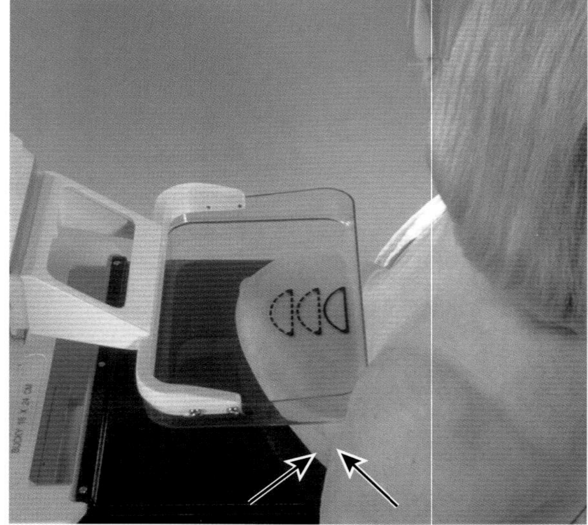

Fig. 18-33. XCCL projection.
Note: Patient is turned so that axillary tissue *(arrows)* is included on the image. Arm and hand are forward for ease in turning body.

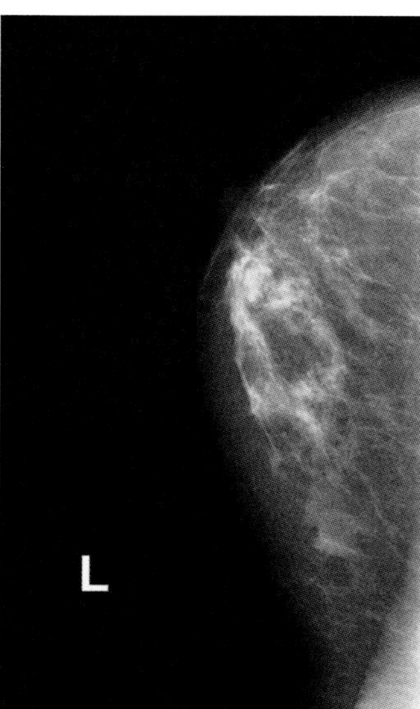

Fig. 18-34. XCCL projection.

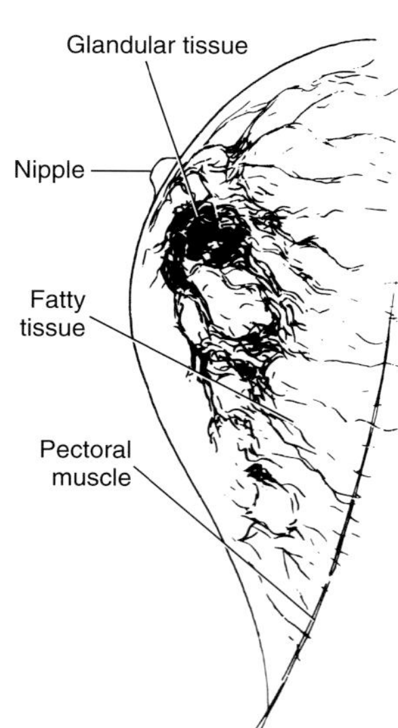

Fig. 18-35. XCCL projection.

IMPLANT DISPLACED (ID) PROCEDURE

Eklund Method*

Warning: Extreme care and precautions must be taken during this implant displaced procedure to prevent rupture of the augmented implant.

Pathology Demonstrated

Projection allows detection and evaluation of breast pathology underlying the implant, plus potential complications to breast augmentation, such as intracapsular or extracapsular leakage of implant.

Patients undergoing breast implant procedures for size and shape enhancement also require routine mammography. However, a slightly different technique is used, as follows:

Mammogram
SPECIAL
• **Mediolateral (ML)**
• **Laterally exaggerated craniocaudal (XCCL)**
• Implant displaced (ID) (Eklund method)

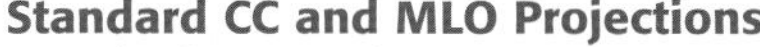

Standard CC and MLO Projections

Standard CC and MLO projections, as previously described, are done first with the implant device in place (Fig. 18-36). Caution must be used with the compression device—**firm compression cannot be accomplished.**

Eklund Method

The Eklund method of "pinching" the breast (Figs. 18-38 and 18-39) is performed after the basic CC and MLO projections. During this procedure, the implant is pushed posteriorly to the chest wall so that the anterior breast tissue can be compressed and visualized in the usual manner (Fig. 18-37).

Exception: The Eklund method can be performed on most patients with implants; however, some implants become encapsulated and only the routine views with the implant in place can be done. An additional projection such as the mediolateral or lateromedial may be helpful to demonstrate all the tissue.

Manual exposure techniques: For those projections done with the implant in place, only **manual exposure techniques should be set** on the generator because the implant will prevent the x-rays from reaching the AEC detector. **This will cause overexposure of the breast,** and the AEC system may possibly go to maximum backup exposure time.

*Eklund GW et al: Improved imaging of the augmented breast, *AJR* 151:469-473, 1988.

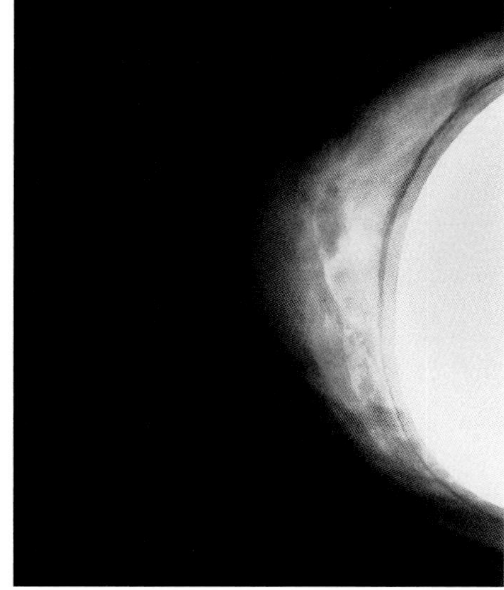

Fig. 18-36. Standard CC projection with implant in place.

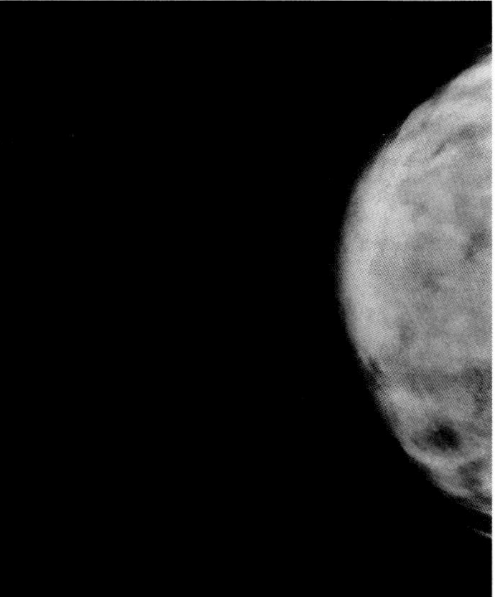

Fig. 18-37. Standard CC projection with implant pushed back. (Same patient as in Fig. 18-36.)

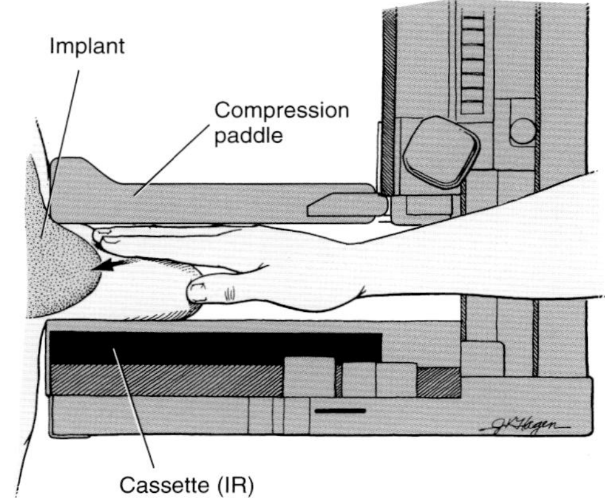

Fig. 18-38. Positioning with Eklund "pinch" technique.

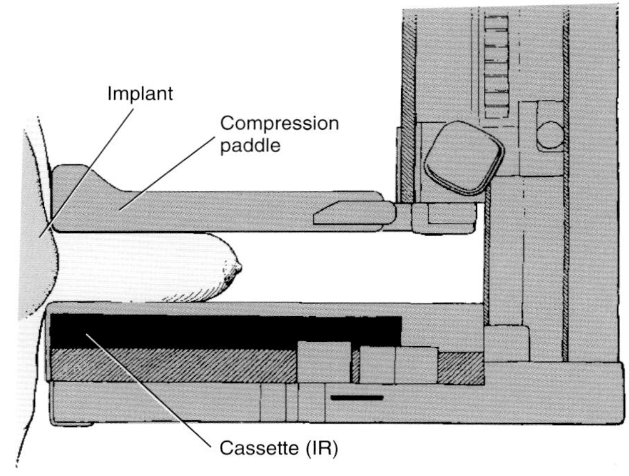

Fig. 18-39. Breast in place for CC projection with implant pushed back.

RADIOGRAPHS FOR CRITIQUE

Each of these radiographic images demonstrates one or more errors that required a repeat. Questions and answers concerning the reasons for these to be repeated are included in the student workbook/lab manuals that accompany this textbook. Answers for the repeatable errors are also provided in Appendix B, at the end of this textbook.

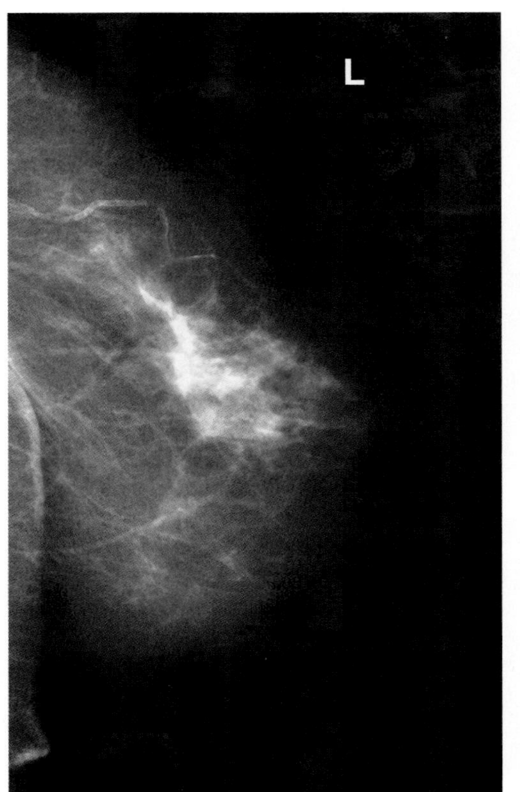

Fig. C18-40. CC projection.

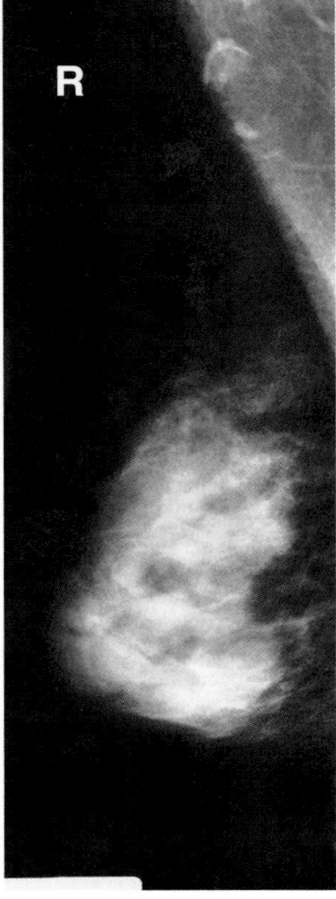

Fig. C18-41. MLO projection.

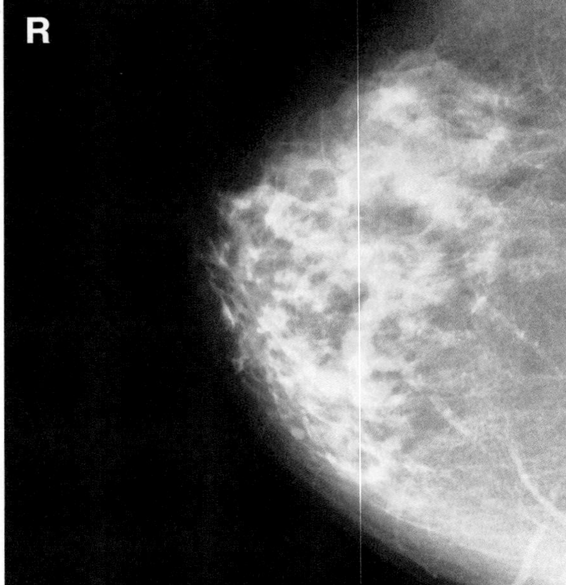

Fig. C18-42. CC projection.

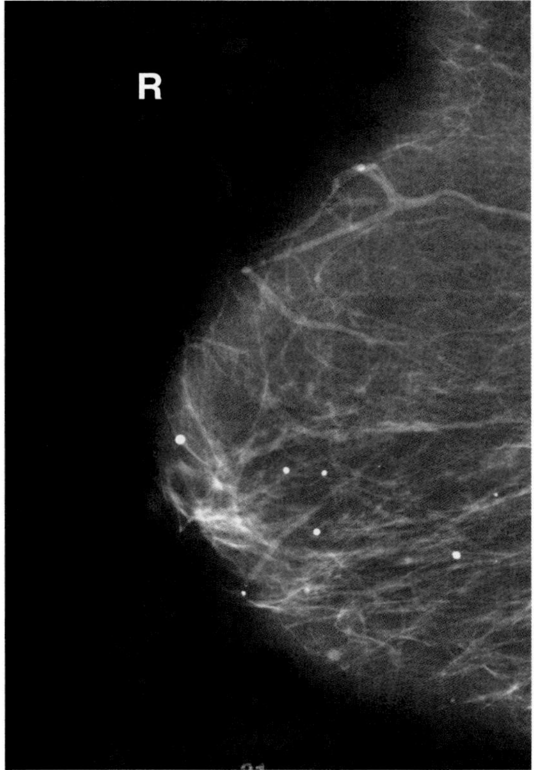

Fig. C18-43. MLO projection.

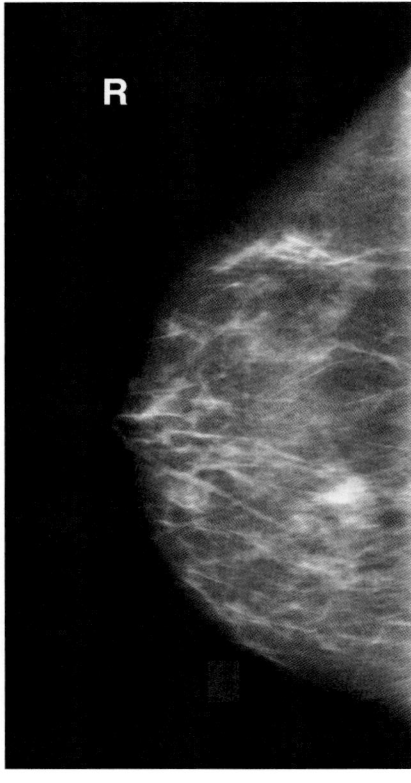

Fig. C18-44. CC projection.

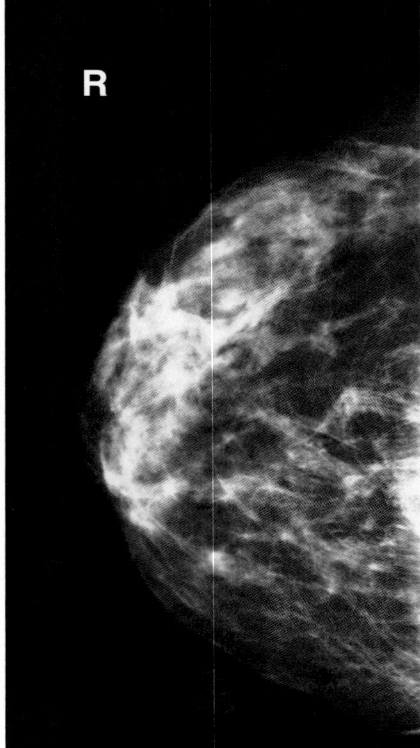

Fig. C18-45. CC projection.

CHAPTER 19

Trauma, Mobile, and Surgical Radiography

CONTRIBUTOR TO PAST EDITIONS Cindy Murphy, RT R, ACR, BHSc

CONTENTS

TERMINOLOGY, PRINCIPLES, AND EQUIPMENT

Introduction

Situations frequently arise in which the radiologic technologist encounters patients who are ill and in a weakened condition or who have experienced severe trauma, both of which require adaptations in positioning and care. This may mean that patients cannot be brought to the radiology department for radiographic procedures as described in other sections of this text. Even if patients are brought to the radiology department, they may be strapped to a backboard with a cervical collar in place or may have one or more splints, indicating possible limb fractures or dislocations. In these cases, the patients cannot be moved into the usual routine positions, and **major adaptation of CR angles and image receptor placement is required.** This may be done with a mobile (portable) x-ray unit taken to the emergency room or to the patient's room. Often all projections must be obtained with the patient in the supine position, requiring the use of stationary grids for the cross-table laterals and/or other adaptations.

This chapter introduces the radiologic technologist to **trauma** and **mobile imaging,** as well as **surgical radiography.** Certain procedures require radiographic imaging during surgery. This requires knowledge and understanding of the sterile environment encountered in surgical suites. Patients are frequently under general anesthesia, and imaging during surgery requires cooperation between the technologist, anesthesiologist, and surgeon, as well as the remainder of the surgical team.

Also described and illustrated in this chapter are commonly used terminology, positioning principles, and methods of adapting the radiographic procedure when routine projections cannot be achieved. Common types of mobile imaging equipment are described, as well as grid use principles and rules essential in trauma, mobile, and surgical radiography.

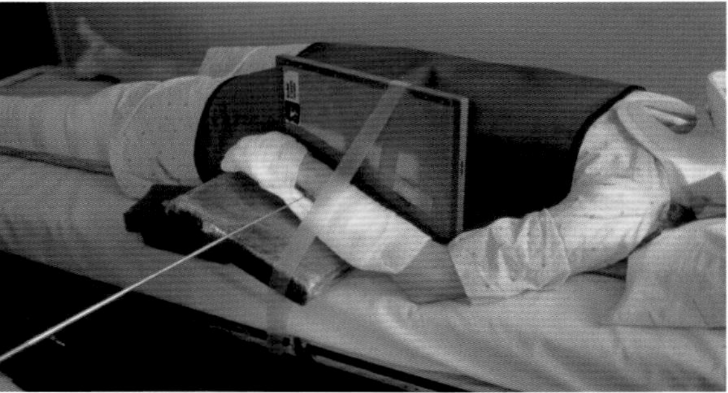

Fig. 19-1. Trauma radiography.

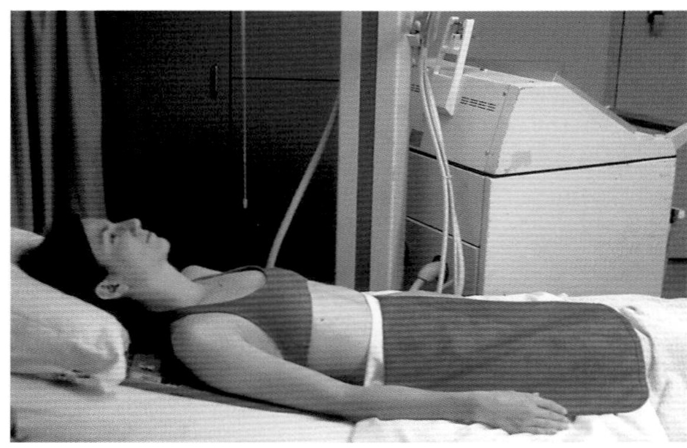

Fig. 19-2. Bedside mobile radiography.

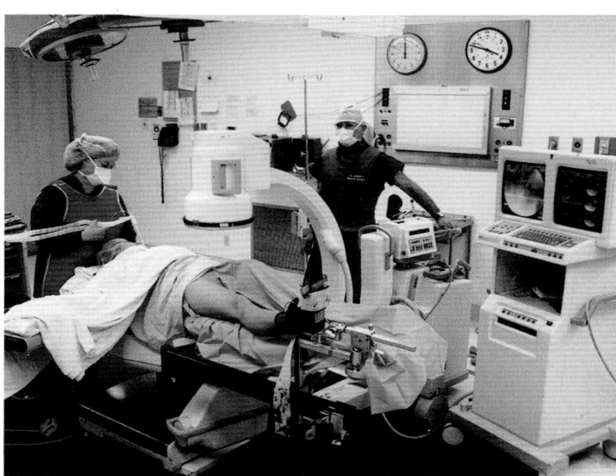

Fig. 19-3. Surgical radiography.

Digital Imaging Considerations

Computed radiography (CR) is especially well suited for trauma and mobile imaging in the emergency room (ER), in the operating room (OR), and for bedside examinations. These procedures are frequently performed under difficult but urgent conditions where opportunities for repeats are limited. The wide exposure latitude and post-processing density adjustments of CR dramatically improve the consistency of these radiographic images and greatly reduce the need for repeat exposures due to technique miscalculations.

Another advantage of CR imaging for trauma and mobile radiographic examinations is the ability to electronically transfer these images simultaneously to more than one location for interpretation or consulting.

19

Correct collimation, accurate centering, and **correct grid use** are important for all digital imaging, as described in earlier chapters of this text. These considerations are also applicable and important with the use of CR digital systems for trauma, mobile, and surgical radiographic procedures.

Alternative Imaging Modalities

COMPUTED TOMOGRAPHY

The increased speed of computed tomography (CT) scanners has contributed to the growth in use of CT for emergency imaging. CT is commonly used to accurately diagnose a wide range of traumatic conditions that affect all body systems, replacing some of the traditionally ordered diagnostic examinations, such as skull radiography. The three-dimensional reconstruction capability with CT is useful to fully assess skeletal trauma.

NUCLEAR MEDICINE

Nuclear medicine is useful in evaluation of specific emergency conditions, such as pulmonary embolus, testicular torsion, and GI bleed. Blood flow to the areas under investigation is assessed through injection of the radionuclide.

ULTRASOUND

Ultrasound is indicated in the early assessment of certain trauma patients, such as those who have had blunt abdominal injury. It is a noninvasive technique used to detect free fluid/blood in the abdomen. Ultrasound is also the modality of choice for imaging emergency conditions of the female reproductive system (e.g., ectopic pregnancy). Ultrasound is also used as required for specific emergency situations when other abdominal organs are imaged.

ANGIOGRAPHY/INTERVENTIONAL PROCEDURES

Angiography is indicated for studies of the aortic arch in the trauma patient, although it is no longer as common because of the increased use of CT for trauma studies. Interventional procedures performed on the trauma patient, as described in Chapter 21, include transcatheter embolizations to occlude hemorrhaging vessels.

Skeletal Trauma and Fracture Terminology

Skeletal trauma and surgical radiography require an understanding of terms that are unique to these situations, such as fracture/dislocation terminology. Knowing the terms that are used in patient histories or on exam requisitions allows the technologist to understand which type of injury or fracture is suspected and which projections are most important. It also helps in knowing how to avoid certain positioning techniques or body positions that may result in additional pain or injury.

Dislocation or luxation *(luk-sa'shun)*

- Dislocation (luxation) occurs when the **bone is displaced from a joint** or when the articular contact of bones that make up a joint is completely lost.*

The most common dislocations encountered in trauma are of the shoulder, fingers or thumb, patella, and hip.

Dislocations can frequently be clinically identified by the abnormal shape or alignment of the body parts, and **any movement of these parts can be painful and must be avoided.** As with fractures, dislocations should be imaged in two planes, 90° to each other, to demonstrate the degree of displacement.

If a bone has relocated itself following the injury, damage may still have occurred, and a minimum of two projections of the affected joint is required to assess for damage and/or possible avulsion fractures.

- ***Subluxation:*** **Partial dislocation** is illustrated in Fig. 19-5, in which a vertebra is displaced posteriorly.

Another example is **nursemaid's elbow ("jerked elbow"),** which is a traumatic **partial dislocation of the radial head of a child,** caused by a hard pull on the hand and wrist of a child by an adult. This frequently is reduced when the forearm is supinated for an AP elbow projection.

Sprain

- **A sprain is a forced wrenching or twisting of a joint, resulting in a partial rupture or tearing of supporting ligaments without dislocation.**

A sprain may result in severe damage to associated blood vessels, tendons, ligaments, or nerves. A severe sprain can be painful and must be handled with great care during the radiographic examination. Severe swelling and discoloration resulting from hemorrhage of ruptured blood vessels frequently accompany a severe sprain. Symptoms are similar to fractures, and radiographs aid in differentiating a sprain from a fracture.

Fracture *(fx)*

- A fracture is a **break in a bone.**

With any possible fracture, the technologist must use extreme caution in moving and positioning the patient so as not to cause further injury or displacement of fracture fragments. The technologist should **never** force a limb or body part into position. If the fracture is obvious, or if severe pain accompanies any movement, positioning should be adapted as needed.

Contusion *(kon-tu'zhun)*

- This is a **"bruise" type of injury** with a possible **avulsion fracture.** An example is a **hip pointer,** a football injury involving a contusion of bone at the iliac crest of the pelvis.

*Manaster BJ: Skeletal radiology, handbooks in radiology, St Louis, 1989, Mosby.

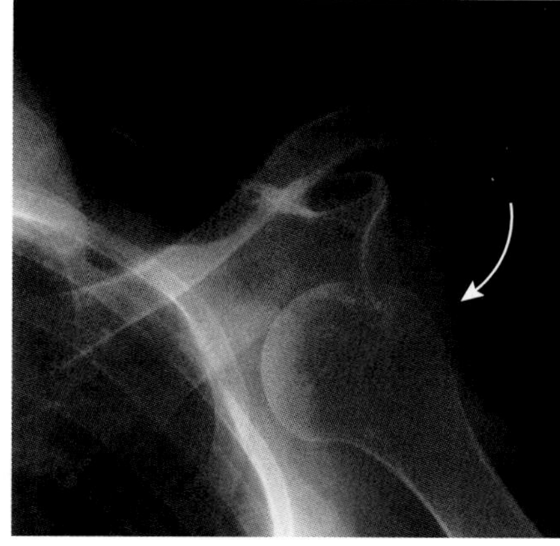

Fig. 19-4. Shoulder dislocation (AP projection).

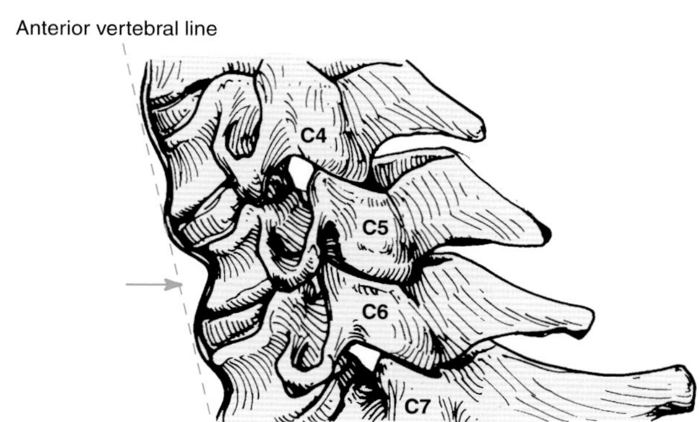

Fig. 19-5. Subluxation of cervical vertebra (C5 vertebra displaced posteriorly).

FRACTURE ALIGNMENT TERMINOLOGY

Apposition (ap″o-zish′un)

- Apposition is an alignment or disalignment describing the **relationship of the long axes of fracture fragments.**

Three types of apposition are as follows:

1. **Anatomic apposition:** Anatomic alignment of ends of fractured bone fragments, wherein the ends of the fragments make end-to-end contact
2. **Lack of apposition (distraction):** The ends of fragments pulled apart and not making contact (such as may occur from excessive traction) (Fig. 19-6).
3. **Bayonet apposition:** A fracture wherein the fragments overlap and the shafts, but not the fracture ends, make contact (Fig. 19-7)

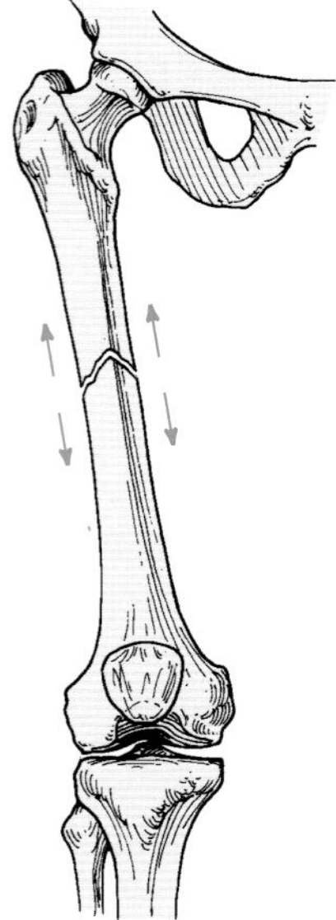

Fig. 19-6. Lack of apposition.

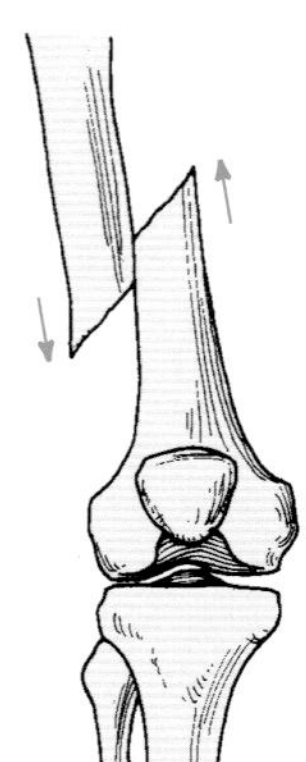

Fig. 19-7. Bayonet apposition.

Angulation

- Angulation refers to the **loss of alignment.**

Three terms describing the type or direction of angulation are as follows:

1. **Apex angulation:** Describes the direction or angle of the apex of the fracture, such as a medial or lateral apex, wherein the point or apex of the fracture points medially or laterally
2. **Varus deformity:** The distal part of the distal fragments angled **toward the midline** of the body, a lateral apex that points away from the midline
3. **Valgus deformity:** The opposite of varus, the apex, directed toward the midline (medial apex), and the distal fragment away **from** midline

Note: *Varus* and *valgus* are also used as inversion and eversion stress movement terms (see Terminology, Chapter 1, p. 26).

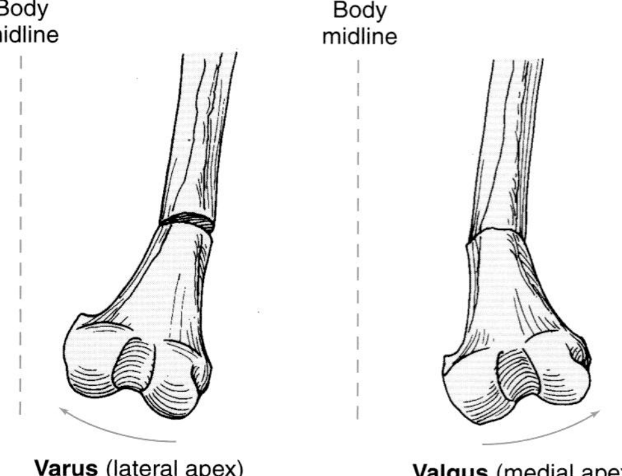

Fig. 19-8. Varus versus valgus deformity.

TYPES OF FRACTURES

Many terms are used in describing fractures. Those terms that technologists are most likely to encounter are as follows:

Simple (closed) fx

A fracture in which the bone **does not break through the skin**

Compound (open) fx (Fig. 19-9)

A fracture in which the **bone protrudes through the skin**

Incomplete (partial) fx

- This fracture **does not traverse through entire bone.** (The bone is not broken into two pieces.) It is most common in children.

Two major types of incomplete fractures are as follows:

1. **Torus fx:** This buckle of the cortex is characterized by localized expansion or torus of the cortex, possibly little or no displacement, and **no complete break in the cortex.**
2. **Greenstick fx *(hickory or willow stick):* Fracture is on one side only.** The cortex on one side of bone is broken, and the other side is bent. When the bone straightens, a faint fracture line in the cortex may be seen on one side of bone and a slight bulging or wrinklelike defect on the opposite side (Fig. 19-10).

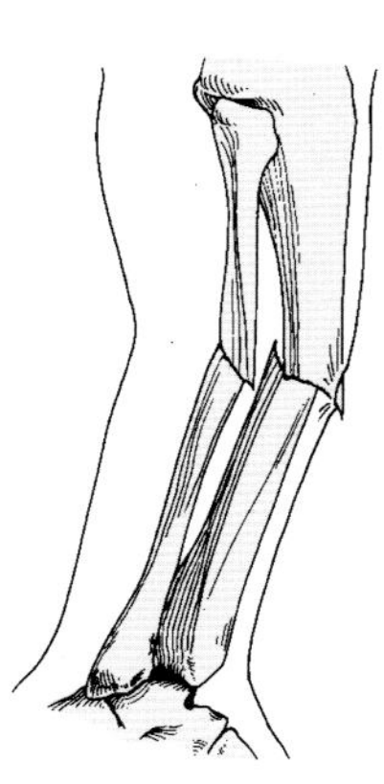

Fig. 19-9. Compound fx (tibia-fibula).

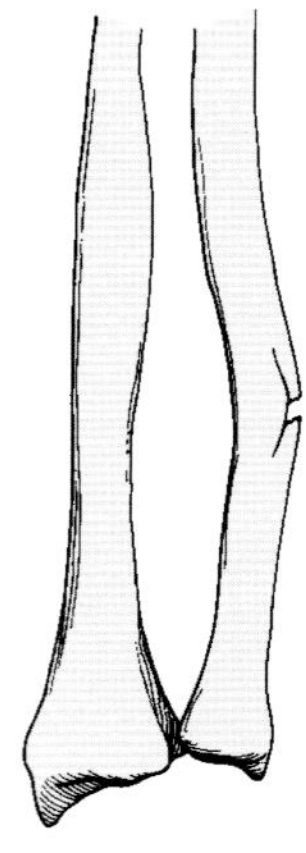

Fig. 19-10. Greenstick fx (ulna).

Complete fx

- In this fracture the **break is complete** and includes the cross-section of bone. The bone is **broken into two pieces.**

Three major types of complete fractures are as follows:

1. **Transverse fx:** Fracture is transverse at a **near right angle** to the long axis of the bone.
2. **Oblique fx:** Fracture passes through bone at an **oblique angle.**
3. **Spiral fx:** In this fracture the bone has been twisted apart and the fracture **spirals** around the long axis (Fig. 19-11).

Comminuted (kom'i-nut-ed) fx

- In this fracture the bone is **splintered or crushed** at the site of impact, resulting in **two or more fragments** (Fig. 19-12).

Following are three types of comminuted fractures that have specific implications for treatment and prognosis, because of the possible substantial disruption of blood.

1. **Segmental fx:** A type of double fracture with **two fracture lines isolating a distinct segment of bone**
2. **Butterfly fx:** A comminuted fracture with **two fragments on each side of a main, wedge-shaped separate fragment;** has some resemblance to the wings of a butterfly
3. **Splintered fx:** A comminuted fracture in which the bone is **splintered into thin, sharp fragments**

Impacted fx

- In this fracture **one fragment is firmly driven into the other,** such as the shaft of the bone being driven into the head or end segment. These most commonly occur at distal or proximal ends of femur, humerus, or radius (Fig. 19-13).

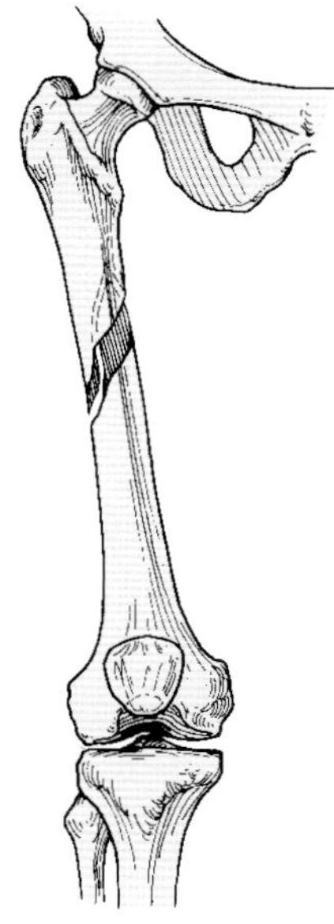

Fig. 19-11. Spiral fx (femur).

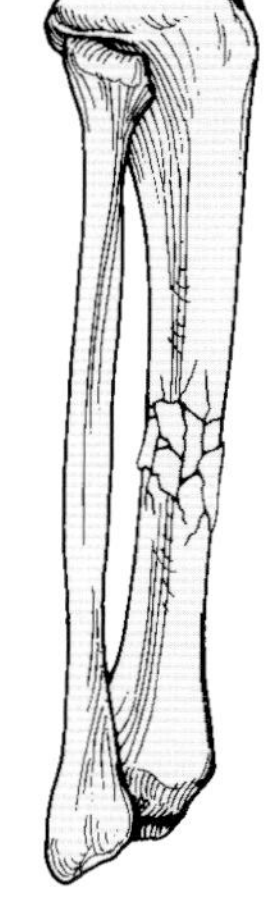

Fig. 19-12. Comminuted fx (tibia).

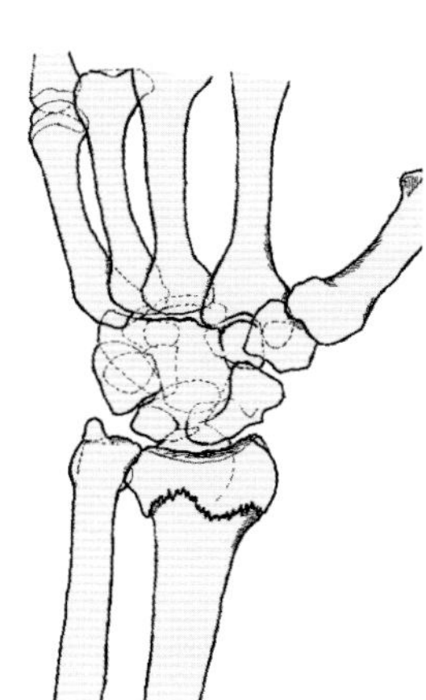

Fig. 19-13. Impacted fx (radius).

Specific "Named" Fractures

Following are some examples and descriptions of "named" fractures, usually named by the type of injury or after the person identifying them.

Barton's fx

- This is an intraarticular fracture of the **posterior lip of the distal radius.**

Baseball (mallet) fx

- This fracture of the **distal phalanx** is caused by a ball striking the end of an extended finger. The distal interphalangeal (DIP) joint is partially flexed, and an avulsion fracture frequently is present at the posterior base of the distal phalanx.

Bennett fx

- This longitudinal fracture, occurring at the **base of the first metacarpal** with the fracture line entering the **carpometacarpal joint,** generally includes posterior dislocation or subluxation.

Boxer's fx

- This fracture most commonly involves the **distal fifth metacarpal** with an apex posterior angulation best demonstrated on the lateral view. It results from punching someone or something.

Colles' (kol'ez) fx

- This fracture of the wrist in which the **distal radius is fractured** with the distal fragment **displaced posteriorly** (apex anterior angulation) results from a fall on an outstretched arm.

Hangman's fx

- This fracture occurs through the pedicles of the axis (C2), with or without displacement of C2 or C3.

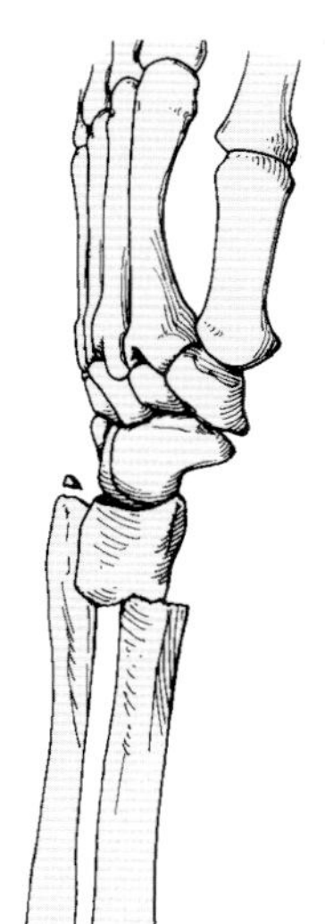

Fig. 19-14. Colles' fx (radius).

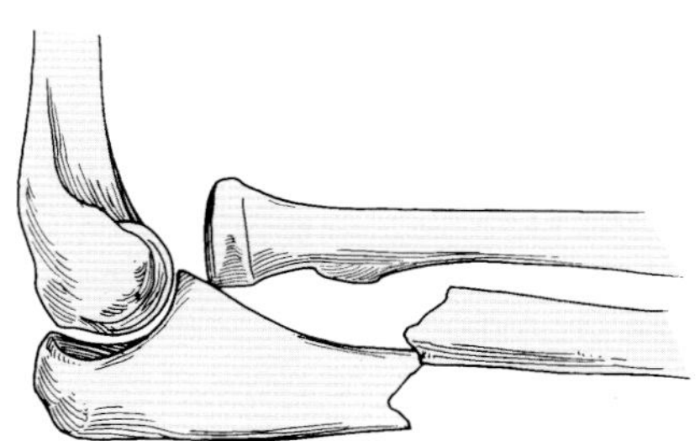

Fig. 19-15. Monteggia's fx (ulna).

Hutchinson's (chauffeur's) fx

- This is an **intraarticular fracture of the radial styloid process.** (The name originates from the time when hand-cranked cars would backfire, with the crank striking the lateral side of the distal forearm.)

Monteggia's (mon-tej'ahz) fx

- This fracture of the **proximal half of the ulna,** along with **dislocation of the radial head,** may result from defending against blows with the raised forearm.

19

Pott's fx

- This old term is used to describe a complete fracture of the **distal fibula** with major injury to ankle joint, including ligament damage and **frequent fracture of distal tibia or medial malleolus.**

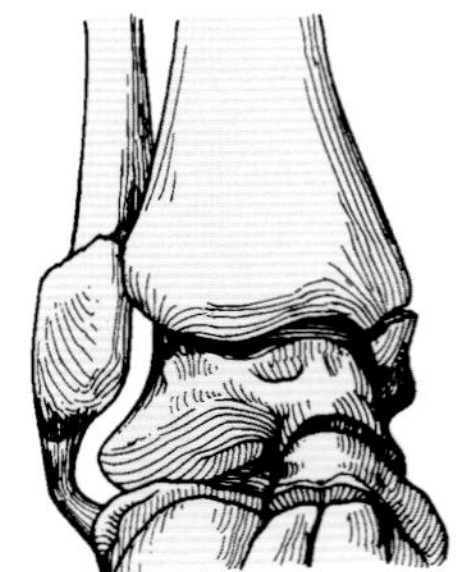

Fig. 19-16. Pott's fx (distal tibia-fibula).

Smith's (reverse Colles') fx

- This is a fracture of the **distal radius with anterior displacement** (apex posterior angulation).

Additional Fracture Types

Avulsion fx

This fracture results from severe stress to a tendon or ligament in a joint region. A **fragment of bone is separated or pulled away** by the attached tendon or ligament.

Blowout and/or tripod fx

These fractures from a **direct blow to the orbit** and/or maxilla and zygoma are described and illustrated in Chapter 13, p. 417.

Chip fx

This fracture involves an **isolated bone fragment.** (This is **not** the same as an avulsion fracture.)

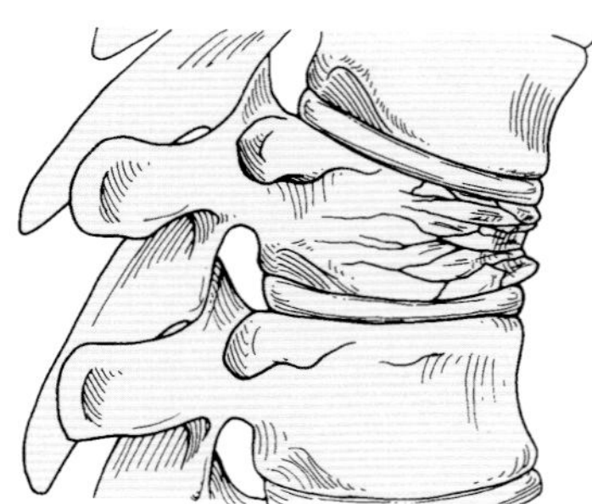

Fig. 19-17. Compression fx (body of vertebra).

Compression fx

This **vertebral fracture is caused by compression-type injury.** The vertebral body collapses or is compressed.

Generally, it is most evident radiographically by a decreased vertical dimension of the **anterior vertebral body.**

Depressed fx (sometimes called a "ping-pong" fx)

In this **fracture of the skull,** a fragment is depressed. Appearance is similar to a ping-pong ball that has been pressed in by the finger, but if the indentation can be elevated again, it can assume its near-original position.

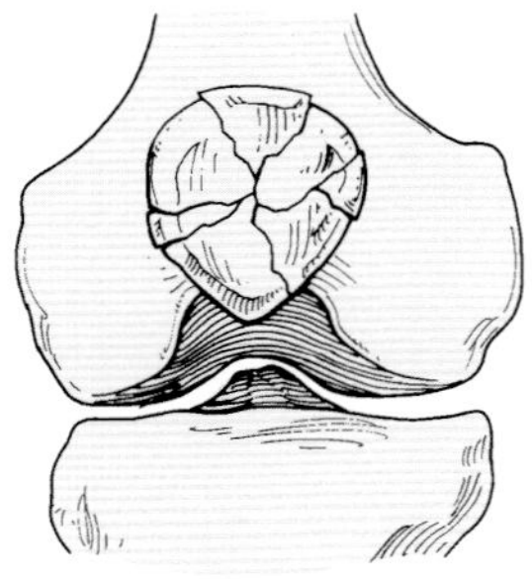

Fig. 19-18. Stellate fx (patella).

Epiphyseal fx

This is a fracture **through the epiphyseal plate,** the point of union of the epiphysis and shaft of a bone.

This is one of the most easily fractured sites in long bones of children. Radiologists commonly use the **Salter-Harris classification** (Salter 1-5) for describing the severity and reasonable indication of prognosis of these fractures.*

Pathologic fx

These fractures are due to **disease process within the bone,** such as osteoporosis, neoplasia, or other bone diseases.

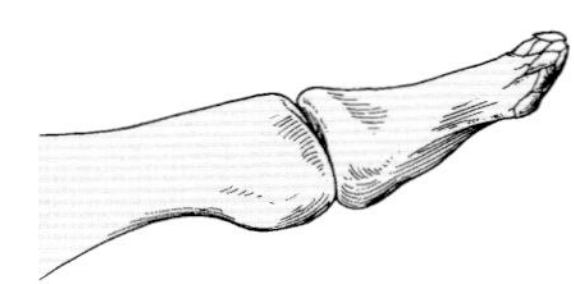

Fig. 19-19. Tuft fx (distal phalanx).

19

Stellate fx

In this fracture the **fracture lines radiate from a central point** of injury with a starlike pattern. The most common example of this type of fracture is at the patella, often caused by knees hitting the dashboard in a motor vehicle accident.

Stress or fatigue fx (sometimes called a "march" fx)

This type of fracture is **nontraumatic in origin.** It results from repeated stress on a bone such as from marching or running. If from marching, these fractures usually are in the midshafts of metatarsals; if from running, they are in the distal shaft of the tibia. Stress fractures are frequently difficult to demonstrate radiographically and may be visible only by subsequent callus formation at the fracture site or by a nuclear medicine bone scan.

Trimalleolar fx

This fracture of the ankle involves both the **medial and lateral malleoli** and the **posterior tip of the distal tibia.**

Tuft or burst fx

This **comminuted fracture of the distal phalanx** may be caused by a crushing blow to the distal finger or thumb.

*Manaster BJ: Skeletal radiology, handbooks in radiology, ed 2, St Louis, 1997, Mosby.

POSTFRACTURE REDUCTION

Closed Reduction Fracture fragments are realigned by manipulation and immobilized by a cast or splint. A **closed reduction** is a **nonsurgical procedure.**

Open Reduction For severe fractures with significant displacement or fragmentation, a surgical procedure is required. The fracture site is exposed, and screws, plates, or rods are installed as needed to maintain alignment of the bony fragments until new bone growth can take place. This is called an **open reduction with internal fixation (ORIF),** as described in the Surgical Radiography section of this chapter.

Follow-up **postreduction radiographs** are generally required for both closed and open reductions. These radiographs must include two projections taken at right angles to each other (Figs. 19-20 and 19-21) to fully assess the fracture reduction.

Fluoroscopy with a mobile C-arm is being used increasingly for open and closed reductions.

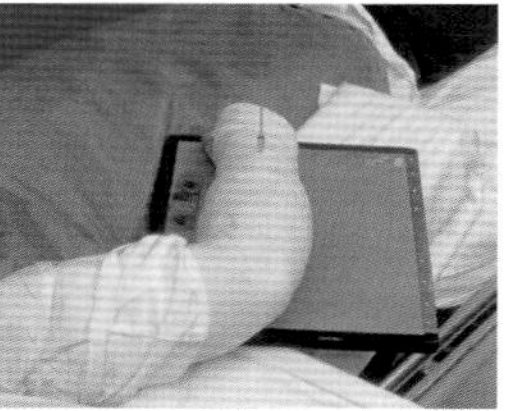

Fig. 19-20. Postreduction PA forearm and wrist.

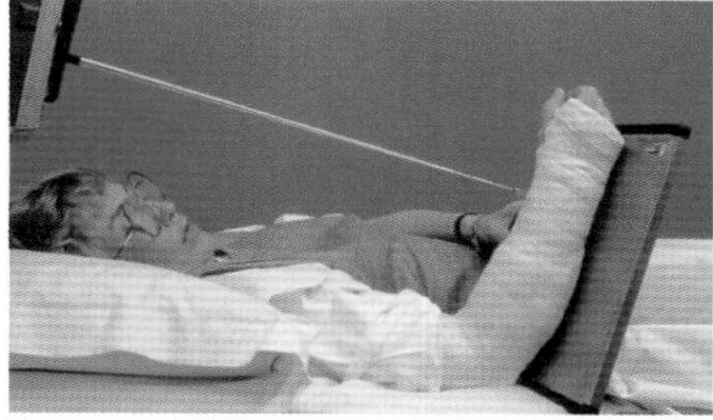

Fig. 19-21. Postreduction lateral forearm and wrist.

Positioning Principles for Trauma and Mobile Radiography

Positioning principles for trauma and mobile radiography are similar to those for routine general radiography, as described in Chapter 1 of this text. The primary difference can be summarized with the word ***adaptation.*** Each trauma patient and situation is unique, and the technologist must evaluate the patient and **adapt CR angles and IR placement as needed.**

PRINCIPLE ONE—TWO PROJECTIONS 90° TO EACH OTHER WITH TRUE CR–PART–IR ALIGNMENT

Principle One states that trauma radiography generally requires **two projections at 90° (or right angles to each other)** while maintaining a true CR–part–IR alignment.

The preferences for the two projections are a **true AP or PA** and a **true lateral** achieved by either turning the body part (standard positioning) **or angling the CR and IR as needed** (trauma adaptation positioning). In this way the **CR–part–IR alignment can be maintained even if the patient cannot be turned or rotated.** An example is shown in Figs. 19-22 and 19-23, in which true AP and lateral foot images are obtained without flexing or moving the lower limb. The AP projection is achieved by angling the CR and IR in relation to the foot, thus maintaining a true CR–part–IR alignment.

This same adaptation principle can be applied to **any body part,** as will be demonstrated throughout this chapter.

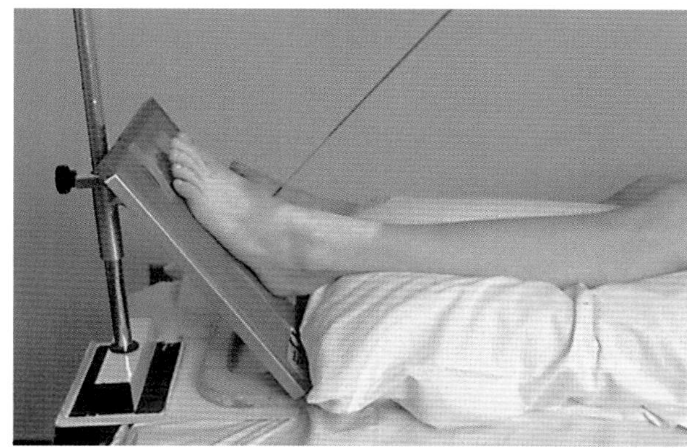

Fig. 19-22. AP foot (trauma adaptation positioning).

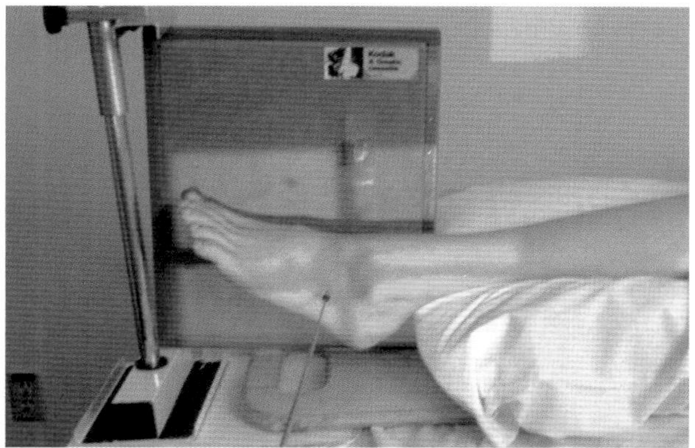

Fig. 19-23. Lateral foot.

Exception to True AP (PA) and Lateral Principle As a result of patient condition, occasionally it may not be possible to maintain this standard CR–part–IR relationship for both the true AP (PA) and lateral projections. It may be impossible because of unavoidable obstructions such as large splints, back supports, traction bars, or other apparatus. The technologist should still attempt two projections as near 90° to each other as possible, even if both projections are partially obliqued. **Only as a last resort should just one projection be taken.** When these exceptions are unavoidable, a note should be made on the patient's history sheet or exam requisition explaining the reason for this variance in routine.

Exception to CR–Part–IR Alignment Generally this principle includes placing the IR at right angles or perpendicular to the CR for minimum part distortion. However, in situations such as that shown in Fig. 19-24 the CR–part relationship can be maintained but not the part-IR relationship. In this example, the oblique cervical spine is obtained with the patient supine and the IR flat on the table under the patient. This will result in some part distortion, but in trauma radiography it may be an acceptable option.

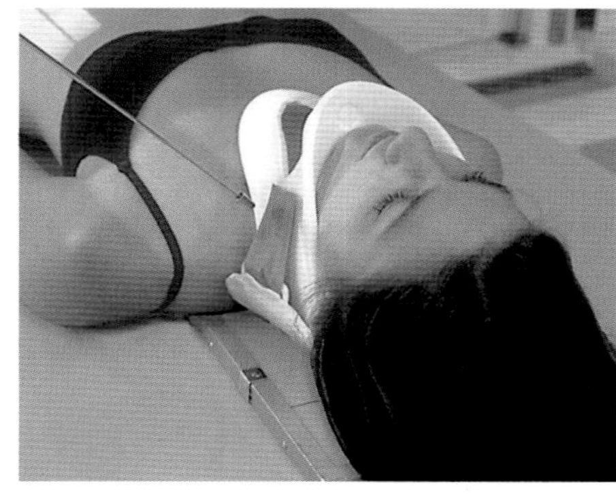

Fig. 19-24. Trauma oblique C-spine exception. IR is not perpendicular to CR.

PRINCIPLE TWO—INCLUDE ENTIRE STRUCTURE OR TRAUMA AREA ON IR

Principle Two of trauma radiography states that it is important that the **entire structure being examined be included on the radiographic image** to ensure that no pathology is missed. This requires selection of sufficiently large image receptors or the use of more than one IR if needed.

Upper and Lower Limbs If an exam request on a trauma patient includes long bones of the upper or lower limbs, **both joints should be included** for possible secondary fractures away from the primary injury. An example is a posttrauma exam request for a leg (tibia-fibula) with the injury to the distal region. This may require a second, smaller IR of the knee to include the proximal tibia-fibula region if the patient's leg is too long to be included on one image. Fractures of the distal tibia may also have a secondary fracture of the proximal fibula. This principle of including both joints is true for AP and lateral projections.

"Always Include a Joint" Rule For **all** upper and lower limb follow-up exams, **always include a minimum of one joint nearest the site of injury.** No exceptions to this rule exist, even if the obvious fracture shown on previous images is in the midshaft region. The joint nearest the fracture site should **always** be included.

Bony Thorax, Chest, and Abdomen Principle Two, including the entire structure or trauma region, applies to these larger body areas also. For example, the abdomen on a large patient may require two IRs placed crosswise to include the entire abdomen. This may also be true for the chest or bony thorax.

Horizontal Beam Lateral Trauma patients often arrive in a supine position, and horizontal beam (cross-table) projections are commonly required for the lateral projections. Care must be taken so that **the divergent x-ray beam does not project the body part off the IR,** especially when the IR is placed on edge directly beside the patient. This is true for the spine, skull, or other parts that rest directly on the tabletop. An example of this is demonstrated in Figs. 19-27 and 19-28 of a horizontal beam lateral skull with and without a possible spine injury. With a questionable spinal injury, the **head and neck cannot be moved or elevated,** and therefore no support or pad can be placed between the head and tabletop. If the IR cassette is placed on edge next to the patient's head, the divergent x-ray beam will project the posterior part of the skull off the IR.

To avoid cutoff of the posterior skull in this example, the patient can be moved to the edge of the table or cart, and the IR placed below the level of the tabletop (Fig. 19-28). This may result in an increase in OID, with resultant magnification. In such situations, this is an acceptable option. Any mAs adjustment required may be calculated using the inverse square law formula.

If cervical spine radiographs have ruled out cervical fracture or subluxation, the head may then be raised and supported by a sponge to prevent posterior skull cutoff (Fig. 19-27).

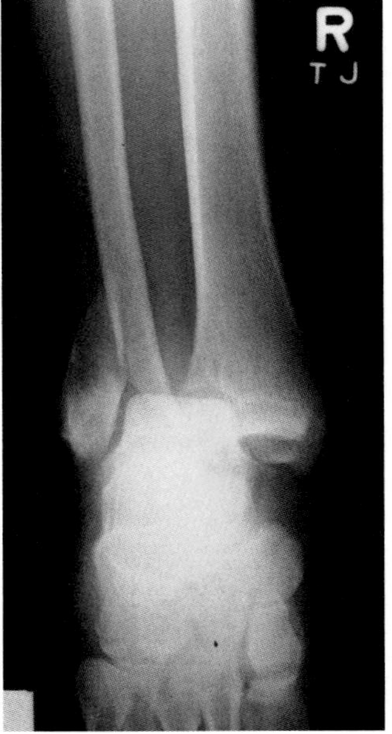

Fig. 19-25. AP distal leg and ankle.

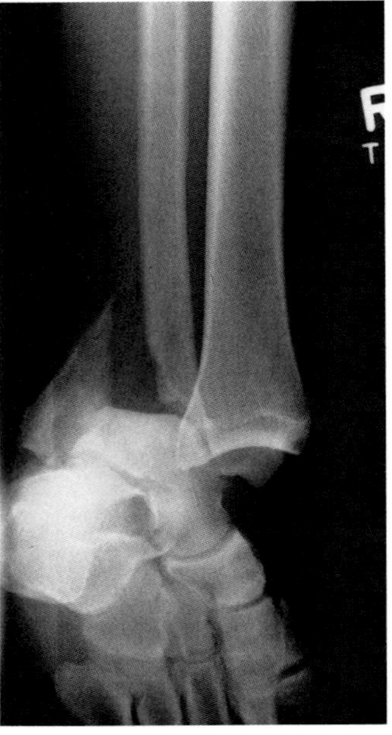

Fig. 19-26. Lateral distal leg and ankle.

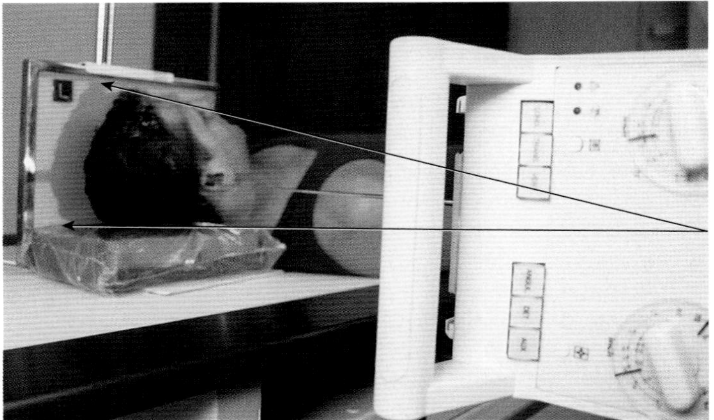

Fig. 19-27. Horizontal beam lateral skull **without** possible spine injury (head raised from tabletop).

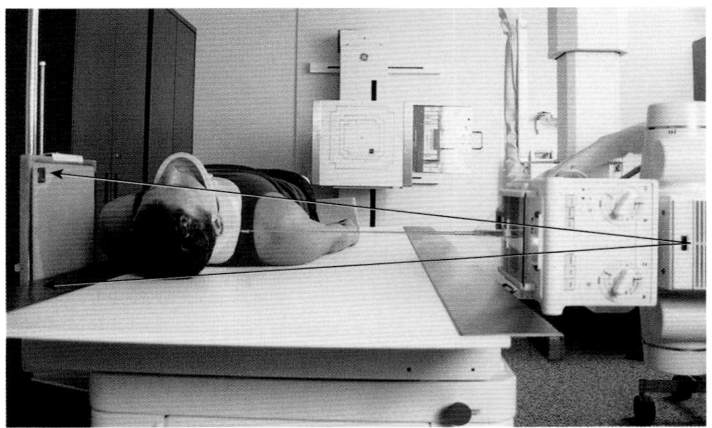

Fig. 19-28. With possible spine injury, head **cannot** be raised or moved (cassette is placed below tabletop level to prevent posterior skull cutoff).

USE OF GRIDS

Grids should generally be used for all body parts measuring more than **10 cm.** This means that except for distal upper and lower limbs and for smaller children, grids are commonly used for trauma or mobile radiographs. Part swelling, splints, and backboards result in additional scatter because of the increase in part thickness, and a higher kV may be required, which makes the use of grids essential.

Preventing grid cutoff is a challenge in trauma and mobile radiography because of required adaptations in CR–part–IR alignments.

Grid Use Rules

Successful use of grids requires an understanding of the principles and rules to prevent grid cutoff, which can occur when these rules are violated. Slight grid cutoff is evident by the areas of decreased density (Fig. 19-29). More severe grid cutoff will completely obliterate all or part of the radiographic image (Fig. 19-30).

Grid cutoff can be avoided by following the rules concerning grid use relating to (1) **CR centering,** (2) **CR angling,** (3) **grid focal range** (minimum and maximum SID range), and (4) **tube side of grid.**

1. CR centering The CR must always be centered along the central axis of the grid. If not, the more the CR is laterally off center from the axis or centerline of the grid, the greater the cutoff that will result. This is demonstrated by comparing Fig. 19-29, in which the CR is about 3 inches (7 cm) off center, with Fig. 19-30, where the CR is about 5 inches (12 cm) off center.

In certain clinical situations in which it is difficult to position the area of interest in the center of the grid, the grid may have to be turned so that the lead strips run perpendicular to the length of the patient to allow accurate centering (e.g., horizontal beam lateral lumbar spine).

Exception: decubitus-type linear grids: An exception to the more common lengthwise focused grid with the lead strips and center axis running lengthwise with the grid is the **decubitus-type** crosswise linear grids. This grid with the lead strips and center axis running crosswise along the shorter dimension of the grid is useful for horizontal beam decubitus type projections. For these the grid is placed lengthwise with the patient, but the CR is centered along the crosswise axis of the grid to prevent grid cutoff.

2. CR angle CR angling must be along the direction of the lead strips. Therefore any time the CR is angled and not perpendicular to the plane of the IR, the grid must be aligned so that the CR angle corresponds to the length of the grid lines. To angle across a grid more than 3 or 4 degrees would result in grid cutoff (Fig. 19-32).

3. Grid focal range Each focused grid has a focal range of minimum and maximum SID to prevent grid cutoff. The focal range is determined by the **grid frequency** (number of grid strips per inch or cm) and the **grid ratio** (height of lead strips compared with the space between them). Portable grids generally have a lower grid frequency and lower grid ratio than fixed grids or Bucky type grids. A common grid ratio for portable grids is **6:1** or **8:1** compared with **12:1** for Bucky grids. This results in a greater focal range for portable grids, but SID limitations still exist to prevent grid cutoff. Each technologist should know the types of portable grids available and the focal range of each.

4. Tube side of grid Each grid has a tube side of the grid marked as such. The lead strips are tilted or focused to allow the x-ray beam to pass through the lead strips unimpeded if the SID is within the focal range and if the grid is correctly placed with the tube side up (facing the table).

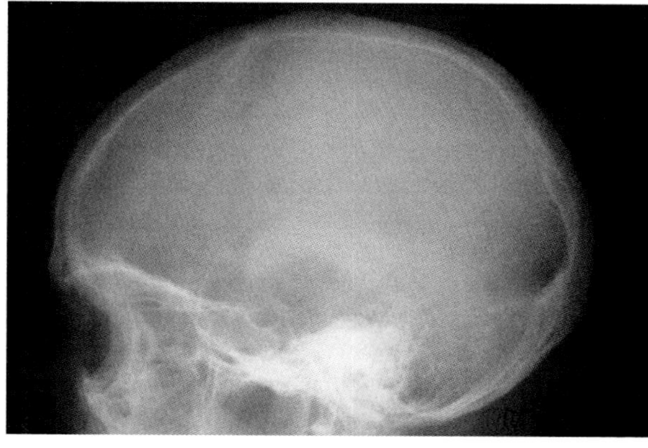

Fig. 19-29. Slight grid cutoff—CR 3 inches off center (appears underexposed).

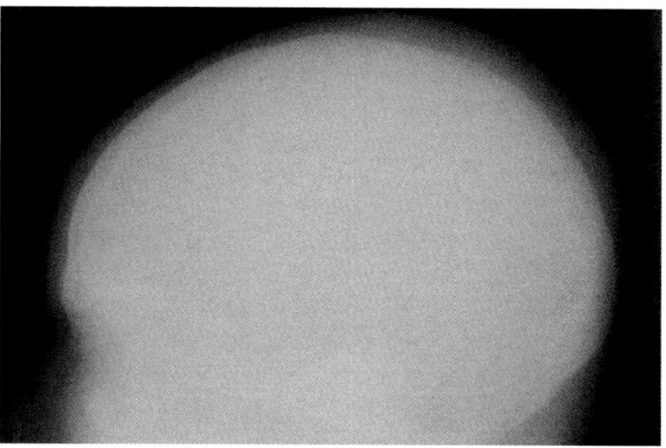

Fig. 19-30. Severe grid cutoff—CR 5 inches off center (appears severely underexposed).

1. CR must be within 1 to 1½ inches (2.5 to 4 cm) of centerline.
2. Angled CR must be along length of centerline.
3. SID must be within grid focal range.

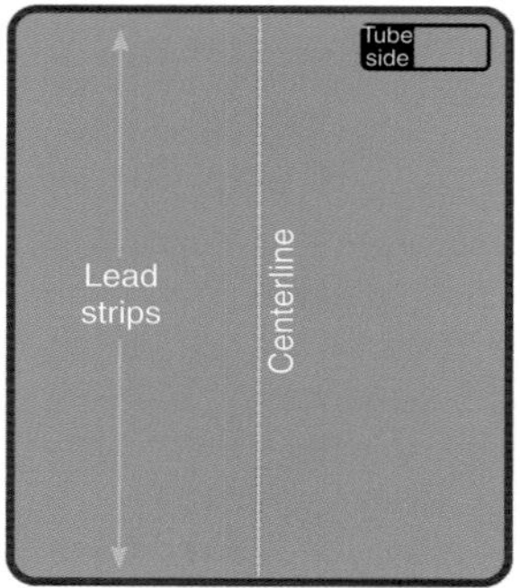

Fig. 19-31. Portable linear focused grid cassette—center axis and lead strips are lengthwise. Exception: decubitus grids, center axis, and lead strips are crosswise.

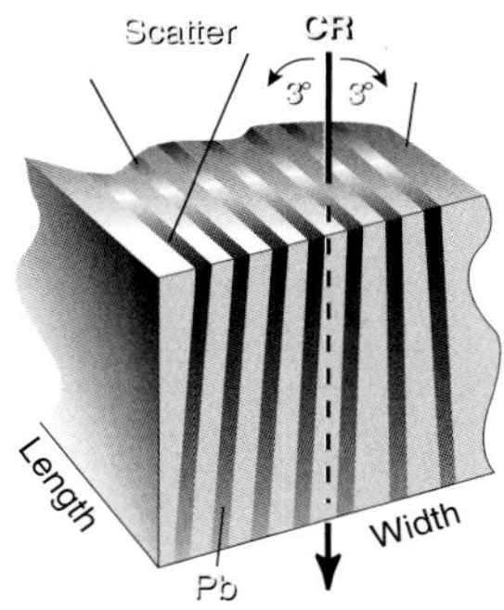

Fig. 19-32. Conventional linear focused grid—limited cross-angle of **3° to 4°**; limited CR angle along **length** of lead strips; limited focal range of **±4 inches** (10 cm) from focal point. (Courtesy Eastman Kodak.)

19

Mobile X-Ray Equipment

A study of trauma and mobile radiography requires an understanding of the functions and operations of the equipment being used. Trauma radiography may be performed either with conventional overhead tube and x-ray table or with **mobile (portable) units** that are brought to the ER, the patient's bedside, or the OR for surgical procedures.

This type of mobile x-ray machine has commonly been called a "portable." However, this is not an accurate term, because *portable* means to be carried or easily movable, and the usual type of mobile units being used today may weigh up to 1000 pounds or more.

TYPES OF MOBILE X-RAY SYSTEMS

Major advances have been made in mobile radiographic and fluoroscopic equipment in recent years. Examples of general types commonly used are described and illustrated.

Battery-Driven, Battery-Operated Mobile X-Ray Units

These systems are powered by 10 to 16 rechargeable, sealed, lead, acid-type 12-volt batteries connected in series. The self-propelled systems of these units are also battery-powered and have variable travel speeds up to an average walking speed of 2½ to 3 mph with a maximum incline of 7°. They have a driving range of up to 10 miles on the level after a full charge.

These units are driven and maneuvered by dual drive motors operating the two drive wheels. They also have a lower speed forward and reverse for maneuvering in close quarters. Parking brakes are automatically engaged when the control levers are not in use and when they are set in the charging mode.

The unit can be plugged in for recharging when not being used and can be recharged at either 110 or 220 volts. With 110-volt, 5-amp outlets, the charging time is about **8 hours** if fully discharged.

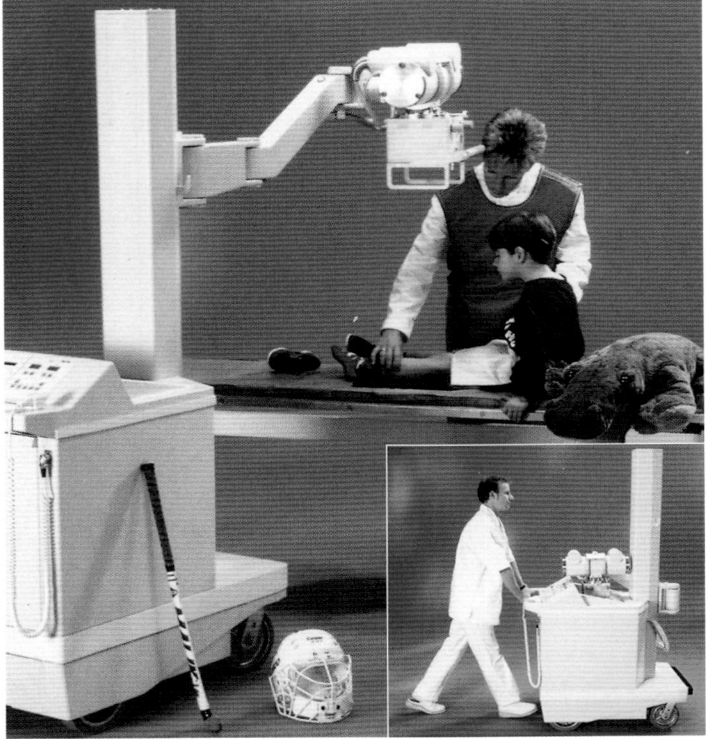

Fig. 19-33. Philips Practix 2000: battery-powered, battery-driven. (Courtesy Philips Medical Systems.)

Standard Power Source, Capacitor-Discharge, Nonmotor-Driven Units

A second type of mobile x-ray unit is available without battery power. These models are much lighter in weight and usually are not motor-driven. They operate with either a 110-volt, 15-amp power source or a 220-volt, 10-amp power source. These units generally incorporate a capacitor-discharge system, which stores electrical charges when plugged in, and then discharges this electrical energy across the x-ray tube when an exposure is initiated. This increases the electrical power (voltage) from the standard 110- or 220-volt power source.

Other systems offer a **dual power source** with both battery power and plug-in electrical power for increased power output. These generally also have a battery-assisted motor drive for easier transporting.

The controls on these units may include some type of optional **programmed memory system** based on anatomic parts, or they may have **operator-selected kV and mAs** technique controls.

Note: These are only two examples of mobile systems available. Other manufacturers offer various modifications, features, and options.

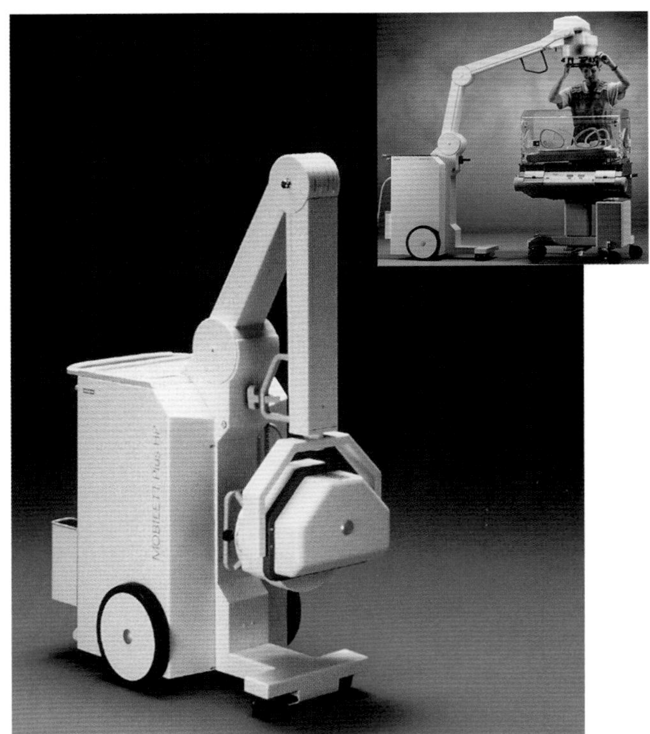

Fig. 19-34. Siemens Mobilett Plus: dual power source, battery, and/or standard power, capacity discharge. (Courtesy Siemens Medical Systems, Inc.)

Radiation Safety With Mobile X-Ray Units

Operator The operator and all persons remaining in the room during the exposure should always be wearing a **lead apron.** In addition, the operator should always be a **minimum of 6 feet (2 m)** from the x-ray tube during all exposures, even if wearing a lead apron.

Patient Lead shielding of radiosensitive organs such as the gonads on children and adults of reproductive age should be available and applied.

Mobile C-Arm Digital Fluoroscopy Systems

A third type of mobile imaging equipment is the C-arm mobile fluoroscopy system. The term *C-arm* is descriptive of this basic design of a mobile fluoroscopy unit, with the x-ray tube at one end of the C-arm and the image intensifier tower at the other end.

Familiarity with the C-arm and the monitor and image controls is essential for the technologist performing ER or OR procedures, where these systems are most commonly used. One must also become familiar with the various types of special beds or carts that are used with the C-arm. For example, a surgical bed used for operative cholangiograms may not accommodate the C-arm x-ray tube under the table in the abdominal area because of the base supports, unless the patient's head is placed at the correct end of the bed or cart, as shown in Fig. 19-35. (This OR procedure is fully described later in this chapter under Surgical Radiographic Procedures.)

Maneuverability The equipment is designed to be very maneuverable, with the C-arm itself attached to an L-shaped arm that can be raised and lowered or extended as needed. The counterbalanced C-arm can also be rotated or tilted for cephalic or caudal angles or rotated into a horizontal beam cross-table position for lateral hip or other lateral projections as needed (Fig. 19-36). It can also be rotated 180° to place the tube on top and the intensifier on the bottom, but **this is not recommended** because it increases the OID, which decreases image resolution and increases scatter radiation. The "tube on top" position also will result in **a significant increase in exposure to the head and neck area** of the surgeon or radiologist because of the exposure pattern of the C-arm in this orientation (see Fig. 19-44).

Overall, the unit is flexible to use and the technologist must be familiar with the variety of built-in joints, extensions, and adjustments. With its three-wheel base, steerable rear wheels, and a swiveling nose wheel, the operator can easily maneuver the unit into almost any possible configuration with reasonable space.

TV monitors and control cart Two monitors are generally used so that the active image can be displayed on one monitor, while the second monitor can be used to "hold an image" for reference purposes. Generally, the active monitor is on the left and the hold monitor on the right. Images can also be rotated or flipped as needed for preferred viewing by the surgeon and/or radiologist.

Uses of C-arm The technologist will use the C-arm unit with various types of procedures in which mobile fluoroscopy and/or still frame imaging is needed. Examples are surgical procedures such as cholangiograms and open reductions of fractures or hip pinnings. Other uses include various types of special procedures and interventional studies.

Images can be stored temporarily with video memory or on hard disks. Optional hard copy printers are also available for printouts. Cine loop capability is also possible, wherein images are recorded in rapid succession and then displayed as a moving (or cine) image, such as for barium swallow or injected contrast media type examinations.

As with other types of digital imaging, image enhancement and manipulation are possible, including overall brightness and contrast controls, magnification, edge enhancement, masking, and digital subtraction studies.

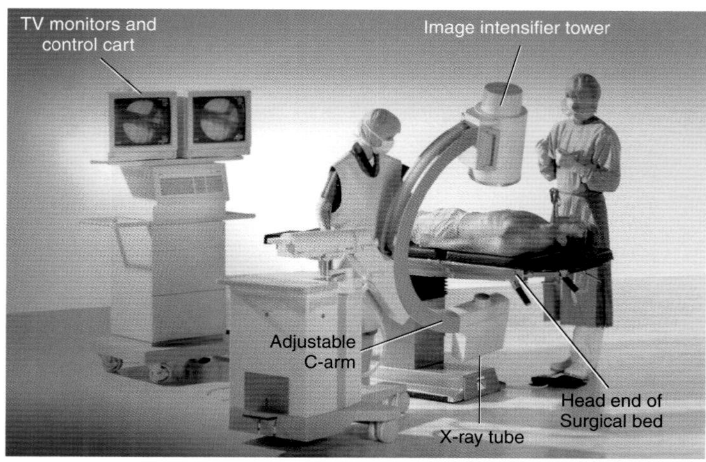

Fig. 19-35. Philips BV29 C-arm with image processor and display stand demonstrating setup for PA projections for surgical and interventional cases. (Courtesy Philips Medical Systems.)

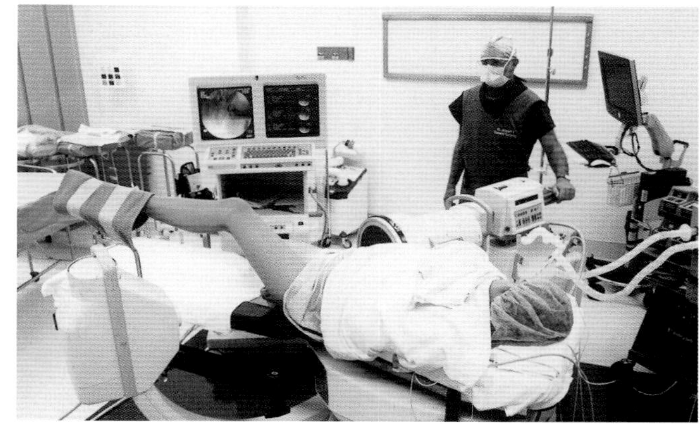

Fig. 19-36. Horizontal setup for lateral hip.

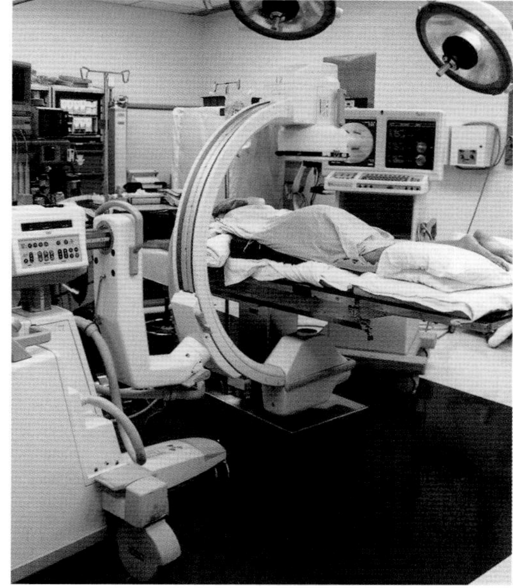

Fig. 19-37. Vertical alignment of C-arm with patient in a prone position. Note that x-ray tube is under surgical table, making this an AP projection.

19

Controls and operation modes The digital C-arm fluoroscopy systems include a variety of operating mode option controls with which the technologist must be familiar. These control panels may be on the TV monitor control cart or, in some cases, on the C-arm unit itself (Fig. 19-38).

The **magnification mode** refers to the ability to magnify the image when requested by surgeons to better visualize structures that they frequently need to view at a distance from the monitor.

The **pulse mode** is used to create a pulsating x-ray beam at timed increments to reduce exposure.

The **snapshot** or **digital spot mode** activates a "digital spot," which results in a higher-quality **computer-enhanced image** as compared with a held fluoro image.

The **film mode** is for exposing standard cassettes placed in the optional holder on the image intensifier. This **cassette holder** can be attached to the image intensifier tower in which regular cassettes are placed for conventional radiographs (Fig. 19-40). In this way the C-arm can also function as a mobile radiography unit without using the digital imaging functions.

Auto/manual exposure control allows for manual exposure control by the operator if desired or the use of AEC controls.

Additional optional modes available on some equipment that allow more complicated procedures are **subtraction** (digital subtraction) and **roadmapping.** Roadmapping is a method of image display wherein a specific fluoro image is held on the screen in combination with continuous fluoro. This is especially useful in interventional procedures requiring placement of catheters and guidewires.

Foot pedal The foot pedal allows the physician or other operator to have hands-free operation of the C-arm. A fully equipped foot pedal has multiple pedals for controlling various functions such as shown in Fig. 19-39. This specific model has four controls. The **scout fluoro** pedal operates unprocessed, or raw, fluoro functions. The **digital process fluoro** activates selected computer-enhanced processing functions such as averaging (fluoro image noise reduction). A third pedal is the **image save** control for saving the last image displayed. When activated, the pedal marked **snapshot** or **boost digital spot** results in a higher-quality computer-enhanced image.

Image Orientation

The flexibility of the C-arm to image a variety of anatomic structures at virtually any conceivable angle from any side or direction **requires correct image orientation each time it is set up for use.** This needs to be done during setup time before the patient is brought into the room to avoid needless exposure to the patient and personnel after the procedure begins. For example, attempting to orient a smaller-size image in the abdominal region, which has few landmarks to indicate top or bottom or right or left, can be very confusing and difficult.

19

Technologists should develop their own method of doing this. One method is to bring the C-arm into the room in the same position and orientation that will be used for the procedure. Place a lead marker *R* on the flat surface of the x-ray tube collimator oriented in the same way the patient will be oriented. The top of the *R* should be to the head end, to be displayed on the patient's right side, to appear anatomically correct on the monitor to the viewer's left. (This is the same orientation as for viewing radiographs, the patient's right to the viewer's left.) An exposure can be made during this setup with an apron or other shielding covering the C-arm to shield other personnel in the room. Viewing and orienting the test image of the *R* on the monitor correctly are important preparations for the procedure.

Sterile Fields

C-arm use in surgical settings requires special attention in maintaining sterile fields, as described later in this chapter under Surgical Radiography. The vertical alignment with the intensifier on top often causes it to be placed over open incisions.

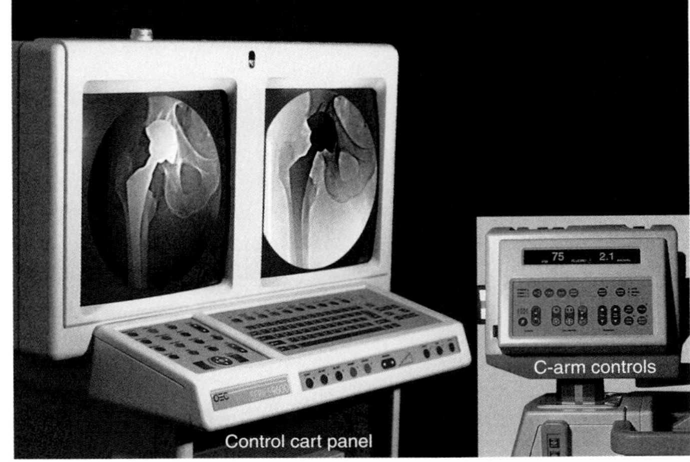

Fig. 19-38. Control panels of OEC 9600 series C-arm.

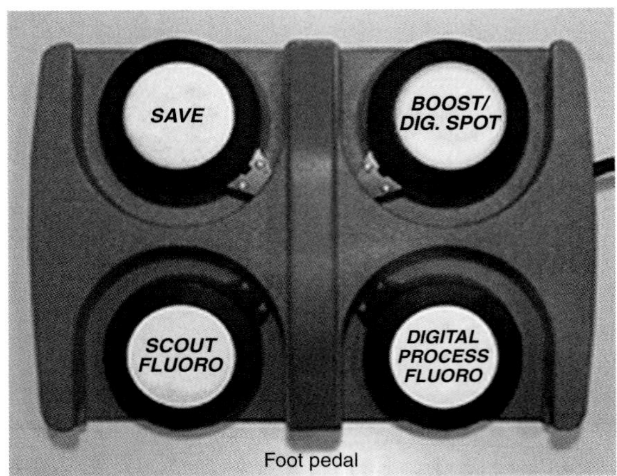

Fig. 19-39. Foot pedal controls.

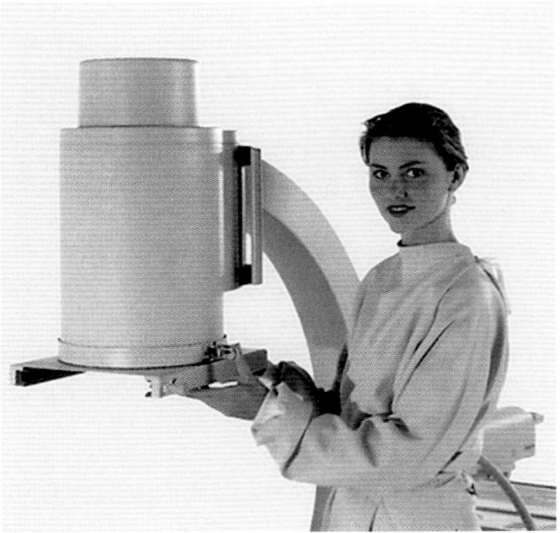

Fig. 19-40. Cassette holder attachment. (Courtesy Philips Medical Systems.)

C-Arm Orientation and Exposure Patterns

Vertical PA Projection CR Assuming the patient is supine, keeping the C-arm PA and directly vertical and perpendicular to the floor minimizes exposure to the neck and facial region (Fig. 19-41). If the C-arm is tilted as much as 30°, as shown in Fig. 19-42, the configuration of the exposure fields changes to significantly increase exposure to the upper body and facial region not shielded by the lead apron. Studies have shown that even a **30° C-arm tilt will increase the dose** to the face and neck region of the average-height operator standing next to the C-arm **by a factor of four.**[†]

Horizontal Projection CR The configuration of the exposure fields with a horizontal beam is demonstrated in Fig. 19-43. Note that the **exposure region on the x-ray tube side of the patient is significantly greater than the region near the intensifier tower.** This should be an important consideration for the surgeon or other operator who may need to stay near the patient.

Vertical AP Projection CR Occasionally the technologist may be asked to reverse the C-arm with the tube on top and the image intensifier on the bottom. This would provide the surgeon more room for manipulation; however, this is **NOT recommended** because of the **significant increase in exposure** to the operator, as shown in Fig. 19-44 (up to 100 times higher dose to the eyes of the operator).

RADIATION PROTECTION

Radiation safety is a special concern with fluoroscopy, especially with the C-arm when used as a mobile unit in an unshielded environment such as the ER or OR. Safety precautions for the C-arm follow the **three cardinal rules** of radiation protection: **distance, time,** and **shielding.**

Distance (most effective means of reducing occupational exposure) As demonstrated by the exposure fields in these drawings, the secondary fields from scatter radiation drop off dramatically with increasing distance from the source (applying the inverse square law).

Before exposures are made the technologist should remind all personnel to stand back as far as possible, even if wearing lead aprons. **Distance is critical in reducing personnel exposure.**

Time Limiting exposure time is also an effective means of radiation protection. This is especially true in fluoroscopy, where fluoro exposure times and resultant scatter radiation can be much greater than with conventional radiographs. This makes the use of the **pulse mode** more important with the C-arm, which allows pulsed fluoroscopy at a rate of only one or two frames per second with the digital recorder holding this image on the monitor between pulses. The technologist should document total fluoro time at the completion of the case.

Shielding In addition to time and distance, correct use of shielding is important. Before any C-arm fluoro procedure begins, the technologist should provide **lead aprons** for all persons remaining in the room during exposures or should provide a mobile lead shield behind which they can stand. For example, in surgical procedures the surgeon, radiologist, anesthesiologist, or other personnel who are remaining in the room and cannot move behind a shield should previously have been given lead aprons to wear under their sterile gowns.

Summary Conscientious radiation protection practices are especially important in trauma and mobile radiography, or in surgery suites where fixed protective barriers do not provide a shielded place to stand during exposures. This is true with all mobile x-ray examinations, but even more so with C-arm mobile fluoroscopy, which potentially results in considerably more scatter radiation to the immediate area and for a longer period of time. The technologist must continually be aware of the three important cardinal rules of radiation protection—**distance, time,** and **shielding.**

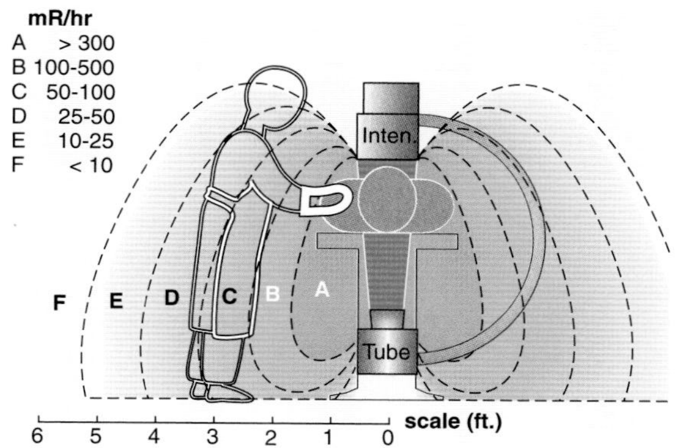

Fig. 19-41. Exposure levels—CR vertical, **PA projection**, intensifier on top.*†
(Least exposure to operator)

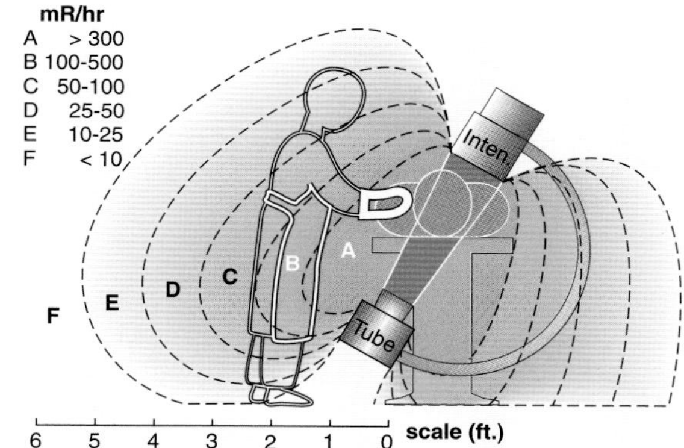

Fig. 19-42. Exposure levels—CR 30° from vertical. *†
(CR angle increases exposure to operator)

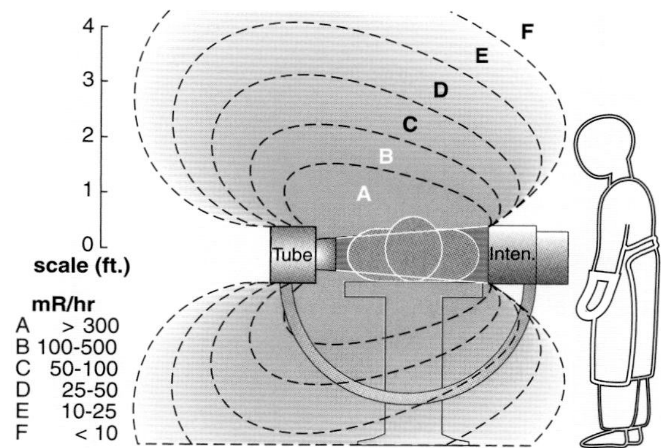

Fig. 19-43. Exposure patterns and levels—CR horizontal.*†
(Least exposure at intensifier side)

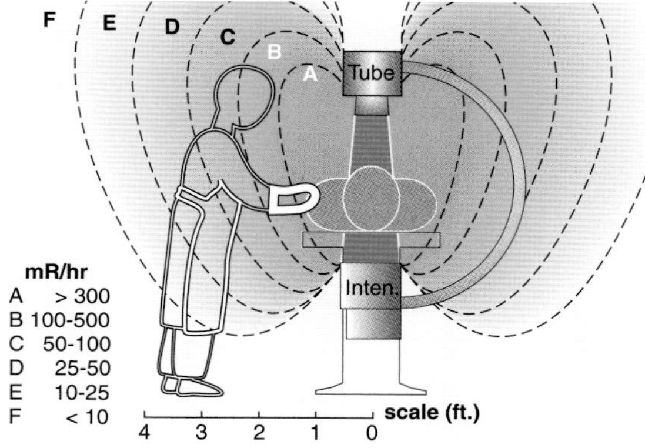

Fig. 19-44. Exposure levels, **AP projection** (tube on top).*†
—**NOT** recommended.

*Technical reference, OEC Medical Systems, Salt Lake City, Utah, 1996.
†Geise RA, Hunter DW: Personnel exposure during fluoroscopy, *Postgrad Radiol* 8, 1988.

19

TRAUMA AND MOBILE POSITIONING

AP CHEST

Warning: With possible spinal injury or severe trauma, do not attempt to move the patient. In these situations the patient will often be on a backboard. Obtain assistance from other medical personnel when placing the IR beneath the board. Some ER stretchers or tables have a tray under the patient in which to place the IR.

Technical Factors

- IR size—35 × 43 cm (14 × 17 inches), **crosswise,** for average to large patients (see Note 1)
- 90-120 kV, depending on whether grid is required (see Note 2)

Shielding Shield pelvic region if patient is of childbearing age.

Positioning (for patient who is able to be moved)

- Enclose IR in a pillow slip or some other type of cover so that it does not make contact with patient's bare skin (for hygiene purposes and for easier IR placement).

Bedside chest: Elevate head end of bed if possible into an erect position. If patient is able to attain only a semierect position, the CR must be angled to maintain the perpendicular relationship with the IR (Fig. 19-46).

- Place top of IR about 1½ to 2 inches (5 cm) above the shoulders, which should center IR to CR.
- Rotate arms internally, if patient's condition allows, to move scapulae out of lung fields.
- Ensure **no rotation** (coronal plane parallel to IR). (Place supports under parts of IR as needed.)

Central Ray

- Direct CR to 3 to 4 inches (7 to 10 cm) below jugular notch.
- Angle CR 3° to 5° caudad, or raise head end of bed slightly to place the CR perpendicular to long axis of sternum (unless grid prevents this). This simulates the PA projection and prevents the clavicles from obscuring the apices of the lungs (Fig. 19-45).
- SID is 48 to 72 inches (122 to 180 cm). Use 72 inches (180 cm) if possible.

Respiration Expose at end of second full inspiration.

Optional lateral chest (not demonstrated here): A lateral image using a horizontal beam CR can be obtained if patient can raise arms at least 90° from body. Place IR parallel to MSP, top of IR 2 inches (5 cm) above level of shoulders. Support patient on radiolucent pad to center chest to IR, and center horizontal CR to level of T7.

Lateral decubitus AP projection: To determine air-fluid levels when patient cannot be elevated sufficiently for erect position, a lateral decubitus can be taken in bed with IR placed behind patient, or on a stretcher in front of IR holder, as shown in Fig. 19-47. Place radiolucent pads under thorax and shoulders, and raise arms above head. CR–part-IR alignment and centering are similar to supine AP with necessary adaptations for decubitus position.

Note 1: Costophrenic angle cutoff is a problem with recumbent chest positions taken with a shorter SID because of the divergence of the x-ray beam. Therefore unless the patient is quite small, a **crosswise IR placement is recommended.**

Note 2: Focused grids are generally difficult to use for mobile chests because of the problems of grid cutoff.

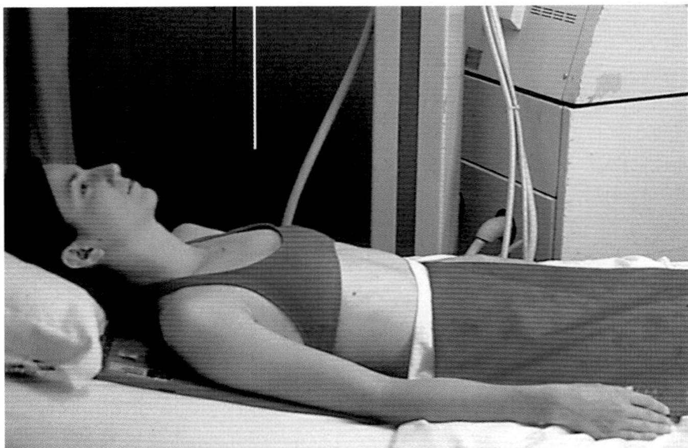

Fig. 19-45. AP supine—bedside (IR crosswise)—CR 3° to 5° caudad, perpendicular to sternum.

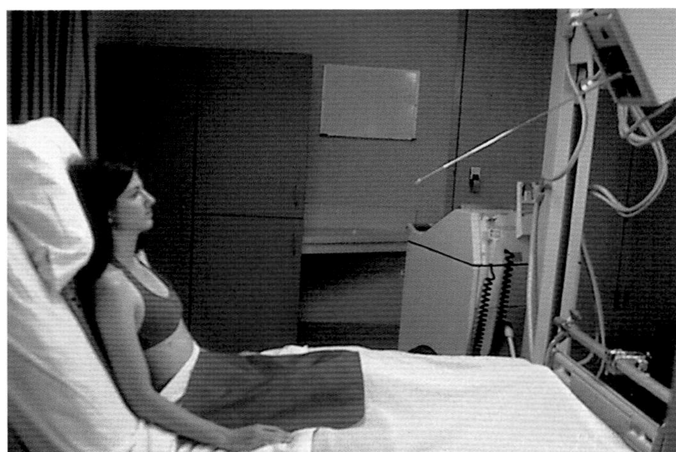

Fig. 19-46. AP semierect—bedside.

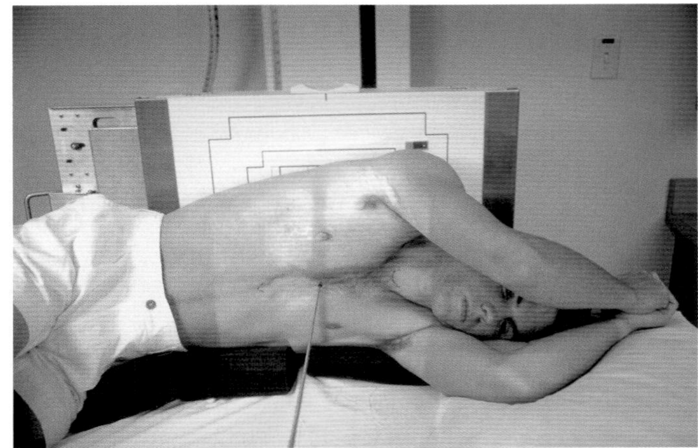

Fig. 19-47. Lateral decubitus (AP), horizontal beam for detecting possible air-fluid levels.

19

AP OBLIQUE AND LATERAL STERNUM

The sternum is nearly impossible to visualize radiographically on a straight AP/PA projection because of the thin, flat bone being superimposed by the thoracic vertebrae. It is possible to visualize the sternum, however, by superimposing it over the homogenous heart shadow. This requires an **LPO position or an equivalent mediolateral CR angle** for a supine patient. (This CR angle results in some undesirable part distortion but may be necessary if the patient cannot be rotated into an oblique position.)

Technical Factors

- IR size—24 × 30 cm (10 × 12 inches) or 30 × 35 cm (11 × 14 inches)
- IR crosswise for supine patient position with a mediolateral angle CR to prevent grid cutoff
- 60-70 kV range with grid
- 2- to 3-second exposure breathing technique commonly used to blur out lung structures and posterior ribs; patients who can cooperate asked to breathe gentle, short breaths for movement of lungs and ribs with little movement of the sternum
- SID of 40 inches (100 cm)

Shielding Shield pelvic region if patient is of childbearing age.

Positioning and Central Ray

AP oblique—LPO (Fig. 19-48):

- If patient cannot be rotated, maintain the CR–part-IR alignment of an LPO position by angling the CR 15° to 20° mediolaterally, from right to left (see Note); or if patient's condition allows, rotate in a 15° to 20° LPO position with CR perpendicular to IR. Ensure grid is correctly aligned if using the CR angle method.
- CR is perpendicular to center of sternum with IR centered to CR.
- Place top of IR about 1½ inches (4 cm) above jugular notch, with IR centered to projected CR.

Respiration See breathing instructions above.

Note: For the oblique sternum, less body rotation or less mediolateral angle CR (>15°) is required on large, deep-chested thorax; more rotation or CR angle (>20°) for smaller thorax.

Lateral, horizontal beam (Fig. 19-49):

- With patient supine, place arms at side, with shoulders drawn back.
- Place grid IR at patient's side parallel to MSP centered to midpoint of sternum (midway between manubrial notch and xiphoid).
- Position horizontal CR to midsternum.
- Expose on full inspiration.

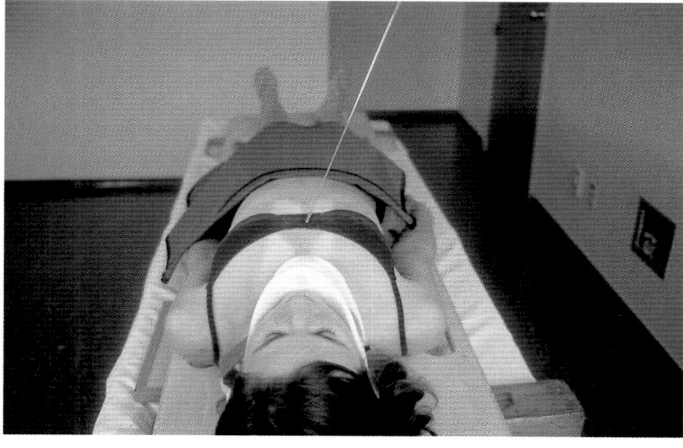

Fig. 19-48. AP supine (oblique) sternum—patient remains supine; 15° to 20° CR mediolateral angle; grid crosswise to prevent cutoff.

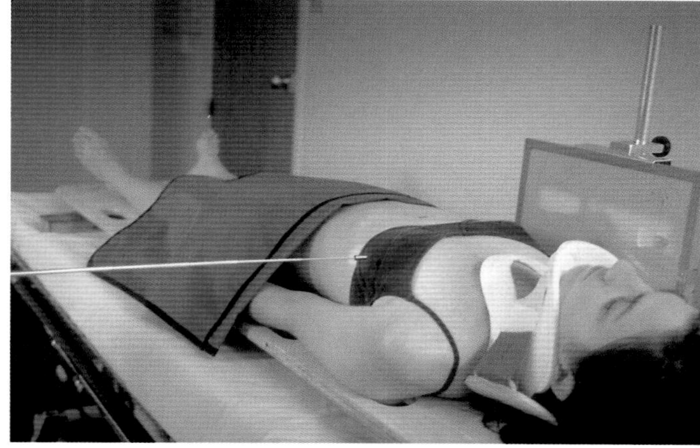

Fig. 19-49. Lateral sternum—horizontal beam CR to midsternum.

19

AP RIBS—ABOVE OR BELOW DIAPHRAGM AND OBLIQUE

If patients are able to assume the erect positions, this is less painful than radiographing ribs in the recumbent position, which places the weight of the body on the site of injury (see Chapter 11). Anterior or posterior obliques would be determined by the affected area. Severe trauma requires adaptation for oblique position with cross-angle CR, as shown in Fig. 19-52. Above or below diaphragm is determined by region of injury.

Remember the importance of including an image of the chest to assess possible lung/thoracic injury resulting from rib fracture. This chest projection, however, may require an erect or lateral decubitus position to detect air-fluid levels, which may not be possible with a trauma patient.

Technical Factors
- IR size—35 × 43 cm (14 × 17 inches), crosswise for bilateral ribs (see Note)
- 65-70 kV range, grid, above diaphragm 75-80 kV range, grid, below diaphragm
- Minimum SID of 40 inches (100 cm)

Shielding Shield pelvic region.

Positioning and Central Ray

AP above or below diaphragm (Figs. 19-50 and 19-51):
- For above diaphragm, place grid IR under patient, centered to thorax bilaterally and to CR.
- Position CR perpendicular to MSP, centered 3 to 4 inches (7 to 10 cm) below jugular notch as for an AP chest.
- For below diaphragm, place bottom of cassette at level of iliac crest.
- Place CR perpendicular to center of IR.

Oblique above or below diaphragm (Fig. 19-52):
- If patient is able, oblique patient 30° to 45°, injured side down.
- Center IR to thorax bilaterally.
- Center IR for above or below diaphragm centering.
- Direct CR perpendicular to center of IR.

Respiration
- Above diaphragm—suspend on inspiration.
  Below diaphragm—suspend on expiration.

Alternative mediolateral of CR (supine immobile patient):
- If patient cannot be rotated, the CR can be angled mediolaterally 30° to 40° with **grid IR crosswise,** centered to include region of injury (Fig. 19-52). The image will be somewhat distorted, however, unless IR is also tilted.

19

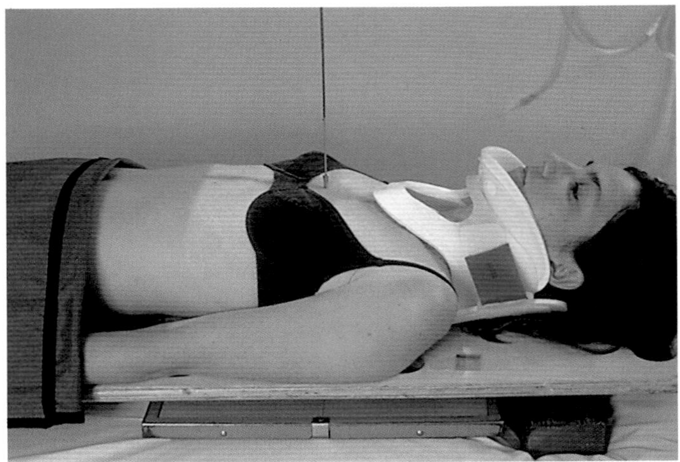

Fig. 19-50. AP ribs above diaphragm.

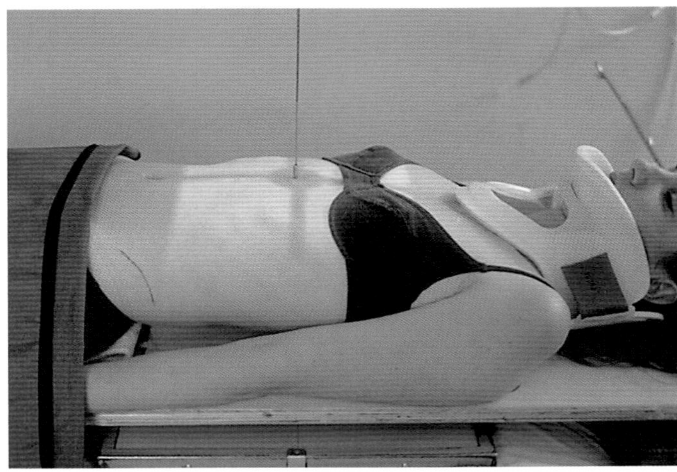

Fig. 19-51. AP ribs below diaphragm.

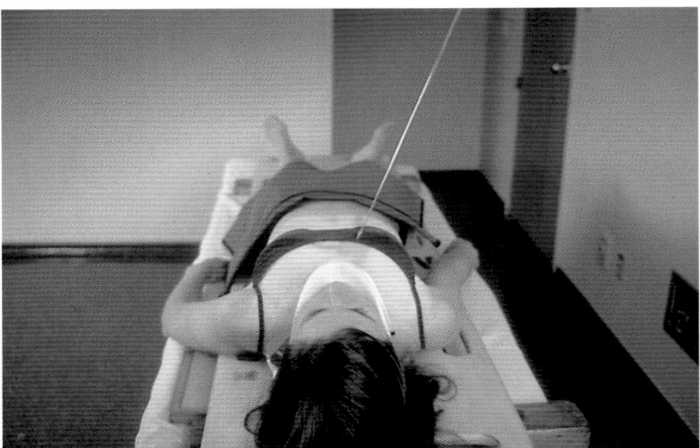

Fig. 19-52. Alternative 30° to 40° mediolateral CR—grid crosswise (results in image distortion unless IR is also tilted).

AP ABDOMEN—SUPINE AND DECUBITUS

Technical Factors
- IR size—35 × 43 cm (14 × 17 inches), lengthwise
- 70-80 kV range, with grid
- Include decubitus and upside markers if applicable
- Minimum SID of 40 inches (100 cm)

Shielding Shield male gonads.

Positioning and Central Ray

AP supine (Fig. 19-53):
- Place IR into pillowcase or cover for easier placement under patient, if taken bedside.
- Align IR lengthwise to MSP.
- Center IR to CR at **level of iliac crest.** Ensure that both sides of upper and lower abdomen are equal distances from lateral IR margins.
- Place supports under parts of IR if needed to ensure that IR is level and perpendicular to CR (prevents patient rotation and grid cutoff on soft bed surfaces).
- Position CR perpendicular to level of iliac crest and to center of IR.

Left lateral decubitus AP (or PA) projection (Fig. 19-54):
- This projection allows determination of air-fluid levels and possible free intraabdominal air when an upright image is not possible. The lateral decubitus can be taken in bed, on a stretcher in the ER, or on a stretcher in radiography room in front of an upright wall Bucky.
- Ensure that **diaphragm and upside of abdomen are included.** Place center of IR 1 to 2 inches (3 to 5 cm) above level of iliac crests.
- Place supports or a positioning board under hips and thorax as needed to center abdomen to IR for both lateral and dorsal decubitus, if done bedside.
- Ensure no rotation and that plane of IR is perpendicular to CR.
- Position **horizontal CR** to center of grid/IR.

Respiration Suspend on expiration.

Note: For lateral decubitus, have patient lie on side for a minimum of **5 minutes** before taking exposure to allow for air to rise to highest position within abdomen.

Dorsal decubitus, lateral position (Fig. 19-55): This is not a common bedside projection. The dorsal decubitus is a useful position to demonstrate a possible abdominal aortic aneurysm or as an alternative to the lateral decubitus position if the patient cannot be moved.

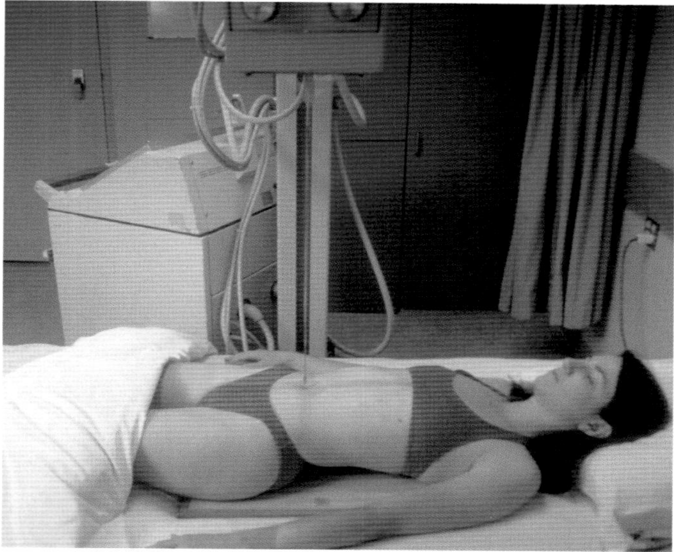

Fig. 19-53. Supine AP—bedside.

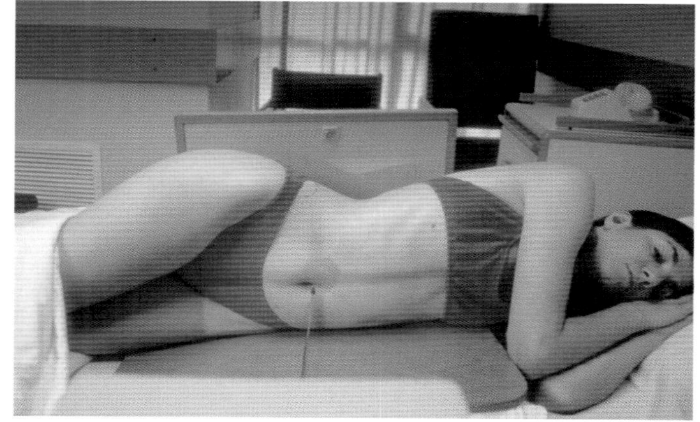

Fig. 19-54. Left lateral decubitus (AP)—bedside.

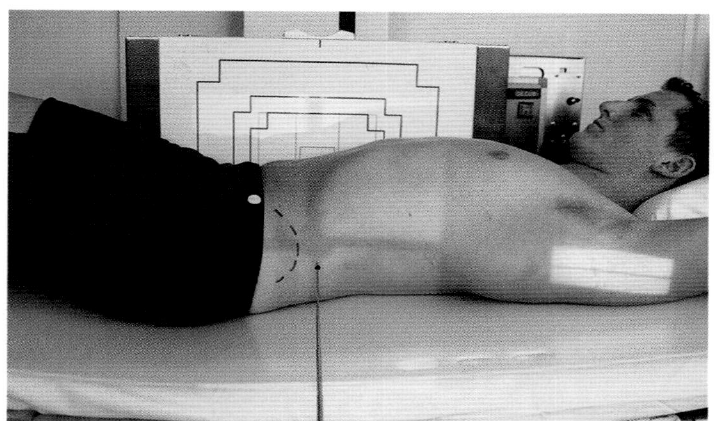

Fig. 19-55. Dorsal decubitus (lateral), on stretcher in front of erect Bucky.

19

AP (PA) OBLIQUE AND LATERAL—FINGERS, THUMB, HAND, AND WRIST

Technical Factors
- IR size—20 × 24 cm (8 × 10 inches) or—24 × 30 cm (10 × 12 inches)
- 50-60 kV range
- Detail screens if using conventional film-screen
- Minimum SID of 40 inches (100 cm)

Shielding Shield pelvic region.

Positioning and Central Ray—Patient Supine

AP—hand and/or wrist (Fig. 19-56):
- Generally, the hand and/or wrist can be positioned as needed on the IR placed on the stretcher or table beside the patient. Move patient to one side of stretcher or table as needed to provide room for IR. If the fingers and hand can be fully extended, AP or PA projections can be readily achieved. Positioning, CR location, and collimation are similar to routine upper limb projections as described in Chapter 5.
- CR is perpendicular to part and IR, centered as follows:
  —Hand, CR to third MP joint
  —Fingers 2 through 4, CR to PIP joint

Alternative AP of fingers (with fingers and hand partially flexed) (Figs. 19-57 and 19-58):
- If patient cannot fully extend fingers, specific AP projections can be done as shown with the **parts of interest placed as near parallel to the IR** as possible.
- Direct CR perpendicular to part of interest and to IR. Angle IR and CR as needed to maintain perpendicular relationship.

PA and lateral thumb (Figs. 19-59 and 19-60):
- If specific injury is to the thumb, a PA projection can be achieved using a radiolucent sponge as demonstrated (Fig. 19-59).
- Lateral positioning of the thumb can also be achieved by angling the CR as needed for a lateral projection (Fig. 19-60). However, some distortion will result using this method.
- Ensure that entire thumb, including all of first metacarpal and trapezium, is included.
- Center CR and IR to first MP joint.

Oblique and lateral—fingers, hand, and/or wrist (Figs. 19-61 and 19-62):
- Obliques and laterals of the fingers, hand, and/or wrist can be achieved by lateral rotation, as with routine positioning of these parts as shown in Chapter 5, or by adjusting CR and IR angles as needed (see lateral wrist, Fig. 19-62).
- Center CR and collimate to specific region of interest.

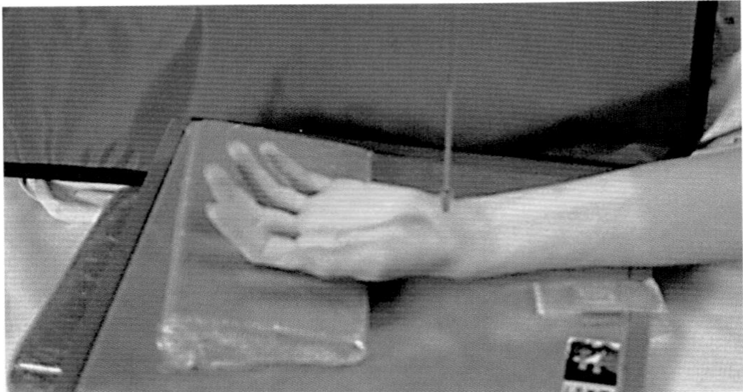

Fig. 19-56. AP hand and/or wrist.

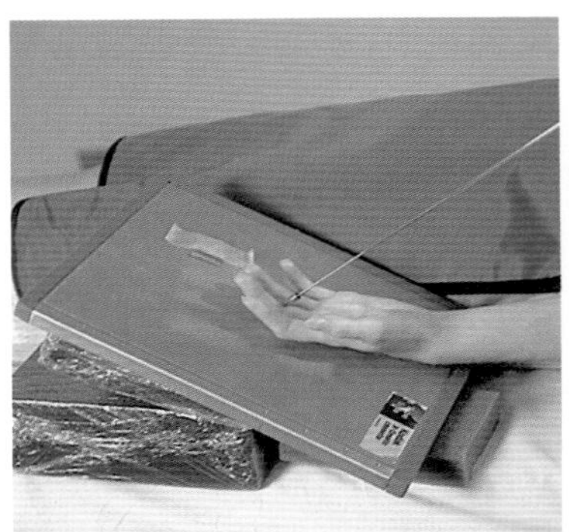

Fig. 19-57. AP hand and fingers for **distal phalanges.**

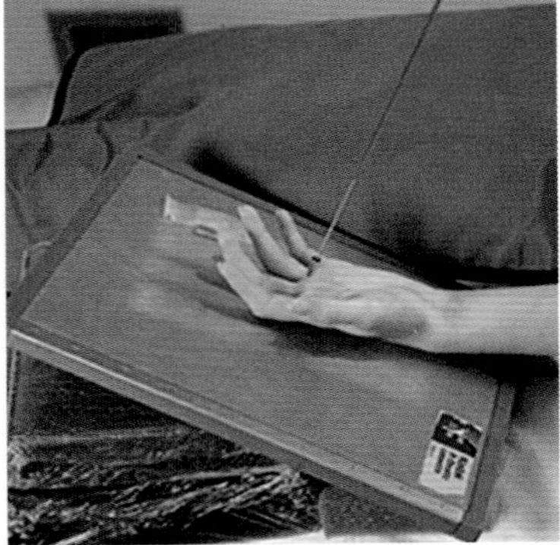

Fig. 19-58. AP hand.

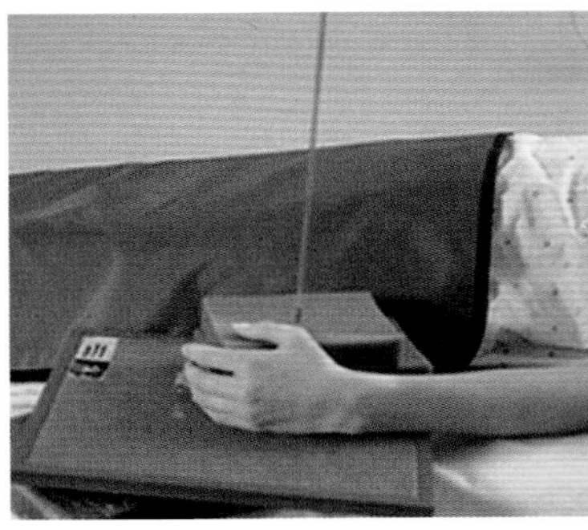

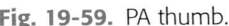

Fig. 19-59. PA thumb.

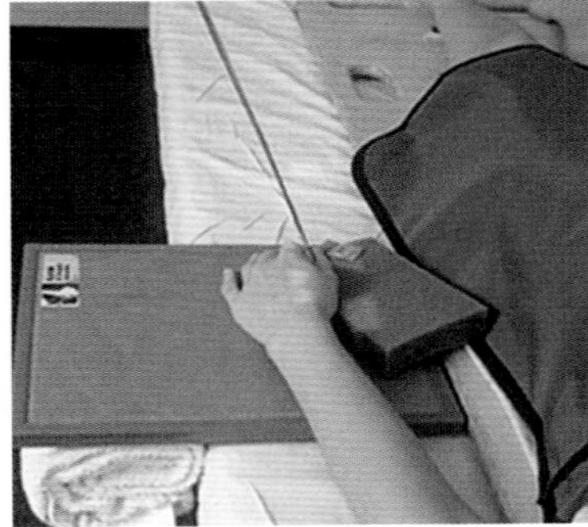

Fig. 19-60. Lateral thumb.

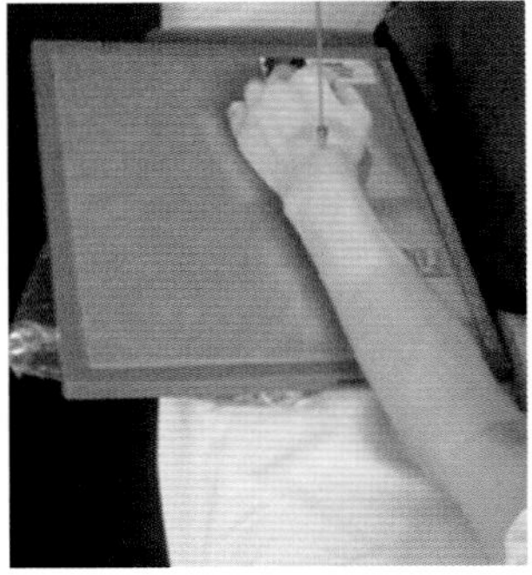

Fig. 19-61. Oblique—Fingers, hand, and/or wrist.

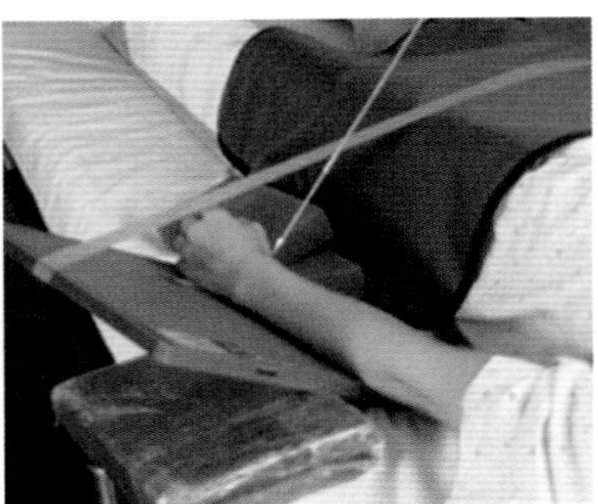

Fig. 19-62. Lateral wrist and hand.

PA (AP) AND LATERAL FOREARM AND WRIST

Include both joints with original trauma images of forearm. Postreduction images may include only the joint nearest fracture site, depending on departmental protocol.

Technical Factors

- IR size—30 × 35 cm (11 × 14 inches) or
  —35 × 43 cm (14 × 17 inches) to include both joints
- 65-70 kV range
- Detail screens if using conventional film-screen
- Minimum SIRD of 40 inches (100 cm)
  Cast conversion: Small to medium cast, +5-7 kV.
  Large cast, 2 × mAs or +8-10 kV.
  Fiberglass +3-4 kV.

Shielding Shield pelvis and chest region.

Positioning and Central Ray—Patient Supine

PA (to include both joints on initial exam) (Fig. 19-63):

- Adjust plane of IR and CR as needed for a true PA; center to midforearm. Collimate to include both elbow and wrist joints.

Lateral (Fig. 19-64):

- With hand pronated as much as possible, use supports to prop up hand and arm as needed for lateral projection with CR–part–IR 90° from PA.

Postreduction forearm and wrist (Figs. 19-65 and 19-66):

- Move patient to one side of stretcher for more room for IR placement for PA and lateral projections.
- PA may be taken as demonstrated. Include either the wrist or elbow, whichever is closest to known fracture site, or both joints if required.
- For lateral, adjust arm, IR, and CR as needed for 90° projection from PA.

Postreduction radiographs: PA and lateral of distal forearm and wrist are shown in Figs. 19-67 and 19-68.

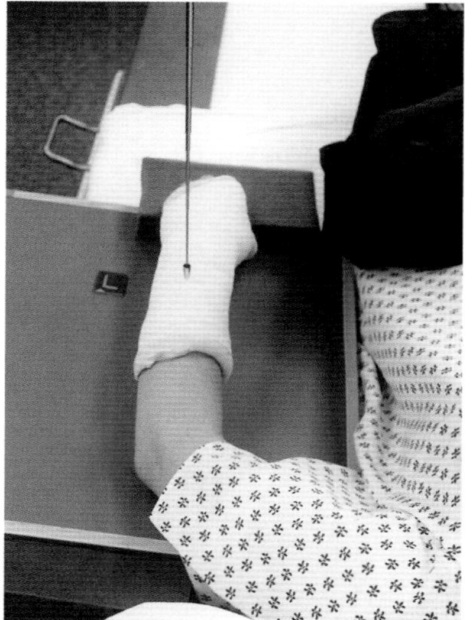

Fig. 19-63. PA forearm to include wrist and elbow

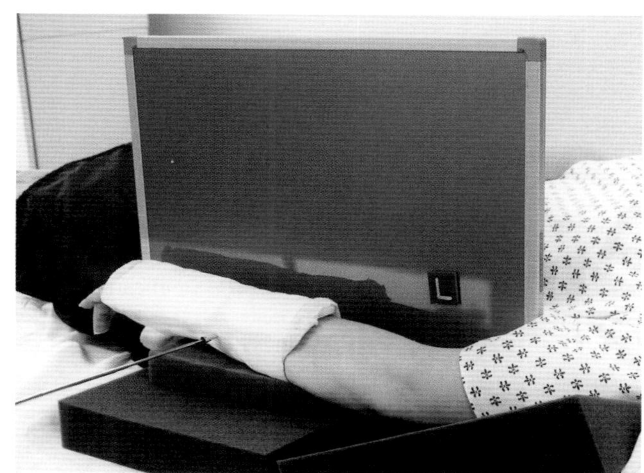

Fig. 19-64. Lateral forearm to include wrist and elbow

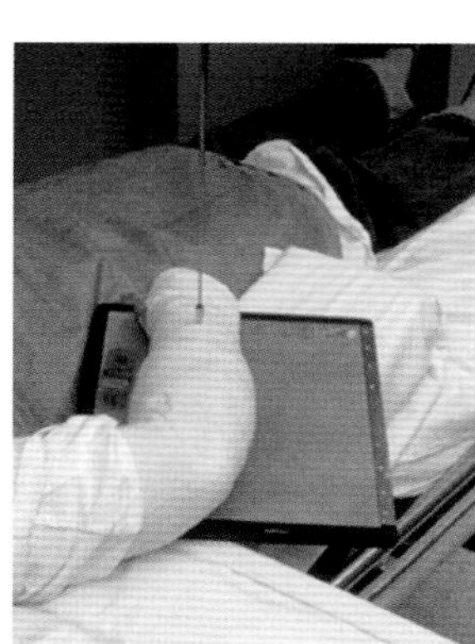

Fig. 19-65. With cast, PA forearm and wrist.

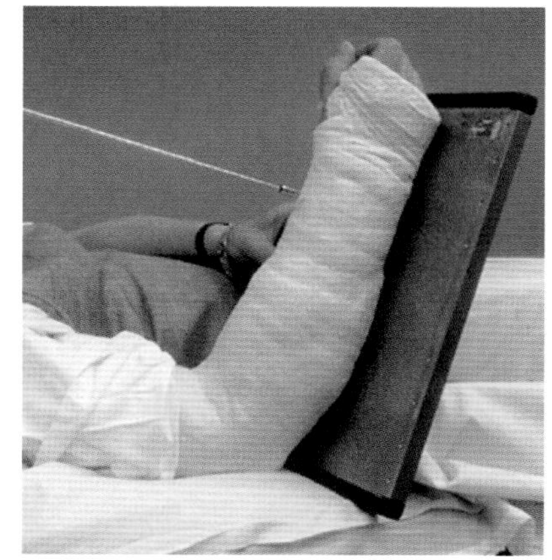

Fig. 19-66. With cast, lateral forearm and wrist (lateromedial).

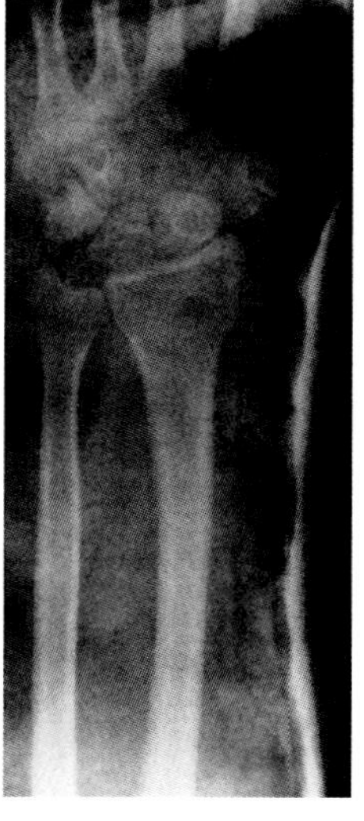

Fig. 19-67. PA wrist.

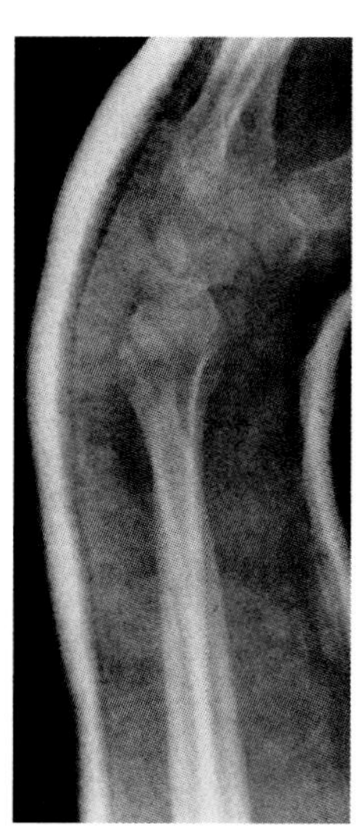

Fig. 19-68. Lateral wrist.

PA, LATERAL (AND OPTIONAL TRAUMA LATEROMEDIALS—COYLE METHOD) ELBOW

As with other trauma radiographic examinations, a minimum of two projections should be obtained of the elbow—an **AP or PA** and a **lateral.** For patients with multiple injuries, including possible trauma to the thorax and/or spine and where the elbow remains partially flexed and the hand pronated, **horizontal beam PA** and **vertical beam lateral** projections may be performed as demonstrated.

If the trauma region includes the proximal humerus or shoulder, the entire humerus to include both elbow and shoulder joints should be examined as shown on the following page, along with a transthoracic lateral.

Technical Factors

- IR size—20 × 24 cm (8 × 10 inches) or —24 × 30 cm (10 × 12 inches)
- 60-70 kV range
- Detail screens if using conventional film/screen
- Minimum SID of 40 inches (100 cm)

Shielding Shield pelvis and chest region.

Positioning and Central Ray

(with Hand Pronated and Elbow Partially Flexed)

PA (Fig. 19-69):

- Place vertical IR between extended arm and patient. (Place shield between IR and thorax.) Place support under arm and hand.
- Direct horizontal beam CR to be **perpendicular to interepicondylar plane** for true PA.

Lateral (Figs. 19-70):

- With arm in similar position as for PA and with elbow partially flexed, place IR under elbow and forearm and angle the CR as needed to be **parallel to interepicondylar plane** (90° from PA).

Trauma axiolaterals: For trauma to the elbow region with potential fractures involving the **radial head** or **coronoid process,** special axiolateral projections of the elbow are shown in Figs. 19-71 and 19-72. These are excellent projections of the trauma elbow when the patient cannot fully extend the elbow for routine medial or lateral obliques. Note the degrees of elbow flexion and the CR angles.

Note: These "Coyle method" trauma axiolateral projections (Figs. 19-71 and 19-72) are further described and demonstrated with radiographic images in Chapter 5 (Upper Limb).

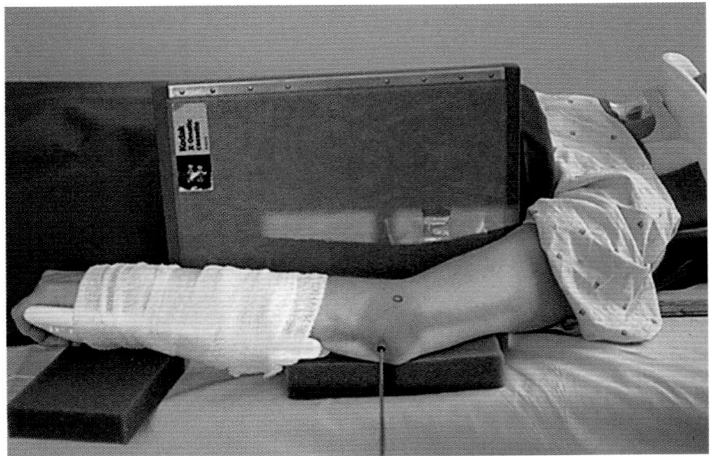

Fig. 19-69. **PA** horizontal beam elbow—CR **perpendicular** to interepicondylar plane.

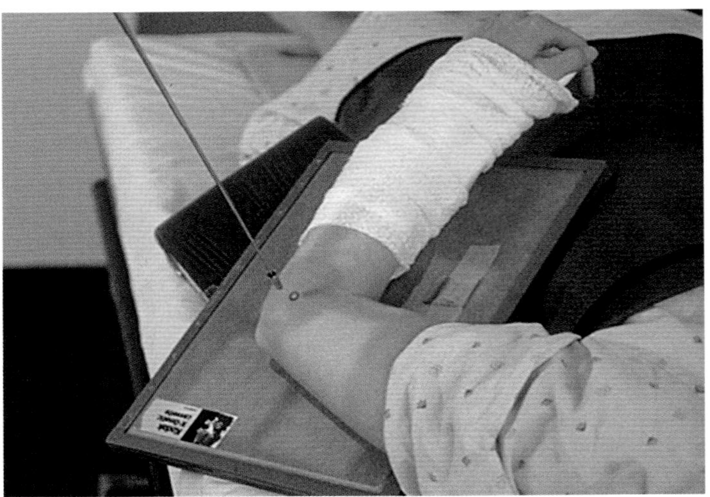

Fig. 19-70. Lateral elbow partially flexed—CR angled as needed to **be parallel** to interepicondylar plane.

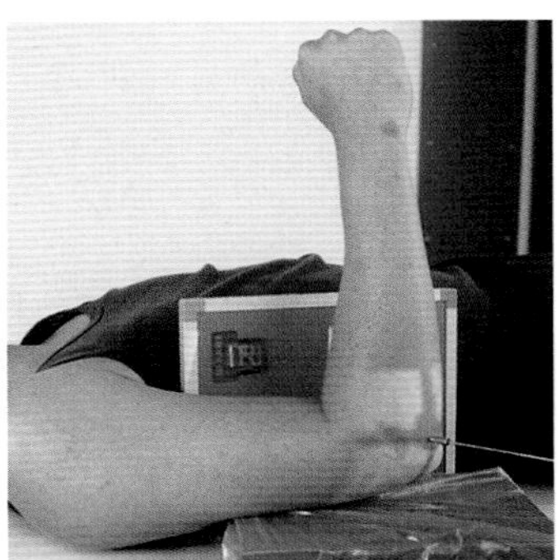

Fig. 19-71 Lateral for **radial head,** elbow flexed **90°**, CR angled 45° proximally (toward shoulder).

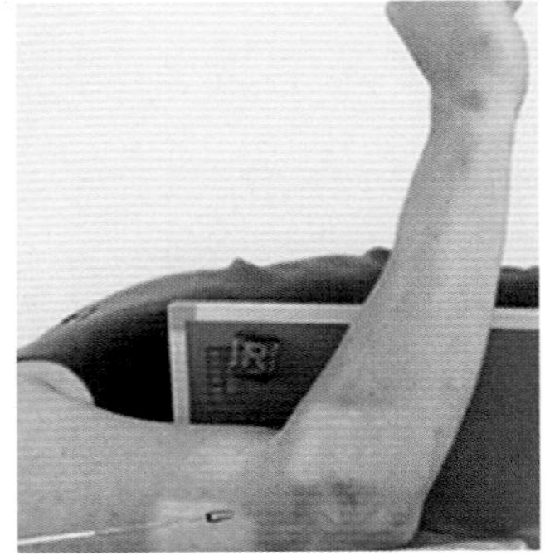

Fig. 19-72 Lateral for **coronoid process,** elbow flexed **80°**, CR angled 45° distally (from shoulder).

AP AND LATERAL HUMERUS

Do not attempt to rotate arm for initial AP and lateral projections if signs and symptoms of fracture or dislocation are present. The AP should include both elbow and shoulder joints, but two lateral images will be required for the initial exam to demonstrate both the proximal and distal humerus.

Depending on departmental protocol, subsequent exams may require that only the joint nearest the injury be included.

Technical Factors

- IR size—35 × 43 cm (14 × 17 inches) or —30 × 35 cm (11 × 14 inches)
- 65-70 kV range
- Large patient over 10 cm: use grid and increase kV accordingly
- 75-80 kV for transthoracic lateral, grid required
- Transthoracic lateral generally taken with 2 to 3 seconds exposure and breathing technique if possible
- Minimum SID of 40 inches (100 cm)

Shielding Shield pelvis and chest region.

Positioning and Central Ray (Patient Supine)

AP (Fig. 19-73):

- With patient supine, carefully place IR under shoulder and arm (large enough IR to include both shoulder and elbow joints).
- Abduct arm slightly and supinate hand if patient's condition allows.
- Center CR to midhumerus.

Lateral—mid- and distal humerus (Fig. 19-74):

- Place vertical IR between arm and thorax with top of IR as far into axilla as possible. Place shield between IR and thorax.
- Flex elbow 90° if possible.
- Position CR horizontal and perpendicular to distal third of humerus and IR.

Lateral—proximal humerus (horizontal beam transthoracic lateral) (Fig. 19-75):

- Place grid IR next to injured shoulder and arm. Align grid lines vertically to prevent grid cutoff if part is not centered to midline of grid.
- Raise opposite arm above head, which also elevates this shoulder.
- Center horizontal CR through thorax to surgical neck and to centerline of grid.
- Have patient lower shoulder of interest.

Note: A 10° to 15° cephalad angle may be required if shoulder of interest cannot be lowered. (Check grid alignment to prevent grid cutoff from cross-angled CR.)

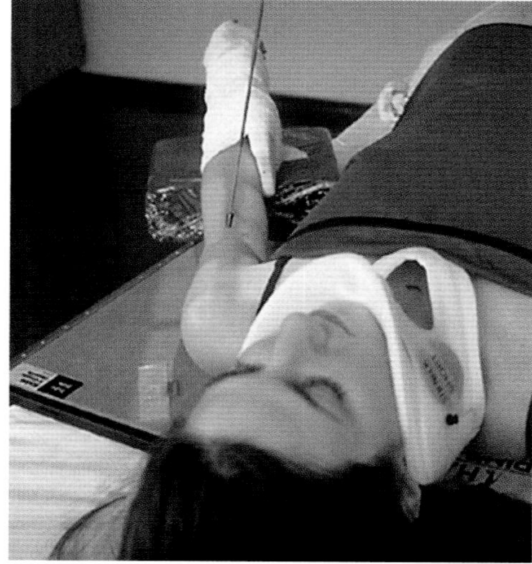

Fig. 19-73. AP humerus—to include both joints.

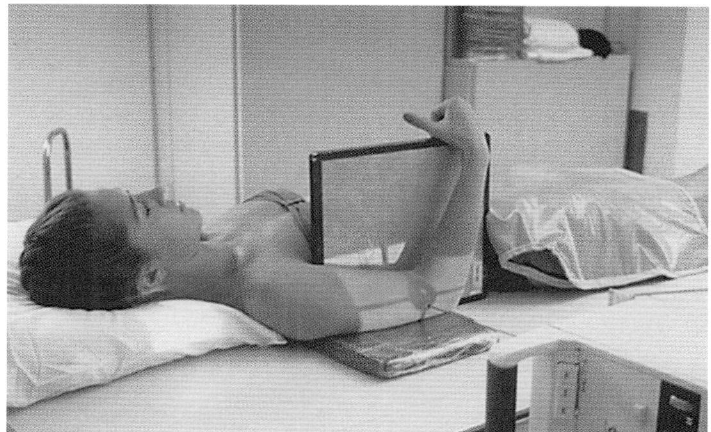

Fig. 19-74. Lateral—mid- and distal humerus to include elbow.

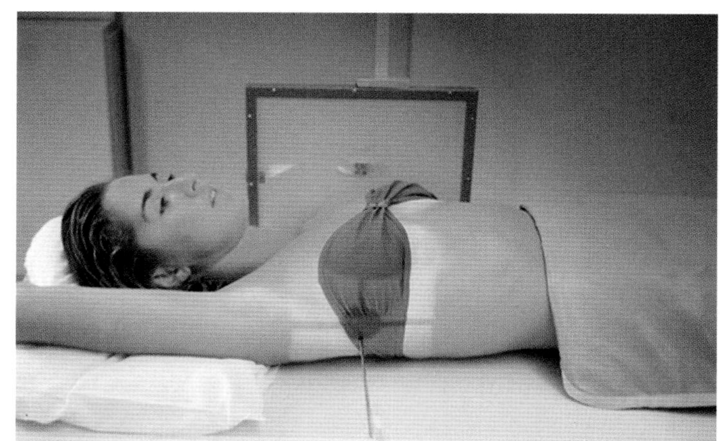

Fig. 19-75. Lateral—transthoracic proximal humerus.

19

AP AND LATERAL—SHOULDER, SCAPULA, AND CLAVICLE

Technical Factors
- IR size—24 × 30 cm (10 × 12 inches)
- 75-80 kV range with grid
- Minimum SID of 40 inches (100 cm)

Shielding Shield pelvis and chest region.

Positioning and Central Ray (Patient Supine)

AP shoulder (Fig. 19-76):
- With patient supine and arm in neutral rotation position at side, center IR (grid IR under patient if on stretcher) centered to shoulder joint and to CR.
- Position CR perpendicular to shoulder joint.

AP scapula (Fig. 19-77):
- With patient supine, gently abduct arm 90° from body if possible and center IR and perpendicular CR to scapula.

Lateral shoulder:
- See transthoracic lateral on preceding page, or take lateral scapular Y projection, as shown in Fig. 19-79 but with CR centered to head of humerus.

Lateral scapular Y—AP oblique (lateromedial scapula) (Figs. 19-78 and 19-79):
- Patient should be in posterior oblique position, with side of interest elevated and arm raised and crossed to opposite shoulder. Palpate borders of scapula, and turn patient until scapula is in profile in lateral position (generally requires about a 25° to 30° posterior oblique body position).
- Project CR perpendicular to IR, or if patient cannot be turned up sufficiently, angle CR as needed to be parallel to scapular blade (place grid crosswise to prevent grid cutoff).
  Note: Some distortion will occur with this medial CR angle if it is needed to achieve a lateral position of the scapula.
- Center CR to midlateral (axillary) border of scapula.

AP and/or AP axial clavicle (Figs. 19-80 and 19-81):
- With patient supine and arm at side, center IR (placed crosswise) to the clavicle.
- Direct CR perpendicular to midclavicle and mid-IR for the AP and 15° to 20° cephalad for the AP axial projection. A greater CR angle (20°) is required on a thin patient and less angle (15°) for a thick patient.

Note: If patient size requires use of a grid for the AP and AP axial projections of the clavicle, align the grid lengthwise to prevent grid cutoff for the axial.

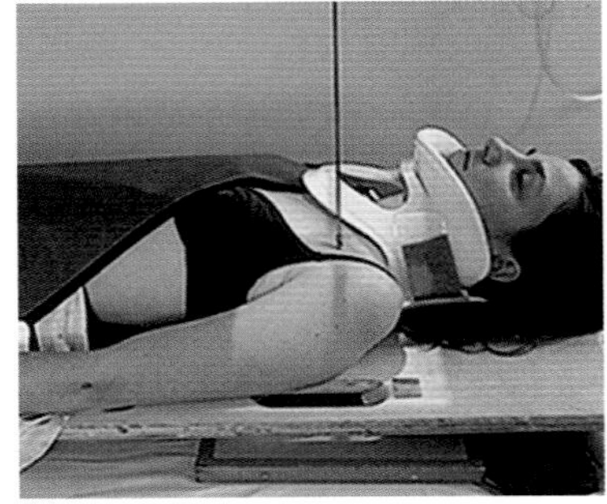

Fig. 19-76. AP shoulder.

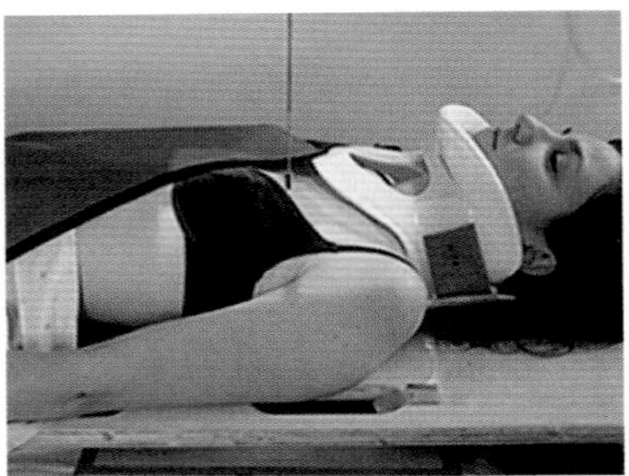

Fig. 19-77. AP scapula.

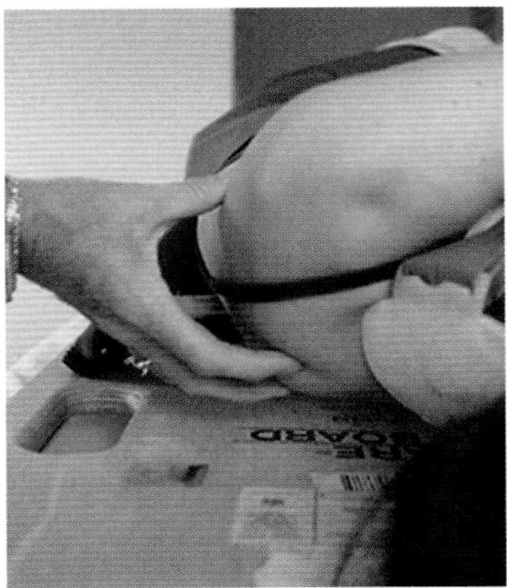

Fig. 19-78. Lateral scapula. Palpate borders of scapula to determine true lateral position.

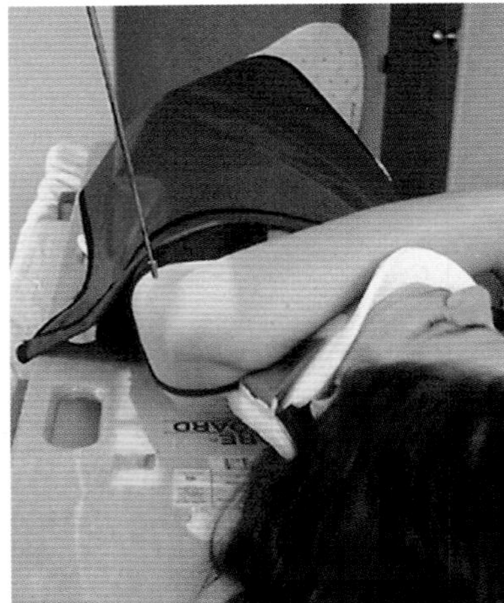

Fig. 19-79. AP oblique, scapular Y—lateromedial projection of scapula.

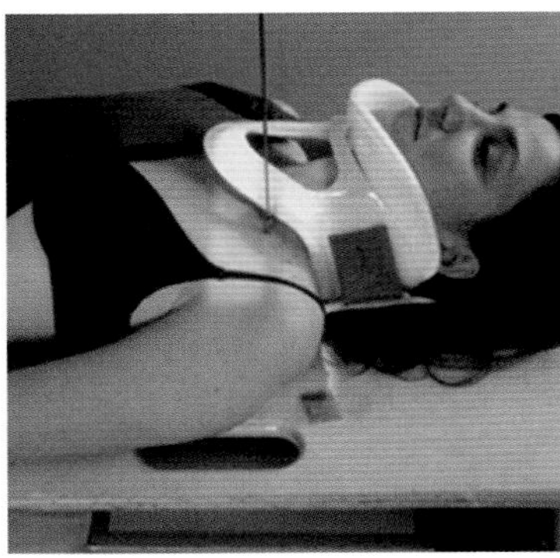

Fig. 19-80. AP clavicle—CR perpendicular.

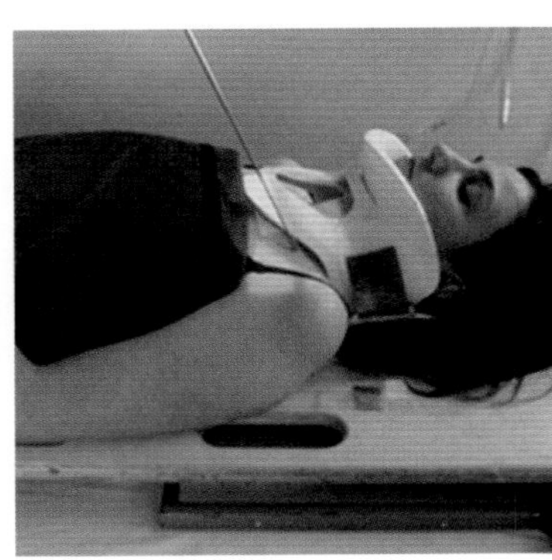

Fig. 19-81. AP axial clavicle—CR 15° to 20° cephalad (grid lines lengthwise).

AP AND LATERAL—TOES AND FOOT

The general trauma rules apply for lower limb radiographic procedures also—namely, a **minimum of two projections taken 90° to each other** should be taken. Therefore the oblique projection is generally not included with these initial trauma examinations unless the proximal metatarsals and tarsals are of special interest and need to be visualized.

Technical Factors

- IR size—24 × 30 cm (10 × 12 inches)
- 60-65 kV range
- Detail screens if using conventional film-screen
- Minimum SID of 40 inches (100 cm)

Shielding Shield gonadal region.

Positioning and Central Ray (Patient Supine, Leg Extended)

AP foot and/or toes (see Note) (Fig. 19-82):

- With patient's leg extended and toes pointing up, place IR vertically against plantar surface of foot. Use IR holder as shown or other means such as a pillow and/or sandbags to hold IR in place.

CR angle: Start with CR perpendicular to IR; then angle CR posteriorly as needed 10° posterior to plantar surface of foot and plane of IR (Fig. 19-82). (This is equivalent to a 10° posterior CR angle for routine AP foot with plantar surface flat on tabletop.)

CR centering: Center CR to **third tarsometatarsal (TMT) joint.** For injuries to specific toes, the entire foot is generally included in trauma cases.

Note: If patient can flex knee and place foot flat on tabletop, routine AP (and oblique) foot projections can be completed as described in Chapter 7.

Lateral foot (lateromedial projection) (Fig. 19-83):

- Place support under foot and ankle with vertical IR against medial surface.
- Direct horizontal CR to base of metatarsals for lateral foot.

Optional Oblique Foot (Fig. 19-84):

- Position foot similar to AP projection and without moving the patient cross-angle the IR 30 to 40° mediolaterally in relationship to plantar surface of foot.
- CR centered to third TMT as for AP foot.

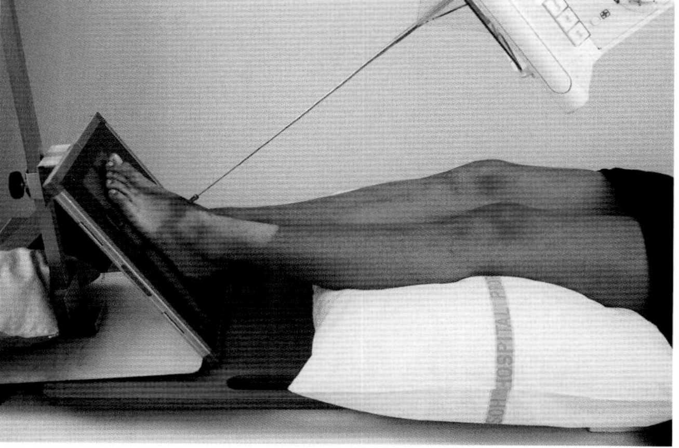

Fig. 19-82. AP foot and/or toes—CR perpendicular to IR.

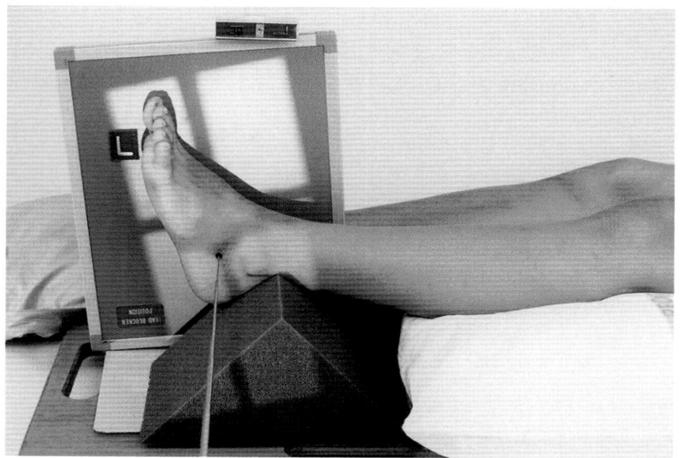

Fig. 19-83. Lateral foot or calcaneus.

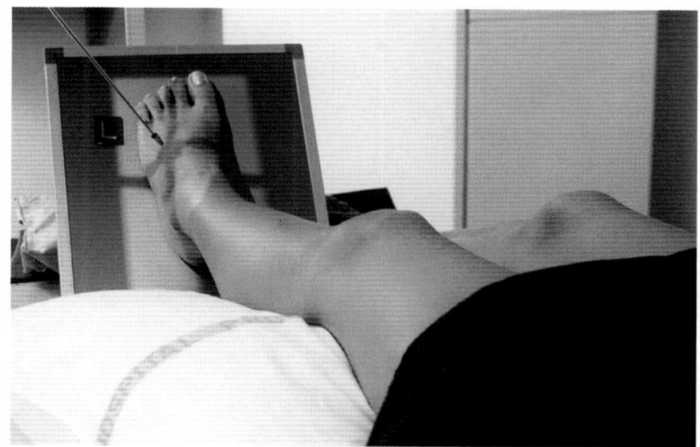

Fig. 19-84. Optional—Oblique foot, CR cross-angled mediolaterally 30 to 40°.

19

AP MORTISE (OR AP) AND LATERAL—ANKLE AND LEG (TIBIA-FIBULA)

The **AP mortise projection** of the ankle is a common projection for trauma or sprains of the ankle joint. (This may be either in place of or in addition to a true AP ankle.) Departmental protocol concerning this should be followed.

The basic **lateral projection** should always be included.

Leg (tibia-fibula): The initial trauma examination should include both ankle and knee joints. Subsequent exams may include only the joint nearest the fracture site, depending on departmental protocol.

Technical Factors

- IR size—24 × 30 cm (10 × 12 inches) for ankle or—35 × 43 cm (14 × 17 inches) for adult leg
- 60-70 kV range
- Detail screens if using conventional film-screens
- Minimum SID of 40 inches (100 cm)

Shielding Shield gonadal region.

Positioning and Central Ray (Patient Supine, Leg Extended)

AP ankle mortise (Fig. 19-85):

- Place IR under ankle, centered to malleoli and CR.
- Angle CR lateromedially as needed to be **perpendicular to the intermalleolar plane.** This requires a 15° to 20° lateromedial angle to the long axis of foot.
- CR is centered to midway between malleoli.

AP ankle (Fig. 19-86):

- Place IR under ankle, centered to malleoli and CR.
- Do not forcefully dorsiflex the foot but allow to remain in a natural position, which aids in demonstrating the base of the fifth metatarsal (a common fracture site) on this ankle projection.
- Position CR parallel to long axis of the foot centered to midway between malleoli.

Lateral ankle (lateromedial projection) (Fig. 19-87):

- Place vertical IR against medial aspect of ankle, centered to malleoli and CR.
- Place support under foot and ankle as needed.
- Direct horizontal CR to lateral malleolus, perpendicular to IR. (Remember, the lateral malleolus will be 15° to 20° more posterior than the medial malleolus on a true lateral ankle.)

AP leg (tibia and fibula) (Fig. 19-88):

- Place large IR under leg to include knee and ankle joints (place diagonally if necessary).
- Center CR to midshaft of leg.

Note: SID may need to be increased to 44 inches (112 cm) for the collimation to cover the 35 × 43 cm (14 × 17 inches) diagonally placed IR.

Lateral leg (lateromedial projection) (Fig. 19-89):

- Place support under knee, leg, and ankle, and support vertical IR against medial surface of leg. Use tape or IR holder to hold IR.
- Direct horizontal CR (or 90° from AP), centered to midshaft of leg.

Note: A large adult patient may require a second smaller IR to include both joints. A general guideline is to use the larger IR nearest the joint of injury and use a smaller IR to include the other joint. This is especially true on this lateral because the IR cannot easily be placed diagonally.

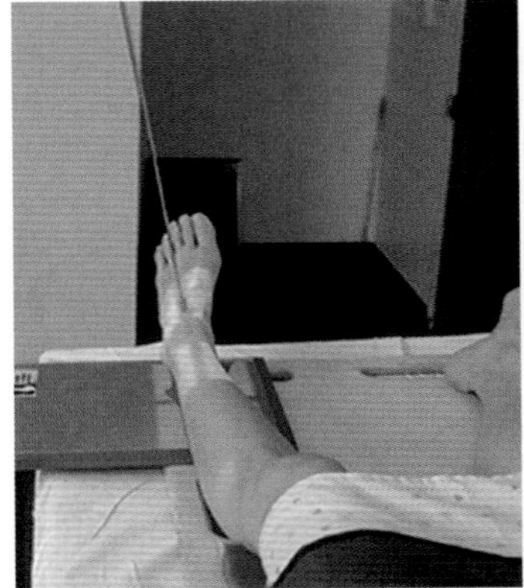

Fig. 19-85. AP mortise projection—CR 15° to 20° lateromedial angle, perpendicular to intermalleolar plane.

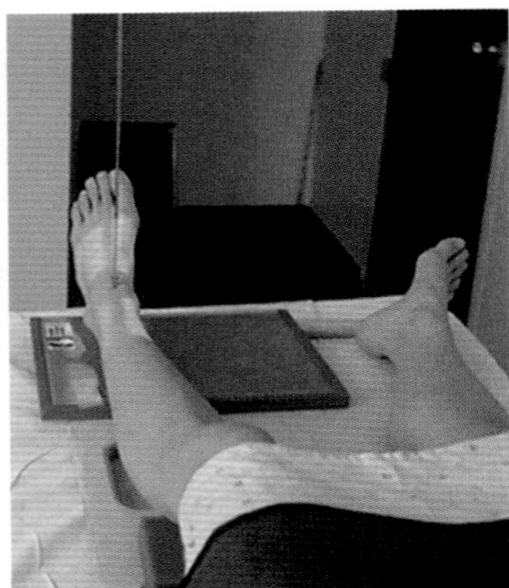

Fig. 19-86. Optional AP ankle—CR perpendicular (parallel to long axis of foot).

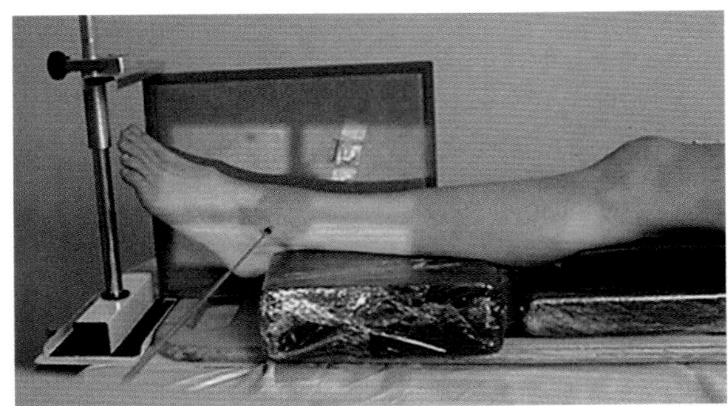

Fig. 19-87. Lateral ankle—CR horizontal.

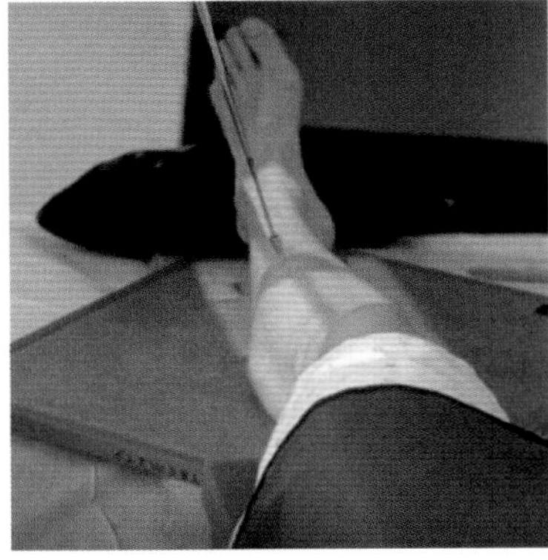

Fig. 19-88. AP leg—CR cross-angled lateromedially (parallel to long axis of foot).

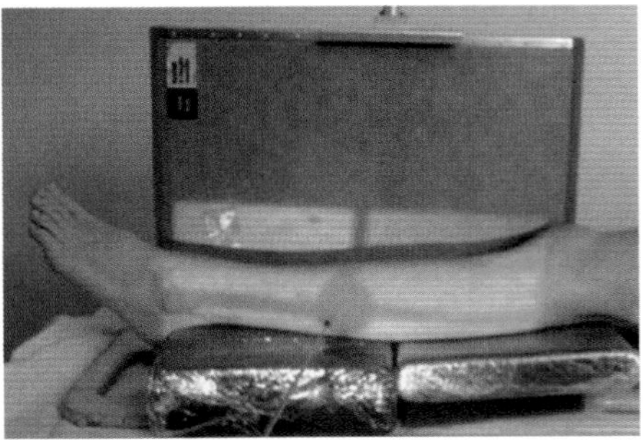

Fig. 19-89. Lateral leg.

19

AP AND LATERAL–KNEE

Technical Factors

- IR size—24 × 30 cm (10 × 12 inches), lengthwise
- 65-70 kV range
- Grid required if knee is larger than 10 cm
- Minimum SID of 40 inches (100 cm)

Shielding Shield gonadal region.

Positioning and Central Ray—Patient Supine, Leg Extended

AP knee (Fig. 19-90):

- Place IR under knee centered to knee joint (¾ inch, or 2 cm, distal to apex of patella).
- Direct CR to knee joint.
- No cephalad CR angle is required for average patient. (Thick thigh and buttocks require 3° to 5° cephalad angle and thin thigh and buttocks a 3° to 5° caudal angle; see Chapter 7)

Lateral knee (Fig. 19-91):

- Place vertical IR against medial aspect of knee centered to level of knee joint (¾ inch, or 2 cm, distal to apex of patella).
- Place support under knee to center leg and knee to IR.
- Direct CR horizontally to be perpendicular to IR.

Note: A horizontal beam true lateral of the knee without knee flexion demonstrates the region of the subpatellar bursa and associated fat pads for possible displacement or presence of fluid level. Effusion (fluid accumulation) is well visualized because of the horizontal ray. Effusion within the articular cavity of the knee is a strong indicator of knee-joint pathology.

This also is a good projection for possible fracture or dislocation of patella.

Optional medial oblique knee—lateromedial CR angle (Fig. 19-92):

This is an optional projection to better demonstrate the **fibular head** and neck unobscured if such is requested.

- Angle CR 45° lateromedially, with grid cassette angled as needed to be near perpendicular to CR. (Place grid crosswise to prevent grid cutoff.)
- Direct CR to knee joint (¾ inch, or 2 cm, distal to apex of patella).
- Place props under leg and knee and support cassette as shown to place IR as near perpendicular to CR as possible to minimize distortion.

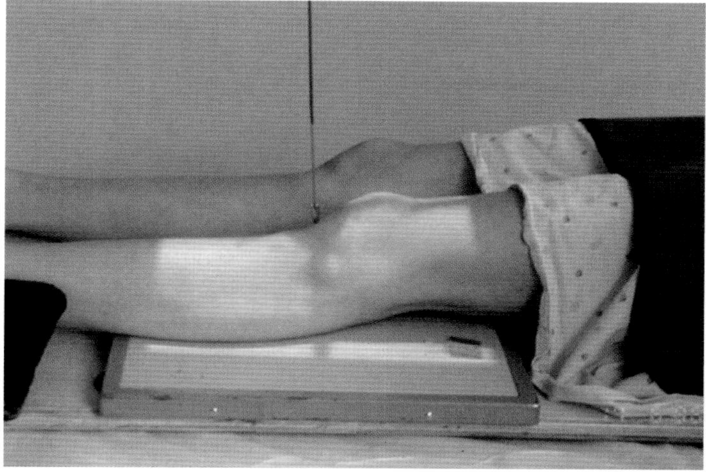

Fig. 19-90. AP knee—CR parallel to long axis of foot, lateromedially. (No cephalic angle is required on average patients.)

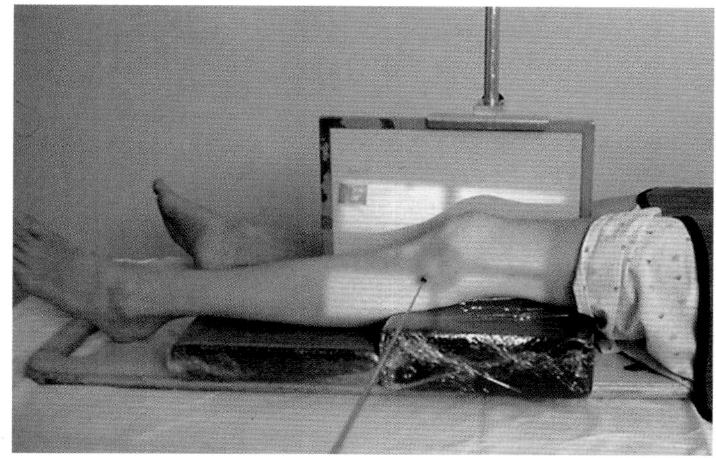

Fig. 19-91. Lateromedial knee—horizontal CR.

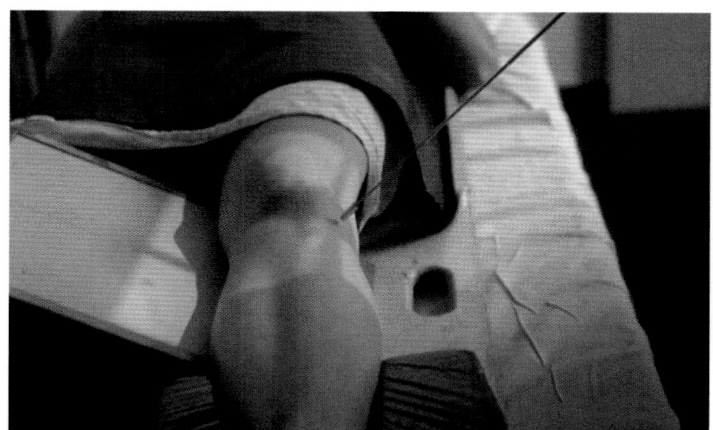

Fig. 19-92. Optional medial oblique knee—CR 45° lateromedial cross-angle; grid crosswise.

AP AND LATERAL—MID- AND DISTAL FEMUR, AP PELVIS, AND PROXIMAL FEMORA

- Ensure that IR and grid are far enough under the proximal tibia/fibula to include this area of anatomy.

Warning: Do not attempt to internally rotate leg if hip fracture is suspected.

Technical Factors
- IR size—35 × 43 cm (14 × 17 inches)
- 70-75 kV range, distal femur
- 75-80 kV range, proximal femur/pelvis
- Minimum SID of 40 inches (100 cm)

Shielding Shield gonadal region on both male and female patients without obscuring essential anatomy. (Ovarian shielding on female patients may not be possible if the area of interest is the pelvic skeletal structures.)

Positioning and Central Ray—Patient Supine, Leg Extended

AP mid- and distal femur (Fig. 19-93):
- Place IR under knee and center femur to ensure that all of knee joint is included, considering the divergence of the x-ray beam.
- Direct CR to mid-IR.
- Collimate closely to femur.

Lateral mid- and distal femur (Fig. 19-94):
- Place vertical grid IR against medial aspect of leg, placed as high proximally as is comfortable for patient. Place support under leg and knee.
- Direct CR horizontally to distal one-third of femur. May require crosswise placement of grid with vertical centerline, as shown in Fig. 19-94 to prevent grid cutoff.
- Collimate closely to femur.

AP pelvis (Fig. 19-95):
- Place pillowcase or cover over grid IR and slide under pelvis, IR crosswise, centered to patient.
- Top of IR will be about 1 inch (2.5 cm) above iliac crest. Ensure **no rotation** and equal distances from ASISs to IR. Rotate feet 15° internally if possible (see Warning above).
- Direct CR perpendicular to center of IR and pelvis.

AP hip (Fig. 19-96):
- Shield gonads for both male and female without obscuring hip region.
- Place IR under hip centered to hip and CR.
- Direct CR perpendicular to IR, centered to hip (2 inches or 5 cm medial to ASIS, at level of greater trochanter).
- Rotate leg 15° internally if possible (see Warning above).

Note: This AP of an individual hip should be taken only as a postreduction or check hip. The initial exam for hip trauma should always first include the AP pelvis to include both hips for comparison.

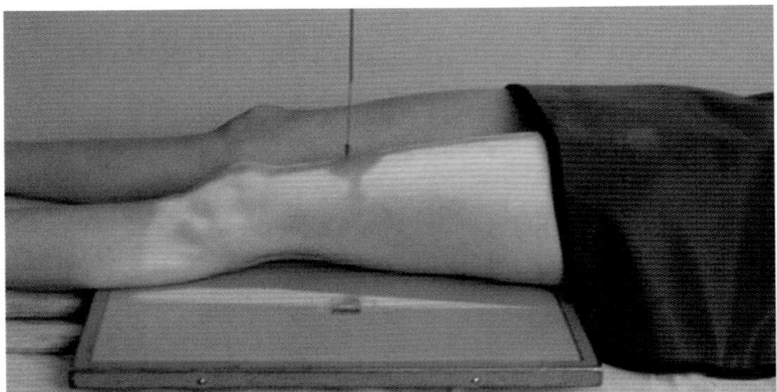

Fig. 19-93. AP mid- and distal femur.

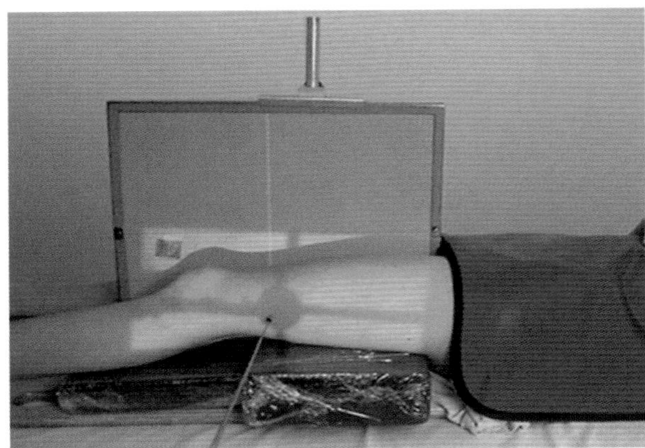

Fig. 19-94. Lateral mid- and distal femur.

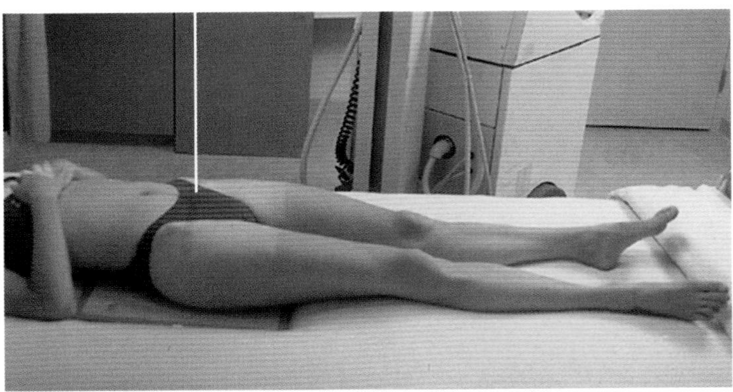

Fig. 19-95. AP pelvis—bedside mobile. (Right leg is not internally rotated in this example.)

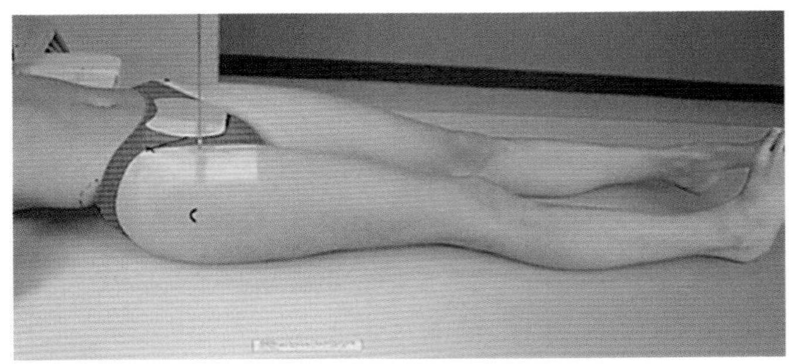

Fig. 19-96. AP hip.

19

LATERAL PROXIMAL FEMUR AND HIP

Inferosuperior Hip—Danelius-Miller Method
Mediolateral Hip—Sanderson Method*

Warning: Do not attempt to rotate or move leg with evidence of fracture.

Technical Factors

- IR size—24 × 30 cm (10 × 12 inches) for hip
  or—35 × 43 cm (14 × 17 inches) for proximal femur and hip
- 70-80 kV range, grid

(Grid lines vertical, unless patient is elevated with hip to near level of center of IR to prevent grid cutoff).

- Minimum SID of 40 inches (100 cm)

Shielding Gonadal shielding generally is not possible.

Positioning and Central Ray—Patient Supine

Inferosuperior lateral hip with unilateral hip injury only—Danelius-Miller method (Fig. 19-97):

- Place vertical IR against patient's side just above iliac crest. Internally rotate leg if possible. Elevate opposite leg.
- Direct horizontal CR perpendicular to femoral neck and to plane of IR. With vertical grid lines, ensure that CR is to centerline of grid IR.

Mediolateral projection for trauma or bedside mobile lateral of hip and proximal femur—Sanderson method (Fig. 19-98):

This is a good projection to demonstrate alignment of hip prosthesis or pin postoperatively. It can be readily obtained in bed or on a stretcher with affected leg relaxed and partially externally rotated. Traction bars or other obstacles do not hinder this projection.

Generally, an AP pelvis or hip is taken first, and as this IR is being removed from under the patient, it can be used to lift the patient **gently.** With the IR about halfway under the patient, it can be used as a lifting device. A folded blanket or towel can then be placed under affected hip and femur. (Patient should be obliqued 20° to 30° from supine.)

- With grid lines vertical, place the grid IR against and partially under the thigh as shown at an angle as needed to be near perpendicular to CR. Support and hold IR in place with 45° support blocks or other supports and/or tape as needed.
- Angle CR mediolaterally as needed to be **near perpendicular to long axis of foot** (90° from AP; see Note). A 10° to 20° cephalad CR angle is possible to better visualize the neck and head if the grid can also be angled sufficiently to prevent grid cutoff.

Note: The amount of CR cross-angle will vary, depending on the external rotation of affected leg.

Summary of Sanderson Method:

- Support is placed under affected hip as patient is lifted gently when removing IR from AP projection.
- With IR partially under hip, angle IR to be parallel to long axis of foot.
- Angle CR mediolaterally to be perpendicular to long axis of foot. (This ensures a true lateral view of the proximal femur with minimal distortion.)

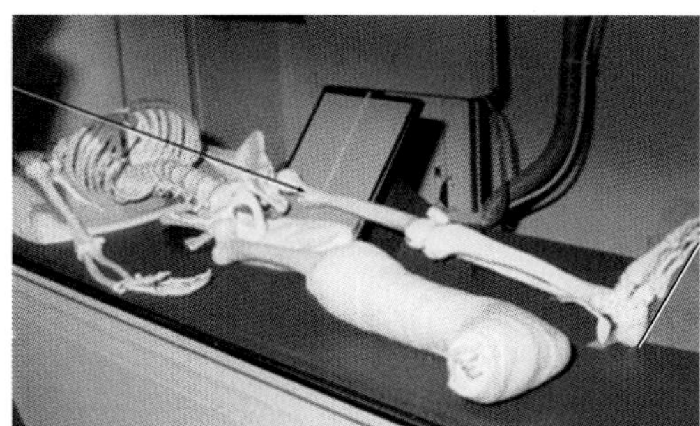

Fig. 19-99. Demonstration of Sanderson method. (Courtesy Jim Sanderson.)

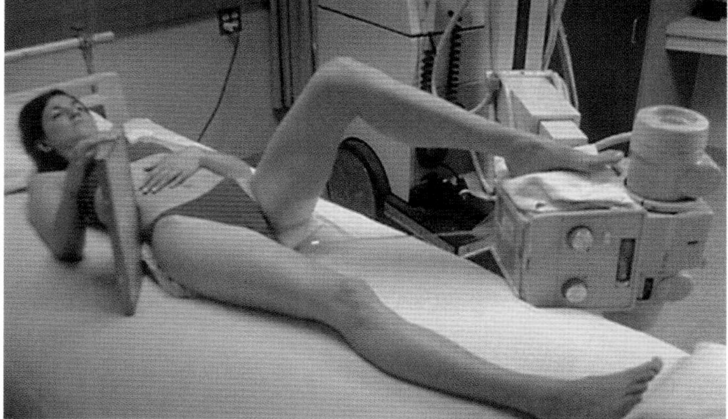

Fig. 19-97. Inferosuperior lateral—bedside mobile, Danelius-Miller method.

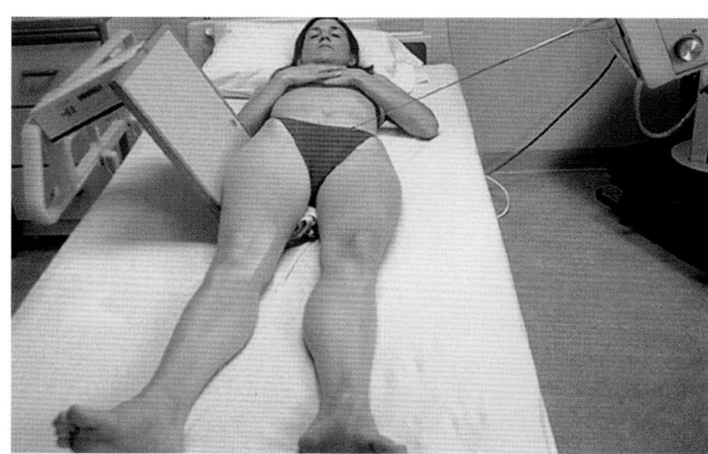

Fig. 19-98. Mediolateral proximal femur and hip—bedside mobile, Sanderson method*; CR cross-angled mediolaterally, perpendicular to long axis of foot.

*James A. Sanderson, Phoenix, Ariz. This method was first demonstrated and described by Sanderson to the author in April 1992.

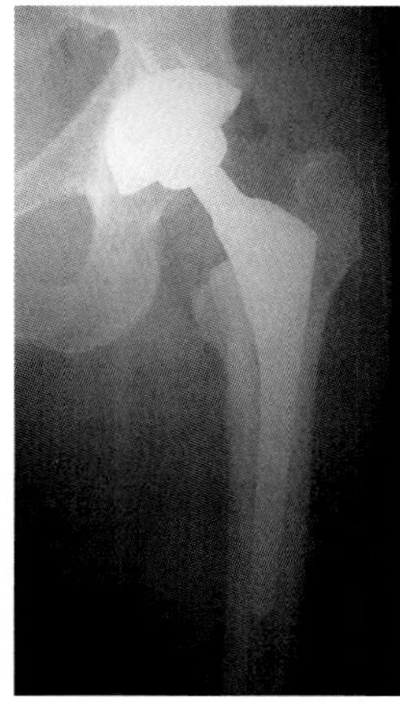

Fig. 19-100. AP hip. (Courtesy Jim Sanderson.)

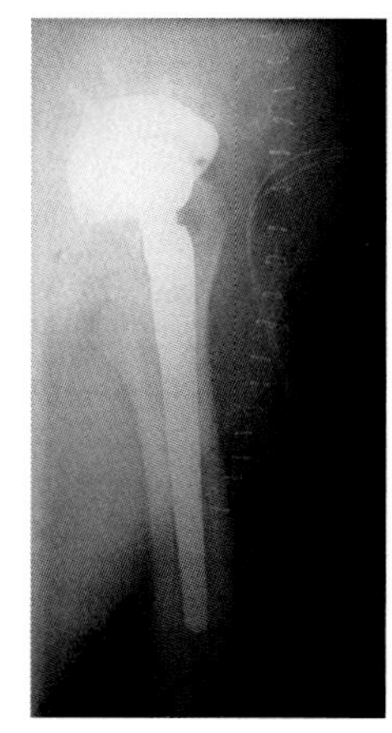

Fig. 19-101. Lat. hip—Sanderson method.

AP AND LATERAL—CERVICAL SPINE

Warning: Do not remove cervical collar or move patient's head or neck until cervical fractures have been ruled out. Generally, this requires an AP and a lateral.

Technical Factors
- IR size—24 × 30 cm (10 × 12 inches)
- 75-80 kV range, grid if required because of patient size

AP:
- Minimum SID of 40 inches (100 cm)

Lateral:
- SID of 60 to 72 inches (150 to 180 cm)

Shielding Shield pelvic region.

Positioning and Central Ray
(Patient supine with potential spinal injury)

AP projection (Fig. 19-102):
- Place IR in Bucky tray or grid IR lengthwise under patient with top of cassette 1 to 2 inches (3 to 5 cm) above level of EAM.
- Angle CR 15° to 20° cephalad, center to exit at the level of C4 (enter at level of lower margin of thyroid cartilage).

AP open mouth—C1 and C2 (Fig. 19-103):
- If condition allows, have patient open mouth as far as possible without moving head or neck.
- CR may be angled if needed to parallel the line from the lower margin of upper teeth to base of skull (mastoid tips).

Optional AP axial C1-C2 region (to demonstrate **dens within foramen magnum** when open mouth projection is not possible and interest is the upper cervical region) (Fig. 19-104):
- Place IR lengthwise, centered to projected CR.
- Angle CR cephalad 35° to 40° or as needed to align CR parallel to a line from symphysis of mandible to base of skull. Center CR to enter just inferior to mandible.

Horizontal beam lateral (C spine) (Fig. 19-105):
- Vertical IR against shoulder, parallel to MSP, with top of IR 12 inches (3 to 5 cm) above level of EAM. Ensure that C7-T1 region is included.
- Have patient relax and depress shoulders as much as possible. If needed, have nonradiology personnel pull down on both arms to further depress shoulders to visualize C7-T1 region. (Supply personnel with lead apron.)
- Direct CR horizontal to C4 (upper thyroid cartilage) and to center of grid to prevent grid cutoff, or turn grid with centerline vertical to prevent grid cutoff if necessary.
- Increase SID to 60 or 72 inches (150 to 180 cm) if equipment and room space allows to decrease beam divergence, which decreases magnification to better visualize C7

Note: The use of grids for a cervical spine examination is determined by departmental protocol and patient size.

Swimmer's lateral (if C7-T1 is not visualized on C-spine lateral) (Fig. 19-106):
- Vertical IR placement is similar to horizontal beam lateral, but elevate arm and shoulder closest to IR and depress opposite shoulder as much as possible.
- Direct CR horizontal, centered to C7-T1 (about 1.5 inches or 4 cm above level of jugular notch). Center the center of grid to CR to prevent grid cutoff (grid lines vertical).

Note: A 5° CR caudal angle may be required if patient cannot depress shoulder opposite IR.

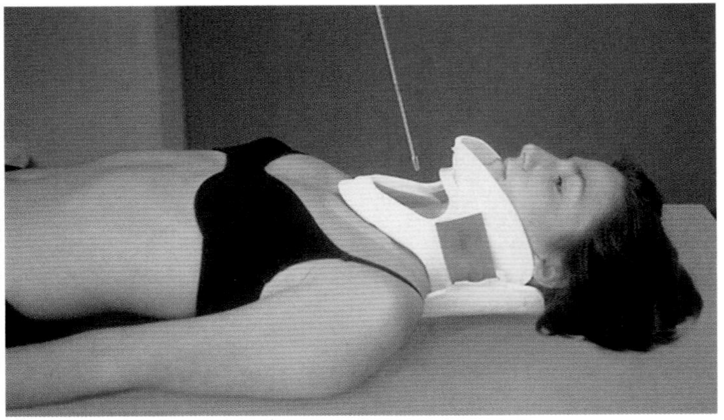

Fig. 19-102. AP cervical—CR 15° to 20° cephalad.

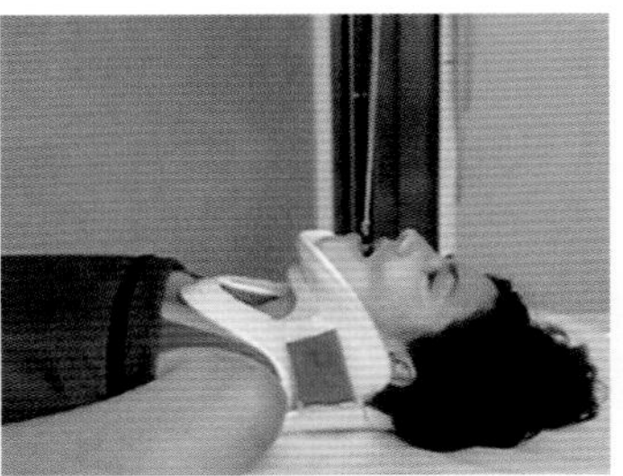

Fig. 19-103. AP open mouth of C1-C2 region if patient can cooperate.

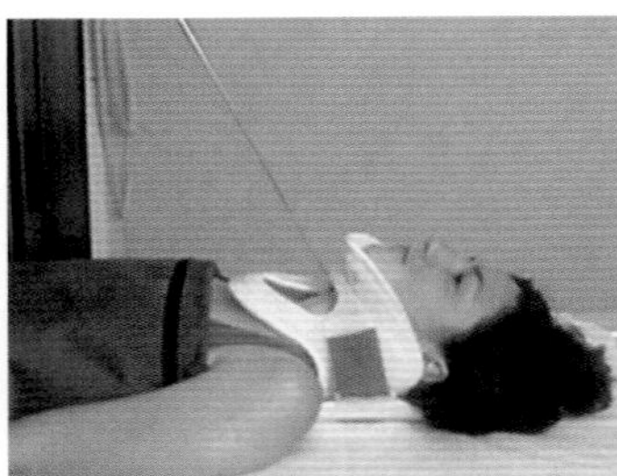

Fig. 19-104. Optional AP C1-C2 region if open mouth AP is not possible—CR 35° to 40° cephalad.

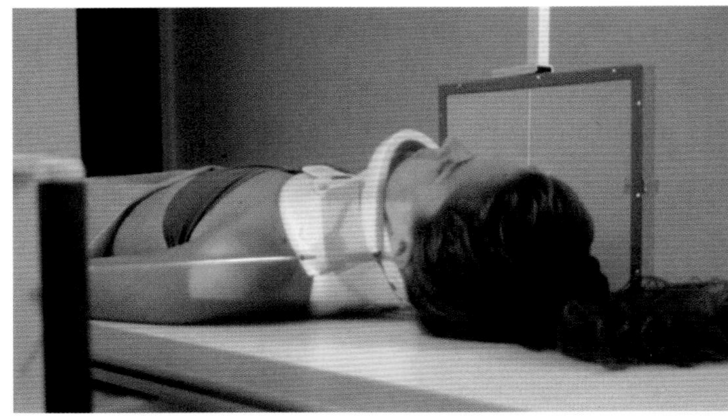

Fig. 19-105. Horizontal beam lateral, C spine.

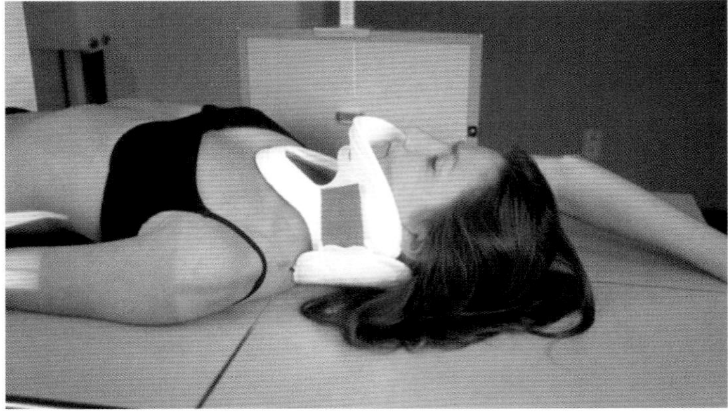

Fig. 19-106. Swimmer's lateral, C7-T1.

19

CERVICAL SPINE—RPO AND LPO TRAUMA OBLIQUES

Two Methods

Supine cervical oblique projections, to visualize pedicles and intervertebral foramina, can be achieved two ways on trauma patients.

Method 1: The IR remains flat on the x-ray table. This is easier and quicker but results in **more distortion** of the pedicles and the intervertebral foramina (Figs. 19-107 and 19-108).

Method 2: With this method the IR is placed under the tabletop angled 45° to be perpendicular to the CR. This method results in **less distortion** but **some magnification.** The increase in OID acts as an air gap and improves image quality (Figs. 19-109 and 19-110).

Technical Factors

- IR size—24 × 30 cm (10 × 12 inches), lengthwise
- Small focal spot
- 70-75 kV range
- SID of 60 inches (150 cm) or 72 inches (180 cm)

Positioning of Patient Supine with Head and Neck Immobilized

Method 1: Place IR lengthwise flat on tabletop under patient and to one side to be centered to projected CR. Angle CR 15° cephalad and 45° medial. Align top of cassette to level of EAM.

Method 2: Angle CR 45° medial and 15° cephalad, and center to level of C4 (level of lower thyroid cartilage). Place IR at a 45° angle just below table height on an adjustable stand or stool.

CR centering: With patient and tabletop completely out of the way and with longitudinal and transverse locks of the tube stand released, angle the CR as needed to achieve the double angle (45° medial angle and 15° cephalic). Center the CR to the center of IR.

The patient and tabletop can then be moved up over the IR into position to center the CR to C4. The CR should remain centered to the IR under the patient and tabletop.

Note: This angulation method can also be adapted to a C-arm type mobile system, in which the IR is attached to the arm with the x-ray tube to maintain a constant perpendicular relationship between the IR and the CR.

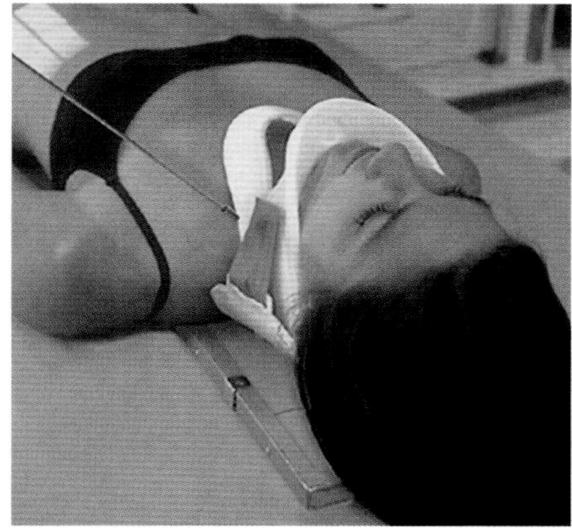

Fig. 19-107. Method 1: Oblique cervical—cassette flat on tabletop.

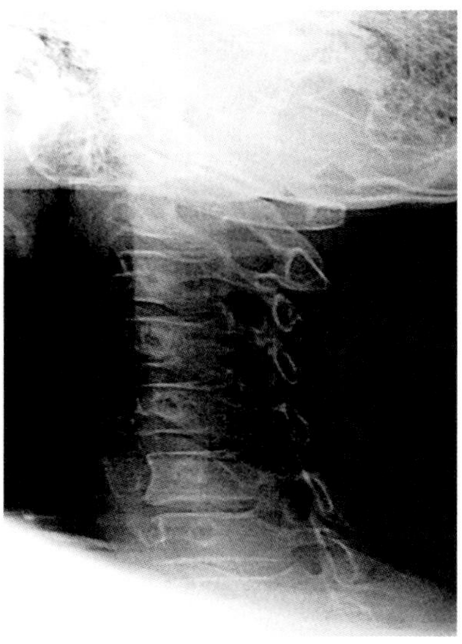

Fig. 19-108. Method 1: Oblique cervical—cassette flat on tabletop. (Courtesy Susan C. Poulin.)

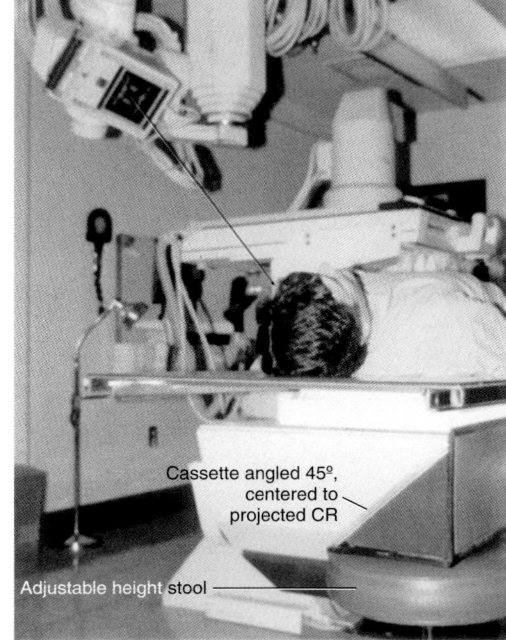

Fig. 19-109. Method two: Oblique cervical—cassette angled 45°. (Courtesy N.J. Martin.)

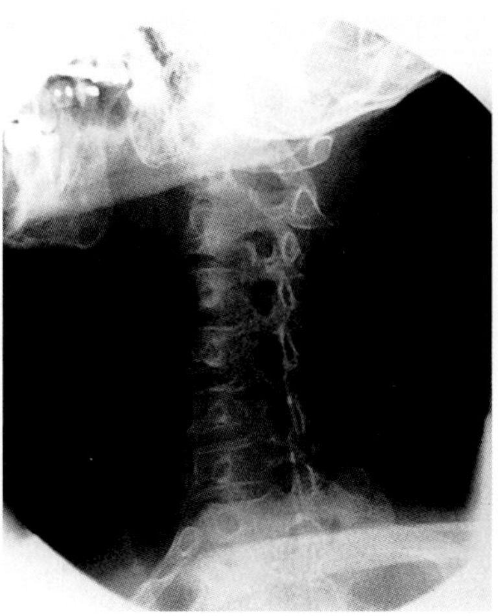

Fig. 19-110. Method two: Oblique cervical—cassette angled 45°. (Courtesy N.J. Martin.)

19

AP AND HORIZONTAL BEAM LATERAL—THORACIC AND LUMBAR SPINE

If patients can be turned on their side, conventional thoracic and lumbar spine images may be obtained, as described in Chapters 9 and 10.

Technical Factors
- IR size—35 × 43 cm (14 × 17 inches), lengthwise
- 75-85 kV range, grid
- Minimum SID of 40 inches (100 cm)

Shielding Shield gonads.

Positioning and Central Ray—Patient Supine

AP thoracic spine (Fig. 19-111):
- Place IR in Bucky, or slide grid under patient with top of IR 3 cm (1½ inch) above shoulders.
- Direct CR perpendicular, to center of IR, at level of T7, 3 to 4 inches (8 to 10 cm) inferior to jugular notch.

AP lumbar spine (Fig. 19-112):
- Position IR as for AP thoracic spine, except IR centered to level of iliac crest. Knees up if patient's condition allows.
- Direct CR perpendicular to center of IR at the level of L4-L5.

Lateral thoracic spine (Fig. 19-113):
- Build up patient/backboard (Fig. 19-113) or move patient to edge of table and place vertical IR below level of tabletop. Use IR holder or tape and/or sandbags to support IR. Center IR to CR at level of T7. Have patient raise arms above head or raise and cross arms above chest so as not to obscure thoracic vertebra.
- Center horizontal CR to vertebral column and to near centerline of grid at level of T7, 3 to 4 inches (8 to 10 cm) inferior to jugular notch.

Lateral lumbar spine (Fig. 19-114):
- Same method as lateral thoracic spine except IR centered to level of iliac crest (L4-L5)
- Horizontal CR centered to vertebral column and to center of grid at level of L4-L5 or the iliac crest

Note: Grid may be placed crosswise to patient as shown in Fig. 19-114 for better centering of CR to near centerline of grid.

A decubitus-type grid with lead strips crosswise can also be used to prevent grid cutoff. This relates to both the horizontal beam thoracic and lumbar spine.

Optional lateral L5-S1 (not shown):
- IR 20 × 24 cm (8 × 10 inches), lengthwise
- Vertical IR centered to 1 inch (2.5 cm) distal to level of iliac crest
- Horizontal CR perpendicular to MSP, centered to IR
- kV increased to 90 to 100 range

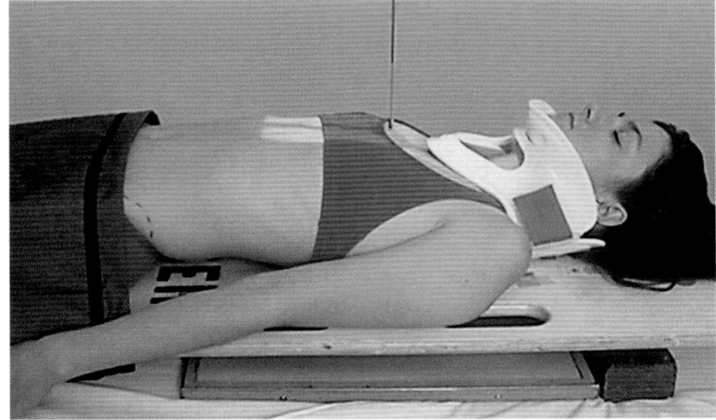

Fig. 19-111. AP thoracic spine.

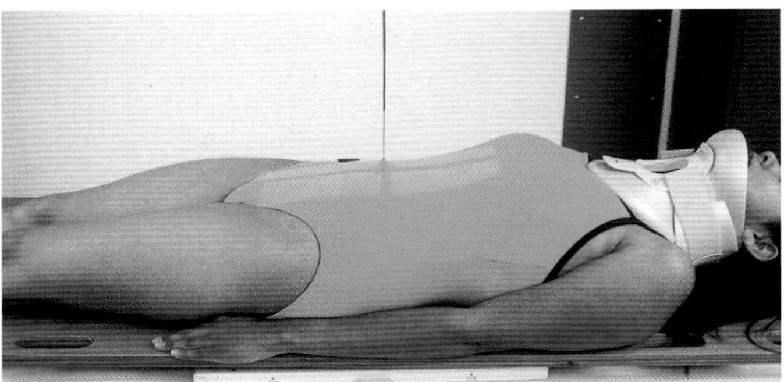

Fig. 19-112. AP lumbar spine.

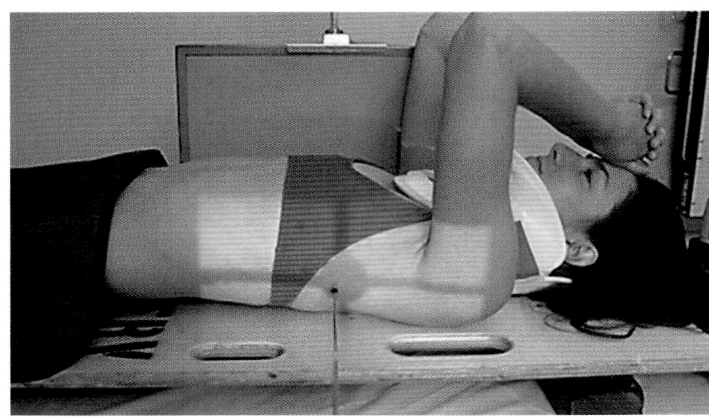

Fig. 19-113. Horizontal beam lateral thoracic spine.

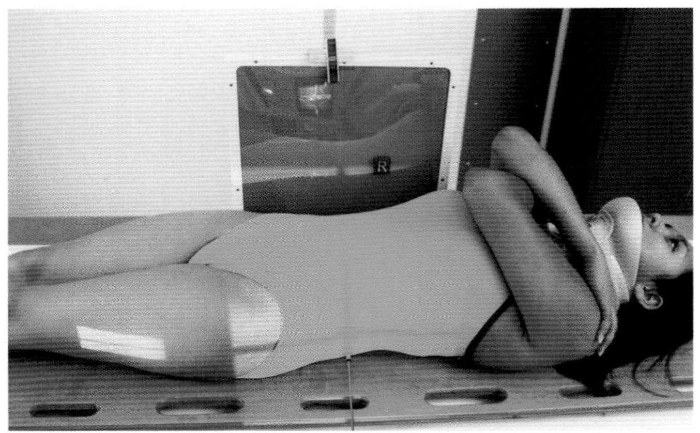

Fig. 19-114. Horizontal beam lateral lumbar spine.

LATERAL TRAUMA SKULL—HORIZONTAL BEAM PROJECTION

Warning: Cervical spine fractures and subluxations/dislocations must be ruled out **before** attempting to move or manipulate the patient's head or neck. This is a good projection for demonstrating sphenoidal effusion (fluid within sphenoid sinus), which may be an indication of intracranial trauma.

Technical Factors

- IR size—24 × 30 cm (10 × 12 inches)
- Grid cassette vertical beside lateral aspect of the cranium
- 70-80 kV range
- Minimum SID of 40 inches (100 cm)
- Small focal spot

Positioning—Patient Supine

- Remove all metal, plastic, or other removable objects from head.
- If patient's head can be manipulated (see Warning above), carefully elevate skull on a radiolucent sponge (Fig. 19-115). If you cannot manipulate head, move patient to edge of table, then place grid IR at least 1 inch (2.5 cm) below tabletop and occipital bone as shown in Fig. 19-116. The divergent beam will then not project posterior skull off the IR.
- Place head in **true lateral position,** relative to IR, with side of interest closest to IR if possible.
- Align MSP parallel with IR and interpupillary line perpendicular to IR.
- Adjust IR to ensure that entire skull will be included on image and center of grid is centered to CR.

Central Ray

- A **horizontal beam** (which is essential for visualization of intracranial air-fluid levels) is directed **perpendicular** to IR.
- Center to a point 2 inches (5 cm) superior to EAM.

Collimation Collimate to outer margins of skull on all sides.

Reminder: On patient with cervical spine injury, **do not** attempt to raise and place support under head, as shown in Fig. 19-115, until cervical pathology has been ruled out with a horizontal beam lateral cervical.

Radiographic Criteria Summary

- Demonstrates superimposed cranial halves with superior detail of the lateral cranium closest to the IR • Also demonstrates the entire sella turcica, including anterior and posterior clinoids and dorsum sellae. • Sella turcica and clivus demonstrated in profile. • **No rotation or tilt** of the cranium as assessed by the following: superimposition of mandibular rami, greater and lesser wings of sphenoid, external auditory meatus (EAMs), and orbital roofs/plates.
- Entire skull is visualized on the image, with the region 5 cm (2 inches) superior to the EAM in the approximate center.
- Sufficient penetration and exposure to visualize bony detail of sellar structures and surrounding skull.

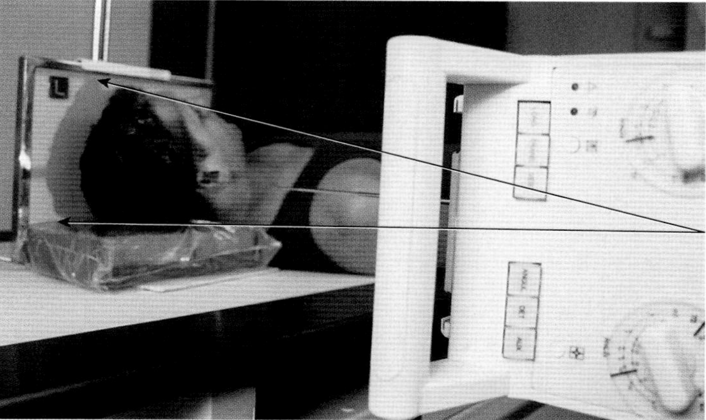

Fig. 19-115. Trauma lateral—**after cervical injury has been ruled out.** Place support under elevated head.

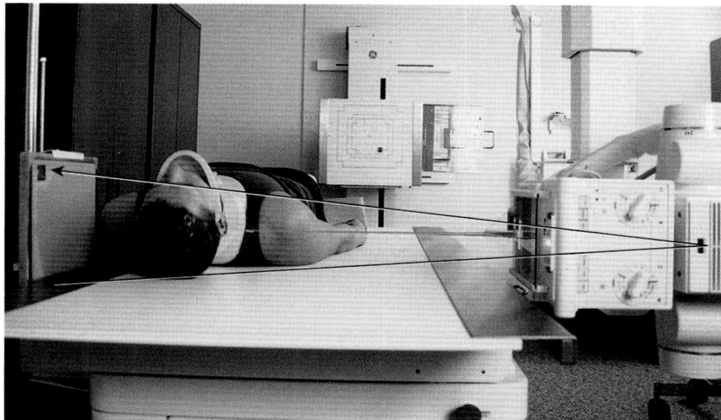

Fig. 19-116. Trauma lateral **without head manipulation.**

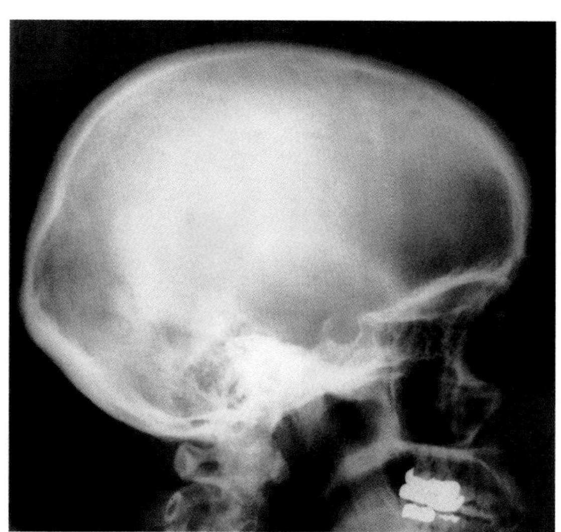

Fig. 19-117. Trauma lateral.

19

AP 0°, AP 15° (REVERSE CALDWELL), AND AP 30° AXIAL (TOWNE)–SKULL

Warning: Cervical spine fractures and subluxations/dislocations must be ruled out before attempting to move or manipulate the patient's head or neck to correct rotation and make adjustments of skull positioning lines.

Exception: If a cervical spine injury has been ruled out, the chin may be depressed to bring the orbitomeatal line perpendicular to the film and the CR can then be adjusted accordingly.

For all three of the projections demonstrated on this page, the patient's head and neck are **not** moved. **The degree of CR angulation is the only variation.**

Technical Factors
- IR size—24 × 30 cm (10 × 12 inches), lengthwise
- Moving or stationary grid
- 70-80 kV range
- Minimum SID of 40 inches (100 cm)
- Small focal spot

Positioning—Patient Supine
- If possible, slide patient onto x-ray table in one movement; do **NOT** move head or neck. You may also use a portable grid placed under patient's head or under the backboard. It is not necessary to remove collar or backboard to obtain these images.
- Remove all metal, plastic, and other removable objects from head.
- Slide patient's entire body to align MSP to midline of table/grid.

Central Ray

AP 0° projection (Figs. 19-118 and 19-121):
- Angle CR **parallel with orbitomeatal line (OML).** With patient in a cervical collar, this is often approximately 10° to 15° caudad, but each patient/situation will be different.
- Center CR to **glabella;** then center IR to projected CR.

AP "reverse Caldwell" projection (Figs. 19-119 and 19-122):
- Angle CR **15° cephalad to OML.** This requires determining the angle of the OML with neck extended as shown; then angle 15° cephalad to the OML.
- Center CR to **nasion;** then center IR to projected CR.

AP axial (Towne) projection (Figs. 19-120 and 19-124):
- Angle CR **30° caudad to OML** or 37° caudad to the infraorbitomeatal line (IOML) (see Note).
- Center CR to pass **midway between EAMs** and exiting the foramen magnum. This centers CR to midsagittal plane 6 cm (2½ inches) above superciliary arch; then center IR to projected CR.

Collimation Collimate to outer margins of skull on all sides.

Note: The CR for the AP axial should not exceed 45° or excessive distortion will hinder the visualization of essential anatomy.

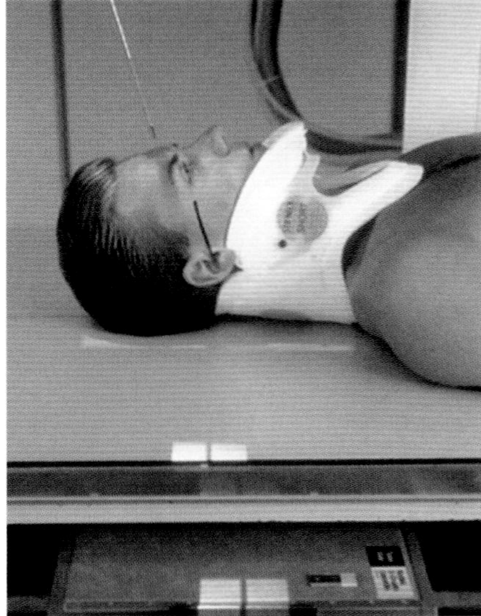

Fig. 19-118. AP 0° to OML—CR parallel to OML, centered to glabella.

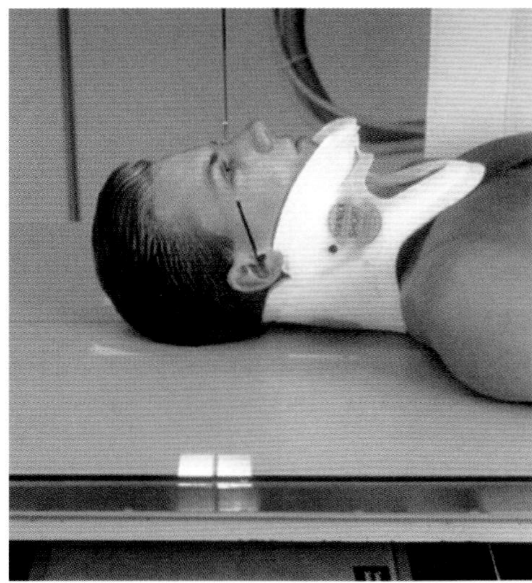

Fig. 19-119. AP 15° reverse Caldwell—CR 15° cephalad to OML, centered to nasion.

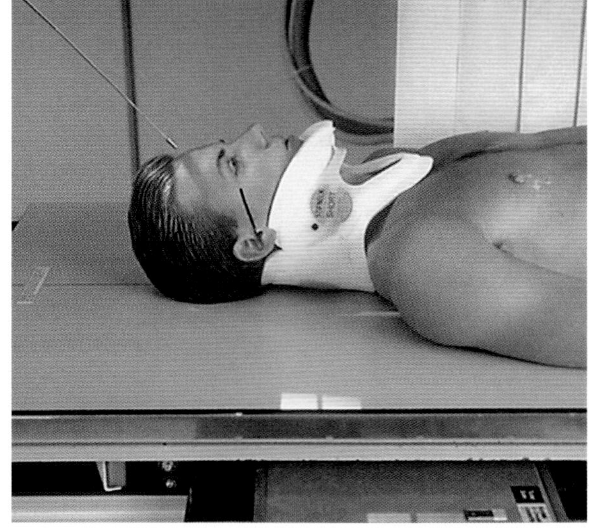

Fig. 19-120. AP axial Towne—CR 30° caudad to OML, centered to midpoint between EAMs.

AP 0°, AP 15° (REVERSE CALDWELL), AND AP 30° AXIAL (TOWNE)—SKULL

AP Versus PA

Trauma skull projections are performed as AP projections, whereas most of the nontrauma projections are PA. This variation will demonstrate reverse anatomic magnification. For example, on a PA projection the orbits, being closest to the IR, will be less magnified than the sagittal and lambdoidal sutures, which are situated farther from the IR. On the AP projection the opposite is true: the orbits are more magnified than the sutures. The PA projection will also demonstrate more distance from the oblique orbital line to the lateral margin of the skull than the AP projection. This is illustrated in Figs. 19-122 and 19-123, which compare an **AP reverse Caldwell** with a standard **PA Caldwell.**

Even though magnification differences exist between the PA and AP projections, causing them to look quite different from one another, the basic radiographic criteria remain the same.

Exposure to neck and thyroid: AP projections of the skull and facial bones obviously increase the exposure to more radiosensitive organs such as the neck and the thyroid regions compared with PA projections. However, benefits outweigh these disadvantages for trauma patients who cannot be turned into a prone position because of possible spinal or other injuries.

Note: If the CR cannot be angled 30° to the OML (before the maximum angle of 45° is reached), the dorsum sella and posterior clinoids will be visualized **superior** to the foramen magnum.

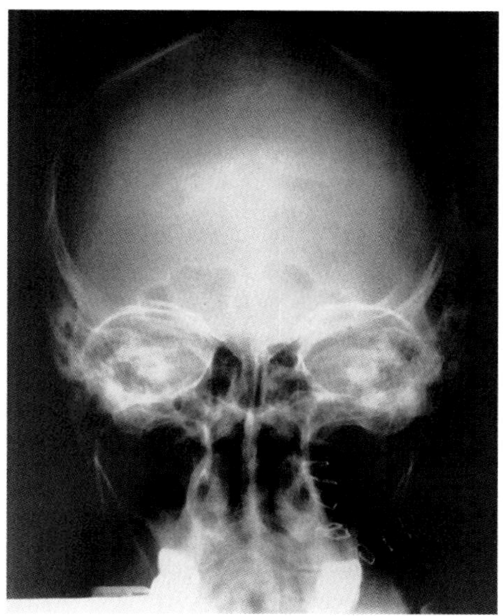

Fig. 19-121. AP 0° to OML.

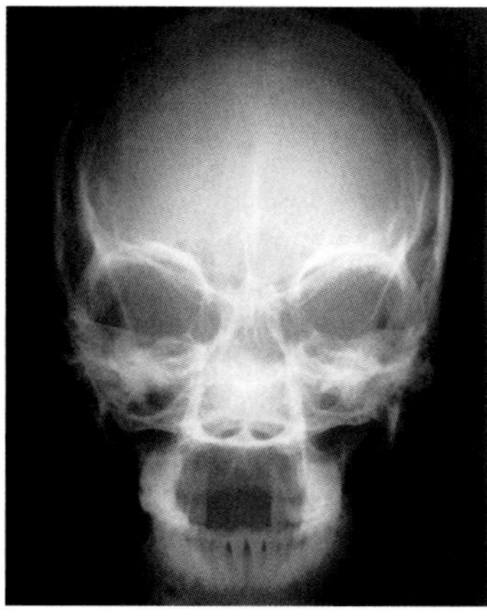

Fig. 19-122. AP "reverse Caldwell"—15° cephalad to OML.

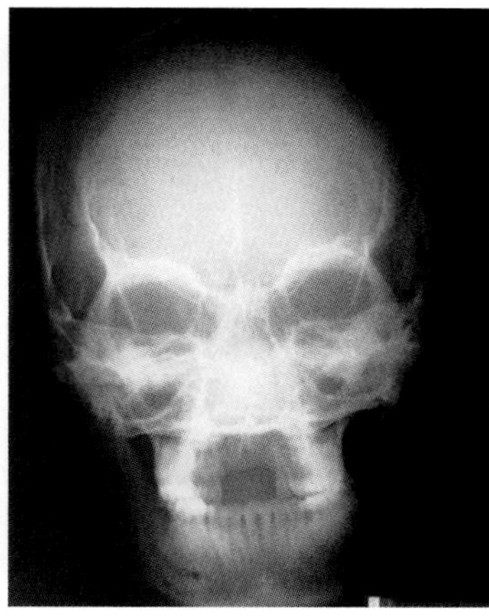

Fig. 19-123. PA Caldwell (15° caudad)—comparison radiograph.

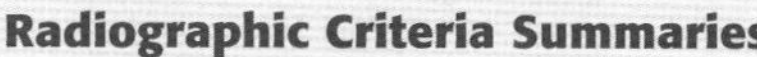

Radiographic Criteria Summaries

Trauma AP 0° Projection:
- Entire skull is visualized on radiograph.
- Petrous ridges superimpose superior orbital region.
- Petrous pyramids fill orbits with internal auditory canals seen horizontally through center of orbits.
- Distance from oblique orbital line to lateral margin of skull on each side is equal.
- Dorsum sellae and anterior clinoids are visualized superior to ethmoid sinuses.
- Sufficient density and contrast are present, without motion, to clearly visualize frontal bone.

Trauma AP "Reverse Caldwell" Projection:
- Entire skull is visualized on radiograph.
- Distance from oblique orbital line to lateral margin of skull on each side is equal.
- Superior orbital fissures are symmetrically visualized within orbits.
- Petrous pyramids and internal auditory canals are projected into the lower one third of orbits.
- Superior orbital margin is visualized without superimposition.
- Sufficient density and contrast are present, without motion, to clearly visualize frontal bone.

Trauma AP Axial (Towne) Projection:
- Entire skull is visualized on radiograph.
- Distance is equal from foramen magnum to lateral margin of skull on each side.
- Dorsum sella and posterior clinoids are projected into foramen magnum. (See Note.)
- Petrous ridges are symmetric and visualized superior to the mastoids.
- Sufficient density and contrast are without motion, to clearly visualize occipital bone.

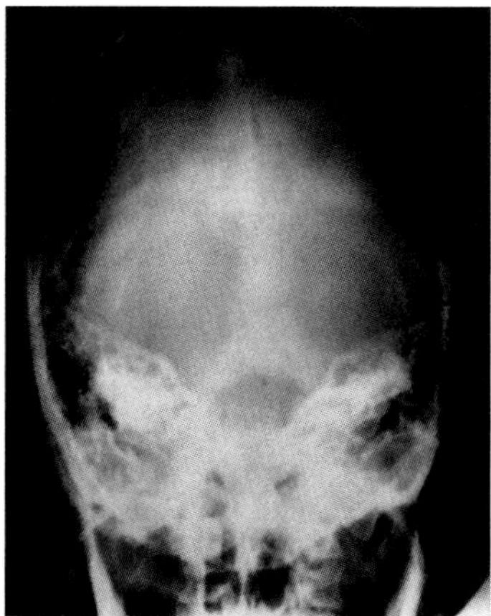

Fig. 19-124. Trauma AP axial "Towne"—30° caudad to OML (max. 45° angle).

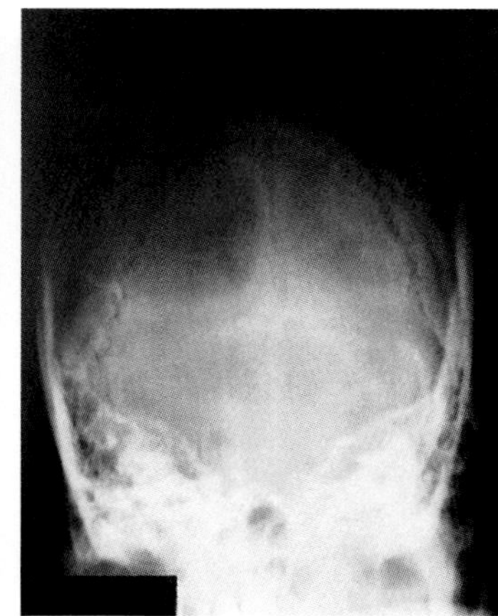

Fig. 19-125. Trauma AP axial—less than 30° caudad to OML.

LATERAL AND ACANTHIOPARIETAL (REVERSE WATERS METHOD)—FACIAL BONES

Warning: Cervical spine fractures and subluxations/dislocations must be ruled out **before** attempting any manipulation of the patient's head or neck. All three of these projections can be achieved without any movement or adjustment of patient's head and neck as demonstrated.

Technical Factors

- IR size—24 × 30 cm (10 × 12 inches), lengthwise
- Grid IR vertical beside lateral aspect of the cranium
- 70-80 kV range
- Small focal spot
- Minimum SID of 40 inches (100 cm)

Positioning—Patient Supine

- If possible, slide patient onto x-ray table in one movement. The head should not be raised to position a grid IR under patient, but if needed it could be placed under the backboard. It is not necessary to remove cervical collar or backboard to obtain these projections.
- Remove all metal, plastic, and other removable objects from head.
- Slide patient's body to bring MSP to midline of table/grid.

Central Ray

Lateral:

- Horizontal beam is essential for visualization of intracranial air-fluid levels.
- Center CR to level **midway between outer canthus and EAM,** which should be in the approximate center of grid.

Acanthioparietal—reverse Waters: This projection best visualizes facial bone structures and the maxilla region by projecting the maxilla and maxillary sinuses above the petrous ridges (see *arrows,* Fig. 19-129).

- Angle CR cephalad as needed to align **CR parallel to mentomeatal line (MML).**
- Center CR to **acanthion;** then center IR to projected CR.

Optional modified acanthioparietal—modified reverse Waters: This projection best demonstrates the floor of orbits and provides a view of entire orbital rims. Petrous ridges are visualized in midmaxillary sinus region (Fig. 19-131).

- Angle CR cephalad as needed to align **CR parallel to lipsmeatal line (LML).**
- Center CR to **acanthion;** then center IR to projected CR.

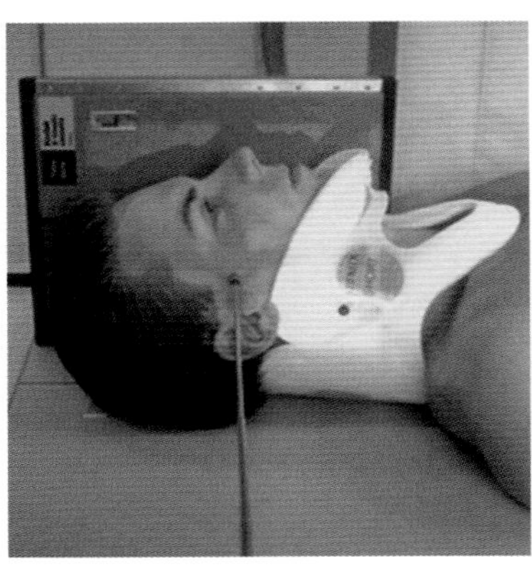

Fig. 19-126. Trauma horizontal beam lateral.

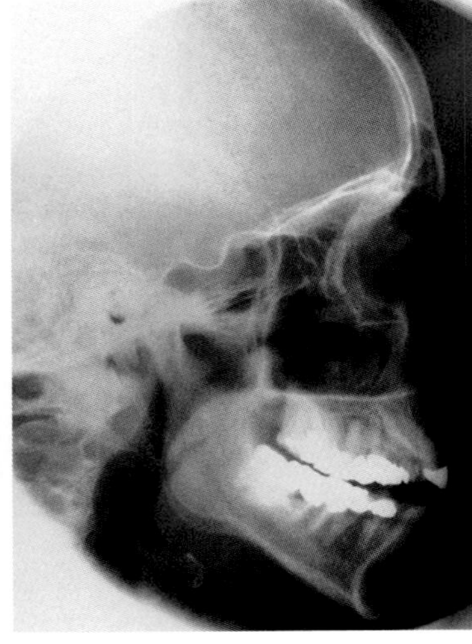

Fig. 19-127. Trauma horizontal beam lateral.

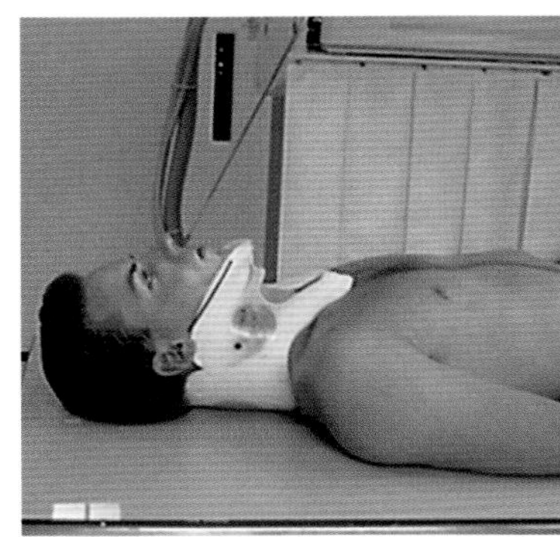

Fig. 19-128. Acanthioparietal (reverse Waters)—CR parallel to MML, centered to acanthion.

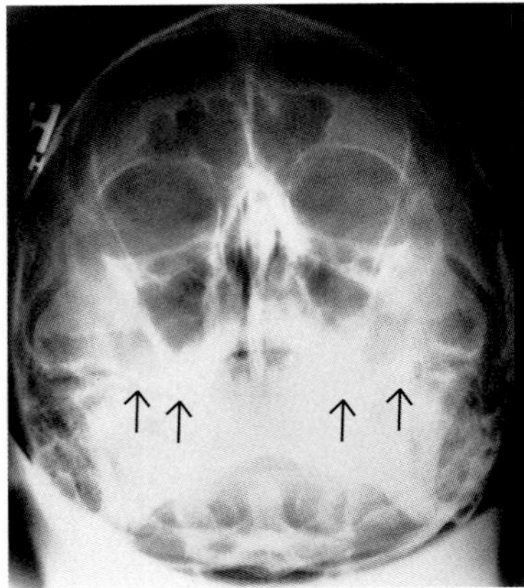

Fig. 19-129. Acanthioparietal (reverse Waters).

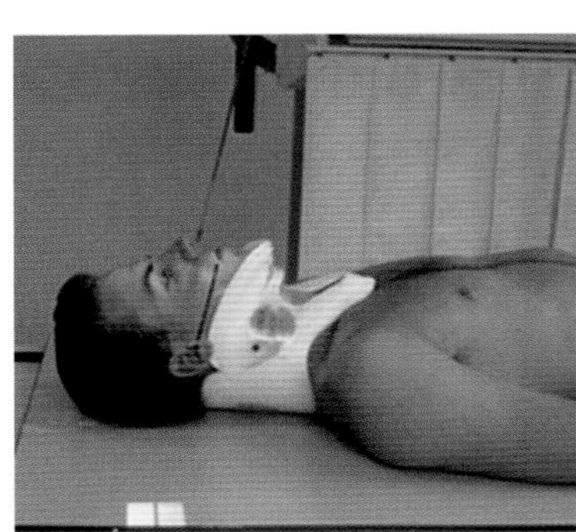

Fig. 19-130. Modified acanthioparietal (modified reverse Waters)—CR parallel to LML, centered to acanthion.

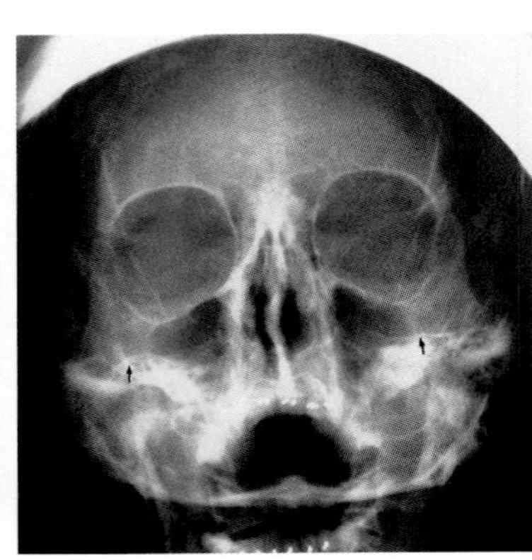

Fig. 19-131. Modified acanthioparietal (modified reverse Waters).

AP, AP AXIAL, AND AXIOLATERAL OBLIQUE—MANDIBLE

Warning: With possible spinal injury, do not attempt to move patient's head or neck. All projections for the mandible can be obtained with the patient supine.

Technical Factors

- IR size—18 × 24 cm (8 × 10 inches), lengthwise, for APs and crosswise for axiolateral obliques
- Grid IR for horizontal beam axiolateral oblique
- 65-75 kV range
- Minimum SID of 40 inches (100 cm)

Positioning—Patient Supine

- Place grid IR under patient's head and shoulders or under backboard. Radiograph may be taken with cervical collar in place.
- Remove all metal, plastic, and other removable objects from head and mandible area.

Central Ray

AP projection (best visualizes rami and lateral body):

- Angle CR caudad as needed to be **parallel to OML.**
- Center CR to midmandible region, approximately at junction of lips.
- Center IR to projected CR.

AP axial (best visualizes condyloid processes, condyles, and temporomandibular joints (TMJs):

- Without manipulating patient's head, angle **CR 35° to 40° caudad to OML.**
- Center CR to pass through region of condyloid processes and condyles, **about 2 inches (5 cm) anterior to EAMs.**
- Center IR to projected CR.

Axiolateral (best visualizes rami, body, and mentum; both sides generally examined):

- Place IR on edge beside face, parallel to MSP with lower edge of IR about 1 inch (2.5 cm) below mentum.
- Depress shoulders if possible and elevate chin (only if cervical fracture/subluxation is **not** a consideration).
- Angle horizontal beam CR 25° to 30° cephalad (from lateral), and angle CR posteriorly 5° to 10° if necessary to clear shoulder. Grid use will not be possible if a double angle is required.
- Center CR to 2 inches (5 cm) inferior to angle of mandible on side away from IR.

Note (axiolateral): Head in true lateral position best demonstrates **ramus** and **proximal body,** and if head can be rotated 10° to 20° toward IR, the **mid- and distal body** and **mentum** region are best visualized.

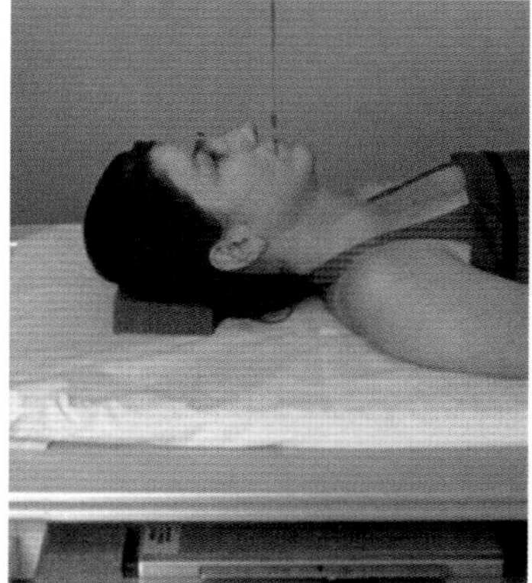
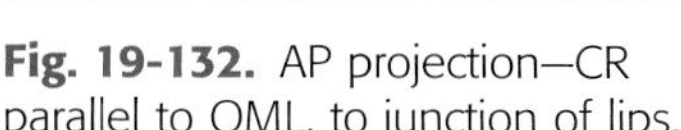

Fig. 19-132. AP projection—CR parallel to OML, to junction of lips.

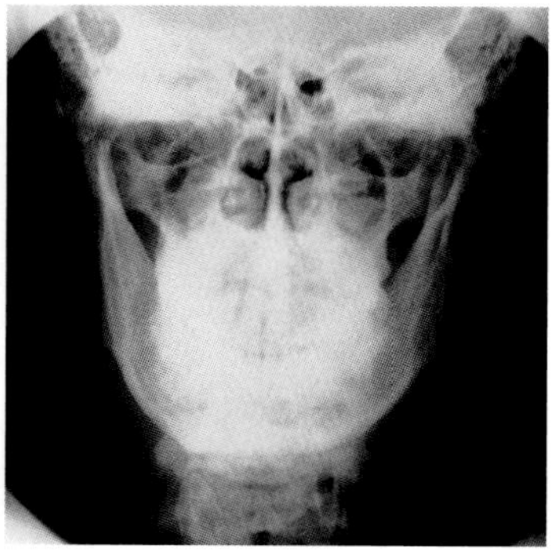

Fig. 19-133. AP projection.

Note: With cervical trauma, do **not** elevate head on sponge as shown (angle CR caudad as needed instead).

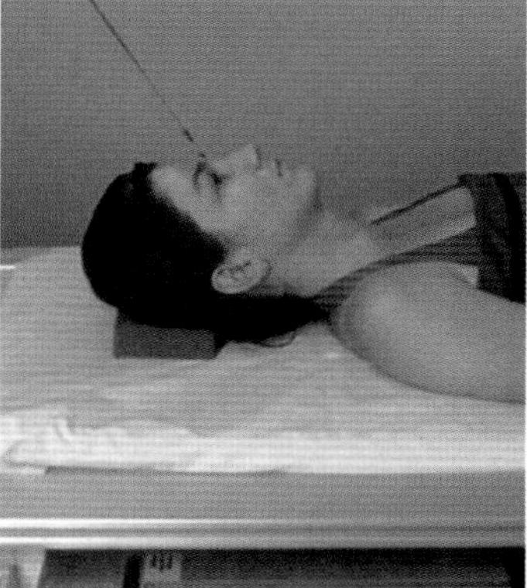

Fig. 19-134. AP axial—CR 35° to 40° caudad to OML.

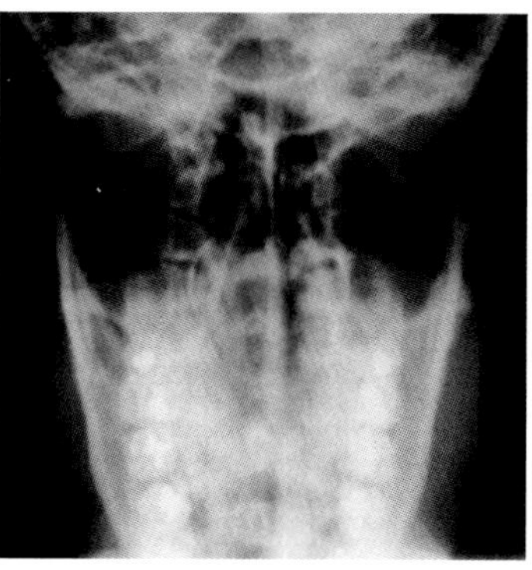

Fig. 19-135. AP axial.

Note: With cervical trauma, do **not** elevate head on sponge as shown (increase CR angle as needed instead).

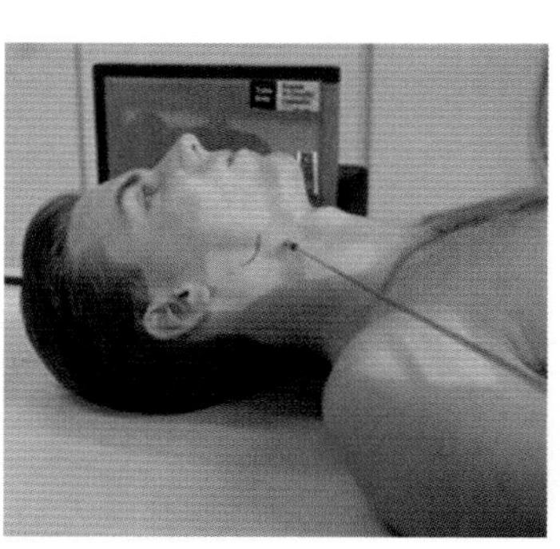

Fig. 19-136. Horizontal beam axiolateral oblique—CR horizontal (or 5° to 10° posteriorly) and 25° to 30° cephalad.

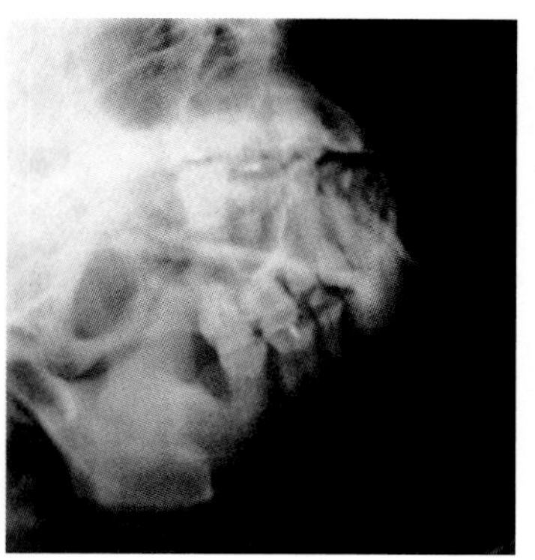

Fig. 19-137. Axiolateral oblique.

19

SURGICAL RADIOGRAPHY

Radiography in surgery may be one of the most demanding challenges encountered by the radiologic technologist. The technologist will be called upon to perform procedures quickly and accurately in a sterile environment, with a minimal number of repeat exposures. Since the patient is often under general anesthesia, the surgeon expects the technologist to perform the procedure without error or delay. These added pressures may create uncertainty and anxiety for the radiography student or recent graduate. However, with a solid knowledge of the surgical procedure and operation of the imaging equipment, the technologist can function very effectively in the surgical suite. Through supervised observations with an experienced surgical technologist, the student can become comfortable and confident in the surgical environment. It is essential that the student technologist be under strict supervision by an experienced technologist in the OR until they have achieved competency for a specific procedure.

Essential Attributes of the Surgical Technologist

While confidence and knowledge of procedures are needed in all aspects of radiography, certain personal attributes, skills, and insights are the trademark of a competent surgical technologist.

CONFIDENCE

Although no one can teach a technologist confidence, it is the first attribute that the other members of the surgical team will expect to see in the technologist. Confidence is judged by the technologist's ease in the use of imaging equipment, ability to problem-solve situations, and respect for the sterile field. The surgical team expects the technologist to be confident in his or her abilities to perform the procedure quickly and accurately with a minimum of repeat exposures. But confidence comes only with experience and knowledge of all aspects of radiography. As the technologist gains more experiences and success in the OR, confidence will grow.

MASTERY

Mastery in all aspects of radiography, including use of the C-arm and mobile radiographic equipment, is essential. The technologist must be able to operate and troubleshoot both conventional and digital equipment. The technologist must also know reliable exposure factors that will work for different sized patients and various procedures.

PROBLEM-SOLVING SKILLS

Even with the best knowledge and preparation, unexpected problems can occur during surgery. C-arms can cease to work, reliable exposure factors may fail to produce a diagnostic image, or the sterile field may be violated. Although it is difficult to predict every situation that may occur in the OR, the surgical technologist must be able to form solutions to these problems quickly. Perhaps the most important skill of the technologist is the ability to immediately problem-solve unforeseen situations.

COMMUNICATION

It is essential that the technologist be an excellent communicator. He or she must communicate with other members of the surgical team any concerns that arise during the procedure. Clear communication between the technologist, surgeon, and anesthesiologist is paramount for most radiographic procedures. For example, during an operative cholangiogram, the technologist must coordinate the exposure with the surgeon injecting the contrast media and the anesthesiologist suspending respiration. Without this team approach, motion may result and the quality of the exposure may be compromised.

The technologist must communicate any radiation safety concerns to the surgical team, including the wearing of aprons, overuse of C-arm real-time imaging, and the placing of hands into the radiation field. In these surgery situations, the technologist is the radiation safety expert and must minimize exposure for the surgical team.

Surgical Team

The composition of the surgical team will vary depending on the surgeon, institutional policy, type of procedure, and other factors. An example of what a typical surgical team may consist of follows.

SURGEON

A physician licensed and trained in either general surgery or a specialty such cardiovascular or orthopedic procedures. The surgeon has the primary responsibility for the surgical procedure and the well-being of the patient prior to, during, and immediately following surgery.

ANESTHESIOLOGIST

A physician anesthesiologist or certified nurse anesthetist who specializes in administering anesthetic drugs to induce and maintain anesthesia to the patient during the surgery. This individual has the responsibility of ensuring the safety of the patient and monitoring physiologic functions and fluid levels of the patient during surgery.

SURGICAL ASSISTANT

A physician, certified surgical technologist, or registered nurse (RN) assistant who assists the surgeon. This person's range of responsibilities may include suctioning, tying and clamping blood vessels, and assisting in cutting and suturing tissue.

CERTIFIED SURGICAL TECHNOLOGIST (CST)

A health professional that prepares the OR by supplying it with the appropriate supplies and instruments. Other CST responsibilities include preparing the patient for surgery and helping to connect surgical equipment and monitoring devices. During surgery, CSTs have the primary responsibility for maintaining the sterile field.

CIRCULATOR

A CST or an RN who assists in the OR by responding to the needs of the scrubbed members within the sterile field before, during, and after the surgical procedure.

SCRUB

A CST or an RN who prepares the sterile field, scrubs and gowns the members of the surgical team, and prepares and sterilizes the instruments before the surgical procedure.

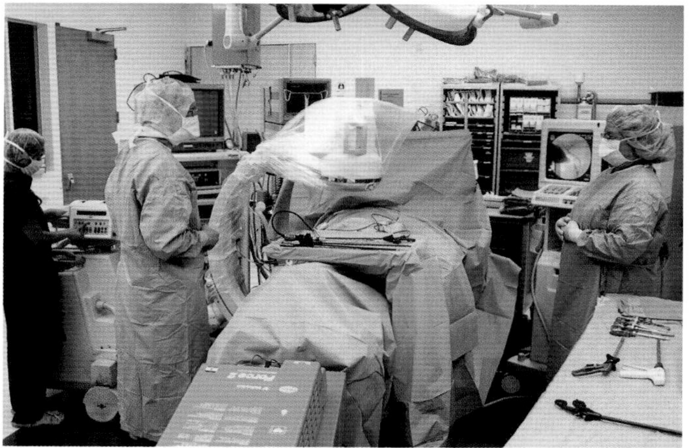

Fig. 19-138. Radiography in the surgical suite.

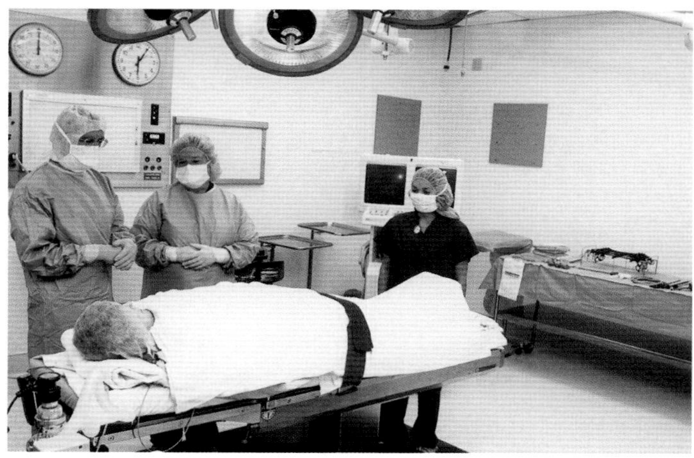

Fig. 19-139. Surgical team—surgeon, certified surgical technologist (CST), and radiologic technologist discussing procedure with patient.

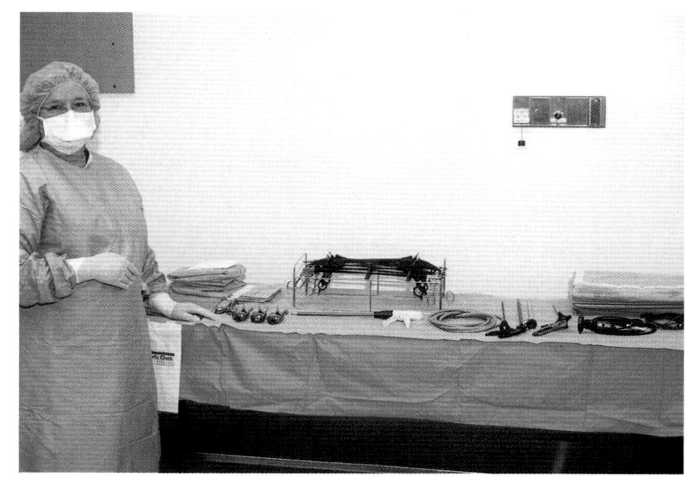

Fig. 19-140. Scrub—preparing and maintaining sterile surgical field.

19

Surgical Suite Environment

The typical surgical suite has two general regions known as **sterile** and **nonsterile** areas.

The **sterile** area includes the patient, surgical field, surgeon and surgical assistants, surgical equipment, tables, and carts. The technologist and imaging equipment must **NOT** violate the sterile area. If the sterile area is violated, the technologist must report this event immediately. Although the violation may have not been noticed by the surgical team, the technologist has a critical responsibility to report it. Often, additional sterile drapes can be used to create a safe and sterile environment once again.

The **nonsterile** area is where the technologist is located, as well as other nonsterile surgical personnel such as the anesthesiologist. The technologist can safely stand and operate imaging equipment within this area. For select procedures, a plastic drape or "shower curtain" may be erected to indicate the dividing point between the sterile and nonsterile areas.

STERILE FIELDS

C-arm use in surgical settings requires special attention to maintaining sterile fields. The top position of the image intensifier often causes it to be placed over open incisions.

Three basic approaches are commonly used to maintain a sterile field, as follows:

The **first** method is **draping the image intensifier, x-ray tube, and C-arm** using a sterile cloth and/or bags with a tension band or adhesive tape holding the cloth or plastic cover in place (Fig. 19-141). Another type of image intensifier cover is called a "snap cover" with a the band that makes a snapping sound when it is released into position (Fig. 19-142). These types of covers also make it possible for the technologist (with guidance from the surgeon) to position the image intensifier precisely as needed over the sterile surgical site for correct centering.

A **second** approach is to temporarily **drape the patient** (or surgery site) with an additional sterile cloth before the undraped C-arm is positioned over the anatomy. Once a satisfactory image has been obtained and the C-arm is removed, the sterile cloth (or drape) is then removed from the patient and discarded. This process is repeated with a new (unused) sterile cloth if it is necessary to use the C-arm again. This approach is used in cases in which the physician does not need to interact with the surgical site during fluoro, or when snap covers are not available.

The **third** method of maintaining a sterile area uses a **"shower curtain."** Hip pinnings or femur roddings require a lateral approach to the surgical incision, making these procedures ideal for the shower curtain. A long horizontal metal bar attached to two vertical suspending rods is placed along the lateral longitudinal axis of the affected side (Fig. 19-143). A large, sterile clear plastic sheet (called a "shower curtain") is suspended from the horizontal bar, which is about 3 feet above the patient. A special opening in the middle of the plastic is attached with a second adhesive strip to the lateral aspect of the hip/proximal femur and is used for access to the incision. The curtain forms a sterile barrier between the doctor and the patient, as the C-arm is positioned for a standard PA and horizontal beam lateral hip from the nonaffected side of the patient.

19

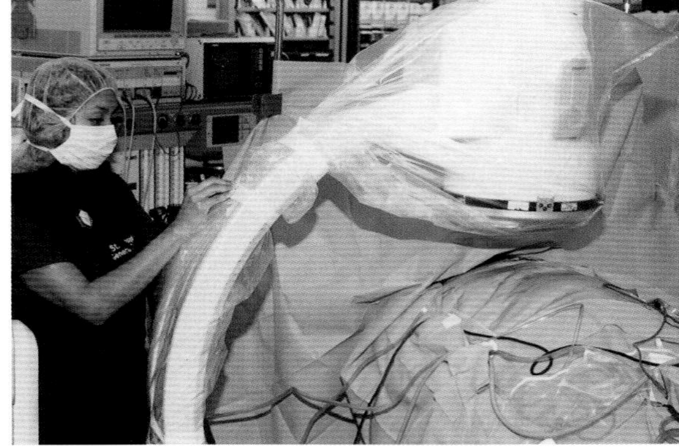

Fig. 19-141. Draping the C-arm with sterile plastic C-arm cover.

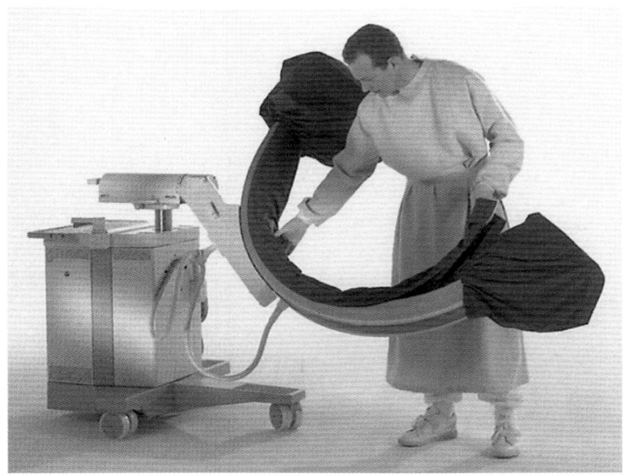

Fig. 19-142. Draping the C-arm and intensifier with snap cover. (Courtesy Philips Medical Systems.)

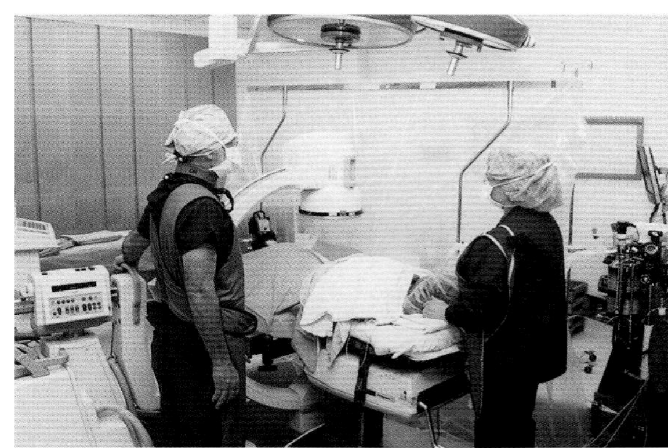

Fig. 19-143. Shower curtain; view from the technologist's (nonsterile) perspective.

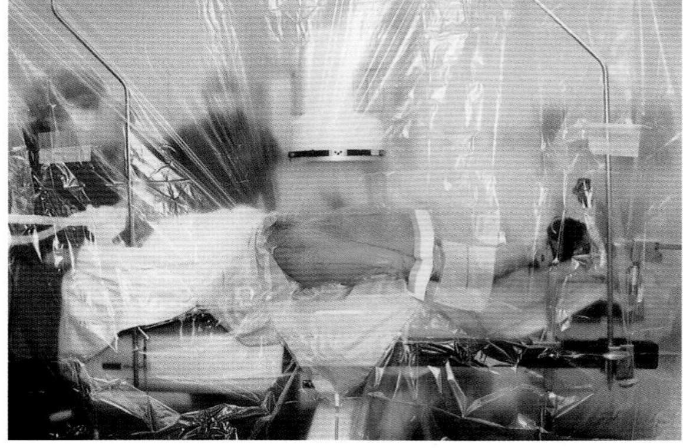

Fig. 19-144. Shower curtain; view from the surgeon's (sterile) perspective.

Surgical Asepsis

ASEPSIS IS THE ABSENCE OF INFECTIOUS ORGANISMS

Unfortunately, it is impossible to remove all infectious organisms from the OR. Surgical asepsis is the practice and procedures to minimize the level of infectious agents present in the surgical environment. By the use of safe practices, wearing proper surgical attire, and exercising care around the surgical incision, the patient's exposure to these infectious agents is greatly minimized. This requires a clear separation of sterile items and areas from nonsterile areas within the surgical suite (Fig. 19-145).

To reduce the risk for infecting the patient during surgery, the following principles of surgical asepsis must be followed:

1. Only sterile items are allowed within the sterile field.
2. If the sterility of an object is in doubt, it must be considered nonsterile.
3. If a sterile drape or cover is touched by a nonsterile object or person, it must be considered contaminated.
4. Nonsterile personnel must not come in contact with a sterile barrier, drape, surgical instrument, or sterile personnel.
5. Any contaminated sterile drape or cover must be reported and replaced by sterile personnel.
6. Sterile gowns are considered sterile from the shoulder to the level of the sterile field, and at the sleeve from the cuff to just above the elbow.
7. OR tables are considered sterile only at the level of the tabletop.
8. Only sterile personnel can touch sterile items.

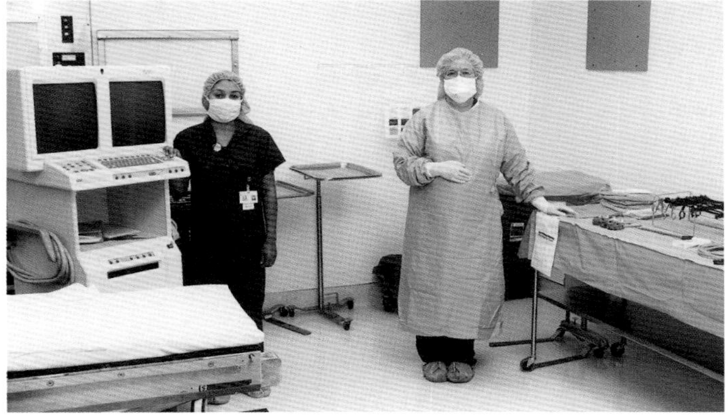

Fig. 19-145. Surgical asepsis—separation of sterile and nonsterile areas.

Surgical Attire

The technologist must change from normal work dress into the appropriate surgical attire before entering the OR. Since the technologist's typical uniform may pose a health concern for the operative patient, proper surgical attire must be worn in all restricted and nonrestricted areas in surgery. Proper surgical attire includes:

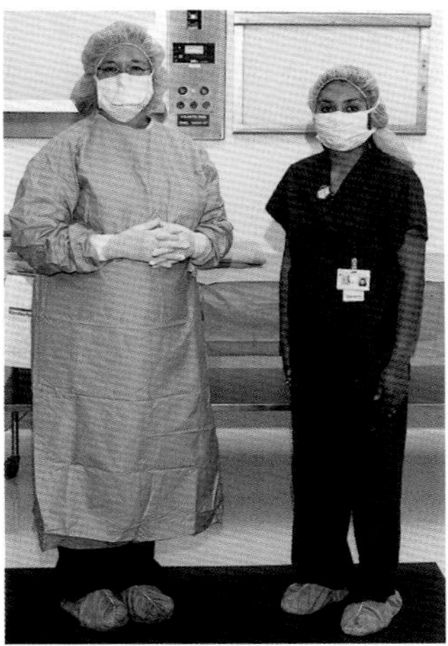

Fig. 19-146. Sterile surgical CST and nonsterile radiologic technologist.

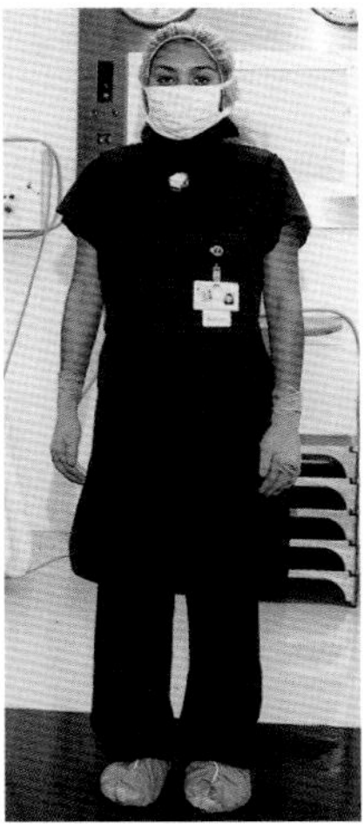

Fig. 19-147. Surgical attire—scrubs, mask, shoe covers, head cover, nonsterile gloves, and protective apron.

SCRUBS

Even if surgical scrubs are normally worn in the general radiology department, the OR technologist must change into approved surgical scrubs. Surgical scrubs should be made of a low-linting material that minimizes bacterial shedding. Two-piece scrubs should fit properly with the top tucked in at the waist. The pant legs of scrub bottom must not drag on the floor. Surgical scrubs must be changed following the procedure and laundered by the hospital. Scrubs must be changed if soiled with blood, perspiration, or food before the wearer reenters the surgical suite.

SCRUB COVER

Scrub covers are button-up or snapped covers worn by the technologist between procedures. They are designed to prevent soiling or cross-contamination of the scrubs while the technologist is outside of the surgical suite. Scrub covers must be removed before entering the surgical suite.

HEAD COVER

A proper-fitting head cover must be worn prior to entering a surgical area. The bouffant and hood type of covers are preferred since they cover the head best. The hood type of cover must be worn for the technologist with a beard or other facial hair. Head covers must be discarded immediately after use and changed for each procedure.

SHOE COVERS

Shoe covers are designed to keep the shoes clean and decrease the amount of soil and bacteria tracked into the surgical suite. They must be changed if they become soiled or torn. They should be worn even in the presurgical and recovery areas.

SHOES

Because of the volume of fluid and presence of sharps in the OR, soft cloth shoes should not be worn. A durable shoe with a closed hard toe and heel will minimize injuries due to falling objects, needles, and cassettes.

MASKS

A surgical mask must be worn to reduce the dispersal of microbial droplets from the technologist during surgery. Masks will also reduce the risk for pathogenic organisms present in the surgical suite being inhaled by the technologist. A single, high-filtration mask is recommended for most procedures. This mask has a pliable nose stripe and two sets of ties to secure it. The nose stripe provides a contoured fit for the wearer and helps prevent fogging for eyeglass wearers. Masks must be changed between procedures or if moisture is detected on the outside of the mask.

PROTECTIVE EYEWEAR

If the technologist is present during a procedure in which blood, body fluids, or tissue debris may strike the eye region, OSHA-approved protective eyewear must be worn. However, this equipment will not be necessary for most of the radiographic procedures performed in surgery.

NONSTERILE GLOVES

When handling contaminated IR cassettes or soiled IR covers or when cleaning equipment following procedures, the technologist must wear nonsterile gloves. Once the gloves are removed, hands must be washed.

Imaging Equipment as Used in Surgery

The technologist must be familiar with the location of power outlets to be used for a procedure. Ideally, all imaging equipment should be in place and checked for correct operation before the procedure.

Although most surgical equipment remains in the surgical area, it must be cleaned and checked frequently for correct operation. Once the procedure has begun, there is no time to troubleshoot equipment or fix problems.

A daily, weekly, and monthly quality control process should be followed on all surgical radiographic equipment. Even a small problem such as a frayed electrical cord must be addressed before it results in an equipment failure.

CLEANING

Portable conventional and C-arm equipment should be cleaned before being brought into the surgical area. An approved antiseptic cleaner should be used to wipe down the equipment. The technologist must wear gloves when cleaning equipment, especially if blood or body fluids are present. A pour type of cleaner rather than an aerosol is recommended to prevent the introduction of air-borne contaminants into the surgical area. Equipment permanently stored in the surgical area must be cleaned weekly or as needed.

Image receptors and grids must be inspected for contamination and cleaned weekly.

OPERATIONAL CHECK

Before imaging equipment is used, an operational check should be performed. A log of any problems and failures should be maintained and monitored.

PROPER EQUIPMENT LOCATION

The technologist must be familiar with the location of power outlets to be used for a procedure. Ideally, all imaging equipment should be in place and checked for correct operation before the procedure.

If C-arm fluoro units are being used, place monitors in clear vision of surgeon. Make sure placement of the C-arm or portable unit is not interfering with normal foot traffic.

IMAGE RECEPTOR PLASTIC COVERS

When an image receptor must be used within the sterile field, it must be placed in a sterile plastic cover. Keep in mind that only the outer surface of the cover is sterile. The inner surface of the cover is nonsterile and comes in contact with the IR. The procedure for placing and removing an IR in a sterile cover is as follows:

1. Sterile surgical personnel hold the plastic cover open with the top cover folded over to maintain sterility of the outer surface and their gloved hands.
2. The technologist carefully slips the IR into the cover.
3. Surgical personnel wrap the top of the cover over and secure it.
4. Once the exposure has been completed, the surgical staff hands the covered IR to the technologist.

Note: The technologist must wear nonsterile gloves when handling the cover because of blood or body fluid exposure.

- The technologist slides the IR onto a nonsterile table or surface, disposes the IR cover, and removes gloves.
- The image is processed.

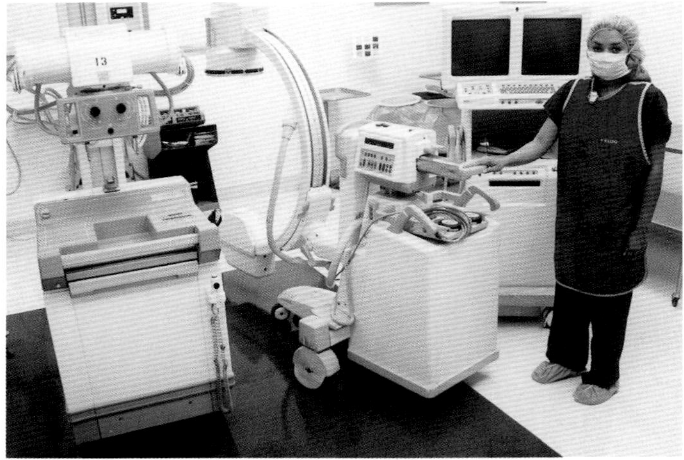

Fig. 19-148. C-arm (mobile fluoroscopy) and conventional mobile radiographic equipment.

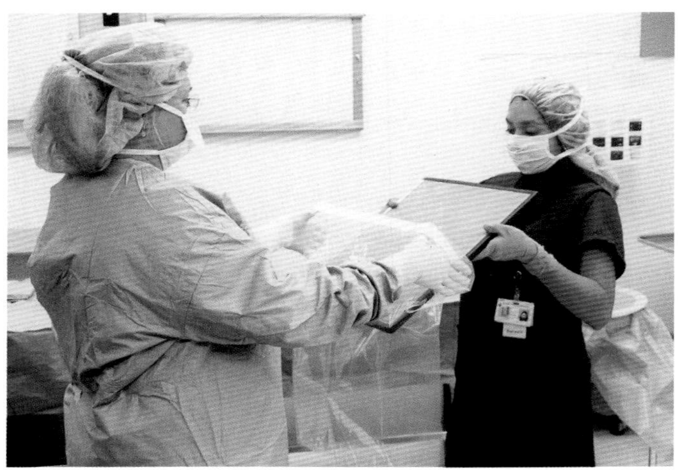

Fig. 19-149 Procedure for placing IR into sterile cover.

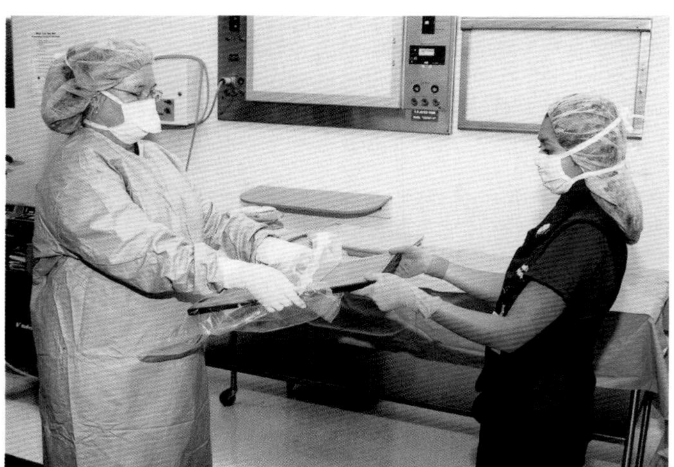

Fig. 19-150 Removing IR from sterile cover.

19

Radiation Protection in the Surgical Suite

Sound radiation protection practices are important for protection of all personnel during mobile imaging as already described. A summary of what this includes in the OR is as follows:

PROTECTIVE APRONS

- Provide adequate number of aprons for all personnel.
- Wear thyroid collar.
- Secure aprons tightly to prevent them from touching sterile field or sterile personnel.
- Clean aprons weekly or as needed with a pour-type cleaner.

USE OF INTERMITTENT FLUOROSCOPY

- Single exposure capacity can greatly reduce fluoroscopy time.
- "Image hold" feature allows last image to remain on monitor.

Minimize Boost Exposures
The "boost" feature on most C-arms provides an improved and brighter image for thick or large anatomy. However, this feature increases radiation, primarily mA, which also increases exposure to the patient and surrounding surgical team by a factor of 3 to 4 times compared with standard fluoroscopy. Use boost feature only when no other alternative or adjustment will improve the image.

Vertical alignment Place vertical alignment of C-arm so the x-ray tube is away from operator's head and neck region. This is achieved by placing the x-ray tube beneath the OR table, reducing the dose to the head and neck region of the surgical team. (See p. 609 for details of C-arm orientation and exposure patterns.)

Minimize Distance Between Anatomy and Image Receptor
Reducing the distance between the anatomy and image intensifier creates a brighter and sharper image with a reduction in radiation to the immediate area.

Coordination of Exposure With Surgical Team
Coordinate exposures between the anesthesiologist, surgeon, and surgical team. For studies such as operative cholangiograms, the injection of contrast media, suspension of patient breathing, and x-ray exposure must be closely coordinated among these team members.

The technologist should clearly announce "x-ray" or "x-ray on" before initiating an exposure to enable nonessential staff to leave the area or get behind lead shields.

Monitor Personal Dosimetry Report Technologists who frequently perform C-arm procedures should closely monitor their personal dosimetry. If they discover excessively high levels, they may need to modify work habits and discuss strategies to reduce dose levels with the department radiation safety officer.

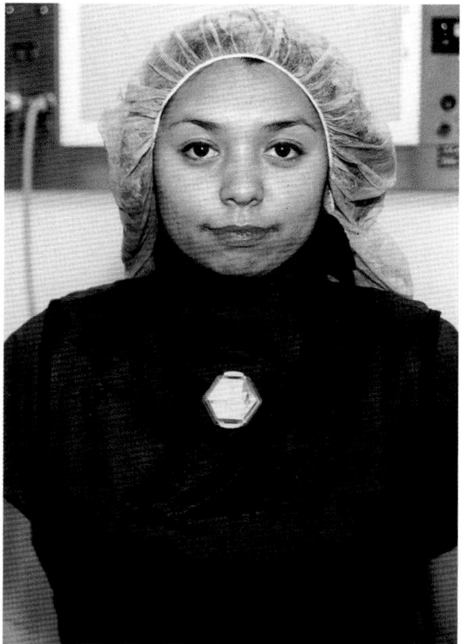

Fig. 19-151. Radiation protection devices—includes protective apron, thyroid shield, and personnel dosimeter.

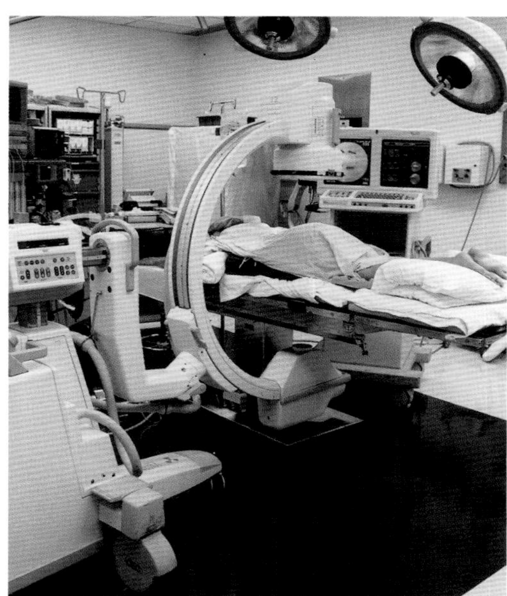

Fig. 19-152. Vertical alignment of C-arm. Note that x-ray tube is under surgical table.

Surgical Radiographic Procedures

OPERATIVE (IMMEDIATE) CHOLANGIOGRAM

Overview of Procedure First performed in 1932, the operative or immediate cholangiogram is performed during surgery to demonstrate anatomy of the biliary ductal system, drainage into the duodenum, and any residual stones in the biliary ducts. In many cases, the patient has a previous history of gallstones, and the surgeon may be concerned about residual stones remaining undetected in one of the biliary ducts.

The operative cholangiogram may be performed before or following surgical removal of the gallbladder. The surgeon places a small catheter into the biliary ducts and injects 6 to 8 ml of iodinated contrast media into the ducts. Once respiration has been suspended, the technologist initiates exposure and produces images using mobile radiographic or C-arm equipment.

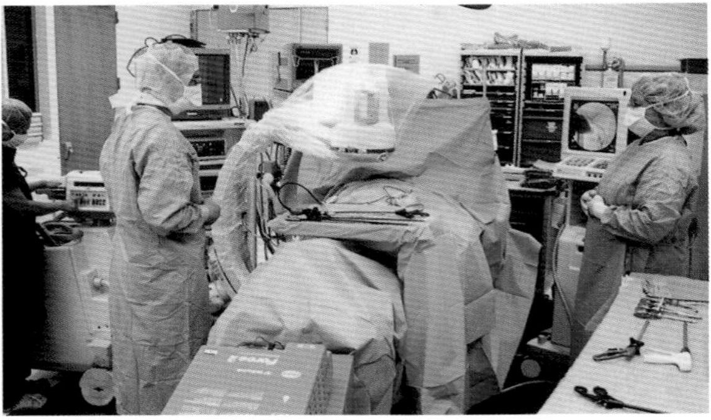

Fig. 19-153. C-arm guided operative cholangiogram.

Equipment Used and Setup C-arm digital fluoroscopic cholangiogram: The C-arm should be set up prior to the beginning of the procedure with the monitors set up in clear view of the surgeon. The C-arm will be positioned in a vertical alignment with the x-ray tube beneath the table. A sterile drape or cover must be placed over the image intensifier. Make sure the C-arm is moved away from the surgical field until needed; then insure that the intensifier portion of the C-arm over the surgical area is covered with a sterile cover during imaging, as shown in Fig. 19-153.

Mobile radiographic cholangiogram: A conventional mobile radiographic unit also can be used for this procedure and should be brought into the surgical suite and positioned carefully near the surgical field. Once the surgical incision has been draped by the surgeon, the x-ray tube is brought in and centered over the anatomy. Often, the surgeon will indicate the centering point by a twist or mark on the sterile towel (Fig. 19-154). The IR is placed in IR holder ("pizza pan") and placed into a special slot underneath the surgical table. The IR and holder are placed into the table near the end of the table closest to the anesthesiologist. Using a handle, the IR is advanced until the IR is centered over the right upper quadrant of the abdomen. With an IR of 35 × 43 cm (14 × 17 inches), the top of the cassette is just below the right axilla.

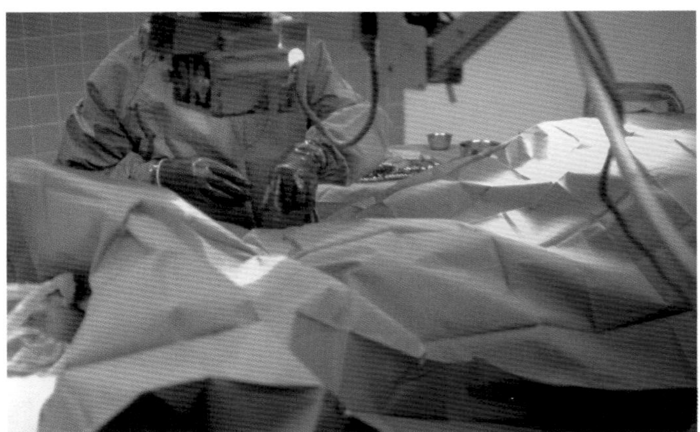

Fig. 19-154. Conventional mobile x-ray unit positioned for AP projection (centering point indicated by surgeon).

Summary of Procedure

1. The technologist changes into surgical attire and ensures that the portable unit or C-arm is functional and clean.
2. Before the patient is surgically prepared, a scout image is taken. The distance the IR is advanced from the head of the table is noted. A special ruler-and-tray setup may be used in the positioning of the IR.
3. The scout image is processed and exposure factors adjusted with IR positioned correctly.
4. Once the catheter is in place, the surgeon injects 6 to 8 ml of contrast media.
5. Images are obtained with the cooperation and synchronization of the surgeon, anesthesiologist, and technologist. The anesthesiologist controls the breathing of the patient.
6. If the OR table is tilted for the oblique positions, the grid cassette is placed crosswise to avoid objectionable grid cutoff.
7. Images are processed and may need to be reviewed by a radiologist. The technologist may convey a written or oral report from the radiologist to the surgeon.

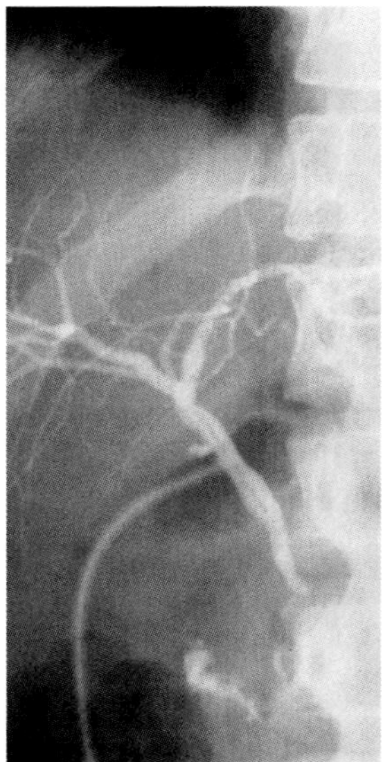

Fig. 19-155. AP projection, biliary ducts.

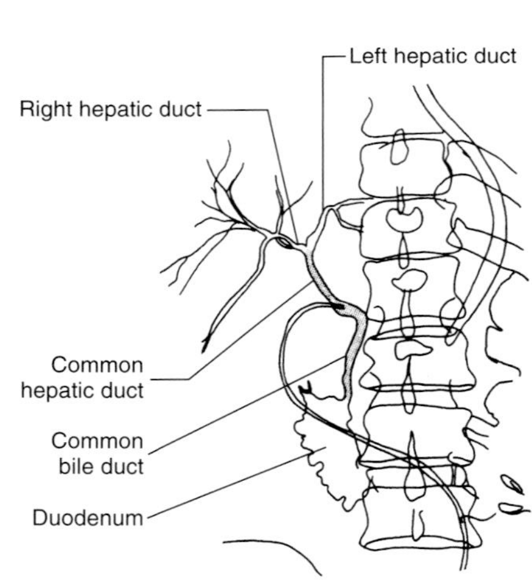

Fig. 19-156. AP projection, biliary ducts.

Images Obtained At least two and preferably three radiographic images are obtained in slightly different positions. Each exposure is preceded by a fractional injection of contrast medium. Positions may include an **AP,** a **slight RPO,** and a **slight LPO.** The RPO is helpful in projecting the biliary ducts away from the spine, especially with a hyposthenic patient.

The C-arm may have to be tilted to project the biliary ducts away from the spine.

Anatomy Demonstrated Contrast-enhanced biliary ducts, including the common bile duct, hepatic ducts, and cystic ducts, are shown. If the cholangiogram is performed before the gallbladder is removed, the gallbladder will be enhanced as well. If stones or biliary duct stenosis are present, opacity of the biliary ducts will be restricted.

19

LAPAROSCOPIC CHOLECYSTECTOMY

Laparoscopic cholecystectomy provides a less invasive approach for the removal of diseased gallbladders. The surgeon makes a small opening in the umbilicus and passes an endoscope into the abdominal cavity. This type of procedure has been used for years in the visual assessment of the abdomen to detect signs of pathology or trauma. It is referred to as a laparoscopic *(lap"ah-ro-skop'ik)* procedure. This technique has been modified to perform cholecystectomy and cholangiography with a minimal amount of surgical trauma to the patient.

Advantages of Laparoscopy Three advantages of laparoscopy are as follows:

1. It can be performed as an outpatient procedure.
2. It is a less invasive procedure. Previous surgical techniques required creation of a large opening to remove the gallbladder. This degree of invasive surgery required that the patient remain in the hospital for at least 2 days.
3. Reduced hospital time (reduced cost). Many patients having the laparoscopic technique can return home the same day and, in certain cases, return to work in 2 to 3 days.

The laparoscopic cholecystectomy, however, is not suited for every patient. More complex disease processes or involved procedures may require the more traditional surgical approach.

RETROGRADE UROGRAPHY

Overview of Procedure Retrograde urography is a nonfunctional examination of the urinary system during which contrast medium is introduced directly retrograde (backward, against the flow) into the pelvicalyceal system via catheterization by a urologist during a minor surgical procedure. Retrograde urography is nonfunctional because the patient's normal physiologic processes are not involved in the procedure. This procedure is frequently performed to determine the location of undetected calculi or other types of obstruction in the urinary system. The procedure may also be performed to study the renal pelvis and calyces for signs of infection or structural defect.

Equipment Used and Setup The procedure usually takes place in outpatient surgery in a dedicated urography room. The urography room generally consists of a combination cystoscopic-radiographic table, which contains a dedicated x-ray tube with a Bucky tray built into the table (Fig. 19-157). If such a table is not available, a mobile radiographic unit or C-arm may be used to image the urinary system. The patient is usually either sedated or anesthetized for this examination. Conventional film-screen or CR image receptors are used for imaging.

Summary of Procedure

1. The patient is placed in the modified lithotomy position, with the legs placed in stirrups, as illustrated in Figs. 19-157 and 19-158.
2. Urologist inserts a cystoscope through the urethra into the bladder. After examining the inside of the bladder, the urologist inserts ureteral catheters into one or both ureters. Ideally, the tip of each ureteral catheter is placed at the level of the renal pelvis.
3. After catheterization a scout radiograph is exposed. The scout radiograph allows the technologist to check technique and positioning and the urologist to check catheter placement. Center IR to level of iliac crest when using a 35- × 43-cm (14- × 17-inch) IR.
4. The second radiograph in the usual retrograde urographic series is a **pyelogram.** The urologist injects 3 to 5 ml of the contrast media directly through the catheter into the renal pelvis of one or both kidneys. Respiration is suspended immediately after injection, and the exposure is made (Fig. 19-159).
5. The third and final radiograph in the usual series is a **ureterogram.** The head end of the table may be elevated for this final radiograph. The urologist withdraws the catheters and simultaneously injects contrast material into one or both ureters. The urologist indicates when to make the exposure.

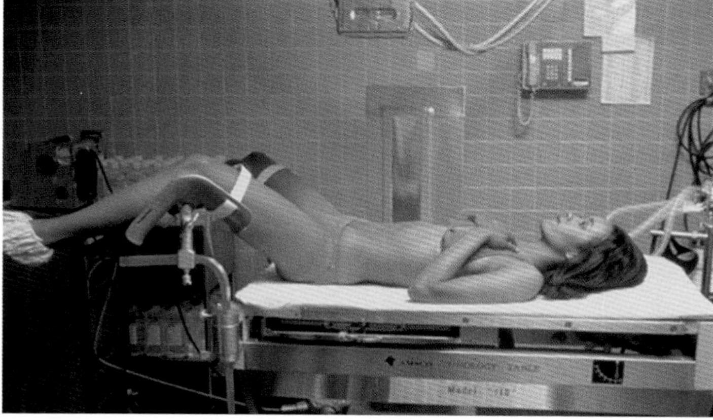

Fig. 19-157. Conventional cystoscopic/radiographic table.

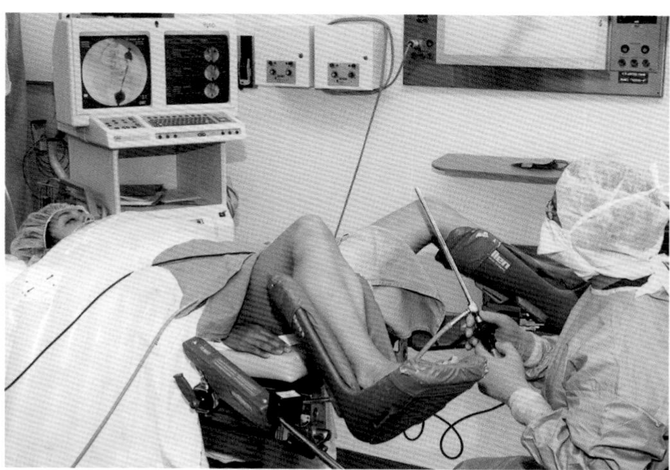

Fig. 19-158. Modified lithotomy position for retrograde urogram.

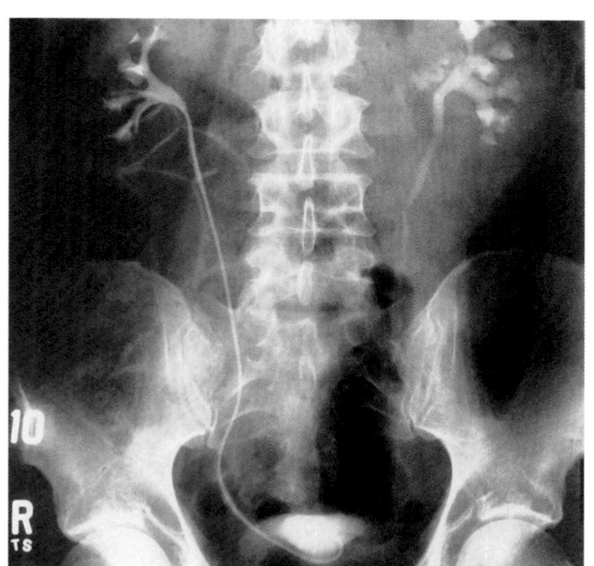

Fig. 19-159. Retrograde urogram—catheter in right ureter, left catheter withdrawn.

This examination is used to directly visualize the internal structures of one or both kidneys and ureters.

Anatomy Demonstrated (Fig. 19-159) A **pyelogram** on the right side with catheter in place best demonstrates the renal pelvis and contrast-filled major and minor calyces. The left side demonstrates the left ureter after the left catheter has been withdrawn; therefore this is called a **ureterogram.**

19

ORTHOPEDIC PROCEDURES

Orthopedic procedures performed in surgery are intended to reestablish the length, shape, and alignment of fractured bones and joints or to restore function and range of motion of joints affected by trauma or disease. Radiography is required for many orthopedic surgical procedures to provide guidance to the surgeon while reducing fractures, inserting various orthopedic devices, or inserting stabilizing rods within long bones.

Technologists have an important role and responsibility during these procedures. They operate the technology that provides the surgeon with "eyes" or vision during the procedure. Either C-arm or mobile radiographic units are used extensively during most orthopedic procedures.

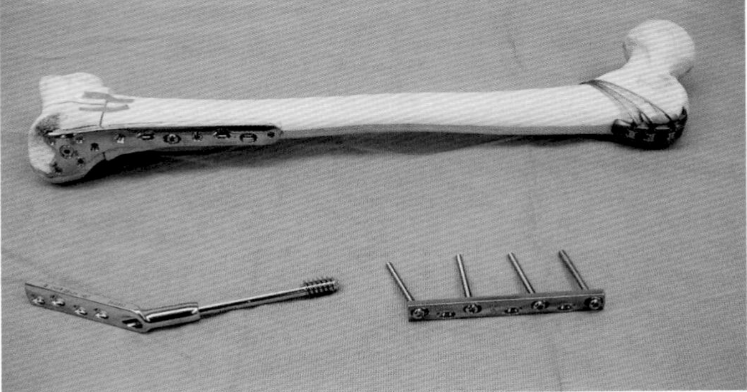

Fig. 19-160. Internal fixation devices.

ORTHOPEDIC SURGICAL TERMINOLOGY AND CONCEPTS

The following terms, procedures, and concepts are common in orthopedic surgery. Knowledge of these terms is essential, because they will frequently be used in the description of various orthopedic surgical procedures.

Closed reduction: Fracture fragments are realigned by manipulation and immobilized by a cast or splint. A closed reduction is a nonsurgical procedure.

Open reduction: For severe fractures with significant displacement or fragmentation, a surgical procedure is required. The fracture site is exposed, and screws, plates, or rods are inserted as needed to maintain alignment of the bony fragments until new bone growth can take place. This surgical procedure is called an **open reduction with internal fixation (ORIF).** Radiographs are frequently taken during such surgical procedures to guide the orthopedic surgeon.

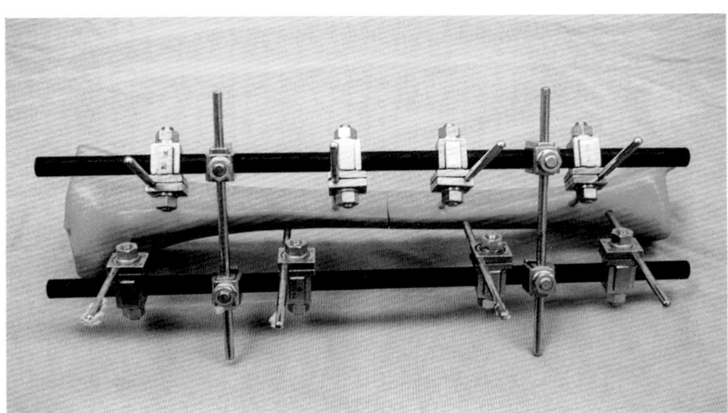

Fig. 19-161. Ilizarov tibial external fixator.

Internal fixation: During open reductions of fractures, a variety of compression plates, screws, pins, intramedullary rods, nails, or wires are applied to reduce or realign the fracture. Based on the age and condition of the individual, the type of procedure performed, and extent of the fracture, these devices are left in place. For other minor surgeries, these fixation devices may be removed later.

External fixation: The use of an external fracture stabilizing device that permits bone healing without the immediate requirement for internal fixation. External fixators can be also used in conjunction with internal fixation procedures. Indications for external fixation include severe open fractures, comminuted closed fractures, arthrodesis, infected joints, and major alignment and length deficits. The Ilizarov device (Fig. 19-161) is a prime example of an external fixator to correct for length deficit. Through a process of tension-stress and distraction, bone length can increase over time through new bone formation. A second external fixation device is shown in Fig. 19-162 for alignment stabilization of the pelvis.

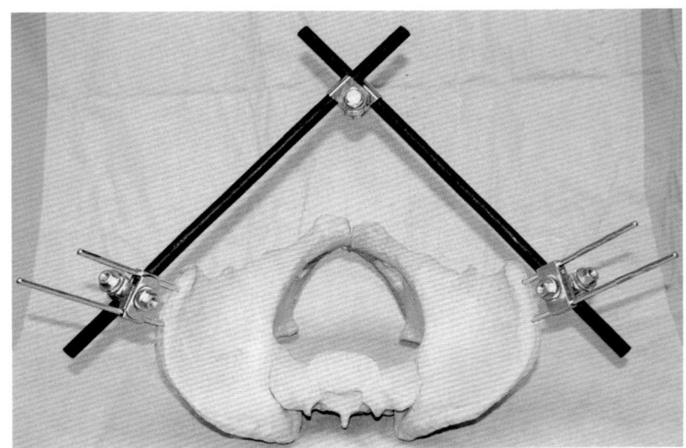

Fig. 19-162. Pelvic external fixator.

Intramedullary fixation: Intramedullary rods and nails are inserted within the shaft of long bones to stabilize fractures. This technique is popular in reducing shaft fractures of the humerus, tibia, and femur. In some cases, the intramedullary rods are a better option than using compression plates and screws to reduce midshaft fractures. Intramedullary fixation devices minimize the amount of tissue exposed during surgery, reduce surgical and healing time, and provide less opportunity for postsurgical infection.

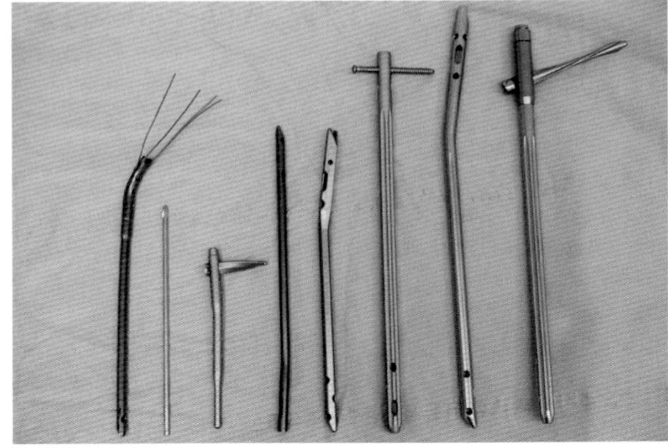

Fig. 19-163. Examples of intramedullary fixators—intramedullary rods and nails.

HIP FRACTURES (PINNING)

Overview of procedure Proximal femur (hip) fractures are classified according to anatomic location. Common hip fractures include **femoral neck** fractures, **intertrochanteric** fractures, and **subtrochanteric** fractures (Fig. 19-164). These fractures require open reduction with internal fixation. The goal of these surgeries is to reduce the fracture, stabilize the fracture, and return use of the lower limb with a minimal loss of blood. Internal fixation devices for hip fractures include the use of cannulated screws, compression screws, lag screw and plate combination, and pins.

During the operative procedure, the patient is placed on a special fracture (orthopedic) table that permits traction of the involved limb and fluoroscopy during the procedure (Fig. 19-166). Based on the type of fracture and the fixation device to be used, the fracture is first reduced through traction and manipulation. An incision is then made at the level of the greater trochanter, and the guide pins are inserted through the fracture, thus stabilizing it. For femoral neck fractures, once the guide pins are aligned, large cannulated screws or some other type of internal fixation pin-type device is inserted through the fracture (Fig. 19-165).

Fluoroscopy is used throughout the procedure to verify the position and location of guide pins and internal fixator. In some cases, the physician may order a postoperative image of the hip and prosthetic device to verify final alignment of the fracture.

Imaging Equipment Used and Setup With the fracture table in place, an isolation drape or "shower curtain" is erected to permit easy access and movement of the C-arm outside of the sterile field (Fig. 19-167). The C-arm must be free to move easily from a PA to a horizontal beam lateral position. A sterile drape is placed over the image intensifier and a nonsterile bag should cover the x-ray tube to prevent blood and Betadine from leaking onto it. The C-arm monitors must be set to provide easy viewing by the surgeon.

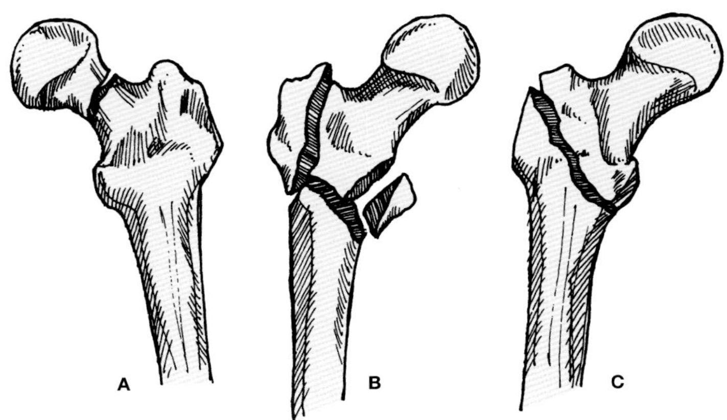

Fig. 19-164. Proximal femur fractures. **A,** Femoral neck. **B,** Comminuted subtrochanteric. **C,** Intertrochanteric. (Modified from Rothrock JC: Alexander's care of the patient in surgery, ed 12, St. Louis, 2003, Mosby.)

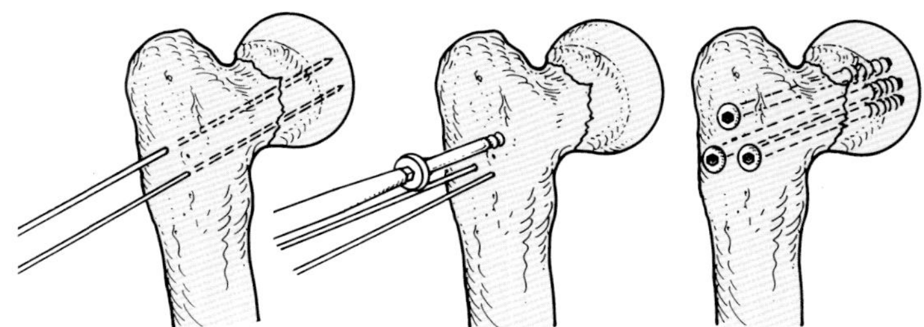

Fig. 19-165. Hip pinning with guidewires and large cannulated screws inserted over guidewires—cannulated screw fixation for nondisplaced femoral neck fractures. (Modified from Rothrock JC: Alexander's care of the patient in surgery, ed 12, St. Louis, 2003, Mosby.)

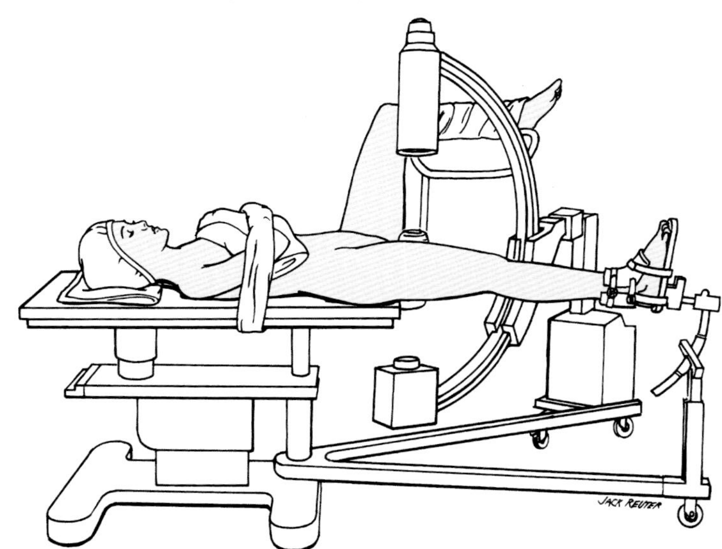

Fig. 19-166. Fracture orthopedic table with C-arm in position. (Modified from Rothrock JC: Alexander's care of the patient in surgery, ed 12, St. Louis, 2003, Mosby.)

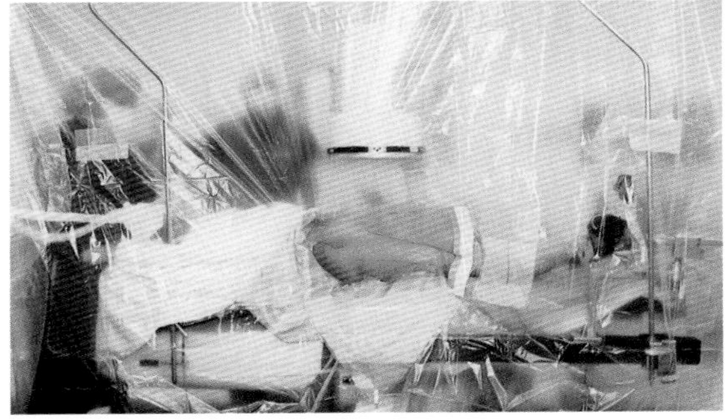

Fig. 19-167. C-arm in PA projection position with intensifier above and tube below and shower curtain in position separating sterile and nonsterile areas.

19

HIP FRACTURES (PINNING)—cont'd

Lateral Hip C-Arm Projection The recommended alignment of the C-arm during a lateral projection hip pinning is to place the x-ray tube inferiorly and the image intensifier superiorly and exteriorly above the hip (Fig. 19-168). This alignment will produce the clearest image of the hip while reducing exposure to the head and neck of the surgeon and surgical personnel (see Fig. 19-43 for radiation exposure patterns for C-arm). However, there may be times when the surgeon will request that the x-ray tube and the intensifier be reversed because the superior position and the size of the image intensifier make it more difficult to perform certain surgical procedures (Fig. 19-169).

Summary of Procedure

1. Fracture is reduced and lower limb is placed in traction to maintain proper alignment of the fracture.
2. Fluoroscopy is used to verify alignment in both AP and lateral perspective.
3. Incision is made just below greater trochanter.
4. Guide pins are inserted thorough fracture site. Location and position of guide pins are verified with fluoroscopy.
5. Bone reamer is used to provide a channel for screw or other internal fixator device.
6. Cannulated, lag, or compression screw assembly is inserted over the guide pins. Position of screw is verified with fluoroscopy in the AP and lateral perspective.
7. Guide pins are removed and traction is released.
8. Surgical wound is closed.
9. Include the entire orthopedic prosthesis for all projections taken postoperatively.

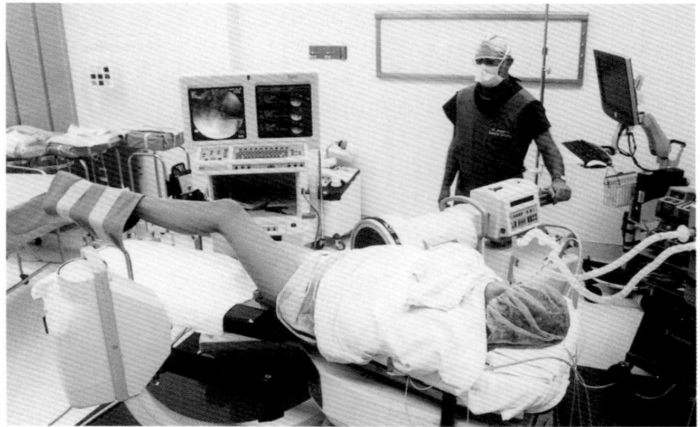

Fig. 19-168. Recommended C-arm alignment for lateral right hip imaging.

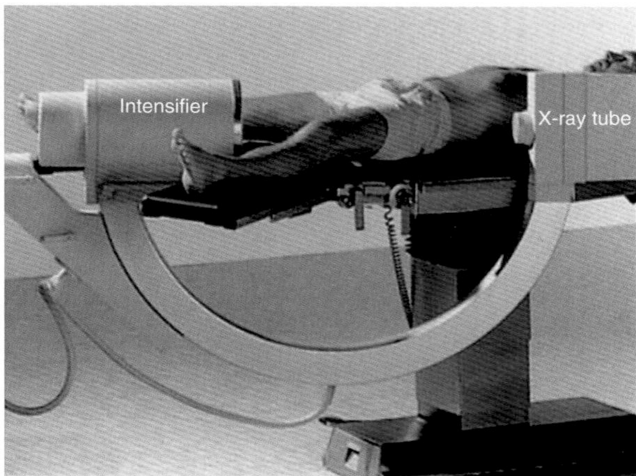

Fig. 19-169. Alternative C-arm alignment if requested by surgeon; not recommended because of increased radiation exposure pattern at tube end.

19

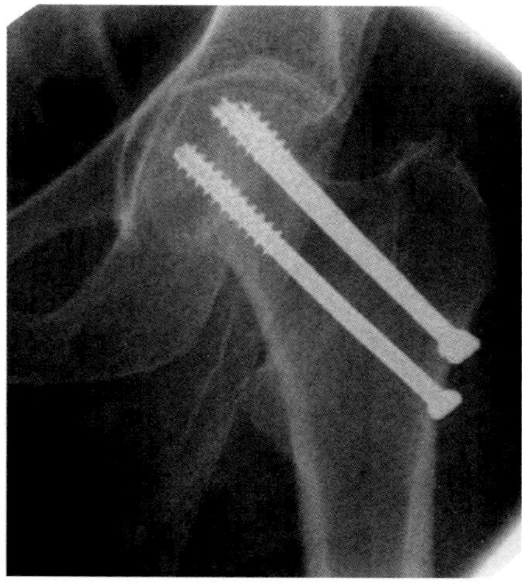

Fig. 19-170. Postoperative radiographic images of hip "pinning" demonstrating internal fixation devices in place—AP projection. (From Ballinger PW, Frank ED: Merrill's atlas of radiographic positions and radiologic procedures, ed 10, St. Louis, 2003, Mosby.)

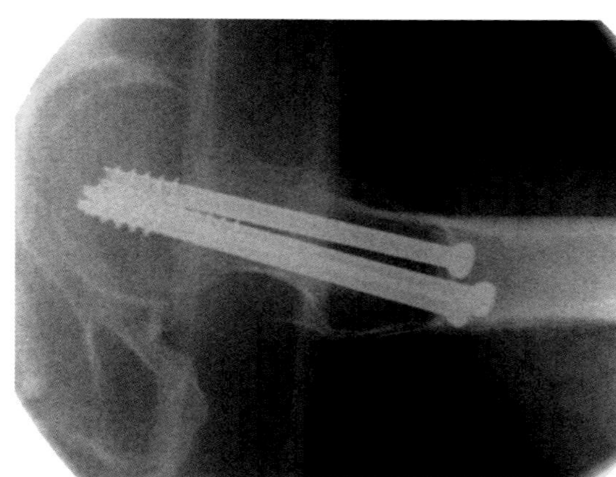

Fig. 19-171. Postoperative radiographic images of hip "pinning" demonstrating internal fixation devices in place—lateral projection. (From Ballinger PW, Frank ED: Merrill's atlas of radiographic positions and radiologic procedures, ed 10, St. Louis, 2003, Mosby.)

TOTAL HIP REPLACEMENT (ARTHOPLASTY)

Overview of Procedure In the case of degenerative disease or chronic trauma to the femoral head and/or acetabulum, a prosthetic hip may be required to return normal function to the patient. These prosthetic appliances vary in composition, design, and components. Metallic alloys are used in the design of newer prosthetic hips, including cobalt-chromium and titanium.

The older Austin-Moore and Thompson endoprosthetics are single-piece devices that take the place of the proximal femur from the head to just below the surgical neck (Fig. 19-172). The newer modular bipolar endoprosthetic hip (Fig. 19-173) also includes a stem inserted into the femoral shaft and the separate alloy femoral head with a polyethylene-lined cup inserted below the bony acetabulum. Once inserted, the three-piece device operates as a single unit. The stem of the prosthesis is either cemented into the medullary cavity or held in place with a combination of compression plates and screws.

Equipment Used and Setup Typically, C-arm fluoroscopy or mobile radiography is not required during a total hip replacement. Postoperative images may be taken in the recovery room with the mobile radiographic unit.

Anatomy Demonstrated The prosthetic device should be seen in its entirety in both the AP and horizontal beam lateral perspectives. Ensure that exposure is adequate to demonstrate the acetabulum.

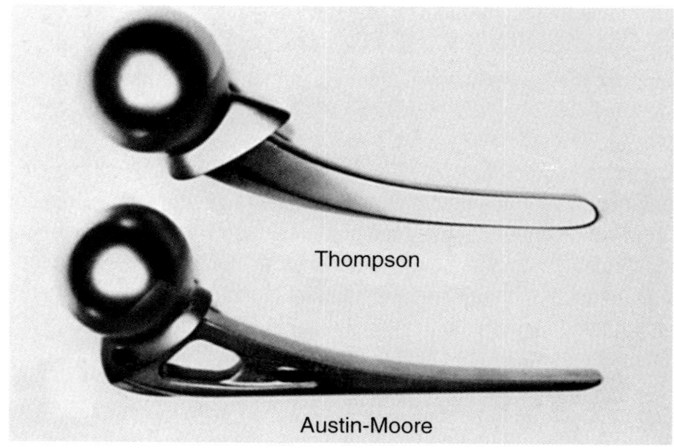

Fig. 19-172. Austin-Moore and Thompson femoral endoprotheses. (Modified from Rothrock JC: Alexander's care of the patient in surgery, ed 12, St. Louis, 2003, Mosby.)

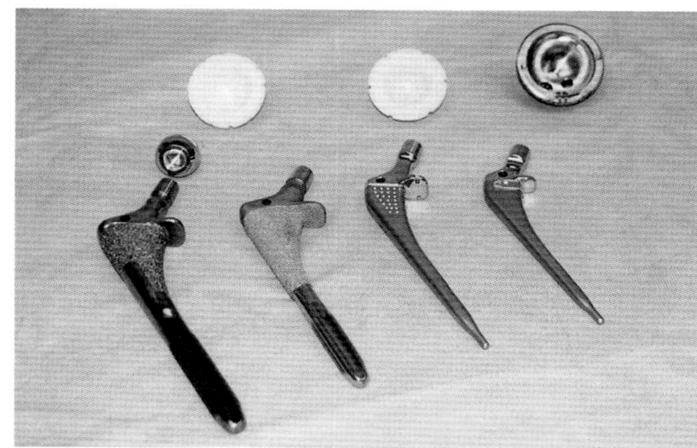

Fig. 19-173. Modular bipolar hip endoprostheses.

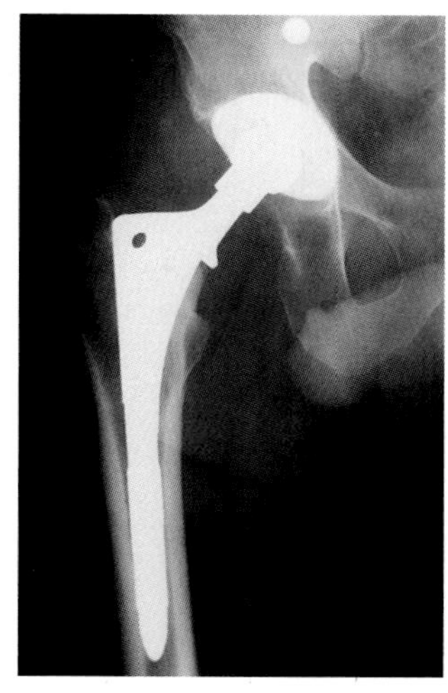

Fig. 19-174. Total hip replacement—AP hip.

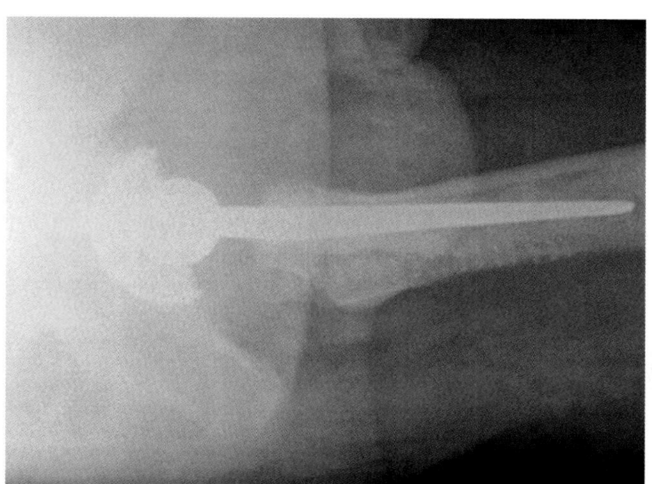

Fig. 19-175. Total hip replacement—lateral hip.

19

LONG BONE INTRAMEDULLARY NAIL OR ROD (INTERNAL FIXATORS)

Overview of Procedure The use of an **intermedullary nail or rod** for femoral, tibial, and humeral shaft fractures has become quite common. These nails or rods are inserted into the intramedullary shaft of the long bone and may be held in place with locking screws.

Intramedullary nails or rods are inserted in either an antegrade or retrograde direction. **Antegrade procedures** will have the nail or rod inserted from the proximal end of the long bone. **Retrograde procedures** will have the internal fixator introduced from the distal aspect of the long bone.

The patient may be placed on a fracture OR table that permits traction of the involved lower limb and use of C-arm fluoroscopy during the procedure. A humeral shaft fracture will not usually require the use of a fracture table. An incision is made either proximal or distal to the long bone. A bone reamer is used to widen the intramedullary cavity. Guidewires are inserted and advanced through the fracture site.

Fluoroscopy is used to verify the location of the guidewire and the alignment of the fracture. Once alignment has been verified, the intramedullary nail or rod is inserted. If locking screws are used, they fix the nail or rod in place. Postoperative images may be taken to document alignment of fracture and proper placement of internal fixator device.

Equipment Used and Setup With the fracture table in place, an isolation drape ("shower curtain") or sterile drape may be erected to permit easy access and movement of the C-arm outside of the sterile field (see Fig. 19-176 for PA projection). The C-arm must be free to move easily from a PA to a horizontal beam lateral position (Fig. 19-177). If a "shower curtain" is not used, a sterile drape is placed over the image intensifier and a nonsterile bag should cover the x-ray tube to prevent blood and Betadine from leaking onto it during the PA projection. The C-arm monitors must be set to provide easy viewing by the surgeon.

Summary of Procedure

1. Incision is made either antegrade or retrograde to long bone.
2. Bone reamer is used to widen the intramedullary cavity to the correct circumference.
3. Guidewire is inserted down the shaft of the long bone through the distal fragment. Position of guidewire is verified with C-arm fluoroscopy in both AP and lateral perspective.
4. Intramedullary nail or rod is inserted over guidewire and manipulated to match the curve of long bone and properly align the fracture.
5. Fluoroscopy is used to verify correct position of internal fixator and reduction of fracture in both AP or PA and lateral perspective.
6. Locking screws may be inserted on proximal and distal ends of long bones to secure the nail or rod.
7. Surgical wound is closed.
8. Postoperative radiographs may be taken to document the final outcome of the procedure.

Anatomy Demonstrated Long bone is demonstrated, with fracture reduced and internal fixator seen in its entirety.

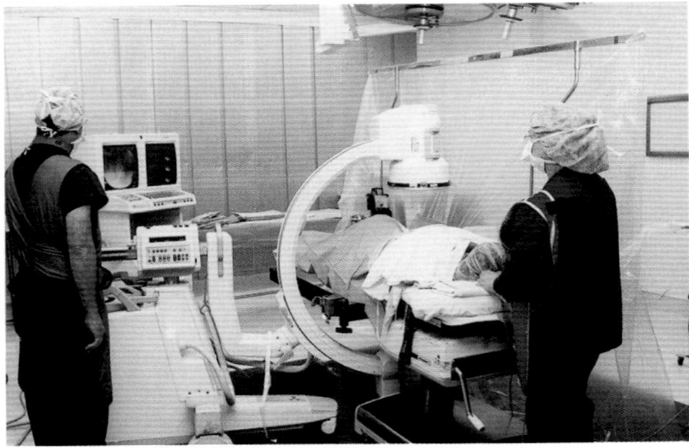

Fig. 19-176. C-arm in place for PA projection with shower curtain in place—tibial nail or femoral intramedullary rod procedure.

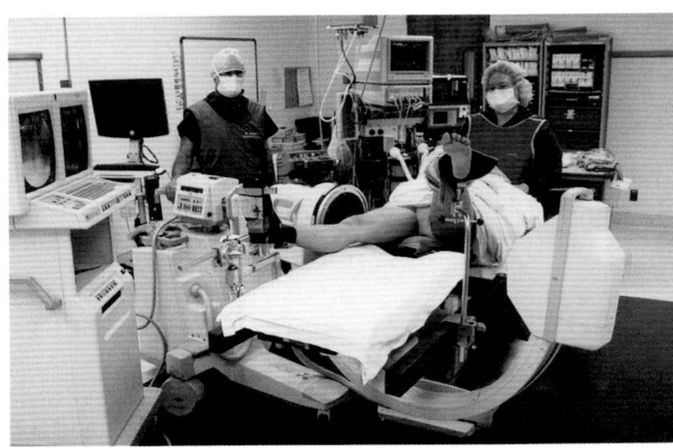

Fig. 19-177. C-arm in place for lateral projection for femoral intramedullary rod procedure.

Spinal Procedures

LAMINECTOMY

Overview of Procedure **Laminectomy** is a surgical procedure performed to alleviate pain caused by neural impingement. The surgery is designed to remove a small portion of the bone or herniated disk material impinging on the nerve root. The surgery is intended to give the nerve root more space by removing the source of impingement or irritation. Based on the number of vertebrae excised during the laminectomy, **spinal fusion** of surgically altered vertebrae may be necessary.

Interbody fusion devices or "cages" are another alternative to the traditional spinal fusion or use of pedicle screws to stabilize the vertebrae. **Interbody fusion cages** are titanium cages filled with bone that are inserted between the vertebral bodies in order to maintain disk space height and fuse the joint, thereby eliminating abnormal movement.

A laminectomy is effective to decrease pain and improve function for patients with lumbar spinal stenosis. **Spinal stenosis** is a condition that primarily afflicts elderly patients; it is caused by degenerative changes that result in enlargement of the facet joints. The enlarged joints then place pressure on the nerves, which may be effectively relieved with a lumbar laminectomy.

Cervical laminectomy is performed to remove bony obstructions such as bone spurs (osteophytes) and herniated disk material that cause pain by impinging on the spinal cord or spinal nerves in the cervical region.

Equipment Used and Setup The laminectomy may require the use of C-arm or mobile radiographic units. The role of radiography is to confirm the correct level for the laminectomy and to provide fluoroscopic guidance if orthopedic plates and/or screws are used during the surgery. The C-arm must be free to move easily from an AP to a horizontal beam lateral position. A sterile drape is placed over the image intensifier, and a nonsterile bag should cover the x-ray tube to prevent blood and Betadine from leaking onto it. The C-arm monitors must be set to provide easy viewing by the surgeon.

Summary of Procedure

Cervical procedure (anterior approach) The patient is placed in a supine position with arms drawn down by the sides of the body. The arms may be placed in traction to ensure visibility of the lower cervical vertebrae.

1. Needle is placed at level of laminectomy. Correct vertebral level is verified by C-arm fluoroscopy in both the AP and lateral perspective. Mobile radiographic unit may be used as well to confirm correct needle placement.
2. The C-arm must be parallel to the vertebra to avoid any distortion of the structures seen.
3. Cervical plates and screws may be used during the procedure to stabilize the vertebrae. C-arm fluoroscopy may be used to guide the placement of the orthopedic appliances.

Lumbar procedure (posterior approach) The patient is prone with bolster under abdomen to flex the spine. Arms are usually above head on arm boards (Fig. 19-178).

1. Needle is placed at level of laminectomy. Correct vertebral level is verified by C-arm fluoroscopy in both the AP and lateral perspective. Mobile radiographic unit may be used as well to confirm correct needle placement.
2. The C-arm must be parallel to the vertebra to avoid any distortion of the structures seen.
3. Pedicle screws, interbody fusion cages, rods, and other appliances may be used during procedure. C-arm fluoroscopy may be used to assist with placement of orthopedic appliances.

Anatomy Demonstrated Spine in AP and lateral perspective at the desired level is shown. The total vertebrae must be demonstrated, including the spinous processes.

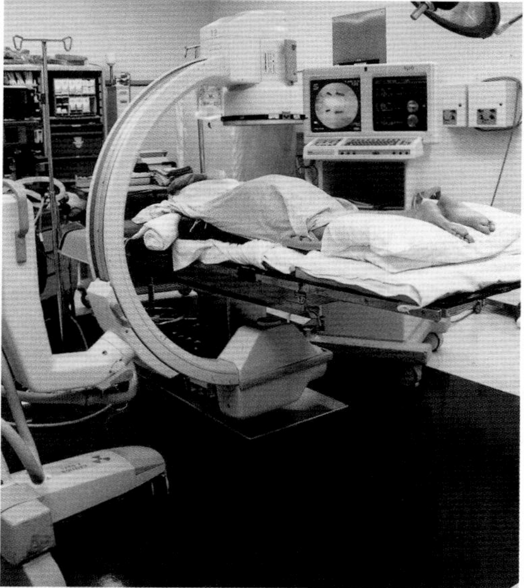

Fig. 19-178. AP projection (patient prone, tube below) for lumbar laminectomy.

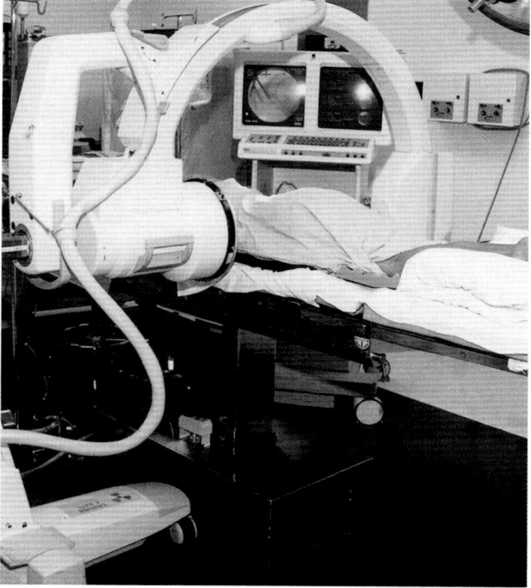

Fig. 19-179. Lateral projection in position for lumbar laminectomy.

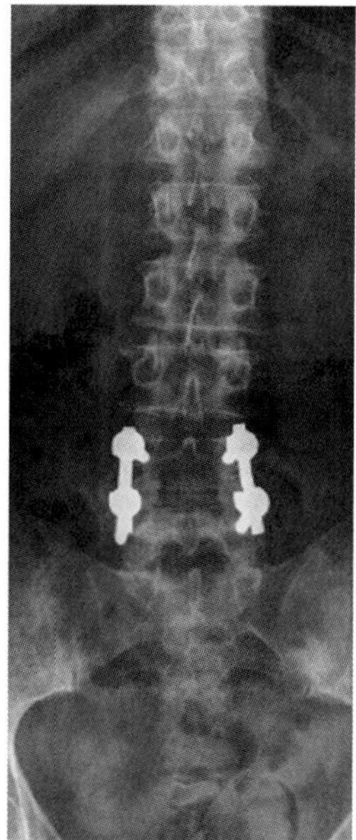

Fig. 19-180. Lumbar laminectomy/fusion—AP projection.

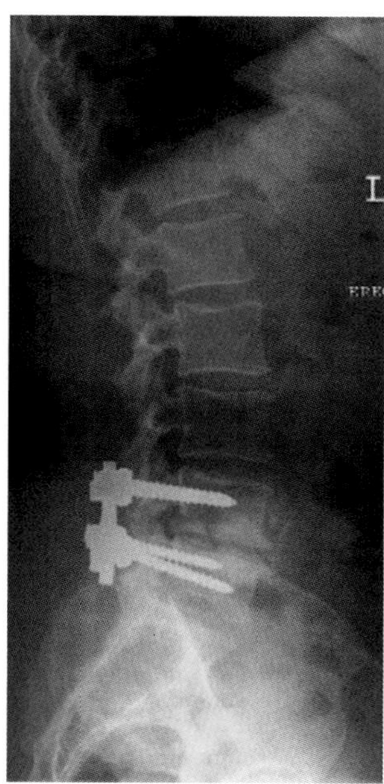

Fig. 19-181. Lumbar laminectomy/fusion—lateral projection.

19

MICRODISKECTOMY

Microdiskectomy is gaining popularity as an alternative to the traditional lumbar laminectomy. First, a laminotomy (opening into the lamina) is performed, which opens up the spinal canal in order to visualize the pinched nerve root.

A high-powered stereoscopic microscope is used to provide illumination and magnification of the impinged nerve and surrounding structures to be visualized clearly through an incision less than 1 inch long. The nerve root is carefully protected with a specialized retractor, and protruding disk fragments, along with any remaining loose or degenerated disk material, are then removed with a small grasping device. The small hole left in the annulus will regenerate in 4 to 6 weeks and fill in with new disk material.

C-arm fluoroscopy may be used in providing an AP and horizontal beam lateral perspective of the spine during the procedure.

SCOLIOSIS CORRECTIVE SURGERY

Scoliosis is an abnormal lateral curvature of the spine. Although a normal lateral curvature of the spine has no negative bearing on the individual, advanced forms of scoliosis may result in deformity of the body, neurologic problems, and unequal lower limb length.

For severe forms of scoliosis, posterior spinal fusion with internal fixation devices inserted may reduce the negative outcome of the scoliosis and provide stability to the spine. Most scoliosis procedures are performed on adolescents to allow for correction of the spine as the individual matures. Devices such as Harrington and Luque rods may be inserted to help reduce abnormal curvature of the spine while providing additional support.

Radiography and C-arm fluoroscopy may be used during the procedure. In certain procedures, both an AP and horizontal beam lateral are taken to confirm correct placement of the rods.

Postoperative images may be taken in the recovery room. It is important to minimize movement of the patient during imaging. A 14 × 17 inch (35 × 43 cm) IR should be used to demonstrate the entire orthopedic device and spine.

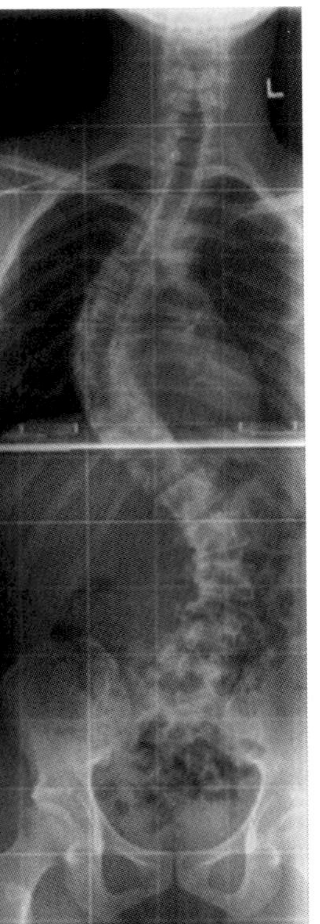

Fig. 19-182. Scoliosis—AP projection.

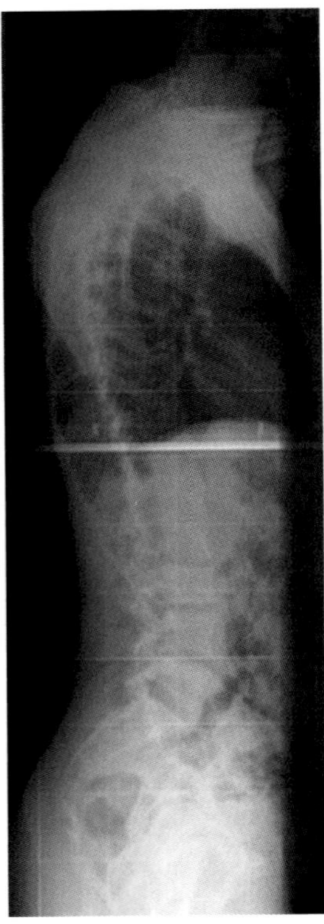

Fig. 19-183. Scoliosis—lateral projection.

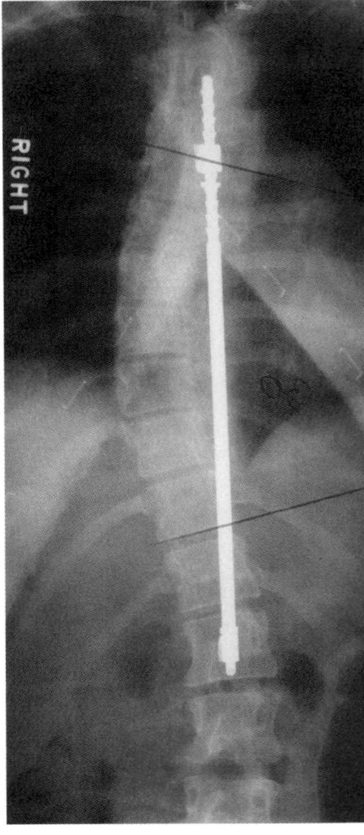

Fig. 19-184. AP with Harrington rod in place.

19

Other Surgical Procedures

PACEMAKER INSERTION

Overview of Procedure Approximately 500,000 Americans have an implantable permanent pacemaker device. A pacemaker implantation is performed under local anesthesia in a hospital by a surgeon assisted by a cardiologist. An insulated wire called a lead is inserted into an incision above the collarbone and guided through a large vein into the chambers of the heart. These electrodes stimulate the heart muscle, causing it to beat at a predetermined rate. This process is referred to as "pacing" of the heart.

The electrodes are often inserted through a vein in the arm or chest and advanced into the right ventricle under fluoroscopic guidance. The pulse generator or battery that provides the electrical sensation to control the heart beat may be external (temporary) or inserted into the superficial tissues of the chest wall.

Equipment Use and Setup A pacemaker or other line insertion procedure can be performed in the surgical suite, outpatient surgery suite, or radiology department. The use of fluoroscopy is essential during the insertion of the electrodes into the right ventricle of the heart.

C-arm mobile fluoroscopy is used in the surgical suite. The C-arm must be free to move easily from an AP to a horizontal beam lateral position. A sterile drape is placed over the image intensifier. The C-arm monitors must be set to provide easy viewing by the cardiologist or surgeon.

Summary of Procedure—Transvenous Approach

1. Venotomy is performed.
2. Under fluoroscopic guidance, the electrode is advanced into the right atrium, through the tricuspid valve, and into the right **ventricle.** The tip of the electrode is advanced until it reaches the right ventricular apex.
3. Pulse generator is inserted in the chest wall.
4. Once the procedure is complete, the patient's vital signs are monitored and a chest x-ray may be taken to ensure that the pacemaker and leads are properly positioned.

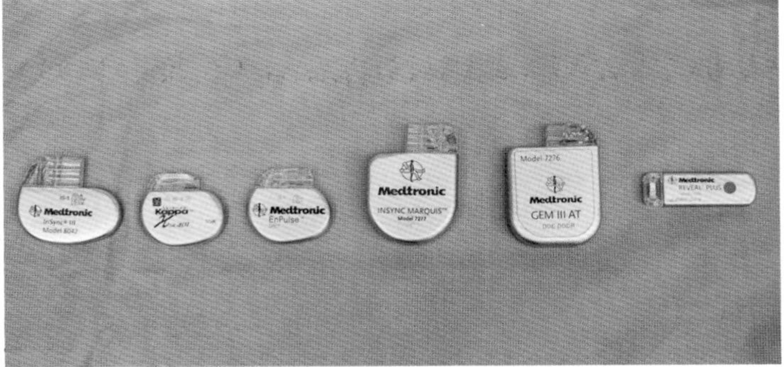

Fig. 19-185. Sample pacemaker pulse generators/batteries.

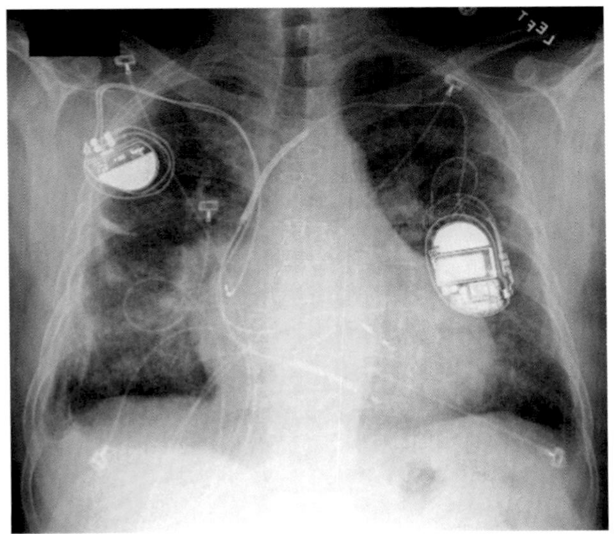

Fig. 19-186. PA chest with pacemaker in place.

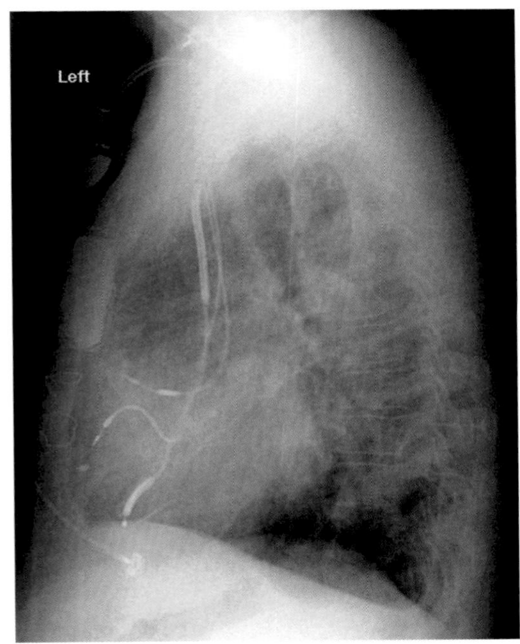

Fig. 19-187. Lateral chest with pacemaker in place.

Glossary of Surgical Abbreviations, Terminology, and Procedures

ACL: Anterior cruciate ligament

Arthrodesis *(ar-thro-de'-sis):* Stiffening of a joint by operative means

Arthopathy *(ar'throp'a-the):* Any disease affecting a joint

Arthroplasty *(ar'thro-plas-te):* Creation of an artificial joint to correct ankylosis

Asepsis *(a-sep'sis):* A state of sterility; condition in which living pathogens are absent

Cancellous screw: Orthopedic screw designed to enter and fix porous and spongy bone

Cannulated screw: Large screw used for internal fixation of nondisplaced fractures of proximal femur

Cardiac pacemaker: An artificial regulator for cardiac rate and rhythm

Cerclage wire: Orthopedic wire that tightens around fracture site to reduce shortening of limb

Cesium *(se'ze-um)* **implants:** The use of radioactive cesium in the treatment of certain malignancies, including prostate cancer

Cholecystectomy *(ko"le-sis-tek'-to-me):* Surgical removal of gallbladder.

Closed reduction: Procedure in which bone fragments are reduced manually without surgical intervention

Cortical screw: Narrow, orthopedic screw designed to enter and fix cortical bone

CR: Closed reduction (cast or traction)

Cystoscope *(sis'to-skop)*: Lighted tubular endoscope used for examination of the urinary bladder

DHS: Dynamic hip screw

Dynamic compression plate: Screw and plate combination to apply forces through the fracture site; used commonly for long bone shaft fractures where stress may be great

ESWL (extracorporeal shock wave lithotripsy): Electrohydraulic shock waves used to break apart calcifications in the urinary system

EX-FIX: External fixation

Fracture (orthopedic) table: A special OR table used for hip pinnings and other orthopedic procedures to provide traction to the involved limb and permit fluoroscopy to be performed during the procedure

Hip pinning: Surgical procedure designed to reduce proximal femoral fractures through the use of various internal fixation devices

HTO: High tibial osteotomy

Ilizarov technique: Procedure using a special external fixator to lengthen long bones as a treatment for severe fracture or congenital deformity

IM-nail: Intramedullary nail

Interbody bone fusion device: Titanium or other alloy cage filled with bone and inserted between the vertebral bodies in order to maintain disk space height and permit fusion of the intervertebral joint

Intramedullary rod: A flexible or rigid device placed within the medullary cavity to reduce a fracture or stabilize a diseased long bone.

Kirschner *(kirsh'ner)* **wire (K-wire):** Unthreaded (smooth) or threaded metallic wire used to reduce fractures of wrist (carpals) and individual bones of the hands and feet; may also be used for skeletal traction

Laparoscopic *(lap"ah-ro-skop'ik)* **cholecystectomy:** Use of a special endoscopic device to visualize and assist with the surgical removal of the gallbladder

Laminectomy *(lam'i-nek' to-me):* A surgical procedure performed to alleviate pain caused by neural impingement by removing an aspect of the lamina in the vertebral arch

Laminotomy *(lam'i-not'o-me):* Surgical opening into one or more lamina of the vertebral arch

Lithotripsy *(lith'o-trip-se):* Crushing of calcification in the renal pelvis, ureter, or urinary bladder by mechanical force or sound waves

Microdiskectomy *(mi'-kro-dis-kek'-to-me):* Microsurgical procedure performed on the spine to remove bony fragments or disk material that may be causing neural impingement

Neural impingement: A condition in which bony changes or a herniated disk produces an impingement of the spinal nerves that pass through the vertebral arch of the vertebra.

Open reduction: To reduce fracture fragments through surgical intervention

Operative (immediate) cholangiogram: Radiographic procedure performed during surgery to visualize and locate undetected stones or obstructions within the biliary ducts

ORIF: Open reduction internal fixation

PCL: Posterior cruciate ligament

Prostheses *(pros'the-sis):* Fabricated (artificial) substitute for a diseased or missing anatomic part.

Reduce: As applied in orthopedic medicine, to align two bone fragments in the correct position as treatment for a fracture

Retrograde urography: A nonfunctional examination of the urinary system during which contrast medium is introduced directly retrograde (backward, against the flow) into the pelvicalyceal system via catheterization by a urologist during a minor surgical procedure

Semitubular plate: Flexible and thin orthopedic plate to fix and connect fractures

Shower curtain: An isolation drape that separates the sterile field from the nonsterile environment; often used to permit the use of C-arm fluoroscopy during a hip pinning procedure

Spinal fusion: Surgical fusion of one vertebra to another, stabilizing them following laminectomy or as treatment for a degenerative condition or fracture

Spinal stenosis: Condition caused by degenerative changes that result in enlargement of the facet joints. This enlargement often leads to impingement of the spinal nerves that pass by them

Strike through: Soaking of moisture through a sterile or nonsterile drape, cover, or protective barrier, permitting bacteria to reach sterile areas

THR/THA: Total hip replacement/total hip appliance

TKR/TKA: Total knee replacement/total knee appliance

Total joint arthroplasty: The use of artificial joint implants to restore motion and function of a joint; for example, the total hip replacement is a common orthopedic procedure performed on patients with degenerative joint disease such as avascular necrosis (AVN) of the proximal femur

Traction: The process of putting a limb, bone, or group of muscles under tension by means of weights and pulleys to align or immobilize the part

CHAPTER 20

Pediatric Radiography

CONTRIBUTORS TO PAST EDITIONS Claudia Calandrino, MPA, RT(R), Jessie R. Harris, RT(R), Cecilie Godderidge, BS, RT(R)

CONTENTS

INTRODUCTION AND PRINCIPLES

The pediatric technologist sees children as special persons to be handled with care and understanding. This requires patience and the necessary time to **talk to** and **make friends** with the child. Explaining instructions to children in a way that they can understand is of great importance in developing trust and cooperation.

AGE OF UNDERSTANDING AND COOPERATION

Children do not all reach a sense of understanding at the same predictable age. This ability varies from child to child, and the pediatric technologist must not assume that children will comprehend what is occurring. Generally, however, by the age of **2 or 3 years,** most children can be talked through a diagnostic radiographic study without immobilization or parental aid. Most important is a sense of trust, which begins at the first meeting between the patient and the technologist; the first impression the child has of the technologist is everlasting and forges the bond of a successful relationship.

Successful radiographic studies are dependent on two things. First and most important is the **technologist's attitude and approach to a child.** Second and also important is the **technical preparation in the room,** which includes certain essential immobilization devices as are described and illustrated in this chapter.

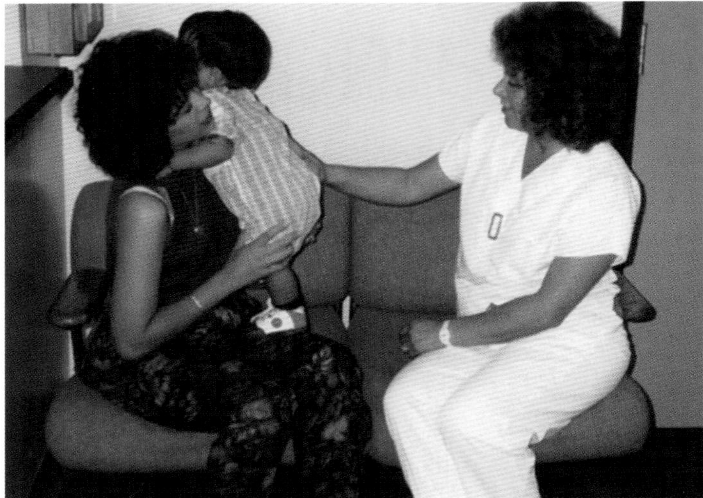

Fig. 20-1. Technologist introducing herself to patient and developing trust.

PREEXAM INTRODUCTION AND CHILD/PARENT EVALUATION

Self-Introduction At the first meeting, most children are accompanied by at least one parent or caregiver. The following steps are important:

- Introduce yourself as the technologist who will be working with this child.
- Find out what information the attending physician has given the parent and patient.
- Explain what you are going to do and what your needs will be.

Tears, fear, and combative resistance are common reactions for a young child. The technologist must take the time to communicate to the parent and child, in language they can understand, exactly what they are going to do. The technologist must try to build an atmosphere of trust in the waiting room before the patient is taken into the radiographic room. This includes discussing the necessity of immobilization as a last resort if the child's cooperation is unattainable.

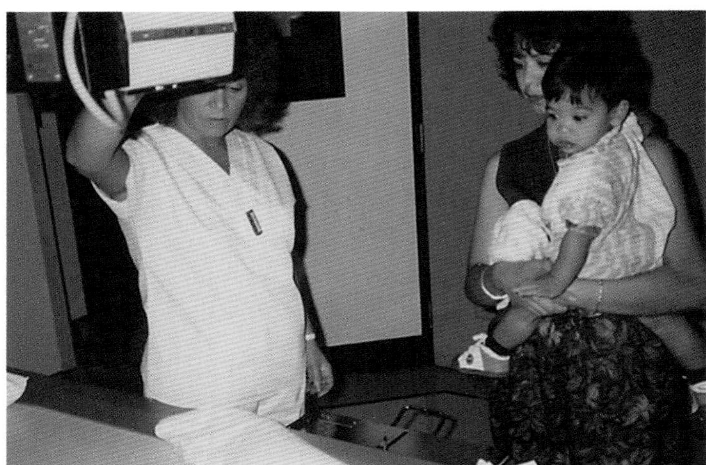

Fig. 20-2. Technologist explaining procedure to patient and parent.

Evaluate Parent's (or Caregiver's) Role This is also the time to evaluate the role of the parent. Three possibilities **(option 3 is required only if parent is pregnant)** are as follows:

1. Parent is in room as an observer, lending support and comfort by their presence.
2. Parent serves as a participator, assisting with immobilization.
3. Parent is asked to remain in the waiting area and not accompany the child into the radiography room.

Sometimes children who act fearful and combative in the waiting room with the parent present will be more cooperative without their presence. This is the time when the technologist's communication skills are tested.

This assessment of the parent's role is important and requires an objective evaluation by the technologist. If it is determined that the parent's anxiety will interfere with the child's cooperation, then option 3 should be chosen. Parents, however, generally do wish to assist in immobilizing the child, and if this option is chosen (if parent is not pregnant and proper shielding is used), the technologist should carefully explain the procedures to both the parent and the patient. This includes instructions to the parent on correct immobilization techniques. Cooperation and the parent's effectiveness in assisting tend to increase with understanding how proper but firm immobilization will improve the diagnostic quality of the image and also will reduce radiation exposure to the patient by reducing the chance of repeats.

REPORTING SUSPECTED CHILD ABUSE

Most medical facilities have a procedure in place to report suspected child abuse. In the past the term used for this was *battered child syndrome (BCS).* The current acceptable term is **nonaccidental trauma (NAT).**

It is generally not the responsibility of the technologist to make a judgment as to whether child abuse has occurred, but rather to **report the facts** as they are seen or suspected. If NAT is suspected, the technologist should discuss this with the radiologist or other supervisor as determined by departmental protocol. Laws vary on technologists' responsibilities, and it is most important that **all technologists know what their responsibilities are concerning this in the state or province in which they are working.**

Immobilization

Pediatric patients in general can include infants through children up to ages 12 to 14. However, older children can be treated more like adults, except for special care in gonadal shielding and reduced exposure factors because of their smaller size. This chapter describes and illustrates radiographing primarily infants and toddlers who require special attention to prevent motion during the exposure.

In general pediatric radiography should **always use as short exposure times and as high mA as possible** to minimize image blurring resulting from patient motion. However, even with short exposure times, preventing motion during exposures is a constant challenge in pediatric radiography, and effective methods of immobilization are essential.

Various types of immobilization devices are available today. These can generally be found in a radiology supply catalog. Examples of these are the **Tam-em board** and **Pigg-O-Stat** as demonstrated. The **Posi-Tot** is another type of immobilization device available commercially. The cost-effectiveness of these devices is dependent on how often the devices are used.

TAM-EM BOARD AND PLEXIGLAS HOLD-DOWN PADDLE (Fig. 20-3)

The **Tam-em board** is shown, along with several short Velcro straps for immobilizing the upper and lower limbs. This is a commercially available immobilization device that is easy to use (see Fig. 20-28).

A **Plexiglas hold-down paddle** is also shown in front of the Tam-em board. This can be cut from a clear sheet of Plexiglas of sufficient thickness for necessary rigidity. It can be used in various applications, such as to hold down upper or lower limbs without obscuring essential anatomy. This can be an aid for parents to use in assisting with immobilization.

PIGG-O-STAT (Fig. 20-4) (See also p. 662, Figs. 20-29 and 20-30)

The **Pigg-O-Stat** is a commonly used immobilization apparatus for erect chest and abdomen procedures on infants and small children up to the approximate age of 2 years. The infant or child is placed on the small bicycle type seat *(A)* with the legs placed down through the opening. This seat is adjustable in height. The arms are then raised above the head, and the two clear plastic body clamps *(B)* are adjusted firmly against each side of the body to prevent movement (see p. 664). Two sizes of these clamps exist, which are easily interchangeable, depending on the size of the child *(B* and *G)*. The cassette is placed in the film holder mount *(C)*.

The entire seat and body clamps are mounted on a swivel base *(D)*, which can be rotated independent of the film holder. This places the patient into the desired position for erect AP, PA, lateral, or oblique projections. The adjustable lead gonadal shield *(E)* is shown in position between the x-ray tube and patient. This shield also contains the necessary film markers. The entire Pigg-O-Stat device is mounted on a stand *(F)* with wheels and locks, which allows it to be easily moved into position and from room to room as needed.

OTHER IMMOBILIZATION FORMS (Fig. 20-5)

The simplest and least expensive form of immobilization is to utilize the equipment and supplies that are commonly found in most departments. **Tape, sheets** or **towels, sandbags, covered radiolucent sponge blocks, compression bands, stockinettes,** and **ace bandages,** if used correctly, are effective in immobilization.

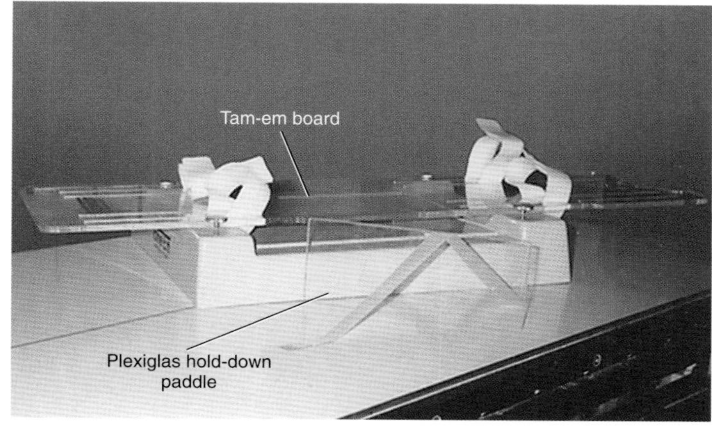

Fig. 20-3. Tam-em board (Plexiglas hold-down paddle).

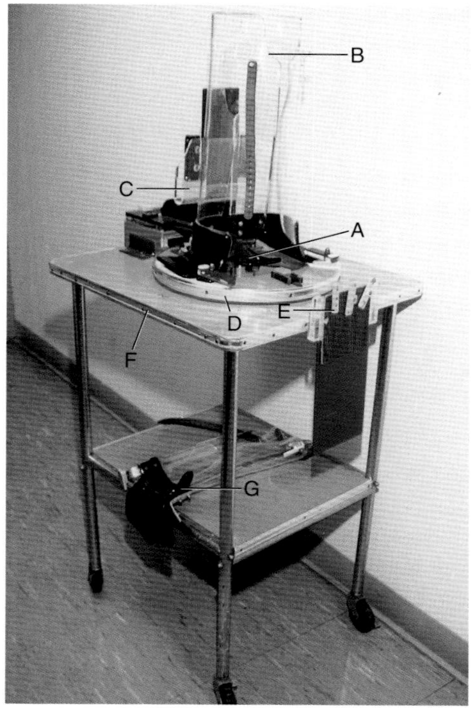

Fig. 20-4. Pigg-O-Stat (set for PA chest).

A. Bicycle type seat
B. Side body clamps
C. Film holder mount
D. Swivel base
E. Adjustable lead shield with markers
F. Mounting stand on wheels
G. Extra set of smaller body clamps

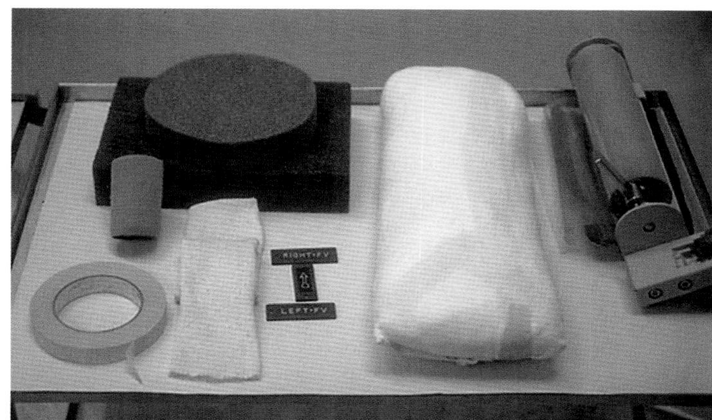

Fig. 20-5. Immobilization aids.

20

SANDBAGS

Sandbags are available for purchase; however, most of these are used as weights or immobilization aids for adults. These bags are not as effective for immobilization of the pediatric patient as those that are made specifically for pediatric purposes.

Strong canvas-type material and children's coarse sterilized playing sand should be used. **Coarse sand is recommended** because if the bag should break open, the sand is more easily cleaned up and the chance of causing artifacts on radiographs is minimized.

Two sandbag sizes are recommended, 8 × 18 inches (20 × 46 cm) and 13 × 20 inches (33 × 50 cm). The sandbag should not be overfilled with sand, which makes the bag stiff; **the bag should be pliable** so that when placed over a patient's limb it will mold to that part.

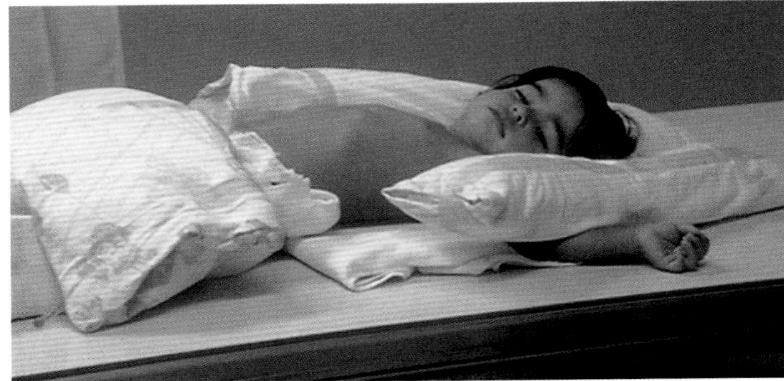

Fig. 20-6. Effective use of sandbags.

TAPE

Various types of "gentle" tape exist for surgical procedures and sensitive skin. Adhesive tape may show on the radiograph and create an artifact that could obscure the anatomic part of interest. Also, some patients have an allergic reaction to adhesive tape. The fragile skin of infants can also be injured by adhesive tape, unless the tape is twisted so that the adhesive surface is not against the skin. Gauze pads placed between skin and adhesive tape can also be used effectively.

STOCKINETTE

If stockinettes are used, they should be tubular. They come in various sizes: 3-inch is recommended for small infants and 4-inch for larger children.

When using the stockinette, double it and place it over the patient's arms, covering the arms up to the shoulders. Not only does this serve to immobilize the arms, but it also acts as a pillow (Fig. 20-8).

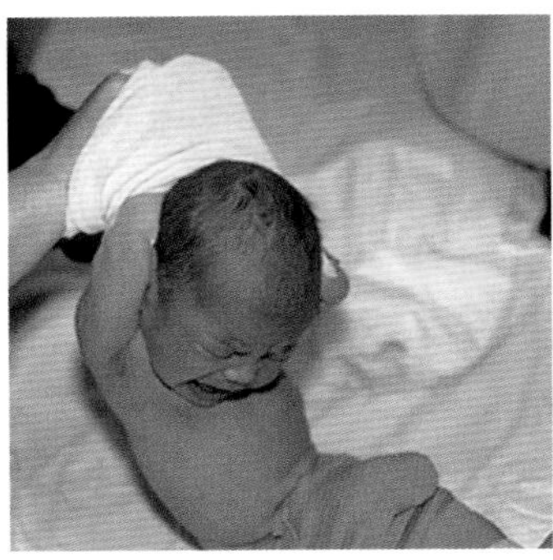

Fig. 20-7. Using stockinette and Ace bandage.

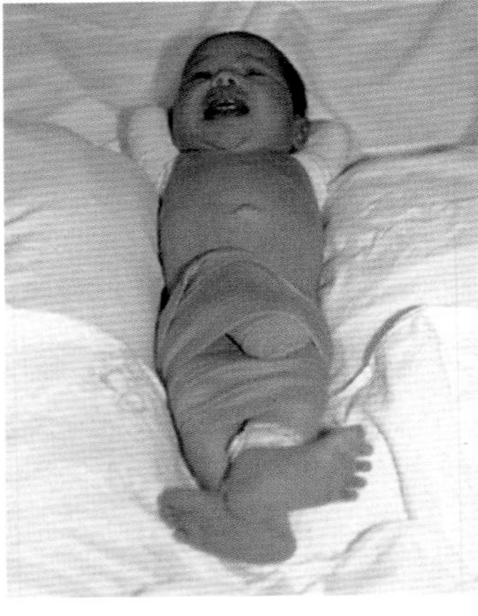

Fig. 20-8. Stockinette and Ace bandage in place.

ACE BANDAGE

A 4-inch ace bandage is best for small infants and young children, whereas a 6-inch bandage works well for older children. These are best used for immobilizing the legs. When starting the wrapping process, begin at the patient's hips and wrap down to the patient's midcalf (Fig. 20-8). Do not wrap too tightly, which would cut off circulation.

COMPRESSION BANDS AND HEAD CLAMPS

Compression or retention bands are also valuable aids for immobilization. Compression bands, however, are more effective with pediatrics when used in combination with sandbags, as demonstrated later in this chapter.

Also available are various types of adjustable head clamps that attach to the tabletop, as shown in Fig. 20-9.

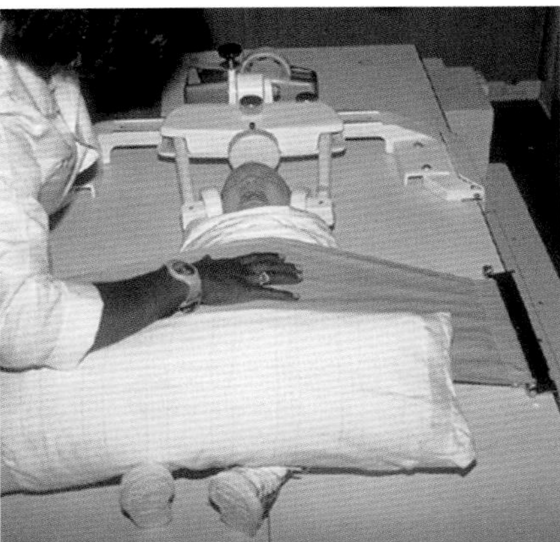

Fig. 20-9. Compression band and head clamps.

WEIGHTED ANGLE BLOCKS AS HEAD CLAMPS

These are heavy steel angle blocks with thick, radiolucent sponge pads attached (Fig. 20-10). They are relatively inexpensive to have made compared with the cost of commercially available head clamps. They are very effective and versatile in immobilization, especially when used in combination with sandbags and/or tape, or if the patient is mummified, as shown in Fig. 20-10.

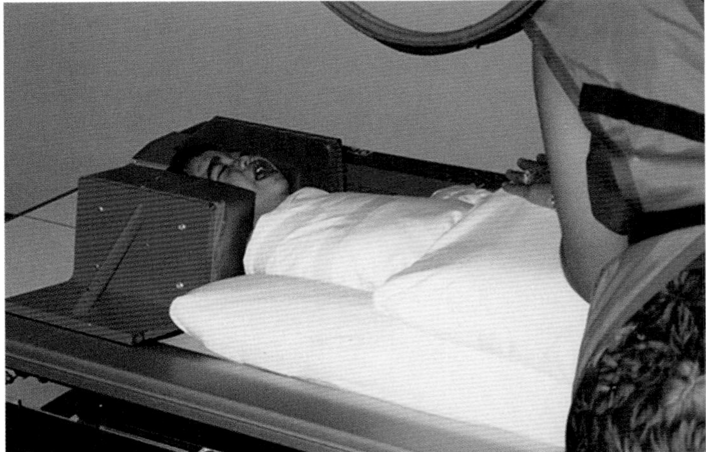

Fig. 20-10. Weighted angle blocks as head clamps (patient "mummified").

"MUMMIFYING," OR WRAPPING WITH SHEETS OR TOWELS

In addition to some type of head clamps, "mummifying" or wrapping is often necessary to immobilize the infant and some children up to 2 or 3 years old for certain radiographic procedures, such as head exams. This is very effective for immobilization if done correctly. Following is a six-step method of how this is done. The room should be set up and prepared before bringing the patient into the room.

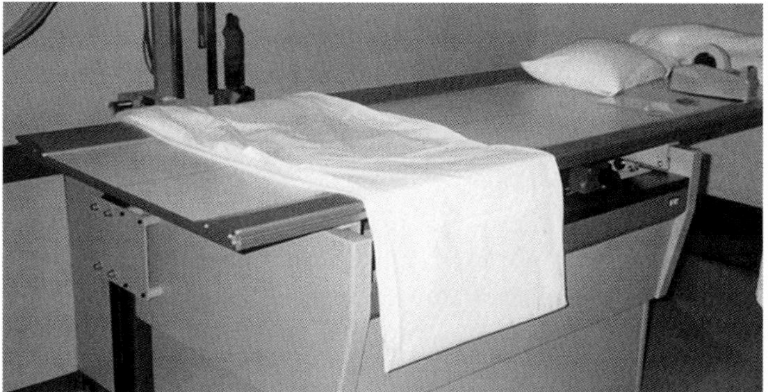

Fig. 20-11. Step 1. Place the sheet on the table folded in half or in thirds lengthwise, depending on the size of the patient.

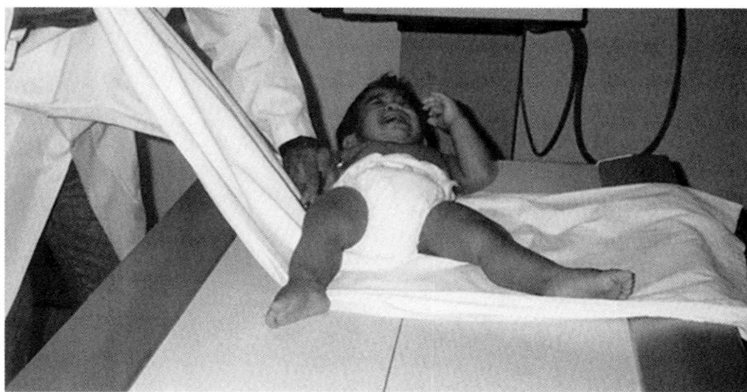

Fig. 20-12. Step 2. Place the patient in the middle of the sheet; then place the patient's right arm along side of his or her body. Take the end of the sheet closest to the technologist and pull the sheet across the patient's body tightly, keeping the arm next to the patient's body.

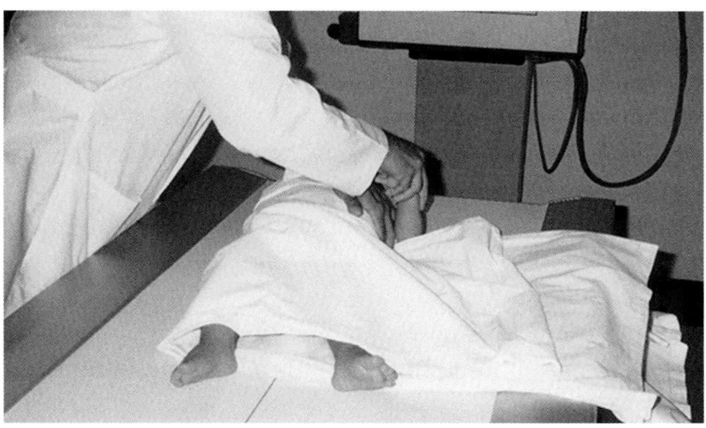

Fig. 20-13. Step 3. Place the patient's left arm along side of his or her body on top of the top sheet. Bring the free sheet over the left arm to the right side of the patient's body and around under the body as needed.

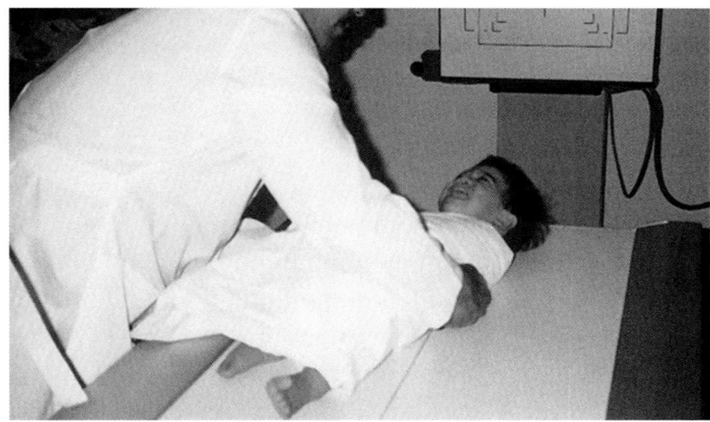

Fig. 20-14. Step 4. Complete the wrapping process by pulling the sheet tightly enough so that the patient cannot free the arms.

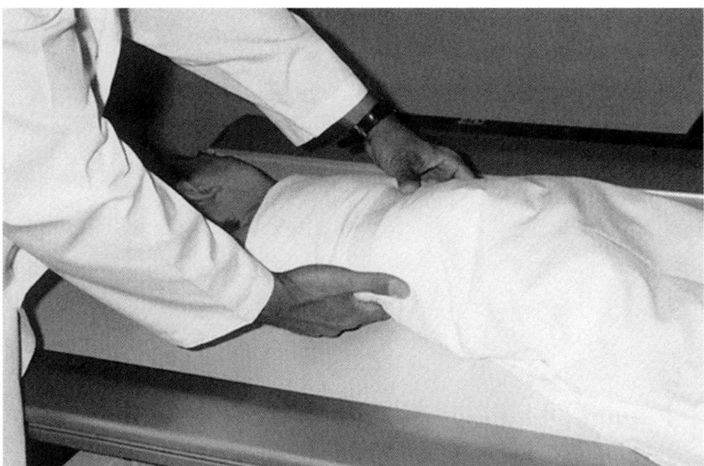

Fig. 20-15. Step 5. Pull the sheet and tape the end of the sheet. Place a long piece of tape from the back of the right wrapped arm to the left wrapped arm over the sheet. This will prevent the patient from breaking out of the sheet.

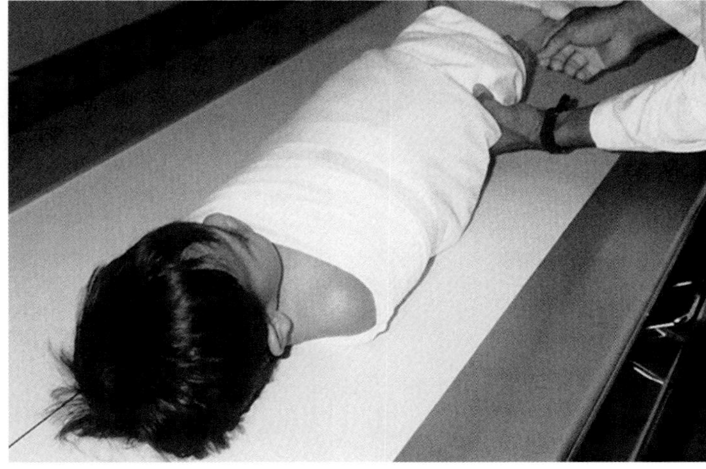

Fig. 20-16. Step 6. Place another piece of tape around the patient's knees. This will keep the patient's lower limbs from becoming free.

BONE DEVELOPMENT (OSSIFICATION)

The bones of infants and small children go through various growth changes from birth through adolescence. The pelvis is an example of ossification changes apparent in children. As shown in Fig. 20-17, the divisions of the hip bone between the ilium, ischium, and pubis are evident. They appear as individual bones separated by a joint space, which is the cartilaginous growth region in the area of the acetabulum.

The heads of the femurs also appear to be separated by a joint space that should not be confused with fracture sites or other abnormalities. These are also normal cartilaginous growth regions.

Most primary centers of bone formation or ossification, such as those involving the midshaft area of long bones, appear before birth. These primary centers become the **diaphysis** (shaft or body) *(D)* of long bones (Figs. 20-18 and 20-19). Each secondary center of ossification involves the ends of long bones and is termed an **epiphysis** *(E)*. This is demonstrated on the PA hand radiograph of a 9-year-old in Fig. 20-18, and the lower limb of a 1-year-old in Fig. 20-19. Note the epiphyses at the ends of the radius and ulna as well as the metacarpals and phalanges (see *small arrows*).

The space between the diaphysis and epiphysis is made up of cartilage and is termed an **epiphyseal plate** *(EP)*. These epiphyseal plates are found between each diaphysis and each epiphysis until skeleton growth is complete upon full maturity, which is normally about 25 years of age.

The epiphyses are the parts of bones that increase in size and appearance as a child grows, as shown on the growth comparison radiographs below (Figs. 20-20 to 20-23). Note in these four knee radiographs the change in size and shape of the epiphyses of the distal femur and proximal tibia and fibula from age 3 to age 12. At age 3 the epiphysis of the fibula is not yet visible, but by 12 years old it becomes obvious (see *arrows*). The size and shape of the larger epiphysis of the proximal tibia and distal femur also change dramatically from age 3 to age 12, as evident on these knee radiographs.

Growth charts are available that list and demonstrate normal growth patterns. Technologists need to be familiar with bone development in infants and children and recognize the appearance of these normal growth stages.

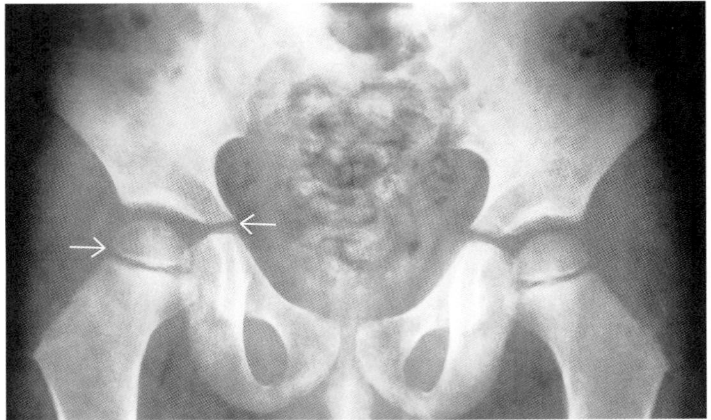

Fig. 20-17. Normal 3-year-old pelvis.

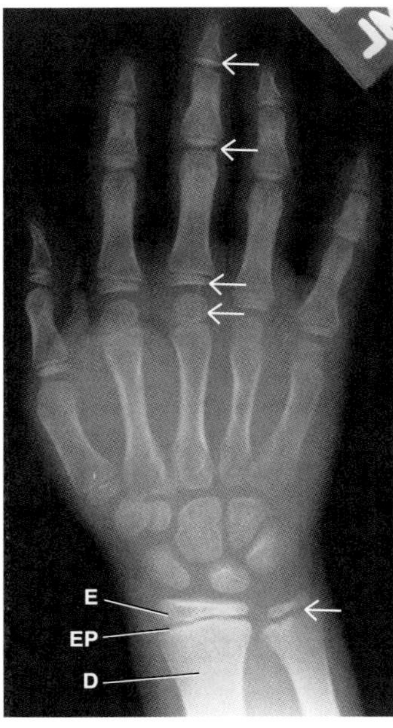

Fig. 20-18. Normal 9-year-old hand.

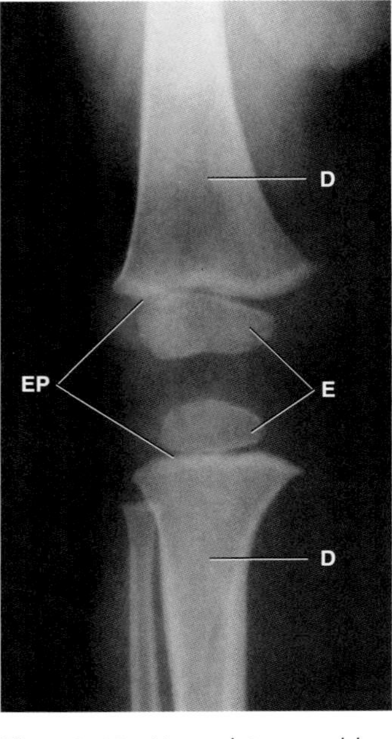

Fig. 20-19. Normal 1-year-old lower limb.

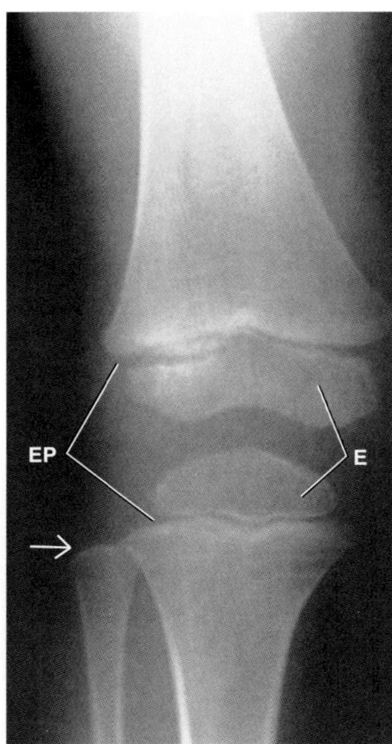

Fig. 20-20. A 3-year-old.

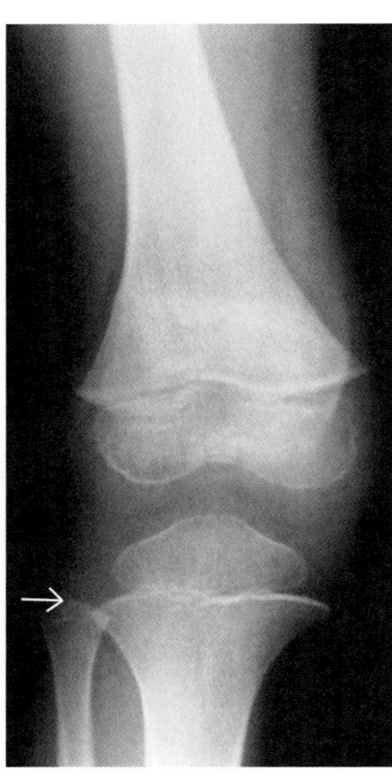

Fig. 20-21. A 4-year-old.

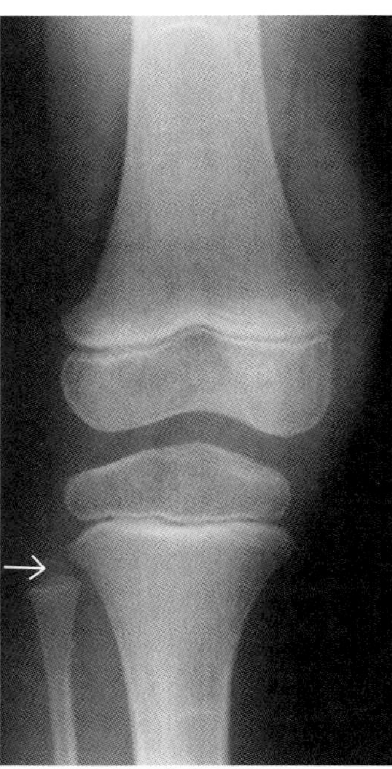

Fig. 20-22. A 6-year-old.

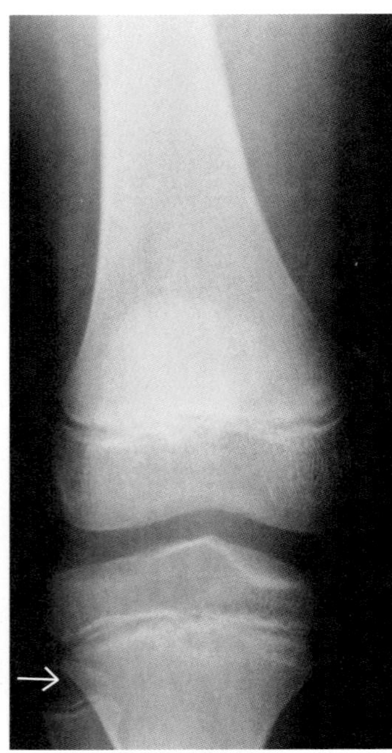

Fig. 20-23. A 12-year-old.

Radiation Protection

MINIMAL REPEATS

Reduction of repeat exposures is critical, especially in young children, whose developing cells are particularly sensitive to the effects of radiation. **Proper immobilization** and **high mA, short exposure time techniques** will reduce the incidence of motion unsharpness. Accurate manual **technique charts with patient body weights** should be used. Radiographic grids should be used only when the body part examined is greater than 10 cm in thickness. Each radiology department should also have a list of specific routines for pediatric imaging exams, including specialized views and limited examination series to ensure that appropriate projections are obtained and no unnecessary exposures are made.

GONADAL PROTECTION

Gonads of the child should **always** be shielded with contact type shields, unless such shields obscure essential anatomy of the lower abdomen or pelvic area. Various shapes and sizes of contact shields are shown in Fig. 20-24.

Because parents often request shielding for their child's gonads, they should also be made aware of other safeguards used for radiation protection such as **close collimation, low dosage techniques,** and a **minimum number of exposures.** To relieve parents' fears, the technologist should explain in as simple language as possible the protection practices and their rationale.

PARENT PROTECTION

If parents are to be in the room, they must be supplied with **lead aprons.** If they are immobilizing the child and their hands are in/or near the primary beam, they should also be given **lead gloves.**

If the mother or other female guardian is within childbearing years and wishes to assist in the procedure, the technologist must **ask whether she is pregnant** before allowing her to remain in the room during the radiographic exposure. If she is pregnant, she should not be allowed in the room and must stay behind the control area.

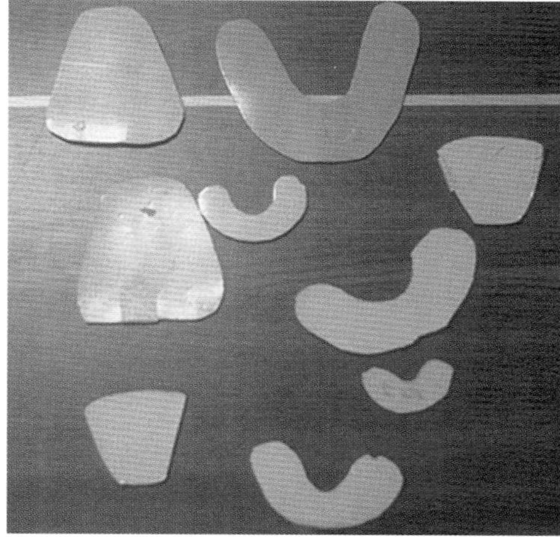

Fig. 20-24. Contact gonad shields.

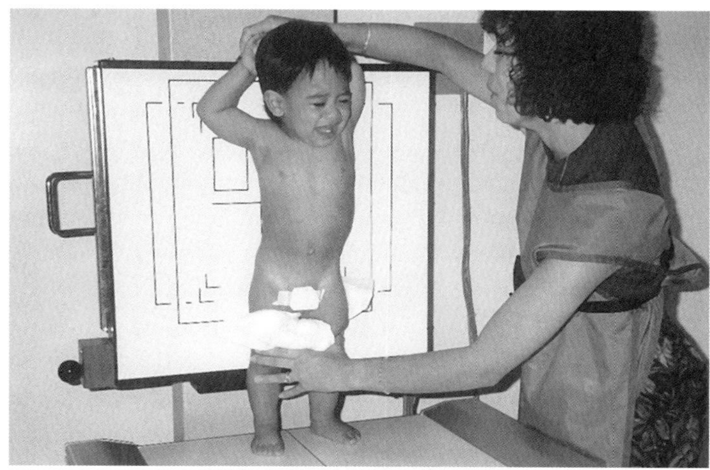

Fig. 20-25. Male gonadal shield in place for erect abdomen. **Note:** Lead gloves should have been provided for the parent holding this patient along with the lead apron.

Preexam Preparation

The following should be completed before the patient is brought into the room:

- The necessary immobilization and shielding paraphernalia should be in place (sandbags, tape, Tam-em board if used, sheets or towels, stockinette, ace bandages, and shielding devices for patient and for parents if assisting).
- Image receptors and markers should be in place and techniques set (if a solo technologist is performing the exam).
- The specific projections should be determined, which may require consultation with the radiologist.
- If two technologists are working together, they should clarify the role each will perform during the procedure. A suggested division of responsibilities is to have the assisting technologist set techniques, make exposures, change the IRs, and process the images while having the primary technologist position the patient, instruct the parents (if assisting) and position the tube, collimation, and required shielding.

CHILD PREPARATION

After the child is brought into room and the procedure is explained to the child and parent's satisfaction, the parent or technologist must then remove any clothing, bandages, and/or diapers from the body parts to be radiographed. This is necessary to prevent these items from casting shadows and creating artifacts on the radiographic image because of low exposure factors used due to the patient's small size.

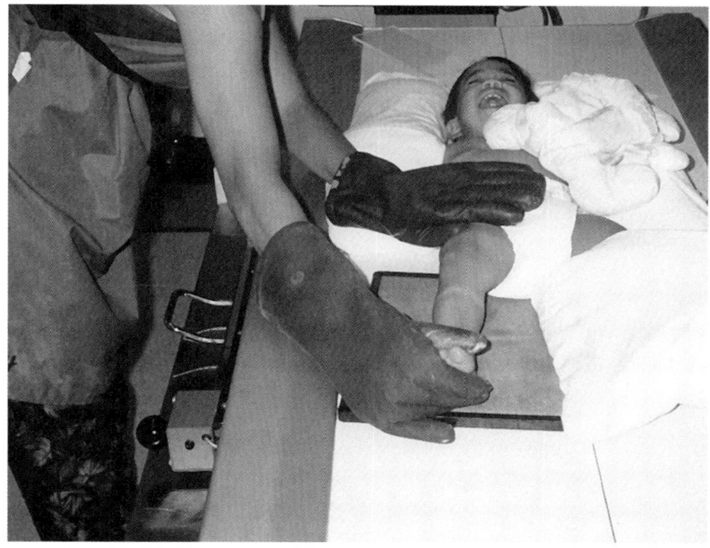

Fig. 20-26. Lead aprons and gloves for parents.

Digital Imaging Considerations

The following guidelines should be followed when using digital imaging systems (CR or DR) for imaging infants and young children (these are described in more detail in Chapter 2 and in preceding chapters for adult patients):

1. **Collimation:** Close collimation is important to ensure that the final image after processing will be of optimal quality.
2. **Accurate centering:** Because of the way the image plate reader scans the exposed imaging plate in CR, it is important that the body part and central ray be accurately centered to the IR.
3. **Exposure factors:** It is important to remember that the ALARA principle must be followed and the lowest exposure factors required to obtain a diagnostic image be used. For children this also means using kV ranges recommended for the age and size of the patient and also using as high mA and short exposure times as possible to minimize the chance for motion unsharpness.
4. **Post-processing evaluation of exposure index values:** After the image is processed and ready for viewing, it must also then be checked for an acceptable exposure index value to verify that the exposure factors used were in the correct range to ensure an optimum quality image with the least possible radiation dose to the patient.

Alternative Modalities

COMPUTED TOMOGRAPHY

Computed tomography (CT) is used for producing cross-sectional images of body parts when slight differences in soft tissue densities must be demonstrated. Examples of this are CT scans of the head, which can visualize various soft tissue pathologies such as blood clots, cerebral edema, or neoplastic processes.

Chest pathology such as parenchymal lung disease can be demonstrated with high-resolution CT, using thin sections.

Spiral/helical CT permits faster scanning without respiratory motion, which is especially advantageous for radiographing the chest in pediatric patients when holding their breath for multiple-level scans becomes a problem. Spiral CT also allows for 3-D reconstruction of images, useful for demonstrating vascular lesions without introducing contrast media (noninvasive), which is a significant advantage with pediatrics.

Higher kV and pitch ratios will reduce patient dose for the pediatric patient.

SONOGRAPHY (ULTRASOUND)

A major advantage of ultrasound for pediatric patients is the lack of ionizing radiation exposure. This is especially important for children and pregnant women. The role of ultrasound in pediatric radiology includes assisting in neurosurgical locations, such as for shunt tube placement or to examine intracranial structures on infants with open fontanelles. Along with clinical evaluation, ultrasound is also frequently the preferred modality for diagnosing acute appendicitis.

Ultrasound is used to diagnose congenital hip dislocations in newborns and young infants. It is effective in diagnosing pyloric stenosis, which frequently can eliminate the need for an upper GI study. It is used on children with sickle cell anemia to image the major blood vessels, and for checking for signs of vascular spasm that may indicate an impending cerebrovascular accident (CVA).

A newer form of ultrasound is **3-D fetal ultrasound,** which aids in earlier diagnosis of potential genetic abnormalities by better visualization of soft tissue such as facial and head features and shapes.

MAGNETIC RESONANCE IMAGING

Longer examination times compared with CT are a major disadvantage with MRI for pediatric use. However, newer rapid imaging techniques, such as echo planar imaging, a very fast MRI technique, allow for thoracic and cardiac evaluations in which breath-holding and vascular motion are a problem, especially with infants and young children.

MRI is an effective tool for evaluating and staging Wilms' tumor. Because the use of iodinated contrast media is not required, it reduces the risk for renal injury for the pediatric patient.

A newer form of MRI, **functional magnetic resonance imaging (fMRI),** is being used along with clinical evaluation to study and diagnose functional brain diseases or disorders. For adults this includes **Alzheimer's** and **Parkinson's diseases.** In children this includes disorders affecting how young children can function at home or in school such as **attention deficit hyperactivity disorder (ADHD), Tourette's syndrome** (multiple motor tics), and **autism** (compulsive and ritualistic behavior). See Chapter 24 for more information on MRI and fMRI.

NUCLEAR MEDICINE

Nuclear medicine procedures are used to measure renal functions and for determining blockage of the ureters and for vesicoureteral reflux (see Chapter 17). Pediatric voiding cystourethrogram (VCUG) exams are less common because of these nuclear medicine procedures.

Pathologic Indications

There are certain pathologies unique to newborns (neonates) and young children with which technologists should be familiar. This is especially important for pediatrics because patients cannot describe their symptoms, and optimal procedures or projection should be performed correctly the first time without repeats. Being familiar with these pathologic indications as noted on patient records provides the technologist information that can determine how the patient should be handled and what precautions should be taken. This information is also important to know what technique adjustments are needed for optimum quality images, and to ensure that the correct procedures or projections are performed.

PEDIATRIC CHEST

1. Aspiration (mechanical obstruction) This is most common in small children when foreign objects are swallowed or aspirated into the air passages of the bronchial tree. (The obstruction is most likely to be in right bronchus because of bronchus size and angle of divergence. See Chapter 3, p. 80.)

2. Asthma Asthma is most common in children and generally is caused by anxiety or allergies. Airways are narrowed by stimuli that don't affect the airways in normal lungs. Breathing is labored, and increase of mucus in lungs may result in some increase in radiodensity of lung fields. (Chest radiographs frequently appear normal, however.)

3. Atelectasis This is a condition rather than a disease, in which collapse of all or a portion of a lung occurs because of an obstruction of the bronchus, or a puncture or "blowout" of an air passageway. With less than normal air in the lung, this region appears more radiodense and may cause the trachea and heart to shift to the affected side.

4. Bronchiectasis In this condition irreversible widening (dilation) of bronchi occurs from acute infection or from congenital structural abnormalities of portions of airways, eventually creating obstruction. It may develop at any age but most often begins in early childhood. Severe conditions may require a slight increase in exposure factors.

5. Croup This condition (primarily in children ages 1 to 3) is caused by a viral infection. It is made evident by labored breathing and a harsh dry cough frequently (but not always) accompanied by fever. It is most commonly treated with antibiotics, but AP and lateral radiographs of neck and upper airway may be requested to demonstrate characteristically smooth but tapered narrowing of upper airway, most obvious on the AP projection.

6. Cystic Fibrosis In this inherited disease, secretions of heavy mucus cause progressive "clogging" of bronchi and bronchioles, which may be demonstrated on chest radiographs as increased radiodensities in specific lung regions.

Symptoms in the lungs are generally not obvious at birth but may develop later. A frequent associated condition in newborns is **meconium ileus** (a type of intestinal obstruction caused by thick meconium). **Meconium** is a dark green secretion of the liver and intestinal glands mixed with some amniotic fluid.

7. Epiglottitis (supraglottitis) This bacterial infection of the epiglottis is most common in children ages 2 to 5 but may also affect adults. Epiglottitis is a **serious condition that can rapidly become fatal** (within hours of onset), resulting from blockage of the airway by the swelling. It usually must be examined in an emergency room by a specialist using a laryngoscope, where the airway can be reopened by inserting an endotracheal tube or by a tracheostomy (opening through front of neck).

A physician or other attendant should accompany the patient during any radiographic procedure to ensure that the airway remains open.

8. Hyaline Membrane Disease (HMD) Now called **respiratory distress syndrome,** or **RDS,** this condition is still commonly known as hyaline membrane disease in infants. This is one of the most common indications for chest radiographs in newborns, especially premature infants.

In this emergency-type condition the alveoli and capillaries of the lung are injured or infected, resulting in leakage of fluid and blood into the spaces between alveoli or into the alveoli themselves. This can be detected radiographically by increased density throughout the lungs in a granular pattern, because the normal air-filled spaces are filled with fluid.

9. Meconium Aspiration Syndrome During the birth process the fetus under stress may pass some meconium stools into the amniotic fluid, which then can be inhaled into the lungs. This may result in some blockage of the airway, causing the air sacs to collapse, which in turn may cause a lung to rupture, creating a pneumothorax or atelectasis.

10. Neoplasia The formation of a neoplasm (tumor or abnormal growth) may occur within the respiratory tract. Symptoms include **hemoptysis** (coughing up blood), a persistent cough, or hoarseness. It is more common in adults but may occur in children.

11. Pneumonia (pneumonitis) This inflammation of the lungs results in **accumulation of fluid** within certain sections of the lungs creating increased radiodensities in these regions. PA and lateral **erect horizontal beam** radiographs make up the most common initial diagnostic exam.

Pneumonia can occur in newborns by a rupture of membranes, allowing the inhalation of amniotic fluid into the lungs.

12. Pneumothorax This accumulation of air in pleural space causes partial or complete collapse of lung. It may be caused by trauma or pathologic condition, causing spontaneous rupture of a weakened area of lung.

It can occur with infants on ventilators, where air will leak from the air sacs into the soft tissue between the lung and heart, a condition called **pneumomediastinum,** which may not be serious unless it leads to pneumothorax.

13. Thyroid Gland Disorders

- **Congenital goiter:** An enlarged thyroid at birth is caused by either an underactive thyroid (hypothyroidism) or an overactive thyroid (hyperthyroidism).
- **Cretinism:** In this neonate form of hypothyroidism, symptoms include jaundice and slowed bone growth or possible dwarfism.
  Radiographic exams include demonstration of ossification centers of long bones to evaluate for retarded bone age. Skull radiographs can demonstrate increased thickness of the cranial vault and also widened sutures with delayed closure.
- **Neonatal Graves' disease:** A life-threatening illness that can occur in infants whose mothers have or have had Graves' disease, this is a form of hyperthyroidism in adults. The enlarged thyroid can press against the airway and close it, causing difficulty in breathing. Chest and upper airway radiographs may be requested to demonstrate this condition.

SUMMARY CHART OF PATHOLOGIC INDICATIONS: PEDIATRIC CHEST

CONDITION OR DISEASE	RADIOGRAPHIC EXAM AND (+) OR (−) EXPOSURE ADJUSTMENT*
1. Aspiration (mechanical obstruction)	AP and lateral chest or AP and lateral upper airway
2. Asthma (in children)	PA and lateral chest
3. Atelectasis (lung collapse)	PA and lateral chest (+) slight increase
4. Bronchiectasis	PA and lateral chest (+) slight increase
5. Croup (viral infection)	PA and lateral chest and AP and lateral upper airway
6. Cystic fibrosis (may develop meconium ileus)	PA and lateral chest (+) slight increase (if severe)
7. Epiglottitis (acute respiratory obstruction)	AP and lateral chest and lateral upper airway
8. Hyaline membrane disease (HMD), or respiratory distress syndrome—RDS (primarily in premature infants)	PA and lateral chest (+) slight increase
9. Meconium aspiration syndrome (newborns)	AP and lateral chest (possible pneumothorax)
10. Neoplasia	PA and lateral chest
11. Pneumonia (accumulation of fluid in lungs)	PA and lateral chest (horizontal beam) (+) moderate increase
12. Pneumothorax (collapse of lung)	PA and lateral erect or lateral decubitus chest (−) slight decrease
13. Thyroid gland disorders –Congenital goiter –Cretinism (long bones, skull) –Neonatal Graves' disease	PA and lateral chest; AP and lateral upper airway, long bone survey

*Exposure adjustments depend on severity or stage of condition for manual exposure settings.

20

PATHOLOGIC INDICATIONS FOR THE PEDIATRIC SKELETAL SYSTEM

1. Craniosteosis (craniosynostosis) A deformity of the skull caused by premature closure of skull sutures. The type of deformity is dependent on which sutures are involved. Most common type involves the sagittal suture resulting in AP (front to back) elongation of the skull.

2. Developmental Dysplasia of Hip (DDH) Older term is *congenital dislocation of hip* (CDH). In this condition the femoral head is separated by the acetabulum in the newborn. The cause of this defect is unknown; it is more common in girls, in infants born in breech (buttocks first), and in infants who have close relatives with this disorder. Ultrasound is commonly used to confirm dysplasia in newborns. It may require frequent hip radiographs later, thus gonadal shielding is important when x-rays are used.

3. Hydrocephalus Hydrocephalus involves enlarged ventricles in which the cerebrospinal fluid produced in the ventricles cannot drain, resulting in a pressure buildup and overall enlargement of the head.

4. Idiopathic Juvenile Osteoporosis This type of osteoporosis (in which bone becomes less dense and more fragile) occurs in children and young adults.

5. Osteochondrodysplasia In this group of hereditary disorders the bones grow abnormally, most often causing dwarfism or short stature.

- **Achondroplasia:** Achondroplasia is the most common form of short-limbed dwarfism. Because this condition results in decreased bone formation in the growth plates of long bones, the upper and lower limbs are usually short with a near normal torso length.

6. Osteochondrosis This group of diseases primarily affects the epiphyseal or growth plates of long bones, resulting in pain, deformities, and abnormal bone growth.

- **Kohler's bone disease:** This disease causes inflammation of bone and cartilage of the navicular bone of the foot. It is most common in males, beginning at ages 3 to 5 years, and rarely lasts more than 2 years.
- **Legg-Calvé-Perthes disease:** This condition leads to abnormal bone growth at the hip (head and neck of femur). It affects children ages 5 to 10 years (head of femur first appears flattened then later appears fragmented). It usually affects only one hip and is more common in males.
- **Osgood-Schlatter disease:** This condition causes inflammation at the tibial tuberosity (tendon attachment). It is most common in 5- to 10-year-old males and usually affects only one leg.
- **Scheuermann's disease:** In this relatively common condition, bone development changes of the vertebrae result in kyphosis (humpback). Scheuermann's disease is more common in boys, beginning in early adolescence.

7. Osteogenesis Imperfecta (OI) In this hereditary disorder the bones are abnormally soft and fragile. Infants with this condition may be born with many fractures, which can result in deformities and/or dwarfism. Sutures of the skull are unusually wide, containing many small wormian bones.

8. Osteomalacia (rickets—infantile osteomalacia) In this condition, developing bones do not harden or calcify, causing skeletal deformities. The most common sign for this is bowed legs, with bowing of the bones of the distal femur and the tibia and fibula as seen on radiographs of the entire lower limbs.

9. Osteomyelitis This infection involves the bone (osteitis) or the bone marrow (myelitis). In children this infection usually occurs first in the long bones of the upper and lower limbs.

Diagnosis: Plain radiographs will not show early signs of this, but with advanced conditions it becomes more apparent as a "patchy" or "moth-eaten" appearance of the shafts of long bones. Early conditions are best seen with radionuclide bone scans, a nuclear medicine procedure. CT or MRI may also demonstrate the affected areas of bone at early stages.

10. Osteopetrosis (marble bones) In this hereditary condition the density of the bones is increased. It may include skull abnormalities. This can be a mild condition causing little disability, or it can be severe, beginning in infancy and often becoming fatal.

Osteopetrosis may be demonstrated prenatally with ultrasound or radiographically with bone survey exams in children and adults. Radiodense bones require an increase in exposure factors.

11. Spina Bifida The posterior aspects of the vertebrae fail to develop, exposing part of the spinal cord. Spina bifida can be discovered before birth by ultrasound and/or by clinical tests of the amniotic fluid. Various degrees of severity exist. Spina bifida can now be demonstrated before birth, using prenatal ultrasound.

- **Meningocele:** A more common and severe form of spina bifida involves the protrusion of the meninges through the undeveloped opening of the vertebrae. This creates a cerebrospinal fluid–filled bulge under the skin called a *meningocele.*
- **Myelocele:** In this most severe type of spina bifida, the spinal cord also protrudes through the opening. This is most serious when occurring in the cervical region and causes major handicaps in physical abilities, deterioration of kidney function, and frequently an associated hydrocephalus (water on the brain).
- **Spina bifida occulta:** Spina bifida occulta is a mild form characterized by some defect or splitting of the posterior arch of the L5-S1 vertebrae without protrusion of the spinal cord or meninges (membranes covering the spinal cord and brain).

12. Talipes (club foot) Talipes is a congenital deformity of the foot that can be diagnosed prenatally using real-time ultrasound. It is also commonly evaluated radiographically as an infant with frontal and lateral projections of each foot. (The kite method is demonstrated later in this chapter.)

The four most common types are as follows:

- **Talipes calcaneus:** Foot dorsiflexed, causing child to walk on heel without support on anterior foot
- **Talipes equinus:** Foot plantar flexed, causing child to walk on toes without support on heel
- **Talipes valgus:** An outward or lateral turning of the foot and heel; child walks on inner portion of foot
- **Talipes varus:** An inward or medial turning of the foot and heel; child walks on outer portion of foot

13. Tumors Malignant bone tumors are much less common in children than adults, as are most cancers. Certain benign bone tumors may be found in adolescents and young adults, but these also are less common in infants and young children.

- **Retinoblastoma:** Retinoblastomas result from cancer of the retina of the eye. They may spread through the optic nerve to the brain. The condition is frequently heritable.

SUMMARY OF PATHOLOGIC INDICATIONS: PEDIATRIC SKELETAL SYSTEM

CONDITION OR DISEASE	RADIOGRAPHIC EXAM AND (+) OR (−) EXPOSURE ADJUSTMENTS*
1. Craniosteosis	AP and lateral skull
2. Developmental dysplasia of hip (DDH), or congenital dislocation of hip (CDH)	Ultrasound, AP hip
3. Hydrocephalus	Prebirth, ultrasound, or AP lateral skull (+) increase based on size
4. Idiopathic juvenile osteoporosis	Bone survey study or AP of bilateral upper or lower limbs (−) slight decrease
5. Osteochondrodysplasias • Achondroplasia	AP survey of long bones (for possible dwarfism)
6. Osteochondroses • Kohler's • Legg-Calvé-Perthes • Osgood-Schlatter • Scheuermann's	AP and lateral of affected parts —Navicular (foot) —Hip —Tibia (proximal) —Spine (kyphosis)
7. Osteogenesis imperfecta (OI)	Bone survey including AP and lateral skull (−) significant decrease, up to 50%
8. Osteomalacia (rickets)	AP lower limbs (−) moderate decrease, depending on severity and age
9. Osteomyelitis	AP and lateral of affected limbs and/or radionuclide bone scans, CT/MRI
10. Osteopetrosis (marble bones)	Bone survey including skull (+) moderateincrease
11. Spina bifida • Meningocele • Myelocele • Spina bifida occulta	Prenatal ultrasound, PA and lateral spine, and CT or MRI of affected region
12. Talipes (club foot) • Talipes calcaneus (up) • Talipes equinus (down) • Talipes valgus (outward) • Talipes varus (inward)	AP and lateral foot (Kite method)
13. Tumors (bone), rare in children	Radiographs of affected region
• Retinoblastoma	AP and lateral skull

*Exposure adjustments depend on severity or stage of condition for manual exposure settings.

PEDIATRIC ABDOMEN

1. Atresias (or clausura) Atresia is a congenital condition that requires surgery because an opening to an organ is absent. One example is an anal atresia (anal imperforate), in which the anal opening is absent at birth. Other examples are biliary, esophageal, duodenal, mitral, and tricuspid atresias.

2. Celiac Disease In this hereditary disorder a certain protein found in wheat (gluten) causes an allergic reaction of the intestinal lining, resulting in improper absorption of fats from the diet.

3. Hematuria Blood in urine, or hematuria, may be caused by various things such as cancer of the kidneys or bladder (intermittent bleeding), kidney stones, kidney cysts, or sickle cell diseases (an inherited blood disease in which the red blood cells are crescent- or sickle-shaped and deficient in oxygen).

4. Hepatitis This condition is caused by infection of the liver with the hepatitis B virus. It usually results from an infected mother during delivery.

5. Hepatomegaly Hepatomegaly, or enlargement of liver, indicates a liver disease such as acute hepatitis, cirrhosis, or bile duct obstruction.

6. Hirschsprung's Disease (congenital megacolon) In this congenital condition of the large intestine, nerves controlling rhythmic contractions are missing. This serious condition results in severe constipation or vomiting. It is usually corrected surgically by connecting the distal portion of the normal part of the large intestine to an opening in the abdominal wall (colostomy).

7. Horseshoe Kidney In this congenital condition the two kidneys are joined together at their lower pelves. The kidneys are malrotated, facing anteriorly, and the ureters attach the kidneys at the anterior rather than the normal medial aspect. This is the most common type of kidney fusion anomaly.

8. Hydronephrosis Hydronephrosis, or an enlarged kidney distended with urine, is caused by an obstruction of urine. It may result from tumors, kidney stones, severe urinary tract infection, or congenital structural abnormalities.

9. Hypospadias In this congenital condition of infant males, the opening of the urethra is to the underside of the penis.

- **Epispadias:** In this condition the urethra lies open as a channel in the penis rather than a closed tube.

10. Inflammatory Bowel Disease (IBD) IBD includes chronic disorders of inflammation of the intestines. The two most common are **Crohn's disease** and **ulcerative colitis,** which have similar symptoms. These may occur at any age but usually occur first at ages 14 to 30.

- **Crohn's disease:** Crohn's disease is an infection of the intestinal wall that may be in either the small or large intestine or both.
- **Ulcerative colitis:** Ulcerative colitis involves only the large intestine and usually starts in the rectum or sigmoid.

11. Intestinal Obstruction In adults, intestinal obstruction is most frequently caused by fibrous adhesions from previous surgery. In newborns or infants it is caused most often by birth defects such as intussusception, volvulus, or meconium ileus.

- **Ileus:** Ileus, which is also called *paralytic ileus* or *adynamic ileus,* is an intestinal obstruction that is **not a mechanical obstruction** (such as a volvulus or an intussusception) but rather an obstruction caused by a lack of contractile movements of the intestinal wall.
- **Intussusception:** Intussusception is a mechanical obstruction caused by the telescoping of a loop of intestine into another loop. It is most common in the region of the distal small bowel (ileus).
- **Meconium ileus:** Meconium ileus is a mechanical obstruction whereby the intestinal contents (meconium) become hardened, creating a blockage.
- **Volvulus:** Volvulus is a mechanical obstruction caused by a twisting of the intestine itself.

12. Meckel's Diverticulum This is a congenital disorder present at birth consisting of a saclike outpouching in the wall of the small intestine (ileum). It is not a serious disorder by itself and usually causes no or few symptoms. It may not be seen on GI studies and is commonly found during abdominal surgery for other reasons or with radionuclide scans.

13. Necrotizing Enterocolitis (NEC) This condition of inflammation of the inner lining of the intestine is due to injury or inflammation. It occurs most often in premature newborns and may lead to tissue death (becomes necrotic) of a portion of intestine. This condition may be confirmed with plain radiographs of the abdomen by the gas produced by bacteria inside the intestinal wall.

14. Peptic Ulcer This erosion of the lining of the stomach or duodenum may occur in newborns, infants, or young children. It is believed to be hereditary.

15. Polycystic Kidney Disease (infantile or childhood) In this inherited renal condition, many cysts form in the kidney, causing enlarged kidneys in infants and children. Generally, it is fatal if it affects both kidneys without dialysis or kidney transplants.

16. Pyelonephritis This bacterial infection of the kidneys is most commonly associated or caused by vesicoureteral reflux of urine from the bladder back into the kidneys.

17. Pyloric Stenosis This narrowing or blocking at the pylorus or stomach outlet occurs in infants, frequently resulting in repeated, forceful vomiting.

18. Tumors (neoplasm) Malignant tumors (cancer) occur less frequently in children than adults and also are more curable in children.

- **Neuroblastoma:** Neuroblastomas are associated with childhood cancer (generally under age 5). They occur in parts of the nervous system, most frequently the adrenal glands. This cancer is the second most common type in children.
- **Wilms' tumor:** Wilms' tumor indicates a cancer of the kidneys of embryonal origin. It usually occurs in children under age 5. The most common of abdominal cancer in infants or children, it typically involves only one kidney.

19. Urinary Tract Infection (UTI) Urinary tract infection frequently occurs in both adults and children and is caused by bacteria, viruses, fungi, or some type of parasite. Bacterial infections in newborns involving the bladder and urethra are most common in males, but after age 1 are more common in females. A common cause of UTI in children is vesicoureteral reflux.

20. Vesicoureteral Reflux This condition causes a backward flow of urine from the bladder into the ureters and kidneys, thereby increasing the chance of spreading infection from the urethra and bladder into the kidneys.

SUMMARY OF PATHOLOGIC INDICATIONS: PEDIATRIC ABDOMEN

CONDITION OR DISEASE	RADIOGRAPHIC EXAM AND (+) OR (−) EXPOSURE ADJUSTMENTS*
1. Atresias (clausura)	AP abdomen and/or GI series
2. Celiac disease	Erect or decubitus abdomen and/or GI series
3. Hematuria	IV urogram (IVU)
4. Hepatitis	AP abdomen
5. Hepatomegaly	AP abdomen
6. Hirschsprung's disease (congenital megacolon)	AP abdomen and/or GI series (frequently requires a colostomy)
7. Horseshoe kidney	IVU and/or ultrasound
8. Hydronephrosis	IVU and/or ultrasound
9. Hypospadias or epispadias (abnormal urethra opening)	Diagnosed clinically or possible urethrogram
10. Inflammatory bowel disease (IBD) • Crohn's disease • Ulcerative colitis	Acute abdomen and/or small bowel and GI series (helical CT and/or MRIcan detect early stages of IBD)
11. Intestinal obstructions Mechanical: • Intussusception • Meconium ileus • Volvulus Nonmechanical: • Ileus (paralytic or adynamic ileus)	Acute abdomen series and small bowel series or barium enema (BE); (−) moderate decrease in exposure depending on severity of bowel distension
12. Meckel's diverticulum	Best seen with radionuclide scan or with small bowel series (SBS)
13. Necrotizing enterocolitis	Acute abdomen series
14. Peptic ulcer	Upper GI series
15. Polycystic kidney disease	IVU, ultrasound, CT, or MRI
16. Pyelonephritis	IVU and/or ultrasound
17. Pyloric stenosis	Upper GI series and/or ultrasound
18. Tumors • Neuroblastoma • Wilms' tumor	Radiographic studies of affected body part, IVU, CT, ultrasound
19. Urinary tract infection (UTI)	IV urogram (IVU) and/or voiding cystourethrogram (VCUG)
20. Vesicoureteral reflux	IVU/VCUG or nuclear medicine

*Exposure adjustments depend on severity or stage of condition for manual exposure setting.

20

RADIOGRAPHIC POSITIONING (CHEST AND SKELETAL SYSTEM)

AP/PA CHEST PROJECTION: CHEST

Chest
BASIC
- AP/PA
- Lateral

Pathology Demonstrated
Pathology involving lung fields, diaphragm, bony thorax, and mediastinum, including the heart and major vessels, is shown.

Note: Patient should be **erect if possible.** Generally, pediatric chest patients, if old enough, should be examined in an erect position using a Pigg-O-Stat or similar erect immobilization device (see next page). Exceptions are infants in an isolette, or those too young to support their heads.

Technical Factors
- IR size—determined by the size of the patient
- IR crosswise (if supine, place cassette under patient)
- Grid not required
- Small focal spot
- 70-80 kV, shortest exposure time possible

R

Shielding Contact lead shielding should be placed over the pelvic area with upper margin to level of iliac crests.

Patient Position—with patient supine
- Patient is supine, arms extended to remove scapula from the lung fields.
- Arms are secured to the table with sandbags or Velcro straps if using Tam-em board.
- Legs extended to prevent rotation of pelvis. Hips and legs are secured by placing sandbags at the level of the hip to the top of the knee. If using Tam-em board, hip and legs are Velcro strapped to the board.
- Utilizing parental assistance (if parent is not pregnant):
  1. Have parent remove child's chest clothing.
  2. Provide parent with lead apron and gloves.
  3. Place child on cassette.
  4. Parent should extend child's arms over head with one hand while keeping head tilted back to prevent superimposing upper lungs. With other hand, hold child's legs at level of the knees, applying pressure as necessary to prevent movement.
  5. Place parent in a position that will not obstruct technologist's view of patient while making exposure.
  6. Place lead gloves over the top of the parent's hands if parent is not wearing the gloves. (It may be easier to hold on to patient if not wearing the gloves.)

Part Position
- Place the patient in the middle of the cassette with the shoulders 2 inches (5 cm) below the top of the cassette.
- Ensure that thorax is **not rotated.**

Central Ray
- CR **perpendicular** to the IR, centered to the midsagittal plane at the **level of midthorax,** which is approximately at the **mammillary (nipple) line**
- SID of 50 to 60 inches (127 to 212 cm); tube raised as high as possible

Collimation Closely collimate on four sides to outer chest margins.

Respiration Make exposure upon second full inspiration. If child is crying, watch respiration and make exposure immediately after the child fully inhales.

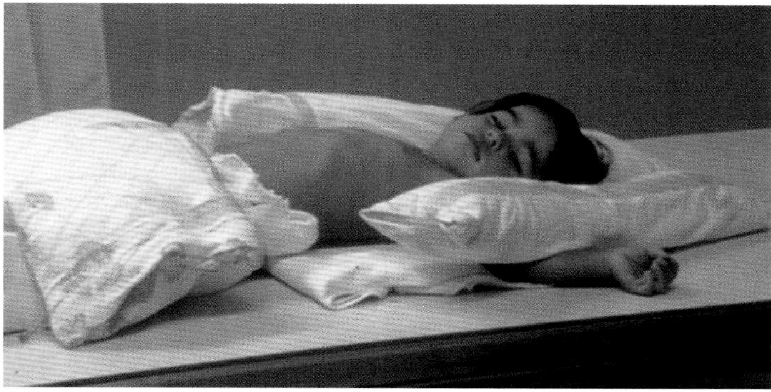

Fig. 20-27. Supine, immobilized with sandbags.

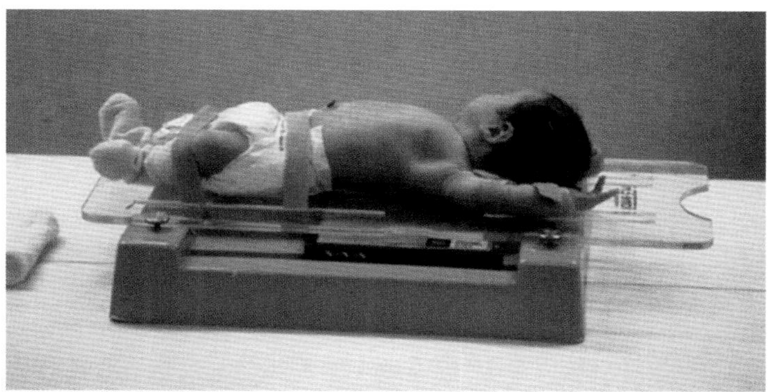

Fig. 20-28. Immobilized with Tam-em board.

Erect PA Chest with Pigg-O-Stat

Patient Position—with patient erect

- Patient is placed on seat with legs down through center opening. Adjust seat to correct height so top of cassette is about 1 inch (2.5 cm) above shoulders.
- Arms are raised, and side body clamps are placed firmly against patient and secured by base adjustment and adjustable strap.
- Lead shield is raised to a level about 1 inch above iliac crest.
- Correct R and L markers and "insp" (inspiration) marker are set to be exposed on lower image (see Fig. 20-29).
- Ensure **no rotation.**

Central Ray

- CR **perpendicular** to IR at **level of midlung fields** (at mammary line)
- SID of 72 inches (180 cm)

Collimation Collimate closely on four sides to outer chest margins.

Respiration If child is crying, watch respiration and make exposure as child fully inhales and holds breath. (Children can frequently hold their breath on inspiration after a practice session.)

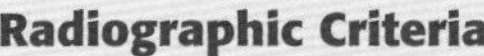

Radiographic Criteria

Structures Shown: • Entire lungs should be included from apices (C12-T1 level) to the costophrenic angles. • The air-filled trachea from T1 down is demonstrated as well as the hilum region markings, heart, and bony thorax.

Position: • Chin is sufficiently elevated to prevent superimposition of apices. • **No rotation,** as evidenced by equal distance from lateral rib margins on each side to the spine and distance from both SC joints to the spine. • **Full inspiration**—visualizes 9 (occasionally 10) posterior ribs above diaphragm on most patients.

Collimation and CR: • Collimation margins on all four sides with equal margins on top and bottom, indicating a correct CR location to midlung fields (T6 or T7).

Exposure Criteria: • Sufficient lung contrast to visualize fine lung markings within lungs. • Faint outlines of ribs and vertebrae visible through heart and mediastinal structures. • No motion, as evidenced by sharp outlines of rib margins, diaphragm, and heart shadows.

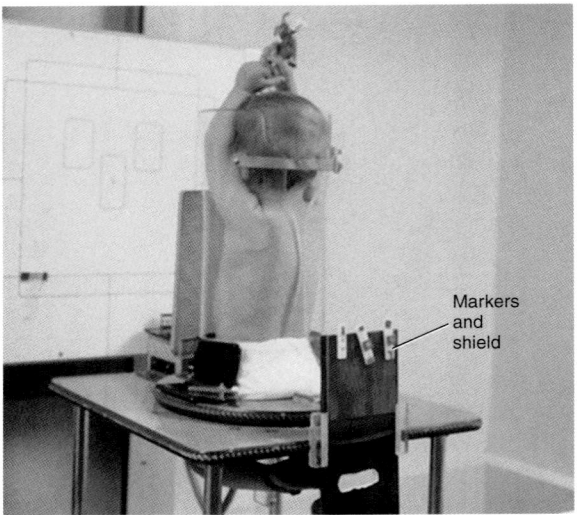

Fig. 20-29. Immobilized by Pigg-O-Stat.

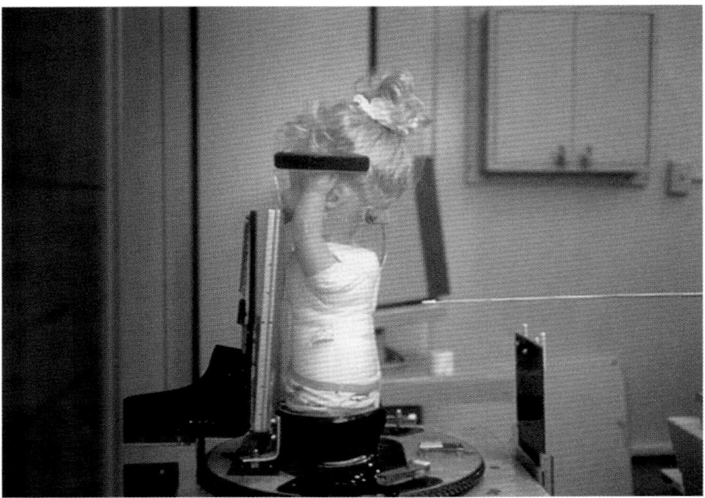

Fig. 20-30. Immobilized by Pigg-O-Stat (view from side).

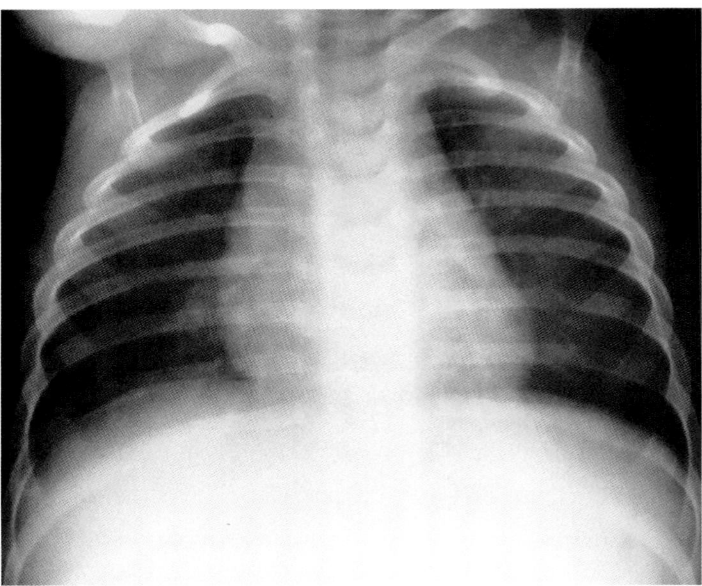

Fig. 20-31. AP (PA) chest. (Some breathing motion is evident; blurred diaphragm.)

LATERAL CHEST POSITION: CHEST

Chest
BASIC
- AP/PA
- Lateral

Pathology Demonstrated

Pathology involving lung fields, trachea, diaphragm, heart, and bony thorax is shown. Horizontal beam projection is needed to visualize air-fluid levels, such as for a hemothorax or pulmonary edema.

Technical Factors

- IR size—determined by the size of patient
- IR lengthwise under patient (unless horizontal beam is taken on Tam-em board)
- Grid not required
- Small focal spot
- 75-80 kV, shortest exposure time possible

Shielding Contact lead shielding should be placed directly over pelvic area with upper margin at the top of the iliac crest.

Patient Position—with patient recumbent

- Patient is lying on side in true lateral (generally left lateral) position with arms extended above head to remove arms from lung field. Bend arms at the elbows for patient comfort and stability with head placed between arms.
- Place one sandbag across arm that is closest to the IR.
- Place a second sandbag over the top of the upside humerus.
- Place a third sandbag between the legs at the level of the knee while bending the legs forward.
- A fourth sandbag is placed across the top of the hips to further immobilize the patient.
- If using Tam-em board, patient position does not change from the AP projection. Turn x-ray tube for horizontal beam projection and place vertical cassette against the lateral wall of the chest as shown (Fig. 20-33).
- If parental assistance is required, perform the following steps:
  1. Place patient on cassette in left lateral position (unless right lateral is indicated).
  2. Bring arms above the head and hold with one hand. Place the other hand across patient's lateral hips to prevent child from rotating or twisting.
  3. Place parent in a position that will not obstruct technologist's view of patient while making exposure.
  4. Place lead gloves over the top of parent's hand if parent is not wearing the gloves.

Part Position

- Place the patient in the middle of the cassette with the shoulders about 2 inches (5 cm) below the top of cassette.
- No rotation should exist; ensure a true lateral position.

Central Ray

- CR **perpendicular** to the IR **centered to the midcoronal plane** at the level of the mammillary (nipple) line
- With use of Tam-em board, the x-ray tube centered in horizontal beam lateral position to midcoronal plane of thorax at level of mammillary line
- SID of 50 to 60 inches (127 to 212 cm)

Collimation Closely collimate on four sides to outer chest margins.

Respiration Make exposure upon second full inspiration. If child is crying, watch respiration and make exposure when the child fully inhales.

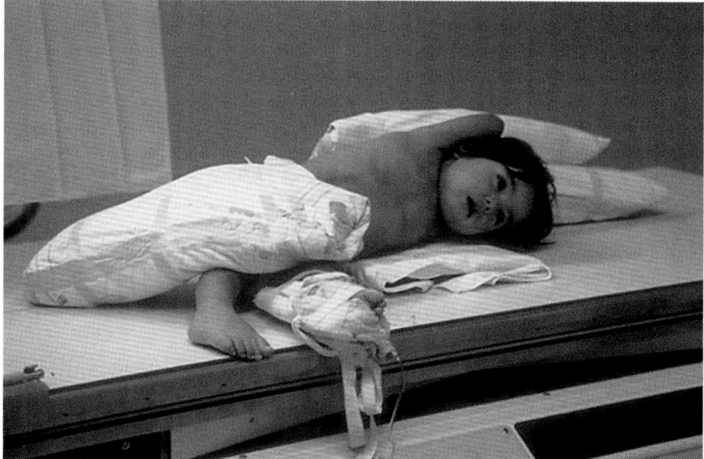

Fig. 20-32. Recumbent lateral chest (with immobilization aids).

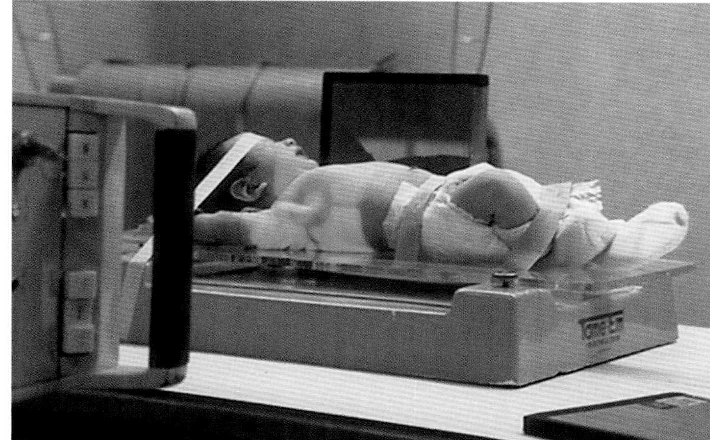

Fig. 20-33. Supine horizontal beam lateral chest (with Tam-em board).

Erect Lateral Chest With Pigg-O-Stat

This can be used with young children up to approximately age 2 (age of patient in Fig. 20-34 is 16 months). The larger-size body clamps are being used on this patient, and the seat is adjusted as low as it will go.

Patient Position—with patient erect

- Patient is placed on seat and adjusted to correct height so top of film holder is about 1 inch (2.5 cm) above shoulders.
- Arms are raised and side body clamps placed firmly against patient and secured by base adjustment and by adjustable strap.
- Lead shield is raised to a level about 1 inch (2.5 cm) above iliac crest.
- Correct R and L markers and inspiration marker are set to be exposed on image.
- Ensure that no rotation exists.

Procedure if lateral follows PA projection: If patient is already in position from the PA projection, then patient and swivel base are turned 90° to lateral position. Lead shield remains in position, and lead marker is changed to indicate correct lateral. Film cassette is placed in film holder mount.

Central Ray

- CR **perpendicular** to IR at **level of midthorax** (mammillary line)
- SID of 72 inches (180 cm)

Collimation Collimate closely on four sides to outer chest margins.

Respiration If child is crying, watch respiration and make exposure as child fully inhales and holds breath.

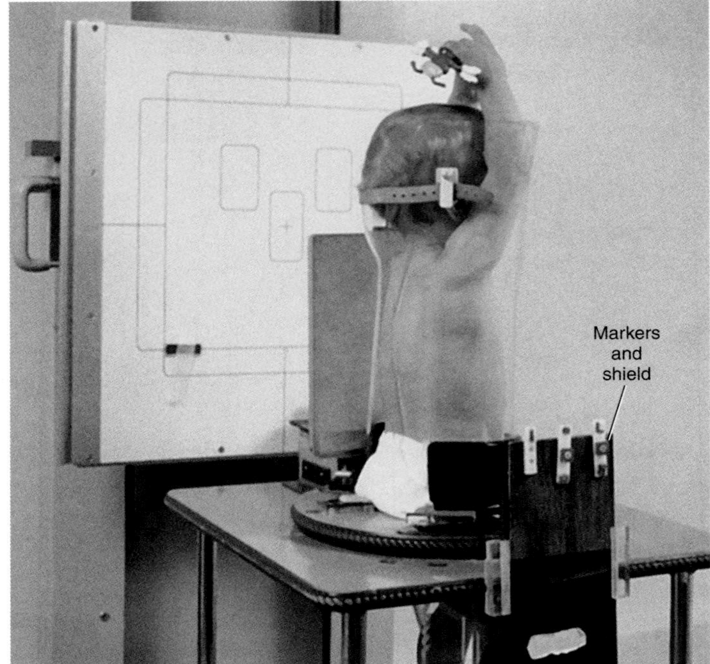

Fig. 20-34. Pigg-O-Stat: left lateral.

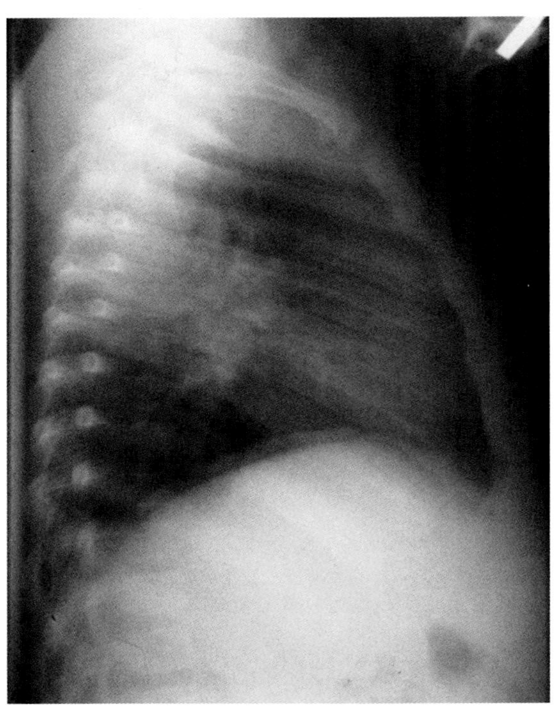

Fig. 20-35. Lateral chest.

Radiographic Criteria

Structures Shown: • Entire lungs from apices to costophrenic angles and from sternum anteriorly to posterior ribs.

Position: • Chin and arms should be elevated sufficiently to prevent excessive soft tissues from superimposing apices. • **No rotation** should exist; bilateral posterior ribs and costophrenic angles should be superimposed.

Collimation and CR: • Collimation borders on four sides with near equal margins on top and bottom with CR to midlung fields.

Exposure Criteria: • No motion is evidenced by sharp outline of diaphragm, rib borders, and lung markings. • Sufficient exposure to faintly visualize rib outlines and lung markings through the heart shadow and upper lung region without overexposing other regions of the lungs.

AP AND LATERAL UPPER LIMBS

Note: Department routines and protocols should be followed as to specific positioning routines for the upper limbs at various ages and for specific diagnostic indicators. The entire upper limb may be included on infants and young children, as shown in Fig. 20-36. For older children with more bone growth in the joint regions (except for general survey exams), individual joints such as the elbow or wrist are radiographed separately, with the CR centered to the joint of interest. For older children, if the area of interest is the hand, generally a PA oblique and lateral hand should be taken, as for an adult.

Upper Limbs
BASIC
- AP
- Lateral

Pathology Demonstrated
Fractures, dislocations, congenital anomalies, or other pathologies involving the upper limbs are shown.

Technical Factors
- IR size determined by the size of patient
- Grid not used for any body part under 10 cm
- Extremity/detail screens used if available
- Small focal spot
- 55-65 kV, shortest exposure time possible

Shielding Secure or place lead shield over entire pelvic area.

Patient Position
- Place patient in the supine position.
- Immobilize patient body part not to be radiographed either on the Tam-em board or with sandbags before the part to be radiographed is positioned.
- When radiographing a long bone, place IR under the limb to be radiographed including both proximal and distal joints.
- When radiographing a joint, place the IR under the joint to be radiographed including a minimum of 1 to 2 inches (2.5 to 5 cm) of proximal and distal long bones.

Part to Be Positioned
- Align the part to be radiographed to the long axis of the IR, or cross-cornered if necessary, to include entire upper limb and both joints.

AP:
- Supinate the hand and forearm into the AP position (with hand and fingers extended).

Lateral:
- If patient is in the supine position, abduct the arm and turn the forearm and wrist into a lateral position.

Immobilization Immobilize the hand, forearm, and humerus with tape or compression band, or have parent immobilize while wearing lead gloves.

Central Ray
- CR perpendicular to the IR directed to the midpoint of the part to be radiographed
- Minimum SID of 40 inches (100 cm)

Collimation Collimate closely on four sides to area of interest.

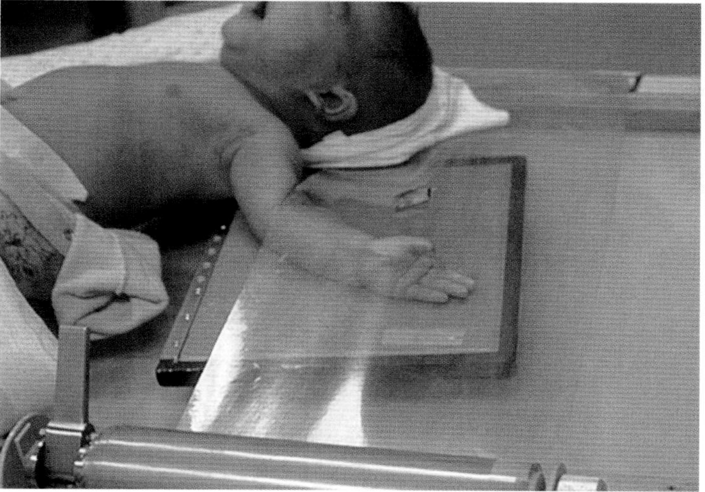

Fig. 20-36. AP upper limb (secured with retention band).

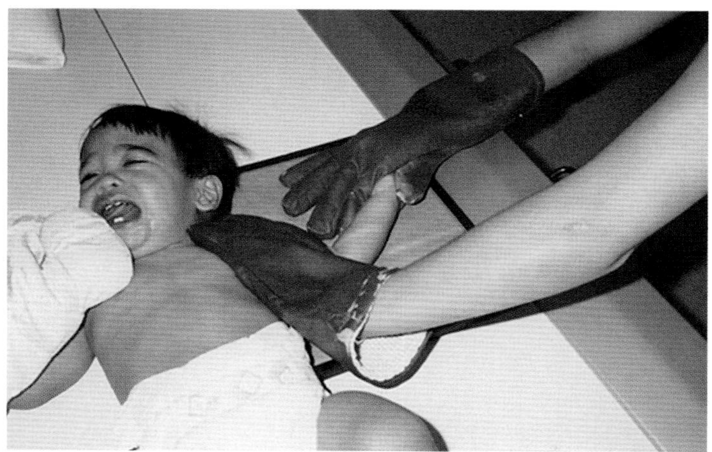

Fig. 20-37. Lateral forearm (parent immobilizing).

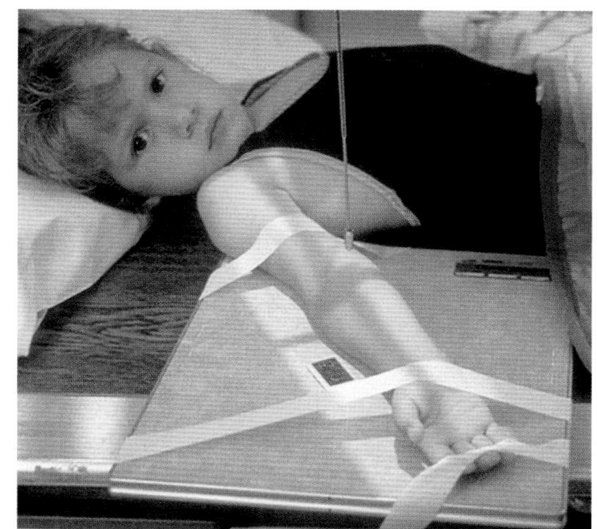

Fig. 20-38. AP forearm: 4-year-old (secured with tape).

Radiographic Criteria

Structures Shown: • See Note at top of preceding page concerning departmental routines and protocols as to how much of the upper limb to include.

Position: • Generally two views 90° from each other should be obtained. (An exception is the hand requiring a PA and oblique.)

Collimation and CR: • Collimation borders should be evident on four sides without cutting off essential anatomy.

Exposure Criteria: • No motion is evidenced by sharp trabecular markings and bone margins. • Optimal exposure demonstrating soft tissue and joint space regions without underexposing the more dense shaft regions of long bones.

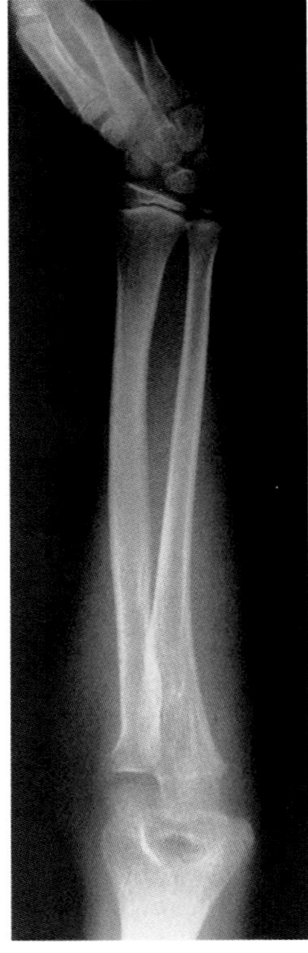

Fig. 20-39. AP forearm: 7-year-old.

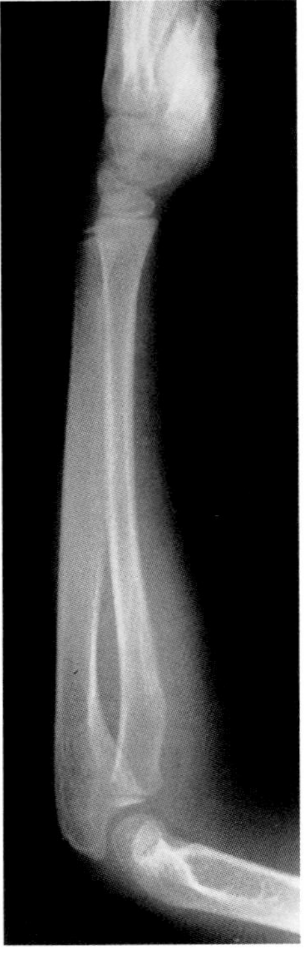

Fig. 20-40. Lateral forearm: 7-year-old.

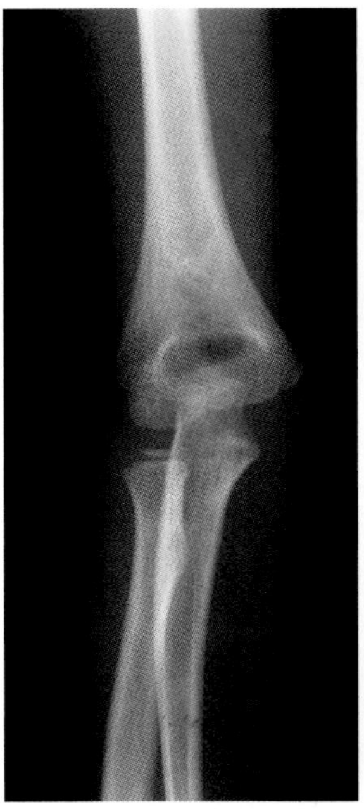

Fig. 20-41. AP elbow: 7-year-old.

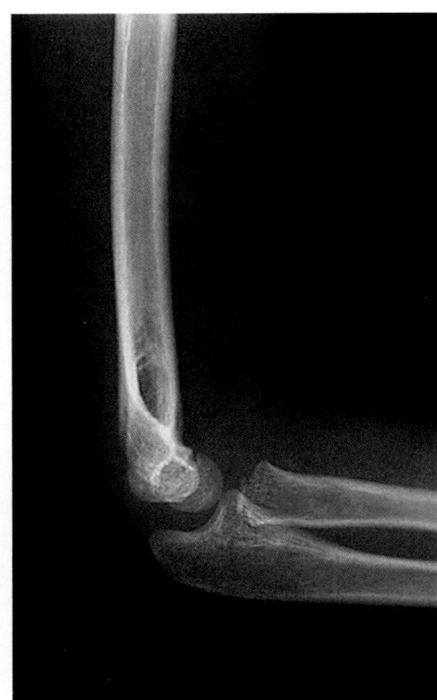

Fig. 20-42. Lateral elbow: 7-year-old.

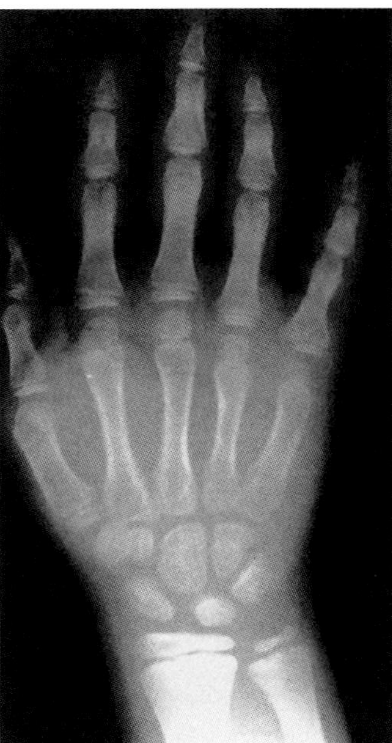

Fig. 20-43. PA hand: 9-year-old.

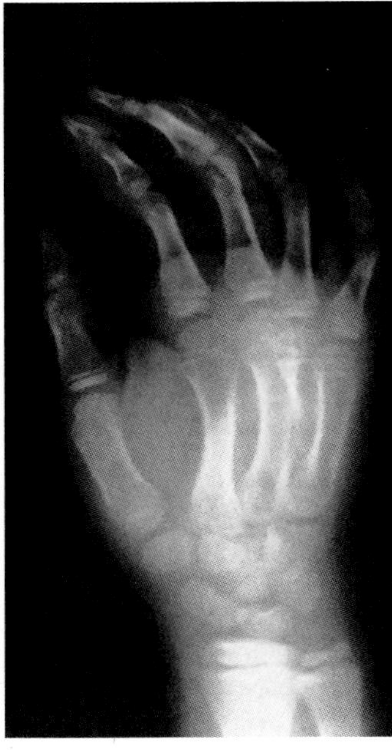

Fig. 20-44. Oblique hand: 9-year-old.

Note: A positioning angle sponge was not used with oblique hand on right; therefore digits are not parallel to IR, resulting in obscured interphalangeal joints.

AP AND LATERAL LOWER LIMBS

Lower Limbs
BASIC
• AP
• Lateral

Pathology Demonstrated

Fractures, dislocations, congenital or other anomalies, and diseases such as Osgood-Schlatter bone disease or osteomalacia are shown.

Technical Factors

- IR size determined by the size of body part to be radiographed, IR crosswise
- Grid not necessary for infants and small children
- 60-65 kV, shortest exposure time possible
- Small focal spot

Shielding Male or female gonadal shields correctly placed so as not to obscure hips and proximal femora

Patient Position and Central Ray

AP and lateral:

- Patient is supine with cassette under patient centered to affected limb or placed diagonally for bilateral limbs if needed to include entire limbs from hips to feet.
- Immobilize with tape and/or compression band, or have parent hold leg in position with one hand on the pelvis above the hip region and one hand holding the foot (wearing lead gloves and apron, Figs. 20-45 and 20-46).
- For lateral, rotate leg externally and immobilize with tape or have parent hold as for AP projection.
- For bilateral limbs, abduct both limbs into "frog-leg" position. Immobilize with tape or compression band across knees and/or ankles.
- CR is perpendicular to mid-area of limbs.
- Minimum SID is 40 inches (100 cm).

Radiographic Criteria

Similar to upper limb criteria on preceding page except for specific positioning criteria for lower limbs as follows:

AP: • Lateral and medial epicondyles of distal femur should appear symmetric and in profile. • Tibia and fibula should appear alongside each other with minimal overlap.

Lateral: • Medial and lateral condyles and epicondyles of distal femur should be superimposed. • Tibia and fibula should appear mostly superimposed.

Note: For young infants, department routines may include entire lower limb, as shown in Figs. 20-45 and 20-46. Also, for infants or young children, bilateral exams may be requested on one IR for a bone survey or for comparison purposes (Figs. 20-47 and 20-48).

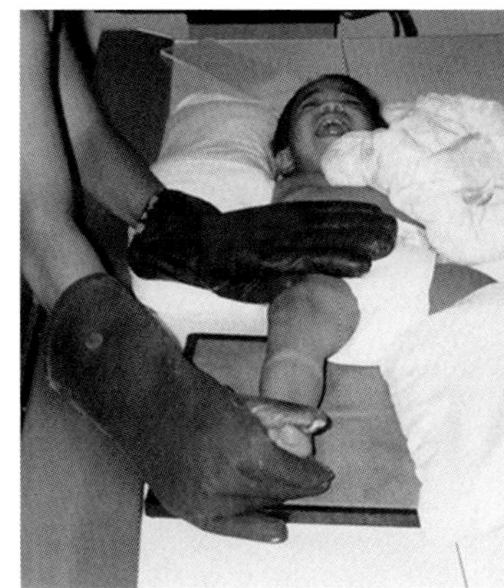

Fig. 20-45. AP leg.

Fig. 20-46. Lateral leg.

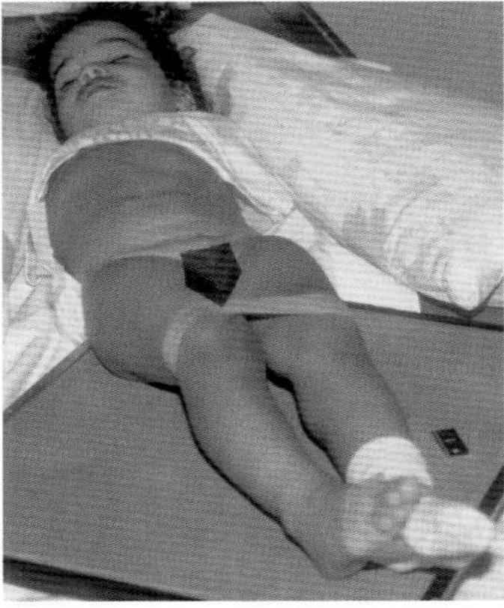

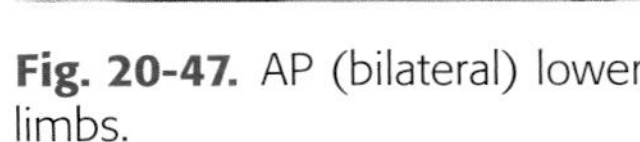

Fig. 20-47. AP (bilateral) lower limbs.

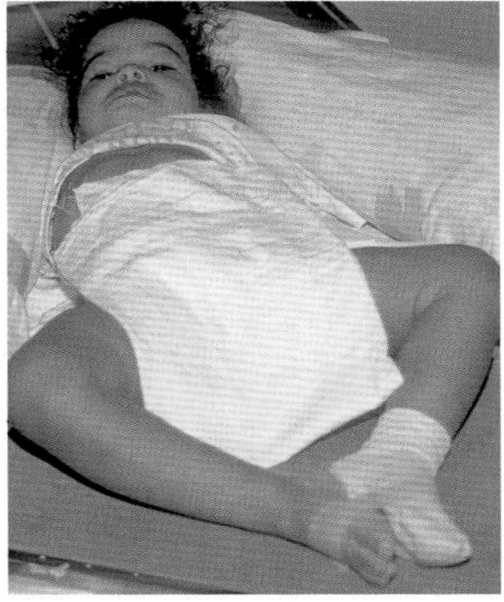

Fig. 20-48. Lateral (bilateral) lower limbs—"frog-leg."

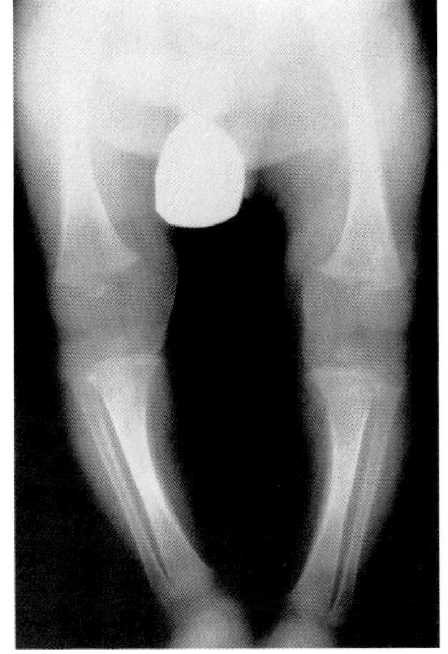

Fig. 20-49. AP (bilateral) lower limbs.

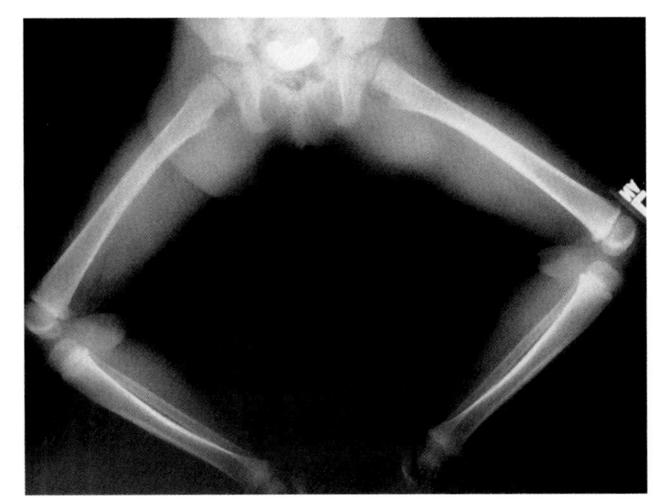

Fig. 20-50. Lateral (bilateral) "frog-leg" for lower limbs.

AP AND LATERAL LEG, AP AND LATERAL FOOT—KITE METHOD

Note: Department routines and protocols should be followed as to specific positioning routines for the lower limbs at various ages and for specific diagnostic indicators. If the specific area of interest is to the **knee, ankle, or foot region,** separate images should be obtained with CR centered to joint of interest (Figs. 20-53 and 20-54).

Leg
BASIC
• AP
• Lateral Foot
BASIC
• AP
• Lateral

Pathology Demonstrated

Fractures, dislocations, congenital deformities, or other anomalies of lower limbs such as Kohler's bone disease or talipes (clubfoot) are shown.

Technical Factors

- IR size determined by the size of the body part to be radiographed
- Grid not necessary for infants and small children
- Small focal spot
- 55-65 kV, shortest exposure time possible

Shielding Place lead gonad shield across pelvis, or specific gonadal shields for male and female, if proximal femurs are to be included.

Patient Position and Central Ray

AP leg:

- With patient supine, immobilize arms and the leg not being radiographed if needed.
- Place cassette under limb being radiographed; include knee and ankle joints.
- Place leg as for a true AP projection, rotating knee internally slightly until the interepicondylar line is parallel to plane of film. The feet and ankles should be in a true anatomic position.
- Immobilize the leg as needed in this position with sandbags, tape, or compression band.
- If parent is being utilized for immobilization, have the parent hold the leg in this position with one hand firmly on the pelvis and the other holding the feet.
- CR is perpendicular to midleg.
- Minimum SID is 40 inches (100 cm).

Lateral leg:

- Rotate patient toward affected side with leg in a frog lateral position, bending knee at an approximate 45° angle.
- Immobilize body parts not being radiographed.
- If parent is helping with immobilization, have parent hold the feet and hips in position.
- Immobilize leg with sandbags, tape, or compression band.
- CR is perpendicular to midleg.
- Minimum SID is 40 inches (100 cm).

Collimation Collimate closely on four sides to area of leg, including knee and ankle.

AP and Lateral Foot

AP foot:

- Seat child on elevated support with knee flexed and foot placed on IR. Use tape to immobilize.
- CR is perpendicular to midfoot.
- Minimum SID is 40 inches (100 cm).

Lateral foot:

- With patient lying or seated on table, rotate leg externally to place foot into lateral position. Use tape to immobilize.
- CR is perpendicular to midfoot.
- Minimum SID is 40 inches (100 cm).

Collimation Collimate closely on four sides to area of foot.

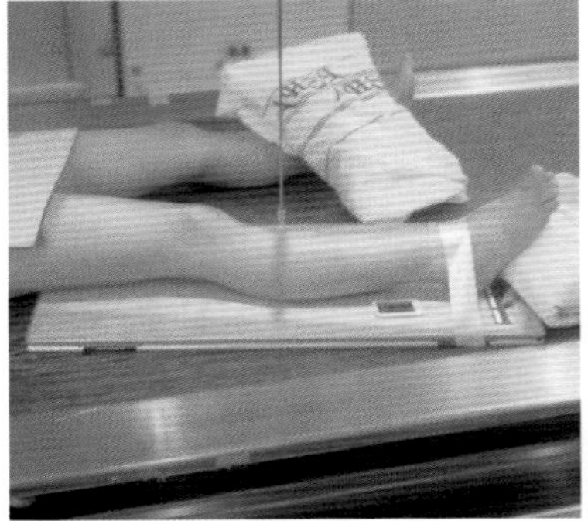

Fig. 20-51. AP leg.

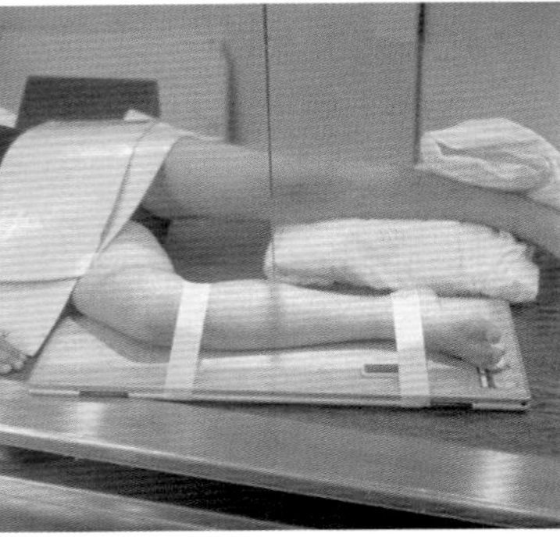

Fig. 20-52. Lateral leg.

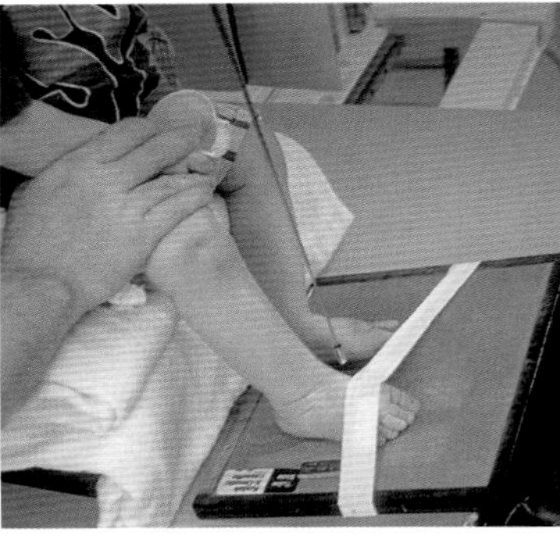

Fig. 20-53. AP foot.

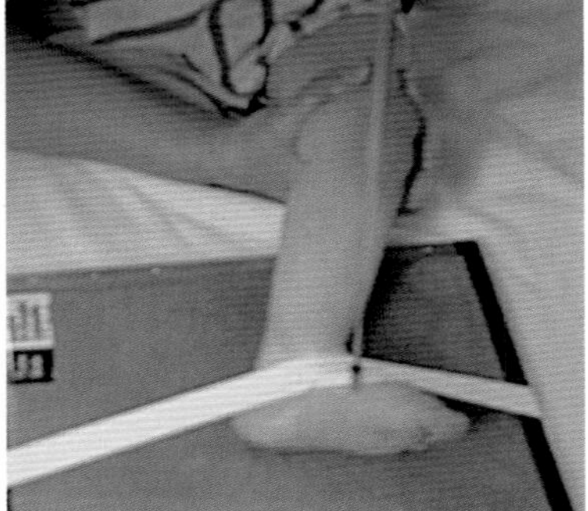

Fig. 20-54. Lateral foot.

(Same patient as Fig. 20-55 below, but 1 year later after corrective treatment had been completed.)

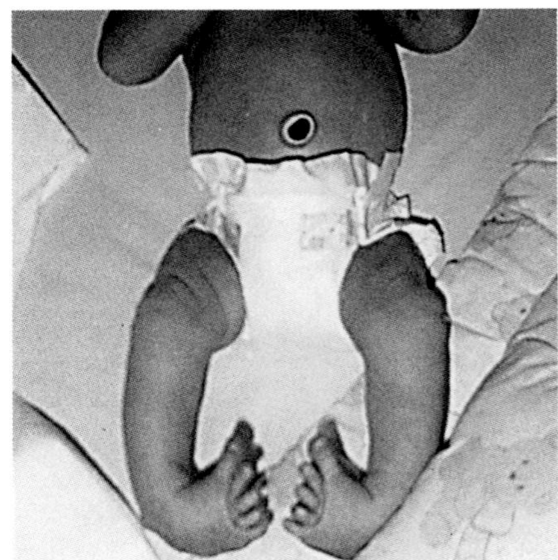

Fig. 20-55. Newborn with clubfeet (talipes varus) before corrective treatment.

Talipes (Congenital Clubfoot)—Kite Method

The foot is positioned for AP and lateral positions as demonstrated, with **no attempt to straighten foot when placing on cassette.** Because of shape distortion (Fig. 20-55), it may be difficult to obtain a true AP and lateral, but two projections 90° from each other should be obtained. Both feet are generally imaged separately for comparison purposes.

AP AND LATERAL PELVIS AND HIPS

Warning: Do not attempt frog-leg hip position on trauma patients until fractures have been ruled out from the AP pelvis projection.

Pelvis and Hips
BASIC
- AP
- Lateral (bilateral frog-leg)

Pathology Demonstrated

Fractures, dislocations, congenital anomalies, or other pathologies involving the pelvis and hips, such as Legg-Calvé-Perthes disease, are shown.

Technical Factors

- IR size determined by the size of body part to be radiographed, IR crosswise
- Moving or stationary grid if more than 9 cm
- Small focal spot
- 60-65 kV, shortest exposure time possible

Shielding

- Before radiographing the patient, discuss the examination with the radiologist. Patient's history may require that a gonad shield not be used if it obscures an area of interest.
- **Female:** Carefully shield the gonadal area. Place the female pediatric shield under the umbilicus and above the pubis. This will avoid covering the hip joints.
- **Male:** Carefully place the upper border of the male pediatric shield at the level of the symphysis pubis.

Patient and Part Position

- Align patient to center of table and/or film holder.
- Immobilize patient so that pelvis is not rotated.
- Immobilize arms with sandbags or Tam-em board.

AP:

- With patient in supine position, position hips for the AP projection by rotating knees and feet internally so that the anterior feet cross each other.
- Immobilize lower limbs in this position with tape and sandbags.

Lateral:

- Abduct the legs by placing the soles of the feet together, knees bent and abducted. Tape soles of feet together, if needed.
- Keep the knees in the lateral position by securing tape to one side of the table crossing over both knees to the other side of the table. This can also be accomplished by using a compression band.

Central Ray

- CR perpendicular to IR, centered at the level of the hips
- Minimum SID of 40 inches (100 cm)

Collimation Collimate closely on four sides to area of interest.

Respiration

- With infants and small children, watch their breathing pattern. When the abdomen is still, make the exposure.
- If the patient is crying, watch for the abdomen to be in full extension.

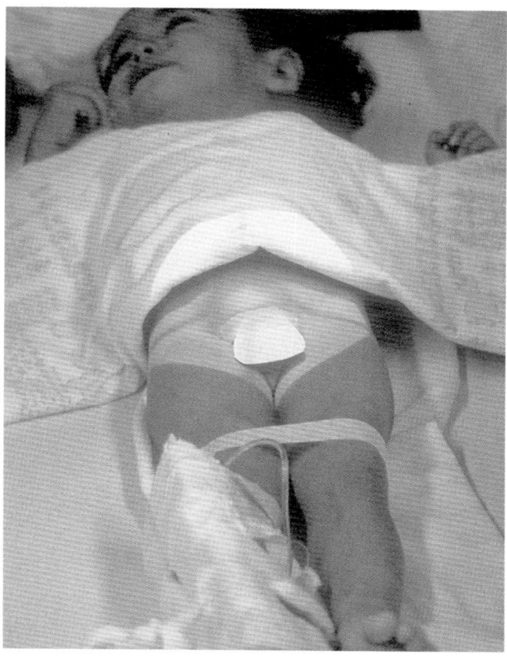

Fig. 20-56. AP pelvis (male gonadal shield taped in place).

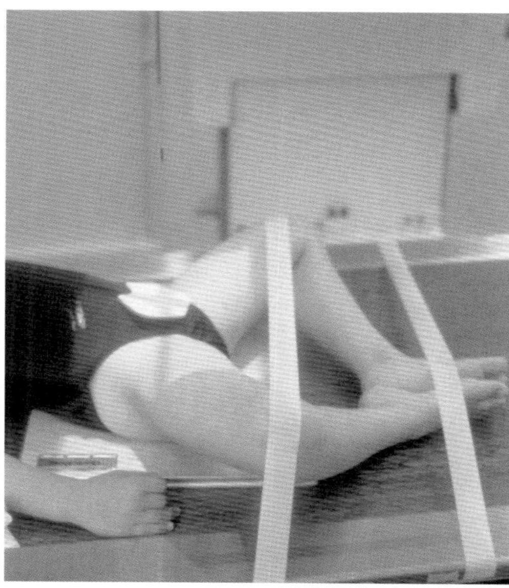

Fig. 20-57. Lateral hips and proximal femora—bilateral frog-leg (female gonadal shield in place).

Radiographic Criteria

Structures Shown: • Sufficiently large IR should be used to include all of pelvis and proximal femurs.

Position: • **No rotation** of pelvis is evidenced by symmetric ala or wings of ilium and by the bilateral obturator foramina.

AP: • **Correct internal rotation** of both legs is evidenced by femoral neck and greater trochanter region seen in profile. (Lesser trochanter should not be visible.)

Lateral: • Proper lateral position of proximal femur regions is evident by superimposition of greater trochanter and neck with lesser trochanters in profile inferiorly.

Collimation and CR: • Minimal collimation borders should be visible on four sides with the center of collimation field (CR) to a point midway between the femoral heads.

Exposure Criteria: • Sharp trabecular markings and bone margins indicate no motion. • Optimal exposure will visualize soft tissue and also bony detail. • An outline of femur heads should be visible through a portion of the acetabulum and ischium.

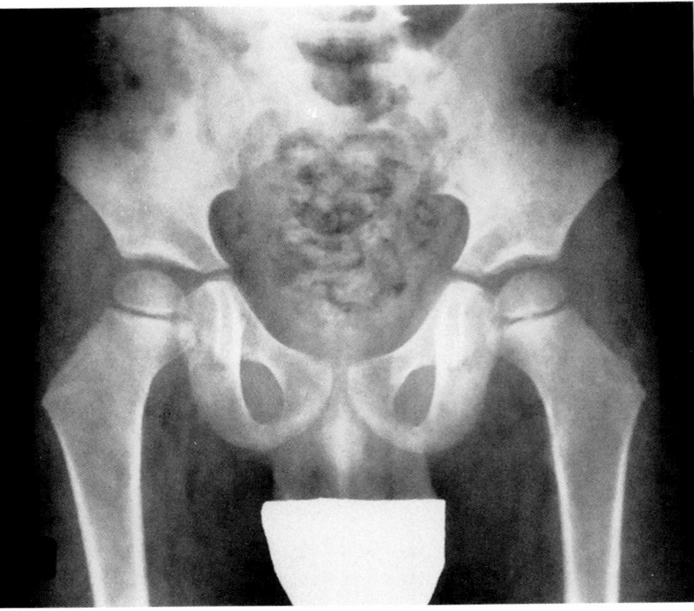

Fig. 20-58. AP hips and proximal femora (male). (Shielding error: Shield should have been placed higher, top of shield at lower margin of symphysis pubis unless pubic bones are an area of interest.)

Note: Correctly placed gonadal shielding should be evident on both male and female patients without obscuring the hip joints (unless contraindicated by radiologist).

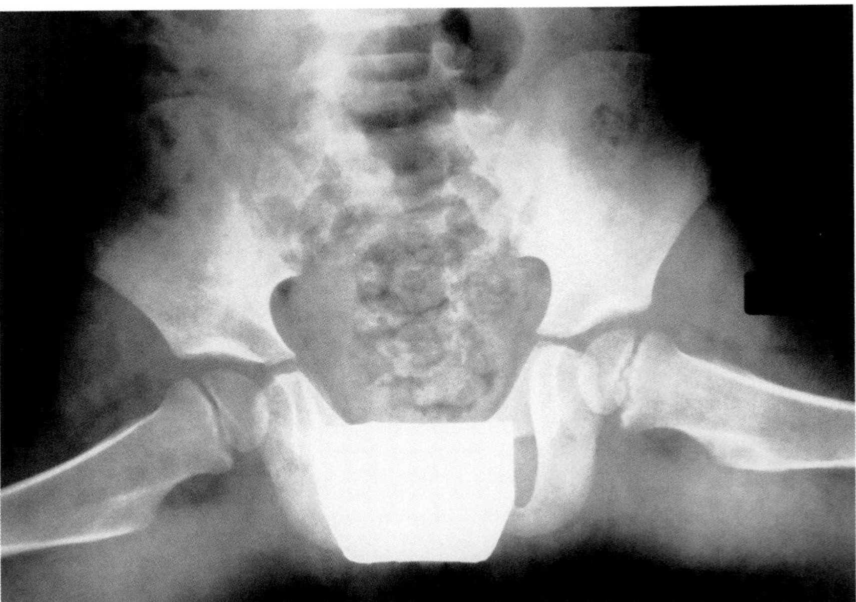

Fig. 20-59. Lateral hips and proximal femora (male). (Shielding error: Shield is placed a little too high on the radiograph; covers up symphysis area and doesn't extend low enough to cover all of genitals.)

AP, AP REVERSE CALDWELL, AND AP TOWNE SKULL PROJECTIONS

Skull (Head)
BASIC
- AP
  AP Caldwell
  AP Towne
- Lateral

Pathology Demonstrated

Fractures, congenital anomalies of cranium including sutures and/or fontanelles, head size, shunt check, bony tumors, or other pathologies of the skull are shown.

Technical Factors

- IR size—infants and small children: 18 × 24 cm (8 × 10 inches), lengthwise
  —children and young adolescents: 24 × 30 cm (10 × 12 inches), lengthwise
- Moving or stationary grid if more than 9 cm
- Small focal spot
- 65-70 kV, shortest exposure time possible

(18) 24
R
24 (30)

Shielding Secure or place lead shield over entire pelvic area.

Patient Position

- Mummify patient's body and limbs if needed.
- Patient is supine, aligned to midline of table/grid.
- If necessary, place sandbags over patient's legs and on each side of mummified body. Compression band can also be used if needed.

Part Position

- Position head with **no rotation.**
- Adjust chin so that **orbitomeatal line (OML) is perpendicular to IR.**
- Immobilize head with head clamps or head supports as demonstrated.
- Tape may also be used if necessary, but turn adhesive side out over patient area so as not to adhere to skin.

Central Ray

- CR **centered to glabella**
  AP skull: **CR parallel to OML**
  AP reverse Caldwell: **CR 15° cephalad to OML**
  AP Towne: **CR 30° caudad to OML**
- IR centered to CR
- Minimum SID of 40 inches (100 cm)

Collimation Collimate closely on four sides to outer margins of skull.

Note: Generally, holding by parent is **not** needed for exams of the head if immobilization devices are used.

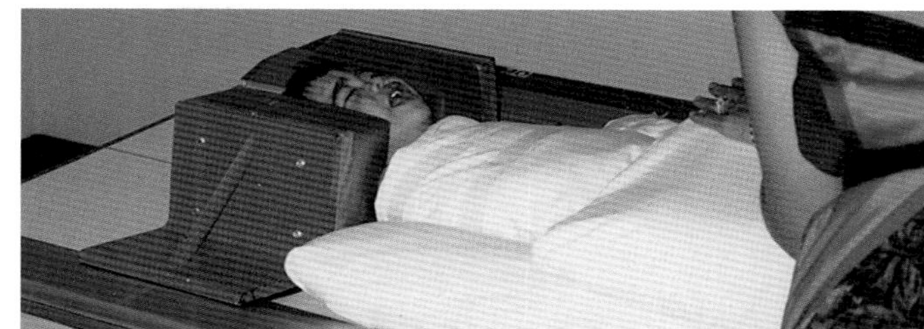

Fig. 20-60. Patient mummified; sandbags and head supports in use.

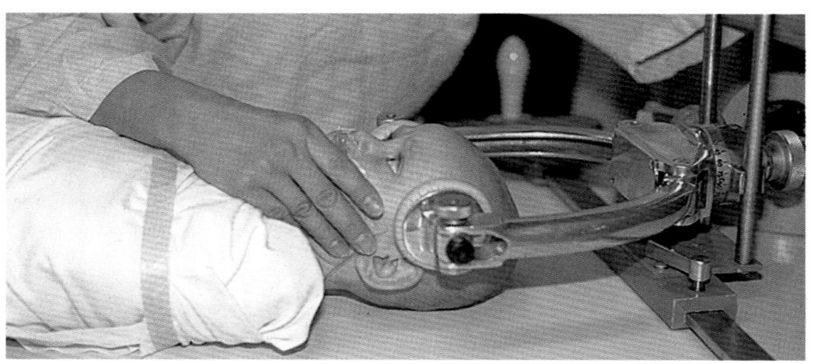

Fig. 20-61. Patient mummified; head clamps in use.

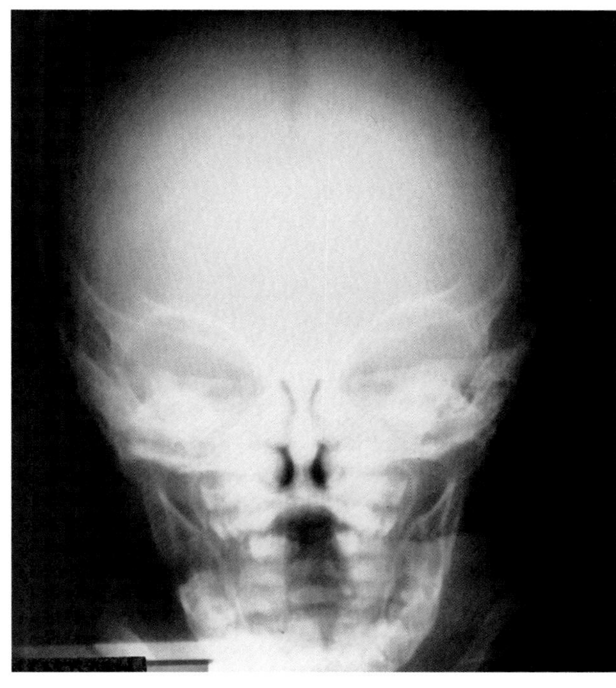

Fig. 20-62. AP skull (CR <10° cephalad to OML).

Radiographic Criteria

Structures Shown: • Entire skull, including cranial and facial bones

Position: • **No rotation** occurs, as evidenced by symmetric orbits at equal distances from outer skull margins. • *AP 0°:* Petrous ridges superimpose superior orbital margins. • *AP with 15° cephalad angle:* Petrous pyramids and internal auditory canals are projected into lower one half to one third of orbits. • *AP Towne with 30° cephalad angle:* Petrous pyramids are projected below the inferior orbital rim, allowing visualization of the entire orbital margin (see Chapter 12, adult AP axial skull). Dorsum sella and posterior clinoids are projected into foramen magnum.

Collimation and CR: • Collimation borders seen on four sides with center (CR) to glabella, midway between supraorbital margins.

Exposure Criteria: • No motion, as evidenced by sharp margins of bony structures. • Penetration and exposure sufficient to visualize the frontal bone and the petrous pyramids through the orbits.

LATERAL SKULL POSITION: SKULL (HEAD)

Pathology Demonstrated
Same pathology is shown as on AP projection on preceding page.

Skull (Head)
BASIC
- AP
- AP Caldwell
- AP Towne
- Lateral

10 (12)
8 (10) R

Technical Factors
- IR size—infants and small children: 18 × 24 cm (8 × 10 inches), crosswise
- IR size—children and young adolescents: 24 × 32 cm (10 × 12 inches), crosswise
- Moving or stationary grid if more than 9 cm
- Small focal spot
- 65-70 kV, shortest exposure time possible

Shielding Secure or place lead shield over pelvic area.

Patient Position
- Mummify patient's body and limbs (may be necessary for infants and for some small children).
- Patient is in semiprone position, centered to midline of table. Place sandbags along patient's back and under elevated side of body.
- If necessary, place sandbag across buttocks and legs (Fig. 20-63). A compression band can be used across sandbags if needed.

Part Position
- Rotate head into true lateral position and maintain by placing a sponge or folded towel under mandible.
- Place weighted support or sponge and sandbag behind head to prevent from pushing the head backward.
- Use compression band across head, or secure tape to each side of table and cross patient's head with adhesive side up to prevent adhering to skin. Sandbags can also be placed over tape to prevent patient from lifting head from tabletop.

Central Ray
- CR **perpendicular** to IR, centered **midway between glabella and occipital protuberance or inion,** 2 inches (5 cm) above EAM
- IR centered to CR
- Minimum SID of 40 inches (100 cm)

Collimation Collimate closely on four sides to outer margins of skull.

Note: For infants, the Tam-em board can be used for skull exams with the lateral taken with horizontal beam, as shown in Fig. 20-64.

Radiographic Criteria

Structures Shown: • Entire cranium and upper cervical region

Position: • **No rotation** is evidenced by superimposed rami of mandible, orbital roofs, and greater and lesser wings of sphenoid. • Sella turcica and clivus are demonstrated in profile without rotation.

Collimation and CR: • Collimate borders on four sides with center (CR) at midway between glabella anteriorly and most posterior margin of occipital bone.

Exposure Criteria: • No motion, as evidenced by sharp margins of bony structures. • Penetration and exposure sufficient to visualize parietal region and the lateral view outline of the sella turcica without overexposing perimeter margins of skull.

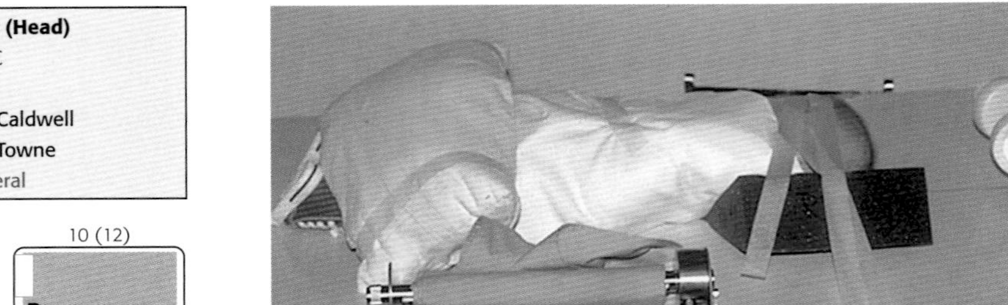

Fig. 20-63. Lateral skull.

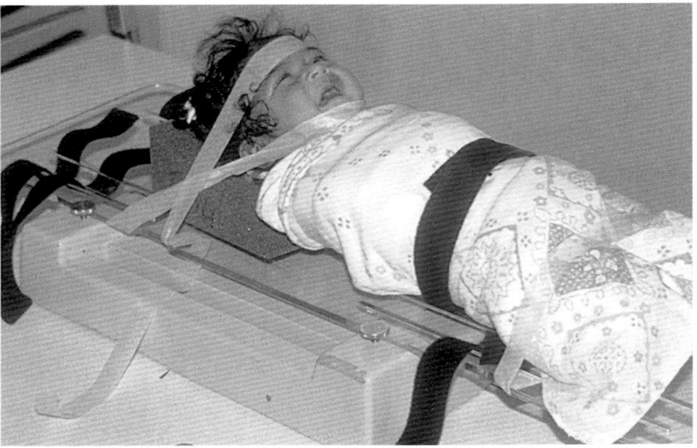

Fig. 20-64. Horizontal beam lateral with Tam-em board.

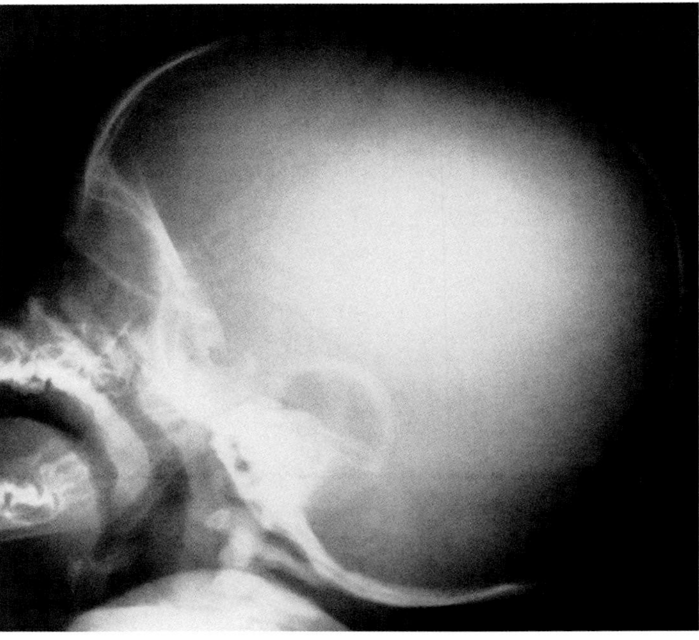

Fig. 20-65. Lateral skull.

RADIOGRAPHIC PROCEDURES OF THE PEDIATRIC ABDOMEN

with Cecilie Godderidge

Differences Between Children and Adults

The difference between children and adults is not only in size but also in the many developmental changes that take place from birth to puberty. The chest and abdomen are almost equal in circumference in the newborn. The pelvis is small and composed more of cartilage than bone. The abdomen is more prominent and the abdominal organs higher in infants than in older children. Accurate centering may be difficult for technologists more used to radiographing adults, using the iliac crest and the anterior superior iliac spine as positioning landmarks, which for all practical purposes are nonexistent in a young child. As a child grows, bone and musculature develop, the body outline and characteristics become distinctive, and familiar landmarks are more easily located.

It is difficult to distinguish on a radiograph between small and large bowels in infants and toddlers, because the haustra of the large bowel are not as apparent as in older children and adults. Also, little intrinsic body fat exists, so an outline of the kidneys, for example, is not as well seen as in adults. Even so, visualization of the soft tissues is important in children, and a good plain radiograph of the abdomen provides valuable diagnostic information. Radiologists commonly say that the gas in the gastrointestinal tract may be the best contrast medium in evaluating the pediatric abdomen.

Precise collimation is important and in children the diaphragm, symphysis pubis, and the outer edges of the abdomen should all be included in a plain supine radiograph. Radiographs of young children tend to look "flat," and less contrast exists than is seen in those of adults. This is to be expected because bones are less dense, there is less fat, muscles are undeveloped, and the range of soft tissues is softer and less defined. Proper exposure factors must be chosen to ensure that subtle changes in soft tissues are not "burned out" at too high a kilovoltage.

Patient Preparation for Contrast Media Procedure

Patient history is important when evaluating the pediatric patient, because this assists the radiologist in deciding the order and type of radiographic procedures to be performed. When it is necessary to withhold feeding for an upper gastrointestinal (GI) study, the examination should be scheduled early in the morning. Children become irritable when hungry, and technologists need to be understanding of the difficulties in having a young child fast and must be supportive of both parent and child before and during fluoroscopic examinations of the GI tract. Having the infant's stomach empty is important not only because this ensures a good diagnostic upper GI study, but also because babies and infants, when hungry, are more likely to drink the barium.

Upper Gastrointestinal Tract (Upper GI, or UGI)

Infants and young children require minimal preparation for upper GI studies. Length of fasting is determined by age; the older the child, the slower the gastric emptying. **Infants under 1 year** should have nothing to eat or drink, or be **NPO, for 4 hours before the exam.** Babies can have an early morning feed at 6:00 a.m. and be scheduled for a barium swallow and UGI at 10:00 a.m. Children **older than 1 year** should be **NPO from 12:00 midnight** for an early morning exam or be **NPO for 6 hours** if the appointment is scheduled for late morning or in the afternoon.

Written instruction should be given to the parent and the reason for "absolutely nothing by mouth" explained and emphasized.

Lower Gastrointestinal System (Lower GI)

Patient history determines the preparation for a lower GI examination. This is usually a single-contrast barium enema in children. Double-contrast enemas are performed less frequently than in adults and are used mainly to diagnose polyps in children.

SUMMARY

Patient Preparation

- Good patient history important
- Early morning scheduling if feeding is withheld (problem of irritability with long fasting)
- Empty stomach required for GI study (hunger increasing likelihood that patient will drink barium)

Upper GI Preparation

Minimum prep required:

Infants to 1-year-olds:

- NPO 4 hours before exam

1 year and older:

- NPO after midnight for early AM exam or
- NPO 6 hours before for late AM or PM exam

Lower GI Preparation

Patient history determines required prep:

(Certain clinical symptoms or diagnoses preclude any prep.)

Infants to 2-year-olds:

- No prep required

2 to 10 years:

- Low-residue meal evening before
- 1 bisacodyl tablet or similar laxative before bedtime evening before
- If no bowel movement in morning, upon advice of physician, Pedi-Fleet enema

10 years to adult:

- Low-residue meal evening before
- 2 bisacodyl tablets or similar laxative evening before
- If no bowel movement in morning, upon advice of physician, Pedi-Fleet enema

IVU Preparation

- No solid food 4 hours before exam (to lessen risk for aspiration from vomiting)
- Drinking of clear liquids encouraged until 1 hour before exam

Courtesy Children's Hospital, Boston, Mass.

Contraindications

Patients with the following clinical symptoms or conditions should not be given laxatives or enemas: **Hirschsprung's disease, extensive diarrhea, appendicitis, obstruction,** and **conditions in which the patient cannot withstand fluid loss.**

Instructions for all other patients are as follows:

Newborn to 2 years: No preparation necessary

Children 2 to 10 years: Low-residue meal the evening before the exam; 1 bisacodyl tablet or similar laxative whole, with water, before bedtime the evening before the examination; if no bowel movement in the morning, a Pedi-Fleet enema possibly given on the advice of a physician

Children 10 years to adult: Low-residue meal the evening before; 2 bisacodyl tablets or similar laxative whole, with water, before bedtime the evening before the examination; if no bowel movement in the morning, a Pedi-Fleet enema possibly given on the advice of a physician

Intravenous Urogram

The preparation of children for an intravenous urogram (IVU) is simple. No solid foods 4 hours before the examination to diminish the risk for aspiration from vomiting. The patient should be encouraged to drink plenty of clear liquids until 1 hour before the examination.

AP PROJECTION (KUB): ABDOMEN

Abdomen
BASIC
- AP (KUB)

OPTIONAL
- AP erect
- Lateral and dorsal decubitus

R

Pathology Demonstrated

Pathology of the abdomen to evaluate gas patterns, soft tissue, possible calcifications, and/or other anomalies or diseases of the abdomen are shown.

Technical Factors

- IR size–determined by the size of patient, IR lengthwise
- 400-speed film-screen combination
- Moving or stationary grid, if more than 10 cm
- 65-85 kV NB to 18 years, shortest exposure time possible

Shielding

- Gonadal shield on all males–size appropriate for age (tape shield in place)
- No gonadal shielding on females

Patient and Part Position

- Patient is supine, aligned to midline of table and/or cassette.
- Immobilize with soft flexible sandbags and compression band.

Newborns and young infants:

- Position the arms away from the body and mold a large flexible sandbag over each arm. Because it is difficult to straighten the little, short legs of infants, place one sandbag under their knees and another over the top to immobilize their legs. Babies, if they feel snug and warm, are usually calm unless they are in pain. If a baby is crying, a pacifier may help and will not interfere with the exam.

Infants and toddlers:

- Restrain the arms the same as for younger infants. Place a sandbag under the knees and tighten a compression band over both femora and knees. Be sure to place padding under the band so that it does not cut into the child's legs. Compression bands on most x-ray tables are designed for adults, so this restraint works best if the spaces between the band and patient are padded with foam sponges or towels.

If parents are providing assistance:

- Provide parent with lead apron and gloves.
- Position tube and cassette and set exposure factors before positioning.
- Position patient so that technologist's view is not obstructed.
- Usually, it is necessary to have a parent hold only the child's arms. The legs can be satisfactorily immobilized as described above.

Central Ray

- With infants and small children, CR and cassette centered **1 inch (2.5 cm) above the umbilicus**
- With older children and adolescents, CR centered at the **level of iliac crest**
- Minimum SID of 40 inches (102 cm)

Respiration

- With **infants and children,** watch the breathing pattern. When the abdomen is still, make the exposure. If the patient is crying, make the exposure as the baby takes a breath to let out a cry.
- Children over 5 years can usually hold their breath after a practice session.

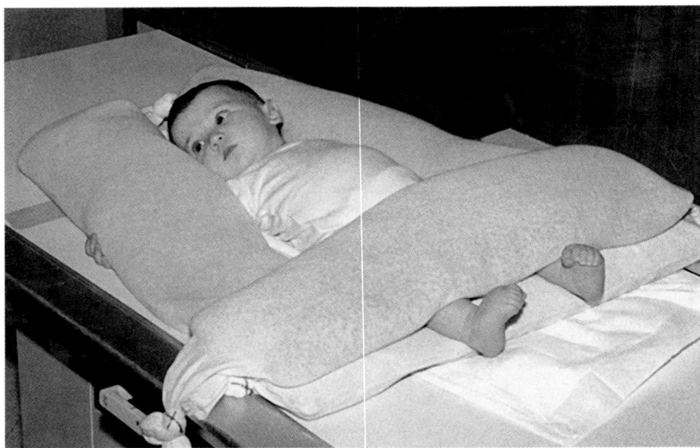

Fig. 20-66. Child immobilized with sandbags for AP abdomen. (Note sandbag under and over lower limbs.)

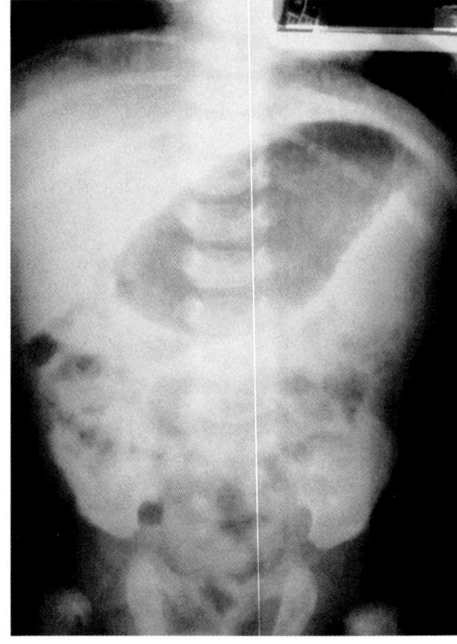

Fig. 20-67. AP abdomen, supine (demonstrates distended air-filled stomach).

Radiographic Criteria

Structures Shown: • Soft tissue border outlines and gas-filled structures such as the stomach and intestines, calcifications (if present), and faint bony skeletal structures are shown.

Position: • The vertebral column is aligned to the center of the radiograph. • **No rotation** should exist: pelvis, hips, and lower rib cage should be symmetric.

Collimation and CR: • Collimation borders from symphysis pubis to diaphragm and to bilateral borders of abdomen.

Exposure Criteria: • No motion should be evident, and diaphragm and gas patterns should appear sharp. • Optimal contrast and exposure will visualize bony structure outlines such as ribs and vertebrae through abdominal contents without overexposing gas-filled structures.

AP ERECT ABDOMEN PROJECTION: ABDOMEN

Abdomen
BASIC
- AP (KUB)

OPTIONAL
- AP erect
- Lateral and dorsal decubitus

Pathology Demonstrated

Pathology of the abdomen, including possible intestinal obstruction by demonstration of air-fluid levels and/or free intraabdominal air, is shown. Generally, this projection is part of a three-way or acute abdomen series (supine, erect, and decubitus).

Technical Factors

- IR size—determined by the size of patient, IR lengthwise
- Moving or stationary grid if more than 10 cm
- 65-85 kV, NB to 18 years, shortest exposure time possible

R

Shielding

- Gonadal shield on all males—size appropriate for age (tape shield in place), no gonadal shielding on females

Patient and Part Position

- Have patient sit or stand with back against upright IR
- Seat younger child on large foam block with legs slightly apart. Immobilize legs with Velcro strap. Ask parent to hold arms away from side or over the child's head. Infants: hold head between arms.
- Children 4 years and older (unless too ill) will stand with assistance.

Tam-em board (not preferred):

- Secure child to board with straps; then firmly secure board to table with compression band and Velcro straps before elevating.

Pigg-O-Stat (preferred):

- Position patient in Pigg-O-Stat as for chest radiograph, with arms over head and back against cassette or upright Bucky.

With parental assistance (if parent is not pregnant):

- Provide parent with lead apron and gloves.
- Position tube and cassette and set exposure factors before positioning.
- Position parent so that technologist's view is not obstructed.

Central Ray

- With infants and small children, center **CR and cassette 1 inch (2.5 cm) above the umbilicus.**
- With older children and adolescents, center **CR at approximately 1 inch (2.5 cm) above the level of the iliac crest,** which should place top collimation border and top of film at **level of the axilla** to include the diaphragm on IR.
- Minimum SID is 40 inches (100 cm).

Respiration

- With infants and children, watch the breathing pattern. When the abdomen is still, make the exposure. If the patient is crying, make the exposure as the baby takes a breath in to let out a cry.
- Children more than 5 years old can usually hold their breath after a practice session.

Radiographic Criteria

Structures Shown: • Entire contents of abdomen, including gas patterns and air fluid levels and soft tissue if not obscured by excessive fluid in distended abdomen, as in Fig. 20-70.

Position: • The vertebral column is aligned to the center of the radiograph. • **No rotation** should exist: pelvis and hips should be symmetric.

Collimation and CR: • Collimation to borders of abdomen from symphysis pubis to diaphragm.

Exposure Criteria: • No motion should be evident, and diaphragm and gas pattern borders should appear sharp. • Bony pelvis and vertebral body outlines should be evident through abdominal contents without overexposing air-filled structures.

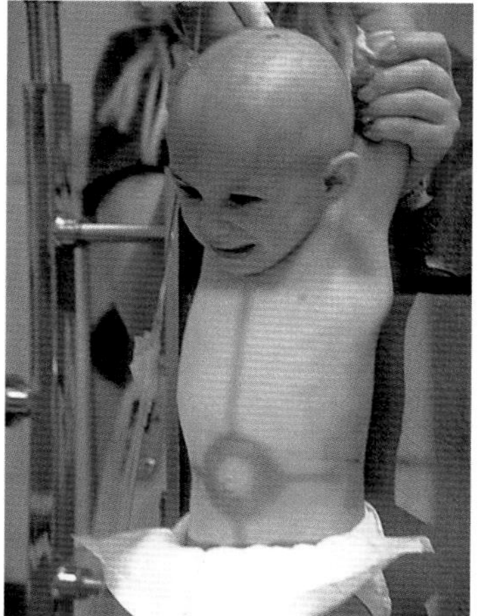

Fig. 20-68. Erect AP abdomen. (Parent holding child should be wearing lead apron and gloves.)

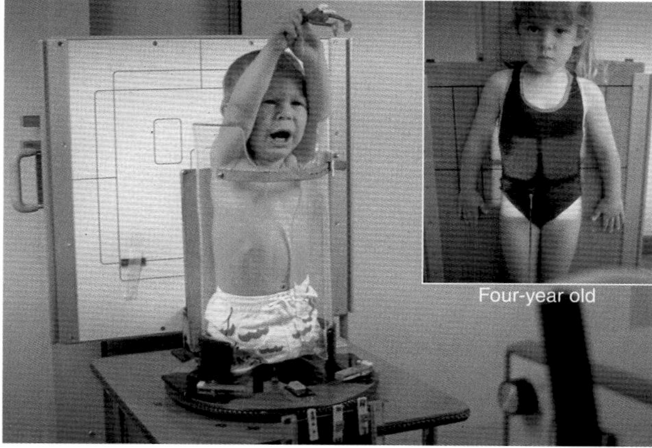

Fig. 20-69. Erect AP abdomen with Pigg-O-Stat. Note top of cassette at axilla to include diaphragm. *Inset* demonstrates 4-year-old child in front of IR.

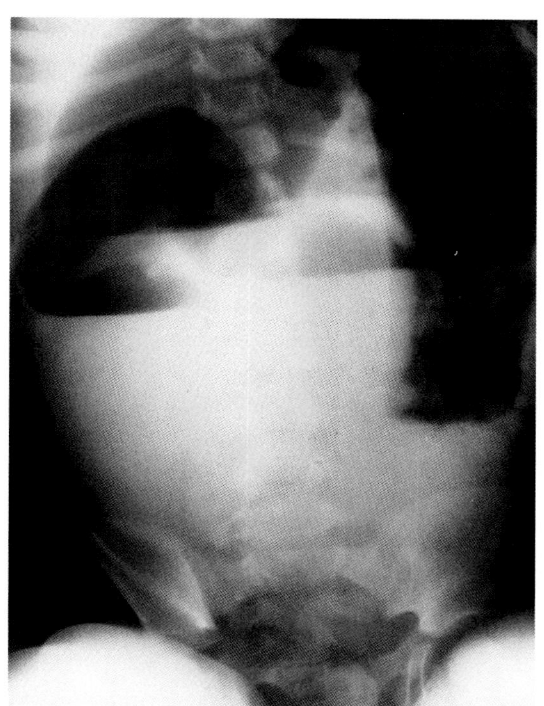

Fig. 20-70. Erect AP abdomen (demonstrates fluid levels and distended air-filled large bowel).

20

LATERAL DECUBITUS AND DORSAL DECUBITUS ABDOMEN

Note: When clinically indicated, a dorsal decubitus abdomen may be performed instead of a right or left lateral decubitus.

Abdomen
BASIC
- AP (KUB)

OPTIONAL
- AP erect
- Lateral and dorsal decubitus

Pathology Demonstrated

Demonstrates air-fluid levels and free air; dorsal decubitus demonstrates the prevertebral region of the abdomen for possible calcifications, masses, or other anomalies.

Technical Factors

- IR size—determined by the size of patient, IR lengthwise
- Moving or stationary grid, if more than 10 cm
- 65-85 kV, newborn to 18 years, shortest exposure time possible

L

Shielding

- Gonadal shield on males
- No gonadal shielding on females

Patient and Part Position

Lateral decubitus:

- Patient on side on a radiolucent foam block with back against IR
- Horizontal CR directed to 1 inch (2.5 cm) superior to umbilicus

Dorsal decubitus:

- Patient is supine on a rectangular radiolucent foam block.
- Legs are immobilized with sandbags as for a supine AP abdomen.
- Gently pull arms above head and ask parent to hold arms and head with newborn or small infant.
- Place IR lengthwise, parallel to the midsagittal plane against side of patient (support with cassette holder device or with sandbags).

Central Ray

- CR **horizontal,** centered to midcoronal plane for dorsal decubitus:
- With infants and small children, CR and IR centered 1 inch (2.5 cm) superior to level of the umbilicus
- With older children and adolescents, CR centered at the level of 1 inch (2.5 cm) superior to the iliac crest
- Minimum SID of 40 inches (100 cm)

Respiration

- With **infants and children,** watch the breathing pattern. When the abdomen is still, make the exposure. If the patient is crying, make the exposure as the baby takes a breath to let out a cry.
- Children more than 5 years old can usually hold their breath after a practice session.

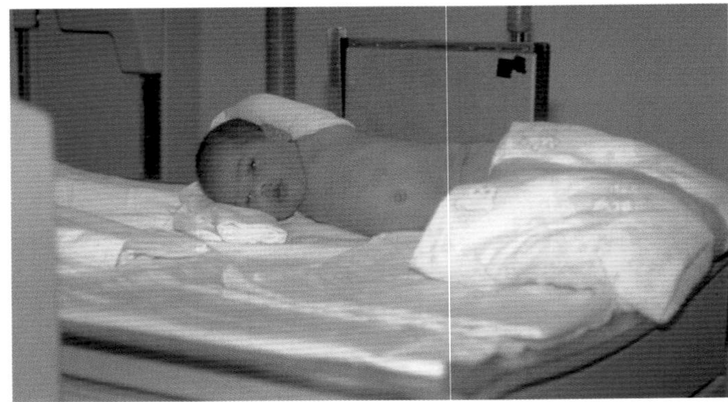

Fig. 20-71. Right lateral decubitus abdomen.

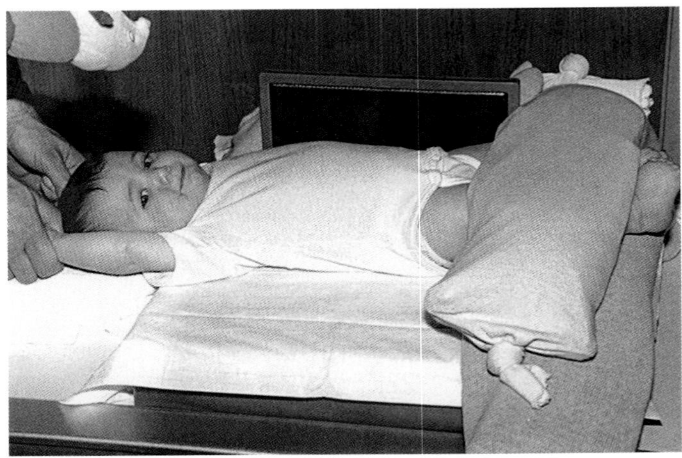

Fig. 20-72. Dorsal decubitus abdomen—left lateral position.

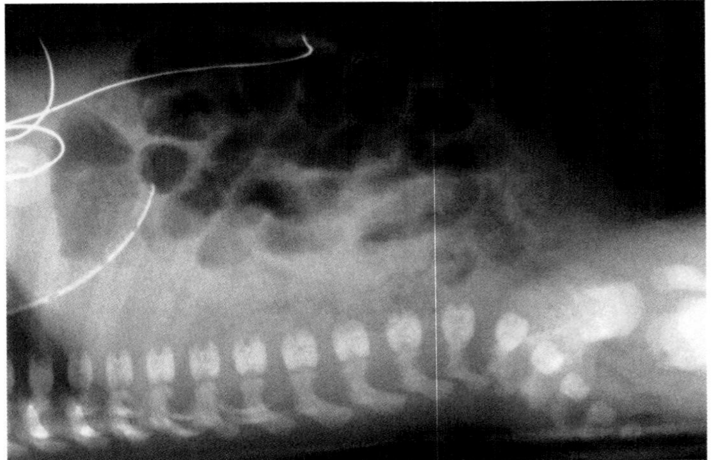

Fig. 20-73. Dorsal decubitus abdomen (demonstrates necrotizing enterocolitis in neonate).

Radiographic Criteria (Dorsal decubitus)

Structures Shown: • Abdominal structures in the prevertebral region as well as air-fluid levels within abdomen; diaphragm included superiorly and pelvis and hips inferiorly.

Position: • **No rotation** should exist: posterior ribs should be superimposed.

Collimation and CR: • At least minimal collimation borders should be visible on four sides, with center of collimation field (CR) to midcoronal plane, midway between diaphragm and symphysis pubis.

Exposure Criteria: • No motion should be evident, and diaphragm and gas patterns should appear sharp. • Abdominal soft-tissue detail should be visible without overexposing gas-filled structures. • Faint rib outlines should be visible through abdominal contents.

20

UPPER GASTROINTESTINAL SYSTEM (UGI) STUDY

Barium Swallow, UGI, and Small Bowel Combination Study

Pathology Demonstrated
Diseases or conditions involving the GI tract (see summary of pathologic indications for the pediatric abdomen, p. 664)

Patient Preparation
- **Infants less than 1 year:** NPO for 4 hours
- **Children more than 1 year:** NPO for 6 hours, or NPO after midnight if exam is scheduled for early morning

Room Preparation The fluoroscopic procedure room should be prepared before the child is brought into the room. The table is placed in the horizontal position and the fluoroscopic controls set. A cotton or disposable sheet should be placed over the table. Depending on the exam, the appropriate barium or contrast medium, feeding bottle, nipple, straw, feeding catheter, and syringe should be ready for use. Suction and oxygen should also be readily available in the event of an emergency.

Shielding A piece of 1-mm lead vinyl is positioned to place under the child's buttocks to shield the gonads from scatter radiation from the "under table" fluoro tube.

Barium Preparation Liquid barium may be used according to a particular manufacturer's instructions. The barium may need to be diluted for younger children and infants. Dilution is usually necessary when using a feeding bottle, and it is helpful to widen the hole in the nipple with a sterile needle or scalpel so that the baby can feed more easily.

The amount of barium given for an upper GI varies with the age of the child. Suggested amounts are as follows*:
- NB to 1 yr—2 to 4 oz
- 1 to 3 yr—4 to 6 oz
- 3 to 10 yr—6 to 12 oz
- More than 10 yr—12 to 16 oz

Patient and Parent Preparation Parents should accompany their child into the procedure room before the study is started. A few minutes spent explaining the exam and how the equipment works is of benefit to both parent and child. The large equipment and strange noises that seem so normal to the technologist are terrifying to many young children. An explanation and demonstration of how the image intensifier is brought down over the chest and abdomen lessen fears that the child might have of being crushed. Children can be shown how they can watch the "milk shake" going down into the stomach on the television monitor.

Barium procedures on children are usually performed with the patient lying down. Parents (if not pregnant) may be given a lead apron and gloves so that they can remain in the room during the fluoroscopic procedure. Holding the child's hand and assisting the technologist in feeding the child reduces anxiety and helps in providing a supportive environment for both parent and child. Continual words of encouragement help the patient with ingestion of the barium.

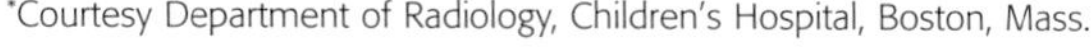

*Courtesy Department of Radiology, Children's Hospital, Boston, Mass.

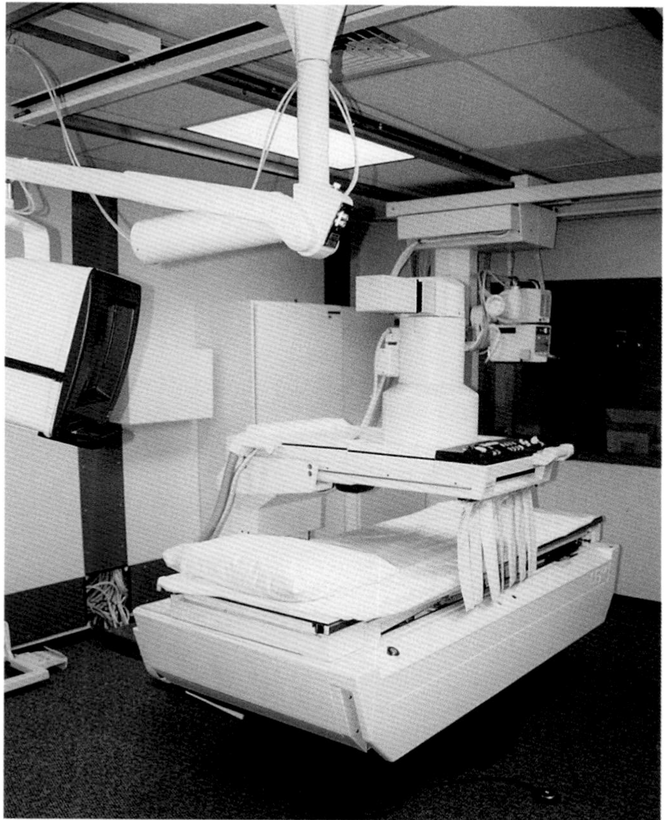

Fig. 20-74. Modern digital R/F equipment for GI study. (Courtesy Philips Medical Systems.)

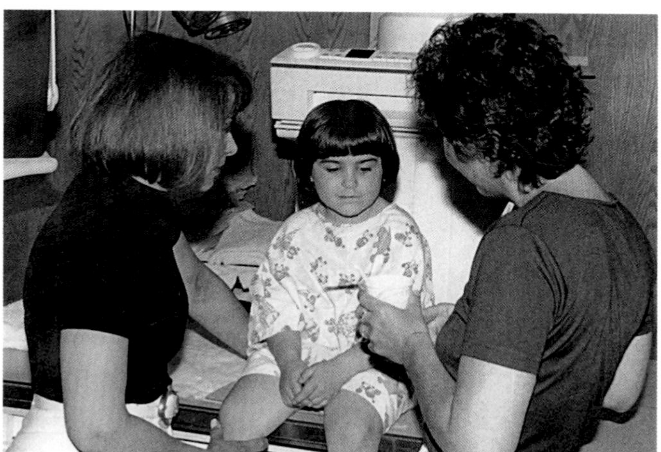

Fig. 20-75. Providing clear explanations to parent and child are beneficial.

Procedure

Pre–GI exams:

- AP supine abdomen (KUB) before a UGI
- PA and lateral chest before a barium swallow

Drinking barium: A baby or infant will drink from a feeding bottle. An older child will usually drink through a straw, which prevents spillage.

In some cases a child may insist on drinking directly from a cup. This entails sitting the child up to drink and then lying down to be fluoroscoped. If the esophagus must be outlined, barium paste can be spooned onto the palate or tongue. Another tactic is to squirt barium into the child's mouth with a 10-ml syringe while gently holding the nose. If a child refuses to swallow the barium, it may be necessary for the radiologist to pass a nasogastric tube into the stomach.

Fluoroscopy Positioning Sequence

Radiologists follow a particular sequence of positions for a UGI starting with the **patient supine.** This is generally followed by a **left lateral, LPO** and **RAO,** then a **right lateral** with the patient turned onto the right side; in this position the stomach empties quickly. It is important to check the location of the duodenojejunal junction to rule out malrotation before the jejunum fills. The final position is **prone.** This is a standard procedure even in patients whose symptoms are not necessarily of malrotation.

Permanent images are recorded during fluoroscopy on spot films of various types, depending on the equipment. With digital fluoroscopy, specific images are captured digitally rather than on spot film cassettes. These digital images can then be displayed on monitors and manipulated later as needed before storage or printing onto film.

Young children generally do not require the usual overhead tube PA and RAO radiographs of the stomach following fluoroscopy that are standard for adults. If these projections are required, the radiologist should be asked to point out the level at which the image should be centered.

Small Bowel Follow-Through

AP or PA abdomen are taken at **20- to 30-minute intervals,** either supine or prone, depending on the age and condition of the patient. Transit time is quite rapid in young children, and the barium may reach the ileocecal region in **1 hour.**

Postprocedure Instructions

Once the examination is complete and the radiographs checked, the patient may eat and drink normally if diet permits. The child should be encouraged to drink plenty of water and fruit juices. The technologist should check that spot films and overheads are placed together in the patient's folder and appropriately labeled; with digital fluoro, the technologist should make sure that the digital images are correctly stored for later retrieval and/or printing. Number of images recorded and fluoroscopic time should be noted on the requisition.

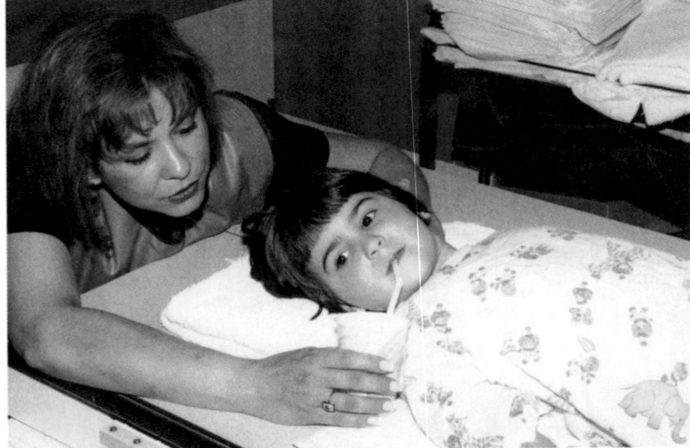

Fig. 20-76. "Drinking" barium just before beginning fluoroscopy.

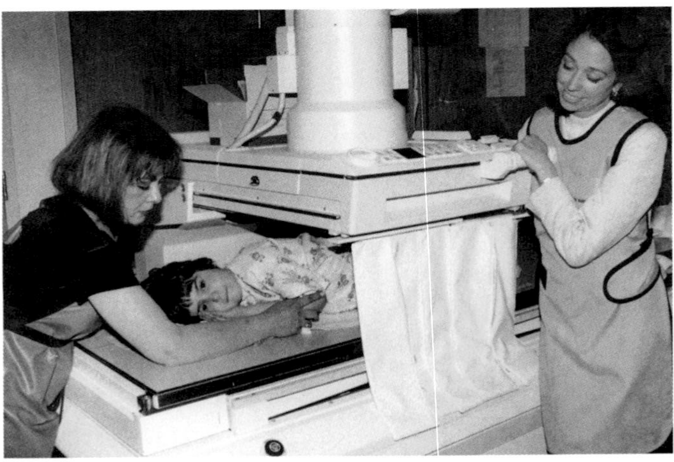

Fig. 20-77. Patient being positioned into an oblique position in preparation for upper GI fluoro. (Parent will step back before fluoro begins.)

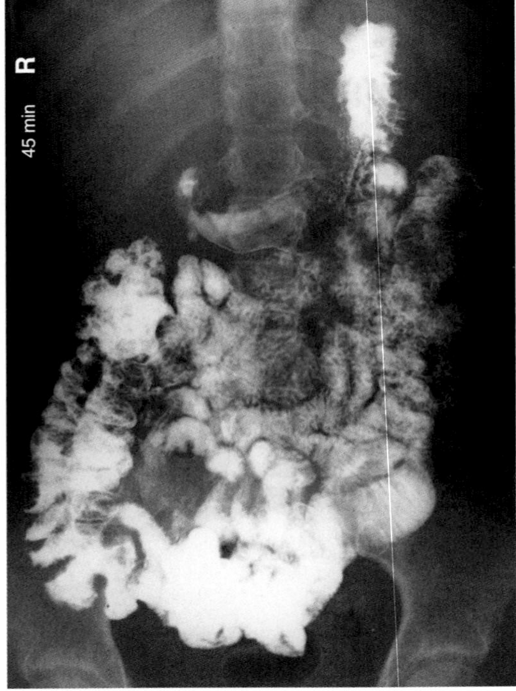

Fig. 20-78. Demonstrates 45-minute small bowel follow-through.

LOWER GASTROINTESTINAL SYSTEM STUDY—BARIUM ENEMA

Single-Contrast, Double-Contrast, and/or Air Enema

Pathology Demonstrated See summary of pathologic indications for pediatric abdomen, p. 660.

Patient Preparation
- **Neonates to 2 yr:** No preparation necessary
- **2 yr to 10 yr:** Low-residue meal the evening before the exam; 1 bisacodyl tablet or similar laxative, whole with water before bedtime; if no bowel movement in the morning, a stimulant enema, such as a Pedi-Fleet enema, given on the advice of a physician
- **10 yr to adult:** Same as for 2 yr to 10 yr, except patient should take 2 bisacodyl tablets with water before bedtime

Contrast and Materials—Barium Enema, Single-Contrast
Children more than 1 yr:
- Disposable enema bag is used with barium sulfate, tubing, and clamp. Add tepid (not cold) water according to manufacturer's instructions.
- **Pediatric flexible enema tip:** Some of these catheters are designed so that they cannot be inserted beyond the rectum. Taping the tube in place will prevent leakage.

Warning: Latex tips must **NOT** be used because of the potential of a life-threatening allergic response to latex. Inflatable balloon-type retention tips must also **NOT** be used as they may perforate the rectum.

Neonates and infants:
- #10 French flexible silicone catheter and a 60-ml syringe; barium injected manually and slowly

All patients:
- Water-soluble lubricating jelly
- Hypoallergenic tape
- Gloves
- Washcloths and towels for clean-up

Contrast and Materials—Barium Enema, Double-Contrast
- High-density barium and air contrast enema kit or enema bag with double-line tip, including tube through which air is introduced
- Air insufflation device
- Remainder of materials same as for a single-contrast barium enema

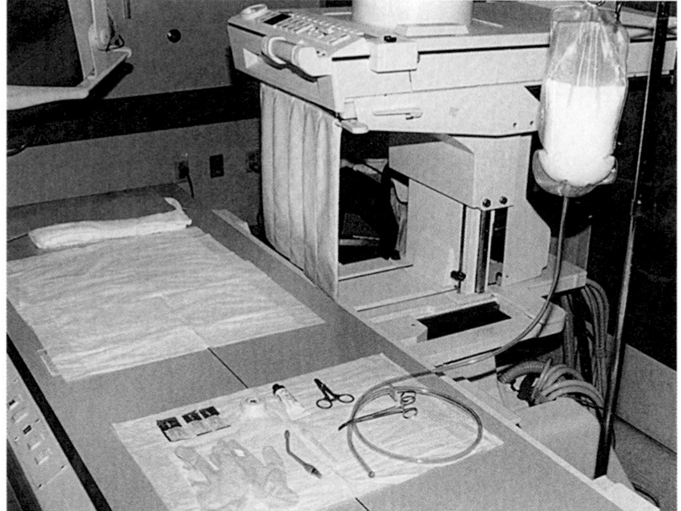

Fig. 20-79. Barium enema room setup with disposable enema bag, tubing, enema tip (use pediatric flexible-type enema tip), and other supplies.

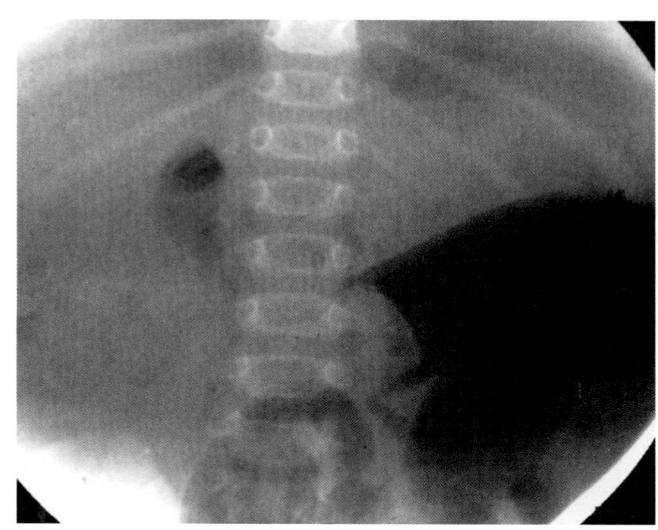

Fig. 20-80. Air enema demonstrating air in the transverse colon, the most common site of intussusception. (From Godderidge C: *Pediatric imaging,* Philadelphia, 1995, WB Saunders.)

Air Enema An air enema is performed under fluoroscopy for the pneumatic reduction of an intussusception. This condition occurs when one portion of the large bowel telescopes into an adjacent portion. The pneumatic reduction is most often performed as an emergency, because the patient is in severe abdominal pain. It is a specialized procedure and must be done carefully to avoid perforation of the bowel. When the procedure is successful, the child's pain dissipates quickly and in many cases the reduction helps prevent an operative procedure. An intussusception may also be reduced by barium enema, depending on the preference of the radiologist.

Materials
- Air insufflation device
- Aneroid air pressure gauge
- Disposable tubing with three-way stopcock
- Flexible enema tip
- Hypoallergenic tape
- Gloves
- Washcloths and towels for clean-up

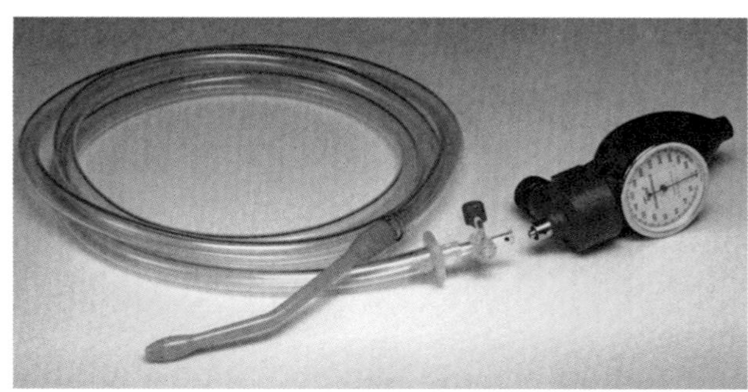

Fig. 20-81. Shields Intussusception Air Reduction System. (Courtesy Custom Medical Products, Maineville, Ohio.)

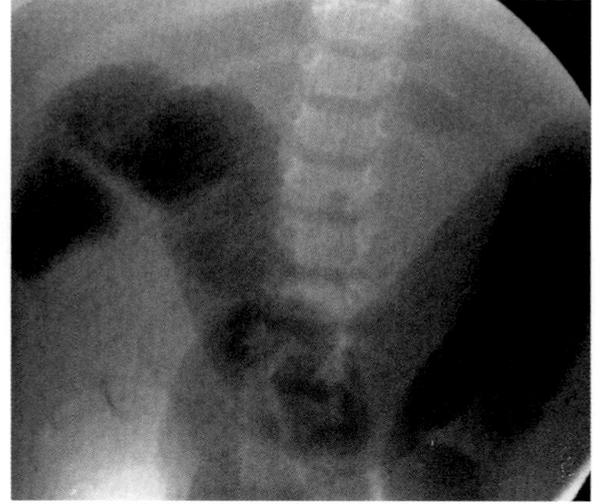

Fig. 20-82. Air enema spot film following the above, showing the air having pushed out the telescoped bowel. (From Godderidge C: *Pediatric imaging,* Philadelphia, 1995, WB Saunders.)

Room Preparation

The room should be prepared as for a UGI with the table horizontal, covered with a disposable or cotton sheet, and the fluoroscopic controls set. The enema bag with barium, tubing, stand, clamp, and tip should be assembled and ready for use. The barium is administered slowly, by gravity, from **3 feet** above the tabletop unless otherwise directed by the radiologist.

Shielding The gonads cannot be shielded during a fluoroscopic examination of the large bowel.

Patient and Parent Preparation The patient and the parent should be brought into the room and the procedure explained clearly and simply. It is particularly important to explain why the tube is being inserted into the rectum and how the barium enhances the bowel on the television screen. Appropriate technology and language should be used in the explanation, depending on the age of the child. A young child most likely will be frightened by having someone touch their buttocks and genital area.

Technologists should be reassuring and supportive and explain to parent and child that the exam does not hurt, though the child may feel a desire to go to the bathroom while the barium is passing into the bowel.

A parent should stay with the child throughout the exam. Talking and giving words of encouragement will help the exam go smoothly.

Procedure

Pre GI exam:

- Preliminary supine AP (KUB) abdomen before beginning fluoroscopy procedure

Fluoroscopy and spot imaging:

- Spot films or digital imaging during fluoroscopy; film or image size depending on age of child and equipment
- Supine or prone abdomen at completion of fluoroscopy
- Right and left lateral decubitus films of the abdomen for double-contrast
- AP supine abdomen postevacuation of barium

Note: Unlike the follow-up images taken for adults, fewer radiographs (sometimes none) are taken at the completion of fluoroscopy.

Postreduction of Intussusception After Air or Barium Enema

- AP supine abdomen; to document that air or barium, depending on the contrast used, has passed through the ileocecal region into the ileum, proving that the intussusception has been reduced (Fig. 20-84)

Postprocedure Tasks Once the examination is complete and the radiographs checked, encourage the patient to drink plenty of water and fruit juices, if diet permits. Ensure that the spot images and overheads are placed together on the patient's folder and are appropriately labeled.

With digital fluoro, ensure that digital images are labeled and stored correctly, ready for further manipulation and viewing and/or printing on film. Record the number of films or images taken and fluoroscopic time.

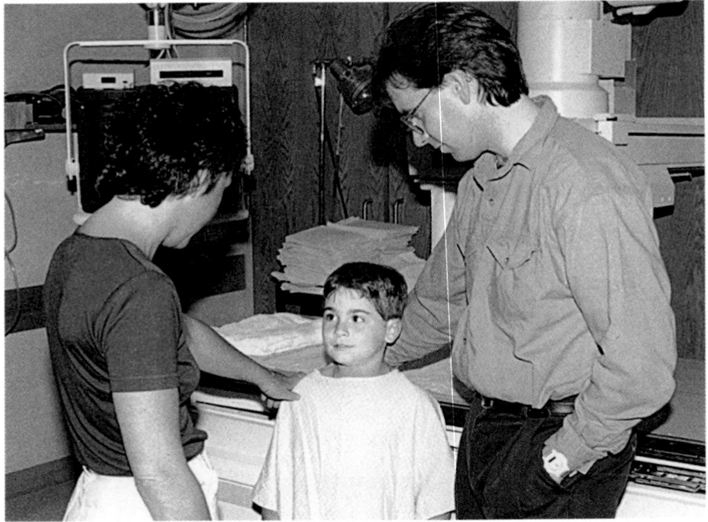

Fig. 20-83. The radiographer providing clear explanations to child and parent.

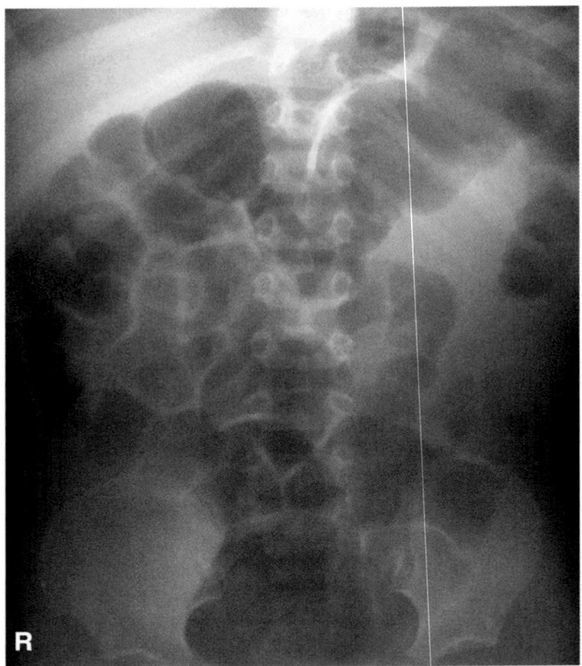

Fig. 20-84. Postreduction of intussusception demonstrating air in terminal ileum. (From Godderidge C: *Pediatric imaging,* Philadelphia, 1995, WB Saunders.)

GENITOURINARY SYSTEM STUDY VOIDING CYSTOURETHROGRAM (VCUG) AND INTRAVENOUS (EXCRETORY) UROGRAM (IVU)

Pathology Demonstrated See summary of diagnostic indications for the pediatric abdomen, p. 660

Technical Factors
- IR size—determined by size of patient
- 400-speed film-screen combination
- Moving or stationary grid if more than 10 cm
- 65-85 kV, NB to 18 years, shortest possible exposure time

Shielding
- Gonadal shielding should always be used on males for plain images of the abdomen and for excretory urography except for voiding films. Shielding is not used during voiding cystourethrography.
- Gonadal shielding cannot be used on females, except when radiographing the kidney area only, because the ovaries of younger children are higher in the abdomen and their location is variable. The lower abdomen may be shielded for the 3-minute radiograph of the kidneys taken during an IVU unless shielding obscures the area of diagnostic interest.

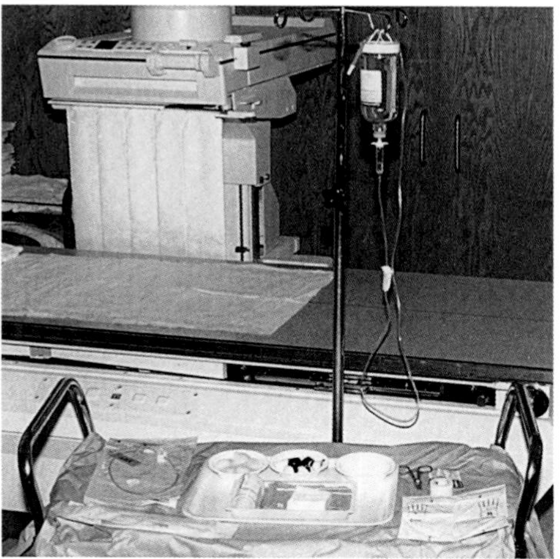

Fig. 20-85. Room setup and materials for VCUG.

Voiding Cystourethrogram (VCUG)

This examination may be performed before an IVU or an ultrasound of the kidneys. One of the most common conditions in young children is **urinary tract infection** (UTI), and this study may be performed to check or evaluate **vesicoureteral reflux,** a common cause of UTI.

Patient Preparation A VCUG requires no special preparation. If the procedure is to be followed by an IVU, the child should follow the preparation for an IVU. This procedure should be described to the patient beforehand, and depending on the age of the child, the timing of this should be left to the parent. Written simple instructions given to the parent will assist them in their explanation.

Contrast Medium and Materials
- Contrast medium for cystography (such as iothalamate meglumine 17.2%)
- IV stand, tubing, and clamp
- Sterile tray with small bowls, sterile gauze, and gloves
- Urine specimen container
- #8 French feeding tube (inflatable balloon-retaining catheters should not be used for children)
- Lidocaine lubricating jelly
- Skin cleanser—antiseptic, wash cloths, and towels
- 10-ml syringe and fistula tip for boys
- Urine receptacle

Room Preparation The table should be in a horizontal position, covered with a disposable or cotton sheet, and the fluoroscopic controls set. The bottle of contrast should be warmed slightly and then hung from an IV stand with tubing and clamp attached. Warmed antiseptic skin cleanser is poured into a small sterile bowl ready for use and the tray covered until the patient is on the table.

Patient and Parent Preparation The patient and parent should be brought into the room and the procedure again explained simply and clearly. The child should be shown the equipment and how it works and be reassured that the image intensifier will not hurt them. The explanation of the procedure should be in language appropriate for the age of the child. "Void" or "voiding" is frequently used by technologists or radiologists, but words such as "tinkle" or "pee" are more likely to be understood by a young child, enabling them to follow instructions. Because so many terms are used for urination, ask the parent what word is used at home.

A VCUG is just as embarrassing and difficult for a young child as it is for an adult. A child who has just been toilet-trained has difficulty in understanding why urinating lying down on a table is acceptable. As much privacy as possible is recommended; allow only those staff in the room who are participating in the exam. If possible, a technologist who is the same sex as the patient should perform the catheterization.

Procedure An older child should be asked to empty the bladder before entering the room. An infant's bladder is drained at catheterization. After cleaning the perineum, the catheter is inserted into the bladder and a urine specimen taken. After running the contrast media to clear air from the tubing, the catheter is attached to the tubing and bottle of contrast and the bladder is slowly filled.

Spot films are taken when the patient's bladder is full and when voiding, because this is when reflux is most likely to occur. A postvoid spot or overhead film is taken of the bladder and kidneys. If reflux occurs, a late film of the abdomen may be taken to check whether the kidneys have emptied. If a patient is being followed for reflux or postoperatively, a radionuclide voiding cystourethrogram, at a reduced radiation dose, may be performed instead of a fluoroscopic procedure.

Postprocedure Tasks Parent and child should be told that when the child first urinates after the procedure, a slight burning sensation may occur and the urine might be pink. Drinking plenty of clear fluids quickly helps to alleviate this problem.

Radiographs should be appropriately labeled and placed in the patient's folder. The amount and type of contrast, number of films, and fluoroscopic time should be recorded. A urine specimen should be sent for culture.

Intravenous (Excretory) Urogram (IVU)

Patient Preparation Preparation for an IVU in children is simple. The patient needs to be hydrated, **NOT** dehydrated, and the child should be encouraged to drink plenty of water and clear fruit juices. No solid foods for 4 hours are eaten before the exam, to diminish the risk for aspiration if the child vomits. Laxatives are not usually recommended for young children for this procedure, because they can cause increased gas and discomfort.

Allergic Response to Contrast Media Although studies of children have found that they have fewer and less severe allergic reactions to iodine-based contrast media than adults, an allergic response is still a possibility. The patient and/or parent must always be asked, before the exam, if the child has asthma or is allergic to iodine, pollens, dust, or any foods and if there is a family history of allergies. Even if the child does not have a history of allergies, caution is mandated if a close relative does. If a patient has had other procedures using iodine-based contrast without incident, it is still possible for an allergic reaction to occur.

Resuscitation equipment and appropriate medications should be immediately available in case a reaction occurs and may consist of the following:

- Diphenhydramine hydrochloride for injection or by mouth
- Epinephrine for injection

Reactions may be slight to severe: warmth and reddening of the skin, nausea, hives, respiratory difficulties, and although rare, cardiac arrest. All personnel, including students, must know how to call a "CODE" should a reaction occur.

Contrast Preparation Low-osmolality, nonionic contrast media are preferred, because although allergic reactions tend to be less severe and occur less frequently in children, many radiology departments prefer not to take the risk. On the other hand, some departments may choose to use nonionic contrast for high-risk patients and high-osmolality contrast for children with no history or family background of allergic response.

DOSAGE ACCORDING TO WEIGHT

		Metric System	
WEIGHT	DOSE	WEIGHT	DOSE
0 to 12 lb	2 ml/lb	0 to 11 kg	3 ml/kg
13 to 25 lb	25 ml	12 to 23 kg	2 ml/kg
26 to 50 lb	1 ml/lb	24 to 45 kg	50 ml
51 to 100 lb	50 ml	>45 kg	1 ml/kg
>100 lb	½ ml/lb		

Courtesy Department of Radiology, Children's Hospital, Boston, Mass. (The metric system doses of ml/kg being used at Children's Hospital are slightly lower doses than the ml/lb doses.)

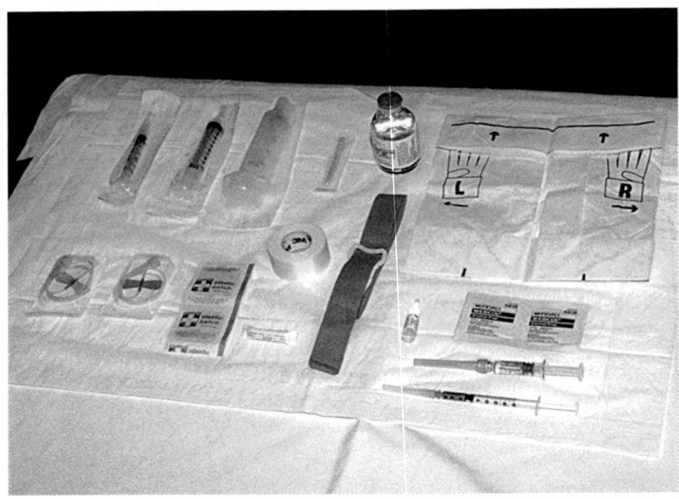

Fig. 20-86. Supplies for injection, IVU.

Materials for Injection

- Syringes: 1, 5, 10, 20, and 50 ml
- Butterfly needles: 19, 23, 25, 27 G
- 16-G straight needle to draw contrast from vial
- Tourniquet
- Gloves
- Mask
- Alcohol swabs
- Band-Aids
- Emesis basin

The contrast medium should be drawn up and ready for use. Cover the tray and syringe before a child is brought into the injection or procedure room. Ensure that the appropriate medications and resuscitation equipment are readily available to respond to an allergic reaction.

20

Patient and Parent Preparation
Children at any age do not like needle sticks. Many adults do not like needles either and may have a problem staying with their child. If at all possible, a parent should stay with the child to hold the child's hand and provide emotional support. The procedure should be explained to the child beforehand and the timing of this should be left to the parent. Usually the best time for very young children is immediately before the procedure.

When explaining a needle stick, do not lie by saying it will not hurt. Suggesting that it is like a bee sting or a pinch in the arm is realistic and less frightening. Babies and very young children may have to be swaddled or "mummified" to immobilize them.

As with any radiographic procedure, the child should be shown the x-ray equipment beforehand and told of the importance of not moving while the exposure is made. Holding a favorite toy or blanket is comforting for many children.

Procedure Fewer radiographs are taken on children than on adults, and in some instances evaluation of kidneys may be made by ultrasound, avoiding the use of ionizing radiation. An imaging sequence may be as follows:

- Preliminary AP supine abdomen (KUB)
- Postinjection (label times accurately):
  - 3-minute of kidneys (shield lower abdomen); tomography used when gas or feces present in the abdomen
  - 15-minute supine or prone abdomen
  - A delayed image may be needed, depending on etiology (factors causing the disease or disorder)
- Gonadal shielding on male patients

Giving a carbonated drink to depress the large bowel and create a radiolucent window to visualize the kidneys is not commonly recommended by pediatric radiologists. The gas passes quickly into the bowel, compounding the problem and causing discomfort to an infant or young child.

Postprocedure Instructions
The child should be told to continue drinking plenty of fluids to clear the contrast medium from the kidneys. Radiographs should be correctly labeled and placed in the patient's folder. The number of images taken, amount of contrast injection, and type of allergic response, if any, should be recorded on the requisition.

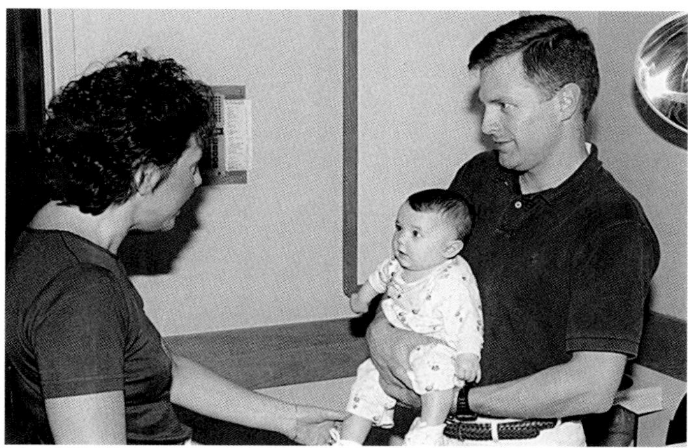

Fig. 20-87. It is important to talk to child and parent.

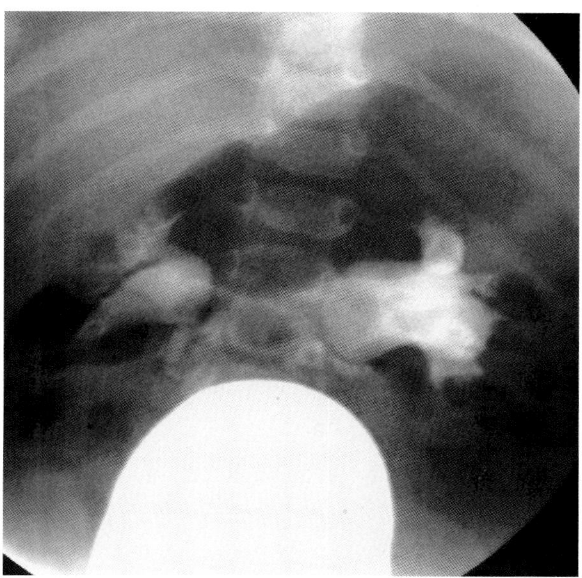

Fig. 20-88. AP demonstrates reflux of both kidneys (18-month-old female).

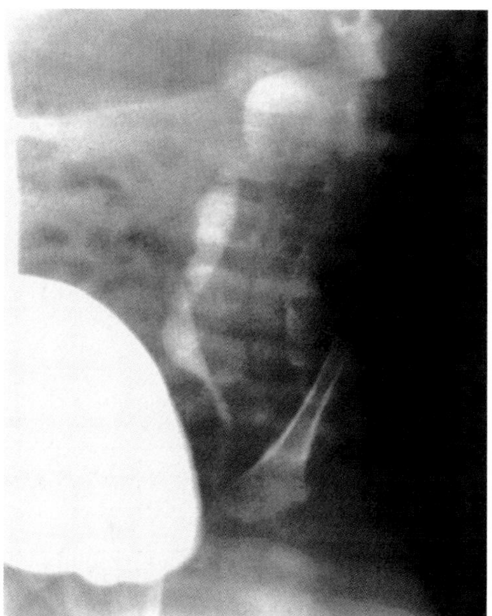

Fig. 20-89. Oblique, reflux of left kidney and ureter. This 18-month-old female is demonstrating vesicoureteral reflux (reflux is most likely to occur during voiding phase of voiding cystourethrogram).

CHAPTER 21

Angiography and Interventional Procedures

CONTRIBUTIONS BY **Cindy Murphy,** RT R, ACR, BHSc

CONTRIBUTORS TO PAST EDITIONS Marianne Tortorici, EdD, RT(R), Patrick Apfel, MEd, RT(R), Barry T. Anthony, RT(R)

CONTENTS

RADIOGRAPHIC ANATOMY

Introduction

DEFINITION

Angiography refers to **the radiographic examination of vessels after injection of a contrast medium.** Because of the relative densities of the soft tissues of the body, contrast medium must be added to visualize the circulatory system. For example, the routine lateral skull radiograph in Fig. 21-1 demonstrates none of the vessels of the **cranial** circulatory system, whereas the lateral carotid arteriogram in Fig. 21-2 clearly differentiates between the brain and blood vessels. This is also true for the circulatory system of other body regions such as the **thorax,** the **abdomen,** and the **upper and lower limbs** (peripheral).

A good understanding of the **vascular anatomy,** as covered in the first part of this chapter, is essential for performing angiography.

DIVISIONS OR COMPONENTS OF THE CIRCULATORY SYSTEM

The **circulatory system** consists of the **cardiovascular** and **lymphatic components.** The cardiovascular portion includes the heart, blood, and vessels that transport the blood.

The **lymphatic element** of the circulatory system is composed of a clear watery fluid called **lymph,** along with **lymphatic vessels and lymphatic nodes.** The cardiovascular and lymphatic components differ in the function and method of transporting their respective fluids within the vessels.

The **cardiovascular,** or blood circulatory, division may further be divided into the **cardio** (circulation within the heart) and **vascular** (blood vessel) components.

The vascular or vessel component is divided into the **pulmonary** (heart to lungs and back) and the general, or **systemic,** system (throughout the body). (See the summary box in the right column.)

CARDIOVASCULAR SYSTEM

The **heart** is the major organ of the cardiovascular system and functions as a pump to maintain circulation of blood throughout the body. The **vascular component** is composed of a network of blood vessels that carry blood from the heart to body tissues and back to the heart again.

Functions Functions of the cardiovascular system include the following:

1. Transportation of oxygen, nutrients, hormones, and chemicals necessary for normal body activity.
2. Removal of waste products through the kidneys and lungs.
3. Maintenance of body temperature and water and electrolyte balance. These functions are performed by the following blood components: red blood cells, white blood cells, and platelets suspended in plasma.

Blood Components **Red blood cells,** or **erythrocytes,** are produced in the red marrow of certain bones and transport oxygen by the protein hemoglobin to body tissues.

White blood cells, or **leukocytes,** are formed in bone marrow and lymph tissue and defend the body against infection and disease. **Platelets,** also originating from bone marrow, repair tears in blood vessel walls and promote blood-clotting.

Plasma, the liquid portion of the blood, consists of 92% water and about 7% plasma protein and salts, nutrients, and oxygen.

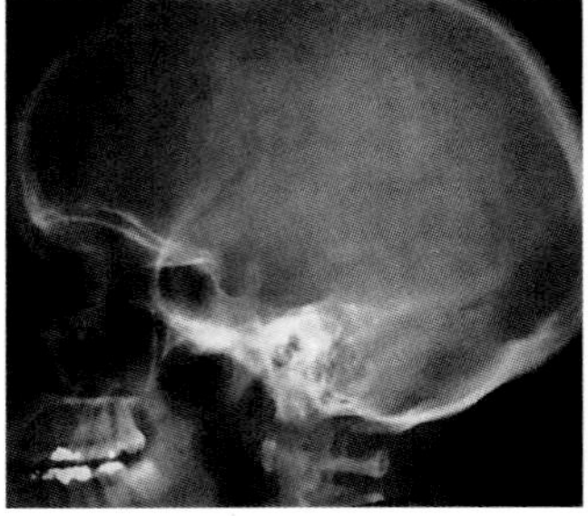

Fig. 21-1. Lateral skull radiograph.

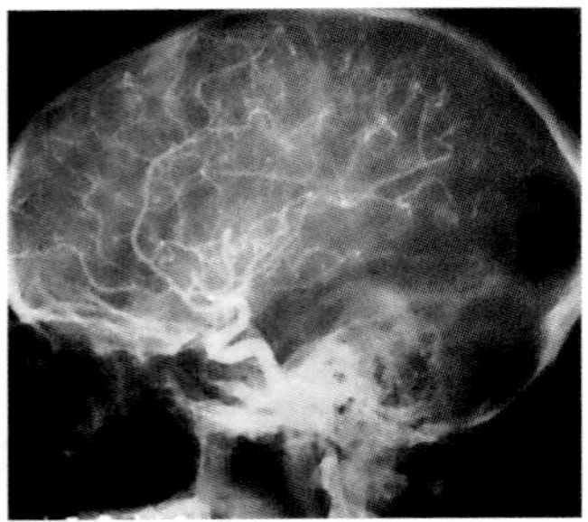

Fig. 21-2. Lateral carotid arteriogram.

SUMMARY OF CIRCULATORY SYSTEM COMPONENTS

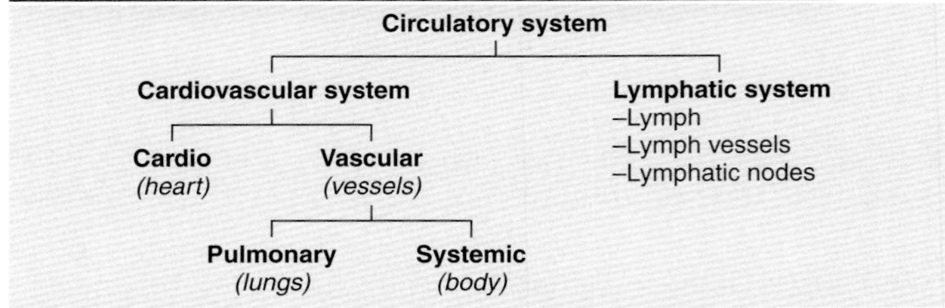

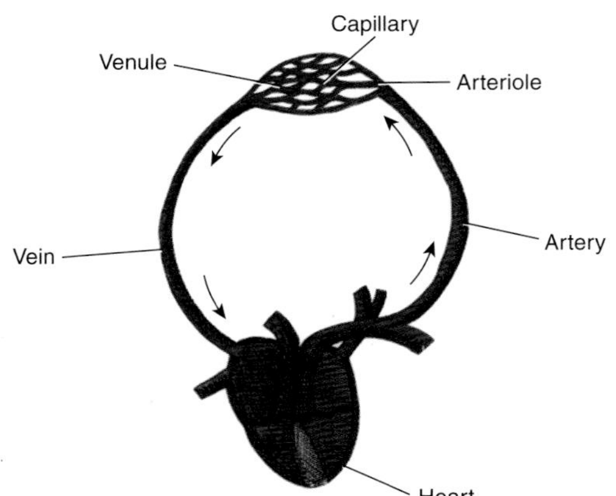

Fig. 21-3. General cardiovascular circulation.

SYSTEMIC CIRCULATION

Arteries

Vessels transporting oxygenated blood from the heart to tissues are called **arteries.** Arteries that originate directly from the heart are large but they subdivide and decrease in size as they extend from the heart to the various parts of the body. The smaller arteries are termed **arterioles.** As the blood travels through the arterioles, it enters the tissues by the smallest subdivision of these vessels, known as **capillaries** (Fig. 21-3).

Veins

The deoxygenated blood returns to the heart through the venous system. The venous system extends from venous capillaries to **venules** to **veins,** increasing in size as it nears the heart.

Pulmonary Circulation

The elements of the blood vessel circuit (veins, venules, capillaries, arterioles, and, arteries), which supply blood to the lungs and back, comprise the **pulmonary circulation** component of the cardiovascular system.

As previously noted, arteries generally carry oxygenated blood away from the heart to the capillaries. Exceptions to this are the **pulmonary arteries,** which carry **deoxygenated blood** to the lungs that has been returned to the heart through the superior and inferior venae cavae.

The **superior** and **inferior venae cavae** (singular, vena cava) empty the returning deoxygenated blood into the **right atrium** of the heart.

The heart pumps this deoxygenated blood from the **right ventricle** through the pulmonary arteries to the lungs, where oxygen and carbon dioxide are exchanged through the small air sacs or alveoli of the lungs. The **oxygenated blood** then returns through the **pulmonary veins** to the **left atrium** of the heart (Fig. 21-4).

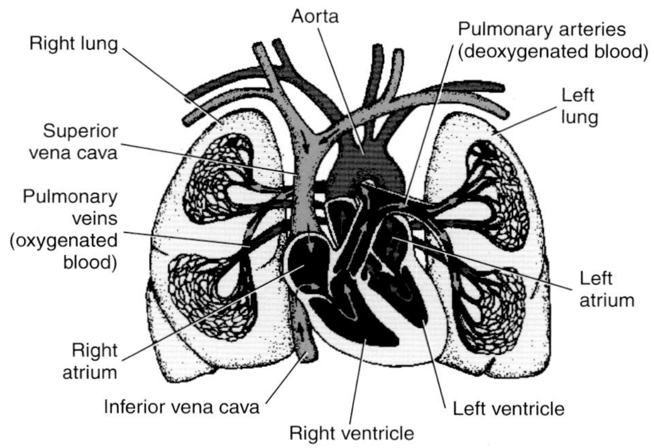

Fig. 21-4. Pulmonary circulation.

General Systemic Circulation

HEART

The heart is a muscular organ that pumps blood throughout the various parts of the body. Anatomically, the heart lies within the mediastinum and rests on the **diaphragm** (Fig. 21-5). Cardiac tissue differs from other muscle tissues of the body in its construction and is termed **myocardium.** The left side of the heart is responsible for the extensive systemic circulation; thus the left muscle wall is about three times as thick as the right side.

The heart itself is divided into four chambers: the **right** and **left atria** and the **right** and **left ventricles.** Each chamber functions to receive and/or pump blood. The blood circulation is a closed system by which unoxygenated blood enters the **right atrium** from all parts of the body, is reoxygenated in the lungs, and is returned to the body by the **left ventricle.**

Blood returning to the heart enters the right atrium through the **superior** and **inferior venae cavae** (Fig. 21-6). Blood in the superior vena cava originates from the head, chest, and upper limbs. The inferior vena cava serves to deliver blood into the right atrium from the abdomen and lower limbs.

From the **right atrium,** blood is pumped through the **tricuspid valve** to the **right ventricle.** The right ventricle contracts, moving the blood through the **pulmonary (pulmonary semilunar) valve** to the **pulmonary arteries** and on to the lungs. While in the lungs, the blood is oxygenated and then returned to the left atrium of the heart by the **pulmonary veins.** As the left atrium contracts, blood is transported through the **mitral (bicuspid) valve** to the left ventricle.

When the left ventricle contracts, the oxygenated blood exits the chamber by the **aortic (aortic semilunar) valve,** flows through the aorta, and is delivered to the various body tissues.

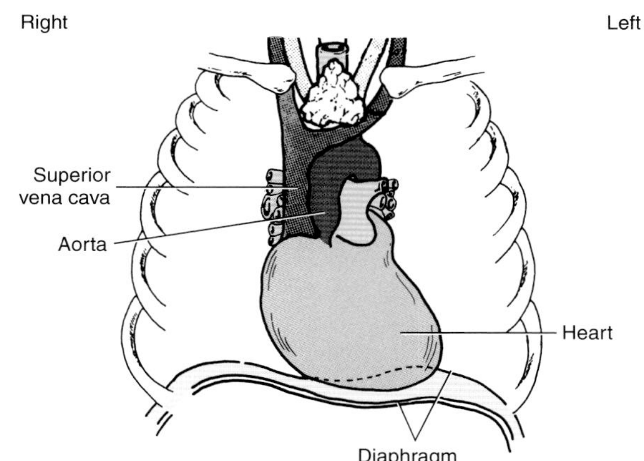

Fig. 21-5. Heart and mediastinal structures.

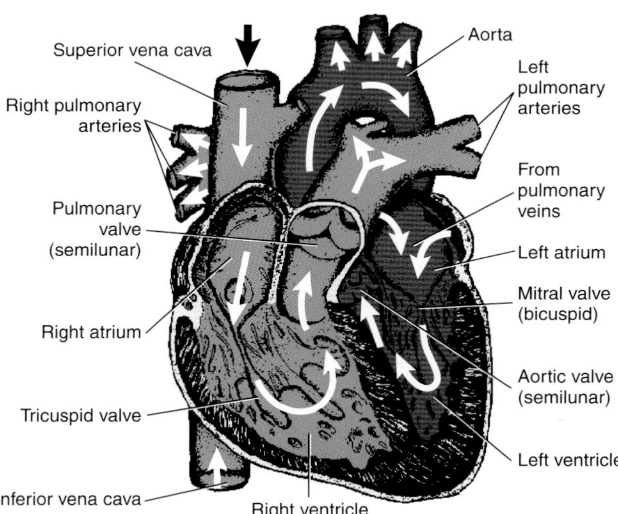

Fig. 21-6. Cross-section of heart.

SUMMARY OF GENERAL SYSTEMIC CIRCULATION

Venae cavae		**Aorta**
↓		↑ (Aortic valve)
Right atrium		**Left ventricle**
↓ (Tricuspid valve)		↑ (Mitral valve)
Right ventricle		**Left atrium**
↓ (Pulmonary valve)		↑ (Pulmonary valves)
Pulmonary arteries →	**Lungs** →	**Pulmonary veins**
(Unoxygenated blood)		(Oxygenated blood)

21

CORONARY ARTERIES

The coronary arteries are the vessels that deliver blood to the heart muscle. The **two coronary arteries** are called the **right** and **left.** Both coronary arteries originate from the **aortic bulb.**

The right coronary artery arises from the right (anterior) sinuses of the aortic bulb, and the left coronary artery originates from the left (posterior) aortic bulb sinus. The **right coronary artery** supplies much of the **right atrium** and the **right ventricle** of the heart.

The **left coronary artery** supplies blood to **both ventricles** and the **left atrium** of the heart. Many interconnections or anastomoses exist between the left and right coronary arteries. Blood returns to the right atrium of the heart by the coronary veins.

CORONARY VEINS

The coronary sinus system returns blood to the right atrium for recirculation. The **coronary sinus** is a large vein on the posterior side of the heart between the atria and ventricles. The coronary sinus has three major branches: the **great, middle,** and **small cardiac veins.**

The **great cardiac vein** receives blood from both ventricles and the left atrium. The **middle cardiac vein** drains blood from the right ventricle, right atrium, and part of the left ventricle. The **small cardiac vein** returns blood from the right ventricle. The coronary sinus drains most of the blood from the heart. Some small veins drain directly into both atria.

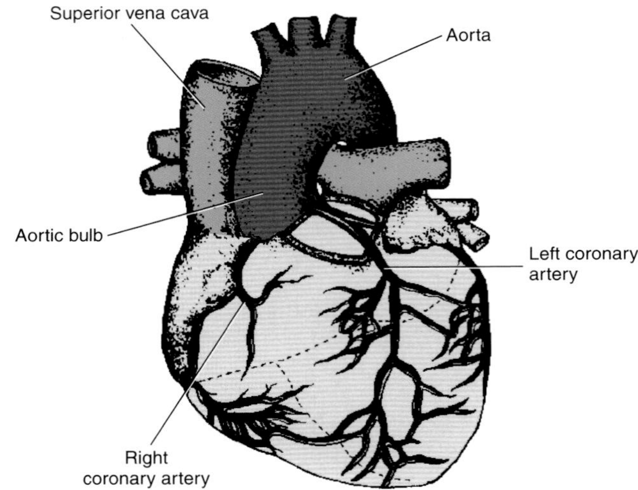

Fig. 21-7. Arteries of the heart (anterior view).

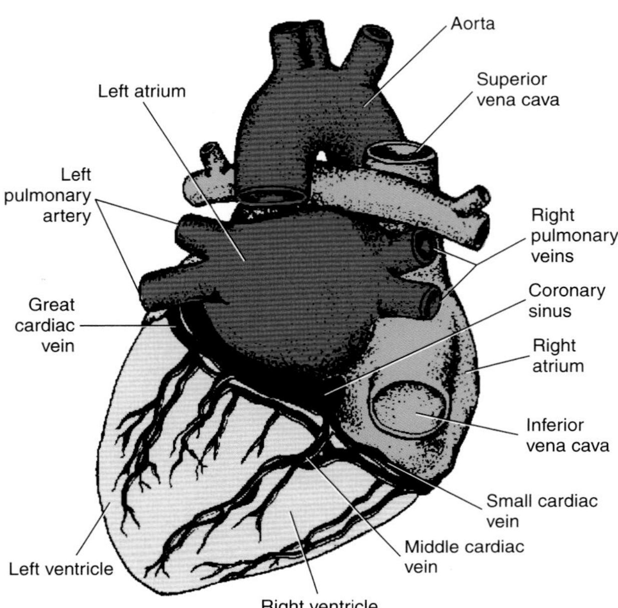

Fig. 21-8. Veins of the heart (posterior view).

Cerebral Arteries

BLOOD SUPPLY TO THE BRAIN

The brain is supplied with blood by major arteries of the systemic circulation. The four major arteries supplying the brain are as follows (Fig. 21-9):

1. **Right common carotid artery**
2. **Left common carotid artery**
3. **Right vertebral artery**
4. **Left vertebral artery**

Major branches of the two common carotids supply the anterior circulation of the brain, and the two vertebrals supply the posterior circulation. Radiographic examination of the neck vessels and entire brain circulation is referred to as a **"four-vessel angiogram"** because these four vessels are collectively and selectively injected with contrast medium. Another common series is the **"three-vessel angiogram"** in which the two carotids and only one vertebral artery are studied.

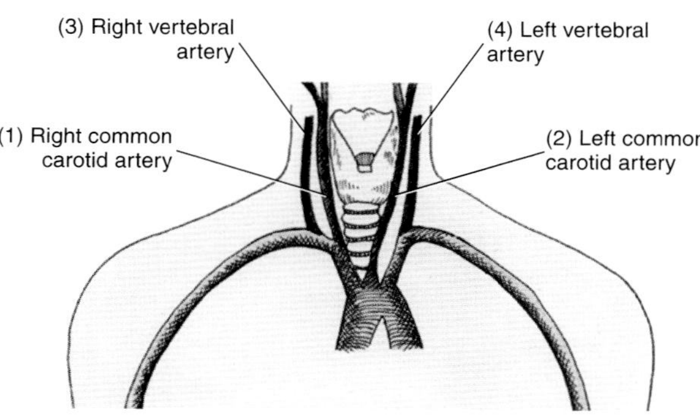

Fig. 21-9. Blood supply to brain—four major arteries.

BRANCHES OF THE AORTIC ARCH

The aorta is the major artery leaving the left ventricle of the heart. Three major branches arise from the **arch** of the **aorta,** and include the following (Fig. 21-10):

1. **Brachiocephalic artery**
2. **Left common carotid artery**
3. **Left subclavian artery**

The brachiocephalic trunk is a short vessel that bifurcates into the **right common carotid artery** and the **right subclavian artery.** This bifurcation occurs directly posterior to the right sternoclavicular joint. The right and left vertebral arteries are branches of the subclavian arteries on each side as described above (see Fig. 21-9). Because the left common carotid artery rises directly from the arch of the aorta, it is slightly longer than the right common carotid artery.

In the cervical region the two common carotids resemble one another. Each common carotid artery passes cephalad from its origin along either side of the trachea and larynx to the level of the upper border of the **thyroid cartilage.** Here, each common carotid artery divides into **external and internal carotid arteries.** The site of bifurcation for each common carotid is at the level of the **third** or **fourth cervical vertebra.**

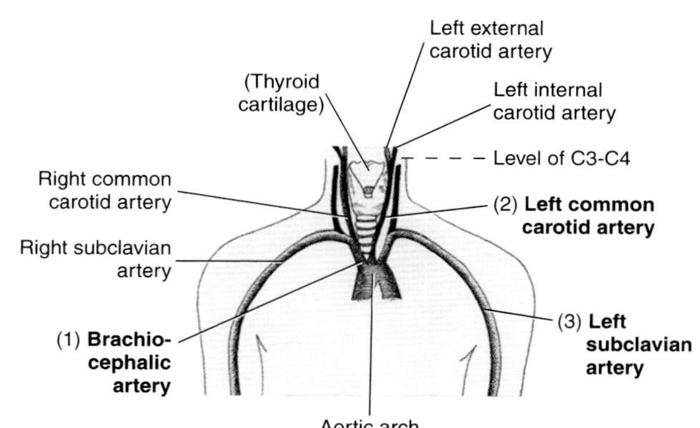

Fig. 21-10. Three branches of aortic arch.

NECK AND HEAD ARTERIES

The major arteries supplying the head, as seen from the right side of the neck, are shown in Fig. 21-11 (only right side vessels are identified on this drawing). The **brachiocephalic trunk artery bifurcates** into the **right common carotid artery** and the **right subclavian artery.**

The right common carotid artery ascends to the level of the fourth cervical vertebra to branch into the **external carotid artery** and the **internal carotid artery** as also described above. Each external carotid artery primarily supplies the anterior neck, the face, and the greater part of the scalp and meninges (brain coverings). Each internal carotid artery supplies the cerebral hemispheres, the pituitary gland, the orbital structures, the external nose, and the anterior portion of the brain.

The **right vertebral artery** arises from the right subclavian artery to pass through the transverse foramina of C6 through C1. Each vertebral artery passes posteriorly along the superior border of C1 before angling upward through the foramen magnum to enter the cranium.

A common carotid arteriogram is shown on the right visualizing the **(A) right internal carotid, (B) right external carotid,** and **(C) right common carotid.**

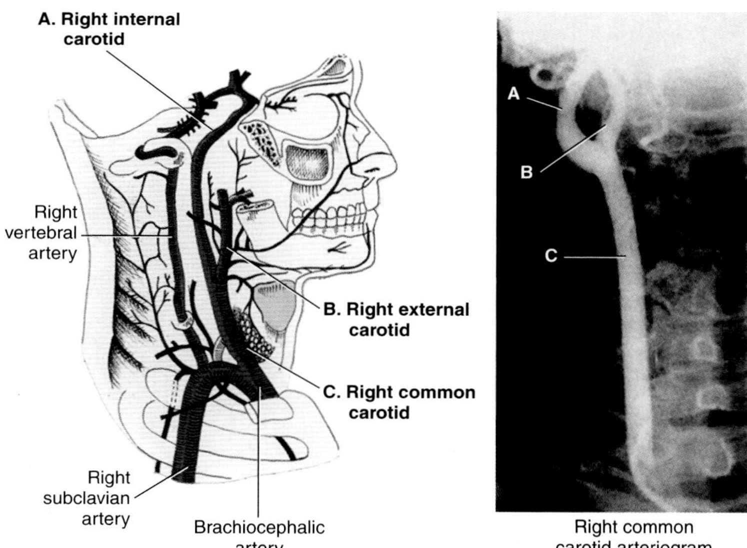

Fig. 21-11. Neck and head arteries.

EXTERNAL CAROTID ARTERY BRANCHES

Four major branches of the external carotid artery include the following:

1. Facial artery
2. Maxillary artery
3. Superficial temporal artery
4. Occipital artery

These do not play a significant role in angiography and will not be demonstrated on drawings.

INTERNAL CAROTID ARTERY

Each **internal carotid artery** ascends to enter the carotid canal in the petrous portion of the temporal bone. Within the petrous pyramid, the artery curves forward and medially. Before supplying the cerebral hemispheres, each internal carotid artery passes through a collection of venous channels around the sella turcica. Each internal carotid artery passes through the dura mater, medial to each anterior clinoid process, to bifurcate into the cerebral branches.

The S-shaped portion of each internal carotid artery is termed the **carotid siphon** and is studied carefully by the radiologist.

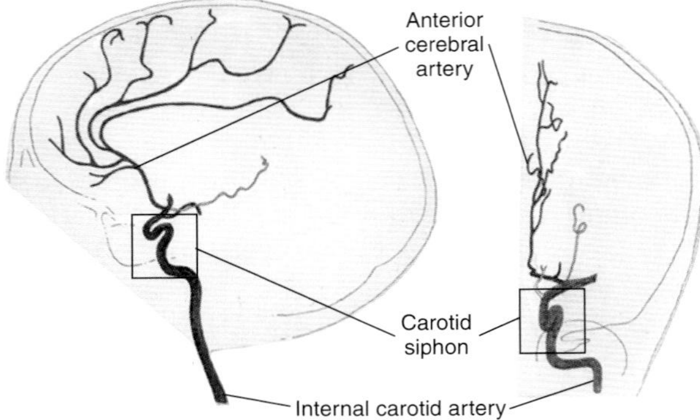

Fig. 21-12. Internal carotid and anterior cerebral artery.

ANTERIOR CEREBRAL ARTERY

The two end branches of each **internal carotid artery** are the **anterior cerebral** (Fig. 21-12) and the **middle cerebral arteries** (Fig. 21-13). Each anterior cerebral artery and its branches supply much of the forebrain near the midline. The anterior cerebral arteries curve around the corpus callosum, giving off several branches to the midportions of the cerebral hemisphere. Each anterior cerebral artery connects to the opposite one and to the posterior brain circulation.

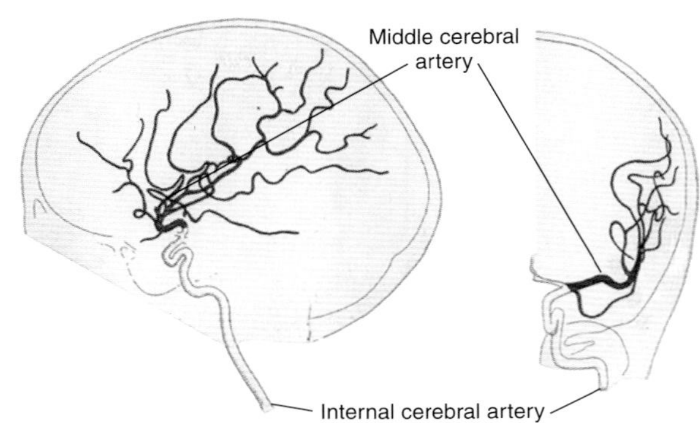

Fig. 21-13. Middle cerebral artery.

MIDDLE CEREBRAL ARTERY

The middle cerebral artery is the largest branch of each internal carotid artery. This artery supplies the **lateral aspects of the anterior cerebral circulation** (Fig. 21-13). As the middle cerebral artery courses toward the periphery of the brain, branches extend upward along the lateral portion of the insula or central lobe of the brain. These small branches supply brain tissue deep within the brain.

INTERNAL CAROTID ARTERIOGRAM

When one internal carotid artery is injected with contrast medium, both the anterior cerebral artery and the middle cerebral artery fill. The arterial phase of a cerebral carotid angiogram is similar to the drawings in Fig. 21-14.

In the frontal view or AP projection, little superimposition of the two vessels occurs because the anterior cerebral courses toward the midline and the middle cerebral extends laterally.

In the lateral position some superimposition obviously exists. Note that the **internal carotid artery supplies primarily the anterior portion of the brain.**

Lateral and AP axial internal carotid internal arteriograms are shown demonstrating the bifurcation of the **carotid artery** into the **anterior** and **middle cerebral arteries.** The S-shaped **carotid siphon region** described above is visualized. Compare the labeled drawing with the radiographs to see whether you can identify the labeled vessels before looking at the answers below.

A. Anterior cerebral artery
B. Middle cerebral artery
C. Carotid siphon region
D. Left internal carotid artery

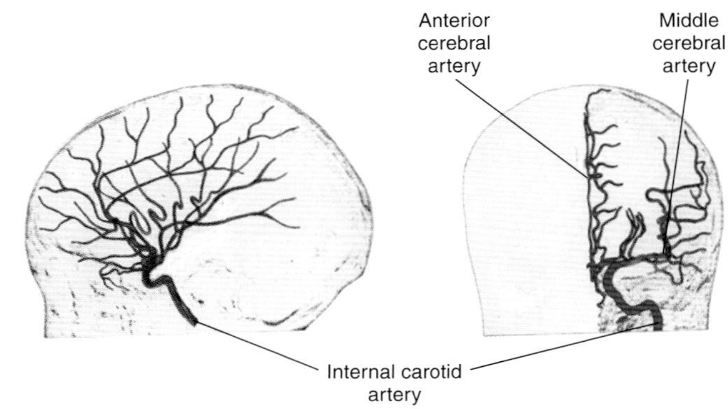

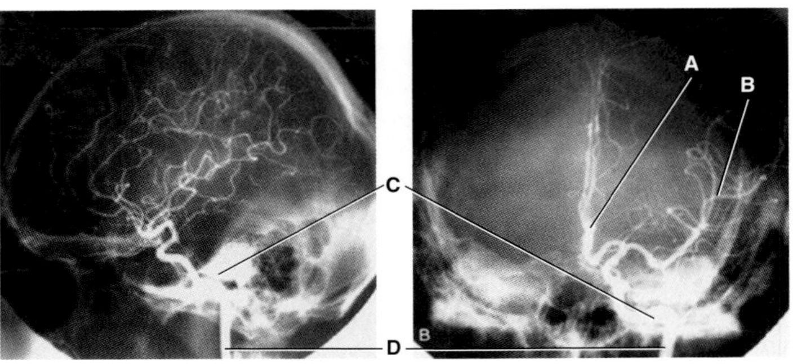

Fig. 21-14. Internal carotid arteriogram; visualizes both anterior and middle cerebral arteries.

VERTEBROBASILAR ARTERIES

The two **vertebral arteries** enter the cranium through the foramen magnum and unite to form the single **basilar artery.** The vertebral arteries and basilar artery and their branches form the vertebrobasilar system. By omitting much of the occipital bone in Fig. 21-15, these arteries are shown along the base of the skull. Several arteries arise from each vertebral artery before their point of convergence to form the basilar artery. These branches supply the spinal cord and the hindbrain. The basilar artery rests on the **clivus,** a portion of the sphenoid bone, and the base of the occipital bone anterior to the foramen magnum and posterior to the dorsum sella.

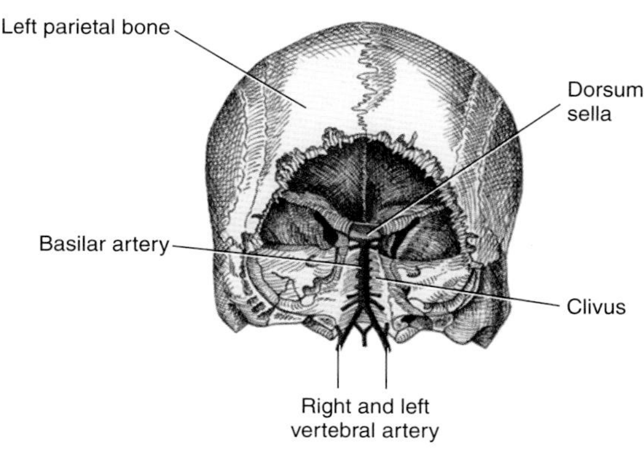

Fig. 21-15. Vertebrobasilar arteries.

CIRCLE OF WILLIS (ARTERIAL CIRCLE)

The blood to the brain is supplied by the internal carotid and vertebral arteries. The posterior brain circulation communicates with the anterior circulation along the base of the brain in the arterial circle, or **circle of Willis** (Fig. 21-16). The five arteries or branches that make up the circle of Willis are (1) the **anterior communicating artery,** (2) the **anterior cerebral arteries,** (3) branches of the **internal carotid arteries,** (4) the **posterior communicating artery,** and (5) the **posterior cerebral arteries.**

Not only are the anterior and posterior circulations connected, but also both sides connect across the midline. Therefore an elaborate anastomosis interconnects the entire arterial supply to the brain. As the basilar artery courses forward toward the circle of Willis, it gives off several branches to the hindbrain and posterior cerebrum. The posterior cerebral arteries are two of the larger branches.

Certain aneurysms may occur in these vessels making up the circle of Willis, and they need to be well demonstrated on cerebral angiographic studies.

The important "master" gland, the **hypophysis** (pituitary gland) and its surrounding bony structure, the **sella turcica,** are located within the circle of Willis. See Fig. 21-15 for the location of the **basilar artery** resting on the **clivus** and the relationship of these structures to the **dorsum sella.**

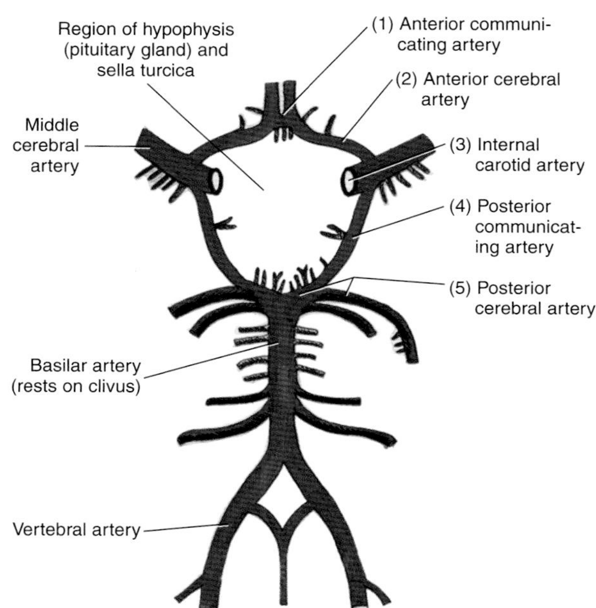

Fig. 21-16. Circle of Willis—five arteries or branches.

VERTEBROBASILAR ARTERIOGRAM

A standard vertebrobasilar arteriogram appears similar to the simplified drawing in Fig. 21-17. The **vertebral arteries, basilar artery,** and **posterior cerebral arteries** can be seen. The several branches to the cerebellum have not been labeled on this drawing.

Lateral and AP vertebrobasilar arteriograms are shown demonstrating a left-side injection with filling of left-side associated vessels. Compare the labeled drawing with the radiographs to see whether you can identify the labeled vessels before looking at the answers below.

A. Posterior cerebral arteries
B. Basilar artery
C. Left vertebral artery
D. Left posterior cerebral artery
E. Right posterior cerebral artery

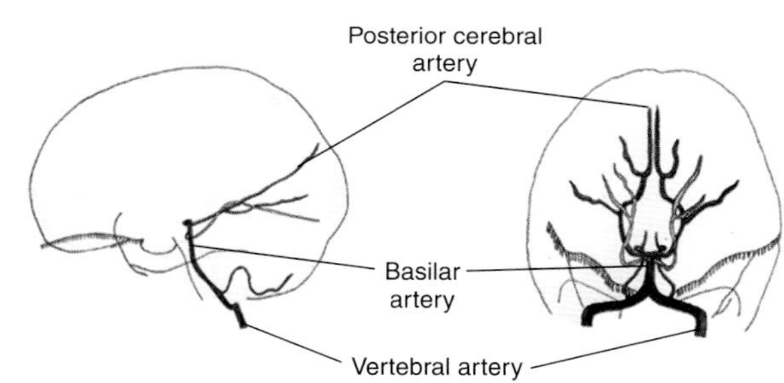

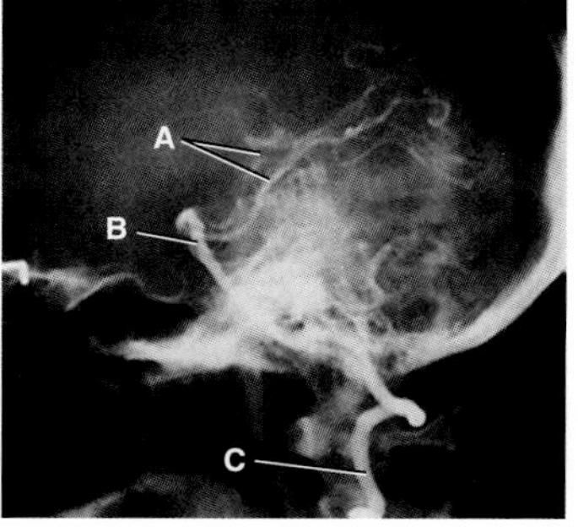

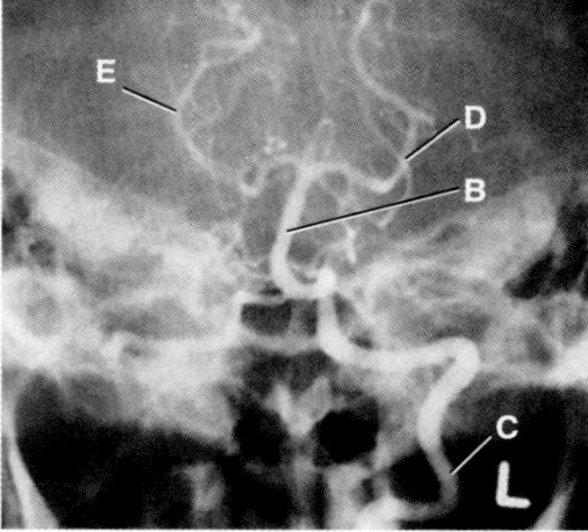

Fig. 21-17. Vertebrobasilar arteriogram.

21

Cerebral Veins

GREAT VEINS OF THE NECK

The **three pairs** of major veins draining the head, face, and neck region shown in Fig. 21-18 include the following:

1. **Right** and **left internal jugular veins**
2. **Right** and **left external jugular veins**
3. **Right** and **left vertebral veins**

Each **internal jugular vein** drains the meninges and brain. In addition, many smaller veins join each internal jugular vein as it passes caudad to eventually become the **brachiocephalic vein** on each side. The right and left brachiocephalic veins join to form the superior vena cava, which returns blood to the right atrium of the heart.

The pair of **external jugular veins** are more superficial trunks that drain the scalp and much of the face and neck. Each external jugular vein joins the respective **subclavian vein.**

The right and left **vertebral veins** form outside the cranium and drain the upper neck and occipital region. Each vertebral vein enters the transverse foramen of C1, descends to C6, and then enters the subclavian vein.

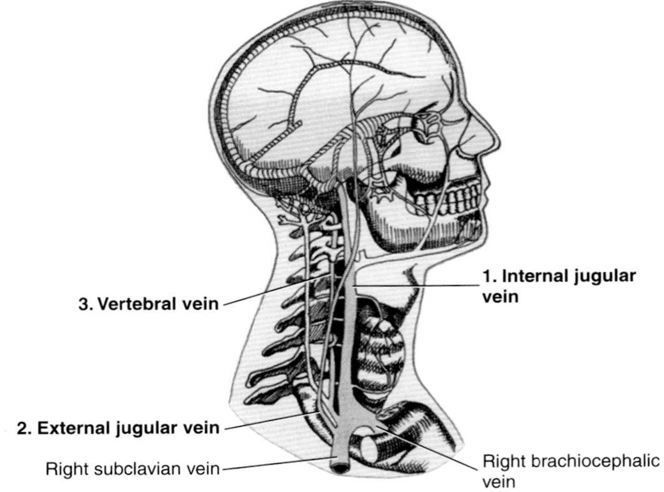

Fig. 21-18. Great veins of neck.

DURA MATER SINUSES

The sinuses of the dura mater are venous channels that drain blood from the brain (Fig. 21-19). The sinuses are situated between the two layers of the dura mater, as described in Chapter 22, which discusses brain coverings and meningeal spaces.

A space between the two layers of the dura, along the superior portion of the longitudinal fissure, contains the **superior sagittal sinus.** The **inferior sagittal sinus** flows posteriorly to drain into the **straight sinus.** The straight sinus and the superior sagittal sinus empty into opposite transverse sinuses.

Each **transverse sinus** curves medially to occupy a groove along the mastoid portion of the temporal bone. The sinus in this region is termed the **sigmoid sinus.** Each sigmoid sinus then curves caudad to continue as the **internal jugular vein** at the jugular foramen.

The **occipital sinus** courses posteriorly from the foramen magnum to join the superior sagittal sinus, straight sinus, and transverse sinuses at their confluence.

The **confluence of sinuses** is located near the internal occipital protuberance. Other major dura mater sinuses drain the area on either side of the sphenoid bone and sella turcica.

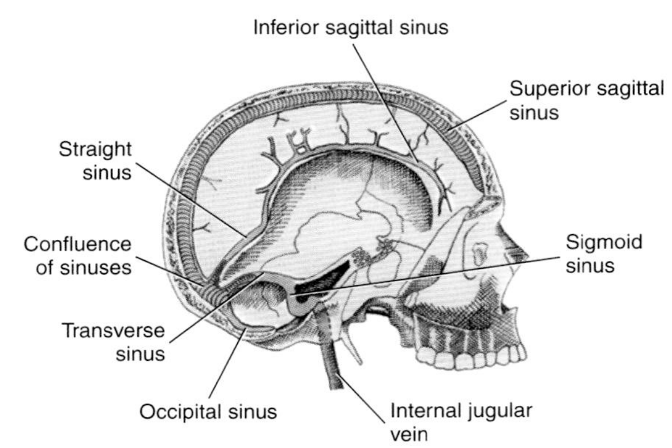

Fig. 21-19. Dura mater sinuses.

CRANIAL VENOUS SYSTEM

The major veins of the entire cranial venous system are labeled in Fig. 21-20. Only the most prominent veins are identified. One group not individually named is the *external cerebral veins,* which along with certain dura mater sinuses drain the outer surfaces of the cerebral hemispheres. Like all veins of the brain, the external cerebral veins possess no valves and are extremely thin because they have no muscle tissue.

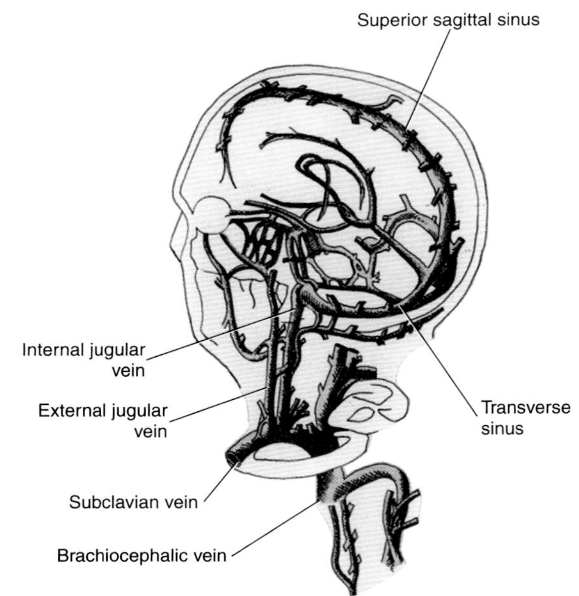

Fig. 21-20. Cranial venous system.

Thoracic Circulatory System

THORACIC ARTERIES

The **aorta** and **pulmonary arteries** are the major arteries located within the chest. The pulmonary arteries supply the lungs with deoxygenated blood (as shown earlier in Fig. 21-4).

The aorta extends from the heart to about the fourth lumbar vertebra and is divided into thoracic and abdominal sections. The **thoracic section** is subdivided into the following **four segments** (Fig. 21-21):

1. **Aortic bulb (root)**
2. **Ascending aorta**
3. **Aortic arch**
4. **Descending aorta**

The **bulb,** or root portion, is at the proximal end of the aorta and is the area from which the coronary arteries originate. Extending from the bulb is the **ascending portion** of the aorta, which terminates at approximately the second sternocostal joint and becomes the **arch.** The arch is unique from the other segments of the thoracic aorta because three arterial branches arise from it: the brachiocephalic artery, the left common carotid artery, and the left subclavian artery. (This is also shown in Fig. 21-10.)

Many variations of the aortic arch exist. Three more common variations sometimes seen in angiography include the following (Fig. 21-22):

A. **Left circumflex aorta** (normal arch with the descending aorta downward and arched to the left)
B. **Inverse aorta** (arch is arched to the right)
C. **Pseudocoarctation** (arched descending aorta)

At its distal end the arch becomes the **descending aorta** (see Fig. 21-21). The descending aorta extends from the isthmus to the level of the twelfth dorsal vertebra. Numerous intercostal, bronchial, esophageal, and superior phrenic arterial branches arise from the descending aorta, not shown in Fig. 21-21. These arteries transport blood to the organs for which they are named.

THORACIC VEINS

The major veins within the chest are the **superior vena cava, azygos,** and **pulmonary veins.** The superior vena cava returns the blood transported from the thorax to the right atrium. The **azygos vein** is the major tributary returning blood from the posterior thoracic wall to the superior vena cava (Fig. 21-23). The azygos vein enters the superior vena cava posteriorly. Blood from the chest enters the azygos vein from the intercostal, bronchial, esophageal, and phrenic veins. Note that a section of the vena cava has been removed on this drawing to better visualize the azygos and intercostal veins.

The superior and **inferior pulmonary veins** return oxygenated blood from the lungs to the left atrium as previously shown. The **inferior vena cava** returns blood from the abdomen and lower limbs to the right atrium (see Figs. 21-4 and 21-6).

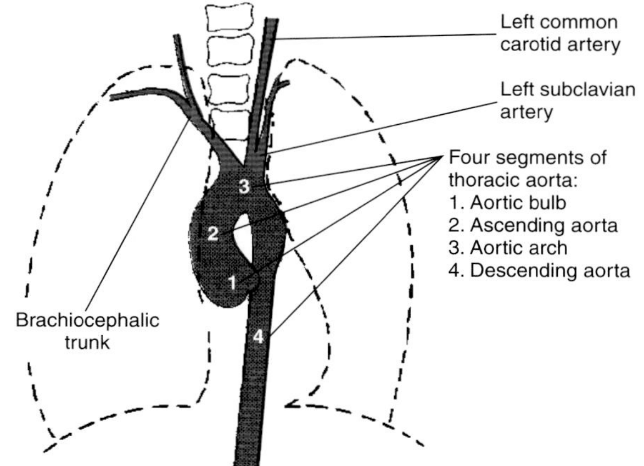

Fig. 21-21. Thoracic aorta.

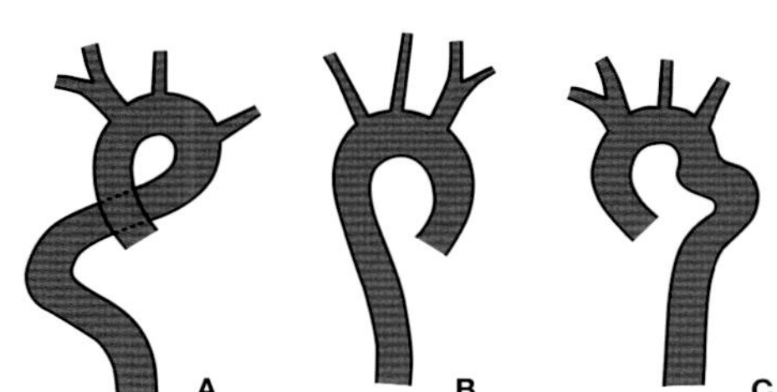

Fig. 21-22. Variations of the arch.

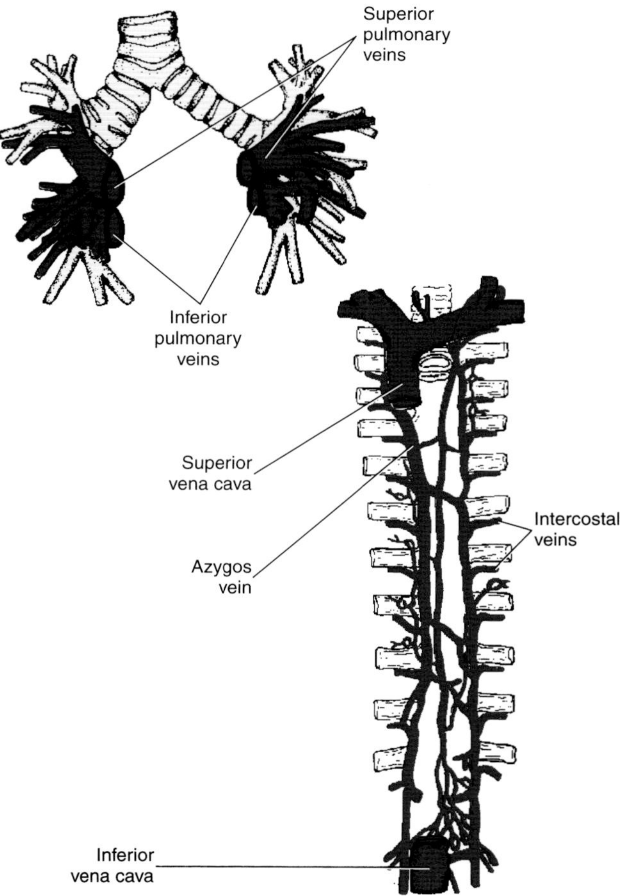

Fig. 21-23. Thoracic veins.

21

Abdominal Circulatory System

ABDOMINAL ARTERIES

The abdominal aorta is the continuation of the thoracic aorta. The abdominal aorta is anterior to the vertebrae and extends from the diaphragm to approximately L4 where it bifurcates into the right and left common iliac arteries. **Five major branches** of the abdominal aorta exist that are of most interest in angiography. Any one of these branches may be selectively catheterized for study of a specific organ.

These are shown in Fig. 21-24 as follows:

1. **Celiac axis artery**
2. **Superior mesenteric artery**
3. **Left renal artery**
4. **Right renal artery**
5. **Inferior mesenteric artery**

The **trunk** of the **celiac axis** arises from the anterior aspect of the aorta just below the diaphragm and about 1.5 cm above the origin of the superior mesenteric artery. Organs supplied with blood by the three large branches of the celiac trunk are the **liver, spleen,** and **stomach.**

The **superior mesenteric artery** supplies blood to the pancreas, most of the small intestine, and portions of the right side of the large intestine (cecum, ascending and about one-half of the transverse colon). It originates from the anterior surface of the aorta at the level of the first lumbar vertebra about 1.5 cm below the celiac artery.

The **inferior mesenteric artery** originates from the aorta at about the third lumbar vertebra (3 or 4 cm above the level of the bifurcation of the common iliac arteries). Blood is supplied to portions of the large intestine (left half of transverse colon, descending colon, sigmoid colon, and most of the rectum) by the inferior mesenteric artery.

The **right** and **left renal arteries** supplying blood to the kidneys originate on each side of the aorta just below the superior mesenteric artery at the level of the disk between the first and second lumbar vertebrae.

The distal portion of the abdominal aorta bifurcates at the level of the fourth lumbar vertebra into the **right** and **left common iliac arteries.** Each common iliac artery then divides into the **internal** and **external iliac arteries.** The internal iliac arteries supply the pelvic organs (urinary bladder, rectum, reproductive organs, and pelvic muscles) with blood.

The lower limbs receive blood from the **external iliac arteries.** The **external** iliac artery is significant in angiography and is used to **study each lower limb.**

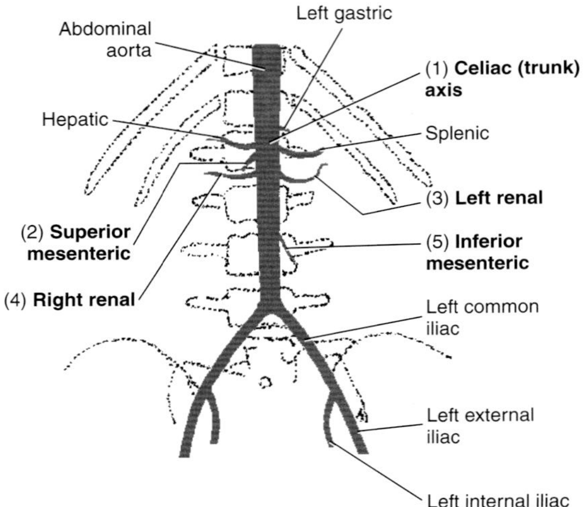

Fig. 21-24. Abdominal arteries.

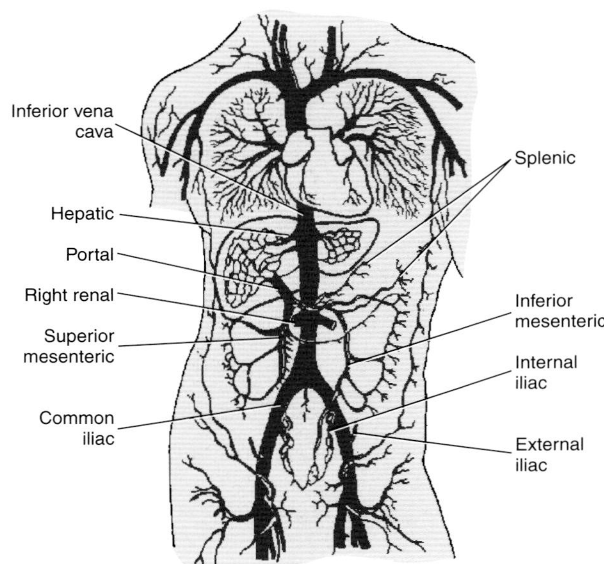

Fig. 21-25. Abdominal veins.

ABDOMINAL VEINS

Blood is returned from structures below the diaphragm (the trunk and lower limbs) to the right atrium of the heart by the **inferior vena cava.** Several radiographically important tributaries to the inferior vena cava exist. These veins include the right and left **common iliacs, internal iliacs, external iliacs, renal veins** (Fig. 21-25), and the **portal system** (Fig. 21-26). The iliacs drain the pelvic area and lower limbs, and the renal veins return blood from the kidneys.

The **superior** and **inferior mesenteric veins** return blood from the small and large intestine through the **portal vein,** the **hepatic veins,** and into the **inferior vena cava.** This is best shown in Fig. 21-26 on the next page.

PORTAL SYSTEM (HEPATOPORTAL SYSTEM)

The portal system includes all the veins that drain blood from the abdominal digestive tract and from the spleen, colon, and small intestine. From these organs, this blood is conveyed to the liver through the **portal vein.** While in the liver, this blood is "filtered" and returned to the inferior vena cava by the hepatic veins. Several major tributaries to the **hepatic veins** exist (Fig. 21-26). The **splenic vein** is a large vein with its own tributaries, which return blood from the spleen.

The **inferior mesenteric vein,** which returns blood from the rectum and from parts of the large intestine, usually opens into the splenic vein, but in about 10% of cases it ends at the angle of union of the splenic and superior mesenteric veins. The **superior mesenteric vein** returns blood from the small intestine and parts of the large intestine. It unites with the splenic vein to form the portal vein.

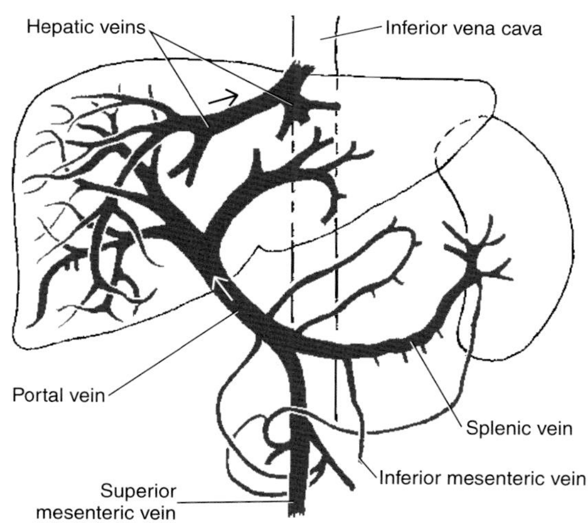

Fig. 21-26. Portal system.

Peripheral Circulatory System

UPPER LIMB ARTERIES

The arterial circulation of the upper limb is generally considered to begin at the **subclavian artery.** The origin of the subclavian artery differs from the right to left side. On the right side, the subclavian arises from the **brachiocephalic artery,** whereas the left subclavian originates directly from the aortic arch.

The subclavian continues to become the **axillary artery,** which gives rise to the **brachial artery.** The brachial artery bifurcates into the **ulnar** and **radial arteries** at approximately the level of the neck of the radius. The radial and ulnar arteries continue to branch until they join together to form **two palmar arches** (deep and superficial). Branches of these arches supply the hand and fingers with blood.

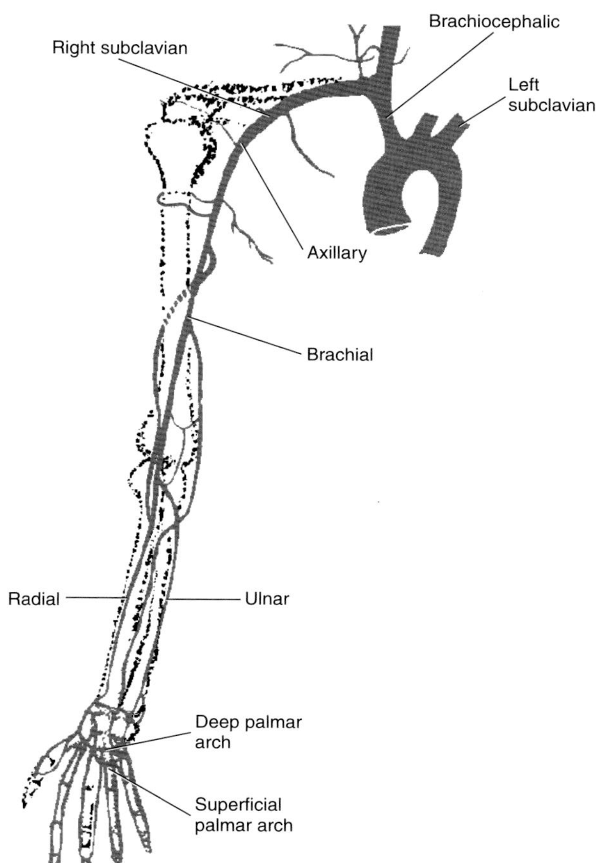

Fig. 21-27. Upper limb arteries.

21

UPPER LIMB VEINS

The venous system of the upper limb may be divided into two sets: the **deep** and the **superficial veins** (Fig. 21-28). They communicate with each other at frequent sites and thus form two parallel drainage channels from any single region. The **cephalic** and **basilic veins** are the primary tributaries of the superficial venous system. Both veins originate in the arch of the hand. Anterior to the elbow joint is the **median cubital vein** (the vein most commonly used to draw blood), which connects the superficial drainage systems of the forearm. The upper basilic vein empties into the large **axillary vein,** which then flows into the **subclavian** and eventually the **superior vena cava.** The lower basilic vein joins the median cubital vein, continuing to the upper basilic vein.

The deep veins include the **two brachial veins** that drain the **radial vein, ulnar vein, and the palmar arches.** The deep brachial veins join the superficial basilic to form the axillary vein, which empties into the subclavian and finally into the **superior vena cava.**

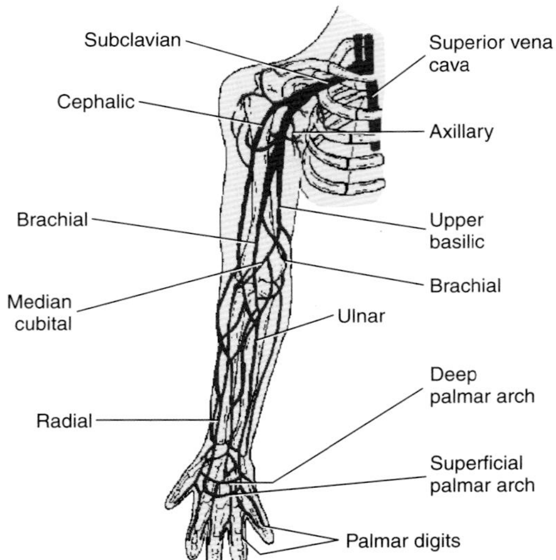

Fig. 21-28. Upper limb veins.

LOWER LIMB ARTERIES

The arterial circulation of the lower limb begins at the **external iliac artery** and ends at the veins of the foot (Fig. 21-29). The first artery to enter the lower limb is the **common femoral artery.** The common femoral artery divides into the **femoral** and **deep femoral arteries.** The femoral artery extends down the leg and becomes the **popliteal artery** at the level of the knee. Branches of the popliteal are the **anterior tibial, posterior tibial,** and **peroneal arteries.**

The **anterior tibial artery** continues as the **dorsalis pedis artery,** with branches to the ankle and foot. The **peroneal artery** and the **posterior tibial artery** supply the calf and plantar surface of the foot.

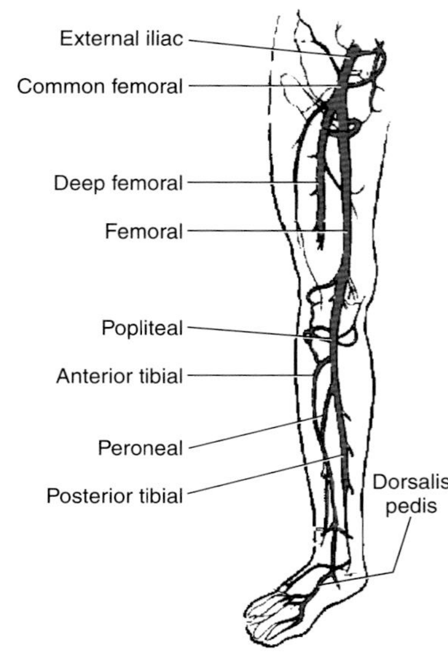

Fig. 21-29. Lower limb arteries.

LOWER LIMB VEINS

The veins of the lower limb are similar to the upper limb in that both have a **superficial** and **deep venous system.** The superficial venous system contains the **great** and **small saphenous veins** and their tributaries and the superficial **veins of the foot.**

The **great saphenous vein** is the longest vein in the body and extends from the foot, along the medial aspect of the leg, to the thigh, where it opens into the **femoral vein.** The **small saphenous** originates in the foot and extends posteriorly along the leg, terminating at the knee, where it empties into the **popliteal vein.**

The **major deep veins** are the **posterior tibial, peroneal, anterior tibial, popliteal,** and **femoral.** The posterior tibial vein and the peroneal vein join after draining the posterior foot and leg. The posterior tibial extends upward and unites with the **anterior tibial vein** to become the **popliteal vein** at the level of the knee. The popliteal continues upward to become the **femoral vein** before becoming the **external iliac vein** (Fig. 21-30).

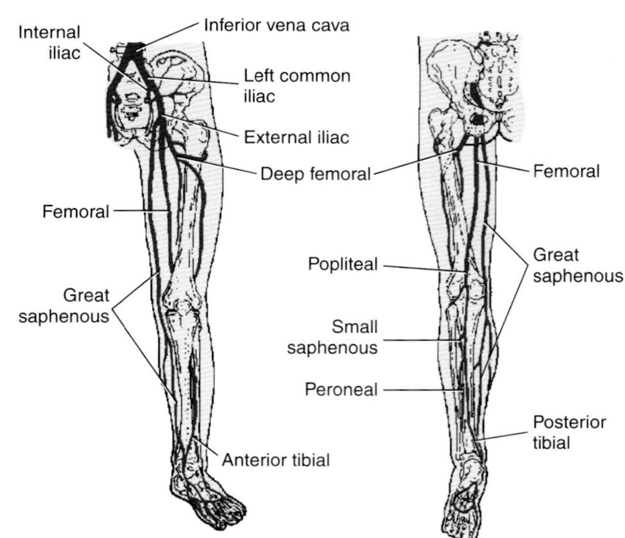

Fig. 21-30. Lower limb veins.

Lymphatic System

LYMPH DRAINAGE

The lymphatic system serves to drain interstitial fluid (fluid in the spaces between the cells) and return it to the venous system. The fluid from the **left side of the body, the lower limbs, pelvis,** and **abdomen** enters the venous system by the **thoracic duct** (largest lymph vessel in body), which drains into the **left subclavian vein** near its junction with the left jugular vein.

The **upper right side of the body, upper limb, head,** and **neck region** drain lymph fluid into the venous system at the junction of the **right jugular** and **right subclavian veins** by the **right lymph duct** (Figs. 21-31 and 21-32).

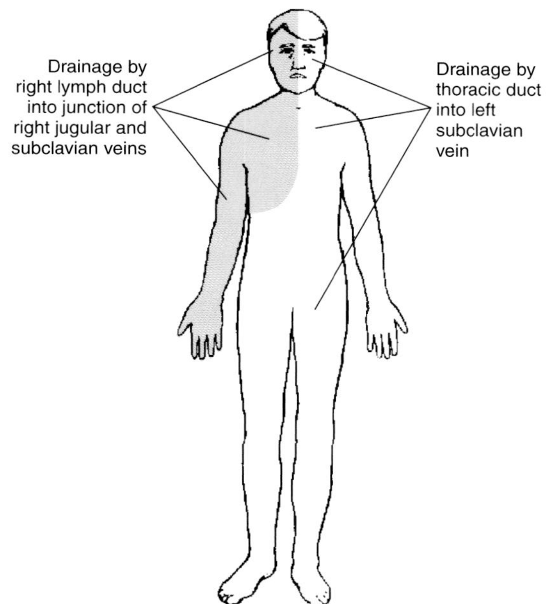

Fig. 21-31. Right and left lymph drainage.

FUNCTIONS

Functions of the lymphatic portion of the circulatory system are as follows:

1. Fights disease by producing lymphocytes and microphages.
2. Returns proteins and other substances to the blood.
3. Filters the lymph in the lymph nodes.
4. Transfers fats from the intestine to the thoracic duct and hence to the blood.

The lymphatic system has no heart pressure to pump lymph fluid to its destination. Rather, fluid is transported by diffusion, peristalsis, respiratory movements, cardiac activities, massage, and muscular activity. The transportation of lymphatic fluid is in one direction only—away from the tissues. The sequence of fluid movement is from lymphatic capillaries to the various lymph vessels, where the fluid enters the lymph nodes and is returned to the venous system by efferent lymphatic vessels.

Lymph nodes tend to form in clusters, although they may appear singularly. Thousands of nodes exist throughout the body, some of which are identified in Fig. 21-32. The major collections of nodes that are seen radiographically are those in the thoracic, abdominal, pelvic, and inguinal regions.

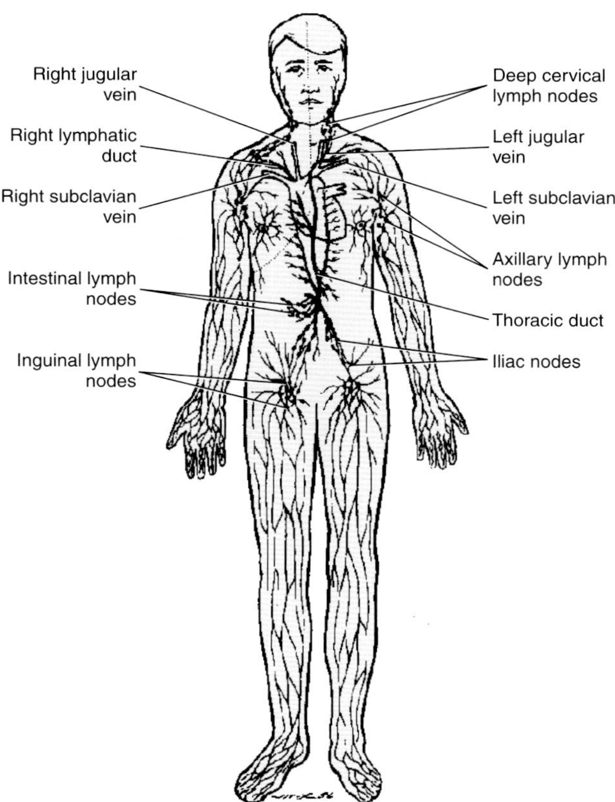

Fig. 21-32. Lymph drainage.

LYMPHOGRAPHY

Lymphography *(lim-fog'rah-fe)* is the general term used to describe radiographic examination of the lymphatic vessels and nodes after injection of a contrast medium; the procedure is described later in this chapter. Computed tomography, however, with its superior contrast resolution, provides excellent visualization of lymph nodes; thus fewer lymphography procedures are being performed.

ANGIOGRAPHIC PROCEDURES

Overview

As defined at the beginning of this chapter, **angiography** refers to **radiologic imaging of vessels after injection of contrast media.** To visualize these low-contrast structures, contrast media is injected by a catheter that is placed in the vessel of interest. Positive contrast media is more commonly used, but there are instances when use of negative contrast media is indicated. Highly specialized imaging equipment is required for these procedures.

Angiography can be more specifically described as follows:

- **Arteriography:** imaging of the arteries
- **Venography:** imaging of the veins
- **Angiocardiography:** imaging of the heart and associated structures
- **Lymphography:** imaging of the lymphatic vessels/nodes

This chapter is intended as an introduction to angiography and interventional procedures and is not inclusive of the variety of techniques, information, and procedures available.

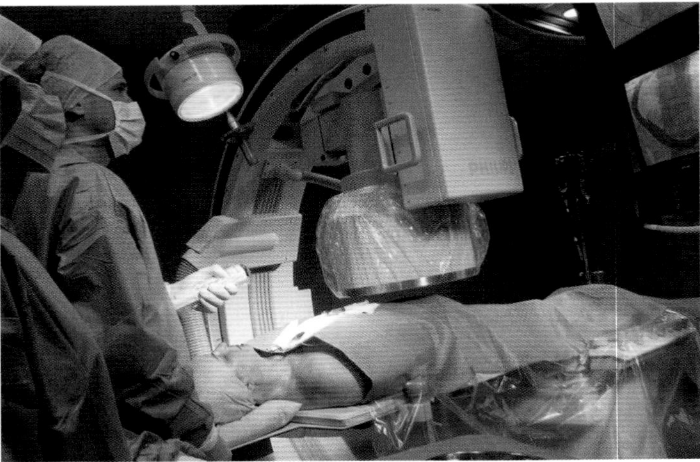

Fig. 21-33. Angiographic procedure. (Courtesy Philips Medical Systems.)

THE ANGIOGRAPHY TEAM

Angiography is performed by a team of health professionals, including (1) a **radiologist** (or other qualified angiographer), (2) a **"scrub" nurse or technologist that assists with sterile and catheterization procedures,** and (3) **a radiologic technologist.** Depending on the departmental protocol and the specific situation, an additional physician, nurse, technologist, and/or a hemodynamic technologist may also be available to assist with the procedure.

Angiography is often an area or specialty practice for technologists and other health professionals. A competent, efficient team is crucial to the success of the procedure.

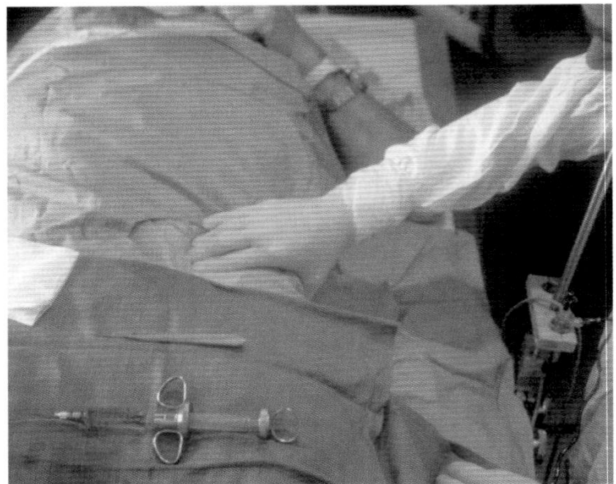

Fig. 21-34. Pulse assessment at femoral artery injection site.

CONSENT AND PREPROCEDURAL PATIENT CARE

A **medical history** should be obtained before the procedure. This should include questions to assess the patient's ability to tolerate the contrast injection (i.e., allergy history, cardiac/pulmonary status, and renal function). The patient will also be interviewed regarding medication history and symptoms. Medication history is important because some medications are anticoagulants and will cause excessive bleeding during and after the procedure. Knowing the medication history is also important when selecting the premedication. Previous laboratory reports and other pertinent data are also reviewed.

A detailed explanation of the procedure will be given to the patient, which is important to ensure full understanding and cooperation. The explanation will include possible risks and complications of the procedure so that the patient is fully informed before signing the consent.

Solid food is withheld for approximately 8 hours before the procedure to reduce the risk for aspiration. However, making sure the patient is well hydrated is important to reduce the risk for contrast-induced renal damage.

Premedication is usually given to patients before the procedure to help them relax. The patient may be made more comfortable on the table by placing a sponge under the knees to reduce strain on the back. Vital signs are obtained and recorded, and pulse in the extremity distal to the selected puncture site is checked. The puncture site is shaved, cleaned, and draped.

Continual communication and monitoring of the patient by the technologist and the rest of the angiography team will greatly alleviate patient discomfort and fear.

VESSEL ACCESS FOR CONTRAST MEDIA INJECTION

To visualize the vessel(s) of interest, a catheter must be introduced to the patient's vasculature through which the contrast media will be injected. A commonly used method for catheterization is the **Seldinger technique.** This technique was developed by Dr. Sven Seldinger in the 1950s and remains popular today. It is a percutaneous (through the skin) technique and can be used for arterial or venous access.

Three vessels are typically considered for catheterization: (1) femoral, (2) brachial, and (3) axillary. The angiographer will make the selection based on the strong presence of a pulse and the absence of vessel disease. The **femoral artery is the preferred site** for an arterial puncture, because of its size and easily accessible location. If a femoral artery puncture is contraindicated because of previous surgical grafts, presence of an aneurysm, or occlusive vascular disease, the brachial or axillary artery may be selected. The **femoral vein** would also be the vessel of choice for venous access.

The following is a step-by-step description of the Seldinger technique:

SELDINGER TECHNIQUE

Step 1—Insertion of needle: The needle with an inner cannula is placed in a small incision and advanced so that it punctures both walls of the vessel.

Step 2—Placement of needle in lumen of vessel: Placement of the needle in the lumen of the vessel is achieved by removing the inner cannula and slowly withdrawing the needle until a steady blood flow returns through the needle.

Step 3—Insertion of guide wire: When the desired blood flow is returned through the needle, the flexible end of a guide wire is inserted through the needle and advanced about 10 cm into the vessel.

Step 4—Removal of needle: After the guide wire is in position, the needle is removed by withdrawing it over that portion of the guide wire remaining outside the patient.

Step 5—Threading of catheter to area of interest: The catheter is then threaded over the guide wire and advanced to the area of interest under fluoroscopic control.

Step 6—Removal of guide wire: When the catheter is located in the desired area, the guide wire is removed from inside the catheter. The catheter then remains in place as a connection between the exterior of the body and the area of interest.

OTHER TECHNIQUES FOR ACCESSING VESSELS

Two less common techniques to access vessels may be used when required. One is called a **cutdown,** which requires a minor surgical procedure to expose the vessel of interest. The second technique is a **translumbar** approach, which requires that the patient be placed in a prone position and a long needle be passed through the abdomen at the level of T12 or L2 into the aorta. These two techniques are not as common and are not illustrated specifically in this chapter.

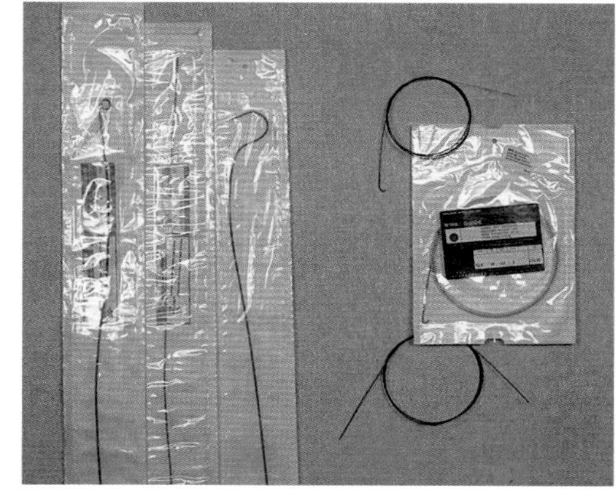

Fig. 21-35. Seldinger technique—catheters and guide wires.

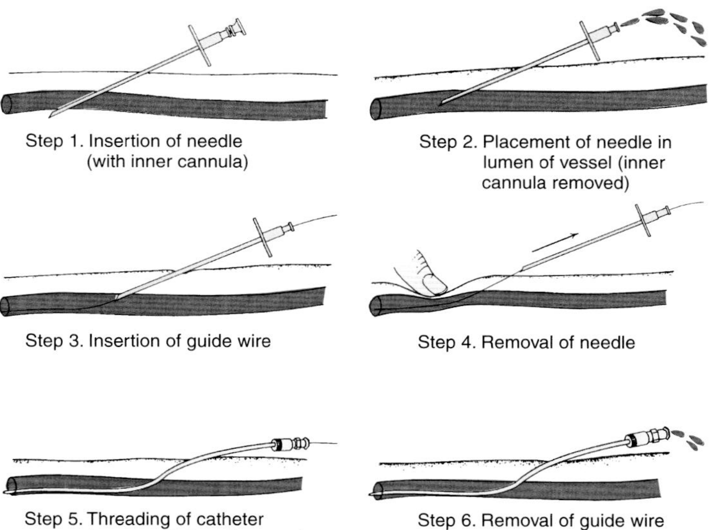
Step 1. Insertion of needle (with inner cannula)
Step 2. Placement of needle in lumen of vessel (inner cannula removed)
Step 3. Insertion of guide wire
Step 4. Removal of needle
Step 5. Threading of catheter to area of interest
Step 6. Removal of guide wire

Fig. 21-36. Six steps of Seldinger technique.

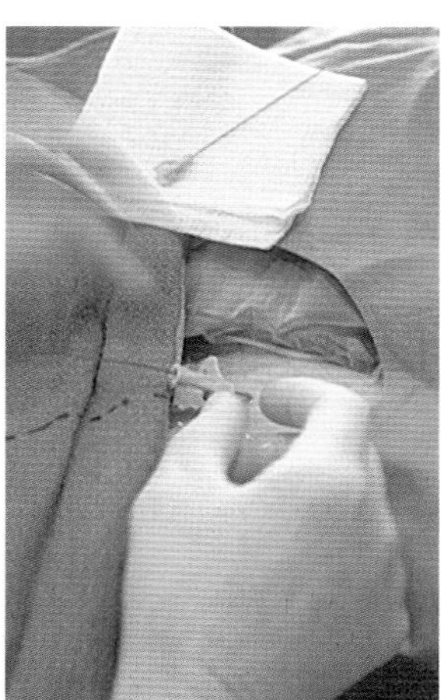

Fig. 21-37. Needle in lumen of artery (Step 2).

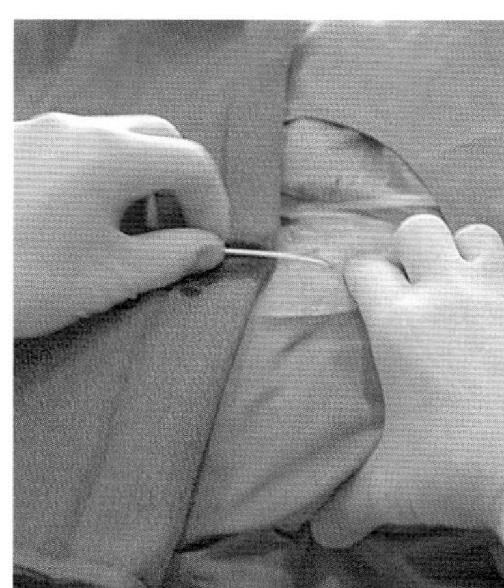

Fig. 21-38. Catheter placement to area of interest (Step 5).

21

VESSEL ACCESS, cont'd

Sterile items shown in Fig. 21-39 have been placed and are ready for the arterial puncture by the radiologist. The three-division manifold shown on the sterile sheet in this photograph is connected by lengths of tubing to (1) a transducer for vessel pressure readings, (2) a heparinized saline drip under pressure, and (3) an appropriate contrast medium. The syringe attached to the lower end of the manifold allows hand injection of medication or contrast medium, and the other end of the manifold attaches to the positioned catheter.

The catheters have different shapes at the distal end to permit easy access to the vessel of interest. The technologist should be familiar with the types, radiopacity, sizes, construction, and tip design of the catheters and guide wires in use. Many such catheters are available (Fig. 21-40).

The catheter should be flushed frequently during the procedure to prevent the formation of blood clots that become emboli.

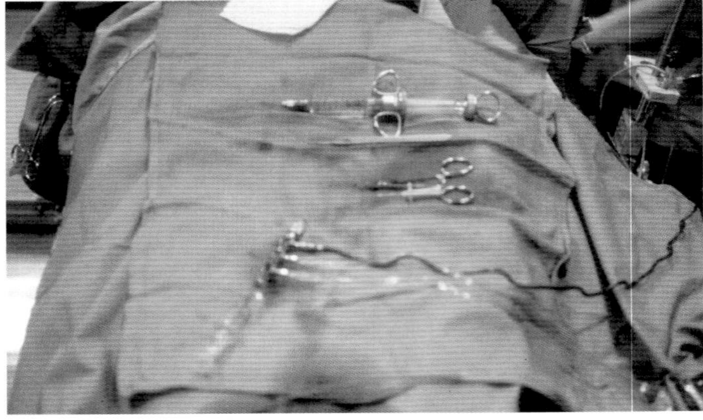

Fig. 21-39. Patient ready for catheter insertion.

ANGIOGRAPHIC TRAY

A sterile tray contains the basic equipment necessary for a Seldinger catheterization of a femoral artery (Fig. 21-41). Basic sterile items include the following:

1. Hemostats
2. Prep sponges and antiseptic solution
3. Scalpel blade
4. Syringe and needle for local anesthetic
5. Basins and medicine cup
6. Sterile drapes and towels
7. Band-Aids
8. Sterile image intensifier cover

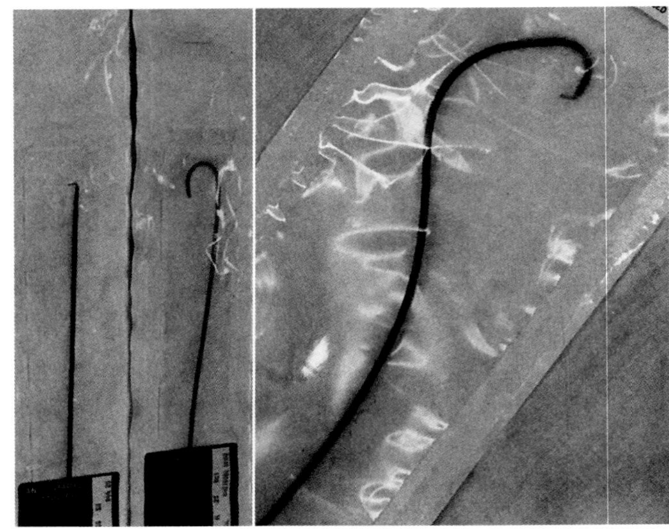

Fig. 21-40. Abdominal angiography catheters.

CONTRAST MEDIA

The contrast media of choice is a water-soluble, nonionic iodinated substance because of its low osmolality and the reduced risk for allergic reaction. The amount required depends on the vessel under examination. As for all procedures that use contrast media, emergency equipment should be readily available and the technologist must be familiar with the protocol in case of allergic reaction by the patient. A full description of contrast media is provided in Chapter 17.

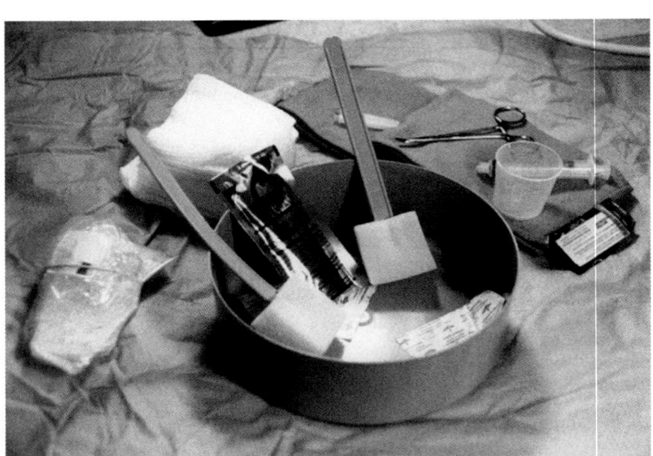

Fig. 21-41. Basic sterile tray.

IMAGING

Once the vessel of interest is catheterized under fluoroscopic guidance, a small hand injection of contrast media will be given to ensure the catheter is in an accurate position (i.e., it is in the vessel lumen and not lodged against the wall). For the imaging series, an electromechanical injector delivers a preset amount of contrast media and images are obtained. The rate of image acquisition is rapid, often in the range of several frames per second. The series will be reviewed to determine what, if any, additional series need(s) be done.

RADIATION PROTECTION

A potential risk exists for increased radiation dose to the health professionals who are members of the angiography team because of the use of fluoroscopy and their proximity to the patient and equipment during the procedure. Conscientious use of **radiation protection devices,** such as lead aprons, thyroid shields, and lead glasses, is required. Ensuring that **fluoroscopy time is the absolute minimum** is also vital to reducing dose.

Precise collimation is important to reduce the dose to the patient and the angiography team. Limiting the amount of secondary radiation produced that will degrade image quality is also essential.

Lead shields may be suspended from the ceiling as an additional means of protecting the angiographer's face and eyes. In addition, angiography units may have specialized beam filtration and pulsed fluoroscopic capabilities to help ensure that dose is kept to a minimum.

CONTRAINDICATIONS

Contraindications for patients to experience angiography include **contrast media allergy, impaired renal function, blood-clotting disorders** or **taking anticoagulant medication,** and **unstable cardiopulmonary/neurologic status.**

RISKS/COMPLICATIONS

Angiographic procedures are not without risk to the patient. Some of the most common risks and complications include the following:

- Bleeding at the puncture site: This can usually be controlled by applying compression.
- Thrombus formation: A blood clot may form in a vessel and disrupt the flow to distal parts.
- Embolus formation: A piece of plaque may be dislodged from a vessel wall by the catheter. A stroke or other vessel occlusion may result.
- Dissection of a vessel: The catheter may tear the intima of a vessel.
- Infection of puncture site: This is caused by contamination of sterile field.
- Contrast reaction: This may be mild, moderate, or severe (see Chapter 17).

If the axillary or brachial artery was used for the catheterization, the additional risk for damage to the nearby nerves and arterial spasm is present. The translumbar approach also has additional risks for the patient, which include hemothorax, pneumothorax, and retroperitoneal hemorrhage.

Rarely, a portion of the guide wire or catheter may break off in a vessel. The fragment becomes an embolus and the patient is at great risk. The fragment may be retrieved using a special type of retrieval catheter (see p. Figs. 21-76 and 21-77, p. 714).

POSTPROCEDURAL CARE

After the angiographic procedure, the catheter is removed and compression is applied to the puncture site. The patient remains on bed rest for a minimum of 4 hours but the head of the bed/stretcher may be elevated approximately 30°. During this time, the patient is monitored and vital signs and the peripheral pulse distal to the puncture site are regularly checked. The extremity is also checked for warmth, color, and numbness to ensure circulation has not been disrupted. Oral fluids are given and analgesics are provided if required.

Patients should be instructed what to do if the puncture site spontaneously begins to bleed: **apply pressure** and **call for help.**

Patients who have had a translumbar approach must follow similar postprocedural guidelines with the exception of external compression. In this case, bleeding is arrested internally, as bleeding into the periaortic musculature provides internal compression.

Recent advances include development of devices to surgically close the puncture site percutaneously. The device used for this is part of the catheter introducer system. At the completion of the procedure, the vessel is sutured using the specialized device attached. This is advantageous to the patient because it reduces the risk for hemorrhage and the angiographer is not required to compress the puncture site for several minutes. This technique is effective even for patients taking anticoagulants.

Procedure Modifications

PEDIATRIC APPLICATIONS

Pediatric patients requiring angiography generally are heavily sedated or under general anesthetic for the procedures, depending on the patient's age and condition. Neonates from special care nurseries are covered with warming blankets during the procedure to maintain their body temperature.

Parents and guardians are not usually permitted in the angiography unit. However, they should be given a thorough explanation of the procedure before signing the consent.

Pediatric patients may suffer from similar pathologies as adult patients. However, angiographic procedures, especially cardiac catheterization, are often indicated to investigate congenital defects.

GERIATRIC APPLICATIONS

Sensory loss (eyesight, hearing, etc.) associated with aging may result in geriatric patients requiring additional patience, assistance, and monitoring throughout the procedure. Geriatric patients also frequently feel nervous and are afraid of falling off the exam table, which is fairly narrow in angiography units. Reassurance and additional care from the technologist throughout the procedure will enable patients to feel secure and comfortable.

A radiolucent mattress of additional padding on the exam table will also provide comfort to geriatric patients. Extra blankets should be available after the procedure to keep them warm.

Older patients may have tremors or difficulty holding steady; use of high mA will result in shorter exposure times that will help to reduce the risk for motion on the images.

21

Angiographic Imaging Equipment

ANGIOGRAPHIC ROOM

An angiographic room is equipped for all types of angiographic and interventional procedures and has a wide variety of needles, catheters, and guide wires close at hand. It is larger than conventional radiographic rooms and has a sink and scrub area and a patient holding area. The room must have outlets for oxygen and suction, and emergency medical equipment must be nearby.

EQUIPMENT REQUIREMENTS

An angiography unit generally requires the following:

- An island-type table that provides access to the patient from all sides. It should have four-way floating capability, adjustable height, and a tilting mechanism.
- An analog-to-digital conversion fluoroscopy imaging system with intensifier; or the newer flat detector digital fluoroscopy acquisition type. Both of these systems are available in C-arm configurations as shown in Figs. 21-42 and 21-43.
- Programmable digital image acquisition system that allows selection and acquisition of the imaging rate and sequence, and processing of the images.
- Specialized x-ray tube(s) with high heat load capacity with rapid cooling to meet the need for high mA, high frame rates, and multiple acquisition series.
- Electromechanical injector for delivery of contrast media (see full description on p. 703).
- Physiologic monitoring equipment that allows monitoring of the patient's venous and arterial pressures and ECG (especially important for angioplasty and cardiac catheterization).
- Image archiving method linked to a picture archiving and communication system (PACS) and/or laser printer.

Older systems use biplane cut-film changers (see Fig. 21-46), but these are largely being replaced by digital systems.

DIGITAL ACQUISITION

As described above, currently there are **two types** of technology available for digital fluoroscopy and image acquisition: (1) **analog-to-digital conversion type** and (2) **flat detectors** (direct digital conversion). These two digital fluoro types are also described in more detail in Chapter 2.

The first type uses image intensifiers (Fig. 21-42). As the radiation passes through the patient and is detected by the image intensifier, the image intensifier converts the x-ray energy to light. It is then transmitted to a television system that converts the light to an electric signal and then sends this signal to an analog-to-digital converter. The signal is then digitized and sent to the digital image processor. The image processor allows the technologist to display, manipulate, and store the images. A digital image of a carotid arteriogram is shown in Fig. 21-44.

The second type of digital acquisition uses flat detectors with direct digital conversion. With this newer system, the digital detector replaces the image intensifier, the video camera, and the digital conversion system (see Fig. 21-43).

DIGITAL SUBTRACTION ANGIOGRAPHY

One advantage of digital technology is the ability to perform **digital subtraction angiography (DSA)** in real time. With digital technology, a highly sophisticated computer "subtracts" or removes certain anatomic structures so that the resultant image demonstrates only the vessel(s) of interest containing contrast media (Fig. 21-45). The subtracted image appears as a reversed image and may demonstrate diagnostic information not apparent on a conventional nonsubtracted image.

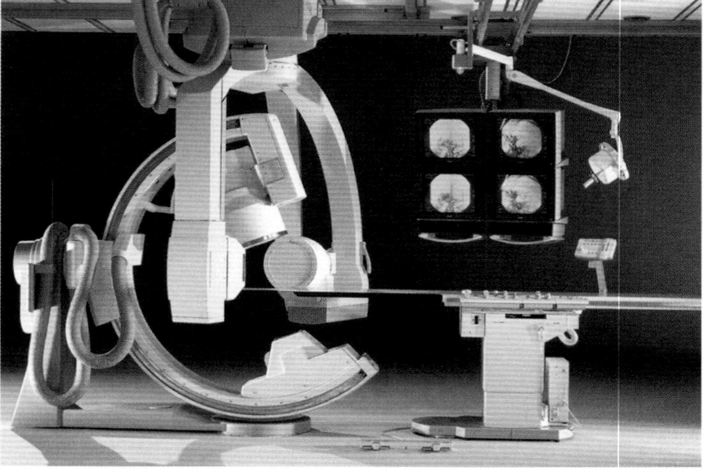

Fig. 21-42. Biplane digital angiographic system. (Courtesy Philips Medical Systems.)

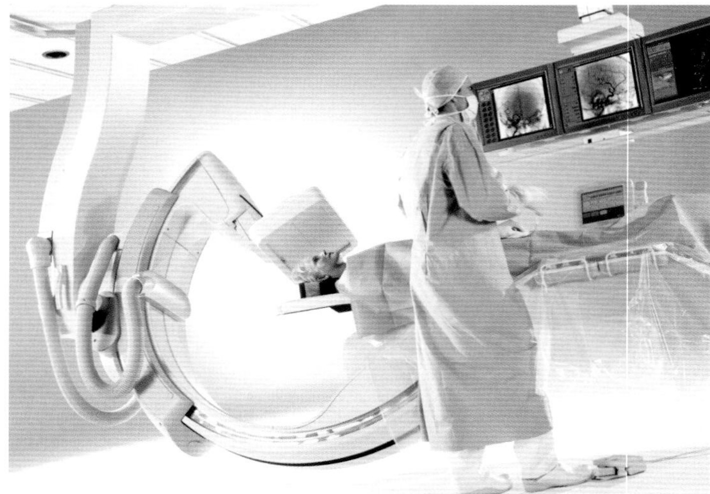

Fig. 21-43. Flat detector digital angiographic system, single plane. (Courtesy Philips Medical Systems.)

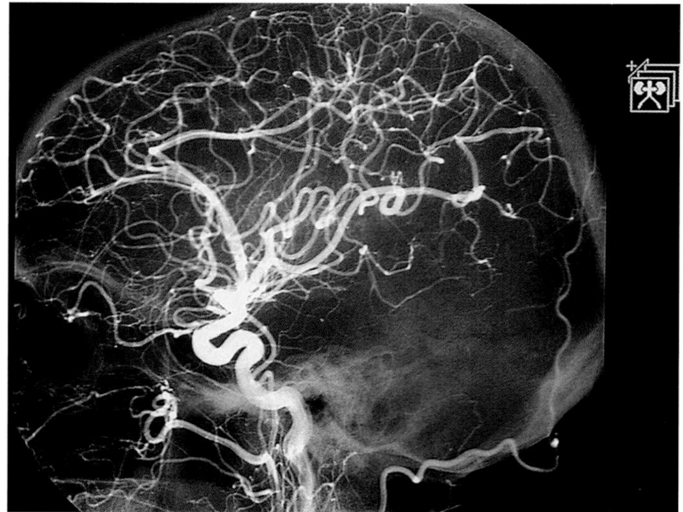

Fig. 21-44. Lateral nonsubtracted carotid arteriogram.

Post-Processing Images Because the images are digital and are stored, a number of **post-processing options** are available to improve or modify the image. Some examples of post-processing functions include **pixel-shifting** or **remasking,** which allows the technologist to improve the quality of the subtracted image. The image may be **magnified, or "zoomed,"** to see specific structures; images may also be **quantitatively analyzed** to measure distances, calculate stenosis, etc. Other options are available. See Chapter 2 for additional information on post-processing of digital images.

Digital acquisition allows the images to be archived directly to a PACS if available, with all the inherent advantages (ease of access to images by specialists, elimination of lost films, simultaneous viewing of images, etc.). If there is no PACS, the images may be printed and archived as hard copies.

CUT FILM CHANGERS

Prior to digital technology, angiography was performed using cut-film changers, in either single or biplane orientation (typical cerebral angiographic procedures were performed using biplane cut film changers) These have largely been replaced with digital equipment, but cut film changers may still be used on occasion and technologists should be familiar with them.

One type of cut film changer is shown in Fig. 21-46. Each cut film changer unit must be independent of the other, and the two should be able to be easily placed at right angles to one another. This arrangement allows exposure of a series of radiographs in both the lateral position and the AP projection with a single injection of contrast medium.

The internal mechanism of the film changer moves film rapidly from the supply compartment to the exposure area and finally to the receiving bin. A program selector operates the film changer during single or serial exposures, regulating filming rate and the duration of each phase of the series. Therefore the program selector controls the number of films per second and the total length of time that exposures are to be made. The program selector is integrated so that the contrast medium injector is synchronized with the imaging process. Chemical processing is required to view the film images.

AUTOMATIC ELECTROMECHANICAL CONTRAST MEDIUM INJECTOR

As contrast media is injected into the circulatory system, it is diluted by blood. The contrast material must be injected with sufficient pressure to overcome the patient's systemic arterial pressure and to maintain a bolus to minimize dilution with blood. To maintain the flow rates necessary for angiography, an automatic electromechanical injector is used. The flow rate is affected by many variables, such as the viscosity of contrast media, length and diameter of the catheter, and injection pressure. Depending on these variables and the vessel to be injected, the desired flow rate can be selected before injection.

A typical automatic digital-type contrast medium injector is shown in Fig. 21-47. Every injector is equipped with syringes, a heating device, a high-pressure mechanism, and a control panel. The syringes in common use are disposable. Reusable syringes must be easily disassembled for sterilization. The heating device warms and maintains the contrast medium at body temperature, reducing the viscosity of the medium. The high-pressure mechanism is usually an electromechanical device consisting of a motor drive that moves a piston into or out of the syringe.

In addition to safety, convenience, ease of use, and reliability of flow rate settings, other features of an automatic mechanical injector include the following: (1) ready light when armed and set for injection, (2) a slow or manual injector control to remove air bubbles from the syringe, and (3) controls to prevent inadvertent injection or excessive pressure or volume injection.

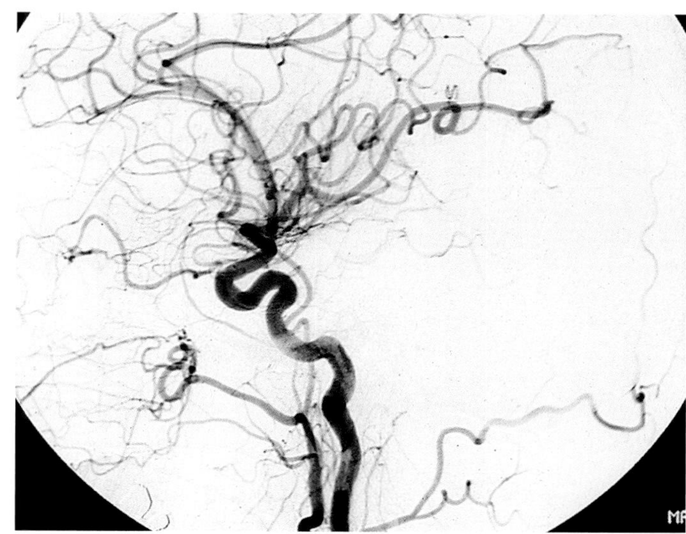

Fig. 21-45. Carotid DSA, lateral view.

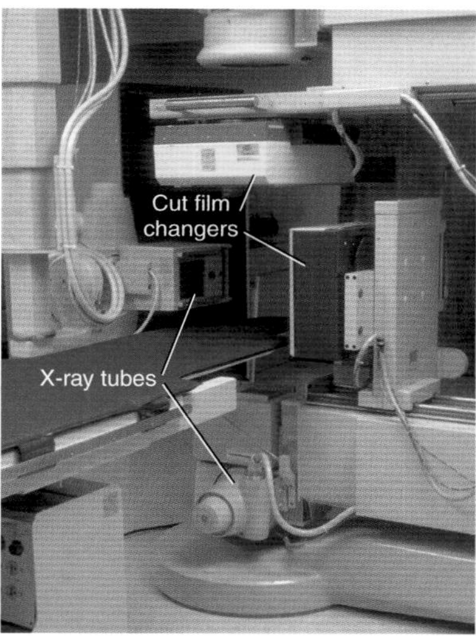

Fig. 21-46. Biplane film changers.

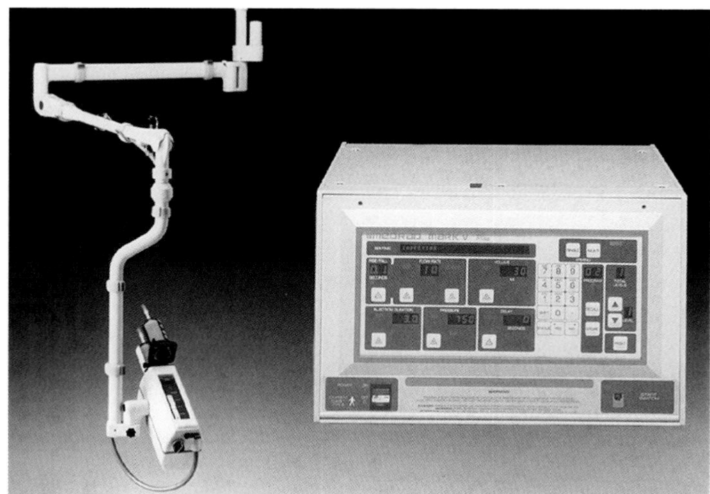

Fig. 21-47. Electromechanical contrast media injector—Medrad Mark V Plus. (Courtesy Medrad Inc., Indianola, PA.)

21

Alternative Modalities or Procedures

In addition to the specific angiographic procedures listed below, alternative modalities and procedures are also available in clinical imaging centers.

COMPUTED TOMOGRAPHY

Volume acquisition, multislice technology, subsecond reconstruction of images, and sophisticated software have made CT a valuable tool in vessel assessment. CT is used to study a wide variety of intracranial, thoracic, abdominal, and peripheral vascular pathologies, such as aortic aneurysms. If equipment specifications permit, CT is also useful in pulmonary embolism diagnosis.

CT angiography (CTA) is a study that provides images of the vascular structures in cross-section, which depending on the capability of the scanner and software, can be reconstructed into a 3D image. Multislice technology has allowed the acquisition of thinner slices thus increasing the resolution of CTA images. CTA provides the advantage of contrast media administered intravenously, eliminating the need for an arterial puncture and catheter insertion.

NUCLEAR MEDICINE

Nuclear medicine technology is often used in conjunction with angiography in investigation of certain cardiovascular pathologies, some of which include pulmonary embolus, GI bleed, renovascular hypertension, and coronary artery disease. Nuclear medicine complements other imaging modalities because it provides primarily physiologic information but little anatomic detail.

ULTRASOUND (SONOGRAPHY)

The role of ultrasound in cardiovascular imaging has increased. Ultrasound may be used to image the patency of vessels and demonstrate thrombus formation, plaque, or stenosis. Color Duplex (color flow Doppler) is also used in ultrasound to demonstrate the presence and absence of flow within a vessel, the direction of flow, and with more sophisticated equipment, the velocity of flow. Echocardiography provides detailed images of the heart for investigation of numerous cardiac conditions, including valve disease, aneurysm, cardiomyopathy, myocardial infarction, and congenital defects.

MAGNETIC RESONANCE ANGIOGRAPHY

Magnetic resonance angiography (MRA) provides highly detailed images of the patient's vasculature. This is advantageous because contrast media is not required and a vessel puncture is avoided.

ROTATIONAL ANGIOGRAPHY

During the contrast injection and while the images are acquired, the C-arm configuration on an angiography unit is rotated up to 180° around the patient. The vascular structure and system are visualized from a wide variety of angles with the single contrast injection. The resultant images may be played back digitally in a *cine loop* mode to provide a dynamic image presentation. Rotational imaging can provide information regarding which vessels require additional investigation or the optimal equipment angle to use for further studies.

THREE-DIMENSIONAL (3D) ROTATIONAL ANGIOGRAPHY

A three-dimensional (3D) image may be produced from the image data acquired during a rotational acquisition. The data are processed by a sophisticated computer system using digital reconstruction techniques similar to those used in computed tomography.

The 3D imaging reconstruction systems are valuable in visualizing complex intracranial vascular pathologies (e.g., arteriovenous malformations or aneurysms with unusual locations or characteristics). Information from 3D images is often useful in planning interventional approaches to these pathologies.

ALTERNATIVE CONTRAST MEDIA: CO_2 AND GADOLINIUM

Alternatives to iodine-based contrast media are required for patients with cardiopulmonary disease, diabetes mellitus, renal insufficiency, or iodinated contrast media allergy.

CO_2 is being used at some centers for selected procedures when iodinated contrast agents are contraindicated. Specialized CO_2 injectors have been developed to provide accurate, well-timed delivery of the gas into the vessels being examined. Some angiographic equipment has specialized digital imaging software to optimize the use of CO_2. The primary limitation of the use of CO_2 as an intravascular contrast agent is the risk for neurotoxicity. Experimental findings have indicated that CO_2 may cause ischemic infarction as a result of gas embolism of cerebral vessels. It has been suggested by the early proponents of this technique that CO_2 should not be used in vessels above the diaphragm.

The limitations of CO_2 as a contrast agent prompted angiographers to seek alternative agents for patients who could not tolerate iodinated contrast media. *Gadolinium,* a popular injectable agent used in MRI, has recently been used in angiography and has shown promise for a variety of vessels. Images obtained are diagnostic, and adverse effects in the patients have not been observed. It should be noted, however, that gadolinium is contraindicated for patients with renal disease.

Specific Angiographic Procedures

The next part of this chapter introduces and briefly describes six more common angiographic procedures that are performed in a typical clinical imaging center. (The specific routines for each of these procedures will be determined by radiologist preferences or department protocol.) The six procedures to be described are:

1. **Cerebral angiography**
2. **Thoracic angiography**
3. **Angiocardiography**
4. **Abdominal angiography**
5. **Peripheral angiography**
6. **Lymphography**

Descriptions of each of these procedures will include the following:

- Purpose
- Pathologic indications
- Catheterization
- Contrast media
- Imaging

CEREBRAL ANGIOGRAPHY

Purpose

Cerebral angiography is a **radiologic study of the blood vessels of the brain.** The primary purpose of cerebral angiography is to provide a vascular "road map" that will enable physicians to localize and diagnose pathology or other anomalies of the brain and neck regions.

Pathologic Indications

Pathologic indications for cerebral angiography include the following:

- Vascular stenosis and occlusions
- Aneurysms
- Trauma
- Arteriovenous malformations
- Neoplastic disease

Catheterization

The femoral approach is preferred for the catheter insertion. The catheter is advanced to the aortic arch, and the vessel to be imaged is selected. Vessels commonly selected for cerebral angiography include the **common carotid arteries, internal carotid arteries, external carotid arteries,** and **vertebral arteries.**

Contrast Media

The amount of contrast required depends on which vessel is being examined, but it usually ranges from 5 to 10 ml.

Imaging

Biplane equipment is preferred for cerebral angiography (Fig. 21-48). The imaging sequence selected must include all phases of the circulation—arterial, capillary, and venous—and will typically be 8 to 10 seconds long.

The projections required depend on the vessels being examined. Following are several examples.

Common Carotid Arteriography

Carotid arteriograms are among the most frequently performed cerebral angiogram studies.

Sometimes before a complete three-vessel or four-vessel carotid angiogram is done, two radiographic views of the neck to visualize each common carotid are taken (Figs. 21-49 and 21-50). The right common carotid artery is demonstrated in the AP projection and the lateral position to examine this artery and its bifurcation into internal and external carotid arteries. The area of bifurcation is studied carefully for occlusive disease (see *arrows*). The left common carotid artery is studied in a similar manner during the examination.

Internal Carotid Arteriography

A second cerebral arteriogram demonstrates the internal carotid arteries. Representative radiographs of the arterial phase of a left internal carotid angiogram are shown in the radiographs of Figs. 21-51 and 21-52. On the AP axial radiograph, the floor of the anterior fossa and the petrous ridges superimpose. This allows visualization of the bifurcation of the internal carotid artery into the anterior and middle cerebral arteries (see anatomy, Figs. 21-12 and 21-13).

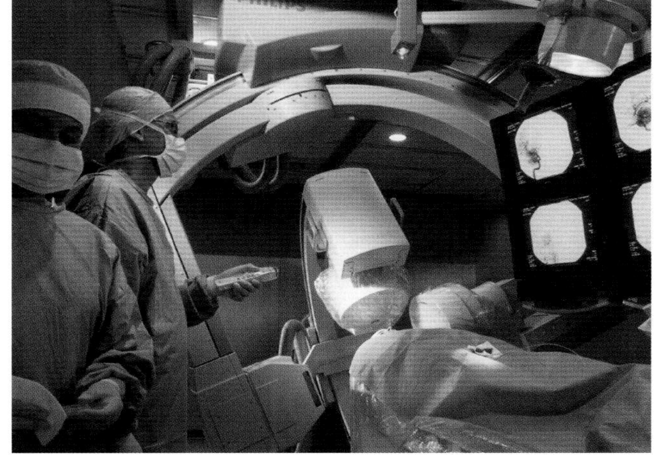

Fig. 21-48. Patient in position for cerebral angiogram. (Courtesy Philips Medical Systems.)

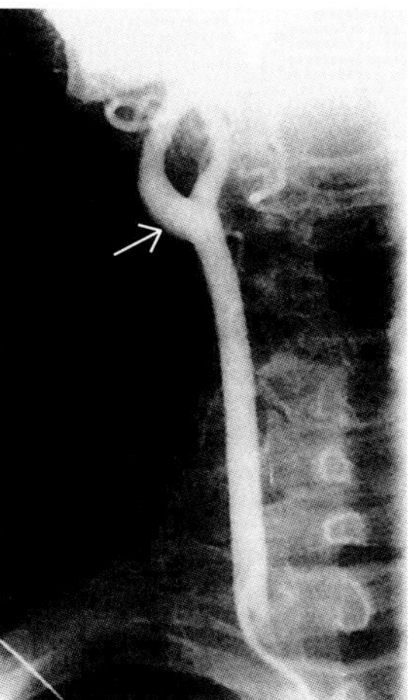

Fig. 21-49. AP. Right common carotid arteriogram.

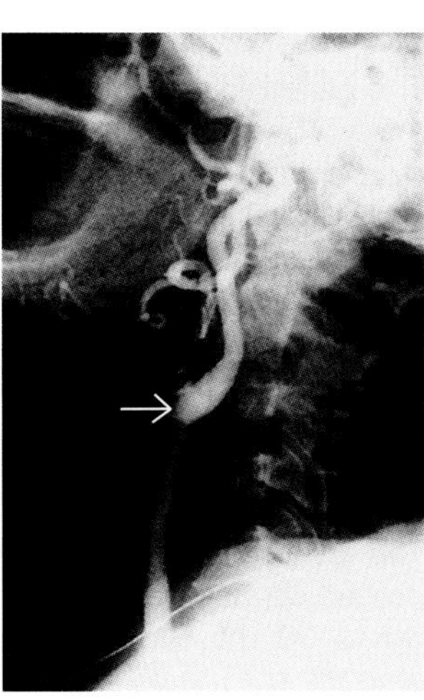

Fig. 21-50. Lateral. Right common carotid arteriogram.

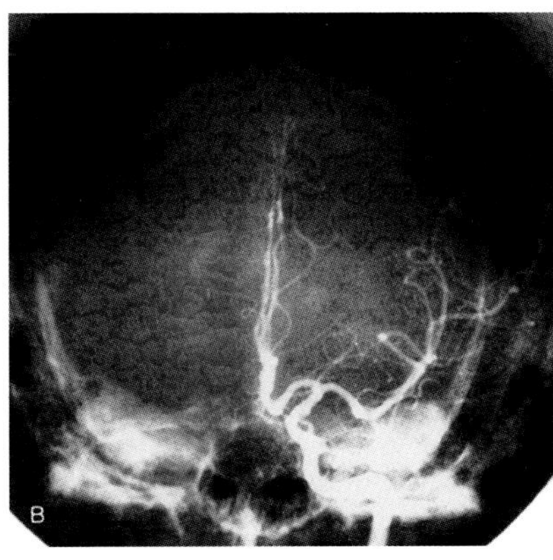

Fig. 21-51. AP axial—left internal carotid arteriogram. (Courtesy M. Tortorici and P. Apfel.)

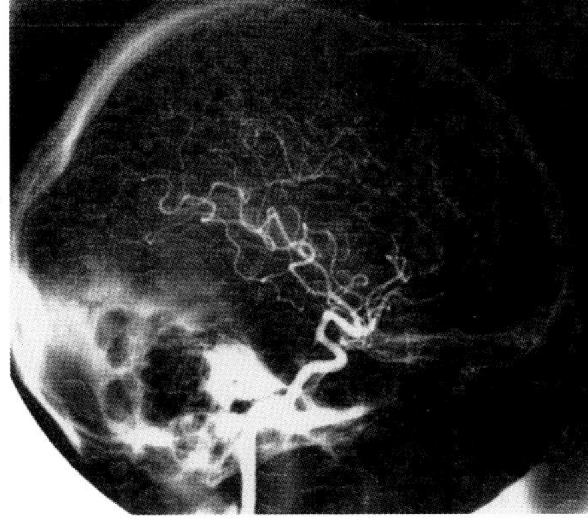

Fig. 21-52. Lateral—left internal carotid arteriogram. (Courtesy M. Tortorici and P. Apfel.)

THORACIC ANGIOGRAPHY

Purpose

Thoracic angiography demonstrates the contour and integrity of the thoracic vasculature. Thoracic aortography is an angiographic study of the **ascending aorta,** the **arch,** the **descending portion of the thoracic aorta,** and the **major branches.**

Pulmonary arteriography is an angiographic study of the pulmonary vessels usually done to investigate for pulmonary embolus. As mentioned earlier, pulmonary angiography is performed less frequently because of the availability of alternative modalities.

Pathologic Indications

Pathologic indications for thoracic and pulmonary angiography include the following:

- Aneurysms
- Congenital abnormalities
- Vessel stenosis
- Embolus
- Trauma

Catheterization

The preferred puncture site for a thoracic aortogram is the femoral artery. The catheter is advanced to the desired location in the thoracic aorta. Selective procedures may be performed by using specially designed catheters to access the vessel of interest.

Because of the location of the pulmonary artery, the femoral vein is the preferred site for catheter insertion. It is advanced along the venous structures, into the inferior vena cava, through the right atrium of the heart into the right ventricle, and into the pulmonary artery. Both pulmonary arteries are typically examined.

Contrast Media

The amount of contrast media injected will vary according to the procedure; however, an average amount for thoracic angiography is 30 to 50 ml. For selective pulmonary angiography, the average amount is 25 to 35 ml.

Imaging

Serial images for thoracic angiography are acquired over several seconds. The imaging rate and sequence depend on many factors including vessel size, patient history, and physician preference.

Respiration is suspended during image acquisition.

Thoracic aortogram Because of the structure of the proximal aorta, an oblique is required to visualize the aortic arch. A 45° LAO is preferred to prevent superimposing the structures and to visualize any anomalies (Figs. 21-53 and 21-54). This is done by manipulating the C-arm, rather than the patient, into the desired obliquity.

Pulmonary arteriogram Fig. 21-55 demonstrates the arterial phase of a pulmonary angiogram (DSA). The imaging sequence is usually extended when imaging the pulmonary artery to visualize the venous phase of circulation.

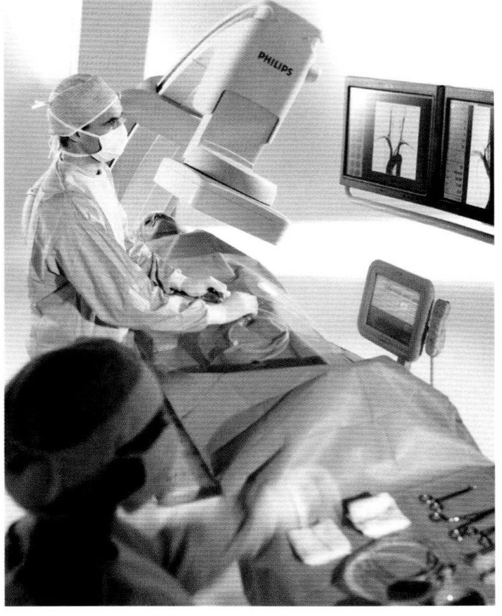

Fig. 21-53. Thoracic aortogram—aortic arch. Catheter is advanced through femoral artery to selected portion of thoracic aorta. (Courtesy Philips Medical Systems.)

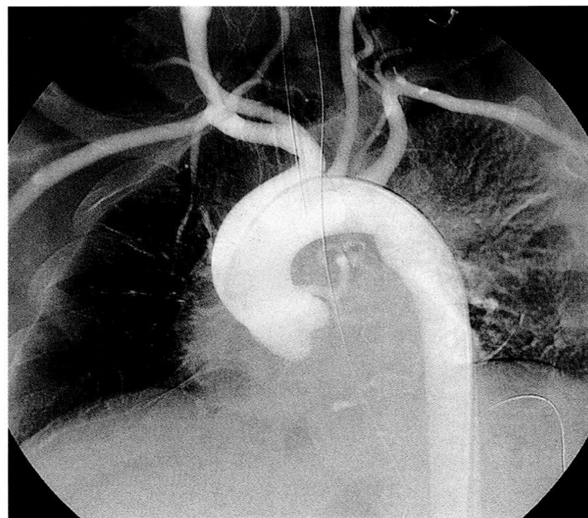

Fig. 21-54. Thoracic aortogram—aortic arch, 45° LAO.

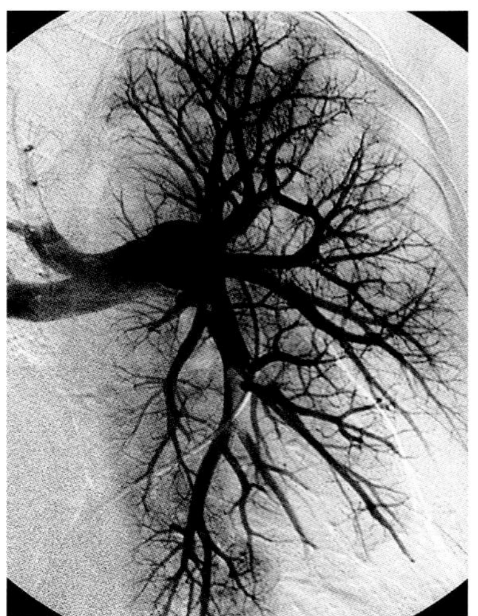

Fig. 21-55 Pulmonary arteriogram (DSA).

ANGIOCARDIOGRAPHY

Purpose

Angiocardiography refers specifically to radiologic imaging of the **heart** and **associated structures. Coronary arteriography** is typically performed at the same time to visualize the **coronary arteries.**

Cardiac catheterization is a more general term used to describe placing a catheter in the heart and includes studies in addition to the radiologic imaging ones, such as obtaining blood samples to measure oxygen saturation (oximetry) and measuring hemodynamic pressures and gradients. Specialized physiologic monitoring equipment is required for these sensitive measurements. For the purposes of this text, the focus will be on the imaging aspect of cardiac catheterization.

Pathologic Indications

Pathologic indications for angiocardiography and coronary arteriography include the following:

- Coronary artery disease and angina
- Myocardial infarct
- Valvular disease
- Atypical chest pain
- Congenital heart anomaly
- Other heart and aorta pathology

Catheterization

As for other angiograms, the femoral artery is the preferred site to catheterize. The catheter is advanced to the aorta and along its length into the left ventricle for the **left ventriculogram.** A pigtail catheter is used because a large volume of contrast media will be injected. For the coronary arteriogram, the catheter is changed and the coronary artery is selected; both right and left coronary arteries are routinely examined. Specially shaped catheters are designed to fit each of the coronary arteries.

After injection of contrast media into the coronary arteries, the catheter is immediately removed to prevent occluding the vessel.

Access to the right side of the heart is obtained by catheterizing the femoral vein and advancing the catheter through the venous structures until the right side of the heart is reached.

Contrast Media

Approximately 40 to 50 ml of nonionic, low-osmolar, water-soluble iodinated contrast media is injected for the ventriculogram. The coronary arteries typically require 7 to 10 ml of contrast media per injection.

Imaging

The imaging rate for angiocardiography is very rapid, in the range of 15 to 30 frames per second, and higher for pediatric patients.

If biplane equipment is available for left ventriculography, RAO and LAO images will be obtained. If equipment is single-plane, routinely a 30° RAO will be obtained (Fig. 21-56). Using the ventriculogram, the **ejection fraction** can be calculated. The ejection fraction is expressed as a percentage and provides an indication of the pumping efficiency of the **left ventricle** (Fig. 21-58).

A series of oblique images is obtained to fully visualize the coronary arteries. Routinely six views of the left coronary artery are obtained, and two views of the right coronary artery are obtained (more views are obtained of the left coronary artery because in most people it and its branches supply blood to the majority of the heart). Use of biplane imaging equipment is advantageous in that it reduces the amount of contrast media required because two oblique projections can be obtained simultaneously. Respiration is suspended for the image acquisition.

The images are archived on compact disc or into a PACS. When played back, the images are viewed in cine mode. If cardiac catheterization examinations are to be archived to a PACS, a system that has been specifically designed for cardiology applications should be used.

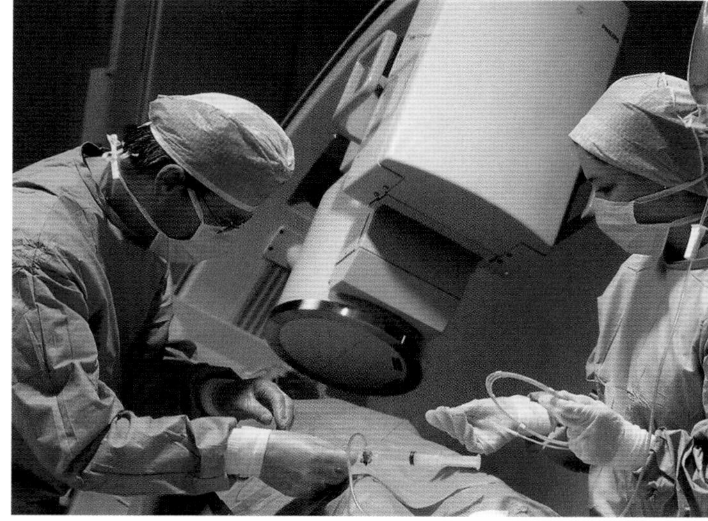

Fig. 21-56. Cardiac catheterization—advancing catheter through femoral artery and aorta to left ventricle. (Courtesy Philips Medical Systems.)

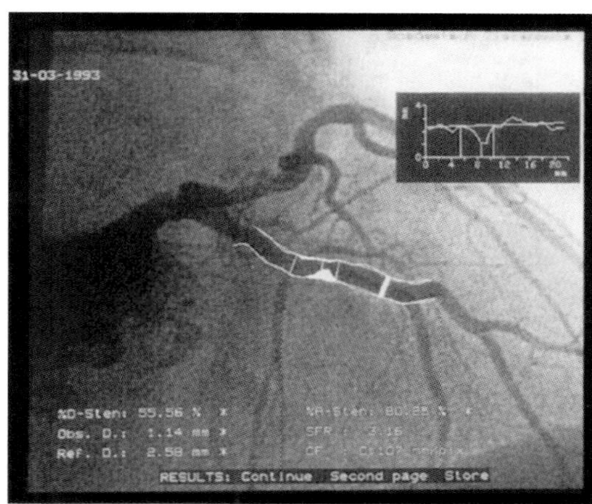

Fig. 21-57. Automated coronary analysis. (Courtesy Philips Medical Systems.)

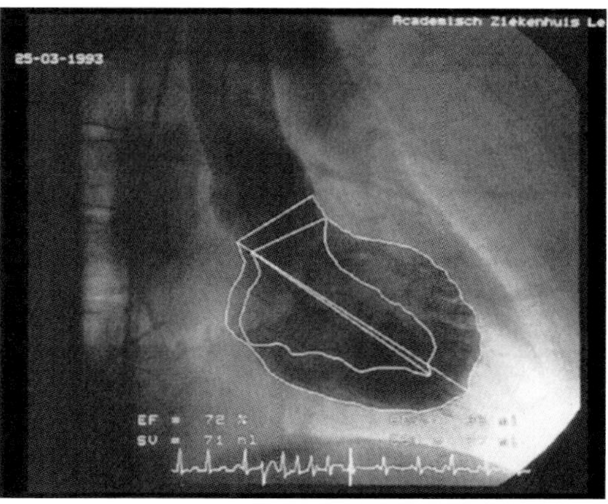

Fig. 21-58. Left ventricle analysis. (Courtesy Philips Medical Systems.)

21

ABDOMINAL ANGIOGRAPHY

Purpose

Abdominal angiography demonstrates the contour and integrity of **abdominal vasculature.** This means that the placement or displacement of abdominal vessels being studied and possible obstructions or vessel tears (e.g., aneurysm ballooning) will be demonstrated. Any displacement of vessels may indicate a space-occupying lesion.

Aortography refers to an angiographic study of the aorta, and selective studies refer to the catheterization of a specific vessel. **Venacavography** demonstrates the superior and/or inferior vena cava.

Pathologic Indications

Pathologic indications for abdominal angiography include the following:

- Aneurysm
- Congenital abnormality
- GI bleed
- Stenosis or occlusion
- Trauma

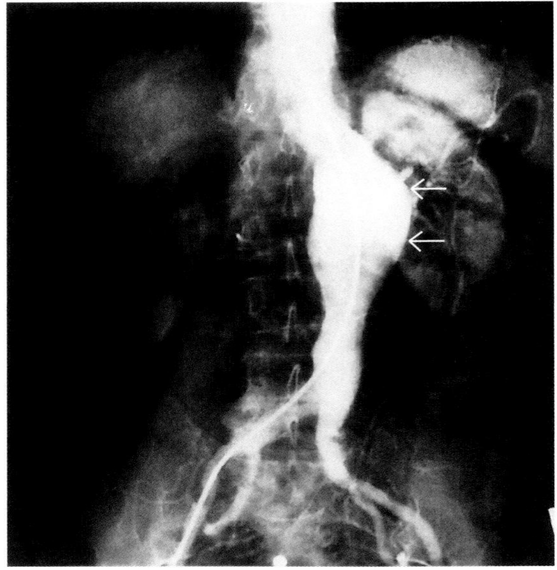

Fig. 21-59. Abdominal angiogram demonstrates an abdominal aneurysm *(arrows).*

Catheterization

For an aortogram, the aorta is typically accessed by the femoral artery. The type and size of catheter required depend on the structure, but a pigtail catheter is usually used because a larger amount of contrast will be delivered such as needed for an abdominal aortogram (Fig. 21-59).

Selective angiographic studies require the use of specially shaped catheters to access the vessel of interest. Common selective studies performed include the celiac axis, the renal arteries (Fig. 21-60), and the superior and inferior mesenteric arteries, which are selected when investigating a GI bleed. A superselective study involves selecting a branch of a vessel. A common example of this is selection of the hepatic or splenic artery, which are two of the branches of the celiac axis.

Catheterization for **venacavography** is obtained by a femoral vein puncture. The catheter is then advanced to the desired level.

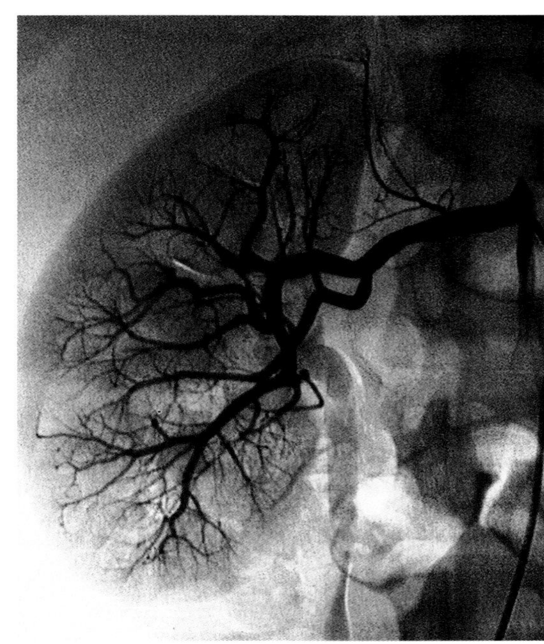

Fig. 21-60. Selective renal angiogram, DSA.

Contrast Media

An average amount of contrast media for an aortogram and a venacavogram is 30 to 40 ml. The amount of contrast media for selective studies varies depending on the vessel under examination. As for other angiographic procedures, the contrast media of choice is nonionic, water-soluble, and iodinated, with low osmolality.

Imaging

Imaging is done with the patient in the supine position; any obliquity required is obtained by manipulating the C-arm. Serial images are acquired, typically over several seconds. The imaging sequence and rate are dependent on many factors, including vessel size, patient history, and physician preference.

Before performing any arterial selective studies, an abdominal angiogram will generally be obtained, preferably including the area from the diaphragm to the aortic bifurcation. Associated branches of the aorta, such as the right and left renal arteries and the superior and inferior mesenteric arteries, will be visualized, as shown on the images in Fig. 21-61.

The imaging sequences for the selective studies are usually extended to visualize the venous phase. Respiration is suspended for the image acquisition.

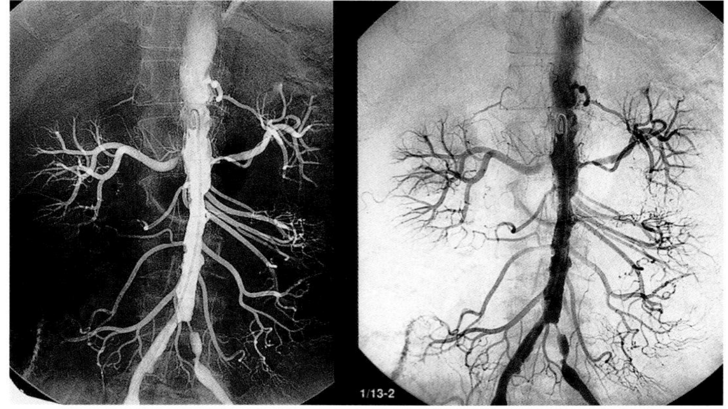

Fig. 21-61. Lower abdomen angiogram, with DSA image on right.

PERIPHERAL ANGIOGRAPHY

Purpose

Peripheral angiography is a radiologic examination of the **peripheral vasculature** after the injection of contrast media. Peripheral angiography may be an **arteriogram** (Fig. 21-62), in which the injection is by a catheter in an artery, or a **venogram,** in which the injection is into a vein of the extremity being examined. It should be noted, however, that venograms are now rarely performed because of the increased sensitivity of ultrasound (color duplex) to demonstrate pathology and will not be discussed further in this chapter.

Pathologic Indications

Pathologic indications for peripheral angiography include the following:

- Atherosclerotic disease
- Vessel occlusion and stenosis
- Trauma
- Neoplasm
- Embolus and thrombus

Catheterization

The Seldinger technique is used to access the femoral artery, or an alternate injection site for a peripheral arteriogram. For a lower limb arteriogram, the catheter is advanced just superior to the aortic bifurcation.

For an upper limb arteriogram, the catheter is advanced along the abdominal and thoracic aorta. For a study of the left upper limb, the left subclavian artery is selected; for a study of the right upper limb, the right subclavian artery is selected from the brachiocephalic trunk.

Contrast Media

The average amount of contrast media required for an upper limb arteriogram is much less than for a lower limb arteriogram. This is because of the difference in part size and the fact that the upper limb exam is unilateral, whereas the lower limb exam is bilateral.

Imaging: Lower Limb

Because variance in blood flow through both lower limbs exists as a result of vessel patency and occlusion, the time of circulation must be determined to ensure contrast is visible in the vessels during imaging. Different methods can be used to time the imaging. It can be done manually by controlling the speed of table movement during acquisition or it can be programmed into the computer.

Using current technology, once the timing of blood flow has been established, the table moves at the predetermined rate and images are acquired in the PA projection. These images can then be reconstructed to provide visualization of the entire lower limb (Fig. 21-63) or viewed individually (Fig. 21-64).

Respiration is suspended for the image acquisition.

Imaging: Upper Limb

Upper limb imaging also requires timing of the blood flow, and a technique similar to the one described previously may be used. The primary difference between upper and lower limb imaging is that the imaging is unilateral for the upper limb, not bilateral as for the lower limb.

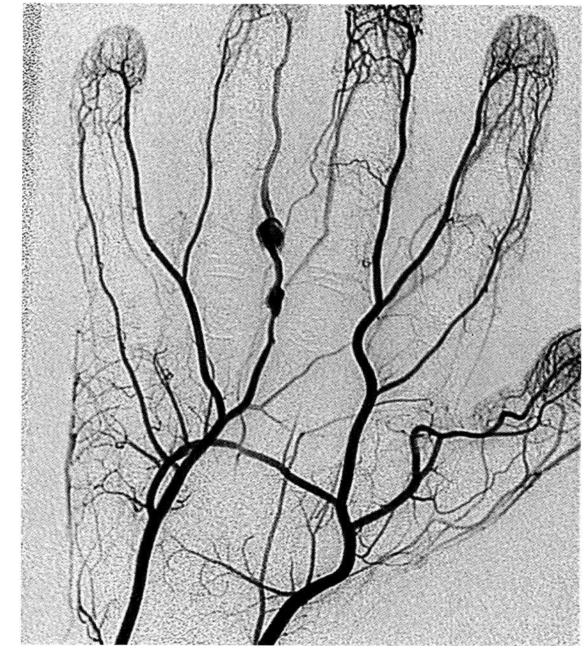

Fig. 21-62. DSA of left hand.

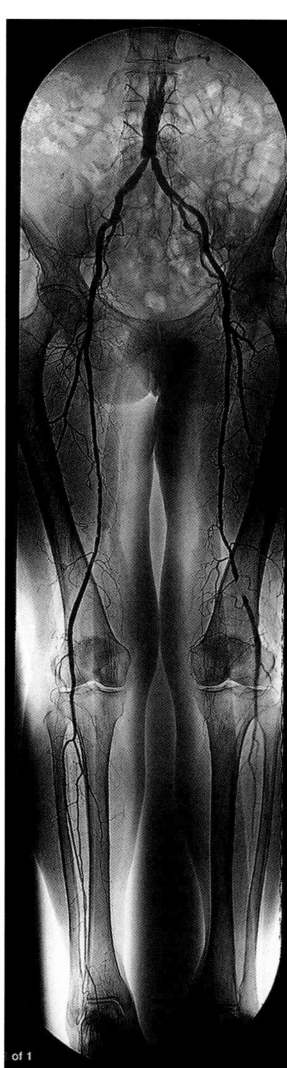

Fig. 21-63. Lower limb arteriogram—entire lower limb.

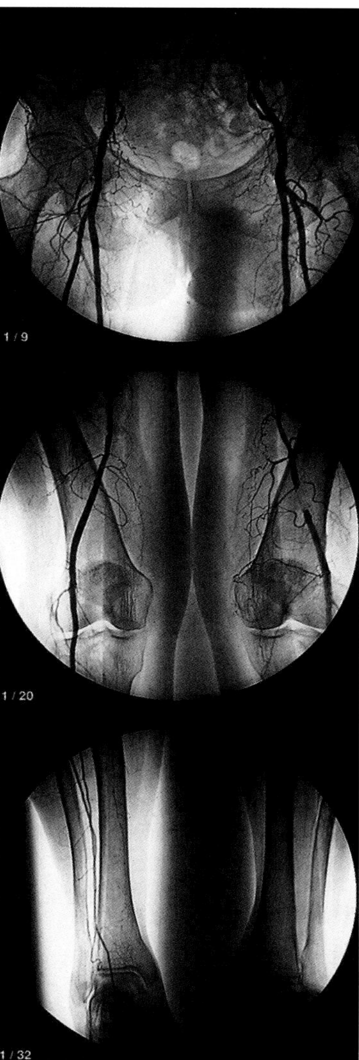

Fig. 21-64. Lower limb arteriogram—spot images.

21

LYMPHOGRAPHY

Purpose

Lymphography is performed to visualize the **lymph vessels** and **nodes.** Lower limb procedures are the most common and will be the ones discussed in this section; however, upper limb procedures may be done.

Although CT has largely replaced lymphography in the assessment of the nodes, lymphography is indicated in certain situations.

Pathologic Indications

Pathologic indications for lymphography include the following:

- Assessment of the lymphatics in the staging of malignancies, especially cervical and prostate cancers
- Assessment of Hodgkin's lymphoma
- Peripheral swelling

Contraindications

Lymphography is contraindicated for patients who have iodine sensitivity, for those with advanced pulmonary disease (the contrast is oil-based and will end up in the lungs via the thoracic duct), and for patients who have recently had radiation therapy to their lungs. Patients with marked tremors are also not candidates for this procedure because the vessels are fragile and the injection time is lengthy.

The Procedure

Lymphography can be performed in any general radiographic room; fluoroscopic capability is not required. As with angiography, the procedure is performed under aseptic conditions.

Lymphatic vessels are not readily visible; therefore a blue dye is injected subcutaneously between the first and second web spaces of the feet. After about 15 to 20 minutes, the feet are prepared and draped for a cutdown procedure. A local anesthetic is given and the cutdown is performed. When the feet are incised, the lymph vessels are visible as thin blue lines because they have picked up the blue dye. A lymphatic vessel in each foot is cannulated and the injection begins. Once the injection is complete, the incision is sutured.

Contrast Media

An automatic injector is used to deliver approximately 6 ml of contrast to each foot. It is delivered slowly, over about 45 minutes, because of the size and fragility of the vessels. It is an oil-based iodinated agent; water-soluble agents are too quickly absorbed for the purpose of this examination.

Imaging

During injection, obtaining an image of the lower leg or thigh to ensure the contrast media is progressing satisfactorily in the lymph vessels is standard procedure.

Approximately 1 hour after injection, a series of images is obtained. This series of images demonstrates the lymphatic vessels (Fig. 21-65). About 24 hours later, another series of images is obtained to visualize the lymph nodes (Fig. 21-66). The contrast media will remain in the lymph nodes for 3 to 4 weeks.

The imaging series focuses on the pelvis and lower abdominal region. AP projections and lateral and oblique positions are used to fully demonstrate the structures.

Risks and Complications

Risks to the patient undergoing lymphography include infections at the incision, oil embolus, and contrast reaction.

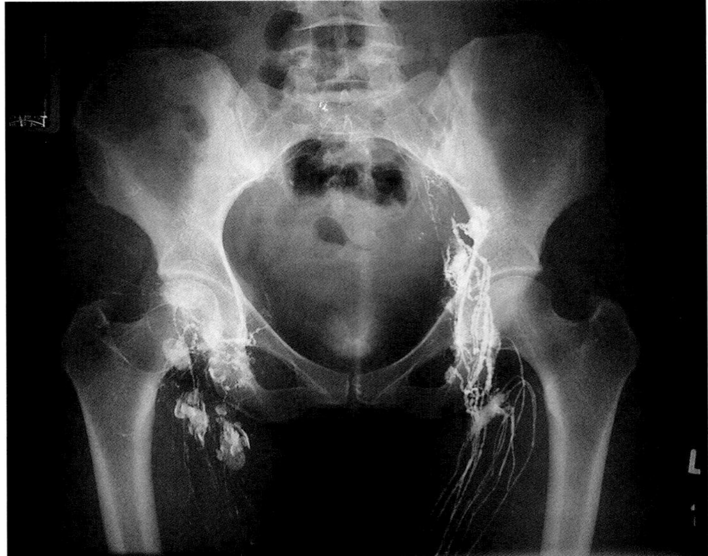

Fig. 21-65. Lymphangiogram—**lymph vessels.**

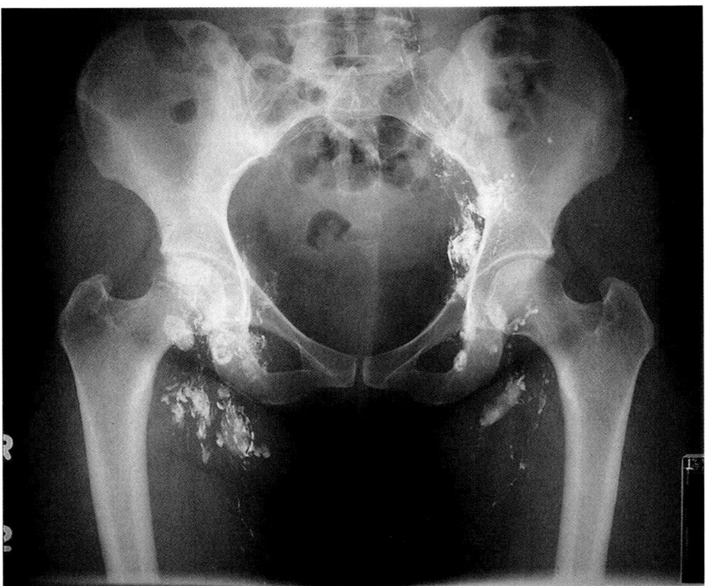

Fig. 21-66. Lymphadenogram—**lymph nodes (glands).**

INTERVENTIONAL IMAGING PROCEDURES

Definition and Purpose

Interventional imaging procedures are **radiologic procedures that intervene in a disease process, providing a therapeutic outcome.** Simply stated, interventional procedures use angiographic techniques for the **treatment of disease** in addition to providing certain diagnostic information.

This is a rapidly growing specialty in medical imaging as interventional procedures have become an increasingly important tool in the management of an ever-growing list of pathologies.

The purpose of these procedures and benefits to the patient and health care system include the following:

- Techniques that are minimally invasive and lower-risk compared with traditional surgical procedures
- Procedures that are less expensive than traditional medical and surgical procedures
- Shorter hospital stays for the patient
- Shorter recovery time because of a safer, less invasive procedure
- Alternatives for patients who are not candidates for surgery

These procedures are typically performed in an angiographic suite under the direction of an interventional radiologist. Fluoroscopic guidance is crucial to follow the path of the required needles and catheters.

The increase in complexity of the type of interventional procedures currently performed has resulted in many angiography units being upgraded to meet operating room specifications. This reduces the risk for infection and allows rapid surgical management in case of complications.

Interventional procedures may be categorized as **vascular** or **nonvascular** procedures.

VASCULAR INTERVENTIONAL PROCEDURES

Embolization

Transcatheter **embolization** is a procedure that uses an angiographic approach to **create an embolus in a vessel,** thus restricting blood flow. A number of clinical indications for this procedure exist, including the following:

- Stop blood blow to a site of pathology.
- Reduce blood flow to a highly vascular structure and tumor before surgery.
- Stop active bleeding at a specific site.
- Deliver a chemotherapeutic agent.

Examples of specific embolization procedures include the following:

Uterine fibroid embolization This is a procedure used to treat symptomatic fibroids. Embolization of the uterine artery can shrink the fibroids and eliminate the associated pain and bleeding, thus replacing a hysterectomy.

Uterine artery embolization The uterine artery may also be embolized to stop life-threatening postpartum bleeding, potentially preventing hysterectomy.

Chemoembolization This is most commonly used for hepatic malignancies. The chemotherapy agent is injected into the tumor vasculature. The survival rate from this procedure is comparable with treatment by a more invasive surgical resection. Investigation is underway regarding the use of this technique for other locally advanced cancers (e.g., lung, breast, brain).

Intracranial endovascular coil embolization This provides an alternative to patients with **brain aneurysms** that are inoperable or of high surgical risk. Using specially designed microcatheters, this procedure employs **detachable coils** to **completely occlude the aneurysmal sac and neck.**

Special catheters are used to place the embolic agent, which may be temporary (e.g., Gelfoam) or permanent (e.g., stainless steel coils), depending on the clinical application of the procedure.

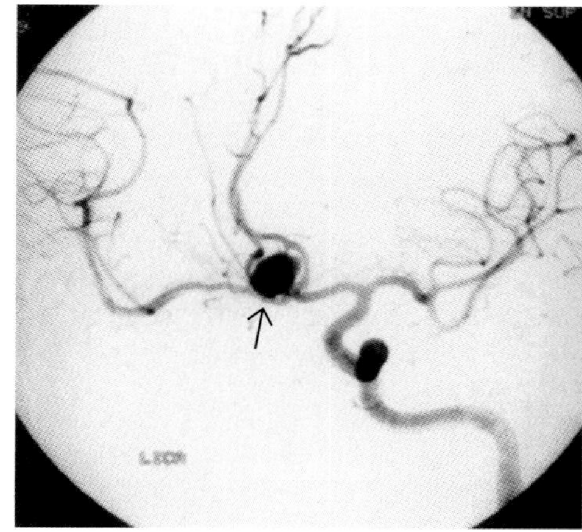

Fig. 21-67. Angiogram (DSA) before embolization procedure. (Courtesy Philips Medical Systems.)

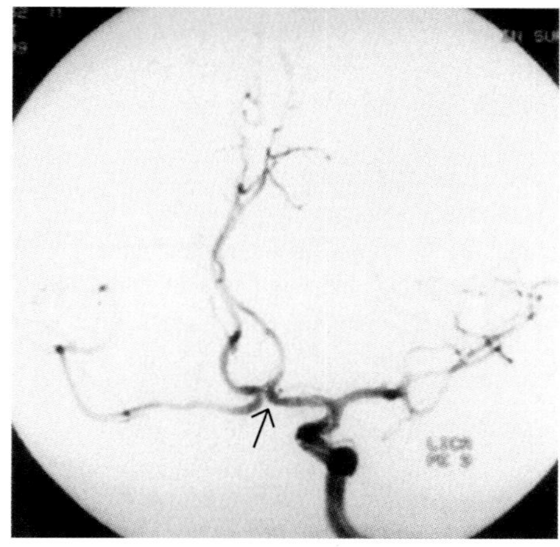

Fig. 21-68. Angiogram (DSA) after embolization procedure (aneurysm occluded). (Courtesy Philips Medical Systems.)

Risks and complications The complications of embolization procedures are similar to other angiographic procedures, including vessel perforation, stroke, and hemorrhage. For these procedures, the added risk for occluding the inappropriate vessel exists. Great care is taken to prevent this.

Examples An example of an embolization procedure used successfully to occlude an aneurysm of the anterior communicating artery is demonstrated in Figs. 21-67 and 21-68 (DSA images). Fig. 21-68 demonstrates the site of the aneurysm (see *arrow*) to be completely occluded after microcatheterization was performed and nine detachable coils were placed into the aneurysm.

21

Percutaneous Transluminal Angioplasty and Stent Placement

Angioplasty Percutaneous transluminal angioplasty (PTA) uses an angiographic approach and specialized catheters to dilate a stenosed vessel. This procedure is a long-standing interventional technique and has an application for a wide variety of vessel types and sizes (e.g., coronary, iliac, renal arteries).

A catheter with a deflated balloon is advanced to the vessel of interest. Hemodynamic pressures proximal and distal to the stenosis are obtained, and a preangioplasty angiogram is performed. The balloon portion of the catheter is placed at the vessel stenosis, and the balloon is inflated. The pressure of the inflation is monitored by a pressure gauge to prevent vessel rupture, and more than one inflation may be required. The duration of the inflations are carefully timed to eliminate damage to distal tissue because the blood supply is temporarily occluded.

The final steps to the procedure include obtaining arterial pressures proximal and distal to the dilated portion of the vessel and a postangioplasty angiogram. This allows the effectiveness of the procedure to be assessed.

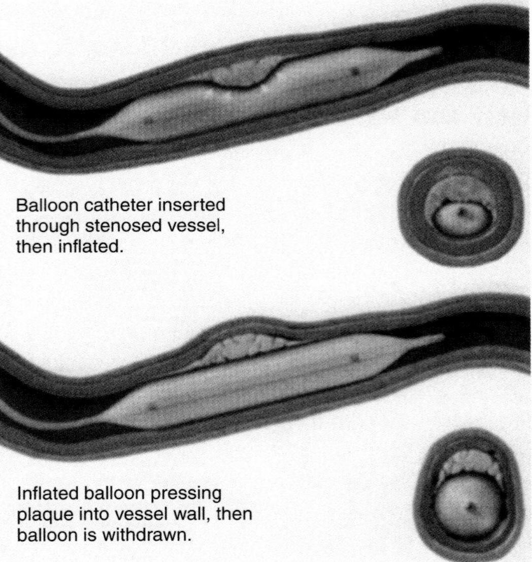

Fig. 21-69. Transluminal angioplasty—balloon catheter. (Courtesy Medi-tech/Boston Scientific Corporation.)

Stent placement To assist in maintaining patency of the vessel, a stent may be inserted across the treated area during the angioplasty. A stent is a **cagelike metal device that is placed in the lumen of a vessel to provide support.** It can be a self-expanding type or a balloon-expandable type. The self-expanding type automatically expands when the stent cover is removed in the vessel, and the balloon-expandable type (the compressed stent covers the balloon on the catheter) is positioned during the balloon-inflation phase of the angioplasty. Use of stents increases the duration of the therapeutic effect of the procedure.

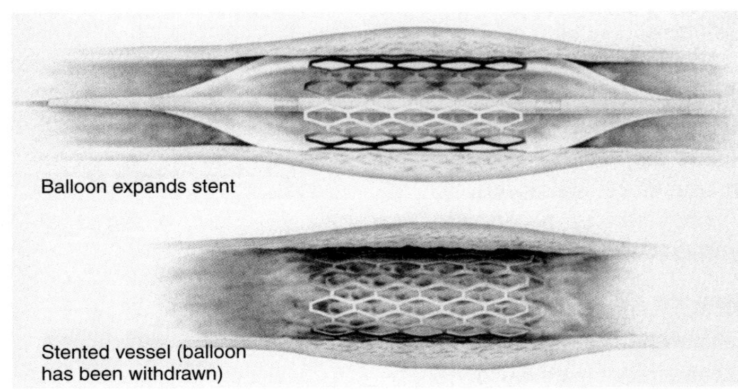

Fig. 21-70. Balloon expanding stent. (Courtesy Cordis Corporation, a Johnson & Johnson Company.)

Drug-eluting stent Recent advances in stent technology include impregnating the stent with a slow-release dose formulation of *paclitaxel.* This drug, an active component of the chemotherapeutic agent Taxol®, **inhibits the regrowth of vascular tissue** within the artery, thus **reducing restenosis.** Clinical trials on use in the coronary arteries have been positive, and drug-eluting stents are now being used in some hospitals.

Risks and complications Risks of transluminal angioplasty include vessel rupture and perforation, embolus, vessel occlusion, and dissection.

Stent-Graft Placement

Stent-grafts are a combination of interventional stents and surgical grafts. The primary clinical indications for stent-graft placement include aortic aneurysms and traumatic vascular injuries (Fig. 21-70). This procedure offers an option for patients who are not candidates for surgical procedures and a lower-risk procedure for patients who are candidates for surgical procedures. These procedures often involve both the interventional radiology team and the vascular surgical team.

Using an angiographic cutdown approach, fluoroscopy is used to follow the progress of a catheter. The stent-graft self-expands after delivery through the catheter, and attached struts anchor it to the vessel wall.

Risks and complications Complications for this procedure include leakage around the stent-graft or migration of the device. Rupture of the vessel is also a risk.

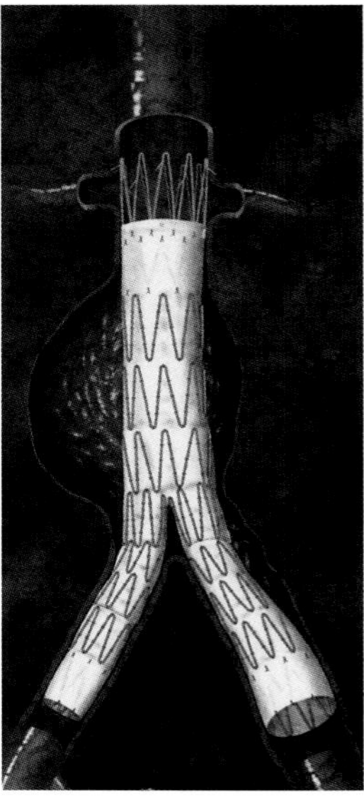

Fig. 21-71. Stent-graft placed for an abdominal aortic aneurysm. (Courtesy Cook Canada, Inc.)

Inferior Vena Cava Filter

An **inferior vena cava filter** is indicated for patients who have recurrent pulmonary emboli or are at high risk for developing them (e.g., posttrauma with pelvic and lower extremity fractures). A filter is placed in the inferior vena cava to trap potentially fatal emboli that originate in the lower limbs. A variety of filter designs are available for this procedure (Fig. 21-72 and Fig. 21-73).

A femoral or jugular vein puncture is used to gain access to the inferior vena cava. An angiographic technique is then used to deploy the filter by a catheter. The filter has struts that anchor it to the walls of the vessel. The filter must be placed inferior to the renal veins to prevent renal vein thrombosis.

Risks and complications Besides the usual angiographic complications (infection, bleeding, etc.), the added risk of the filter migrating into the heart and lungs exists. The filter may also become occluded in the long term.

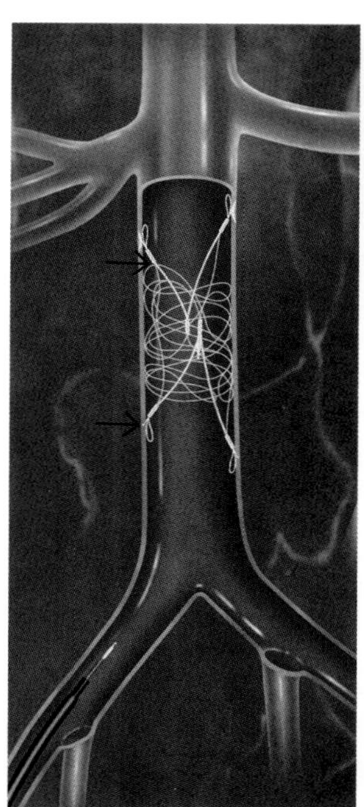

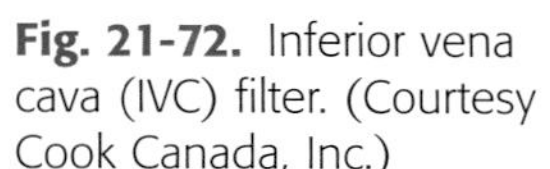

Fig. 21-72. Inferior vena cava (IVC) filter. (Courtesy Cook Canada, Inc.)

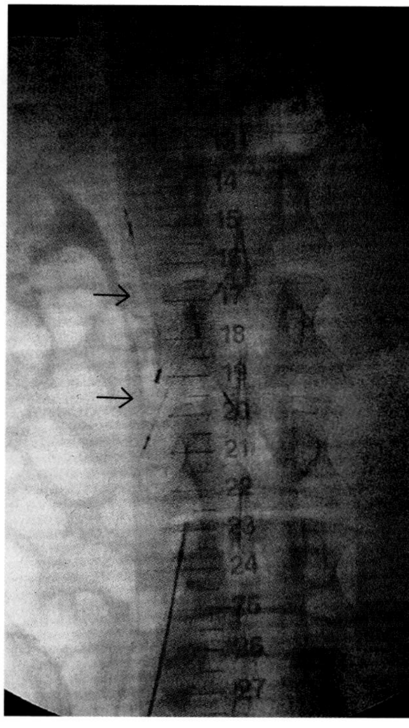

Fig. 21-73. Radiograph with IVC filter in place.

Insertion of Venous Access Devices

The placement of venous access devices has become a common procedure in vascular and interventional units because the insertion of the catheter may be followed under fluoroscopy. These venous catheters are used for administering chemotherapy or large amounts of antibiotics, for frequent blood tests, and for total parenteral nutrition (TPN). The catheters may remain in place for several months, depending on the type being used and the clinical indication. The three most common devices inserted include the following:

- **Peripherally inserted central catheter** (PICC line) may remain in place for up to 6 months. The proximal catheter tip is positioned near the right atrium, and the distal end remains exposed and must be covered.
- **Hickman line** is usually used for TPN and for patients having bone marrow transplantation. The catheter tip is positioned near the right atrium, and the distal end is tunneled under the skin.
- **Subcutaneous port** is the most permanent and the most expensive. The catheter tip is placed near the right atrium, and the injection port for chemotherapy is just beneath the chest wall.

The lines are inserted under strict aseptic conditions because the patient is often immunocompromised. Access to the venous system is usually through the cephalic vein or the jugular vein.

Risks and complications Complications include infection, thrombosis, and pneumothorax.

Transjugular Intrahepatic Portosystemic Shunt

A transjugular intrahepatic portosystemic shunt (TIPS) is a vascular interventional procedure developed to treat variceal bleeding (caused by portal hypertension), refractory ascites, and cirrhosis. TIPS is useful in managing a variety of patients, ranging from those with end-stage liver disease to those awaiting liver transplantation. This procedure creates an artificial passageway to allow portal venous circulation to bypass the normal route through the liver (Fig. 21-74).

The portal system is accessed through the right jugular vein. A sheath is inserted to protect vessels from needle and catheter manipulations. Using fluoroscopic guidance and a transjugular needle, the needle is advanced, following the venous structures until it reaches the **hepatic vein.** The needle is then advanced **through** an **intrahepatic vein, through the liver, to the portal vein.** A guide wire is advanced through the needle, which is removed, so that a balloon (angioplasty) catheter may be advanced. The balloon on the catheter is then inflated to create a tract through the liver. A metallic stent is placed across the tract that has been formed to maintain its patency.

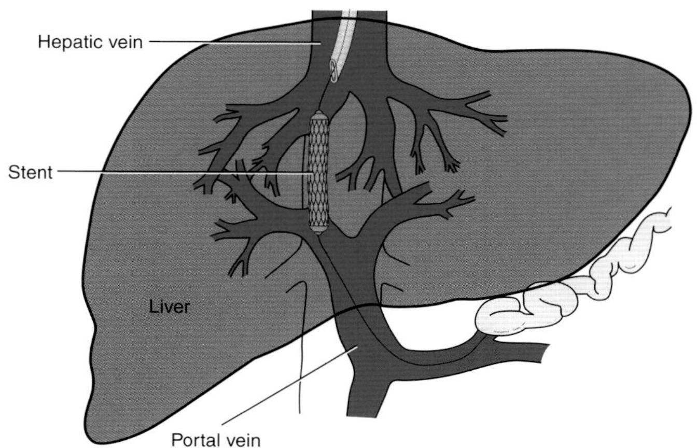

Fig. 21-74. Intrahepatic stent placement in a TIPS procedure.

Risks and complications Primary complications of the procedure include hemorrhage and thrombus formation. Later, risk for stenosis or occlusion of the TIPS exists, so patient progress is monitored closely. Increased incidence of hepatic encephalopathy after this procedure also exists. Because much of the blood is bypassing the liver, the blood contains a higher than normal level of toxins. This affects the brain and may cause confusion, disorientation, and in extreme cases, coma. In severe cases of hepatic encephalopathy, the TIPS may have to be occluded.

Research is ongoing to find methods to increase the long-term effectiveness of TIPS. Possible adjuncts to the procedure include anticoagulation therapy and development of a stent-graft.

Thrombolysis

If diagnostic angiographic studies demonstrate that a vessel is blocked by a thrombus (clot), a **thrombolysis** procedure may be indicated. If blood-clotting coagulation laboratory studies support this procedure, a thrombolysis may be performed, wherein the clot or thrombus is lysed (disintegrated) by passing a guide wire and catheter through the clot or as far into the clot as possible.

A dissolving agent is then injected through the catheter into the region of the thrombus. Various types of catheters may be used for this, such as a pulse spray type or an infusion type (Fig. 21-75).

The pulse spray method involves hand injection with a syringe, whereas the infusion method generally involves a slow injection process using a pump to slowly infuse the dissolving agent over a period of hours or even several days. The catheter may be advanced during this time as the thrombus is being dissolved.

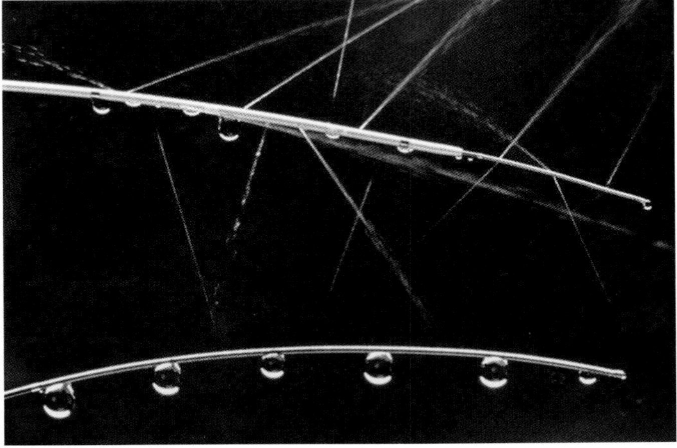

Fig. 21-75. Thrombolysis pulse spray and infusion catheters. (Courtesy Medi-tech/Boston Scientific Corporation.)

Risks and complications Possible complications with this procedure include bleeding and partially dissolved clots moving on to block other smaller vessels.

Infusion Therapy

The infusion of therapeutic drugs may be by a systemic or a superselective approach. Treatment duration ranges from a few days to several weeks. The type of approach and the duration of infusion therapy are determined by the pathology present, the area to be treated, the patient's condition, and the results of previous therapeutic methods. Vasoconstrictors, vasodilators, chemotherapeutic drugs, and radioactive materials are employed for infusion therapy.

Vasoconstrictors are used to help control bleeding. A common vasoconstricting drug currently employed is vasopressin (Pitressin), which may be administered intravenously or intraarterially. Vasodilators are useful in the treatment of vascular spasms or constriction. Currently, sodium nitroprusside is employed for vascular spasms, and papaverine relieves nonocclusive mesenteric vascular ischemia.

Infusion of drugs for chemotherapeutic reasons is used in patients with advanced nonresectable malignancies. The percentage of patients responding to chemotherapy varies greatly.

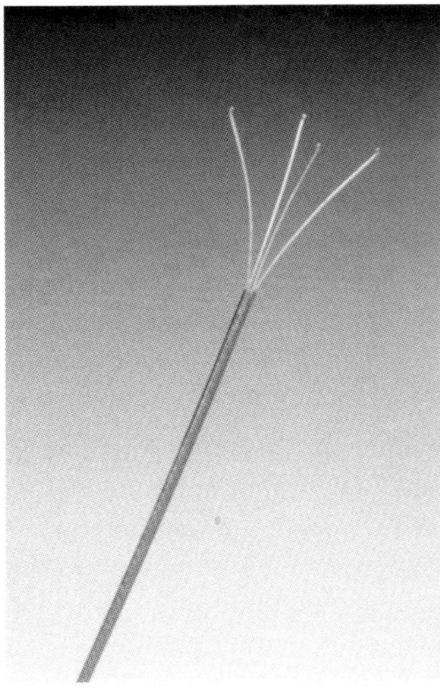

Fig. 21-76. Retrieval instruments—grasping forceps. (Courtesy Medi-tech/Boston Scientific Corporation.)

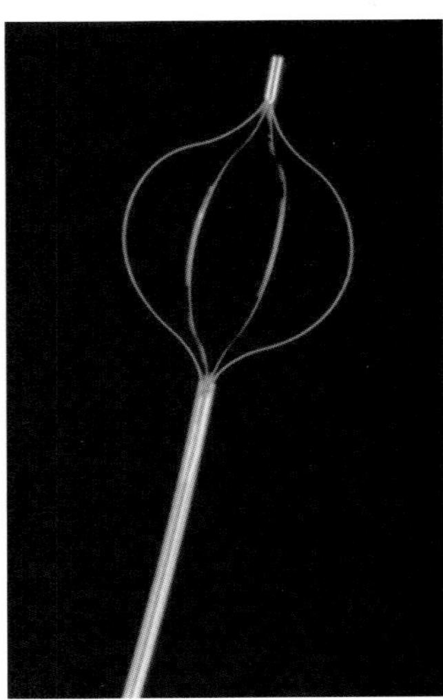

Fig. 21-77. Retrieval basket. (Courtesy Medi-tech/Boston Scientific Corporation.)

Extraction of Vascular Foreign Bodies

Most foreign bodies found in the vascular system are limited to calculi, fragments of vascular catheters or guide wires, pacemaker electrodes, and shunts. Some common instruments used to retrieve the foreign bodies include loop snares, ureteral stone basket catheters, and endoscopic grasping forceps. To remove foreign bodies with a loop snare or a basket catheter, the catheter is inserted beyond the foreign body and then withdrawn to catch the foreign body.

Risks and complications Care should be taken to avoid tearing the vascular intima lining when removing foreign bodies that are adhered to the vessel; these must be removed surgically.

NONVASCULAR INTERVENTIONAL PROCEDURES

Percutaneous Vertebroplasty and Kyphoplasty

Vertebroplasty Percutaneous vertebroplasty is used to treat patients who have vertebral pain and instability caused by osteoporosis, spinal metastases, compression fractures, or vertebral angiomas. A percutaneous injection of acrylic cement into the vertebral body under fluoroscopic guidance contributes to stabilization of the spine and long-term pain relief (Figs. 21-78 and 79).

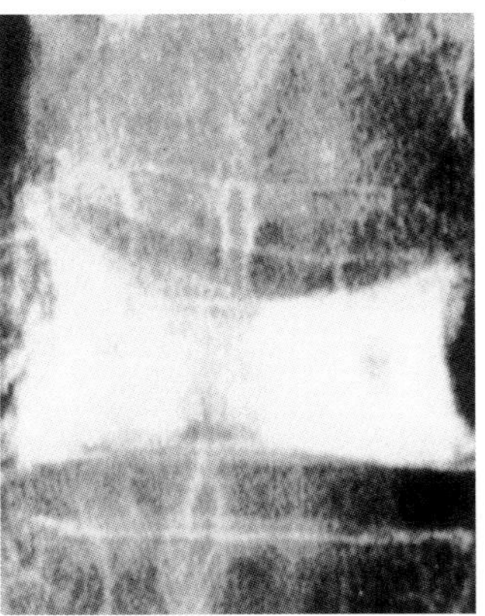

Fig. 21-78. Vertebroplasty of T10 vertebral body. (Courtesy Philips Medical Systems.)

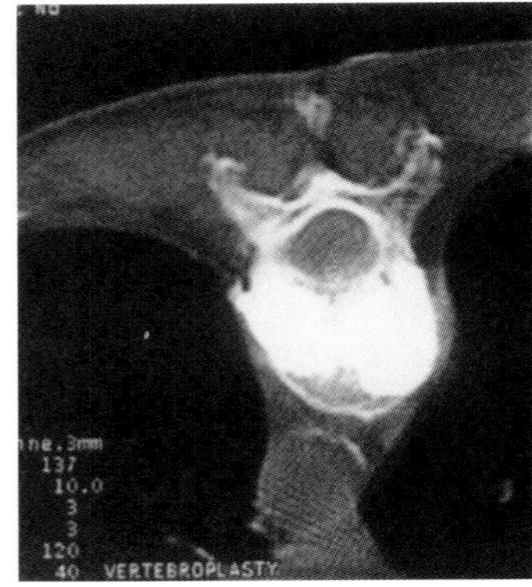

Fig. 21-79. CT demonstrating cement deposition throughout vertebral body. (Courtesy Philips Medical Systems.)

Kyphoplasty The vertebroplasty technique has more recently been modified, leading to a procedure known as *kyphoplasty.* Through small incisions, a kyphoplasty balloon is inserted into a collapsed vertebral body. The balloon is inflated, intending to restore the collapsed portion of the vertebrae (Fig. 21-80). Acrylic cement is then injected to stabilize the vertebrae.

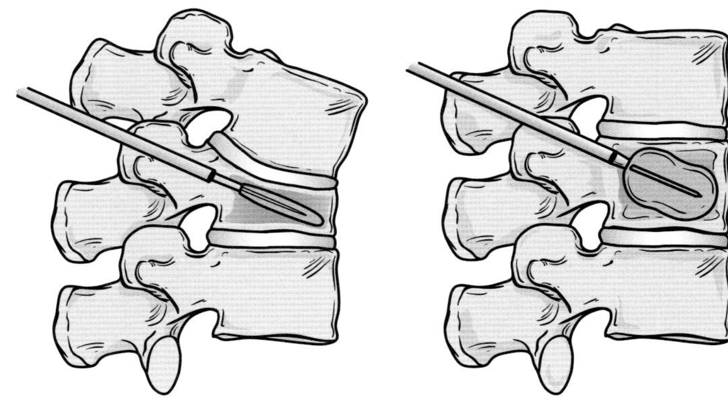

Fig. 21-80. Kyphoplasty drawings illustrate vertebrae before and after balloon is inflated.

Risks and complications Complications of vertebroplasty include leakage of the cement into adjacent structures, which may require emergency surgery. A less common complication is pulmonary embolus, causing migration of the cement into perivertebral veins.

The complications from kyphoplasty are less than for vertebroplasty since less cement is required and it is injected in a more controlled fashion.

Enteric Stenting

Using guide wires and catheters, stents are advanced into the colon under fluoroscopic (and sometimes endoscopic) guidance (Fig. 21-81). This procedure is used preoperatively to reduce postoperative complications in the case of bowel obstructions and as a palliative measure for colonic strictures because of inoperable neoplastic disease. Placement of the stent allows for decompression of the obstructed bowel and relief of severity of patient symptoms (Fig. 21-82).

Stents may also be inserted into the biliary tract to open blocked ducts and in the esophagus to relieve obstructions.

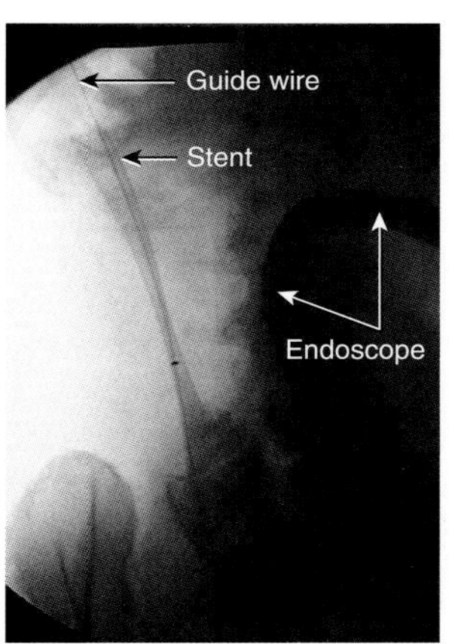

Fig. 21-81. Image during stenting procedure, showing endoscope, guide wire, and stent.

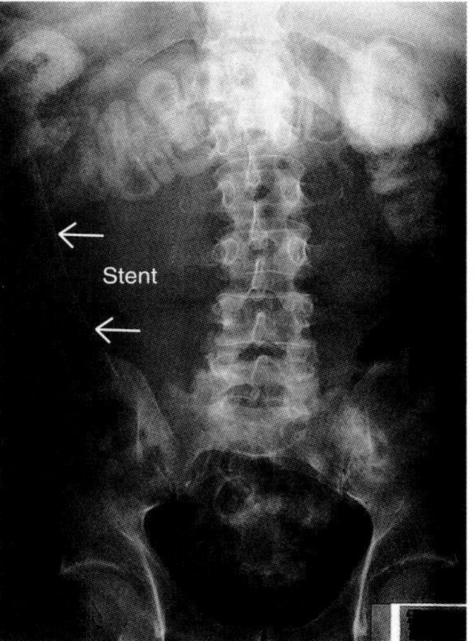

Fig. 21-82. Abdomen (KUB) 2 days postprocedure, illustrating some opening of stricture and gastrografin passing through stent into portions of large bowel.

Risks and complications Complications and risks of the procedure include migration of the stent, perforation, and bleeding.

Nephrostomy

Nephrostomy may be performed for diagnostic or therapeutic reasons and is useful in treating several types of kidney pathologies or disorders. Nephrostomy is useful as a diagnostic procedure for renal function assessment, a urine culture, brush biopsy, Whitaker test to determine cause of urinary tract dilation, nephroscopy, and failed retrograde pyelography. Therapeutic reasons for performing nephrostomy include stone diversion, chemolysis, and abscess drainage.

In this procedure, a catheter (Fig. 21-83) is introduced through the skin and kidney parenchyma to the renal pelvis or other target area (Fig. 21-84). After proper catheter placement, the specific intervention such as drainage and stone removal occurs.

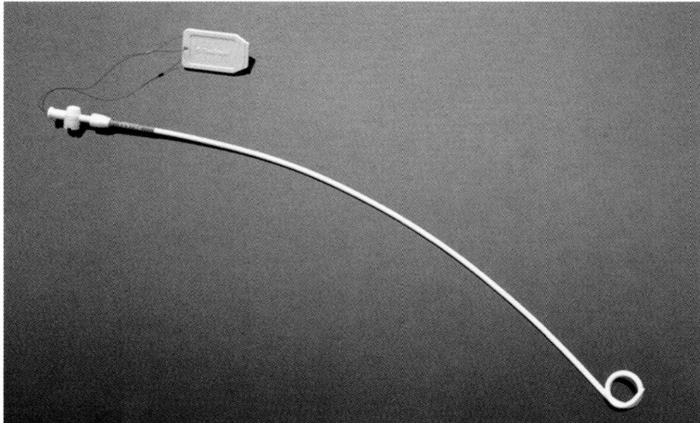

Fig. 21-83. Nephrostomy drainage catheter. (Courtesy Medi-tech/ Boston Scientific Corporation.)

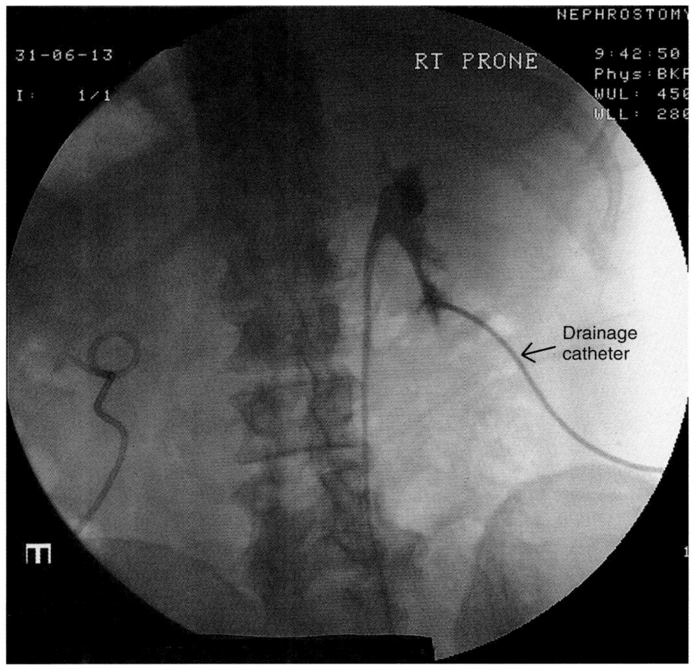

Fig. 21-84. Nephrostomy catheter inserted into renal pelvis.

21

Percutaneous Biliary Drainage

Percutaneous biliary drainage (PBD) can be used for many reasons, such as internal or external drainage, stone removal, dilation of obstructed bile duct, and biopsy. The most common use of PBD is as a palliative procedure for unresectable malignant disease. Less popular uses include the treatment of biliary obstruction, suppurative cholangitis, postoperative or posttraumatic biliary leakage, and stone removal.

Patients undergoing PBD tend to have infected bile. To avoid the spread of infection, antibiotics should be administered at least 1 hour before the procedure.

A common use of PBD is internal or external drainage. External treatment usually involves placement of the catheter in the duodenum. Internal drainages use a stent or catheter. Often an external drain is in place for a couple of days and then the catheter is capped, resulting in internal drainage.

Percutaneous Abdominal Abscess Drainage

Percutaneous abdominal drainage (PAD) has a 70% to 80% success rate. It is indicated when abdominal or pelvic abscess cannot be readily treated by simple incision and when the location of the abscess is in a safe place for needle entry. If present, foreign bodies should be removed because they serve as foci of infection. If no improvement is seen in 24 to 48 hours, another treatment method may be considered.

Needle aspiration Needle placement is performed under CT or sonography. Sonography is better for superficial abscess, for abscess in solid material, and when the abscess is not surrounded by bowel. The advantage of sonography is that it allows for continuous monitoring. The procedure requires a 20- or 22-gauge needle to be positioned in the abscess, through which fluid is withdrawn for immediate Gram's stain and other tests. If the fluid is purulent, the drainage procedure continues. If the material is sterile, the fluid is withdrawn and the needle is removed. The fluid is removed using gravity or a special suction pump. The gravity method is preferred because suction may erode the abscess wall or cause the wall to adhere to the catheter.

Catheter drainage Catheter drainage using the Seldinger over-the-wire technique may be used for inserting the catheter. An example of this is the Van Sonnenberg Sump drain-type catheter illustrated in Fig. 21-85. If a sump pump type of arrangement is used, a double-lumen type catheter is required, in which room air can flow into the abscess region while the suction is being applied. This simultaneous drainage and venting prevents suction, which will cause the abscess material to cling to the walls of the catheter, blocking the drainage holes. The "pig tail" type of design at the end of the catheter shown in Fig. 21-85 aids in retention or accidental withdrawal.

The catheter is removed when no more symptoms exist or the signs of infection disappear (normal WBC), when no more drainage occurs, or when a postprocedural CT or ultrasound is normal.

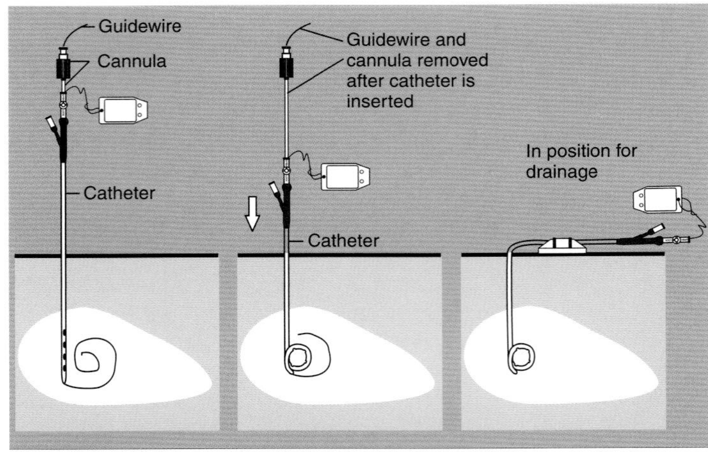

Fig. 21-85. Over-the-wire (Seldinger) technique with Van Sonnenberg Sump drain catheter. (Courtesy Medi-tech/Boston Scientific Corporation.)

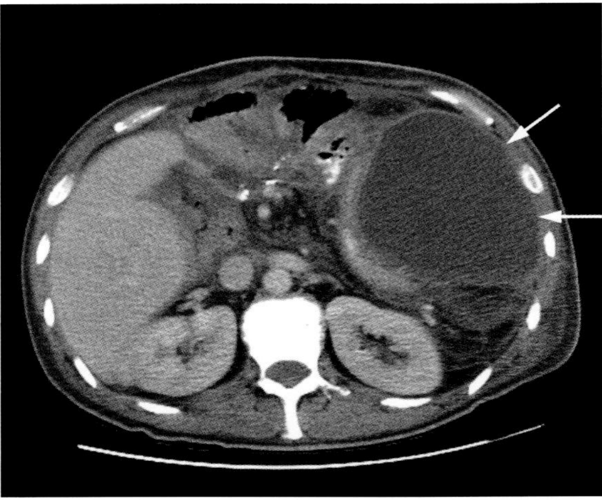

Fig. 21-86. Before drainage of abdominal abscess (see arrows to large dark area on your right).

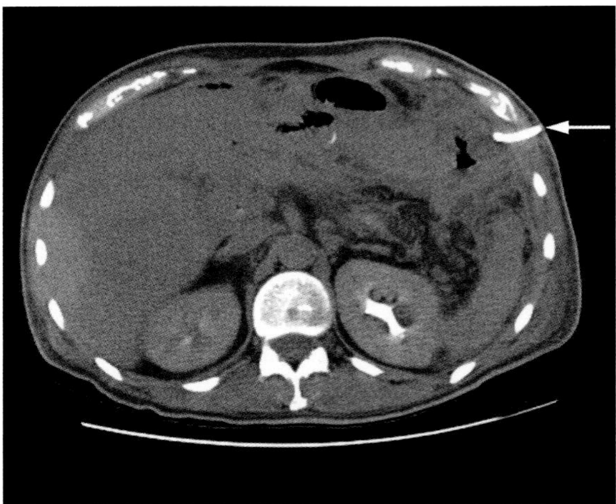

Fig. 21-87. After drainage of abscess (see arrow to drainage tube).

Percutaneous Needle Biopsy

Percutaneous needle biopsy is performed when primary or metastatic malignancy is suspected. A biopsy is useful in providing information about the stage and extent of the disease, confirming whether a tumor recurrence occurs, and diagnosing infection.

To perform a biopsy, a site and depth of the pathology are determined. Correct positioning of the needle may be achieved by monitoring needle introduction with sonography, CT, or fluoroscopy. Sonography is the modality of choice for lesions in organs that differ significantly in echogenicity from adjacent structures—as long as the lesion is not surrounded by gas, fat, or calcified structures, such as liver, kidney, and pelvic organs. CT is good for small, deep lesions, especially those surrounded by large vessels or bowel. The disadvantage of CT is the time needed for placement of the needle, scanning, and repositioning. Fluoroscopy is best for lesions that differ significantly in radiopacity from surrounding tissue, such as pulmonary pleura, osseous lesions, and lymph nodes filled with contrast medium.

A tissue sample is obtained by advancing the needle to the target and alternately moving it vertically 1 to 2 cm and rotating it. The needle is then removed, and the sample is prepared for immediate examination. At least four samples should be taken to include the center and peripheral areas.

Research indicates the following accuracy rates for biopsy:

Lung: 85% to 90%

Liver, kidney, and pancreas: 70% to 90%

Lymph node: 50% to 75%

Percutaneous Gastrostomy

Percutaneous gastrostomy is performed for extended feeding (greater than 4 weeks) of patients unable to eat, for gastric decompression, or for dilation of upper GI tract when the oral approach fails. Individuals who may be candidates for gastrostomy include those with impaired swallowing because of neurologic disease or obstructing oropharyngeal and esophageal tumors; burn patients; trauma patients; cancer patients suffering from anorexia; or patients with pharyngeal or esophageal fistulae.

In this procedure, preexaminations are performed to ensure that no organ is located over the puncture site to avoid puncturing these organs. A nasogastric tube is placed in the stomach to inflate the stomach with 500 to 1000 ml of air. The puncture site is at the upper or middle area of the stomach. A tube is placed and secured in the stomach. Once the tube is positioned, the patient is suctioned for 24 hours, after which feeding begins.

References

Alternative modalities and procedures

Kerns SR, Hawkins IF, Sabatelli FW: Current status of carbon dioxide angiography, Radiol Clin North Am 33(1):15-29, 1995.

Moret J, Kembers R, Op de Beek, J et al: 3D rotational angiography: clinical value in endovascular treatment, Medicamundi 42(3): 8-14, 1998.

Wagner HJ, Kalinowski M, Klose Kj, Alfke H: The use of gadolinium chelates for x-ray subtraction angiography, Invest Radiol 36(5):257-265, 2001.

Wilson MA: Textbook of nuclear medicine, Philadelphia, 1998, Lippincott-Raven.

Interventional angiography

Binkert CA, Ledermann H, Jost R, et al: Acute colonic obstruction: clinical aspects and cost-effectiveness of preoperative and palliative treatment with self-expanding metallic stents—a preliminary report, Radiology 206:199-204, 1998.

Clark T: TIPS: current roles and trends, Appl Radiol 10-15, 1998.

Katzen BT, Becker GJ, Mascioli CA, et al: Creation of a modified angiography (endovascular) suite for transluminal endograft placement and combined interventional-surgical procedures, J Vasc Interv Radiol (2) 161-167, 1996.

Padovani B, Kasriel O, Brunner P, Peretti-Viton P: Pulmonary embolism caused by acrylic cement: a rare complication of percutaneous vertebroplasty, Am J Neuroradiol 20(3):375-377, 1999.

Soulen MC, Shlansky-Goldbert RD: Powerful forces reshape practice of interventional radiology, Diagn Imaging 20:37-51, 1998.

Teng RM: Endovascular grafting for aneurysmal disease and trauma, Appl Radiol 26-31, 1998.

Tortorici MR, Apfel PJ: Advanced radiographic and angiographic procedures with an introduction to specialized imaging, Philadelphia, 1995, FA Davis.

Vanninen R, Koivisto T, Saari T, Hernesniemi J, et al: Ruptured intracranial aneurysms: acute endovascular treatment with electrolytically detachable coils—a prospective randomized study, Radiology 211:325-336, 1999.

Weil A, Chiras J, Simon JM, et al: Spinal metastases: indications for and result of percutaneous injection of acrylic surgical cement, Radiology 199:241-247, 1996.

CHAPTER 22

Computed Tomography

CONTRIBUTIONS BY **Cindy Murphy,** RT R, ACR, BHSc
CONTRIBUTORS TO PAST EDITIONS Barry T. Anthony, RT(R), James D. Lipcamon, RT(R)

CONTENTS

RADIOGRAPHIC ANATOMY

This chapter covers computed tomography (CT) procedures of three body divisions: (1) the **cranium (brain)** and **spinal cord,** (2) the **thorax,** or **chest,** and (3) the **abdomen** and **pelvis.** The gross anatomy for these body divisions needs to be mastered before studying the detailed sectional anatomy as seen on CT images.

The anatomy of these body divisions has been described and demonstrated in previous chapters, except for the anatomy of the central nervous system, which includes the brain and spinal cord as follows:

Gross Anatomy of the Central Nervous System—Brain and Spinal Cord

The anatomy related to **cranial or head CT** includes the bony anatomy of the skull and facial bones, as described in **Chapters 12 and 13.** The anatomy of the **central nervous system** (CNS), as seen on head and spine CT images, includes the **brain** and **spinal cord.**

NEURONS

Neurons, or nerve cells, are the specialized cells of the nervous system that conduct electrical impulses. Each neuron is composed of an **axon,** a **cell body,** and one or more **dendrites.**

Dendrites are processes that conduct impulses **toward** the neuron cell body. An axon is a process **leading away from** the cell body.

A **multipolar motoneuron** is shown in Fig. 22-1. This type of neuron is typical of the neurons conducting impulses from the spinal cord to muscle tissue. A multipolar neuron is one **with several dendrites and a single axon.**

The **dendrites** and **cell bodies** make up the **gray matter** of the brain and spinal cord, and the large myelinated **axons** make up the **white matter,** as is seen on later drawings and CT scans.

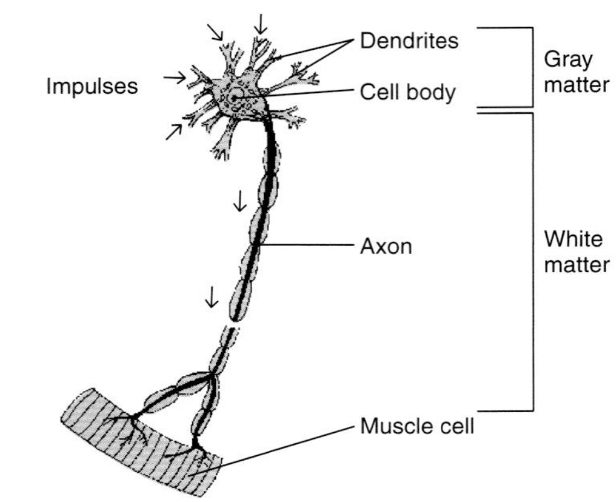

Fig. 22-1. Multipolar motoneuron (several dendrites, one axon).

DIVISIONS OF THE CENTRAL NERVOUS SYSTEM

One must know the general gross anatomy of the brain and central nervous system before learning sectional anatomy as seen on tomographic sections or slices.

The central nervous system can be divided into two main divisions: (1) the **brain,** which occupies the cavity of the cranium, and (2) the solid **spinal cord,** which extends inferiorly from the brain and is protected by the bony vertebral column. The solid spinal cord terminates at the lower border of **L1,** with a tapered area called the **conus medullaris** *(ko'nus med'u-lar-is).* Nerve root extensions of the spinal cord, however, continue down to the first coccyx segment. The subarachnoid space continues down to sacrum segment two (S2).

Summary of Spinal Cord Anatomy The drawing in Fig. 22-2 demonstrates three anatomic factors of the brain and spinal cord important radiographically, as follows:

1. The **conus medullaris** is the distal tapered ending of the spinal cord at the **lower level of L1.**
2. The **subarachnoid space,** containing cerebrospinal fluid (CSF), a clear, colorless watery liquid, surrounds both the spinal cord and the brain and continues down to the lower **second segment of the sacrum (S2).**
3. A common **lumbar puncture site,** as required for a spinal tap or for removal of CSF and the injection of contrast media for a myelogram, is **between the spines of L3 and L4.** The needle can enter the subarachnoid space without the danger of striking the spinal cord, which ends at the lower level of L1 vertebra.

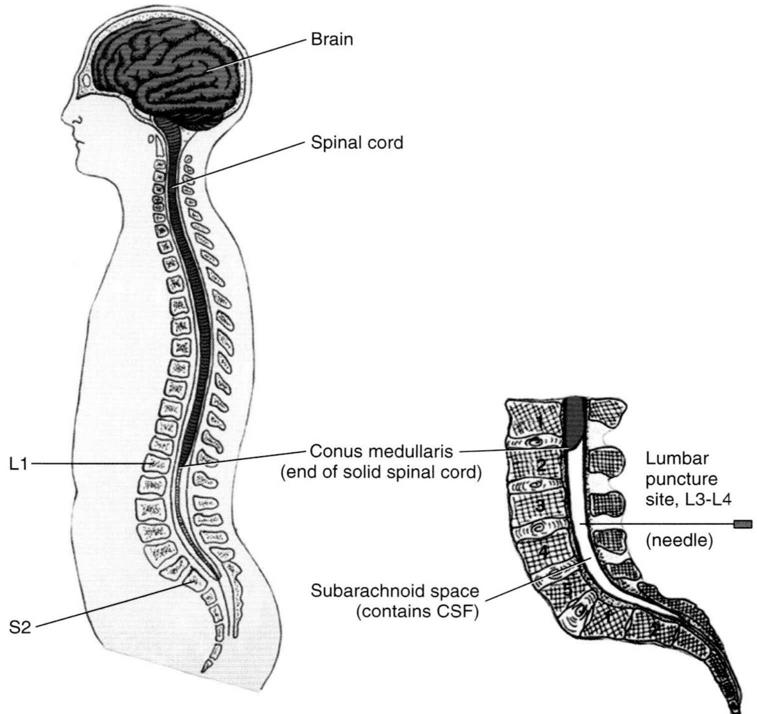

Fig. 22-2. Central nervous system (CNS).

Brain and Spinal Cord Coverings—Meninges

Both the brain and spinal cord are enclosed by **three** protective coverings or membranes termed **meninges** (Fig. 22-3). Starting externally these are the (1) **dura mater** *(du'rah ma'ter),* (2) **arachnoid** *(ah-rak'noid),* and (3) **pia mater** *(pi'ah ma'ter).*

Dura mater: The outermost membrane is the **dura mater,** which means "hard" or "tough mother." This strong, fibrous brain covering has an **inner** and **outer layer.** The outer layer of the dura mater is tightly fused to the inner layer, except for spaces that are provided for large venous blood channels called **venous sinuses** or **dura mater sinuses.** The outer layer adheres closely to the inner table of the **cranium,** or skull. The inner layers of dura mater below these sinuses join to form the **falx cerebri,** as seen on CT scans extending down into the longitudinal fissure between the two cerebral hemispheres (seen on a later drawing, Fig. 22-6).

Pia mater: The innermost of these membranes is the pia mater, literally meaning "tender mother." This membrane is very thin and highly vascular and lies next to the brain and spinal cord. It encloses the entire surface of the brain, dipping into each of the fissures and sulci.

Arachnoid: Between the pia mater and dura mater is a delicate avascular membrane called the **arachnoid** mater. Delicate, thread-like trabeculae attach the arachnoid membrane to the pia mater, thus its name, meaning "spider mother."

MENINGEAL SPACES (Fig. 22-3)

Immediately exterior to each meningeal layer is a space or potential space. Therefore there are three of these spaces or potential spaces—the (1) **epidural space,** (2) **subdural space,** and (3) **subarachnoid space.**

Epidural space: Exterior to the dura mater, between the dura and the inner table of the skull, is a potential space termed the *epidural space.*

Subdural space: Beneath the dura mater, between the dura and the arachnoid, is a narrow space called the *subdural space,* which contains a thin film of fluid and various blood vessels. Both the epidural and the subdural spaces are potential sites for hemorrhage after trauma to the head.

Subarachnoid space: Beneath the arachnoid membrane, between the arachnoid and the pia mater, is a comparatively wide space termed the *subarachnoid space.* The subarachnoid spaces of the brain and spinal cord are normally filled with **cerebrospinal fluid (CSF).**

THREE DIVISIONS OF THE BRAIN

The brain can be divided into three general areas: (1) the **forebrain,** (2) the **midbrain,** and (3) the **hindbrain.** These three divisions of the brain are further divided into specific areas and structures, as shown on the midsagittal sectional drawing in Fig. 22-4 and in the summary chart of brain divisions on the right. Each of these divisions will be described in more detail later in this chapter.

BRAIN STEM

The combination of **midbrain, pons,** and **medulla oblongata** makes up the **brain stem,** which passes through the large opening at the base of the skull, the foramen magnum, to become the **spinal cord.**

Secondary terms for these brain divisions are included in parentheses in the summary chart on the right.

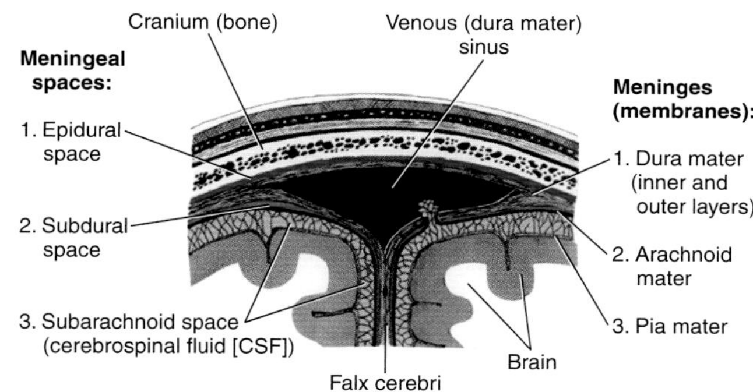

Fig. 22-3. Meninges and meningeal spaces.

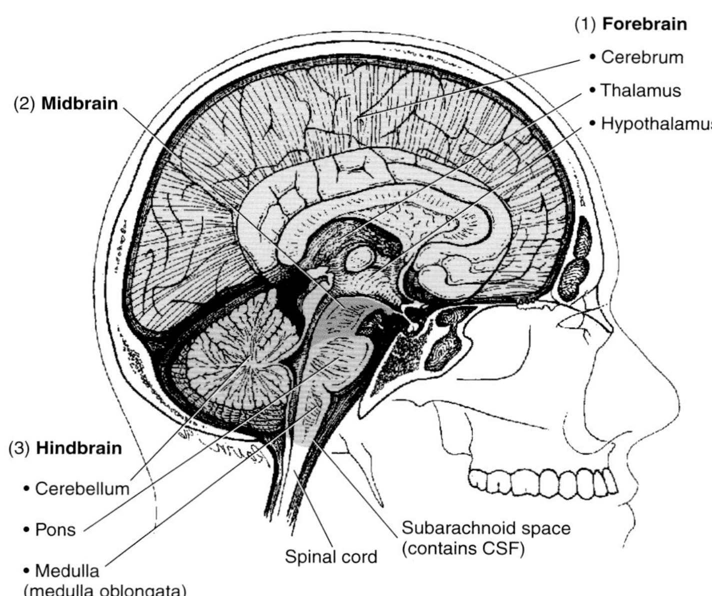

Fig. 22-4. Brain (midsagittal section).

SUMMARY OF BRAIN DIVISIONS

1. Forebrain *(Prosencephalon)*	**Cerebrum**	*(Telencephalon)*
	Thalamus	*(Diencephalon)*
	Hypothalamus	*(Diencephalon)*
2. Midbrain *(Mesencephalon)*	**Midbrain**	Brain stem
3. Hindbrain *(Rhombencephalon)*	**Pons**	Brain stem
	Medulla	Brain stem
	Cerebellum	

Forebrain

The first part of the forebrain to be studied is the large **cerebrum.**

CEREBRUM

A sagittal section through the head and neck leaving the brain and upper spinal cord intact is demonstrated in Fig. 22-5, showing the relative size of the various structures, including the **five lobes** of the cerebrum. The surface layer of the entire cerebrum, about 2 to 4 mm in thickness, directly under the bony skull cap is called the **cerebral cortex.** As can be seen, the total cerebrum occupies the majority of the cranial cavity.

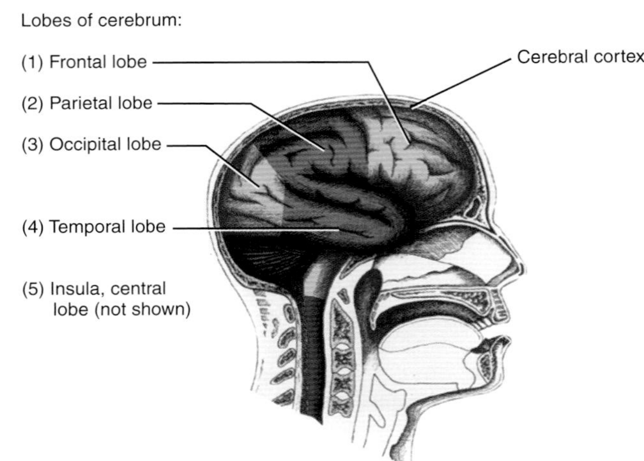

Fig. 22-5. Demonstrates four lobes located in each cerebral hemisphere.

22

Five Lobes of Each Cerebral Hemisphere Each side of the cerebrum is termed a ***cerebral** (ser'e-bral) **hemisphere*** and is divided into five lobes. The four lobes seen in Figs. 22-5 and 22-6 lie beneath the cranial bones of the same name. The **frontal lobe** lies under the frontal bone, with the **parietal lobe** under the parietal bone. Similarly, the **occipital lobe** and the **temporal lobe** lie under their respective cranial bones. The fifth lobe, termed the **insula,** or **central lobe,** is more centrally located and cannot be seen on these views.

CEREBRAL HEMISPHERES

The top of the brain is shown in Fig. 22-6. The cerebrum is partially separated by a deep **longitudinal fissure** in the midsagittal plane. This fissure divides the cerebrum into right and left cerebral hemispheres. Parts of the **frontal, parietal,** and **occipital lobes** are again visualized on this top-view drawing.

The surface of each cerebral hemisphere is marked by numerous grooves and convolutions, which are formed during the rapid embryonic growth of this portion of the brain. Each convolution or raised area is termed a **gyrus.** Two such gyri that be identified on CT sectional radiographs are an **anterior central (precentral) gyrus** and a **posterior central (postcentral) gyrus,** as shown on each side of the **central sulcus.** A sulcus is a shallow groove, and the central sulcus, which divides the frontal and parietal lobes of the cerebrum, is a landmark used to identify specific sensory areas of the cortex.

A deeper groove is called a **fissure,** such as the deep **longitudinal fissure** separating the two hemispheres.

The **corpus callosum,** located deep within the longitudinal fissure and not visible on this drawing, consists of an arched mass of transverse fibers (white matter) connecting the two cerebral hemispheres.

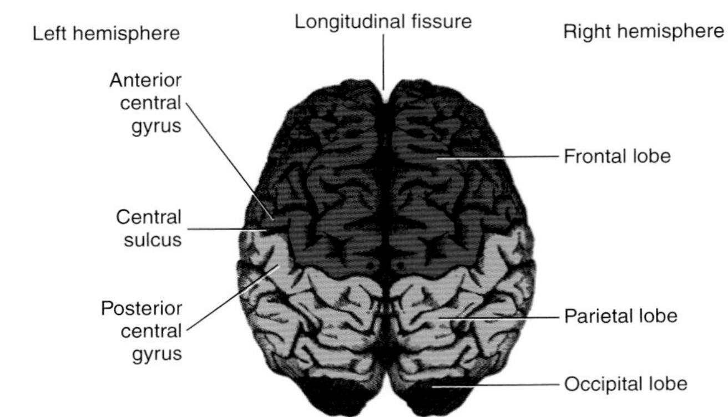

Fig. 22-6. Cerebral hemispheres (top view) demonstrating the frontal, parietal, and occipital lobes and the relative differences among a gyrus, sulcus, and fissure.

CEREBRAL VENTRICLES

A thorough understanding of the cerebral **ventricles** is important for cranial CT because they are readily identified on sectional CT radiographs. The ventricular system of the brain is connected to the subarachnoid space. There are **four cavities** in the ventricular system. These four cavities are filled with CSF and interconnect through small tubes.

The ventricular system contains **four** major cavities.

The **right and left lateral ventricles** are located in the right and left cerebral hemispheres. The **third ventricle** is a single ventricle located centrally and inferior to the lateral ventricles. The **fourth ventricle** is also a single ventricle located centrally, just inferior to the third ventricle.

CSF is formed in the lateral ventricles in specialized capillary beds called **choroid plexuses,** which filter the blood to form CSF. According to *Gray's Anatomy,* about 140 ml of CSF is present within and around the entire CNS, even though up to 500 ml of CSF is formed daily, with the balance being reabsorbed into the venous circulatory system. CSF is believed to serve some nutrient role during development, but in the adult it serves a protective role for the CNS.

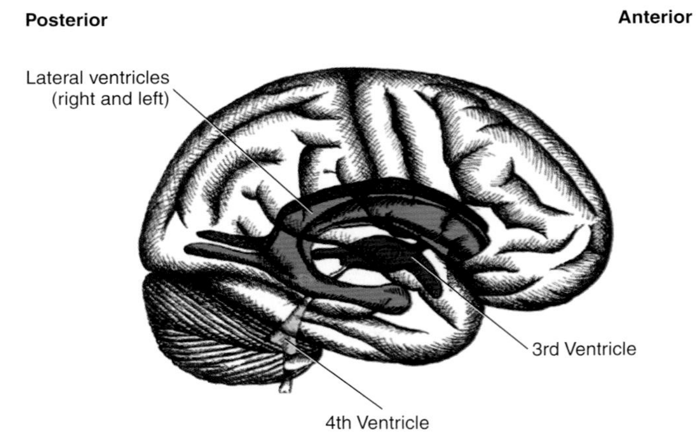

Fig. 22-7. Cerebral ventricles.

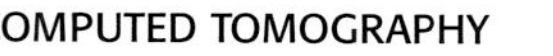

LATERAL VENTRICLES

Each lateral ventricle is composed of four parts. The superior and lateral views in Fig. 22-8 demonstrate that each of the lateral ventricles has a centrally located **body** and three projections, or horns, extending from the body. The **anterior,** or **frontal, horn** is toward the front. The **posterior,** or **occipital, horn** is toward the back, and the **inferior,** or **temporal, horn** extends inferiorly.

The two lateral ventricles are located on each side of the midsagittal plane within the cerebral hemispheres and are mirror images of each other. Certain pathologic processes, such as a space-occupying lesion or "mass lesion," alter the symmetric appearance of the ventricular system, as seen on CT radiographs.

THIRD VENTRICLE

Each of the lateral ventricles connects to the third ventricle through an **interventricular foramen.** The **third ventricle** is located in the midline and is roughly four-sided in shape. It lies just below the level of the bodies of the two lateral ventricles. The **pineal** *(pin'e-al)* **gland** is attached to the roof of the posterior part of the third ventricle directly above the cerebral aqueduct, which causes a recess in the posterior part of this ventricle. (The pineal gland is also shown on a later drawing in Fig. 22-15 in relationship to the thalamus portion of the forebrain.)

FOURTH VENTRICLE

The cavity of the third ventricle connects posteroinferiorly with the **fourth ventricle** through a passage known as the **cerebral aqueduct.** The diamond-shaped fourth ventricle connects with a wide portion of the subarachnoid space called the **cisterna cerebellomedullaris** (see Figs. 22-9 and 22-12).

On each side of the fourth ventricle is a lateral extension termed the **lateral recess,** which also connects with the subarachnoid space through an opening or foramen.

SUPERIOR VIEW OF VENTRICLES

A superior view of the ventricles is shown in Fig. 22-10. This view demonstrates the relationship of the **third and fourth ventricles** to the two **lateral ventricles.** The third ventricle is seen on this view only as a narrow, slitlike structure lying in the midline between and below the bodies of the lateral ventricles.

The **cerebral aqueduct** is clearly shown connecting the third ventricle to the fourth ventricle.

The **lateral recess** is shown on each side of the fourth ventricle, providing a communication with the subarachnoid space.

The **body, inferior horn,** and **anterior** and **posterior horns** of each of the lateral ventricles are again well demonstrated on this top view.

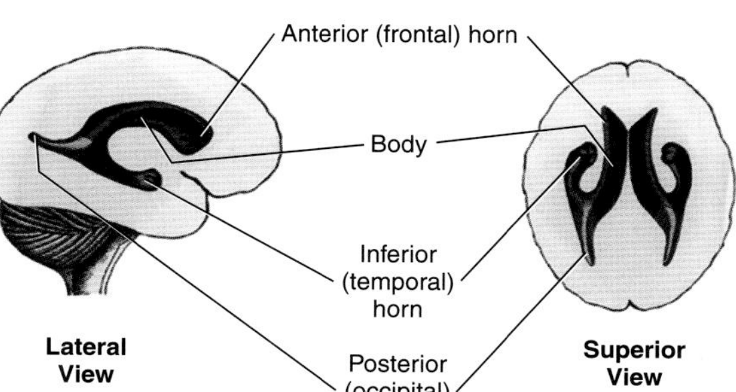

Fig. 22-8. Lateral ventricles.

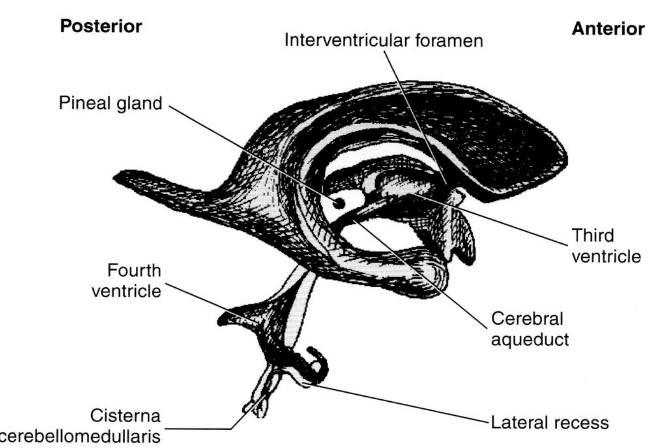

Fig. 22-9. Third and fourth ventricles (lateral view).

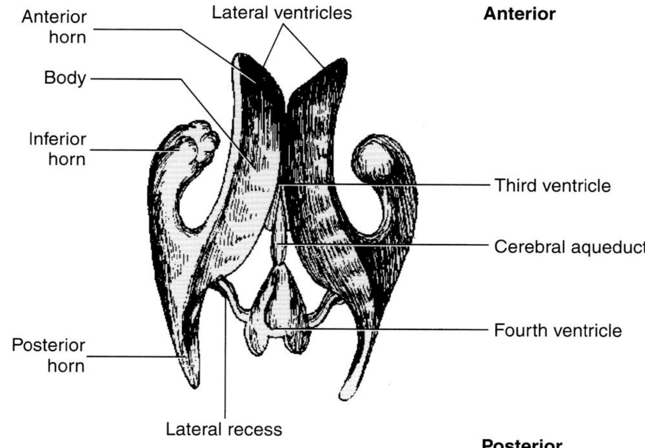

Fig. 22-10. Ventricles (superior view).

22

ANTERIOR VIEW OF VENTRICLES

An anterior view of the ventricles within the brain is shown in Fig. 22-11. The **interventricular foramina** connect the body of each lateral ventricle to the third ventricle. This view emphasizes the fact that the **third** and **fourth ventricles** are midline structures. The **anterior horn, body,** and **inferior horn** of each lateral ventricle are shown on this drawing as they would appear on a frontal projection. The region of the **lateral recess** connecting the fourth ventricle to the subarachnoid space is also shown.

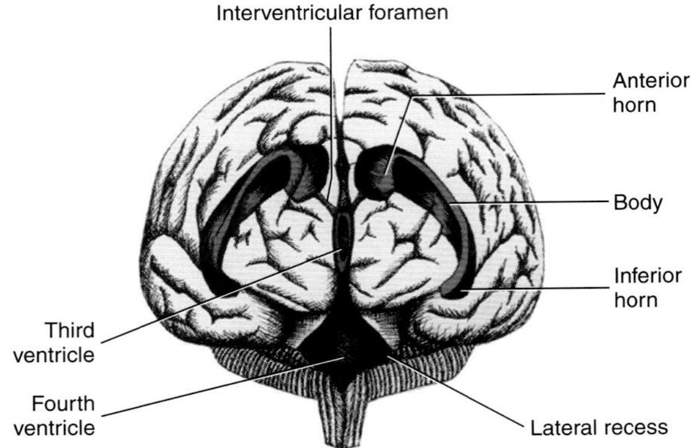

Fig. 22-11. Ventricles (anterior view).

SUBARACHNOID CISTERNS

22

As already noted, CSF is normally manufactured within each lateral ventricle. It then passes through the third ventricle into the fourth. After CSF leaves the **fourth ventricle,** it completely surrounds the brain and spinal cord by filling the **subarachnoid space,** as shown by the red dotted areas in Fig. 22-12. Any blockage along the pathway leading from the ventricles to the subarachnoid space may cause excessive accumulation of CSF within the ventricles, a condition known as *hydrocephalus.*

There are various larger areas within the subarachnoid space or system called **cisterns,** the largest being the **cistern cerebellomedullaris** (cisterna magna), located inferiorly to the fourth ventricle and the cerebellum.

Cisternal Puncture The cistern cerebellomedullaris is the site for a **cisternal puncture** by a needle inserted into this cistern between C1 and the occipital bone to introduce anesthesia into the subarachnoid space. This location is a secondary puncture site, with the L3-L4 space being a primary lumbar puncture site as shown in a previous drawing (Fig. 22-2).

The **cisterna pontis** is located just inferior and anterior to the **pons.** Each of the larger black "dots" in these drawings indicates specific cisterns that are usually named according to their locations. The **chiasmatic cistern,** shown on the top-view drawing of the brain (Fig. 22-13), is so called because of its relationship to the optic chiasma, the site of crossings of optic nerves, as will be identified in later drawings.

Various other cisterns lie along the base of the brain and brain stem. Because the midbrain is totally surrounded by fluid-filled cisterns, this area can be well seen on a CT scan.

The CSF-filled subarachnoid space and ventricular system are important in CT because these areas can be differentiated from tissue structures.

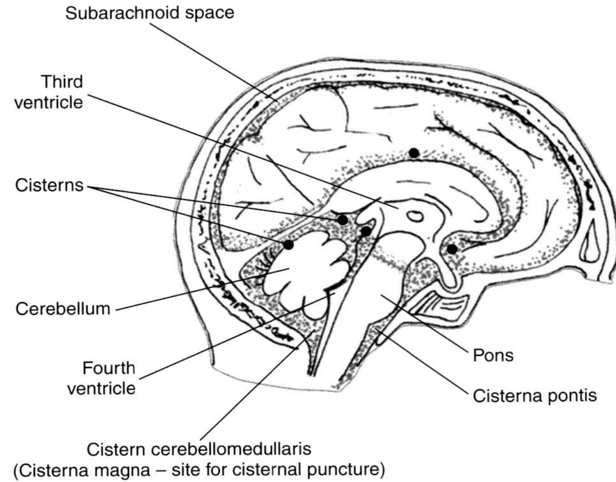

Fig. 22-12. Subarachnoid cisterns—side view.

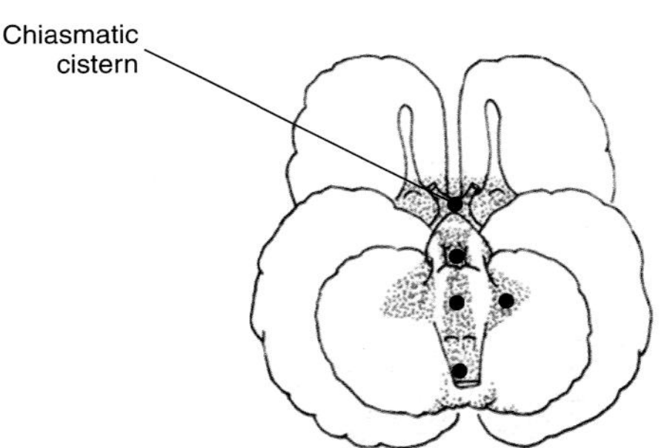

Fig. 22-13. Subarachnoid cisterns—top view.

THALAMUS

Following the large cerebrum, the second part or the forebrain is the **thalamus** (Figs. 22-14 and 22-15). The thalamus is a relatively small oval structure (about 1 inch, or 2.5 cm, in length) located just above the midbrain and under the corpus callosum. It consists of two oval masses of primarily gray matter or nuclei that **form part of the walls of the third ventricle,** just superior to the midbrain.

These groups of nuclei (gray matter) of the thalamus serve as relay stations for most of the sensory impulses as they pass from the spinal cord and midbrain structures into the cerebral cortex. Thus the thalamus serves as **an interpretation center** for certain sensory impulses, such as **pain, temperature,** and **touch,** as well as **certain emotions** and **memory.**

The thalamus and hypothalamus together make up the diencephalon portion of the forebrain, as described previously.

HYPOTHALAMUS

The third and final division of the forebrain is the **hypothalamus** (Figs. 22-14 and 22-15). *Hypo* means "under," thus its location **under the thalamus.** The hypothalamus forms **the floor and lower walls of the third ventricle.** Three significant structures associated with the hypothalamus are the **infundibulum** *(in"fun-dib'u-lum),* **posterior pituitary gland,** and **optic chiasma** *(ki-as'mah).*

The infundibulum is a conical process projecting downward and ending in the posterior lobe of the pituitary gland. The infundibulum plus the posterior pituitary are known as the **neurohypophysis** *(nu"ro-hi-pof'i-sis).*

The **optic chiasma** (Fig. 22-14) is so named because it resembles the Greek letter X (chi). It is located superior to the pituitary gland and anterior to the third ventricle.

The hypothalamus is small in size, but it **controls important body activities** through a link with the endocrine system. Most of these activities are related to **homeostasis,** the tendency or ability of the body to stabilize its normal body states.

Midbrain and Hindbrain

The **midbrain** is seen as a short, constricted portion of the upper brain stem connecting the forebrain to the hindbrain.

The **hindbrain** consists of the **cerebellum, pons,** and **medulla.** As seen in the drawing in Fig. 22-15, the cerebellum is the largest portion of the hindbrain and the second largest portion of the entire brain. The hindbrain is described in detail on the following page.

BRAIN STEM

The brain stem includes the **midbrain** and the **pons** and **medulla.** The pons is a prominent oval structure inferior to the midbrain. The medulla is the final portion of the brain stem, located at the level of the foramen magnum, the opening at the base of the skull. Thus the brain stem is composed of midbrain, pons, and medulla and connects the forebrain to the spinal cord.

PITUITARY AND PINEAL GLANDS

Two important midline structures are the pituitary and pineal glands. The **pineal gland** was demonstrated in its relationship to the third ventricle in Fig. 22-9. This small gland (approximately 5 mm, or ¼ inch, in length) is an **endocrine gland,** which secretes hormones that aid in regulating certain secretory activities.

The important **pituitary gland,** also called the **hypophysis** *(hi-pof'i-sis),* is referred to as the **"master" gland** because it regulates so many body activities. It is located in and protected by the **sella turcica** of the sphenoid bone and is attached to the hypothalamus of the brain by the **infundibulum** (shown in Figs. 22-14 and 22-15). This gland, which is also relatively small, about 1.3 cm (or ½ inch) in diameter, is divided into anterior and posterior lobes. The hormones secreted by this master gland control a wide range of body functions, including growth and reproductive functions.

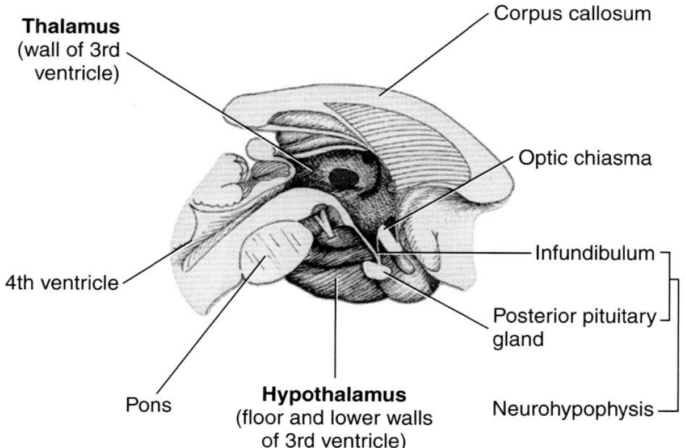

Fig. 22-14. Thalamus and hypothalamus (midsagittal section).

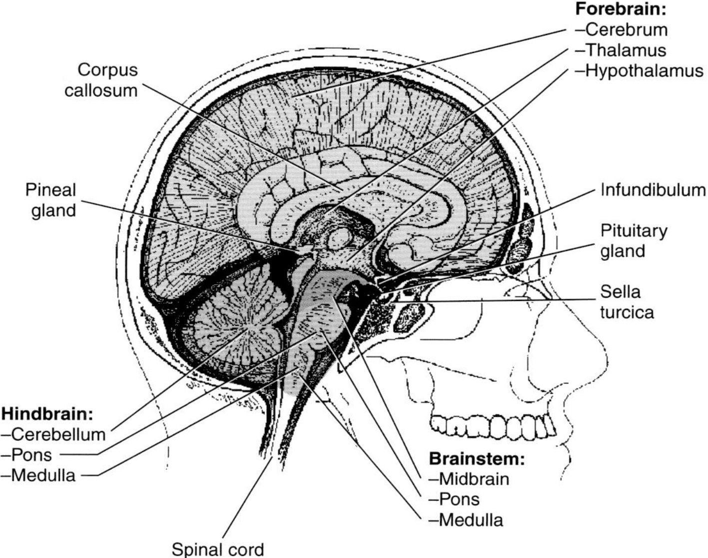

Fig. 22-15. Brain (midsagittal section).

22

CEREBELLUM

The last part of the brain to be described is the **cerebellum** (Fig. 22-16), which occupies the major portion of the inferior and posterior cranial fossa. In the adult the size proportion between the cerebrum and cerebellum is about 8 to 1.

The cerebellum is shaped somewhat like a butterfly and consists of **right** and **left hemispheres** united by a narrow median strip, the **vermis.** Toward the superior end of the anterior surface is the wide, shallow **anterior cerebellar notch.** The fourth ventricle is located within the anterior cerebellar notch, separating the pons and medulla from the cerebellum.

Inferiorly, along the posterior surface the cerebellar hemispheres are separated by the **posterior cerebellar notch.** An extension of the dura mater, termed the **falx cerebelli,** is located within the posterior cerebellar notch.

The cerebellum primarily **coordinates the important motor functions** of the body, such as **coordination, posture,** and **balance.**

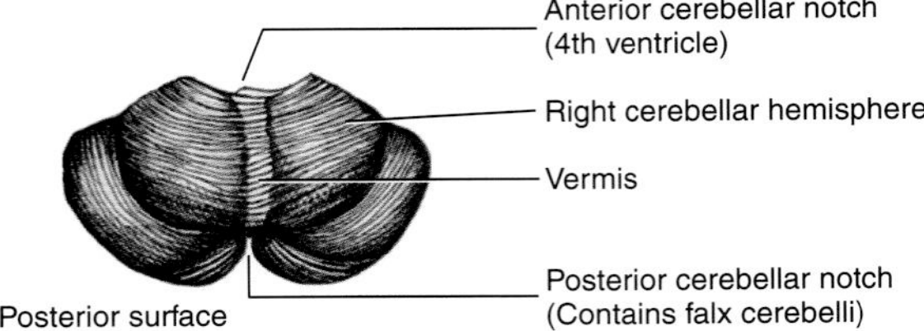

Fig. 22-16. Cerebellum.

22

Gray Matter and White Matter

The CNS can be divided by appearance into white matter and gray matter. **White matter** in the brain and spinal cord is composed of **tracts,** which consist of bundles of **myelinated axons.** Myelinated axons are those axons wrapped in a myelin sheath, a fatty substance having a creamy-white color. Thus axons comprise the majority of the white matter.

The **gray matter** is composed mainly of **neuron dendrites** and **cell bodies.** A section of brain tissue through the cerebral hemispheres is shown in Fig. 22-17. At this level of the brain, gray matter forms the **outer cerebral cortex,** whereas the brain tissue under the cortex is white matter. This underlying mass of white substance is termed the **centrum semiovale.** Deep within the cerebrum, inferior to this level, is more gray matter termed the **cerebral nuclei,** or **basal ganglia.**

Because a cranial CT scan can differentiate between white and gray matter, a section through the cerebral nuclei provides a wealth of diagnostic information. The horizontal or axial section of the right cerebral hemisphere shown in Fig. 22-18 demonstrates those areas that can usually be visualized. Areas of white matter include the **corpus callosum** and **centrum semiovale.** Gray matter areas include the **cerebral nuclei, thalamus,** and **cerebral cortex.**

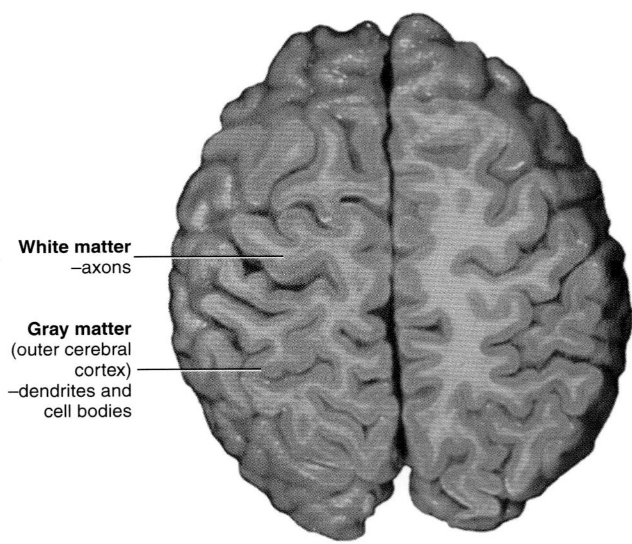

Fig. 22-17. Brain section demonstrating white and gray matter.

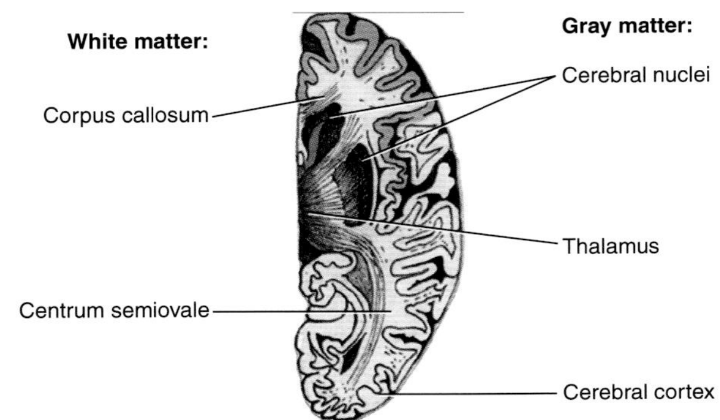

Fig. 22-18. White and gray matter.

SUMMARY—WHITE MATTER VERSUS GRAY MATTER

White Matter White matter consists of **myelinated axons** commonly identified on CT brain sections as light- or white-appearing tissue. It is most commonly seen on sectional scans of the cerebral hemispheres as subcortical white masses of **centrum semiovale,** which are fibers connecting the gray matter of the cerebral cortex with the deep, more caudal parts of the midbrain and spinal cord.

The second major white matter structure is the **corpus callosum,** a band of fibers connecting the right and left cerebral hemispheres deep within the longitudinal fissure.

Gray Matter The thin outer layer of the folds of the **cerebral cortex** is gray matter, made up of dendrites and cell bodies.

Other gray matter of the brain includes more central brain structures, such as the **cerebral nuclei** or **basal ganglia,** located deep within the cerebral hemispheres, and the groups of **nuclei** making up the **thalamus.**

CEREBRAL NUCLEI (BASAL GANGLIA)

The **cerebral nuclei,** or basal ganglia, are paired collections of gray matter deep within each cerebral hemisphere (Fig. 22-19). There are four specific areas or groupings of these cerebral nuclei, as shown on this cutaway drawing. These are the (1) **caudate nucleus,** (2) **lentiform nucleus,** composed of putamen and globus pallidus, (3) **claustrum** (not visible on this drawing), and (4) **amygdaloid nucleus** or body.

The relationship of the **brain stem** and **cerebellum** to three of the cerebral nuclei and to the **thalamus** is shown in this drawing. The cerebral nuclei are bilaterally symmetric collections of gray matter located on **both sides of the third ventricle.**

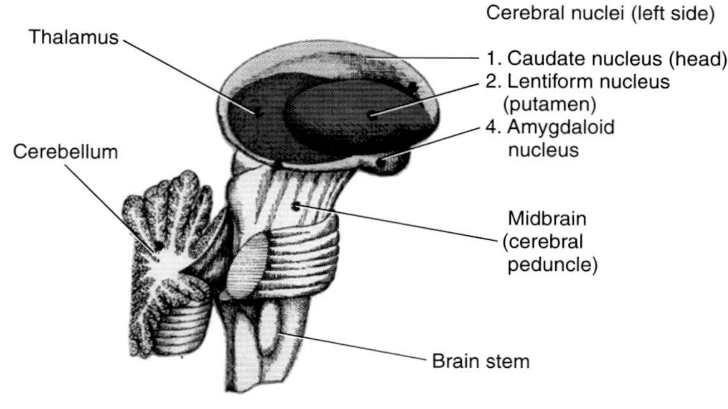

Fig. 22-19. Midsagittal view of cerebral nuclei (basal ganglia) deep within the cerebrum.

BRAIN—INFERIOR SURFACE

This drawing of the inferior surface of the brain demonstrates the **infundibulum, pituitary gland,** and **optic chiasma,** which are anterior to the **pons** and **midbrain** (Fig. 22-20). Extending forward from the optic chiasma are the large **optic nerves,** and extending posterolaterally are the **optic tracts.** A portion of the **corpus callosum** is shown to be located deep within the longitudinal fissure.

CRANIAL NERVES

The 12 pairs of cranial nerves are attached to the base of the brain and leave the skull through various foramina. Identifying all these cranial nerves on radiographs or drawings is generally beyond the scope of anatomy required of technologists.

Technologists, however, should know all the names and general functions described below. They are numbered in order from anterior to posterior with roman numerals. The **smallest** of cranial nerves are **IV,** the **trochlear nerves,** and the **largest** are **V,** the **trigeminal nerves.**

The mnemonic **On Old Olympus' Towering Tops, A Finn** and **German Viewed Some Hops** gives the first letter of each of the 12 pairs of cranial nerves, using two of the older terms as listed in parentheses and underlined, as shown below in the summary chart.

Fig. 22-20. Brain (inferior surface).

SUMMARY OF CRANIAL NERVES

I.	**Olfactory nerve** (smell)	On
II.	**Optic nerve** (vision)	Old
III.	**Oculomotor nerve** (eye movement)	Olympus'
IV.	**Trochlear nerve** (eye movement)	Towering
V.	**Trigeminal nerve** (mixed sensory and motor with three branches)	Tops
VI.	**Abducens nerve** (eye movement)	A
VII.	**Facial nerve** (sensory and motor)	Finn
VIII.	**Vestibulocochlea** (Acoustic) **nerve** (hearing)	And
IX.	**Glossopharyngeal nerve** (taste and swallowing)	German
X.	**Vagus nerve** (sensory and motor)	Viewed
XI.	**Accessory** (Spinal accessory) **nerve** (swallowing)	Some
XII.	**Hypoglossal nerve** (tongue, speech and swallowing)	Hops

ORBITAL CAVITY

The orbital cavities are often filmed as a routine part of cranial CT. The orbital cavity as dissected from the front includes the **bulb** of the eye and numerous associated structures, as illustrated in Fig. 22-21. Orbital contents include the **ocular muscles, nerves** (including the large optic nerve), **blood vessels, orbital fat, lacrimal gland,** and **lacrimal sac and duct.**

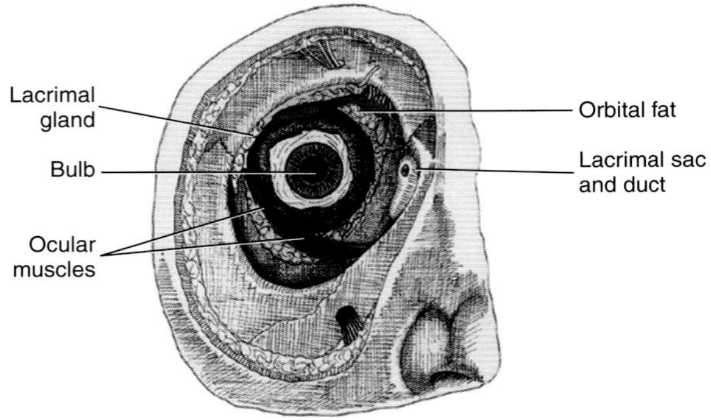

Fig. 22-21. Orbital cavity.

ORBITAL CAVITIES (SUPERIOR VIEW)

The orbital cavities are exposed from above, as shown in Fig. 22-22, by removal of the orbital plate of the frontal bone. The right orbit illustrates the normal fullness of the orbital cavity. The **lacrimal gland** in the upper outer quadrant, **orbit fat,** and **ocular muscles** help fill the entire cavity. The **internal carotid artery** is seen entering the base of the skull. At this point the internal carotid artery has already given off an artery that supplies the orbital contents.

The left orbital cavity, with fat and some muscles removed, illustrates the course of the larger **optic nerve** as it emerges from the bulb to course medially to the **optic chiasma.** Orbital tumors and foreign bodies can be readily detected through CT of the orbits.

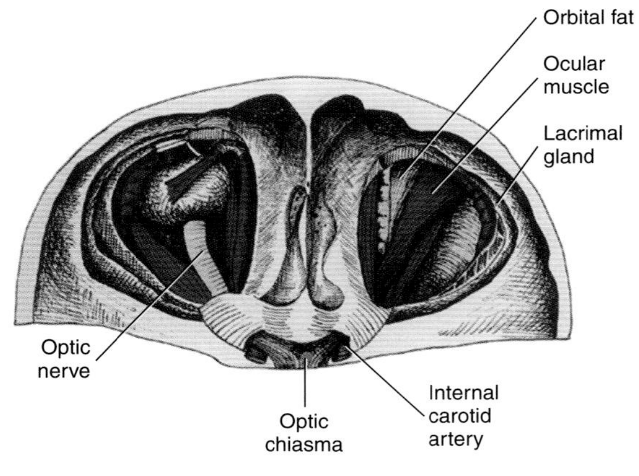

Fig. 22-22. Orbital cavities (superior view).

VISUAL PATHWAY

Axons leaving each eyeball travel via the **optic nerves** to the **optic chiasma.** Within the optic chiasma, some fibers cross to the opposite side and some remain on the same side, as shown in Fig. 22-23. After passing through the optic chiasma, the fibers form an **optic tract.** Each optic tract enters the brain and terminates in the **thalamus.**

In the thalamus, fibers synapse with other neurons, axons of which form the **optic radiations,** which then pass to the **visual centers** in the cortex of the occipital lobes of the cerebrum. Because of the partial crossing of fibers, sight can be affected in various ways, depending on the location of a lesion in the visual pathway. An example is **hemianopia,** which causes blindness or defective vision in only half the visual field of each eye.

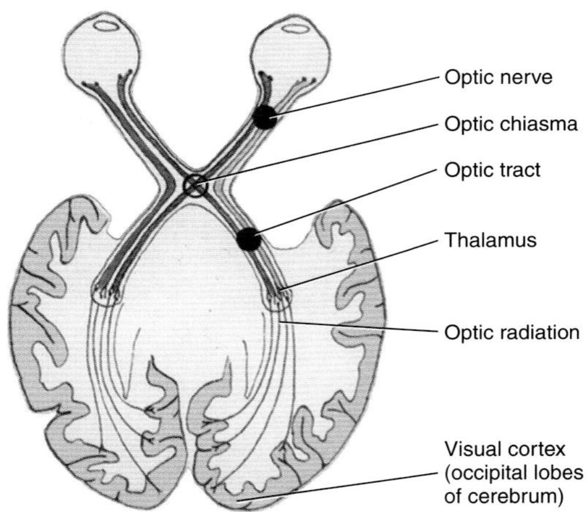

Fig. 22-23. Visual pathway.

BASIC PRINCIPLES

Basic Principles of Computed Tomography

INTRODUCTION

The radiographic term **tomography** is derived from the Greek word *tomos,* meaning "section." CT provides sectional anatomic images in either the **axial, sagittal,** or **coronal plane,** using a complex computer and mechanical imaging system. The concept of CT imaging may be simplified by comparing a procedure to imaging a loaf of bread; conventional radiography captures images of the loaf as a whole, whereas CT takes the loaf and images it in individual *slices* (also called sections, or cuts), which are viewed independently. Refer to Fig. 22-24 for an illustration of this example; the AP abdomen is the "loaf," and the CT image on the right is the "slice."

A CT unit utilizes an x-ray tube and a detector array to gather anatomic data from a patient. These data are reconstructed into an image. Because of the complexity of the procedures and the equipment, CT is often an area of specialty practice for technologists.

This chapter provides an introduction to CT equipment, imaging principles, and clinical applications; additional study on the topic will be required for competence in performing CT procedures.

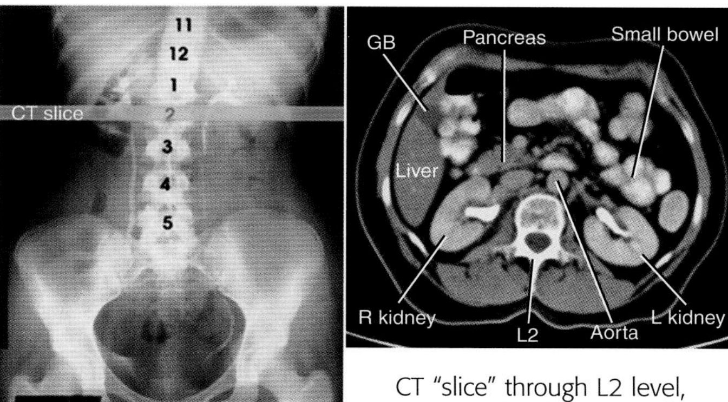

AP abdomen ("loaf").

CT "slice" through L2 level, midkidneys.

Fig. 22-24. Example of CT scan of the abdomen at level of kidneys, L2.

EVOLUTION OF CT

Since the introduction of clinical CT scanning in the early 1970s, systems have evolved through four generations. The difference between each generation is primarily related to the number and arrangement of the *detectors,* the devices that measure the attenuation of the transmitted x-ray beam.

First- and Second-Generation Scanners The **first-generation** scanners used a pencil-thin x-ray beam with **one detector.** It required a $4\frac{1}{2}$-minute exposure time to gather enough information for one slice from a 180° rotation of the tube and detector. These scanners were only capable of head CT.

Second-generation scanners were greatly improved and provided a fan-shaped x-ray beam with **30 or more detectors.** Exposure times were shorter, at about 15 seconds per slice, or 10 minutes for a 40-slice exam.

Third-Generation Scanner The **third-generation** scanner (Fig. 22-25) includes a bank of up to **960 detectors** opposite the x-ray tube that together rotate around the patient in a complete **360° cycle** to demonstrate one slice of tissue. Scanning times were reduced significantly as compared with first- and second-generation scanners.

Fourth-Generation Scanner **Fourth-generation** scanners were developed during the 1980s and possess a **fixed ring** of 4800 or more detectors, completely surrounding the patient in a full circle within the gantry. A single x-ray tube rotates through a 360° arc during data collection. Throughout the continuous rotary motion, short bursts of radiation are provided by a pulsed, rotating-anode x-ray tube providing shorter scan times of as little as 1 minute for an entire exam (similar to a third-generation scanner). It is important to note that fourth-generation technology is not more advanced or more desirable than third-generation technology; it is simply different.

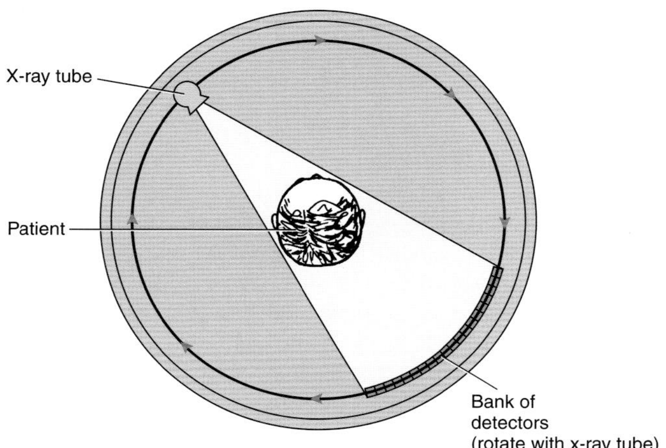

Fig. 22-25. Third-generation scanner; 360° **simultaneous rotation of x-ray tube and detectors.**

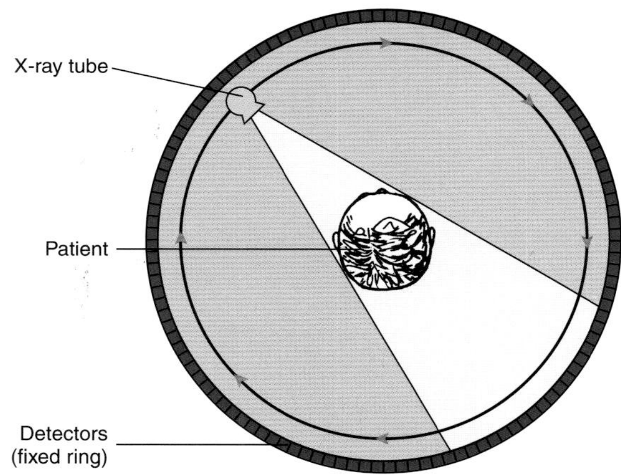

Fig. 22-26. Fourth-generation scanner; detectors on **fixed ring.**

22

VOLUME CT SCANNERS

X-ray tube movement in early CT scanners was restricted by high-tension cables. The x-ray tube would rotate 360° in one direction to obtain one slice; the CT table would advance a set amount; then the x-ray tube would rotate 360° in the opposite direction and obtain the next slice. The development of slip-ring technology in the early 1990s allowed CT technology to move beyond single-slice acquisition.

Slip rings replaced the high tension cables and allowed for **continuous rotation of the x-ray tube,** which when combined with patient movement through the gantry acquired data in a helical or spiral fashion (see Fig. 22-27). The general term to describe this acquisition of a volume of data is *volume scanning.* The terms *helical* and *spiral scanning* are sometimes used to refer to this scanning technique, but these are vendor-specific terms. Volume CT systems are either **third- or fourth-generation** scanners, depending on the manufacturer, and are also capable of single-slice acquisition.

22

Advantages There are several advantages of volume scanning over single-slice scanning.

- **Multiplanar reconstruction (MPR):** Volumetric data allow more accurate reconstruction of patient data into alternative planes (coronal, sagittal, three-dimensional), thus the name *multiplanar reconstruction.*
- **Shorter scan times:** The scan times are shorter since the patient moves continuously through the gantry.
- **Artifacts reduced:** The artifacts caused by patient motion are reduced.

MULTISLICE CT SCANNERS

Third- and fourth-generation scanners developed before 1992 were single-slice scanners capable of imaging only one slice at a time. By late 1998, several CT manufacturers announced that new **multislice technology scanners** were available that were capable of imaging **four slices simultaneously.** These scanners imaged four slices per x-ray tube rotation. The drawing in Fig. 22-28 illustrates the usual single-detector bank scanner on the left with the four multidetector array bank type on the right.

Multislice CT has continued to progress rapidly, largely because of the advances in computer technology. Currently, multislice scanners are available that can image as many as 64 slices per x-ray tube rotation.

Advantages There are several advantages of multislice CT over single-slice or volume CT.

- **Shorter acquisition time:** A state of the art 64-slice system can acquire up to 160 images per second versus a 1-slice per second scanner. This faster imaging is advantageous for procedures that require a single breath hold or in cases in which patient motion is a problem. It also makes procedures that require shorter exposure times possible (e.g., cardiac CT).
- **Decreased amount of contrast media:** A decreased amount of intravenous contrast media can be used due to the increased acquisition speed of multislice scanners.
- **Improved spatial resolution:** Submillimeter slice thickness is possible as a result of multislice technology. This is especially advantageous for examinations of the inner ear and other complex structures. Also, a decreased amount of contrast media is required because of the increased speed of image acquisition.
- **Improved image quality:** Image quality for CT angiography and 3D/MPR is improved as a result of the acquisition of thinner slices.

Disadvantages One disadvantage of multislice scanners is an **increase in cost,** sometimes 30% to 50% higher. Another potential problem involves reviewing and archiving large-volume cases (e.g., data for a 3D reconstruction may consist of more than 1000 images).

CT SYSTEM TERMINOLOGY

As CT technology has evolved, so have the terms used to describe it. Initially *computer-assisted tomography* and *computerized axial tomography* (*CAT*) were used, but as the technology advanced, the accepted term became *computed tomography* (*CT*). Although the term *CAT scan* may still be heard, it is not strictly accurate, because CT images are now available in the sagittal and coronal planes, as well as the axial plane.

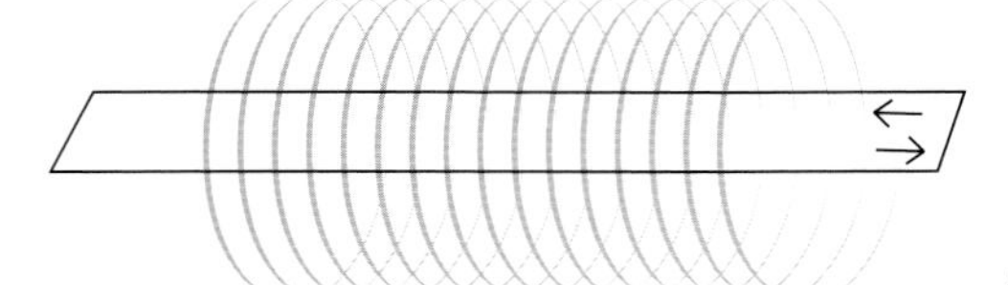

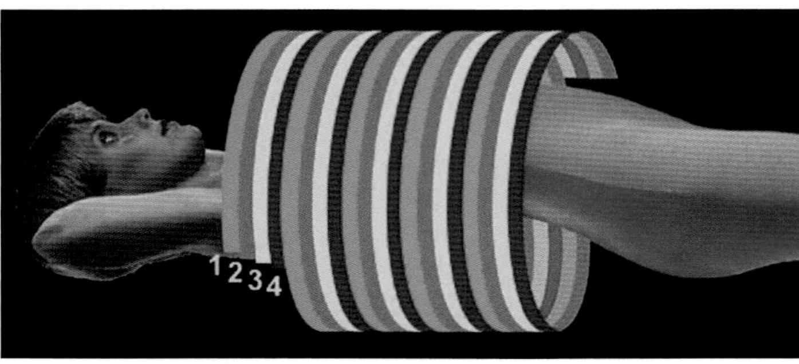

Fig. 22-27. Volume (spiral) multislice scan; 360° continuous rotation of tube and detectors while patient moves in and/or out. (**A** courtesy GE Medical Systems; **B** courtesy Philips Medical Systems.)

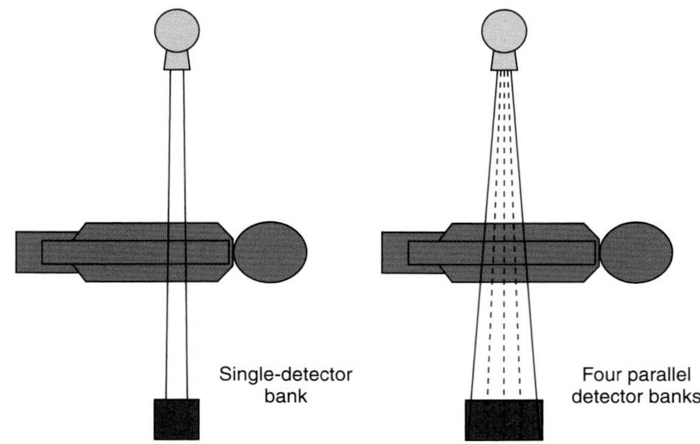

Fig. 22-28. Comparison of single- and multislice scanner concepts.

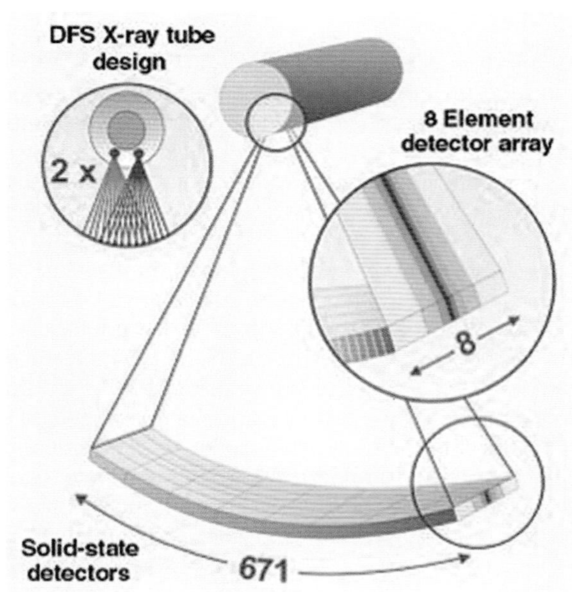

Fig. 22-29. An illustration of a dual-focus x-ray tube with an 8-element detector array, resulting in 16 slices per rotation.

CT SYSTEM COMPONENTS

CT systems can be fixed or mobile, depending on the application required. Mobile CT scanners (Fig. 22-30) have an application for trauma or intraoperative imaging, as well as serving as an auxiliary or backup system within an imaging department. They are also useful in military field hospitals and for imaging patients on strict isolation.

CT systems consist of three major components—the **gantry,** the **computer,** and the **operator console.** These systems include highly complex computing and imaging devices. The following section is intended as a broad introduction to a very technical topic.

The Gantry

The gantry consists of the **x-ray tube,** the **detector array,** and the **collimators.** The gantry can typically be angled up to 30 degrees in each direction, as required for CT scanning of the head or spine. The central opening in the gantry is the **aperture.** The CT **table** (sometimes called the **patient couch**) is electronically linked to the gantry for controlled movement during the scan. The patient anatomy within the aperture is the area being scanned at that time.

The x-ray tube The x-ray tube is similar to a general radiographic tube in construction and operation; however, there are often design modifications required to ensure that the tube is able to withstand additional heat capacity due to increased exposure times.

The detector array Detectors are solid-state, composed of photodiodes coupled with scintillation crystal materials (cadmium tungstate or rare earth oxide ceramic crystals). Solid-state detectors convert the transmitted x-ray energy into light, which is then converted into electrical energy, and into a digital signal. The detector array affects patient dose and the efficiency of the CT unit.

The collimator assembly Collimation in CT is important because it reduces patient dose and improves image quality. CT uses **two collimators—prepatient** (at the x-ray tube) and **postpatient** (at the detector)—which shape and limit the beam. The postpatient collimator determines the slice thickness.

The Computer

The CT computer requires **two types** of highly sophisticated software—one for the **operating system** and the other for **applications.** The operating system (often Microsoft Windows–based) manages the hardware, whereas the applications software manages preprocessing, image reconstruction, and a wide variety of postprocessing operations.

The CT computer must possess staggering speed and memory capacity. For instance, consider that for one CT slice (image) with a 512 × 512 matrix, the computer must simultaneously perform 262,144 mathematical calculations per slice; then consider that current multislice scanners are capable of 160 slices per second.

The Operator Console

The components of the operator console include a keyboard, a mouse, and single or dual monitors, depending on the system (see Fig. 22-32). The operator console allows the technologist to control the parameters of the examination, called the *protocol,* and view and/or manipulate the images generated. The protocol is predetermined for each procedure, and includes factors such as kilovoltage, milliamperage, pitch, field of view, slice thickness, table indexing, reconstruction algorithms, and display windows. These parameters may be modified by the technologist, if required, based on patient presentation and/or clinical history.

Networking and Archiving

Networking of computer workstations is common, a setup in which workstations are situated in other locations for use by the radiologist or technologist. These workstations may be within the imaging department or in remote areas with electronic transmission of data.

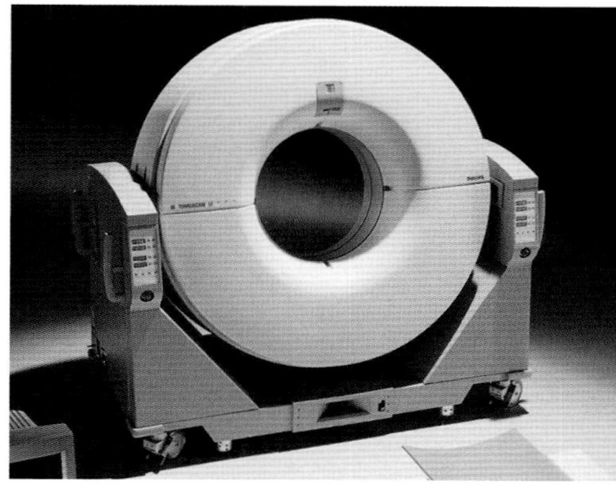

Fig. 22-30. Mobile CT unit. (Courtesy Philips Medical Systems.)

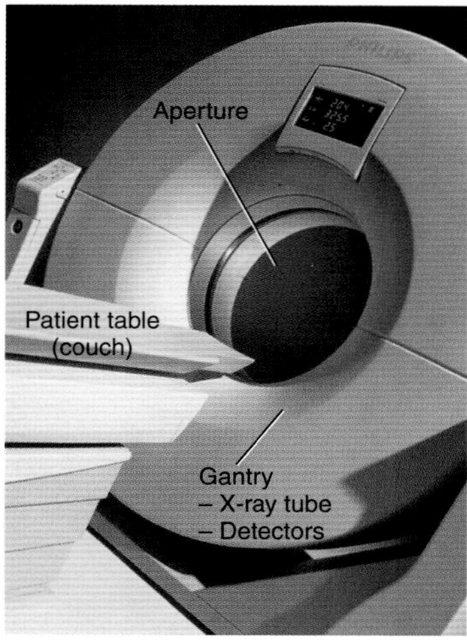

Fig. 22-31. CT scanning unit—patient table (couch) and gantry. (Courtesy Philips Medical Systems.)

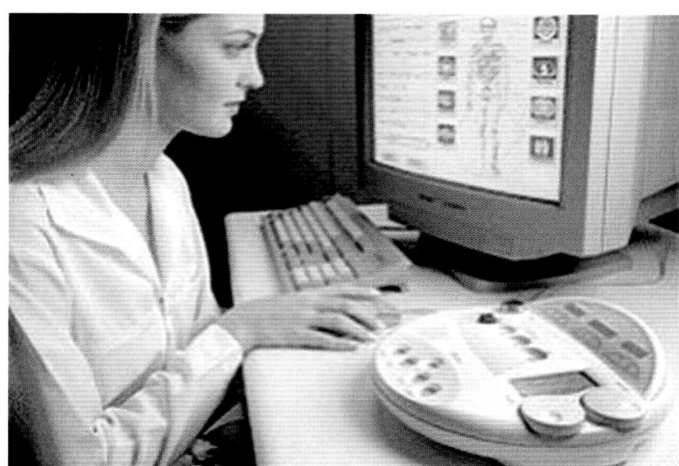

Fig. 22-32. Operator-control console. (Courtesy Philips Medical Systems.)

Image archiving for most modern CT systems is maintained in a picture archiving and communication system (PACS). Those that are not stored in a PACS may use a combination of optical disks and hard disk drives for high-capacity permanent storage of data. If a PACS is not available, laser printers are often used to print a hardcopy of the examination for storage. Interpretation of the examination, however, is generally performed by the radiologist on a high-resolution workstation.

22

IMAGE RECONSTRUCTION

As in conventional radiography, CT images display a variety of shades of gray. The incident radiation is differentially attenuated by the patient, and the remnant radiation is measured by the detectors. Low-density structures (lungs/air-filled structures) will attenuate very little of the x-ray beam, whereas higher-density structures (bones, contrast media) attenuate all or nearly all of the x-ray beam. The attenuation information exits the detectors in analog form, which is then converted to a digital signal by an analog-to-digital converter. The digital values are used in the next step, which is reconstruction of the image using a series of reconstruction algorithms.

Volume Element (Voxel)

The display matrix of the digital image is composed of rows and columns of tiny blocks called *pixels* (picture elements). Each of the pixels is a two-dimensional representation of the three-dimensional volume of tissue in the CT slice. These three-dimensional tissue volumes are called **volume elements,** or *voxels.* Voxels have height, width, and depth. The depth of a voxel is determined by the slice thickness, as selected by the technologist. Each voxel is represented by a pixel in the two-dimensional reconstructed image.

As stated previously, multislice CT allows submillimeter slice thicknesses, whereby voxels have equal dimensions in all three axes (height, width, and depth—or x, y, and z planes). Data sets from these voxels are said to be *isotropic.* Isotropic data sets allow optimal MPR and 3D images with equal spatial resolution in all planes. Isotropic imaging is especially useful where high-resolution MPR images are required, such as in CT angiography, inner ear imaging, and skeletal imaging.

Any CT image, such as in Fig. 22-35, is composed of a large number of pixels representing various degrees of attenuation, depending on the anatomic density of the tissue in the voxel being represented.

Attenuation (Differential Absorption) of Each Voxel

Each voxel in the tissue slice is assigned a number by the computer that is proportional to the degree of x-ray attenuation of that tissue volume. In CT, data from differential absorption of tissues in each voxel are collected and processed by the processing unit of the computer.

Converting Three-Dimensional Voxels to Two-Dimensional Pixels

Once the degree of attenuation of each voxel is determined, the three-dimensional tissue slice is displayed on the computer monitor as a **two-dimensional image.** Each voxel of tissue is represented on the computer display as a pixel. The number of pixels capable of being displayed is determined by the manufacturer.

Fig. 22-35 demonstrates an example of a two-dimensional display of a slice of brain tissue created by the attenuation or differential absorption of these tissues. CSF within the ventricles results in less attenuation of the voxels of these tissues than the dense bony regions of the cranium or the calcified tumor region to the left (our right) of the ventricles that appears white or very light gray.

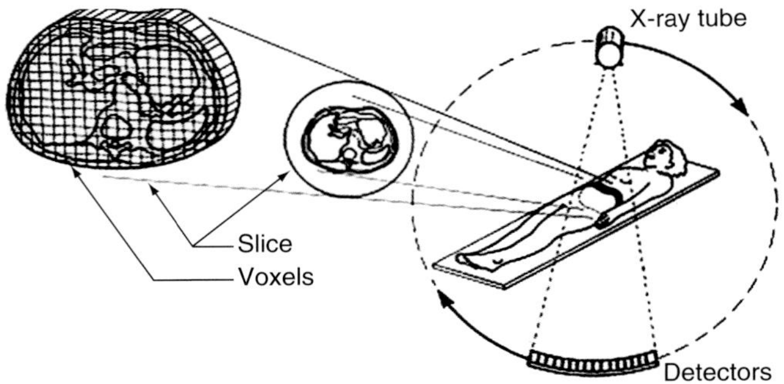

Fig. 22-33. CT image reconstruction—*voxels* (three-dimensional) to *pixels* (two-dimensional display).

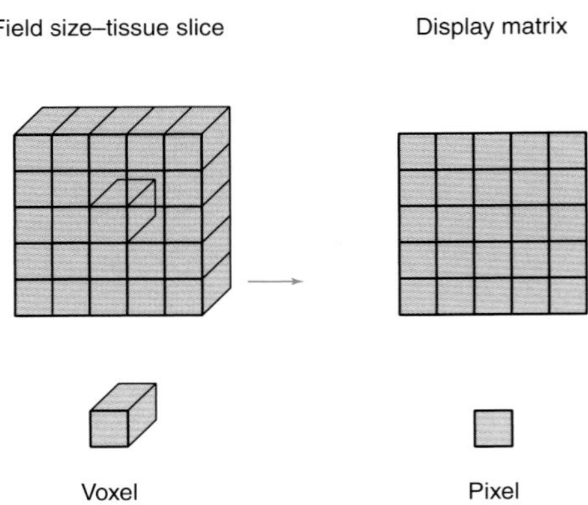

Fig. 22-34. CT image—voxels and pixels.

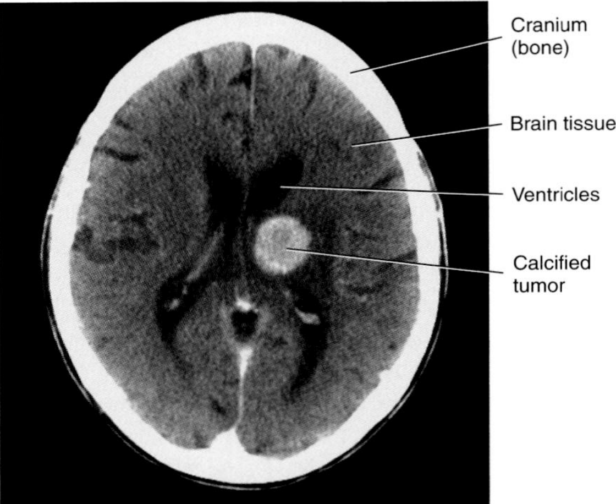

Fig. 22-35. Cranial CT (axial slice).

Computed Gray Scale and CT Numbers

After the CT computer (through thousands of mathematic calculations) determines the degree of attenuation (called the *linear attenuation coefficient*) for each voxel, the values are then converted to another numeric scale called **CT numbers,** which are used in the display matrix. Originally, these CT numbers were called *Hounsfield units,* after Godfrey Hounsfield*, an English scientist who in 1970 produced the first head CT scan.

Shades of gray are then assigned to the CT numbers. The baseline for CT numbers is **water,** which is assigned the CT number value of **0.** Scanners are calibrated so that water is always valued as 0. Dense cortical bone has a value of +1000, or up to +3000, and air (which produces the least amount of attenuation) has the value of −1000. Between these two extremes are tissues and substances that possess various CT numbers according to their attenuation. Different shades of gray are assigned specific CT numbers to create the displayed image. To the right is a table that lists common tissue types or structures and their associated CT numbers and appearances.

As seen on the chest CT scan in Fig. 22-36, bone, soft tissue, muscle, and fat all appear differently on a CT image because of their attenuation and the resultant CT number. Dense tissues, such as **bone,** appear white. **Contrast media–filled structures** also appear white. **Air,** which is not dense compared with tissues, appears black. **Fat, muscle,** and **organs,** which fall between the densities of bone and air, appear as varying shades of gray.

Window Width and Window Level (Window Center)

Window width (WW) refers to the range of CT numbers that are displayed as shades of gray. Wide window indicates more CT numbers as a group (long scale or low contrast). Therefore **WW controls the displayed image contrast** (wide window, low contrast as in chest imaging; narrow window, high contrast as in cranial imaging).

Window level (WL) controls image brightness, or determines the CT number that will be the center of the window width. WL is usually determined by the tissue density that occurs most frequently within an anatomic structure.

Pitch with volume scanners

The x-ray tube/detector array and patient are in continuous motion during a volume acquisition. The amount of anatomy covered during a particular scan is determined by the *pitch.* Pitch is a ratio reflecting the relationship between table speed and slice thickness. The formula for pitch is:

$$\text{Pitch} = \frac{\text{Couch movement (mm/sec) per } 360^\circ \text{ rotation of tube}}{\text{Collimation}}$$

A **1:1 pitch** indicates that table speed and slice thickness are equal. A 1.5:1 pitch would be created if table speed equaled 15 mm per second with a slice thickness of 10 mm. A 2:1 pitch increases the risk that pathology may be missed as a result of undersampling of the anatomy. A 0.5:1 ratio would increase patient dose because of oversampling of the anatomy.

Pitch is determined by the radiologist according to the nature of the study or the pathologic indications.

*Godfrey Hounsfield and Alan Cormack won the Nobel Prize in medicine in 1979 for their work on computed tomography.

TISSUE TYPE AND CT NUMBERS

TISSUE TYPE	CT NUMBERS	APPEARANCE
Cortical bone	+1000	White
Muscle	+50	Gray
White matter	+45	Light gray
Gray matter	+40	Gray
Blood	+20	Gray*
CSF	+15	Gray
Water	**0 (Baseline)**	
Fat	−100	Dark gray to black
Lung	−200	Dark gray to black
Air	−1000	Black

*White if iodinated contrast media is present.

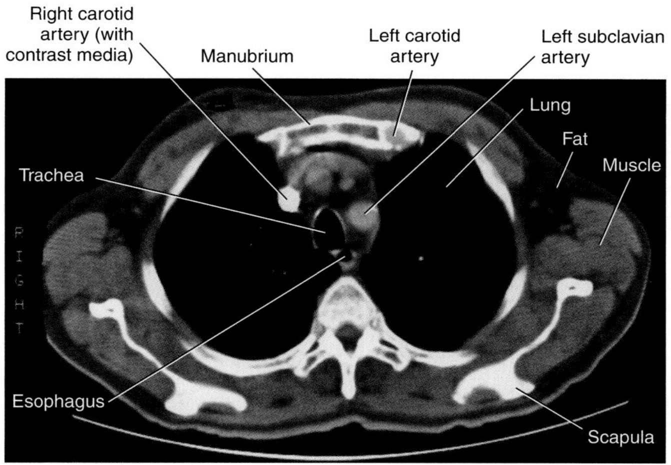

Fig. 22-36. Axial section through level of inferior manubrium.

Image Reconstruction Summary

During a CT procedure the tube and detector array rotates around the patient. Thousands of measurements are taken to determine the radiation attenuation value (the linear attenuation coefficient) for each tissue volume element (voxel). Once the linear attenuation coefficient has been determined, the data are converted into CT numbers for display purposes. On the monitor a two-dimensional image is displayed as a matrix of picture elements (pixels), with each pixel representing the CT number of a specific volume element (voxel) in the CT slice. The window width and level may then be adjusted to alter the image appearance.

Clinical Application of CT

CT VERSUS CONVENTIONAL RADIOGRAPHY

CT is widely used today. When compared with conventional radiography, CT has several advantages as follows:

- **Anatomic structures are visualized with no superimposition.** Three-dimensional anatomic information is presented as a series of thin slices of the internal structure of the part in question.
- **CT images have increased contrast resolution.** The CT system is more sensitive in tissue-type differentiation when compared with conventional radiography so that differences in tissue types can be more clearly delineated and studied. Conventional radiography can display tissues that have at least a 10% difference in density, whereas CT can detect tissue density differences as low as 1% or less. This detection aids in differential diagnosis of pathologies; for example, a solid mass can be distinguished from a cyst, or (in some cases) a benign neoplasm may be distinguished from a malignant neoplasm.
- **MPR—multiplanar reconstruction:** Acquired data may be reconstructed and viewed in alternate planes with no additional radiation exposure to the patient.
- **Manipulation of attenuation data:** Tissue attenuation data collected by the detectors may be manipulated and measured by the computer. Lesions visualized on the image may be measured, and the recorded numerical value (CT number) of the lesion may be viewed to assess its composition (fat, calcium, water, etc.)

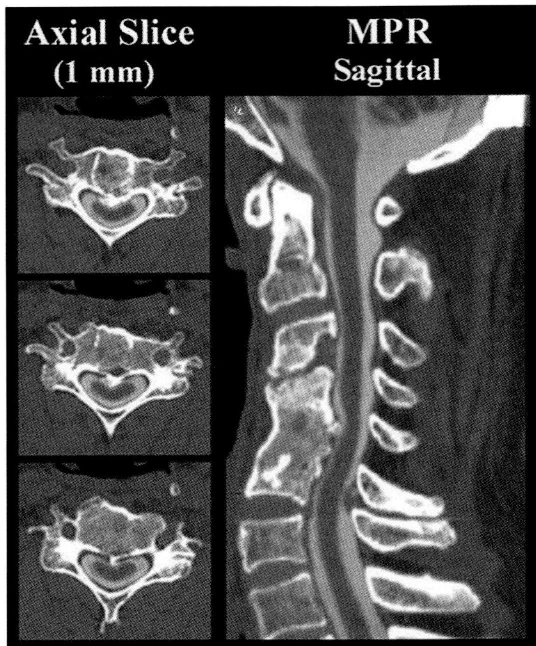

Fig. 22-37. Example of multiplanar-MPR (multislice) volume scan of cervical spine in axial and sagittal slices. Demonstrates superior contrast resolution compared to conventional radiography.

PATIENT COMMUNICATION AND CONSENT

The CT procedure must be fully explained to the patient. The explanation should include the nature of the exam and what the patient can expect, how long it will take, the need to remain still, and reassurance that the technologist will be monitoring the patient throughout the procedure. Breathing instructions should also be given and can be rehearsed if required. If a clinical history has not already been provided by the referring physician, the technologist should take one.

The equipment can appear intimidating to a patient and a thorough explanation by the technologist can alleviate fears and ensure a successful diagnostic procedure.

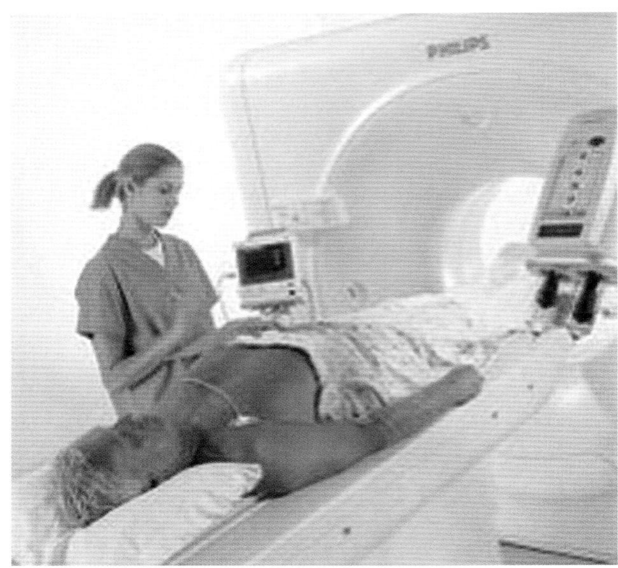

Fig. 22-38. Patient being prepared for CT examination.

THE PROCEDURE

Following the explanation of the procedure, the patient is positioned on the CT table. This position (supine vs. prone; head-first vs. feet-first) depends on the examination being performed. A preliminary image of the area being examined is obtained. This preliminary image is called a **scanogram,** scout, or topogram, depending on the brand of CT equipment used; the term scanogram will be used in this chapter. The technologist uses the scanogram to select the range of the CT scan. Additional parameters important to the examination are contained in the selected protocol and include kilovoltage, milliamperage, pitch, field of view, slice thickness, table indexing, reconstruction algorithms, and display windows.

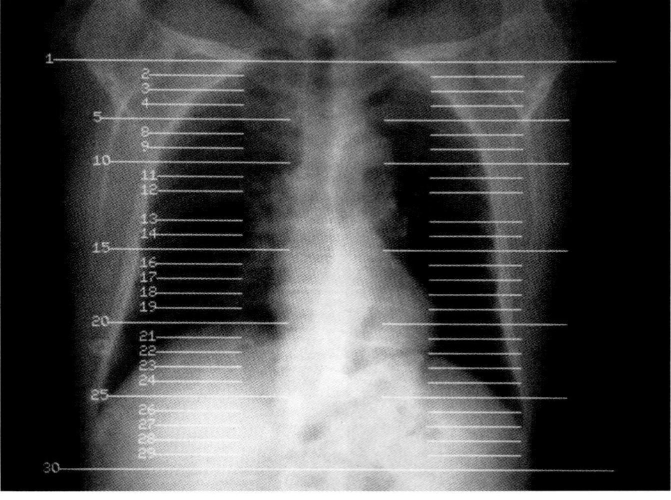

Fig. 22-39. Chest scanogram, with slices indicated.

Viewing CT Images

When CT images are viewed, the patient's right is placed to the viewer's left, as in conventional radiography. Axial scans are viewed as though the viewer were facing the patient and looking at the scan from the foot end of the patient.

Intravenous Contrast Media

An intravenous injection of iodinated contrast media is frequently required in CT to distinguish between normal tissue and pathology. Refer to Chapter 17 for information regarding venipuncture, contrast media contraindications, and reactions.

Contrast Media and Blood-Brain Barrier

Estimates are that 50% to 90% of all head CTs require an intravenous injection of contrast media. The contrast media used are similar to that used for intravenous urography. These iodinated contrast media are usually administered as bolus injections but may also be introduced slowly via an intravenous infusion.

The brain is well supplied with blood vessels that carry oxygen and nutrients. Oxygen must be in constant supply because total oxygen deprivation for the short time of 4 minutes can lead to permanent brain cell damage. Similarly, glucose must be continually available because carbohydrate storage in the brain is limited. Glucose, oxygen, and certain ions pass readily from the circulatory blood into extracellular fluid, then into brain cells. Other substances found in the blood normally enter brain cells quite slowly. Still others, however, such as proteins, most antibiotics, and contrast media, do not pass at all from the normal cranial capillary system into brain cells.

The brain tissue is different from other tissues in that it possesses a natural barrier to the passage of certain substances. This natural phenomenon is termed the **blood-brain barrier.** Therefore contrast medium appearing outside the normal vascular system is an indication that something is wrong.

Radiation Dose

As for all imaging procedures, adherence to the ALARA principle is required to reduce dose to patients and personnel.

Patient dose It should be noted that radiation dose for CT procedures is higher than that of a conventional radiographic examination of the same part. Patient dose is related to pitch: a lower pitch results in a higher dose (slice overlap). Thinner slices also result in a higher dose.

Technologist/personnel dose Anyone who must remain in the CT exam room during an examination must wear protective lead apparel. The highest radiation exposure is nearest the patient because of the scatter produced in the patient—if possible, it is desirable to maintain maximum distance from the source.

Patient lead shielding of radiosensitive organs should also be used if such shielding does not cover essential anatomy.

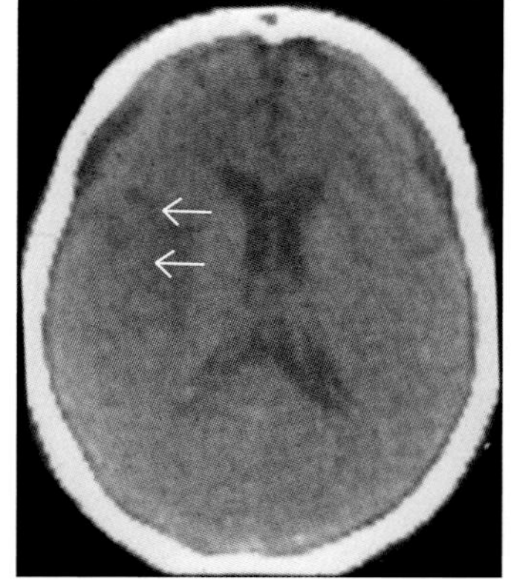

Fig. 22-40. Positive CT (gliomatous tumor) without contrast media.

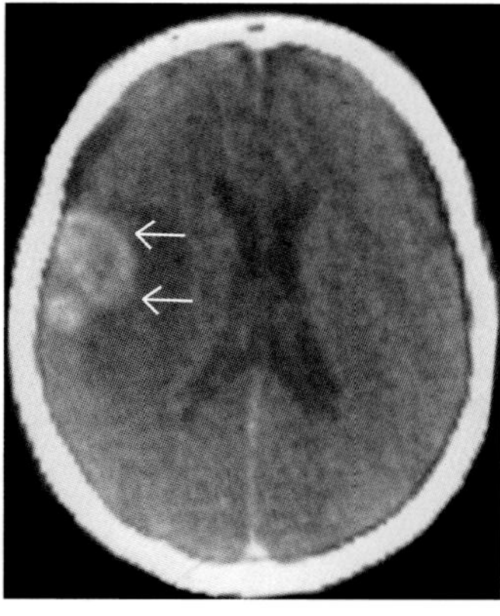

Fig. 22-41. Same patient, CT with contrast media.

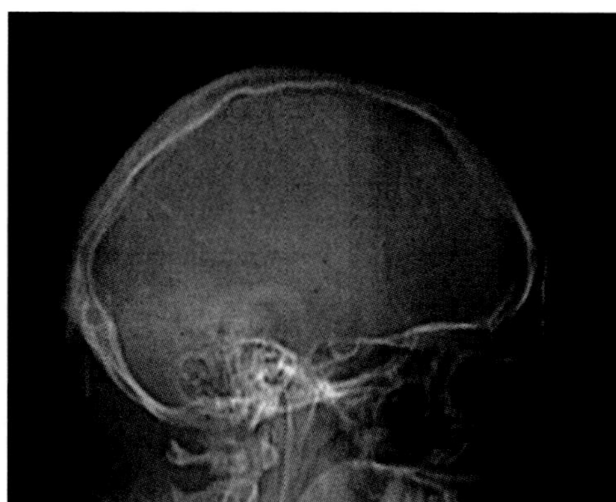

Fig. 22-42. Scanogram for head CT without slice lines visualized on this image.

22

Cranial Computed Tomography—Head CT

INTRODUCTION

Plain radiographic images provide a two-dimensional image of the bony skull only, whereas injury and pathology of the head often involve the brain and associated soft tissues. CT is a vital tool in evaluation of the patient because it can differentiate among blood clots, white/gray matter, CSF, cerebral edema, and neoplasms.

The term "head CT" refers to CT imaging of the brain. There are also specific CT procedures for investigation of pathology of orbits, the sella turcica, sinuses, temporal bones, and TMJs. This section will focus on CT imaging of the brain.

THE HEAD CT PROCEDURE

The basic principles of skull positioning in conventional radiography also apply to CT; however, specific positioning for head CT will vary, depending on radiologist preferences and department protocols.

Metallic items (earrings, bobby pins, etc.) and dentures must be removed. The patient is placed supine on the CT table and positioned so that there is no rotation or tilt of the head in order to accurately assess any bilateral asymmetry due to pathology. The head is then immobilized.

A scanogram must be obtained prior to the procedure to allow the technologist to determine the range of the scan—for a routine head CT, the procedure includes the area from the skull base to the vertex, in 5- to 10-mm slices. Gantry/beam angulation is also determined from the scanogram. Typically for head CT, the beam is aligned parallel to a line passing from the nasion to the skull.

Head CT images are viewed with **two sets of window settings**—one set allows optimal **visualization of the brain** ("brain windows") with lower contrast; the other set displays optimal **bony detail** ("bone windows") with higher contrast (Figs. 22-43 and 22-44).

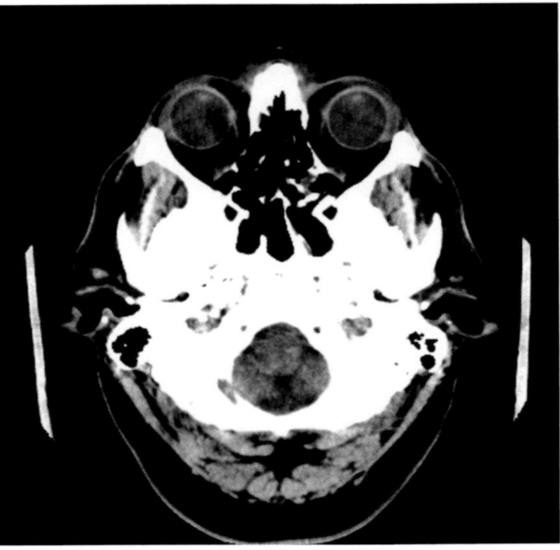

Fig. 22-43. Optimal visualization of brain—brain windows (lower contrast).

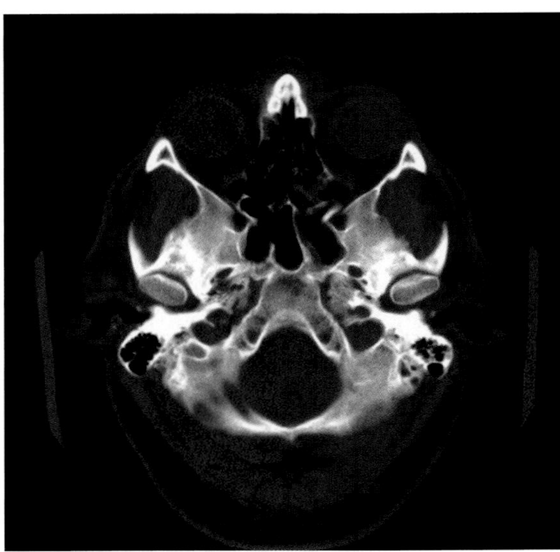

Fig. 22-44. Optimal bony detail—bone windows (higher contrast).

SECTIONAL ANATOMY

Axial Sections of the Brain

Included here are three sample axial slices of the brain. These include the structures labeled on the CT axial scan. The drawings on the right indicate the level of that CT scan and should help the reader identify the labeled structures as seen in the axial (cross-sectional) views.

A good learning exercise for the sectional anatomy portions of this chapter is to try to identify as many labeled structures as possible before checking the answers listed below.

Axial Section 1 (Figs. 22-45 and 22-46)

Axial section 1 is the most superior of the axial sections and is termed the **extreme hemispheric level.** Parts labeled are as follows:

A. Anterior portion or the superior sagittal sinus
B. Centrum semiovale (white matter of the cerebrum)
C. Longitudinal fissure (region of falx cerebri)
D. Sulcus
E. Gyrus
F. Posterior portion of superior sagittal sinus

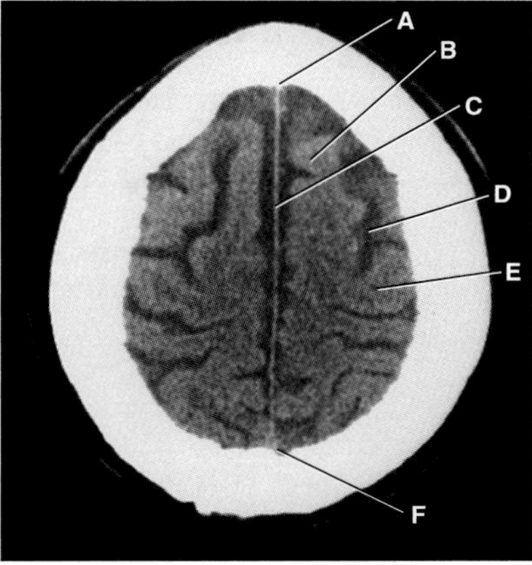

Fig. 22-45. CT axial section 1.

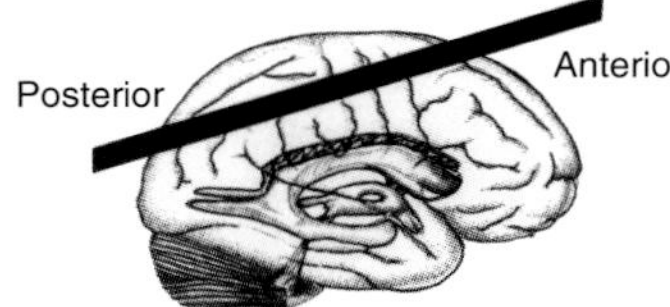

Fig. 22-46. Section 1.

Axial Section 4 (Figs. 22-47 and 22-48)

This scan is of the typical fourth axial section, which is of the **mid-ventricular level.** The region of the deep-lying cerebral nuclei is visible at this level in the scan.

Those structures labeled are as follows:

A. Anterior of corpus callosum (genu)
B. Anterior horn of the left lateral ventricle
C. Region of caudate nucleus
D. Region of thalamus
E. Third ventricle
F. Pineal gland or body (slightly calcified)
G. Posterior (occipital) horn of the left lateral ventricle

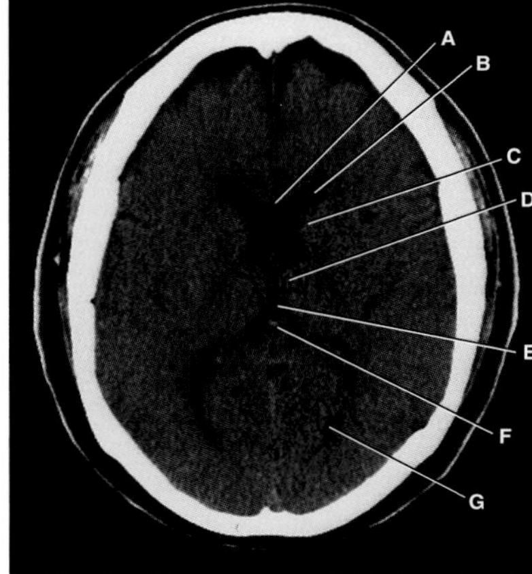

Fig. 22-47. CT axial section 4.

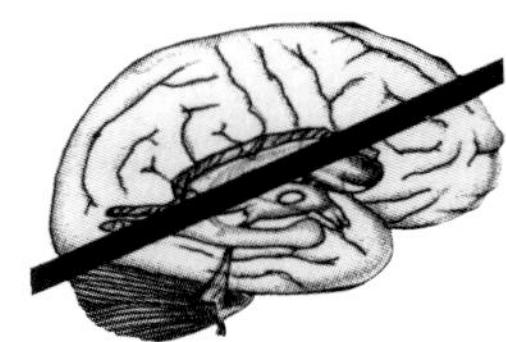

Fig. 22-48. Axial section 4.

Axial Section 5 (Figs. 22-49 and 22-50)

The typical axial section 5 scan visualizes the brain tissue through the **mid-third ventricle.**

Those parts labeled are as follows:

A. Anterior corpus callosum (genu)
B. Anterior horn of right lateral ventricle
C. Third ventricle
D. Region of pineal gland
E. Internal occipital protuberance

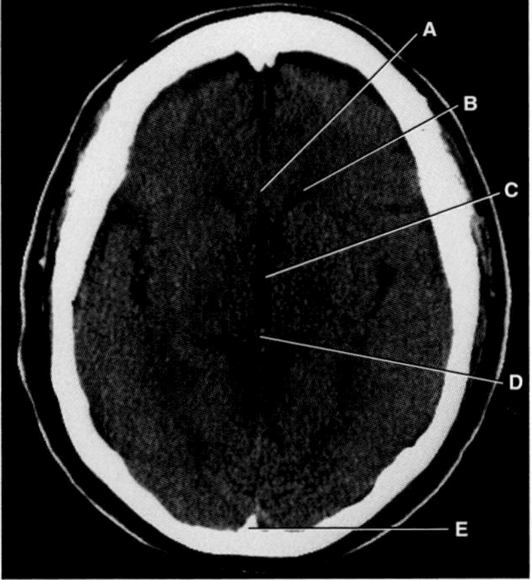

Fig. 22-49. CT axial section 5.

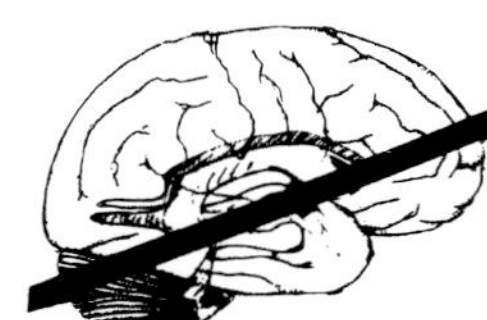

Fig. 22-50. Axial section 5.

PATHOLOGIC INDICATIONS

Any suspected disease process involving the brain is an indication for head CT. Some of the more common indications include:

- **Tumors:** metastatic lesions, meningioma, glioma
- **Circulatory pathology:** cerebrovascular accident (CVA), aneurysm, arteriovenous malformation (AVM)
- **Inflammatory/infectious conditions**: meningitis, abscess
- **Degenerative disorders:** brain atrophy
- **Trauma:** epidural and subdural hematoma, fracture
- **Congenital abnormalities**
- **Hydrocephalus**

22

EXAMPLES OF POSITIVE HEAD CT IMAGES

Glioma An example of a positive CT is shown in Figs. 22-51 and 22-52. This particular lesion is a **glioma** *(gli-o'mah),* a type of brain tumor. A noncontrast CT slice is shown in Fig. 22-51. A contrast-enhanced version of the same slice appears in Fig. 22-52. Contrast enhancement is necessary for all suspected neoplasia because of possible breakdown of the normal blood-brain barrier, as described under the discussion of contrast media and the blood-brain barrier.

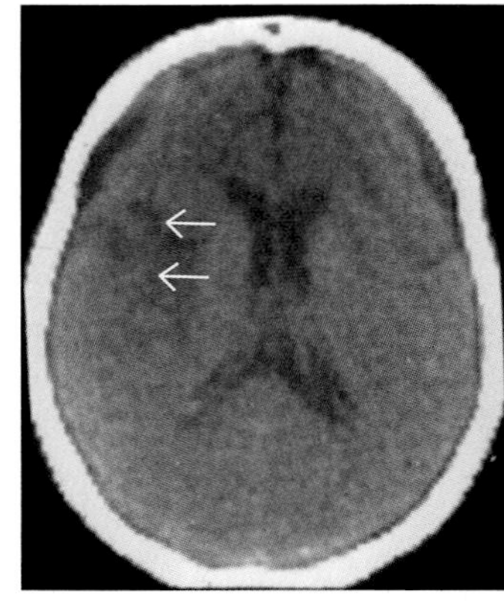

Fig. 22-51. Positive CT (gliomatous tumor) without contrast media.

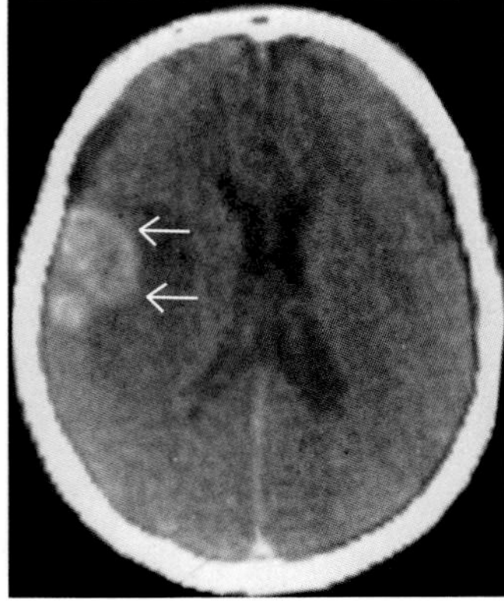

Fig. 22-52. CT with contrast media.

Subdural Hematoma and Hydrocephalus Two additional positive examples of cranial CTs are illustrated in Figs. 22-53 and 22-54. A large bilateral subdural hematoma is shown in Fig. 22-53. A **subdural hematoma** involves a collection of blood under the dura mater that is caused by trauma to the skull. This blood pooling causes compression and damage to brain tissue, resulting in drowsiness or loss of consciousness. This condition, whether acute or chronic, can be diagnosed without contrast enhancement with CT.

Fig. 22-54 demonstrates an example of **hydrocephalus,** caused by blockage to drainage of CSF from ventricles, which results in enlargement of ventricles and compression of the brain. Note the enlarged ventricles and how well they visualize on the CT.

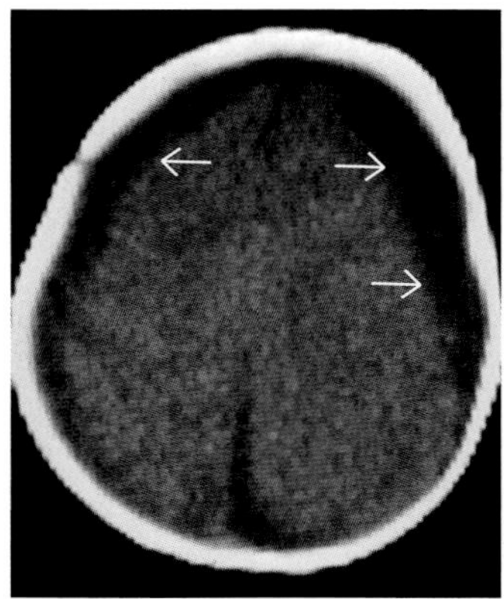

Fig. 22-53. Subdural hematoma.

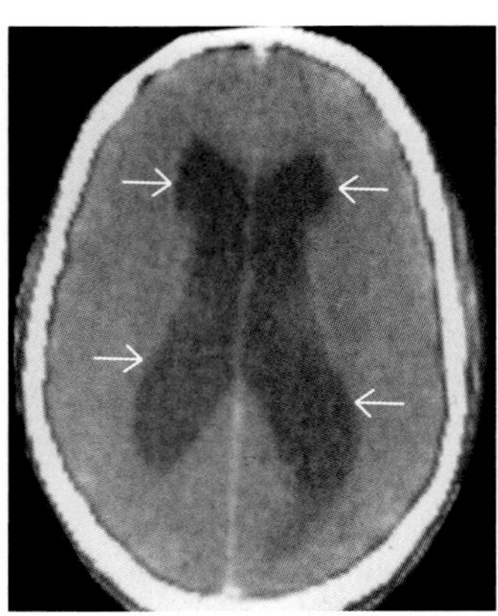

Fig. 22-54. Hydrocephalus.

Thoracic Computed Tomography—Chest CT

INTRODUCTION

The primary purpose of thoracic computed tomography is to **serve as a diagnostic adjunct to conventional chest radiography.** Conventional chest radiography, because of its cost effectiveness, still remains the primary screening tool in patients suspected of having chest pathology. However, virtually any abnormality discovered with conventional imaging will be investigated using CT. The superior contrast resolution and cross-sectional imaging afforded by CT make it a valuable modality for the investigation of new pathology and the management and evaluation of previously diagnosed conditions.

PROCEDURE FOR CT OF THE CHEST

Jewelry and metallic objects must be removed before the patient is placed supine on the table with the arms elevated. A **scanogram** is obtained to allow the technologist to determine the range of the scan for the procedure. Routine chest CT includes scanning from the apices to the lung bases, often in 7- to 10-mm slices, whereas high-resolution chest CT includes acquisition of thinner slices, from 2 to 3 mm, obtained at specified points in the chest. Fig. 22-55 illustrates a routine chest CT with the location of the first slice selected at the apices *(line 1)* and the final slice selected at the bases *(line 30)*. If the primary concern is pulmonary malignancy, however, scanning continues to the adrenal glands because a number of pulmonary malignancies metastasize here. Chest CT performed for various types of aneurysm will have specific protocols.

Soft tissue masses frequently compress the esophagus. To help distinguish the esophagus from surrounding soft tissue, the patient may be asked to swallow radiopaque esophageal creams to coat the mucosa and opacify the esophagus.

Faster acquisition times have increased the application of chest CT as artifacts due to respiratory and cardiac motion have been minimized. Additionally, assuming the patient is able to hold his or her breath, volume scanning has virtually eliminated anatomic misregistration, which occurred when the patient took a separate inspiration for each slice in conventional CT.

Patients undergoing chest CT are coached by the technologist to hyperventilate prior to the procedure—they take two or three deep breaths and are then asked to hold their breath for the 20 to 30 seconds required for the scan.

Chest CT images are viewed with **two sets of window settings**—one set allows optimal **visualization of the lung** ("lung windows") with low contrast, and the other set displays **mediastinal detail** ("mediastinum windows") with high contrast (see Figs. 22-56 and 22-57).

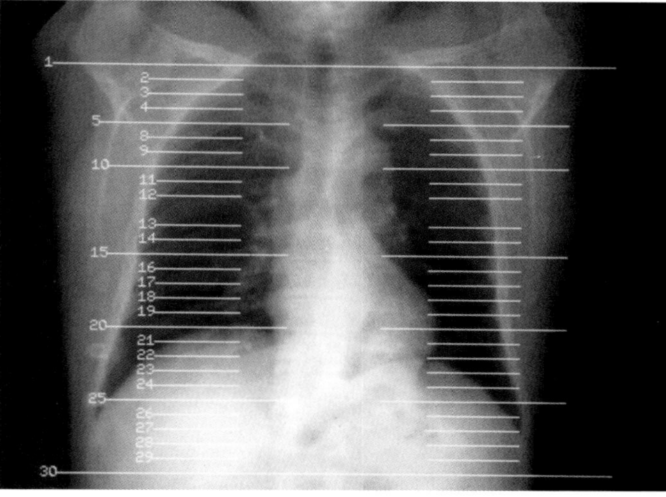

Fig. 22-55. Chest scanogram with slices indicated.

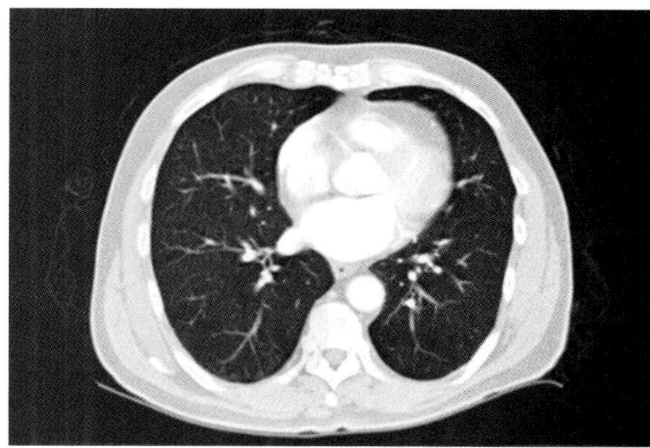

Fig. 22-56. Optimal visualization of lungs—lung windows (low contrast).

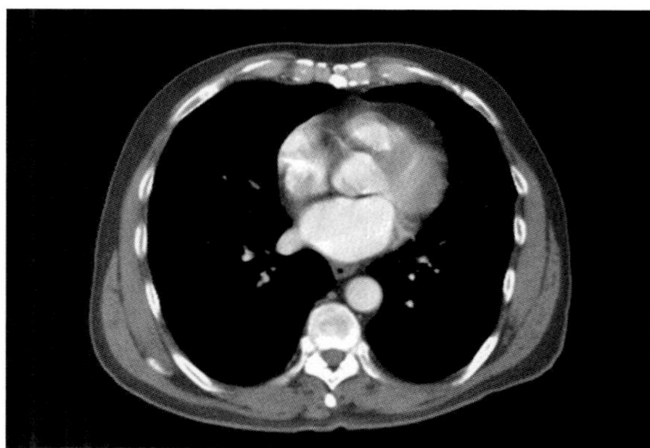

Fig. 22-57. Optimal visualization of mediastinal detail—mediastinal windows (higher contrast).

SECTIONAL CHEST ANATOMY

The anatomy of the thorax is covered thoroughly in **Chapter 3** (for general chest anatomy), **Chapter 11** (for the bony thorax), and **Chapter 21** (for the heart and circulatory system). Mastery of the anatomy in these chapters is recommended before continuing with the study of sectional anatomy of the chest.

Axial Sections of the Chest

Five sample chest CT axial slices of 10-mm thickness are shown. Chest radiographs and model photographs are shown on the right of each CT image, with the scan level shaded in green to help orient the reader to the anatomic structures visualized at that level.

The examination for these scans was obtained with bolus injections of intravenous contrast.

CONTRAST MEDIA

The use of intravenous contrast media is important for visualization of structures within the mediastinum. Department protocols and/or radiologist preferences determine the specific type, volume, and injection sites.

22

Axial Section 1 (Fig. 22-58)

Axial section 1 represents a section at **the level of the sternal notch.**

Parts labeled are as follows:

A. Right internal jugular vein
B. Right common carotid artery
C. Trachea
D. Sternum
E. SC joint
F. Clavicle
G. Left internal jugular vein
H. Left subclavian artery
I. Left common carotid artery
J. T2-T3 vertebrae
K. Right subclavian artery
L. Spine and acromion process of scapula
M. Head of humerus

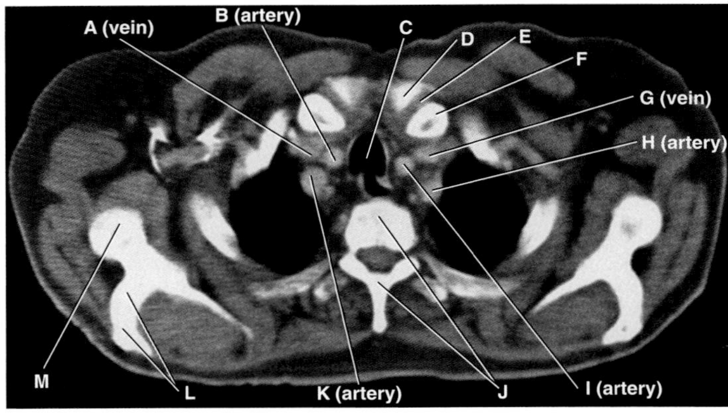

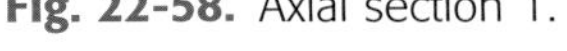

Fig. 22-58. Axial section 1.

Axial Section 3 (Fig. 22-59)

Axial section 3 represents a section through the **inferior portion of the manubrium.**

Parts labeled are as follows:

A. Right brachiocephalic vein (with contrast medium)
B. Brachiocephalic artery (innominate)
C. Manubrium of sternum
D. Left brachiocephalic vein
E. Left common carotid artery
F. Left subclavian artery
G. Esophagus
H. T3-T4 vertebrae
I. Trachea

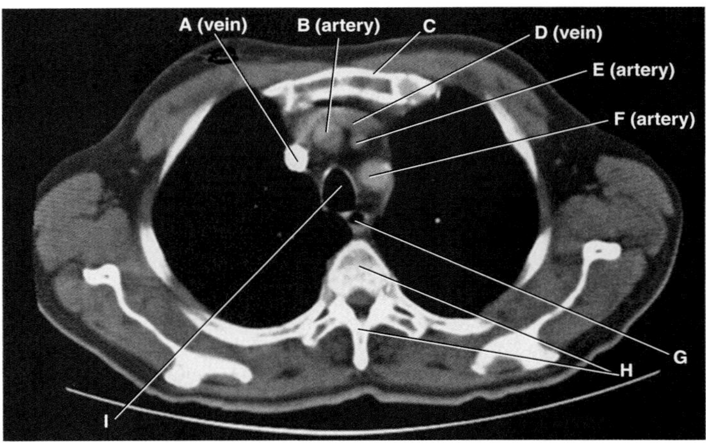

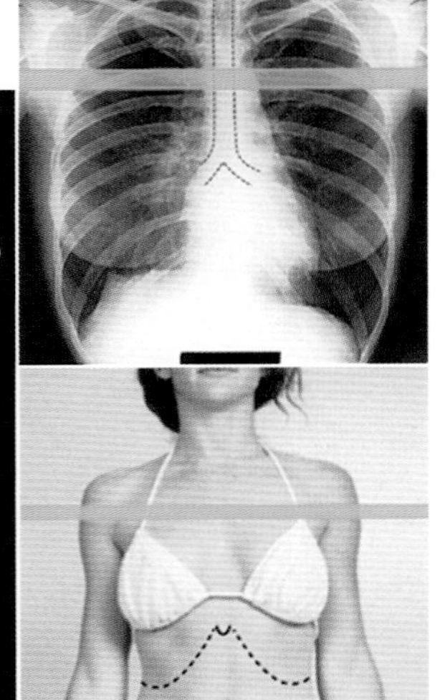

Fig. 22-59. Axial section 3

Axial Section 5 (Fig. 22-60)

Axial section 5 represents a section at the level of the **aortopulmonary window.** This is a space located between the ascending aorta and pulmonary artery.

Parts labeled are as follows:

A. Superior vena cava
B. Ascending aorta
C. Body of sternum
D. Aortopulmonary window
E. Esophagus
F. Descending aorta
G. T4-T5 vertebrae
H. Trachea

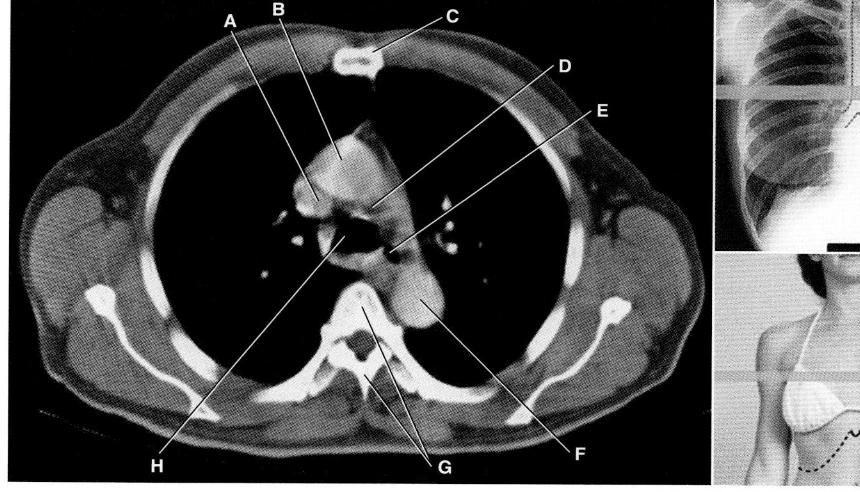

Fig. 22-60. Axial section 5.

Axial Section 7 (Fig. 22-61)

Axial section 7 was taken at a level of **1 cm below the carina.**

Parts labeled are as follows:

A. Superior vena cava
B. Ascending aorta
C. Main pulmonary artery
D. Left pulmonary vein
E. Left pulmonary artery
F. Descending aorta
G. T6-T7 vertebrae
H. Azygos vein
I. Esophagus
J. Right pulmonary artery

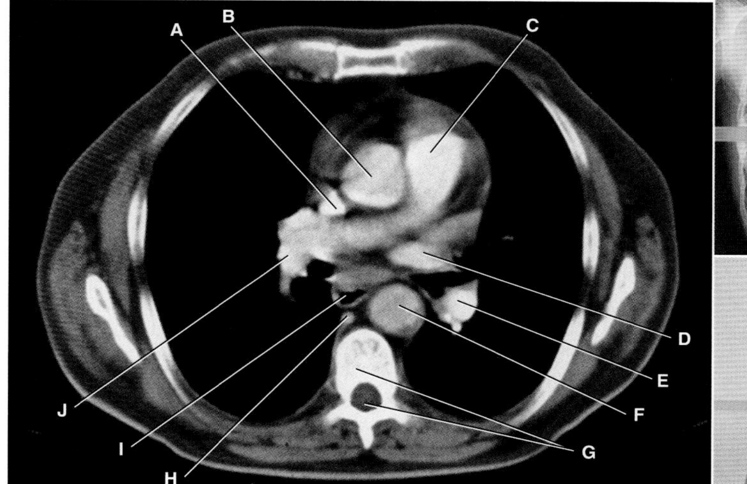

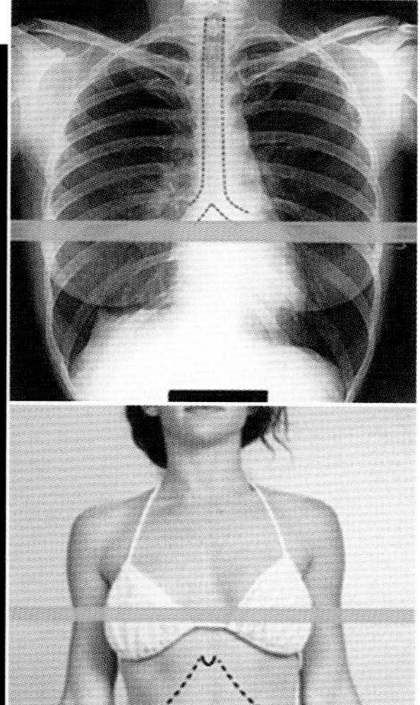

Fig. 22-61. Axial section 7.

Axial Section 10 (Fig. 22-62)

At this level of axial section 10 **through the base of the heart,** the small circled area *(C)* is the tricuspid valve between the right ventricle and the right atrium.

Parts labeled are as follows:

A. Inferior vena cava
B. Right atrium
C. Tricuspid valve
D. Pericardium
E. Right ventricle
F. Interventricular septum
G. Left ventricle
H. Left atrium
I. Descending aorta
J. T9-T10 vertebrae
K. Esophagus
L. Right hemidiaphragm and upper liver

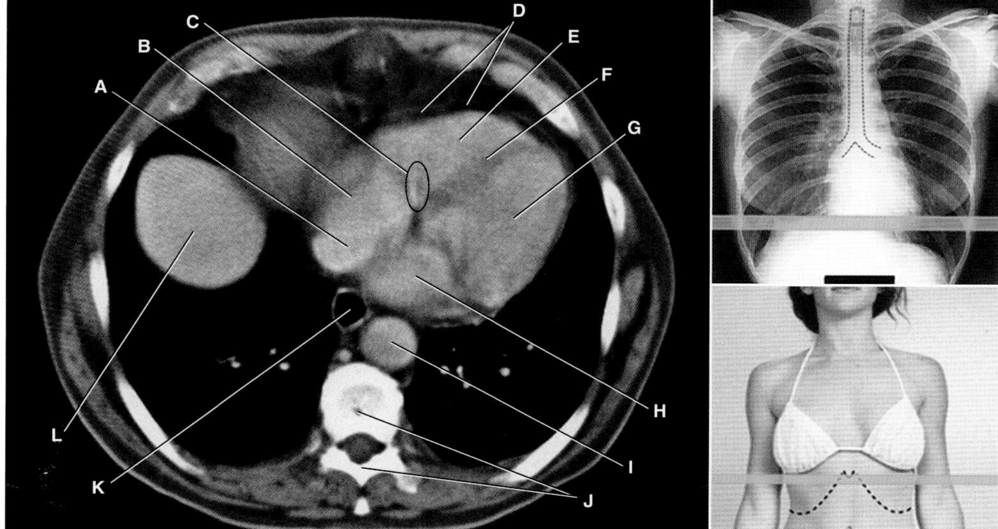

Fig. 22-62. Axial section 10.

PATHOLOGIC INDICATIONS

Common pathologic indications for CT of the chest are:

- **Tumors:** metastatic lesions, mediastinal and hilar neoplasia, carcinoma
- **Circulatory pathology:** aneurysms, aortic dissection, pulmonary embolus
- **Inflammatory/infectious conditions:** abscess, empyema
- **Trauma:** mediastinal or lung injury
- **Pericardial disease:** pericardial effusion
- **Disease processes of the chest:** asbestosis, sarcoidosis, emphysema

EXAMPLE OF THORACIC PATHOLOGY (Figs. 22-63 and 22-64)

These figures demonstrate how thoracic CT can be used to provide diagnostic information on a mediastinal mass.

The AP chest projection (Fig. 22-63) of a 53-day-old male demonstrates mediastinal widening *(arrows)* of unknown cause. A CT axial scan (Fig. 22-64) shows a well-circumscribed, homogeneous mass in the posterior mediastinum. From the attenuation value of this mass, which is slightly above water, this mass was determined to be a **bronchogenic cyst.**

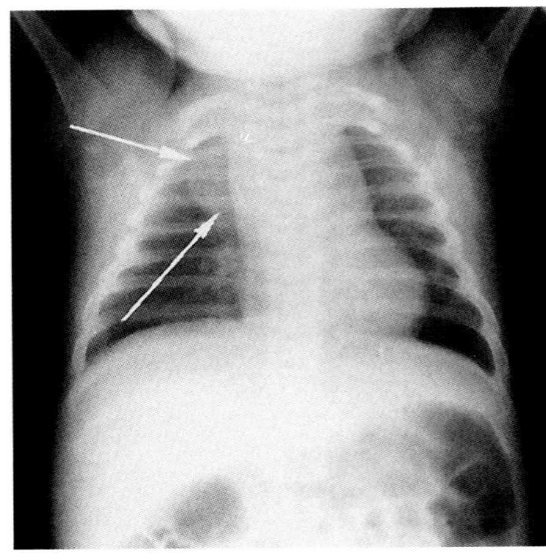

Fig. 22-63. AP chest projection.

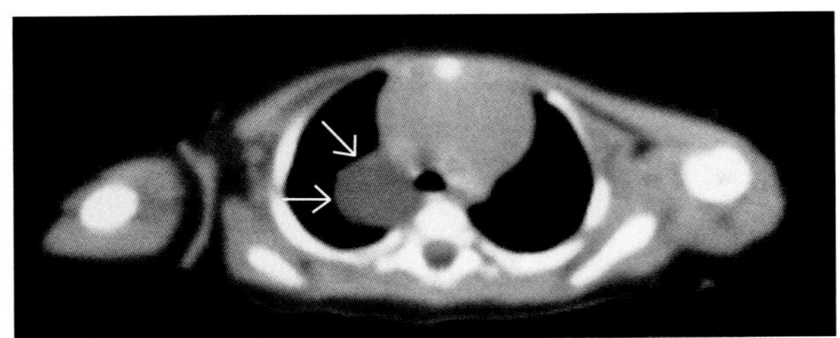

Fig. 22-64. CT axial image—bronchogenic cyst.

Abdominal and Pelvic Computed Tomography—Abdomen and Pelvis CT

INTRODUCTION

With the advent of CT the ability to diagnose abdominal and pelvic morphology has been significantly enhanced. Because of its speed and accuracy, CT has become an effective management and treatment tool for abdominal and pelvic disease and has been especially useful in malignancy cases. The use of standard diagnostic tests, such as intravenous urography (IVU) and endoscopic retrograde cholangiopancreatography (ERCP) has been greatly reduced because of the superior contrast resolution of the CT examination.

PROCEDURE FOR CT OF THE ABDOMEN AND PELVIS

Metallic objects from the abdomen/pelvis area must be removed before the patient is placed supine on the table with the arms elevated. A **scanogram** is obtained to allow the technologist to determine the range of the scan for the procedure. A routine abdomen CT protocol typically includes scanning from the diaphragm to the iliac crests in 7- to 10-mm slices, and a routine pelvis CT protocol often includes scanning from the iliac crests to the symphysis pubis, also in 7- to 10-mm slices. Any suspicious areas visualized may then be scanned using thinner slices.

Faster exposure times have improved the quality of CT images as artifacts due to peristaltic motion have been reduced. Additionally, assuming the patient is able to hold their breath, volume scanning has virtually eliminated anatomic misregistration, which occurred when the patient took a different inspiration for each slice in conventional CT.

Patients undergoing abdomen/pelvis CT are coached by the technologist to hyperventilate prior to the procedure—they take two or three deep breaths and are then asked to hold their breath for the 20 to 30 seconds required for the scan. Depending on the scanner and the patient condition, a complete abdomen and pelvis scan may require two volume acquisitions—one for the abdomen and one for the pelvis. The patient may be given a short break between the two exposures in order to catch their breath. Remember, 30 seconds is a long time to hold your breath—try it!!

The pitch required for the scan is identified in the protocol; it is based on the exam requested and the clinical history. Pitch is related to the table speed and the thickness of the slice as described previously in this chapter on p. 733. Correct selection of pitch is vital to ensure that the anatomy is optimally imaged.

CONTRAST MEDIA

To distinguish the GI tract from adjacent structures, **oral** and/**or rectal contrast media are required** in abdomen and pelvis CT. Unopacified portions of the small and large bowel may be misdiagnosed as lymph nodes, abscesses, or masses.

Oral contrast media must be ingested before the exam in a manner that allows the contrast media to be distributed throughout the GI tract. Typically the patient ingests oral contrast at three intervals: (1) the night before the exam, (2) 1 hour before the exam, and (3) immediately before the exam. The reason for this pattern is that the contrast taken the night before will be in the large bowel, that taken 1 hour before will be in the small bowel, and that taken immediately before the exam will be in the stomach. Contrast media may be instilled rectally if oral contrast has not reached the rectum.

There are **two types** of positive contrast agents used to opacify the gastrointestinal tract: **barium sulfate suspensions** and **nonionic water-soluble solutions.** Each has been proven effective with specific applications.

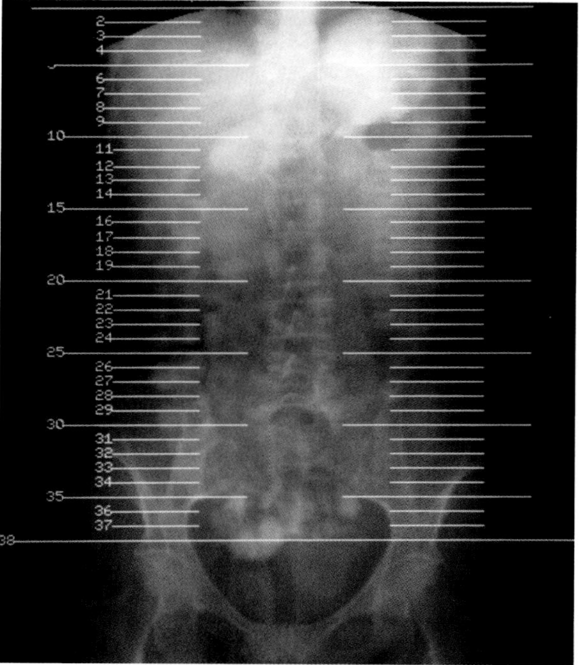

Fig. 22-65. Localizing (pilot) scan for abdomen and pelvis (solid while line representing the slice location).
Note: A routine complete abdomen and pelvis sonogram should extend down to the symphysis pubis.

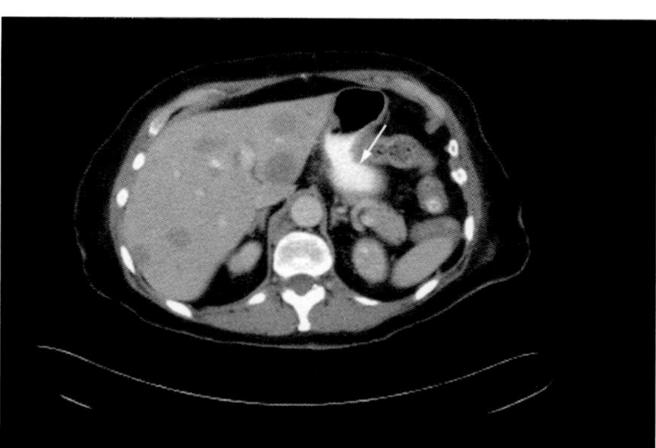

Fig. 22-66. Liver metastasis with oral contrast media ingested as seen in the stomach (see *arrow*).

22

ARTIFACTS AND BARIUM SULFATE SUSPENSIONS

There are numerous flavored barium sulfate suspensions made especially for abdominal CT. To be useful in abdominal CT, barium sulfate suspensions must be of **low concentrations** (1% to 3%) to prevent streak artifacts on the image. **Beam-hardening** (streak) artifacts may also result if there has been a delay in imaging following ingestion of the contrast; much of the water will be absorbed, leaving dense residual barium. Additionally, if the patient has had a recent barium enema, dense barium may be present in the bowel. Fig. 22-67 illustrates the beam-hardening artifacts that will occur if the barium is too dense.

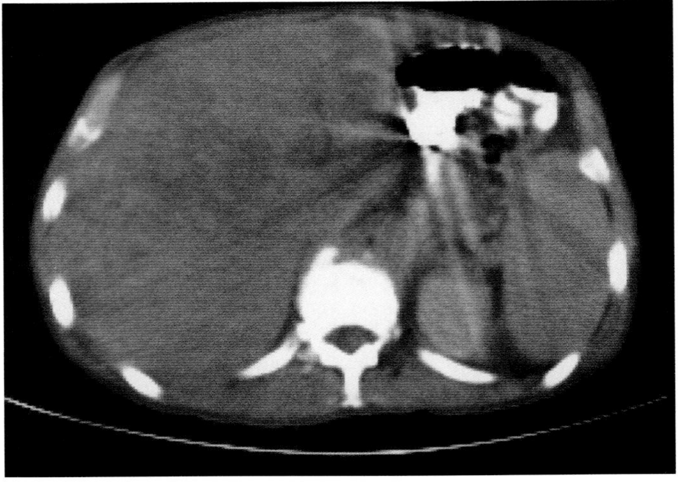

Fig. 22-67. Beam-hardening artifacts with too dense barium.

INTRAVENOUS CONTRAST MEDIA

Nonionic, iodinated intravenous contrast media is frequently required for abdominal CT, particularly for evaluation of the liver and pancreas. Vessel opacification throughout the abdomen is helpful in differentiating vessels from masses and in assessing vessel pathology and integrity.

SECTIONAL ABDOMEN AND PELVIS ANATOMY

The anatomy of the abdomen and bony pelvis is covered in **Chapters** 4 and **8,** respectively, with additional anatomy of digestive, biliary, and urinary systems discussed in **Chapters 14, 15, 16,** and **17.** Mastery of the anatomy in these chapters is recommended before continuing with the study of sectional anatomy of the abdomen and pelvis.

Axial Sections of the Abdomen

Five sample CT 10-mm axial slices of the abdomen are shown. The examination was obtained using a 50-ml bolus injection followed by a 100-ml drip infusion of intravenous contrast. An oral preparation of water-soluble contrast solution was also used.

Axial Section 1 (Fig. 22-68)

Axial section 1 is through the **upper portion of the liver.** The liver is divided into 2 lobes—the right *(A)* and left *(B)* lobes.

The labeled parts are as follows:

A. Right lobe of liver
B. Left lobe of liver
C. Stomach (lower body)
D. Stomach (fundus and upper body region)
E. Spleen
F. T10 and T11 vertebrae
G. Abdominal aorta
H. Inferior vena cava

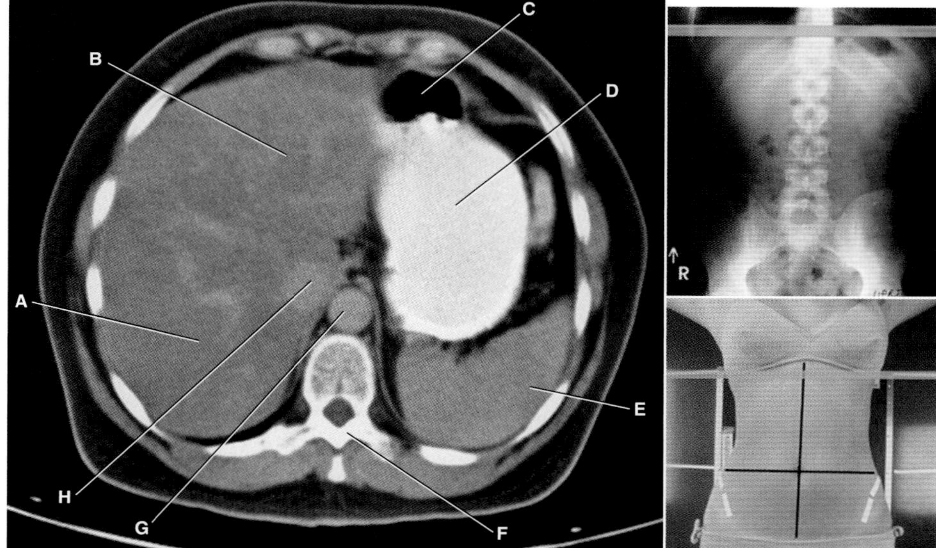

Fig. 22-68. Axial section 1. Remember from Chapter 14 that the lower body region of the stomach is air-filled in the supine position, and the fundus and upper portion of the stomach are barium-filled because these structures are posterior in position.

Axial Section 3 (Fig. 22-69)

The scan of axial section 3 is at the level of the **pancreatic tail** *(F).* The pancreatic tail is in its general position, anterior to the left kidney. Note the excellent visualization of the adrenal gland and its inverted V shape *(I).*

The parts as labeled are as follows:

A. Right lobe of liver, posterior segment
B. Gallbladder
C. Left lobe of liver
D. Stomach (lower body)
E. Colon (descending)
F. Pancreatic tail
G. Spleen
H. Upper lobe of left kidney
I. Left adrenal gland
J. T11-T12 vertebrae
K. Inferior vena cava
L. Upper lobe of right kidney

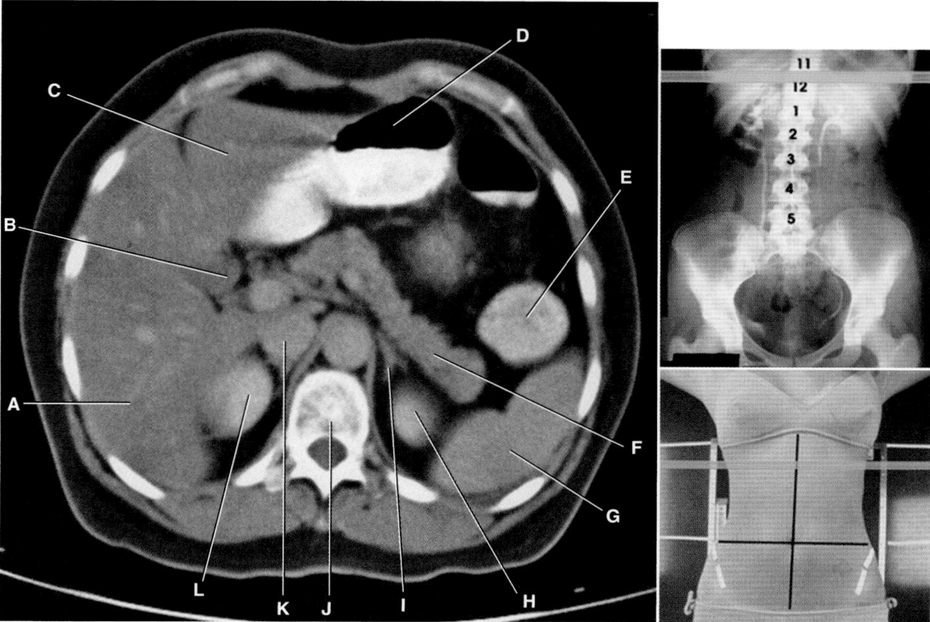

Fig. 22-69. Axial section 3.

Axial Section 5 (Fig. 22-70)

This scan of axial section 5 was taken at the level of the **second portion of the duodenum** *(C)*. The head of the pancreas *(L)* is well outlined by the duodenum. If the second portion of the duodenum is inadequately opacified, it can be confused for a pancreatic tumor.

The parts as labeled are as follows:

A. Right lobe of liver
B. Gallbladder
C. Second portion of duodenum
D. Left lobe of liver
E. Stomach (pylorus)
F. Small intestine (jejunum)
G. Colon (descending)
H. Left kidney
I. Abdominal aorta
J. L1 vertebra
K. Inferior vena cava
L. Head of pancreas

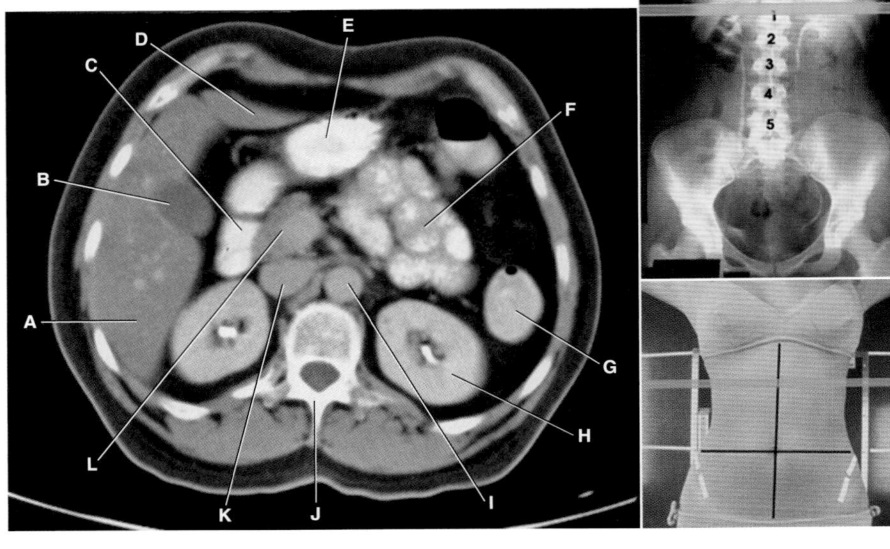

Fig. 22-70. Axial section 5.

Axial Section 7 (Fig. 22-71)

This scan of axial section 7 was taken through the **midportion of the kidneys.** There is excellent visualization of both the right and left (G) renal pelvis.

The parts as labeled are as follows:

A. Inferior lobe of the liver
B. Uncinate process of the pancreas
C. Gallbladder
D. Colon (ascending and/or transverse)
E. Jejunum
F. Descending colon
G. Renal pelvis of left kidney
H. Abdominal aorta
I. L2 vertebra
J. Inferior vena cava

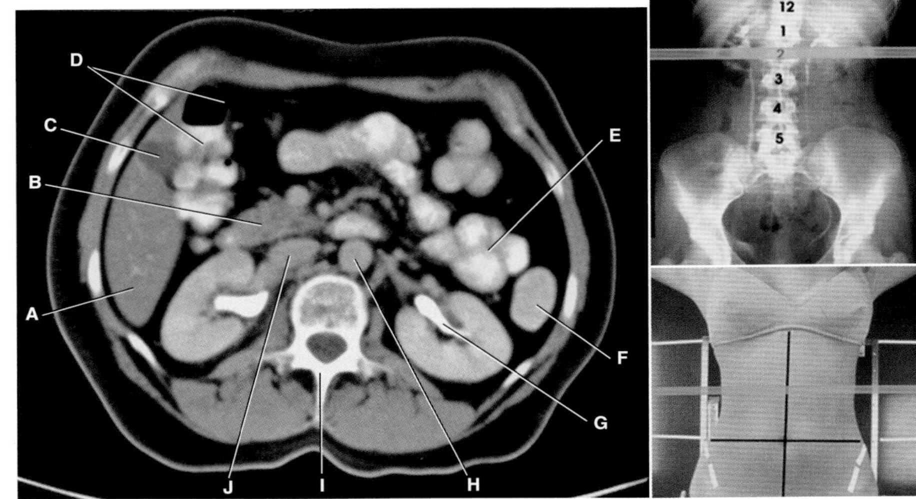

Fig. 22-71. Axial section 7.

Axial Section 8 (Fig. 22-72)

This scan of axial section 8 is **2-cm caudal to the renal pelvis** of the kidneys and demonstrates the contrast-filled **ureters** medial to the kidneys.

The parts as labeled are as follows:

A. Inferior lobe of the liver
B. Ascending colon
C. Inferior vena cava
D. Aorta
E. Jejunum
F. Descending colon
G. Left kidney
H. Left ureter
I. L2-L3 vertebrae
J. Psoas major muscle
K. Right ureter

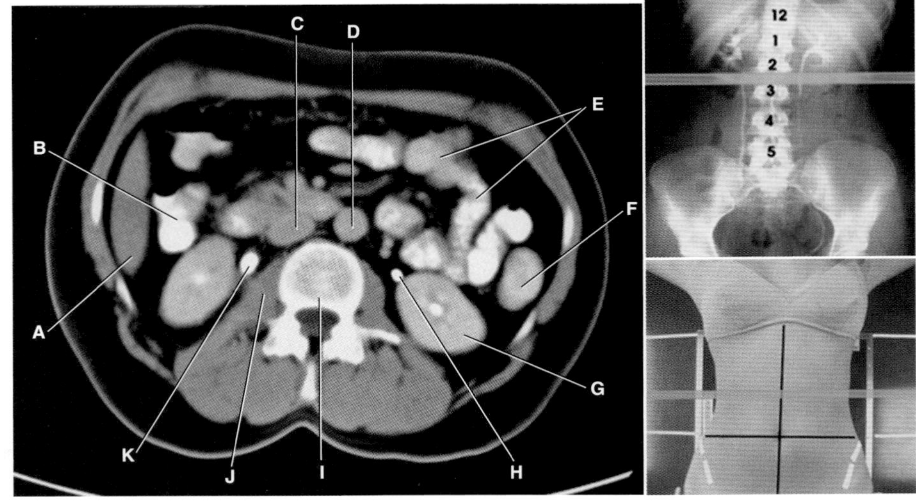

Fig. 22-72. Axial section 8.

22

Axial Sections of the Pelvis

Three sample CT axial slices of 10-mm thickness are shown. The pelvis CT on the male patient was obtained with a 150-ml drip infusion of intravenous contrast. Intravenous contrast was not used for the female patient examination due to a medical history of renal failure. Gastrointestinal opacification was obtained through oral and rectal administration of barium sulfate for both patients.

Axial Section 1, Male Pelvis (Fig. 22-73)

Axial section 1 is **2-cm caudal to the iliac crest.** This is a male pelvis.

The labeled parts are as follows:

A. Gluteus medius muscle
B. Right iliac wing
C. Ascending colon
D. Psoas major muscle
E. Left superior articular process of sacrum
F. L5 vertebra

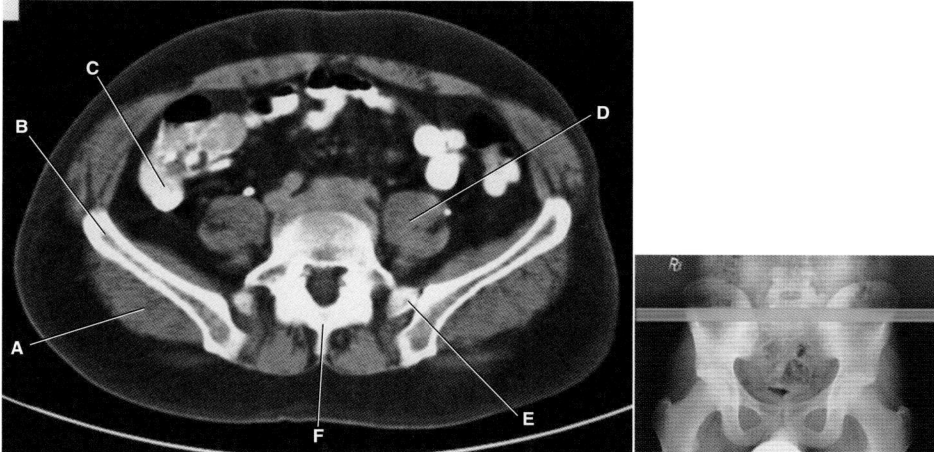

Fig. 22-73. Axial section 1, male.

Axial Section 5, Male (Fig. 22-74)

Axial section 5 is at the level of the **acetabular roof** *(B).* The paired oval-shaped seminal vesicles *(D)* are seen posterior to the bladder *(C).* This obviously is a male pelvis.

The labeled parts are as follows:

A. Gluteus maximus muscle
B. Body of ilium (acetabular roof)
C. Bladder
D. Seminal vesicles
E. Rectum
F. Distal sacrum

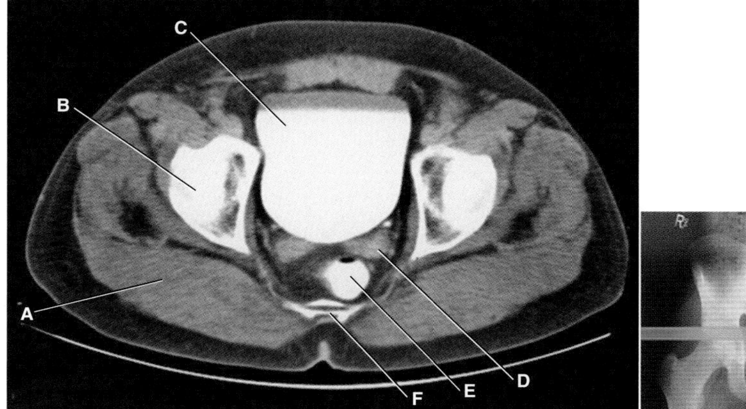

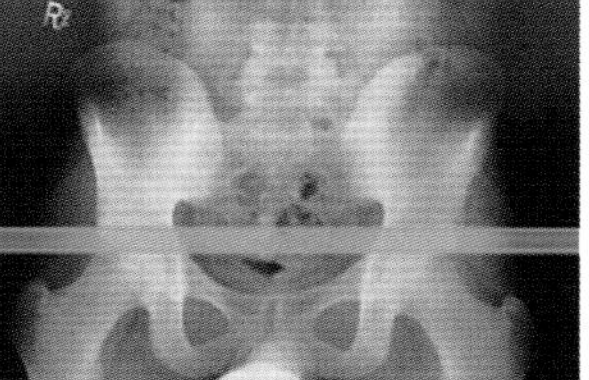

Fig. 22-74. Axial section 5, male.

Axial Section 10, Female (Fig. 22-75)

This scan of axial section 10 at the **symphysis pubis** *(D)* of this female pelvis gives excellent visualization of the vagina *(E)* due to insertion of a tampon for added contrast.

The labeled parts are as follows:

A. Ischial tuberosity
B. Distal femoral head and neck
C. Pubic bone
D. Symphysis pubis
E. Vagina (with tampon inserted)
F. Rectum

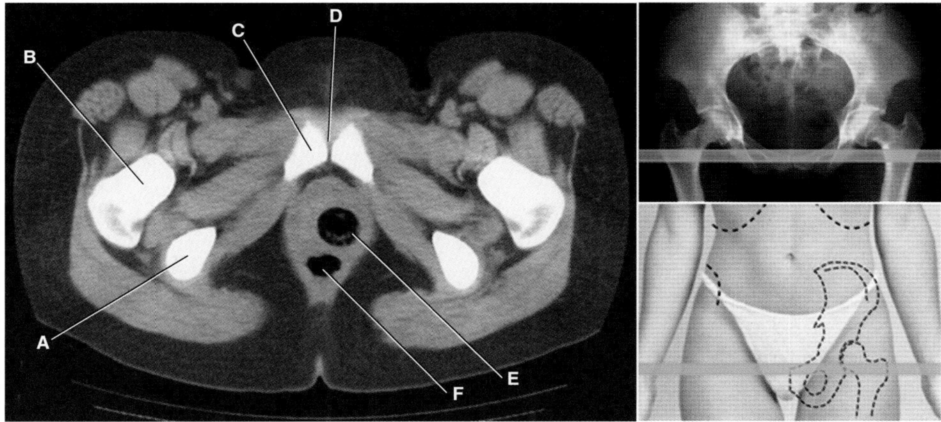

Fig. 22-75. Axial section 10, female.

PATHOLOGIC INDICATIONS AND EXAMPLES

Abdomen

- **Tumors:** lymphoma, metastatic lesions of the liver (Fig. 22-76), pancreas, kidney, adrenals, GI tract, or spleen
- **Inflammatory/infectious conditions: pancreatitis, abscess**
- **Renal stones**
- **Trauma**
- **Lymphadenopathy**
- **Circulatory pathology:** aneurysm, hemangioma, thrombosis

Pelvis

- **Tumors:** prostate, cervix, urinary bladder, and ovary
- **Inflammatory/infectious conditions:** abscess
- **Trauma:** fractures (Fig. 22-77)

EXAMPLES OF ABDOMINAL PATHOLOGY VISUALIZED BY CT

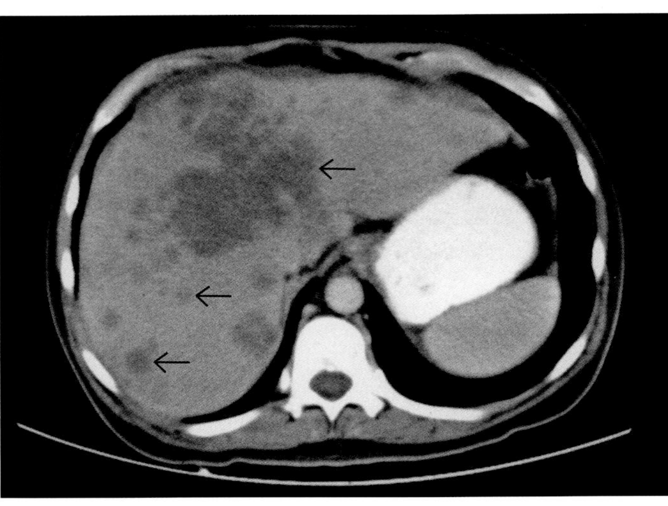

Fig. 22-76. Liver metastasis—multiple low-density lesions of variable size are visible within the liver tissue, representing metastatic disease.

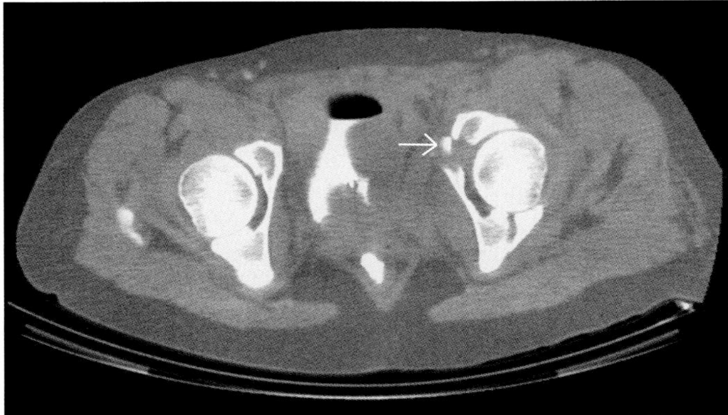

Fig. 22-77. Left acetabular fracture—scan of an 18-year-old female shows fracture of the anterior segment of the acetabulum.

Additional CT Procedures

NECK CT

Neck CT allows visualization of complex low-contrast anatomy. Common pathologic indications include:

- **Congenital abnormalities**
- **Trauma**
- **Infection/abscess,**
- **Tumors of the nasopharynx, oropharynx, parotid gland, and larynx.**

Before the procedure begins, metallic objects must be removed and the patient is positioned supine on the table. A scanogram, or scout image, is obtained to determine the range of the exam, usually from the skull base to the thoracic inlet, using 5-mm slices. The patient should be instructed to refrain from swallowing and any form of upper airway movement (talking, gum chewing, breathing, etc.). To help distinguish the esophagus from surrounding soft tissue, the patient may be asked to swallow low-density radiopaque esophageal paste. Intravenous contrast media is frequently indicated in neck CT to determine the extent of soft-tissue tumors and to visualize vascular structures. The Valsalva maneuver may be required.

MUSCULOSKELETAL CT

Musculoskeletal CT demonstrates bone destruction and soft tissue. Upper and lower limbs and extremities, shoulders, and hips may be examined (the hip examination is similar to a pelvis CT). When extremities are imaged, it is desirable to image both extremities for comparison purposes.

Common **pathologic indications** include:

- **Trauma**
- **Tumor**

The protocol will be determined by the clinical history, using the patient's plain radiographs as a reference. A scanogram, or scout image, is required to establish the parameters of the scan. When reviewing the CT images, both **soft-tissue window settings** and **bone window settings** should be used. Images may be reconstructed into alternate planes or 3D if required. Intravenous contrast media may be helpful in assessing tumors, and an intraarticular injection of air (as for an arthrogram) may be required to study joints.

SPINE CT

Common **pathologic indications** for spine CT include:

- Disk herniation
- Infection
- Spinal stenosis
- Tumor
- Trauma/fracture

Spine CT images are often reformatted into alternate planes (see Fig. 22-78).

A scanogram, or scout image, is required to establish the parameters of the scan. Slice thickness ranges from 3 to 5 mm.

Specialized CT Procedures

THREE-DIMENSIONAL (3D) RECONSTRUCTION

A data set obtained in a volume acquisition may be reconstructed into a 3D image if the required software and hardware are available. Clinical application includes assessment of trauma to the face, spine, pelvis, shoulder, and knee; evaluation of congenital abnormalities of the skull; and further investigation of the CNS, pulmonary structures, and vasculature (see Fig. 22-79 for example).

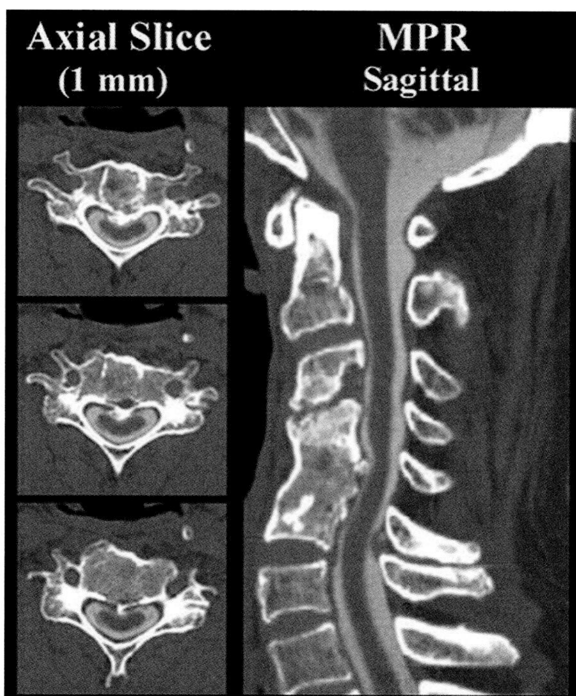

Fig. 22-78. Cervical spine CT, axial and sagittal planes.

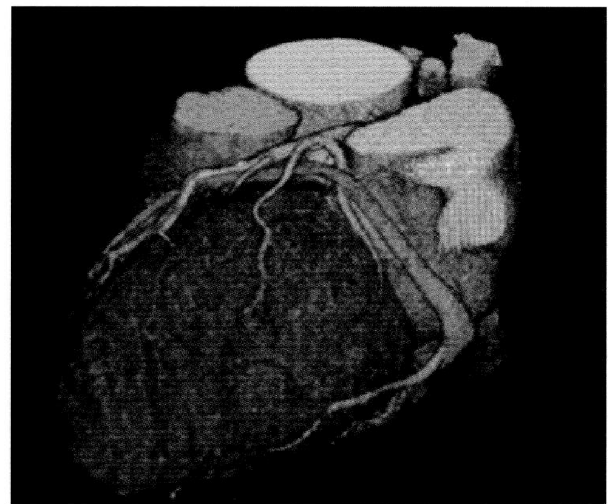

Fig. 22-79. Heart—example of 3D reconstruction.

CT (VIRTUAL) ENDOSCOPY

The most recent application of 3D imaging is for **virtual endoscopy.** 3D reconstruction software is used to simulate endoscopic views, typically bronchoscopy, laryngoscopy, and colonoscopy. This technique requires high contrast between the lumen and surrounding tissues so that the internal surfaces of the structure of interest can be identified for image formatting. Most endoscopic applications rely on air as the contrast medium of choice. Anatomic structures can be visualized in a variety of formats.

Virtual colonoscopy (Fig. 22-80) is the most widely used CT endoscopic application at this time. It is useful in the investigation of colonic polyps and as a diagnostic tool for patients who are not candidates for conventional colonoscopy. The procedure requires that patients undergo a standard bowel preparation. To provide the required contrast, air is instilled in the bowel through a rectal tube before the procedure; then the patient is scanned in both the supine and prone positions to allow visualization of all bowel structures. Risks for the procedure are related to the bowel preparation, rectal tube insertion, and colon insufflation; however, feedback from patients typically indicates that they find the virtual endoscopy procedure less uncomfortable and painful than conventional colonoscopy.

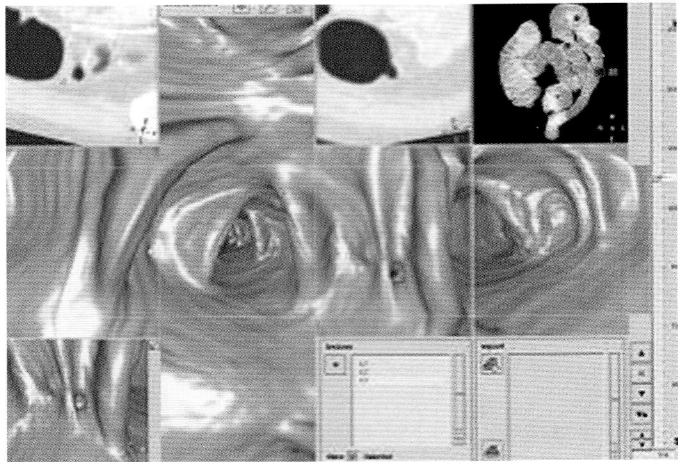

Fig. 22-80. Virtual colonoscopy—CT endoscopic procedure. (Courtesy Philips Medical Systems.)

22

CT FLUOROSCOPY

Dynamic images in CT are available, similar to dynamic images in conventional fluoroscopy. The patient/table is stationary, with the body section being imaged in the gantry aperture. Partially reconstructed images can be obtained and displayed at the rate of 6 to 8 images per second. Technical advances have provided improved image quality and speed—and will continue to do so.

CT fluoro has an application for biopsies and CT interventional procedures, such as abscess drainage, where the availability of real-time images allows for accurate placement of needles. It is important for the operator to adhere to radiation safety guidelines; that is, lead aprons, thyroid shields, and lead goggles must be worn, and special needle holders must be used to keep the operator's hands out of the beam. Special filters are also used to reduce the patient skin dose.

INTERVENTIONAL CT (Fig. 22-81)

The two most common interventional CT procedures are percutaneous biopsy and abscess drainage.

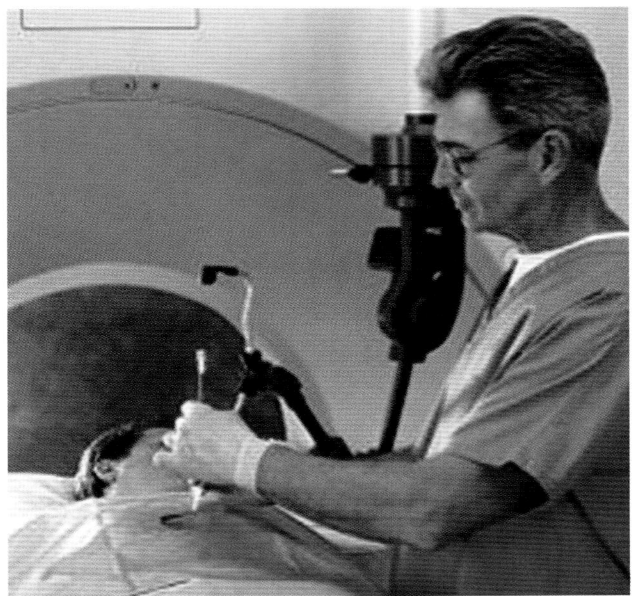

Fig. 22-81. Interventional CT procedures such as for biopsy or abscess drainage. (Courtesy Philips Medical Systems.)

Percutaneous Biopsy

Core biopsy and aspiration biopsy performed under CT guidance are less invasive than a surgical biopsy procedure and have a high accuracy rate. Depending on the site to biopsy, the patient may be positioned either supine, prone, or lateral. The patient is scanned to localize the tumor, the area is prepped and anesthetized, and the needle is placed. The area is again scanned to ensure the needle is correctly placed (CT fluoro is helpful here); the needle tip can be accurately visualized within a tumor (Fig. 22-82). The specimen is obtained and sent to the laboratory.

Possible complications from the procedure include infection, hemorrhage, pneumothorax (from a transpleural puncture for a proximal liver tumor), and pancreatitis (if performing a pancreatic biopsy).

Percutaneous Abscess Drainage

Abscesses are potentially life-threatening for the patient and must be treated. CT allows accurate localization of the abscess and placement of a needle into the abscess.

For a percutaneous abscess drainage, the patient is scanned to localize the abscess, the area is prepped and anesthetized, and the needle is placed. The area is again scanned to ensure the needle is correctly placed (CT fluoro is helpful here). When the needle is in optimal position, a guide wire is placed, followed by a catheter. The catheter is sutured into place, and the abscess drains for approximately 24 to 48 hours. The success rate of CT percutaneous abscess drainage is 85%.

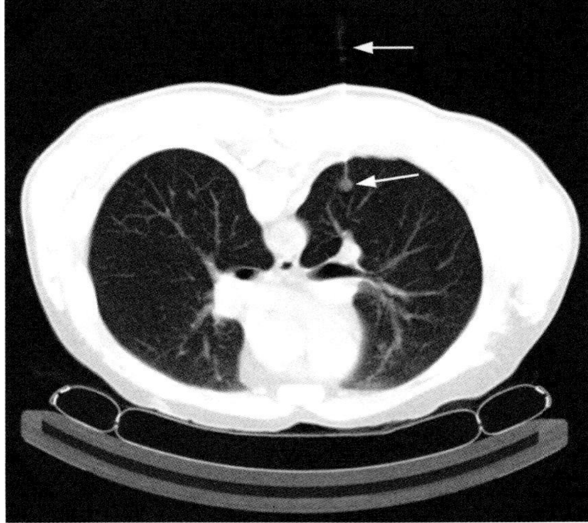

Fig. 22-82. CT lung biopsy, needle inserted in lesion *(arrow)*. (Courtesy Philips Medical Systems.)

Glossary of CT Terms

Artifact: Undesirable feature or density in the image not representative of anatomy.

Computed tomography (CT): A radiographic examination that displays sectional anatomic images in the axial, sagittal, or coronal planes.

CT number: A number representing the attenuation value for each pixel, relative to water.

Gantry: The component of a CT system that houses the x-ray tube, detectors, and collimators.

Isotropic: Having the same value of a property, in all directions; used to describe voxels that have the same value (size) in all directions (cubic).

Linear attenuation coefficient: Numerical expression of the decrease in radiation intensity following transmission through matter.

Matrix: Series of rows and columns (of pixels) that give form to the digital image.

Multiplanar reconstruction (MPR): Method by which images acquired in the axial plane may also be reconstructed in the coronal or sagittal plane.

Networking: Hardware and software that allow computers to be connected for the purpose of sharing resources and interacting.

Pixel: Picture element; an individual matrix box; each pixel is assigned a CT number.

Protocol: A predetermined procedure; in CT, protocol refers to the parameters of an exam.

Scanogram: The preliminary image of a CT exam that is used to plan the range of the scan. Depending on the vendor, it may also be called a *topogram,* or a *scout.*

Slice: Section of the object being scanned.

Slip rings: A device that transmits electrical energy and allows continuous rotation of the x-ray tube for volumetric acquisition.

Volume scanning: Refers to acquisition of a volume of CT data; the patient moves through the gantry with uninterrupted rotation and output of the x-ray tube. May also be referred to as *helical* or *spiral scanning.*

Voxel: Volume element; corresponds to a three-dimensional tissue volume, having height, width, and depth. Each pixel represents a voxel when viewing an image.

Windowing: Adjustment of the window level and window width (brightness and image contrast) by the user.

Window level: Controls the brightness of an image within a certain range.

Window width: Controls the gray level of an image (the contrast).

Workstation: A computer that serves as a digital postprocessing station and/or an image review station.

CHAPTER 23

Additional Diagnostic Procedures

CONTRIBUTIONS TO BONE DENSITOMETRY BY **Charles R. Wilson,** PhD, FAAPM, FACR, **Brenda K. Hoopingarner,** MS, RT(R)

CONTRIBUTORS TO PAST EDITIONS Brenda K. Hoopingarner, MS, RT(R), Marianne Tortorici, EdD, RT(R), Patrick Apfel, MEd, RT(R)

CONTENTS

ARTHROGRAPHY

Introduction

Arthrography *(ar-throg'rah-fe)* is a **contrast-media study of synovial joints and related soft tissue structures.** The joints include the hip, knee, ankle, shoulder, elbow, wrist, and temporomandibular joints (TMJs).

Some physicians prefer arthrography for examination of these joints; others prefer magnetic resonance imaging (MRI) in place of, or in addition to, arthrography, especially for the knee and shoulder.

With arthrography the technique of examination is similar for all the joints, with variations occurring primarily because of anatomic differences. Arthrogram studies of the TMJs are occasionally performed—examples are shown in Figs. 23-1 and 23-2, where contrast media is seen in the TMJ space in lateral open- and closed-mouth positions. The mandibular condyle can be seen outlined by the contrast medium within the TMJ joint capsule *(small arrows).*

Arthrograms of the shoulder and knee are the most common arthrography procedures being performed today and are described and illustrated in this chapter.

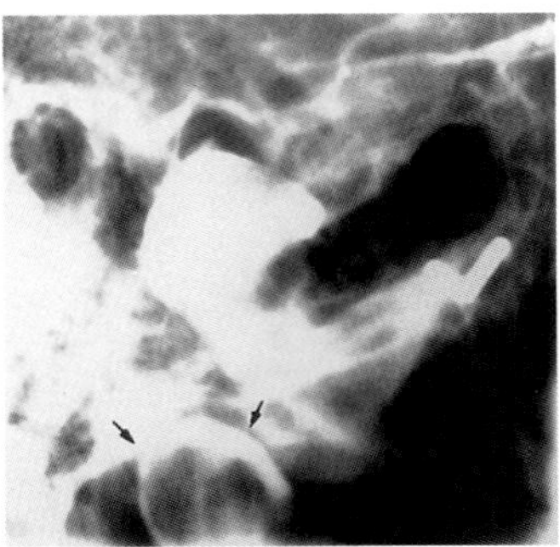

Fig. 23-1. Closed mouth.

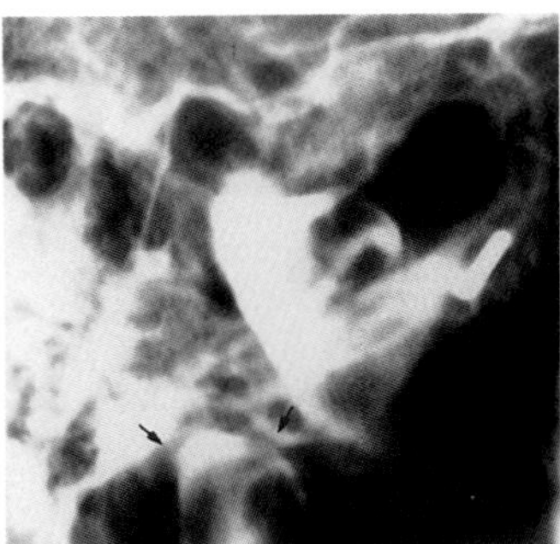

Fig. 23-2. Open mouth.

TMJ arthrograms.

Knee Arthrography

ANATOMY

The anatomic structures demonstrated during arthrography of the knee are presented in Chapter 7.

PURPOSE

Knee arthrography is performed to **demonstrate and assess the knee joint and associated soft-tissue structures for pathologic processes.** The structures of major interest include the **joint capsule; menisci;** and **collateral, cruciate,** and other **minor ligaments.** These structures are visualized through the introduction of a contrast medium into the joint capsule with fluoroscopic spot filming and/or conventional radiographic filming or with digital fluoroscopy/imaging.

PATHOLOGIC INDICATIONS

Knee arthrography is indicated when **tears of the joint capsule, menisci,** or **ligaments are suspected.** The knee is a joint subject to considerable stress, especially during sports activities. Therefore many of the pathologic processes seen in the knee are due to **trauma.**

An example of a **nontraumatic pathologic process** indicating arthrography is a **Baker's cyst,** which communicates with the joint capsule in the popliteal area.

CONTRAINDICATIONS

In general, arthrography of any joint is contraindicated when the patient is known to be allergic to an iodine-based contrast medium or to local anesthetics.

PATIENT PREPARATION

Any arthrographic procedure should be thoroughly explained before the examination proceeds to preclude unnecessary anxiety on the part of the patient. The patient should be advised of any complications and must sign an informed consent form.

MAJOR EQUIPMENT

The major equipment for knee arthrography varies with the method of imaging. Image acquisition is obtained during fluoroscopy and can be conventional spot films or digital images. The radiographic room used must be equipped so that horizontal-beam radiography can be accomplished.

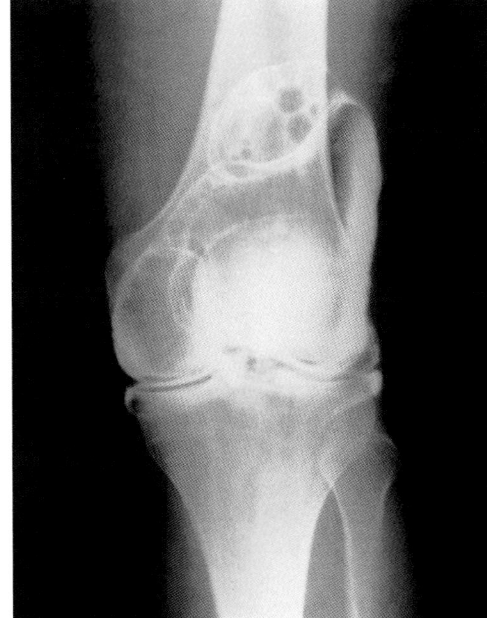

Fig. 23-3. AP knee during arthrogram.

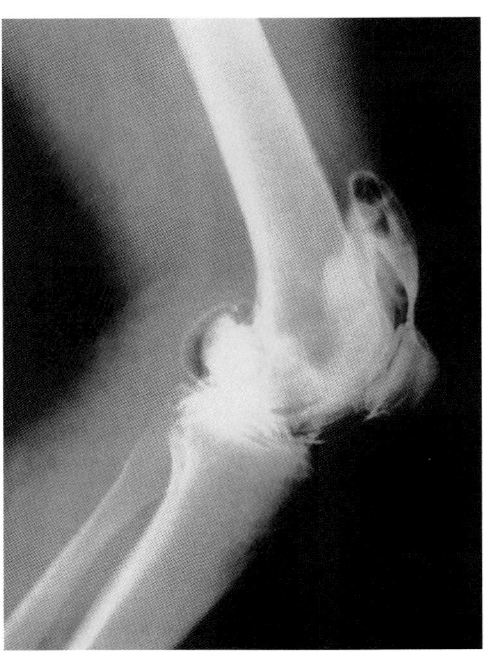

Fig. 23-4. Lateral knee during arthrogram.

ACCESSORY EQUIPMENT

Accessory equipment for examination of the knee varies according to the method of imaging, except for those items needed for the contrast injection and preparation of the injection site. These items are basically the same for any arthrogram tray (Fig. 23-5).

Arthrogram tray: Generally, a **disposable tray** is used for the procedure, which is an aseptic procedure. Such a tray should contain **prep sponges, gauze sponges, a fenestrated drape, one 50-ml** and **two 10-ml syringes, a flexible connector, several hypodermic needles** (usually 18-, 20-, 21-, and 25-gauge) and a **5-ml ampule of local anesthetic,** such as xylocaine. Additionally, **sterile gloves** and **antiseptic solution** (such as Betadine), **a razor,** and the contrast media are needed. For knee arthrography, a **2- to 3-inch wide Ace bandage** is also required.

The injection site is prepared by shaving the area with a razor and cleansing the site, using the prep sponges and basin containing the antiseptic solution. The area is dried with the gauze sponges and draped with the fenestrated drape (a drape with a central opening). The positive contrast medium is drawn up for injection later (approximately 5 ml) with a 10-ml syringe and 18-gauge needle. The physician injects the skin, underlying tissues, and the joint capsule with the local anesthetic using a 10-ml syringe with a 21- or 25-gauge needle.

NEEDLE PLACEMENT AND INJECTION PROCESS

A retropatellar, lateral, or medial approach may be used during needle placement. The actual site of injection is the preference of the physician.

With the site prepared, draped, and anesthetized, the physician introduces the 20-gauge needle, mounted on a 10-ml syringe, through the skin and underlying tissues into the joint space. Joint fluid is aspirated. If it is normal in appearance (that is, clear and tinged yellow), it may be discarded. If it appears abnormal (cloudy), it should be sent to the laboratory for assessment.

With all the fluid aspirated, the positive contrast medium (drawn up earlier) is injected into the joint through the 20-gauge needle, which has been left in place for the injection. If the study is a dual-contrast exam, the 50-ml syringe is used to inject the negative contrast medium.

Once the contrast medium is injected, the needle is removed and the Ace bandage wrapped around the distal femur to obliterate the area of the suprapatellar bursae.

CONTRAST MEDIA

Knee arthrography can be accomplished by use of a radiolucent (negative) medium, a radiopaque (positive) medium, or a combination of both media (dual-contrast). The dual-contrast study seems to be the method of choice. For this study a very small amount (approximately 5 ml) of a relatively low-density positive medium is used, along with 80 to 100 ml of a negative medium such as carbon dioxide, oxygen, or room air.

With the media injected the knee is gently flexed, which produces a thin, even coating of the soft tissue structures with the positive medium.

Fluoroscopic or Overhead Imaging Either fluoroscopic or overhead imaging is used. Image receptors include 18 × 24 cm (8 × 10 inch) cassettes or fluoroscopy image receptors. A table-mounted patient restraining device arranged as a sling around the knee area should be available (Fig. 23-6). The sling is used to provide lateral or medial stress to "open up" the appropriate area of the joint to better visualize the meniscus during fluoroscopy. Overhead (vertical-beam) radiography is the least used imaging method. Fluoroscopy is more common and requires a fluoroscopic tube with a small (fractional) focal spot to provide the detail necessary to adequately visualize the menisci.

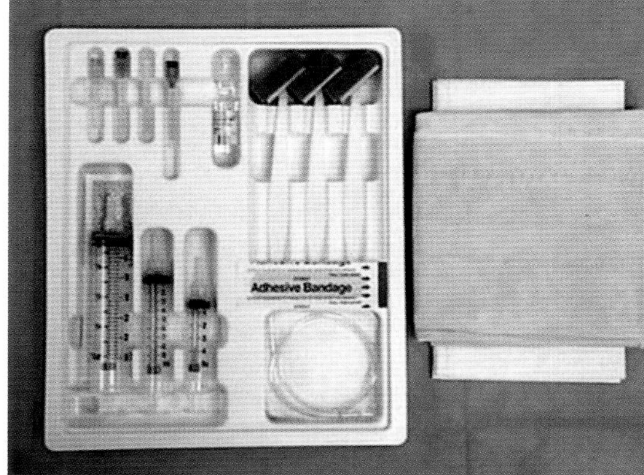

Fig. 23-5. Arthrogram tray.

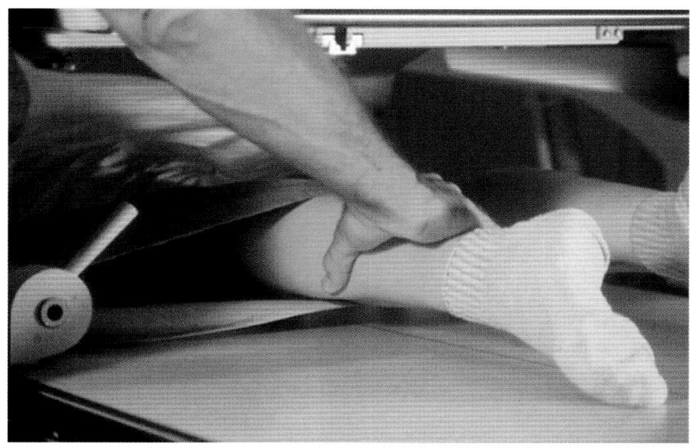

Fig. 23-6. Knee arthrogram (sling around knee in place).

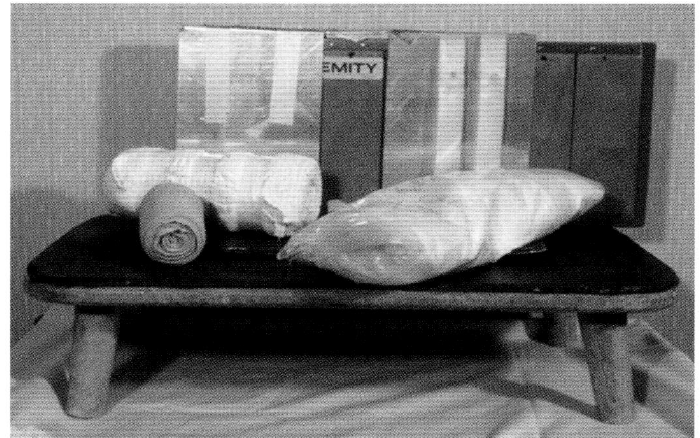

Fig. 23-7. Accessory equipment for horizontal-beam radiograph of knee.

Horizontal-Beam Radiography Horizontal-beam radiography is another common form of imaging, as described and illustrated on p. 757. This procedure requires a 35 × 43 cm (14 × 17 inch or 7 × 17 inch) image receptor, a lead diaphragm, a low small table or stand to support the knee, a firm pillow, and a 5-lb sandbag (Figs. 23-7 and 23-12).

POSITIONING ROUTINES

Radiographic Routines

The routine positioning and procedure for knee arthrography varies with the method of examination, such as fluoroscopy, conventional radiography, or a combination of both.

Fluoroscopy/Spot Filming or Digital Fluoroscopy/Imaging

During fluoroscopy the radiologist usually takes a series of closely collimated views of **each meniscus,** rotating the leg approximately **20° between each exposure.** The result is a spot film with nine exposures of each meniscus, which demonstrates the meniscus in profile throughout its diameter (Fig. 23-9).

If digital fluoroscopy and imaging are used. the images are stored on a computer's hard drive for final viewing and storage or printing to hard copy.

Radiographic Criteria

- Each meniscus should be clearly visualized in varying profiles on each of the nine exposed areas of the image receptor. Additional exposures may be necessary to demonstrate pathologic processes.
- The meniscus being visualized should be in the center of the collimated field.
- Correct exposure and adequate penetration should be evident to visualize the meniscus and contrast media.
- The meniscus under examination should be appropriately marked as M (medial) or L (lateral) with small lead markers (smaller than usual right and left markers to lessen the chance of obscuring anatomy).
- The patient ID marker should be clear, and the R or L marker should be visualized without superimposition of the anatomy.

Conventional "Overhead" Projections

23

In addition to the spot films or digital fluoroscopy imaging, routine AP and lateral radiographs of the entire knee, utilizing the radiographic tube, are usually included (Figs. 23-10 and 23-11). These images are obtained after removal of the Ace bandage from the distal femur.

Radiographic Criteria

- The AP and lateral images should demonstrate the entire articular capsule as outlined by the combination of negative and positive contrast media.
- Positioning criteria should be similar to the conventional AP and lateral knee, as described in Chapter 7.
- The patient ID marker should be clear, and the R or L marker should be visualized without superimposing anatomy.

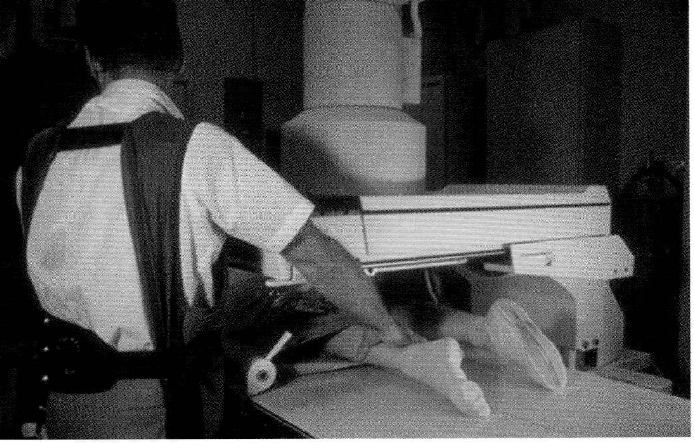

Fig. 23-8. Fluoroscopic spot filming (left knee).

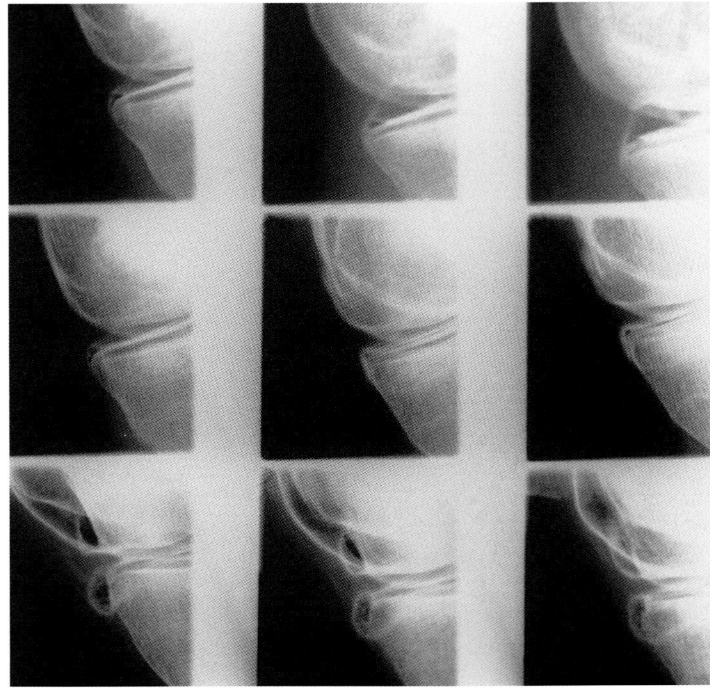

Fig. 23-9. Fluoroscopic spot film (approx. 20° rotation between exposures).

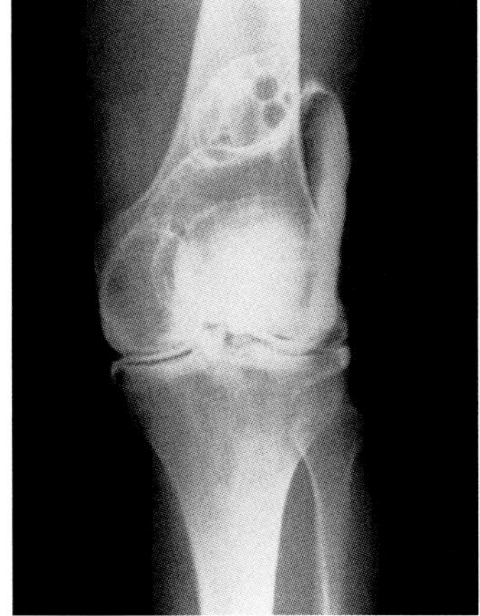

Fig. 23-10. AP knee.

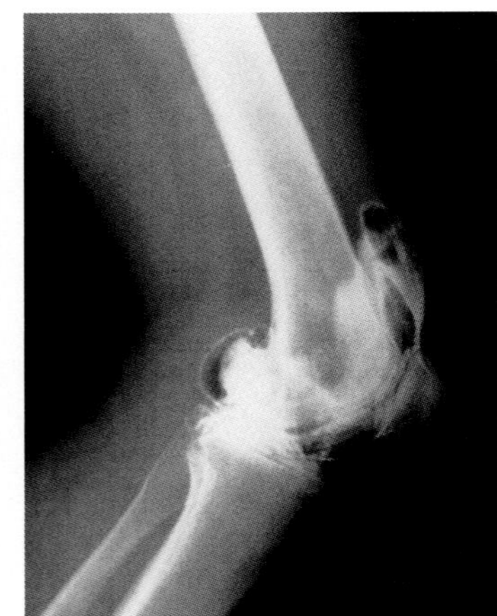

Fig. 23-11. Lateral knee.

Horizontal-Beam Projections

Horizontal-beam radiography is another common method of imaging for knee arthrography and requires some special equipment (Fig. 23-12), including the following:

- Six views of each meniscus
- Low, small table or stand for use during radiographing of the lateral meniscus; a firm pillow
- 5-lb sandbag

These last two items are used to open up the appropriate area of the joint space to visualize the lateral and medial menisci.

Each meniscus is radiographed on one image receptor with the patient's leg **rotated 30° between each exposure.** The resulting radiograph demonstrates **six views of each meniscus,** in profile, throughout its diameter (Fig. 23-13).

Radiographic Criteria

- Each meniscus should be demonstrated in a different profile in six exposures.
- Collimated fields should not overlap.
- The joint/meniscus should be centered to the collimated field.
- Correct exposure and adequate penetration should exist to visualize the meniscus and contrast media.
- The patient ID marker should be clear, and the R or L marker should be visualized without superimposing anatomy.

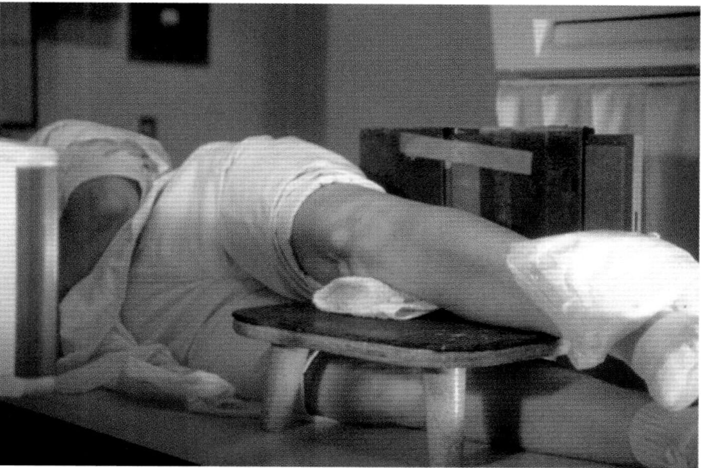

Fig. 23-12. Horizontal-beam projection.

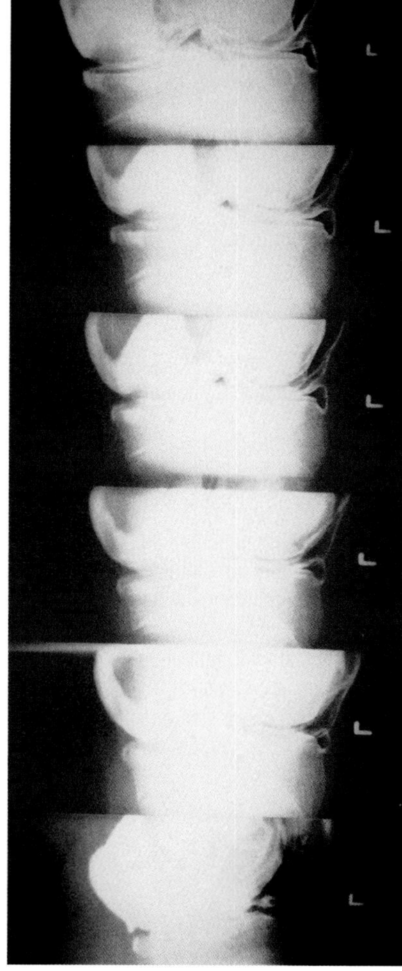

Fig. 23-13. Six views of lateral meniscus (AP on top to lateral on bottom).

23

Shoulder Arthrography

PURPOSE

Arthrography of the shoulder utilizes either a single- or double-contrast injection to **demonstrate the joint capsule, rotator cuff** (formed by conjoined tendons of four major shoulder muscles), **long tendon of the biceps muscle,** and **articular cartilage.**

EQUIPMENT AND PROCEDURES

A radiographic/fluoroscopic room is needed for the procedure, similar to that of a knee arthrogram. Contrast injection is monitored under fluoroscopic control, and conventional imaging is done with the overhead x-ray tube. Equipment and supplies needed include a standard disposable arthrogram tray and a $2\frac{1}{2}$- to $3\frac{1}{2}$-inch spinal needle.

NEEDLE PLACEMENT AND INJECTION PROCESS

The injection site, directly over the joint, is prepared as in any arthrographic procedure (Fig. 23-14). Once the area is anesthetized, the physician uses fluoroscopy to guide the needle into the joint space. Because the joint is quite deep, a spinal needle must be used. A small amount of contrast medium is injected to determine whether the bursa has been penetrated. Once the contrast medium has been fully instilled, filming begins.

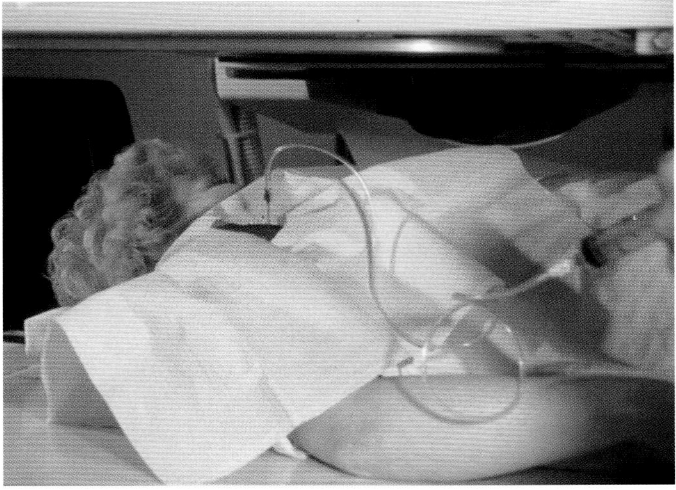

Fig. 23-14. Needle placement.

CONTRAST MEDIA

Arthrography of the shoulder can be accomplished with either a single-, positive-contrast medium or a combination of positive- and negative- (dual-) contrast media. For a single-contrast study, 10 to 12 ml of a positive medium, such as Omnipaque, is used. For a dual-contrast study, 3 to 4 ml of the positive medium and 10 to 12 ml of a negative medium (for example, room air) are used.

A dual-contrast study is believed by some practitioners to better demonstrate specific areas, such as the inferior portion of the rotator cuff, when the views are done with the patient upright.

ROUTINE POSITIONING AND IMAGING SEQUENCE

Routine radiography varies, and imaging can be done with the patient upright or supine. A suggested imaging sequence can include **scout AP projections,** with **internal and external rotation** as standard, and a **glenoid fossa, transaxillary,** or **bicipital groove projection** (per departmental routine or as indicated).

Once the contrast medium has been injected, the views are repeated (Fig. 23-15). If the radiographs appear normal, the patient is directed to exercise the shoulder and the radiographs are repeated a second time. Caudad angulations of 15° to 23° may be used on the AP projections per specific department routines.

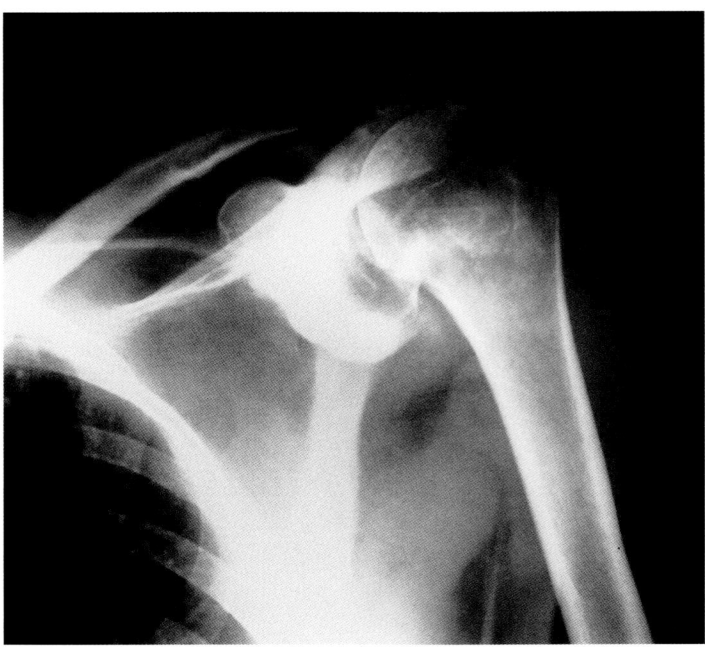

Fig. 23-15. AP shoulder with contrast media.

HYSTEROSALPINGOGRAPHY

Introduction

The **hysterosalpingogram** *(his"tar-o-sal"pin-go'gram)* **(HSG)** primarily demonstrates the **uterus** and **uterine** (fallopian) **tubes** of the female reproductive system. The female pelvic organs and their relationship to the abdominal peritoneal cavity are described in Chapter 17. More detailed anatomy of the uterus and uterine tubes, which is demonstrated with hysterosalpingography and should be understood by technologists, is described in the following discussion.

Anatomy

The anatomic considerations for hysterosalpingography include the principal organs of the **female reproductive system,** including the **vagina, uterus, uterine tubes,** and **ovaries.** Emphasis is placed on the uterus and uterine tubes. Additional anatomic considerations include the subdivisions, layers, and supporting structures of the female organs. The female reproductive organs are located within the **true pelvis.** The differentiation between the true and false pelvis is defined by a plane through the brim or inlet plane of the pelvis, as described in Chapter 8.

Uterus: The **uterus** is the central organ of the female pelvis. It is a pear-shaped, hollow, muscular organ bordered posteriorly by the rectosigmoid colon and anteriorly by the urinary bladder (Fig. 23-16). The size and shape of the uterus vary, depending on the patient's age and reproductive history. The uterus is positioned most commonly in the midline of the pelvis in an anteflexed position supported chiefly by the various ligaments. The position may vary with bladder or rectosigmoid distention, age, and posture.

The uterus is subdivided into four divisions: (1) the **fundus,** (2) the **corpus** (body), (3) the **isthmus,** and (4) the **cervix** (neck) (Fig. 23-17). The **fundus** is the rounded, superior portion of the uterus. The **corpus** (body) is the larger central component of the uterine tissue. The narrow, constricted segment, often described as the lower uterine segment that joins the cervix at the **internal os,** is the **isthmus.** The **cervix** is the distal cylindric portion projecting into the **vagina,** ending as the **external os.**

The uterus is composed of inner, middle, and outer layers. The inner lining is the **endometrium,** which lines the **uterine cavity** and undergoes cyclic changes in correspondence to the woman's menstrual cycle. The middle layer, the **myometrium,** consists of smooth muscle and constitutes the majority of the uterine tissue. The outer surface of the uterus is the **serosa,** lined with peritoneum and forming a capsule around the uterus.

Uterine tubes: The **uterine** (fallopian) **tubes** communicate with the uterine cavity from a superior lateral aspect between the body and fundus. This region of the uterus is referred to as the **cornu.** The uterine tubes are approximately 10 to 12 cm in length and 1 to 4 mm in diameter. They are subdivided into four segments. The proximal portion of the tube is the **interstitial** segment, which communicates with the uterine cavity. The **isthmus** is the constricted portion of the tube, where it widens into the central segment termed the **ampulla,** which arches over the bilateral **ovaries.** The most distal end, the **infundibulum,** contains fingerlike extensions termed **fimbriae,** one of which is attached to each ovary. The ovum passes through this **ovarian fimbria** into the uterine tube, where—if it is fertilized—it then passes into the uterus for implantation and development.

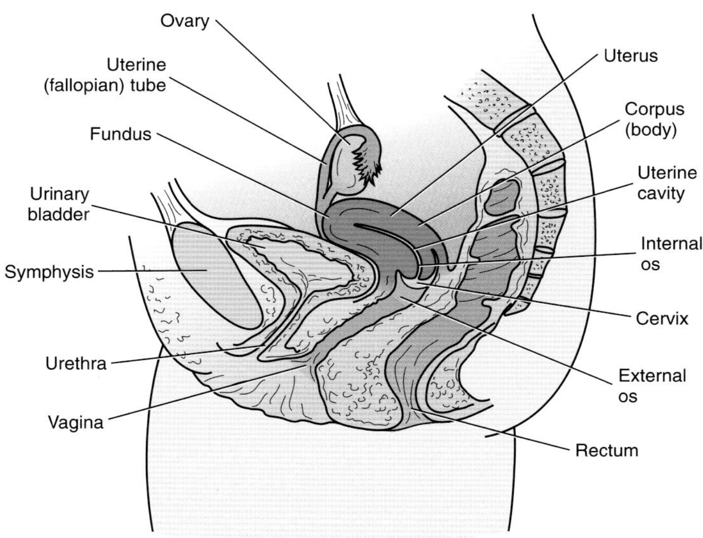

Fig. 23-16. Female reproductive organs—sagittal section.

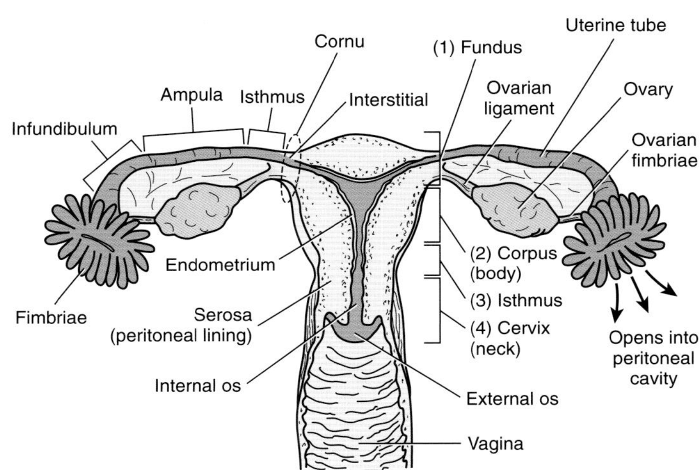

Fig. 23-17. Uterus—frontal view.

The distal infundibulum portion of the uterine tubes containing the fimbriae **opens into the peritoneal cavity.**

Definition and Purpose

Hysterosalpingography is the **radiographic demonstration of the female reproductive tract with a contrast medium.** The radiographic procedure best demonstrates the **uterine cavity** and **patency** (degree of openness) **of the uterine tubes.** The uterine cavity is outlined by injection of a contrast medium through the cervix. The shape and contour of the uterine cavity are assessed to detect any uterine pathologic process. As the contrast agent fills the uterine cavity, patency of the uterine tubes can be demonstrated as the contrast flows through the tubes and spills into the peritoneal cavity.

23

Pathologic Indications

Infertility assessment: One of the most common indications for HSG is in the **assessment of female infertility.** The procedure is performed to diagnose any **functional** or **structural defects.** A blockage of one or both uterine tubes may inhibit fertilization from occurring. In some cases, HSG can be a **therapeutic tool.** The injection of the contrast media may dilate or straighten a narrowed, tortuous, or occluded uterine tube.

Demonstration of intrauterine pathology: Although ultrasound is generally the modality of choice, HSG may also be performed when patient symptoms indicate the presence of **intrauterine pathologic processes.** Abnormal uterine bleeding, pelvic pain, and pelvic fullness are typical symptoms patients exhibit. **Lesions** demonstrated can include endometrial polyps, uterine fibroids, and intrauterine adhesions. HSG is also used to diagnose pelvic masses, fistulas, habitual spontaneous abortions, and congenital defects.

A third indication is the **evaluation of the uterine tube after tubal ligation** or **reconstructive surgery.**

Contraindications

Hysterosalpingography is contraindicated with **pregnancy.** To avoid the possibility that the patient may be pregnant, the examination is typically performed 7 to 10 days after the onset of menstruation.

Other contraindications include **acute pelvic inflammatory disease** and **active uterine bleeding.**

Patient Preparation

Departmental protocol should determine patient preparation requirements. These procedures may include proper bowel preparations to ensure adequate visualization of the reproductive tract unobstructed by bowel gas and/or feces. Preparation may include a mild laxative, suppositories, and/or a cleansing enema before the procedure. In addition, the patient may be instructed to take a mild pain reliever before the examination to alleviate some of the discomfort associated with cramping.

To prevent displacement of the uterus and uterine tubes, the patient should be instructed to empty her bladder immediately before the examination.

The procedure and possible complications should be explained to the patient and informed consent obtained. In some instances the physician may also perform a manual pelvic examination before the radiographic procedure.

Major Equipment

The major equipment for an HSG is a radiographic fluoroscope room (Fig. 23-18). Newer equipment may include digital fluoroscopy capabilities. Ideally the table should have the capability to tilt the patient to a Trendelenburg position if needed. If available, gynecologic stirrups should be attached to the table to assist the patient in the lithotomy position.

Accessory and Optional Equipment

Routinely a sterile, disposable HSG tray is used (Fig. 23-19). The general contents of the tray include a **vaginal speculum, basin, cotton balls, medicine cup, sterile gauze, sterile drapes, sponge-holding forceps, 10-ml syringes, 16-** and **18-gauge needles, extension tubing,** and **lubricating jelly.** In addition to the HSG tray, sterile **gloves,** an **antiseptic solution,** a **cannula** or **balloon catheter,** and **contrast media** are also necessary.

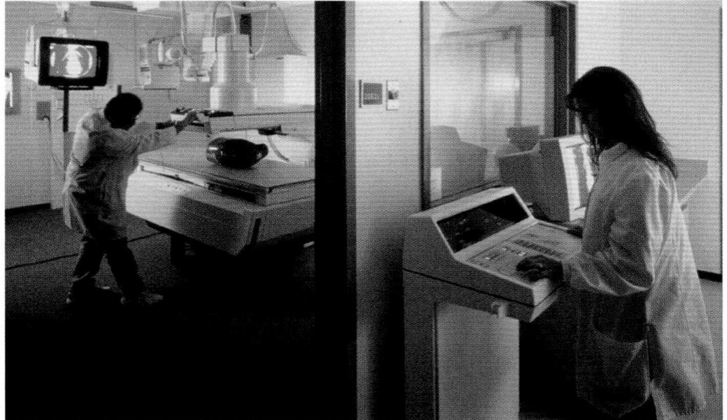

Fig. 23-18. Radiographic/fluoroscopic room with digital and spot film capabilities. (Courtesy Gateway Community College, Phoenix, Ariz; Bill Timmerman Photography.)

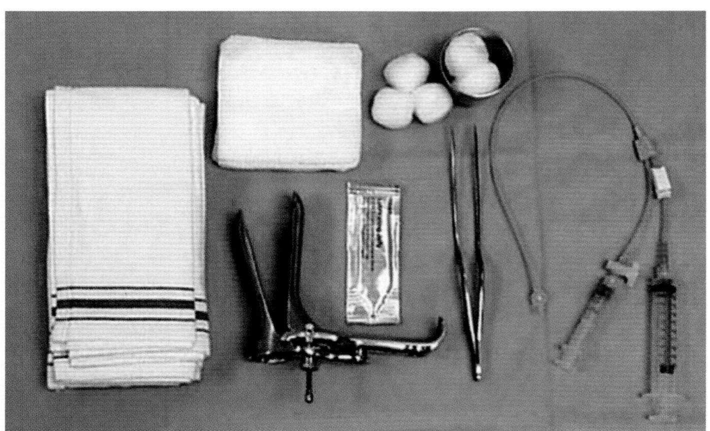

Fig. 23-19. HSG tray.

An additional instrument that may be requested by the physician is a **tenaculum** (an instrument with a hooklike end for gathering and holding tissues and structures in place).

Contrast Media

Two categories of radiopaque (positive) iodinated contrast media are used in HSG. Either an oil-based or water-soluble nonionic contrast medium is used, based on physician preference. **Most commonly preferred** today is the **water-soluble** contrast medium. It is easily absorbed by the patient, does not leave a residue within the reproductive tract, and provides adequate visualization. This medium does, however, cause pain when injected within the uterine cavity, and the pain may persist for several hours after the procedure. In contrast, the oil-based medium may be well tolerated by the patient and it is extremely opaque, allowing for maximal visualization of uterine structures. However, it has a very slow absorption rate and may persist in the body cavities for an extended period of time.

The amount of contrast medium to be introduced into the reproductive tract is recommended by the manufacturer and is variable, depending on the category of contrast media chosen. On the average, approximately 5 ml is necessary to fill the uterine cavity and an additional 5 ml is needed to demonstrate uterine tube patency.

23

Cannula/Catheter Placement and Injection Process

At the beginning of the procedure, the patient lies supine on the table in the lithotomy position. If gynecologic stirrups are unavailable, the patient bends her knees and places her feet at the end of the table. The patient is draped with sterile towels, and with sterile technique a vaginal speculum is inserted into the vagina. The vaginal walls and cervix are cleansed with an antiseptic solution. A cannula or balloon catheter is then inserted into the cervical canal. Dilation with a balloon catheter helps to occlude the cervix, preventing contrast medium from flowing out of the uterine cavity during the injection phase. A tenaculum may be necessary to aid in the insertion and fixation of the cannula or catheter.

Once cervical placement of the cannula or catheter is obtained, the physician may remove the speculum and place the patient in a slight Trendelenburg position. This position facilitates the flow of contrast media into the uterine cavity. A syringe filled with contrast is attached to the cannula or balloon catheter. Using fluoroscopy, the physician slowly injects the contrast medium into the uterine cavity. If the uterine tubes are patent (open), contrast media will flow from the distal ends of the tubes into the peritoneal cavity.

Positioning Routines

RADIOGRAPHIC ROUTINES

The routine positioning for hysterosalpingography varies with the method of examination. Fluoroscopy, conventional radiography, or a combination of both may be used.

FLUOROSCOPY/SPOT FILMING OR DIGITAL FLUOROSCOPY/IMAGING

Imaging of the reproductive tract is most commonly acquired with the use of spot-film fluoroscopy, or more recently, digital fluoroscopy. Typically, a collimated scout image is obtained with fluoroscopy. During the injection of the contrast medium, a series of collimated images may be taken while the uterine cavity and uterine tubes are filling (Fig. 23-21). After injection of the contrast media, an additional image may be taken to document spillage of the contrast into the peritoneum (Fig. 23-22). The patient most commonly remains in the supine position during imaging, but additional images may be taken with the patient in an LPO or RPO position to adequately visualize pertinent anatomy.

CONVENTIONAL RADIOGRAPHY

An overhead AP scout image may be obtained on a 24 × 30 cm (10 × 12 inch) IR. The central ray and IR are centered to a point 2 inches (5 cm) superior to the symphysis pubis. If fluoroscopy is unavailable, fractional injection of the contrast medium is implemented with a radiograph performed after each fraction to document filling of the uterine cavity, the uterine tubes, and contrast medium within the peritoneum. Additional images as determined by the radiologist may include LPO or RPO positions.

RADIOGRAPHIC CRITERIA

- The pelvic ring as seen on an AP projection should be centered within the collimation field.
- The cannula or balloon catheter should be demonstrated within the cervix.
- An opacified uterine cavity and uterine tubes are demonstrated centered to the IR.
- Contrast medium is seen within the peritoneum if one or both uterine tubes are patent.
- Appropriate density and short-scale contrast demonstrate anatomy and contrast medium.
- The patient ID marker should be clear, and the R or L marker should be visualized without superimposing anatomy.

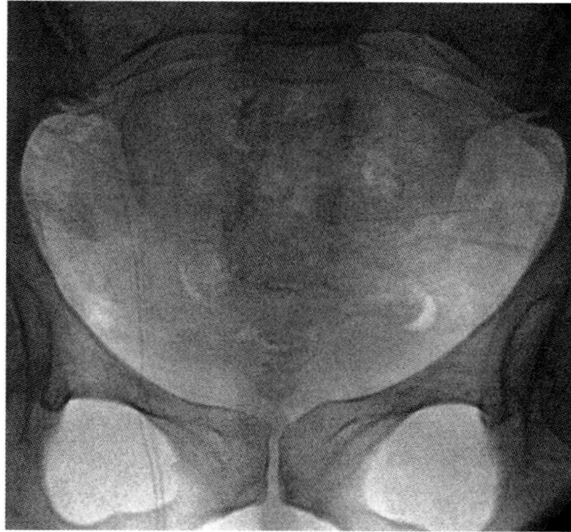

Fig. 23-20. Scout projection of pelvis.

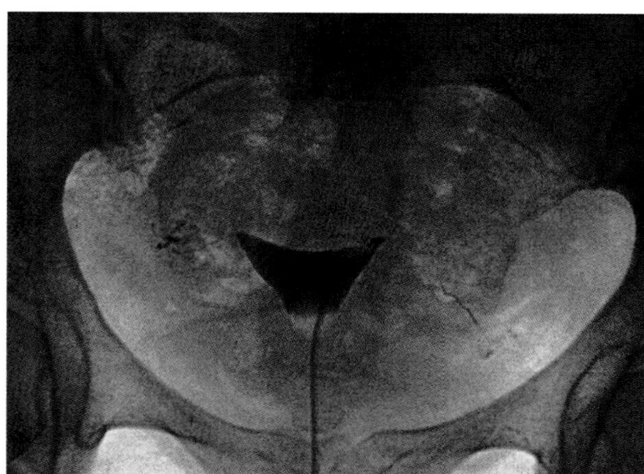

Fig. 23-21. Contrast media being injected into uterine cavity.

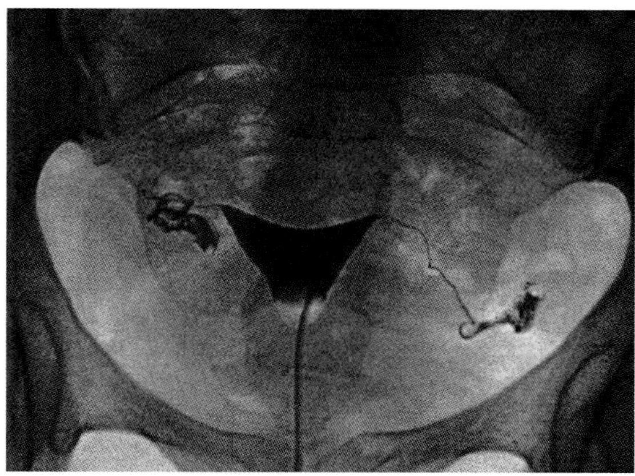

Fig. 23-22. Contrast media exiting distal uterine tubes into peritoneal cavity.

23

MYELOGRAPHY

Note: The myelogram procedure has largely been replaced by non-invasive MRI or CT procedures, but technologists should still be proficient in performing it when requested.

Anatomy

The bony anatomy related to **myelography** *(mi"e-log'rah-fe)* of the cervical, thoracic, and lumbar level of the spine is presented in Chapters 9 and 10. Additional spinal cord and related brain anatomy is demonstrated in Chapter 22.

Definition and Purpose

A **myelogram** *(mi'e-lo-gram)* is a **radiographic study of the spinal cord and its nerve root branches with a contrast medium.**

The spinal cord and nerve roots are outlined by injection of a contrast medium into the subarachnoid space of the spinal canal. The shape and contour of the contrast medium are assessed to detect possible pathologic processes. Because most conditions demonstrated by this procedure occur in the lumbar and cervical areas, myelography of these areas of the spine is most common.

Pathologic Indications

Myelography is performed when patient symptoms indicate the presence of a **lesion that may either be present within the spinal canal or protruding into the canal.** If the pathologic process impinges on the spinal cord, patient symptoms may include pain and numbness, often in the upper or lower limbs. The most common lesions demonstrated by myelography include **herniated nucleus pulposus (HNP), which is the most common clinical indication for myelography, cancerous or benign tumors, cysts,** and (in the case of trauma) **possible bone fragments.** If a lesion is present, myelography serves to identify the extent, size, and level of the pathologic process.

Another important feature of myelography is the identification of **multiple lesions.**

Contraindications

Myelography is contraindicated as follows:

Blood in the cerebrospinal fluid (CSF): The presence of blood in the CSF indicates probable irritation within the spinal canal, which can be aggravated by the contrast medium.

Arachnoiditis (inflammation of the arachnoid membrane): Myelography is contraindicated in the case of arachnoiditis because the contrast medium may increase the severity of the inflammation.

Increased intracranial pressure: In cases of elevated intracranial pressure, tapping of the subarachnoid space with needle insertion may cause severe complications to the patient as the pressure equalizes between the areas of brain and spinal cord.

Recent lumbar puncture *(within 2 weeks of the current procedure):* Performing myelography on a patient who has had a recent lumbar puncture may result in the contrast medium extravasating outside the subarachnoid space through the hole left by the previous puncture.

Patient Preparation

Patients scheduled for myelography may be apprehensive about the procedure. To reduce anxiety and relax the patient an injectable sedative/muscle relaxant is usually administered 1 hour before the examination. The type and amount of premedication used are determined by the radiologist performing the procedure.

Before the examination, the physician should explain the procedure and possible complications to the patient, and an informed consent should be signed by the patient.

Major Equipment

The major equipment for myelography includes a radiographic/fluoroscopic room with a 90°/45° (or 90°/90°) tilting table, shoulder braces, and a footrest with myelography ankle restraints (Fig. 23-23). Shoulder braces and the ankle restraints are used to secure the patient during the procedure, which may require tilting of the table in the Trendelenburg position (head lower than feet). Using the shoulder rests and ankle restraints together rather than separately is advised. The footrest is used to support the patient when the table is moved to the upright position.

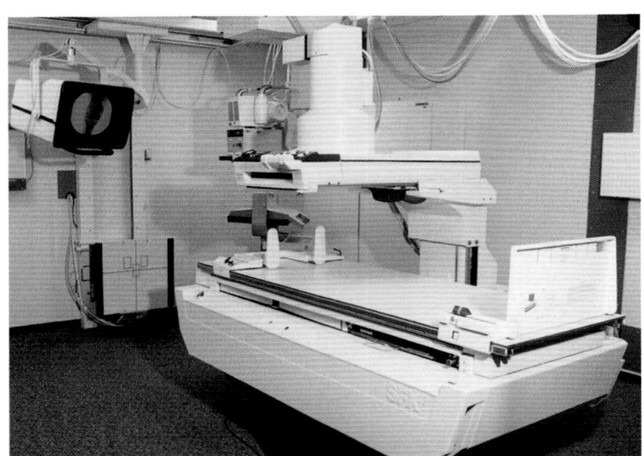

Fig. 23-23. Myelography-equipped room.

23

Accessory and Optional Equipment

The accessory equipment for myelography includes **grid cassettes with holders** for horizontal-beam radiography, a **myelography tray, sterile gloves,** an **antiseptic solution, appropriate laboratory requisitions,** and a **large position sponge or pillow.** The number and sizes of grid cassettes used depend on the level of the spinal canal being examined.

The myelography tray is generally a commercial prepackaged, sterilized, disposable unit (Fig. 23-24). A typical tray should contain the following: a **razor,** a **basin** and **prep sponges, sterile drapes, sterile gauze, 5-ml** and **20-ml syringes, 25-gauge** and **22-gauge needles, 18-gauge spinal needle,** a **single-dose vial of local anesthetic,** and **three test tubes.**

Needle Placement and Injection Process

Introduction of contrast medium for myelography is accomplished through a puncture of the subarachnoid space. There are generally two locations for the puncture site: the **lumbar** (L3-L4) and **cervical** (C1-C2) areas. Of the two locations the lumbar area is safer, easier on the patient, and most commonly used for the procedure. A cervical puncture is indicated if the lumbar area is contraindicated, or if pathologic condition indicates a complete blockage of the vertebral canal above the lumbar area, obstructing the flow of contrast medium to the upper spinal region.

After the puncture site is selected, the radiologist may use fluoroscopy to facilitate needle placement.

There are generally two body positions for a **lumbar puncture.** The patient may be **prone,** with a firm pillow or large positioning block placed under the abdomen to flex the spine (Fig. 23-25) or may lie in a **left lateral position** with the spine flexed. Flexion of the spine widens the interspinous space, which facilitates introduction of the spinal needle.

For a **cervical puncture** the patient may be seated in an **erect position** (Fig. 23-26) or **prone,** with the head flexed to open the interspinous space.

In both types of punctures the technologist prepares the injection site for this sterile procedure by shaving any hair present with the razor and cleaning the skin, using the basin, the sponges, and an antiseptic solution. The area is then dried with gauze pads and covered with a fenestrated drape. The local anesthetic is administered with the 5-ml syringe, with either the 22- or 25-gauge needle. With the area anesthetized, the spinal needle is introduced through the skin and underlying tissues into the subarachnoid space.

The location of the needle in the subarachnoid space is verified by an unobstructed back flow of CSF, which generally is allowed to flow through the needle. Allowing free flow of the CSF rather than drawing it out with a syringe reduces the risk for spinal cord trauma at the distal end of the needle within the canal. A sample of CSF is collected at this time and sent to the laboratory for analysis. The amount of CSF collected is dictated by the amount needed for the laboratory tests ordered. When the CSF is collected, the spinal needle is left in place for the contrast medium injection.

The contrast medium is injected through the spinal needle into the subarachnoid space, using the 20-ml syringe. Once the injection is completed, the needle is removed. A Band-Aid is applied to the puncture site, and images are acquired.

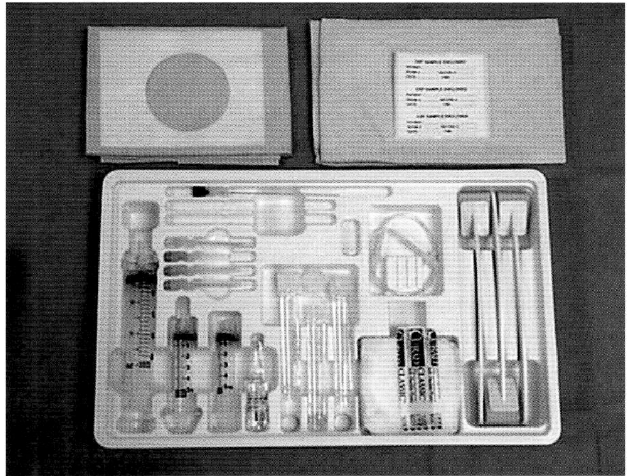

Fig. 23-24. Myelogram tray.

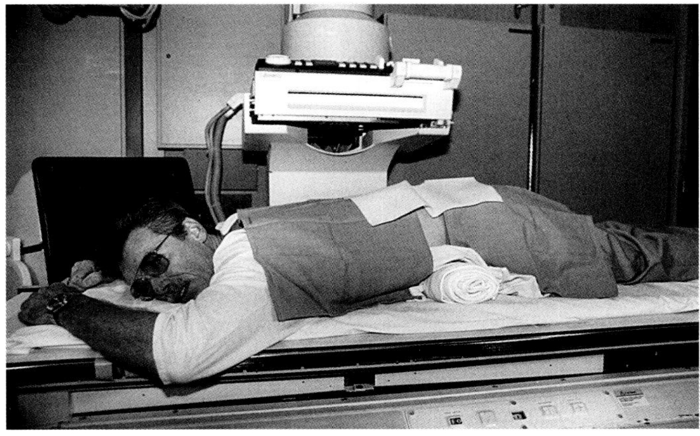

Fig. 23-25. Prone position for lumbar puncture.

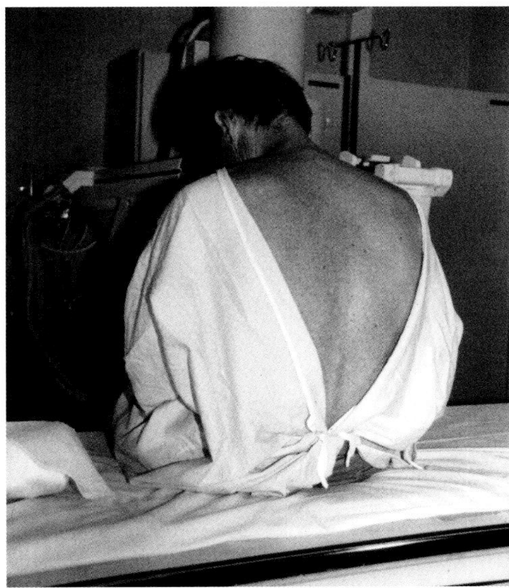

Fig. 23-26. Erect position for cervical (C1-C2) puncture.

Contrast Media

The best type of contrast medium for myelography is one that is miscible (mixes well) with the CSF, easily absorbed, nontoxic, and inert (nonreactive) and has good radiopacity. No one type of contrast medium meets all these criteria. In the past, air or gas (radiolucent) and oil-based iodinated (radiopaque) media have been used for myelography. Currently, however, primarily **nonionic, water-soluble iodine-based media** are used because of the relatively low osmolality (see Chapter 17).

Water-soluble contrast media provides excellent radiographic visualization of the nerve roots, is easily absorbed into the vascular system, and is excreted by the kidneys. Absorption begins approximately 30 minutes after injection with good radiopacity up to about 1 hour after injection. After 4 to 5 hours the contrast medium has a hazy radiographic effect, and it is radiographically undetectable after 24 hours.

Dosages: Dosage for myelographic contrast media is recommended by the manufacturer and varies with the concentration of the medium used and the area of the spine under examination. In general, a range of approximately **6 to 17 ml** is used.

Care should be taken to prevent the contrast medium from entering the area of the head. For example, during examination of the cervical area with the patient prone or in Trendelenburg position, the chin is hyperextended to prevent the medium from flowing into the cranial region of the subarachnoid space.

Positioning Routines

FLUOROSCOPY/SPOT FILMING OR DIGITAL FLUOROSCOPY/IMAGING

During fluoroscopy the table (and patient) is tilted from erect through Trendelenburg positions. This movement facilitates the flow of contrast medium to the area under examination.

Under fluoroscopic control, once the contrast medium has reached the desired area, the radiologist may image the patient in a variety of positions from prone to supine and in anterior or posterior oblique positions (Figs. 23-27 and 23-28). Images may be obtained using conventional or digital technology, depending on the equipment available. After fluoroscopy the technologist takes conventional radiographs that are appropriate for the area under examination, as requested by the radiologist.

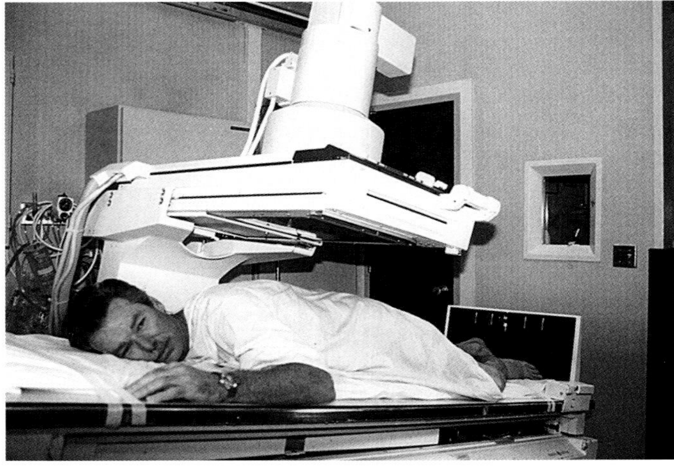

Fig. 23-27. Left posterior oblique for spot filming of lumbar myelogram. (X-ray tube is under table, making this a posterior oblique, AP projection.)

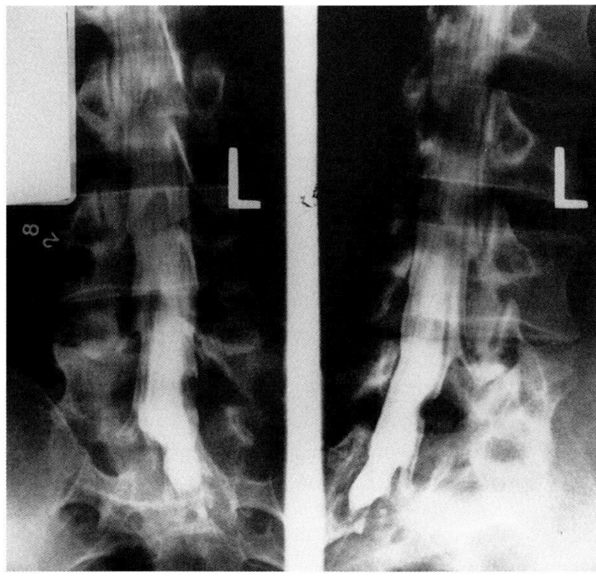

Fig. 23-28. Spot films of lumbar myelogram (RPO and LPO).

CONVENTIONAL RADIOGRAPHIC MYELOGRAPHY ROUTINES (AFTER FLUOROSCOPY)

Although department radiographic routines for myelography may vary significantly, the following positions/projections represent suggested **basic** routines for the different levels of the spinal column. Additional positions/projections that may be considered routine or special are also included.

Before routine radiography begins, the radiologist adjusts the table tilt as needed to concentrate the contrast medium to the level of the spinal cord being radiographed.

CERVICAL REGION

Horizontal-Beam Lateral (Fig. 23-29) The patient is prone, with the arms extended along the sides of the body and the shoulders depressed. The chin is extended and resting on a small positioning sponge or folded linen for comfort and to maintain extension. The central ray is directed to the level of C4-C5. The field should be collimated to reduce scatter radiation. Respiration is suspended during the exposure.

Swimmer's Lateral—Horizontal Beam (Fig. 23-30) The patient is prone, with the chin extended. For a right lateral the right arm is extended along the right side of the body, with that shoulder depressed. The left arm is flexed (i.e., stretched superior to the head). The central ray is directed to the level of C7. The field is collimated to reduce scatter radiation. Respiration is suspended during the exposure.

Note: Additional positions may include anterior obliques.

THORACIC REGION

Right Lateral Decubitus Position—AP or PA Projection With Horizontal Beam (Fig. 23-31) The patient is positioned in a true right lateral, with the right arm flexed, superior to the head. The left arm is extended and resting along the left side of the body. To maintain the alignment of the spine parallel to the tabletop, the patient may rest the head on the arm. If needed, a small positioning sponge or folded linen may be placed between the head and the arm to maintain alignment. The central ray is directed to the level of T7. Collimation of the field is to the area of interest to reduce scatter radiation. Respiration is suspended during the exposure.

Left Lateral Decubitus Position—AP or PA Projection With Horizontal Beam (Fig. 23-32) The patient is positioned in a true left lateral position, with the left arm raised and flexed above the head. The right arm is extended down, resting on the right side of body as shown. The spine remains parallel to the tabletop. The central ray is directed to T7 with close collimation to reduce scatter radiation. Respiration is suspended during the exposure.

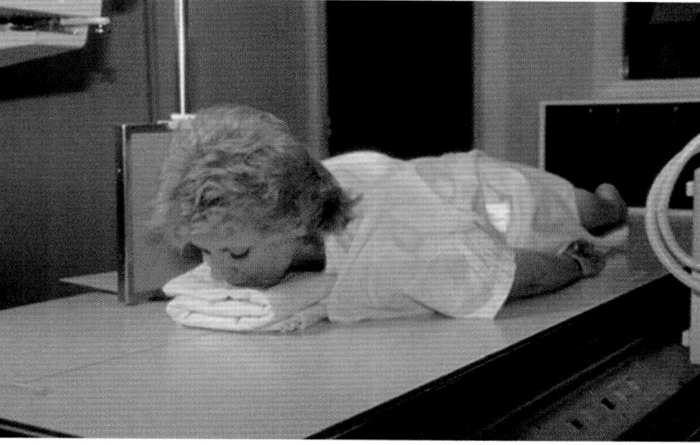

Fig. 23-29. Cervical region—horizontal-beam lateral.

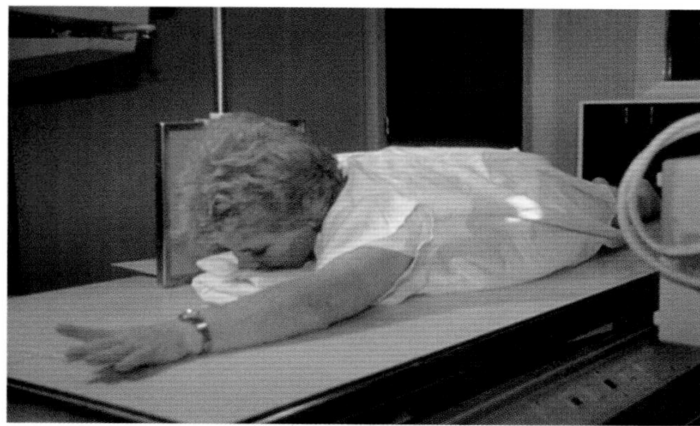

Fig. 23-30. Cervical region (C7 to T1 region)—swimmer's (horizontal-beam) lateral.

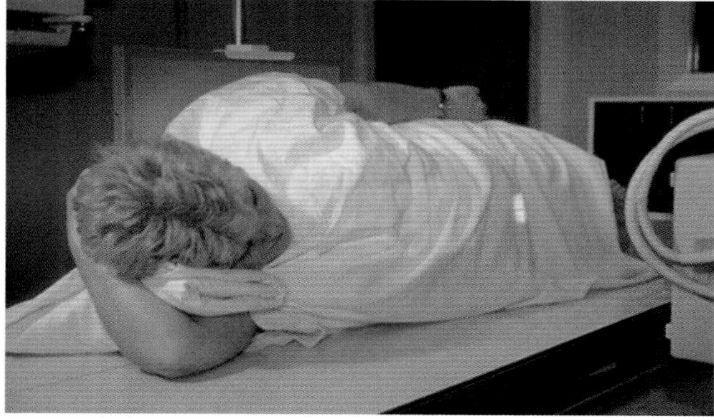

Fig. 23-31. Thoracic region—right lateral decubitus (AP horizontal-beam projection).

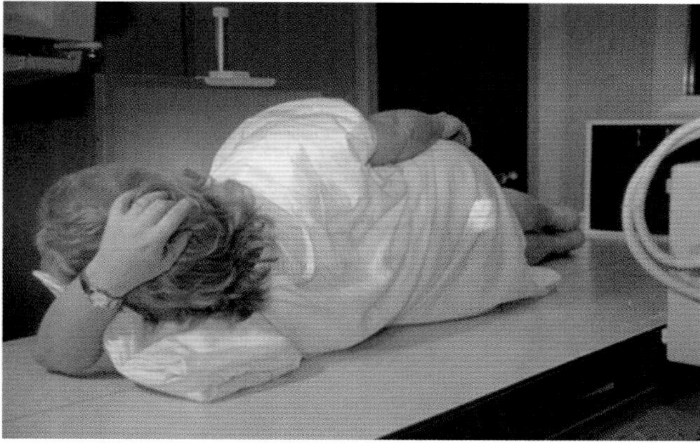

Fig. 23-32. Thoracic region—left lateral decubitus (PA horizontal-beam projection).

Right or Left Lateral—Vertical Beam (Fig. 23-33) The patient is positioned in a true lateral, with the knees flexed. Both arms are semiflexed. The alignment of the spine should be maintained parallel to the tabletop. The patient may rest the head on the hands, or a small positioning sponge or folded linen may be placed between the hands and the head to maintain alignment of the spine. The central ray is directed to the level of T7. The field is collimated to reduce scatter radiation. Respiration is suspended during the exposure.

Additional positions may include a supine (AP projection) and lateral with a horizontal beam.

Note: A supine AP and horizontal-beam lateral are not generally recommended, because in the supine position, pooling of the contrast medium occurs in the midthoracic region as a result of the usual thoracic curvature. This pooling, of course, is more prominent in some patients. Therefore to best demonstrate the entire spinal canal of the thoracic region, **AP and PA projections** should be taken in both the **right and left lateral decubitus positions,** in addition to the **vertical-beam lateral position** as described and illustrated.

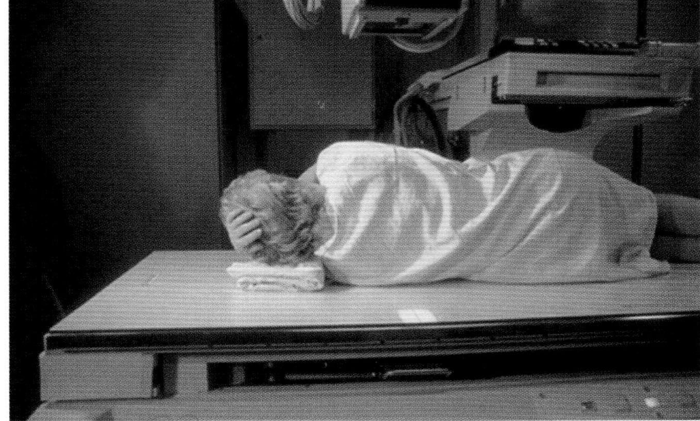

Fig. 23-33. Thoracic region—left vertical beam lateral.

LUMBAR REGION

Semierect Lateral—Horizontal Beam (Fig. 23-34) The patient is positioned prone, with the arms flexed superior to the head. The table and patient are semierect. The radiologist, under fluoroscopic control, adjusts the angulation of the table to concentrate the contrast medium in the lumbar area.

The central ray is directed to L3. Collimation to the area of interest is important to reduce scatter radiation. Respiration is suspended during the exposure.

Additional positions may include obliques with either a vertical or horizontal beam and a supine AP projection.

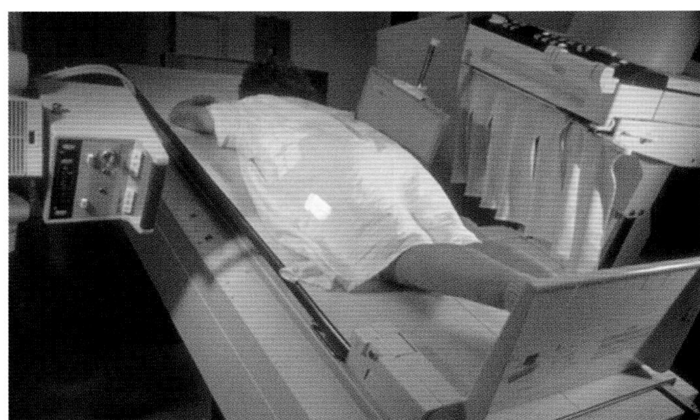

Fig. 23-34. Lumbar region—semierect transabdominal (horizontal-beam right lateral).

Radiographs

RADIOGRAPHIC CRITERIA (FOR ALL LEVELS OF THE SPINAL COLUMN)

- The appropriate level of the spinal column, with contrast present, should be demonstrated.
- Correct exposure and adequate penetration should exist to demonstrate anatomy and contrast medium.
- The patient ID markers and anatomic markers (right or left) should be clearly visualized without superimposing anatomy.
- Collimation should be evident.

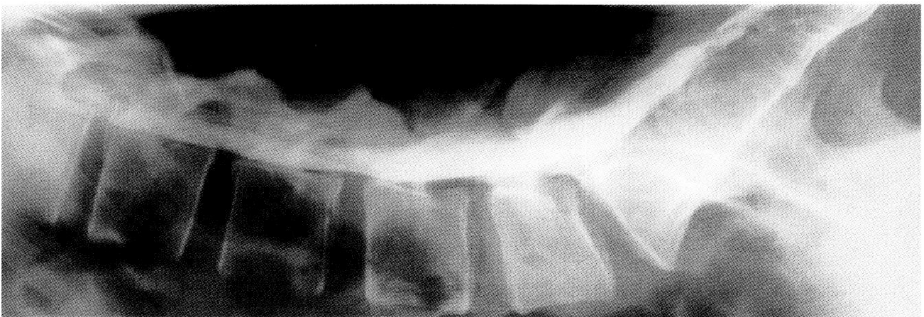

Fig. 23-35. Lumbar—transabdominal (horizontal-beam) lateral.

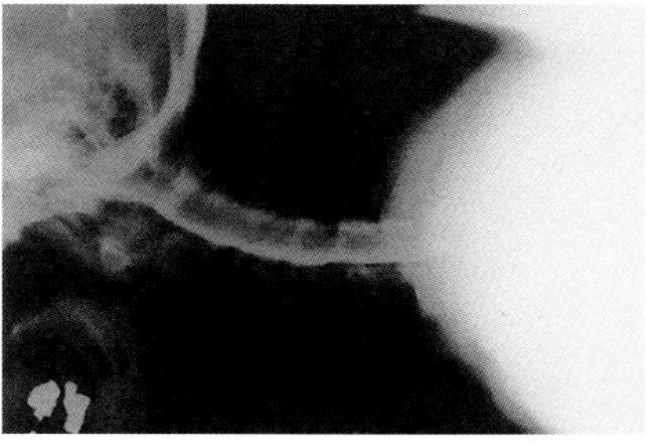

Fig. 23-36. Transcervical (horizontal-beam) lateral.

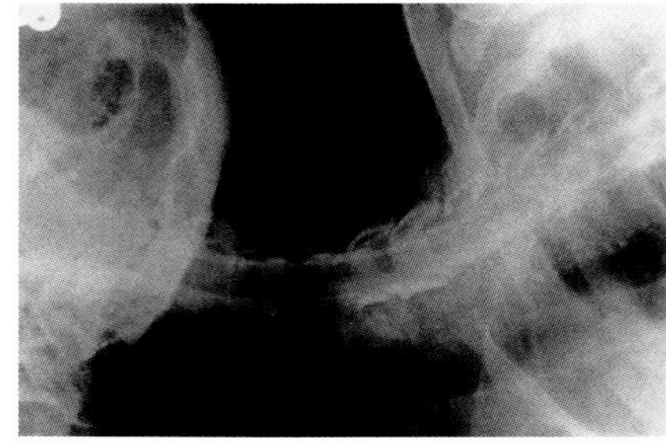

Fig. 23-37. Swimmer's (horizontal-beam) lateral.

SIALOGRAPHY

Introduction and Survey Results

Radiographic examination of the salivary glands and associated ducts by contrast-enhanced conventional sialogram procedures has largely been replaced with CT or MRI studies where these modalities are available. However, technologists should still be able to perform this procedure, as described in this chapter, when requested.

Anatomy

The accessory organs of digestion located within and adjacent to the oral cavity include the teeth and **salivary glands.** The salivary glands secrete the majority of the saliva found within the oral cavity that helps to dissolve foods and facilitate digestion. The glands are located adjacent to the oral cavity and communicate with the mouth via the **ducts.** Each gland is composed of numerous, small lobules that comprise large lobes of the gland. Saliva is secreted into the oral cavity by the ductal system of each gland. The small lobules contain small ductules that combine to form large branches, which eventually unite to form the major duct that empties into the oral cavity. The anatomy specific to sialography includes the **salivary glands** and **associated ducts** of each of the **three major pairs of glands.**

Parotid: The **parotid glands** are positioned anterior and inferior to the ear. They are the **largest** of the salivary glands and consist of a superficial and deep component. The superficial component is located directly anterior and inferior to the ear. It is adjacent to the mandibular ramus, with the posterior surface of the gland extending to the external auditory meatus.

The major duct supplying saliva from the parotid gland is the **parotid duct,** which is also known as **Stensen's duct.** This duct is approximately 5 to 7 cm in length and courses anteriorly and medially to pierce the fat pad of the cheek. It then communicates with the oral cavity at an opening opposite the second molar tooth.

Submandibular: The **submandibular,** or **submaxillary, gland** is the second largest salivary gland. Its primary location is medial and inferior to the body of the mandible. It also is composed of a superficial and deep component. The superficial portion lies anterior and inferior to the angle of the mandible and extends anteriorly along the body of the mandible.

The small, deep portion extends and curves around the mylohyoid muscle (muscle of the tongue and floor of the mouth). Arising from this deep portion is the **submandibular,** or **submaxillary duct,** more commonly known as **Wharton's duct.** It is approximately 5 cm in length and courses anteriorly and medially to the mandible. It opens into the oral cavity via a small, fleshy protuberance at the sides of the base of the frenulum of the tongue. (The frenulum is the central vertical fold of membrane under the tongue.)

Sublingual: The smallest of the salivary glands is the narrow, elongated **sublingual** gland. It is located beneath the mucous membrane of the floor of the mouth directly beneath the sublingual fold. The gland lies medial to the body of the mandible and extends posteriorly from the side of the frenulum to the submandibular gland. Unique to the sublingual gland are approximately **12 small ducts,** called the **ducts of Rivinus,** which help transport saliva to the oral cavity. These small ducts originate along the superior portion of the gland to open into the floor of the mouth at the sublingual fold. One or two of these ducts, **Bartholin's duct(s),** are larger in size and may connect with the submandibular duct.

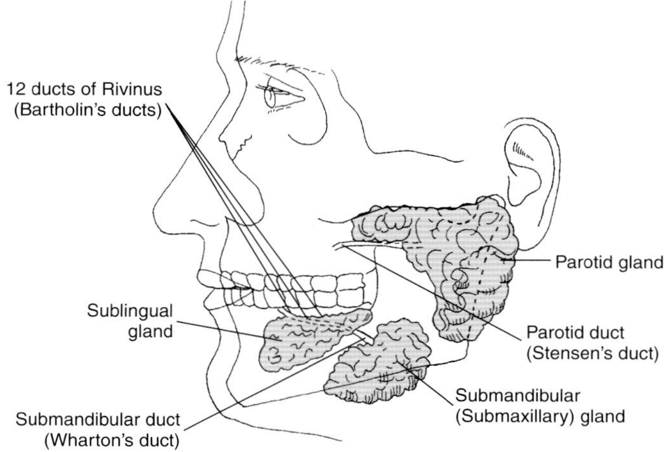

Fig. 23-38. Salivary glands and ducts.

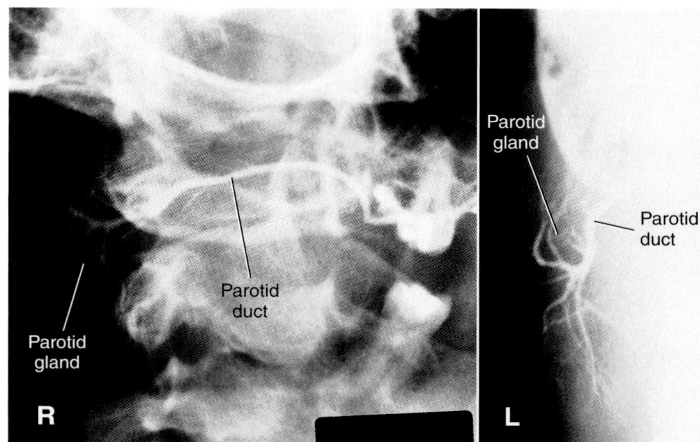

Fig. 23-39. Parotid gland and duct.

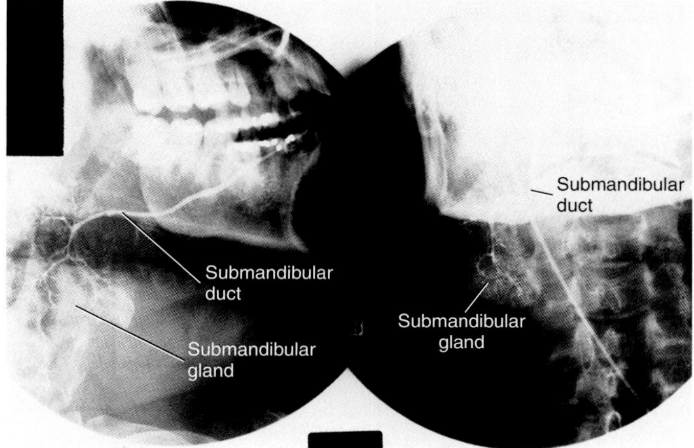

Fig. 23-40. Submandibular gland and duct.

23

Definition and Purpose

Sialography *(si″a-log′ra-fe)* is the radiographic examination of the salivary ducts and associated parenchymal tissue of salivary glands after the injection of a contrast medium. The **purpose** of a sialographic procedure is to **opacify the salivary duct of interest and associated glandular tissue to demonstrate potential pathologic processes.** The administration of contrast fills the salivary duct and flows distal to the intraglandular ductules to outline the salivary gland. Because of the close proximity of the three pairs of salivary glands, only one of the salivary ducts and its gland can be imaged at a time.

Pathologic Indications

Sialography is performed when a patient's symptoms indicate a potential **pathologic process of the salivary duct or gland.** Swelling and recurrent pain are typical symptoms patients exhibit. The pathologic process demonstrated can include **obstruction of the ductal system** by **calculi, strictures,** or **tumors** located within the duct.

Sialectasia (dilation of a duct) can be assessed, as well as the extent of a possible **fistula.** Sialography is essential in preoperative cases of known salivary gland pathologic conditions.

Contraindications

Sialography is contraindicated with **severe inflammation** or **infection** of the salivary duct and gland. In addition, because the procedure involves the administration of a contrast medium, any patients with a history of known allergy to iodinated contrast media would be contraindicated.

Patient Preparation

The patient should be instructed to remove any dentures or other removable orthodontics. All radiopaque items, such as jewelry, should be removed from the head and neck region. The procedure and possible complications should be explained to the patient before the examination and informed consent obtained.

23

Major Equipment

The major equipment for a sialography procedure is a radiographic fluoroscope. In certain instances, conventional or computed tomography (CT) may be performed in conjunction with this procedure. Access to a radiographic room with conventional tomographic capabilities or a CT unit may be necessary.

Accessory Equipment

The majority of supplies essential for this procedure can be found in a typical radiography department. Some facilities may have a prepackaged sialography tray (Fig. 23-41). The necessary supplies are a **3-ml syringe, cotton swabs, sterile gauze, extension tubing, adhesive tape,** and a **cannula.** The cannula selection depends on physician preference. A blunt-tipped cannula or modified butterfly setup may be the choice. The gauge size depends on the size of the duct. The number of ducts to be localized also influences the supplies needed. Additional supplies would include **sterile disposable gloves,** a **topical anesthetic,** and the preferred contrast media.

In some instances the physician may request a lemon slice or package of lemon juice for the patient to express some saliva for localization of the orifice of the selected duct. In addition, an overhead lamp can be used for better illumination of the orifice.

Cannula/Catheter Placement and Injection Process

The procedure begins with localization of the orifice of the selected duct. To achieve this, the physician may either palpate the salivary gland or ask the patient to suck on a lemon slice. Once it is located, the duct may be accessed with a lacrimal probe or a double-ended blunt dilator for cannulization. To ensure that no air is injected into the duct, the selected cannula should be filled with the contrast medium before its insertion into the duct. A modified butterfly needle or sialography catheter is then placed within the duct.

Before the injection process, the cannula and any tubing should be immobilized. This immobilization is accomplished by placement of sterile gauze pads between the cannulated site and the tongue and/or by instruction of the patient to close the mouth around the tubing. The extension tubing and contrast-filled syringe may then be secured to the shoulder or chest with adhesive tape.

Once immobilized, the contrast medium can then be introduced. Utilizing fluoroscopy, the physician slowly injects the contrast medium into the duct. After any filming sequence, the procedure concludes with the patient excreting the contrast medium from the salivary duct. As done before the examination, this task is accomplished when the patient is instructed to suck on a lemon slice.

Contrast Media

A radiopaque (positive) iodinated contrast media is used in sialography. Patient indications for the sialographic procedure and selection of imaging modality influence the type of contrast media to be implemented. The physician decides whether an oil-based or water-soluble contrast media is indicated. An oil-based contrast media is best indicated when imaging is to be accomplished with tomography. It is highly opaque, has a very slow excretion rate, and provides optimal visualization of ducts and the parenchymal tissue. If calculi of the salivary gland or duct are suspected, an oil-based media is not the best choice because it is very radiopaque and may inhibit the visualization of a stone. **In most instances a water-soluble contrast media is routinely used.** Indications for water-soluble contrast selection would include the presence of ductal stones and strictures. Additionally, if the possibility of extravasation of the contrast media or possible retention in the duct exists, a water-soluble media would be considered.

The amount of contrast material injected into a single salivary duct is recommended by the manufacturer and is variable, depending on the anatomy of interest. The physician administers the contrast medium to adequately fill the duct with approximately 1 to 2 ml.

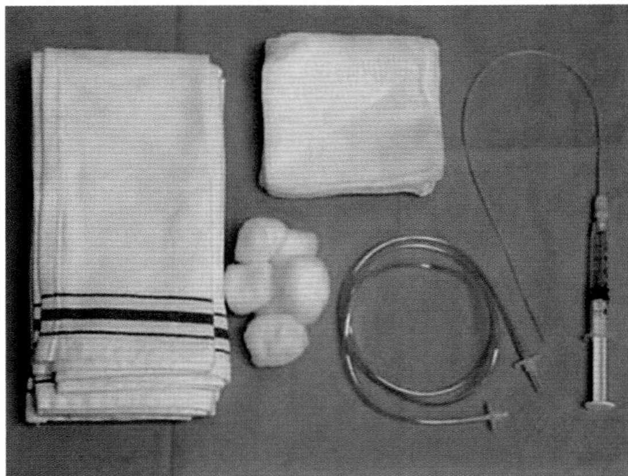

Fig. 23-41. Sialography tray of supplies.

Positioning Routines

RADIOGRAPHIC ROUTINES

The routine positioning for a sialographic examination varies with the method of imaging. Fluoroscopy, conventional radiography, CT, or a combination of imaging modalities may be used.

FLUOROSCOPY/SPOT FILMING OR DIGITAL FLUOROSCOPY/IMAGING

The use of spot film/fluoroscopy, or the more recent digital fluoroscopy, is the method of imaging most commonly used during the injection process. A series of collimated images may be taken as the contrast fills the salivary duct of interest. The patient most commonly remains in the supine position during filming, with rotation of the head in various positions to adequately visualize the salivary duct and gland of interest.

CONVENTIONAL RADIOGRAPHY

Preliminary radiographs may be taken before the examination to demonstrate any obvious conditions. In cases of a suspected calculus these scout images are necessary to determine whether an apparent calculus is present before selection of the appropriate contrast material. After fluoroscopic imaging, radiographs may be obtained. Routine radiographs vary by imaging department and by the salivary gland and duct to be visualized. Imaging can be done with the patient erect, supine, or prone as established by department routine.

The imaging sequence for preliminary and postprocedural imaging may include AP or PA, lateral, modified lateral, or lateral oblique mandible projections. Delayed imaging may be requested to visualize any retention of contrast within the duct. The functional emptying capability of the gland can then be assessed.

RADIOGRAPHIC CRITERIA

- The selected salivary duct is opacified, and the associated glandular tissue is demonstrated centered to the IR.
- Appropriate technique is used with short-scale contrast to demonstrate anatomy and contrast medium.
- The patient ID marker should be clear, and the R or L marker should be visualized without superimposing anatomy.

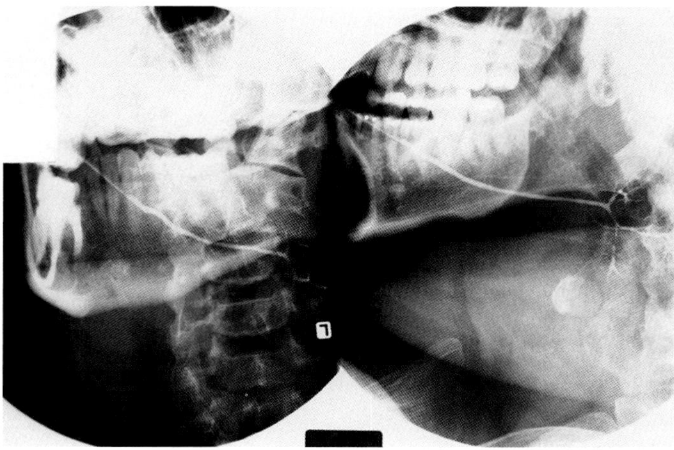

Fig. 23-42. Demonstration of fluoroscopic spot images of submandibular duct and gland.

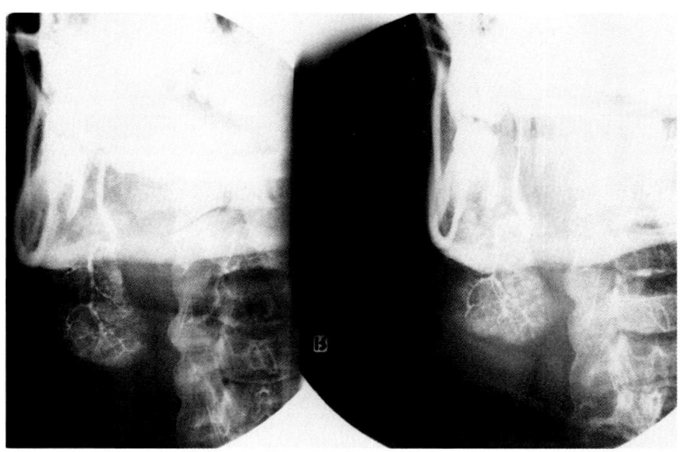

Fig. 23-43. Lateral oblique position demonstrating mandibular gland.

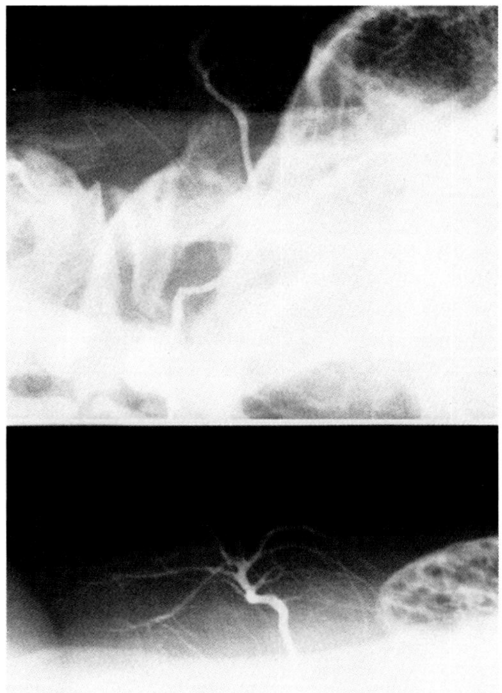

Fig. 23-44. Spot fluoroscopic images during filling of parotid duct and gland.

ORTHOROENTGENOGRAPHY

Long Bone Measurement

COMPUTED TOMOGRAPHY (CT) SCANOGRAMS

One way limb length discrepancies can be determined is with CT scanograms, in which CT cursors are placed over the respective joints of either the upper or lower limbs and measurements obtained. However, this procedure requires the use of specialized and more costly equipment and is not as commonly performed as orthoroentgenograms, which utilize conventional radiography, as described in this chapter.

ORTHOROENTGENOGRAMS

The term **orthoroentgenogram** *(or'tho-rent-gen'o-gram)* is a combination of the prefix *ortho* and the term *roentgenogram* (another term for radiograph). *Ortho* means **straight,** or at **right angles to.** Thus *orthoroentgenogram* literally means **"a straight or right-angle radiograph."** This is a very appropriate term because this procedure is performed utilizing a straight or right-angle CR to radiograph the long bones without magnification to determine accurate and comparative long bone measurements.

As described in Chapter 1, in the section about principles of image formation, the usual long bone radiograph results in significant magnification and elongation because of the divergent x-ray beam. This feature is more pronounced with large images, especially with some distance between the body part and the IR, as occurs when the IR is in the Bucky tray for an AP femur to include the hip or knee (Fig. 23-45). The distance *A* equals the magnification or elongation of the distal femur occurring with this AP projection.

If the "straight" or "right angle" CR in Figs. 23-45 and 23-46 were centered directly over the joints, there would theoretically be no elongation on radiographs of these long bones. This elongation is in essence what the orthoroentgenogram procedure of the lower or upper limb does by using multiple exposures on one IR, with the CR centered directly over the limb joints. A long ruler with metallic markings is placed on the tabletop directly beside or under each limb. The respective length of the bones of each limb can be measured by subtraction of the numeric value as visualized on the ruler at one end of the bone from the reading at the other end (Fig. 23-47).

PATHOLOGIC INDICATIONS—LIMB LENGTH DISCREPANCIES

The orthoroentgenogram is occasionally performed on **adults** for **leg length discrepancies** that may be a cause of back pain or other symptoms. However, this procedure is more common for **children** who sometimes **develop differences in the length of their limbs** during periods of bone growth. This difference is most common for the lower limbs but can also occur with the upper limbs.

Orthoroentgenography is a common and accurate way to diagnose and monitor limb length discrepancies. If the condition is too severe, it can be corrected by either shortening one limb or lengthening the other. Limb shortening can be done with an operation called **epiphysiodesis** *(ep"i-fiz"e-od' e-sis),* a premature fusion of the epiphysis that retards the growth of that limb. Limb lengthening can also be done surgically by cutting and lengthening the shorter limb and stabilizing it until new bone growth occurs.

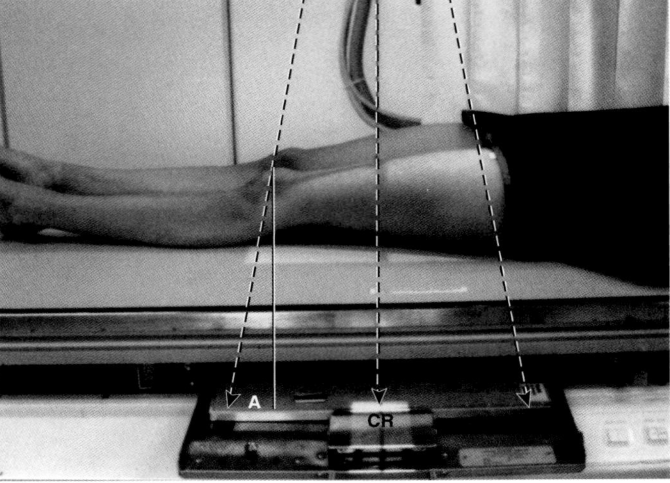

Fig. 23-45. Conventional AP distal femur demonstrating extensive image elongation of distal femur region.

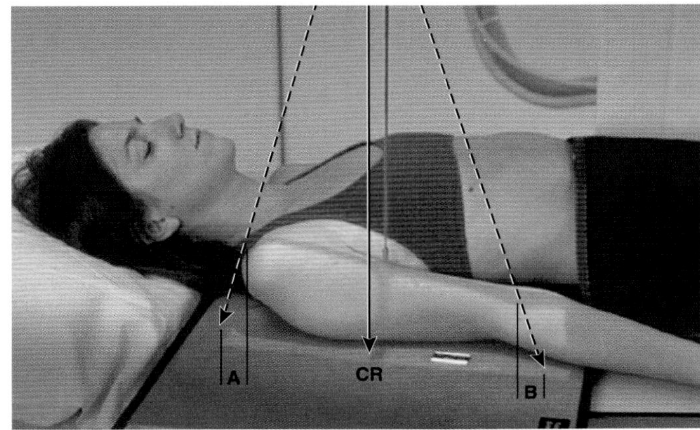

Fig. 23-46. Conventional AP humerus demonstrating some image elongation in regions *A* and *B.*

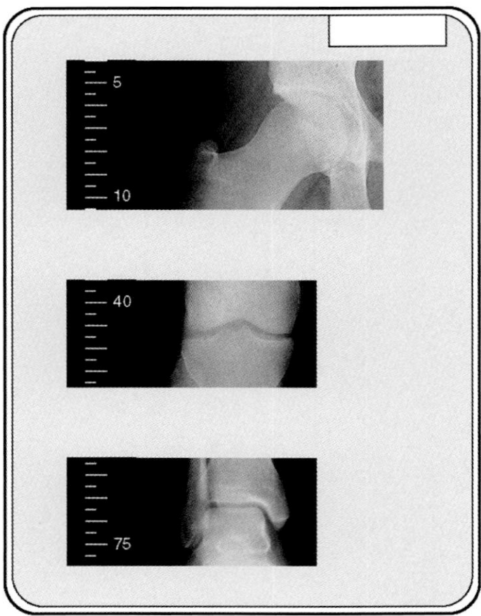

Fig. 23-47. Orthoroentgenogram of lower limb—three exposures on one film; CR centered to joints; metallic ruler placed beside limb.

23

LOWER LIMB MEASUREMENT (UNILATERAL OR BILATERAL ON SAME IR)

This exam for the lower limbs is commonly performed on each limb separately, and measurements are compared for limb length discrepancies. It can also be done bilaterally by placement of a ruler under each limb (or one ruler midway between them) and radiographing of both limbs simultaneously on a larger IR placed lengthwise. This method requires centering of the CR midway between the limbs at the level of the respective joints.

More precise measurements are possible, however, if each limb is radiographed separately because of the more centrally located CR. The selection of method should be determined by departmental protocol, but some references suggest that if the lower limb length discrepancy is more than 1 inch (2.5 cm), the limbs should be radiographed separately.*

Technical Factors

24 (30) (35)

R

30 (35) (43)

- IR size—24 × 30 cm, 30 × 35 cm, or 35 × 43 cm, depending on age or size of patient and whether taken unilaterally on one IR or bilaterally on same IR, placed lengthwise
- 70-80 kV, Bucky grid with cassette in Bucky tray so that it can be moved between exposures without movement of patient or ruler
- Requires long **"Bell-Thompson" type of ruler** with metallic markings

Shielding Carefully place appropriate-size ovarian or testes shield so that neither **hips nor ruler** is obscured.

Positioning and Central Ray—Unilateral Exposure

- Position patient supine, with leg extended and feet up. Center hip and entire leg to be examined to CR, and ensure **no rotation** of pelvis.
- Place ruler directly beside or under the limb. Ensure that ruler is placed high enough lengthwise so that the exposure at both ends includes calibrated reading portions of the ruler.
- Immobilize the foot and/or leg if needed to **ensure no movement of leg or ruler between exposures.** The ruler can be taped to the tabletop.

AP Hip

- Center **head and neck** (approximately ¾ inch or 2 cm above level of symphysis pubis or at upper level of greater trochanter) to perpendicular CR.
- Center upper portion of IR to CR. (Ensure that three exposure areas of the hip, knee, and ankle do not overlap.)
- Perform narrow collimation field to include head, neck, and greater trochanter regions. Ensure that upper margin of femoral head is included on IR for total femur length measurement.

AP Knee

- Center **knee joint** (¾ inch or 2 cm distal to apex of patella) to perpendicular CR.
- Ensure narrow collimation field, centered to mid-IR region.
- Reduce exposure factors from hip to knee technique.

AP Ankle

- Center **ankle joint** (midway between malleoli) to perpendicular CR.
- Ensure narrow collimation field, centered to lower third of IR.
- Reduce exposure factors to an ankle grid technique.

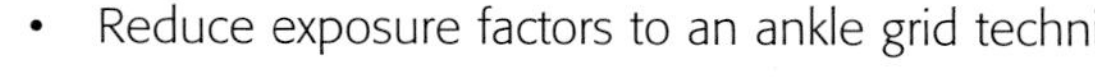

*Godderidge C: Pediatric imaging, Philadelphia, 1995, WB Saunders.

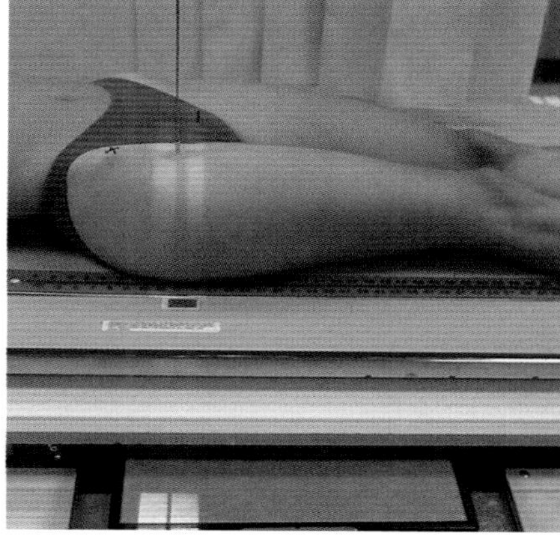

Fig. 23-48. Unilateral—AP hip.

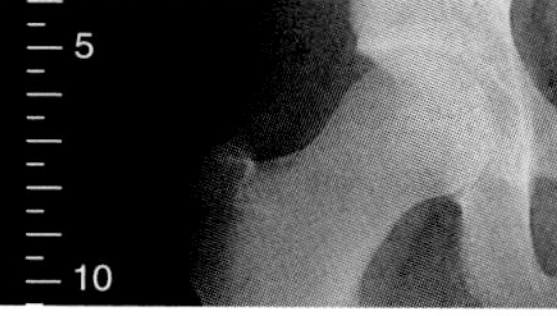

Fig. 23-49. AP hip.

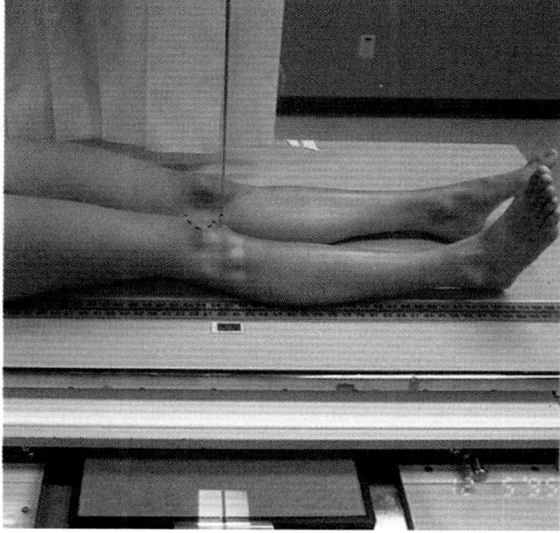

Fig. 23-50. Unilateral—AP knee.

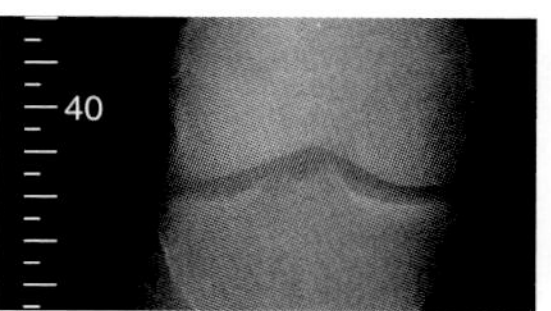

Fig. 23-51. AP knee.

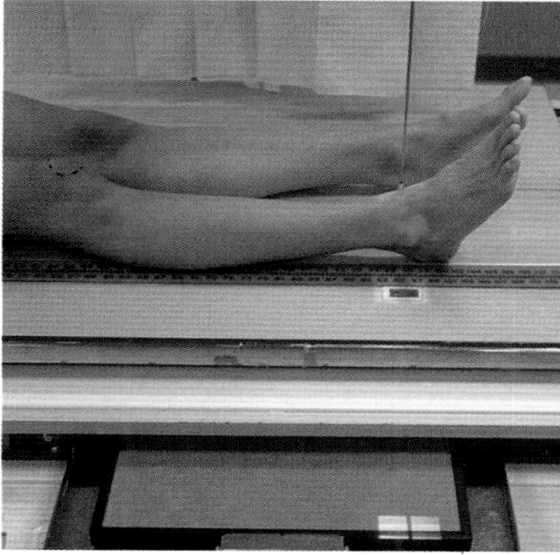

Fig. 23-52. Unilateral—AP ankle.

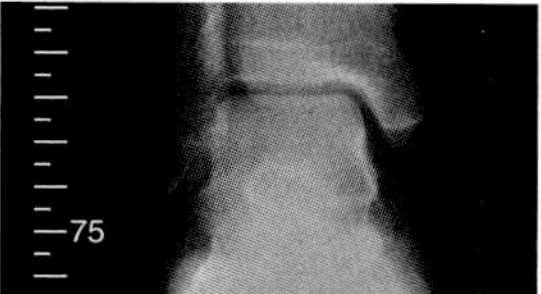

Fig. 23-53. AP ankle.

UPPER LIMB MEASUREMENT

Discrepancy of long bone lengths of the upper limbs is less common than that of the lower limbs, but the procedure is similar, with three exposures made at the shoulder, elbow, and wrist joints, respectively. Each side is radiographed separately. The ruler is placed under each limb, and it is important that neither the arm nor the ruler be moved between exposures.

Technical Factors

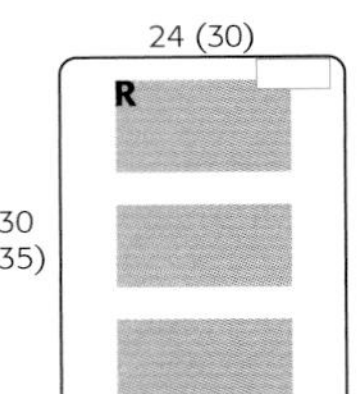

- IR size—24 × 30 cm (10 × 12 inches), lengthwise or
  30 × 35 cm (11 × 14 inches), depending on age and size of patient
- 60-70 kV range; grid with IR in Bucky tray
- Ruler placed lengthwise under the outer edge of arm and shoulder

Shielding Shield pelvis, and also breast region on females.

Positioning and Central Ray

- Position patient supine, arm extended and hand supinated.
- Center shoulder, elbow, and wrist, respectively, to CR.

AP Shoulder

- Center **midshoulder joint** (approximately 2 inches, or 5 cm, inferior and medial to superolateral border of shoulder) to perpendicular CR.
- Ensure that ruler is placed high enough to include calibrated reading portion of ruler in exposure field.
- Ensure narrow collimation field to include entire humeral head, centered to upper portion of film. (Ensure that collimator fields do not overlap.)

AP Elbow

- Center **midelbow joint** to perpendicular CR.
- Ensure narrow collimation field to elbow joint region, centered to midportion of IR.

AP Wrist

- Center **midwrist joint** region to perpendicular CR.
- Ensure narrow collimation field to wrist joint, centered to lower portion of IR.

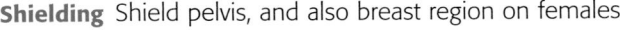

Fig. 23-54. AP shoulder.

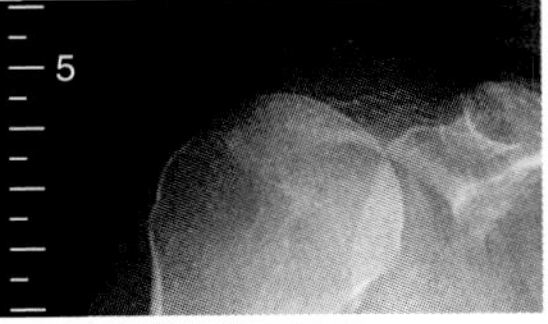

Fig. 23-55. AP shoulder.

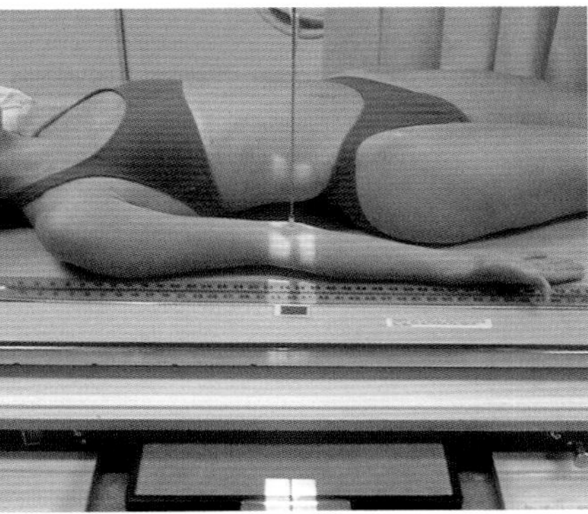

Fig. 23-56. AP elbow.

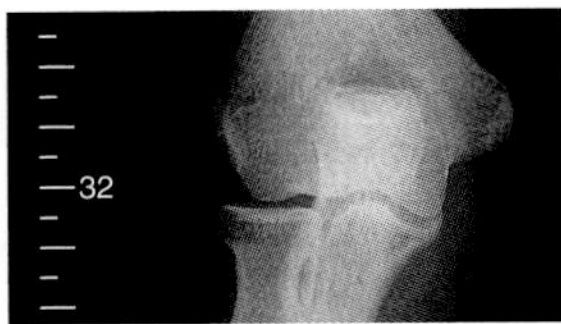

Fig. 23-57. AP elbow.

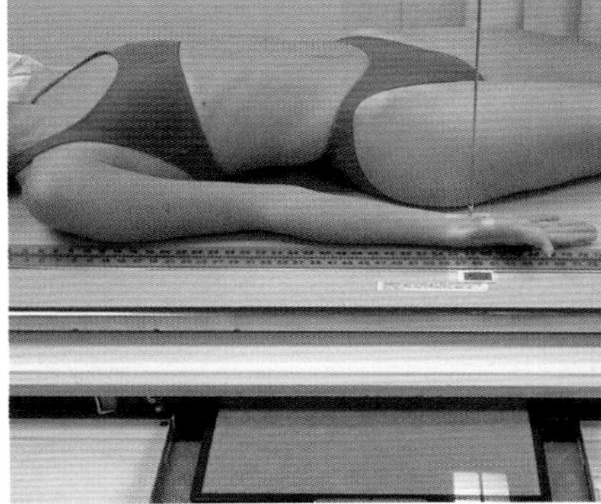

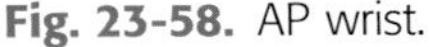

Fig. 23-58. AP wrist.

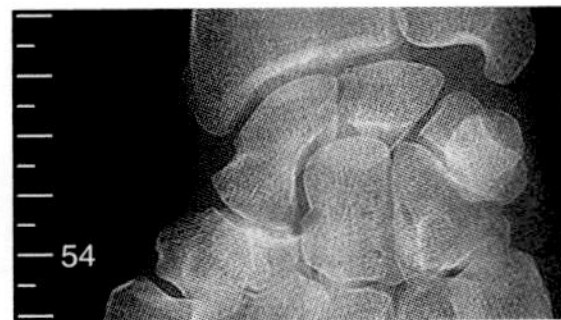

Fig. 23-59. AP wrist.

CONVENTIONAL TOMOGRAPHY

Note: Most conventional tomographic procedures have been replaced with specialized CT, but conventional linear tomograms are still being performed in many departments for certain procedures such as intravenous urograms (IVUs), where overlying structures may obscure essential anatomy. Therefore technologists should understand the principles of the conventional linear tomogram as described in this chapter to be able to set up and perform such procedures when requested.

Definition and Purpose

Tomography is a special type of imaging used to **obtain a diagnostic image of a specific layer of tissue or object that is superimposed by other tissues or object(s).** This image is accomplished by use of accessory equipment that allows the x-ray tube and image receptor (IR) to move about a fulcrum point during the exposure. The resulting radiograph is called a **tomogram** and demonstrates a clear image of an object lying in a specific plane, blurring the structures located above and below the specific plane. Fig. 23-60 illustrates a patient in position on the x-ray table for a tomogram of the thoracic region. A basic linear tomographic equipment setup is shown in position behind the patient, connecting the x-ray tube to the Bucky tray containing the image receptor. The basic principles of conventional tomography are described, beginning with terminology.

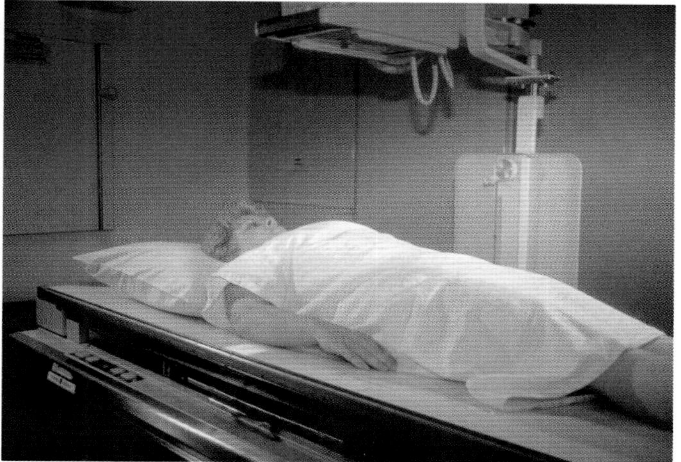

Fig. 23-60. Linear tomographic unit.

Terminology

Because the tomogram represents a section of the body, this type of imaging is sometimes termed **body section radiography.** The International Commission on Radiological Units and Measures (ICRU) in 1962 established the term ***tomography*** to describe all forms of body section radiography.

Because terminology may differ, following is a list of terms and their definitions as used in this textbook.

Tomogram: The radiograph produced by the tomographic process.
Fulcrum: The pivot point between the x-ray tube and the IR
Fulcrum level: Distance, measured in centimeters or inches, from the tabletop to the fulcrum
Objective plane (focal plane): The plane in which the object is clear and in focus
Sectional thickness: The thickness of the objective or focal plane (variable, controlled by exposure angle and tube movement)
Exposure angle: The angle resulting from the x-ray beam movement
Tube movement (or shift): The distance the tube travels
Amplitude: The speed of tube movement measured in inches or centimeters per second
Blur: The area of distortion of objects outside the objective plane
Blur margin: The outer edge of the blurred object

These terms are used and illustrated in this chapter.

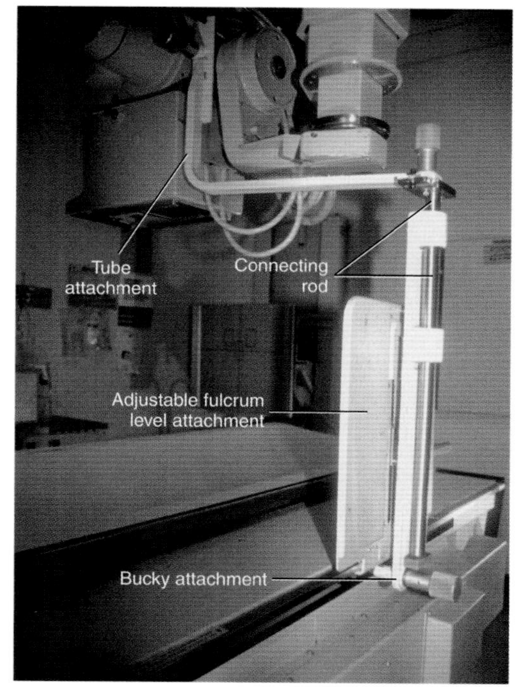

Fig. 23-61. Linear (unidirectional) tomographic equipment.

Linear Unidirectional Tube Trajectory

A linear or unidirectional tomogram type equipment setup is shown in Fig. 23-61. This procedure uses a basic x-ray table with the Bucky tray and overhead tube connected by a metal connecting arm or rod. This rod passes through an adjustable fulcrum level attachment (Fig. 23-62). This attachment is used to manually or electrically adjust the height of the fulcrum level.

Tube movement is achieved by a motor attached to the unit. Because the tube moves along the longitudinal axis of the table, the longitudinal tube lock must be opened (unlocked). The Bucky tray and tube angle locks must also be opened to permit these items to move freely.

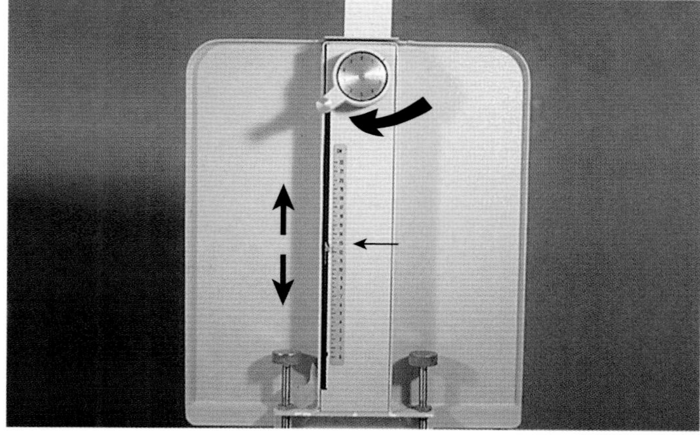

Fig. 23-62. Adjustable fulcrum level attachment.

23

Control Panel

The tomographic unit is operated by its own control panel. The options on the control panel vary from unit to unit. Common features of the control apparatus regulate the following:

- Tube travel speed (in inches or cm/sec) for those units with variable amplitude
- Objective plane (focal plane thickness or sectional thickness)
- Tube center
- Fulcrum level

Some units are designed so that all features except the fulcrum level adjustment are on a control apparatus located in the x-ray room control area. In these units, it is common for the fulcrum level to be the adjustable type located directly on the fulcrum attachment connected to the x-ray table (see Fig. 23-62). Other units may also have the exposure angle selector located in the x-ray table area rather than in the control booth area.

Fulcrum and Blurring Principle

Fulcrum The fulcrum is **the pivot point through which the x-ray tube and IR move.** This pivot point is important because all structures located in its plane (objective plane) and parallel to the tube trajectory or travel remain sharp and in focus because they are in the same position (structures not moving) on the IR during the exposure (see point B in Fig. 23-63). Conversely, all objects located outside the objective plane, either above or below, are projected from one point on the IR to another. For example, see point A in Fig. 23-63 as the tube and IR move from position 1 to position 2. Point A starts out on the left edge of the IR in position 1 but ends up on the right edge in position 2, resulting in movement or blurring of objects at point A.

Point C below the fulcrum level also in the same way is blurred as it is projected from one edge of the IR to the other edge. (Point C is on the right edge of the IR in position 1 and finally ends up on the left edge of the IR in position 2.)

Blurring Principle The amount of movement of these structures is determined by the distance of the object from the fulcrum. Consequently, the objects that remain stationary (do not move) appear well defined (sharp) on the tomogram, whereas those objects above and below the fulcrum move and therefore are blurred. This result is referred to as the ***tomographic blurring principle.***

DETERMINING FULCRUM LEVEL AND CENTERING

With general knowledge of relative location of organs or structures of interest, the technologist can approximate the area of specific interest and center to this area. The initial scout tomogram would be taken with the fulcrum set at the estimated level or plane of the specific area of interest. For example, on a nephrotomogram (sometimes taken during an IVU exam) centering is to the area of the kidneys, and the fulcrum level for the initial scout image would therefore be to the level of the kidneys (anteriorly-posteriorly). This centering and fulcrum level setting is described for a nephrotomogram procedure in Chapter 17 (Urinary System).

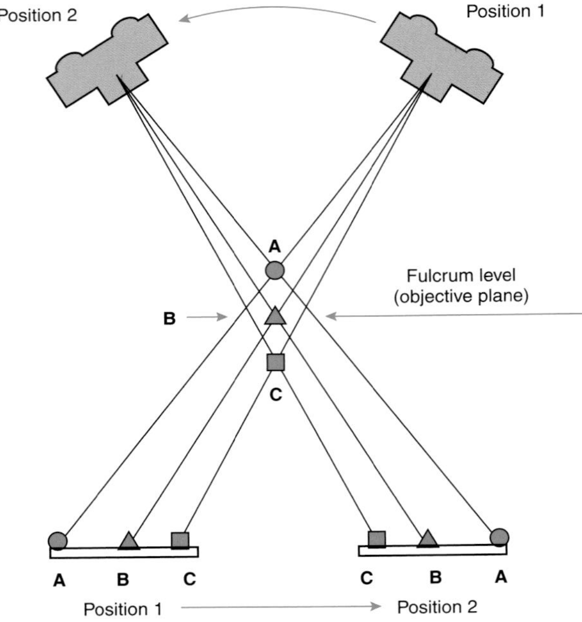

Fig. 23-63. Tomographic "blurring" principle. (From Tortorici M: Concepts in medical radiographic imaging, Philadelphia, 1992, WB Saunders.)

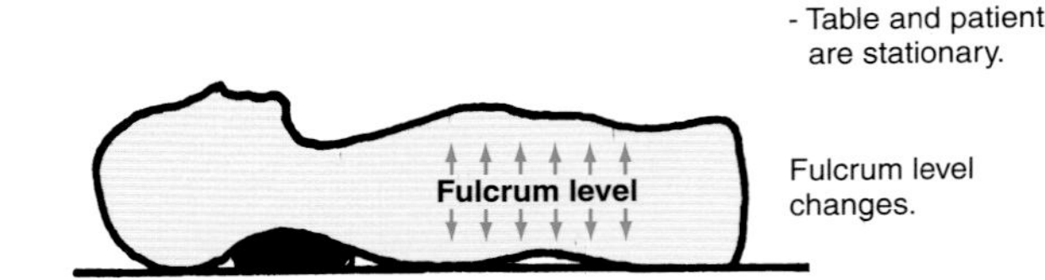

Fig. 23-64. Variable fulcrum. (From Tortorici M: Concepts in medical radiographic imaging, Philadelphia, 1992, WB Saunders.)

23

Blur

Blur was defined as **the area of distortion of objects outside the objective plane.** In tomography the structures that superimpose the object of interest are blurred. These blurred objects or structures within the patient are either above or below the level of interest at the fulcrum level.

INFLUENCING AND CONTROLLING FACTORS

Three factors that determine the amount of blurring are as follows:

(1) Distance of Object From Objective Plane *(d)* (Figs. 23-65 and 23-66) If all factors except *d* remain constant, then as *d* increases, movement or blurring increases. This increase is demonstrated by comparison of Figs. 23-65 and 23-66, wherein the exposure angle remains constant at 30°, but *d* changes (distance from fulcrum plane to objects above and below). Fig. 23-65, with a greater *d* distance, has greater movement of objects A and C on the IR from position 1 to position 2; therefore it has increased blurring.

This discussion demonstrates that those objects within the body that are farther from the focal plane have greater movement and therefore increased blurring.

(2) Exposure Angle (Θ) (Fig. 23-66 and 67) If only **Θ**, the exposure angle, is increased and other factors remain constant, then the movement or blurring increases. This observation is demonstrated by comparison of Fig. 23-67 at a 60° exposure angle with the 30° angle of Fig. 23-66. The 60° exposure angle increases the movement of objects A and C, even if *d* remains fixed, thereby increasing the blurring.

Summary: This demonstrates that as **the distance of the object from the objective plane increases,** and/or as **the exposure angle increases,** an increase in the amount of blurring occurs. The net effect of this increased blurring is a **thinner focal plane** (objective plane) as described and demonstrated in Fig. 23-68.

(3) Object Image Receptor Distance (OID) The third factor affecting blurring is the distance of the object from the image receptor (IR). **As the distance from the IR increases, blurring increases.** This increase in blurring may not be an adjustable or controllable variable if it is determined by body part thickness or by the general location or distance of the part being radiographed in relationship to the film. However, the body part may be placed on the table in such a way as to increase the OID. For example, the head can be placed in a lateral position, with the upside being examined rather than the downside.

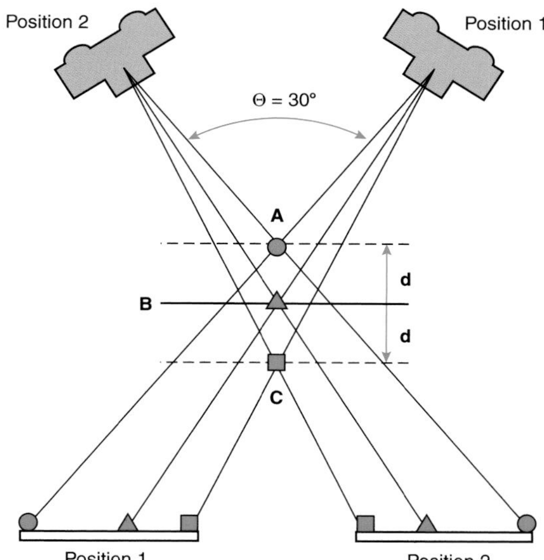

Fig. 23-65. Increase in *d* = increase in movement or blurring. (From Tortorici M: Concepts in medical radiographic imaging, Philadelphia, 1992, WB Saunders.)

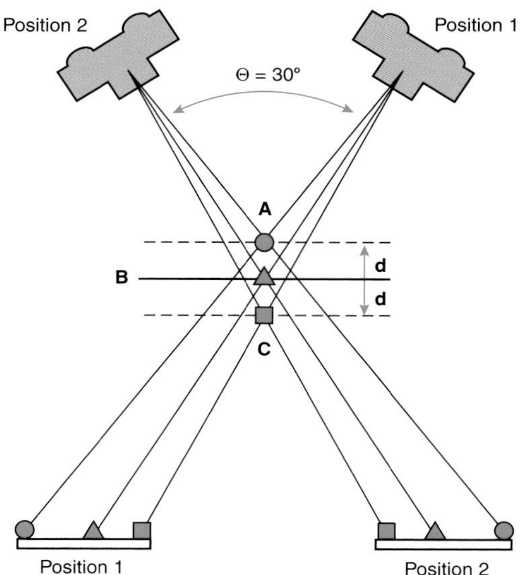

Fig. 23-66. Decrease in *d* = decrease in movement or blurring. (From Tortorici M: Concepts in medical radiographic imaging, Philadelphia, 1992, WB Saunders.)

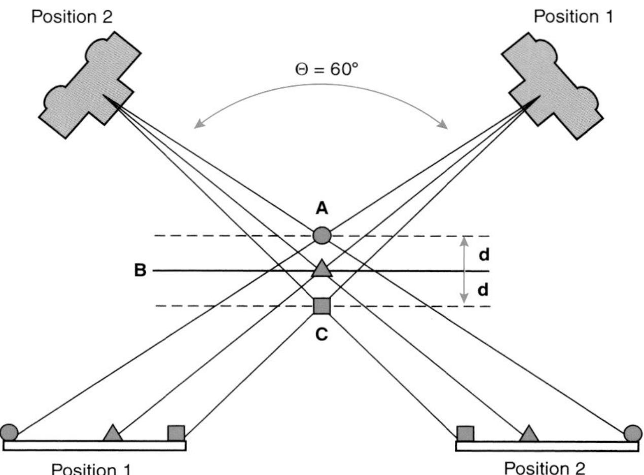

Fig. 23-67. Increase in exposure angle = increase in movement and increase in blurring. (From Tortorici M: Concepts in medical radiographic imaging, Philadelphia, 1992, WB Saunders.)

23

SECTIONAL THICKNESS (OBJECTIVE PLANE THICKNESS)

The more blurring that occurs, the thinner the objective plane. The primary factor affecting sectional thickness (a factor that is under the control of the operator) is the exposure angle (Fig. 23-68). It is advantageous to adjust the thickness of the objective plane to correspond to the object being imaged. Small objects are best imaged by use of a thin objective plane with greater exposure angle, whereas large objects, such as the lung, should use a thick objective plane with less exposure angle.

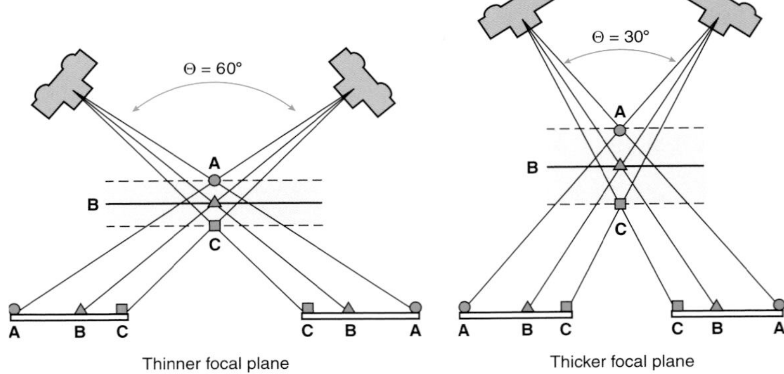

Fig. 23-68. Sectional thickness (objective plane thickness). (From Tortorici M: Concepts in medical radiographic imaging, Philadelphia, 1992, WB Saunders.)

Variations of Conventional Tomography

Various techniques and imaging modalities have evolved from the fundamental principles of conventional tomography. Following is a brief discussion of several tomographic applications.

BREATHING TECHNIQUE

With breathing technique the **patient moves and the IR and tube remain stationary.** This technique is easily performed on a regular conventional radiographic unit and requires no special equipment. The objective is to blur out structures (by the patient's moving them) that superimpose the object of interest. Examples of this are the lateral thoracic spine, oblique sternum, and transthoracic lateral of the proximal humerus (Fig. 23-69). For these examinations the patient continues breathing during the exposure, which blurs the ribs and pulmonary markings. Exposure times must be long enough (2 to 3 seconds) to allow sufficient movement of body parts during the exposure.

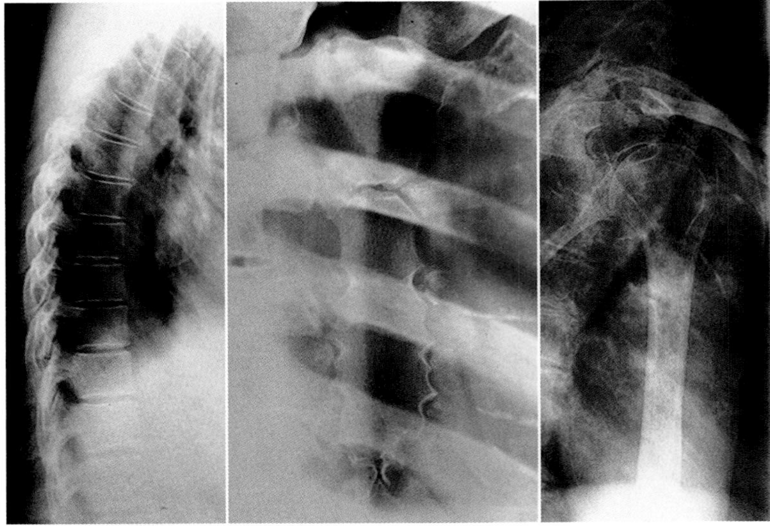

Fig. 23-69. Autotomogram (breathing technique).

PANTOMOGRAPHY (PANOREX)

Pantomography is used for a curved body part, most commonly the mandible, and for dental (teeth) purposes. An example of this application is the **panorex unit,** as illustrated in Figs. 23-70 and 23-71. In pantomography the patient is stationary, and the tube and film move.

The beam restrictor of a pantomographic unit has a thin, narrow slit (*small white arrows,* Fig. 23-70), which is essential for elimination of the diverging x-rays that normally produce penumbra blurring. This procedure results in a pantomogram, which has an image similar to a conventional radiograph (Fig. 23-72).

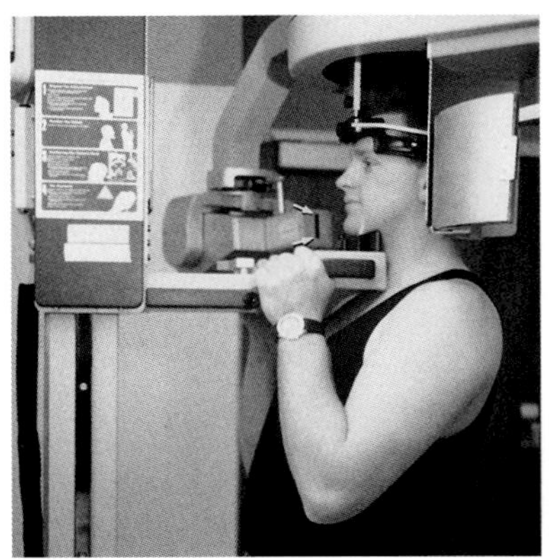

Fig. 23-70. Panorex unit.

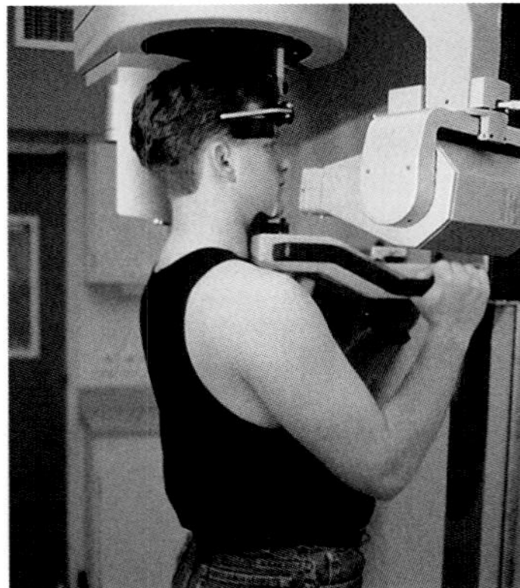

Fig. 23-71. Panorex unit.

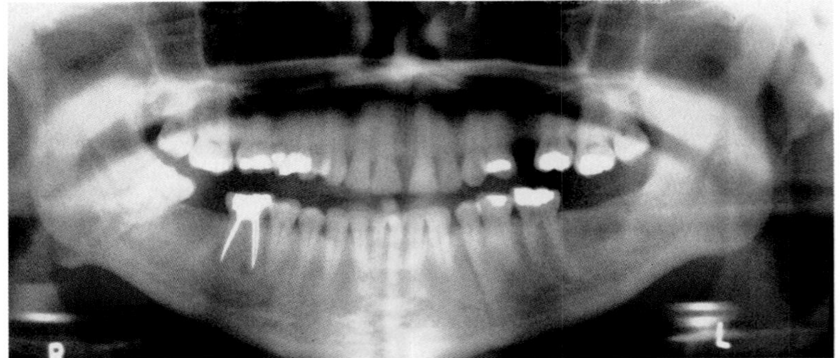

Fig. 23-72. Pantomogram (panorex) of mandible.

BONE DENSITOMETRY

Introduction

Bone densitometry is a specialty that uses various methods in assessing **bone mineral density (BMD)** for diagnosis of **osteoporosis.** An estimated 28 million people in the United States have osteoporosis or are at risk for developing the disease. The medical, economic, and social costs associated with the health problems of patients with osteoporosis are alarming, reaching 14 billion dollars per year. The importance of early detection and diagnosis has increased the interest in bone densitometry techniques. Advanced applications of bone densitometry have significantly affected diagnosis and management of this disease process.

History

Before the development of dedicated bone densitometry methods, standard radiographs of the dorsal and lumbar spine were evaluated to detect any visible changes within the bone density. It proved to be a very subjective method. A loss of 30% to 50% of trabecular bone may produce the first visible changes on radiographs.* Thus detection of osteoporosis radiographically is typically delayed until late in the course of the disease. Dedicated bone densitometry equipment is the best objective method to measure bone mass loss in early stages.

Composition of Bone

To understand the underlying principle of bone densitometry, the technologist must have a basic understanding of bone composition and how the osteoporotic process occurs. Bone is a living tissue that is constantly undergoing change to meet the body's metabolic and physiologic needs.

OSTEOCLASTS AND OSTEOBLASTS

Osteoclasts and osteoblasts are the principal osteocytes (bone cells) responsible for bone remodeling. **Osteoclasts remove bone, causing bone resorption,** whereas **osteoblasts build or replace bone tissue.** The rate at which this process is accomplished contributes to the bone density. When we are young and actively growing, osteoblasts build or replace our bone tissue. Typically, about the age of 35, more bone is removed than replaced, resulting in a gradual decrease in bone. Increasing age results in bones of the skeleton becoming thinner and weaker. With the loss of bone density, there is an increased incidence of fractures of the hip, spine, wrist, and other bones from little or minimal trauma. Early detection through bone densitometry can lead to intervention before associated skeletal fractures occur.

BMC VERSUS BMD

Bone mineral content (BMC) is a measurement of the **quantity or mass of bone measured in grams (g).** BMD is the **ratio of BMC to area,** and the calculated quantity units are **g/cm^2.** T-scores and Z-scores, which are used in bone densitometry and described later in this chapter, are determined using the quantity **bone mineral density,** sometimes referred to simply as **bone density.**

*Sturtridge W, Lentle B, Hanley DA: The use of bone density measurement in the diagnosis and management of osteoporosis, Can Med Assoc J 155(suppl):924-929, 1996.

Purpose

Bone densitometry is used to:

- Measure BMD
- Detect bone loss
- Establish the diagnosis of osteoporosis
- Assess an individual's risk for fracture
- Assess the response to osteoporosis therapy

Bone densitometry is accomplished by a variety of methods and techniques utilizing ionizing radiation and a relatively new technique incorporating the use of ultrasound. These methods and techniques will be described later in this chapter.

Clinical and Pathologic Indications

The *Bone Mass Measurement Act* (BMMA) of 1998 (formerly called the Balanced Budget Act [BBA] of 1997) provided Medicare coverage of medically necessary bone densitometry after July 1, 1998. Bone densitometry is indicated for individuals who meet specific medical criteria within at least one of the five following categories:

1. A woman who has been determined by a physician or a qualified practitioner to be **estrogen-deficient** and at clinical risk for osteoporosis based on her medical history and other findings, which include:
   - Lack of adequate estrogen replacement therapy
   - Family history of osteoporotic fractures
   - Body weight of less than the 25th percentile
   - History of anorexia
   - History of amenorrhea for a period of at least 1 year before the age of 45
   - History of, or current, gastrointestinal tract malabsorption
   - Hyperthyroidism or excessive thyroid replacement therapy doses
   - Heparin use for longer than 1 month
2. An individual with **vertebral abnormalities,** as demonstrated by an x-ray, to be indicative of osteoporosis, osteopenia, or vertebral fracture.
3. An individual receiving or planning to receive **glucocorticoid therapy** equivalent to or greater than 7.5 mg of prednisone per day for more than 3 months and long-term glucocorticoid therapy for a condition such as rheumatoid arthritis, asthma, chronic active hepatitis, chronic obstructive lung disease, and inflammatory bowel disease.
4. An individual with primary **hyperparathyroidism** or additional endocrine disorders.
5. An individual being monitored to assess the response to or efficacy of an FDA-approved **osteoporosis drug therapy.**

BMD and Fracture Risk

Bone strength and bone density are very much related. Individuals with low BMD also have an increased risk for fragility fracture. Numerous studies have demonstrated that the age-adjusted relative risk for fracture increases approximately twofold for each decrease of one standard deviation (SD) in BMD. The ability to predict future fractures with BMD is better than that of serum cholesterol to predict cardiovascular disease. The relationship between fracture risk and BMD is continuous, and there is no BMD threshold above which fragility fractures do not occur.

When measured at any site, BMD shows approximately the same fracture risk for each standard deviation decrease in the BMD. Obtaining a BMD of the proximal femur is, however, better at predicting fractures of the hip compared with other measurement sites. The relative risk is 2.7 for each SD decrease in the BMD of the hip. This means that a woman whose BMD is two SD below the mean for her age is over 7 times (2.7 × 2.7) more likely to have a hip fracture than a woman of the same age whose BMD is equal to the mean.

Clinical Risk Factors for Fracture

Many other risk factors for osteoporotic fracture have been identified. In addition to a low BMD, **age** is a strong predictor of fracture. There is a relative age-associated risk that doubles for each 5 to 10 years. Other risk factors are:

- Sex (female greater risk than male)
- Sex hormone level
- Low body weight
- The presence of previous fragility fractures
- Family history of hip fracture
- Premature menopause, primary or secondary amenorrhea
- Asian or Caucasian ethnicity
- Cigarette smoking
- Excessive alcohol consumption
- Neuromuscular disorders
- Chronic steroid use
- Poor visual acuity
- Long-term disability
- Low dietary calcium intake
- Vitamin D deficiency

ASSESSMENT OF FRACTURE RISK

Fracture risk prediction is enhanced with the **combination of the BMD and clinical risk factors.** Individuals with multiple clinical risk factors have a higher risk for fracture than those with fewer clinical risk factors at a given BMD. Those with low BMD have a greater risk for fracture than those with higher BMD for a given number of clinical risk factors. Patients with low BMD and multiple clinical risk factors are at the greatest risk for fracture. **Fracture risk should be based on both the BMD and the presence of clinical risk factors.**

WORLD HEALTH ORGANIZATION DIAGNOSTIC CRITERIA FOR DIAGNOSIS OF OSTEOPOROSIS

With the development of DXA units capable of highly precise and accurate measurements of BMD, the paradigm for diagnosing osteoporosis has shifted from the occurrence of the fragility fracture to that of the risk for suffering a fragility fracture in the future. This shift in emphasis from the presence of a fracture to the risk for fracture is evident in the internationally agreed upon description of osteoporosis as **a systemic skeletal disease characterized by low bone mass and microarchitectural deterioration of bone tissue, with a consequent increase in bone fragility and susceptibility to fracture.**

Instead of actually calculating a fracture risk, the World Health Organization (WHO) in 1994 recommended the use of BMD for the diagnosis of osteoporosis. Osteoporosis in postmenopausal Caucasian women is defined as a BMD value more than **2.5 SDs** below the average for a young normal population (i.e., a T-score of <-2.5). The **T-score** is simply the number of SDs the individual's BMD is from the mean BMD of a young normal populatin of the same sex and ethnic background.

An individual's T-score is then used to classify the individual as normal, osteopenic, or osteoporotic. **Normal** is defined as a T-score of no lower than −1.0; **osteopenic** is a T-score lower than −1.0 but higher than −2.5; and **osteoporotic** is a T-score −2.5 or lower. An additional classification **of severely osteoporotic** is given to those individuals with a T-score −2.5 or lower with one or more fragility fractures present.

SUMMARY OF INDIVIDUAL T-SCORE CLASSIFICATIONS

TERM	T-SCORE	DESCRIPTION
Normal	No lower than −1.0	Bone mass of no less than −1.0
Osteopenia	Lower than −1.0 but higher than −2.5	A condition of lower than normal bone mass
Osteoporosis	−2.5 or lower	A disorder defined by a reduction in the amount of bone mass less than −2.5
Severe osteoporosis	−2.5 or lower	A disorder with reduced bone mass of −2.5 or lower combined with one or more fragility fractures present

Osteoporosis Management

The U.S. Food and Drug Administration (FDA) has approved the use of osteoporosis drugs for treatment and prevention of osteoporosis. These drugs can either (1) **inhibit bone resorption** (antiresorptive agents) or (2) **stimulate bone formation** (anabolic agents). Those that inhibit bone resorption are estrogen, selective estrogen receptor modulators (SERMS), calcitonin, and a number of biphosphonates. Parathyroid hormone is the best stimulator of bone formation.

Following is a brief discussion of the benefits of each of the common osteoporosis agents:

ESTROGEN

Estrogen replacement therapy (ERT) has been shown to reduce bone loss, increase bone density in both the spine and hip, and reduce the risk for hip and spinal fractures in postmenopausal women.

Mode of action: Antiresorption.

SELECTIVE ESTROGEN RECEPTOR MODULATORS (SERMS)

Raloxifene (Evista®) is a drug that prevents bone loss at the spine, hip, and total body and reduces fractures.

Mode of action: Antiresorption.

BIPHOSPHONATES

Alendronate (Fosamax®) and risedronate (Actonel®) reduce bone loss, increase bone density in both the spine and hip, and reduce the risk for both spine and hip fractures.

Mode of action: Antiresorption.

CALCITONIN

This agent, brand name Miacalcin®, is a naturally occurring nonsex hormone involved in calcium regulation and bone metabolism. It slows bone loss, increases spinal bone density, and relieves the pain associated with bone fractures. It reduces the risk for spinal fractures and may reduce hip fracture risk as well.

Mode of action: Antiresorption.

PARATHYROID HORMONE

Parathyroid hormone 1-35 analog (teriparatide, brand name Forteo®) stimulates bone formation and reduces risk for vertebral fractures. The route of treatment is a daily subcutaneous injection.

Mode of action: Antiresorption.

SUMMARY OF OSTEOPOROSIS DRUGS OR AGENTS

TYPE	DRUGS OR AGENTS
Antiresorptive agents (inhibit bone resorption)	• Estrogen—estrogen replacement therapy (ERT) • Selective estrogen receptor modulators (SERMS) Raloxifene (Evista®) • Biphosphonates • Calcitonin (Miacalcin®) –Alendronate (Fosamax®) –Risedronate (Actonel®)
Anabolic agents (stimulate bone formation)	• Parathyroid hormone –Teriparatide (Forteo®)

Contraindications

Bone densitometry is contraindicated if quality control procedures and standardizations are not maintained to ensure accurate results. Other limitations include a bone mass that is too low or a body part that is too thick in the area of interest. Anatomic malformations of the anatomic site, such as those exhibited with the spine, may also provide less accurate results. Examples of this would include severe scoliosis or kyphosis.

As with any radiographic examination, the pregnant patient should not be scanned, and the standards established to prevent inadvertent exposure to the fetus should be maintained. Additionally, the patient should be scheduled at least a week after the date of any prior radiographic contrast examination or with administration of any isotopes for a nuclear medicine study.

Patient Preparation

The patient is instructed to wear loose clothing with no dense objects (e.g., belt, zipper) in the abdomen and pelvic area. Departmental protocol may require the patient to undress and wear a gown during the procedure to ensure an artifact-free acquisition.

Major Equipment Methods and Techniques

Different types of scanners are available, employing various methods and techniques to determine BMD or content. From a historical perspective, the early developed techniques provided a foundation from which more recent advanced techniques have been developed. Bone densitometry includes the use of:

- Radiographic absorptiometry (RA)
- Single-energy photon absorptiometry (SPA)
- Dual-energy photon absorptiometry (DPA)
- Single-energy x-ray absorptiometry (SXA)
- **Dual-energy x-ray absorptiometry (DXA)**
- **Quantitative computed tomography (QCT)**
- **Quantitative ultrasound (QUS)**

The last three methods listed above are in more common use and are described in this chapter.

DUAL-ENERGY X-RAY ABSORPTIOMETRY

Dual-energy x-ray absorptiometry *(ab-sorp"she-om'a-tre)* (DXA) is a common technique employed in current practice. The physical basis of DXA incorporates the **use of both a high and a low x-ray energy range to account for maximal attenuation differences in bone and soft tissue.** This action may be accomplished through the use of an energy switching system or filters. Energy switching systems are altered between a specific high and low kilovoltage. Filters used in conjunction with discriminating detector systems separate the x-ray beam into effective high and low energies.

The first such systems used a single pencil-beam type of x-ray beam and detector. Newer DXA systems include a **fan-beam construction** with an **array of detectors,** or most recently a **C-arm method.** Such newer units are faster and, depending on the beam construction, scanning can be accomplished within a few minutes.

Radiation Dose The radiation dose the patient receives is much lower than that in conventional radiography. Current guidelines of medical exposure for this system define the exposure units in microSieverts (μSv) (1 rem = $10^{-4\ \mu Sv}$). Effective doses from bone density exams range from approximately 1 to 30 μSv.* The dose range for QCT is slightly higher, approximately 50 to 60 μSv. Thus x-ray absorptiometry examinations offer diagnostic information at a very low risk compared with the potential benefit.

DXA, as with other ionizing densitometry techniques, begins with a **scout or pilot radiographic image** to determine correct positioning and evaluate for the presence of artifacts before data acquisition (Fig. 23-74). The selected site is then analyzed, and a **bone mineral report** is collected. This report typically contains the **bone mineral image, bone density measurements and compared standards, patient information,** and **quality control data** (Fig. 23-75). The information collected is then compared with historical databases of bone density to determine the presence of osteoporosis.

Z-score The two standards used to compare the patient's bone density measurements are the Z-score and the T-score. The **Z-score** standard **compares the patient with an average individual of the same age and sex.**

T-score The **T-score compares the patient with an average young, healthy individual with peak bone mass.**† These values can help assess the presence or extent of osteoporosis risk for future fracture.

*Kalender WA: Effective dose values in bone mineral measurements by photon absorptiometry and computed tomography, Osteoporosis Int 2:82-87, 1992.

†Genant HK, Guglielmi G, Jergas M: Bone densitometry and osteoporosis, New York, 1998, Springer-Verlag.

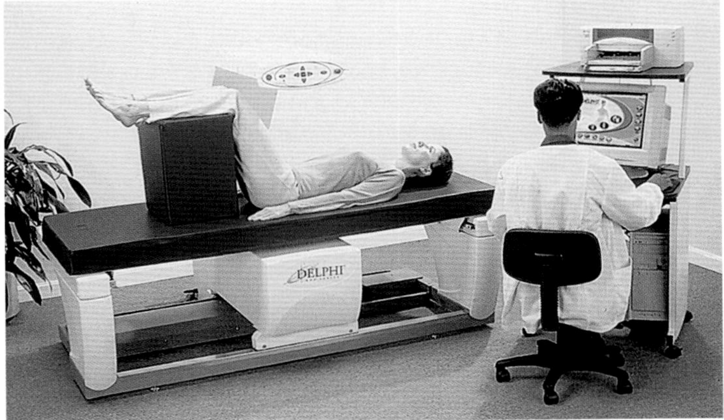

Fig. 23-73. DXA system. (Courtesy Hologic Inc., Bedford Mass.)

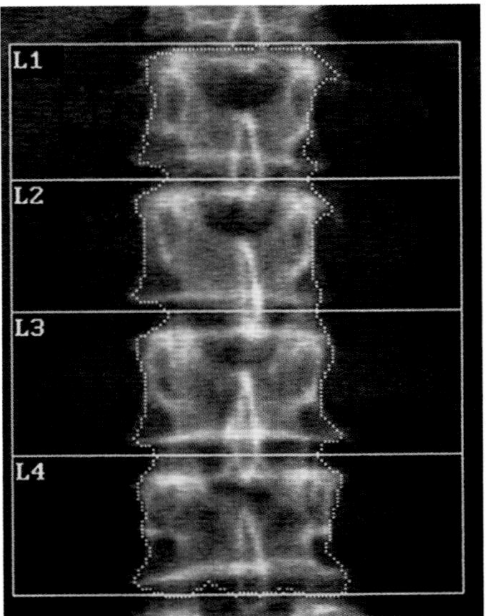

Fig. 23-74. DXA scout image. (Courtesy Hologic Inc., Bedford, Mass.)

Results Summary:

Total BMD:	**0.797 g/cm²**		
Peak reference:	**76%**	T score:	**-2.3**
Age matched:	**94%**	Z score:	**-0.4**

Region	Area [cm²]	BMC [g]	BMD [g/cm²]	T score	%PR	Z score	%AM
L1	10.47	6.18	0.591	-3.0	64%	-1.4	79%
L2	11.77	9.47	0.805	-2.0	78%	-0.2	97%
L3	12.15	10.37	0.853	-2.1	79%	-0.2	98%
L4	15.03	13.37	0.889	-2.1	80%	-0.1	99%
Total	49.43	39.39	0.797	-2.3	76%	-0.4	94%

Fig. 23-75. Bone mineral density report. (Courtesy Hologic Inc., Bedford Mass.)

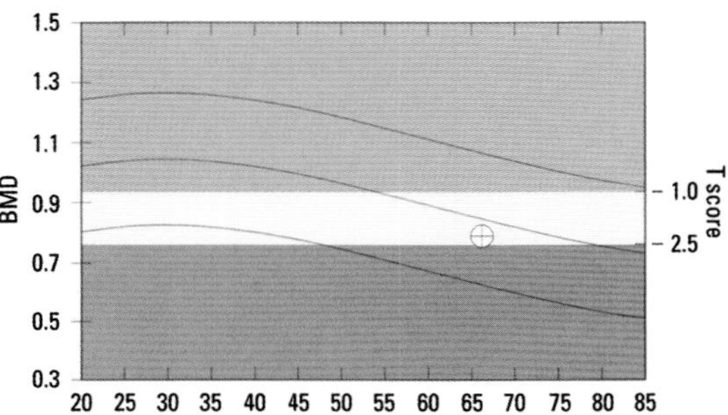

Fig. 23-76. Age–BMD chart. (Courtesy Hologic Inc., Bedford, Mass.)

QUANTITATIVE COMPUTED TOMOGRAPHY (QCT)

The basis of this technique is again related to the attenuation of ionizing radiation as it passes through the tissues of the selected site, most often a central site. The process also involves first obtaining a scout image to localize the area to be analyzed. Then either an **8- to 10-mm slice** is obtained through four separate vertebral bodies or **20 to 30 continuous 5-mm slices** are obtained over 2 or 3 vertebral bodies between T12 and L5 (see sample scan; Fig. 23-77).

A calibration standard is routinely scanned at the same time for correlation, and image analysis software averages the values from all bones. Unique to QCT, this software enables the determination of BMD measurement of both **trabecular** and **cortical bone.** It also allows three-dimensional or **volumetric analysis** of data.

QCT is a technique widely accepted and used to obtain BMD. However, the cost of this method is higher and the radiation dose the patient receives also is higher, approaching 60 +μSv.

With increased interest in peripheral scanning, small-scale models of CT equipment have been developed to assess bone density of peripheral bone (pQCT).

QUANTITATIVE ULTRASOUND (QUS)

Quantitative ultrasound is a **nonionizing technique** used to assess BMD in **peripheral site selections.** The technique offers relatively quick and simple measurements, with no radiation exposure to the patient. QUS is used in peripheral sites with minimal soft tissue covering. The most common site selection is the **os calcis** (heel) (see Fig. 23-79).

An ultrasound beam is directed through the specified site. The velocity and attenuation of sound demonstrate modifications as it passes through variations in the structural components or density of the tissue being evaluated. As the technology is refined, QUS may replace existing peripheral techniques.

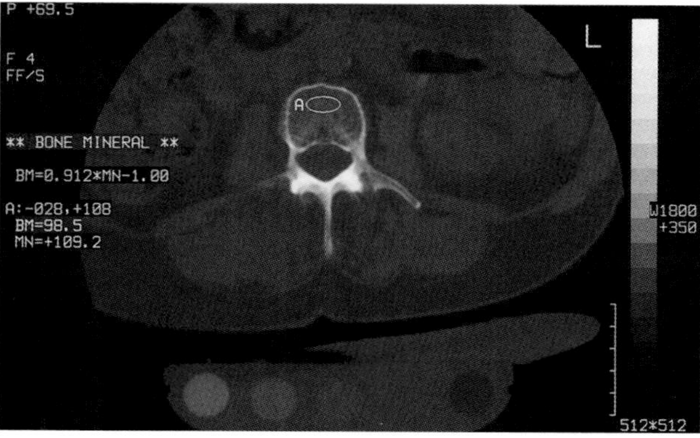

Fig. 23-77. QCT scan through L1 with calibration phantom.

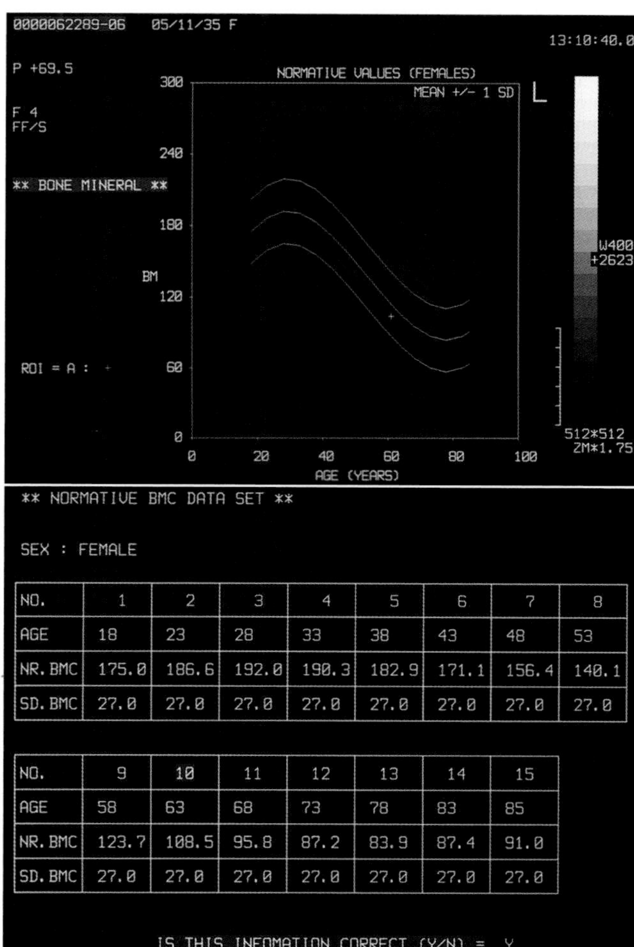

NO.	1	2	3	4	5	6	7	8
AGE	18	23	28	33	38	43	48	53
NR. BMC	175.0	186.6	192.0	190.3	182.9	171.1	156.4	140.1
SD. BMC	27.0	27.0	27.0	27.0	27.0	27.0	27.0	27.0

NO.	9	10	11	12	13	14	15
AGE	58	63	68	73	78	83	85
NR. BMC	123.7	108.5	95.8	87.2	83.9	87.4	91.0
SD. BMC	27.0	27.0	27.0	27.0	27.0	27.0	27.0

Fig. 23-78. Top, Bone mineral (BM) report from QCT scans. **Bottom,** BM female value chart.

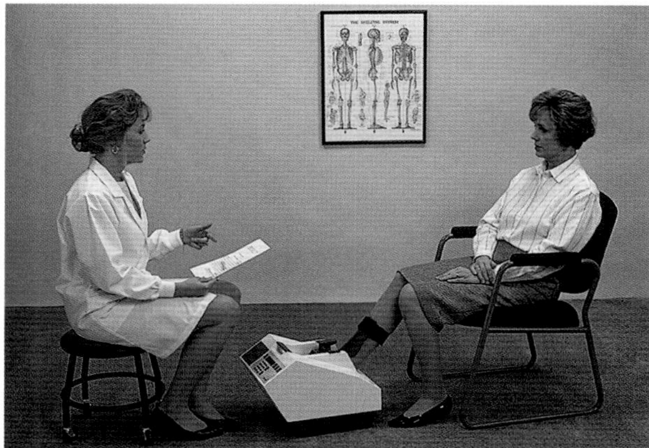

Fig. 23-79. QUS unit assessing os calcis. (Courtesy Hologic Inc., Bedford, Mass.)

Site Selection and Method

Bone mineral analysis can be performed in various locations of the body or from the whole-body scan acquisition. The site selected for analysis may be determined by the patient's clinical history and associated risk factors. If **trabecular bone** is being evaluated, for example, **QCT may be the method of choice.** In addition, QCT is the only technique that provides three-dimensional analysis, thus providing a true volumetric measurement.

The technique to be employed may be influenced by the site selected. Considering current applications, most often **central/axial site** selection is performed with **DXA** or **QCT.**

Peripheral site selection may be performed with **SXA, DXA, pQCT,** or **QUS.**

POSITIONING (FOR DXA IMAGING)

Positioning considerations of DXA are described in more detail because this is the prevalent densitometric technique used. Positioning adjustments may be necessary in special situations, with anatomic variations or abnormalities as per departmental protocol.

Spine DXA imaging of the **spine** is most often obtained for evaluation of risk for future vertebral fracture. The patient is placed in a supine position, with the midsagittal plane aligned with the midplane of the table. The technologist then places support beneath the patient's legs to position the patient at a 90° angle to reduce lordotic curvature (Fig. 23-80).

The spine should be straight and aligned to the scan field as can be assessed from the scout radiographic image. If necessary, modification in positioning can be performed. The image should be evaluated to ensure an artifact-free acquisition. The region included should be from **T12 to the iliac crest** for analysis to be obtained from either L1 or L2 through L4 (Fig. 23-81). Any abnormal vertebral body is usually not considered in the assessment of the BMD.

Hip Imaging of the **hip** with DXA is most valuable to predict future hip fracture. Again, the patient is placed in a supine position, with the midsagittal plane aligned with the midplane of the table. The patient's legs are extended, and shoes are removed. The hip selected for analysis should be determined by any prior fractures or congenital disease of the hip. For example, if there is any prior history of a left hip fracture, then the right hip should be selected. If there is no prior history of such factors, then either hip may be scanned.

The leg is then positioned as it would be for **a true AP projection of the hip.** It should be rotated internally, approximately 15° to 20° to place the femoral neck parallel to the imaging surface. An immobilizing support device is typically available with the DXA unit that allows for correct positioning. The device aids the patient in retaining this position, ensuring consistency for subsequent studies.

Once the scout image is obtained, it is evaluated for proper positioning and for external artifacts. The scan should include the proximal femur, with the midline of the femoral body parallel to the lateral edge of the scan (Fig. 23-82).

Body Habitus Body habitus plays a role in how this bone mineral analysis is performed. For example, if a patient has very little soft tissue in the hip area (such as a thin elderly person), it may be difficult to get an accurate soft-tissue analysis. Therefore the technologist must be aware of the body habitus and soft-tissue variations of each patient to ensure an appropriate amount of soft tissue for an adequate scan analysis.

Severe variance from normal may require selecting a different scanning mode in order to acquire an adequate amount of data for analysis.

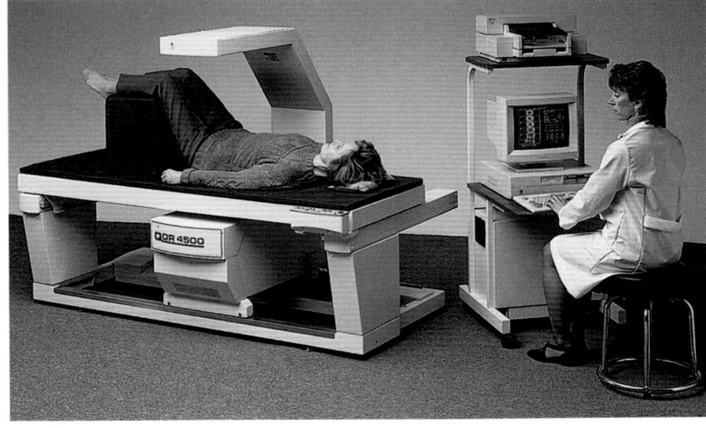

Fig. 23-80. Positioning for scout of spine. (Courtesy Hologic Inc., Bedford, Mass.)

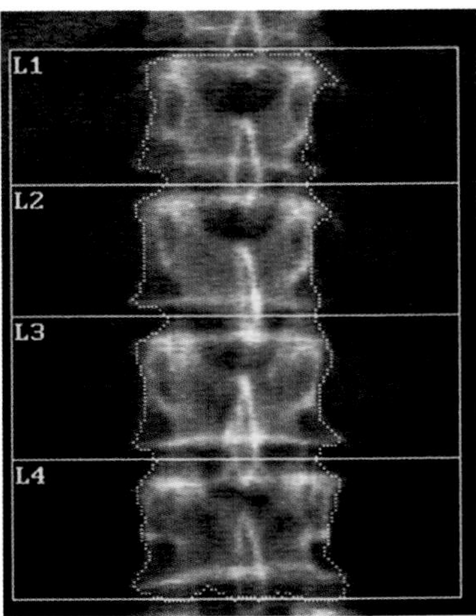

Fig. 23-81. Scout image of spine. (Courtesy Hologic Inc., Bedford, Mass.)

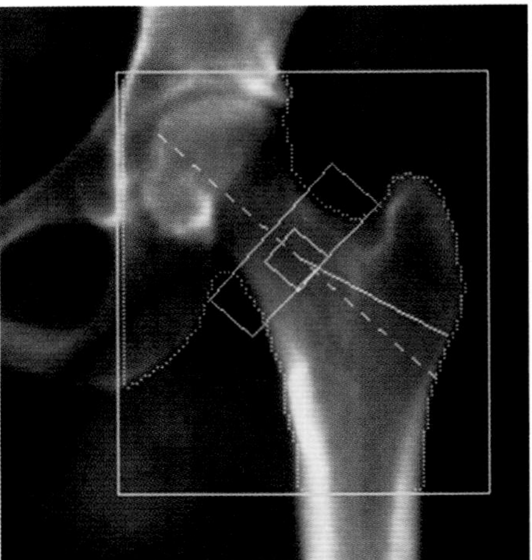

Fig. 23-82. Scout image of proximal femur. (Courtesy Hologic Inc., Bedford, Mass.)

DXA PRECISION AND ACCURACY

Precision *Precision,* commonly referred to as "reproducibility," is **the ability of a DXA system to obtain consistent BMD values of repeated measurements of the same patient.** In order to monitor bone loss or the efficacy of treatment, precision (i.e., small variations in measurements) is essential. Precision determines the least significant change in BMD that can be statistically recognized as a real change in BMD and not simply be random errors of measurement.

Clinical DXA precision is influenced by a combination of the short- and long-term variability of the scanner, patient motion during scanning, body habitus, and operator-related factors such as patient positioning and placement of the regions of interest being analyzed. Patient- and operator-related sources of variability are more important than the scanner variability itself. Operator-related factors have the most influence on the overall precision of DXA measurements.

Precision is characterized by the standard deviation of a set of measurements, or the coefficient of variation (the standard deviation divided by the mean and expressed as a percentage). The precision of DXA is different for the various clinical measurement sites. The commonly used sites indicate **precision of the total hip as 1%,** the **spine 1.5%-2.5%,** and the **femoral neck about 2%-3%.** The least significant change in BMD that can be recognized with 95% confidence is 2.8 × the coefficient of variation. Thus, if a DXA scanner and operator having a combined precision of 1% are used to scan a patient on two occasions 1 year apart, the difference between the two readings must exceed 2.8% for the referring physician to be confident that a change in BMD since the baseline measurement has actually occurred. If the precision were 2%, a change of more than 5.6% would have to have occurred.

As you see, the poorer the precision, the larger the change in BMD that is required for the change to be recognized as real. Since the rate of change of bone in normal individuals or patients being treated is small, **good measurement precision is essential for detecting changes in BMD.** Achieving the best DXA precision requires the operator to carefully position the patient for scanning, consistently analyze the scan, and routinely perform instrument quality control.

Accuracy Accuracy is defined as **how well the measured value reflects the true or actual value of the object measured.** Accuracy is the difference between the true and measured values compared with the true value of the quantity measured expressed in percentage points. Typically, the accuracy of a DXA unit is better than 10% and is sufficient for the clinical assessment of fracture risk and the diagnosis of osteoporosis. Scanners made by different manufacturers are calibrated differently, and the BMD of a patient measured, using DXA units of different manufacturers, may differ by as much as 15%, depending on the skeletal site scanned. Even if identical DXA scanners made by the same manufacturer are used to scan a patient, the measured BMD of the patient may differ by several percentage points.

Although cross-calibration techniques can reduce the differences between DXA units made by different manufacturers to less than several percentage points, it is not recommended that follow-up scans intended to monitor serial changes in BMD be performed on different manufacturers' scanners—nor is it recommended to use a different DXA scanner, even if produced by the same manufacturer. This is because the goal is to monitor a patient's BMD longitudinally, if indicated. Fortunately, most clinical situations do not involve comparison BMD values of the same individual measured on different densitometers. The more common situation is the comparison of two readings of the same individual made at different times using the same DXA unit. In this scenario, the precision of the measurement is more important than accuracy.

Summary Bone densitometry requires a high level of technical expertise if the system's potential is to be realized. Both precision and accuracy are required. Follow-up scans monitoring BMD changes should be performed using the same DXA scanner. Patient positioning, technique employed, and scan settings must be precise according to baseline studies and must be reproduced for any follow-up procedures to ensure true diagnostic comparisons.

The use of bone densitometry as a diagnostic tool will continue to expand as the technology advances, complemented by improvements in osteoporosis management.

CHAPTER 24

Additional Diagnostic and Therapeutic Modalities

CONTRIBUTIONS TO PET BY **Daniel J. Bandy,** MS, CNMT
CONTRIBUTORS TO PAST EDITIONS Joan Radke, BS, RT(R), E. Russell Ritenour, PhD

CONTENTS

Introduction

The intent of this chapter is to introduce students to five related imaging modalities: (1) **nuclear medicine,** (2) **positron emission tomography** (PET), (3) **radiation oncology**—therapy, (4) **ultrasound imaging**—sonography, and (5) **magnetic resonance imaging**—MRI.

In today's health care facilities, workers are expected to become more **"cross-functional"** in their duties and responsibilities. In radiology, for example, the technologist is expected to be flexible and skilled in a wide range of procedures with possible cross-training and certification in more than one modality. All imaging technologists should understand at least the basic principles and the possible procedures and exams that can be performed in each of these modalities.

This chapter not only provides the student and technologist with necessary information on these five modalities and their functions but also will help in determining whether additional training in one or more of the modalities is desired. Advanced clinical training, along with additional study and certification, is available in each of these modalities.

NUCLEAR MEDICINE (NM)

Definition and Introduction

Nuclear medicine involves the use of radioactive materials called **radiopharmaceuticals** in the study and treatment of various medical conditions and diseases.

Specific radiopharmaceuticals termed **tracers** are introduced into the body by injection, inhalation, and/or orally to evaluate specific organs and metabolic functions. These tracers concentrate in specific organs that permit them to emit gamma radiation that is measured by a **gamma or scintillation camera.** Based on the intensity of the signal, the function of a particular organ can be determined.

Single photon emission computed tomography (SPECT), introduced in 1979, provides three-dimensional views of anatomy. SPECT uses one to three gamma camera detectors that rotate 360° around the patient to collect signals being emitted by the body. This information is then reconstructed by a computer in a variety of sectional perspectives that produce slice images (scans) of anatomy.

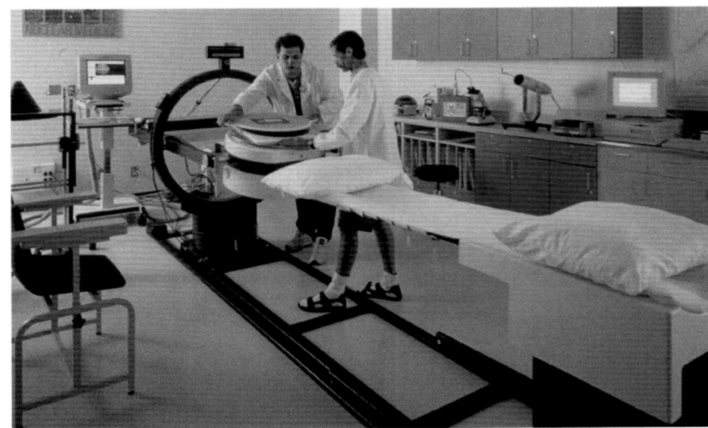

Fig. 24-1. SPECT nuclear medicine camera. (Courtesy Gateway Community College, Bill Timmerman Photography.)

Clinical Applications

Nuclear medicine applications are growing through advances in digital imaging and more efficient radiopharmaceuticals. Because select radionuclides will concentrate in specific organs or tissues, different types of **radionuclide tracers** can be used to evaluate these organs, organ systems, and various physiologic functions. One of the most commonly used radionuclides is **technetium 99m** (99mTc). Different forms of technetium are used for studies of the brain, heart, kidney, liver, and skeletal system.

Bone Scan

Bone scintigraphy is a study of the skeletal system that uses a form of 99mTc injected intravenously. The technetium is absorbed by the bone and provides a survey study of the skeletal system for abnormal musculoskeletal conditions such as metastasis, stress fractures, or other bony injuries. Technologists may need to perform closely collimated radiographs of skeletal "hot spots" as determined by bone scans.

Genitourinary Studies

Nuclear **genitourinary** studies provide both an anatomic and functional evaluation of the kidneys. This modality is excellent for the assessment of a kidney transplant.

Brain Scan

Brain perfusion-SPECT studies will evaluate the brain for various neurologic conditions, including stroke, Alzheimer's disease, and Parkinson's disease (see Fig. 24-2 for sample brain scans).

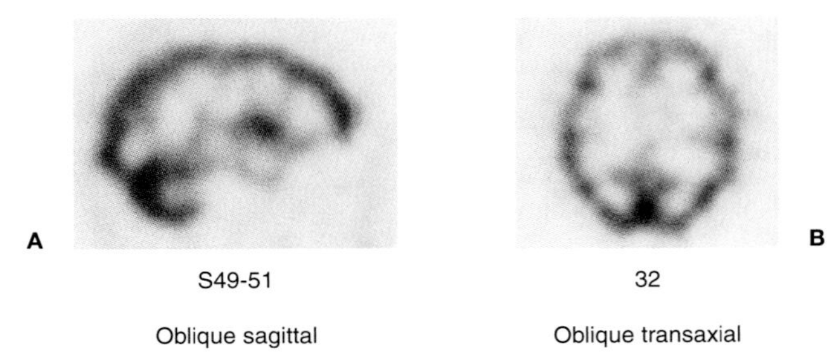

Fig. 24-2. A, Oblique sagittal SPECT brain scan. **B,** Oblique transaxial SPECT brain scan. (Courtesy Bernadette Hanko.)

Gastrointestinal Studies

Gastrointestinal studies using radiopharmaceuticals are numerous. Through oral administration or intravenous injections, procedures such as gastric emptying, hepatobiliary scans, gastroesophageal reflux studies, and liver and spleen scans can be performed. In many cases, both the anatomic appearance and organ function can be evaluated.

One common gastrointestinal study performed with nuclear medicine is the **Meckel's diverticulum scan.** A Meckel's diverticulum is a congenital defect or sac in the wall of the ileum. Although most Meckel's diverticula are asymptomatic, they may begin to bleed or become infected. Nuclear medicine is considered the gold standard in pinpointing the location of this defect.

Heart (Cardiac) Studies

One of the most common SPECT procedures is a **myocardial perfusion-thallium** study, in which radioactive **thallium** or **Cardiolite** is injected intravenously and perfused through the heart. The patient is then directed to exercise on a treadmill or is given a **vasodilator,** an agent that causes dilation of blood vessels, resulting in increased blood flow. The action of exercise, or the vasodilator, will demonstrate the degree of perfusion of the thallium or Cardiolite throughout the heart muscle. This procedure combined with a second resting scan may show myocardial perfusion defects in the ventricular wall, or signs of **myocardial infarct,** a "heart attack" resulting from sudden restricted blood flow, causing death of heart muscle (myocardium).

Lung Studies

The **lung ventilation/perfusion** study is a common nuclear medicine procedure to rule out pulmonary emboli, chronic obstructive pulmonary disease (COPD), and lung cancer. During the ventilation phase of the lung scan, the patient inhales xenon-133 gas during the onset of the procedure. Images are obtained quickly to determine whether abnormalities in the lung are present (Fig. 24-3). A **lung perfusion** study is then performed. The lung ventilation study must precede the lung perfusion study. Radioactive albumin is injected intravenously during this phase of the lung scan. The perfusion phase of the study reveals the presence of any pulmonary emboli.

To aid in the early detection of **lung cancer,** the Food and Drug Administration (FDA) has approved a radiolabeled peptide termed **"Neo Tect"** to help determine whether a pulmonary lesion is benign or malignant. Lesions under 1 cm can be detected with this procedure.

Thyroid Uptake Study

Thyroid uptake measurements are obtained to evaluate the functions of the thyroid gland (Fig. 24-4). The radiopharmaceutical sodium iodide (^{131}I) is taken orally, with a follow-up reading of the thyroid taken at predetermined intervals, such as 6 hours and 24 hours. A **hyperthyroid** (overactive thyroid) will result in a higher uptake reading, which may indicate Graves' disease (toxic multiple nodular goiter, also known as Plummer's disease). A lower thyroid reading indicates a **hypothyroid** (thyroid with reduced activity). This condition is much more common in women than in men.

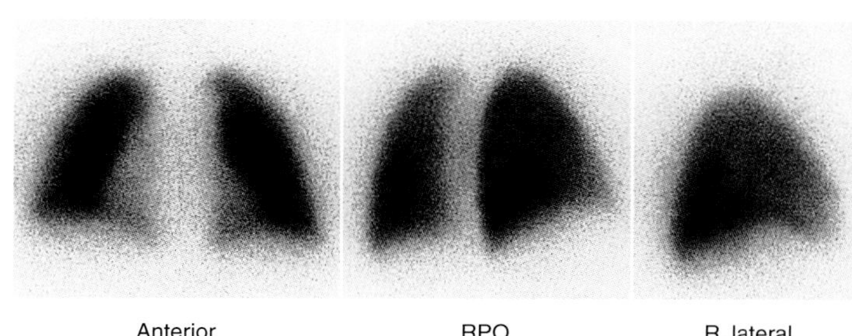

Fig. 24-3. Lung perfusion scan. **A,** Anterior. **B,** Oblique-RPO. **C,** Right lateral. (Courtesy Bernadette Hanko.)

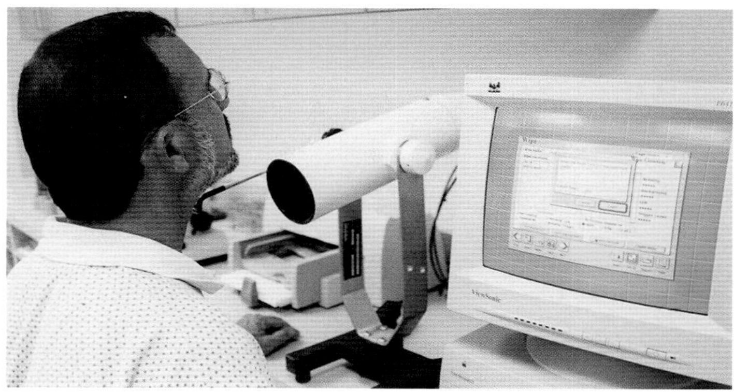

Fig. 24-4. Thyroid uptake measurement.

Nuclear Medicine Team

Nuclear medicine procedures are performed by a team of professionals including the following:

1. *Nuclear medicine technologist:* This technologist has a good background in radiation physics, anatomy and physiology, radiation safety, computers, and imaging procedures. Responsibilities include the handling, assessment, and administration of radionuclides. Patient safety is paramount in nuclear medicine, and it is essential that the correct amount of radionuclide be given to the patient. Excessive levels of radionuclide introduced to the patient may injure the target organ.

   Once images have been produced, the nuclear medicine technologist must perform statistical analysis of the data and digitally process the images.

   In the case of spills of radionuclides, the technologist will need to determine the location of spills, decontaminate the area, and properly dispose of contaminated materials.
2. *Nuclear medicine physician:* This radiologist has received additional training in the performance and interpretation of nuclear medicine procedures. The nuclear medicine radiologist is licensed to acquire and use radioactive materials.
3. *Medical nuclear physicist:* This individual has received advanced training in nuclear physics, computers, and radiation safety. Responsibilities of the nuclear physicist include handling and preparing radioactive materials and calibration and maintenance of imaging equipment. The physicist often serves as the department's radiation safety officer.

Glossary of Nuclear Medicine Terms*

Alpha particle: A helium nucleus, consisting of 2 protons and 2 neutrons.

Attenuation: Process by which radiation is reduced in intensity when passing through some material.

Becquerel (Bq): Unit of radioactivity in SI (International System of Units).

Beta emission: Release of high-energy beta particles by disintegration of certain radioactive nuclides.

Beta particle: Ionizing radiation with characteristics of an electron emitted from the nucleus of a radioactive atom.†

Biologic half-life: Time required for an organism to eliminate half of an administered dose of any substance by normal processes.

Collimator: A device for confining the elements of a beam within an assigned solid angle.

Contamination (radioactive): Deposition of radioactive material in any place where its presence may be harmful.

Count: External indication of a device designed to enumerate ionizing events.

Curie (Ci): Traditional or standard unit of radioactivity.

Cyclotron: Device for accelerating charged particles in a spiral fashion to high energies by means of an alternating electric field.

Daughter: Synonym for a product of decay.

Decay: The spontaneous transformation of a radionuclide resulting in decrease of the number of radioactive events in a sample.

Disintegration (nuclear): Spontaneous nuclear transformation characterized by the emission of energy and/or mass from the nucleus.

Dose: The amount of test substance added to any given reference standard.

Electron capture: Method of radioactive decay involving the capture of an orbital electron by its nucleus.

Equilibrium: Stage in a reaction in which the concentration of the reactive species is no longer changing.

Gamma rays: High-energy, short-wavelength electromagnetic radiation emanating from the nucleus of a nuclide.

Half-life: Time required for disintegration of half of a radioactive nuclide's original energy.

In vitro: Outside of the patient; occurring or being in an artificial environment such as a test tube or culture plate.

In vivo: Inside of the patient; describes a process or reaction occurring within the patient.

Ion: An atom or chemical radical bearing an electrical charge that is either positive or negative.

Isotope: Nuclides of the same element having different atomic mass (neutrons) but the same atomic number (protons).

Microcurie (μCi): A unit of radioactivity equal to one-millionth of a curie.

Millicurie (mCi): A unit of radioactivity equal to one-thousandth of a curie.

Parent: Radionuclide that yields another nuclide during disintegration.

Proportional counter: Gas-filled radiation detector.

Radioactivity: Spontaneous disintegration of an unstable atomic nucleus, resulting in the emission of ionizing radiation.

Radionuclide: Type of atom whose nucleus disintegrates spontaneously.

Radiopharmaceutical: Group of radioactive drugs used in the diagnosis and treatment of disease.

Scintillation: Emission of light flashes from certain materials as a result of interaction with ionizing radiation.

Single photon emission computed tomography (SPECT): Imaging system that utilizes one to three gamma detectors to produce tomographic images of an organ or structure.

Technetium 99m: A common radioisotope of technetium used for studies of the brain, thyroid, lungs, liver, and spleen.

Tracer: Test substance labeled with a marker such as a radioactive isotope or a fluorescent compound.

*Early PJ, Sodee DB, Principles and practice of nuclear medicine, ed 2, St. Louis, 1995, Mosby, Inc.
†Bushong SC: Radiologic science for the technologist, ed 7, St. Louis, 2001, Mosby, p. 584.

POSITRON EMISSION TOMOGRAPHY (PET)

Definition and Description

Positron emission tomography (PET) is a unique, **three-dimensional, tomographic imaging technique capable of demonstrating the biochemical function of the body's organs and tissue.** This is different from other imaging devices (x-ray, CT, ultrasound, MRI), which primarily show **structures** of the body.

Information obtained from PET procedures is important because the biochemical metabolism and function of organs and tissues can determine whether they are diseased or healthy. Often PET can detect abnormal function before the onset of symptoms. This ability to detect disease in the early stages and to measure responses to therapy during treatment can help physicians plan the most appropriate care for the patient.

COMPARISON WITH NUCLEAR MEDICINE

PET is similar to nuclear medicine in that radioactive compounds or "tracers" are administered to a patient by injection or inhalation. Once these tracers are inside the body, the PET scanner is able to determine how organs and tissues function. The PET scanner itself does not produce any radiation. It detects the radiation emitted from the tracer within the patient's anatomy. By using special computers, a three-dimensional (3D) tomographic image of the distribution of a radioactive tracer in the body is produced.

USE OF POSITRONS

Unlike nuclear medicine, PET uses radioactive compounds that emit **positrons** during the radioactive decay process. When a PET radioactive compound undergoes radioactive decay, it emits a positron from the nucleus. As soon as the positron comes to rest, it combines with an electron; then, in a process called *annihilation,* the masses of the positron and the electron are converted into **two 511-keV photons, which are emitted 180 degrees from each other,** which are then detected by detector arrays surrounding the patient (Fig 24-6).

Pet Scanner The PET scanner is composed of many individual detectors arranged in series of circular arrays designed to simultaneously detect the 511-keV photons in order to create its image. This detection process is also called *"coincidence imaging."*

POSITRON-EMITTING ELEMENTS

Although there are many positron-emitting elements, PET primarily uses **oxygen, nitrogen, carbon,** and **fluorine.** The first three of these naturally occurring elements are known as the "basic building blocks of life" and thus are easily incorporated into a wide variety of biochemical compounds. The last, fluorine, can be substituted for the hydrogen atom present in numerous biochemical compounds. When attached to other compounds to form a specific radioactive tracer, these elements can ultimately measure vital processes at the cellular level such as glucose metabolism, oxygen utilization, and tissue perfusion. A given compound acts as a tracer of a specific biochemical process.

Some common compounds used in PET imaging are ^{18}F-FDG* (glucose metabolism), ^{15}O-water and ^{13}N-ammonia (blood flow/perfusion), and ^{11}C-methionine (amino acid metabolism).

Cyclotron

PET requires a specialized device called a ***cyclotron*** to produce the positron-emitting elements. The cyclotron accelerates subatomic particles such as protons or deuterons in a circular orbit to very high energies and then directs them into a nonradioactive target material. The end result is the production of a radioactive material. The specific radioactive material produced is dependent on three things: (1) the type of target material, (2) the particle being accelerated, and (3) the energy to which the particles are accelerated.

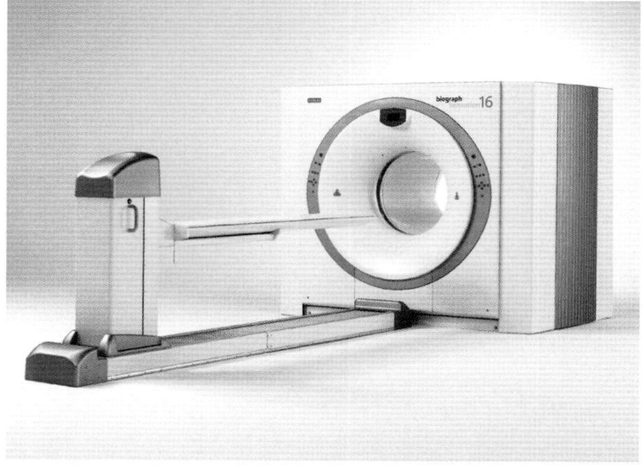

Fig. 24-5. PET Imaging System-ECAT). (Courtesy CTI Molecular Imaging Inc., Knoxville, Tenn.)

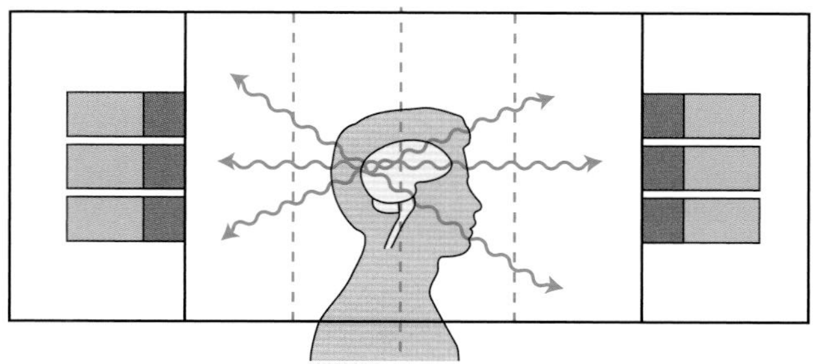

Fig. 24-6. Positron emission and detector array. Side view of PET scanner illustrating possible directions of 511-keV emitted photons. (From Ballinger PW, Frank ED: Merrill's atlas of radiographic procedures, ed 10, St. Louis, Mosby, 2003.)

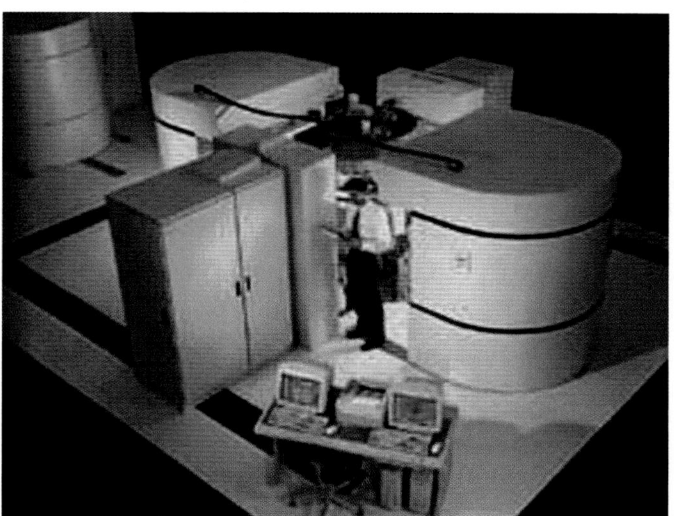

Fig. 24-7. PET medical cyclotron with radiation shields retracted to show internal components. (Courtesy CTI Molecular Imaging Inc., Knoxville, Tenn.)

Most PET tracers have **very short half-lives** (120 seconds to 110 minutes), and therefore the PET scanner must be in close proximity to a cyclotron. If a PET center is using only ^{18}F-FDG,* which has a 110-minute half-life, the tracer can be shipped from an offsite cyclotron production facility. However, if shorter-lived tracers using ^{11}C, ^{15}O, or ^{13}N are required, the cyclotron must be located at the site of the PET scanner. Currently, there are cyclotrons located in most major metropolitan areas as well as universities.

*The superscripted "18" refers to the atomic mass of this particular isotope of fluorine.

24

Clinical Applications

ONCOLOGY (STUDY OF TUMORS)

PET is a valuable tool for assessing the metabolism of tumors. In general, malignant cells have a high rate of metabolism because of their unregulated growth and thus readily use sugar as a fuel source. The glucose analog, FDG, is also taken up readily by active tumors. PET scans for this application are generally done as a whole body survey to determine the initial sites of cancers and to see whether cancer has spread to other areas of the body. An increase in glycolysis (increase use of sugar by the cells) in a specific organ or region of the body is an indicator of malignancy. PET may be used for the initial diagnosis and staging of a malignancy and also as a follow-up technique to determine the response to treatment.

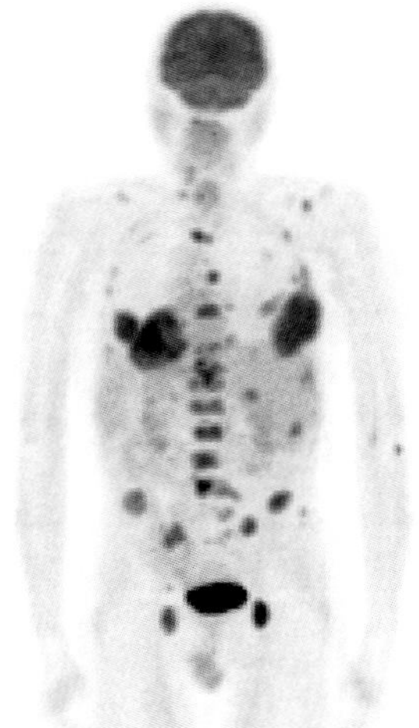

Fig. 24-8. Coronal view of a whole-body PET scan. Darker areas indicated increased uptake of ^{18}F-FDG. It is normal to see activity in the brain because this organ naturally consumes a great deal of glucose. In addition, activity in the bladder is normal due to urinary excretion of the tracer. All the other sites of increased activity represent metastatic disease.

CARDIOLOGY

Coronary Artery Disease Coronary artery disease (CAD) begins when blood flow to the heart is obstructed. Chest pain, heart attack, and even death may occur as a result of this disease. PET can be used to assess how CAD affects the normal functioning of the heart. In these studies, an ammonia tracer (^{13}N-ammonia) is used to investigate whether certain areas of the heart are not receiving sufficient blood flow (Fig. 24-9).

Additional studies using the FDG sugar tracer can tell clinicians whether these same areas will be able to resume normal function if blood flow is restored. Using these images, clinicians can get a more complete picture of the scope of disease, and help identify patients who may or may not benefit from other procedures that reroute blood to areas of the heart that are in need.

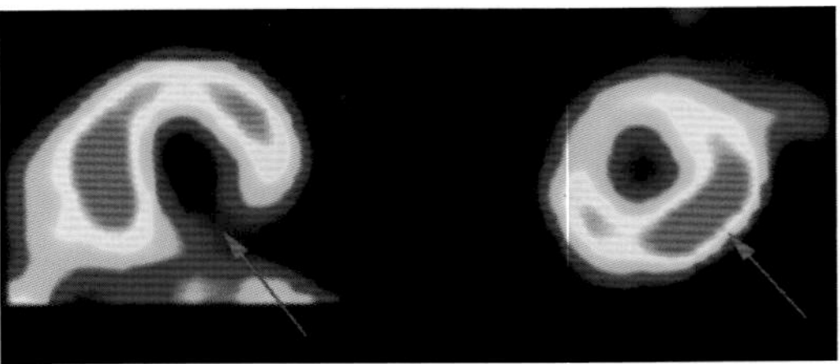

Fig. 24-9. Demonstrates short-axis images of the heart using ^{13}N-ammonia *(left)* and ^{18}FDG *(right)* to assess perfusion and glucose metabolism, respectively. The perfusion images reveal a defect in the inferior-lateral area of the heart evident by decreased function (see *arrows*). The FDG images have increased glucose metabolism in this same region. This "mismatched" pattern is indicative of viable myocardium.

NEUROLOGY

Epilepsy PET can be used to investigate the location of seizure sites in epileptic patients who are not responding to drug therapy. This is accomplished by measuring changes in how the brain uses the sugar tracer (FDG) in the affected areas. PET can detect seizure sites in the brain regardless of whether or not a patient is experiencing one at the time of scanning. During a seizure, the image that is created demonstrates an increase in sugar utilization at the seizure site. On the other hand, if a patient is seizure-free at the time of scanning, the image shows a decrease in sugar utilization in the area of the seizure site. With results of these types of PET scans, surgeons can identify the affected seizure site in order to remove it.

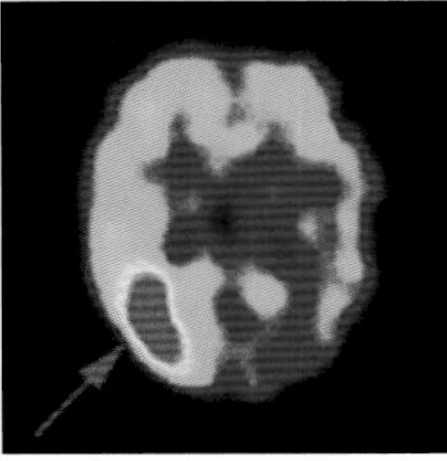

Fig. 24-10. ^{18}F-FDG PET scan of a 6-month-old male with infantile spasms. The PET scan shows increased glucose (FDG) uptake *(arrow)* relative to surrounding brain areas. This is indicative of an active seizure focus.

Brain Mapping Lesions are described as abnormalities involving tissues or organs as a result of disease or injury. When lesions are found in areas of the brain that are vital to the performance of behaviors such as language, memory, vision, and movement, neurosurgery carries the risk for permanent disability. PET brain mapping techniques are able to minimize the risk for injuring a key motor or sensory region of the brain by evaluating patients prior to surgery in order to characterize the location of these vital areas.

24

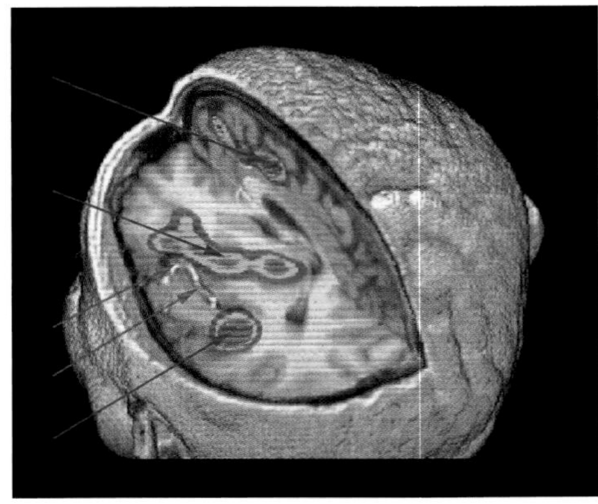

Fig. 24-11. Increases in cerebral blood flow during a language activation exam *(blue arrows)* relative to an arterial venous malformation (AVM-*red arrows*).

CNS Tumor Imaging PET can be used to characterize central nervous system tumors in the same manner as it is used for imaging tumors elsewhere in the body. Actively growing brain tumors will concentrate FDG. In addition to FDG, another tracer, ^{11}C-methionine, can be used to assess amino acid metabolism. This agent is much more sensitive to the presence of even low-grade tumors. By combining a ^{11}C-methionine scan followed by FDG, it is possible to detect the presence of tumor and determine how aggressive it is.

Evaluation of Dementia PET scanning is also capable of evaluating and characterizing various types of dementias such as Alzheimer's disease. Using FDG, PET can measure glucose metabolism in the brain. During the normal aging process, glucose metabolism naturally decreases uniformly throughout the brain. In patients with Alzheimer's disease, glucose metabolism is dramatically decreased in several key areas of the brain. PET can help confirm the diagnosis of Alzheimer's disease and also monitor the effect of treatment.

PET/CT FUSION TECHNOLOGY (COREGISTRATION)

Anatomic and Functional Image Coregistration PET can also be combined with other imaging modalities to enhance the diagnosis of a specific condition. The most common example of this is the hybrid PET/CT combination known as **PET/CT fusion technology.** Since images produced by a PET scanner primarily demonstrate the biochemical functions occurring in the body, it is often helpful to have the corresponding structural information obtained by CT or MRI. New technology incorporating a PET scanner with a CT scanner has created the ability to **acquire functional PET and anatomic CT images simultaneously.** These two image data sets can be displayed as a single volume in which PET data are directly merged onto the CT image. This permits direct, accurate localization of pathology found on a PET scan. In addition, the hybrid PET/CT units permit the attenuation correction to be performed by the CT scanner. The CT-based attenuation correction is much quicker and also negates the need for dedicated sealed sources, which are required in nonhybrid PET scanners.

There are also computer software programs available that are able to coregister a PET scan with an MRI or CT acquired on an independent system. This precludes the need for a dedicated hybrid system such a combination PET/CT system. However, the use of these software applications is not as accurate in coregistering the image sets because of the differences in patient position between the two imaging systems.

PET/CT Fusion (Coregistration) Applications (Fig. 24-15) Recently new instrumentation incorporating PET scanners with traditional CT scanners has allowed physicians to receive not only the functional PET image but also the anatomic CT image as a single-image set. This new technique will aid physicians in localizing areas of pathology with a higher degree of accuracy in order to better treat the patient.

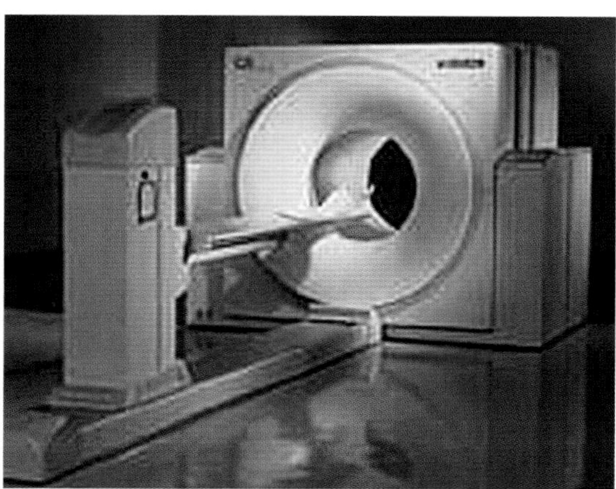

Fig. 24-14. Hybrid scanner featuring combined PET/CT capability. (Courtesy CTI Molecular Imaging Inc., Knoxville, Tenn.)

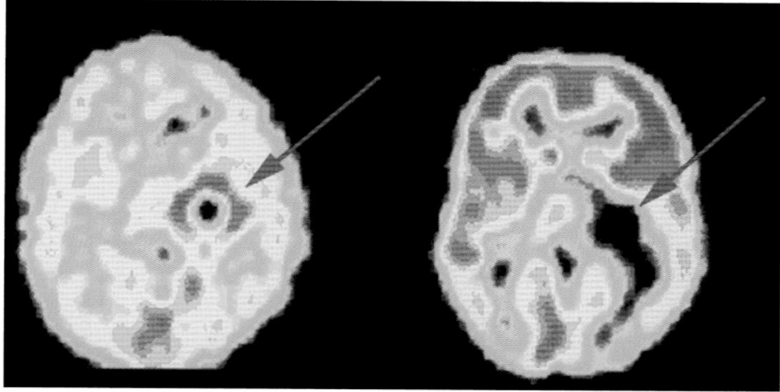

Fig. 24-12. Tumor imaging using ^{11}C-methionine *(left)* and ^{18}FDG *(right)* in a patient being evaluated for a newly discovered brain tumor. The ^{11}C-methionine demonstrates a rim of hyperactivity with a "cold" cystic center *(arrow, left image).* The ^{18}FDG on the right shows little or no uptake in the same region *(arrow).* This pattern is indicative of a low-grade tumor. ^{11}C-methionine is used to determine the presence or extent of tumor, whereas ^{18}FDG is used to determine the grade of the tumor.

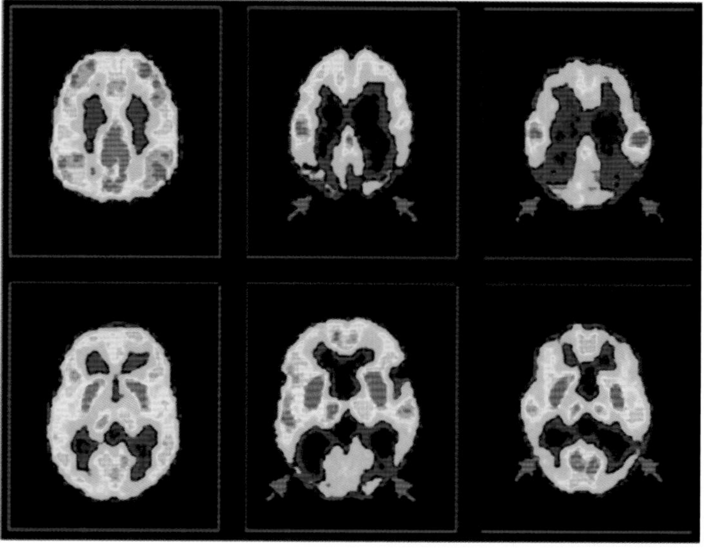

Fig. 24-13. Columns A, B, and C represent FDG brain studies of three individuals; normal patient (column A), patient with mild dementia (column B), and severe dementia (column C). Within each column, the top image and bottom image represent superior and midbrain slices of an ^{18}FDG brain study, respectively. Note the characteristic decreases in glucose metabolism *(blue shade)* in the posterior-parietal regions indicated by the arrows.

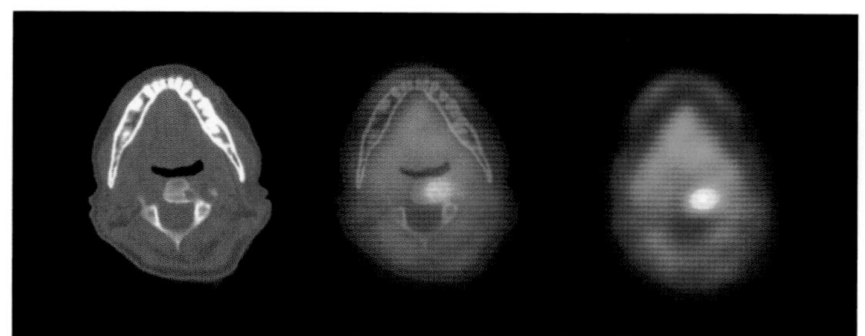

Fig. 24-15. From left to right: CT, coregistered PET/CT, and PET scans demonstrating increased uptake of ^{18}F fluorodopa in a patient with suspected recurrence of medullary thyroid cancer. There is a small lesion on CT that corresponds to the functional increase on the PET. With this technology it is possible to determine whether cancer is present and also accurately determine its anatomic location. This specific example fuses PET and CT that were acquired on separate machines using fusion software.

RADIATION ONCOLOGY (THERAPY)

Definition and Introduction

Radiation oncology, commonly termed *radiation therapy,* or *radiotherapy,* involves the use of **ionizing radiation for treatment of cancer** and some benign diseases. Cancer is second only to heart-related diseases in causing death in the United States and Canada.

Surgery, chemotherapy, and radiotherapy are the methods of cancer treatment. Radiation is frequently combined with chemotherapy if a tumor is too complex or is entrenched in other tissue and cannot be removed surgically. Surgery, when it is possible, is commonly followed with either chemotherapy or radiotherapy, or a combination of both. Unfortunately, in certain cases, the cancer is too advanced or complex to respond to any method of treatment. In these cases, radiotherapy may be used for palliative treatment to shrink tumors and reduce pressure and pain for a better quality of life.

Brachytherapy and Teletherapy

Two types of radiation treatment exist: the **internal** radiation type termed **brachytherapy** and the **external** beam types termed **teletherapy.**

Internal radiation, or brachytherapy, involves the insertion of low-intensity radioactive nuclides inside the body placed in close proximity to the tumor or cancerous tissue. Prostate cancer is one common candidate for this type of treatment.

Teletherapy is the application of external beam radiation, which historically has been of three types: **x-ray-type** units, **cobalt-60 gamma ray units,** and **linear accelerators.**

Cobalt-60 units emitting high-energy **gamma rays** of about **1.25 meV** were the standard for many years for deeper-depth tissue treatment. The x-ray and the cobalt types may still be used in some locations, but they have largely been replaced with **linear accelerators,** which have both lower- and higher-energy capabilities, from **4 million volts to as high as 30 million volts** (4 to 30 MeV). Based on the type of tumor being treated, a combination of brachytherapy and teletherapy may be used.

Linear Accelerators

The linear accelerator that emits x-rays or beam of electrons is capable of producing **high-energy x-rays** when a target (anode) is placed in the path of the accelerating high-energy stream of electrons emitted from the filament (cathode). The energy range of emitted x-rays is controlled by high voltage applied to the accelerating electron beam striking the target or anode, in a similar manner to that of a general diagnostic-type x-ray tube.

This same equipment, by removing the anode or target out of the electron beam, is also capable of projecting a **beam of electrons** of selected energies directly onto the site of tissue being treated. The energy of this emitted electron beam is controlled by the applied voltage.

The projection of these electrons directly on the cancerous tissue is more effective in the treatment of shallow or superficial tissue than higher-energy x-rays or gamma rays. Electron beam–type energy will penetrate tissue only to the depth of the superficial cancer and therefore will not affect or damage the deeper underlying healthy tissue.

Deep-seated cancers, however, are best treated by high-energy x-rays as produced by the linear accelerator or high-energy gamma rays emitted from cobalt units. This high-energy radiation is distributed directly to the cancerous tissue lying deep within body parts with the least possible damage to surrounding normal tissue.

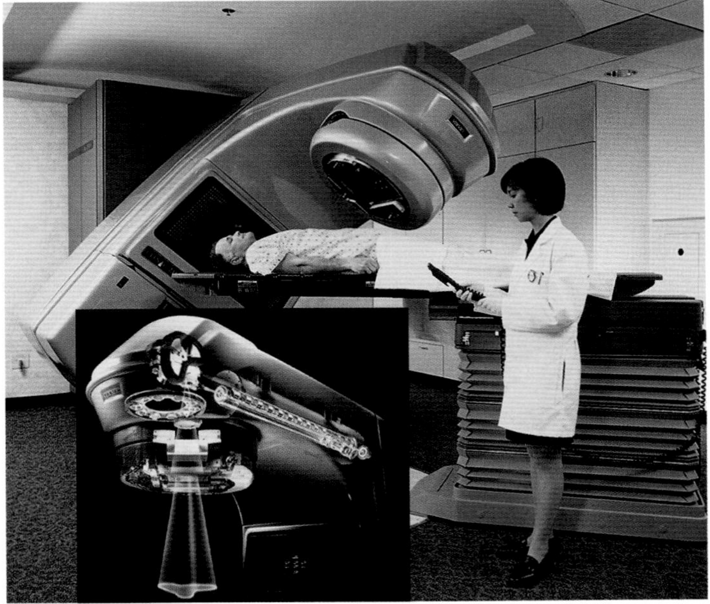

Fig. 24-16. Linear accelerator—high-energy x-rays or low-energy electron beam. *Inset* demonstrates internal parts. (Courtesy Varian Medical Systems, Palo Alto, Calif.)

SIMULATION

Simulation is an important first step in determining the area and volume of tissue to be treated. This is achieved by using radiographic images obtained with a diagnostic type x-ray-fluoroscopy machine and/or CT or MRI images of the affected regions to be treated. This information is loaded into a sophisticated computer program to help determine the various angles and treatment depth. Discreet skin markings are mostly replacing the obvious, permanent tattoos once required for radiation therapy treatments. If the treatment area is the exposed head or neck region, markings are made on a specially designed closely fit mask.

Radiation Oncology Team

The team of workers in radiation oncology and their general responsibilities are as follows:

1. *Radiation therapist:* This technologist is responsible for scheduling, administering radiation treatments, and maintaining records. Radiation therapists are responsible for obtaining preliminary radiographs of affected regions. They may be required to use fluoroscopy to determine the treatment field dimensions, after which markings of such are made on the patient's skin.

   These therapists must possess good communication skills and have special empathy and understanding for patients to effectively interact with them and other members of the health care team, knowing that the patients they see on a regular basis have a potentially terminal disease.
2. *Radiation oncologist:* This medical doctor specialist prescribes the treatment needed and the area to be treated.
3. *Medical dosimetrist:* This person educated in dosimetry outlines the plan for obtaining the desired dosage to the cancerous tissue as determined by the oncologist.
4. *Medical radiation physicist:* This medical health physicist advises the oncologist and dosimetrist on treatment techniques and dosage calculations. This person is also responsible for the maintenance and calibration of the equipment.

ULTRASOUND IMAGING (SONOGRAPHY)

Definition and Introduction

Ultrasound (sonography) is an imaging technique that uses **high-frequency sound waves to produce images of organs and structures in the body.** These images are produced by recording the reflections (echoes) of ultrasonic waves directed into the body.

The technical terms for ultrasound commonly used in imaging and recording are **sonography** (*sonic,* meaning sound) or **ultrasonography** (ultra high frequency). The term **echosonography** may also be used for this imaging process.

Sound wave frequencies heard by the human ear are called *audible sound.* Sound waves with frequencies higher than audible sound ("ultra high" or **ultrasonic**) are called **ultrasound,** meaning high-frequency sound waves that are above audible sound. The range of sound waves heard by the human ear is approximately 20 Hz to 20 kHz (20 to 20,000 cycles per second). For medical ultrasound, the range of sound waves used is from **1 to 17 MHz** (1 to 17 million cycles per second). Sound waves of this frequency are **transmissible only in liquids and solids,** not in air or gas.

Ultrasound imaging is painless and harmless, because there is no ionizing radiation involved. Studies have revealed no adverse biologic effects associated with the use of ultrasound. This makes it a safe and preferred imaging modality for certain radiosensitive exams such as obstetrics, in which the fetus is spared any radiation exposure.

History

The birth of ultrasound can be traced back to World War I or shortly after with the development of **sonar,** which was further developed during World War II. Sonar is a technique of sending sound waves through water and observing the returning echoes to identify submerged objects. After the war, medical researchers explored and developed ways to apply these concepts to medical diagnosis.

A-mode: The first **A-mode** ultrasound unit was built in Japan in the early 1950s. A-mode ultrasound images represent anatomy by a series of "blips" seen on a monitor. The height of these blips represents the intensity of the returning echo.

B-mode: Later in the 1950s, researchers in the United States, Japan, and Europe introduced two-dimensional, gray scale ultrasound devices termed **B-mode.** The use of **gray scale** allows the intensity of returning echoes to be represented by varying degrees of grayness. A videoscan converter amplifies and processes these echoes and displays them on a gray scale monitor.

Real-time dynamic: In the 1970s improvements in the electronics and the introduction of computers produced **real-time** or **dynamic imaging,** which allows physicians and technologists to view the anatomy during the actual scan.

Doppler: **Doppler** ultrasound was first used in Japan to study vascular structures and the behavior of flowing blood. Later, in the 1980s, advances in technology resulted in **color-flow Doppler ultrasound,** which depicts blood flow in various colors to indicate speed and direction.

Digital system: Newer digital systems were first introduced in the early 1990s. They convert the ultrasound image to a digital format for processing, manipulation, viewing, and storage. The image can then also be transmitted to remote sites as can all digital type images.

Newer high-definition digital systems are now available, which offer a significant **increase in dynamic range,** the total range of signals from the strongest to the weakest that can be received and recorded by these systems.

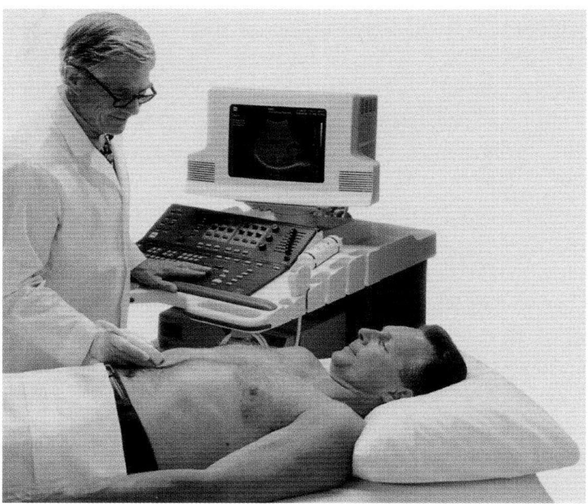

Fig. 24-17. Ultrasound examination of the abdomen. (Courtesy Philips Medical System and ATL Ultrasound.)

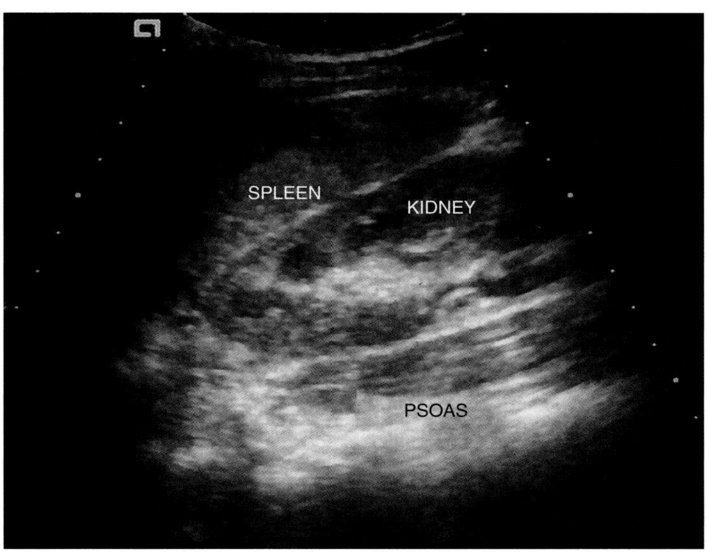

Fig. 24-18. Abdomen—spleen, kidney, and psoas muscle. (Courtesy Shpetin Tlegrafi, New York University.)

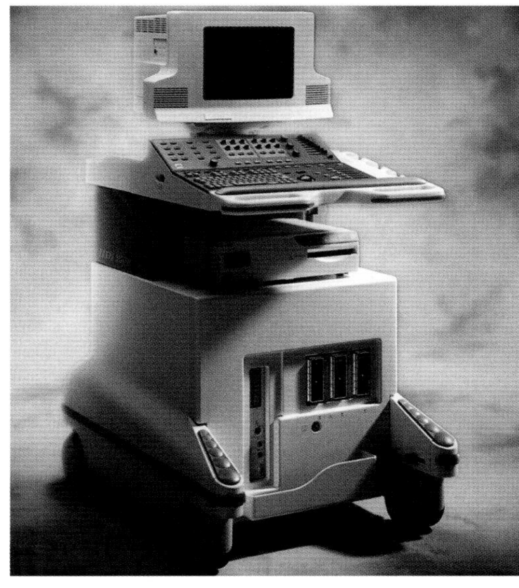

Fig. 24-19. HDI® (high-definition imaging) digital ultrasound system. (Courtesy Philips Medical Systems and ATL Ultrasound, Bothell, Wash.)

24

Principles of Ultrasound

Transducer: A transducer converts energy from one form to another. An ultrasound transducer **converts electrical energy to ultrasonic energy.** This transducer contains a special ceramic material that creates the high-frequency sound when an electrical current is passed through it, causing it to vibrate. This process is termed the **piezoelectric effect** *(pi-e"zo-e-lek'trik).* This term, meaning "pressure electric," describes the property of certain crystals (such as quartz) expanding and contracting in response to the application of an electrical field.

During an ultrasound exam the transducer, which produces the ultrasonic waves, is placed directly on top of the skin, which has a gel applied to it. This gel ensures no loss of signal exists as a result of air trapped between the face of the transducer and skin surface.

Different frequency transducers are available for specific purposes. For example, a 5.0- to 7.0-MHz **higher-frequency** type transducer is used for an average or small abdomen, resulting in **higher resolution** but **lower penetration.** For a larger patient, a **lower frequency transducer** of 3.5 MHz will **decrease resolution** but **increase penetration.** Intraluminal transducers of up to **17 MHz** are used when minimal penetration is required for the **highest resolution.**

Echoes: Once the sound waves are produced, they are directed into the body. They travel through the body until striking a tissue barrier that reflects the sound wave to the transducer. These sound waves that are reflected by internal structures back to the transducer are termed **echoes.** Thus the transducer **acts as both a transmitter and a receiver;** it both sends and receives these echo waves and converts them to electrical voltages. During the imaging process the transducer sends out a short burst of ultrasound energy followed by a silent period as it listens for the returning echo. This is called a **pulsed system** of imaging rather than a continuous wave type ultrasound energy more commonly used in therapeutic ultrasound systems.

These returned echoes are then measured and depicted on the viewing monitor as varying shades of gray according to their intensity and the time it takes for these echoes to return to the transducer.

Ultrasound images: These images can be viewed directly on a monitor as a **real-time image,** and/or recorded on a film or videotape for later viewing and storage. Newer digital units convert these images to a digital format for processing and storage as already described.

Each image is a representation of a **slice or thin section of anatomy** displayed as a two-dimensional image somewhat similar to CT or MR images although much different in appearance.

Plane of orientation: The plane of orientation produced varies according to how the transducer is held. A **transverse scan** will produce an image that resembles an axial or transverse CT scan. A **longitudinal scan** produces a sagittal type of perspective.

Limitations and Advantages

Ultrasound has certain limitations and advantages compared with other imaging modalities. Bone and air-filled structures prove to be barriers to ultrasound's high-frequency sound waves. Therefore anatomy surrounded by bone is difficult for ultrasound to visualize.

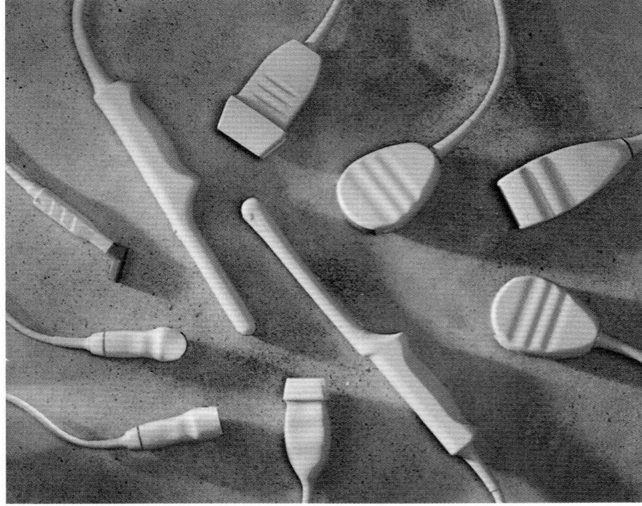

Fig. 24-20. Example of transducer types. (Courtesy Philips Medical Systems and ATL Ultrasound.)

Large amounts of gas trapped within the intestine will also limit the effectiveness of ultrasound of the abdomen. Ultrasound, however, excels in differentiating **between solid and cystic** (fluid-filled) structures in the body. Ultrasound also has the advantage of **dynamic evaluation of joint structures** during joint movements, which MRI, CT, or radiographic arthrogram studies cannot provide.

Ultrasound has become the "gold standard" for studies of the **pancreas, liver, gallbladder,** and **uterus.** Because ultrasound does not use any ionizing radiation, it is safe to use for studies of the pelvis and fetus during pregnancy and has replaced x-ray examinations such as pelvimetry for determining pelvic outlet measurements and fetal position.

Ultrasound Imaging Team

1. *Sonographer:* The role of the sonographer is somewhat different from the technologist, nuclear medicine technologist, or radiation therapist. Although all four professionals must be highly competent in anatomy, physiology, specialized equipment, and procedures, the sonographer must also **provide an initial interpretation** of the images. The sonographer must have a deep understanding of pathophysiology and sectional anatomy to provide a complete assessment of a particular structure or system.

   As with other imaging technologists, sonographers must also possess excellent communication skills to gain a complete history from the patient and communicate impressions and findings accurately to the radiologist.
2. *Radiologist:* Most board-certified radiologists can interpret ultrasound images. In some cases, a department will have a **sonologist,** an MD who specializes in ultrasound. The sonologist works closely with the sonographer to ensure that a correct and complete study has been achieved. The radiologist or sonologist will confirm and document the findings of the sonographer.

Clinical Applications

Differences in tissue types are demonstrated by varying degrees of gray on the monitor or recording medium. Many soft-tissue structures will produce **internal echoes,** which often indicate vascular and ductile structures.

LIVER AND GALLBLADDER

A **liver scan** produces an image of the liver with various internal echoes. The liver is an example of an echogenic structure with varying internal echoes representing biliary ducts and branches of the hepatic and portal veins.

Cystic structures are demonstrated by an "echo-free" (or anechoic) region surrounded by a well-defined margin or border. The **gallbladder** is an excellent example of a fluid-filled, or anechoic, structure. A stone within the gallbladder or biliary ducts can be demonstrated by the acoustic interface or "shadowing" that is produced. The region behind the stone will produce a shadow or an area void of signal.

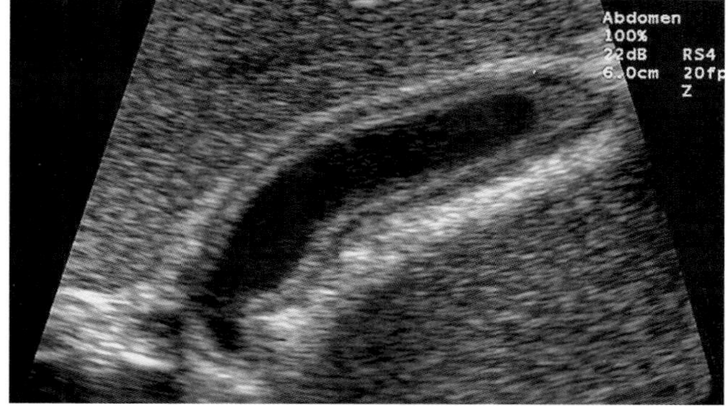

Fig. 24-21. Gallbladder (thickened walls).

GENERAL ABDOMEN

Numerous applications exist for ultrasound of the abdomen. In addition to the gallbladder and liver, the **spleen, pancreas,** and **kidneys** can be examined. Because ultrasound can differentiate between cystic and solid masses, it can detect abnormal collections of fluid and can provide guidance during biopsies. To offset the artifact created by a gas-filled stomach, fluids or contrast agents can be given to the patient before the procedure.

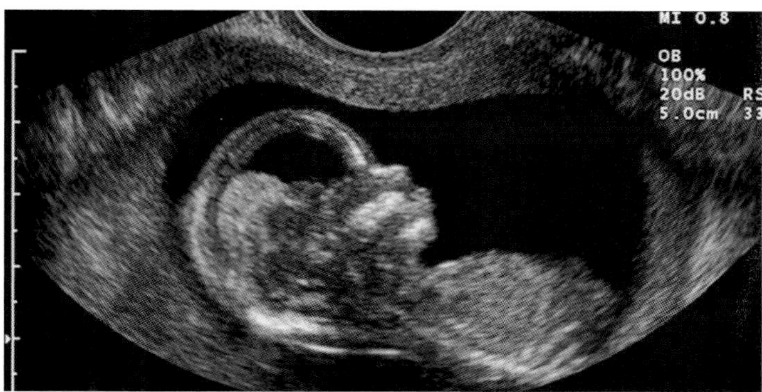

Fig. 24-22. Single-fetus pregnancy. (Courtesy Siemens Medical Systems, Inc, Iselin, NJ.)

Gynecology and Obstetrics Gynecologic and obstetric applications of ultrasound are vast. Transvaginal studies are popular because they produce more diagnostic images of the uterus and ovaries than conventional scanning. Masses within the uterus and surrounding region are well defined with ultrasound. Abnormal accumulations of fluid surrounding the uterus can be easily detected.

Ultrasound has become the most common means for evaluation of the fetus and the pregnant abdomen. Congenital defects of the fetus can be detected with the use of ultrasound. Early indications of **spina bifida, hydrocephaly,** and **heart defects** can be visualized before birth.

Using ultrasound guidance, a needle can withdraw some of the amniotic fluid within the uterus for genetic analysis. This analysis is performed to determine whether any genetic conditions may be present in the fetus. This procedure is termed an **amniocentesis.** The early diagnosis of these conditions may permit the physician to take steps to correct or monitor a condition before birth.

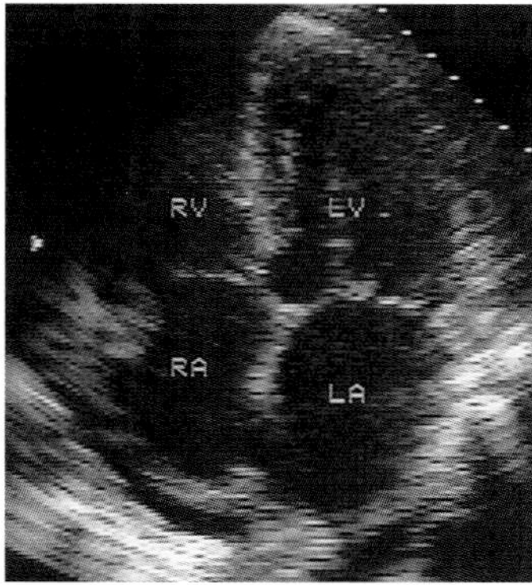

Fig. 24-23. Heart chambers. (From Hagen-Ansert: Textbook of diagnostic ultrasonography, ed 5, St. Louis, 2001, Mosby.)

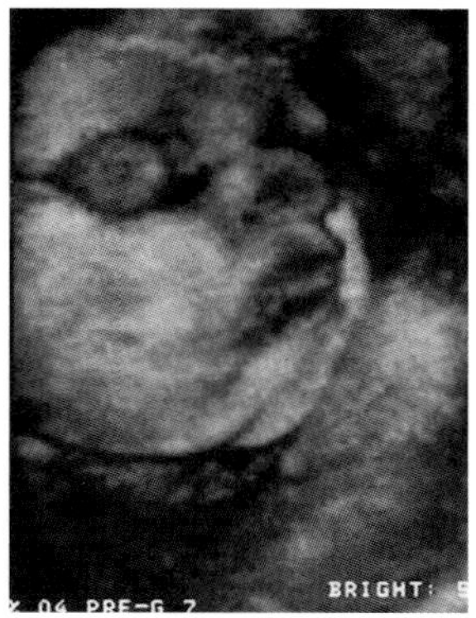

Fig. 24-24. Three-dimensional image of face (third-trimester fetus). (From Hagen-Ansert: Textbook of diagnostic ultrasonography, ed 5, St. Louis, 2001, Mosby.)

HEART

Echocardiography is an ultrasound study of the heart. The echocardiography will detect **pericardial effusion,** provide information of the four chambers, and diagnose **septal defects** and **heart valve disease.** These studies can measure the ejection fraction, stroke volume, and valve leaf motion within the heart.

BREAST

Because ultrasound can be used to differentiate between a **cystic** or **solid mass,** it is therefore often used as an adjunct to radiographic mammography for this purpose.

EYE

Ultrasound is used in ophthalmology for detection of retinal detachment, vitreous hemorrhage, or intraocular foreign bodies.

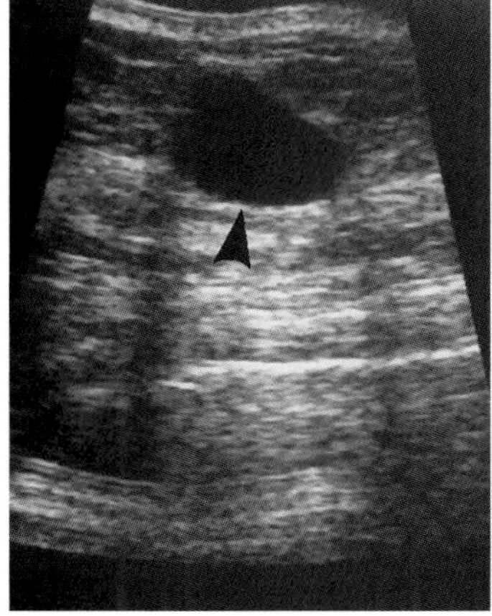

Fig. 24-25. Cyst in breast *(arrow).*

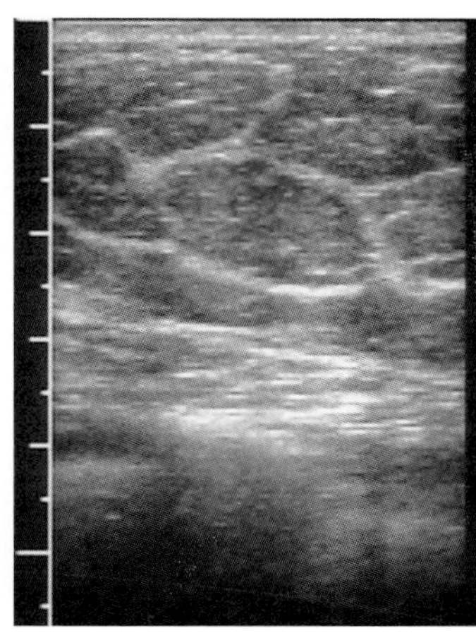

Fig. 24-26. Normal breast tissue. (Courtesy Robert Kuo.)

24

VASCULAR STRUCTURES

Doppler ultrasound permits the study of **vascular structures** and the **flow of blood** within them. A Doppler transducer transmits a fixed ultrasound frequency into a moving object (flowing blood). As a result of this interaction, a shift in the transmitted frequency is reflected back to the transducers. This "shift in frequency" produces an effect called **Doppler shift.** Doppler shift helps to determine the direction and velocity of the flowing blood. Color can be added to the data received by the transducer to indicate the direction of the flowing blood. This color coding must not be confused with arterial versus venous blood flow. It indicates direction of blood flow in relation to the transducer, not the source of the blood flow.

Using the color-flow technique, areas of stricture, restricted flow, or plaque formation can be detected within a vessel. Aneurysms, deep vein thrombus, and vascular malformations can be demonstrated with Doppler ultrasound. Doppler ultrasound is replacing conventional venography of the lower limb. It provides an efficient way to detect deep vein thrombi in the lower leg without the use of iodinated contrast media.

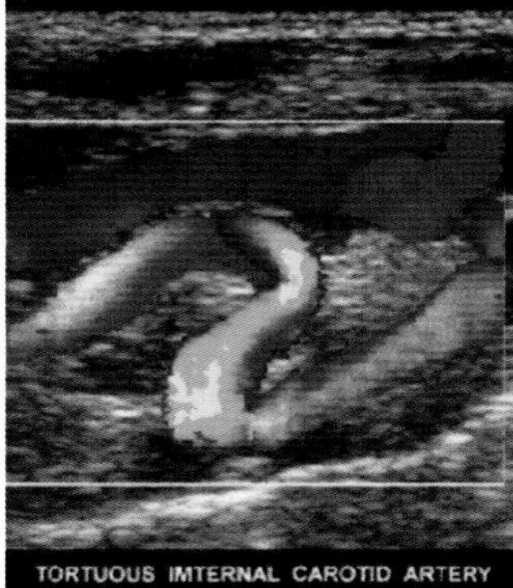

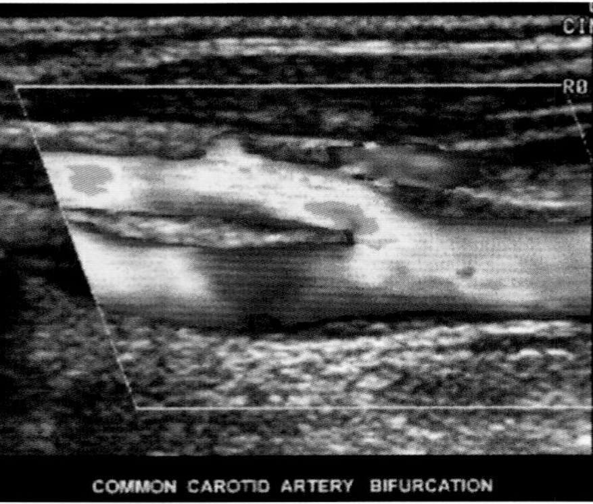

Fig. 24-27. Color flow image of blood vessels. (From Hagen-Ansert: Textbook of diagnostic ultrasonography, ed 5, St. Louis, 2001, Mosby.)

MUSCULOSKELETAL TESTING AND DIAGNOSIS

A newer use of ultrasound in the United States is **musculoskeletal imaging** of the joints, such as the shoulder, wrist, hip, knee, and ankle. These exams are noninvasive and provide for dynamic evaluation of soft tissues within the joints in conditions such as rotator cuff tears, bursa injuries, or disruption and damage to nerves, tendons, and ligaments. These musculoskeletal procedures can be used as an adjunct to, or screening for, more expensive MRI studies. Ultrasound has the advantage of dynamic evaluation during joint movements and is therefore becoming a valuable additional diagnostic tool in sports medicine.

GLOSSARY OF SONOGRAPHY TERMS

Acoustic shadow: Loss of acoustic signal of structures situated behind object that blocks or interferes with the signal; for example, the shadow produced by a calculus located within the gallbladder.

Anechoic: An anatomic structure or region of the body that does not produce any echoes.

Artifact: An echo that does not represent a real object and/or anatomic structure.

Backscatter: That aspect of acoustic energy reflected back toward the source of origin.

B-mode: Abbreviation for brightness modulation mode; basis for all gray-scale ultrasound images; echoes converted into bright dots that vary in intensity according to the strength of the echo.

Color-flow Doppler: An ultrasound technique that measures the velocity and direction of blood within a vessel; changes in velocity and direction seen as different shades of red and blue.

Doppler effect: Alteration in frequency or wavelength of sound waves reflected from moving structures or medium.

Doppler ultrasound: Application of the Doppler effect to ultrasound to detect frequency and velocity shifts of a moving structure or medium; used for blood flow studies of the body.

Echo: Measurement of the intensity of acoustic energy received from anatomic structures.

Echogenic: An anatomic structure or region of the body that possesses echo-producing structures.

Frequency: The number of ultrasound waves per second.

Gray scale: The display of various levels of echo brightness or intensities represented in shades of gray.

Hyperechoic: An anatomic structure or region of the body that produces more echoes than normal.

Hypoechoic: An anatomic structure or region of the body that produces fewer echoes than normal.

Isoechoic: An anatomic structure or region of the body that produces a similar degree of echoes as that of the surrounding tissue.

Pulse echo sonography: Ultrasound techniques using a single transducer to send short bursts of ultrasound into the body and alternatively listening for echoes.

Real-time imaging: Ultrasound images that demonstrate dynamic motion or changes within a structure in real time.

Reflection: Acoustic energy reflected from a structure that interferes with the expected path of the acoustic wave.

Sonar: Abbreviation for "sound navigation and ranging"; a naval instrument used to detect objects under the water.

Sonography: The process of generating images with ultrasound.

Through transmission: Process of imaging by transmitting the acoustic signal through an object or structure and picking up the transmitted energy on its far surface.

Transducer: A device that contains specific types of crystals that undergo mechanical stress to produce an ultrasound wave; serves as a sender and receiver of the ultrasound signal.

Two-dimensional image: An image that possesses both width and height.

Ultrasound: Sound waves that exceed a frequency level of 20,000 cycles per second (20 kHz); for diagnostic ultrasound, uses sound frequencies between 1 and 17 mHz.

Velocity of sound: The rate at which sound passes through a particular medium; varies greatly among structures containing gas, air, fat, and bone.

Wave: Acoustic energy that travels through a medium.

Wavelength: The distance between each ultrasound wave.

MAGNETIC RESONANCE IMAGING (MRI)

Definition and Introduction

Magnetic resonance imaging (MRI; also commonly abbreviated as MR imaging) can be defined as **the use of magnetic fields and radio waves to obtain a mathematically reconstructed image.** This image represents differences among various tissues of the patient in the **number of nuclei** and in the **rate at which these nuclei recover** from stimulation by radio waves in the presence of a magnetic field.

It has become increasingly popular to refer to radiology departments as **diagnostic imaging centers.** This new terminology is due in part to the increased use of MRI. The need for technologists to have a basic knowledge of MRI becomes more important as MRI continues to improve in its ability to show disease processes.

With increases in the number of MRI scanners available, technologists will continue to be called on to assume staff positions in the MRI section of the radiology field. Many students of radiologic technology will have the opportunity to observe and participate in patient examinations using MRI, and all technologists should know the basic principles of MRI and how they differ from x-ray production and radiographic imaging.

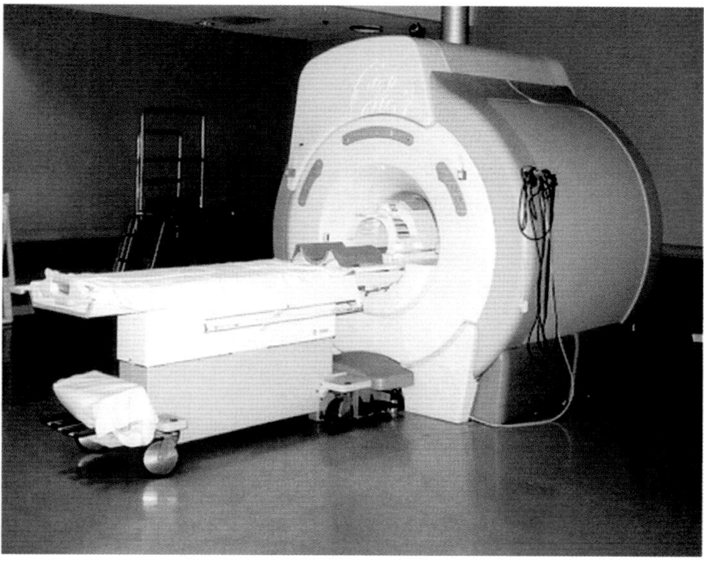

Fig. 24-28. Modern MRI unit, short-bore design (Courtesy Philips Medical Systems.)

Comparison With Radiography

X-rays are electromagnetic waves and as such can be described in terms of their wavelength, frequency, and the amount of energy that each "wave packet," or photon, carries. A typical x-ray photon used in medical imaging may have a wavelength of 10^{-11} meters, a frequency of 10^{19} hertz (Hz, cycles/sec), and energy of **60,000 electron volts (eV)** (Fig. 24-30).

Imaging with x-rays is possible because the photon has enough energy to ionize atoms. The pattern of photons transmitted through the patient constitutes a radiographic image that may then be captured by an image receptor such as film. The fact that x-ray photons have enough energy to ionize atoms implies that some small biologic hazard is associated with a radiographic examination.

It is possible to obtain an image of the body through the use of electromagnetic waves having energies far below that required to ionize atoms, thereby reducing (if not eliminating) the threat of biologic harm to the patient. The technique of MRI makes use of the **radio portion** of the electromagnetic spectrum, in which photons have relatively long wavelengths of 10^{3} to 10^{-2} meters with frequencies of only 10^{5} to 10^{10} Hz. A typical photon used in MRI has an energy of only $\mathbf{10^{-7}}$ **eV** (a tenth of a millionth of an electron volt). (See Fig. 24-30.)

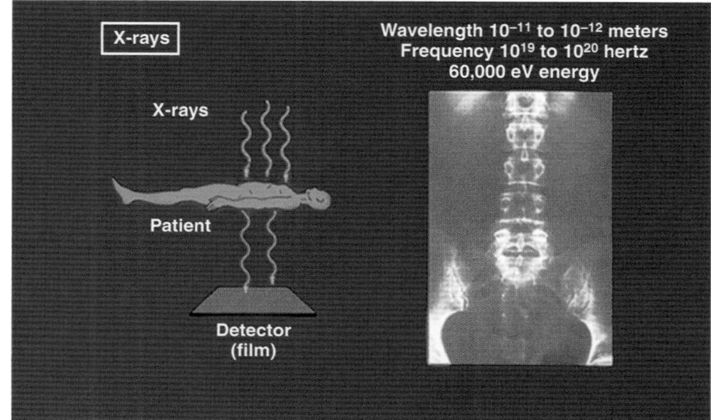

Fig. 24-29. Typical x-ray—**60,000 eV** energy (implies some biologic hazard).

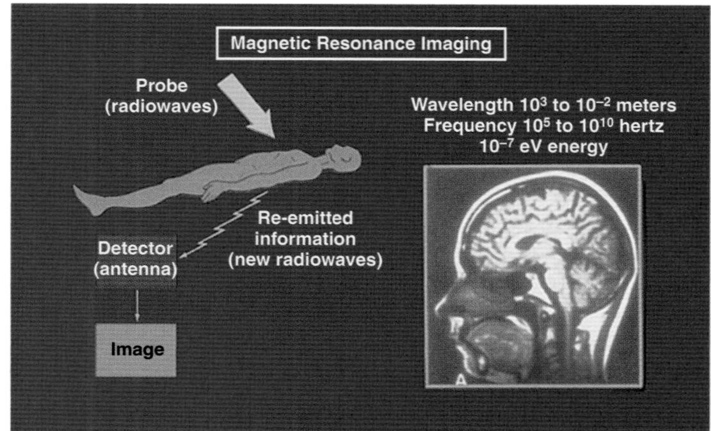

Fig. 24-30. MRI—0.0000001 (10^{-7}) eV energy.

24

Comparison With Computed Tomography

In clinical applications MRI is often compared with CT because MRI, like CT, displays images in sections. CT scanners acquire data that are manipulated by the computer to form axial or transverse sections (Fig. 24-32). Coronal and sagittal views can also be reconstructed with both CT and MRI.

MRI does not require the use of ionizing radiation as with a CT procedure. With a CT scan, patient dose can be significant based on the number of images taken and the region of body examined. Although CT does an excellent job in demonstrating bony anatomy, MRI can demonstrate soft-tissue anatomy that may be obscured during a CT procedure.

Bone does not produce an MRI signal; therefore it does not limit the view of soft-tissue anatomy surrounded by it. The posterior fossa (base) of the brain and spinal cord are two regions of the body that are better demonstrated with MRI than with CT.

Although CT and MRI have their distinct advantages and disadvantages, they both serve the physician well in diagnosing pathology and trauma.

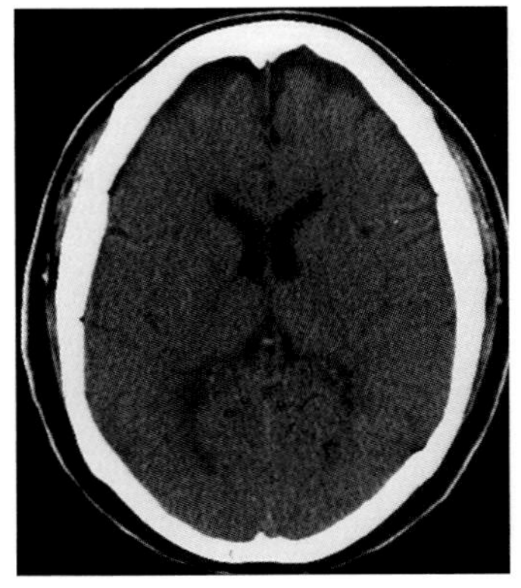

Fig. 24-31. CT axial section.

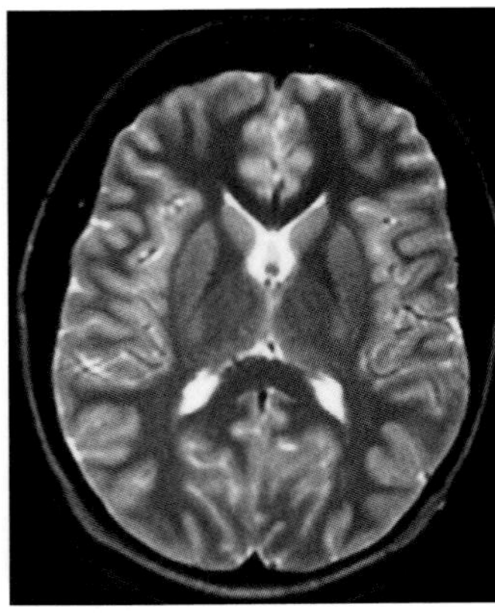

Fig. 24-32. MRI axial section.

Clinical Applications

MRI and CT technologists must possess an in-depth knowledge of anatomy (including sectional anatomy) for accurate viewing of images obtained from various planes or sections. A thorough knowledge of bony landmarks, organs, and vessel placement will enable technologists to appropriately interpret images to determine whether the scans have adequately covered the region of interest.

MRI technologists are also required to have an understanding of how technical factors affect signal production. These technical factors affect the contrast and spatial resolution. Therefore the technologist is required to use these technical factors for optimum image quality.

CT shows an improvement in soft-tissue contrast over conventional film-screen imaging. This ability to show soft-tissue contrast is referred to as **contrast resolution.** The MR imaging system is more sensitive to the molecular nature of tissue and thus allows excellent contrast resolution, as shown on these MRI sections. For example, MRI is sensitive to the slight difference in tissue composition of normal gray and white matter of the brain. Therefore MRI is replacing CT as the study of choice for diseases involving the CNS, especially for examination of white matter pathology.

Whereas CT and conventional radiography measure the attenuation of the x-ray beam, MRI uses a technique that stimulates the body to produce a radiofrequency signal and uses an antenna or receiver coil to measure this signal.

Diagnosis of diseases such as those involving the CNS can be made with MRI by making comparisons between the signal produced in normal tissue and the signal produced in abnormal tissue.

Because no ionizing radiation is used, MRI is deemed safer than CT in terms of biologic tissue damage. Even though the MRI scanner does not use ionizing radiation, safety considerations must be identified and understood, as demonstrated on the following pages.

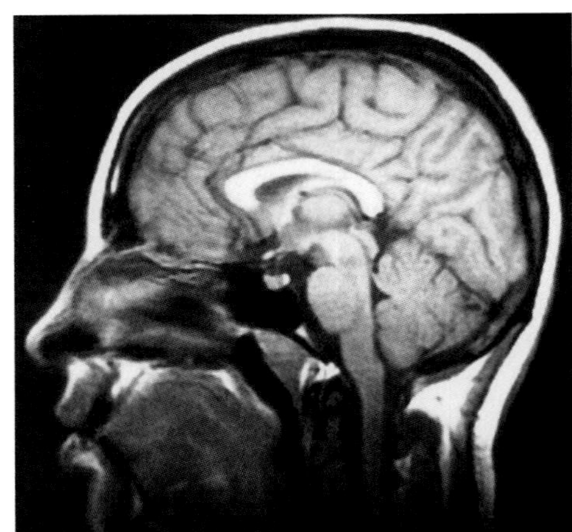

Fig. 24-33. MRI sagittal section.

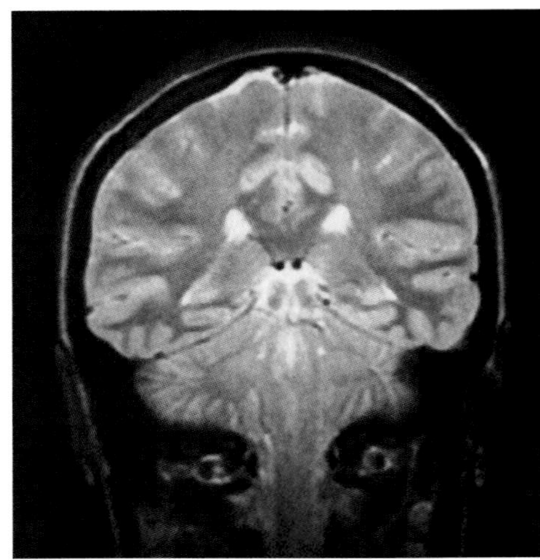

Fig. 24-34. MRI coronal section.

24

Physical Principles of MRI

Certain **nuclei** in the body will **absorb and reemit radio waves** of specific frequencies when those nuclei are under the influence of a magnetic field. These reemitted radio signals contain information about the patient that is captured by a **receiver** or **antenna.** The electrical signal from the antenna is transmitted through an "analog-to-digital" (A to D) converter and then to a computer, where an image of the patient is reconstructed mathematically.

The main components of the MRI system are shown in Fig. 24-35.

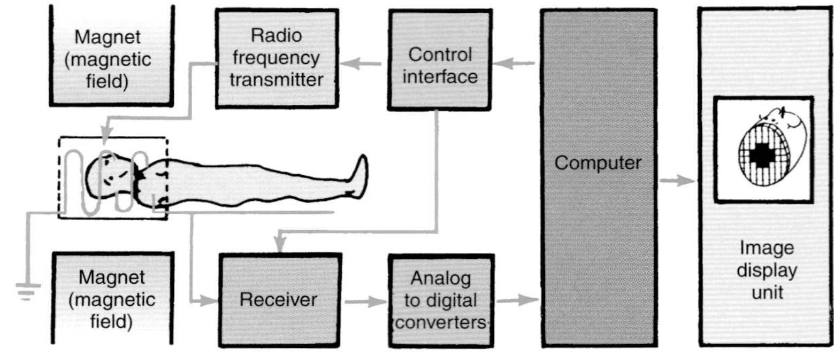

Fig. 24-35. MRI schematic.

THE INTERACTION OF NUCLEI WITH MAGNETIC FIELDS (THE BASIS OF MRI)

Radiographic imaging involves the interaction of x-rays with the electrons surrounding the nuclei of atoms, whereas MRI involves the **interaction of radio waves** (and static magnetic fields) **with the nuclei alone.** Not all nuclei respond to magnetic fields. A list of the nuclei found in the body that are magnetic themselves (those having odd numbers of protons or neutrons) and thus suitable for magnetic resonance studies is shown on the right. Although theoretically a number of such suitable nuclei exist, at present most imaging is performed with **hydrogen nuclei (single protons).**

One reason for this preference is that a great deal of hydrogen is present in most tissues. This is evident by the fact that there are two hydrogen atoms in each water molecule and the body is roughly 85% water. Hydrogen is also contained within many other molecules. Thus a typical cubic centimeter of the body may contain approximately 1022 hydrogen atoms, each of which is capable of sending and receiving radio signals. Other nuclei do not exist in such abundance and therefore will not provide such a strong signal.

NUCLEI SUITABLE FOR MRI

1 **1**	**H**	**–Hydrogen**
13 6	C	–Carbon
14 7	N	–Nitrogen
17 8	O	–Oxygen
39 19	K	–Potassium
19 9	F	–Fluorine
23 11	Na	–Sodium
31 15	P	–Phosphorus

Nuclei that are magnetic (odd number of protons or neutrons). Hydrogen most abundant in body.

PRECESSION

MRI is possible because a magnetic nucleus will **precess** about a strong **static (unchanging) magnetic field.** The phenomenon of precession **occurs whenever a spinning object is acted upon by an outside force.** Three examples of precession are shown in Fig. 24-36. A spinning top, when acted upon by the force of gravity, precesses, or wobbles about the line defined by the direction of gravitational force. In MRI application, a spinning proton (hydrogen nucleus) precesses when placed in a strong magnetic field. A third example is the earth itself, which precesses because of the interplay between the forces of the sun and the planets.

The **rate of precession** of a proton in a magnetic field **increases as the strength of magnetic field increases.** The rate of precession of protons in an MRI system is difficult to imagine. Protons in a low field system may precess at 5,000,000 cycles per second (see Fig. 24-36). The spinning top is shown to precess at a rate of one cycle per second, and the earth at only 0.004 cycles per century.

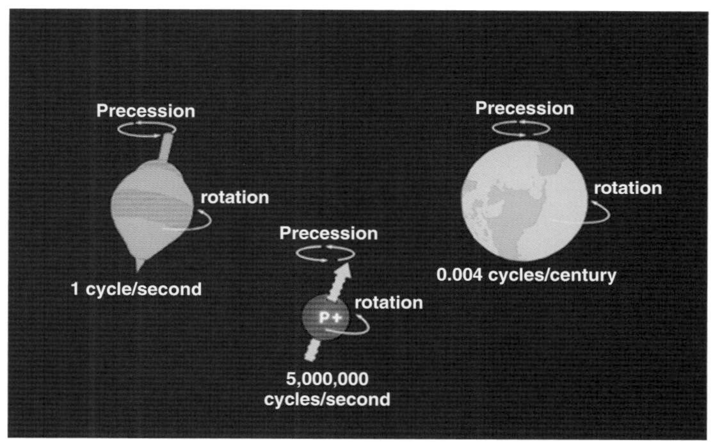

Fig. 24-36. Examples of precession.

SENDING A RADIO SIGNAL TO PRECESSING NUCLEI

After the static magnetic field has been applied, the precession of nuclei in the patient can be further influenced by radio waves, because a radio wave contains a time-varying magnetic field. One effect of the radio wave is to cause the nucleus to precess at a greater angle. **The longer the radio wave is applied to the patient, the greater the angle of precession.** In the example shown in Fig. 24-37, the radio wave has been applied long enough to cause the nucleus to change from near vertical (parallel to the static magnetic field) to horizontal (at right angles to the static magnetic field). However, even this duration of the radio waves sufficient to change the precession of the nuclei to a near horizontal position seems short in relation to events in everyday life. We say that the radio wave is applied to the patient in a "pulse" that may last for a fraction of a second during the "send" phase of the MRI process.

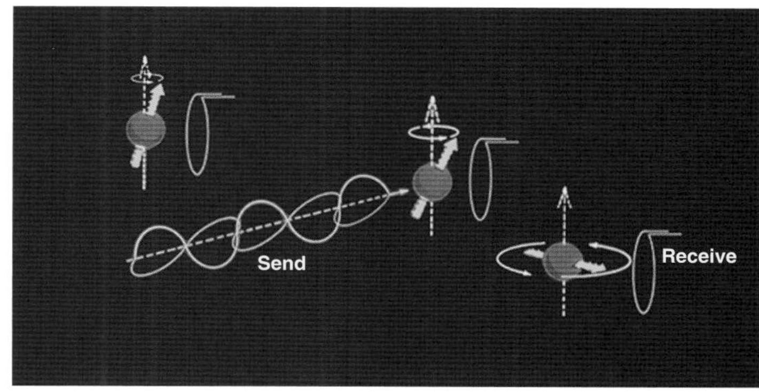

Fig. 24-37. Radio waves increase angle of precession.

RESONANCE

Radio waves affect the precessing nuclei, because the **time-varying magnetic field** of the radio wave changes at the **same rate** as the nuclei precess. This means that as the nucleus rotates, the magnetic field appears at just the proper time to have maximum effect in "pushing" the nucleus away from the static magnetic field. This timing of a force and a periodically changing system is an example of the concept of **"resonance."**

Another common example of resonance is the pushing of a child on a swing. When we push a child on a swing, we naturally push the child in "resonance." That is, we apply force to the swing at a frequency that matches the frequency with which the swing returns to us. We know that applying our energy at any other frequency has no useful effect. Thus the principle of resonance explains why we use radiofrequency waves applied in pulses for MR imaging. **Radio waves** (because of their specific wavelength) **are in resonance with the precessing nuclei.** This explains the use of radio waves in MRI rather than other electromagnetic waves such as microwaves or visible light, which because of their wavelength would not be in resonance with the precessing nuclei.

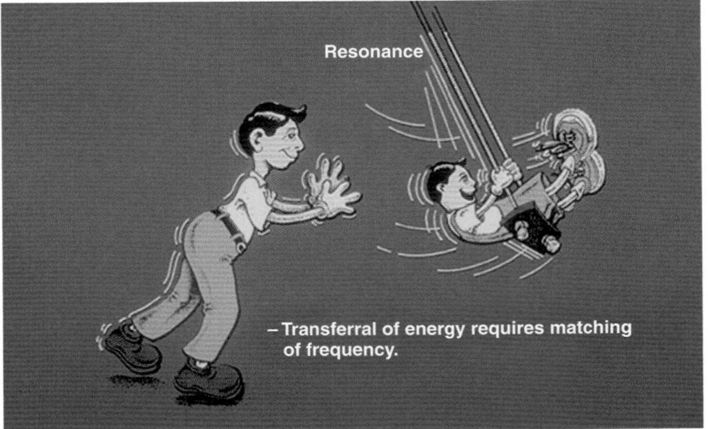

Fig. 24-38. Example of resonance.

RECEIVING THE MRI SIGNAL FROM BODY TISSUES

Because the nucleus is itself a tiny magnet, as it rotates, it emits electromagnetic waves. These emitted waves from nuclei within body tissue are picked up by an antenna or **receiver coil** during the "receive" phase of the MRI process (Fig. 24-39). This electric signal obtained from the receiver coil is sent to a computer. The image of the patient is then reconstructed by the computer. Various mathematic techniques may be used to build up an image from the received radio waves. Some techniques are similar to those used in CT.

The received signal is described relative to random superimposed signals that are also picked up by the antenna. These random signals are called "noise." **The signal-to-noise ratio** (SNR, or S/N) **is used to describe the relative contribution of the true signal from the tissue and random noise.**

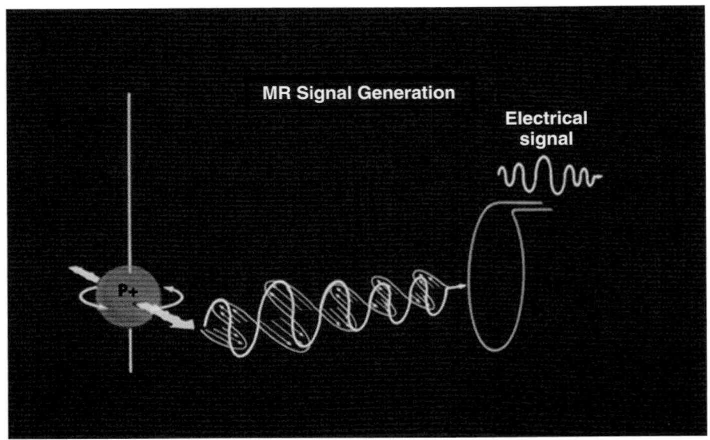

Fig. 24-39. MRI signal generation and receiver coil sending electrical signal to computer.

RELAXATION

When the radiofrequency pulse that was sent to the nuclei is over, the nuclei are precessing together in phase. As soon as the radiofrequency pulse is turned off, the nuclei begin to return to a more random configuration in a process called **relaxation.** As the nuclei relax, the MRI signal received from the precessing nuclei diminishes.

The **rate of relaxation** gives us information about normal tissue and pathologic process in the tissues. Thus relaxation influences the appearance of the MR image. Relaxation may be divided into two categories, as shown in Fig. 24-40. These are commonly referred to as **T1** and **T2 relaxation.**

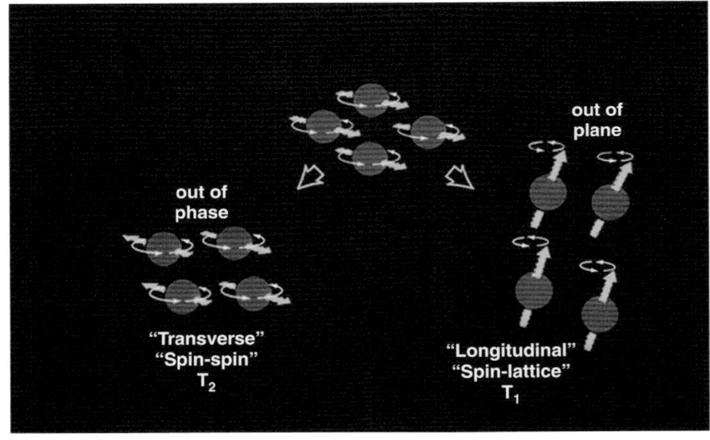

Fig. 24-40. Two categories of relaxation.

T1 Relaxation This relaxation category occurs when the spins (excited nuclei) begin to precess at **smaller and smaller angles,** that is, from a near horizontal or transverse precession to a more vertical (see Fig. 24-41). This process, referred to as **longitudinal or spin lattice** type relaxation (T1), causes the **MRI signal to decrease in strength.** We define the time required for this signal to decrease to 37% of its maximum value as T1 (see Fig. 24-41).

T2 Relaxation When spins begin to precess **out of phase** with each other, the result is referred to as **transverse, or spin-spin,** relaxation. This is known as T2 relaxation. Note in Fig. 24-42 that the nuclei along the top of the graph are shown to be "in phase" at the beginning, but they go out of phase as indicated by the direction of the *arrows.* As this T2 relaxation occurs, the **MRI signal will decrease in strength.** The time required for the MRI signal to decrease to 37% of its maximum value is defined as T2 (see Fig. 24-41).

The rate of these two types of relaxation changes, T1 and T2, following exposure to the radiofrequency (applied in resonance) constitutes the primary basis from which the MR image is reconstructed. However, a third factor, **spin density,** also plays a minor role in determining the appearance of the MR image.

Spin Density A stronger signal will be received if the **quantity** of hydrogen nuclei that are present in a given volume of tissue **is increased.** However, this quantity, called the "proton density," or **"spin density,"** is a minor contributor to the appearance of an MR image because the tissues imaged by proton (hydrogen nucleus) do not differ markedly in spin density. A more important consideration, as discussed above, is that the nuclei that comprise **different tissues** within the body **respond at different relaxation rates.**

SUMMARY

The **MRI signal strength,** as received by an antenna or receiver coil, is used to define the **brightness of each point of the image of the patient.** Thus the differences among T1, T2, and spin density of tissues produce differences in relative brightness of points in the image.

The **primary factors** that determine the signal strength and therefore the brightness of each part of the image or the image contrast are **spin density** and **T1 and T2 relaxation rates.** Other factors such as flowing blood or the presence of contrast material also play a role but are beyond the scope of this introductory discussion.

MRI is a fundamentally different way of looking at the body compared with other imaging modalities. For example, in radiography, the physical density (grams per ml) and atomic number of tissues help determine the appearance of the image. The rate of recovery of atoms from their interactions with x-rays is not important in radiography. In MRI, however, the **rate of recovery of nuclei** after the application of radio waves (relaxation rate) is the most important factor in determining the MR image. This provides the basis for the MR image as seen in Fig. 24-43. High tissue density such as in dense **bone structure** does **not** result in image contrast in MR imaging. Cortical bone does not produce an MR signal due to the hydrogen nuclei being tightly bound with the bony matrix. As seen on this sagittal head MRI scan, soft tissues such as **gray and white matter** of the brain, the brain stem, and the corpus callosum are clearly visualized because of the response of nuclei in these tissues as described above.

The **strength of the MRI signal** is determined by the number of nuclei per unit volume **(spin density)** and the orientation of the nuclei with respect to the static magnetic field **(T1 relaxation)** and with respect to each other **(T2 relaxation).**

The **location of origin** within the patient of the MRI signal may be determined by the **frequency** of the MRI signal. The application of gradient magnetic fields assures us that the frequency of the MRI signal will vary from one location to another within the patient and that the computer may therefore produce a unique image of the patient.

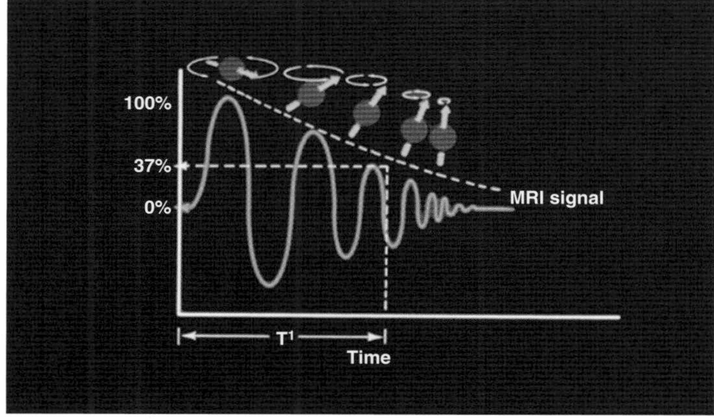

Fig. 24-41. T1 relaxation (longitudinal or spin lattice).

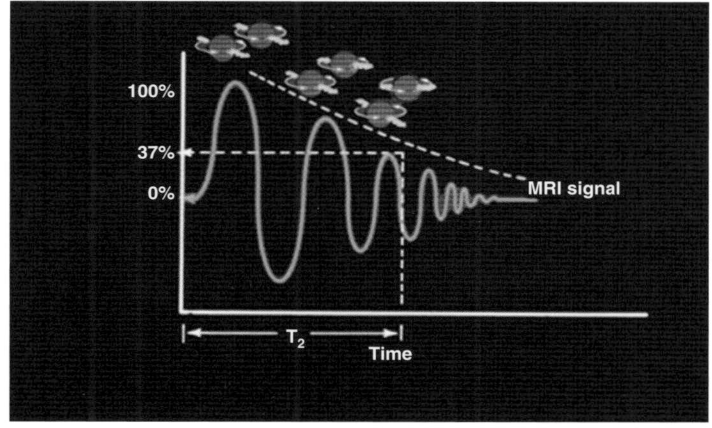

Fig. 24-42. T2 relaxation (transverse or spin-spin).

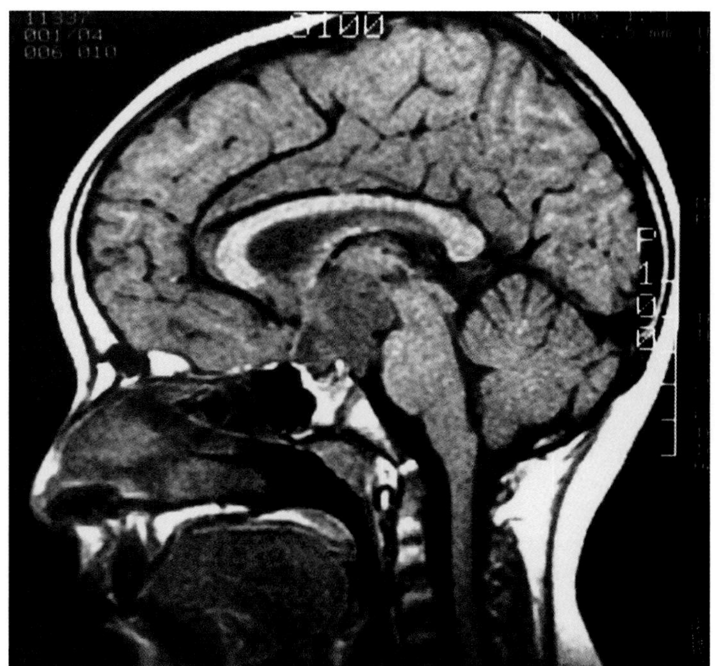

Fig. 24-43. Sagittal head MRI (T1-weighted image).

24

MAGNETS

The most visible and probably the most often discussed component of the MRI system is the magnet. The **magnet provides the powerful static** (constant strength) **magnetic field** about which the nuclei precess. Several types of MRI system magnets exist, and they share a common purpose, that of creating a very strong magnetic field measured in units of **Tesla*** *(tes'la),* abbreviated as T. Field strengths most commonly used clinically vary from 0.1 to 3.0 Tesla. In comparison, the earth's magnetic field is approximately 0.00005 Tesla (Fig. 24-45).

Static field strengths surrounding the magnet, called *fringe magnetic fields,* are sometimes measured in **Gauss†** *(gous).* One Tesla equals 10,000 Gauss.

Resistive Magnets The resistive magnet works on the principle of the electromagnet. A magnetic field is created by passing an electric current through a coil of wire. Resistive magnets require **large amounts of electric power,** many times greater than that required for typical radiographic equipment, to provide the high currents necessary for the production of high-strength magnetic fields. The cost of this electric power must be considered as part of the cost of operation of the unit.

In addition, the high electric currents produce heat, which must be dissipated with a cooling system. The heat is produced by the resistance of the wire to the flow of electricity. This resistance acts as a type of "friction" that produces heat and ultimately limits the amount of current that can be produced. Typical resistive systems produce magnetic field strengths of up to **0.3 Tesla.**

Permanent Magnets A second type of magnet that can be used with MRI is the **permanent magnet.** The high operating costs associated with the other two types of magnets (namely, the electric power and cryogens) are avoided in the permanent magnet system. Certain materials can be given permanent magnetic properties. For MRI use, certain very large permanent magnets may be made with field strengths up to **0.3 Tesla,** the same as the resistive-type magnet.

A disadvantage of this type of magnet is the inability to turn off the power of the magnetic field. If metal objects accidentally become lodged in the bore of the magnet, they must be removed against the full power of the magnetic field.

Superconducting Magnets The third and **most common type** of large magnet in use is the **superconducting magnet,** which also uses the principle of the **electromagnet.** In addition, it uses a property that is demonstrated by some materials at **extremely low temperatures,** the property of ***superconductivity.*** A superconductive material is a material that has lost all resistance to electric current. When this occurs, large electric currents may be maintained with essentially no use of electric power. Thus the electric costs of running a superconducting magnet are negligible.

24

A significant factor, however, is the cost of providing these low-temperature cooling materials, called **cryogens** *(kri'o-jen).* The two cryogens commonly employed are **liquid nitrogen** (−195.8° C) and **liquid helium** (−268.9° C).

High magnetic field strengths are possible with the superconducting magnet, with values as high as **2.0** or **3.0 Tesla** for clinical use.

The strong magnetic field allows for a high signal-to-noise ratio, which optimizes brain mapping and real-time brain acquisitions.

Flared, Short-Bore Design Fig. 24-45 demonstrates a modern superconducting magnet with a flared and short bore (60 cm) to help relieve the anxiety and possible claustrophobia of patients. (The outward design and appearance of these systems are similar for either the 1.5 or the 3.0 T models.)

*Nikola Tesla, 1856-1943, U.S. researcher (born in Croatia) in electromagnetic phenomena. A *Tesla (T)* is a unit of magnetic flux density equal to 1 weber per square meter (SI unit of measurement).

†Carl F. Gauss, German physicist, 1777-1855. A Gauss is a measurement of magnetic flux density in lines of flux per square centimeter (GCS unit of measurement).

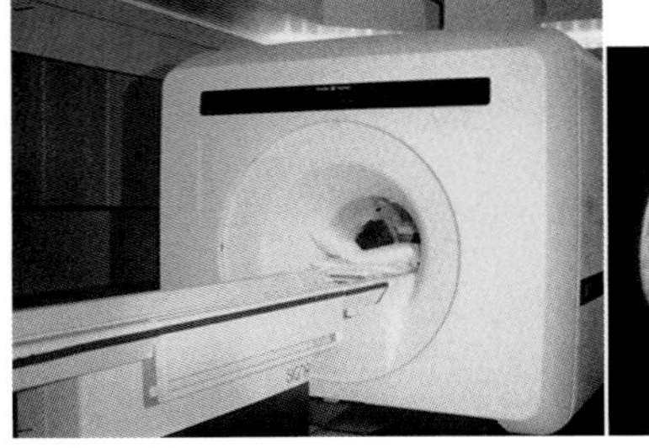

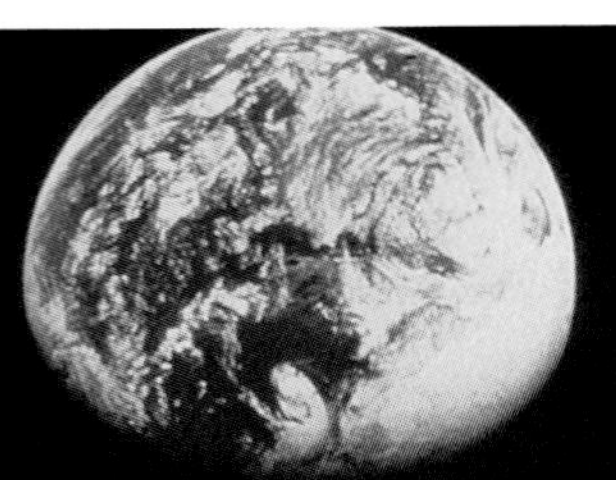

Fig. 24-44. Magnetic field strength comparisons. **MRI**—0.1 to 3.0 Tesla (1000 to 30,000 Gauss); **Earth**—0.00005 Tesla (0.5 Gauss).

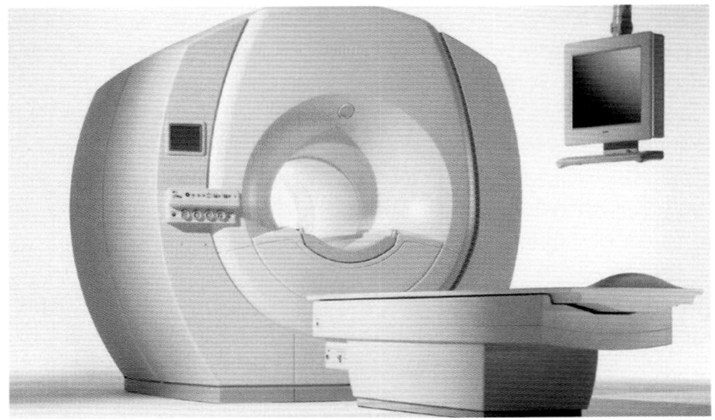

Fig. 24-45. Example of a superconducting magent with a flared short-bore design, 1.5 to 3 Tesla. (Courtesy Philips Medical Systems.)

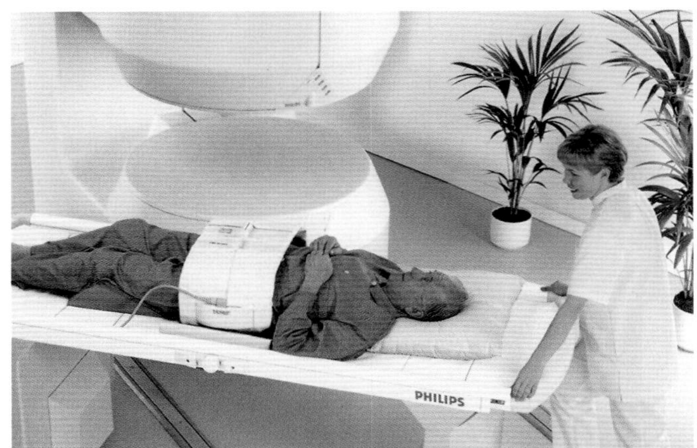

Fig. 24-46. Open MRI system, resistive magnet type, 0.23 T. (Courtesy Philips Medical Systems.)

Open MRI System A totally open MRI system is shown in Fig. 24-46. This is a 0.23-T **resistive magnet type** unit. Certain other manufacturers have similar-size **open permanent-type** magnets. One company now has an **open superconducting type** available, and several similar open larger units of up to 1.0 T are being designed.

All of these smaller open-type units are slower, thus requiring longer exam times, and are restricted to basic MRI functions. These open types are useful for children or adults with severe claustrophobic fears who cannot tolerate the close confines of the larger, more enclosed type systems.

New High-Field Strength Systems Some newer superhigh-field strength magnets of up to **7 Tesla** weighing 30 tons are in use in certain research facilities where researchers are studying and diagnosing CNS diseases, such as multiple sclerosis, epilepsy, depression, Alzheimer's, and Parkinson's. The detail and resolution of such high-field strength systems are improved to the extent that molecular imaging is possible, wherein early chemical changes within the brain due to these diseases can be studied.

Clinical Applications

CONTRAINDICATIONS

Certain absolute contraindications exist to patient MRI scanning, as shown on the right.

Although not an absolute contraindication, **pregnancy** is often considered a contraindication. When an MRI examination is indicated for a pregnant patient, an informed consent should be obtained and clinically documented. Pregnant women will not be scanned in most MRI departments.

ABSOLUTE CONTRAINDICATIONS TO MRI*

- Pacemakers
- Ferromagnetic aneurysm clips
- Metallic fragments in the eye
- Cochlear implants
- Starr-Edwards pre-6000 model prosthetic heart valve
- Internal drug infusion pumps
- Neurostimulators
- Bone-growth stimulators

*Shellock FG, Crues JV: Safety consideration in magnetic resonance imaging, *MRI Decisions* 2:25, 1988.

PATIENT PREPARATION

Each person involved in patient scheduling and preparation plays a key role in a successful MRI exam. A brief form or brochure explaining the exam may be given when the appointment is scheduled. Gaining the patient's confidence is a major concern, because the more relaxed and comfortable the patient is, the more likely a successful exam. Sufficient time must be allowed to inquire about the patient's history, explain the exam in detail, ask patient to **remove all metal, analog watches, and credit cards.** Ensure that the patient is comfortable. Information to be included when preparing a patient for an MRI scan may include explanations of the following:

1. A description about the MRI unit
2. The importance of lying still
3. The knocking sound the patient will hear*
4. The length of time a sequence will last
5. The two-way communication system and the monitoring that will take place
6. The lack of ionizing radiation
7. The importance of removing all ferrous (iron-based) metal (prosthetic devices, such as artificial hips, are usually constructed of nonferrous materials)

RELIEVING PATIENT ANXIETY

The aperture or bore of the magnet (gantry) into which the patient is positioned on the scanning couch or table for MR imaging is shown in Fig. 24-47. This may be a rather narrow and confining space, and some patients with claustrophobic tendencies may become anxious or even alarmed by this. Some controversy exists over whether to tell the patient claustrophobia is possible, but in general, it is considered better not to mention the potential for claustrophobia. The MRI technologist, however, must be prepared if the patient mentions claustrophobia, in which case, steps can be taken to ensure the patient has as little anxiety as possible. Claustrophobia may occur quite spontaneously once the patient is in the magnet. The following options may be used to reduce anxiety and gain a successful examination:

1. Music and relaxation techniques; patients close their eyes and think of something pleasant.
2. Move the patient slowly into the magnet.
3. Allow a family member in the room during the exam. The family member can hold the patient's foot or hand, reminding the patient that the scanner is open on both ends.
4. Keep in constant communication with the patient during the scan. It is highly recommended that claustrophobic patients **NOT** be firmly restrained during the scan. Such action will often lead to increased anxiety.

In some situations, sedation may be required. The type of sedation and contraindications vary depending on department routines. The patient must be closely monitored if sedated and must not be allowed to travel home alone after sedation.

*__Certain pulse sequences generate a high-volume knocking noise__ that is associated with the gradient coils turning off and on. The patient must be informed of this, and ear protection may be required during these sequences.

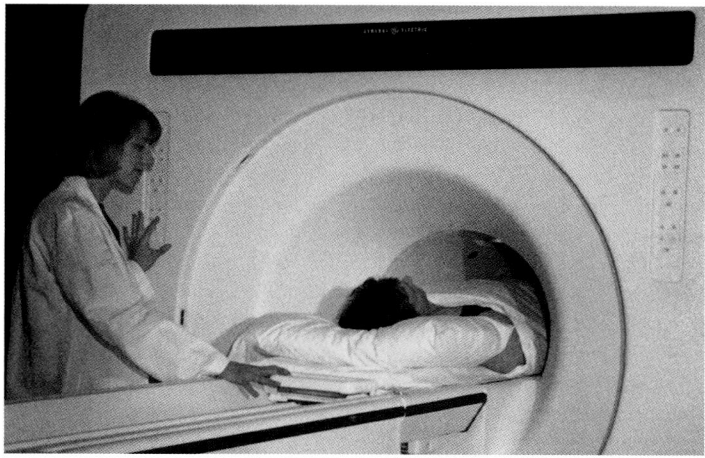

Fig. 24-47. Relieving patient anxiety (claustrophobia may occur).

PATIENT MONITORING

Monitoring of the patient may require frequent reassurance during the scan or during the breaks between pulse sequences. If reassurance is given during the examination, the patient must be reminded not to move or talk during data acquisition.

Monitoring of the sedated patient is difficult because of the length of the bore of the magnet. The key concerns are whether patients are breathing and whether they have enough oxygen. Observing respirations is generally sufficient to ensure breathing, but a pulse oximeter may be needed to verify an adequate exchange of O_2 and CO_2. Magnetic field and radiofrequency interference can cause problems in the operation of such monitoring equipment and therefore present some limitations.

Summary The major concerns in preparing a patient for an MRI examination are as follows:

1. Screening for contraindications
2. Explaining the exam (reducing patient anxiety and fear)
3. Removing all metal
4. Ensuring patient comfort

Basic Safety Considerations

Safety concerns for the technologist, patient, and medical personnel must be recognized. These concerns are due to **the interaction of the magnetic fields with metallic objects and tissues.** During an MRI scan, patients as well as other personnel in the immediate area are exposed to **static, gradient-induced** (time-varying), and **radiofrequency (RF) magnetic fields.**

Safety concerns of MRI, resulting from the interaction of these magnetic fields with tissues and metallic objects, are as follows:

1. Potential hazard of projectiles
2. Electrical interference with implants
3. Torquing of certain metallic objects
4. Local heating of tissues and metallic objects
5. Electric interference with the normal function of nerve cells and muscle fibers

Each of these five safety concerns will be discussed beginning with the potential hazards of projectiles.

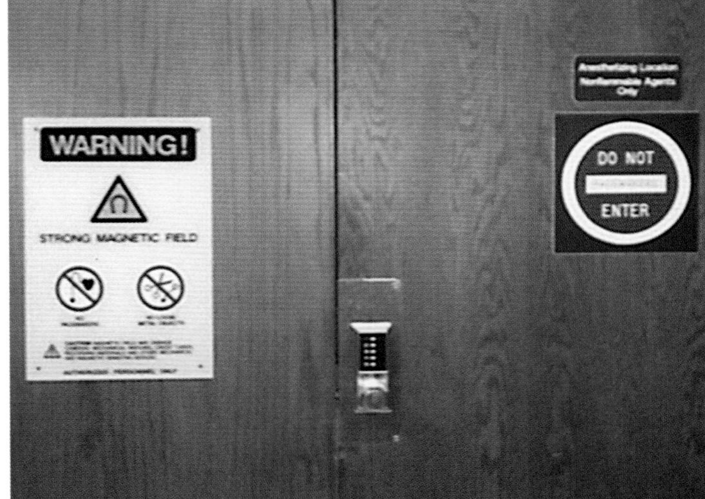

Fig. 24-48. Warning posters and door security.

POTENTIAL HAZARD OF PROJECTILES

A static magnetic field surrounds the magnet and is referred to as the **fringe magnetic field.** Certain items are not allowed inside these fringe fields, and monitoring is essential before allowing anyone to enter the magnet room. Warning posters and door security systems need to be in use to prevent unauthorized personnel from entering restricted areas within the fringe magnetic field.

The fringe magnetic fields are generally measured in Gauss (G). The fringe field strength is inversely proportional to the cube of the distance from the bore of the magnet; therefore the danger of projectiles becomes greater as one moves closer to the magnet. For example, on a 1.5-Tesla imaging system, a ferromagnetic object 3 feet away will have a force 10 times that of gravity; at 7 feet the force would equal that of gravity (Fig. 24-49). If a small ferromagnetic object were released close to the magnet, it could become lethal, since it would attain a terminal velocity of 40 miles per hour by the time it reached the center of the magnet.*

In the event of a code (respiratory or cardiac arrest), the patient must first be removed from the scan room and all personnel advised of the routine procedure of response to eliminate the possibility of metallic objects becoming dangerous projectiles.

As a rule, patient equipment such as O_2 tanks, IV pumps, patient monitoring equipment, wheelchairs, and carts are **not allowed** inside the **50-Gauss line,** although some special equipment has been designed to be used specifically within the MRI examination area.

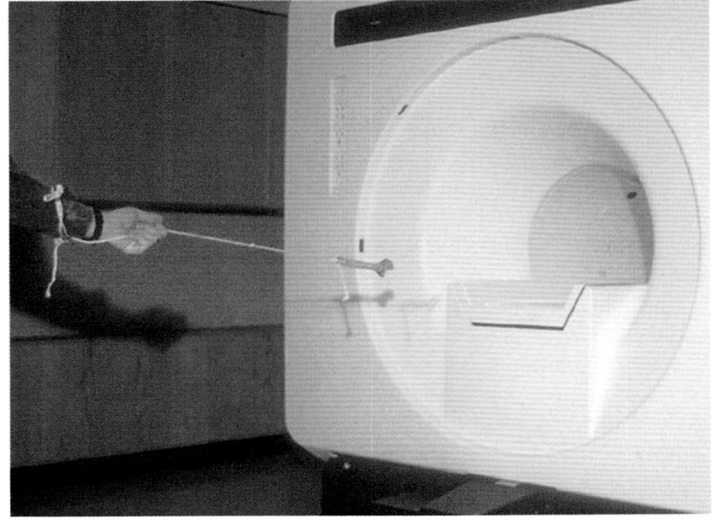

Fig. 24-49. Demonstration of potential hazard of projectiles. A metallic object (wrench) is shown in midair suspension as it is strongly attracted toward the magnet. If not securely held back by the rope, it would become a dangerous projectile. (This demonstration is not recommended without adequate precautions and safety measures.)

ELECTRICAL INTERFERENCE WITH ELECTROMECHANICAL IMPLANTS

A second major concern is possible damage to **electronic components** and function of **cardiac pacemakers;** therefore these are not allowed within the **5-Gauss line.** Besides the static magnetic field causing possible damage to cardiac pacemakers, the RF pulses may induce voltage in the pacemaker leads.

Other devices that may be adversely affected by MRI are **cochlear implants, neurostimulators, implanted drug infusion pumps,** and **bone growth stimulators.** Objects such as **magnetic tapes, credit cards,** and **analog watches** may also be affected and should therefore be kept outside the **10-Gauss line.**

*Williams KD, Drayer BP: *BNI Quarterly* 5:1, 1989.

TORQUING OF METALLIC OBJECTS

The third safety concern involves **metallic objects** such as surgical clips located inside or on the patient's body and their interaction with the static field. The magnetic field may cause torquing, or a twisting movement, of the ferromagnetic objects and damage to the tissue surrounding the surgical site.

The most important contraindication in this category is for patients with intracranial aneurysm clips. Various aneurysm clips have been shown to exhibit torquing when exposed to the static magnetic field used in MRI. Aneurysm clips would be considered a contraindication unless the exact type is known and has been proven to be nonferromagnetic.*

Caution is recommended for all patients with recent placement of surgical clips. Stapedial replacement prostheses may be considered a contraindication. Patients with metallic foreign objects such as bullets, shrapnel, and especially intraocular metallic objects must be carefully screened. Conventional screening radiographs may be indicated.

LOCAL HEATING OF TISSUES AND METALLIC OBJECTS

A fourth area of concern is **local heating of tissues and large metallic objects** inside the patient's body. The RF pulses that pass through the patient's body cause tissue heating. This heating is measured in W/kg (watts per kilogram) and is referred to as the specific absorption ratio, or **SAR.** Technologists must be concerned with SAR limits, although MRI scanners may be equipped to regulate the parameters so that SAR limits are not exceeded. Often the technologist must enter the patient's weight for this calculation to be made.

The amount of heat produced is dependent on the number of slices, the flip angle, the number of signal averages, the TR, and the tissue type. The body is able to dispel the heat through the normal circulatory and evaporative processes. At the RF levels used in MR, no biologically detrimental tissue heating has been shown to occur. This, however, is one reason **pregnant women are not routinely scanned.** The increase in fetal temperature may be harmful. The effects of this for MRI have not been fully documented.

ELECTRIC INTERFERENCE WITH NORMAL FUNCTIONS OF NERVE CELLS AND MUSCLE FIBERS

Rapidly changing gradient-induced magnetic fields may cause **electric current in tissues.** These may be great enough to interfere with the normal function of nerve cells and muscle fibers. Examples of this include sensations of flashes of light and ventricular fibrillation. The maximum gradient magnetic field change allowed in MRI is at least 10 times lower than the threshold value for fibrillation and has therefore not been considered a serious problem.

Occupational Hazards

To date, no long-term biologic adverse effects have been documented for technologists working in the MRI department. As a precaution, some MRI centers have recommended that technologists who are pregnant remain outside the scan room when the gradients are pulsing. Radiobiologists continue to investigate the possibility and occurrence of adverse effects as a result of electromagnetic fields.

*Heiken JP, Brown JJ. Manual of clinical magnetic resonance imaging, ed 2, New York, 1991, Raven Press.

Patient History

A thorough patient history must be obtained before scanning. When contrast is indicated, an allergy history must be obtained. A patient information form is given to the patient before the exam in preparation for the upcoming questions. The patient is questioned regarding surgical, accidental, and occupational histories. If an implant is unknown, the exam may have to be delayed until an exact description can be obtained. Certain occupations, such as machinist, often require a screening radiograph of the orbits be taken before an MRI scan.

Conventional radiographs may also need to be obtained first. Limb braces that may be ferromagnetic must be removed before entering the scanning room because they could become dangerous projectiles. Permanent eyeliner and other types of eye makeup may contain metallic fragments and can cause discomfort.

SAMPLE MRI INFORMATION FORM

You have been referred to the Magnetic Resonance Imaging Center for an examination that your physician feels may provide useful diagnostic information about your physical condition. Magnetic resonance (MR) imaging is a technique that will provide pictures of the interior of your body. This examination consists of placing you inside a large magnet. Radio signals will be transmitted into your body. This will cause your body to emit weak radio signals, which are picked up by an antenna and formed into a picture or image by a computer. The examination will take about an hour. The only discomforts will be from lying still in the confined center of the magnet for a length of time, and the level of noise involved in the examination.

Examining you could be hazardous if you have certain metal in your body from either surgery or an accident.

Please inform us if you have undergone inner ear surgery or have any of the following apparatuses or conditions:

- *Cardiac pacemaker*
- *Electronic implant*
- *Aneurysm clip in the brain*
- *Metallic fragments*
- *Metal in and/or removed from your eye(s)*
- *Eye prostheses*
- *Pregnancy*

Nothing should enter the examination room that can be attracted to a magnet. You may or may not receive an injection of a contrast agent to improve the diagnostic capability of the examination. This agent is injected into one of your veins. Most patients experience no unusual effects from this injection.

Your radiologist will be happy to answer any specific questions you may have about the procedure, either before or at the time of the study. At this time, please empty all of your pockets and remove your watch, earrings, necklaces, chains, and anything in your hair that contains metal. You may be asked to change into a hospital gown.

Your name: ____________________ Your weight: __________

(Courtesy University of Iowa Hospitals and Clinics.)

24

Contrast Agents

Contrast agents have become increasingly popular for MRI examinations. A popular contrast agent is **gadolinium-DTPA (Gd-DTPA).*** It is typically given in a dose of 0.2 ml/kg (body weight) with the injection rate not to exceed 10 ml/min. The injection may be followed by a saline flush. The patient may experience a sensation at the injection site and should be observed during and after the injection for possible reaction. Gd-DTPA has lower toxicity and has fewer side effects than iodinated contrast.

The major route of excretion of contrast agents is through the kidneys; therefore **renal failure would be a contraindication** for its use. **Pregnancy** may also be a contraindication for the use of Gd-DTPA.

Gd-DTPA improves visualization of small tumors and tumors of isointensity during a scan of a normal brain. The most frequent use of Gd-DTPA is in evaluation of the central nervous system. Gd-DTPA is useful for evaluation of **meningiomas, acoustic neuroma, schwannomas, chordomas,** and **pituitary tumors.** (See p. 810 for definitions.)

This contrast medium often helps differentiate primary disease (tumor) from secondary effects (edema). Furthermore, it helps in the evaluation of metastasis, infection, inflammatory processes, and subacute cerebral infarcts. In the spine, Gd-DTPA increases sensitivity in detecting primary and secondary tumors and can help differentiate scarring from recurrent disk disease in the postoperative spine.

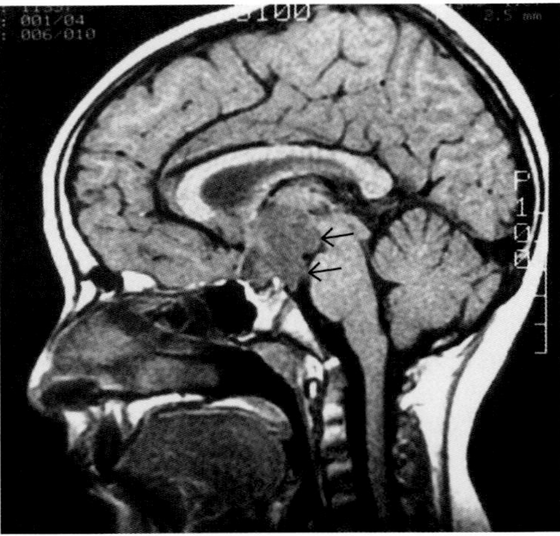

Fig. 24-50. Without contrast agent (T1-weighted image). (Pathology appears gray; see *arrows.*)

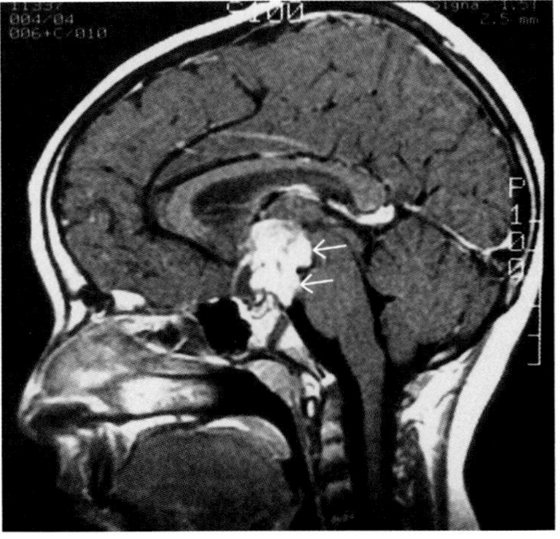

Fig. 24-51. With contrast agent, Gd-DTPA (T1-weighted image). (Pathology appears as "bright" areas in central brain, see *arrows.*)

Appearance of Anatomy

SUMMARY OF T1- AND T2-WEIGHTED IMAGES

Although T1 and T2 relaxation occur simultaneously, they are independent of each other. The T1 of most biologic tissue is in the range of 200 to 2000 msec. The T2 relaxation in most tissues falls in the 20 to 300 msec range, although water has a T2 of about 2000 msec.

These differences in relaxation times enable the computer to distinguish among different types of tissues. Remember that the appearance of a specific type of tissue on MR images is not related to x-ray beam attenuation as with CT imaging, because x-ray energy is not used. Rather, **MR imaging reflects the rate and strength of the signal being emitted during relaxation by the stimulated nuclei of specific tissues.** Listed in the table below are the appearances of various tissues for **T1-** and **T2-weighted** imaging.

Bone, in general, does not produce a signal in either T1 or T2 relaxation and therefore appears black on an MR image. This is due to the tightly bound hydrogen protons found in cortical bone. Red bone marrow, however, can be displayed as gray with T1-weighted imaging.

In the case of **air,** the stimulated nuclei do not produce a signal within the time allotted for either T1 and T2 imaging; therefore they also appear black. Flowing blood or cerebrospinal fluid (CSF) within a vessel passes beyond the receiving coils before the signal can be collected with T1-weighted imaging. Therefore areas of cortical bone, air, flowing blood, or CSF will be displayed as regions of blackness without signal with T1 imaging.

However, some of these tissue types, such as CSF and water, appear bright with longer T2-weighted imaging, as seen by comparing the T1 and T2 images on the right.

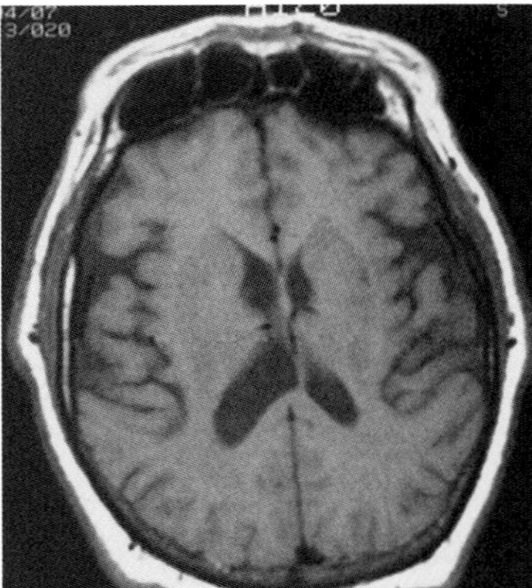

Fig. 24-52. T1-weighted image.

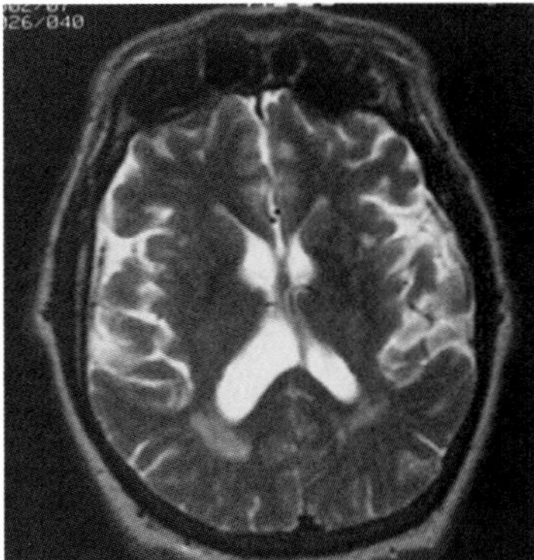

Fig. 24-53. T2-weighted image.

*Gadolinium *(gad"o-lin'e-um)* is a rare element that is metallic and very magnetic; symbol, Gd-DTPA (diethylene-triaminepentaacetic acid).

APPEARANCE OF T1- AND T2-WEIGHTED IMAGES

TISSUE TYPE	T1	T2
Cortical bone	Dark	Dark
Red bone marrow	Light gray	Dark gray
Air	Dark	Dark
Fat	Bright	Dark
White brain matter	Light gray	Dark gray
Gray brain matter	Dark gray	Light gray
CSF/water	Dark	Bright
Muscle	Dark gray	Dark gray
Vessels	Dark	Dark

Sample MRI Examinations

The more common MRI examinations involving the **brain, spine, limbs** and **joints,** and **abdomen** and **pelvis** are described on the following pages.

An increasing number of software choices are available for selection, depending on the patient and pathologic considerations. Both T1- and T2-weighted images are acquired, allowing for a complete examination and diagnosis.

The main goal of MRI software is **good quality images in an acceptable time limit.** When choosing software options, attention is given so that the scan time, resolution, signal-to-noise ratio (S/N), and number of slices are within acceptable limits.

BRAIN IMAGING

MRI is highly effective in demonstrating key tissues of the brain, including gray matter, white matter, nerve tissue, basal ganglia, ventricles, and the brain stem. Pathologic conditions best demonstrated with MRI include white matter diseases (multiple sclerosis and other demyelinating disorders), neoplasm, infectious diseases (including those associated with AIDS and herpes), hemorrhagic disorders, CVA, and ischemic disorders.

Comparisons With CT MRI has proven to have superior soft-tissue contrast resolution and multiplanar imaging capabilities as compared with CT. As opposed to CT, MRI involves no ionizing radiation. MRI is superior to CT in detecting small changes in tissue water content. Furthermore, because of its lack of bone artifact, MRI is preferred over CT for imaging the posterior fossa and brain stem.

In cases in which small calcifications are important to identify, CT is chosen over MRI because MRI is generally insensitive to small calcifications. CT and conventional radiography have remained the combined study of choice for brain imaging to diagnose fractures of the cranium. The very ill patient with monitoring and life support equipment is often imaged in CT as is the trauma patient. This is due to the faster examination time, tolerance to patient motion, ability to monitor the patient adequately, ability to show acute blood and fractures, and issues related to the physical components of life support equipment.

T1-weighted Images T1-weighted images demonstrate general brain structure. Gd-DTPA T1-weighted studies are best utilized to improve detection and to characterize brain lesions.

T2-weighted Images T2-weighted images are effective in demonstrating pathology and the edema associated with the abnormality. Conditions demonstrated on T2-weighted images include infarction, trauma, inflammation, degeneration, neoplasm, and bleeding.

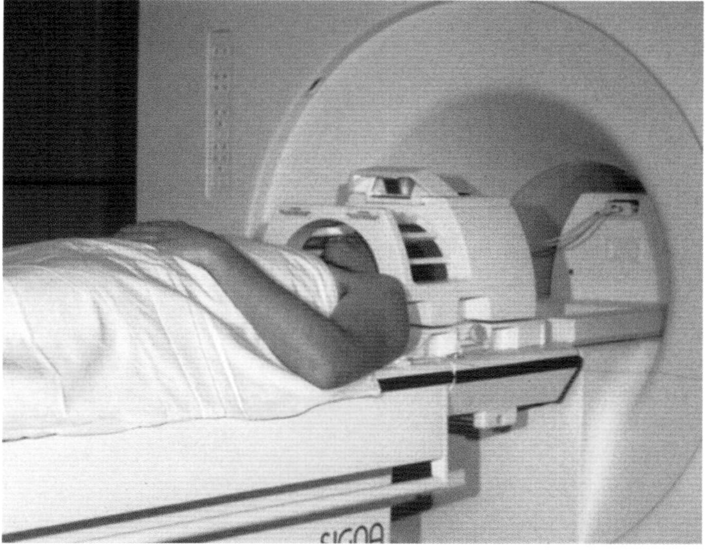

Fig. 24-54. Patient positioned in head coil (patient and coil will be moved into magnet center).

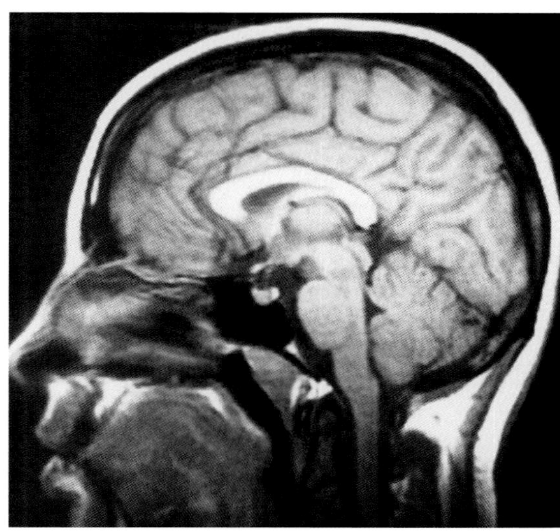

Fig. 24-55. Sagittal section (T1).

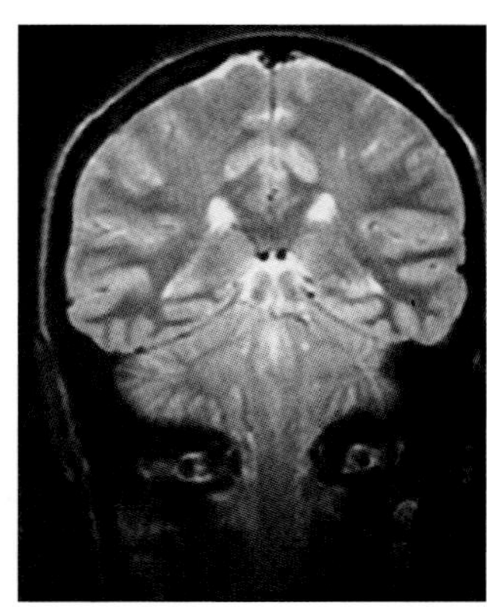

Fig. 24-56. Coronal section (T2).

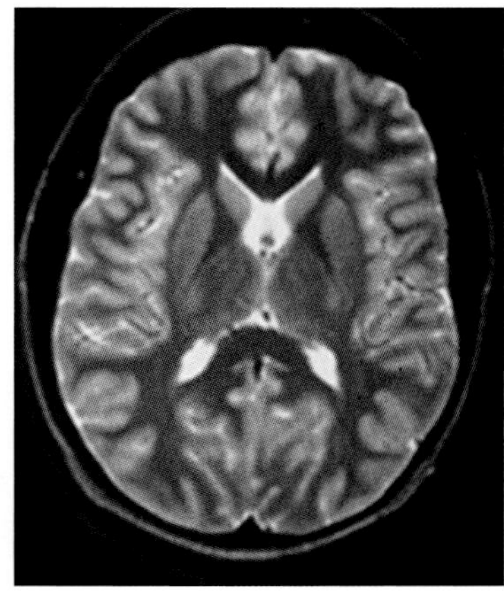

Fig. 24-57. Axial section (T2).

SPINE IMAGING

Comparison With CT The major advantages of MRI over CT are that MRI does not require the use of intrathecal (injected within the subarachnoid space) contrast material to evaluate the spinal cord and subarachnoid space and that it covers large areas of the spine in a single sagittal view. CT, however, remains essential for evaluation of significant spinal trauma.

Even though the need for myelography has decreased, it is still useful in selected cases. Myelography combined with CT is useful when patient motion or severe scoliosis renders MRI suboptimal. **CT myelography** provides valuable information on the location and extent of a herniated intervertebral disk.

T1-weighted Images T1-weighted images are useful to show anatomic details such as nerve roots outlined by fat, information requiring disks, vertebra, facet joints, and adequacy of intervertebral foramina. They are also useful in evaluation of cysts, syrinx, and lipomas.

T2-weighted Images T2-weighted images are required in the evaluation of disk disease, cord abnormalities, tumor, and inflammatory changes. Gradient echo (GE) or spin-echo images using T2 weighting produce a myelographic effect showing sharp contrast between spinal cord and CSF.

JOINT AND LIMB IMAGING

T1-weighted Images T1-weighted images are useful for showing anatomic detail and for evaluating articular cartilage, ligaments, and tendons. T1-weighted images are also useful in depicting osteonecrosis.

T2-weighted Images T2-weighted images are useful to show tumors, inflammatory changes, and the edema surrounding ligament and tendon tears. T2-weighted images are also useful for showing bone marrow disorders, bony tumors, and extent of lesions in muscles.

Note: MRI is a primary method of evaluating internal derangements of the knee, meniscal abnormalities in the temporomandibular joint (TMJs), avascular necrosis of the hip and other bony regions, soft-tissue masses, and bone marrow abnormalities. Evaluation of soft-tissues shoulder derangements with MRI has proved to be highly effective.

ABDOMEN AND PELVIS IMAGING

T1-weighted Images T1-weighted images are useful for demonstrating anatomic detail and to identify tumors containing fat and hemorrhage.

T2-weighted Images T2-weighted images are useful to demonstrate changes in water content in the tissue associated with tumors and other abnormalities.

Physiologic Gating

Note: In the past, MRI evaluation of the abdomen was limited because of artifacts caused by respiratory, cardiac, and peristaltic motion. However, MRI systems using respiratory and cardiac gating have greatly reduced scan times to approximately that of CT, which now allows MR imaging of these body systems.

Gating is a technique to collect MRI signals during a specific point during the respiratory or cardiac cycle to avoid motion artifact. With **cardiac gating**, the signal collection occurs at the same point of the cardiac cycle. Heartbeat can be monitored by ECG, and the pulse sequence can be initiated consistently at the same point of cardiac activity. Other segments of the cardiac cycle are ignored and not added during the image reconstruction process.

Scans of the lungs and abdominal structures can be "gated" to avoid motion artifact in a similar manner.

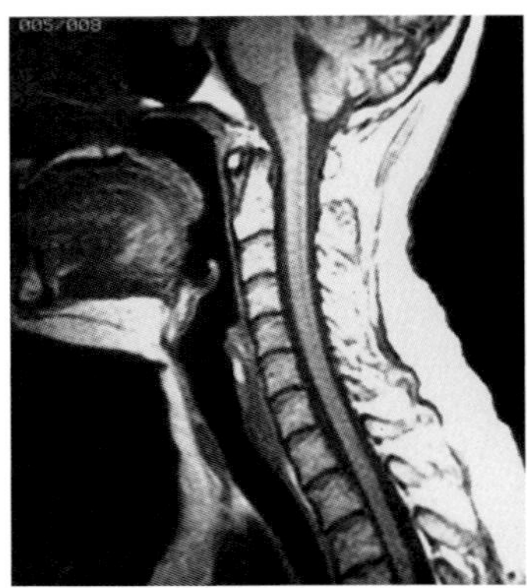

Fig. 24-58. C spine—sagittal section (T1).

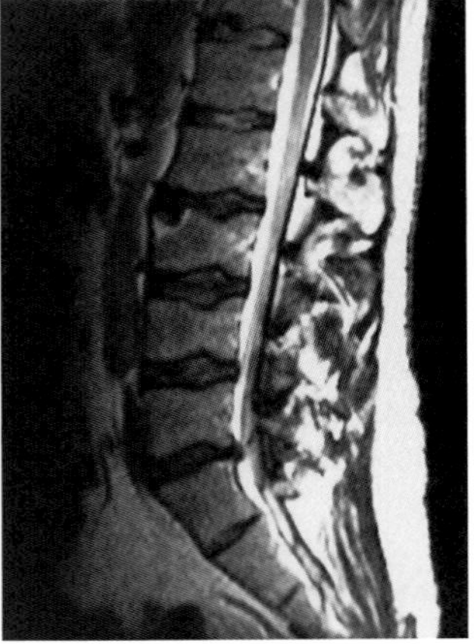

Fig. 24-59. L spine—sagittal section (T2).

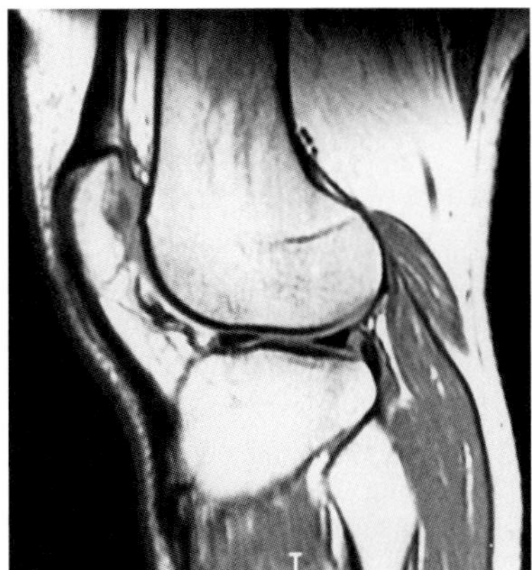

Fig. 24-60. Knee—sagittal section (proton density).

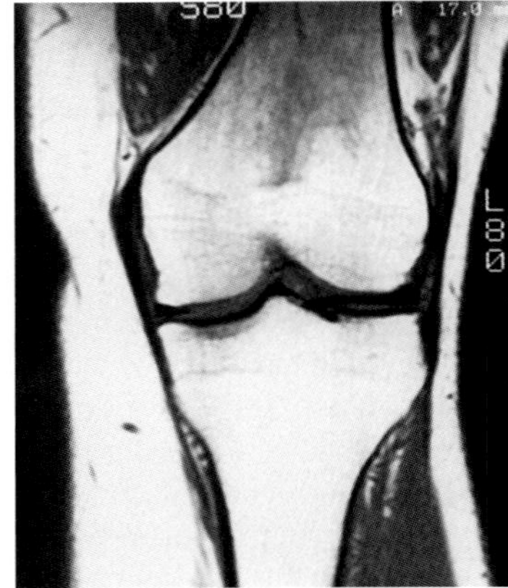

Fig. 24-61. Knee—coronal section (T1).

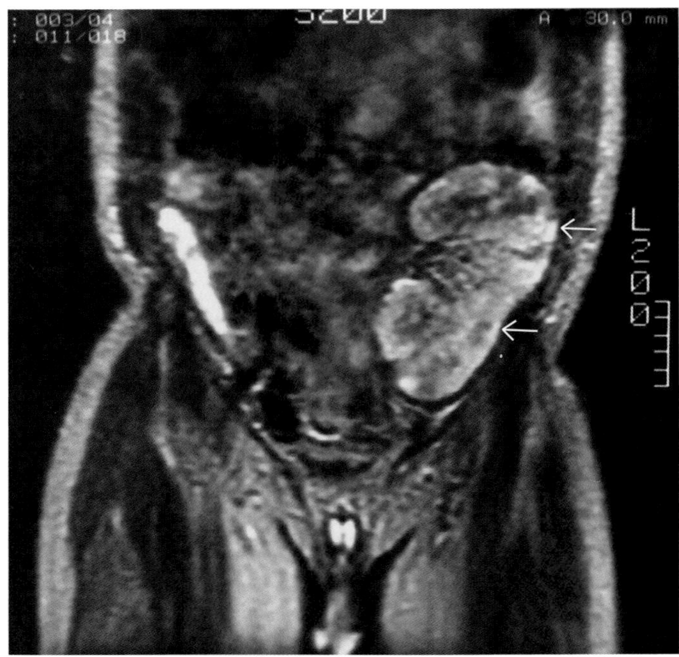

Fig. 24-62. Coronal section (T2). (After left kidney transplant; see *arrows.*)

FUNCTIONAL MRI (fMRI)

Functional MRI (fMRI) provides the ability to **study both the anatomy and specific functions** of the brain. First introduced in the mid-1990s, fMRI permits physicians and researchers to observe brain function and measure certain cognitive tasks. Furthermore, fMRI has created opportunities to advance our understanding of brain organization, as well as establish new standards for assessing neurologic status and neurosurgical risk.

Functional MRI is based on changes in blood flow to the local vasculature that accompanies neural activity in the brain. Neural activity is measured by a **blood oxygen level–dependent signal.** Blood flow to specific brain tissues increases or decreases during certain neural activities. **fMRI** procedures measure the shift in a component of blood termed **deoxygenated hemoglobin** during these activities. **Deoxygenated hemoglobin possesses paramagnetic qualities that enable fMRI to track shifts** in blood flow that occur with neurologic activity.

fMRI is best used for studying processes that can be rapidly turned on and off, such as language, vision, movement, hearing, and memory. Functional MRI is increasing our knowledge of how people learn, shifts in mood and behavior, and human cognition or problem solving. It is equally effective in identifying critical regions of the brain associated with chronic pain. By understanding which region of the brain is associated with chronic pain, physicians are able to select treatment that will be most effective in reducing pain.

Advantages of fMRI Over PET

fMRI, like other imaging techniques such as PET, can be used to find out what the brain is doing when individuals perform specific tasks or are exposed to specific stimuli. However, fMRI has certain advantages over PET. These advantages include the following:

1. fMRI does not require injections of radioactive isotopes. This means there is no radiation exposure with fMRI and no added risk to the patient associated with the intravenous injection.
2. Scan times with fMRI can be very short as compared with PET. PET requires multiple acquisitions, which extends scan times.
3. Spatial resolution of the fMRI image is generally about 1.5 × 1.5 mm, which exceeds the resolution currently available in PET or SPECT images. PET and SPECT cannot match the spatial and temporal resolution of fMRI.

Functional MRI has a bright future in neurosurgical planning and assessment of risk for individual patients, the treatment of chronic pain, localization of seizure regions within the brain, and improved understanding of the physiology of neurologic disorders. The number of medical and research centers with fMRI capability continues to grow.

Glossary of Terms*

PATHOLOGIC INDICATIONS

Acoustic neuroma (nu-ro'mah): A tumor growing from nerve cells and nerve fibers involving the sense of hearing.

Chordoma (kor-do' mah): A malignant tumor arising from the embryonic remains of the notochord (the rod-shaped body defining the primary axis of the embryonic body).

Meningioma (me-nin-je-o'mah): A hard, slow-growing vascular tumor occurring primarily along the meningeal vessels and superior longitudinal sinus, invading the dura and skull and causing erosion and thinning of the skull.

Osteonecrosis (os"te-o-ne-kro'sis): A death or necrosis of bone.

Pituitary tumors: Tumors involving the pituitary gland.

Schwannoma (shwon-no'mah): A new growth of the white substance of Schwann cells (nerve sheath).

TERMS RELATED TO MRI

Artifacts: False features of an image caused by patient instability or equipment deficiencies.†

Averaging (signal averaging): An SNR-enhancing technique in which the same MRI signal is repeatedly acquired two or more times and then combined and averaged.‡

Bipolar flow-encoding gradients: Gradients whose polarity is inverted to encode velocities as changes of phase—a technique used in phase-contrast angiography.‡

Cine: In MRI, acquisition of multiple images at different times in a cycle (e.g., the cardiac cycle and subsequent sequential display of the images in a manner that simulates motion).‡

Coil: Single or multiple loops of wire designed either to produce a magnetic field from current flowing through the wire or to detect a changing magnetic field by voltage induced in the wire.†

Contrast resolution: Ability of an imaging process to distinguish adjacent soft tissues from one another. This is the principal advantage of MRI.†

Cryogen: Atmospheric gases such as nitrogen and helium that have been cooled sufficiently to condense into a liquid.

Field of view (FOV): The area (usually expressed in cm) of the anatomy being imaged; a function of acquisition matrix times pixel size.‡

Filling factor: Measure of the geometric relationship of the RF coil and the body; affects the efficiency of irradiating the body and detecting MRI signals, thereby affecting the signal-to-noise ratio. High filling factor requires fitting the coil close to the body.†

*Unless otherwise noted, all definitions are from Dorland's illustrated medical dictionary, ed 28, Philadelphia, 1994, WB Saunders.

†Bushong, SC: Magnetic resonance imaging: physical and biological principles, ed 2, St. Louis, 1995, Mosby.

‡Signa Applications Guide: Vascular magnetic resonance imaging, vol 3, GE Medical Systems, Cat #E8804DB, 1990.

Flip angle: Amount of rotation of the net magnetization vector produced by an RF pulse, with respect to the direction of the static magnetic field B_o.†

Flow-related enhancement: A process by which the signal intensity of moving tissues, such as blood, can be increased compared with the signal of stationary tissue; occurs when unsaturated, fully magnetized spins replace saturated spins between RF pulses.‡

Fourier transform (FT): Mathematical procedure to separate the frequency components of a signal from its amplitudes as a function of time; used to generate the spectrum from the FID; essential to most imaging techniques.†

FOV: See field of view.

Free induction decay (FID): If transverse magnetization (Mxy) of the spins is produced, a transient MR signal will result, which will decay with a characteristic time constant T2. This decaying signal is the FID.†

Fringe field: Stray magnetic field that exists outside the imager.†

Gating: An MRI technique used to minimize motion artifacts, in which conventional electrocardiography or photopulse sensing is used to trigger the acquisition of image data. Gating times the data acquisition to physiologic motion.‡

Gauss (G): Unit of magnetic flux density in the older CGS system. Currently preferred (SI) unit is the Tesla (T). 1 T equals 10,000 G.†

Gradient coils: Current-carrying coils designed to produce a desired gradient magnetic field. Proper design of the size and configuration of the coils is necessary to produce a controlled and uniform gradient.†

Gradient-induced magnetic field: A magnetic field that changes in strength in a given direction; necessary to select a region for imaging (slice selection) and for encoding the location of the MRI signal.

Gradient moment nulling: Application of gradients to correct phase errors caused by velocity, acceleration, or other motion. First-order gradient nulling is the same as flow compensation.‡

Gradient pulse: Briefly applied gradient magnetic field.†

Inversion recovery (IR): RF pulse sequence for MRI wherein the net magnetization is inverted and returns to equilibrium with the emission of an NMR signal.†

Magnetic field gradient: Device for varying the strength of the static magnetic field at different spatial locations; used for slice selection and determining the spatial locations of the protons being imaged; also used for velocity encoding and flow compensation and in place of RF pulses during gradient echo acquisitions to rephase spins; commonly measured in gauss per centimeters.‡

Partial saturation (PS): Excitation technique applying repeated 90° RF pulses at times on the order of or shorter than T1. Although PS is commonly referred to as saturation recovery, this latter term is properly reserved for the particular case of partial saturation when the 90° RF pulses are far enough apart in time that the return of nuclear spins to equilibrium is complete.†

Phase contrast (PC) angiography: A 2D or 3D imaging technique that relies on velocity-induced phase shifts to distinguish flowing blood from stationary tissues. Two or more acquisitions with opposite polarity of the bipolar flow-encoding gradients are subtracted to produce an image of the vasculature.‡

Phase encoding: The act of localizing an MRI signal by applying a gradient to alter the phase of spins before signal readout.‡

Pixel: Picture element; the smallest discrete part of a digital image display.†

Precession: Comparatively slow gyration of the axis of a spinning body so as to trace out a cone; caused by the application of a torque tending to change the direction of the rotation axis.†

Presaturation: See **saturation.**

Proton density: See **spin density.**

Pulse sequences: Set of RF or gradient magnetic field pulses and time spacings between these pulses.†

Radiofrequency (RF): Electromagnetic radiation just lower in energy than infrared. RF used in MRI is commonly in the 10- to 100-MHz range.†

Radiofrequency (RF) pulse: A burst of RF energy that if at the correct Larmor frequency, will rotate the macroscopic magnetization vector by a specific angle, dependent on the pulse's amplitude and duration.‡

Receiver coil: Coil of the RF receiver; detects the NMR signal.†

Relaxation time: After excitation, the nuclear spins will tend to return to their equilibrium position, in accordance with these time constants.†

Rephasing gradient: Gradient magnetic field applied briefly after a selective excitation pulse, in the opposite direction to the gradient used for the selective excitation; gradient reversal resulting in a rephasing of the spins, forming a spin echo.†

RF coil: Used for transmitting RF pulses and/or receiving NMR signals.†

RF magnetic fields: Electromagnetic radiation just lower in energy than infrared; RF magnetic fields applied during pulse sequences.

Saturation: Repeated application of radiofrequency pulses in a time that is short compared with the T1 of the tissue, producing incomplete realignment of the net magnetization with the static magnetic field.‡

Saturation recovery (SR): Particular type of partial saturation pulse sequence in which the preceding pulses leave the spins in a state of saturation so that recovery to equilibrium is complete by the time of the next pulse.†

Signal averaging: Method of improving SNR by averaging several FIDs or spin echoes.†

†Bushong, SC: Magnetic resonance imaging: physical and biological principles, ed 2, St. Louis, 1995, Mosby.

‡Signa Applications Guide: Vascular magnetic resonance imaging, vol 3, GE Medical Systems, Cat #E8804DB, 1990.

Signal-to-noise ratio (SNR or S/N): The relative contributions to a detected signal of the true signal and random superimposed signals or noise; can be improved by averaging several NMR signals, by sampling larger volumes, or by increasing the strength of the B_o magnetic field.†

Spin density (SD): Density of resonating nuclear spins in a given region; one of the principal determinants of the strength of the NMR signal from that region.†

Spin echo: Reappearance of an NMR signal after the FID has disappeared; the result of the effective reversal of the dephasing of the nuclear spins.†

Spin echo imaging: Any one of many MRI techniques in which the spin echo NMR signal rather than the FID is used.†

Static magnetic fields: The regions surrounding a magnet; produces a magnetizing force on a body within it.

T1: Spin lattice, or longitudinal relaxation time; the characteristic time constant for spins to tend to align themselves with the external magnetic field.†

T2: Spin-spin, or transverse relaxation time; the characteristic time constant for loss of phase coherence among spins oriented at an angle to the main magnetic field owing to interactions between the spins; never exceeds T1.†

TE echo time: Time between middle of 90° RF pulse and middle of spin echo.

Tesla (T): Preferred (SI) unit of magnetic flux density or magnetic field intensity; 1 Tesla is equal to 10,000 gauss, the older (CSG) unit; 1 Tesla also equals 1 newton/amp-m.†

Time-of-flight (TOF) angiography: 2D or 3D imaging technique that relies primarily on flow-related enhancement to distinguish moving from stationary spins in creating MRI angiograms. Blood flow into the slice, not having experienced RF pulses, appears brighter than stationary tissue.†

Time-varying magnetic field: See **gradient-induced magnetic field.**

Torque: Force that causes or tends to cause a body to rotate; vector quantity given by the product of the force and the position vector where the force is applied.†

TR: Repetition time; the time between successive excitations of a slice (i.e., the time from the beginning of one pulse sequence to the beginning of the next). In conventional imaging, TR is a fixed value equal to a user-selected value; in cardiac-gated studies, however, TR can vary from beat to beat, depending on the patient's heart rate.‡

Turbulence: In a flowing fluid, velocity components that fluctuate randomly, causing spin dephasing and signal loss.‡

Two-dimensional Fourier transform imaging (2DFT): Form of sequential plane imaging using Fourier transform imaging.†

Voxel: Volume element; the element of 3D space corresponding to a pixel for a given slice thickness.†

References for MRI

BOOKS

Berquist TH: MRI of the musculoskeletal system, 4th ed, Philadelphia, 2000, Lippincott, Williams & Wilkins.

Brant-Zawadski M, Norman D: Magnetic resonance imaging of the CNS, Philadelphia, 1987, Lippincott, Williams & Wilkins.

Bushong SC: Magnetic resonance imaging physical and biological principles, 3rd ed, St. Louis, 2003, Mosby.

Heiken JP, Brown JJ: Manual of clinical magnetic resonance imaging, ed 2, Philadelphia 1991, Lippincott, Williams & Wilkins.

Kaiser R: MRI of the spine: a guide to clinical applications, New York, 1990, Thieme Medical Publishers.

Lufkin RB: The MRI manual, 2e, St. Louis, 1997, Mosby.

Maravilla KR, Cohen WA: MRI, atlas of the spine, Philadelphia, 1991, Lippincott, Williams & Wilkins.

Partain CL et al: Magnetic resonance imaging, volume 1, ed 2, Philadelphia, 1998, WB Saunders.

Runge VM: Clinical magnetic resonance imaging, Philadelphia, 2002, WB Saunders.

Start DD, Bradley WG, editors: Magnetic resonance imaging, St. Louis, 1987, Mosby.

PERIODICALS

Brant-Zawadski M: MR imaging of the brain, Radiology 166:187-192, 1988.

Drayer BP et al: MRI in the diagnosis of disk space infection, *BNI Quarterly* 5(2):14-18, 1989.

GE Medical Systems: Signa applications guide, vascular magnetic resonance imaging, vol. 3, 1990.

Marqulis, Higgins, Kaufman, Crooks: Clinical magnetic resonance imaging, San Francisco, 1983, Radiology Research and Education Foundation.

Shellock FG, Crues JV: Safety considerations in magnetic resonance imaging, *MRI Decisions* 2:25, 1988.

Shellock F, Emanual MD: Policies, guidelines, and recommendations for MR imaging safety and patient management, *SMRI Report J Magn Reson Imaging* 1:97-101, 1991.

Shellock F: MR imaging of metallic implants and materials: a compilation of the literature 151:811-814 *AJR* Oct 1988.

Underwood R, Firmin D: Magnetic resonance of the cardiovascular system, London, 1991, Blackwell Scientific Publications.

References for Ultrasound

Ballinger PW, Frank ED: Merrill's atlas of radiographic positions and radiologic procedures, ed 10, St. Louis, 2003, Mosby.

Hedrick WR, Hykes DL, Starchman DE: Ultrasound physics and instrumentation, ed 3, St. Louis, 1995, Mosby.

Hendee WR, Ritenour ER: Medical imaging physics, ed 3, St. Louis, 1992, Mosby.

Zwiebel WJ, Sohaey R: Introduction to ultrasound, Philadelphia, 1998, WB Saunders.

Bibliography

Ballinger PW, Frank ED: Merrill's atlas of radiographic positions and radiologic procedures, ed 9, vols 1, 2, 3, St. Louis, 1999, Mosby.

Berkow R, Beer M, Fletcher A: The Merck manual of medical information, Whitehouse Station, NJ, 1997, Merck Research Laboratories.

Bushong SC: Radiologic science for technologists, ed 6, St. Louis, 1997, Mosby.

Cahill DR, Orland MJ: Atlas of human cross-sectional anatomy, Philadelphia, 1984, Lea & Febiger.

Carlton RR, Adler AM: Principles of radiographic imaging, ed 2, Albany, 1996, Delmar.

Carroll QB: Fuchs's principles of radiographic exposure, processing, and quality control, ed 4, Springfield, Ill, 1990, Charles C Thomas.

Clark KC: Positioning in radiography, ed 11, London, 1986, Ilford Ltd, William Heinemann Medical Books.

Compere W: Radiographic atlas of the temporal bone, book 1, ed 1, St. Paul, Minn, 1964, HM Smyth.

Cornuelle AG, Gronefeld DH: Radiographic anatomy & positioning, Stanford, 1998, Appleton & Lange.

Cullinan AM: Optimizing radiographic positioning, Philadelphia, 1992, JB Lippincott.

Eisenberg RL, Dennis CA, May CR: Radiographic pathology, ed 2, St. Louis, 1995, Mosby.

Gerhart P, Van Kaich G: Total body computed tomography, ed 2, Stuttgart, 1979, Georg Thieme.

Godderidge C: Pediatric imaging, Philadelphia, 1995, WB Saunders.

Gray H: Anatomy of the human body, ed 30, Philadelphia, 1985, Lea & Febiger.

Hedrick WR, Hykes DL, Starchman DE: Ultrasound physics and instrumentation, ed 3, St. Louis, 1995, Mosby.

Hendee WR, Ritenour ER: Medical imaging physics, ed 3, St. Louis, 1992, Mosby.

Linn-Watson TA: Radiographic pathology, Philadelphia, 1996, WB Saunders.

Long BW, Rafert JA: Orthopaedic radiography, Philadelphia, 1995, WB Saunders.

Manaster BJ: Handbook of skeletal radiology, ed 2, St. Louis, 1997, Mosby.

McQuillen-Martensen K: Radiographic critique, Philadelphia, 1996, WB Saunders.

Meschan I: An atlas of anatomy basic to radiology, ed 1, Philadelphia, 1975, Lea & Febiger.

Meschan I: Radiographic positioning and related anatomy, ed 2, Philadelphia, 1978, WB Saunders.

Netter FH: Atlas of human anatomy, ed 2, East Hanover, 1997, Novartis.

Norman D, Korobkin M, Newton T, editors: Computed tomography, ed 1, St. Louis, 1977, Mosby.

Statkiewicz MA, Ritenour ER: Radiation protection in medical radiography, ed 3, St. Louis, 1998, Mosby.

Tortora GR, Anagnostakos NP: Principles of anatomy and physiology, ed 4, New York, 1984, Harper & Row.

Tortorici M: Administration of imaging pharmaceuticals, Philadelphia, 1996, WB Saunders.

Tortorici M: Medical imaging, Philadelphia, 1996, WB Saunders.

Tortorici MR, Apfel PJ: Advanced radiographic and angiographic procedures with an introduction to specialized imaging, Philadelphia, 1995, FA Davis.

Watkins GL, Moore TF: Atypical orthopaedic radiographic procedures, St. Louis, 1993, Mosby.

Woodburne RT, Burkel WE: Essentials of human anatomy, ed 8, New York, 1988, Oxford University Press.

APPENDIX 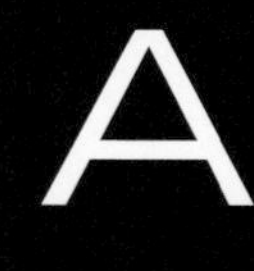

Survey Results

Initial Survey

In November 1989 the first questionnaire was sent to all accredited radiologic technology programs in the United States and to each of their clinical affiliates. The purpose of this survey was to determine a national standard or norm for procedures and specific projections or positions for which all students should demonstrate competency before graduation. Based on the tabulated results of this survey, these basic procedures and minimal routines were then included in this positioning textbook, with the recommendation that they be taught by all schools nationwide to prepare students to function effectively in any region of the United States after graduation.

Updated Survey: May 1995

In May 1995, as an initial step in planning and preparing for the fourth edition of this textbook, a second survey was conducted to provide updated information on the minimal standard of routine (basic) and special (optional) projections. In an effort to provide information as accurate as possible for minimal routines that should be included and taught by all schools, this time only those responses completed by the clinical facilities themselves were included in the final survey tabulation. The purpose of this decision was to determine what the clinical facilities wanted, which should be the same as what the college educators are teaching. A total of 637 completed questionnaires were received and totaled. These responses were divided into hospital-based and college-based programs. The differences between these programs were not significant. The difference in the size of the hospitals or clinical facilities also was not significant.

Expanded Survey: March 2000

In preparation for the fifth edition, the survey was again conducted and expanded to include Canada. This time questionnaires were sent out to the educational institutions (college- and hospital-based programs), and respondents were asked to provide a summary of all their clinical affiliates in their response on the survey. A total of 338 completed questionnaires were received and tabulated.

All projections or positions checked by 18% to 20% or more of respondents are considered essential and are therefore included in this text as either basic or special projections. A few exceptions were made to include newer special projections that, in the author's opinion, were significant enough to be included. Examples of such exceptions are the apical oblique for the shoulder and the mediolateral projection for the hip (Sanderson method) as first described in Chapter 19 of the fourth edition.

Several new projections were added to the fifth edition on the basis of questionnaire response. These included the AP thumb with 10° CR angle (Robert method), AP bilateral oblique hands (ball-catcher, Norgard method), the posterior oblique for the acetabulum (Judet method), the AP axial inlet pelvis projection (modified Lilienfeld method), and the AP axial (Pillar) vertebral arch projection.

APPENDIX 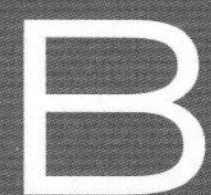

Answer Key: Radiographs for Critique

The following answers identify the repeatable errors for the critique radiographs at the end of the textbook chapters. (More complete critique exercises, with answers for these same radiographs, are included in the student workbooks.)

Chapter 3: Chest (p. 107)

A. PA chest (Fig. C3-91)
Repeatable error—Criterion 1, **Structures Shown:** Left costophrenic angle is cut off. Image receptor should have been placed crosswise to ensure inclusion of costophrenic angles on the radiograph.

B. PA chest (Fig. C3-92)
Repeatable error—Criterion 1, **Structures Shown:** An extra left anatomic side marker is obscuring a portion of the right lung. (An anatomic side marker is present and correctly placed.)

C. Lateral chest (Fig. C3-93)
Repeatable error—Criterion 2, **Positioning:** Excessive rotation is evident by posterior ribs (+ ¼ inch, or 1 cm). Right side is anterior (right diaphragm is discernible because of association of gastric bubble with the higher [right] diaphragm).

Left marker is not evident (may be present but is not visible here).

Note: Many departments will request that the radiograph be repeated if anatomic marker is not clearly visible.

D. PA chest (Fig. C3-94)
Repeatable error—Criterion 1, **Structures Shown:** Bra artifact is present in lung field. Bra also creates increased breast shadows in lung field.

E. Lateral chest (Fig. C3-95)
Repeatable errors (two)—Criterion 2, **Positioning:** Rotation is present. Shoulders are more rotated than hips (+ ½ inch, or 1.25 cm, rotation can be measured on actual radiograph along the posterior ribs). This radiograph should be repeated; however, in some departments it may be acceptable if this is the only error.

Criterion 4, **Exposure Criteria:** Motion is present, evident by blurring of the diaphragm and lower lung field (more visible on actual radiograph).

Chapter 4: Abdomen (p. 128)

A. Left lateral decubitus abdomen (Fig. C4-48)
Repeatable error—Criterion 3, **Collimation and CR:** Diaphragm is cut off. Free air caused by trauma or pathology may be trapped beneath the diaphragm and would be visualized. The CR is centered too low (RUQ is cut off), and collimation is not evident.

B. AP supine abdomen (Fig. C4-49)
Repeatable error—Criterion 3, **Collimation and CR:** Upper abdomen (including the tops of kidneys) is cut off. Even though the CR is centered correctly to the iliac crest, the image receptor is not centered to CR; it is too low. Unequal and excessively close side collimation is also evident.

C. AP supine abdomen (Fig. C5-50)
Repeatable errors (two)—Criterion 3, **Collimation and CR:** Upper abdomen is cut off because CR and IR are centered too low. Only lower collimation is visible because of poor CR-to-IR centering.

Criterion 4, **Exposure Criteria:** Motion is present (evident by blurring of abdominal structures, including gas shadow margins). Shorter exposure time and/or more complete breathing instructions are needed.

D. AP supine abdomen (Fig. C4-51)
Repeatable error—Criterion 3, **Collimation and CR:** Region of the bladder is cut off. CR and IR are centered too high, even for an erect abdomen.

Chapter 5: Upper Limb (p. 179)

A. PA hand (Fig. C5-174)
Repeatable error—Criterion 4, **Exposure Criteria:** Exposure factors selected are acceptable, but streaking artifacts are seen on radiograph (may be printing artifacts or chemical artifacts resulting from processing).

Note: Some rotation is evident, but most departments will not require a repeat.

B. Lateral hand (Fig. C5-175)
Repeatable error—Criterion 2, **Positioning:** The hand is rotated medially (excessive pronation of hand toward IR). The radius and ulna are not directly superimposed, and the metacarpals are not all superimposed.

Note: Anatomic markers are not evident on some of these images; they may be visible elsewhere on the radiographs but are not shown on these printed copies.

C. AP external (lateral) oblique elbow (Fig. C5-176)
Repeatable error—Criterion 2, **Positioning:** The arm is insufficiently rotated laterally. Radial tuberosity is partially superimposed; the capitulum is not sufficiently elongated and not in complete profile. (The upper limb must be rotated more laterally or externally.)

D. PA wrist (Fig. C5-177)
Note: This demonstrates radial **deviation** for the ulnar side carpals (the opposite of the ulnar **deviation** for scaphoid).

Repeatable error—Criterion 3, **Collimation and CR:** The lateral aspect of pisiform is cut off because of CR centering and collimation errors.

E. PA oblique hand (Fig. C5-178)
Repeatable error—Criterion 4, **Exposure Criteria:** Hand is underexposed. (The soft tissue is too evident, and the trabecular markings of bones are not visible.)

F. Lateral elbow (Fig. C5-179)
Repeatable error—Criterion 2, **Positioning:** Elbow is overflexed (beyond 90°) and not a true lateral; too much distance exists between parts of concentric circles 1 and 2, and the trochlear notch space is not open. (Compare with Figs. 5-138 and 5-139.)

Chapter 6: Proximal Humerus and Shoulder Girdle (p. 208)

A. AP clavicle (Fig. C6-85)
Repeatable error—Criterion 2, **Positioning:** The body is rotated toward the right, superimposing sternal end over the spine. This creates overall distortion of the clavicle and associated joints. CR and IR are also centered too low, creating additional distortion.

B. AP apical oblique axial shoulder (Garth method) (Fig. C6-86)
Repeatable errors (two)—Criterion 1, **Structures Shown:** All pertinent anatomy is demonstrated but severely distorted because of excessive CR angle.

Criterion 3, **Collimation and CR:** Excessive CR angulation has resulted in distortion of anatomy (see p. 187 for correct appearance of this projection). Excessive OID could also have added to this distortion.

C. AP scapula (Fig. C6-87)
Repeatable errors (two)—Criterion 1, **Structures Shown:** Lower margin of scapula is cut off. Repeatable error could also be considered under Criterion 4 or 3.

Criterion 4, **Exposure Criteria:** The scapula is underexposed.

Criterion 3, **Collimation and CR:** CR and IR must be centered lower to include the entire scapula.

D. AP shoulder and proximal humerus (Fig. C6-88) (AP projection, external rotation)
Repeatable error—Criterion 3, **Collimation and CR:** The majority of the shoulder girdle is cut off and not demonstrated. Collimation is evident on one side only, indicating incorrect centering. CR and IR centering are too far lateral.

Chapter 7: Lower Limb (p. 259)

A. Bilateral tangential patella (Fig. C7-146)
Repeatable errors (two)—Criterion 1, **Structures Shown:** A portion of each patella is superimposed over the intercondylar sulcus of the femur. Error may also be considered under Criteria 2 and 3, **Positioning** and **Collimation and CR.** Excessive flexion of knee most likely led to superimposition of patella over femur (overflexion of lower limb will draw patella into intercondylar sulcus). If CR is not parallel to the patellofemoral joint space, it will narrow the opening. (This error may have contributed to the poor visibility of the posterior aspect of the patella.)

Criterion 4, **Exposure Criteria:** This radiograph appears underexposed, which may be partially the result of incorrect positioning and CR angle.

B. AP foot (Fig. C7-147)
Repeatable error—Criterion 1, **Structures Shown:** Proximal metatarsals and all tarsals are totally obscured. Metatarsophalangeal joints are not open, and fourth and fifth metatarsals are partially superimposed. (Compare with Fig. 7-57, p. 232).

Error could also be considered under Criterion 2, **Positioning,** and Criterion 3, **Collimation and CR.** Part centering is acceptable but superimposed, and obscured anatomy indicates foot was not extended (plantar flexion) sufficiently and was rotated slightly externally. Collimation is evident, but insufficient CR angle can also lead to the distortion and closure of joint spaces and the obscuring of proximal metatarsals and tarsals.

C. Lateral ankle (Fig. C7-148)
Repeatable error—Criterion 2, **Positioning:** Rotation of anterior foot toward IR is excessive (overrotation).

Error could also be considered under Criterion 1, **Structures Shown,** because the anterior tubercle is obscured and the joint space between tibia and talus is not open (compare with correctly positioned lateral ankle in Fig. 7-88, p. 241).

D. AP knee (Fig. C7-149)
Repeatable error—Criterion 3, **Collimation and CR:** Incorrect CR angle results in narrowing and closing of joint space. (This may not be a repeatable error in some departments, depending on departmental protocol or other factors.)

E. Lateral knee (Fig. C7-150)
Repeatable error—Criterion 2, **Positioning:** Note appearance of adductor tubercle, which identifies the medial condyle as being more posterior. Excessive rotation away from IR is evident, along with overflexion of knee.

Error could also be considered under Criterion 1, **Structures Shown.** All pertinent anatomy is included, but patellofemoral joint is not open and patella is superimposed over lateral condyle as a result of rotation.

F. Lateral knee (Fig. C7-151)
Repeatable error—Criterion 2, **Positioning:** Rotation toward the IR is excessive. Overrotation is evident by observing that the outline of the adductor tubercle on the medial condyle is anterior to the lateral condyle.

Chapter 8: Proximal Femur and Pelvic Girdle (p. 286)

A. AP pelvis (Fig. C8-76)
Repeatable error—Criterion 1, **Structures Shown:** Both hands of patient are superimposed over hips, obscuring hip detail. (Note wristwatch on left wrist.)

B. Unilateral frog-leg (Fig. C8-77)
Repeatable error—Criterion 1, **Structures Shown:** Distal part of orthopedic prosthesis is cut off. It must be seen in its entirety.

C. AP pelvis (Fig. C8-78)
Repeatable error—Criterion 2, **Positioning:** Pelvis is rotated toward the left (note the elongation of the left ilium). Lesser trochanters are visible, and femoral necks are severely foreshortened, indicating that the legs were not rotated internally for a true AP projection. Note that the radiograph is incorrectly placed for viewing: the patient's right should be to the viewer's left.

D. Bilateral frog-leg (Fig. C8-79)
Repeatable error—Criterion 1, **Structures Shown:** Left hip (assuming it is the left side, although the side marker is not visible) is obscured by artifact (patient's hand is superimposed). Note that gonadal shielding is also misplaced.

Chapter 9: Cervical and Thoracic Spine (p. 320)

A. AP open mouth (Fig. C9-91)
Repeatable error—Criterion 1, **Structures Shown:** Upper aspect of dens is obscured by base of skull. Error may also be considered under Criterion 2, **Positioning,** because overextension of the skull has superimposed the base of skull over dens.

B. AP open mouth (Fig. C9-92)
Repeatable error—Criterion 1, **Structures Shown:** Upper aspect of dens and joint spaces are obscured by front incisors.
Error may also be considered under Criterion 2, **Positioning.** Overflexion of skull superimposes front incisors over top of dens.

C. AP axial projection (Fig. C9-93)
Repeatable error—Criterion 1, **Structures Shown:** Vertebral bodies and intervertebral joint spaces are distorted. Base of skull is superimposed over upper cervical spine.
Error could also be considered under Criterion 2, **Positioning.** Overextension of skull and/or excessive CR cephalic angle probably led to poor definition of vertebral bodies and joint spaces.

D. Oblique position (Fig. C9-94)
Repeatable error—Criterion 1, **Structures Shown:** Intervertebral joint spaces and foramina are not clearly demonstrated. The mandible is superimposed over upper cervical spine.
Error could also be considered under Criterion 2, **Positioning.** Body appears to be underrotated (appearance of upper rib cage suggests underrotation rather than overrotation). This error has resulted in narrowing and obscuring of the intervertebral foramina.
Insufficient or **incorrect CR angulation** (foreshortened appearance of cervical spine) may also have led to closure of disk spaces.

E. Lateral (trauma) position (Fig. C9-95)
Repeatable error—Criterion 1, **Structures Shown:** Aspects of C1 and dens are cut off. C7-T1 is not demonstrated.
Error could also be considered under Criterion 2, **Positioning,** and Criterion 3, **Collimation and CR.** Shoulders must be depressed. CR and IR are centered too low, which has resulted in upper cervical spine being cut off.

F. Lateral (nontrauma) position (Fig. C9-96)
Repeatable error—Criterion 1, **Structures Shown:** Only six cervical vertebra are demonstrated. C7 is totally superimposed by shoulders.

Chapter 10: Lumbar Spine, Sacrum, and Coccyx (p. 347)

A. Lateral lumbar spine (Fig. C10-78)
Repeatable error—Criterion 1, **Structures Shown:** Posterior elements of upper lumbar spine are cut off.
Error could also be considered under Criterion 2, **Positioning,** or Criterion 3, **Collimation and CR.** Patient is centered too far posterior, and CR and IR centerings are too anterior, leading to posterior elements being cut off.

B. AP lumbar spine (Fig. C10-79)
Repeatable errors (two)—Criterion 1, **Structures Shown:** Metallic artifacts obscure aspects of the lumbar spine.
Criterion 4, **Exposure Criteria:** Radiograph is overexposed.

C. Lateral L5-S1 (Fig. C10-80)
Repeatable errors (two)—Criterion 3, **Collimation and CR:** L5-S1 joint space is not open. Waist support or CR caudal angle is needed.
Criterion 4, **Exposure Criteria:** The region of L5-S1 joint space is underexposed.

D. Oblique lumbar spine (Fig. C10-81)
Repeatable errors (two)—Criterion 1, **Structures Shown:** Posterior elements of upper lumbar spine are cut off.
Criterion 2, **Positioning:** The upper aspect of lumbar spine is overobliqued (eyes of "Scotty dog," representing the pedicles, are too far posterior and not centered to body).

E. Oblique lumbar spine (Fig. C10-82)
Repeatable error—Criterion 2, **Positioning:** The lumbar spine is underobliqued (pedicles or eyes of "Scotty dog" are too far anterior).

Chapter 11: Bony Thorax—Sternum and Ribs (p. 366)

A. Ribs above diaphragm (Fig. C11-43)
There are no answers for this mystery critique radiograph. (See workbook for explanation.)

B. Oblique sternum (Fig. C11-44)
Repeatable error—Criterion 2, **Positioning:** Sternum is overobliqued and too far away from the spine (rotated beyond heart shadow). Sternum is also distorted.

C. Ribs below diaphragm (Fig. C11-45)
Repeatable error—Criterion 1, **Structures Shown:** Right lower ribs are cut off. Also, only the lower three pairs of ribs are demonstrated, indicating that the diaphragm is too low because of poor expiration. (Image receptor should have been placed crosswise to prevent cut-off of lateral margins of ribs.)

D. Lateral sternum (Fig. C11-46)
Repeatable error—Criterion 1, **Structures Shown:** Lower aspect of sternum is cut off.
Error could also be considered under Criterion 3, **Collimation and CR.** CR and IR are centered too high, leading to the lower sternum being cut off.

Chapter 12: Skull and Cranial Bones (p. 399)

A. Lateral (Fig. C12-83)
Repeatable errors (two)—Criterion 1, **Structures Shown:** Foreign bodies (earrings) obscure essential anatomy.
Criterion 4, **Exposure Criteria:** In most departments, this would be sufficiently underexposed to be repeatable.

B. Lateral skull (Fig. C12-84)
Repeatable error—Criterion 2, **Positioning:** The skull is tilted and rotated. (Note the separation of the orbital plates from the tilt and separation of the greater wings of the sphenoid, the rami of the mandible, and the EAMs, all indicating rotation.) The vertex of the skull also appears to be just slightly cut off (region of skull trauma), indicating a **collimation and CR** error.

C. AP axial (Towne) (C12-85)
Repeatable error—Criterion 3, **Collimation and CR:** CR is overangled. The anterior arch of C1 (rather than the dorsum sellae) is projected into the foramen magnum.

D. AP skull (Fig. C12-86)
Note: This is an AP projection, as evident by the large size of the orbits resulting from magnification due to increased OID (compare with radiograph in Fig. C12-87).
Repeatable errors—Criterion 2, **Positioning,** or Criterion 3, **Collimation and CR:** The petrous ridges are not projected into the lower one third of orbits. More flexion of neck or less CR angulation is required. The skull is also slightly rotated (note distance between orbits and lateral margins of skull).

E. PA skull (Fig. C12-87)
This is a PA 15° Caldwell projection.
Repeatable error—Criterion 1, **Structures Shown:** Patient ID marker and side marker are obscuring skull.
This error could also be considered under Criterion 5, **Markers.** Anatomic side marker is evident but placed over skull; patient ID marker is over upper right cranium. Both of these (Criteria 1 and 5) are repeatable errors

Chapter 13: Facial Bones and Paranasal Sinuses (p. 443–Facial Bones)

A. PA Waters (C13-135)
Repeatable errors (two)—Criterion 2, **Positioning:** Skull is underextended, which results in the petrous ridges being projected into the lower maxillary sinuses. Skull is also rotated.

Criterion 4, **Exposure Criteria:** Facial bone region appears to be overexposed and underdeveloped, resulting in poor radiographic contrast. (This could also be caused by "fogging" or other processing problems.)

B. SMV mandible (C13-136)
Repeatable error—Criterion 2, **Positioning:** Skull is underextended, or CR angle is incorrect, or both. (IOML was not parallel to IR and not perpendicular to CR.) Mandible is foreshortened, and rami are projected into temporal bone.

C. Optic foramina, Rhese method (C13-137)
Repeatable error—Criterion 2, **Positioning:** Skull is rotated excessively toward a PA. The skull is rotated more than 53° from the lateral position. This results in the optic foramen being projected into the middle lower aspect of the orbit. (See Fig. 13-85, p. 428, for correctly positioned parietoorbital, Rhese method radiographs with the optic foramina projected into lower outer quadrants of orbits.)

D. Optic foramina, Rhese method (C13-138)
Repeatable error—Criterion 2, **Positioning:** Skull appears to be overextended. (The AML was not perpendicular.) This projects the optic foramina into the infraorbital rim structure. Skull also appears to be underrotated, toward a lateral position.

E. Lateral facial bones (C13-139)
Repeatable error—Criterion 2, **Positioning:** Skull is rotated. (Note the separation of rami of mandible, greater wings of sphenoid, and orbits.)

Chapter 13: Facial Bones and Paranasal Sinuses (p. 444–Sinuses)

A. Parietoacanthial transoral (open-mouth Waters) (C13-140)
Repeatable error—Criterion 2, **Positioning:** Skull is underextended (chin not elevated sufficiently), leading to petrous ridges being projected into lower aspect of maxillary sinuses. The base of the skull is superimposed over sphenoid sinus.

B. Parietoacanthial (Waters) (C13-141)
Repeatable error—Criterion 2, **Positioning:** Skull is underextended and severely rotated. This results in petrous ridges being projected into the lower aspect of maxillary sinuses. Artifacts appear to be external hair pins or clips.

C. Submentovertex (SMV) sinuses (C13-142)
Repeatable errors (two)—Criterion 2, **Positioning:** Skull is grossly underextended and tilted (also some rotation).

Criterion 3, **Collimation and CR:** Collimation would have been adequate if centering had been correct. CR centering is off laterally, leading to the anatomy being cut off. Mandible is superimposed over sinuses.

D. Submentovertex (SMV) sinuses (C13-143)
Repeatable error—Criterion 2, **Positioning:** Skull is underextended and slightly rotated to the right. Earrings were not removed.

Chapter 18: Mammography (p. 595)

A. CC projection (Fig. C18-40)
Repeatable error—Criterion 1, **Structures Shown:** Folds of fatty tissue superimpose breast tissue.

B. MLO projection (Fig. C18-41)
Repeatable error—Criterion 1, **Structures Shown:** Pertinent muscle is not seen all the way to the nipple level, and outer tissue is not compressed. Lower part of breast is not sufficiently pulled away from chest wall onto IR.

C. CC projection (Fig. C18-42)
Repeatable error—Criterion 2, **Positioning:** Part of lateral posterior breast is cut off. Medial posterior breast also is not included, and shoulder is superimposed over the lateral posterior tissue.

D. MLO projection (Fig. C18-43)
Repeatable error—Criterion 1, **Structures Shown:** Posterior medial breast is cut off, and no pectoral muscle is visible. Breast is not pulled out away from chest wall. (White specks are calcium, not dust artifacts.)

E. CC projection (Fig. C18-44)
Repeatable error—Criterion 1, **Structures Shown:** Motion is present, which obliterates all detail.

F. CC projection (Fig. C18-45)
Repeatable error—Criterion 1, **Structures Shown:** Hair artifacts are evident on posterior breast tissue, which obscures breast tissue detail.

Index

Page numbers followed by f indicate figures; t, tables; b, boxes.

H

J

V